Toronto Notes 2017

Comprehensive medical reference and review for the
Medical Council of Canada Qualifying Exam Part I and the
United States Medical Licensing Exam Step 2

33rd Edition

Editors-in-Chief:
Jieun Kim and Ilya Mukovozov

*Wherever the art of medicine is loved,
there is also a love of humanity.*

– Hippocrates

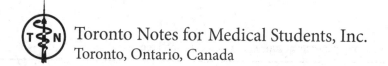

Toronto Notes for Medical Students, Inc.
Toronto, Ontario, Canada

Thirty-third Edition

Cover illustration: David Moratto
Cover design layout: Jieun Kim
Illustrations: Biomedical Communications, University of Toronto

Notice:
THIS PUBLICATION HAS NOT BEEN AUTHORED, REVIEWED, OR OTHERWISE SUPPORTED BY THE MEDICAL COUNCIL OF CANADA NOR DOES IT RECEIVE ENDORSEMENT BY THE MEDICAL COUNCIL AS REVIEW MATERIAL FOR THE MCCQE PART I. THIS PUBLICATION HAS NOT BEEN AUTHORED, REVIEWED, OR OTHERWISE SUPPORTED BY THE NATIONAL BOARD OF MEDICAL EXAMINERS U.S.A. NOR DOES IT RECEIVE ENDORSEMENT BY THE NATIONAL BOARD AS REVIEW MATERIAL FOR THE USMLE.

The editors of this edition have taken every effort to ensure that the information contained herein is accurate and conforms to the standards accepted at the time of publication. However, due to the constantly changing nature of the medical sciences and the possibility of human error, the reader is encouraged to exercise individual clinical judgement and consult with other sources of information that may become available with continuing research. The authors, editors, and publisher are not responsible for errors or omissions or for any consequences from application of the information in this textbook, atlas, or software and make no warranty, expressed or implied, with respect to the currency, completeness, or accuracy of the contents of the publication. In particular, the reader is advised to check the manufacturer's insert of all pharmacologic products before administration.

FEEDBACK AND ERRATA
We are constantly trying to improve the *Toronto Notes* and welcome your feedback. If you have found an error in this edition please do not hesitate to contact us. As well, we look forward to receiving any comments regarding any component of the *Toronto Notes* package and website.

Please send your feedback to: torontonotes.production@gmail.com

Alternatively, send mail to: Toronto Notes for Medical Students
Editors-in-Chief
c/o The Medical Society
1 King's College Circle, Room 2260
Toronto, Ontario M5S 1A8
Canada
email: torontonotes2017@gmail.com
Tel: 1-416-946-3047   Fax: 1-416-978-8730

Library of Congress Cataloging-in-Publication Data is available upon request

Dedicated to all

past and present contributors

and

supporters of Toronto Notes

who have made the production of the 2017 edition possible!

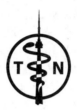

The *Toronto Notes* is dedicated to helping fund many charitable endeavours and medical student initiatives at the University of Toronto's Faculty of Medicine. Programs that have received *Toronto Notes* funding include:

Community Affairs Projects
- Saturday Program for Inner City High School and Grade 8 students
- St. Felix Mentorship Program for Inner City children
- Parkdale Mentorship Program for Grade 10-12 students
- WoodGreen Community Centre
- Let's Talk Science
- Growing Up Healthy

Annual Faculty Showcase Events
- Bruce Tovee Lecture Series
- Daffydil, in support of the Canadian Cancer Society
- Earthtones Benefit Concert
- Convocation and Ceremonies

Medical School Clubs
- Books with Wings
- Women in Medicine
- University of Toronto International Health Program
- Complementary and Alternative Medicine
- Peer Support for Students
- History of Medicine Society
- Faculty of Medicine Yearbook

Scholarships and Bursaries
- Nishant Fozdar Memorial Award
- Graduating Medical Class Scholarships and Bursaries

NOTE:

Many of you have wondered about the *Toronto Notes* logo, which is based on the rod of Asclepius, the Greek god of medicine. The rod of Asclepius consists of a single serpent entwined around a staff. This icon symbolizes both rebirth, by way of a snake shedding its skin, and also authority, by way of the staff.

In ancient Greek mythology, Asclepius was the son of Apollo and a skilled practitioner of medicine who learned the medical arts from the centaur Chiron. Asclepius' healing abilities were so great that he was said to be able to bring back people from the dead. These powers displeased the gods, who punished Asclepius by placing him in the sky as the constellation Orphiuchus.

The rod of Asclepius is at times confused with the caduceus, or wand, of Hermes, a staff entwined with two serpents and often depicted with wings. The caduceus is often used as a symbol of medicine or medical professionals, but there is little historical basis for this symbolism.

As you may have guessed, our logo uses the rod of Asclepius that is modified to also resemble the CN Tower – our way of recognizing the university and community in which we have been privileged to learn the art and science of medicine.

Thomas O'Brien, MD
Class of 2009
M.D. Program, University of Toronto

Preface – From the Editors

Dear Readers,

As the Editors-in-Chief of *Toronto Notes 2017*, we are proud to present this updated edition.

Toronto Notes began humbly in 1985 from a set of student notes circulated among medical students at the University of Toronto. Over time, Toronto Notes has grown into one of the premier study resources for generations of Canadian medical trainees. This rich history solidified our commitment to publish a comprehensive study resource for medical students engaged in clinical rotations and studying for both the Canadian MCCQE Part 1 and USMLE Step 2.

For the past 32 years we have remained committed to our original vision. The 2017 edition of *Toronto Notes* contains significant improvements including:

1. A new emphasis on *'Approaches to Common Clinical Presentations'* in addition to traditional content organized by disease.
2. A completely revised Psychiatry chapter incorporating the DSM-V in a quick-to-reference and readable format.
3. The Toronto Notes Quiz App, which is available for free on iTunes and Google Play. This app contains hundreds of questions allowing users to test themselves on the content contained within *Toronto Notes*.
4. A significantly improved interactive eBook with many new high-quality colour images.
5. A brand-new Clinical Handbook that is more concise, has numerous new figures, and features approaches to hundreds of common clinical situations.

Toronto Notes 2017 is produced by Toronto Notes for Medical Students Inc., which is a non-for-profit organization supporting various charity organizations in the city of Toronto. This year Toronto Notes for Medical Students has supported organizations including medical school clubs, community outreach groups, student bursaries and scholarships, and the Canadian Cancer Society. Your purchase of Toronto Notes 2017 is much appreciated by these well-deserving groups.

We would like to highlight the exceptional work of our team, composed of over 150 medical students, medical illustrators/artists, and faculty members at the University of Toronto Faculty of Medicine. Without the tireless effort expended by these individuals the production of *Toronto Notes 2017* would not have been possible. In particular, we would like to highlight the work of the executive team, all of whom made personal sacrifices in balancing their clinical and academic duties with the responsibilities asked of them: our production managers, Tina Binesh Marvasti and Sydney McQueen, our associate editors, Narayan Chattergoon, Desmond She, Claudia Frankfurter, Inna Gong, Dhruvin Hirpara, and Sneha Raju, and our EBM editors, Arnav Agarwal, Quynh Huynh, Robert Vanner, Brittany Prevost, Simran Mundi, and Valerie Lemieux. We also want to highlight the work of Rajkumari Chatterjee from University of Toronto Bookstore, who has contributed to the production of Toronto Notes for the past ten years, and has been instrumental in the annual launch of the Toronto Notes Ebook. Lastly, we would like to thank our partners at Type & Graphics Inc., particularly Enrica Aguilera, for their assistance during the production of *Toronto Notes 2017*.

We hope that *Toronto Notes 2017* enhances your medical knowledge and allows you to perform better on both your clinical rotations and licensing exams. We continue to encourage feedback – this year, we have read and incorporated every piece of feedback we received regarding the previous edition of Toronto Notes. On behalf of the *Toronto Notes 2017* team, we wish you success in your studies and academic endeavours.

Sincerely,

Jieun Kim, *MSc, MD/PhD Candidate* and
Ilya Mukovozov, *MSc, PhD, MD Candidate*
Editors-in-Chief, *Toronto Notes 2017*
MD Program, University of Toronto

Acknowledgements

We would like to acknowledge the exceptional work of all previous Toronto Notes (formerly MCCQE Notes) Editors-in-Chief and their editorial teams. The 33rd edition of this text was made possible with their contributions.

2016 (32nd ed.): Zamir Merali and Justin D. Woodfine

2015 (31th ed.): Justin Hall and Azra Premji

2014 (30th ed.): Miliana Vojvodic and Ann Young

2013 (29th ed.): Curtis Woodford and Christopher Yao

2012 (28th ed.): Jesse M. Klostranec and David L. Kolin

2011 (27th ed.): Yingming Amy Chen and Christopher Tran

2010 (26th ed.): Simon Baxter and Gordon McSheffrey

2009 (25th ed.): Sagar Dugani and Danica Lam

2008 (24th ed.): Rebecca Colman and Ron Somogyi

2007 (23rd ed.): Marilyn Heng and Joseph Ari Greenwald

2006 (22nd ed.): Carolyn Jane Shiau and Andrew Jonathan Toren

2005 (21st ed.): Blair John Normand Leonard and Jonathan Chi-Wai Yeung

2004 (20th ed.): Andrea Molckovsky and Kashif S. Pirzada

2003 (19th ed.): Prateek Lala and Andrea Waddell

2002 (18th ed.): Neety Panu and Sunny Wong

2001 (17th ed.): Jason Yue and Gagan Ahuja

2000 (16th ed.): Marcus Law and Brian Rotenberg

1999 (15th ed.): Sofia Ahmed and Matthew Cheung

1998 (14th ed.): Marilyn Abraham and M Appleby

1997 (13th ed.): William Harris and Paul Kurdyak

1996 (12th ed.): Michael B. Chang and Laura J. Macnow

1995 (11th ed.): Ann L. Mai and Brian J. Murray

1994 (10th ed.): Kenneth Pace and Peter Ferguson

1993 (9th ed.): Joan Cheng and Russell Goldman

1992 (8th ed.): Gideon Cohen-Nehemia and Shanthi Vasudevan

All former Chief Editors from 1991 (7th ed.) to 1985 (1st ed.)

Student Contributors

Faculty Contributors, University of Toronto

All contributing professors have been appointed at the University of Toronto.

David Adam, MD, FRCPC
Division of Dermatology
Department of Medicine
St. Michael's Hospital

Iqbal Ahmed, MD, FRCSC
Department of Ophthalmology
and Vision Science
University of Toronto

Ruby Alvi, MD, CCFP, MHSc
Department of Family
and Community Medicine
University of Toronto

Meyer Balter, MD, FRCPC
Division of Respiratory Medicine
Department of Medicine
Mount Sinai Hospital

Abdollah Behzadi, MD, MBA, FRCSC, FACS
Division of Thoracic Surgery
Department of Surgery
University of Toronto

Nirit Bernhard, MSc, MD, FRCPC
Department of Pediatrics
Hospital for Sick Children

Katherine Bingham, MD, MPH, CCFP-EM
Faculty of Medicine
University of Toronto

Matthew Binnie, MD
Division of Respirology
University Health Network
St. Michael's Hospital

Ari Bitnun, MD, MSc, FRCPC
Division of Infectious Diseases
The Hospital for Sick Children

Andrea Boggild, MSc, MD, FRCPC
Tropical Disease Unit and
Division of Infectious Diseases
University Health Network
Toronto General Hospital

Arthur Bookman, MD, FRCPC
Division of Rheumatology
Department of Medicine
University Health Network
Toronto Western Hospital

Mark Boulos, MD, MSc, CSCN(EEG), FRCPC
Division of Neurology and Sleep Medicine
Department of Medicine
Sunnybrook Health Sciences Centre

John Byrne, MD, MB, BCh, BAO
Division of Vascular Surgery
Department of Surgery
University of Toronto

Simon Carette, MD, FRCPC
Division of Rheumatology
Department of Medicine
Mount Sinai Hospital

Vicky Chau, MD, MScCH, FRCPC
Division of Geriatric Medicine
Department of Medicine
University Health Network

Alice Cheung, MD, FRCPC
Division of Endocrinology and Metabolism
Department of Medicine
St. Michael's Hospital

Chi-Ming Chow, MDCM, MSc, FRCPC
Division of Cardiology
Department of Medicine
St. Michael's Hospital

Allison Chris, MD, MSc, FRCPC
Division of Clinical Public Health
Dalla Lana School of Public Health

Maria Cino, HonBSc, MSc, MD, FRCPC
Division of Gastroenterology
University Health Network
Toronto Western Hospital

Alfonso Fasano, MD, PhD, FRCPC
Division of Neurology
University Health Network
Toronto Western Hospital

Mark Freedman, MD, FRCPC
Department of Emergency Medicine
Sunnybrook Health Sciences Centre

Natasha Gakhal, MD, FRCPC
Division of Rheumatology
Department of Medicine
Women's College Hospital

Barry J. Goldlist, MD, FRCPC
Division of Geriatric Medicine
Department of Medicine
University Health Network

David Hall, MD, PhD, FRCPC
Divisions of Respirology and Critical Care
Medicine
Department of Medicine
University of Toronto
St. Michael's Hospital

Jeremy Hall, MD, FRCSC
Division of Orthopedic Surgery
Department of Surgery
St. Michael's Hospital

Philip C. Hébert, MA, PhD, MD, FCFPC
Department of Family and
Community Medicine
Joint Centre for Bioethics
Sunnybrook Health Sciences Centre

Sender Herschorn, MDCM, FRCSC
Division of Urology
Department of Surgery
Sunnybrook Health Sciences Centre and
Women's College Hospital

Jonathan C. Irish, MD, MSc, FRCSC
Department of Otolaryngology -
Head and Neck Surgery
University Health Network

Nasir Jaffer, MD, FRCPC
Division of Abdominal Imaging
Department of Medical Imaging
Joint Department of Medical Imaging
University of Toronto

David Juurlink, BPhm, MD, PhD, FRCPC
Division of Clinical Pharmacology
and Toxicology
Departments of Medicine and Pediatrics
Sunnybrook Health Sciences Centre

Gabor Kandel, MD, FRCPC
Division of Gastroenterology, Department of
Medicine
St. Michael's Hospital

Sari L. Kives, MD, FRCSC
Department of Obstetrics and Gynecology
St. Michael's Hospital and
The Hospital for Sick Children

Wai-Ching Lam, MD, FRCSC
Department of Ophthalmology and
Vision Science
University Health Network
Toronto Western Hospital

Chloe Leon, MD, FRCPC
Division of Brain and Therapeutics
Department of Psychiatry
Centre for Addiction and Mental Health

Armando Lorenzo, MD, FRCSC
Division of Urology
Department of Surgery
The Hospital for Sick Children

Todd Mainprize, MD, FRCSC
Department of Neurosurgery
Sunnybrook Health Sciences Centre

Faculty Contributors, University of Toronto

Eric Massicotte, MD, MSc, FRCSC
Department of Neurosurgery
University Health Network
Toronto Western Hospital

Michael McDonald, MD, FRCPC
Division of Cardiology and
The Multi-Organ Transplant Program
Department of Medicine
University Health Network
Toronto General Hospital

Adam C. Millar, MD, MScCH
Division of Endocrinology and Metabolism
Department of Medicine
Mount Sinai Hospital

Azadeh Moaveni, MD, CCFP
Department of Family and
Community Medicine
University Health Network
Toronto Western Hospital

Ally Murji, MD, MPH, FRCS(C)
Department of Obstetrics and Gynecology
Mount Sinai Hospital

Melinda Musgrave, MD, PhD, FRCSC
Division of Plastic and Reconstructive Surgery
Department of Surgery
St. Michael's Hospital

Sharon Naymark, MD, FRCPC
Department of Pediatrics
St. Joseph's Health Centre

George Oreopoulos, MD, MSc, FRCSC
Division of Vascular Surgery
Department of Surgery
University Health Network

Richard Pittini, MD, MEd, FRCSC, FACOG
Department of Obstetrics and Gynaecology
University of Toronto
Sunnybrook Health Sciences Centre

Susan Poutanen, MD, MPH, FRCPC
Department of Microbiology
University Health Network and
Mount Sinai Hospital

Ramesh Prasad, MBBS, MSc, FRCPC
Division of Nephrology
Department of Medicine
St. Michael's Hospital

Mary Preisman, MD, FRCPC
Department of Psychiatry
Mount Sinai Hospital

Evan Propst, MD, MSc, FRCSC
Division of Head and Neck Surgery
Department of Otolaryngology
The Hospital for Sick Children

Angela Punnett, MD, FRCPC
Department of Pediatrics
The Hospital for Sick Children

Amanda Selk, MD, FRCSC
Department of Obstetrics and Gynecology
Mount Sinai Hospital

Marisa Sit, MD, FRCSC
Department of Ophthalmology
and Vision Science
University Health Network
Toronto Western Hospital

Michelle Sholzberg, MDCM, MSc, FRCPC
Division of Hematology
Department of Medicine
St. Michael's Hospital

Kevin Skarratt, MD, FRCPC
Department of Emergency Medicine
Sunnybrook Health Sciences Centre

Elizabeth Slow, MD, PhD, FRCP
Division of Neurology
University Health Network

Peter Tai, MD, FRCPC
Division of Neurology
University Health Network
Toronto Western Hospital

Diana Tamir, MD, FRCPC
Department of Anesthesia and
Pain Management
University Health Network

Gemini Tanna, MD, FRCPC
Division of Nephrology
Department of Medicine
Sunnybrook Health Sciences Centre

Piero Tartaro, MD, FRCPC
Division of Gastroenterology
Department of Medicine
Sunnybrook Health Sciences Centre

Fernando Teixeira, MD, FRCPC
Department of Emergency Medicine
St. Michael's Hospital

Martina Trinkaus, MD, FRCPC
Division of Hematology
Department of Medicine
St. Michael's Hospital

Herbert P. von Schroeder, MD, MSc, FRCSC
Divisions of Orthopedic Surgery and
Plastic Surgery
Department of Surgery
University Health Network

Oshrit Wanono, MD, FRCPC
Division of Child and Adolescent Psychiatry
Department of Psychiatry
Centre for Addiction and Mental Health

Kyle R. Wanzel, MD, MEd, FRCSC
Division of Plastic Surgery
St. Joseph's Health Centre

Jeffrey Wassermann, MD, FRCPC
Department of Anesthesia
St. Michael's Hospital

Alice Wei, MD CM, MSc, FRCSC
Division of General Surgery
Department of Surgery
University Health Network

Michael J. Weinberg, MD, MSc, FRCS(c)
Division of Plastic Surgery
Department of Surgery
University of Toronto
Trillium Health Centre

Fay Weisberg, MD, FRCSC
Division of Reproductive Endocrinology
and Infertility
Department of Obstetrics and Gynecology
University of Toronto

Anna Woo, MD CM, SM, DABIM, FRCPC
Division of Cardiology
Department of Medicine
University Health Network
Toronto General Hospital

Jensen Yeung, MD, FRCPC
Division of Dermatology
Department of Medicine
Women's College Hospital

Eugene Yu, MD, FRCPC
Division of Neuroradiology
Department of Medical Imaging
University Health Network

Table of Contents

How to Use This Book

This book has been designed to remain as one book or to be taken apart into smaller booklets. Identify the beginning and end of a particular section, then carefully bend the pages along the perforated line next to the spine of the book. Then tear the pages out along the perforation.

The layout of *Toronto Notes* allows easy identification of important information. These items are indicated by icons interspersed throughout the text:

Icon	Icon Name	Significance
	Key Objectives	This icon is found next to headings in the text. It identifies key objectives and conditions as determined by the Medical Council of Canada or the National Board of Medical Examiners in the USA. If it appears beside a dark title bar, all subsequent subheadings should be considered key topics.
	Clinical Pearl	This icon is found in sidebars of the text. It identifies concise, important information which will aid in the diagnosis or management of conditions discussed in the accompanying text.
	Memory Aid	This icon is found in sidebars of the text. It identifies helpful mnemonic devices and other memory aids.
	Clinical Flag	This icon is found in sidebars of the text. It indicates information or findings that require urgent management or specialist referral.
	Cross-Reference	This icon is found in sidebars of the text. It indicates a cross-reference for information that is discussed in a separate chapter.
	Evidence Based Medicine	This icon is found in sidebars of the text. It identifies key research studies for evidence-based clinical decision making related to topics discussed in the accompanying text.
	Colour Photo Atlas	This icon is found next to headings in the text. It indicates topics that correspond with images found in the Colour Photo Atlas available online (www.torontonotes.ca).
	Radiology Atlas	This icon is found next to headings in the text. It indicates topics that correspond to images found in the Radiology Atlas available online (www.torontonotes.ca).
	Online Resources	This icon is found next to headings in the text. It indicates topics that correspond with electronic resources such as Functional Neuroanatomy or ECGs Made Simple, available online (www.torontonotes.ca).

Chapter Divisions

To aid in studying and finding relevant material quickly, each chapter is organized in the following general framework:

Basic Anatomy/Physiology Review
- features the high-yield, salient background information students are often assumed to have remembered from their early medical school education

Common Differential Diagnoses
- aims to outline a clinically useful framework to tackle the common presentations and problems faced in the area of expertise

Diagnoses
- the bulk of the book
- etiology, epidemiology, pathophysiology, clinical features, investigations, management, complications, and prognosis

Common Medications
- a quick reference section for review of medications commonly prescribed

Common Unit Conversions

To convert from the conventional unit to the SI unit, **multiply** by conversion factor
To convert from the SI unit to the conventional unit, **divide** by conversion factor

	Conventional Unit	Conversion Factor	SI Unit
ACTH	pg/mL	0.22	pmol/L
Albumin	g/dL	10	g/L
Bilirubin	mg/dL	17.1	μmol/L
Calcium	mg/dL	0.25	mmol/L
Cholesterol	mg/dL	0.0259	mmol/L
Cortisol	μg/dL	27.59	nmol/L
Creatinine	mg/dL	88.4	μmol/L
Creatinine clearance	mL/min	0.0167	mL/s
Ethanol	mg/dL	0.217	mmol/L
Ferritin	ng/mL	2.247	pmol/L
Glucose	mg/dL	0.0555	mmol/L
HbA1c	%	0.01	proportion of 1.0
Hemaglobin	g/dL	10	g/L
HDL cholesterol	mg/dL	0.0259	mmol/L
Iron, total	μg/dL	0.179	μmol/L
Lactate (lactic acid)	mg/dL	0.111	mmol/L
LDL cholesterol	mg/dL	0.0259	mmol/L
Leukocytes	x 10^3 cells/mm^3	1	x 10^9 cells/L
Magnesium	mg/dL	0.411	mmol/L
MCV	$μm^3$	1	fL
Platelets	x 10^3 cells/mm^3	1	x 10^9 cells/L
Reticulocytes	% of RBCs	0.01	proportion of 1.0
Salicylate	mg/L	0.00724	mmol/L
Testosterone	ng/dL	0.0347	nmol/L
Thyroxine (T_4)	ng/dL	12.87	pmol/L
Total Iron Binding Capacity	μg/dL	0.179	μmol/L
Triiodothyronine (T_3)	pg/dL	0.0154	pmol/L
Triglycerides	mg/dL	0.0113	mmol/L
Urea nitrogen	mg/dL	0.357	mmol/L
Uric acid	mg/dL	59.48	μmol/L

Celsius → Fahrenheit	F = (C x 1.8) + 32
Fahrenheit → Celsius	C = (F – 32) x 0.5555
Kilograms → Pounds	1 kg = 2.2 lbs
Pounds → Ounces	1 lb = 16 oz
Ounces → Grams	1 oz = 28.3 g
Inches → Centimetres	1 in = 2.54 cm

Commonly Measured Laboratory Values

Test	Conventional Units	SI Units
Arterial Blood Gases		
pH	7.35-7.45	7.35-7.45
PCO_2	35-45 mmHg	4.7-6.0 kPa
PO_2	80-105 mmHg	10.6-14 kPa
Serum Electrolytes		
Bicarbonate	22-28 mEq/L	22-28 mmol/L
Calcium	8.4-10.2 mg/dL	2.1-2.5 mmol/L
Chloride	95-106 mEq/L	95-106 mmol/L
Magnesium	1.3-2.1 mEq/L	0.65-1.05 mmol/L
Phosphate	2.7-4.5 mg/dL	0.87-1.45 mmol/L
Potassium	3.5-5.0 mEq/L	3.5-5.0 mmol/L
Sodium	136-145 mEq/L	136-145 mmol/L
Serum Nonelectrolytes		
Albumin	3.5-5.0 g/dL	35-50 g/L
ALP	35-100 U/L	35-100 U/L
ALT	8-20 U/L	8-20 U/L
Amylase	25-125 U/L	25-125 U/L
AST	8-20 U/L	8-20 U/L
Bilirubin (direct)	0-0.3 mg/dL	0-5 µmol/L
Bilirubin (total)	0.1-1.0 mg/dL	2-17 µmol/L
BUN	7-18 mg/dL	2.5-7.1 mmol/L
Cholesterol	<200 mg/dL	<5.2 mmol/L
Creatinine (female)	10-70 U/L	10-70 U/L
Creatinine (male)	25-90 U/L	25-90 U/L
Creatine Kinase – MB fraction	0-12 U/L	0-12 U/L
Ferritin (female)	12-150 ng/mL	12-150 µg/L
Ferritin (male)	15-200 ng/mL	15-200 µg/L
Glucose (fasting)	70-110 mg/dL	3.8-6.1 mmol/L
HbA1c	<6%	<0.06
LDH	100-250 U/L	100-250 U/L
Osmolality	275-300 mOsm/kg	275-300 mOsm/kg
Serum Hormones		
ACTH (0800h)	<60 pg/mL	<13.2 pmol/L
Cortisol (0800h)	5-23 µg/dL	138-635 nmol/L
Prolactin	<20 ng/mL	<20 ng/mL
Testosterone (male, free)	9-30 ng/dL	0.31-1 pmol/L
Thyroxine (T_4)	5-12 ng/dL	64-155 nmol/L
Triiodothyronine (T_3)	115-190 ng/dL	1.8-2.9 nmol/L
TSH	0.5-5 µU/mL	0.5-5 µU/mL
Hematologic Values		
ESR (female)	0-20 mm/h	0-20 mm/h
ESR (male)	0-15 mm/h	0-15 mm/h
Hemoglobin (female)	12.3-15.7 g/dL	123-157 g/L
Hemoglobin (male)	13.5-17.5 g/dL	140-174 g/L
Hematocrit (female)	36-46%	36-46%
Hematocrit (male)	41-53%	41-53%
INR	1.0-1.1	1.0-1.1
Leukocytes	$4.5\text{-}11 \times 10^3$ cells/mm^3	$4.5\text{-}11 \times 10^9$ cells/L
MCV	88-100 µm^3	88-100 fL
Platelets	$150\text{-}400 \times 10^3$/mm^3	$150\text{-}400 \times 10^9$/L
PTT	25-35 s	25-35 s
Reticulocytes	0.5-1.5% of RBC	$20\text{-}84 \times 10^9$/L

ELOM | Ethical, Legal, and Organizational Medicine

Patrick Steadman, Zafir Syed, and **Stephanie Zhou**, chapter editors
Narayan Chattergoon and **Desmond She**, associate editors
Arnav Agarwal and **Quynh Huynh**, EBM editors
Dr. Philip C. Hébert, staff editor

Acronyms 2

The Canadian Health Care System 2
Overview of Canadian Health Care System
Legal Foundation
History of the Canadian Health Care System
Health Care Expenditure and Delivery in Canada
Physician Licensure and Certification
Role of Professional Associations

Ethical and Legal Issues in Canadian Medicine . . . 5
Introduction to the Principles of Ethics
Confidentiality
Consent and Capacity
Negligence
Truth-Telling
Ethical Issues in Health Care
Reproductive Technologies
End-of-Life Care
Physician Competence and Professional Conduct
Research Ethics
Physician-Industry Relations
Resource Allocation
Conscientious Objection

References 16

Further information on these topics can be found in the Objectives of the Considerations of the Legal, Ethical and Organizational Aspects of the Practice of Medicine (CLEO) – which can be downloaded free of charge from the Medical Council of Canada website at http://mcc.ca/wp-content/uploads/CLEO.pdf

Canadian law applicable to medical practice varies between jurisdictions and changes over time.
Criminal law is nationwide, but non-criminal (civil) law varies between provinces. This section is meant to serve only as a guide. Students and physicians should ensure that their practices conform to local and current laws.

Acronyms

AE	adverse event	FMEQ	Fédération médicale étudiante du Québec	OMA	Ontario Medical Association
ART	advanced reproductive technologies	FRCPC	Fellow of the Royal College of Physicians of Canada	OTC	over the counter
RDoC	Resident Doctors of Canada	FRCSC	Fellow of the Royal College of Surgeons of Canada	PHO	Provincial Housestaff Organization
CFMS	Canadian Federation of Medical Students	GA	gestational age	PIPEDA	Personal Information Protection and Electronic Documents Act
CFPC	College of Family Physicians of Canada	GDP	gross domestic product	POA	power of attorney
CMA	Canadian Medical Association	HCCA	Health Care Consent Act	PTMA	Provincial/Territorial Medical Association
CME	continuing medical education	IVF	*in vitro* fertilization	RCPSC	Royal College of Physicians and Surgeons of Canada
CMPA	Canadian Medical Protective Association	LMCC	Licentiate of the Medical Council of Canada	SDM	substitute decision-maker
CPSO	College of Physicians and Surgeons of Ontario	MCC	Medical Council of Canada		
EMR	electronic medical record	OECD	Organization for Economic Co-operation and Development		

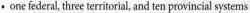

The Canadian Health Care System

Overview of Canadian Health Care System

Principles of the Canada Health Act
1. Public Administration: provincial health insurance programs must be administered by public authorities
2. Comprehensiveness: provincial health insurance programs must cover all necessary diagnostic, physician, and hospital services
3. Universality: all eligible residents must be entitled to health care services
4. Portability: emergency health services must be available to Canadians who are outside their home province, paid for by the home province
5. Accessibility: user fees, charges, or other obstructions to insured health care services are not permitted

- one federal, three territorial, and ten provincial systems
- major complexities involved in establishment of Canadian health policy include geographical diversity, socioeconomic divisions, and international pressures
- financed by both the public (70%) and private (30%) sectors
- each provincial plan must cover all medically necessary health services delivered in hospitals and by physicians; may choose to cover services such as home care and prescription drugs
- non-insured health services and fees are either covered by private insurance or by the individual
- workers' compensation funds cover treatment for work-related injuries and diseases

Table 1. Division of Government Responsibilities in Health Care

Federal Government	Provincial Government
Marine hospitals and quarantine (Constitution Act, 1867)	Establishment, maintenance and management of hospitals, asylums, charities, and charitable institutions (*Constitution Act*, 1867)
Health care services for Aboriginal people, federal government employees (RCMP and armed forces), immigrants, and civil aviation personnel	Licensing of physicians, nurses and other health professionals
Investigations into public health	Determining the standards for licensing all hospitals
Regulation of food and drugs	Administering provincial medical insurance plans
Inspection of medical devices	Financing health care facilities
Administration of health care insurance	Delivery of certain public health services
General information services related to health conditions and practices	
Role in health derived from government's constitutional powers over criminal law (basis for legislation such as *Food and Drugs Act and Controlled Substances Act*), spending, and 'peace, order, and good government'	

Legal Foundation

The federal government can reduce its contributions to provinces that violate the key principles of the Canada Health Act

- the legal foundation of the Canadian health system is based on two constitutional documents:
  1. *Constitution Act* (1867): deals primarily with the jurisdictional power between federal and provincial governments
  2. *The Canadian Charter of Rights and Freedoms* (1982): does not guarantee a right to health care but, given government's decision to finance health care, they are constitutionally obliged to do so consistently with the rights and freedoms outlined in the Charter (including the right to equality, physicians' mobility rights, etc.)

- and two statutes:
  1. *Canada Health Act* (1984): outlines the national terms and conditions that provincial health systems must meet in order to receive federal transfer payments
  2. *Canada Health and Social Transfer Act* (1996): federal government gives provinces a single grant for health care, social programs, and post-secondary education; division of resources at provinces' discretion

History of the Canadian Health Care System

1867   British North America Act (now Constitution Act) establishes Canada as a confederacy
- "establishment, maintenance, and management of hospitals" under provincial jurisdiction

1965   *Royal Commission on Health Services* (Hall Commission) recommends federal leadership and financial support with provincial government operation

1984	*Canada Health Act* passed by federal government

- replaces Medical Care Act (1966) and Hospital Insurance and Diagnostic Services Act (1957)
- provides federal funds to provinces with universal hospital insurance
- maintains federal government contribution at 50% on average, with poorer provinces receiving more funds
- medical insurance must be 'comprehensive, portable, universal, and publicly administered'
- bans extra-billing by new fifth criterion: accessibility

1996   *Canada Health and Social Transfer Act* passed by federal government
- federal government gives provinces a single grant for health care, social programs, and post-secondary education; division of resources at provinces' discretion

2001   *Kirby and Romanow Commissions* appointed

Kirby Commission (final report, October 2002)
- examines history of health care system in Canada, pressures and constraints of current health care system, role of federal government, and health care systems in foreign jurisdictions

Romanow Commission (final report, November 2002)
- dialogue with Canadians on the future of Canada's public health care system

2004   *First Ministers' Meeting on the Future of Health Care* produces a 10 year plan
- priorities include reductions in waiting times, development of a national pharmacare plan, and primary care reform

2005   *Chaoulli v. Québec*, Supreme Court of Canada decision
- rules that Québec's banning of private insurance is unconstitutional under the Québec Charter of Rights, given that patients do not have access to those services under the public system in a timely way

2011   First progress report by the Health Council reviews progress (2004 First Ministers' 10 year plan)
- significant reductions in wait times for specific areas (such as cancer, joint replacement and sight restoration), but may have inadvertently caused increases in wait times of other services
- despite large investments into EMRs, Canada continues to have very low uptake, ranking last in the Commonwealth Fund International Health Policy survey, with only 37% use among primary care physicians
- little progress in creating a national strategy for equitable access to pharmaceuticals; however, there has been some success in increasing pharmacists' scope of practice, reducing generic drugs costs, and implementing drug info systems
- increases in funding to provinces at 6% per annum until the 2016-2017 fiscal year; from then onwards, increases tied to nominal GDP at a minimum of 3% per annum

2012   Second progress report by the Health Council reviews progress towards 2004 First Ministers' 10 year plan
- funding is sufficient; however, more innovation is needed including incentivizing through models of remuneration
- 46 recommendations made to address the lack of progress

2014   Expiry of current *10 Year Health Care Funding Agreement* between federal and provincial governments

2015   Negotiations underway for a new Health Accord with a $3 billion investment over four years to homecare and mental health services by the elected Liberal government

Health Care Expenditure and Delivery in Canada

- projected total health care expenditure in 2014 was $214.9 billion, 11% of the GDP, approximately $6,045 CDN per person

Sources of Health Care Funding
- 71% of total health expenditure in 2015 came from public-sector funding with 66% coming from the provincial and territorial governments and 5% from other parts of the public sector: federal direct government, municipal, and social security funds. 29% is from private sources including out of pocket (14%), private insurance (12%) and other (3%)
- public sector covers services offered on a either a fee for service, capitation, or alternate payment plan in physicians' offices and in hospitals
- public sector does not cover services provided by privately practicing health professionals (e.g. dentists, chiropractors, optometrists, massage therapists, osteopaths, physiotherapists, podiatrists, psychologists, private duty nurses, and naturopaths), prescription drugs, OTC drugs, personal health supplies, and use of residential care facilities

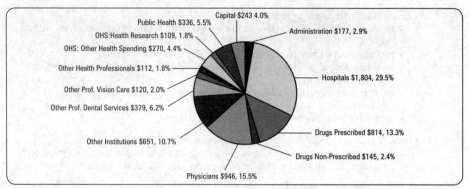

Figure 1. Total health expenditure by use of funds, Canada, 2015 (percentage share and billions of dollars)
Source: https://secure.cihi.ca/free_products/nhex_trends_narrative_report_2015_en.pdf

Delivery of Health Care
- hospital services in Canada are publicly funded but delivered through private, not-for-profit institutions owned and operated by communities, religious organizations, and regional health authorities
- other countries, such as the United States (a mix of public and private funding, as well as private for-profit and private not-for-profit delivery) and the United Kingdom (primarily public funding and delivery) have different systems of delivery

Physician Licensure and Certification

- physician certification is governed nationally, while the medical profession in Canada self-regulates under the authority of provincial legislation
- self-regulation is based on the premise that the licensing authority must act first and foremost in the interest of the public

Table 2. Key Physician Certification and Licensing Bodies in Canada

Certifying Body	Description
MCC	Certifies physicians with the LMCC The LMCC is acquired by passing the MCC Qualifying Examination Parts I and II
RCPSC	Certifies specialists who complete an accredited residency program and pass the appropriate exam Voluntary membership of the RCPSC is designated FRCPC or FRCSC
CFPC	Certifies family physicians who complete an accredited residency program and pass the Certification Examination in Family Medicine

Licensing Body	Description

CPSO	Membership to the provincial licensing authority is mandatory
	Licensing authority functions include:
	    Provide non-transferable licensure to physicians
	    Maintaining ethical, legal, and competency standards and developing policies to guide doctors
	    Investigating complaints against doctors
	    Disciplining doctors guilty of professional misconduct or incompetence
	    At times of license investiture and renewal, physicians must disclose if they have a condition (such as HIV positivity, drug addiction, or other illnesses that may impact their ability to practice safely)

- the RCPSC and CFPC are responsible for monitoring ongoing CME and professional development
- certification by the LMCC plus either the RCPSC or CFPC is a minimum requirement for licensure by most provincial licensing authorities

Role of Professional Associations

Table 3. Key Professional Associations

Association	Description
CMA	Provides leadership to doctors and advocates for access to high quality care in Canada Represents physician and population concerns at the national level Membership is voluntary
OMA and Other PTMAs	Negotiates fee and benefit schedules with provincial governments Represents the economic and professional interests of doctors Membership is voluntary
CMPA	Physician-run organization that protects the integrity of member physicians Provides legal defence against allegations of malpractice or negligence Provides risk management and educational programs Membership is voluntary
RDoC and PHO	Upholds economic and professional interests of residents across Canada Facilitates discussion amongst PHOs regarding policy and advocacy items
CMFS and FMÉQ	Medical students are represented at their universities by student bodies, which collectively form the CFMS or FMÉQ The FMÉQ membership includes that of francophone medical schools

Ethical and Legal Issues in Canadian Medicine

Introduction to the Principles of Ethics

- ethics addresses
    1. principles and values that help define what is morally right and wrong
    2. rights, duties and obligations of individuals and groups
- the practice of medicine assumes there is one code of professional ethics for all doctors and that they will be held accountable by that code and its implications
- the doctor-patient relationship is formed on trust, which is recognized in the concept of fiduciary duty/responsibility of physician towards patient
- a fiduciary duty is a legal duty to act solely in another party's interest; one may not profit from the relationship with principals unless he/she has the principal's express consent

Table 4. The Four Principles Approach to Medical Ethics

Principle	Definition
Autonomy	Recognizes an individual's right and ability to decide for himself/herself according to his/her beliefs and values Not applicable in situations where informed consent and choice are not possible or may not be appropriate
Beneficence	The patient-based 'best interests' standard that combines doing good, avoiding harm, taking into account the patient's values, beliefs, and preferences, so far as these are known Autonomy should be integrated with the physician's conception of a patient's medically-defined best interests The aim is to minimize harmful outcomes and maximize beneficial ones Paramount in situations where consent/choice is not possible or may not be appropriate
Non-Maleficence	Obligation to avoid causing harm; *primum non nocere* ("First, do no harm") A limit condition of the Beneficence principle
Justice	Fair distribution of benefits and harms within a community, regardless of geography or privilege Concept of fairness: Is the patient receiving what he/she deserves – his/her fair share? Is he/she treated the same as equally situated patients? How does one set of treatment decisions impact others? Basic human rights, such as freedom from persecution and the right to have one's interests considered and respected

Autonomy vs. Competence
Autonomy: the right that patients have to make decisions according to their beliefs and preferences
Competence: the ability or capacity to make a specific decision for oneself

CMA Code of Ethics

- The CMA developed a Code of Ethics that acts as a common ethical framework for Canadian physicians. The Code of Ethics is:
    - prepared by physicians for physicians and applies to physicians, residents, and medical students
    - based on the fundamental ethical principles of medicine
    - sources include the Hippocratic Oath, developments in human rights, recent bioethical discussion
    - CMA policy statements address specific ethical issues not mentioned by the code (e.g. abortion, transplantation, and euthanasia)

The CMA Code of Ethics is a quasi-legal standard for physicians; if the law sets a minimal moral standard for doctors, the Code augments these standards

Confidentiality

Overview of Confidentiality

- a full and open exchange of information between patient and physician is central to a therapeutic relationship
- privacy is the right of patients (which they may forego) while confidentiality is the duty of doctors (which they must respect barring patient consent or the requirements of the law)
- if inappropriately breached by a doctor, he/she can be sanctioned by the hospital, court, or regulatory authority
- based on the ethical principle of patient autonomy, patients have the right to the following:
    - control of their own information
    - the expectation that information concerning them will receive proper protection from unauthorized access by others (see *Privacy of Medical Records*, ELOM6)
- confidentiality may be ethically and legally breached in certain circumstances (e.g. the threat of harm to others)
- unlike the solicitor-client privilege, there is no 'physician-patient privilege' by which a physician, even a psychiatrist, can promise the patient absolute confidentiality
- physicians should seek advice from their local health authority or the CMPA before disclosing HIV status of a patient to someone else
    - many jurisdictions make mandatory not only the reporting of serious communicable diseases (e.g. HIV), but also the reporting of those who harbour the agent of the communicable disease
    - physicians failing to abide by such regulations could be subject to professional or civil actions
- the legal duty to maintain patient confidentiality is imposed by provincial health information legislation and precedent-setting cases in the common law

Legal Aspects of Confidentiality
Advice should always be sought from provincial licensing authorities and/or legal counsel when in doubt

CMA Code of Ethics
"Disclose your patients' personal health information to third parties only with their consent, or as provided for by law, such as when the maintenance of confidentiality would result in a significant risk of substantial harm to others or, in the case of incompetent patients, to the patients themselves. In such cases take all reasonable steps to inform the patients that the usual requirements for confidentiality will be breached"

Statutory Reporting Obligations

- legislation has defined specific instances where public interest overrides the patient's right to confidentiality; varies by province, but may include
  1. suspected child abuse or neglect – report to local child welfare authorities (e.g. Children's Aid Society)
  2. fitness to drive a vehicle or fly an airplane – report to provincial Ministry of Transportation (see <u>Geriatric Medicine</u>, GM11)
  3. communicable diseases – report to local public health authority (see <u>Population Health and Epidemiology</u>, PH24)
  4. improper conduct of other physicians or health professionals – report to College or regulatory body of the health professional (sexual impropriety by physicians is required reporting in some provinces)
  5. vital statistics must be reported; reporting varies by province (e.g. in Ontario, births are required to be reported within 30 days to Office of Registrar General or local municipality; death certificates must be completed by a MD then forwarded to municipal authorities)
  6. reporting to coroners (see *Physician Responsibilities Regarding Death*, ELOM14)
- physicians who fail to report in these situations are subject to prosecution and penalty, and may be liable if a third party has been harmed

Duty to Protect/Warn

- the physician has a duty to protect the public from a known dangerous patient; this may involve taking appropriate clinical action (e.g. involuntary detainment of violent patients for clinical assessment), informing the police, or warning the potential victim(s) if a patient expresses an intent to harm
- first established by a Supreme Court of California decision in 1976 (*Tarasoff v. Regents of the University of California*); supported by Canadian courts
- obliged by the CMA Code of Ethics and recognized by some provincial/territorial regulatory authorities
- concerns of breaching confidentiality should not prevent the MD from exercising the duty to protect; however, the disclosed information should not exceed that required to protect others
- applies in a situation where
  1. there is a clear risk to identifiable person(s);
  2. there is a risk of serious bodily harm or death; and
  3. the danger is imminent (i.e. more likely to occur than not)

Disclosure for Legal Proceedings

- disclosure of health records can be compelled by a court order, warrant, or subpoena

Privacy of Medical Records

- privacy of health information is protected by professional codes of ethics, provincial and federal legislation, the *Canadian Charter of Rights and Freedoms*, and the physician's fiduciary duty
- the federal government created the PIPEDA in 2000 which established principles for the collection, use, and disclosure of information that is part of commercial activity (e.g. physician practices, pharmacies, private labs)
- PIPEDA has been superseded by provincial legislation in many provinces, such as the *Ontario Personal Health Information Protection Act*, which applies more specifically to health information

Duties of Physicians with Regard to the Privacy of Health Information

- inform patients of information-handling practices through various means (e.g. posting notices, brochures and pamphlets, and/or through discussions with patients)
- obtain the patient's expressed consent to disclose information to third parties
  - under Ontario privacy legislation, the patient's expressed consent need not be obtained to share information between health care team members involved in the "circle of care." However, the patient may withdraw consent for this sharing of information and may put parts of the chart in a "lock box"
- provide the patient with access to their entire medical record; exceptions include instances where there is potential for serious harm to the patient or a third party
- provide secure storage of information and implement measures to limit access to patient records
- ensure proper destruction of information that is no longer necessary
- regarding taking pictures or videos of patients, findings, or procedures, in addition to patient consent and privacy laws, trespassing laws apply in some provinces

Consent and Capacity

Ethical Principles Underlying Consent and Capacity

- consent is the autonomous authorization of a medical intervention by a patient
- usually the principle of respect for patient autonomy overrides the principle of beneficence
- where a patient cannot make an autonomous decision (i.e. incapable), it is the duty of the SDM (or the physician in an emergency) to act on the patient's known prior wishes or, failing that, to act in the patient's best interests
- there is a duty to discover, if possible, what the patient would have wanted when capable
- central to determining best interests is understanding the patient's values, beliefs, and cultural or religious background
- more recently expressed wishes take priority over remote ones

- patient wishes may be verbal or written
- patients found incapable to make a specific decision should still be involved in that decision as much as possible
- agreement or disagreement with medical advice does not determine findings of capacity/incapacity
- however, patients opting for care that puts them at risk of serious harm that most people would want to avoid should have their capacity carefully assessed

Four Basic Requirements of Valid Consent

1. Voluntary
- consent must be given free of coercion or pressure (e.g. from parents or other family members who might exert 'undue influence')
- the physician must not deliberately mislead the patient about the proposed treatment

2. Capable
- the patient must be able to understand and appreciate the nature and effect of the proposed treatment

3. Specific
- the consent provided is specific to the procedure being proposed and to the provider who will carry out the procedure (e.g. the patient must be informed if students will be involved in providing the treatment)

4. Informed
- sufficient information and time must be provided to allow the patient to make choices in accordance with his/her wishes, including
  - the nature of the treatment or investigation proposed and its expected effects
  - all significant risks and special or unusual risks
  - alternative treatments or investigations and their anticipated effects and significant risks
  - the consequences of declining treatment
  - risks that are common sense need not be disclosed (i.e. bruising after venipuncture)
  - answers to any questions the patient may have
- the reasonable person test – the physician must provide all information that would be needed "by a reasonable person in the patient's position" to be able to make a decision
- disclose common adverse events (>1/200 chance of occurrence) and serious risks (e.g. death), even if remote
- it is the physician's responsibility to make reasonable attempts to ensure that the patient understands the information
- physicians should not withhold information about a legitimate therapeutic option based on personal conscience (e.g. not discussing the option of emergency contraception)

4 Basic Elements of Consent
- Voluntary
- Capable
- Specific
- Informed

Administration of treatment for an incapable patient in an emergency situation is applicable if the patient is:
- Experiencing extreme suffering
- At risk of sustaining serious bodily harm if treatment is not administered promptly

Patients may also ask to waive the right to choice (e.g. "You know what's best for me, doctor") or delegate their right to choose to someone else (e.g. a family member)

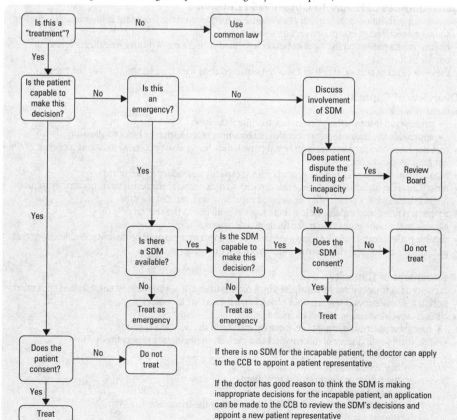

If there is no SDM for the incapable patient, the doctor can apply to the CCB to appoint a patient representative

If the doctor has good reason to think the SDM is making inappropriate decisions for the incapable patient, an application can be made to the CCB to review the SDM's decisions and appoint a new patient representative

Figure 2. Ontario consent flowchart   CCB = consent and capacity board; SDM = substitute decision-maker
Adapted by Hébert P from Sunnybrook Health Sciences Centre Consent Guidelines

The Supreme Court of Canada expects physicians to disclose the risks that a "reasonable" person would want to know. In practice, this means disclosing minor risks that are common as well as serious risks that happen infrequently, especially those risks that are particularly relevant to a particular patient (e.g. hearing loss for a musician)

Obtaining Legal Consent

- consent of the patient must be obtained before any medical intervention is provided; consent can be
  - verbal or written, although written is usually preferred
    - a signed consent form is only evidence of consent – it does not replace the process for obtaining valid consent
      - what matters is what the patient understands and appreciates, not what the signed consent form states
  - implied (e.g. a patient holding out their arm for an immunization) or expressed
- consent is an ongoing process and can be withdrawn or changed after it is given, unless stopping a procedure would put the patient at risk of serious harm
- *HCAA of Ontario* (1996) covers consent to treatment, admission to a facility, and personal assistance services (e.g. home care)

Exceptions to Consent

1. Emergencies

- treatment can be provided without consent where a patient is experiencing severe suffering, or where a delay in treatment would lead to serious harm or death and consent cannot be obtained from the patient or their SDM
- emergency treatment should not violate a prior expressed wish of the patient (e.g. a signed Jehovah's Witness card)
- if patient is incapable, MD must document reasons for incapacity and why situation is emergent
- patients have a right to challenge a finding of incapacity as it removes their decision-making ability
- if a SDM is not available, MD can treat without consent until the SDM is available or the situation is no longer emergent

Major Exceptions to Consent
- Emergencies
- Public and Mental Health Legislation
- Communicable diseases

2. Legislation

- Mental Health legislation allows for:
  - the detention of patients without their consent
  - psychiatric outpatients may be required to adhere to a care plan in accordance with Community Treatment Orders (see Psychiatry, PS51)
  - Public Health legislation allows medical officers of health to detain, examine, and treat patients without their consent (e.g. a patient with TB refusing to take medication) to prevent transmission of communicable diseases

3. Special Situations

- public health emergencies (e.g. an epidemic or communicable disease treatment)
- warrant for information by police

Consequences of Failure to Obtain Valid Consent

- treatment without consent is battery (an offense in tort), even if the treatment is life-saving (excluding situations outlined in exceptions section above)
- treatment of a patient on the basis of poorly informed consent may constitute negligence, also an offense in tort
- the onus of proof that valid consent was not obtained rests with the plaintiff (usually the patient)

Consent
- Treatment without consent = battery, including if NO consent or if WRONG procedure
- Treatment with poor or invalid consent = negligence

Overview of Capacity

- capacity is the ability to
  - understand information relevant to a treatment decision
  - appreciate the reasonably foreseeable consequences of a decision or lack of a decision
- capacity is specific for each decision (e.g. a person may be capable to consent to having a chest x-ray, but not for a bronchoscopy)
- capacity can change over time (e.g. temporary incapacity secondary to delirium)
- most Canadian jurisdictions distinguish capacity to make healthcare decisions from capacity to make financial decisions; a patient may be deemed capable of one, but not the other
- a person is presumed capable unless there is good evidence to the contrary
- capable patients are entitled to make their own decisions
- capable patients can refuse treatment even if it leads to serious harm or death; however, decisions that put patients at risk of serious harm or death require careful scrutiny

CPSO Policy on Capacity
Capacity is an essential component of valid consent, and obtaining valid consent is a policy of the CMA and other professional bodies

Assessment of Capacity

- capacity assessments must be conducted by a physician and, if appropriate, in consultation with other healthcare professionals (e.g. another physician, a mental health nurse)
- clinical capacity assessment may include
  - specific capacity assessment (i.e. capacity specific to the decision at hand)
    1. effective disclosure of information and evaluation of patient's reason for decision
    2. understanding of
       - his/her condition
       - the nature of the proposed treatment
       - alternatives to the treatment
       - the consequences of accepting and rejecting the treatment
       - the risks and benefits of the various options

Capacity Assessment
Test for understanding: can the patient recite what you have disclosed?
Test for appreciation: are his/her beliefs responsive to evidence?
Refer to: *JAMA* The Rational Clinical Examination "Does This Patient Have Medical Decision-Making Capacity?"

3. for the appreciation needed for decision making capacity, a person must
  – acknowledge the condition that affects him/herself
  – be able to assess how the various options would affect him or her
  – be able to reach a decision and adhere to it, and make a choice, not based primarily upon delusional belief
- general impressions
- input from psychiatrists, neurologists, etc.
- employ "Aid to Capacity Evaluation"
- a decision of incapacity may warrant further assessment by psychiatrist(s), legal review boards (e.g. in Ontario, the Consent and Capacity Review Board), or the courts
- judicial review is open to patients if found incapable

Treatment of the Incapable Patient in a Non-Emergent Situation
- obtain informed consent from SDM
- an incapable patient can only be detained against his/her will to receive treatment if he/she meets criteria for certification under the Mental Health Act (see Psychiatry, PS51); in such a situation:
  - document assessment in chart
  - notify patient of assessment using appropriate Mental Health Form(s) (Form 42 in Ontario)
  - notify Rights Advisor

Substitute Decision-Makers
- SDMs must follow the following principles when giving informed consent:
  - act in accordance with wishes previously expressed by the patient while capable
  - if wishes unknown, act in the patient's best interest, taking the following into account
    1. values and beliefs held by the patient while capable
    2. whether well-being is likely to improve with vs. without treatment
    3. whether the expected benefit outweighs the risk of harm
    4. whether a less intrusive treatment would be as beneficial as the one proposed
  - the final decision of the SDM may and should be challenged by the MD if the MD believes the SDM is not abiding by the above principles

Instructional Advance Directives
- allow patients to exert control over his/her care once they are no longer capable
- the patient sets out his/her decisions about future health care, including who he/she would allow to make treatment decisions on his/her behalf and what types of interventions he/she would want
- takes effect once the patient is incapable with respect to treatment decisions
- in Ontario, a person can appoint a power of attorney for personal care to carry out his/her advance directives
- patients should be encouraged to review these documents with their family and physicians and to reevaluate them often to ensure they are current with their wishes

POWERS OF ATTORNEY
- all Guardians and Attorneys have fiduciary duties for the dependent person

Definitions
- **Power of Attorney for Personal Care**
  - a legal document in which one person gives another the authority to make personal care decisions (health care, nutrition, shelter, clothing, hygiene, and safety) on their behalf if they become mentally incapable
- **Guardian of the Person**
  - someone who is appointed by the Court to make decisions on behalf of an incapable person in some or all areas of personal care, in the absence of a POA for personal care
- **Continuing Power of Attorney for Property**
  - a legal document in which a person gives another the legal authority to make decisions about their finances if they become unable to make those decisions
- **Guardian of Property**
  - someone who is appointed by the Public Guardian and Trustee or the Courts to look after an incapable person's property or finances
- **Public Guardian and Trustee**
  - acts as a SDM of last resort on behalf of mentally incapable people who do not have another individual to act on their behalf
- **Pediatric Aspects of Capacity Covered**
  - no age of consent in all provinces and territories except Québec; consent depends on patient's decision-making capacity
  - Québec has a specific age of consent, but common law and case law deem underage legal minors capable, allowing them to make their own choices
  - infants and children are assumed to lack mature decision-making capacity for consent but they should still be involved (i.e. be provided with information appropriate to their comprehension level)

Aid to Capacity Evaluation
- Ability to understand the medical problem
- Ability to understand the proposed treatment
- Ability to understand the alternatives (if any) to the proposed treatment
- Ability to understand the option of refusing treatment or of it being withheld or withdrawn
- Ability to appreciate the reasonably foreseeable consequences of accepting the proposed treatment
- Ability to appreciate the reasonably foreseeable consequences of refusing the proposed treatment
- Ability to make a decision that is not substantially based on delusions or depression
Adapted from Etchells et al. 1996

Most provinces have legislated hierarchies for SDMs; the hierarchy in Ontario is:
- Legally appointed guardian
- Appointed attorney for personal care, if a power of attorney confers authority for treatment consent (see *Powers of Attorney*)
- Representative appointed by the Consent and Capacity Board
- Spouse or partner
- Child (age 16 or older) or parent (unless the parent has only a right of access)
- Parent with only a right of access
- Sibling
- Other relative(s)
- Public guardian and trustee

There is no age of consent in Ontario Capacity is assessed on an individual basis

Other Types of Capacity Not Covered by the HCCA
- Testamentary (ability to make a will)
- Fitness (ability to stand trial)
- Financial (ability to manage property – Form 21 of the Mental Health Act)
- Personal (ability to care for oneself on a daily basis)

- adolescents are usually treated as adults
- preferably, assent should still be obtained from patient, even if not capable of giving consent
- in the event that the physician believes the SDM is not acting in the child's best interests, an appeal must be made to the local child welfare authorities
- under normal circumstances, parents have right of access to the child's medical record

Negligence

Ethical Basis
- the doctor-patient relationship is formed on trust, which is recognized in the concept of fiduciary duty/responsibility of physician towards patient
- negligence or malpractice is a form of failure on the part of the physician in fulfilling his/her fiduciary duty in providing appropriate care and leading to harm of the patient (and/or abuse of patient's trust)

Legal Basis
- physicians are legally liable to their patients for causing harm (tort) through a failure to meet the standard of care applicable under the circumstances
- standard/duty of care is defined as one that would reasonably be expected under similar circumstances of an ordinary, prudent physician of the same training, experience, specialization, and standing
- liability arises from physician's common law duty of care to his/her patients in the doctor/patient relationship (or, in Québec, from the Civil Code provisions regarding general civil liability)
- action(s) in negligence (or civil liability) against a physician must be launched by a patient within a specific prescribed period required by the respective province in which the actions occurred

Truth-Telling

Ethical Basis
- helps to promote and maintain a trusting physician-patient relationship
- patients have a right to be told important information that physicians have regarding their care
- enables patients to make informed decisions about health care and their lives

Legal Basis
- required for valid patient consent (see *Consent and Capacity*, ELOM6)
    - goal is to disclose information that a reasonable person in the patient's position would need in order to make an informed decision ("standard of disclosure")
- withholding information can be a breach of fiduciary duty and duty of care
- obtaining consent on the basis of misleading information can be seen as negligent

Evidence about Truth-Telling
- most patients want to know what is wrong with them
- although many patients want to protect family members from bad news, they themselves would want to be informed in the same situation
- truth-telling improves adherence and health outcomes
- informed patients are more satisfied with their care
- negative consequences of truth-telling can include decreased emotional well-being, anxiety, worry, social stigmatization, and loss of insurability

Challenges in Truth-Telling
Medical Error
- medical error may be defined as 'preventable adverse events (AEs)' caused by the patient's medical care and not the patient's underlying illness; some errors may be identified before they harm the patient, so not all error is truly 'adverse'
- many jurisdictions and professional associations expect and require physicians to disclose medical error; that is, any event that harms or threatens to harm patients must be disclosed to the patient or the patient's family and reported to the appropriate health authorities
- physicians should disclose to patients the occurrence of AEs or errors caused by medical management, but should not suggest that they resulted from negligence because:
    - negligence is a legal determination
    - error is not equal to negligence (see *Negligence*)
- disclosure allows the injured patient to seek appropriate corrective treatment promptly
    - physicians should avoid simple attributions as to cause and sole responsibility of others or oneself
    - physicians should offer apologies or empathic expressions of regret (e.g. "I wish things had turned out differently") as these can increase trust and are not admissions of guilt or liability
    - *Apology Acts* across Canada protect apologies, both as expressions of regret and admissions of responsibility, from being used as evidence of liability and negligence

Errors of care are compatible with non-negligent care if they are ones that a reasonably cautious and skilled MD could make (i.e. mistakes can be made due to 'honest error')

Four basic elements for action against a physician to succeed in negligence:
1. A duty of care owed to the patient (i.e. doctor/patient relationship must be established)
2. A breach of the standard of care
3. Some harm or injury to the patient
4. The harm or injury must have been caused by the breach of the duty of care

CPSO Policy on Truth-Telling
Physicians should provide patients with whatever information that will, from the patient's perspective, have a bearing on medical decision-making and communicate that information in a way that is comprehensible to the patient

Adverse Event
An unintended injury or complication from health care management resulting in disability, death, or prolonged hospital stay

Open Disclosure of AEs: Transparency and Safety in Health Care
Surg Clin North Am 2012;92(1):163-177
Health care providers have a fiduciary duty to disclose AEs to their patients. Professional societies codify medical providers' ethical requirement to disclose AEs to patients in accordance with the four principles of biomedical ethics. Transparency and honesty in relationships with patients create opportunities for learning that lead to systems improvements in health care organizations. Disclosure invariably becomes a component of broad systems improvement and is closely linked to improving patient safety.

Examples of Warning of Impending Bad News
"I have something difficult to tell you…"
"This may come as a shock to you, but the tests indicate…"
"There is no easy way for me to tell you this, so I will tell you straight away that you have a serious problem…"

Breaking Bad News
- 'bad news' may be any information that reveals conditions or illnesses threatening the patient's sense of well-being
- caution patients in advance of serious tests about possible bad findings
- give warnings of impending bad news and make sure you provide time for the patient
- poorly done disclosure may be as harmful as non-disclosure
- truth-telling may be a process requiring multiple visits
- adequate support should be provided along with the disclosure of difficult news
- SPIKES protocol was developed to facilitate "breaking bad news"

Protocol to Break Bad News: SPIKES
S **Setting** the scene and listening skills
P **Patient's** perception of condition and seriousness
I **Invitation** from patient to give information
K **Knowledge** – giving medical facts
E **Explore** emotions and empathize
S **Strategy** and summary
Source: Baile WF, Buckman R. 2000

Arguments Against Truth-Telling
- may go against certain cultural norms and expectations
- may lead to patient harm and increased anxiety
- 10-20% of patients prefer not to be informed
- medical uncertainty may result in the disclosure of uncertain or inaccurate information

Exceptions to Truth-Telling
- a patient may waive his/her right to know the truth about their situation (i.e. decline information that would normally be disclosed) when
  - the patient clearly declines to be informed
  - a strong cultural component exists that should be respected and acknowledged
  - the patient may wish others to be informed and make the medical decisions for him/her
- the more weighty the consequences for the patient from non-disclosure, the more carefully one must consider the right to ignorance
- 'emergencies': an urgent need to treat may legitimately delay full disclosure; the presumption is that most people would want such treatment and the appropriate SDM cannot be found
- 'therapeutic privilege'
  - withholding of information by the clinician in the belief that disclosure of the information would itself lead to severe anxiety, psychological distress or physical harm to the patient
  - clinicians should avoid invoking therapeutic privilege due to its paternalistic overtones and is a defence of non-disclosure that is rarely accepted anymore
  - it is often not the truth that is unpalatable; it is how it is conveyed that can harm the patient

Truth-Telling in Discussing Prognosis in Advanced Life-Limiting Illnesses
Palliat Med 2007;21(6):507-517
Many physicians express discomfort at having to broach the topic of prognosis, including limited life expectancy, and may withhold information or not disclose prognosis. A systematic review of 46 studies relating to truth-telling in discussing prognosis with patients with progressive, advanced life-limiting illnesses and their caregivers showed that although the majority of physicians believed that patients and caregivers should be told the truth about the prognosis, in practice, many either avoid discussing the topic or withhold information. Reasons include perceived lack of training, stress, no time to attend to the patient's emotional needs, fear of a negative impact on the patient, uncertainty about prognostication, requests from family members to withhold information and a feeling of inadequacy or hopelessness regarding the unavailability of further curative treatment.
Evidence suggests that patients can discuss the topic without it having a negative impact on them.

Ethical Issues in Health Care

Managing Controversial and Ethical Issues in Practice
- discuss in a non-judgmental manner
- ensure patients have full access to relevant and necessary information
- identify if certain options lie outside of your moral boundaries and refer to another physician if appropriate
- consult with appropriate ethics committees or boards
- protect freedom of moral choice for students or trainees
Source: MCC-CLEO *Objectives* 1998

Reproductive Technologies

Overview of the Maternal-Fetal Relationship
- in general, maternal and fetal interests align
- in some situations, a conflict between maternal autonomy and the best interests of the fetus may arise

Ethical Issues and Arguments
- principle of reproductive freedom: women have the right to make their own reproductive choices
- coercion of a woman to accept efforts to promote fetal well-being is an unacceptable infringement of her personal autonomy

Legal Issues and Arguments
- the law upholds a woman's right to life, liberty, and security of person, and does not recognize fetal rights; key aspects of the mother's rights include
  - if a woman is competent and refuses medical advice, her decision must be respected even if the fetus will suffer
  - the fetus does not have legal rights until it is born alive and with complete delivery from the body of the woman

Royal Commission on New Reproductive Technologies (1993) recommendations:
1. medical treatment must never be imposed upon a competent pregnant woman against her wishes
2. no law should be used to confine a pregnant woman in the interest of her fetus
3. the conduct of a pregnant woman in relation to her fetus should not be criminalized
4. child welfare should never be used to control a woman's behaviour during pregnancy
5. civil liability should never be imposed upon a woman for harm done to her fetus during pregnancy

Payment of gamete donors is currently illegal in Canada. The ART Act is, however, not being enforced currently as it does not clarify whether ART falls under the jurisdiction of the federal or provincial government

The fetus does not have legal rights until it is born alive and with complete delivery from the body of the woman

Once outside the mother's body, the neonate becomes a member of society with all the rights and protections other vulnerable persons receive.
- Non-treatment of a neonate born alive is only acceptable if <22 wk GA
- 23-25 wk GA: treatment should be a consensual decision between physician and parents
- 25 wk GA and more: neonate should receive full treatment unless major anomalies or conditions incompatible with life are present
Source: *Paed Child Health* 2012:443

Examples involving the use of established guidelines
- a woman is permitted to refuse HIV testing during pregnancy, even if vertical transmission to fetus results
- a woman is permitted to refuse Caesarean section in labour that is not progressing, despite evidence of fetal distress

Advanced Reproductive Technologies: Ethically Appropriate Actions
- Educate patients and address contributors to infertility (e.g. stress, alcohol, medications, etc.)
- Investigate and treat underlying health problems causing infertility
- Wait at least 1 yr before initiating treatment with ART (exceptions – advanced age or specific indicators of infertility)
- Educate and prepare patients for potential negative outcomes of ART

Advanced Reproductive Therapies
- includes non-coital insemination, hormonal ovarian stimulation, and IVF
- topics with ethical concerns
  - donor anonymity vs. child-centred reproduction (i.e. knowledge about genetic medical history)
  - preimplantation genetic testing for diagnosis before pregnancy
  - use of new techniques without patients appreciating their experimental nature
  - embryo status – the Supreme Court of Canada maintains that fetuses are "unique" but not persons under law; this view would likely apply to embryos as well
  - access to ART
  - private vs. public funding of ART
  - social factors limiting access to ART (e.g. same-sex couples)
  - the 'commercialization' of reproduction

Fetal Tissue
- pluripotent stem cells can currently be derived from human embryonic and fetal tissue
- potential uses of stem cells in research
  - studying human development and factors that direct cell specialization
  - evaluating drugs for efficacy and safety in human models
  - cell therapy: using stem cells grown *in vitro* to repair or replace degenerated/destroyed/malignant tissues (e.g. Parkinson's disease)
  - genetic treatment aimed at altering somatic cells (e.g. myocardial or immunological cells) is acceptable and ongoing

The Tri-Council Policy Statement
1. Genetic treatment aimed at altering germ cells is prohibited in Canada and elsewhere
2. Embryo research is permitted up to 14 d post-fertilization
3. Embryos created for reproductive purposes that are no longer required may be used
4. Gamete providers must give free and informed consent for research use
5. No commercial transactions in the creation and use of the embryos are permitted
6. Creation of embryos solely for research purposes is prohibited
7. Human cloning is strictly prohibited
8. Risks of coercion must be minimized (i.e. the fertility treatment team may not be pressured to generate more embryos than necessary)
9. One may only discuss the option of using fetal tissue for research after free and informed choice to have a therapeutic abortion has been made by the patient
10. Physicians responsible for fertility treatment may not be part of a stem cell research team

Induced Abortion
- CMA definition of induced abortion: the active termination of a pregnancy before fetal viability (fetus >500 g or >20 wk GA)
- CMA policy on induced abortion
  1. induced abortion should not be used as an alternative to contraception
  2. counselling on contraception must be readily available
  3. full and immediate counselling services must be provided in the event of unwanted pregnancy
  4. there should be no delay in the provision of abortion services
  5. no patient should be compelled to have a pregnancy terminated
  6. physicians should not be compelled to participate in abortion – if morally opposed, the physician should inform the patient so she may consult another physician
  7. no discrimination should be directed towards either physicians who do not perform or assist at induced abortions or physicians who do
  8. induced abortion should be uniformly available to all women in Canada and health care insurance should cover all the costs (note: the upper limit of GA for which coverage is provided varies between provinces)
  9. elective termination of pregnancy after fetal viability may be indicated under exceptional circumstances

Ethical and Legal Concerns and Arguments
- no law currently regulates abortion in Canada
- it is a woman's medical decision to be made in consultation with whom she wishes; there is no mandatory role for spouse/family
- 2nd and even 3rd trimester abortions are not illegal in Canada, but are usually only carried out when there are serious risks to the woman's health, or if the fetus has died *in utero* or has major malformations (e.g. anencephaly)

Prenatal/Antenatal Genetic Testing
- uses
  1. to confirm a clinical diagnosis
  2. to detect genetic predisposition to a disease
  3. allows preventative steps to be taken and helps patient prepare for the future
  4. gives parents the option to terminate a pregnancy or begin early treatment
- ethical dilemmas arise because of the sensitive nature of genetic information; important considerations of genetic testing include:
  - the individual and familial implications
  - its pertinence to future disease
  - its ability to identify disorders for which there are no effective treatments or preventive steps
  - its ability to identify the sex of the fetus
- ethical issues and arguments regarding the use of prenatal/antenatal genetic testing include:
- obtaining informed consent is difficult due to the complexity of genetic information
- doctor's duty to maintain confidentiality vs. duty to warn family members
- risk of social discrimination (e.g. insurance) and psychological harm

Legal Aspects
- no current specific legislation exists
- testing requires informed consent
- no standard of care exists for clinical genetics, but physicians are legally obligated to inform patients that prenatal testing exists and is available
- a physician can breach confidentiality terms in order to warn family members about a condition if harm can possibly be prevented via treatment or prevention (e.g. familial adenomatous polyposis, Gastroenterology, G34)

Genetic Testing: Ethically Appropriate Actions
- thorough discussion and realistic planning with patient before testing is done
- genetic counselling for delivery of complex information

End-of-Life Care

Overview of Palliative and End-of-Life Care
- focus of care is comfort and respect for person nearing death and maximizing quality of life for patient, family, and loved ones
- appropriate for any patient at any stage of a serious or life-limiting illness
- may occur in a hospital, hospice, in the community, or at home
- often involves an interdisciplinary team of caregivers
- addresses the medical, psychosocial, and spiritual dimensions of care

Euthanasia and Physician-Assisted Suicide
- **euthanasia**: a deliberate act undertaken by one person with the intention of ending the life of another person to relieve that person's suffering, where the act is the cause of death
- **physician-assisted suicide**: the act of intentionally killing oneself with the assistance of a physician who deliberately provides the knowledge and/or the means

Common Ethical Arguments/Opinions
- patient has the right to make autonomous choices about the time and manner of their own death
- belief that there is no ethical difference between the acts of euthanasia/assisted suicide and forgoing life-sustaining treatments
- belief that these acts benefit terminally ill patients by relieving suffering
- patient autonomy has limits
- death should be the consequence of the morally justified withdrawal of life-sustaining treatments only in cases where there is a fatal underlying condition, and it is the condition (not the withdrawal of treatment) that causes death

Legal Aspect
- in Canada, euthanasia is no longer a punishable offence under the Criminal Code of Canada
- in the *Carter v. Canada* decision of February 2015, physician-assisted suicide ruled to be not criminal, with the decision taking effect in 2016, now postponed to June 2016
- until June 2016, applicants for assistance in dying (MAID - 'Medical Aid in Dying') must obtain court sanction (as an exemption to the Criminal Code)

Criteria for MAID
- grievously and irreversibly ill / injured
- suffering intolerable to the patient
- not treatable by means acceptable to the patient
- adult, competent patient, clear and freely given consent

Acceptable Use of Palliative and End-of-Life Care
- the use of palliative sedation with opioids in end-of-life care, knowing that death may occur as an unintended consequence (principle of double effect) is distinguished from euthanasia and assisted suicide where death is the primary intent
- the appropriate withdrawal of life-support is distinguished from euthanasia and assisted suicide as it is seen as allowing the underlying disease to take its 'natural course' but this distinction may be more theoretical than real
- consent for withdrawal of life-support must be sought from SDMs, as ruled in Cuthbertson v. Rasouli in 2013, as palliative care would be instituted and consent for that would require SDM consent
- refusals of care by the patient that may lead to death as well as requests for a hastened death, ought to be carefully explored by the physician to rule out any 'reversible factors' (e.g. poor palliation, depression, poverty, ill-education, isolation) that may be hindering authentic choice

Surrogate mothers cannot be paid or offered compensation beyond a reimbursement of their expenses
Source: Assisted Human Reproduction Act, 2004

No one under age 18 can donate sperm or eggs, except for the purpose of creating a child that the donor plans to raise himself/herself (e.g. young patients receiving radiation therapy for cancer that may cause infertility)
Source: Semen Regulations of the Food and Drug Act, 1996

Know the Difference
Palliative care assists patients who are dying, but unlike euthanasia or physician-assisted suicide, it does not aim directly at or intend to end the person's life

Euthanasia: Ethically Appropriate Actions
- Respect competent decisions to forgo treatment
- Provide appropriate palliative measures
- Decline requests for euthanasia and assisted suicide
- Try to assess reasons for such requests from patients to see if there are 'reversible factors' (such as depression, pain, loneliness, anxiety) that can be treated

Mental Health Outcomes of Family Members of Patients Who Request Physician Aid in Dying
J Pain Symptom Manage 2009;38(6):807-815
Surveyed 95 family members of patients who had explicitly requested aid in dying, including 59 whose loved one received a lethal prescription and 36 whose loved one died by lethal ingestion. For comparison purposes, family members of patients who died of cancer or amyotrophic lateral sclerosis also were surveyed.
Among those whose family member requested aid in dying, whether or not the patient accessed a lethal prescription had no influence on subsequent depression, grief, or mental health services use; however, family members of patients who received a lethal prescription were more likely to believe that their loved one's choices were honored and less likely to have regrets about how the loved one died. Comparing family members of those who requested aid in dying to those who did not revealed no differences in primary mental health outcomes of depression, grief, or mental health services use. Family members of patients who requested aid in dying felt more prepared and accepting of the death than comparison family members.
Pursuit of aid in dying does not have negative effects on surviving family members and may be associated with greater preparation and acceptance of death.

Physician Responsibilities Regarding Death

- physicians are required by law to complete a medical certificate of death unless the coroner needs notification; failure to report death is a criminal offence
- *Coroner's Act*, 1990 (specific to Ontario, similar in other provinces) requires physicians to notify a coroner or police officer if death occurs
  - due to violence, negligence, misconduct, misadventure, or malpractice
  - during pregnancy or is attributable to pregnancy
  - suddenly and unexpectedly
  - from disease which was not treated by a legally qualified medical practitioner
  - from any cause other than disease
  - under suspicious circumstances
- coroner investigates these deaths, as well as deaths that occur in psychiatric institutions, jails, foster homes, nursing homes, hospitals to which a person was transferred from a facility, institution or home, etc.
- in consultation with forensic pathologists and other specialists, the coroner establishes:
  - the identity of the deceased
  - where and when the death occurred
  - the medical cause of death
  - the means of death (i.e. natural, accidental, suicide, homicide, or undetermined)
- coroners do not make decisions regarding criminality or legal responsibility
  unclear as yet whether physicians who object to MAID on grounds of conscience will have to refer to willing physicians and also unclear what patients seeking MAID in religious affiliated hospitals will do

Notify Coroner if Death Occurs due to:
- Violence, negligence, misconduct
- Pregnancy
- Sudden or unexpected causes
- Disease not treated
- Cause other than disease
- Suspicious circumstances

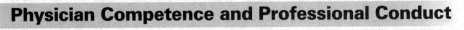

Physician Competence and Professional Conduct

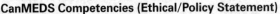

CanMeds Competencies
- Communicator
- Collaborator
- Health Advocate
- Leader
- Professional
- Scholar
- Medical Expert

CanMEDS Competencies (Ethical/Policy Statement)
- a framework of professional competencies established by the MCC as objectives for the MCC Qualifying Exam
- further information on MCC objectives can be found at www.mcc.ca

Legal Considerations
- physicians' conduct and competence are legally regulated to protect patients and society via mandatory membership to provincial governing bodies (e.g. the CPSO)
- physicians are legally required to maintain a license with the appropriate authority, and are thus legally bound to outlined policies on matters of conduct within his/her medical practice
- the ultimate constraint on MD behaviour as regards to unprofessionalism is 'conduct unbecoming a physician', such as inappropriate behaviour with colleagues, conflicts of interest, untruthfulness, unethical billing practices, and sexual impropriety with patients

Common Policies on Physician Conduct
- physicians must ensure that patients have access to continuous on-call coverage and are never abandoned
- sexual conduct with patients, even when consented to by the patient, is a serious matter that can lead to accusations of battery by the patient and provincial governing body. Important notes on this topic include:
  - inappropriate sexual conduct includes intercourse, undue touching, references to sexual matters, sexual jokes, and physician presence when capable patients undress or dress
  - in specified situations, physicians may have a personal relationship with a patient provided a year has passed since the last therapeutic contact
  - physicians are permanently prohibited from personal relationships with patients whom they saw for psychotherapy
  - in Ontario, physicians must report any colleagues of whom they have information regarding sexual impropriety (as per CPSO Code of Ethics)
- physicians must maintain adequate records for each patient, which include:
  - demonstration that care has been continuous and comprehensive
  - minimal standards for record-keeping, including readability, diagnosis, differential diagnosis, appropriate tests and referrals, and a coherent patient record, including drugs, a Cumulative Patient profile, all aspects of charting that are required for safe patient care (full standards available at www.cpso.on.ca). Another physician should be able to take over the safe care of the patient based on the record
  - records stored for 10 years in most jurisdictions
  - although the medical record is the property of the physician or an institution, the patient or the patient's delegate must be allowed full access to information in the medical record in a reasonable period of time, and can charge a reasonable fee, upon (usually written) request
- in the hospital, physicians must ensure their own competence, respect hospital by-laws and regulations, practice only within the limits of granted privileges, cooperate with other hospital personnel, and maintain adequate hospital records

CPSO Policy: Treating Self and Family Members
Physicians will not diagnose or treat themselves or family members except for minor conditions or in emergencies and then only if no other physician is readily available

CPSO Policy: Ending the Physician-Patient Relationship
Discontinuing services that are needed is an act of professional misconduct unless done by patient request, alternative services are arranged, or adequate notice has been given

CMA Code of Ethics
Report any unprofessional conduct by colleagues to the appropriate authority

Research Ethics

- involves the systematic analysis of ethical dilemmas arising during research involving human subjects to ensure that:
  - study participants are protected
  - clinical research is conducted to serve the interests of the participants and/or society as a whole
- major ethical dilemmas arise when a physician's obligation to the patient comes into conflict with other obligations and incentives
- any exceptions to disclosure for therapeutic consent do not apply in an experimental situation
- important ethical principles to consider when conducting research on human subjects were laid out in the *Declaration of Helsinki, the Belmont Report,* and the *Tri-Council Policy Statement: Ethical Conduct on Research Involving Human Subjects*

Table 5. Ethical Principles for Research Involving Human Subjects

Patient's participation in research should not put him/her at a known or probable disadvantage with respect to medical care (i.e. cannot deny participants in research 'known effective care', such as randomizing some depressed patients to a placebo arm with no treatment)

Participant's voluntary and informed choice is usually required, except in special circumstances (i.e. chart reviews without patient contact, or emergency situations for which there is no accepted or helpful standard of care and the proposed intervention is not likely to cause more harm than such patients already face)

Access to the treatment that is considered standard (i.e. placebo-controlled trials are generally acceptable where patients all receive still receive the standard of care, or, if not, are informed about the placebo arm and what that entails)

Must employ a scientifically valid design to answer the research question (ensured via peer review, expert opinion)

Must demonstrate sufficient value to justify any risk posed to participants

Must be conducted honestly (i.e. carried out as stated in the approved protocol)

Findings must be reported promptly and accurately without exaggeration, to allow practicing clinicians to draw reasonable conclusions

Patients must not be enticed into risky research by the lure of money and investigators must not trade the interests of patients for disproportionate recompense by a sponsor; both participants and investigators are due fair recompense for their time and efforts

Any significant interventional trial ought to have a data safety monitoring board that is independent of the sponsor and can ensure safety of the ongoing trial

Physician-Industry Relations

- health care delivery in Canada involves collaboration between physicians and the pharmaceutical and health supply industries in the areas of research, education, and clinical evaluation packages (i.e. product samples)
- physicians have a responsibility to ensure that their participation in such collaborative efforts is in keeping with their duties to their patients and society
- gifts or free products from the pharmaceutical industry are usually inappropriate
  - sponsorship for travel and fees for conference attendance may be accepted only where the physician is a conference presenter and not just in attendance
  - physicians receiving such sponsorship must disclose this at presentations and/or in written articles

Resource Allocation

- definition: the distribution of goods and services to programs and people
- physicians have the duty to inform patients about therapeutic options even if they are not available
- physicians must make health care resources available to patients in a manner which is fair and equitable, without bias or discrimination
  - need and benefit are morally relevant criteria for resource allocation
  - gender, sexual orientation, religion, level of education, or age alone are morally irrelevant criteria
- ethical dilemmas that arise when deciding how best to allocate resources
  - fair chances versus best outcome: favouring best outcome vs. giving all patients fair access to limited resources (e.g. transplant list prioritization)
  - priorities problem: how much priority should the sickest patients receive?
  - aggregation problem: modest benefits to many vs. significant benefits to few
  - democracy problem: when to rely on a fair democratic process to arrive at a decision

Guidelines for Appropriately Allocating Resources
- the physician's primary obligation is to:
  - protect and promote the welfare and best interests of his/her patients
  - choose interventions known to be beneficial on the basis of evidence of effectiveness
  - seek the tests or treatments that will accomplish the diagnostic or therapeutic goal for the least cost
  - advocate for one's patients, but avoid manipulating the system to gain unfair advantage for them
  - resolve conflicting claims for scarce resources justly, on the basis of morally relevant criteria such as need and benefit, using fair and publicly defensible procedures
  - inform patients of the impact of cost constraints on care, but in a sensitive way
  - seek resolution of unacceptable shortages at the level of hospital management or government

Guiding Principles for Research Ethics
- Respect for persons: informed consent
- Beneficence: harm vs. benefit
- Justice: avid exploitation/unjustified exclusion

Informed Consent for Research
- Purpose of study
- Sum of funding
- Name and probability of harm and benefits
- Nature of physician's participation including compensation
- Proposals for research must be submitted to a research ethics board

Randomization is allowed even if there is an efficacious standard if, for example, there are drawbacks to it (such as it doesn't work for all, has side effects, and is not wanted by all patients). In such cases, there must be a good safety net established to make sure subjects in the placebo arm do not deteriorate (i.e. there must be a safety monitoring plan for such studies)

CMA and CPSO Guidelines for Ethically Appropriate Physician-Industry Relations
- The primary goal should be the advancement of the health of Canadians
- Relationships should be guided by the CMA Code of Ethics
- The physician's primary obligation is to the patient
- Physicians should avoid any self-interest in their prescribing and referral practices
- Physicians should always maintain professional autonomy, independence, and commitment to the scientific method

Professional Considerations
Elderly Patient
- Identify their resuscitation options (CPR or DNR), if applicable
- Check for documentation of advance directives and POA where applicable
- For further details, see Geriatric Medicine, GM12
Pediatric Patient
- Identify the primary decision-maker (parents, guardian, wards-of-state, emancipated)
- Regarding capacity assessment see Pediatric Aspects of Capacity Covered by the HCCA, ELOM9
- Be wary of custody issues if applicable
Terminally Ill or Palliative Patient
- Consider the SPIKES approach to breaking bad news
- What are his/her goals of care (i.e. disease vs. symptom management)?
- Identify advance directives, POA, or SDM, if applicable (see ELOM9)
- Check for documentation of resuscitation options (CPR or DNR) and likelihood of success
- For further details, see Geriatric Medicine, GM12
Incapable Patient
- If not already present, perform a formal capacity assessment
- Identify if the patient has a SDM or who has their POA
- Check the patient's chart for any Mental Health Forms (e.g. Form 1) or any forms they may have on their person (e.g. Form 42)

Conscientious Objection

Patients Refusing Treatment

- in accordance with the principle of autonomy, it is generally acceptable for competent patients to refuse medical interventions for themselves or others, although exceptions may occur
- if parents or SDMs make decisions that are clearly not in the "best interests" of an incapable child, physicians may have ethical grounds for administering treatment, depending on the acuity of the clinical situation
  - in high-acuity scenarios (e.g. refusing blood transfusion based on religious grounds for a child in hemorrhagic shock), physicians have a stronger obligation to act in the child's best interests
  - in lower acuity scenarios (e.g. refusing childhood immunization in a developed nation) there is a stronger obligation to respect the autonomy of the decision-makers
  - pursuing traditional First Nations healing (in conjunction or in the place of standard biomedical therapy) is legally considered a constitutionally protected right, which can be made by a SDM, as ruled in *Hamilton Health Sciences v. DH* in 2014

Physicians Refusing to Provide Treatment

- physicians may refuse to provide treatment or discontinue relationships with patients, but must ensure these patients can access services elsewhere (e.g. a pediatrician who refuses to treat an unvaccinated child should refer the family to another practice)

References

Bioethics
Bioethics for Clinicians Series. CMAJ.
Chenier NM. Reproductive technologies: Royal Commission final report. 1994. Available from: http://publications.gc.ca/Collection-R/LoPBdP/MR/mr124-e.htm.
CMA Code of Ethics, Canadian Medical Association. Available from: http://www.cma.ca.
Etchells E, Sharpe G, Elliott C, et al. Bioethics for clinicians. CMAJ 1996;155:657-661.
Gilmour J, Harrison C, Asadi L, et al. Childhood immunization: When physicians and parents disagree. Pediatrics 2011;128:S167-174.
Hébert P. Doing right: A practical guide to ethics for physicians and medical trainees, 3rd ed. Toronto: Oxford University Press, 2014.
Hébert PC, Hoffmaster B, Glass K, et al. Bioethics for clinicians. CMAJ 1997;156:225-228.

Governing Organizations
Canadian Medical Association. Available from: http://www.cma.ca.
College of Physicians and Surgeons of Ontario. Available from: http://www.cpso.on.ca.
College of Physicians and Surgeons of Ontario. CPSO policy statements. Available from: http://www.cpso.on.ca/policies/mandatory.htm.
Ontario Medical Association. Available from: http://www.oma.org.
Royal College of Physicians and Surgeons of Ontario. CanMEDS 2005 framework. Available from: http://www.royalcollege.ca/shared/documents/canmeds/the_7_canmeds_roles_e.pdf.
WHO. World Health Report 2005. Available from: http://www.who.int/whr/en.

Health Care Delivery
Baile WF, Buckman R, Lenzi R, et al. SPIKES: A six-step protocol for delivering bad news: application to the patient with cancer. Oncologist 2000;5:302-311.
Baker GR, Norton PG, Flintoft V, et al. The Canadian adverse events study: The incidence of adverse events among hospital patients in Canada. CMAJ 2004;70:1678-1686.
Canadian Institute for Health Information. National health expenditure trends 1975 to 2014. Ottawa; CIHI, 2014.
Collier R. Steps forward no guarantee that health targets will be met, council says. CMAJ 2011;183:e619-620.
Devereaux PJ, Choi PT, Lacchetti C, et al. A systematic review and meta-analysis of studies comparing mortality rates of private for-profit and private not-for-profit hospitals. CMAJ 2002;166:1399-1406.
Kirby M. The Kirby Commission: The health of Canadians – the federal role. 2002. Available from: http://www.parl.gc.ca/37/2/parlbus/commbus/senate/Com-e/soci-e/rep-e/repoct02vol6-e.htm.
National Center for Health Statistics, Center for Disease Control and Prevention. Available from: http://www.cdc.gov/nchs.
National Center for Health Statistics. With special feature on medical technology. Hyattsville (US), 2010.
Naylor CD. Health care in Canada: Incrementalism under fiscal duress. Health Affair 1999;18:9-26.
OECD. Health Data. 2008. Available from: http://www.oecd.org.
PBS. Healthcare crisis: Healthcare timeline. 2012. Available from: http://www.pbs.org/healthcarecrisis/.
Romanow R. The Romanow report: Royal commission on the future of health care in Canada. 2002. Available from: http://www.hc-sc.gc.ca/hcs-sss/alt_formats/hpb-dgps/pdf/hhr/romanow-eng.pdf.
Shah CP. Public health and preventive medicine in Canada, 5th ed. Toronto: Elsevier Canada, 2003:357-360,426.
News release: The Senate Committee on Social Affairs, Science and Technology tables its report on the review of the 2004 health accord. 2012. Available from: http://www.parl.gc.ca/Content/SEN/Committee/411/soci/press/27mar12B-e.htm.

Important Acts/Charters
Canada Health Act - R.S.C., 1985, c. C-6.
Canadian Public Health Association and WHO. Ottawa charter for health promotion. Ottawa: Health and Welfare Canada, 1986.
Health Care Consent Act - S.O., 1996, c. 2, Sched. A.
Health Protection and Promotion Act - R.S.O., 1990, c. 7; O. Re.g. 559/91, amended to O. Re.g. 96/03.

Law
Carter v. Canada (Attorney General), 2015 SCC 5.
Cuthbertson v. Rasouli, 2013 SCC 53, [2013] 3 S.C.R. 341.
Devereaux PJ, Heels-Ansdell D, Lacchetti C, et al. Canadian health law and policy. Markham: LexisNexis, 2007.
Ferris LE, Barkun H, Carlisle J, et al. Defining the physician's duty to warn: consensus statement of Ontario's medical expert panel on duty to Inform. CMAJ 1998;158:1473-1479.
Hamilton Health Sciences Corp. v. D.H., 2014 ONCJ 603 (CanLII).
Medical Council of Canada. Objectives of the considerations of the legal, ethical and organizational aspects of the practice of medicine. 1999. Available from: http://www.mcc.ca.
Ontario Medical Association. Physician privacy toolkit. 2004. Available from: http://www.oma.org/phealth/privacymain.htm.
Ontario's Office of the Chief Coroner. Available from: http://www.mpss.jus.gov.on.ca.

Research Ethics
Canadian Medical Association. Policy: Guidelines for physicians in interactions with industry. 2012. Available from: http://policybase.cma.ca/dbtw-wpd/Policypdf/PD08-01.pdf.
Government of Canada: Interagency panel on research ethics. Tri-council policy statement: Ethical conduct on research involving humans. 2014. Available from: http://www.pre.ethics.gc.ca/eng/policy-politique/initiatives/tcps2-eptc2/Default/.

Anesthesia and Perioperative Medicine

Simon Feng, Madelaine Kukko, and **Michael Poon,** chapter editors
Naryan Chattergoon and **Desmond She,** associate editors
Arnav Agarwal and **Quynh Huynh,** EBM editors
Dr. Diana Tamir and **Dr. Jeff Wassermann,** staff editors

Acronyms

2,3-BPG	2,3-Bisphosphoglycerate	FiO2	fraction of oxygen in inspired air
ACC	American College of Cardiology	FFP	fresh frozen plasma
ACh	acetylcholine	FRC	functional residual capacity
AChE	acetylcholinesterase	GA	general anesthetic
ACV	assist-control ventilation	GERD	gastroesophageal reflux disease
AHA	American Heart Association	Hb(i)	initial hematocrit
ALS	amyotrophic lateral sclerosis	Hb(f)	final hematocrit
ARDS	acute respiratory distress syndrome	Hct	hematocrit
atm	atmosphere	HES	hydroxyethyl starch
CCS	Canadian Cardiovascular Society	ICP	intracranial pressure
CK	creatine kinase	ICS	inhaled corticosteroids
CO	cardiac output	IOP	intraocular pressure
CSF	cerebrospinal fluid	LA	local anesthetic
CVP	central venous pressure	LABA	long-acting β-agonist
DIC	disseminated intravascular coagulation	LES	lower esophageal sphincter
ETCO2	End-Tidal CO2	LMA	laryngeal mask airway
ETT	endotracheal tube	LOC	level of consciousness

MAC	minimum alveolar concentration	PPV	positive pressure ventilation
MAP	mean arterial pressure	RSI	rapid sequence induction
MH	malignant hyperthermia	SABA	short-acting β-agonist
MS	multiple sclerosis	SCh	succinylcholine
NMJ	neuromuscular junction	SIADH	syndrome of inappropriate antidiuretic hormone
NYHA	New York Heart Association		
OCS	oral costicosteroids	SNS	sympathetic nervous system
OR	operating room	SV	stroke volume
PaCO2	arterial partial pressure of carbon dioxide	SVR	systemic vascular resistance
		TBW	total body water
PaO2	arterial partial pressure of oxygen	TIVA	total intravenous anesthetic
PC	patient-controlled	TURP	transurethral resection of prostate
PCA	patient-controlled analgesia	V/Q	ventilation/perfusion
PCV	pressure-controlled ventilation	VT	ventricular tachycardia
PEEP	positive end-expiratory pressure	VTE	venous thromboembolism
PNS	parasympathetic nervous system		
PONV	post-operative nausea and vomiting		

Overview of Anesthesia

- anesthesia: lack of sensation/perception
- **approach to anesthesia**

6 As of General Anesthesia
Anesthesia
Anxiolysis
Amnesia
Areflexia (muscle relaxation - not always required)
Autonomic stability
Analgesia

1. pre-operative assessment
2. patient optimization

3. plan anesthetic
   various types of anesthesia
   pre-medication
   airway management
   monitors
   induction
   maintenance
   emergence
   extubation

4. post-operative care

Types of Anesthesia

- **general**
  - general anesthesia (GA)
  - total IV anesthesia (TIVA)
- **regional**
  - spinal, epidural
  - peripheral nerve block
  - IV regional
- **local**
  - local infiltration
  - topical

Note that different types of anesthesia can be combined (general + regional)

Pre-Operative Assessment

Purpose
- identify concerns for medical and surgical management of patient
- allow for questions to help allay any fears or concerns patient and/or family may have
- arrange further investigations, consultations and treatments for patients not yet optimized
- plan and consent for anesthetic techniques

History and Physical

History
- age, gender
- indication for surgery
- surgical/anesthetic Hx: previous anesthetics, any complications, previous intubations, medications, drug allergies, post-operative N/V
- FHx: abnormal anesthetic reactions, malignant hyperthermia, pseudocholinesterase deficiency (see *Uncommon Complications*, A28)

- PMHx
  - CNS: seizures, TIA/strokes, raised ICP, spinal disease, aneurysm
  - CVS: angina/CAD, MI, CHF, HTN, valvular disease, dysrhythmias, peripheral vascular disease (PVD), conditions requiring endocarditis prophylaxis, exercise tolerance, CCS/NYHA class (Cardiology and Cardiac Surgery, C35 sidebar for *NYHA Classification*)
  - respiratory: smoking, asthma, COPD, recent upper respiratory tract infection, sleep apnea
  - GI: GERD, liver disease, NPO status
  - renal: insufficiency, dialysis, chronic kidney disease
  - hematologic: anemia, coagulopathies, blood dyscrasias
  - MSK: conditions associated with difficult intubations – arthritides (e.g. rheumatoid arthritis), cervical tumours, cervical infections/abscesses, trauma to cervical spine, previous cervical spine surgery, Trisomy 21, scleroderma, conditions affecting neuromuscular junction (e.g. myasthenia gravis)
  - endocrine: DM, thyroid disorders, adrenal disorders
  - other: morbid obesity, pregnancy, ethanol/other drug use

Physical Exam

- weight, height, BP, pulse, respiratory rate, oxygen saturation
- focused physical exam of the CNS, CVS, and respiratory systems
- general assessment of nutrition, hydration, and mental status
- airway assessment is done to determine intubation difficulty (no single test is specific or sensitive) and ventilation difficulty
  - cervical spine stability and neck movement – upper cervical spine extension, lower cervical spine flexion ("sniffing position")
  - Mallampati classification
  - "3-2-1 rule"
    - thyromental distance (distance of lower mandible in midline from the mentum to the thyroid notch); <3 finger breadths (<6 cm) is associated with difficult intubation
    - mouth opening (<2 finger breadths is associated with difficult intubation)
    - anterior jaw subluxation (<1 finger breadth is associated with difficult intubation)
  - tongue size
  - dentition, dental appliances/prosthetic caps, existing chipped/loose teeth – pose aspiration risk if dislodged and must inform patients of rare possibility of damage
  - nasal passage patency (if planning nasotracheal intubation)
  - assess potential for difficult ventilation
- examination of anatomical sites relevant to lines and blocks
  - bony landmarks and suitability of anatomy for regional anesthesia (if relevant)
  - sites for IV, central venous pressure (CVP), and pulmonary artery (PA) catheters

Evaluation of Difficult Airway

LEMON
Look – obesity, beard, dental/facial abnormalities, neck, facial/neck trauma
Evaluate – 3-2-1 rule
Mallampati score
Obstruction – stridor, foreign bodies
Neck mobility

To Assess for Ventilation Difficulty

BONES
Beard
Obesity (BMI>26)
No teeth
Elderly (age>55)
Snoring Hx (sleep apnea)

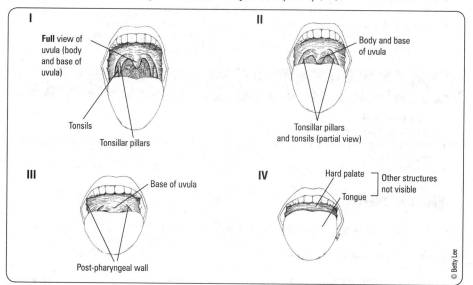

I – Full view of uvula (body and base of uvula); Tonsils; Tonsillar pillars

II – Body and base of uvula; Tonsillar pillars and tonsils (partial view)

III – Base of uvula; Post-pharyngeal wall

IV – Hard palate; Tongue; Other structures not visible

© Betty Lee

Figure 1. Mallampati classification of oral opening

Pre-Operative Investigations

Impact of Anesthesia Management Characteristics on Severe Morbidity and Mortality
Anesth 2005;102:257-268
Study: Case-control study of patients undergoing anesthesia.
Patients: 807 cases and 883 controls were analyzed among a cohort of 869,483 patients undergoing anesthesia between 1995-1997. Cases were defined as patients who either remained comatose or died within 24 h of receiving anesthesia. Controls were defined as patients who neither remained comatose nor died within 24 h of receiving anesthesia.
Intervention: General, regional, or combined anesthesia to patients undergoing a surgical procedure.
Main Outcome: Coma or death within 24 h of receiving anesthesia.
Results: The incidence of 24 h post-operative death was 8.8 per 10,000 anesthetics (95% CI 8.2-9.5) and the incidence of coma was 0.5 (95% CI 0.3-0.6). Anesthesia management risk factors that were associated with a decreased risk of morbidity and mortality were equipment check with protocol and documentation, directly available anesthesiologist with no change during anesthesia, 2 persons present at emergence of anesthesia, reversal of muscle relaxation, and post-operative pain medication.

- routine pre-operative investigations are only necessary if there are comorbidities or certain indications

Table 1. Suggested Indications for Specific Investigations in the Pre-Operative Period

Test	Indications
CBC	Major surgery requiring group and screen or cross and match; chronic cardiovascular, pulmonary, renal, or hepatic disease; malignancy; known or suspected anemia; bleeding diathesis or myelosuppression; patient >1 yr of age
Sickle Cell Screen	Patients from geographic areas with high prevalence of sickle cell disease and/or genetically predisposed patients (hemoglobin electrophoresis if screen is positive)
INR, aPTT	Anticoagulant therapy, bleeding diathesis, liver disease
Electrolytes and Creatinine	Hypertension, renal disease, DM, pituitary or adrenal disease; vascular disease, digoxin, diuretic, or other drug therapies affecting electrolytes
Fasting Glucose Level	DM (repeat on day of surgery)
Pregnancy (β-hCG)	Women of reproductive age
ECG	Heart disease, DM, other risk factors for cardiac disease; subarachnoid or intracranial hemorrhage, cerebrovascular accident, head trauma
Chest Radiograph	Patients with new or worsening respiratory symptoms/signs

Guidelines to the Practice of Anesthesia Revised Edition 2013. Supplement to the *Canadian Journal of Anesthesia*, Vol 60, Dec. 2013. Reproduced with permission © Canadian Anesthesiologists' Society

American Society of Anesthesiology Classification

Aspirin® in Patients undergoing Non-Cardiac Surgery
NEJM 2014;370:1494-1503
Purpose: This study evaluated the effect of low-dose ASA on the risk of death or non-fatal MI in 10,010 patients undergoing non-cardiac surgery. Patients were randomized into two groups in a double-blind process.
Methods: RCT in which ASA or placebo to be taken shortly before surgery and in the early post-operative period. The primary outcome was a composite of death or non-fatal MI.
Results: Death or non-fatal MI occurred in 7.0% in the ASA group and 7.1% in the placebo group. Major bleeding was more common in the ASA group than the placebo group.
Conclusion: Administration of ASA before surgery and throughout the early post-surgical period had no significant effect on the incidence of death or MI but increased the risk of major bleeding.

- common classification of physical status at the time of surgery
- a gross predictor of overall outcome, NOT used as stratification for anesthetic risk (mortality rates)
- **ASA 1**: a healthy, fit patient
- **ASA 2**: a patient with mild systemic disease
    - e.g. controlled Type 2 DM, controlled essential HTN, obesity, smoker
- **ASA 3**: a patient with severe systemic disease that limits activity
    - e.g. stable CAD, COPD, DM, obesity
- **ASA 4**: a patient with incapacitating disease that is a constant threat to life
    - e.g. unstable CAD, renal failure, acute respiratory failure
- **ASA 5**: a moribund patient not expected to survive 24 h without surgery
    - e.g. ruptured abdominal aortic aneurysm (AAA), head trauma with increased ICP
- **ASA 6**: declared brain dead, a patient whose organs are being removed for donation purposes
- for emergency operations, add the letter E after classification (e.g. ASA 3E)

Pre-Operative Optimization

- in general, prior to elective surgery
    - any fluid and/or electrolyte imbalance should be corrected
    - extent of existing comorbidities should be understood and these conditions should be optimized prior to surgery
    - medications may need adjustment

Medications

- pay particular attention to cardiac and respiratory medications, opioids and drugs with many side effects and interactions
- **pre-operative medications to consider**
    - prophylaxis
        - risk of GE reflux: sodium citrate and/or ranitidine and/or metoclopramide 30 min-1 h prior to surgery
        - risk of infective endocarditis, GI/GU interventions: antibiotics
        - risk of adrenal suppression: steroid coverage
        - anxiety: consider benzodiazepines
        - COPD, asthma: bronchodilators
        - CAD risk factors: nitroglycerin and β-blockers
- **pre-operative medications to stop**
    - oral antihyperglycemics: stop on morning of surgery
    - ACE inhibitors and angiotension receptor blockers: may stop on morning of surgery (controversial)

- warfarin (consider bridging with heparin), anti-platelet agents (e.g. clopidogrel)
  - discuss perioperative use of ASA, NSAIDs with surgeon (± patient's cardiologist/internist)
  - in patients undergoing non-cardiac surgery, starting or continuing low-dose aspirin in the perioperative period does not appear to protect against post-operative MI or death, but increases the risk of major bleeding
    - note: this does not apply to patients with bare metal stents or drug-eluting coronary stents
- **pre-operative medications to adjust**
  - insulin (consider insulin/dextrose infusion or holding dose), prednisone, bronchodilators

Hypertension

- BP <180/110 is not an independent risk factor for perioperative cardiovascular complications
- target SBP <180 mmHg, DBP <110 mmHg
- assess for end-organ damage and treat accordingly

Coronary Artery Disease

- ACC/AHA Guidelines (2014) recommend that at least 60 days should elapse after a MI before a non-cardiac surgery in the absence of a coronary intervention
  - this period carries an increased risk of re-infarction/death
  - if operative procedure is essential and cannot be delayed then invasive intra- and post-operative ICU monitoring is required to reduce the above risk
- mortality with perioperative MI is 20-50%
- perioperative β-blockers
  - may decrease cardiac events and mortality (controversial, as recent data suggests stroke risk)
  - continue β-blocker if patient is routinely taking it prior to surgery
  - consider initiation of β-blocker in
    - patients with CAD or indication for β-blocker
    - intermediate or high risk surgery, especially vascular surgery

Respiratory Diseases

- smoking
  - adverse effects: altered mucus secretion and clearance, decreased small airway calibre, and altered immune response
  - abstain at least 8 wk pre-operatively if possible
  - if unable, abstaining even 24 h pre-operatively has been shown to increase oxygen availability to tissues
- asthma
  - pre-operative management depends on degree of baseline asthma control
  - increased risk of bronchospasm from intubation
    - administration of short course (up to 1 wk) pre-operative corticosteroids and inhaled β2-agonists decreases the risk of bronchospasm and does not increase the risk of infection or delay wound healing
  - avoid non-selective β-blockers due to risk of bronchospasm
  - cardioselective β-blockers (metoprolol, atenolol) do not increase risk of bronchospasm in the short-term
  - delay elective surgery for poorly controlled asthma (increased cough or sputum production, active wheezing)
  - delay elective surgery by a minimum of 6 wk if patient develops URTI
- COPD
  - anesthesia, surgery (especially abdominal surgery, in particular upper abdominal surgery) and pain predispose the patient to atelectasis, bronchospasm, pneumonia, prolonged need for mechanical ventilation, and respiratory failure
  - pre-operative ABG is needed for all COPD stage II and III patients to assess baseline respiratory acidosis and plan post-operative management of hypercapnea
  - cancel/delay elective surgery for acute exacerbation

Aspiration

- increased risk of aspiration with
  - decreased LOC
  - trauma
  - meals within 8 h
  - suspected sphincter incompetence (GERD, hiatus hernia, nasogastric tube)
  - increased abdominal pressure (pregnancy, obesity, bowel obstruction, acute abdomen)
  - laryngeal mask vs. endotracheal tube (ETT)

Effects of Extended-Release Metoprolol Succinate in Patients undergoing Non-Cardiac Surgery (POISE Trial): A Randomized Controlled Trial
Lancet 2008;371:1839-1847
Purpose: To investigate the role of β-blockers (metoprolol) perioperatively in patients with known vascular disease undergoing non-cardiac surgery.
Methods: Patients from 190 centres in 23 countries were eligible if they were age >45, undergoing non-cardiac surgery, and were known to have significant vascular disease. Patients were randomized to either the metoprolol group or placebo. Participants received metoprolol (or placebo) 100 mg 2-4 h prior to surgery, 6 h after surgery, and then 20 mg daily for 30 d. The primary endpoint was a composite of cardiovascular death, non-fatal myocardial infarction, and non-fatal cardiac arrest. Analysis was by intention to treat.
Results: 8,351 patients were recruited into the study, with 8,331 completing the 30 d course. Use of metoprolol was found to significantly reduce the risk of cardiovascular death, non-fatal MI, or non-fatal cardiac arrest vs. placebo (hazard ratio 0.84, p<0.05) but significantly increased the rate of stroke (hazard ratio 2.17, p<0.01) and overall risk of death (hazard ratio 1.33, p<0.05).
Conclusion: Use of perioperative β-blockers (metoprolol) in patients with known vascular disease provides both risks and benefits, and these must be considered for each patient individually.

β-blockers
- β1-receptors are located primarily in the heart and kidneys
- β2-receptors are located in the lungs
- Non-selective β-blockers block β1 and β2-receptors (labetalol, carvedilol, nadolol). Caution is required with non-selective β-blockers, particularly in patients with respiratory conditions where β2 blockade can result in airway reactivity

- management
  - reduce gastric volume and acidity
  - delay inhibiting airway reflexes with muscular relaxants
  - employ rapid sequence induction (see *Rapid Sequence Induction*, A15)

Fasting Guidelines

Fasting Guidelines Prior to Surgery (Canadian Anesthesiologists' Society)
- **8 h** after a meal that includes meat, fried or fatty foods
- **6 h** after a light meal (such as toast or crackers) or after ingestion of infant formula or non-human milk
- **4 h** after ingestion of breast milk
- **2 h** after clear fluids (water, black coffee, tea, carbonated beverages, juice without pulp)

Hematological Disorders

- history of congenital or acquired conditions (sickle cell anemia, factor VIII deficiency, ITP, liver disease)
- evaluate hemoglobin, hematocrit and coagulation profiles when indicated (Table 1)
- anemia
  - pre-operative treatments to increase hemoglobin (erythropoietin or pre-admission blood collection in certain populations)
- coagulopathies
  - discontinue or modify anticoagulation therapies (warfarin, clopidogrel, ASA) in advance of elective surgeries
  - administration of reversal agents if necessary: vitamin K, FFP, prothrombin complex concentrate, recombinant activated factor VII

Endocrine Disorders

- diabetes mellitus
  - clarify type 1 vs. type 2
  - clarify treatment – oral anti-hyperglycemics and/or insulin
  - assess glucose control with history and HbA1c; well controlled diabetics have more stable glucose levels intraoperatively
  - end organ damage: be aware of damage to cardiovascular, renal, and nervous systems, including autonomic neuropathy
  - formulate intraoperative glucose management plan based on type (1 vs. 2), glucose control, and extent of end organ damage
- hyperthyroidism
  - can experience sudden release of thyroid hormone (thyroid storm) if not treated or well-controlled preoperatively
  - treatment: β-blockers and pre-operative prophylaxis
- adrenocortical insufficiency (Addison's, exogenous steroid use)
  - consider intraoperative steroid supplementation

Obesity and Obstructive Sleep Apnea

- assess for co-morbid conditions in obese patient (independent risk factor for CVD, DM, OSA, cholelithiasis, HTN)
- previously undiagnosed conditions may require additional testing to characterize severity
- both obesity and OSA increase risk of difficult ventilation, intubation and post-operative respiratory complications
  - risk may be magnified with both diseases present

Monitoring

Canadian Guidelines to the Practice of Anesthesia and Patient Monitoring
- an anesthetist present: "the only indispensable monitor"
- a completed pre-anesthetic checklist: including ASA class, NPO policy, Hx and investigations
- a perioperative anesthetic record: HR and BP every 5 min, O$_2$ saturation, End Tidal CO$_2$, dose and route of drugs and fluids
- continuous monitoring: see *Routine Monitors for All Cases*

Routine Monitors for All Cases
- pulse oximeter, BP monitor, electrocardiography and capnography are required for general anesthesia and sedation (Ramsey Sedation Scale 4-6), agent-specific anesthetic gas monitor when inhalational anesthetic agents are used
- the following must also be available: temperature probe, peripheral nerve stimulator, stethoscope, appropriate lighting, spirometer

Pre-Anesthetic Checklist

SAMMM
Suction: connected and working
Airways: laryngoscope and blades, ETT, syringe, stylet, oral and nasal airways, tape, bag, and mask
Machine: connected, pressures okay, all meters functioning, vaporizers full
Monitors: available, connected, and working
Medications: IV fluids and kit ready, emergency medicines in correct location and accessible

Elements to Monitor
- anesthetic depth
  - inadequate: blink reflex present when eyelashes lightly touched, HTN, tachycardia, tearing or sweating
  - excessive: hypotension, bradycardia
- oxygenation: pulse oximetry, fraction of inspired O_2 (FiO₂)
- ventilation: verify correct position of ETT, chest excursions, breath sounds, ETCO₂ analysis, end tidal inhaled anesthesia analysis
- circulation: pulse, rhythm, BP, telemetry, oximetry, CVP, pulmonary capillary wedge pressure
- temperature
- hourly urine output

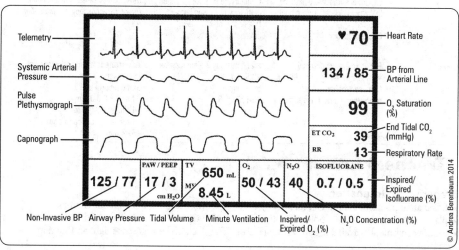

Figure 2. Typical anesthesia monitor

Airway Management

Airway Anatomy

- resistance to airflow through nasal passages accounts for approximately 2/3 of total airway resistance
- pharyngeal airway extends from posterior aspect of the nose to cricoid cartilage
- glottic opening (triangular space formed between the true vocal cords) is the narrowest segment of the laryngeal opening in adults
- the glottic opening is the space through which one visualizes proper placement of the ETT
- the trachea begins at the level of the thyroid cartilage, C6, and bifurcates into the right and left main bronchi at T4-T5 (approximately the sternal angle)

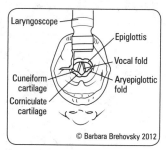

Figure 3. Landmarks for intubation

Methods of Supporting Airways

1. non-definitive airway (patent airway)
   - jaw thrust/chin lift
   - oropharyngeal and nasopharyngeal airway
   - bag mask ventilation
   - LMA
2. definitive airway (patent and protected airway)
   - ETT
   - surgical airway (cricothyrotomy or tracheostomy)

Table 2. Methods of Supporting the Airway

	Bag and Mask	Laryngeal Mask Airway (LMA)	Endotracheal Tube (ETT)
Advantages/ Indications	Basic Non-invasive Readily available	Easy to insert Less airway trauma/irritation than ETT Frees up hands (vs. face mask) Primarily used in spontaneously ventilating patient	Indications for intubation (5 Ps) **P**atent airway **P**rotects against aspiration **P**ositive pressure ventilation **P**ulmonary toilet (suction) **P**harmacologic administration also hemodynamic instability
Disadvantages/ Contraindications	Risk of aspiration if decreased LOC Cannot ensure airway patency Inability to deliver precise tidal volume Operator fatigue	Risk of gastric aspiration PPV <20 cm H_2O needed Oropharyngeal/retropharyngeal pathology or foreign body Does not protect against laryngospasm or gastric aspiration	Insertion can be difficult Muscle relaxant usually needed Most invasive – see *Complications During Laryngoscopy and Intubation*, A9
Other	Facilitate airway patency with jaw thrust and chin lift Can use oropharyngeal/ nasopaharyngeal airway	Sizing by body weight (approx) 40-50 kg: 3 50-70 kg: 4 70-100 kg: 5	Auscultate to avoid endobronchial intubation Sizing (approx): Male: 8.0-9.0 mm Female: 7.0-8.0 mm Pediatric Uncuffed (>age 2): (age/4) + 4 mm

Equipment for Intubation

MDSOLES
Monitors
Drugs
Suction
Oxygen source and self-inflating bag with oropharyngeal and nasopharyngeal airways
Laryngoscope
Endotracheal tubes (appropriate size and one size smaller)
Stylet, **S**yringe for tube cuff inflation

Medications that can be Given Through the ETT

NAVEL
Naloxone
Atropine
Ventolin
Epinephrine
Lidocaine

Tracheal Intubation

Preparing for Intubation
- failed attempts at intubation can make further attempts more difficult due to tissue trauma
- plan, prepare, and assess for potential difficulties (see *Pre-Operative Assessment*, A2)
- ensure equipment is available and working (test ETT cuff, check laryngoscope light and suction, machine check)
- pre-oxygenate/denitrogenate: patient breathes 100% O_2 for 3-5 min or for 4-8 vital capacity breaths
- may need to suction mouth and pharynx first

Proper Positioning for Intubation
- align the three axes (mouth, pharynx, and larynx) to allow visualization from oral cavity to glottis
    - "sniffing position": flexion of lower C-spine (C5-C6), bow head forward, and extension of upper C-spine at atlanto-occipital joint (C1), nose in the air
    - contraindicated in known/suspected C-spine fracture/instability
- laryngoscope tip placed in the epiglottic vallecula in order to visualize cord

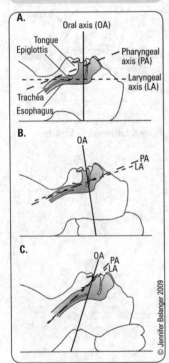

Figure 5. Anatomic considerations in laryngoscopy
A. Neutral position
B. C-spine flexion
C. C-spine flexion with atlanto-occipital extension

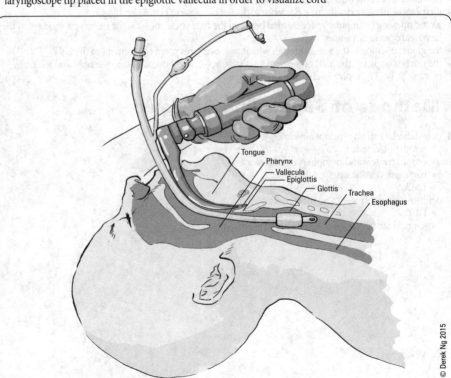

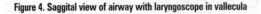

Figure 4. Saggital view of airway with laryngoscope in vallecula

Tube Insertion
- laryngoscopy and ETT insertion can incite a significant sympathetic response via stimulation of cranial nerves 9 and 10 due to a "foreign body reflex" in the trachea, including tachycardia, dysrhythmias, myocardial ischemia, increased BP, and coughing
- a malpositioned ETT is a potential hazard for the intubated patient
  - if too deep, may result in right endobronchial intubation, which is associated with left-sided atelectasis and right-sided tension pneumothorax
  - if too shallow, may lead to accidental extubation, vocal cord trauma, or laryngeal paralysis as a result of pressure injury by the ETT cuff
- the tip of ETT should be located at the midpoint of the trachea at least 2 cm above the carina and the proximal end of the cuff should be placed at least 2 cm below the vocal cords
  - approximately 20-23 cm mark at the right corner of the mouth for men and 19-21 cm for women

Confirmation of Tracheal Placement of ETT
- direct
  - visualization of ETT passing through cords
  - bronchoscopic visualization of ETT in trachea
- indirect
  - $ETCO_2$ in exhaled gas measured by capnography – a mandatory method for confirming the ETT is in the airway
  - auscultate for equal breath sounds bilaterally and absent breath sounds over epigastrium
  - bilateral chest movement, condensation of water vapour in ETT visible during exhalation and no abdominal distention
  - refilling of reservoir bag during exhalation
  - CXR (rarely done): only confirms position of the tip of ETT and not that ETT is in the trachea
- esophageal intubation suspected when
  - $ETCO_2$ zero or near zero on capnograph
  - abnormal sounds during assisted ventilation
  - impairment of chest excursion
  - hypoxia/cyanosis
  - presence of gastric contents in ETT
  - breath sounds heard when auscultating over epigastrium/LUQ
  - distention of stomach/epigastrium with ventilation

Complications During Laryngoscopy and Intubation
- dental damage
- laceration (lips, gums, tongue, pharynx, vallecula, esophagus)
- laryngeal trauma
- esophageal or endobronchial intubation
- accidental extubation
- insufficient cuff inflation or cuff laceration: results in leaking and aspiration
- laryngospasm (see *Extubation*, A20 for definition)
- bronchospasm

Difficult Airway

- difficulties with bag-mask ventilation, supraglottic airway, laryngoscopy, passage of ETT through the cords, infraglottic airway or surgical airway
- algorithms exist for difficult airways (*Can J Anesth* 2013;60:1119-1138; *Anesthesiology* 2003;98:3273; *Anesthesiology* 2013;118:251-270), see *ACLS Guidelines* (Figures 14, A29 and 15, A30)
- pre-operative assessment (history of previous difficult airway, airway examination) and pre-oxygenation are important preventative measures
- if difficult airway expected, consider
  - awake intubation
  - intubating with bronchoscope, trachlight (lighted stylet), fibre optic laryngoscope, glidescope, etc.
- if intubation unsuccessful after induction
  1. CALL FOR HELP
  2. ventilate with 100% O_2 via bag and mask
  3. consider returning to spontaneous ventilation and/or waking patient
- if bag and mask ventilation inadequate
  1. CALL FOR HELP
  2. attempt ventilation with oral airway
  3. consider/attempt LMA
  4. emergency invasive airway access (e.g. rigid bronchoscope, cricothyrotomy, or tracheostomy)

Differential Diagnosis of Poor Bilateral Breath Sounds after Intubation

DOPE
Displaced ETT
Obstruction
Pneumothorax
Esophageal intubation

Predicting Difficult Intubation in Apparently Normal Patients
Anesth 2005;103:429-437
Purpose: To assess widely available bedside tests and widely used laryngoscopic techniques in the prediction of difficult intubations.
Study: Meta-analysis.
Patients: 35 studies encompassing 50,760 patients.
Definitions: Difficult intubation was defined usually as Cormack–Lehane grade of 3 or greater, but some authors reported the requirement of a special technique, multiple unsuccessful attempts, or a combination of these as the accepted standard for difficult intubation.
Results: The overall incidence of difficult intubation was 5.8% (95% CI 4.5-7.5%) for the overall patient population, 6.2% (95% CI 4.6-8.3%) for normal patients excluding obstetric and obese patients, 3.1% (95% CI 1.7-5.5%) for obstetric patients, and 15.8% (95% CI 14.3-17.5%) for obese patients Mallampati score: SN:49% SP:86% PLR:3.7 NLR:0.5; thyromental distance: SN:20% SP:94% PLR:3.4 NLR:0.8; sternomental distance: SN:62% SP:82% PLR:5.7 NLR:0.5; mouth opening: SN:22% SP:97% PLR: 4.0 NLR:0.8; Wilson risk-sum: SN:46% SP:89% PLR:5.8 NLR:0.6; combination Mallampati and thyromental distance: SN:36% SP:87% PLR:9.9 NLR:0.6.
Conclusions: A combination of the Mallampati score and thyromental distance is the most accurate at predicting difficult intubation. The PLR (9.9) is supportive of the test as a good predictor of difficult intubation.
PLR: positive likelihood ratio; **NLR:** negative likelihood ratio; **SN:** sensitivity; **SP:** specificity

Oxygen Therapy

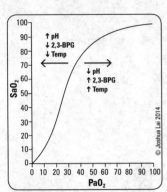

Figure 6. HbO₂ saturation curve

- in general, the goal of oxygen therapy is to maintain arterial oxygen saturation (SaO_2) > at a minimum, 90%
- small decrease in saturation below SaO_2 of 90% corresponds to a large drop in arterial partial pressure of oxygen (PaO_2)
- in intubated patients, oxygen is delivered via the ETT
- in patients not intubated, there are many oxygen delivery systems available; the choice depends on oxygen requirements (FiO_2) and the degree to which precise control of delivery is needed
- cyanosis can be detected at SaO_2 <85%, frank cyanosis at SaO_2 = 67%

Low Flow Systems
- provide O_2 at flows between 0-10 L/min
- acceptable if tidal volume 300-700 mL, respiratory rate (RR) <25, consistent ventilation pattern
- dilution of oxygen with room air results in a decrease in FiO_2
- an increase in minute ventilation (tidal volume x RR) results in a decrease in FiO_2
- e.g. nasal cannula (prongs)
    - well tolerated if flow rates <5-6 L/min; drying of nasal mucosa at higher flows
    - nasopharynx acts as an anatomic reservoir that collects O_2
    - delivered oxygen concentration (FiO_2) can be estimated by adding 4% for every additional litre of O_2 delivered
    - provides FiO_2 of 24-44% at O_2 flow rates of 1-6 L/min

Composition of Air
78.1% nitrogen
20.9% oxygen
0.9% argon
0.04% carbon dioxide

Reservoir Systems
- use a volume reservoir to accumulate oxygen during exhalation thus increasing the amount of oxygen available for the next breath
- simple face mask
    - covers patient's nose and mouth and provides an additional reservoir beyond nasopharynx
    - fed by small bore O_2 tubing at a rate of at least 6 L/min to ensure that exhaled CO_2 is flushed through the exhalation ports and not rebreathed
    - provides FiO_2 of 55% at O_2 flow rates of 10 L/min
- non-rebreather mask
    - a reservoir bag and a series of one-way valves prevent expired gases from re-entering the bag
    - during the exhalation phase, the bag accumulates with oxygen
    - provides FiO_2 of 80% at O_2 flow rates of 10-15 L/min

High Flow Systems
- generate flows of up to 50-60 L/min
- meet/exceed patient's inspiratory flow requirement
- deliver consistent and predictable concentration of O_2
- Venturi mask
    - delivers specific FiO_2 by varying the size of air entrapment
    - oxygen concentration determined by mask's port and NOT the wall flow rate
    - enables control of gas humidity
    - FiO_2 ranges from 24-50%

Ventilation

Changes in peak pressures in ACV and tidal volumes in PCV may reflect changes in lung compliance and/or airway resistance – patient may be getting better or worse

- ventilation is maintained with PPV in patients given muscle relaxants
- assisted or controlled ventilation can also be used to assist spontaneous respirations in patients not given muscle relaxants as an artificial means of supporting ventilation and oxygenation

Mechanical Ventilation
- indications for mechanical ventilation
    - apnea
    - hypoventilation/acute respiratory acidosis
    - intraoperative positioning limiting respiratory excursion (e.g. prone, Trendelenburg)
    - required hyperventilation (to lower ICP)
    - deliver positive end expiratory pressure (PEEP)
    - increased intrathoracic pressure (e.g. laparoscopic procedure)
- complications of mechanical ventilation
    - airway complications
        - tracheal stenosis, laryngeal edema
        - alveolar complications
        - ventilator-induced lung injury (barotrauma, volutrauma, atelectatrauma), ventilator-associated pneumonia (nosocomial pneumonia), inflammation, auto-PEEP, patient-ventilator asynchrony
        - cardiovascular complications
        - reduced venous return (secondary to increased intrathoracic pressure), reduced cardiac output, hypotension

Positive End Expiratory Pressure (PEEP)
- Positive pressure applied at the end of ventilation that helps to keep alveoli open, decreasing V/Q mismatch
- Used with all invasive modes of ventilation

Tracheostomy
- Tracheostomy should be considered in patients who require ventilator support for extended periods of time
- Shown to improve patient comfort and give patients a better ability to participate in rehabilitation activities

- neuromuscular complications
    - muscle atrophy
    - increased intracranial pressure
- metabolic
    - decreased CO_2 due to hyperventilation
    - alkalemia with over correction of chronic hypercarbia

Ventilator Strategies
- mode and settings are determined based on patient factors (e.g. ideal body weight, compliance, resistance) and underlying reason for mechanical ventilation
- hypoxemic respiratory failure: ventilator provides supplemental oxygen, recruits atelectatic lung segments, helps improve V/Q mismatch, and decreases intrapulmonary shunt
- hypercapnic respiratory failure: ventilator augments alveolar ventilation; may decrease the work of breathing, allowing respiratory muscles to rest

Modes of Ventilation
- assist-control ventilation (ACV) or volume control (VC)
    - every breath is delivered with a pre-set tidal volume and rate or minute ventilation
    - extra controlled breaths may be triggered by patient effort; if no effort is detected within a specified amount of time the ventilator will initiate the breath
- pressure control ventilation (PCV)
    - a minimum frequency is set and patient may trigger additional breaths above the ventilator
    - all breaths delivered at a preset constant inspiratory pressure
- synchronous intermittent mandatory ventilation (SIMV)
    - ventilator provides controlled breaths (either at a set volume or pressure depending on whether in VC or PCV, respectively)
    - patient can breathe spontaneously (these breaths may be pressure supported) between controlled breaths
- pressure support ventilation (PSV)
    - patient initiates all breaths and the ventilator supports each breath with a pre-set inspiratory pressure
    - useful for weaning off ventilator
- high-frequency oscillatory ventilation (HFOV)
    - high breathing rate (up to 900 breaths/min in an adult), very low tidal volumes
    - used commonly in neonatal and pediatric respiratory failure
    - occasionally used in adults when conventional mechanical ventilation is failing
- non-invasive positive pressure ventilation (NPPV)
    - achieved without intubation by using a nasal or face mask
    - BiPAP: increased pressure (like PSV) on inspiration and lower constant pressure on expiration (i.e. PEEP)
    - CPAP: delivers constant pressure on both inspiration and expiration

Table 3. Causes of Abnormal End Tidal CO_2 Levels

Hypocapnea (Decreased CO_2)	Hypercapnea (Increased CO_2)
Hyperventilation	Hypoventilation
Hypothermia (decreased metabolic rate)	Hyperthermia and other hypermetabolic states
Decreased pulmonary blood flow (decreased cardiac output)	Improved pulmonary blood flow after resuscitation or hypotension
Technical issues	Technical issues
Incorrect placement of sampling catheter	Water in capnography device
Inadequate sampling volume	Anesthetic breathing circuit error
	Inadequate fresh gas flow
	Rebreathing
	Exhausted soda lime
	Faulty circuit absorber valves
V/Q mismatch	Low bicarbonate
Pulmonary thromboembolism	
Incipient pulmonary edema	
Air embolism	

Monitoring Ventilatory Therapy
- Pulse oximetry, end-tidal CO_2 concentration
- Regular arterial blood gases
- Assess tolerance regularly

Patients who develop a pneumothorax while on mechanical ventilation require a chest tube

Causes of Intraoperative Hypoxemia
Inadequate oxygen supply
e.g. breathing system disconnection, obstructed or malpositioned ETT, leaks in the anesthetic machine, loss of oxygen supply
Hypoventilation
Ventilation-perfusion inequalities e.g. atelectasis, pneumonia, pulmonary edema, pneumothorax
Reduction in oxygen carrying capacity
e.g. anemia, carbon monoxide poisoning, methemoglobinemia, hemoglobinopathy
Leftward shift of the hemoglobin-oxygen saturation curve
e.g. hypothermia, decreased 2,3-BPG, alkalosis, hypocarbia, carbon monoxide poisoning
Right-to-left cardiac shunt

A Comparison of Four Methods of Weaning Patients from Mechanical Ventilation
NEJM 1995;332:345-350
Study: Prospective, randomized, multicentre trial.
Participants: 130 of 546 patients who received mechanical ventilation and were considered ready for weaning but had respiratory distress during a 2 h trial of spontaneous breathing.
Intervention: One of four weaning techniques following standardized protocol.
Outcome: Median duration of weaning.
Results: The median duration of weaning for intermittent mandatory ventilation, pressure-support ventilation, intermittent (multiple) trials of spontaneous breathing, and once-daily trial of spontaneous breathing was 5 d, 4 d, and 3 d, respectively. The rate of successful weaning was higher with once-daily trial of spontaneous breathing than with intermittent mandatory ventilation (rate ratio 2.83; 95% CI 1.36-5.89; p<0.006) or pressure-support ventilation (ratio 2.05; 95% CI 1.04-4.04; p<0.04). There was no significant difference in the rate of success between once-daily trials and multiple trials of spontaneous breathing.
Conclusions: Once-daily or multiple trials of spontaneous breathing led to extubation more quickly than intermittent mandatory or pressure-support ventilation.

Intraoperative Management

Temperature

Causes of Hypothermia (<36.0°C)

Impact of Hypothermia (<36°C)
- Increased risk of wound infections due to impaired immune function
- Increases the period of hospitalization by delaying healing
- Reduces platelet function and impairs activation of coagulation cascade increasing blood loss and transfusion requirements
- Triples the incidence of VT and morbid cardiac events
- Decreases the metabolism of anesthetic agents prolonging post-operative recovery

- intraoperative temperature losses are common (e.g. 90% of intraoperative heat loss is transcutaneous), due to
  - OR environment (cold room, IV fluids, instruments)
  - open wound
- prevent with forced air warming blanket and warmed IV fluids

Causes of Hyperthermia (>37.5-38.3°C)
- drugs (e.g. atropine)
- blood transfusion reaction
- infection/sepsis
- medical disorder (e.g. thyrotoxicosis)
- malignant hyperthermia (see *Uncommon Complications*, A28)
- over-zealous warming efforts

Heart Rate

Cardiac Arrest
- pulseless arrest occurs due to 4 cardiac rhythms divided into shockable and non-shockable rhythms
  - shockable: ventricular fibrillation (VF) and ventricular tachycardia (VT)
  - non-shockable: asystole and pulseless electrical activity (PEA)
- for VF/VT, key to survival is good early CPR and defibrillation
- for asystole/PEA, key to survival is good early CPR and exclusion of all reversible causes
- reversible causes of PEA arrest (5 Hs and 5 Ts)
  - 5 Hs: **h**ypothermia, **h**ypovolemia, **h**ypoxia, **h**ydrogen ions (acidosis), **h**ypo/**h**yperkalemia
  - 5 Ts: **t**amponade (cardiac), **t**hrombosis (pulmonary), **t**hrombosis (coronary), **t**ension pneumo**t**horax, **t**oxins (overdose/poisoning)
  - when a patient sustains a cardiac arrest during anesthesia, it is important to remember that there are other causes on top the Hs and Ts to consider (i.e. local anesthetic systemic toxicity (LAST), excessive anesthetic dosing and others)
- for management of cardiac arrest, see *ACLS Guidelines* (Figure 16), A31

Intraoperative Tachycardia
- tachycardia = HR >150 bpm; divided into narrow complex supraventricular tachycardias (SVT) or wide complex tachycardias
- SVT: sinus tachycardia, atrial fibrillation/flutter, accessory pathway mediated tachycardia, paroxysmal atrial tachycardia
- wide complex tachycardia: VT, SVT with aberrant conduction
- causes of sinus tachycardia
  - shock/hypovolemia/blood loss
  - anxiety/pain/light anesthesia
  - full bladder
  - anemia
  - febrile illness/sepsis
  - drugs (e.g. atropine, cocaine, dopamine, epinephrine, ephedrine, isoflurane, isoproterenol, pancuronium) and withdrawal
  - Addisonian crisis, hypoglycemia, transfusion reaction, malignant hyperthermia
- for management of tachycardia, see *ACLS Guidelines* (Figure 17), A32

Intraoperative Bradycardia
- bradycardia = HR <50 bpm; most concerning are 2nd degree (Mobitz type II) and 3rd degree heart block, which can both degenerate into asystole
- causes of sinus bradycardia
  - increased parasympathetic tone vs. decreased sympathetic tone
  - must rule out hypoxemia
  - arrhythmias (see <u>Cardiology and Cardiac Surgery</u>, C16)
  - baroreceptor reflex due to increased ICP or increased BP
  - vagal reflex (oculocardiac reflex, carotid sinus reflex, airway manipulation)
  - drugs (e.g. SCh, opioids, edrophonium, neostigmine, halothane, digoxin, β-blockers)
  - high spinal/epidural anesthesia
- for management of bradycardia, see *ACLS Guidelines* (Figure 18), A32

Blood Pressure

Causes of Intraoperative Hypotension/Shock
- shock: condition characterized by inability of cardiovascular system to maintain adequate end-organ perfusion and delivery of oxygen to tissues
a) hypovolemic/hemorrhagic shock
  - most common form of shock, due to decrease in intravascular volume
b) obstructive shock
  - obstruction of blood into or out of the heart
  - increased JVP, distended neck veins, increased systemic vascular resistance, insufficient cardiac output (CO)
  - e.g. tension pneumothorax, cardiac tamponade, pulmonary embolism (and other emboli – i.e. fat, air)
c) cardiogenic shock
  - increased JVP, distended neck veins, increased systemic vascular resistance, decreased CO
  - e.g. myocardial dysfunction, dysrhythmias, ischemia/infarct, cardiomyopathy, acute valvular dysfunction
d) septic shock
  - see Infectious Diseases, ID21
e) spinal/neurogenic shock
  - decreased sympathetic tone
  - hypotension without tachycardia or peripheral vasoconstriction (warm skin)
f) anaphylactic shock
  - see Emergency Medicine, ER38
g) drugs
  - vasodilators, high spinal anesthetic interfering with sympathetic outflow
h) other
  - transfusion reaction, Addisonian crisis, thyrotoxicosis, hypothyroid, aortocaval syndrome
  - see Hematology, H52 and Endocrinology, E33

Intraoperative Shock

SHOCKED
Sepsis or Spinal shock
Hypovolemic/Hemorrhagic
Obstructive
Cardiogenic
anaphylactiK
Extra/other
Drugs

BP = CO x SVR, where CO = SV x HR
SV is a function of preload, afterload, and contractility

Causes of Intraoperative Hypertension
- inadequate anesthesia causing pain and anxiety
- pre-existing HTN, coarctation, or preeclampsia
- hypoxemia/hypercarbia
- hypervolemia
- increased intracranial pressure
- full bladder
- drugs (e.g. ephedrine, epinephrine, cocaine, phenylephrine, ketamine) and withdrawal
- allergic/anaphylactic reaction
- hypermetabolic states: malignant hyperthermia, neuroleptic malignant syndrome, serotonin syndrome (see Psychiatry, PS44), thyroid storm, pheochromocytoma (see Endocrinology, E25)

Fluid Balance and Resuscitation

- total requirement = maintenance + deficit + ongoing loss
- in surgical settings this formula must take into account multiple factors including pre-operative fasting/decreased fluid intake, increased losses during or before surgery, fluid shifting during surgery, fluids given with blood products and medications

What is the Maintenance?
- average healthy adult requires approximately 2500 mL water/d
  - 200 mL/d GI losses
  - 800 mL/d insensible losses (respiration, perspiration)
  - 1500 mL/d urine (beware of renal failure)
- 4:2:1 rule to calculate maintenance requirements (applies to crystalloids only)
  - 4 mL/kg/h first 10 kg
  - 2 mL/kg/h second 10 kg
  - 1 mL/kg/h for remaining weight >20 kg
- increased requirements with fever, sweating, GI losses (vomiting, diarrhea, NG suction), adrenal insufficiency, hyperventilation, and polyuric renal disease
- decreased requirements with anuria/oliguria, SIADH, highly humidified atmospheres, and CHF
- maintenance electrolytes
  - Na^+: 3 mEq/kg/d
  - K^+: 1 mEq/kg/d
- 50 kg patient maintenance requirements
  - fluid = 40 + 20 + 30 = 90 mL/h = 2160 mL/d = 2.16 L/d
  - Na^+ = 150 mEq/d (therefore 150 mEq / 2.16 L/d ≈ 69 mEq/L)
  - K^+ = 50 mEq/d (therefore 50 mEq / 2.16 L/d ≈ 23 mEq/L)
- above patient's requirements roughly met with 2/3 D5W, 1/3 NS
  - 2/3 + 1/3 at 100 mL/h with 20 mEq KCl per litre

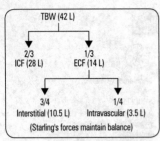

Figure 7. Total body water division in a 70 kg adult

What is the Deficit?
- patients should be adequately hydrated prior to anesthesia
- total body water (TBW) = 60% or 50% of total body weight for an adult male or female, respectively (e.g. for a 70 kg adult male TBW = 70 x 0.6 = 42 L)
- total Na^+ content determines ECF volume; $[Na^+]$ determines ICF volume
- hypovolemia due to volume contraction
  - extra-renal Na^+ loss
    - GI: vomiting, NG suction, drainage, fistulae, diarrhea
    - skin/resp: insensible losses (fever), sweating, burns
    - vascular: hemorrhage
  - renal Na^+ and H_2O loss
    - diuretics
    - osmotic diuresis
    - hypoaldosteronism
    - salt-wasting nephropathies
  - renal H_2O loss
    - diabetes insipidus (central or nephrogenic)
  - hypovolemia with normal or expanded ECF volume
    - decreased CO
    - redistribution
      - hypoalbuminemia: cirrhosis, nephrotic syndrome
      - capillary leakage: acute pancreatitis, rhabdomyolysis, ischemic bowel, sepsis, anaphylaxis
- replace water and electrolytes as determined by patient's needs
- with chronic hyponatremia, correction must be done gradually over >48 h to avoid central pontine myelinolysis

Table 4. Signs and Symptoms of Dehydration

Percentage of Body Water Loss	Severity	Signs and Symptoms
3%	Mild	Decreased skin turgor, sunken eyes, dry mucous membranes, dry tongue, reduced sweating
6%	Moderate	Oliguria, orthostatic hypotension, tachycardia, low volume pulse, cool extremities, reduced filling of peripheral veins and CVP, hemoconcentration, apathy
9%	Severe	Profound oliguria or anuria and compromised CNS function with or without altered sensorium

What are the Ongoing Losses?
- losses from Foley catheter, NG, surgical drains
- third-spacing (other than ECF, ICF)
  - pleura, GI, retroperitoneal, peritoneal
  - evaporation via exposed viscera, burns
- blood loss
- ongoing loss due to surgical exposure and evaporative losses

IV Fluids

- replacement fluids include crystalloid and colloid solutions
- IV fluids improve perfusion but NOT O_2 carrying capacity of blood

Initial Distribution of IV Fluids
- H_2O follows ions/molecules to their respective compartments

Crystalloid Infusion
- salt-containing solutions that distribute only within ECF
- maintain euvolemia in patient with blood loss: 3 mL crystalloid infusion per 1 mL of blood loss for volume replacement (i.e. 3:1 replacement)
- if large volumes are to be given, use balanced fluids such as Ringer's lactate or Plasmalyte*, as too much normal saline (NS) may lead to hyperchloremic metabolic acidosis

Colloid Infusion (see Blood Products, A15)
- includes protein colloids (albumin and gelatin solutions) and non-protein colloids (dextrans and starches e.g. hydroxyethol starch [HES])
- distributes within intravascular volume
- 1:1 ratio (infusion:blood loss) only in terms of replacing intravascular volume
- HES colloids remain in intravascular space (metabolized by plasma serum amylase and renally excreted); two available in Canada: Voluven* and Pentaspan*
- the use of HES solutions is controversial because of recent RCTs and meta-analyses highlighting their renal (especially in septic patients) and coagulopathic side effects, as well as a lack of specific indications for their use
  - colloids are being used based on mechanistic and experimental evidence but there is a paucity of definitive studies investigating their safety and efficacy; routine use of colloids should be avoided

Colloids vs. Crystalloids for Fluid Resuscitation in Critically Ill Patients
Cochrane DB Syst Rev 2012;6:CD000567
Purpose: To evaluate the effects of colloids compared to crystalloids for fluid resuscitation, specifically when used in critically ill patients.
Methods: A meta-analysis was performed looking at randomized controlled trials comparing colloid vs. crystalloid use in patients requiring volume replacement. Pregnant women and neonates were excluded. Primary outcome was overall mortality.
Results: Results were broken down based on specific colloid. For albumin (or plasma protein fraction) the relative risk (RR) was 1.01 (95% CI 0.93-1.10) as compared to crystalloid. For hydroxyethyl starch the RR was 1.10 (95% CI 0.91-1.32). Modified gelatin had a RR of 0.91 (95% CI 0.49-1.72) and Dextran had a RR of 1.24 (95% CI 0.94-1.65). For colloids mixed in a hypertonic crystalloid as compared to isotonic crystalloid the RR was 0.88 (91% CI 0.71-1.06).
Conclusions: There is no evidence that use of colloids improves survival in trauma patients, burn patients, or post-operative patients when compared to crystalloid solutions. Given the increased cost of colloids as compared to crystalloids, it is recommended that crystalloids be the fluid of choice in these patients.

Table 5. IV Fluid Solutions

		ECF	Ringer's Lactate	0.9% NS	0.45% NS in D5W	D5W	2/3 D5W + 1/3 NS	Plasmalyte
mEq/L	Na$^+$	142	130	154	77	-	51	140
	K$^+$	4	4	-	-	-	-	5
	Ca^{2+}	4	3	-	-	-	-	-
	Mg^{2+}	3	-	-	-	-	-	3
	Cl$^-$	103	109	154	77	-	51	98
	HCO$_3^-$	27	28*	-	-	-	-	27
mOsm/L		280-310	273	308	154	252	269	294
pH		7.4	6.5	5.0	4.5	4.0	4.3	7.4

*Converted from lactate

Table 6. Colloid HES Solutions

	Concentration	Plasma Volume Expansion	Duration (h)	Maximum Daily Dose (mL/kg)
Voluven®	6%	1:1	4-6	33-50
Pentaspan®	10%	1:1.2-1.5	18-24	28

Blood Products

- see Hematology, H52

Induction

Routine Induction vs. Rapid Sequence Induction

- routine induction is the standard in general anesthesia, however a RSI is indicated in patients at risk of regurgitation/aspiration (see *Aspiration*, A5)
- RSI uses pre-determined doses of induction drugs given in rapid succession to minimize the time patient is at risk for aspiration (i.e. from the time when they are asleep without an ETT until the time when the ETT is in and the cuff inflated)

Table 7. Comparison of Routine Induction vs. RSI

Steps	Routine Induction	RSI
1. Equipment Preparation	Check equipment, drugs, suction, and monitors; prepare an alternative laryngoscope blade and a second ETT tube one size smaller	Check equipment, drugs, suction, and monitors; prepare an alternative laryngoscope blade and a second ETT tube one size smaller; suction on
2. Pre-Oxygenation/Denitrogenation	100% O$_2$ for 3 min or 4-8 vital capacity breaths	100% O$_2$ for 3 min or 4-8 vital capacity breaths
3. Pre-Treatment Agents	Use agent of choice to blunt physiologic responses to airway manipulation 3 min prior to laryngoscopy	Use agent of choice to blunt physiologic responses to airway manipulation; if possible, give 3 min prior to laryngoscopy, but can skip this step in an emergent situation
4. Induction Agents	Use IV or inhalation induction agent of choice	Use pre-determined dose of fast acting induction agent of choice
5. Muscle Relaxants	Muscle relaxant of choice given after the onset of the induction agent	Pre-determined dose of fast acting muscle relaxant (e.g. SCh) given IMMEDIATELY after induction agent
6. Ventilation	Bag-mask ventilation	DO NOT bag ventilate – can increase risk of aspiration
7. Cricoid Pressure	Backwards upwards rightwards pressure (BURP) on thyroid cartilage to assist visualization if indicated	Sellick maneuver, also known as cricoid pressure, to prevent regurgitation and assist in visualization (2 kg pressure with drowsiness, 3 kg with loss of consciousness)
8. Intubation	Intubate, inflate cuff, confirm ETT position	Intubate once paralyzed (~45 s after SCh given), inflate cuff, confirm ETT position; cricoid pressure maintained until ETT cuff inflated and placement confirmed
9. Secure Machines	Secure ETT, and begin manual/machine ventilation	Secure ETT, and begin manual/machine ventilation

Calculating Acceptable Blood Losses (ABL)
- Blood volume
  term infant   80 mL/kg
  adult male   70 mL/kg
  adult female 60 mL/kg
- Calculate estimated blood volume (EBV) (e.g. in a 70 kg male, approx. 70 mL/kg)
  EBV = 70 kg x 70 mL/kg = 4900 mL
- Decide on a transfusion trigger, i.e. the Hb level at which you would begin transfusion, (e.g. 70 g/L for a person with Hb(i) = 150 g/L)
  Hb(f) = 70 g/L
- Calculate
  $$ABL = \frac{Hb(Hi) - Hb(Hf)}{Hb(Hi)} \times EBV$$
  $$= \frac{150 - 70}{150} \times 4900$$
  $$= 2613 \text{ mL}$$
- Therefore in order to keep the Hb level above 70 g/L, RBCs would have to be given after approximately 2.6 L of blood has been lost

Transfusion Infection Risks

Virus	Risk per 1 unit pRBCs
HIV	1 in 21 million
Hepatitis C virus	1 in 13 million
Hepatitis B virus	1 in 7.5 million
HTLV	1 in 1-1.3 million
Symptomatic Bacterial Sepsis	1 in 40,000 from platelets and 1 in 250,000 from RBC
West Nile virus	No cases since 2003

Source: Callum JL, Pinkerton PH. Bloody Easy. Fourth Edition ed. Toronto: Sunnybrook and Women's College Health Science Centre; 2016

Induction Agents

Solubility of Volatile Anesthetics in Blood Least Soluble to Most Soluble
Nitrous oxide < desflurane < sevoflurane < isoflurane < halothane

- induction in general anesthesia may be achieved with intravenous agents, volatile inhalation agents, or both

Intravenous Agents
- see Table 8
- IV induction agents are non-opioid drugs used to provide hypnosis, amnesia and blunt reflexes
- these are initially used to draw the patient into the maintenance phase of general anesthesia rapidly, smoothly and with minimal adverse effects
  - examples include propofol, sodium thiopental (not available in North America), or ketamine
  - a continuous propofol infusion may also be used for the maintenance phase of GA

Table 8. Intravenous Induction Agents

	Propofol (Diprivan®)	Thiopental (sodium thiopental, sodium thiopentone)	Ketamine (Ketalar®, Ketaject®)	Benzodiazepines (midazolam [Versed®], diazepam [Valium®], lorazepam [Ativan®])	Etomidate
Class	Alkylphenol – hypnotic	Ultra-short acting thiobarbiturate – hypnotic	Phencyclidine (PCP) derivative – dissociative	Benzodiazepines – anxiolytic	Imadazole derivative - hypnotic
Action	Inhibitory at GABA synapse Decreased cerebral metabolic rate and blood flow, decreased ICP, decreased SVR, decreased BP, and decreased SV	Decreased time Cl– channels open, facilitating GABA and suppressing glutamic acid Decreased cerebral metabolism and blood flow, decreased CPP, decreased CO, decreased BP, decreased reflex tachycardia, decreased respiration	May act on NMDA, opiate, and other receptors Increased HR, increased BP, increased SVR, increased coronary flow, increased myocardial O₂ uptake CNS and respiratory depression, bronchial smooth muscle relaxation	Causes increased glycine inhibitory neurotransmitter, facilitates GABA Produces antianxiety and skeletal muscle relaxant effects Minimal cardiac depression	Decreases concentration of GABA required to activate receptor CNS depression Minimal cardiac or respiratory depression
Indications	Induction Maintenance Total intravenous anesthesia (TIVA)	Induction Control of convulsive states, obstetric patients	Major trauma, hypovolemia, obstetric bleeding, severe asthma because sympathomimetic	Used for sedation, amnesia, and anxiolysis	Induction Poor cardiac function, severe valve lesions, uncontrolled hypertension
Caution	Patients who cannot tolerate sudden decreased BP (e.g fixed cardiac output or shock)	Allergy to barbiturates Uncontrolled hypotension, shock, cardiac failure Porphyria, liver disease, status asthmaticus, myxedema	Ketamine allergy TCA medication (interaction causes HTN and dysrhythmias) History of psychosis Patients who cannot tolerate HTN (e.g. CHF, increased ICP, aneurysm)	Marked respiratory depression	Post-operative nausea and vomiting Venous irritation
Dosing	IV induction: 2.5-3.0 mg/kg (less with opioids) Unconscious <1 min Lasts 4-6 min t₁/₂ = 55 min Decreased post-operative sedation, recovery time, N/V	IV induction: 3-5 mg/kg Unconscious about 30 s Lasts 5 min Accumulation with repeat dosing – not for maintenance t₁/₂ = 5-10 h Post-operative sedation lasts hours	IV induction 1-2 mg/kg Dissociation in 15 s, analgesia, amnesia, and unconsciousness in 45-60 s Unconscious for 10-15 min, analgesia for 40 min, amnesia for 1-2 h t₁/₂ = ~3 h	Onset less than 5 min if given IV Duration of action long but variable/somewhat unpredictable	IV induction 0.3 mg/kg Onset 30-60 seconds Lasts 4-8 minutes
Special Considerations	0-30% decreased BP due to vasodilation Reduce burning at IV site by mixing with lidocaine	Combining with rocuronium causes precipitates to form	High incidence of emergence reactions (vivid dreaming, out-of-body sensation, illusions) Pretreat with glycopyrrolate to decrease salivation	Antagonist: flumazenil (Anexate®) competitive inhibitor, 0.2 mg IV over 15 s, repeat with 0.1 mg/min (max of 2 mg), t₁/₂ of 60 min Midazolam also has amnestic (antegrade) effect and decreased risk of thrombophlebitis	Adrenal suppression after first dose, cannot repeat dose or use as infusion Myoclonic movements during induction

Volatile Inhalational Agents
- examples include sevoflurane, desflurane, isoflurane, enflurane, halothane, and nitrous oxide
- see Table 9

Table 9. Volatile Inhalational Agents

	Sevoflurane	Desflurane	Isoflurane	Enflurane	Halothane	Nitrous oxide (N₂O)*
MAC (% gas in O₂)	2.0	6.0	1.2	1.7	0.8	104
CNS	Increased ICP	Increased ICP	Decreased cerebral metabolic rate Increased ICP	ECG seizure-like activity Increased ICP	Increased ICP and cerebral blood flow	—
Resp	Respiratory depression (severely decreased TV, increased RR), decreased response to respiratory CO₂ reflexes, bronchodilation					—
CVS	Less decrease of contractility, stable HR	Tachycardia with rapid increase in concentration	Decreased BP and CO, increased HR, theoretical chance of coronary steal**	Stable HR, decreased contractility	Decreased BP, CO, HR, and conduction Sensitizes myocardium to epinephrine-induced arrhythmias	Can cause decreased HR in pediatric patients with existing heart disease
MSK	Muscle relaxation, potentiation of other muscle relaxants, uterine relaxation					

*Properties and Adverse Effects of N₂O
Due to its high MAC, nitrous oxide is combined with other anesthetic gases to attain surgical anesthesia. A MAC of 104% is possible in a pressurized chamber only
Second Gas Effect
Expansion of closed spaces: closed spaces such as a pneumothorax, the middle ear, bowel lumen and ETT cuff will markedly enlarge if N₂O is administered
Diffusion hypoxia: during anesthesia, the washout of N₂O from body stores into alveoli can dilute the alveolar [O₂], creating a hypoxic mixture if the original [O₂] is low
**Coronary steal: isoflurane causes small vessel dilation which may compromise blood flow to areas of the heart with fixed perfusion (e.g. stents, atherosclerosis)

MAC (Minimum Alveolar Concentration)

- the alveolar concentration of a volatile anesthetic at one atmosphere (atm) of pressure that will prevent movement in 50% of patients in response to a surgical stimulus (e.g. abdominal incision)
- potency of inhalational agents is compared using MAC
- 1.2-1.3 times MAC will often ablate response to stimuli in the general population
- MAC values are roughly additive when mixing N₂O with another volatile agent; however, this only applies to movement, not other effects such as BP changes (e.g. 0.5 MAC of a potent agent + 0.5 MAC of N₂O = 1 MAC of potent agent)
- MAC-intubation: the MAC of anesthetic that will inhibit movement and coughing during endotracheal intubation, generally 1.3 MAC
- MAC-block adrenergic response (MAC-BAR): the MAC necessary to blunt the sympathetic response to noxious stimuli, generally 1.5 MAC
- MAC-awake: the MAC of a given volatile anesthetic at which a patient will open their eyes to command, generally 0.3-0.4 of the usual MAC

Muscle Relaxants and Reversing Agents

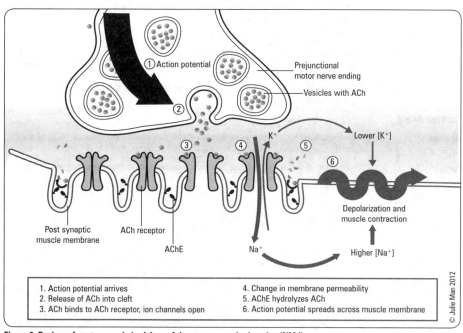

1. Action potential arrives
2. Release of ACh into cleft
3. ACh binds to ACh receptor, ion channels open
4. Change in membrane permeability
5. AChE hydrolyzes ACh
6. Action potential spreads across muscle membrane

© Julie Man 2012

Figure 8. Review of anatomy and physiology of the neuromuscular junction (NMJ)

Plasma Cholinesterase
Plasma cholinesterase is produced by the liver and metabolizes SCh, ester local anesthetics, and mivacurium. A prolonged duration of blockade by SCh occurs with:
(a) decreased quantity of plasma cholinesterase, e.g. liver disease, pregnancy, malignancy, malnutrition, collagen vascular disease, hypothyroidism
(b) abnormal quality of plasma cholinesterase, e.g. normal levels but impaired activity of enzymes, genetically inherited

Muscle Relaxants

- two types of muscle relaxants
    1. depolarizing muscle relaxants: succinylcholine (SCh)
    2. non-depolarizing muscle relaxants: rocuronium, mivacurium, vecuronium, cistracurium, pancuronium
- block nicotinic cholinergic receptors in NMJ
- provides skeletal muscle paralysis, including the diaphragm, but spares involuntary muscles such as the heart and smooth muscle
- never use muscle relaxants without adequate preparation and equipment to maintain airway and ventilation
- muscle relaxation produces the following desired effects
    1. facilitates intubation
    2. assists with mechanical ventilation
    3. prevents muscle stretch reflex and decreases muscle tone
    4. allows access to the surgical field (intracavitary surgery)
- nerve stimulator (i.e. train of four) is used intraoperatively to assess the degree of nerve block; no twitch response seen with complete neuromuscular blockade
- see Tables 10 and 11, for more details including mechanism of action

Table 10. Depolarizing Muscle Relaxants (Non-Competitive): Succinylcholine (SCh)

Mechanism of Action	Mimics ACh and binds to ACh receptors causing prolonged depolarization; initial fasciculation may be seen, followed by temporary paralysis secondary to blocked ACh receptors by SCh
Intubating Dose (mg/kg)	1-1.5
Onset	30-60 s – rapid (fastest of all muscle relaxants)
Duration	3-5 min – short (no reversing agent for SCh)
Metabolism	SCh is hydrolyzed by plasma cholinesterase (pseudocholinesterase), found only in plasma and not at the NMJ
Indications	Assist intubation Increased risk of aspiration (need rapid paralysis and airway control (e.g. full stomach), hiatus hernia, obesity, pregnancy, trauma) Short procedures Electroconvulsive therapy (ECT) Laryngospasm

Side Effects	1. SCh also stimulates muscarinic cholinergic autonomic receptors (in addition to nicotinic receptors; may cause bradycardia, dysrhythmias, sinus arrest, increased secretions of salivary glands (especially in children)
	2. Hyperkalemia
	Disruption of motor nerve activity causes proliferation of extrajunctional (outside NMJ) cholinergic receptors
	Depolarization of an increased number of receptors by SCh may lead to massive release of potassium out of muscle cells
	Patients at risk
	  3rd degree burns 24 h-6 mo after injury
	  Traumatic paralysis or neuromuscular diseases (e.g. muscular dystrophy)
	  Severe intra-abdominal infections
	  Severe closed head injury
	  Upper motor neuron lesions
	3. Can trigger MH (see Malignant Hyperthermia, A28)
	4. Increased ICP/intraocular pressure/intragastric pressure (no increased risk of aspiration if competent lower esophageal sphincter)
	5. Fasciculations, post-operative myalgia – may be minimized if small dose of non-depolarizing agent given before SCh administration

Contraindications	
Absolute	Known hypersensitivity or allergy, positive history of malignant hyperthermia, myotonia (m. congenita, m. dystrophica, paramyotonia congenital), high risk for hyperkalemic response
Relative	Known history of plasma cholinesterase deficiency, myasthenia gravis, myasthenic syndrome, familial periodic paralysis, open eye injury

Table 11. Non-Depolarizing Muscle Relaxants (Competitive)

Mechanism of Action	Competitive blockade of postsynaptic ACh receptors preventing depolarization				
Classification	Short		Intermediate		Long
	Mivacuronium	Rocuronium	Vecuronium	Cisatracurium	Pancuronium
Intubating Dose (mg/kg)	0.2	0.6-1.0	0.1	0.2	0.1
Onset (min)	2-3	1.5	2-3	3	3-5
Duration (min)	15-25	30-45	45-60	40-60	90-120
Metabolism	Plasma cholinesterase	Liver (major) Renal (minor)	Liver	Hofmann Eliminations	Renal (major) Liver (minor)
Indications	Assist intubation, assist mechanical ventilation in some ICU patients, reduce fasciculations and post-operative myalgias secondary to SCh				
Side Effects					
Histamine Release	Yes	No	No	No	No
Other	—	—	—	—	Tachycardia
Considerations	Increased duration of action in renal or liver failure	Quick onset of rocuronium allows its use in rapid sequence induction Cisatracurium is good for patients with renal or hepatic insufficiency			Pancuronium if increased HR and BP desired

Reversing Agents

- neostigmine, pyridostigmine, edrophonium
- reversal agents are acetylcholinesterase inhibitors
  - inhibits enzymatic degradation of ACh; increases amount of ACh at nicotinic and muscarinic receptors, displacing non-depolarizing muscle relaxant
  - administer reversal agents when there has been some recovery of blockade (i.e. muscle twitch)
  - can only reverse the effect of non-depolarizing muscle relaxants
- anticholinergic agents (e.g. atropine, glycopyrrolate) are simultaneously administered to minimize muscarinic effect of reversal agents (i.e. bradycardia, salivation and increased bowel peristalsis)

Table 12. Reversal Agents for Non-Depolarizing Relaxants

Cholinesterase Inhibitor	Neostigmine	Pyridostigmine	Edrophonium
Onset and Duration	Intermediate	Longest	Shortest
Mechanism of Action	Inhibits enzymatic degradation of ACh, increases ACh at nicotinic and muscarinic receptors, displaces non-depolarizing muscle relaxants Muscarinic effects of reversing agents include unwanted bradycardia, salivation, and increased bowel peristalsis*		
Dose	0.04-0.08 mg/kg	0.1-0.4 mg/kg	0.5-1 mg/kg
Recommended Anticholinergic	Glycopyrrolate	Glycopyrrolate	Atropine
Dose of Anticholinergic (per mg)	0.2 mg	0.05 mg	0.014 mg

*Atropine and glycopyrrolate are anticholinergic agents administered during the administration of reversal agents to minimize muscarinic effects

Analgesia

- options include opioids (e.g. morphine, fentanyl, hydromorphone), NSAIDS, acetaminophen, ketamine, gabapentin, local, and regional anesthetic (see Table 15, A25)

Maintenance

- general anesthesia is maintained using volatile inhalation agents and/or IV agents (i.e. propofol infusion)
- analgesia (usually IV opioids) and muscle relaxants are also given as needed

Extubation

- criteria: patient must no longer have intubation requirements (see Table 2, A8)
  - patency: airway must be patent
  - protection: airway reflexes intact
  - patient must be oxygenating and ventilating spontaneously
- general guidelines
  - ensure patient has normal neuromuscular function (peripheral nerve stimulator monitoring) and hemodynamic status
  - ensure patient is breathing spontaneously with adequate rate and tidal volume
  - allow ventilation (spontaneous or controlled) with 100% O_2 for 3-5 min
  - suction secretions from pharynx, deflate cuff, remove ETT on inspiration (vocal cords abducted)
  - ensure patient is breathing adequately after extubation
  - ensure face mask for O_2 delivery available
  - proper positioning of patient during transfer to recovery room (supine, head elevated)

Complications of Extubation

- early extubation: aspiration, laryngospasm
- late extubation: transient vocal cord incompetence, edema (glottic, subglottic), pharyngitis, tracheitis

Laryngospasm
- defined as forceful involuntary spasm of laryngeal muscles caused by stimulation of superior laryngeal nerve (by oropharyngeal secretions, blood, extubation)
- causes partial or total airway obstruction
- more likely to occur in semi-conscious patients
- prevention: extubate while patient is still deeply under anesthesia or fully awake
- treatment: apply sustained positive pressure with bag-mask ventilation with 100% oxygen, low-dose propofol (0.5-1.0 mg/kg) optional, low-dose succinylcholine (approximately 0.25 mg/kg) and reintubation if hypoxia develops

Regional Anesthesia

Benefits of Regional Anesthesia
- Reduced perioperative pulmonary complications
- Reduced perioperative analgesia requirements
- Decreased PONV
- Reduced perioperative blood loss
- Ability to monitor CNS status during procedure
- Improved perfusion
- Lower incidence of VTE
- Shorter recovery and improved rehabilitation
- Pain blockade with preserved motor function

- local anesthetic agent (LA) applied around a peripheral nerve at any point along the length of the nerve (from spinal cord up to, but not including, the nerve endings) for the purpose of reducing or preventing impulse transmission
- no CNS depression (unless overdose of local anesthetic); patient remains conscious
- regional anesthetic techniques categorized as follows:
  - epidural and spinal anesthesia (neuraxial anesthesia)
  - peripheral nerve blocks
  - IV regional anesthesia (e.g. Bier block)

Patient Preparation
- sedation may be indicated before block
- monitoring should be as extensive as for general anesthesia

Epidural and Spinal Anesthesia

Landmarking Epidural/Spinal Anesthesia
Spinous processes should be maximally flexed
L4 spinous processes found between iliac crests
Common sites of insertion are L3-L4 and L4-L5

- most useful for surgeries performed below level of umbilicus

Anatomy of Spinal/Epidural Area
- spinal cord extends to L2, dural sac to S2 in adults
- nerve roots (cauda equina) from L2 to S2
- needle inserted below L2 should not encounter cord, thus L3-L4, L4-L5 interspace commonly used
- structures penetrated (outside to inside)
  - skin
  - subcutaneous fat
  - supraspinous ligament
  - interspinous ligament
  - ligamentum flavum (last layer before epidural space)
  - dura + arachnoid for spinal anesthesia

Classic Presentation of Dural Puncture Headache
- Onset 6 h-3 d after dural puncture
- Postural component (worse when sitting)
- Occipital or frontal localization
- ± tinnitus, diplopia

Table 13. Epidural vs. Spinal Anesthesia

	Epidural	Spinal
Deposition Site	LA injected in epidural space (space between ligamentum flavum and dura) Initial blockade is at the spinal roots followed by some degree of spinal cord anesthesia as LA diffuses into the subarachnoid space through the dura	LA injected into subarachnoid space in the dural sac surrounding the spinal cord and nerve roots
Onset	Significant blockade requires 10-15 min Slower onset of side effects	Rapid blockade (onset in 2-5 min)
Effectiveness	Effectiveness of blockade can be variable	Very effective blockade
Difficulty	Technically more difficult; greater failure rate	Easier to perform due to visual confirmation of CSF flow
Patient Positioning	Position of patient not as important; specific gravity not an issue	Hyperbaric LA solution – position of patient important
Specific Gravity/Spread	Epidural injections spread throughout the potential space; specific gravity of solution does not affect spread	LA solution may be made hyperbaric (of greater specific gravity than the cerebrospinal fluid by mixing with 10% dextrose, thus increasing spread of LA to the dependent (low) areas of the subarachnoid space)
Dosage	Larger volume/dose of LA (usually > toxic IV dose)	Smaller dose of LA required (usually < toxic IV dose)
Continuous Infusion	Use of catheter allows for continuous infusion or repeat injections	None
Complications	Failure of technique Hypotension Bradycardia if cardiac sympathetics blocked (only if ~T2-4 block), e.g. "high spinal" Epidural or subarachnoid hematoma Accidental subarachnoid injection can produce spinal anesthesia (and any of the above complications) Systemic toxicity of LA (accidental intravenous) Catheter complications (shearing, kinking, vascular or subarachnoid placement) Infection Dural puncture	Failure of technique Hypotension Bradycardia if cardiac sympathetics blocked (only if ~T2-4 block), e.g. "high spinal" Epidural or subarachnoid hematoma Post-spinal headache (CSF leak) Transient paresthesias Spinal cord trauma, infection
Combined Spinal-Epidural	Combines the benefits of rapid, reliable, intense blockade of spinal anesthesia together with the flexibility of an epidural catheter	

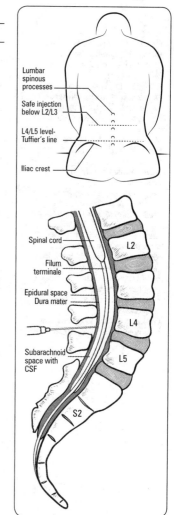

Figure 9. Landmarks for placement of epidural/spinal

Contraindications to Spinal/Epidural Anesthesia
- absolute contraindications
  - lack of resuscitative drugs/equipment
  - patient refusal
  - allergy to local anesthetic
  - infection at puncture site or underlying tissues
  - coagulopathies/bleeding diathesis
  - raised ICP
  - sepsis/bacteremia
  - severe hypovolemia
  - cardiac lesion with fixed output states (severe mitral/aortic stenosis)
  - lack of IV access
- relative contraindications
  - pre-existing neurological disease (demyelinating lesions)
  - previous spinal surgery, severe spinal deformity
  - prolonged surgery
  - major blood loss or maneuvers that can compromise reaction

Peripheral Nerve Blocks

- deposition of LA around the target nerve or plexus
- ultrasound guidance and peripheral nerve stimulation (needle will stimulate target nerve/plexus) may be used to guide needle to target nerve while avoiding neural trauma or intraneural injection
- most major nerves or nerve plexi can be targeted (brachial plexus block, femoral nerve block, sciatic nerve block, etc.)
- performed with standard monitors
- approximately 2-4 per 10,000 risk of late neurologic injury
- resuscitation equipment must be available

Contraindications to Peripheral Nerve Blockade
- absolute contraindications
    - allergy to LA
    - patient refusal
- relative contraindications
    - certain types of pre-existing neurological dysfunction (e.g. ALS, MS, diabetic neuropathy)
    - local infection at block site
    - bleeding disorder

Local Anesthesia

Local Anesthetic Agents

- see Table 14, for list of LA agents

Definition and Mode of Action
- LA are drugs that block the generation and propagation of impulses in excitable tissues: nerves, skeletal muscle, cardiac muscle, brain
- LA bind to receptors on the cytosolic side of the Na^+ channel, inhibiting Na^+ flux and thus blocking impulse conduction
- different types of nerve fibres undergo blockade at different rates

Absorption, Distribution, Metabolism
- LA readily crosses the blood-brain barrier (BBB) once absorbed into the bloodstream
- ester-type LA (procaine, tetracaine) are broken down by plasma and hepatic esterases; metabolites excreted via kidneys
- amide-type LA (lidocaine, bupivicaine) are broken down by hepatic mixed-function oxidases (P450 system); metabolites excreted via kidneys

Selection of LA
- choice of LA depends on
    - onset of action: influenced by pKa (the lower the pKa, the higher the concentration of the base form of the LA, and the faster the onset of action)
    - duration of desired effects: influenced by protein binding (longer duration of action when protein binding of LA is strong)
    - potency: influenced by lipid solubility (agents with high lipid solubility penetrate the nerve membrane more easily)
    - unique needs (e.g. sensory blockade with relative preservation of motor function by bupivicaine at low doses)
    - potential for toxicity

Table 14. Local Anesthetic Agents

	Maximum Dose	Maximum Dose with Epinephrine	Potency	Duration
chloroprocaine	11 mg/kg	14 mg/kg	Low	15-30 min
lidocaine	5 mg/kg	7 mg/kg	Medium	1-2 h
bupivacaine	2.5 mg/kg	3 mg/kg	High	3-8 h
ropivacaine	2.5 mg/kg	3 mg/kg	High	2-8 h

Reduction of Post-Operative Mortality and Morbidity with Epidural or Spinal Anaesthesia: Results from Overview of Randomized Trials
BMJ 2000;321:1-12
Purpose: To obtain reliable estimates of the effects of neuraxial blockade with epidural or spinal anesthesia on post-operative morbidity and mortality after various surgeries with or without general anesthesia.
Study: Systematic review of all trials with randomization to intraoperative neuraxial blockade vs. control group.
Patients: 141 trials including 9,559 patients.
Main Outcomes: All cause mortality, MI, PE, DVT, transfusion requirements, pneumonia, other infections, respiratory depression, and renal failure
Results: With neuraxial blockade, overall mortality was reduced by about one third. Neuraxial blockade reduced the risk of PE by 55%, DVT by 44%, transfusion requirements by 50%, pneumonia by 39%, and respiratory depression by 59%. There were also reductions in MI and renal failure. These mortality reductions are irrespective of surgical group, type of blockade (epidural or spinal), or whether neuraxial blocker was combined with general anesthetic.
Conclusions: Neuraxial blockade reduces post-operative mortality and other serious complications.

Systemic Toxicity

- see Table 16, A25 for maximum doses, potency, and duration of action for common LA agents
- occurs by accidental intravascular injection, LA overdose, or unexpectedly rapid absorption

CNS Effects
- CNS effects first appear to be excitatory due to initial block of inhibitory fibres, then subsequent block of excitatory fibres
- effects in order of appearance
  - numbness of tongue, perioral tingling, metallic taste
  - disorientation, drowsiness
  - tinnitus
  - visual disturbances
  - muscle twitching, tremors
  - unconsciousness
  - convulsions, seizures
  - generalized CNS depression, coma, respiratory arrest

CVS Effects
- vasodilation, hypotension
- decreased myocardial contractility
- dose-dependent delay in cardiac impulse transmission
  - prolonged PR, QRS intervals
  - sinus bradycardia
- CVS collapse

Treatment of Systemic Toxicity
- early recognition of signs, get help
- 100% O_2, manage ABCs
- diazepam or sodium thiopental may be used to increase seizure threshold
- manage arrhythmias (see *ACLS Guidelines*, A31-32)
- Intralipid® 20% to bind local anesthetic in circulation

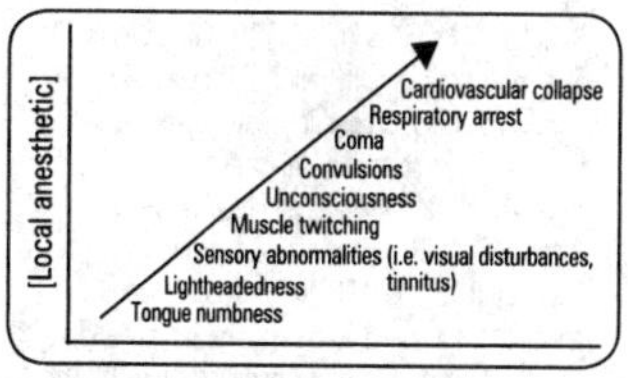

Figure 10. Local anesthetic systemic toxicity

Local Infiltration and Hematoma Blocks

Local Infiltration
- injection of tissue with LA, producing a lack of sensation in the infiltrated area due to LA acting on nerves
- suitable for small incisions, suturing, excising small lesions
- can use fairly large volumes of dilute LA to infiltrate a large area
- low concentrations of epinephrine (1:100,000-1:200,000) cause vasoconstriction, thus reducing bleeding and prolonging the effects of LA by reducing systemic absorption

Where Not to Use LA with Epinephrine
"Ears, Fingers, Toes, Penis, Nose"

Fracture Hematoma Block
- special type of local infiltration for pain control during manipulation of certain fractures
- hematoma created by fracture is infiltrated with LA to anesthetize surrounding tissues
- sensory blockade may only be partial
- no muscle relaxation

Topical Anesthetics

- various preparations of local anesthetics available for topical use, may be a mixture of agents (EMLA cream is a combination of 2.5% lidocaine and prilocaine)
- must be able to penetrate the skin or mucous membrane

Post-Operative Care

- pain management should be continuous from OR to post-anesthetic care unit (PACU) to hospital ward and home

Common Post-Operative Anesthetic Complications

Nausea and Vomiting
- hypotension and bradycardia must be ruled out
- pain and surgical manipulation also cause nausea
- often treated with dimenhydrinate (Gravol®), metoclopramide (Maxeran®; not with bowel obstruction), prochlorperazine (Stemetil®), ondansetron (Zofran®), granisetron (Kytril®)

Drugs for Preventing Post-Operative Nausea and Vomiting
Cochrane DB Syst Rev 2006;3:CD004125
Purpose: To evaluate the efficacy of antiemetics in preventing PONV.
Methods: A meta-analysis was performed looking at randomized controlled trials comparing an antiemetic to either a second antiemetic or placebo. Trials looking at dosing and/or timing of medication administration were also included. PONV was used as the primary outcome.
Results: 737 studies involving 103,237 patients. Eight drugs significantly reduced the occurence of PONV, namely: droperidol, metoclopramide, ondansetron, tropisetron, dolasetron, dexamethasone, cyclizine, and granisetron. Relative risk (RR) versus placebo varied between 0.60, and 0.80. Side effects included a significant increase in drowsiness for droperidol (RR 1.32) and headache for ondansetron (RR 1.16). The cumulative number needed to treat was 3.57.
Conclusion: Antiemetic medication is effective for reducing the occurrence of PONV. However, further investigation needs to be done to determine whether antiemetics can cause more severe (and likely rare) side effects, which could alter how liberally they are used.

Confusion and Agitation
- ABCs first – confusion or agitation can be caused by airway obstruction, hypercapnea, hypoxemia
- neurologic status (Glasgow Coma Scale, pupils), residual paralysis from anesthetic
- pain, distended bowel/bladder
- fear/anxiety/separation from caregivers, language barriers
- metabolic disturbance (hypoglycemia, hypercalcemia, hyponatremia – especially post-TURP)
- intracranial cause (stroke, raised intracranial pressure)
- drug effect (ketamine, anticholinergics, serotonin)
- elderly patients are more susceptible to post-operative delirium

Respiratory Complications
- susceptible to aspiration of gastric contents due to PONV and unreliable airway reflexes
- airway obstruction (secondary to reduced muscle tone from residual anesthetic, soft tissue trauma and edema, or pooled secretions) may lead to inadequate ventilation, hypoxemia, and hypercapnia
- airway obstruction can often be relieved with head tilt, jaw elevation, and anterior displacement of the mandible. If the obstruction is not reversible, a nasal or oral airway may be used

Hypotension
- must be identified and treated quickly to prevent inadequate perfusion and ischemic damage
- reduced cardiac output (hypovolemia, most common cause) and/or peripheral vasodilation (residual anesthetic agent)
- first step in treatment is usually the administration of fluids ± inotropic agents

Hypertension
- pain, hypercapnia, hypoxemia, increased intravascular fluid volume, and sympathomimetic drugs can cause hypertension
- sodium nitroprusside or β-blocking drugs (e.g. esmolol and metoprolol) can be used to treat hypertension

Pain Management

Definitions
- pain: perception of nociception, which occurs in the brain
- nociception: detection, transduction, and transmission of noxious stimuli

Pain Classifications
- temporal: acute vs. chronic
- mechanism: nociceptive vs. neuropathic

Acute Pain

- pain of short duration (<6 wk) usually associated with surgery, trauma, or acute illness; often associated with inflammation
- usually limited to the area of damage/trauma and resolves with healing

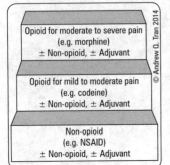

Figure 12. WHO analgesia ladder

- Opioid for moderate to severe pain (e.g. morphine) ± Non-opioid, ± Adjuvant
- Opioid for mild to moderate pain (e.g. codeine) ± Non-opioid, ± Adjuvant
- Non-opioid (e.g. NSAID) ± Non-opioid, ± Adjuvant

© Andrew Q. Tran 2014

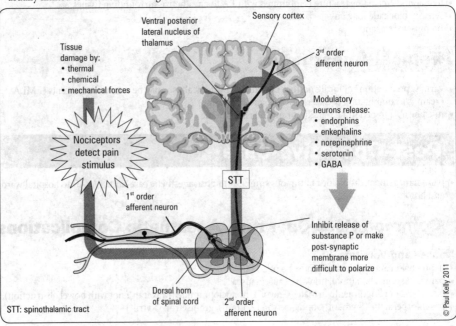

Figure 11. Acute pain mechanism

STT: spinothalamic tract

© Paul Kelly 2011

Pharmacological Management of Acute Pain
- ask the patient to rate the pain out of 10, or use visual analog scale, to determine severity
- pharmacological treatment guided by WHO analgesia ladder
- patient controlled analgesia (PCA)
  - involves the use of computerized pumps that can deliver a constant infusion and bolus breakthrough doses of parenterally-administered opioid analgesics
  - limited by lockout intervals
  - most commonly used agents: morphine and hydromorphone
  - see Table 17, A26 for suggested infusion rate, PCA dose and lockout intervals

Table 15. Commonly Used Analgesics

	Acetaminophen	NSAIDs	Opioids
Examples	Tylenol®	Aspirin®, ibuprofen, naproxen ketorolac (IV)	Oral: codeine, oxycodone, morphine, hydromorphone Parenteral: morphine, hydromorphone, fentanyl
Indications	First-line for mild acute pain	Mild-moderate pain	Oral: moderate acute pain Parenteral: moderate-severe acute pain
Mechanism of Action	Unclear, hypothesized cyclooxygenase-2 (COX-2) inhibition Unclear, hypothesized modulation of endogenous cannabinoid system	Non-selective COX-1 and 2 inhibition reducing proinflammatory prostaglandin synthesis	Dampens nociceptive transmission between 1st and 2nd order neurons in the dorsal horn Activates ascending modulatory pathways resulting in release of inhibitory neurotransmitters Inhibits peripheral inflammatory response and hyperalgesia Affects mood and anxiety – alleviates the affective component of perceived pain
Dosing/ Administration	Limited by analgesic ceiling beyond which there is no additional analgesia Opioid-sparing Max dose of 4 g/24 h	Limited by analgesic ceiling beyond which there is no additional analgesia Opioid-sparing Significant inter-individual variation in efficacy	No analgesic ceiling (except for codeine) Can be administered intrathecally (spinal block) or by continuous infusion
Side Effects/ Toxicity	Considered relatively safe Liver toxicity in elevated doses	Gastric ulceration/bleeding Decreased renal perfusion Photosensitivity Premature closure of the ductus arteriosus in pregnancy	Respiratory depression Constipation and abdominal pain Sedation N/V Pruritus Confusion (particularly in the elderly) Dependence

Table 16. Opioids

Agent	Relative Dose to 10 mg Morphine IV	Moderate Dose	Onset	Duration	Special Considerations
Codeine	200 mg PO	15-30 mg PO	Late (30-60 min)	Moderate (4-6 h)	Primarily post-operative use, not for IV use
Meperidine (Demerol®)	75 mg IV	2-3 mg/kg IV	Moderate (10 min)	Moderate (2-4 h)	Anticholinergic, hallucinations, less pupillary constriction than morphine, metabolite build up may cause seizures
Morphine	10 mg IV 20 mg PO	0.2-0.3 mg/kg IV 0.4-0.6 mg/kg PO	Moderate (5-10 min)	Moderate (4-5 h)	Histamine release leading to decrease in BP
Oxycodone Controlled Release (Oxyneo®)	15 mg PO	10-20 mg PO (no IV)	Late (30-45 min)	Long (8-12 h)	Do not split, crush, or chew tablet
Oxycodone Regular Tablet (Oxy IR®)	15 mg PO (no IV)	5-15 mg PO	Moderate (15 min)	Moderate (3-6 h)	Percocet® = oxycodone 5 mg + acetaminophen 325 mg
Hydromorphone (Dilaudid®)	2 mg IV 10 mg PO	40-60 µg/kg IV 2-4 mg PO	Moderate (15 min)	Moderate (4-5 h)	
Fentanyl	100 µg IV	2-3 µg/kg IV	Rapid (<5 min)	Short (0.5-1 h)	Transient muscle rigidity in very high doses
Remifentanil	100 µg IV	0.5-1.5 µg/kg IV	Rapid (1-3 min)	Ultra short (<10 min)	Only use during induction and maintenance of anesthesia

In general, parenteral route is 2-3x more potent than oral

Cautionary Use of NSAIDs in Patients with
- Asthma
- Coagulopathy
- GI ulcers
- Renal insufficiency
- Pregnancy, 3rd trimester

Common Side Effects of Opioids
- N/V
- Constipation
- Sedation
- Pruritus
- Abdominal pain
- Urinary retention
- Respiratory depression
When prescribing opioids, consider:
- Breakthrough dose
- Anti-emetics
- Laxative

PCA Parameters
- Loading dose
- Bolus dose
- Lockout interval
- Continuous infusion (optional)
- Maximum 4 h dose (limit)

Advantages of PCA
- Improved patient satisfaction
- Fewer side effects
- Accommodates patient variability
- Accommodates changes in opioid requirements

Patient Controlled Opioid Analgesia vs. Conventional Opioid Analgesia for Post-Operative Pain
Cochrane DB Syst Rev 2006;4:CD003348
Purpose: To evaluate the efficacy of patient controlled analgesia (PCA) as compared to conventional 'as-needed' analgesia administration providing pain relief in post-operative patients.
Methods: Meta-analyses of randomized controlled trials comparing PCA vs. conventional administration of opioid analgesia. Assessment employed a visual analog scale (VAS) for pain intensity along with overall analgesic consumption, patient satisfaction, length of stay, and adverse side effects.
Results: 55 studies with a total of 2,023 patients receiving PCA and 1,838 patients with standard as-needed opioid administration. PCA provided significantly better pain control through 72 h post-operatively, but patients consumed significantly more opioids (>7 mg morphine/24 h, p<0.05) Significantly more patients reported pruritus in the PCA group compared to control with a number needed to harm of 13. No significant difference in overall length of stay in hospital, sedation level, N/V, or urinary retention.
Conclusions: PCA is more effective than standard as-needed administration for reducing post-operative pain. However, patients using PCA consume more opioids overall and have more pruritus.

Table 17. Opioid PCA Doses

Agent	PCA Dose	PCA Lockout Interval	PCA 4 h Maximum
Morphine	1 mg	5 min	30 mg
Hydromorphone	0.2 mg	5 min	6 mg
Fentanyl	25-50 μg	5 min	400 μg

Opioid Antagonists (naloxone, naltrexone)
- indication: opioid overdose (manifests primarily at CNS, e.g. respiratory depression)
- mechanism of action: competitively inhibit opioid receptors, predominantly μ receptors
  - naloxone is short-acting ($t_{1/2}$ = 1 h); effects of narcotic may return when naloxone wears off; therefore, the patient must be observed closely following its administration
  - naltrexone is longer-acting ($t_{1/2}$ = 10 h); less likely to see return of opioid effects
- side effects: relative overdose of naloxone may cause nausea, agitation, sweating, tachycardia, hypertension, re-emergence of pain, pulmonary edema, seizures (essentially opioid withdrawal)

Neuropathic Pain

- see Neurology, N41

Chronic Pain

- chronic pain: greater than 3 mo, or recurrent pain that occurs at least 3 times throughout three month period
- pain of duration or intensity that persists beyond normal tissue healing and adversely affects functioning
- may have nociceptive and neuropathic components; dysregulation of analgesic pathways implicated
- in the perioperative period, consider continuing regular long-acting analgesics and augmenting with regional techniques, adjuvants, additional opioid analgesia and non-pharmacological techniques

Obstetrical Anesthesia

Anesthesia Considerations in Pregnancy
- airway
  - possible difficult airway as tissues becomes edematous and friable especially in labour
- respiratory
  - decreased FRC and increased O_2 consumption cause more rapid desaturation during apnea
- cardiovascular system
  - increased blood volume > increased RBC mass results in mild anemia
  - decreased SVR proportionately greater than increased CO results in decreased BP
  - prone to decreased BP due to aortocaval compression – therefore for surgery, a pregnant patient is positioned in left uterine displacement using a wedge under her right flank
- central nervous system
  - decreased MAC due to hormonal effects
  - increased block height due to engorged epidural veins
- gastrointestinal system
  - delayed gastric emptying
  - increased volume and acidity of gastric fluid
  - decreased LES tone
  - increased abdominal pressure
  - combined, these lead to an increased risk of aspiration – therefore for surgery, a pregnant patient is given sodium citrate 30 cc PO immediately before surgery to neutralize gastric acidity

Options for Analgesia during Labour
- psychoprophylaxis – Lamaze method
  - patterns of breathing and focused attention on fixed object
- systemic medication
  - easy to administer, but risk of maternal or neonatal respiratory depression
  - opioids most commonly used if delivery is not expected within 4 h
- inhalational analgesia
  - easy to administer, makes uterine contractions more tolerable, but does not relieve pain completely
  - 50% nitrous oxide
- neuraxial anesthesia
  - provides excellent analgesia with minimal depressant effects
  - hypotension is the most common complication
  - maternal BP monitored q2-5 min for 15-20 min after initiation and regularly thereafter
  - epidural usually given as it preferentially blocks sensation, leaving motor function intact

The Effect of Epidural Analgesia on Labour, Maternal, and Neonatal Outcomes: A Systematic Review
Am J Obstet Gynecol 2002;186:S69-77
Study: Meta-analysis of 14 studies with 4,324 women.
Selection Criteria: RCTs and prospective cohort studies between 1980-2001 comparing epidural analgesia to parenteral opioid administration during labour.
Types of Participants: Healthy women with uneventful pregnancies.
Intervention: Participants were randomized to either epidural analgesia or parenteral opioid administration during labour.
Outcomes and Results: Maternal – there were no differences between the 2 groups in first-stage labour length, incidence of Cesarean delivery, incidence of instrumented vaginal delivery for dystocia, nausea, or mid-to-low back pain post-partum. However, second-stage labour length was longer (mean=15 min) and there were greater reports of fever and hypotension in the epidural group. Also, lower pain scores and greater satisfaction with analgesia were reported among the epidural group. There was no difference in lactation success at 6 wk and urinary incontinence was more frequent in the epidural group immediately post-partum, but not at 3 mo or 1 yr (evidence from PC studies only) Neonatal – there were no differences between the 2 groups for incidence of fetal heart rate abnormalities, intrapartum meconium, poor 5-min Apgar score, or low umbilical artery pH. However, the incidence of poor 1-min Apgar scores and need for neonatal naloxone were higher in the parenteral opioid group.
Conclusions: Epidural analgesia is a safe intrapartum method for labour pain relief and women should not avoid epidural analgesia for fear of neonatal harm, Cesarean delivery, breastfeeding difficulties, long-term back pain, or long-term urinary incontinence.

Nociceptive Pathways in Labour and Delivery
Labour
- Cervical dilation and effacement stimulates visceral nerve fibres entering the spinal cord at T10-L1
Delivery
- Distention of lower vagina and perineum causes somatic nociceptive impulses via the pudendal nerve entering the spinal cord at S2-S4

Options for Caesarean Section
- neuraxial: spinal or epidural
- general: used if contraindications or time precludes regional blockade

Pediatric Anesthesia

Respiratory System
- in comparison to adults, anatomical differences in infants include:
  - large head, short trachea/neck, large tongue, adenoids, and tonsils
  - narrow nasal passages (obligate nasal breathers until 5 mo)
  - narrowest part of airway at the level of the cricoid vs. glottis in adults
  - epiglottis is longer, U shaped and angled at 45°; carina is wider and is at the level of T2 (T4 in adults)
- physiologic differences include
  - faster RR, immature respiratory centres which are depressed by hypoxia/hypercapnea (airway closure occurs in the neonate at the end of expiration)
  - less oxygen reserve during apnea – decreased total lung volume, vital and functional reserve capacity together with higher metabolic needs
  - greater V/Q mismatch – lower lung compliance due to immature alveoli (mature at 8 yr)
  - greater work of breathing – greater chest wall compliance, weaker intercostals/diaphragm, and higher resistance to airflow

Cardiovascular System
- blood volume at birth is approximately 80 mL/kg; transfusion should be started if >10% of blood volume lost
- children have a high HR and low BP
- CO is dependent on HR, not stroke volume because of low heart wall compliance; therefore, bradycardia severe compromise in CO

Temperature Regulation
- vulnerable to hypothermia
- minimize heat loss by use of warming blankets, covering the infant's head, humidification of inspired gases, and warming of infused solutions

Central Nervous System
- MAC of halothane is increased compared to the adult (0.75% adult, 1.2% infant, 0.87% neonate)
- NMJ is immature for the first 4 wk of life and thus there is an increased sensitivity to non-depolarizing relaxants
- parasympathetics mature at birth, sympathetics mature at 4-6 mo thus autonomic imbalance
- infant brain is 12% of body weight and receives 34% of CO (adult: 2% body weight and 14% CO)

Glucose Maintenance
- infants less than 1 yr old can become seriously hypoglycemic during pre-operative fasting and post-operatively if feeding is not recommenced as soon as possible
- after 1 yr, children are able to maintain normal glucose homeostasis in excess of 8 h

Pharmacology
- higher dose requirements because of higher TBW (75% vs. 60% in adults) and greater volume of distribution
- barbiturates/opioids more potent due to greater permeability of BBB
- muscle relaxants
  - non-depolarizing
    - immature NMJ, variable response
  - depolarizing
    - must pre-treat with atropine or may experience profound bradycardia and/or sinus node arrest due to PNS > SNS (also dries oral secretions)
    - more susceptible to arrhythmias, hyperkalemia, rhabdomyolysis, myoglobinemia, masseter spasm and malignant hyperthermia

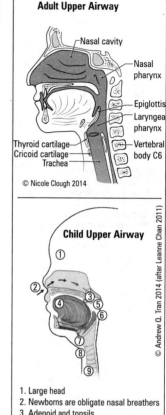

Adult Upper Airway

- Nasal cavity
- Nasal pharynx
- Epiglottis
- Laryngeal pharynx
- Vertebral body C6
- Thyroid cartilage
- Cricoid cartilage
- Trachea

© Nicole Clough 2014

Child Upper Airway

© Andrew Q. Tran 2014 (after Leanne Chan 2011)

1. Large head
2. Newborns are obligate nasal breathers
3. Adenoid and tonsils
4. Larger tongue in proportion to mouth
5. Smaller pharynx
6. Larger and more flaccid epiglottis
7. Larynx is more superior and anterior
8. Narrowest point at cricoid cartilage
9. Trachea is more narrow and less rigid

Figure 13. Comparison of pediatric vs. adult airway

To increase alveolar minute ventilation in neonates, increase respiratory rate, not tidal volume.
Neonate: 30-40 breaths/min
Age 1-13: (24 – [age/2]) breaths/min

ETT Sizing in Pediatrics
Diameter (mm) of tracheal tube in children after 1 year = (age/4) + 4
Length (cm) of tracheal tube = (age/2) + 12

Uncommon Complications

Malignant Hyperthermia

- hypermetabolic disorder of skeletal muscle
- due to an uncontrolled increase in intracellular Ca^{2+} (because of an anomaly of the ryanodine receptor which regulates Ca^{2+} channel in the sarcoplasmic reticulum of skeletal muscle)
- autosomal dominant inheritance
- incidence of 1-5 in 100,000, may be associated with skeletal muscle abnormalities such as dystrophy or myopathy
- anesthetic drugs triggering MH include
  - all inhalational agents except nitrous oxide
  - depolarizing muscle relaxants: SCh

Signs of Malignant Hyperthermia
- Unexplained rise in ET_{CO2}
- Increase in minute ventilation
- Tachycardia
- Rigidity
- Hyperthermia (late sign)

Clinical Picture
- onset: immediate or hours after contact with trigger agent
  - increased oxygen consumption
  - increased ET_{CO2} on capnograph
  - tachycardia/dysrhythmia
  - tachypnea/cyanosis
  - diaphoresis
  - hypertension
  - increased temperature (late sign)
- muscular symptoms
  - trismus (masseter spasm) common but not specific for MH (occurs in 1% of children given SCh with halothane anesthesia)
  - tender, swollen muscles due to rhabdomyolysis
  - trunk or total body rigidity

Complications
- coma
- DIC
- rhabdomyolysis
- myoglobinuric renal failure/hepatic dysfunction
- electrolyte abnormalities (e.g. hyperkalemia) and secondary arrhythmias
- ARDS
- pulmonary edema
- can be fatal if untreated

Prevention
- suspect MH in patients with a family history of problems/death with anesthetic
- avoid all trigger medications, use vapour free equipment, use regional anesthesia if possible
- central body temp and ET_{CO2} monitoring

Basic Principles of MH Management

"Some Hot Dude Better Get Iced Fluids Fast"
Stop all triggering agents, give 100% O_2
Hyperventilate
Dantrolene 2.5 mg/kg every 5 min
Bicarbonate
Glucose and insulin
IV fluids; cool patient to 38°C
Fluid output; consider furosemide
Tachycardia: be prepared to treat VT

Malignant Hyperthermia Management (Based on Malignant Hyperthermia Association of the U.S. [MHAUS] Guidelines, 2008)
1. notify surgeon, discontinue volatile agents and succinylcholine, hyperventilate with 100% oxygen at flows of 10 L/min or more, halt the procedure as soon as possible
2. dantrolene 2.5 mg/kg IV, through large-bore IV if possible
   - repeat until there is control of signs of MH; up to 30 mg/kg as necessary
3. bicarbonate 1-2 mEq/kg if blood gas values are not available for metabolic acidosis
4. cool patients with core temperature >39°C
   - lavage open body cavities, stomach, bladder, rectum; apply ice to surface; infuse cold saline IV
   - stop cooling if temperature is <38°C to prevent drift to <36°C
5. dysrhythmias usually respond to treatment of acidosis and hyperkalemia
   - use standard drug therapy except Ca^{2+} channel blockers as they may cause hyperkalemia and cardiac arrest in presence of dantrolene
6. hyperkalemia
   - treat with hyperventilation, bicarbonate, glucose/insulin, calcium
   - bicarbonate 1-2 mEq/kg IV, calcium chloride 10 mg/kg or calcium gluconate 10-50 mg/kg for life-threatening hyperkalemia and check glucose levels hourly
7. follow ET_{CO2}, electrolytes, blood gases, creatine kinase (CK), core temperature, urine output/colour with Foley catheter, coagulation studies
   - if CK and/or potassium rises persistently or urine output falls to <0.5 mL/kg/h, induce diuresis to >1 mL/kg/h urine to avoid myoglobinuric renal failure
8. maintain anesthesia with benzodiazepines, opioids, and propofol
9. transfer to ICU bed

Abnormal Pseudocholinesterase

- pseudocholinesterase hydrolyzes SCh and mivacurium
- individuals with abnormal pseudocholinesterase will have prolonged muscular blockade
- SCh and mivacurium are contraindicated in those with abnormal pseudocholinesterase
- if SCh or mivacurium are given accidentally, treat with mechanical ventilation until function returns to normal (do not use cholinesterase inhibitors rebound neuromuscular blockade once drug effect is terminated)

Appendices

Difficult Tracheal Intubation in Unconscious Patient

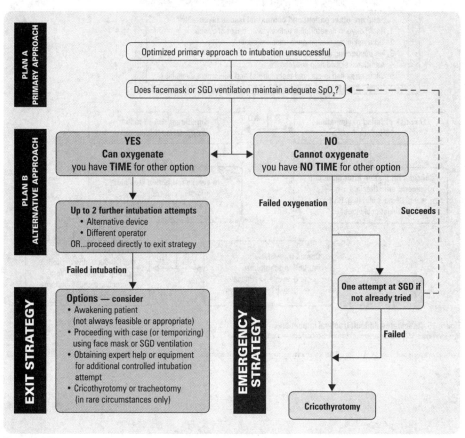

Figure 14. Difficult tracheal intubation encountered in the unconscious patient
SGD = supraglottic device

Reprinted with permission. Law JA, et al. The difficult airway with recommendations for management – Part 1 – Difficult tracheal intubation encountered in an unconscious/induced patient. *Can J Anesth* 2013;60:1089–1118.

Difficult Tracheal Intubation

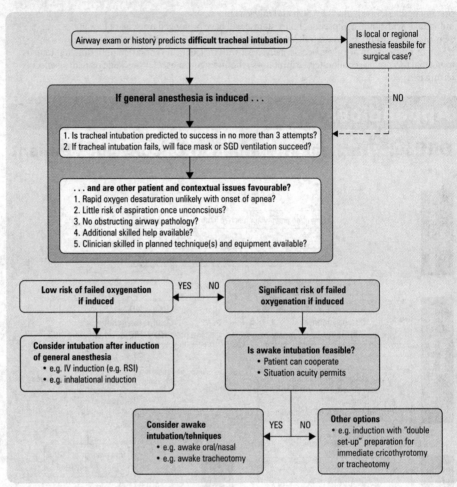

Figure 15. Anticipated difficult tracheal intubation

IV = intravenous; RSI = rapid sequence induction/intubation; SGD = supraglottic device

Reprinted with permission: Law JA, et al. The difficult airway with recommendations for management – Part 2 – The anticipated difficult airway. *Can J Anesth* 2013;60:1119-1138.

Advanced Cardiac Life Support Guidelines

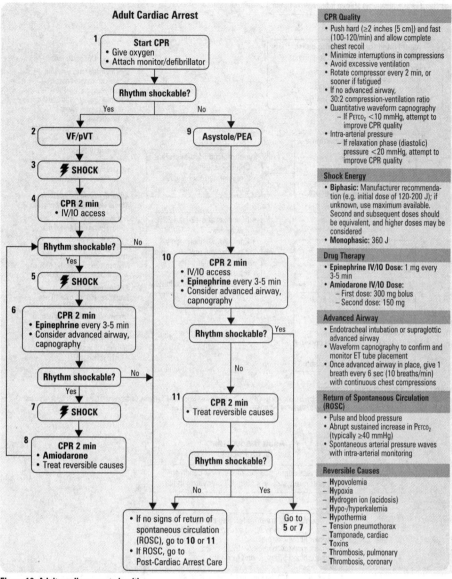

Figure 16. Adult cardiac arrest algorithm
Reprinted with permission: Link, M. S., Berkow, L. C., Kudenchuk, P. J., Halperin, H. R., Hess, E. P., Moitra, V. K., ... & White, R. D. (2015). Part 7: Adult Advanced Cardiovascular Life Support 2015 American Heart Association Guidelines Update for Cardiopulmonary Resuscitation and Emergency Cardiovascular Care. *Circulation 2015*, 132(18 suppl 2), S444-S464. ©2015 American Heart Association, Inc.

Appendices

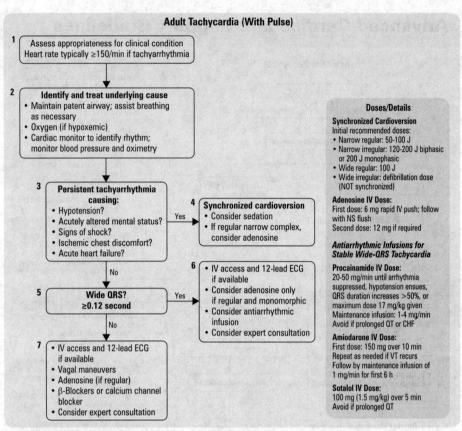

Figure 17. Adult tachycardia algorithm
Reprinted with permission: 2015 American Heart Association Guidelines for Cardiopulmonary Resuscitation and Emergency Cardiovascular Care, Part 8: Adult Advanced Cardiovascular Life Support. *Circulation* 2010;122(suppl 3):S729-S767 ©2015 American Heart Association, Inc.

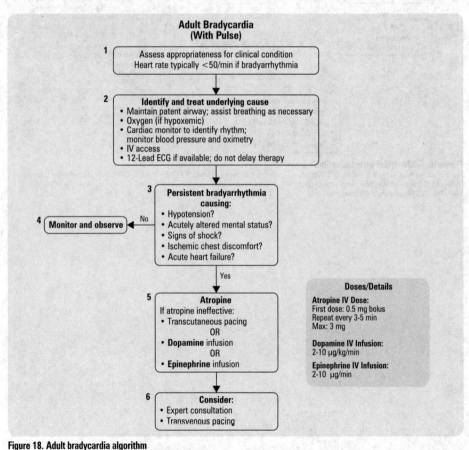

Figure 18. Adult bradycardia algorithm
Reprinted with permission: 2015 American Heart Association Guidelines for Cardiopulmonary Resuscitation and Emergency Cardiovascular Care, Part 8: Adult Advanced Cardiovascular Life Support. *Circulation* 2010;1229(suppl 3):S729-S767 ©2015 American Heart Association, Inc.

References

Arbous MS, Meursing AE, van Kleef JW, et al. Impact of anesthesia management characteristics on severe morbidity and mortality. Anesthesiology 2005;102:257-268.

Barash P, Cullen BF, Stoelting RK, et al. Clinical anesthesia, 6th ed. Philadelphia: Lippincott, 2009.

Bell RM, Dayton MT, Lawrence PF. Essentials of surgical specialties. Philadelphia: Lippincott, 2000. Anesthesiology 1-67.

Blanc VF, Tremblay NA. The complications of tracheal intubation: a new classification with review of the literature. Anesth Analg 1974;53:202-213.

Carlisle J, Stevenson CA. Drugs for preventing post-operative nausea and vomiting. Cochrane DB Syst Rev 2006;Issue 3.

Collins VJ. Physiologic and pharmacologic bases of anesthesia. Philadelphia: Lippincott, 1996.

Craft TM, Upton PM. Key topics in anesthesia, clinical aspects, 3rd ed. Oxford: BIOS Scientific, 2001.

Duke J. Anesthesia secrets, 4th ed. Philadelphia: Mosby, 2010.

Frank SM, Fleisher LA, Breslow MJ, et al. Perioperative maintenance of normothermia reduces the incidence of morbid cardiac events: a randomized clinical trial. JAMA 1997;227:1127-1134.

Fleisher LA, Beckman JA, Brown KA, et al. ACC/AHA 2007 Guidelines on perioperative cardiovascular evaluation for non-cardiac surgery: executive summary. Circulation 2007;116:1971-1996.

Hebert PC, Wells G, Blajchman MA, et al. A multicenter, randomized, controlled clinical trial of transfusion requirements in critical care. NEJM 1999;340:409-417.

Henderson JJ, Popat MT, Latto IP, et al. Difficult Airway Society guidelines for management of the unanticipated difficult intubation. Anaesthesia 2004;59:675-694.

Hudcova J, McNicol E, Quah C, et al. Patient controlled opioid analgesia versus conventional opioid analgesia for post-operative pain. Cochrane DB Syst Rev 2006;Issue 4.

Kalant H, Grant D, Mitchell J. Principles of medical pharmacology, 7th ed. New York: Oxford University Press, 2006.

Law JA, Broemling N, Cooper RM, et al. The difficult airway with recommendations for management –Part 1 – Difficult tracheal intubation encountered in an unconscious/induced patient. Can J Anesth 2013;60:1089-1118.

Law JA, Broemling N, Cooper RM, et al. The difficult airway with recommendations for management –Part 2 – The anticipated difficult airway. Can J Anesth 2013;60:1119-1138.

Lee A, Fan LTY. Stimulation of the wrist acupuncture point P6 for preventing post-operative nausea and vomiting. Cochrane DB Syst Rev 2009;Issue 2.

Leighton BL, Halpern SH. The effects of epidural analgesia on labour, meternal, and neonatal outcomes: a systemic review. Am J Obstet Gynecol 2002;186:569-577.

Lette J, Waters D, Bernier H, et al. Preoperative and long-term cardiac risk assessment predictive value of 23 clinical descriptors, 7 multivariate scoring systems, and quantitative dipyridamole imaging in 360 patients. Ann Surg 1992;216:192-204.

Levine WC, Allain RM, Alston TA, et al. Clinical anesthesia procedures of the Massachusetts General Hospital, 8th ed. Philadelphia: Lippincott, 2010.

Liccardi G, Salzillo A, DeBlasio F, et al. Control of asthma for reducing the risk of bronchospasm in asthmatics undergoing general anesthesia and/or intravascular administration of radiographic contrast media. Curr Med Res Opin 2009;25:1621-1630.

MacDonald NE, O'Brien SF, Delage G. Canadian Paediatric Society Infectious Diseases and Immunization Committee: Transfusion and risk of infection in Canada Update 2012. Paediatr Child Health 2012;17:e102-e111.

Malignant Hyperthermia Association of the United States. Available from http://www.mhaus.org.

Mangano DT, Browner WS, Hollenberg M, et al. Long-term cardiac prognosis following non-cardiac surgery. JAMA 1992;268:233-240.

Mangano DT, Layug EL, Wallace A, et al. Effect of atenolol on mortality and cardiovascular morbidity after non-cardiac surgery. NEJM 1996;335:1713-1720.

Merchant R, Chartrand D, Dain S, et al. Guidelines to the practice of anesthesia - Revised edition 2014. Can J Anaesth 2014;61:46-59.

Miller RD, Eriksson LI, Fleisher LA, et al. Miller's anesthesia, 7th ed. Philadelphia: Churchill Livingstone, 2000.

Morgan GE, Mikhail MS, Murray MJ. Clinical anesthesiology, 4th ed. New York: McGraw-Hill Medical, 2005.

Neumar RW, Otto CW, Link MS, et al. American Heart Association guidelines for cardiopulmonary resuscitation and emergency cardiovascular care science. Circulation 2010;122:5729-5760.

Palda VA, Detsky AS. Perioperative assessment and management of risk from coronary artery disease. Ann Intern Med 1997;127:313-328.

Perel P, Roberts I, Pearson M. Colloids versus crystalloids for fluid resuscitation in critically ill patients. Cochrane DB Syst Rev 2012;Issue 4.

POISE Study Group. Effects of extended-release metoprolol succinate in patients undergoing non-cardiac surgery (POISE Trial): a randomized controlled trial. Lancet 2008;371:1839-1847.

Poldermans D, Boersma E, Bax JJ, et al. The effect of bisoprolol on perioperative mortality and myocardial infarction in high-risk patients undergoing vascular surgery. NEJM 1999;341:1789-1794.

Posner KL, Van Norman GA, Chan V. Adverse cardiac outcomes after non-cardiac surgery in patients with prior percutaneous transluminal coronary angioplasty. Anesth Analg 1999;89:553-560.

Rao TL, Jacobs KH, El-Etr AA. Reinfarction following anaesthesia in patients with myocardial infarction. Anaesthesiology 1983;59:499-505.

Roberts JR, Spadafora M, Cone DC. Proper depth placement of oral endotracheal tubes in adults prior to radiographic confirmation. Acad Emerg Med 1995;2:20-24.

Rodgers A, Walker N, Schug S, et al. Reduction of post-operative mortality and morbidity with epidural or spinal anesthesia: Results from overview of randomized trials. BMJ 2000;321:1-12.

Salpeter SR, Ormiston TM, Salpeter EE. Cardioselective betablockers for chronic obstructive pulmonary disease. Cochrane DB Syst Rev 2005;Issue 4.

Salpeter S, Ormiston T, Salpeter E. Cardioselective betablockers for reversible airway disease. Cochrane DB Syst Rev 2002;Issue 4.

Sessler DI. Complications and treatment of mild hypothermia. Anesthesiology 2001;95:531-543.

Shiga T, Wajima Z, Inoue T, et al. Predicting difficult intubation in apparently normal patients. Anesthesiology 2005;103:429-437.

Sullivan P. Anesthesia for medical students. Ottawa: Doculink International, 1999.

Zwillich CW, Pierson DJ, Creagh CE, et al. Complications of assisted ventilation. Am J Med 1974;57:16

Notes

C

Cardiology and Cardiac Surgery

Sean Cai, Shun Chi Ryan Lo, and Zain Sohail, chapter editors
Claudia Frankfurter and Inna Gong, associate editors
Brittany Prevost and Robert Vanner, EBM editors
Dr. Chi-Ming Chow, Dr. Michael McDonald, and Dr. Anna Woo, staff editors

Acronyms

AAA	abdominal aortic aneurysm	CVD	cerebrovascular disease	LMWH	low molecular weight heparin	RAO	right anterior oblique
ABI	ankle-brachial index	CXR	chest x-ray	LV	left ventricle	RBB	right bundle branch
ACEI	angiotensin converting enzyme inhibitor	DCM	dilated cardiomyopathy	LVAD	left ventricular assist device	RBBB	right bundle branch block
ACS	acute coronary syndrome	DM	diabetes mellitus	LVEF	left ventricular ejection fraction	RBW	routine blood work
AFib	atrial fibrillation	DOAC	direct oral anticoagulant	LVH	left ventricular hypertrophy	RV	right ventricle
AR	aortic regurgitation	DVT	deep vein thrombosis	MAT	multifocal atrial tachycardia	RVAD	right ventricular assist device
ARB	angiotensin receptor blocker	ECASA	enteric coated ASA	MI	myocardial infarction	RVH	right ventricular hypertrophy
ARDS	acute respiratory distress syndrome	ECG	electrocardiogram	MPI	myocardial perfusion imaging	SA	sinoatrial
AS	aortic stenosis	Echo	echocardiogram	MR	mitral regurgitation	SCD	sudden cardiac death
ASA	acetylsalicylic acid (Aspirin®)	EPS	electrophysiology studies	MRA	MRI angiography	SEM	systolic ejection murmur
ASD	atrial septal defect	EtOH	ethanol/alcohol	MS	mitral stenosis	SLE	systemic lupus erythematosus
AV	atrioventricular	GERD	gastroesophageal reflux disease	NSR	normal sinus rhythm	STEMI	ST elevation myocardial infarction
AVM	arteriovenous malformation	HCM	hypertrophic cardiomyopathy	NSTEMI	non-ST elevation myocardial infarction	SV	stroke volume
AVNRT	atrioventricular nodal re-entrant tachycardia	HFPEF	heart failure with preserved ejection fraction	OS	opening snap	SVC	superior vena cava
				PAC	premature atrial contraction	SVR	systemic vascular resistance
AVRT	atrioventricular re-entrant tachycardia	HFREF	heart failure with reduced ejection fraction	PCI	percutaneous coronary intervention	SVT	supraventricular tachycardia
BBB	bundle brunch block			PCWP	pulmonary capillary wedge pressure	TAA	thoracic aortic aneurysm
BNP	brain natriuretic peptide	HTN	hypertension	PDA	patent ductus arteriosus	TB	tuberculosis
BP	blood pressure	HR	heart rate	PE	pulmonary embolism	TEE	transesophageal echocardiography
BiVAD	biventricular assist device	ICD	implantable cardioverter-defibrillator	PFO	patent foramen ovale	TIA	transient ischemic attack
CABG	coronary artery bypass graft	IE	infective endocarditis	PIV	posterior-interventricular artery	TR	tricuspid regurgitation
CAD	coronary artery disease	JVP	jugular venous pressure	PMI	point of maximal impulse	TTE	transthoracic echocardiography
CCB	calcium channel blocker	LA	left atrium	PND	paroxysmal nocturnal dyspnea	UA	unstable angina
CHF	congestive heart failure	LAE	left atrial enlargement	PUD	peptic ulcer disease	VAD	ventricular assist device
CI	cardiac index	LBB	left bundle branch	PVC	premature ventricular contraction	VFib	ventricular fibrillation
CO	cardiac output	LBBB	left bundle branch block	PVD	peripheral vascular disease	VT	ventricular tachycardia
COPD	chronic obstructive pulmonary disease	LICS	left intercostal space	RA	right atrium	VTE	venous thromboembolism
CTA	CT angiography	LLSB	left lower sternal border	RAE	right atrial enlargement	WPW	Wolff-Parkinson-White

Basic Anatomy Review

Coronary Circulation

- conventional arterial supply to the heart arises from the right and left coronary arteries, which originate from the root of the aorta
  - right coronary artery (RCA)
    - acute marginal branches
    - atrioventricular (AV) nodal artery
    - posterior interventricular artery (PIV) = posterior descending artery (PD)
  - left main coronary artery (LCA):
    - left anterior descending artery (LAD)
      - septal branches
      - diagonal branches
    - left circumflex artery (LC)
      - obtuse marginal branches
- dominance of circulation
  - right-dominant circulation: PIV and at least one posterolateral branch arise from RCA (80%)
  - left-dominant circulation: PIV and at least one posterolateral branch arise from LC (15%)
  - balanced circulation: dual supply of posteroinferior LV from RCA and LC (5%)
- the sinoatrial (SA) node is supplied by the SA nodal artery, which may arise from the RCA (60%) or LCA (40%)
- most venous blood from the heart drains into the RA through the coronary sinus, although a small amount drains through Thebesian veins into all four chambers, contributing to the physiologic R-L shunt

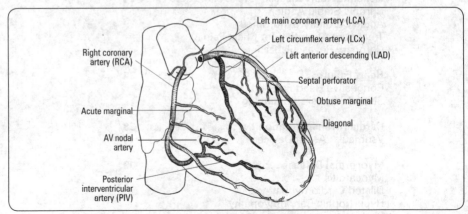

Figure 1. Anatomy of the coronary arteries (right anterior oblique projection)

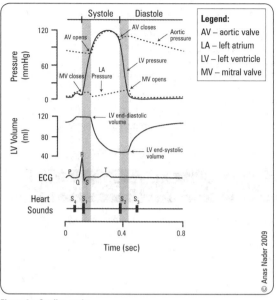

Figure 2a. Cardiac cycle
Grey shaded bars indicate isovolumic contraction (left) and isovolumic relaxation (right)

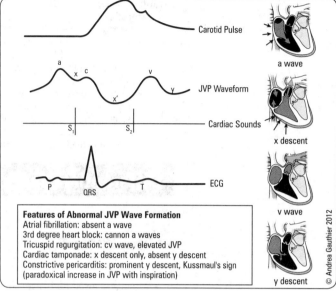

Features of Abnormal JVP Wave Formation
Atrial fibrillation: absent a wave
3rd degree heart block: cannon a waves
Tricuspid regurgitation: cv wave, elevated JVP
Cardiac tamponade: x descent only, absent y descent
Constrictive pericarditis: prominent y descent, Kussmaul's sign (paradoxical increase in JVP with inspiration)

Figure 2b. JVP waveform

Cardiac Anatomy

- **layers of the heart**
  - endocardium, myocardium, epicardium, visceral pericardium, pericardial cavity, parietal pericardium
- **valves**
  - semilunar valves:
    - aortic valve, 3 valve leaflets: separates LV and ascending aorta
    - pulmonic valve, 3 valve leaflets: separates RV and main pulmonary artery (PA)
  - atrioventricular valves: subvalvular apparatus present in the form of chordae tendinae and papillary muscles
    - tricuspid valve, 3 valve leaflets: separates RA and RV
    - mitral/bicuspid valve, 2 valve leaflets: separates LA and LV
- **conduction system**
  - SA node governs pacemaking control
  - anterior-, middle-, and posterior-internal nodal tracts carry impulses in the right atrium and along Bachmann's bundle in the left atrium
  - atrial impulses converge at the AV node
    - the AV node is the only conducting tract from the atria to the ventricles because of electrical isolation by the annulus fibrosis (except when accessory pathways are present)
  - the bundle of His bifurcates into left and right bundle branches (LBB and RBB)
  - LBB further splits into anterior and posterior fascicles
  - RBB and fascicles of LBB give off Purkinje fibres which conduct impulses into the ventricular myocardium

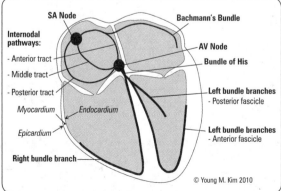

Figure 3. Conduction system of the heart

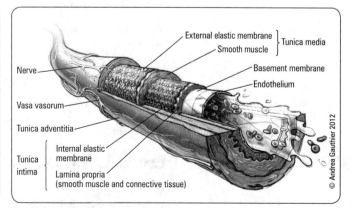

Figure 4. Blood vessel structure

- **cardiovascular innervation**
  - sympathetic nerves
    - innervate the SA node, AV node, ventricular myocardium and vasculature
    - SA node (β1) fibres increase pacemaking activity (chronotropy - HR)
    - cardiac muscle (β1) fibres increase contractility (inotropy - SV)
    - stimulation of β1- and β2-receptors in the skeletal and coronary circulation causes vasodilatation
  - parasympathetic nerves
    - innervate the SA node, AV node, atrial myocardium but few vascular beds
    - basal vagal tone dominates the tonic sympathetic stimulation of the SA node and AV node resulting in slowing of pacemaker activity and conduction (i.e. reduced dromotropy – if only affecting AV node conduction)
    - parasympathetics have very little impact on total peripheral vascular resistance

Differential Diagnoses of Common Presentations

Note: **bold** text indicates most common, underlined text indicates life threatening condition

Chest Pain

- cardiac
  - MI/angina, myocarditis, pericarditis/Dressler's syndrome
- pulmonary
  - PE, pneumothorax/hemothorax, tension pneumothorax, pneumonia, empyema, pulmonary neoplasm, bronchiectasis, TB
- gastrointestinal
  - esophageal: **GERD**, esophageal rupture, spasm, esophagitis, ulceration, achalasia, neoplasm, Mallory-Weiss syndrome
  - other structures: PUD, gastritis, pancreatitis, biliary colic
- mediastinal
  - lymphoma, thymoma
- vascular
  - dissecting aortic aneurysm, aortic rupture
- surface structures
- costochondritis
- rib fracture
- skin (bruising, herpes zoster)
- breast
- anxiety/psychosomatic

Loss of Consciousness

- **hypovolemia**
- **vasovagal**
- cardiac
  - structural or obstructive causes
    - ACS, AS, HCM, cardiac tamponade, constrictive pericarditis
  - arrhythmias (see *Arrhythmias*, C16)
- respiratory
  - massive pulmonary embolism, pulmonary hypertension, hypoxia, hypercapnia
- neurologic
  - stroke/TIA (esp. vertebrobasilar insufficiency), migraine, seizure
- metabolic
  - anemia, hypoglycemia
- drugs
  - antihypertensives, antiarrhythmics, diuretics
- autonomic dysfunction
  - diabetic neuropathy
- psychiatric
  - panic attack

Local Edema

- inflammation/infection
- venous or lymphatic obstruction
  - thrombophlebitis/deep vein thrombosis, venous insufficiency, chronic lymphangitis, lymphatic tumour infiltration, filariasis

Generalized Edema

- increased hydrostatic pressure/fluid overload
  - heart failure, pregnancy, drugs (e.g. CCBs), iatrogenic (e.g. IV fluids)
- decreased oncotic pressure/hypoalbuminemia
  - **liver cirrhosis**, nephrotic syndrome, malnutrition
- increased capillary permeability
  - severe sepsis
- hormonal
  - hypothyroidism, exogenous steroids, pregnancy, estrogens

Palpitations

- cardiac
  - **arrhythmias** (PAC, PVC, SVT, <u>VT</u>), **valvular heart disease**, <u>HCM</u>
- endocrine
  - thyrotoxicosis, pheochromocytoma, hypoglycemia
- systemic
  - **anemia**, fever
- drugs
  - stimulants and anticholinergics
- psychiatric
  - panic attack

Dyspnea

- cardiovascular
  - acute MI, CHF/LV failure, aortic/mitral stenosis, aortic/mitral regurgitation, arrhythmia, cardiac tamponade, constrictive pericarditis, left-sided obstructive lesions (e.g. left atrial myxoma), elevated pulmonary venous pressure
- respiratory
  - airway disease
    - asthma, COPD exacerbation, upper airway obstruction (anaphylaxis, foreign body, mucus plugging)
  - parenchymal lung disease
    - ARDS, pneumonia, interstitial lung disease
  - pulmonary vascular disease
    - PE, pulmonary HTN, pulmonary vasculitis
  - pleural disease
    - pneumothorax, pleural effusion
- neuromuscular and chest wall disorders
  - C-spine injury
    - polymyositis, myasthenia gravis, Guillain-Barré syndrome, kyphoscoliosis
- anxiety/psychosomatic
- hematological/metabolic
  - anemia, acidosis, hypercapnia

Cardiac Diagnostic Tests

Electrocardiography Basics

Description
- a graphical representation (time versus amplitude of electrical vector projection) of the electrical activity of the heart
- on the ECG graph
  - the horizontal axis represents time (at usual paper speed 25 mm/s)
    - 1 mm (1 small square) = 40 msec
    - 5 mm (1 large square) = 200 msec
  - the vertical axis represents voltage (at usual standard gain setting 10 mm/mV)
    - 1 mm (1 small square) = 0.1 mV
    - 10 mm (2 large squares) = 1 mV
- leads
  - standard 12-lead ECG
    - limb leads: I, II, III, aVL, aVR, aVF
    - precordial leads: V1-V6 (V1-V2 septal, V3-V4 anterior, V5-V6 lateral)
  - additional leads
    - right-sided leads: V3R-V6R (useful in RV infarction and dextrocardia)
  - lateral = I, aVL, V5, V6; inferior = II, III, aVF; anterior = V1-V4

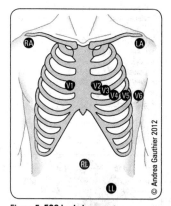

Figure 5. ECG lead placement

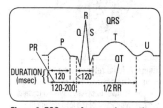

Figure 6. ECG waveforms and normal values

Indications
- detect myocardial injury, ischemia, and the presence of prior infarction
- palpitations, syncope, antiarrhythmic drug monitoring
- arrhythmia surveillance in patients with documented or potentially abnormal rhythms
- surveillance of non-sustained arrhythmias that can lead to prophylactic intervention

Contraindications
- no absolute contraindications except patient refusal or electrode latex adhesive allergy

Approach to ECGs

Introduction
Below, we are presenting both the Classical Approach and the newer PQRSTU Approach to provide students with different ways to view the ECG. Despite methodological differences, the rigor and final result is the same. These two approaches should help you better understand the concepts of ECG interpretation and equip you with the necessary skills to interpret ECGs in exam scenarios and clinical practice

Classical Approach to ECGs

RATE
- normal = 60-100 bpm (atrial rate: 150-250 bpm = paroxysmal tachycardia, 250-350 bpm = atrial flutter, >350 bpm = AFib)
- regular rhythm
  - to calculate the rate, divide 300 by number of large squares between 2 QRS complexes (there are 300 large squares in 1 min: 300 x 200 msec = 60 sec)
  - or remember 300-150-100-75-60-50-43 (rate falls in this sequence with the number of large squares between 2 QRS complexes)
- irregular rhythm
  - rate = 6 x number of R-R intervals in 10 s (the "rhythm strips" are 10 sec recordings)
- atrial escape rhythm = 60-80 bpm; junctional escape rhythm = 40-60 bpm; ventricular escape rhythm = 20-40 bpm

RHYTHM
- regular: R-R interval is the same across the tracing
- irregular: R-R interval varies across the tracing
- regularly irregular: repeating pattern of varying R-R intervals e.g. A. Flutter
- irregularly irregular: R-R intervals vary erratically e.g. A. Fib, V. Fib
- normal sinus rhythm (NSR)
  - P wave precedes each QRS; QRS follows each P wave
  - P wave axis is normal (positive in 2 out of the 3 following leads I, II, aVF)
  - rate between 60-100 bpm

AXIS
- mean axis indicates the direction of the mean vector
- can be determined for any waveform (P, QRS, T)
- the standard ECG reported QRS axis usually refers to the mean axis of the frontal plane – it indicates the mean direction of ventricular depolarization forces
- QRS axis in the frontal plane
  - normal axis: -30° to 90° (i.e. positive QRS in leads I and II)
  - left axis deviation (LAD): axis <-30°
  - right axis deviation (RAD): axis >90°
- QRS axis in the horizontal plane is not routinely calculated
  - transition from negative to positive is usually in lead V3

Rate Calculations
- Examples, practice

For more examples and practice visit www.ecgmadesimple.com

Classical Approach to ECG
- Rate
- Rhythm
- Axis
- Conduction abnormalities
- Hypertrophy/chamber enlargement
- Ischemia/infarction
- Miscellaneous ECG changes

Differential Diagnosis for Left Axis Deviation (LAD)
- Left anterior hemiblock
- Inferior MI
- WPW
- RV pacing
- Normal variant
- Elevated diaphragm
- Lead misplacement
- Endocardial cushion defect

Differential Diagnosis for Right Axis Deviation (RAD)
- RVH
- Left posterior hemiblock
- Pulmonary embolism
- COPD
- Lateral MI
- WPW
- Dextrocardia
- Septal defects

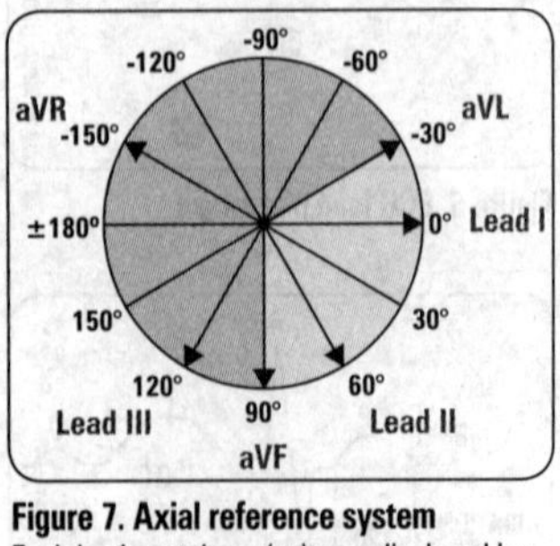

Figure 7. Axial reference system
Each lead contains a (+) area displayed by the bold arrows. Impulses traveling toward the positive region of the lead results in an upward deflection in that lead. Normal QRS axis is between -30° and +90°

Table 1. Conduction Abnormalities

Left Bundle Branch Block (LBBB)	Right Bundle Branch Block (RBBB)
Complete LBBB QRS duration >120 msec Broad notched R waves in leads V4, and V5, and usually I, aVL Deep broad S waves in leads V1-2 Secondary ST-T changes (-ve in leads with broad notched R waves, +ve in V1-2) are usually present LBBB can mask ECG signs of MI	**Complete RBBB** QRS duration >120 msec Positive QRS in lead V1 (rSR' or occasionally broad R wave) Broad S waves in leads I, V5-6 (>40 msec) Usually secondary T wave inversion in leads V1-2 Frontal axis determination using only the first 60 msec

Left Anterior Fascicular Block (LAFB) (Left Anterior Hemiblock)	Left Posterior Fascicular Block (LPFB) (Left Posterior Hemiblock)	Bifascicular Block
Left Axis Deviation (-30° to -90°) Small q and prominent R in leads I and aVL Small r and prominent S in leads II, III, and aVF	**Right Axis Deviation (110° to 180°)** Small r and prominent S in leads I and aVL Small q and prominent R in leads II, III, and aVF	RBBB pattern Small q and prominent R The first 60 msec (1.5 small squares) of the QRS shows the pattern of LAFB or LPFB Bifascicular block refers to impaired conduction in two of the three fascicles, most commonly a RBBB and left anterior hemiblock; the appearance on an ECG meets the criteria for both types of blocks

Nonspecific Intraventricular Block

- QRS duration >120 msec
- absence of definitive criteria for LBBB or RBBB

Table 2. Hypertrophy/Chamber Enlargement

Left Ventricular Hypertrophy (LVH)	Right Ventricular Hypertrophy (RVH)

S in V1 + R in V5 or V6 >35 mm above age 40, (>40 mm for age 31-40, >45 mm for age 21-30)
R in aVL >11 mm
R in I + S in III >25 mm
Additional criteria
  LV strain pattern (asymmetric ST depression and T wave inversion in leads I, aVL, V4-V6)
  Left atrial enlargement
N.B. The more criteria present, the more likely LVH is present.
If only one voltage criteria present, it is called minimal voltage criteria for LVH which could be a normal variant
	Right axis deviation
	R/S ratio >1 or qR in lead V1
	RV strain pattern: ST segment depression and T wave inversion in leads V1-2

Left Atrial Enlargement (LAE)	**Right Atrial Enlargement (RAE)**
Biphasic P wave with the negative terminal component of the P wave in lead V1 ≥1 mm wide and ≥1 mm deep P wave >100 msec, could be notched in lead II ("P mitrale")	P wave >2.5 mm in height in leads II, III, or aVF ("P pulmonale")

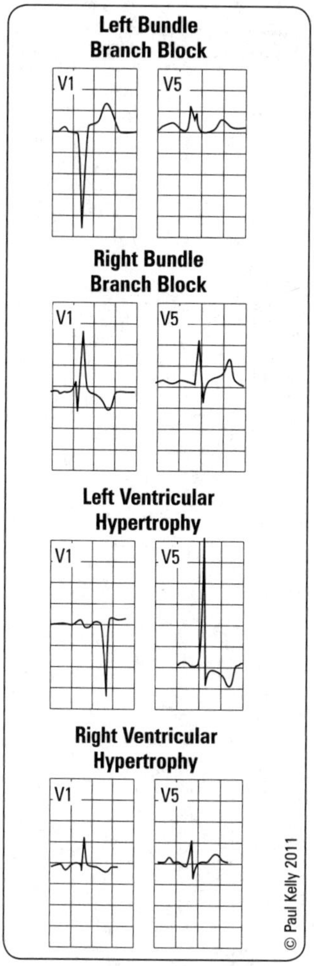

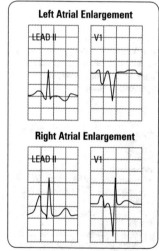

Figure 8. Complete LBBB, RBBB, LVH, and RVH (please see online examples for the full range of waveforms and the text for additional characteristics)

© Paul Kelly 2011

ISCHEMIA/INFARCTION

- look for the anatomic distribution of the following ECG abnormalities (see Table 3, C8)
- ischemia
  - ST segment depression
  - T wave inversion (most commonly in V1-V6)
- injury/infarct
  - transmural (involving the epicardium)
  - ST elevation in the leads facing the area injured/infarcted
  - subendocardial
  - marked ST depression in the leads facing the affected area
  - may be accompanied by enzyme changes and other signs of MI

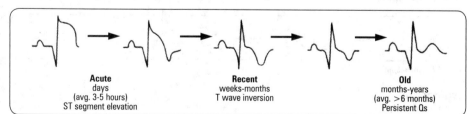

Acute
days
(avg. 3-5 hours)
ST segment elevation

Recent
weeks-months
T wave inversion

Old
months-years
(avg. >6 months)
Persistent Qs

Figure 10. Typical ECG changes with infarction

Figure 9. LAE, RAE (please see online examples and the text for characteristics)

- ST elevation: at least 1 mm in 2 adjacent limb leads or at least 1-2 mm in adjacent precordial leads in STEMI (signifies complete occlusion and transmural ischemic injury) vs. diffuse pattern in early pericarditis vs. transient ST elevation in patients with coronary artery spasm (e.g. Prinzmetal angina) which can be slight or prominent (>10 mm)

- "typical" sequential changes of evolving MI
  1. hyperacute T waves (tall, symmetric T waves) in the leads facing the infarcted area, with or without ST elevation
  2. ST elevation (injury pattern) in the leads facing the infarcted area
     - usually in the first hours post infarct
     - in acute posterior MI, there is ST depression in V1-V3 (reciprocal to ST elevation in the posterior leads, that are not recorded in the standard 12-lead ECG) - get a 15-lead ECG
  3. significant Q waves: >40 msec or >1/3 of the total QRS and present in at least 2 consecutive leads in the same territory (hours to days post-infarct)
     - Q waves of infarction may appear in the very early stages, with or without ST changes
     - non-Q wave infarction: there may be only ST or T changes despite clinical evidence of infarction
  4. inverted T waves (one day to weeks after infarction)
- completed infarction
  - abnormal Q waves (Q waves may be present in leads III and aVL in normal individuals due to initial septal depolarization)
  - duration >40 msec (>30 msec in aVF for inferior infarction)
  - Q/QRS voltage ratio is >33%
  - present in at least 2 consecutive leads in the same territory
  - abnormal R waves (R/S ratio >1, duration >40 msec) in V1 and occasionally in V2 are found in posterior infarction (usually in association with signs of inferior and/or lateral infarction)

Table 3. Areas of Infarction/Ischemia (right dominant anatomy)

Vessel Usually Involved	Infarct Area (LAD and LC)	Leads (LAD and LC)
Left anterior descending (LAD)	Anteroseptal	V1, V2
	Anterior	V3, V4
	Anterolateral	I, aVL, V3-6
	Extensive anterior	I, aVL, V1-6
Right coronary artery (RCA)	Inferior	II, III, aVF
	Right ventricle	V3R, V4R (right sided chest leads)
	Posterior MI (assoc. with inf. MI)	V1, V2 (prominent R waves)
Left circumflex (LCX)	Lateral	I, aVL, V5-6
	Isolated posterior MI	V1, V2 (prominent R waves)

MISCELLANEOUS ECG CHANGES

Electrolyte Disturbances
- hyperkalemia
  - mild to moderate (K^+ 5-7 mmol/L): tall peaked T waves
  - severe (K^+ >7 mmol/L): progressive changes whereby P waves flatten and disappear, QRS widens and may show bizarre patterns, axis shifts left or right, ST shift with tall T waves, eventually becomes a "sine wave" pattern
- hypokalemia
  - ST segment depression, prolonged QT interval, low T waves, prominent U waves (U>T)
  - enhances the toxic effects of digitalis
- hypercalcemia
  - shortened QT interval (more extracellular Ca^{2+} means shorter plateau in cardiac action potential)
- hypocalcemia
  - prolonged QT interval (less extracellular Ca^{2+} means longer plateau in cardiac action potential)

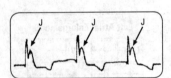

Figure 13. Osborne J waves of a hypothermic patient

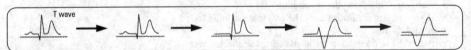

Figure 11. Hyperkalemia

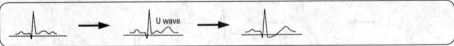

Figure 12. Hypokalemia

Pacemakers
- Demand pacemaker has discharge (narrow vertical spike on ECG strip) prior to widened QRS
- Atrial pacemaker has discharge prior to P wave
- Triggered pacemaker has discharge following the P wave but prior to the widened QRS
- Atrial and ventricular pacing have discharge before the P wave and widened QRS wave

Hypothermia
- sinus bradycardia
- when severe, prolonged QRS and QT intervals
- AFib with slow ventricular response and other atrial/ventricular dysrhythmias
- Osborne J waves: "hump-like" waves at the junction of the J point and the ST segment

Pericarditis
- early: diffuse ST segment elevation ± PR segment depression, upright T waves
- later: isoelectric ST segment, flat or inverted T waves
- ± tachycardia

Drug Effects

- digitalis
  - therapeutic levels may be associated with "digitalis effect"
    - ST downsloping or "scooping"
    - T wave depression or inversion
    - QT shortening ± U waves
    - slowing of ventricular rate in AFib
    - toxic levels associated with
    - arrhythmias: paroxysmal atrial tachycardia (PAT) with conduction block, severe bradycardia in AFib, accelerated junctional rhythms, PVCs, ventricular tachycardia (see *Arrhythmias*, C16)
    - "regularization" of ventricular rate in AFib due to a junctional rhythm and AV dissociation
- amiodarone, quinidine, phenothiazines, tricyclic antidepressants, antipsychotics, some antihistamines, some antibiotics: prolonged QT interval, U waves

Digitalis Side Effects
Palpitations, fatigue, visual changes (yellow vision), decreased appetite, hallucinations, confusion, and depression

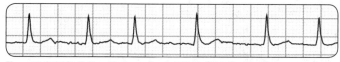

Figure 14. Atrial fibrillation, ST change due to digitalis ("digitalis effect")

Pulmonary Disorders

- *cor pulmonale* (often secondary to COPD)
  - low voltage, right axis deviation (RAD), poor R wave progression in precordial leads
  - RAE and RVH with strain
  - multifocal atrial tachycardia (MAT)
- massive pulmonary embolism (PE)
  - sinus tachycardia and A. Fib/atrial flutter are the most common arrhythmias
  - RAD, RVH with strain
  - most specific sign is S1Q3T3 (S in I, Q and inverted T wave in III) but rather uncommon

Alternative PQRSTU Approach to ECGs

Note: the information seen in this alternative approach – the PQRSTU Approach – is the same as the information in the Classical Approach; it is just organized in a different way based on the anatomy of the ECG

PQRSTU approach to ECGs
P wave
P-R interval
QRS complex
ST segment
T wave
Q-T interval
U wave

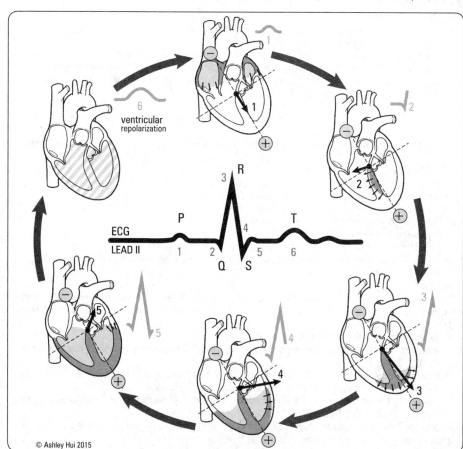

© Ashley Hui 2015

Figure 15. ECG correlations with heart activity

P WAVE
- the P wave represents atrial contraction; best leads: II, VI
  - lead II: the P wave should be rounded, <120 msec and <2.5 mm in height
  - lead VI: the P wave is biphasic with a negative phase slightly greater than the positive phase
- atrial flutter: sawtooth P wave (Hint: flip the ECG upside-down to see it better if unclear)
- atrial fibrillation: absent P wave, may have fibrillatory wave, irregular rhythm
- right atrial enlargement: tall P wave (>2.5 mm) in II or V1 (P pulmonale)
- left atrial enlargement: negative deflection >1 mm deep or >1 mm wide in V1, wide (>100 msec) notched P wave in II may be present (P mitrale)

P-R INTERVAL
- the P-R interval shows the delay between atrial and ventricular contraction that is mediated by the AV node; the magnitude of the delay is referred to as "dromotropy"
- positive dromotropy increases conduction velocity (e.g. epinephrine stimulation), negative dromotropy decreases velocity (e.g. vagal stimulation)
- P-R interval should be 120-200 msec
- long P-R interval (>200 msec)
  - heart block
    - first degree: fixed, prolonged P-R interval
    - second degree Mobitz I/Wenckebach: steadily prolonging P-R interval to eventual dropped beat
    - second degree Mobitz II/Hay: fixed P-R interval with ratio of beat to dropped beat (e.g. for every 3 beats, there is one dropped beat [3:1])
    - third degree/complete: variable P-R intervals, P-P and R-R intervals individually constant but not in sync
  - atrial flutter
  - sinus bradycardia (normal to have long P-R if heart rate slow)
  - hypokalemia
  - "trifascicular" block -1st degree AV block with LAHF and complete RBBB
- short P-R interval (<120 msec)
  - pre-excitation syndrome (delta wave: upswooping of the P-R segment into the QRS complex indicating pre-excitation)
    - accessory pathways
    - WPW
  - low atrial rhythm

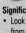

Significant ECG Changes
- Look for ST changes starting at 60 msec from J point
- J point = the junction between the QRS complex and the ST segment
- ST elevation: at least 1 mm in 2 adjacent limb leads, or at least 1-2 mm in adjacent precordial leads
- ST depression: downsloping or horizontal
- Q Wave: pathological if Q wave ≥1 small square (≥40 msec) or >33% of the total QRS

QRS COMPLEX
- the QRS is where ventricular contraction is visualized
- rate: check the R-R interval to see if it matches the P-P interval
- amplitude: check for hypertrophy (see Table 2, C7)
- narrow width (<120 msec) QRS means that the His-Purkinje system is being used
- wide width (>120 msec) QRS means that the His-Purkinje system is being bypassed or is diseased
  - BBB, VT, ventricular hypertrophy, cardiomyopathy, WPW, ectopic ventricular beat, hyperkalemia, drugs (e.g. TCAs, antiarrhythmics)
- Q wave: the first downward deflection of the QRS complex
  - significant Q wave: >40 msec or >33% of total QRS amplitude; indicate myocardial necrosis (new or historical)
- R and S wave abnormalities typically show pathology in terms of BBB or intraventricular abnormalities

Insignificant Q Wave
- Septal depolarization by the left bundle
- Seen in leads I, II, III, aVL, V5, V6
- <40 msec

ST SEGMENT
- located between QRS complex and the beginning of T wave
  - corresponds to the completion of ventricular depolarization
- normally at the same level as "baseline/TP segment"
- ST elevation: please see the infarct section above
- ST depression: ischemia
  - ischemia which causes ST depression can result in myocardial damage (NSTEMI)
  - lateral ST depression (leads I, aVL, V5, V6) may actually indicate a STEMI in the right heart

T WAVE
- this is the repolarization phase of the ventricles (repolarization of the atria are obscured by the QRS complex)
- typically positive (except in aVR and V1) on ECG but normal isolated negative T waves may be present (esp. in V1 and V2)
- pathology when T wave variation occur in consecutive leads
  - inversion: BBB, ischemia, hypertrophy, drugs (e.g. digitalis), pulmonary embolism (lead III as part of S1Q3T3 sign)
  - elevation: infarction (STEMI, Prinzmetal, hyperacute), hyperkalemia (wider, peaked)
  - flattened: hypokalemia, pericarditis, drugs (e.g. digitalis), pericardial effusion
  - variations: T wave alterans; beat-to-beat variations due to PVC overlap (R on T phenomenon which may precipitate VT or VFib)
- appropriate T wave discordance: in BBB, T wave deflection should be opposite to that of the terminal QRS deflection (i.e. T wave negative if ends with R or R'; positive if ends with S)
  - inappropriate T wave concordance suggests ischemia or infarction

Q-T INTERVAL

- this represents the duration of ventricular depolarization and repolarization and is often difficult to interpret
- corrected QT (QTc) is often used instead in practice to correct for the repolarization duration; $QTc = QT \div \sqrt{RR}$
- normal QTc is 360-450 msec for males and 360-460 for females
  - increased (>450 msec for males and >460 for females): risk of Torsades de Pointes (a lethal tachyarrhythmia)
    - genetic Long QT Syndrome (often a channelopathy)
    - drugs: antibiotics, SSRIs, antipsychotics, antiarrhythmics
    - electrolytes: low Ca^{2+}, low Mg^{2+}, low K^+
    - others: hypothyroidism, hypothermia, cardiomyopathy
  - decreased (<360 msec): risk of VFib
    - electrolytes: high Ca^{++}
    - drugs: digoxin
    - others: hyperthyroidism

U WAVE

- origin unclear but may be repolarization of Purkinje fibres or delayed/prolonged repolarization of the myocardium
- more visible at slower heart rates
- deflection follows T wave with <25% of the amplitude
- variations from norm could indicate pathologic conditions:
  - prominent (>25% of T wave): electrolyte (low K+), drugs (digoxin, antiarrhythmics)
  - inverted (from T wave): ischemia, volume overload

Cardiac Biomarkers

- provide diagnostic and prognostic information in acute coronary syndromes and in heart failure

Table 4. Cardiac Enzymes

Enzyme	Peak	Duration Elevated	DDx of Elevation
Troponin I, Troponin T	1-2 d	Up to 2 wk	MI, CHF, AFib, acute PE, myocarditis, chronic renal insufficiency, sepsis, hypovolemia
CK-MB	1 d	3 d	MI, myocarditis, pericarditis, muscular dystrophy, cardiac defibrillation, chronic renal insufficiency, etc.

- check troponin I at presentation and 8 h later ± creatine kinase-MB (CK-MB; depends on local laboratory protocol)
- new CK-MB elevation can be used to diagnose re-infarction
- other biomarkers of cardiac disease
  - AST and LDH also increased in MI (low specificity)
  - BNP and NT-proBNP: secreted by ventricles in response to increased end-diastolic pressure and volume
    - DDx of elevated BNP: CHF, AFib, PE, COPD exacerbation, pulmonary HTN

Ambulatory ECG

- **description**
  - extended ambulatory ECG of 24 or 48 h or 14 or 30 d duration
  - provides a view of only two or three leads of electrocardiographic data over an extended period of time
  - permits evaluation of changing dynamic cardiac electrical phenomena that are often transient and of brief duration
  - **continuous loop:** a small, lightweight, battery operated recorder that records two or three channels of electrocardiographic data
    - patient activated event markers
    - minimum of 24-48 h
  - **implantable device:** subcutaneous monitoring device for the detection of cardiac arrhythmias
    - typically implanted in the left pectoral region and stores events when the device is activated automatically according to programmed criteria or manually with magnet application
    - can be used for months to years
- **indications**
  - evaluation of cardiac rhythm abnormalities
  - has also been used for assessing pacemaker and implantable cardioverter-defibrillator function, evidence of myocardial ischemia, late potentials, and heart rate variability
- **contraindications**
  - no absolute contraindications
  - patient refusal
  - allergies (sensitivities to latex adhesive)
- **risks:** no absolute risks

Differential Diagnosis of ST Segment Changes

ST Elevation I HELP A PAL
Ischemia with reciprocal changes
Hypothermia (Osborne waves)
Early repolarization (normal variant, need old ECGs to confirm)
LBBB
Post-MI
Acute STEMI
Prinzmetal's (Vasospastic) angina
Acute pericarditis (diffuse changes)
Left/right ventricular aneurysm

ST Depression WAR SHIP
WPW syndrome
Acute NSTEMI
RBBB/LBBB
STEMI with reciprocal changes
Hypertrophy (LVH or RVH) with strain
Ischemia
Post-MI

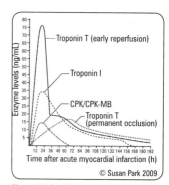

Figure 16. Cardiac enzymes

Use of B-Type Natriuretic Peptide in the Evaluation and Management of Acute Dyspnea (BASEL)
NEJM 2004;350:647-54
Study: Prospective, RCT.
Population: 452 patients (mean age 71 yr 58% male) with acute dyspnea; patients with severe renal disease or cardiogenic shock were excluded.
Intervention: Assessment including measurement of B-type natriuretic peptide or standard assessment.
Outcome: Time to discharge and total cost of treatment.
Results: Median time to discharge was significantly shorter in the intervention group when compared with the control group (8.0 vs. 11.0 d, p=0.001). Total cost was also significantly lower in the intervention group ($5410 vs. $7264, p=0.006). In addition, the measurement of B-type natriuretic peptide significantly reduced the need for admission to hospital and intensive care. The 30-d mortality rates were similar (10% vs. 12%, p=0.45).
Conclusions: In patients with acute dyspnea, measurement of B-type natriuretic peptide improves clinical outcomes (need for hospitalization or intensive care) and reduces time to discharge and total cost of treatment.

Echocardiography

Transthoracic Echocardiography (TTE)
- **description**: ultrasound beams are directed across the chest wall to obtain images of the heart
- **indications**
  - evaluation of LVEF, wall motion abnormalities, myocardial ischemia and complications of MI
  - evaluation of chamber size, wall thickness, valve morphology, proximal great vessel morphology, pericardial effusion
  - evaluation of unexplained hypotension, murmurs, syncope, congenital heart disease

Transoesophageal Echocardiography (TEE)
- **description**: invasive procedure used to complement transthoracic echocardiography
  - ultrasound probe inserted into the esophagus to allow for better resolution of the heart and structures
  - better visualization of posterior structures, including left atrium, mitral and aortic valves, inter-atrial septum
- **indications**
  - should be performed as the initial test in certain life-threatening situations, (e.g. aortic dissection) when other tests contraindicated (e.g. CT angiography in patient with renal failure)
  - intracardiac thrombi, tumours, valvular vegetations (infective endocarditis), aortic dissection, aortic atheromas, prosthetic valve function, shunt, technically inadequate transthoracic study
  - evaluation for left atrial/left atrial appendage thrombus in a patient with atrial fibrillation/atrial flutter to facilitate clinical decision making regarding electrical cardioversion or ablation
- **risks**
  - serious complications are extremely rare (<1 in 5,000)
  - esophageal perforation
  - gastrointestinal bleeding
  - pharyngeal hematoma

Stress Echocardiography (SE)
- **description**: echocardiography using either exercise (treadmill or bicycle) or pharmacologic agents (dobutamine) as the stress mechanism
- **indications**
  - useful alternative to other stress imaging modalities
  - when ECG cannot be interpreted appropriately
  - intermediate pre-test probability with normal/equivocal exercise ECG
  - post-ACS when used to decide on potential efficacy of revascularization
  - to evaluate the clinical significance of valvular heart disease
  - evaluation of myocardial viability, dyspnea of possible cardiac origin, mitral valve disease, aortic stenosis, mitral regurgitation, pulmonary hypertension, patients with hypertrophic cardiomyopathy (for LVOT obstruction)
  - dobutamine
    - pharmacologic stress for patients who are physically unable to exercise; same indications as exercise stress echo
    - low dose dobutamine stress echo can be used to assess myocardial viability and for assessing aortic stenosis with LV systolic dysfunction
- **contraindications**
  - contraindications to exercise testing
  - contraindications to dobutamine stress echocardiography: tachyarrhythmias and systemic hypertension
  - AAA has been considered as a relative contraindication to exercise testing or dobutamine stress echocardiography

Contrast Echocardiography with Agitated Saline Contrast
- **description**: improves resolution and provides real-time assessment of intracardiac blood flow
  - conventional agent is agitated saline (contains microbubbles of air)
  - allows visualization of right heart and intracardiac shunts, most commonly patent foramen ovale (PFO) and intrapulmonary shunt

Contrast Echocardiography with Transpulmonary Contrast Agents
- **description**: newer contrast agents are capable of crossing the pulmonary bed and achieving left heart opacification following intravenous injection; these contrast agents improve visualization of endocardial borders and enhance evaluation of LV ejection fraction and wall motion abnormalities (in patients with technically inadequate echocardiograms), and intracardiac mass
- **risks**
  - risk of non-fatal MI and death are rare
  - ultrasound contrast agents may cause back pain, headache, urticaria, and anaphylaxis

Stress Testing

EXERCISE TESTING

- **description:** cardiovascular stress test that uses treadmill or bicycle exercise with electrocardiographic and blood pressure monitoring
- **indications**
- patients with intermediate (10-90%) pretest probability of CAD based on age, gender, and symptoms
- ST depression <1 mm at rest, no left bundle branch block, no digoxin or estrogen use
- exercise test results stratify patients into risk groups
  1. low risk patients can be treated medically without invasive testing
  2. intermediate risk patients may need additional testing in the form of exercise imaging studies or cardiac catheterization
  3. high risk patients should be referred for cardiac catheterization
- **contraindications**
  - acute myocardial infarction (within two days)
  - unstable angina pectoris
  - uncontrolled arrhythmias causing symptoms of hemodynamic compromise
  - symptomatic severe valvular stenosis
  - uncontrolled symptomatic heart failure
  - active endocarditis or acute myocarditis or pericarditis
  - acute aortic dissection
  - acute pulmonary or systemic embolism
  - acute non-cardiac disorders that may affect exercise performance or may be aggravated by exercise
  - termination of exercise testing
    - patient's desire to stop
    - drop in systolic blood pressure of >10 mmHg from baseline despite an increase in workload, when accompanied by other evidence of ischemia
    - moderate to severe angina
    - ST elevation (>1 mm) in leads without diagnostic Q-waves (other than V1 or aVR)
    - increasing nervous system symptoms (e.g. ataxia, dizziness, or near syncope)
    - signs of poor perfusion (cyanosis or pallor)
    - technical difficulties in monitoring ECG or systolic blood pressure
    - sustained ventricular tachycardia
- **risks:** death, myocardial infarction, arrhythmia, hemodynamic instability, and orthopedic injury (<1-5/10,000 supervised tests)

NUCLEAR CARDIOLOGY

- **description**
  - myocardial perfusion imaging (MPI) with ECG-gated single photon emission computed tomography (SPECT), using radiolabelled tracer
  - evaluates myocardial viability, detects ischemia, and assesses perfusion and LV function simultaneously
  - predicts the likelihood of further cardiac event rates independent of the patient's history, examination, resting ECG, and stress ECG
  - often denoted as MIBI scan with reference to radiolabelled tracer (sestamibi)
  - stress with either treadmill or IV vasodilator stress (dipyridamole, adenosine, regadenoson)
  - images of the heart obtained during stress and at rest 3-4 h later
  - tracers
    - Thallium-201 (^{201}Tl, a K$^+$ analogue)
    - Technetium-99 (^{99}Tc)-labeled tracer (sestamibi/Cardiolite® or hexamibi/Myoview®)
- **indications**
  - exercise MPI
    - when ECG cannot be interpreted appropriately
    - intermediate pre-test probability with normal/equivocal exercise ECG
    - in patients with previous imaging whose symptoms have changed
    - to diagnose ischemia
  - dipyridamole/adenosine MPI
  - to diagnose CAD in possible ACS patients with non-diagnostic ECG and negative serum biomarkers
  - when ECG is cannot be interpreted appropriately due to LBBB or V-paced rhythm among patients unable to exercise, with the same indications as exercise MPI
- **contraindications**
  - contraindications to exercise testing
  - vasodilators (i.e. adenosine, regadenoson, and dipyridamole) are contraindicated in patients with hypotension, sick sinus syndrome, high-degree AV block (in the absence of backup pacemaker capability), and reactive airways disease
  - pregnancy
- **risks:** radiation exposure

STRESS ECHOCARDIOGRAPHY

- see *Echocardiography*, C12

Most Commonly Used Treadmill Stress Test Protocols
- The Bruce Protocol: 7 stage test with each stage lasting 3 min. With each successive stage, the treadmill increases in both speed (2.7 km/h to 9.6 km/h) and grade (10% with a 2% increase per stage up to 22%)
- The Modified Bruce, Modified Naughton Protocol: for older individuals or those with limited exercise capacity

Important Contraindications to Exercise Testing
- Acute MI, aortic dissection, pericarditis, myocarditis, PE
- Severe AS, arterial HTN
- Inability to exercise adequately

Important Prognostic Factor
Duke Treadmill Score (DTS)
Weighted Index Score
- Treadmill exercise time using standard Bruce protocol
- Maximum net ST segment deviation (depression or elevation)
- Exercise-induced angina provides diagnostic and prognostic information (such as 1 yr mortality)
DTS = exercise time – (5 x MaxST) – (4 x angina index)
Angina index: 0 (no angina), 1 (angina but not exercise-limiting), 2 (exercise-limiting angina)
DTS ≥5: 0.25% 1 yr mortality
DTS 4 to -10: 1.25% 1 yr mortality
DTS ≤ -11: 5.25% 1 yr mortality
Ann Intern Med 1987;106:793-800

Patients with normal imaging (nuclear perfusion or stress echo) studies at peak stress have a <1%/yr incidence of death or nonfatal MI and are thus often spared further invasive evaluation

Cardiac Catheterization and Angiography

Right Heart Catheterization (Swan-Ganz Catheter)
- **description:** also known as pulmonary artery catheterization
  - obtain direct measurements of central venous, right-sided intracardiac, pulmonary artery, and pulmonary artery occlusion pressures
  - can estimate cardiac output, systemic and pulmonary vascular resistance as well as mixed venous oxyhemoglobin saturation, oxygen delivery, and oxygen uptake
  - right atrial, right ventricular, and pulmonary artery pressures are recorded
  - can also be used to measure the Cardiac Index (CI)
    - CI = CO/body surface area
    - cardiac index is a measure of cardiac function
    - <1.8 L/min/m² usually means cardiogenic shock
    - 2.6-4.2 L/min/m² is considered normal
  - pulmonary capillary wedge pressure (PCWP)
    - obtained by advancing the catheter to wedge in the distal pulmonary artery
    - records pressure measured from the pulmonary venous system
    - in the absence of pulmonary venous disease reflects left atrial pressure
- **indications**
  - unexplained or unknown volume status in shock
  - severe cardiogenic shock (e.g. acute valvular disease, suspected pericardial tamponade)
  - suspected or known pulmonary artery hypertension
  - severe underlying cardiopulmonary disease (e.g. congenital heart disease, left-to-right shunt, severe valvular disease, pulmonary hypertension) and undergoing corrective or other surgery
- **contraindications**
  - lack of consent
  - infection at the insertion site
  - the presence of a right ventricular assist device
  - insertion during cardiopulmonary bypass
- **risks**
  - complications for diagnostic catheterization <1%
  - inadequate diagnostic procedures occur in <1% of cases
  - complications of insertion: atrial and/or ventricular arrhythmias (~3% of patients)
  - catheter misplacement or knotting (uncommon)
  - perforation of a cardiac chamber and rupture of a cardiac valve or the pulmonary artery (rare)
  - complications of catheterization: pulmonary artery rupture, pulmonary infarction, thromboembolic events, infection, and data misinterpretation
  - within 24 h of catheterization: death, MI, or stroke (0.2% to 0.3% of patients)

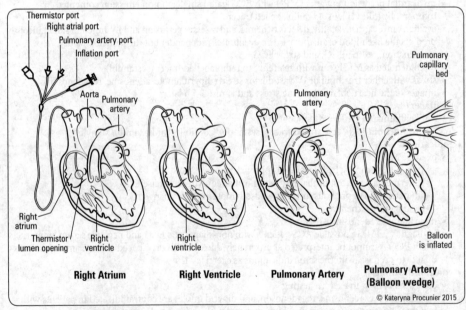

Figure 17. Swan-Ganz catheter placement

Left Heart Catheterization

- **description**
  - accomplished by introducing a catheter into the brachial or femoral artery and advancing it through the aorta, across the aortic valve, and into the left ventricle
  - evaluates mitral and aortic valvular defects and myocardial disease
  - systolic and end-diastolic pressure tracings recorded
  - LV size, wall motion and ejection fraction can be assessed by injecting contrast into the LV (left ventriculography) via femoral/radial artery catheterization
  - cardiac output (measured by the Fick oxygen method or the indicator dilution method)
- **indications**
  - identification of the extent and severity of CAD and evaluation of left ventricular function
  - assessment of the severity of valvular or myocardial disorders (e.g. aortic stenosis or insufficiency, mitral stenosis or insufficiency, and various cardiomyopathies) to determine the need for surgical correction
  - collection of data to confirm and complement noninvasive studies
  - determination of the presence of CAD in patients with confusing clinical presentations or chest pain of uncertain origin
- **contraindications**
  - severe uncontrolled hypertension
  - ventricular arrhythmias
  - acute stroke
  - severe anemia
  - active gastrointestinal bleeding
  - allergy to radiographic contrast
  - acute renal failure
  - uncompensated congestive failure (so that the patient cannot lie flat)
  - unexplained febrile illness or untreated active infection
  - electrolyte abnormalities (e.g. hypokalemia)
  - severe coagulopathy
- **risks**
  - complications for diagnostic catheterization <1%
  - inadequate diagnostic procedures occur in <1% of cases
  - within 24 h of catheterization: death, MI, or stroke (0.2% to 0.3% of patients)

Chambers	Pressure (systolic; mmHg)
Right atrium/central venous	1-8
Right ventricle	1-8 (15-30)
Pulmonary artery	4-12 (15-30)
Left atrium/ pulmonary capillary wedge	4-12
Left ventricle end diastolic	4-12

Coronary Angiography

- **description**
  - radiographic visualization of the coronary vessels after injection of radiopaque contrast media
  - coronary vasculature accessed via the coronary ostia
- **indications**
  - to define the coronary anatomy and the degree of luminal obstruction of the coronary arteries
  - to determine the presence and extent of obstructive CAD
  - to assess the feasibility and appropriateness of various forms of therapy, such as revascularization by percutaneous or surgical interventions
  - can also be used when the diagnosis of CAD is uncertain and CAD cannot be reasonably excluded by noninvasive techniques
- **contraindications:** severe renal failure (due to contrast agent toxicity – must check patient's renal status)
- **risks:** major complications <2%, but increased in patients with pre-existing renal failure (especially in diabetic patients)

ACC/AHA 2011 Recommended Indications for Coronary Angiography
- Disabling (CCS classes III and IV) chronic stable angina despite medical therapy
- High-risk criteria on clinical assessment or non-invasive testing
- Serious ventricular arrhythmia or CHF
- Uncertain diagnosis or prognosis after non-invasive testing
- Inability to undergo non-invasive testing

Coronary Angiography
Gold standard for localizing and quantifying CAD

Hemodynamically significant stenosis is defined as 70% or more narrowing of the luminal diameter

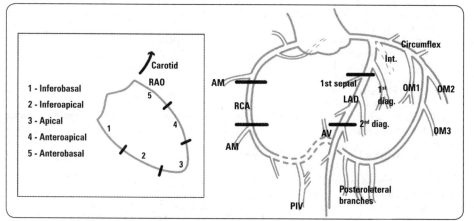

Figure 18. Coronary angiogram schematic
AM = acute marginal; LAD = left anterior descending; OM = obtuse marginal; RCA = right coronary artery

Diagnostic Catheterization
- complications for diagnostic catheterization <1%
- inadequate diagnostic procedures occur in fewer than 1% of cases
- provocative pharmacological agents can be used to unmask pathology
  - fluid loading may unmask latent pericardial constriction
  - afterload reduction or inotropic stimulation may be used to increase the outflow tract gradient in HCM
  - coronary vasoreactive agents (e.g. methylergonovine, acetylcholine)
  - a variety of pulmonary vasoreactive agents in primary pulmonary HTN (e.g. oxygen, calcium channel blockers, adenosine, nitric oxide, or prostacyclin)

Contrast-Enhanced CT Coronary Angiography

- **description:** fast ECG-synchronized multi-slice CT image acquisition in the heart to enable non-invasive imaging of the coronary arterial tree
- **indications:** often used to assess coronary artery and previous graft stenosis/viability that could not be seen during coronary angiography
- sensitivity = 85%, specificity = 90% for the diagnosis of obstructive coronary disease with >50% stenosis
- **contraindications:** allergy to contrast dye; severe renal dysfunction
- **risks:** radiation exposure

Magnetic Resonance Imaging

- **description:** offers high spatial resolution, eliminates the need for iodinated contrast, and does not involve exposure to ionizing radiation
- **indications:** valuable in assessment of congenital cardiac anomalies, abnormalities of the aorta, assessment of viable myocardium, and assessment of cardiomyopathies
- **contraindications:** metallic foreign bodies/implants
- **risks:** hazards posed by certain metallic devices inside patients

CARDIAC DISEASE

Arrhythmias

Mechanisms of Arrhythmias

Alterations in Impulse Formation

A. Abnormal Automaticity
- automaticity is a property of certain cardiomyocytes to spontaneously depolarize to their threshold voltage to generate action potentials in a rhythmic fashion
- under normal circumstances only cells in the specialized conduction system (SA node, AV node, and ventricular conduction system) exhibit natural automaticity. These cells are pacemaking cells. The automaticity of these cells can become abnormally increased or decreased
- in disease (e.g. post-MI ventricular ischemia) cells in the myocardium outside the conduction system may inappropriately acquire the property of automaticity and contribute to abnormal depolarization. If these ectopic generators depolarize at a rate greater than the SA node, they assume pacemaking control and become the source of abnormal rhythm
- automaticity can be influenced by:
  - neurohormonal tone (sympathetic and parasympathetic stimulation)
  - abnormal metabolic conditions (hypoxia, acidosis, hypothermia)
  - electrolyte abnormalities
  - drugs (e.g. digitalis)
  - local ischemia/infarction
  - other cardiac pathology
- this mechanism is responsible for the accelerated idioventricular rhythm and ventricular tachycardia that often occurs 24-72 h post MI

B. Triggered Activity due to Afterdepolarizations

1. Early Afterdepolarizations
- occur in the context of action potential prolongation
- consequence of the membrane potential becoming more positive during repolarization (e.g. not returning to baseline)
- result in self-maintaining depolarizing oscillations of action potential, generating a tachyarrhythmia (e.g. new baseline voltage is greater than threshold, which automatically triggers a new action potential after the refractory period ends)
- basis for the degeneration of QT prolongation, either congenital or acquired, into Torsades de Pointes

Sinus Arrhythmia (SA)
- Normal P waves, with variation of the P-P interval by >120 msec due to varying rate of SA node

Respiratory SA
- Seen more often in young adults (<30 yr old)
- Normal, results from changes in autonomic tone during respiratory cycle
- Rate increases with inspiration, slows with expiration

Non-Respiratory SA
- Seen more often in the elderly
- Can occur in the normal heart; if marked may be due to sinus node dysfunction (e.g. in heart disease, or after digitalis toxicity)
- Usually does not require treatment

2. Delayed Afterdepolarizations
- occur after the action potential has fully repolarized, but before the next usual action potential, thus called a delayed afterdepolarization
- commonly occurs in situations of high intracellular calcium (e.g. digitalis intoxication, ischemia) or during enhanced catecholamine stimulation (e.g. "twitchy" pacemaker cells)

Alterations in Impulse Conduction

A. Re-Entry Circuits
- the presence of self-sustaining re-entry circuit causes rapid repeated depolarizations in a region of myocardium (see Figure 26, C20, for an example in the context of AV nodal re-entrant tachycardia)
  - e.g. myocardium that is infarcted/ischemic will consist of non-excitable and partially excitable zones which will promote the formation of re-entry circuits

B. Conduction Block
- ischemia, fibrosis, trauma, and drugs can cause transient, permanent, unidirectional or bidirectional block
- most common cause of block is due to refractory myocardium (cardiomyocytes are in refractory period or zone of myocardium unexcitable due to fibrosis)
- if block occurs along the specialized conduction system distal zones of the conduction system can assume pacemaking control
- conduction block can lead to bradycardia or tachycardia when impaired conduction leads to re-entry phenomenon

C. Bypass Tracts
- normally the only conducting tract from the atria to the ventricles is the AV node into the His-Purkinje system
- congenital/acquired accessory conducting tracts bypass the AV node and facilitate premature ventricular activation before normal AV node conduction
- see *Pre-Excitation Syndromes*, C21

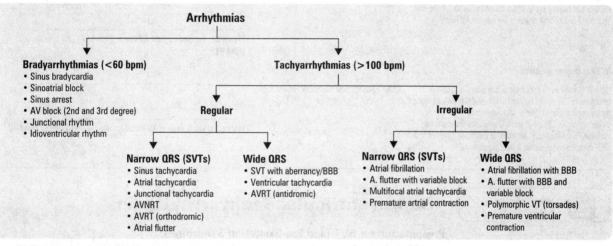

Figure 19. Clinical approach to arrhythmias

Bradyarrhythmias
• Examples

Bradyarrhythmias

1. SA NODAL DYSFUNCTION

A. Sinus Bradycardia

P axis normal (P waves positive in I and aVF)
Rate <60 bpm ; marked sinus bradycardia (<50 bpm)
May be seen in normal adults, particularly athletes, and in
elderly individuals
Increased vagal tone or vagal stimulation; drugs (β-blockers,
calcium channel blockers, etc.); ischemia/infarction

Atropine; pacing for sick sinus syndrome

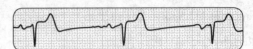
Figure 20. Sinus bradycardia

2. AV CONDUCTION BLOCKS

A. First Degree AV Block

Prolonged PR interval (>200 msec)
Frequently found among otherwise healthy adults

No treatment required

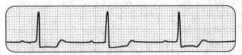
Figure 21. First degree AV block

B. Second Degree AV Block: Type I (Mobitz I)

A gradual prolongation of the PR interval precedes the failure
of conduction of a P wave (Wenckebach phenomenon)
AV block is usually in AV node (proximal) triggers (usually
reversible): increased vagal tone (e.g. following surgery),
RCA-mediated ischemia

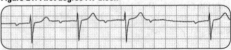
**Figure 22. Second degree AV block with Wenckebach phenomenon
(Mobitz I) (4:3 conduction) (lead V1)**

B. Second Degree AV Block: Type II (Mobitz II)

The PR interval is constant; there is an abrupt failure of
conduction of a P wave
AV block is usually distal to the AV node (i.e. bundle of His);
increased risk of high grade or 3rd degree AV block

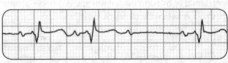
**Figure 23. Second degree AV block (Mobitz II) (3:2 conduction)
(lead V1)**

B. Third Degree AV Block

Complete failure of conduction of the supraventricular
impulses to the ventricles; ventricular depolarization initiated
by an escape pacemaker distal to the block
Wide or narrow QRS, P-P and R-R intervals are constant,
variable PR intervals; no relationship between P waves and
QRS complexes (P waves "marching through")

Management (see *Electrical Pacing*, C24)

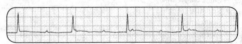
Figure 24. Third degree AV block (complete heart block) (lead II)

Tachyarrhythmias
• Examples

Supraventricular Tachyarrhythmias

Presentation for SVT (and Pre-Excitation Syndromes)
• presentation can include: palpitations, dizziness, dyspnea, chest discomfort, presyncope/syncope
• may precipitate CHF, hypotension, or ischemia in patients with underlying disease
• untreated tachycardias can cause cardiomyopathy (rare, potentially reversible with treatment of SVTs)
• includes supraventricular and ventricular rhythms

Supraventricular Tachyarrhythmias
• tachyarrhythmias that originate in the atria or AV junction
• this term is used when a more specific diagnosis of mechanism and site of origin cannot be made
• characterized by narrow QRS, unless there is pre-existing bundle branch block or aberrant ventricular
  conduction (abnormal conduction due to a change in cycle length)

1. Sinus Tachycardia
• sinus rhythm with rate >100 bpm
• occurs in normal subjects with increased sympathetic tone (e.g. exercise, emotions, pain), alcohol use,
  caffeinated beverages, drugs (e.g. β-adrenergic agonists, anticholinergic drugs, etc.)
• etiology: fever, hypotension, hypovolemia, anemia, thyrotoxicosis, CHF, MI, shock, PE, etc.
• treatment: treat underlying disease; consider β-blocker if symptomatic, calcium channel blocker if
  β-blockers contraindicated

2. Premature Beats
- premature atrial contraction
  - ectopic supraventricular beat originating in the atria
  - P wave morphology of the PAC usually differs from that of a normal sinus beat
- junctional premature beat
  - ectopic supraventricular beat that originates in the vicinity of the AV node
  - P wave is usually not seen or an inverted P wave is seen and may be before or closely follow the QRS complex (referred to as a retrograde, or "traveling backward" P wave)
- treatment usually not required

3. Atrial Flutter
- rapid, regular atrial depolarization from a macro re-entry circuit within the atrium (most commonly the right atrium)
- atrial rate 250-350 bpm, usually 300 bpm
- AV block usually occurs; it may be fixed (2:1, 3:1, 4:1, etc.) or variable
- etiology: CAD, thyrotoxicosis, mitral valve disease, cardiac surgery, COPD, PE, pericarditis
- ECG: sawtooth flutter waves (most common type of flutter) in inferior leads (II, III, aVF); narrow QRS (unless aberrancy); commonly see HR of 150
- in atrial flutter with 2:1 block, carotid sinus massage (first check for bruits), Valsalva maneuver, or adenosine may decrease AV conduction and bring out flutter waves
- treatment of acute atrial flutter
  - acute and if unstable (e.g. hypotension, CHF, angina): electrical cardioversion
  - if unstable (e.g. hypotension, CHF, angina): electrical cardioversion
  - if stable
    1. rate control: β-blocker, diltiazem, verapamil, or digoxin
    2. chemical cardioversion: sotalol, amiodarone, type I antiarrhythmics, or electrical cardioversion
  - anticoagulation guidelines same as for patients with AFib
- treatment of long-term atrial flutter: antiarrhythmics, catheter radiofrequency (RF) ablation (success rate dependent on site of origin of atrial flutter – i.e. whether right-sided isthmus-dependent or left-sided origin)

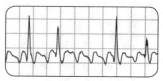

Figure 25. Atrial flutter with variable block

4. Multifocal Atrial Tachycardia (MAT)
- irregular rhythm caused by presence of 3 or more atrial foci (may mimic AFib)
- atrial rate 100-200 bpm – 3 or more distinct P wave morphologies and PR intervals vary, some P waves may not be conducted
- occurs more commonly in patients with COPD, and hypoxemia; less commonly in patients with hypokalemia, hypomagnesemia, sepsis, theophylline, or digitalis toxicity
- treatment: treat the underlying cause; calcium channel blockers may be used (e.g. diltiazem, verapamil), β-blockers may be contraindicated because of severe pulmonary disease
- no role for electrical cardioversion, antiarrhythmics, or ablation

5. Atrial Fibrillation
- see *CCS Atrial Fibrillation Guidelines 2014* for details (free mobile app – iCCS available on iOS and Android)
- most common sustained arrhythmia
- incidence increases with age (10% of population >80 yr old)
- symptoms: palpitations, fatigue, syncope, may precipitate or worsen heart failure
- classification
  - lone: occurs in persons younger than 60 yr and in whom no clinical or echocardiographic causes are found
  - nonvalvular: not caused by valvular disease, prosthetic heart valves, or valve repair
  - paroxysmal: episodes that terminate spontaneously
  - persistent: AFib sustained for more than 7 d or AFib that terminates only with cardioversion
  - permanent/chronic: continuous AFib that is unresponsive to cardioversion or in which clinical judgement has led to a decision not to pursue cardioversion
  - recurrent: two or more episodes of AFib
  - secondary: caused by a separate underlying condition or event (e.g. myocardial infarction, cardiac surgery, pulmonary disease, hyperthyroidism)
  - may be associated with thromboembolic events (stroke risk can be assessed by CHADS2 score in nonvalvular AFib; CHA2DS2-VASc if the former gives a score of 0 or 1)
- initiation
  - single circuit re-entry and/or ectopic foci act as aberrant generators producing atrial tachycardia (350-600 bpm)
  - impulses conduct irregularly across the atrial myocardium to give rise to fibrillation
  - in some cases, ectopic foci have also been mapped to the pulmonary vein ostia and can be ablated
- maintenance
  - the tachycardia causes atrial structural and electrophysiological remodelling changes that further promote AFib; the longer the patient is in AFib the more difficult it is to convert back to sinus rhythm
- consequences
  - the AV node irregularly filters incoming atrial impulses producing an irregular ventricular response of <200 bpm and the tachycardia leads to suboptimal cardiac output
  - fibrillatory conduction of the atria promotes blood stasis increasing the risk of thrombus formation – AFib is an important risk factor for stroke

Atrial Fibrillation – AFFIRM Trial
NEJM 2002;347:1825-1833
Study: Randomized, multicentre trial with mean follow-up of 3.5 yr.
Population: 4,060 patients (mean age 70 yr, 61% male, 89% white) with AF and a high risk of stroke or death.
Intervention: Rate control (β-blockers, calcium channel blockers, or digoxin alone or in combination) vs. rhythm control (antiarrhythmic drug chosen by the treating physician).
Primary Outcome: All cause mortality.
Results: There was no difference in mortality or disabling stroke, anoxic encephalopathy, major bleeding, and cardiac arrest between the two groups. There were more incidents of hospitalizations (80.1% vs. 73%, p<0.001) and adverse events (Torsades de Pointes (12 vs. 2, p=0.007), pulseless or bradycardic arrest (9 vs. 1, p=0.01), pulmonary event (108 vs. 24, p<0.001), gastrointestinal event (127 vs. 35, p<0.001), prolonged QT interval (31 vs. 4, p≤0.001), bradycardia (105 vs. 64, p=0.001) in the rhythm-control group.
Conclusion: Rate-control was as effective as rhythm-control in AF and was better tolerated. There were more hospitalization incidents in the rhythm-control group.

Lenient versus Strict Rate Control in Patients with Atrial Fibrillation
NEJM 362:1363-1373
Study: Randomized, multi-centre Netherlands prospective study, follow up for at least 2 yr
Population: 614 patients with permanent atrial fibrillation.
Intervention: Lenient control (resting HR <110 bpm) or strict control (resting HR <80 bpm)
Primary Outcomes: Death from cardiovascular causes, hospitalization for heart failure, and stroke, systemic embolism, bleeding, and life-threatening arrhythmic events.
Results: Goal of the study was to establish whether lenient control was equivalent to strict control for prevention of primary outcomes. Resulting hazard ratios were not significantly different between the treatment groups (P = 0.001). Frequencies of hospitalization and adverse effects were also similar. More patients were able to maintain lenient targets (97.7%) compared to strict targets (67%).
Conclusion: Lenient control was equivalent to strict control for prevention of primary outcomes in patients with atrial fibrillation. Furthermore, lenient control was more easily achieved.

Rivaroxaban for Stroke Prevention in AFib – ROCKET-AF Trial
NEJM 2011;365:883-891
Study: Prospective, non-inferiority, double blind, RCT, median follow-up of 1.9 yr.
Population: 14,264 patients with AFib (mean CHADS2=3.5). Patients either had previous thromboembolism or ≥3 risk factors.
Intervention: Patients were randomized to receiving rivaroxaban or warfarin.
Outcome: Composite of strokes and systemic thromboembolic event (STE).
Results: The hazard ratio of the primary outcome for rivaroxaban compared to warfarin was 0.88; 95% CI 0.74-1.03; p<0.001 for noninferiority; p=0.12 for superiority. Furthermore, the hazard ratio for major and non-major, but clinically relevant, bleeding was 1.03; 95% CI 0.96-1.11; p=0.44). There were also significant reductions in intracranial hemorrhage (0.5% vs. 0.7%, p=0.02) and fatal bleeding (0.2% vs. 0.5%, p=0.003) for rivaroxaban.
Conclusions: In patients with AFib, rivaroxaban is non-inferior to warfarin for stroke prevention and major and non-major bleeding.

Rivaroxaban for Stroke Prevention in AFib – ROCKET-AF Trial
NEJM 2011;365:883-891
Study: Prospective, non-inferiority, double blind, RCT, median follow-up of 1.9 yr.
Population: 14,264 patients with AFib (mean CHADS2=3.5). Patients either had previous thromboembolism or ≥3 risk factors.
Intervention: Patients were randomized to receiving rivaroxaban or warfarin.
Outcome: Composite of strokes and systemic thromboembolic event (STE).
Results: The hazard ratio of the primary outcome for rivaroxaban compared to warfarin was 0.88; 95% CI 0.74-1.03; p<0.001 for noninferiority; p=0.12 for superiority. Furthermore, the hazard ratio for major and non-major, but clinically relevant, bleeding was 1.03; 95% CI 0.96-1.11; p=0.44). There were also significant reductions in intracranial hemorrhage (0.5% vs. 0.7%, p=0.02) and fatal bleeding (0.2% vs. 0.5%, p=0.003) for rivaroxaban.
Conclusions: In patients with AFib, rivaroxaban is non-inferior to warfarin for stroke prevention and major and non-major bleeding.

Table 5. CHADS2 Risk Prediction for Non-Valvular AFib and Refer to AHA/ACC/HRS AFib Guidelines 2014 for more details

Risk Factor	Points	CHADS2 Score	Stroke Risk (%/Yr)
Congestive Heart Failure	1	0	1.9 (low)
Hypertension	1	1	2.8 (low-mod)
Age >75	1	2-3	4.0-5.9 (mod)
Diabetes	1	4-6	8.5-18.2 (high)
Stroke/TIA (prior)	2		

JAMA 2001;285:2864-70 and Can J Cardiol 2014 Oct;30(10):1114-30.

- **ECG findings**
  - no organized P waves due to rapid atrial activity (350-600 bpm) causing a chaotic fibrillatory baseline
  - irregularly irregular ventricular response (typically 100-180 bpm), narrow QRS (unless aberrancy or previous BBB)
  - wide QRS complexes due to aberrancy may occur following a long-short cycle sequence ("Ashman phenomenon")
  - loss of atrial contraction, thus no "a" wave seen in JVP, no S4 on auscultation

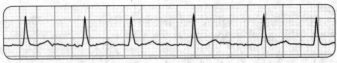

Figure 26. Atrial fibrillation (lead II)

- **management** (adapted from CCS Atrial Fibrillation Guidelines 2012 & 2014)
  - **major objectives (RACE):** all patients with AF (paroxysmal, persistent, or permanent), should be stratified using a predictive index for stroke risk and for the risk of bleeding, and most patients should receive either an oral anticoagulant or ASA (see below)
    1. **R**ate control: β-blockers, diltiazem, verapamil (in patients with heart failure: digoxin, amiodarone)
    2. **A**nticoagulation: use either warfarin or direct oral anticoagulant (DOACs) e.g. apixaban, dabigatran, rivaroxaban to prevent thromboembolism
       - for patients with non-valvular AF (NVAF): oral anticoagulant (OAC) is recommended for most patients aged > 65 years or CHADS2 >= 1. ASA 81 mg is recommended only for patients with none of the risk outlined in the CCS algorithm (age <65 and no CHADS2 risk factors) who have arterial disease (coronary, aortic, or peripheral). Novel oral anticoagulant (NOAC) is to be used in preference to warfarin
    3. **C**ardioversion (electrical)
       - if AFib <24-48 h, can usually cardiovert without anticoagulation
       - if AFib >24-48 h, anticoagulate for 3 wk prior and 4 wk after cardioversion due to risk of unstable intra-atrial thrombus
       - if patient unstable (hypotensive, active angina due to tachycardia, uncontrolled heart failure) should cardiovert immediately
    4. **E**tiology
       - HTN, CAD, valvular disease, pericarditis, cardiomyopathy, myocarditis, ASD, post-operative, PE, COPD, thyrotoxicosis, sick sinus syndrome, alcohol ("holiday heart")
       - may present in young patients without demonstrable disease ("lone AFib") and in the elderly without underlying heart disease
  - studies of patients with AFib suggest that there is no difference in long-term survival when treating patients with a rhythm-control versus rate-control strategy
  - however, many patients with a significant underlying structural heart lesion (e.g. valve disease, cardiomyopathy) will not tolerate AFib well (since may be dependent on atrial kick) and these patients should be cardioverted (chemical or electrical) as soon as possible
  - **newly discovered AFib**
    - anticoagulants may be beneficial if high risk for stroke
    - if the episode is self-limited and not associated with severe symptoms, no need for antiarrhythmic drugs
    - if AFib persists, 2 options
      1. rate control and anticoagulation (as indicated above)
      2. cardioversion (as above)
  - recurrent or permanent AFib
    - if episodes are brief or minimally symptomatic, antiarrhythmic drugs may be avoided; rate control and anticoagulation are appropriate
    - patients who have undergone at least one attempt to restore sinus rhythm may remain in AFib after recurrence; permanent AFib may be accepted (with rate control and antithrombotics as indicated by CHADS2 score) in certain clinical situations
    - if symptoms are bothersome or episodes are prolonged, antiarrhythmic drugs should be used
      - no or minimal heart disease: flecainide, propafenone, or sotalol
      - LV dysfunction: amiodarone
      - CAD: β-blockers, amiodarone

6. AV NODAL RE-ENTRANT TACHYCARDIA (AVNRT)
- re-entrant circuit using dual pathways (fast conducting β-fibres and slow conducting α-fibres) within or near the AV node; often found in the absence of structural heart disease – cause is commonly idiopathic, although familial AVNRT has been reported
- sudden onset and offset
- fast regular rhythm: rate 150-250 bpm
- usually initiated by a supraventricular or ventricular premature beat
- AVNRT accounts for 60-70% of all paroxysmal SVTs
- retrograde P waves may be seen but are usually lost in the QRS complex (see Figure 27)
- treatment
  - acute: Valsalva maneuver or carotid sinus pressure technique, adenosine is first choice if unresponsive to vagal maneuvers; if no response, try metoprolol, digoxin, diltiazem, electrical cardioversion if patient hemodynamically unstable (hypotension, angina, or CHF)
  - long-term: 1st line – β-blocker, diltiazem, digoxin; 2nd line – flecainide, propafenone; 3rd line – catheter ablation

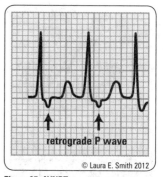

Figure 27. AVNRT

N.B. Refer to ECG Made Simple for further discussion and an animation of the mechanism (www.ecgmadesimple.com)

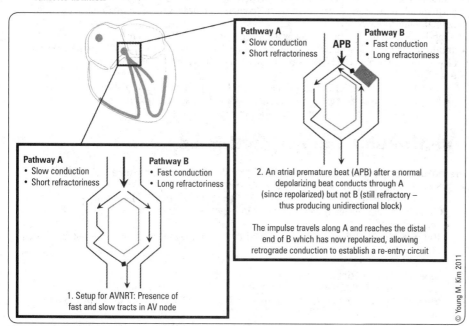

Pathway A
- Slow conduction
- Short refractoriness

Pathway B
- Fast conduction
- Long refractoriness

APB

2. An atrial premature beat (APB) after a normal depolarizing beat conducts through A (since repolarized) but not B (still refractory – thus producing unidirectional block)

The impulse travels along A and reaches the distal end of B which has now repolarized, allowing retrograde conduction to establish a re-entry circuit

Pathway A
- Slow conduction
- Short refractoriness

Pathway B
- Fast conduction
- Long refractoriness

1. Setup for AVNRT: Presence of fast and slow tracts in AV node

© Young M. Kim 2011

Figure 28. Mechanism for AVNRT

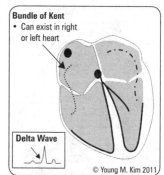

Bundle of Kent
- Can exist in right or left heart

Delta Wave

© Young M. Kim 2011

Figure 29. Accessory pathway conduction in WPW. Early ventricular activation leads to the appearance of a delta wave (slurred upstroke of the QRS) on the ECG before usual conduction across the AV node

Pre-Excitation Syndromes

- refers to a subset of SVTs mediated by an accessory pathway which can lead to ventricular pre-excitation

Wolff-Parkinson-White Syndrome
- congenital defect present in 1.5-2/1,000 of the general population
- an accessory conduction tract (Bundle of Kent; can be in right or left atrium) abnormally allows early electrical activation of part of one ventricle
- impulses travel at a greater conduction velocity across the Bundle of Kent thereby effectively 'bypassing' AV node
- since the ventricles are activated earlier, the ECG shows early ventricular depolarization in the form of initial slurring of the QRS complex – the so-called "delta wave"
- atrial impulses that conduct to the ventricles through both the Bundle of Kent and the normal AV node/His-Purkinje system generate a broad "fusion complex"
- ECG features of WPW
  - PR interval <120 msec
  - delta wave: slurred upstroke of the QRS (the leads with the delta wave vary with site of bypass)
  - widening of the QRS complex due to premature activation
  - secondary ST segment and T wave changes
  - tachyarrhythmias may occur – most often AVRT and AFib

Arrhythmias

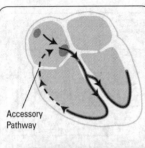

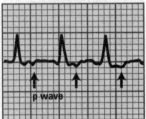

Accessory Pathway

Orthodromic AVRT

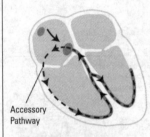

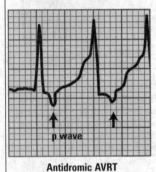

Accessory Pathway

p wave

Antidromic AVRT

© Laura E. Smith 2012

Figure 30. Orthodromic vs. antidromic AVRT

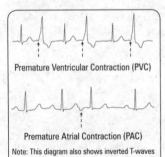

Premature Ventricular Contraction (PVC)

Premature Atrial Contraction (PAC)

Note: This diagram also shows inverted T-waves

© Caitlin LaFlamme 2009

Figure 31. PVC (with bigeminy pattern) and PAC. Note the difference between the normal QRS/T wave and the PVC-generated QRS/T wave

AFib in WPW Patients
- AFib is the index arrhythmia in up to 20% of patients with WPW syndrome
  - it is usually intermittent rather than persistent or permanent
- rapid atrial depolarizations in AFib are conducted through the bypass tract which is not able to filter impulses like the AV node can
- consequently the ventricular rate becomes extremely rapid (>200 bpm) and the QRS complex widens
- treatment: electrical cardioversion, IV procainamide, or IV amiodarone
  - do not use drugs that slow AV node conduction (digoxin, β-blockers) as this may cause preferential conduction through the bypass tract and precipitate VF
  - long-term: ablation of bypass tract if possible

AV Re-Entrant Tachycardia
- re-entrant loop via accessory pathway and normal conduction system
- initiated by a premature atrial or ventricular complex
- **orthodromic AVRT:** stimulus from a premature complex travels up the bypass tract (V to A) and down the AV node (A to V) with narrow QRS complex (no delta wave because stimulus travels through normal conduction system)
- comprises 95% of the reentrant tachycardias associated with WPW syndrome
- **antidromic AVRT:** more rarely the stimulus goes up the AV node (V to A) and down the bypass tract (A to V); wide and abnormal QRS as ventricular activation is only via the bypass tract
- treatment
  - acute: similar to AVNRT except avoid long-acting AV nodal blockers (e.g. digoxin and verapamil)
  - long-term: for recurrent arrhythmias ablation of the bypass tract is recommended
  - drugs such as flecainide and procainamide can be used

Ventricular Tachyarrhythmias

Premature Ventricular Contraction (PVC) or Ventricular Premature Beat (VPB)
- QRS width >120 msec, no preceding P wave, bizarre QRS morphology
- origin: LBBB morphology of VT = RV origin; RBBB morphology of VT = LV origin
- PVCs may be benign but are usually significant in the following situations
  - consecutive (≥3 = VT) or multiform (varied origin)
  - PVC falling on the T wave of the previous beat ("R on T phenomenon"): may precipitate ventricular tachycardia or VF

Accelerated Idioventricular Rhythm
- ectopic ventricular rhythm with rate 50-100 bpm
- more frequently occurs in the presence of sinus bradycardia and is easily overdriven by a faster supraventricular rhythm
- frequently occurs in patients with acute MI or other types of heart disease (cardiomyopathy, hypertensive, valvular) but it does not affect prognosis and does not usually require treatment

Ventricular Tachycardia (VT)
- 3 or more consecutive ectopic ventricular complexes
  - rate >100 bpm (usually 140-200)
  - ventricular flutter: if rate >200 bpm and complexes resemble a sinusoidal pattern
  - "sustained VT" if it lasts longer than 30 s
  - ECG characteristics: wide regular QRS tachycardia (QRS usually >140 msec)
  - AV dissociation; bizarre QRS pattern
  - also favour Dx of VT: left axis or right axis deviation, nonspecific intraventricular block pattern, monophasic or biphasic QRS in V1 with RBBB, QRS concordance in V1-V6
  - occasionally during VT supraventricular impulses may be conducted to the ventricles generating QRS complexes with normal or aberrant supraventricular morphology ("ventricular capture") or summation pattern ("fusion complexes")
- **monomorphic VT**
  - identical complexes with uniform morphology
  - more common than polymorphic VT
  - typically result from intraventricular re-entry circuit
  - potential causes: chronic infarct scarring, acute MI/ischemia, cardiomyopathies, myocarditis, arrhythmogenic right ventricular dysplasia, idiopathic, drugs (e.g. cocaine), electrolyte disturbances
- **polymorphic VT**
  - complexes with constantly changing morphology, amplitude, and polarity
  - more frequently associated with hemodynamic instability due to faster rates (typically 200-250 bpm) vs. monomorphic VT
  - potential causes: acute MI, severe or silent ischemia, and predisposing factors for QT prolongation
- treatment
  - sustained VT (>30 s) is an emergency, requiring immediate treatment
  - hemodynamic compromise: electrical cardioversion
  - no hemodynamic compromise: electrical cardioversion, lidocaine, amiodarone, type Ia agents (procainamide, quinidine)

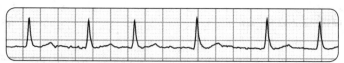

Figure 32. Ventricular tachycardia (monomorphic)

Table 6. Wide Complex Tachycardia: Clues for Differentiating VT vs. SVT with Aberrancy*

Clinical Clues		ECG Clues	
Presenting symptoms	Not helpful	AV dissociation	VT
History of CAD and previous MI	VT	Capture or fusion beats	VT
Physical exam		QRS width >140 msec	VT
Cannon "a" waves Variable S1	VT	Extreme axis deviation (left or right superior axis)	VT
Carotid sinus massage/adenosine terminates arrhythmia	SVT**	Positive QRS concordance (R wave across chest leads)	VT
		Negative QRS concordance (S wave across chest leads)	May suggest VT
		Axis shift during arrhythmia	VT (polymorphic)

*If patient >65 yr and previous MI or structural heart disease, then chance of VT >95%
**May terminate VT in some patients with no structural heart disease

Torsades de Pointes
- a variant of polymorphic VT that occurs in patients with baseline QT prolongation – "twisting of the points"
- looks like usual VT except that QRS complexes "rotate around the baseline" changing their axis and amplitude
- ventricular rate >100 bpm, usually 150-300 bpm
- etiology: predisposition in patients with prolonged QT intervals
  - congenital long QT syndromes
  - drugs: e.g. class IA (quinidine), class III (sotalol), phenothiazines (TCAs), erythromycin, quinolones, antihistamines
  - electrolyte disturbances: hypokalemia, hypomagnesemia
  - nutritional deficiencies causing above electrolyte abnormalities
- treatment: IV magnesium, temporary pacing, isoproterenol and correct underlying cause of prolonged QT, electrical cardioversion if hemodynamic compromise

Arrhythmias that May Present as a Wide QRS Tachycardia
- VT
- SVT with aberrant conduction (rate related)
- SVT with preexisting BBB or nonspecific intraventricular conduction defect
- AV conduction through a bypass tract in WPW patients during an atrial tachyarrhythmia (e.g. atrial flutter, atrial tachycardia)
- Antidromic AVRT in WPW patients (see *Pre-Excitation Syndromes*, C21)

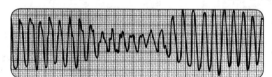

Figure 33. Torsades de pointes

Ventricular Fibrillation (VFib)
- chaotic ventricular arrhythmia, with very rapid irregular ventricular fibrillatory waves of varying morphology
- terminal event, unless advanced cardiac life-support (ACLS) procedures are promptly initiated to maintain ventilation and cardiac output, and electrical defibrillation is carried out
- most frequent cause of sudden death
- refer to ACLS algorithm for complete therapeutic guidelines

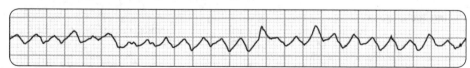

Figure 34. Ventricular fibrillation

Sudden Cardiac Arrest

Definition
- unanticipated, non-traumatic cardiac death in a stable patient which occurs within 1 h of symptom onset; VFib is most common cause

Etiology
- primary cardiac pathology
  - ischemia/MI
  - LV dysfunction
  - severe ventricular hypertrophy
  - HCM
  - AS
  - congenital heart disease e.g. arrhythmogenic right ventricular dysplasia
  - mutations in cardiac ion channels e.g. long QT syndrome, Brugada syndrome

Management
- acute: resuscitate with prompt CPR and defibrillation
- investigate underlying cause (cardiac catheterization, electrophysiologic studies, echo)
- treat underlying cause
- antiarrhythmic drug therapy: amiodarone, β-blockers
- implantable cardioverter defibrillator (ICD)
- refer to ACLS guidelines (see Anesthesia and Perioperative Medicine, A31)

Electrophysiology Studies

- invasive test for the investigation and treatment of cardiac rhythm disorders using intracardiac catheters
- provide detailed analysis of the arrhythmia mechanism and precise site of origin when ECG data are nondiagnostic or unobtainable
- bradyarrhythmias: define the mechanisms of SA node dysfunction and localize site of AV conduction block
- tachyarrhythmias: map for possible ablation or to assess inducibility of VT

Electrical Pacing

- the decision to implant a pacemaker usually is based on symptoms of a bradyarrhythmia or tachyarrhythmia in the setting of heart disease

Pacemaker Indications
- SA node dysfunction (most common): symptomatic bradycardia ± hemodynamic instability
- common manifestations include: syncope, presyncope, or severe fatigue
- SA node dysfunction is commonly caused by: intrinsic disease within the SA node (e.g. idiopathic degeneration, fibrosis, ischemia, or surgical trauma), abnormalities in autonomic nervous system function, and drug effects
- AV nodal-infranodal block: Mobitz II, complete heart block

Pacemaker Complications
- complications related to surgical implantation include venous access (pneumothorax, hemothorax, air embolism), pacemaker leads (perforation, malposition), pocket hematomas and infection
- complications specific to the pacemaker include a failure to pace, failure to sense, pulse generator failure, pacemaker syndrome and pacemaker mediated tachycardia

Pacing Techniques
- temporary: transvenous (jugular, subclavian, femoral) or external (transcutaneous) pacing
- permanent: transvenous into RA, apex of RV, or both
- can sense and pace atrium, ventricle, or both
- new generation: rate responsive, able to respond to physiologic demand
- biventricular

Implantable Cardioverter Defibrillators

- sudden cardiac death (SCD) usually results from ventricular fibrillation (VFib), sometimes preceded by monomorphic or polymorphic ventricular tachycardia (VT)
- ICDs detect ventricular tachyarrhythmias and are highly effective in terminating VT/VFib and in aborting SCD
- mortality benefit vs. antiarrhythmics in secondary prevention
- benefit seen in patients with ischemic and non-ischemic cardiomyopathy, depressed left ventricular ejection fraction (LVEF), prolonged QRS
- see Heart Failure, C34 for current treatment recommendations

CCS Consensus Conference 2003: Assessment of the Cardiac Patient for Fitness to Drive and Fly – Executive Summary
Can J Cardiol 2004;20:1313-1323
In both primary and secondary prevention ICD patients with private driving licenses, no restrictions to drive directly following implantation or an inappropriate shock are warranted. However, following an appropriate shock these patients are at an increased risk to cause harm to other road users and therefore should be restricted to drive for a period of 2 and 4 mo, respectively. In addition, all ICD patients with commercial driving licenses have a substantial elevated risk to cause harm to other road users during the complete follow-up after both implantation and shock and should therefore be restricted to drive permanently.
(A complete set of easy to access CCS Drive and Fly guidelines is available in the iCCS App available for iOS and Android platforms)

Systematic Review: Implantable Cardioverter Defibrillators for Adults with Left Ventricular Systolic Dysfunction
Ann Intern Med 2007;147:251-262
Study: Meta-review of 12 RCTs used for ICD efficacy, 5 RCTs and 48 observational studies for effectiveness, and 21 RCTs and 43 observational studies for safety review.
Population: 8,516 patients for ICD efficacy, 26,840 patients for effectiveness, and 86,809 patients for safety review with left ventricular ejection fraction ≤0.35.
Intervention: ICD implantation.
Outcomes: All-cause mortality and adverse events.
Results: ICDs reduced all-cause mortality by 20% (95% CI, 10%-29%; I2=44.4%) with greatest reduction (54%) in sudden cardiac death (CI 37%-63%; I2=0%). Observational studies had a reduced relative risk of 0.54 for all-cause mortality versus RCTs (CI 0.43-0.58, I2=60.4%). Rates of success of ICD implantation were 99% (CI 98.8%-99.3%) with a 1.2% (CI 0.9%-1.5%) chance of peri-implantation death. Post-implantation complications (per 100 patient yr) were: 1.4 (CI 1.2-1.6) device malfunctions; 1.5 (CI 1.3-1.8) lead problems; 0.6 (CI 0.5-0.8) implant site infection and 19.1 (CI 16.5-22.0) inappropriate discharges in RCTs versus a rate of 4.9 (CI 4.5-5.3) inappropriate discharges in observational studies.
Conclusion: ICDs are safe and effective in reducing mortality in adult patients with LV systolic dysfunction but carry significant risks of inappropriate discharges. Differences between RCTs and observational studies show that improved risk stratification of patients may further improve outcomes and reduce adverse events.

Catheter Ablation

Techniques
- radiofrequency (RF) ablation: a low-voltage high-frequency form of electrical energy (similar to cautery); RF ablation produces small, homogeneous, necrotic lesions approximately 5-7 mm in diameter and 3-5 mm in depth
- cryoablation: new technology which uses a probe with a tip that can decrease in temperature to -20°C and -70°C. Produces small, necrotic lesions similar to RF ablation; when brought to -20°C, the catheter tip reversibly freezes the area; bringing the tip down to -70°C for 5 min permanently scars the tissue
  - advantage: can "test" areas before committing to an ablation
  - disadvantage: takes much longer than RF (5 min per cryoablation vs. 1 min per RF ablation)

Indications
- paroxysmal SVT
  - AVNRT: accounts for more than half of all cases
- accessory pathway (orthodromic reciprocating tachycardia): 30% of SVT
  - re-entrant rhythm, with an accessory AV connection as the retrograde limb
  - corrected by targeting the accessory pathway
- atrial flutter: reentry pathway in right atrium
- AFib: potential role for pulmonary vein ablation
- ventricular tachycardia: focus arises from the right ventricular outflow tract and less commonly originates in the inferoseptal left ventricle near the apex (note: majority of cases of VT are due to scarring from previous MI and cannot be ablated)

Major Complications
- 1% of patients
- death: 0.1-0.2%
- cardiac: high grade AV block requiring permanent pacemaker (less risk with cryoablation), tamponade, pericarditis
- vascular: hematoma, vascular injury, thromboembolism, TIA/stroke
- pulmonary: PE

Ischemic Heart Disease

Epidemiology
- most common cause of cardiovascular morbidity and mortality
- Canadian-led INTERHEART study showed that 9 modifiable risk factors accounted for >90% of MI
- atherosclerosis and thrombosis are the most important pathogenetic mechanisms
- M:F = 2:1 with all age groups included (Framingham study), 8:1 for age <40, 1:1 for age >70
  - according to the Framingham Heart Study, men develop coronary heart disease at a rate double that of women for age <60; incidence in women triples shortly after menopause
- peak incidence of symptomatic IHD is age 50-60 (men) and 60-70 (women)
- for primary prevention of ischemic heart disease see Family Medicine, FM7

Table 7. Risk Factors and Markers for Atherosclerotic Heart Disease

Non-Modifiable Risk Factors	Modifiable Risk Factors	Markers of Disease
Age	Hyperlipidemia*	Elevated lipoprotein(a)
Male, postmenopausal female	HTN*	Hyperhomocysteinemia
Family history (FHx) of MI*	DM*	Elevated high-sensitivity C-reactive
First degree male relative <55	Cigarette smoking*	protein (hsCRP)
First degree female relative <65	Psychosocial stress	Coronary artery calcification
	Obesity	Carotid IMT/plaque
	Sedentary lifestyle	Ankle-brachial index
	Heavy alcohol intake	

* Major risk factor

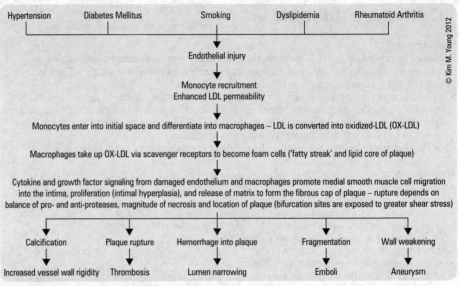

Figure 35. Pathophysiology of atherosclerosis

Chronic Stable Angina

Definition
- symptom complex resulting from an imbalance between oxygen supply and demand in the myocardium

Etiology and Pathophysiology
- factors that decrease myocardial oxygen supply
  - decreased luminal diameter: atherosclerosis, vasospasm
  - decreased duration of diastole: tachycardia (decreased duration of diastolic coronary perfusion)
  - decreased hemoglobin: anemia
  - decreased SaO_2: hypoxemia
  - congenital anomalies
- factors that increase myocardial oxygen demand
  - increased heart rate: hyperthyroidism
  - increased contractility: hyperthyroidism
  - increased wall stress: myocardial hypertrophy, aortic stenosis

Signs and Symptoms
- typical: (1) retrosternal chest pain, tightness or discomfort radiating to left (± right) shoulder/arm/neck/jaw, associated with diaphoresis, nausea, anxiety; (2) predictably precipitated by the "3 Es": exertion, emotion, eating; (3) brief duration, lasting <10-15 min and typically relieved by rest and nitrates
- atypical/probable angina (meets 2 of the above); non-cardiac chest pain (meets <1 of the above)
- Levine's sign: clutching fist over sternum when describing chest pain
- anginal equivalents: dyspnea, acute LV failure, flash pulmonary edema

Clinical Assessment
- history including directed risk factor assessment and physical exam
- labs: Hb, fasting glucose, fasting lipid profile
- ECG (at rest and during episode of chest pain if possible)
- CXR (suspected heart failure, valvular disease, pericardial disease, aortic dissection/aneurysm, or signs or symptoms of pulmonary disease)
- stress testing (see *Stress Testing*, C13) or angiography
- echo
- to assess systolic murmur suggestive of aortic stenosis, mitral regurgitation, and/or HCM
- to assess LV function in patients with Hx of prior MI, pathological Q waves, signs or symptoms of CHF

Differential Diagnosis
- see *Differential Diagnosis of Common Presentations*, C4

Chronic stable angina is most often due to a fixed stenosis caused by an atheroma
Acute coronary syndromes are the result of plaque rupture

Canadian Cardiovascular Society (CCS) Functional Classification of Angina
- **Class I:** ordinary physical activity (walking, climbing stairs) does not cause angina; angina with strenuous, rapid, or prolonged activity
- **Class II:** slight limitation of ordinary activity: angina brought on at >2 blocks on level or climbing >1 flight of stairs or by emotional stress
- **Class III:** marked limitation of ordinary activity: angina brought on at <2 blocks on level or climbing <1 flight of stairs
- **Class IV:** inability to carry out any physical activity without discomfort; angina may be present at rest

Treatment of Chronic Stable Angina

1. General Measures
- goals: to reduce myocardial oxygen demand and/or increase oxygen supply
- lifestyle modification (diet, exercise)
- treatment of risk factors: statins (see Endocrinology, E5, Family Medicine, FM9 for target lipid guidelines), antihypertensives, etc
- pharmacological therapy to stabilize the coronary plaque to prevent rupture and thrombosis

2. Antiplatelet Therapy (first-line therapy)
- ASA
- clopidogrel when ASA absolutely contraindicated

3. β-blockers (first-line therapy – improve survival in patients with hypertension)
- increase coronary perfusion and decrease demand (HR, contractility) and BP (afterload)
- cardioselective agents preferred (e.g. metoprolol, atenolol) to avoid peripheral effects (inhibition of vasodilation and bronchodilation via β2 receptors)
- avoid intrinsic sympathomimetics (e.g. acebutolol) which increase demand

4. Nitrates (symptomatic control, no clear impact on survival)
- decrease preload (venous dilatation) and afterload (arteriolar dilatation), and increase coronary perfusion
- maintain daily nitrate-free intervals to prevent tolerance (tachyphylaxis)

5. Calcium Channel Blockers (CCBs, second-line or combination)
- increase coronary perfusion and decrease demand (HR, contractility) and BP (afterload)
- caution: verapamil/diltiazem combined with β-blockers may cause symptomatic sinus bradycardia or AV block

6. ACE Inhibitors (ACEI, not used to treat symptomatic angina)
- angina patients tend to have risk factors for CV disease which warrant use of an ACEI (e.g. HTN, DM, proteinuric renal disease, previous MI with LV dysfunction)
- benefit in all patients at high risk for CV disease (concomitant DM, renal dysfunction, or
- LV systolic dysfunction)
- angiotensin II receptor blockers (ARBs) can be used when ACEI contraindicated

7. Invasive Strategies
- revascularization (see *Coronary Revascularization*, C31 and COURAGE trial sidebar)

Optimal Medical Therapy with or without PCI for Stable Coronary Disease. COURAGE Trial
NEJM 2007;356:1503-1516
Study: Randomized, controlled trial with median follow-up of 4.6 yr.
Population: 2,287 patients who had objective evidence of myocardial ischemia and significant stable coronary artery disease.
Intervention: Patients were randomized to receive intensive pharmacologic therapy and lifestyle intervention with or without percutaneous coronary intervention (PCI).
Outcome: Primary outcome was all-cause mortality and nonfatal myocardial infarction (MI). Secondary outcome had additional events of stroke, all MI, and hospitalization for unstable angina with negative biomarkers.
Results: There was no significant difference in primary (unadjusted hazard ratio: 1.05; p=0.62) or secondary outcomes (hazard ratio: 1.05; p=0.62) between the PCI and non-PCI intervention groups. The PCI group had significantly lower rates of subsequent revascularization at 4.6 yr of follow-up (hazard ratio 0.60, p<0.001) and was more angina-free in the first 4 yr of follow-up.
Conclusions: PCI as an adjunct in initial management in patients with significant stable coronary artery disease does not reduce mortality, MI, stroke, or hospitalization for ACS, but does provide angina relief and reduced risk of revascularization.

VARIANT ANGINA (PRINZMETAL'S ANGINA)
- myocardial ischemia secondary to coronary artery vasospasm, with or without atherosclerosis
- uncommonly associated with infarction or LV dysfunction
- typically occurs between midnight and 8 am, unrelated to exercise, relieved by nitrates
- typically ST elevation on ECG
- diagnosed by provocative testing with ergot vasoconstrictors (rarely done)
- treat with nitrates and CCBs

SYNDROME X
- typical symptoms of angina but normal angiogram
- may show definite signs of ischemia with exercise testing
- thought to be due to inadequate vasodilator reserve of coronary resistance vessels
- better prognosis than overt epicardial atherosclerosis

Acute Coronary Syndromes

Definition
- ACS includes the spectrum of UA, NSTEMI, and STEMI; this distinction aids in providing the appropriate therapeutic intervention
  - MI is defined by evidence of myocardial necrosis. It is diagnosed by a rise/fall of serum markers plus any one of
  - symptoms of ischemia (chest/upper extremity/mandibular/epigastric discomfort; dyspnea)
  - ECG changes (ST-T changes, new BBB or pathological Q waves)
  - imaging evidence (myocardial loss of viability, wall motion abnormality, or intracoronary thrombus)
  - if biomarker changes are unattainable, cardiac symptoms combined with new ECG changes is sufficient
  - NSTEMI meets criteria for myocardial infarction without ST elevation or BBB
  - STEMI meets criteria for myocardial infarction characterized by ST elevation or new BBB

- **UA** is clinically defined by any of the following
  - accelerating pattern of pain: increased frequency, increased duration, decreased threshold of exertion, decreased response to treatment
  - angina at rest
  - new-onset angina
  - angina post-MI or post-procedure (e.g. percutaneous coronary intervention [PCI], coronary artery bypass grafting [CABG])

Investigations

- history and physical
  - note that up to 30% of MIs are unrecognized or "silent" due to atypical symptoms – more common in women, DM, elderly, post-heart transplant (because of denervation)
- ECG
- CXR
- labs
  - serum cardiac biomarkers for myocardial damage (repeat 8 h later) (see *Cardiac Biomarkers*, C11)
  - CBC, INR/PTT, electrolytes and magnesium, creatinine, urea, glucose, serum lipids
  - draw serum lipids within 24-48 h because values are unreliable from 2-48 d post-MI

MANAGEMENT OF ACUTE CORONARY SYNDROMES

1. General Measures
  - ABCs: assess and correct hemodynamic status first
  - bed rest, cardiac monitoring, oxygen
  - nitroglycerin SL followed by IV
  - morphine IV

2. Anti-Platelet and Anticoagulation Therapy
  - see also *CCS Antiplatelet Guidelines 2012* for details (free mobile apps available on iOS and Android platforms in the CCS app stores)
  - ASA chewed
  - NSTEMI
    - ticagrelor in addition to ASA or if ASA contraindicated, subcutaneous low molecular weight heparin or IV unfractionated heparin (UFH) (LMWH preferable, except in renal failure or if CABG is planned within 24 h)
    - clopidogrel used if patient ineligible for ticagrelor
  - if PCI is planned: ticagrelor or prasugrel and consider IV GP IIb/IIIa inhibitor (e.g. abciximab)
    - clopidogrel used if patient ineligible for ticagrelor and prasugrel
    - prasugel contraindicated in those with a history of stroke/TIA, and avoidance of or lower dose is recommended for those >75 yr old or weighing under 60 kg (TRITON-TIMI 38)
  - anticoagulation options depend on reperfusion strategy:
    - primary PCI: UFH during procedure; bivalirudin is a possible alternative
    - thrombolysis: LMWH (enoxaparin) until discharge from hospital; can use UFH as alternative because of possible rescue PCI
    - no reperfusion: LMWH (enoxaparin) until discharge from hospital
  - continue LMWH or UFH followed by oral anticoagulation at discharge if at high risk for thromboembolic event (large anterior MI, AFib, severe LV dysfunction, CHF, previous DVT or PE, or echo evidence of mural thrombus)

3. β-blockers
  - STEMI: contraindications include signs of heart failure, low output states, risk of cardiogenic shock, heart block, asthma or airway disease; initiate orally within 24 h of diagnosis when indicated
  - if β-blockers are contraindicated or if β-blockers/nitrates fail to relieve ischemia, non-dihydropyridine calcium channel blockers (e.g. diltiazem, verapamil) may be used as second-line therapy in the absence of severe LV dysfunction or pulmonary vascular congestion (calcium channel blockers do not prevent MI or decrease mortality)

4. Invasive Strategies and Reperfusion Options
  - UA/NSTEMI: early coronary angiography ± revascularization if possible is recommended with any of the following high-risk indicators:
    - recurrent angina/ischemia at rest despite intensive anti-ischemic therapy
    - CHF or LV dysfunction
    - hemodynamic instability
    - high (≥3) TIMI risk score (tool used to estimate mortality following an ACS)
    - sustained ventricular tachycardia
    - dynamic ECG changes
    - high-risk findings on non-invasive stress testing
    - PCI within the previous 6 mo
    - repeated presentations for ACS despite treatment and without evidence of ongoing ischemia or high risk features
    - note: thrombolysis is NOT administered for UA/NSTEMI

TIMI Risk Score for UA/NSTEMI

Characteristics	Points
Historical	
Age ≥65 yr	1
≥3 risk factors for CAD	1
Known CAD (stenosis ≥50%)	1
Aspirin® use in past 7 d	1
Presentation	
Recent (≤24 h) severe angina	1
ST-segment deviation ≥0.5 mm	1
Increased cardiac markers	1

Risk Score = Total Points
If TIMI risk score ≥3, consider early LMWH and angiography
TIMI = thrombolysis in myocardial infarction
UA = unstable angina
JAMA 2000;284:835-842

- STEMI
  - after diagnosis of STEMI is made, do not wait for results of further investigations before implementing reperfusion therapy
  - goal is to re-perfuse artery: thrombolysis ("EMS-to-needle") within 30 min or primary PCI ("EMS-to-balloon") within 90 min (depending on capabilities of hospital and access to hospital with PCI facility)
  - thrombolysis
    - preferred if patient presents ≤12 h of symptom onset, and <30 min after presentation to hospital, has contraindications to PCI, or PCI cannot be administered within 90 min
  - PCI
    - early PCI (≤12 h after symptom onset and <90 min after presentation) improves mortality vs. thrombolysis with fewer intra-cranial hemorrhages and recurrent MIs
    - primary PCI: without prior thrombolytic therapy – method of choice for reperfusion in experienced centres (*JAMA* 2004;291:736-739)
    - rescue PCI: following failed thrombolytic therapy (diagnosed when following thrombolysis, ST segment elevation fails to resolve below half its initial magnitude and patient still having chest pain)

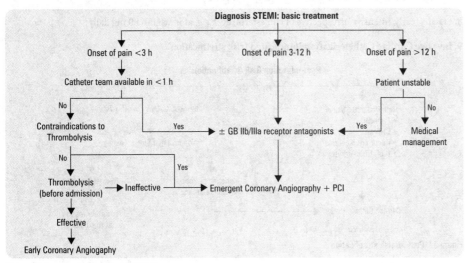

Figure 36. Reperfusion strategy in STEMI

Table 8. Contraindications for Thrombolysis in STEMI

Absolute	Relative
Prior intracranial hemorrhage	Chronic, severe, poorly controlled HTN
Known structural cerebral vascular lesion	Uncontrolled HTN (sBP >180, dBP >110)
Known malignant intracranial neoplasm	Current anticoagulation
Significant closed-head or facial trauma (≤3 mo)	Noncompressible vascular punctures
Ischemic stroke (≤3 mo)	Ischemic stroke (≥3 mo)
Active bleeding	Recent internal bleeding (≤2-4 wk)
Suspected aortic dissection	Prolonged CPR or major surgery (≤3 wk)
	Pregnancy
	Active peptic ulcer disease

Long-Term Management of ACS
- risk of progression to MI or recurrence of MI or death is highest within 1 mo
- at 1-3 mo after the acute phase, most patients resume a clinical course similar to that in patients with chronic stable coronary disease
- pre-discharge workup: ECG and echo to assess residual LV systolic function
- drugs required in hospital to control ischemia should be continued after discharge in all patients
- other medications for long-term management of ACS are summarized below

1. General Measures
- education
- risk factor modification

2. Antiplatelet and Anticoagulation Therapy
- see also *CCS Antiplatelet Guidelines 2012* for details (free mobile apps available on iOS and Android platforms in the CCS app stores)
- ECASA 81 mg daily
- ticagrelor 90 mg twice daily or prasugrel 10 mg daily (at least 1 mo, up to 9-12 mo, if stent placed at least 12 mo)
- clopidogrel 75 mg daily can be used as alternatives to ticagrelor and prasugrel when indicated
- ± warfarin x 3 mo if high risk (large anterior MI, LV thrombus, LVEF <30%, history of VTE, chronic AFib)

Is this Patient Having a Myocardial Infarction? From The Rational Clinical Examination
JAMA 2009; http://www.jamaevidence.com/content/3484335
Study: Systematic review of articles assessing the accuracy and precision of the clinical exam in the diagnosis of an acute myocardial infarction.
Results: In patients with normal or non-diagnostic ECG, no established CAD, and prolonged or recurrent chest pain typical of their usual discomfort, radiation of pain to the shoulder OR both arms had the highest positive likelihood ratio (+LR) of 4.1 (95% CI 2.5-6.5) and a negative likelihood ratio (-LR) of 0.68 (95% CI 0.52-0.89). Radiation to right arm had a +LR of 3.8 (95% CI 2.2-6.6) and –LR of 0.86 (95% CI 0.77-0.96), vomiting had a +LR of 3.5 (95% CI 2.0-6.2) and –LR of 0.87 (95% CI 0.79-0.97), while radiation to left arm only had a +LR of 1.3 (95% CI 0.93-1.8) and a –LR of 0.9 (95% CI 0.76-1.1).
Conclusions: The most compelling features that increase likelihood of an MI are ST-segment and cardiac enzyme elevation, new Q-wave, and presence of an S3 heart sound. In patients where the diagnosis of MI is uncertain, radiation of pain to the shoulder OR both arms, radiation to the right arm, and vomiting had the best predictive values, while radiation to the left arm is relatively non-diagnostic.

Complications of MI

CRASH PAD
Cardiac **R**upture
Arrhythmia
Shock
Hypertension/Heart failure
Pericarditis/Pulmonary emboli
Aneurysm
DVT

Resting LVEF is a useful prognostic factor

Enoxaparin vs. Unfractionated Heparin with Fibrinolysis for ST-elevation Myocardial Infarction
NEJM 2006;354:1477-1488
Study: Prospective multicentre RCT.
Patients: 20,479 patients (median age 60 yr, 77% male) with STEMI who were scheduled to undergo fibrinolysis.
Intervention: Patients were randomized to receive either enoxaparin or weight based unfractionated heparin in addition to thrombolysis and standard therapies.
Primary Outcome: Death or recurrent nonfatal MI 30 d post-event.
Results: The composite primary outcome occurred less often in the enoxaparin group compared with those who received unfractionated heparin (9.9% vs. 12.0%, p<0.001, NNT=47). Taken separately, there was a trend toward reduced mortality (6.9% vs. 7.5%, p=0.11) and a significant reduction in nonfatal reinfarction (3.0% vs. 4.5%, p<0.001) in the enoxaparin group. The risk of major bleeding was significantly increased in the enoxaparin group (2.1% vs. 1.4%, p<0.001, NNH=142).
Conclusion: In patients with STEMI receiving thrombolysis, enoxaparin is superior to unfractionated heparin in preventing recurrent nonfatal MI and may lead to a small reduction in mortality.

3. **β-Blockers** (e.g. metoprolol 25-50 mg bid or atenolol 50-100 mg daily)

4. **Nitrates**
   - alleviate ischemia but do not improve outcome
   - use with caution in right-sided MI patients who have become preload dependent

5. **Calcium Channel Blockers** (NOT recommended as first line treatment, consider as alternative to β-blockers)

6. **Angiotensin-Converting Enzyme Inhibitors**
   - prevent adverse ventricular remodelling
   - recommended for asymptomatic high-risk patients (e.g. diabetics), even if LVEF >40%
   - recommended for symptomatic CHF, reduced LVEF (<40%), anterior MI
   - use ARBs in patients who are intolerant of ACEI; avoid combing ACE and ARB

7. **± Aldosterone Antagonists**
   - if on ACEI and β-blockers and LVEF <40% and CHF or DM
   - significant mortality benefit shown with eplerenone by 30 d

8. **Statins** (early, intensive, irrespective of cholesterol level; e.g. atorvastatin 80 mg daily)

9. **Invasive Cardiac Catheterization if indicated** (risk stratification)

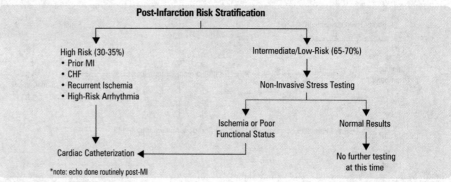

Figure 37. Post-MI risk stratification

Prognosis following STEMI
- 5-15% of hospitalized patients will die
  - risk factors
    - infarct size/severity
    - age
    - comorbid conditions
    - development of heart failure or hypotension
- post-discharge mortality rates
  - 6-8% within first year, half of these within first 3 mo
  - 4% per year following first yr
  - risk factors
    - LV dysfunction
    - residual myocardial ischemia
    - ventricular arrhythmias
    - history of prior MI

Table 9. Complications of Myocardial Infarction

Complication	Etiology	Presentation	Therapy
Arrhythmia			
1. Tachycardia	Sinus, AFib, VT, VFib	First 48 h	See *Arrhythmias*, C16
2. Bradycardia	Sinus, AV block	First 48 h	
Myocardial Rupture			
1. LV free wall	Transmural infarction	1-7 d	Surgery
2. Papillary muscle (→ MR)	Inferior infarction	1-7 d	Surgery
3. Ventricular septum (→ VSD)	Septal infarction	1-7 d	Surgery
Shock/CHF	Infarction or aneurysm	Within 48 h	Inotropes, intra-aortic balloon pump
Post-Infarct Angina	Persistent coronary stenosis Multivessel disease	Anytime	Aggressive medical therapy PCI or CABG
Recurrent MI	Reocclusion	Anytime	Aggressive medical therapy PCI or CABG
Thromboembolism	Mural/apical thrombus DVT	7-10 d, up to 6 mo	Anticoagulation
Pericarditis	Inflammatory	1-7 d	ASA
Dressler's Syndrome	Autoimmune	2-8 wk	

Treatment Algorithm for Chest Pain

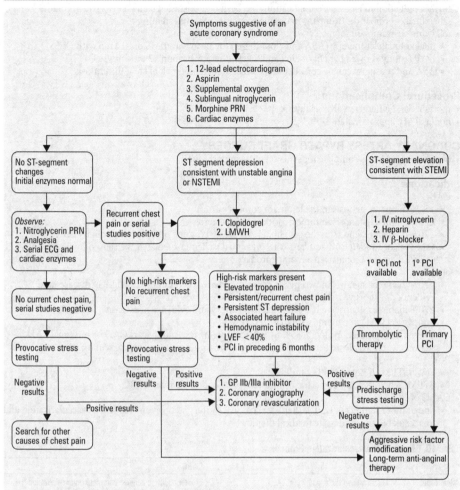

ECG = electrocardiogram; LMWH = low-molecular-weight heparin; NSTEMI = non-ST-segment elevation myocardial infarction;
PCI = percutaneous coronary intervention; STEMI = ST-segment elevation myocardial infarction

Figure 38. Treatment algorithm for patients with symptoms suggestive of an acute coronary syndrome
Adapted from: Andreoli TE, et al. Cecil Essentials of Medicine, 8th ed. 2011. Elsevier. With permission from Elsevier

Intensive vs. Moderate Lipid Lowering with Statins after Acute Coronary Syndromes
NEJM 2004;350:1495-1504
Study: Prospective, double blind, RCT; mean follow-up of 2 yr.
Population: 4,162 patients who had been hospitalized for an ACS within the preceding 10 d.
Intervention: Patients were randomized to receiving pravastatin 40 mg or atorvastatin 80 mg daily.
Primary Outcome: Composite of death from any cause, myocardial infarction, documented unstable angina requiring rehospitalization, revascularization (performed at least 30 d after randomization), and stroke.
Results: High dose atorvastatin was associated with a 16% hazard ratio reduction (p=0.005; 95% CI 5-26%) in the primary outcome compared to standard dose pravastatin.
Conclusions: In patients who recently experienced an ACS, high dose statin therapy provides greater protection against death and major cardiovascular events than standard dose therapy.

Coronary Revascularization

PERCUTANEOUS CORONARY INTERVENTION
- interventional cardiology technique aimed at relieving significant coronary stenosis
- main techniques: balloon angioplasty, stenting
- less common techniques: rotational/directional/extraction atherectomy

Indications
- medically refractory angina
- NSTEMI/UA with high risk features (e.g. high TIMI risk score, see sidebar C28)
- primary/rescue PCI for STEMI

Balloon Angioplasty and Intracoronary Stenting
- coronary lesions dilated with balloon inflation
- major complication is restenosis (approximately 15% at 6 mo), felt to be due to elastic recoil and neointimal hyperplasia
- majority of patients receive intracoronary stent(s) to prevent restenosis
  - bare metal stent (BMS) versus drug-eluting stents: PRAMI trial demonstrated stenting non-culprit lesions results in 14% absolute risk reduction of cardiac death, nonfatal MI, or refractory angina
  - coated with antiproliferative drugs (sirolimus, paclitaxel, everolimus)
  - reduced rate of neointimal hyperplasia and restenosis compared to BMS (5% vs. 20%)
  - complication: late stent thrombosis (5 events per 1,000 stents implanted)

Treatment of NSTEMI

BEMOAN
β-blocker
Enoxaparin
Morphine
O₂
ASA
Nitrates

Adjunctive Therapies
- ASA and heparin decrease post-procedural complications
- further reduction in ischemic complications has been demonstrated using GPIIb/IIIa inhibitors (abciximab, eptifibatide, tirofiban) in coronary angiography and stenting
- following stent implantation
  - dual antiplatelet therapy (ASA and clopidogrel) for 1 mo with BMS or ≥12 mo with DES
  - DAPT study showed benefit of dual antiplatelet therapy beyond 12 mo
  - ASA and prasugrel can be considered for those at increased risk of stent thrombosis

Procedural Complications
- mortality and emergency bypass rates <1%
- nonfatal MI: approximately 2-3%

CORONARY ARTERY BYPASS GRAFT SURGERY
- objective of CABG is complete reperfusion of the myocardium

Indications
- CABG
  - ≥50% diameter stenosis in the left main coronary artery
  - ≥70% diameter stenosis in three major coronary arteries
  - ≥70% diameter stenosis in the proximal LAD artery plus one other major coronary artery
  - survivors of sudden cardiac arrest with presumed ischemia-mediated VT caused by significant (≥70% diameter) stenosis in a major coronary artery
- other
  - ≥70% diameter stenosis in two major coronary arteries (without proximal LAD disease) and evidence of extensive ischemia
  - ≥70% diameter stenosis in the proximal LAD artery and evidence of extensive ischemia
  - multivessel CAD in patients with diabetes
  - LV systolic dysfunction (LVEF 35% to 50%) and significant multivessel CAD or proximal LAD stenosis where viable myocardium is present in the region of intended revascularization
- PCI
  - UA/NSTEMI if not a CABG candidate
  - STEMI when PCI can be performed more rapidly and safely than CABG
- CABG or PCI
  - one or more significant (≥70% diameter) coronary artery stenosis amenable to revascularization and unacceptable angina despite medical therapy

Percutaneous Coronary Intervention vs. Coronary-Artery Bypass Grafting for Severe Coronary Artery Disease: The SYNTAX Trial
NEJM 2009;360;961-972
Study: Prospective RCT.
Population: 1,800 patients with untreated three-vessel or left main coronary artery disease and anatomically equivalent for both Percutaneous Intervention (PCI) and Coronary Artery Bypass Graft (CABG).
Intervention: PCI vs. CABG.
Outcome: Composite of death from any cause, stroke, MI, or repeat revascularization in 12 mo post-intervention.
Results: Incidence of primary outcome was lower in the CABG intervention vs. PCI (12.4% vs. 17.8%, p=0.002, NNT=19). PCI was associated with significantly higher rates of repeat revascularization (13.5% vs. 5.9%, p<0.001) and cardiac death (3.7% vs. 2.1%, p=0.05), while CABG had higher rates of stroke (2.2% vs. 0.6%, p=0.03).
Conclusions: In patients with three-vessel or left main coronary artery disease CABG is superior to PCI in preventing major adverse cardiovascular and cerebrovascular events within 12 mo of intervention.

Table 10. Choice of Revascularization Procedure

	PCI	CABG
Advantages	Less invasive technique Decreased periprocedural morbidity and mortality Shorter periprocedural hospitalization	Greater ability to achieve complete revascularization Decreased need for repeated revascularization procedures
Indications	Single or double-vessel disease Inability to tolerate surgery	Triple-vessel or left main disease DM Plaque morphology unfavourable for PCI

Table 11. Conduits for CABG

Graft	Occlusion/Patency Rate	Considerations
Saphenous Vein Grafts (SVG)	At 10 yr, 50% occluded, 25% stenotic, 25% angiographically normal	Used when arterial grafts are not available or many grafts are required, such as triple or quadruple bypass
Left Internal Thoracic/Mammary Artery (LITA/LIMA) (LIMA to LAD)	90-95% patency at 15 yr	Most preferred option because of excellent patency Improved event-free survival (angina, MI) Decreased late cardiac events No increase in operative risk
Right Internal Thoracic/Mammary Artery (RITA/RIMA)	Pedicled RIMA patency comparable to LIMA Free RIMA patency less	Used in bilateral ITA/IMA grafting Patients receiving bilateral ITAs/IMAs have less risk of recurrent angina, late MI, angioplasty
Radial Artery (free graft)	85-90% patency at 5 yr	Prone to severe vasospasm post-operatively due to muscular wall
Right Gastroepiploic Artery	80-90% patency at 5 yr	Primarily used as an in situ graft to bypass the RCA Use limited because of the fragile quality of the artery, other technical issues, increased operative time (laparotomy incision), and incisional discomfort with associated ileus
Complete Arterial Revascularization		For younger patients (<60 yr of age) Is preferred due to longer term graft patency
Redo Bypass Grafting		Operative mortality 2-3x higher than first operation 10% perioperative MI rate Reoperation undertaken only in symptomatic patients who have failed medical therapy and in whom angiography has documented progression of the disease Increased risk with redo-sternotomy secondary to adhesions which may result in laceration to aorta, RV, IMA/ITA, and other bypass grafts

Operative Issues
- left ventricular (LV) function is an important determinant of outcome of all heart diseases
- patients with severe LV dysfunction usually have poor prognosis, but surgery can sometimes dramatically improve LV function
- assess viability of non-functioning myocardial segments in patients with significant LV dysfunction using delayed thallium myocardial imaging, stress echocardiography, PET scanning, or MRI

CABG and Antiplatelet Regimens
- please refer to CCS guidelines – 2012 update on antiplatelet therapy – for more information if possible
- prior to CABG, clopidogrel and ticagrelor should be discontinued for 5 d and prasugrel for 7 d before surgery
- dual antiplatelet therapy should be continued for 12 mo in patients with ACS within 48-72 h after CABG
- ASA (81 mg) continued indefinitely (can be started 6 h after surgery)
- patients requiring CABG after PCI should continue their dual antiplatelet therapy as recommended in the post-PCI guidelines

Table 12. Risk Factors for CABG Mortality and Morbidity (decreasing order of significance)

Risk Factors for CABG Mortality	Risk Factors for CABG Post-Operative Morbidity or Increased Length of Stay
Urgency of surgery (emergent or urgent)	Reoperation
Reoperation	Emergent procedure
Older age	Pre-operative intra-aortic balloon pump (IABP)
Poor left ventricular function (see below)	CHF
Female gender	CABG + valve surgery
Left main disease	Older age
Others include catastrophic conditions (cardiogenic shock, ventricular septal rupture, ongoing CPR), dialysis-dependent renal failure, end-stage COPD, DM, cerebrovascular disease, and peripheral vascular disease	Renal dysfunction
	COPD
	DM
	Cerebrovascular disease

Safety and Efficacy of Drug-Eluting and Bare Metal Stents
Circulation 2009;119;3198-3206
Study: Meta-analysis of RCTs and observational studies. 22 RCTs and 34 observational studies.
Population: 9,470 and 182,901 patients in RCTs and observational studies respectively who underwent percutaneous coronary intervention.
Intervention: Drug-Eluting Stents (DES) versus Bare Metal Stents (BMS).
Outcome: All-cause mortality, myocardial infarction (MI), and target vessel revascularization (TVR).
Results: No difference in mortality was found between DES vs. BMS by RCTs, while observational studies showed significantly lower mortality rates in DES-treated patients (hazard ratio (HR) 0.78, p<0.001). No difference in MI incidence was found in RCTs, while lower incidences of MI were found in observational studies (HR 0.87, p=0.014). DES has a significantly lower TVR rate in both RCT (HR 0.45, p<0.001) and observational studies (HR 0.46, p<0.001).
Conclusions: DES significantly reduces rates of TVR compared to BMS. Although there is no difference in mortality or MI incidence as found by RCTs, observational studies suggest lowered mortality and MI rates in patients with DES over BMS.

Procedural Complications
- CABG using cardiopulmonary bypass (CPB)
  - stroke and neurocognitive defects (microembolization of gaseous and particulate matter)
  - immunosuppression
  - systemic inflammatory response leading to
    - myocardial dysfunction
    - renal dysfunction
    - neurological injury
    - respiratory dysfunction
    - coagulopathies

OFF-PUMP CORONARY ARTERY BYPASS SURGERY

Procedure
- avoids the use of CPB by allowing surgeons to operate on a beating heart
  - stabilization devices (e.g. Genzyme Immobilizer®) hold heart in place allowing operation while positioning devices (Medtronic Octopus® and Starfish® system) allow the surgeon to lift the beating heart to access the lateral and posterior vessels
  - procedure is safe and well tolerated by most patients; however, this surgery remains technically more demanding

Indications
- used in poor candidates for CPB who have: calcified aorta, poor LVEF, severe peripheral vascular disease (PVD), severe COPD, chronic renal failure, coagulopathy, transfusion objections (e.g. Jehovah's Witness), good target vessels, anterior/lateral wall revascularization, target revascularization in older, sicker patients
- **absolute contraindications:** hemodynamic instability, poor quality target vessels including intramyocardial vessels, diffusely diseased vessels, and calcified coronary vessels
- **relative contraindications:** cardiomegaly/CHF, critical left main disease, small distal targets, recent or current acute MI, cardiogenic shock, LVEF <35%

Outcomes
- OPCAB decreases in-hospital morbidity (decreased incidence of chest infection, inotropic requirement, supraventricular arrhythmia), blood product transfusion, ICU stay, length of hospitalization, and CK-MB and troponin I levels
- no significant difference in terms of survival at 2 yr, frequency of cardiac events (MI, PCI, CHF, recurrent angina, redo CABG), or medication usage compared to on-pump CABG

Heart Failure

- see also *CCS Heart Failure Guidelines 2012* for details (free mobile apps available on iOS and Android platforms in the CCS app stores) as well as the CCS Heart Failure Guidelines Compendium available at CCS.ca

Congestive Heart Failure

Does this Dyspneic Patient in the Emergency Department have Congestive Heart Failure?
JAMA 2005;294:1944-1956

	LR + (95% CI)	LR – (95% CI)
Initial clinical judgment	4.4 (1.8-10.0)	0.45 (0.28-0.73)
Past Medical History		
Heart failure	5.8 (4.1-8.0)	0.45 (0.38-0.53)
Myocardial infarction	3.1 (2.0-4.9)	0.69 (0.58-0.82)
Coronary artery disease	1.8 (1.1-2.8)	0.68 (0.48-0.96)
Symptoms		
Paroxysmal nocturnal dyspnea	2.6 (1.5-4.5)	0.7 (0.54-0.91)
Orthopnea	2.2 (1.2-3.9)	0.65 (0.45-0.92)
Dyspnea on exertion	1.3 (1.2-1.4)	0.48 (0.35-0.67)
Physical Exam		
Third heart sound	11 (4.9-25)	0.88 (0.83-0.94)
Jugular venous distension	5.1 (3.2-7.9)	0.66 (0.57-0.77)
Rales	2.8 (1.9-4.1)	0.51 (0.37-0.70)
Lower extremity edema	2.3 (1.5-3.7)	0.64 (0.47-0.87)
Chest Radiograph		
Pulmonary venous congestion	12 (6.8-21)	0.48 (0.28-0.83)
Interstitial edema	12 (5.2-27)	0.68 (0.54-0.85)
Cardiomegaly	3.3 (2.4-4.7)	0.33 (0.23-0.48)
ECG		
Atrial fibrillation	3.8 (1.7-8.8)	0.79 (0.65-0.96)
Any abnormal finding	2.2 (1.6-3.1)	0.64 (0.47-0.88)

Dichotomies of Heart Failure
- Forward vs. backward
- Left-sided vs. right-sided
- Systolic vs. diastolic dysfunction
- Low output vs. high output

Use Ejection Fraction to Grade LV Dysfunction
- Grade I (EF >60%) (Normal)
- Grade II (EF = 40-59%)
- Grade III (EF = 21-39%)
- Grade IV (EF ≤20%)

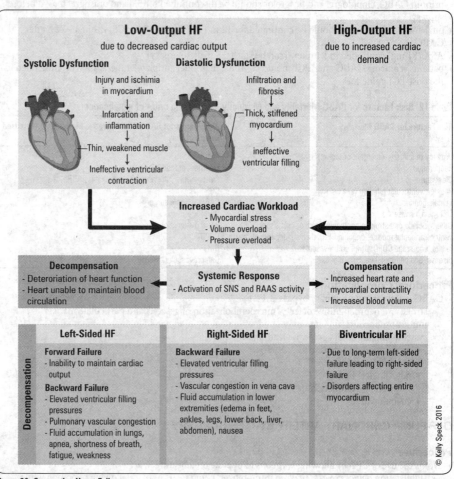

Figure 39. Congestive Heart Failure

© Kelly Speck 2016

Table 13. Signs and Symptoms of Left vs. Right Heart Failure

	Left Failure	Right Failure
Low Cardiac Output (Forward)	Fatigue Syncope Systemic hypotension Cool extremities Slow capillary refill Peripheral cyanosis Pulsus alternans Mitral regurgitation S3	Left failure symptoms if decreased RV output leads to LV underfilling Tricuspid regurgitation S3 (right-sided)
Venous Congestion (Backward)	Dyspnea, orthopnea, PND Cough Crackles	Peripheral edema Elevated JVP with abdominojugular reflux, and Kussmaul's sign Hepatomegaly Pulsatile liver

Pathophysiology
- most common causes are ischemic heart disease, hypertension and valvular heart disease
- myocardial insult causes pump dysfunction/impaired filling leading to myocardial remodelling
  - pressure overload (e.g. AS or HTN) leads to compensatory hypertrophy (concentric remodelling) and eventually interstitial fibrosis
  - volume overload (e.g. AI) leads to dilatation (eccentric remodelling)
  - both processes lead to maladaptive changes contributing to disease process
- results in decreased volume cardiac output resulting in activation of the SNS and RAAS
- Na^+ and water retention, increasing preload and afterload, tachycardia
  - perpetuates cycle of increasing cardiac demand and decompensation

Heart Failure with Reduced Ejection Fraction
- impaired myocardial contractile function → decreased LVEF and SV → decreased CO

Volume Overload and Eccentric Remodelling is the Typical Phenotype
- findings: apex beat displaced, S3, cardiothoracic ratio >0.5, decreased LVEF, LV dilatation
- causes
  - ischemic (e.g. extensive CAD, previous MI)
  - non-ischemic
    - HTN
    - DM
    - alcohol (and other toxins)
    - myocarditis
    - dilated cardiomyopathy (multiple causes – see *Dilated Cardiomyopathy*, C40)

Heart Failure with Preserved Ejection Fraction
- previously known as "diastolic heart failure"
- concentric remodelling with a "stiff" left ventricle is the typical phenotype
- 1/2 of patients with heart failure have preserved EF; confers similar prognosis to HRrEF; more common in the elderly and females
- reduced LV compliance causes increased LV filling pressures, increased LA pressure/volume, and pulmonary congestion
- findings: HTN, apex beat sustained, S4, normal-sized heart on CXR, LVH on ECG/echo, normal EF
- causes
  - transient: ischemia (relaxation of myocardium is active and requires ATP)
  - permanent
    - severe hypertrophy (HTN, aortic stenosis, HCM)
    - restrictive cardiomyopathy (e.g. amyloid)
    - MI

High-Output Heart Failure
- caused by demand for increased cardiac output
- often exacerbates existing heart failure or decompensates a patient with other cardiac pathology
- differential diagnosis: anemia, thiamine deficiency (beriberi), hyperthyroidism, A-V fistula or L-R shunting, Paget's disease, renal disease, hepatic disease

Precipitants of Symptomatic Exacerbations
- consider natural progression of disease vs. new precipitant
- always search for reversible cause
- differential diagnosis can also be organized as follows:
  - new cardiac insult/disease: MI, arrhythmia, valvular disease
  - new demand on CV system: HTN, anemia, thyrotoxicosis, infection, etc.
  - medication non-compliance
  - dietary indisretion e.g. salt intake
  - obstructive sleep apnea

Investigations
- identify and assess precipitating factors and treatable causes of CHF
- blood work: CBC, electrolytes (including calcium and magnesium), BUN, creatinine, fasting blood glucose, HbA1c, lipid profile, liver function tests, serum TSH ± ferritin, BNP, uric acid
- ECG: look for chamber enlargement, arrhythmia, ischemia/infarction
- CXR: cardiomegaly, pleural effusion, redistribution, Kerley B lines, bronchiolar-alveolar cuffing
- echo: systolic function (LVEF), diastolic function (E/A ratio, E/e'), cardiac dimensions, wall motion abnormalities, RVSP (from TR jet), valvular disease, pericardial effusion
- radionuclide angiography: LVEF
- myocardial perfusion scintigraphy (thallium or sestamibi SPECT)

A Validated Clinical and Biochemical Score for the Diagnosis of Acute Heart Failure: the ProBNP Investigation of Dyspnea in the Emergency Department (PRIDE) Acute Heart Failure Score
Am Heart J 2006;151:48-54

Predictor	Possible Score
Age >75 yr	1
Orthopnea present	2
Lack of cough	1
Current loop diuretic use (before presentation)	1
Rales on lung exam	1
Lack of fever	2
Elevated NT-proBNP (>450 pg/mL if <50 yr, >900 pg/mL if >50 yr)	4
Interstitial edema on chest x-ray	2
Total	/14

Likelihood of heart failure
    Low = 0-5
    Intermediate = 6-8
    High = 9-14

Brain natieuretic peptide (BNP) is secreted by ventricles due to LV stretch and wall tension. Cardiomyocytes secrete BNP precursor that is cleaved into proBNP. After secretion into ventricles, proBNP is cleaved into the active C-terminal portion and the inactive NT-proBNP. The above scoring algorithm developed by Baggish et al. is commonly used. A score of <6 has a negative predictive value of 98%, while scores ≥6 had a sensitivity of 96% and specificity of 84% (p<0.001) for the diagnosis of acute heart failure.

New York Heart Association (NYHA) Functional Classification of Heart Failure
- **Class I:** ordinary physical activity does not cause symptoms of HF
- **Class II:** comfortable at rest, ordinary physical activity results in symptoms
- **Class III:** marked limitation of ordinary activity; less than ordinary physical activity results in symptoms
- **Class IV:** inability to carry out any physical activity without discomfort; symptoms may be present at rest

Five Most Common Causes of CHF
- CAD (60-70%)
- HTN
- Idiopathic (often dilated cardiomyopathy)
- Valvular (e.g. AS, AR, and MR)
- Alcohol (dilated cardiomyopathy)

Precipitants of Heart Failure

HEART FAILED
Hypertension (common)
Endocarditis/environment (e.g. heat wave)
Anemia
Rheumatic heart disease and other valvular disease
Thyrotoxicosis
Failure to take meds (very common)
Arrhythmia (common)
Infection/Ischemia/Infarction (common)
Lung problems (PE, pneumonia, COPD)
Endocrine (pheochromocytoma, hyperaldosteronism)
Dietary indiscretions (common)

Heart Failure

The most common cause of right heart failure is left heart failure

Measuring NT-Pro BNP
BNP is secreted by ventricles due to LV stretch and wall tension

Cardiomyocytes secrete BNP precursor that is cleaved into proBNP

After secretion into ventricles proBNP is cleaved into the active C-terminal portion and the inactive NT-proBNP portion

NT-proBNP levels (pg/mL)	
Age	HF very likely
<50	>450
50-75	>900
>75	>1800

Limitations: Age, body habitus, renal function, pulmonary embolism

Features of Heart Failure on CXR

HERB-B
Heart enlargement (cardiothoracic ratio >0.50)
Pleural **E**ffusion
Re-distribution (alveolar edema)
Kerley **B** lines
Bronchiolar-alveolar cuffing

Patients on β-blocker therapy who have acute decompensated heart failure should continue β-blockers where possible (provided they are not in cardiogenic shock or in severe pulmonary edema)

Can the Clinical Examination Diagnose Left-Sided Heart Failure in Adults?
From The Rational Clinical Examination
JAMA 2009; http://www.jamaevidence.com/content/3478992
Study: Systematic review of articles assessing the accuracy and precision of the clinical exam in the diagnosis of CHF.
Results: The diagnosis of left ventricular dysfunction in patient after an MI based on the presence of radiographic pulmonary venous congestion with edema, rales one-third up the lung fields in the absence of a chronic pulmonary disease, or a 3rd heart sound had a positive likelihood ratio (+LR) of 3.1 (95% CI 1.7-5.8) and a negative likelihood ratio (-LR) of 0.62 (95% CI 0.46-0.83). In inpatients the combination of clinical findings, ECG, and CXR had a +LR of 2.0 (95% CI 1.6-2.5) and a –LR of 0.41 (95% CI 0.30-0.56). Female sex (+LR, 1.6 [95% CI 1.2-2.2]) and sBP ≥160 mmHg (+LR, 1.8 [95% CI 1.3-2.6]) were most indicative for diastolic dysfunction. Heart rate ≥100/min (+LR 0.43 [95% CI 0.28-0.65]) and left atrial ECG abnormality (+LR 0.42 [95% CI 0.26-0.63]) were most indicative for systolic dysfunction.
Conclusions: Patients with signs, symptoms, and risk factors for systolic dysfunction should receive an ECG and CXR. Female sex and sBP >160 mmHg are suggestive of diastolic dysfunction; heart rate ≥100/min and left atrial ECG abnormality suggest systolic dysfunction.

Acute Treatment of Pulmonary Edema
- treat acute precipitating factors (e.g. ischemia, arrhythmias)
- **L** – Lasix® (furosemide) 40-500 mg IV
- **M** – morphine 2-4 mg IV: decreases anxiety and preload (venodilation)
- **N** – nitroglycerin: topical/IV/SL - use with caution in preload-dependent patients (e.g. right HF or RV infarction) as it may precipitate CV collapse
- **O** – oxygen: in hypoxemic patients
- **P** – positive airway pressure (CPAP/BiPAP): decreases preload and need for ventilation when appropriate
- **P** – position: sit patient up with legs hanging down unless patient is hypotensive
- in ICU setting or failure of LMNOPP, other interventions may be necessary
  - nitroprusside IV
  - hydralazine PO
  - sympathomimetics
    - dopamine
      - low dose: selective renal vasodilation (high potency D1 agonist)
      - medium dose: inotropic support (medium potency β1 agonist)
      - high dose: increases SVR (low potency β1 agonist), which is undesirable
    - dobutamine
      - β1-selective agonist causing inotropy, tachycardia, hypotension (low dose) or hypertension (high dose); most serious side effect is arrhythmia, especially AF
    - phosphodiesterase inhibitors (milrinone)
      - inotropic effect and vascular smooth muscle relaxation (decreased SVR), similar to dobutamine
- consider pulmonary artery catheter to monitor pulmonary capillary wedge pressure (PCWP) if patient is unstable or a cardiac etiology is uncertain (PCWP >18 indicates likely cardiac etiology)
- mechanical ventilation as needed
- rarely used, but potentially life-saving measures:
  - intra-aortic balloon pump (IABP) - reduces afterload via systolic unloading and improves coronary perfusion via diastolic augmentation
  - left or right ventricular assist device (LVAD/RVAD)
  - cardiac transplant

Long-Term Management
- overwhelming majority of evidence-based management applies to HFREF
- currently no proven pharmacologic therapies shown to reduce mortality in HFPEF; control risk factors (e.g. hypertension)

Conservative Measures
- symptomatic measures: oxygen in hospital, bedrest, elevate the head of bed
- lifestyle measures: diet, exercise, DM control, smoking cessation, decrease alcohol consumption, patient education, sodium and fluid restriction
- multidisciplinary heart failure clinics: for management of individuals at higher risk, or with recent hospitalization

Non-Pharmcological Management
- from CCS guidelines (2013 update)
- cardiac rehabilitation: participation in a structured exercise program for NYHA class I-III after clinical status assessment to improve quality of life (HF-ACTION trial)

Pharmacological Therapy

1. Renin-angiotensin-aldosterone blockade
- ACEI: standard of care – slows progression of LV dysfunction and improves survival
  - all symptomatic patients functional class II-IV
  - all asymptomatic patients with LVEF <40%
  - post-MI
- angiotensin II receptor blockers
  - second-line to ACEI if not tolerated, or as adjunct to ACEI if β-blockers not tolerated
    - combination with ACEI is not routinely recommended and should be used with caution as it may precipitate hyperkalemia, renal failure, the need for dialysis and increase (CHARM, ONTARGET)
  - combination angiotensin II receptor blockers with neprilysin inhibitors (ARNI) is a new class of medication that has morbidity and mortality benefit over ACEI alone; it has been recommended to replace ACEI or ARBs for patients who have persistent symptoms (PARADIGM HF)

2. β-blockers: slow progression and improve survival
- class I-III with LVEF <40%
- stable class IV patients
- carvedilol improves survival in class IV HF (COMET)
- note: should be used cautiously, titrate slowly because may initially worsen CHF

3. **Mineralocorticoid receptor (aldosterone) antagonists:** mortality benefit in symptomatic heart failure and severely depressed ejection fraction
   - spironolactone or eplerenone symptomatic heart failure in patients already on ACEI, beta blocker and loop diuretic
   - note: potential for life threatening hyperkalemia
     - monitor K^+ after initiation and avoid if Cr >220 μmol/L or K^+ >5.2 mmol/L

4. **Diuretics:** symptom control, management of fluid overload
   - furosemide (40-500 mg daily) for potent diuresis
   - metolazone may be used with furosemide to increase diuresis
   - furosemide, metolazone, and thiazides oppose the hyperkalemia that can be induced by β-blockers, ACEI, ARBs, and aldosterone antagonists

5. **Digoxin and cardiac glycosides:** digoxin improves symptoms and decreases hospitalizations, no effect on mortality
   - indications: patient in sinus rhythm and symptomatic on ACEI, or CHF and AFib
   - patients on digitalis glycosides may worsen if these are withdrawn

6. **Antiarrhythmic drugs:** for use in CHF with arrhythmia
   - can use amiodarone, β-blocker, or digoxin

7. **Anticoagulants:** warfarin for prevention of thromboembolic events
   - prior thromboembolic event or AFib, presence of LV thrombus on echo

Procedural Interventions
- resynchronization therapy: symptomatic improvement with biventricular pacemaker
- consider if QRS >130 msec, LVEF <35%, and persistent symptoms despite optimal therapy
- greatest benefit likely with marked LV enlargement, mitral regurgitation, QRS >150 msec,
- ICD: mortality benefit in 1° prevention of sudden cardiac death
  - prior MI, optimal medical therapy, LVEF <30%, clinically stable
  - prior MI, non-sustained VT, LVEF 30-40%, EPS inducible VT
- LVAD/RVAD (see *Ventricular Assist Devices*, C38)
- cardiac transplantation (see *Cardiac Transplantation*, C38)
- valve repair if patient is surgical candidate and has significant valve disease contributing to CHF (see *Valvular Heart Disease*, C43)

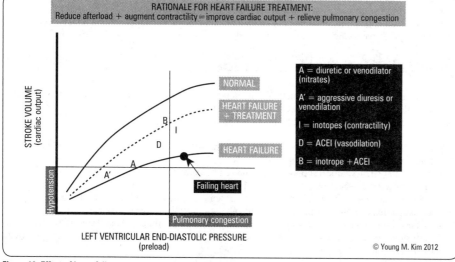

RATIONALE FOR HEART FAILURE TREATMENT:
Reduce afterload + augment contractility = improve cardiac output + relieve pulmonary congestion

A = diuretic or venodilator (nitrates)
A' = aggressive diuresis or venodilation
I = inotopes (contractility)
D = ACEI (vasodilation)
B = inotrope + ACEI

© Young M. Kim 2012

Figure 40. Effect of heart failure treatment on the Frank-Starling curve

Sleep-Disordered Breathing

- 45-55% of patients with CHF have sleep disturbances, including Cheyne-Stokes breathing and sleep apnea (central or obstructive)
- associated with a worse prognosis and greater LV dysfunction
- nasal continuous positive airway pressure (CPAP) is effective in treating symptoms of sleep apnea with secondary beneficial effects in cardiac function and symptoms

Chronic Treatment of CHF
- ACEI*
- β-blockers*
- ± Mineralocorticoid receptor antagonists*
- Diuretic
- ± Inotrope
- ± Antiarrhythmic
- ± Anticoagulant
*Mortality benefit

Influence of Ejection Fraction on Cardiovascular Outcomes in a Broad Spectrum of Heart Failure Patients
Circulation 2005;112:3738-3744
Purpose: Understand the relationship between ejection fractions and cardiovascular risk in patients with heart failure.
Methods: 7,599 patients from the CHARM study (Candesartan in Heart failure: Assessment of Reduction in Mortality and morbidity; RCT comparing placebo vs. candesartan in patients with NYHA class II to IV). Compared LVEF to cardiovascular outcomes and causes of death.
Results: All-cause mortality increased by 39% per 10% reduction in LVEF below 45% (Hazard ratio 1.39, 95% CI 1.32-1.46). For LVEF >45%, ejection fraction does not further contribute to assessment of cardiovascular risk in HF patients.
Conclusions: At LVEF <45%, lower ejection fractions were associated with poorer cardiovascular outcomes.

LVEF	CHF Hospitalization	All-Cause Mortality
≤22%	14.9%	15.4%
23-32%	10.9%	10.8%
33-42%	7.2%	7.4%
43-52%	5.7%	5.2%
>52%	6.9%	5.7%

Higher New York Heart Association Classes and Increased Mortality and Hospitalization in Patients with Heart Failure and Preserved Left Ventricular Function
Am Heart J 2006;151:444-450
Purpose: To establish the association between NYHA class and outcomes with heart failure and preserved systolic function.
Methods: Retrospective follow-up study (median 38.5 mo) of 988 patients with heart failure with ejection fracture >45%. Estimated risks of various outcomes using Cox proportional hazard models.
Results: Adjusted hazard ratio for all-cause mortality for NYHA class II, III, IV patients was 1.54, 2.56, and 8.46, respectively. Adjusted hazard ratio for all-cause hospitalization for NYHA class II, III, IV patients was 1.23, 1.71, and 3.4, respectively.
Conclusions: Higher NYHA classes were associated with poorer outcomes in patients with heart failure and preserved systolic function. Proportions of NYHA I, II, III, and IV patients who died of all causes during the study were 14.3%.

NYHA	Proportion of All-Cause Hospitalization	Proportion of All-Cause Mortality
I	60.7%	14.3%
II	65.2%	21.3%
III	77.7%	35.9%
IV	75.0%	58.3%

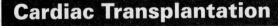

Cardiac Transplantation

- treatment for end-stage heart disease; due to ischemic or non-ischemic cardiomyopathy
- worldwide 1 yr survival is 85-90%, 5 yr survival about 60%, annual mortality rate of 4%
- matching is according to blood type, body size and weight (should be within 25%), and HLA tissue matching (if time allows)

Indications for Surgery
- severe cardiac disability despite maximal medical therapy (e.g. recurrent hospitalizations for CHF, NYHA III or IV, peak metabolic oxygen consumption <14 mL/kg/min in absence of β-blocker)
- symptomatic cardiac ischemia refractory to conventional treatment (e.g. unstable angina not amenable to CABG or PCI with LVEF <30%; recurrent, symptomatic ventricular arrhythmias)
- exclusion of all surgical alternatives to cardiac transplantation

Prerequisites
- psychosocial stability
- medically compliant and motivated
- relative contraindications: incurable malignancy, major systemic illness, irreversible major organ disease, active systemic infection, obesity, irreversible pulmonary HTN (pulmonary vascular resistance [PVR] >6 Wood units), severe COPD (FEV1 <1 L) or active drug addiction or alcoholism

Complications
- rejection
    - common, <5% have serious hemodynamic compromise
    - gold standard to detect rejection: endomyocardial biopsy
    - risk of acute rejection is greatest during the first 3 mo after transplant
- infection
    - leading cause of morbidity and mortality after cardiac transplantation
    - risk peaks early during the first few months after transplantation and then declines to a low persistent rate
- allograft CAD
    - approximately 50% develop graft CAD within 5 yr of transplantation
    - most common cause of late death following transplantation
- malignancy
    - develops in 15% of cardiac transplant recipients due to immunosuppressive medication
    - second most common cause of late death following transplantation
    - cutaneous neoplams most common, followed by non-Hodgkin's lymphoma and lung cancer
- immunosuppressive medication side effects (prednisone, cyclosporine, tacrolimus, sirolimus)

Ventricular Assist Devices

- work to unload the ventricle while maintaining output; also results in decreased myocardial oxygen consumption permitting recovery of the myocardium that is not irreversibly injured
- can support the left (LVAD), right (RVAD), or both ventricles (BiVAD)
- indications
    - bridge to transplantation, bridge to decision (for transplant), or long term permanent therapy ("destination therapy")
    - post-operative mechanical support when unable to separate from cardiopulmonary bypass despite inotropic and intra-aortic balloon pump (IABP) support
    - IABP is a catheter based device inserted into the femoral artery and advanced to the descending aorta that decreases myocardial O_2 demand and increases blood flow to coronary arteries
    - inflation of the balloon occurs during diastole to increase ascending aorta and coronary artery perfusion pressure; deflation occurs at systole to reduce intra-aortic pressure thus reducing afterload
- post-operative cardiogenic shock

Effects of Donor Pre-Treatment with Dopamine on Survival After Heart Transplantation: A Cohort Study of Heart Transplant Recipients Nested in a Randomized Controlled Multicentre Trial
J Am Coll Cardiol 2010;58:1768-1777
Treatment of brain-dead donors with dopamine of 4 µg/kg/min will not harm cardiac allografts but appears to improve the clinical course of the heart allograft recipient.

REMATCH Trial
NEJM 2001;345:1435-1443
Increased survival of 23% vs. 8% with LVAD vs. medical management of heart failure after 2 yr. Heartmate VAD has a biologic surface therefore does not require long-term anticoagulation but higher risk of infection

Canadian Cardiovascular Society Focused Position Statement Update on Assessment of the Cardiac Patient for Fitness to Drive: Fitness following Left Ventricular Assist Device Implantation
Can J Cardiol 2012;28:137-140
Patients with a continuous flow, NYHA class I-III, LVAD that are stable 2 mo post LVAD implantation qualify for private driving only and are disqualified from commercial driving.

Myocardial Disease

Definition of Cardiomyopathy
- intrinsic or primary myocardial disease not secondary to congenital, hypertensive, coronary, valvular, or pericardial disease
- functional classification: dilated, hypertrophic, or restrictive
- LV dysfunction 2° to MI often termed "ischemic cardiomyopathy", is not a true cardiomyopathy (i.e. primary myocardial disorder) since the primary pathology is obstructive CAD

Table 14. Summary Table for CHF and Myocardial Disease

Heart Failure Reduced Ejection Fraction		Heart Failure Preserved Ejection Fraction		
Dilated Cardiomyopathy	Secondary Causes	Hypertrophic Cardiomyopathy	Restrictive Cardiomyopathy	Secondary Causes
Idiopathic, infectious (e.g. myocarditis), alcohol, familial, collagen vascular disease, etc.	CAD, MI, DM, valvular (e.g. AR, MR)	Genetic disorder affecting cardiac sarcomeres (most common cause of sudden cardiac death in young athletes)	Amyloidosis, sarcoidosis, scleroderma, hemochromatosis, Fabry's, Pompe's Disease, Loeffler's, etc.	HTN, DM, valvular (e.g. AS), post-MI, transiently by ischemia, etc.

Cardiomyopathy

HARD
Hypertrophic cardiomyopathy
Arrhythmogenic right ventricular cardiomyopathy
Restrictive cardiomyopathy
Dilated cardiomyopathy

Myocarditis

Definition
- inflammatory process involving the myocardium ranging from acute to chronic; an important cause of dilated cardiomyopathy

Etiology
- idiopathic
- infectious
  - viral (most common): parvovirus B19, influenza, coxsackie B, echovirus, poliovirus, HIV, mumps
  - bacterial: *S. aureus, C. perfringens, C. diphtheriae, Mycoplasma, Rickettsia*
  - fungi
  - spirochetal (Lyme disease – *Borrelia burgdorferi*)
  - Chagas disease (*Trypanosoma cruzi*), toxoplasmosis
- toxic: catecholamines, chemotherapy, cocaine
- hypersensitivity/eosinophilic: drugs (antibiotics, diuretics, lithium, clozapine), insect/snake bites
- systemic diseases: collagen vascular diseases (SLE, rheumatoid arthritis, others), sarcoidosis, autoimmune
- other: giant cell myocarditis, acute rheumatic fever

Signs and Symptoms
- constitutional symptoms
- acute CHF - dyspnea, tachycardia, elevated JVP
- chest pain – due to pericarditis or cardiac ischemia
- arrhythmias
- systemic or pulmonary emboli
- pre-syncope/syncope/sudden death

Investigations
- ECG: non-specific ST-T changes ± conduction defects
- blood work
  - increased CK, troponin, LDH, and AST with acute myocardial necrosis ± increased WBC, ESR, ANA, rheumatoid factor, complement levels
  - blood culture, viral titres and cold agglutinins for Mycoplasma
- CXR: enlarged cardiac silhouette
- echo: dilated, hypokinetic chambers, segmental wall motion abnormalities
- cardiovascular magnetic resonance: functional and morphological abnormalities as well as tissue pathology (gadolinium enhancement)
- myocardial biopsy

Management
- supportive care
- restrict physical activity
- treat CHF
- treat arrhythmias
- anticoagulation
- treat underlying cause if possible

Prognosis
- often unrecognized, and may be self-limited
- myocarditis treatment trial showed 5 yr mortality between 25-50%
- giant cell myocarditis, although rare can present with fulminant CHF and be rapidly fatal, with 5 yr mortality >80%
- sudden death in young adults
- may progress to dilated cardiomyopathy

Dilated Cardiomyopathy

Definition
- unexplained dilation and impaired systolic function of one or both ventricles

Major Risks Factors for DCM
Alcohol, cocaine, family history

Etiology
- idiopathic (presumed viral or idiopathic) ~50% of DCM
- alcohol
- familial/genetic
- uncontrolled tachycardia (e.g. persistent rapid AFib)
- collagen vascular disease: SLE, polyarteritis nodosa, dermatomyositis, progressive systemic sclerosis
- infectious: viral (coxsackie B, HIV), Chagas disease, Lyme disease, Rickettsial diseases, acute rheumatic fever, toxoplasmosis
- neuromuscular disease: Duchenne muscular dystrophy, myotonic dystrophy, Friedreich's ataxia
- metabolic: uremia, nutritional deficiency (thiamine, selenium, carnitine)
- endocrine: hyper/hypothyroidism, DM, pheochromocytoma
- peripartum
- toxic: cocaine, heroin, organic solvents
- drugs: chemotherapies (doxorubicin, cyclophosphamide), anti-retrovirals, chloroquine, clozapine, TCA
- radiation

Abnormal Labs in DCM
- High BNP
- High Cr
- High LFTs
- Low bicarbonate
- Low Na$^+$

Signs and Symptoms
- may present as
  - CHF
  - systemic or pulmonary emboli
  - arrhythmias
  - sudden death (major cause of mortality due to fatal arrhythmia)

Investigations
- blood work: CBC, electrolytes, Cr, bicarbonate, BNP, CK, troponin, LFTs, TSH, TIBC
- ECG: variable ST-T wave abnormalities, poor R wave progression, conduction defects (e.g. BBB), arrhythmias (non-sustained VT)
- CXR: global cardiomegaly (globular heart), signs of CHF, pleural effusion
- echo: chamber enlargement, global hypokinesis, depressed LVEF, MR and TR, mural thrombi
- endomyocardial biopsy: not routine, used to rule out a treatable cause
- coronary angiography: in selected patients to exclude ischemic heart disease

Management
- treat underlying disease: e.g. abstinence from alcohol
- treat CHF: see *Heart Failure*, C34
- thromboembolism prophylaxis: anticoagulation with warfarin
  - indicated for: AFib, history of thromboembolism or documented thrombus
- treat symptomatic or serious arrhythmias
- immunize against influenza and S. pneumoniae
- consider surgical options (e.g. LVAD, transplant, volume reduction surgery) in appropriate candidates with severe, drug refractory disease
- consider ICD among patients with a LVEF <30%

Prognosis
- depends on etiology
- better with reversible underlying cause, worst with infiltrative diseases, HIV, drug-induced
- cause of death usually CHF (due to pump failure) or sudden death 2° to ventricular arrhythmias
- systemic emboli are significant source of morbidity
- 20% mortality in 1st yr, 10% per year after

Hypertrophic Cardiomyopathy

- see *2011 ACCF/AHA Guideline for the Diagnosis and Treatment of Hypertrophic Cardiomyopathy* for details

Definition
- defined as unexplained ventricular hypertrophy
- various patterns of HCM are classified, but most causes involve pattern of septal hypertrophy

Etiology and Pathophysiology
- histopathologic features include myocyte disarray, myocyte hypertrophy, and interstitial fibrosis
- cause is felt to be a genetic defect involving one of the cardiac sarcomeric proteins (>400 mutations associated with autosomal dominant inheritance, incomplete penetrance)
- prevalence of 1/500-1/1,000 in general population
- generally presents in early adulthood

Hemodynamic Classification
- hypertrophic obstructive cardiomyopathy (HOCM): dynamic LV outflow tract (LVOT) obstruction, either at rest or with provocation, defined as LVOT gradient of at least 30 mmHg
    - dynamic i.e. obstruction (and the murmur) is reduced with maneuvers that increase preload, and augmented with maneuvers that reduce preload
- non-obstructive HCM: no LVOT obstruction
- many patients have diastolic dysfunction (impaired ventricular filling secondary to LV hypertrophy which decreases compliance)

Signs and Symptoms
- clinical manifestations: asymptomatic (common, therefore screening is important), SOB on exertion, angina, presyncope/syncope (due to LV outflow obstruction or arrhythmia), CHF, arrhythmias, SCD
- pulses: rapid upstroke, "spike and dome" pattern in carotid pulse (in HCM with outflow tract obstruction)
- precordial palpation: PMI localized, sustained, double impulse, 'triple ripple' (triple apical impulse in HOCM), LV lift
- precordial auscultation: normal or paradoxically split S2, S4, harsh systolic diamond-shaped murmur at LLSB or apex, enhanced by squat to standing or Valsalva (murmur secondary to LVOT obstruction as compared to AS); often with pansystolic murmur due to mitral regurgitation

Investigations
- ECG/Holter monitor: LVH, high voltages across precordium, prominent Q waves (lead I, aVL, V5, V6), tall R wave in V1, P wave abnormalities
- transthoracic echocardiography and echo-Doppler study: asymmetric septal hypertrophy (less commonly apical), systolic anterior motion (SAM) of mitral valve and MR; LVOT gradient can be estimated by Doppler measurement
- genetic studies (± magnetic resonance imaging) can be helpful when echocardiography is inconclusive for diagnosis
- cardiac catheterization (only when patient being considered for invasive therapy)

Management
- avoid factors which increase obstruction (e.g. volume depletion)
    - avoidance of all competitive sports
- treatment of obstructive HCM
    - medical agents: β-blockers, disopyramide, verapamil (started only in monitored setting), phenylephrine (in setting of cardiogenic shock)
    - avoid nitrates, diuretics, and ACEI as they increase LVOT gradient and worsen symptoms
- patients with obstructive HCM and drug-refractory symptoms
    - surgical myectomy
    - alcohol septal ablation - percutaneous Intervention that ablates the hypertrophic septum with 100% ethanol via the septal artery
    - dual chamber pacing (rarely done)
- treatment of patients at high risk of sudden death : ICD
- first-degree relatives (children, siblings, parents) of patients with HCM should be screened (physical, ECG, 2D echo) every 12-18 mo during during adolescence, then serially every 5 yr during adulthood

Prognosis
- potential complications: AFib, VT, CHF, sudden cardiac death (1% risk/yr; most common cause of SCD in young athletes)
    - major risk factors for sudden death (consider ICD placement)
    - history of survived cardiac arrest/sustained VT
    - family history of multiple premature sudden deaths
    - other factors associated with increased risk of sudden cardiac death
        - syncope (presumed to be arrhythmic in origin)
        - non-sustained VT on ambulatory monitoring
        - marked ventricular hypertrophy (maximum wall thickness ≥30 mm)
        - abnormal BP in response to exercise (in patients <40 yr old with HCM)

RCM vs. Constrictive Pericarditis (CP)
Present similarly but CP is treatable with surgery

Restrictive Cardiomyopathy

Definition
- impaired ventricular filling with preserved systolic function in a non-dilated, non-hypertrophied ventricle secondary to factors that decrease myocardial compliance (fibrosis and/or infiltration)

Etiology
- infiltrative: amyloidosis, sarcoidosis
- non-infiltrative: scleroderma, idiopathic myocardial fibrosis
- storage diseases: hemochromatosis, Fabry's disease, Gaucher's disease, glycogen storage diseases
- endomyocardial
  - endomyocardial fibrosis, Loeffler's endocarditis, or eosinophilic endomyocardial disease
  - radiation heart disease
  - carcinoid syndrome (may have associated tricuspid valve or pulmonary valve dysfunction)

Clinical Manifestations
- CHF (usually with preserved LV systolic function), arrhythmias
- elevated JVP with prominent x and y descents, Kussmaul's sign
- S3, S4, MR, TR
- thromboembolic events

Investigations
- ECG: low voltage, non-specific, diffuse ST-T wave changes ± non-ischemic Q waves
- CXR: mild cardiac enlargement
- Echo: LAE, RAE; specific Doppler findings with no significant respiratory variation
- cardiac catheterization: increased end-diastolic ventricular pressures
- endomyocardial biopsy: to determine etiology (especially for infiltrative RCM)

Management
- exclude constrictive pericarditis
- treat underlying disease: control HR, anticoagulate if AFib
- supportive care and treatment for CHF, arrhythmias
- heart transplant: might be considered for CHF refractory to medical therapy

Prognosis
- depends on etiology

Valvular Heart Disease

- see *Guidelines on the Management of Valvular Heart Disease. JACC* Jun 10;63(22):2438-88 for details

Infective Endocarditis

- see <u>Infectious Diseases</u>, ID16
- American Heart Association (AHA) 2007 guidelines recommend IE prophylaxis
  - only for patients with
    - prosthetic valve material
    - past history of IE
    - certain types of congenital heart disease
    - cardiac transplant recipients who develop valvulopathy
  - only for the following procedures
    - dental
    - respiratory tract
    - procedures on infected skin/skin structures/MSK structures
    - not GI/GU procedures specifically

Rheumatic Fever

- see <u>Pediatrics</u>, P58

Prognosis

- acute complications: myocarditis (DCM/CHF), conduction abnormalities (sinus tachycardia, AFib), valvulitis (acute MR), acute pericarditis (not constrictive pericarditis)
- chronic complications: rheumatic valvular heart disease – fibrous thickening, adhesion, calcification of valve leaflets resulting in stenosis/regurgitation, increased risk of IE ± thromboembolism
- onset of symptoms usually after 10-20 yr latency from acute carditis of rheumatic fever
- mitral valve most commonly affected

Valve Repair and Valve Replacement

- indication for valve repair or replacement depends on the severity of the pathology; typically recommended when medical management has failed to adequately improve the symptoms or reduce the risk of morbidity and mortality
- pathologies that may require surgical intervention include congenital defects, infections, rheumatic heart disease as well as a variety of valve diseases associated with aging
- valve repair: balloon valvuloplasty, surgical valvuloplasty (commissurotomy, annuloplasty), chordae tendineae shortening, tissue patch
- valve replacement: typically for aortic or mitral valves only; mitral valve repair is favoured in younger individuals; percutaneous techniques being established

Choice of Valve Prosthesis

Table 15. Mechanical Valve vs. Bioprosthetic Valve

Mechanical Valve	Bioprosthetic Valve
Good durability	Limited long-term durability (mitral < aortic)
Less preferred in small aortic root sizes	Good flow in small aortic root sizes
Increased risk of thromboembolism (1-3%/yr): requires long-term anticoagulation with coumadin	Decreased risk of thromboembolism: long-term anticoagulation not needed for aortic valves
Target INR Aortic valves: 2.0-3.0 (mean 2.5) Mitral valves: 2.5-3.5 (mean 3.0)	Some recommendation for limited anticoagulation for mitral valves
Increased risk of hemorrhage: 1-2%/yr	Decreased risk of hemorrhage

Mitral Valve Repair vs. Replacement for Severe Ischemic Mitral Regurgitation
NEJM 2014;370:23-32
Purpose: Ischemic mitral regurgitation is associated with significant mortality risk. The purpose of this study was to compare the effectiveness and safety of repairing versus replacing the mitral valve in patients with severe chronic ischemic mitral regurgitation.
Study Design: RCT with 251 patients with severe ischemic mitral regurgitation were randomly assigned to mitral valve repair or chordal-sparing replacement. The primary endpoint was the left ventricular end-systolic volume index (LVESVI) at 12 mo.
Results: There were no significant between-group differences in LVESVI, in the rate of major adverse cardiac or cerebrovascular events, in functional status, or in quality of life at 12 mo. The rate of moderate or severe mitral regurgitation recurrence at 12 mo was significantly higher in the repair group than in the replacement group (32.6% vs. 2.3%, respectively).
Conclusions: No significant difference in left ventricular reverse modelling or survival at 12 mo between patients who underwent mitral valve repair or replacement. Replacement provided more durable correction of mitral regurgitation, but there were no significant differences in clinical outcomes.

Summary of Valvular Disease

Table 16. Valvular Heart Disease

Aortic Stenosis (AS)

Etiology
Congenital (bicuspid, unicuspid valve), calcification (wear and tear), rheumatic disease

Definition
Normal aortic valve area = 3-4 cm²
Mild AS 1.5 to 3 cm²
Moderate AS 1.0 to 1.5 cm²
Severe AS <1.0 cm²
Critical AS <0.5 cm²

Pathophysiology
Outflow obstruction → increased EDP → concentric LVH → LV failure → CHF, subendocardial ischemia

Symptoms
Exertional angina, syncope, dyspnea, PND, orthopnea, peripheral edema

Physical Exam
Narrow pulse pressure, brachial-radial delay, pulsus parvus et tardus, sustained PMI
Auscultation: crescendo-decrescendo SEM radiating to R clavicle and carotid, musical quality at apex (Gallavardin phenomenon), S4, soft S2 with paradoxical splitting, S3 (late)

Investigations
ECG: LVH and strain, LBBB, LAE, AFib
CXR: post-stenotic aortic root dilatation, calcified valve, LVH, LAE, CHF
Echo: reduced valve area, pressure gradient, LVH, reduced LV function

Treatment
Asymptomatic: serial echos, avoid exertion
Symptomatic: avoid nitrates/arterial dilators and ACEI in severe AS
Surgery if: symptomatic or LV dysfunction

Surgical Options
Valve replacement: aortic rheumatic valve disease and trileaflet valve
– prior to pregnancy (if AS significant)
– balloon valvuloplasty (in very young)

Interventional Options
Percutaneous valve replacement (transfemoral or transapical approach) is an option in selected patients who are not considered good candidates for surgery

Aortic Regurgitation (AR)

Etiology
Supravalvular: aortic root disease (Marfan's, atherosclerosis and dissecting aneurysm, connective tissue disease)
Valvular: congenital (bicuspid aortic valve, large VSD), IE
Acute Onset: IE, aortic dissection, trauma, failed prosthetic valve

Pathophysiology
Volume overload → LV dilatation → increased SV, high sBP and low dBP → increased wall tension → pressure overload → LVH (low dBP → decreased coronary perfusion)

Symptoms
Usually only becomes symptomatic late in disease when LV failure develops
Dyspnea, orthopnea, PND, syncope, angina

Physical Exam
Waterhammer pulse, bisferiens pulse, femoral-brachial sBP >20 (Hill's test wide pulse pressure), hyperdynamic apex, displaced PMI, heaving apex
Auscultation: early decrescendo diastolic murmur at LLSB (cusp pathology) or RLSB (aortic root pathology), best heard sitting, leaning forward, on full expiration, soft S1, absent S2, S3 (late)

Investigations
ECG: LVH, LAE
CXR: LVH, LAE, aortic root dilatation
Echo/TTE: quantify AR, leaflet or aortic root anomalies
Cath: if >40 yr and surgical candidate – to assess for ischemic heart disease
Exercise testing: hypotension with exercise

Treatment
Asymptomatic: serial echos, afterload reduction (e.g. ACEI, nifedipine, hydralazine)
Symptomatic: avoid exertion, treat CHF
Surgery if: NYHA class III-IV CHF; LV dilatation and/or LVEF <50% with/without symptoms

Surgical Options
Valve replacement: most patients
Valve repair: very limited role
Aortic root replacement (Bentall procedure):
– when ascending aortic aneurysm present, valved conduit used

Mitral Stenosis (MS)

Etiology
Rheumatic disease most common cause, congenital (rare)

Definition
Severe MS is mitral valve area (MVA) <1.5 cm²

Pathophysiology
MS → fixed CO and LAE → increased LA pressure → pulmonary vascular resistance and CHF; worse with AFib (no atrial kick), tachycardia (decreased atrial emptying time) and pregnancy (increased preload)

Symptoms
SOB on exertion, orthopnea, fatigue, palpitations, peripheral edema, malar flush, pinched and blue facies (severe MS)

Physical Exam
AFib, no "a" wave on JVP, left parasternal lift, palpable diastolic thrill at apex
Auscultation: mid-diastolic rumble at apex, best heard with bell in left lateral decubitus position following exertion, loud S1, OS following loud P2 (heard best during expiration), long diastolic murmur and short A2-OS interval correlate with worse MS

Investigations
ECG: NSR/AFib, LAE (P mitrale), RVH, RAD
CXR: LAE, CHF, mitral valve calcification
Echo/TTE: shows restricted opening of mitral valve
Cath: indicated in concurrent CAD if >40 yr (male) or >50 yr (female)

Treatment
Avoid exertion, fever (increased LA pressure), treat AFib and CHF, increase diastolic filling time (β-blockers, digitalis)
Surgery if: NYHA class III-IV CHF and failure of medical therapy

Invasive Options
Percutaneous balloon valvuloplasty: young rheumatic pts and good leaflet morphology (can be determined by echo), asymptomatic pts with moderate-severe MS, pulmonary HTN
Contraindication: left atrial thrombus, moderate MR
Open Mitral Commissurotomy: if mild calcification + leaflet/chordal thickening
– restenosis in 50% pts in 8 yr
Valve replacement: indicated in moderate-severe calcification and severely scarred leaflets

Mitral Regurgitation (MR)

Etiology
Mitral valve prolapse, congenital cleft leaflets, LV dilatation/aneurysm (CHF, DCM, myocarditis), IE abscess, Marfan's syndrome, HOCM, acute MI, myxoma, mitral valve annulus calcification, chordae/papillary muscle trauma/ischemia/rupture (acute), rheumatic disease

Pathophysiology
Reduced CO → increased LV and LA pressure → LV and LA dilatation → CHF and pulmonary HTN

Symptoms
Dyspnea, PND, orthopnea, palpitations, peripheral edema

Physical Exam
Displaced hyperdynamic apex, left parasternal lift, apical thrill
Auscultation: holosystolic murmur at apex, radiating to axilla ± mid-diastolic rumble, loud S2 (if pulmonary HTN), S3

Investigations
ECG: LAE, left atrial delay (bifid P waves), ± LVH
CXR: LVH, LAE, pulmonary venous HTN
Echo: etiology and severity of MR, LV function, leaflets
Swan-Ganz Catheter: prominent LA "v" wave

Treatment
Asymptomatic: serial echos
Symptomatic: decrease preload (diuretics), decrease afterload (ACEI) for severe MR and poor surgical candidates; stabilize acute MR with vasodilators before surgery
Surgery if: acute MR with CHF, papillary muscle rupture, NYHA class III-IV CHF, AF, increasing LV size or worsening LV function, earlier surgery if valve repairable (>90% likelihood) and patient is low-risk for surgery

Surgical Options
Valve repair: >75% of pts with MR and myxomatous mitral valve prolapse – annuloplasty rings, leaflet repair, chordae transfers/shorten/replacement
Valve replacement: failure of repair, heavily calcified annulus
Advantage of repair: low rate of endocarditis, no anticoagulation, less chance of re-operation

© Anas Nader 2011

Table 16. Valvular Heart Disease (continued)

Tricuspid Stenosis (TS)

Etiology
Rheumatic disease, congenital, carcinoid syndrome, fibroelastosis; usually accompanied by MS

Pathophysiology
Increased RA pressure → right heart failure → decreased CO and fixed on exertion

Symptoms
Peripheral edema, fatigue, palpitations

Physical Exam
Prominent "a" waves in JVP, +ve abdominojugular reflux, Kussmaul's sign, diastolic rumble 4th left intercostal space

Investigations
ECG: RAE
CXR: dilatation of RA without pulmonary artery enlargement
Echo: diagnostic

Treatment
Preload reduction (diuretics), slow HR
Surgery if: only if other surgery required (e.g. mitral valve replacement)

Surgical Options
Valve Replacement:
– if severely diseased valve
– bioprosthesis preferred

Pulmonary Stenosis (PS)

Etiology
Usually congenital, rheumatic disease (rare), carcinoid syndrome

Pathophysiology
Increased RV pressure → RV hypertrophy → right heart failure

Symptoms
Chest pain, syncope, fatigue, peripheral edema

Physical Exam
Systolic murmur at 2nd left intercostal space accentuated by inspiration, pulmonary ejection click, right-sided S4

Investigations
ECG: RVH
CXR: prominent pulmonary arteries enlarged RV
Echo: diagnostic

Treatment
Balloon valvuloplasty if severe symptoms

Surgical Options
Percutaneous or open balloon valvuloplasty

Tricuspid Regurgitation (TR)

Etiology
RV dilatation, IE (particularly due to IV drug use), rheumatic disease, congenital (Ebstein anomaly), carcinoid

Pathophysiology
RV dilatation → TR further RV dilatation → right heart failure

Symptoms
Peripheral edema, fatigue, palpitations

Physical Exam
"cv" waves in JVP, +ve abdominojugular reflux, Kussmaul's sign, holosystolic murmur at LLSB accentuated by inspiration, left parasternal lift

Investigations
ECG: RAE, RVH, AFib
CXR: RAE, RV enlargement
Echo: diagnostic

Treatment
Preload reduction (diuretics)
Surgery if: only if other surgery required (e.g. mitral valve replacement)

Surgical Options
Annuloplasty (i.e. repair, rarely replacement)

Pulmonary Regurgitation (PR)

Etiology
Pulmonary HTN, IE, rheumatic disease, tetrology of Fallot (post-repair)

Pathophysiology
Increased RV volume → increased wall tension → RV hypertrophy → right heart failure

Symptoms
Chest pain, syncope, fatigue, peripheral edema

Physical Exam
Early diastolic murmur at LLSB, Graham Steell (diastolic) murmur 2nd and 3rd left intercostal space increasing with inspiration

Investigations
ECG: RVH
CXR: prominent pulmonary arteries if pulmonary HTN; enlarged RV
Echo: diagnostic

Treatment
Rarely requires treatment; valve replacement (rarely done)

Surgical Options
Pulmonary valve replacement

Mitral Valve Prolapse (MVP)

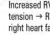

Etiology
Myxomatous degeneration of chordae, thick, bulky leaflets that crowd orifice, associated with Marfan's syndrome, pectus excavatum, straight back syndrome, other MSK abnormalities; <3% of population

Pathophysiology
Mitral valve displaced into LA during systole; no causal mechanisms found for symptoms

Symptoms
Prolonged, stabbing chest pain, dyspnea, anxiety/panic, palpitations, fatigue, presyncope

Physical Exam
Ausculation: mid-systolic click (due to billowing of mitral leaflet into LA; tensing of redundant valve tissue); mid to late systolic murmur at apex, accentuated by Valsalva or squat-to-stand maneuvers

Investigations
ECG: non-specific ST-T wave changes, paroxysmal SVT, ventricular ectopy
Echo: systolic displacement of thickened mitral valve leaflets into LA

Treatment
Asymptomatic: no treatment; reassurance
Symptomatic: β-blockers and avoidance of stimulants (caffeine) for significant palpitations, anticoagulation if AFib

Surgical Options
Mitral valve surgery (repair favoured over replacement) if symptomatic and significant MR

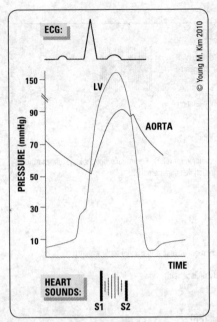

Figure 41. Hemodynamics of aortic stenosis
Stenosis across the aortic valve results in the generation of a significant pressure gradient between the left ventricle and the aorta and a crescendo-decrescendo murmur during systolic contraction. The stenosis decreases the intensity of aortic valve closure hence diminishing S2

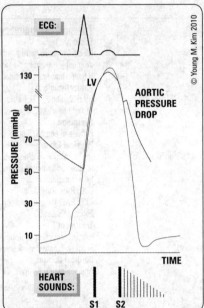

Figure 42. Hemodynamics of aortic regurgitation
Regurgitation across the aortic valve during diastole causes the aortic pressure to rapidly decrease and a decrescendo murmur can be heard at the onset of diastole (after S2 is audible). The presence of regurgitant blood from the aorta increases left-ventricular end-diastolic volume

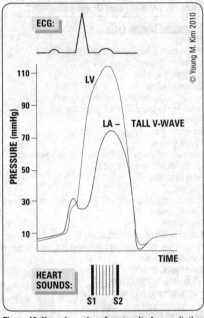

Figure 43. Hemodynamics of acute mitral regurgitation
During systolic contraction, blood regurgitates from the left ventricle into the left atrium across the incompetent mitral valve resulting in an audible holosystolic murmur between S1 and S2. The portion of left ventricular end diastolic volume that regurgitates into the left atrial myocardium increases left atrial pressures resulting in a tall V-wave (in the JVP)

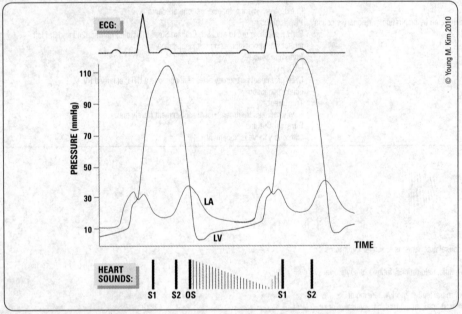

Figure 44. Hemodynamics of mitral stenosis
First note that the left atrial pressure exceeds the left ventricular pressure during diastole due to mitral stenosis and the consequent generation of a pressure gradient across the left atrium and left ventricle. In diastole the stenotic mitral valve opens which corresponds to the opening snap (OS) and the passage of blood across the mitral stenosis results in an audible decrescendo murmur. Left atrial contraction prior to S1 increases the pressure gradient resulting in accentuation of the murmur before S1 is audible

Pericardial Disease

Acute Pericarditis

Etiology of Pericarditis/Pericardial Effusion
- idiopathic is most common: presumed to be viral
- infectious
  - viral: Coxsackie virus A, B (most common), echovirus
  - bacterial: *S. pneumoniae, S. aureus*
  - TB
- fungal: histoplasmosis, blastomycosis
- post-MI: acute (direct extension of myocardial inflammation, 1-7 d post-MI), Dressler's syndrome (autoimmune reaction, 2-8 wk post-MI)
- post-cardiac surgery (e.g. CABG), other trauma
- metabolic: uremia (common), hypothyroidism
- neoplasm: Hodgkin's, breast, lung, renal cell carcinoma, melanoma
- collagen vascular disease: SLE, polyarteritis, rheumatoid arthritis, scleroderma
- vascular: dissecting aneurysm
- other: drugs (e.g. hydralazine), radiation, infiltrative disease (sarcoid)

Signs and Symptoms
- diagnostic triad: chest pain, friction rub and ECG changes (diffuse ST elevation and PR depression with reciprocal changes in aVR)
- pleuritic chest pain: alleviated by sitting up and leaning forward
- pericardial friction rub: may be uni-, bi-, or triphasic; evanescent and rare
- ± fever, malaise

Investigations
- ECG: initially diffuse elevated ST segments ± depressed PR segment, the elevation in the ST segment is concave upwards → 2-5 d later ST isoelectric with T wave flattening and inversion
- CXR: normal heart size, pulmonary infiltrates
- Echo: performed to assess for pericardial effusion

Acute Pericarditis Triad
- Chest pain
- Friction rub
- ECG changes

Treatment
- treat the underlying disease
- anti-inflammatory agents (high dose NSAIDs/ASA, steroids use controversial), analgesics
- colchicine reduces the rate of incessant/recurrent pericarditis (ICAP *N Engl J Med* 2013; 369:1522-1528)

Complications
- recurrent episodes of pericarditis, atrial arrhythmia, pericardial effusion, tamponade, constrictive pericarditis

Pericardial Effusion

Etiology
- transudative (serous)
- CHF, hypoalbuminemia/hypoproteinemia, hypothyroidism
- exudative (serosanguinous or bloody)
  - causes similar to the causes of acute pericarditis
  - may develop acute effusion secondary to hemopericardium (trauma, post-MI myocardial rupture, aortic dissection)
- physiologic consequences depend on type and volume of effusion, rate of effusion development, and underlying cardiac disease

Signs and Symptoms
- may be asymptomatic or similar to acute pericarditis
- dyspnea, cough
- extra-cardiac (esophageal/recurrent laryngeal nerve/tracheo-bronchial/phrenic nerve irritation)
- JVP increased with dominant "x" descent
- arterial pulse normal to decreased volume, decreased pulse pressure
- auscultation: distant heart sounds ± rub
- Ewart's sign

Ewart's Sign
Bronchial breathing and dullness to percussion at the lower angle of the left scapula in pericardial effusion due to effusion compressing left lower lobe of lung

Investigations
- ECG: low voltage , flat T waves, electrical alternans (classic, but not sensitive to exclude effusion)
  - be cautious in diagnosing STEMI in a patient with pericarditis and an effusion - antiplatelets may precipitate hemorrhagic effusion
- CXR: cardiomegaly, rounded cardiac contour
- ER: bedside ultrasound with subxiphoid view showing fluid in pericardial sac
- Echo (procedure of choice): fluid in pericardial sac
- pericardiocentesis: definitive method of determining transudate vs. exudate, identify infectious agents, neoplastic involvement

Treatment
- mild: frequent observation with serial echos, treat underlying cause, anti-inflammatory agents
- severe: treat as in tamponade (see *Cardiac Tamponade*)

Cardiac Tamponade

Etiology
- major complication of rapidly accumulating pericardial effusion
- cardiac tamponade is a clinical diagnosis
- any cause of pericarditis but especially trauma, malignancy, uremia, proximal aortic dissection with rupture

Pathophysiology
- high intra-pericardial pressure → decreased venous return → decreased diastolic ventricular filling → decreased CO → hypotension and venous congestion

Signs and Symptoms
- tachypnea, dyspnea, shock, muffled heart sounds
- pulsus paradoxus (inspiratory fall in systolic BP >10 mmHg during quiet breathing)
- JVP "x" descent only, blunted "y" descent
- hepatic congestion/peripheral edema

Investigations
- ECG: electrical alternans (pathognomonic variation in R wave amplitude), low voltage
- echo: pericardial effusion, compression of cardiac chambers (RA and RV) in diastole
- cardiac catheterization

Treatment
- pericardiocentesis: Echo-guided
- pericardiotomy
- avoid diuretics and vasodilators (these decrease venous return to already under-filled RV → decrease LV preload → decrease CO)
- IV fluid may increase CO
- treat underlying cause

Constrictive Pericarditis

Etiology
- chronic pericarditis resulting in fibrosed, thickened, adherent, and/or calcified pericardium
- any cause of acute pericarditis may result in chronic pericarditis
- major causes are idiopathic, post-infectious (viral, TB), radiation, post-cardiac surgery, uremia, MI, collagen vascular disease

Signs and Symptoms
- dyspnea, fatigue, palpitations
- abdominal pain
- may mimic CHF (especially right-sided HF)
  - ascites, hepatosplenomegaly, edema
- increased JVP, Kussmaul's sign (paradoxical increase in JVP with inspiration), Friedreich's sign (prominent "y" descent)
- BP usually normal (and usually no pulsus paradoxus)
- precordial examination: ± pericardial knock (early diastolic sound)
- see Table 17 for differentiation from cardiac tamponade

Investigations
- ECG: non-specific – low voltage, flat T wave, ± AFib
- CXR: pericardial calcification, effusions
- echo/CT/MRI: pericardial thickening, ± characteristic echo-Doppler findings
- cardiac catheterization: equalization of end-diastolic chamber pressures (diagnostic)

Treatment
- medical: diuretics, salt restriction
- surgical: pericardiectomy (only if refractory to medical therapy)
- prognosis best with idiopathic or infectious cause and worst in post-radiation; death may result from heart failure

Classic Quartet of Tamponade
- Hypotension
- Increased JVP
- Tachycardia
- Pulsus paradoxus

Beck's Triad
- Hypotension
- Increased JVP
- Muffled heart sounds

DDx Pulsus Paradoxus
- Constrictive pericarditis (rarely)
- Severe obstructive pulmonary disease (e.g. asthma)
- Tension pneumothorax
- PE
- Cardiogenic shock
- Cardiac tamponade

Table 17. Differentiation of Constrictive Pericarditis vs. Cardiac Tamponade

Characteristic	Constrictive Pericarditis	Cardiac Tamponade
JVP	"y" > "x"	"x" > "y"
Kussmaul's sign	Present	Absent
Pulsus paradoxus	Uncommon	Always
Pericardial knock	Present	Absent
Hypotension	Variable	Severe

Common Medications

Table 18. Commonly Used Cardiac Therapeutics

Drug Class	Examples	Mechanism of Action	Indications	Side Effects	Contraindications
ANGIOTENSIN CONVERTING ENZYME INHIBITORS (ACEI)					
	enalapril (Vasotec®), perindopril (Coversyl®), ramipril (Altace®), lisinopril (Zestril®)	Inhibit ACE-mediated conversion of angiotensin I to angiotensin II (AT II), causing peripheral vasodilation and decreased aldosterone synthesis	HTN, CAD, CHF, post-MI, DM	Dry cough, 10% hypotension, fatigue, hyperkalemia, renal insufficiency, angioedema	Bilateral renal artery stenosis, pregnancy, caution in decreased GFR
ANGIOTENSIN II RECEPTOR BLOCKERS (ARBs)					
	candesartan, irbesartan, valsartan	Block AT II receptors, causing similar effects to ACEI	Same as ACEI, although evidence is generally less for ARBs; often used when ACEI are not tolerated	Similar to ACEI, but do not cause dry cough	Same as ACEI
DIRECT RENIN INHIBITORS (DRIs)					
	aliskiren	Directly blocks renin thus inhibiting the conversion of angiotensinogen to angiotensin I; this also causes a decrease in AT II	HTN (exact role of this drug remains unclear)	Diarrhea, hyperkalemia (higher risk if used with an ACEI), rash, cough, angioedema, reflux, hypotension, rhabdomyolysis, seizure	Pregnancy, severe renal impairment
β-BLOCKERS					
β1 antagonists β1/β2 antagonists α1/β1/β2 antagonists β1 antagonists with intrinsic sympathomimetic activity	atenolol, metoprolol, bisoprolol propranolol labetalol, carvedilol acebutalol	Block β-adrenergic receptors, decreasing HR, BP, contractility, and myocardial oxygen demand, slow conduction through the AV node	HTN, CAD, acute MI, post-MI, CHF (start low and go slow), AFib, SVT	Hypotension, fatigue, light-headedness, depression, bradycardia, hyperkalemia, bronchospasm, impotence, depression of counterregulatory response to hypoglycemia, exacerbation of Raynaud's phenomenon, and claudication	Sinus bradycardia, 2nd or 3rd degree heart block, hypotension, WPW Caution in asthma, claudication, Raynaud's phenomenon, and decompensated CHF
CALCIUM CHANNEL BLOCKERS (CCBs)					
Benzothiazepines Phenylalkylamines (non-dihydropyridines)	diltiazem verapamil	Block smooth muscle and myocardial calcium channels causing effects similar to β-blockers Also vasodilate	HTN, CAD, SVT, diastolic dysfunction	Hypotension, bradycardia, edema Negative inotrope	Sinus bradycardia, 2nd or 3rd degree heart block, hypotension, WPW, CHF
Dihydropyridines	amlodipine (Norvasc®), nifedipine (Adalat®), felodipine (Plendil®)	Block smooth muscle calcium channels causing peripheral vasodilation	HTN, CAD	Hypotension, edema, flushing, headache, light-headedness	Severe aortic stenosis and liver failure
DIURETICS					
Thiazides	hydrochlorthiazide, chlorthalidone, metolazone	Reduce Na+ reabsorption in the distal convoluted tubule (DCT)	HTN (drugs of choice for uncomplicated HTN)	Hypotension, hypokalemia, polyuria	Sulfa allergy, pregnancy
Loop diuretics	furosemide (Lasix®)	Blocks Na+/K+-ATPase in thick ascending limb of the loop of Henle	CHF, pulmonary or peripheral edema	Hypovolemia, hypokalemic metabolic alkalosis	Hypovolemia, hypokalemia
Aldosterone receptor antagonists	spironolactone, eplenerone	Antagonize aldosterone receptors	HTN, CHF, hypokalemia	Edema, hyperkalemia, gynecomastia	Renal insufficiency, hyperkalemia, pregnancy
INOTROPES					
	digoxin (Lanoxin®)	Inhibit Na+/K+-ATPase, leading to increased intracellular Na+ and Ca2+ concentration and increased myocardial contractility Also slows conduction through the AV node	CHF, AFib	AV block, tachyarrhythmias, bradyarrhythmias, blurred or yellow vision (van Gogh syndrome), anorexia, N/V	2nd or 3rd degree AV block, hypokalemia, WPW

Table 18. Commonly Used Cardiac Therapeutics (continued)

Drug Class	Examples	Mechanism of Action	Indications	Side Effects	Contraindications
ANTICOAGULANTS					
Coumarins	warfarin (Coumadin®)	Antagonizes vitamin K, leading to decreased synthesis of clotting factors II, VII, IX, and X	AFib, LV dysfunction, prosthetic valves	Bleeding (by far the most important side effect), paradoxical thrombosis, skin necrosis	Recent surgery or bleeding, bleeding diathesis, pregnancy
Heparins	Unfractionated heparin LMWHs: dalteparin, enoxaparin, tinzaparin	Antithrombin III agonist, leading to decreased clotting factor activity	Acute MI/ACS; when immediate anticoagulant effect needed	Bleeding, osteoporosis, heparin-induced thrombocytopenia (less in LMWHs)	Recent surgery or bleeding, bleeding diathesis, thrombocytopenia, renal insufficiency (for LMWHs)
Direct thrombin inhibitors	dabigatran, melagatran	Competitive, direct thrombin inhibitor; thrombin enables fibrinogen conversion to fibrin during the coagulation cascade, thereby preventing thrombus development	AFib	Bleeding, GI upset	Severe renal impairment, recent surgery, active bleeding
Direct Factor Xa inhibitors	rivaroxaban apixaban edoxaban	Direct, selective and reversible inhibition of factor Xa in both the intrinsic and extrinsic coagulation pathways	AFib	Bleeding, GI upset, elevated liver enzymes	Hepatic disease, active bleeding, bleeding diathesis, pregnancy, lactation
ANTIPLATELETS					
Salicylates	ASA (Aspirin®)	Irreversibly acetylates platelet COX-1, preventing thromboxane A2-mediated platelet aggregation	CAD, acute MI, post-MI, post-PCI, CABG	Bleeding, GI upset, GI ulceration, impaired renal perfusion	Active bleeding or PUD
Thienopyridines	clopidogrel (Plavix®), ticlopidine (Ticlid®) prasugrel (Effient®)	P2Y12 antagonist (block platelet ADP receptors	Acute MI, post-MI, post-PCI, CABG	Bleeding, thrombotic thrombocytopenic purpura, neutropenia (ticlopidine)	Active bleeding or PUD
Nucleoside analogues	ticagrelor (Brillinta®)	P2Y12 antagonist (but different binding site than thienopyridines)			
GPIIb/IIIa inhibitors	eptifibatide, tirofiban, abciximab	Block binding of fibrinogen to Gp IIb/IIIa	Acute MI, particularly if PCI is planned	Bleeding	Recent surgery or bleeding, bleeding diathesis
THROMBOLYTICS					
	alteplase, reteplase, tenecteplase, streptokinase	Convert circulating plasminogen to plasmin, which lyses cross-linked fibrin	Acute STEMI	Bleeding	See Table 8, C29
NITRATES					
	nitroglycerin	Relax vascular smooth muscle, producing venous and arteriolar dilation	CAD, MI, CHF (isosorbide dinitrate plus hydralazine)	Headache, dizziness, weakness, postural hypotension	Concurrent use of cGMP phosphodiesterase inhibitors, angle closure glaucoma, increased intracranial pressure
LIPID LOWERING AGENTS					
Statins	atorvastatin (Lipitor®), pravastatin (Pravachol®), rosuvastatin (Crestor®), simvastatin (Zocor®), lovastatin (Meracor®)	Inhibit HMG-CoA reductase, which catalyzes the rate-limiting step in cholesterol synthesis	Dyslipidemia (1° prevention of CAD), CAD, post-MI (2° prevention of CV events)	Myalgia, rhabdomyolysis, abdominal pain	Liver or muscle disease
Cholesterol absorption inhibitor	ezetimibe (Ezetrol®)	inhibits gut absorption of cholesterol	Decreases LDL but does not reduce mortality	Myalgia, rhabdomyolysis, abdominal pain	Liver or renal impairment
Miscellaneous	fibrates, bile acid sequestrates, nicotinic acid		Primarily in familial hypercholesterolemia	GI side effects common	
Investigational	PSCK9 inhibitor	monoclonal antibody	hypercholesterolemia		

Antiarrhythmics

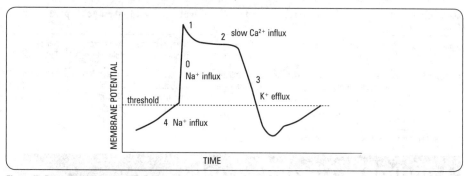

Figure 45. Representative cardiac action potential

Table 19. Antiarrhythmic* Drugs (Vaughan-Williams Classification)

Class	Agent	Indications	Side Effects	Mechanism of Action
Ia	quinidine procainamide disopyramide	SVT, VT	Torsades de Pointes (all Ia), diarrhea Lupus-like syndrome Anticholinergic effects	Moderate Na^+ channel blockade Slows phase 0 upstroke Prolongs repolarization, slowing conduction
Ib	lidocaine mexiletine	VT	Confusion, stupor, seizures GI upset, tremor	Mild Na^+ channel blockade Shortens phase 3 repolarization
Ic	propafenone flecainide encainide	SVT, VT AFib	Exacerbation of VT (all Ic) Negative inotropy (all Ic) Bradycardia and heart block (all Ic)	Marked Na^+ channel blockade Markedly slows phase 0 upstroke
II	propranolol metoprolol, etc.	SVT, AFib	Bronchospasm, negative inotropy, bradycardia, AV block, impotence, fatigue	β-blocker Decreases phase 4 depolarization
III	amiodarone** sotalol	SVT, VT AFib SVT, VT, AFib	Amiodarone: Photosensitivity, pulmonary toxicity, hepatotoxicity, thyroid disease, increased INR Amiodarone and Sotalol: Torsades de Pointes, bradycardia, heart block, β-blocker side effects	Blocks K^+ channel Prolongs phase 3 repolarization, which prolongs refractory period
IV	verapamil diltiazem	SVT AFib	Bradycardia, AV block Hypotension	Calcium channel blocker Slows phase 4 spontaneous depolarization, slowing AV node conduction

*All antiarrhythmics have potential to be proarrhythmic   **Amiodarone has class I, II, III, and IV properties

Table 20. Actions of α and β Adrenergic Receptors

	α RECEPTORS		β RECEPTORS	
Target System	α1	α2	β1	β2
Cardiovascular	Constriction of vascular smooth muscle Constriction of skin, skeletal muscle, and splanchnic vessels	Same as α1	Increased myocardial contractility Accelerate SA node Accelerate ectopic pacemakers	Decreased vascular smooth muscle tone
	Increased myocardial contractility Decreased heart rate	Peripherally act to modulate vessel tone Vasoconstrict and dilate; oppose α1 vasoconstrictor activity		
Respiratory				Bronchodilation
Dermal	Pilomotor smooth muscle contraction Apocrine constriction			
Ocular	Radial muscle contraction		Ciliary muscle relaxation	
Gastrointestinal	Inhibition of myenteric plexus Anal sphincter contraction			
Genitourinary	Pregnant uterine contraction Penile and seminal vesicle ejaculation Urinary bladder contraction	Smooth muscle wall relaxation	Stimulation of renal renin release	Bladder wall relaxation Uterine relaxation
Metabolic	Stimulate liver gluconeogenesis and glycogenolysis at the liver	Same as α1 Fat cell lipolysis	Fat cell lipolysis Glycogenolysis	Gluconeogenesis Fat cell lipolysis

Adapted from the Family Practice Notebook (www.fpnotebook.com/NEU194.htm)

Table 21. Commonly Used Drugs that Act on α and β Adrenergic Receptors

Mechanism of Action	α RECEPTORS			β RECEPTORS		
	α1	α1 and α2	α2	β1	β1 and β2	β2
Agonist	Phenylephrine Methoxamine	Epinephrine Norepinephrine	Clonidine Methyldopa	Norepinephrine Dobutamine	Isoproterenol Epinephrine	Albuterol Terbutaline
Antagonist	Prazosin Phenoxybenzamine	Phentolamine	Yohimbine Mirtazipine	Metoprolol Acebutolol Alprenolol Atenolol Esmolol	Propranolol Timolol Nadolol Pindolol Carvedilol	Butoxamine

Adapted from the Family Practice Notebook (http://www.fpnotebook.com/NEU194.htm)

Landmark Cardiac Trials

Trial	Reference	Results
ISCHEMIC HEART DISEASE		
ASCOT-LLA	*Lancet* 2003; 361:1149-58	In hypertensive patients with risk factors for CHD and average or below-average cholesterol, atorvastatin reduced nonfatal MI, fatal CHD, fatal/nonfatal stroke, coronary events but not all-cause mortality
CAPRIE	*Lancet* 1996; 348:1329-39	In atherosclerotic vascular disease clopidogrel reduced the primary combined endpoint of stroke, MI, or vascular death and improved PAD compared to ASA
CARE	*NEJM* 1996; 335:1001-9	Pravastatin reduced MI and stroke in patients with previous MI and average cholesterol
COURAGE	*NEJM* 2007; 356:1503-16	Compared with optimal medical therapy alone PCI + medical therapy did not reduce all-cause mortality and non fatal MI, and it did not reduce the incidence of major cardiovascular events
CURE	*NEJM* 2001; 345:494-502	Clopidogrel plus ASA reduced death from CV causes, non fatal MI, or stroke but increased bleeding complications
EUROPA	*Lancet* 2003; 362:782-88	With stable CAD and no CHF perindopril reduced cardiovascular death, MI, and total mortality
HOPE	*NEJM* 2000; 342:154-60	In high-risk patients without low LVEF or CHF ramipril reduced rates of death, MI, stroke, revascularization, new diagnosis of DM and complications due to DM; vitamin E had no effect on outcomes
HPS	*Lancet* 2002; 360:7-22	In high-risk patients with various cholesterol values simvastatin reduced all-cause mortality, coronary deaths, and major vascular events
INTERHEART	*Lancet* 2004; 364:937-52	Nine modifiable risk factors account for 90% of myocardial infarction
IMPROVE-IT	*N Engl J Med* 2015 Jun 3. [Epub ahead of print]	Ezetimibe added to statin reduces mortality in ACS patients
JUPITER	*NEJM* 2008; 359:2195-2207	With low to normal LDL-C and elevated hsCRP treatment with rosuvastatin significantly reduced major cardiovascular events; NNT with rosuvastatin for 2 yr to prevent one primary endpoint = 95
SYNTAX	*NEJM* 2009; 360:961-972	CABG has lower rate of major cardiac or cerebrovascular events; the rate of stroke was increased with CABG, whereas the rate of repeat revascularization was increased with PCI
TNT	*NEJM* 2005; 352:1425-35	Lipid-lowering therapy with atorvastatin 80 mg/d in patients with stable CHD provides clinical benefit beyond atorvastatin 10 mg/d
WHI	*JAMA* 2002; 288:321-333	Estrogen plus progestin therapy is associated with increased risks of cardiovascular disease and breast cancer but decreased risks of hip fracture and colorectal cancer in postmenopausal women
MYOCARDIAL INFARCTION		
BHAT	*JAMA* 1982; 247:1707-14	In acute MI propranolol reduced all-cause mortality, cardiovascular death, and sudden death from atherosclerotic heart disease
COURAGE	*NEJM* 2007; 356:1503-16	Compared with optimal medical therapy alone PCI + medical therapy did not reduce all-cause mortality and non fatal MI, and it did not reduce the incidence of major cardiovascular events
DAPT	*NEJM* 2014; 371: 2155-66	Dual antiplatelet therapy beyond one year confers additional benefit

Trial	Reference	Results
MYOCARDIAL INFARCTION		
ISIS-2	*Lancet* 1988; 2:349-60	Early therapy with streptokinase and ASA in patients with MI individually and in combination significantly reduced all-cause mortality and in combination demonstrated additive effect
ISIS-4	*Lancet* 1995; 345:669-85	In patients with suspected or definite acute MI early treatment with captopril reduced all-cause mortality at 35 d and during long-term follow up
OASIS-5	*NEJM* 2006; 354:1464-76	Compared to enoxaparin, fondaparinux reduced mortality rates, major bleeds at 9 and MI at 30 and 180 d
PEGASUS-TIMI 54	*NEJM* 2015 EPUB	Ticagrelor on top of ASA reduces CV events and in patients with a history of MI
PLATO	*NEJM* 2009: 361:1045-57	ACS patients with either STEMI or NSTEMI, regardless of reperfusion strategy, ticagrelor reduced mortality, MI and stroke without increased bleeding compared to clopidogrel
PROVE IT – TIMI 22	*NEJM* 2004; 350:1495-1504	In patients hospitalized for ACS high-dose atorvastatin reduced all-cause mortality, MI, unstable angina, revascularization, and stroke compared with pravastatin
TRITON-TIMI 38	*NEJM* 2007; 357:2001-15	In ACS patients scheduled for PCI, prasugrel reduced ischemic events but increased major bleeding compared to clopidogrel; no change in mortality
HEART FAILURE		
AIRE	*Lancet* 1993; 342:821-8	Ramipril commenced 3-10 d after MI and continued for a mean 15-month period significantly reduced all-cause mortality in patients with non-severe CHF
CHARM	*Lancet* 2003; 362:759-66	Candesartan reduced overall mortality, cardiovascular death, and CHF hospitalizations
CIBIS II	*Lancet* 1999; 353:9-13	Bisoprolol reduced all-cause mortality, cardiovascular death, all-cause hospitalization, and CHF hospitalization
COMET	*Lancet* 2003; 362:7-13	Carvedilol was associated with a reduction in all cause mortality compared with metoprolol
CONSENSUS	*NEJM* 1987; 316:1429-35	Enalapril reduced all-cause mortality, death due to progression of heart failure
COPERNICUS	*NEJM* 2001; 344:1651-8	Carvedilol in addition to standard treatment significantly reduced the risk of death or hospitalization in patients with severe CHF
I-PRESERVE	*NEJM* 2008; 359:2456-2467	In patients with CHF and normal LVEF treatment with ARB (irbesartan) did not improve mortality or cardiovascular morbidity compared to placebo
MERIT-HF	*Lancet* 1999; 353:2001-7	Metoprolol CR/XL daily in addition to optimum standard therapy improved survival in clinically stable patients equating to prevention of 1 death per 27 patients treated per year
PARADIGM-HF	*NEJM* 2014; 371:993-1004	Novel drug (LCZ696 containing valsartan and a neprilysin inhibitor (prevents degradation of natriuretic peptides) reduces hospitalization and mortality
RALES	*NEJM* 1999; 341:709-17	In severe CHF (class III/IV) and LVEF <35% spironolactone reduced all-cause mortality, sudden death, and death due to progression of heart failure
SAVE	*NEJM* 1992; 327:669-77	Patients with LV dysfunction post-MI long-term captopril over 3.5 yr reduced the risk of death due to cardiovascular causes, recurrent MI, development of severe CHF, and CHF hospitalization
SCD-HeFT	*NEJM* 2005; 352:225-237	In mild-to-moderate CHF shock-only ICD significantly reduces risk of death; amiodarone had no benefit compared with placebo in treating patients with mild-to-moderate CHF
SOLVD	*NEJM* 1991; 325:293-302	In stable chronic CHF with decreased LVEF (<0.35) long-term enalapril reduced death due to all causes and death or hospitalization due to CHF
TRACE	*NEJM* 1995; 333:1670-6	In patients with LV dysfunction post-MI long-term trandolapril reduced the risk of death or progression to severe CHF and reduced risk of sudden death
V-HeFT II	*NEJM* 1991; 325:303-10	In chronic CHF enalapril reduced mortality more than hydralazine-isosorbide for at least 2 yr; treatment with either enalapril or hydralazine-isosorbide increased LVEF
DIABETES		
CARDS	*Lancet* 2004; 264:685-96	Atorvastatin reduces the risk of cardiovascular events in patients with type 2 DM
ONTARGET	*NEJM* 2008; 358:1547-59	In patients with vascular disease or DM without CHF telmisartan is equally as effective as ramipril, with telmisartan causing a reduced risk of cough and angioedema, and an increased risk of hypotensive symptoms; combination therapy offers no advantage

Trial	Reference	Results
ARRHYTHMIA		
AFFIRM	*NEJM* 2002; 347:1825-33	No significant difference in mortality rates between rate or rhythm control of AFib
AF-CHF	*NEJM* 2008; 358:2667-77	In patients with AFib and CHF there is no significant difference in mortality rates from cardiovascular causes between rate and rhythm control
ARISTOTLE	*NEJM* 2011: 365:981-92	AF patients treated with apixaban had a lower incidence of stroke, major bleeding and mortality compared to warfarin
ENGAGE AF-TIMI48	*NEJM* 2013: 369:2093-2104	AF patients treated with edoxaban had similar rates of stroke and lower rates of major bleeding compared to warfarin
RE-LY	*NEJM* 2009: 361:1139-51	AF patients treated with dabigatran had a lower incidence of stroke compared to warfarin, with similar rates of major bleeding
ROCKET-AF	*NEJM* 2011; 365:883-891	In patients with AFib rivoxabarin is non-inferior to warfarin for stroke prevention, and major and non-major bleeding
HYPERTENSION		
HYVET	*NEJM* 2008; 358:1887-98	In hypertensive patients >80 yr treatment with indapamide, with or without perindopril, showed a trend towards reduced relative risk of fatal or non-fatal stroke
SIPLICITY-HTN 3	*NEJM* 2014: 370:1393-1401	Renal denervation does not reduce blood pressure in patients with resistant hypertension compared to sham procedure
SPRINT	*NEJM* 2015: 373:2103-2116	In patients with high risk of cardiovascular events excluding diabetes, strict systolic BP control (<120 mmHg) is associated with fewer cardiovascular events and lower all-cause mortality
UKHDS (UKPDS)	*BMJ* 1998; 317:703-13	Hypertensive patients with DM and tight BP control at <150/85 mmHg by use of ACEI or β-blocker reduced risk of diabetic complications and death related to DM and reduced risk of end-organ damage
VALUE	*Lancet* 2004; 363:2022-2031	Valsartan group had higher incidence of MI than amlodipine group, whereas amlodipine had a higher incidence of new-onset DM

References

Ischemic Heart Disease
Cannon CP, Braunwald E, McCabe CH, et al. Intensive versus moderate lipid lowering with statins after acute coronary syndromes. NEJM 2004;350:1495-504.
Lindahl B, Toss H, Siegbahn A, et al. Markers of myocardial damage and inflammation in relation to long-term mortality in unstable coronary artery disease. NEJM 2000;343:1139-1147.
Pitt B, Remme W, Zannad F, et al. Eplerenone, a selective aldosterone blocker, in patients with left ventricular dysfunction after myocardial infarction. NEJM 2003;348:1309-1321.
Rauch U, Osende JI, Fuster V, et al. Thrombus formation on the atherosclerotic plaques: pathogenesis and clinical consequences. Ann Intern Med 2001;134:224-238.
Spinler S, Rees C. Review of prasugrel for the secondary prevention of atherothrombosis. J Manag Care Pharm 2009;15:383-95.
The Arterial Revascularization Therapies Study Group. Comparison of coronary-artery bypass surgery and stenting for the treatment of multivessel disease. NEJM 2001;344:1117-1124.
Turpie AGG, Antman EM. Low-molecular-weight heparins in the treatment of acute coronary syndromes. Arch Intern Med 2001;161:1484-1490.
Yeghiazarians Y, Braunstein JB, Askari A, et al. Review article: unstable angina pectoris. NEJM 2000;342:101-114.

Cardiomyopathies
Feldman AM, McNamara D. Myocarditis (review). NEJM 2000;343:1388-1398.

Guidelines
2013 ACCF/AHA guideline for the management of ST-elevation myocardial infarction. JACC 2013; 61:e78-140.
2012 ACCF/AHA/ACP/AATS/PCNA/SCAI/STS Guideline for the diagnosis and management of patients with stable ischemic heart disease. JACC 2012;60:e44-e164.
ACC/AHA guidelines for percutaneous coronary intervention. Circulation 2001;103:3019-3041.
ACC/AHA 2002 guideline update for the management of patients with unstable angina and non-ST-segment elevation myocardial infarction. Available from: http://www.acc.org.
ACCF/AHA 2009 focused update on the guidelines for the diagnosis and management of heart failure in adults. Circulation 2009;119:1977-2016.
ACC/AHA guidelines for the management of patients with ST-elevation myocardial infarction: a report of the American College of Cardiology/American Heart Association Task Force on Practice Guidelines (Committee to Revise the 1999 Guidelines for the Management of Patients with Acute Myocardial Infarction). Circulation 2004;110:e82-292.
American College of Cardiology (clinical guidelines, etc). Available from: http://www.acc.org.
Antman EM, Anbe DT, Armstrong PW, et al. ACC/AHA guidelines for the management of patients with ST-elevation myocardial Infarction – summary: a report of the American College of Canadian Cardiovascular Society (CCS) mobile guidelines. Available from: http://www.ccs.ca/mobile.Free.
Aurigemma GP, Gaasch WH. Clinical practice, diastolic heart failure. NEJM 2004;351:1097.
Beard JD. Chronic lower limb ischemia. BMJ 2000;320:854-857.
Canadian Cardiovascular Society 2005 Consensus Conference Peripheral Arterial Disease (Draft). Available from: http:// www.ccs.ca.
Cardiology. American Heart Association Task Force on practice guidelines. Circulation 2004;110-588.
Cardiology Online. Available from: http:// www.theheart.org.
CCS focused 2012 update of the CCS atrial fibrillation guidelines: recommendations for stroke prevention and rate/rhythm control. Can J Cardiol 2012;28:125-136.
CCS. The use of antiplatelet therapy in the outpatient setting: CCS guidelines. Can J Cardiol 2011;27:S1-S59.
CCS. 2012 heart failure management guidelines update: Focus on acute and chronic heart failure. Can J Cardiol 2013;29:168-181.
CCS. 2001 Canadian cardiovascular society consensus guideline update for the management and prevention of heart failure. Can J Cardiol 2001;17(suppE):5-24.
CCS 2000 Consensus Conference: Women and ischemic heart disease. Can J Cardiol 2000:17(suppl D).
Harrington RA, Becker RC, Ezekowitz M, et al. Antithrombotic therapy for coronary artery disease: the seventh ACCP conference on antithrombotic and thrombolytic therapy. Chest 2004;126(3 suppl):513s-584s.
Heart valve repair. Available from: http:// www.heartvalverepair.net.
May J, White GH, Harris JP. The complications and downside of endovascular therapies. Adv Surg 2001;35:153-172.
Rutherford RB. Vascular surgery, 4th ed. Toronto: WB Saunders, 1995. Chapter: Atherogenesis and the medical management of atherosclerosis. p222-234.
Schmieder FA, Comerota AJ. Intermittent claudication: magnitude of the problem, patient evaluation, and therapeutic strategies. Am J Card 2001;87(Suppl):3D-13D.
Simpson C, Dorian P, Gupta A, et al. Assessment of the cardiac patient for fitness to drive and fly: executive summary. Can J Cardiol 2004;20:1313-1323.
Task Force on the Diagnosis and Treatment of Peripheral Artery Diseases of the European Society of Cardiology (ESC). Eur Heart J 2011;32:2851-2906.
Thygesen K, Alpert JS, Jaffe AS, et al. Third universal definition of myocardial infarction. Eur Heart J 2012;33:2551-2567.
Way LW, Doherty GM (editors). Current surgical diagnosis and treatment, 11th ed. Lange Medical Books/McGraw-Hill, 2004.
Welsh RC, Travers A, Huynh T, et al. Canadian Cardiovascular Society Working Group: providing a perspective on the 2007 focused update of the ACC/AHA 2004 guidelines for the management of ST elevation myocardial infarction. Can J Cardiol 2009;25:25-32.
Yang SC, Cameron DE (editors). Current therapy in thoracic and cardiovascular medicine. McGraw-Hill, 2004.

Ambulatory ECG
Kadish AH, Buxton AE, Kennedy HL. ACC/AHA clinical competence statement on electrocardiography and ambulatory electrocardiography: a report of the ACC/AHA/ACP-ASIM task force on clinical competence. Circulation 2001;104:3169-3178.
Krahn A, Klein G, Skane A, et al. Insertable loop recorder use for detection of intermittent arrhythmias. Pacing and Clinical Electrophysiol 2004;27:657-564.
Zimetbaum P, Josephson M. The evolving role of ambulatory arrhythmia monitoring in general clinical practie. Ann Intern Med 1999;130:848-856.

Stress Testing
Gibbons RJ, Balady GJ, Beasley JW, et al. ACC/AHA Guidelines for Exercise Testing. A report of the American College of Cardiology/American Heart Association Task Force on Practice Guidelines (Committee on Exercise Testing). JACC 1997;30:260-315.

Echocardiography
Cheitlin M. ACC/AHA/ASE 2003 guideline update for the clinical application of echocardiograohy: summary article. J Am Soc Echocardiography 2003;16:1091-1110.
Gowda R, Khan I, Sacchi T, et al. History of the evolution of echocardiography. Int J Cardiol 2004;97:1-6.
Heatlie G, Giles M. Echocardiography and the general physician. Postgrad Med J 2004;80:84-88.
Picano E. Stress echocardiography: a historical perspective. AJM 2003;114:126-130.

Nuclear Cardiology
Beller G, Zaret B. Contributions of nuclear cardiology to diagnosis and prognosis of patients with coronary artery disease. Circulation 2000;101:1465-1478.
Lee TH, Boucher CA. Noninvasive tests in patients with stable coronary artery disease (review). NEJM 2000;344:1840-1845.
Sabharwal N, Lahiri A. Role of myocardial perfusion imaging for risk stratification in suspected or known coronary artery disease. Heart 2003;89:1291-1297.

MR
Danias P, Roussakis A, Ioannidis J. Cardiac imaging diagnostic performance of coronary magnetic resonance angiography as compared against conventional x-ray angiography: a meta-analysis. J Am Col Cardiol 2004;44:1867-1876.
Kim WY, Danias PG, Stuber M, et al. Coronary magnetic resonance angiography for the detection of coronary stenoses. NEJM 2001;345:1863-1869.

CT
Miller JM, Rochitte CE, Dewey M, et al. Diagnostic performance of coronary angiography by 64-row CT. NEJM 2008;359:2324-2336.
Schoepf J, Becker C, Ohnesorge B, et al. CT of coronary artery disease. Radiology 2004;232:18-37.
Somberg J. Arrhythmia therapy. Am J Therapeutics 2002;9:537-542.

Cath/EPS

Conti J. ACC 2005 Annual session highlight. Cardiac arrhythmias. J Am Coll Cardiol 2005;45:B30-B32.

Hayes D, Furman S. Cardiac pacing: how it started, where we are, where we are going. J Cardiovasc Electrophysiology 2004;15:619-627.

Keane D. New catheter ablation techniques for the treatment of cardiac arrhythmias. Card Electrophysiol Rev 2002;6:341-348.

Packer D. Evolution of mapping and anatomic imaging of cardiac arrhythmias. J Cardio Electrophysiol 2004;15:839-854.

Ryan TJ, Faxon DP, Gunnar RM, et al. Guidelines for percutaneous transluminal coronary angioplasty. A report of the American College of Cardiology/American Heart Association Task Force on assessment of diagnostic and therapeutic cardiovascular procedures (subcommittee on percutaneous transluminal coronary angioplasty). Circulation 1988;78:486-502.

Skanes A, Klein G, Krahn A, et al. Cryoablation: potentials and pitfalls. J Cardiovasc Electrophysiol 2004;15:528-534.

Wellens J. Cardiac arrhythmias: the quest for a cure. J Am Coll Cardiol 2004;44:1155-1163.

Zipes D. The year in electrophysiology. J Am Coll Cardiol 2004;43:1306-1324.

Zipes DP, DiMarco JP, Gillete PC, et al. ACC/AHA task force report guidelines for clinical intracardiac electrophysiological and catheter ablation procedures. JACC 1995;26:555-573.

Arrhythmias

Bernstein AD. The NASPE/BPEG pacemaker code. Tex Heart Inst J 1991;18:299-300.

Camm AJ, Kirchof P, Lip GYH, et al. Task Force for the Management of Atrial Fibrillation of the European Society of Cardiology (ESC). Guidelines for the management of atrial fibrillation. Eur Heart J 2010;31:2369-2429.

Gutierrez C, Blanchard DG. Atrial fibrillation: diagnosis and treatment. Am Fam Phys 2011;83:61-68.

Garcia TB, Miller GT. Arrhythmia Recognition: The Art of Interpretation. Sudbury: Jones & Bartlett, 2004.

Thijssen J, Borleffs CJ, van Rees JB, et al. Driving restrictions after implantable cardioverter defibrillator implantation: an evidence-based approach. Eur Heart J 2011;32:2678-2687.

Lip GYH, Nieuwlaat R, Pisters R, et al. Refining clinical risk stratification for predicting stroke and thromboembolism in atrial fibrillation using a novel risk factor-based approach: the Euro heart survey on atrial fibrillation. Chest 2010;137:263-72.

Patel MR, Mahaffey KW, Garg J, et al. Rivaroxaban versus warfarin in nonvalvular atrial fibrillation. NEJM 2011;365:883-891.

Prystowsky EN, Topol EJ, Califf RM, et al. (editors). Textbook of cardiovascular medicine, 3rd ed. Philadelphia: Lippincott Williams & Wilkins, 2007. Chapter: Electrophysiology and pacing.

Percutaneous Angiography/PCI

Baim D. New devices for percutaneous coronary intervention are rapidly making bypass surgery obsolete. Curr Opin Cardiol 2004;19:593-597.

Bashore TM, Bates ER, Berger PB, et al. ACC/SCA&I expert concensus document. American College of Cardiology/Society for Cardiac Angiography and Interventions Clinical Expert Consensus Document on Cardiac Catheterization Laboratory Standards. J Am Coll Cardiol 2001;37:2170-214.

Guidelines for percutaneous transluminal coronary angioplasty: a report of the American College of Cardiology/Am Heart Association Task Force on Assessment of Diagnostic and Therapeutic Cardiovascular Procedures Subcommittee on percutaneous transluminal coronary angioplasty. J Am Coll Cardiol 1988;12:529-545.

O'Neil W, Dixon S, Grines C. The year in interventional cardiology. J Am Coll Cardiol 2005;45:1117-1134.

Serruys PW, Morice MC, Kappetain AP, et al. Percutaneous coronary intervention versus coronary-artery bypass grafting for severe coronary artery disease. NEJM 2009;360:961-972.

Cardiovascular Surgery

Alexander P, Giangola G. Deep venous thrombosis and pulmonary embolism: diagnosis, prophylaxis, and treatment. Ann Vasc Surg 1999;13:318-327.

American College of Cardiology. Available from: http://www.acc.org.

Beard JD. Chronic lower limb ischemia. BMJ 2000;320:854-857.

Bojar RM. Manual of perioperative care in cardiac surgery, 3rd ed. Massachusetts: Blackwell Science, 1999.

Cardiology Online. Available from: http://www.theheart.org.

Cheng DCH, David TE. Perioperative care in cardiac anesthesia and surgery. Austin: Landes Bioscience, 1999.

Coulam CH, Rubin GD. Acute aortic abnormalities. Semin Roentgenol 2001;36:148-164.

Crawford ES, Crawford JL, Veith FJ, et al. (editors). Vascular surgery: principles and practice, 2nd ed. Toronto: McGraw-Hill, 1994. Chapter: Thoracoabdominal aortic aneurysm.

Fuchs JA, Rutherford RB (editors). Vascular surgery, 4th ed. Toronto: WB Saunders, 1995. Chapter: Atherogenesis and the medical management of atherosclerosis. p222-234.

Freischlag JA, Veith FJ, Hobson RW, et al. (editors). Vascular surgery: principles and practice, 2nd ed. Toronto: McGraw-Hill, 1994. Chapter: Abdominal aortic aneurysms.

Hallett JW Jr. Abdominal aortic aneurysm: natural history and treatment. Heart Dis Stroke 1992;1:303-308.

Hallett JW Jr. Management of abdominal aortic aneurysms. Mayo Clin Proc 2000;75:395-399.

Harlan BJ, Starr A, Harwin FM. Illustrated handbook of cardiac surgery. New York: Springer-Verlag, 1996.

Heart Valve Repair. Available from: http://www.heartvalverepair.net.

Hiratzka LF, Bakris GL, Beckman JA, et al. 2010 ACCF/AHA/AATS/ACR/ASA/SCA/SCAI/SIR/STS/SVM guidelines for the diagnosis and management of patients with thoracic aortic disease. J Am Coll Cardiol 2010;55:e27-e129.

May J, White GH, Harris JP. The complications and downside of endovascular therapies. Adv Surg 2001;35153-35172.

Pitt MPI, Bonser RS. The natural history of thoracic aortic aneurysm disease: an overview. J Card Surg 1997;12(Suppl):270-278.

Powell JT, Brown LC. The natural history of abdominal aortic aneurysms and their risk of rupture. Adv Surg 2001;35:173-185.

Rabi D, Clement F, McAlister F, et al. Effect of perioperative glucose-insulin-potassium infusions on mortality and atrial fibrillation after coronary artery bypass grafting: a systematic review and meta-analysis. Can J Cardiol 2010;26:178-184.

Rosen CL, Tracy JA. The diagnosis of lower extremity deep venous thrombosis. Em Med Clin N Am 2001;19:895-912.

Schmieder FA, Comerota AJ. Intermittent claudication: magnitude of the problem, patient evaluation, and therapeutic strategies. Am J Card 2001;87(Suppl):3D-13D.

Verma S, Szmitko PE, Weisel RD, et al. Clinician update: should radial arteries be used routinely for coronary artery bypass grafting? Circulation 2004;110:e40-e46.

Way LW, Doherty GM. Current surgical diagnosis and treatment, 11th ed. Lange Medical Books/McGraw-Hill, 2004.

Van Gelder, IC, Groenveld, HF, Crijns, HJ et al. Lenient versus strict rate control in patients with atrial fibrillation. NEJM;362:1363-1373

Yang SC, Cameron DE. Current therapy in thoracic and cardiovascular medicine. McGraw-Hill, 2004.

Clinical Pharmacology

Pamela Leung and **Teja Voruganti**, chapter editors
Narayan Chattergoon and **Desmond She**, associate editors
Arnav Agarwal and **Quynh Huynh**, EBM editors
Dr. David Juurlink, staff editor

Acronyms

ACE	angiotensin converting enzyme	CSF	cerebrospinal fluid	NDC	National Drug Code	RCT	randomized controlled trial
ACh	acetylcholine	CSFa	certain safety factor	NE	norepinephrine	TBW	total body water
ADR	adverse drug reaction	CYP	cytochrome P450 protein	Po/w	partition coefficient of a drug	TDM	therapeutic drug monitoring
ARB	angiotensin receptor blocker	DIN	drug identification number	PD	pharmacodynamics	TI	therapeutic index
BBB	blood brain barrier	F	bioavailability	PDE	phosphodiesterase	Vd	volume of distribution
Cl	clearance	GFR	glomerular filtration rate	Pgp	p-glycoprotein		
Cr	creatinine	HH	Henderson Hasselbalch	PK	pharmacokinetics		

General Principles

Drug Nomenclature

- **chemical name**: describes chemical structure; consistent in all countries (e.g. N-(4-hydroxyphenyl) acetamide is acetaminophen)
- **DIN or NDC**: DIN assigned by Health Canada; NDC assigned by FDA (US)
- **non-proprietary name**: approved name (post-phase III trial), official name (listed in pharmacopoeia), or generic name (off-patent) such as acetaminophen
- **proprietary (trade) name**: the brand name or registered trademark (e.g. Tylenol®)

Phases of Clinical Drug Testing

At the time of drug launch, only data from phases I-III are available; thus, effectiveness and safety may be unknown because real-world patients and usage patterns often differ from those in premarket phases

- **pre-clinical**: testing a drug in a controlled environment (lab) on animal or human cells before human testing to discern the PK and toxicological profile
- **phase I**: first administration to healthy human volunteers, following animal studies; to determine PK and PD
- **phase II**: first administration to patients, small sample sizes; to determine initial safety and efficacy, dose range, PK, and PD
- **phase III**: large sample sizes, often double-blinded RCT; comparative (new drug vs. placebo or standard of care) to establish safety and efficacy
- **phase IV**: post-marketing surveillance, wide distribution; to determine effects of long-term use, rare ADRs, ideal dosing, and effects in real-world practice

Drug Administration

- choice of route of administration depends on: drug properties, local and systemic effects, desired onset and/or duration of action, and patient characteristics

Common Latin Abbreviations

q	each, every
OD/bid/tid/qid	once/twice/three/four times a day
hs	at bedtime
ac/pc/cc	before/after/with meals
prn	as necessary
gtt	drops
ung	ointment
ud	as directed
od/os/ou	right/left/each eye
ad/as/au	right/left/each ear

Table 1. Routes of Drug Administration

Route	Advantage	Disadvantage
Oral (PO)	Convenient, easy to administer Large surface area for absorption Inexpensive relative to parenteral administration	Incomplete absorption Hepatic first-pass effect Potential GI irritation
Buccal/Sublingual (SL)	Rapid onset of action No hepatic first-pass effect	Must be lipid-soluble, non-irritating Short duration of action
Rectal (PR)	Almost no hepatic first-pass effect Use when NPO, vomiting, or unconscious	Inconvenient, irritation at site of application Erratic absorption
Intravenous (IV)	No hepatic first-pass effect Slow infusion or rapid onset of action Easy to titrate dose	Hard to remove once administered Risk of infection, bleeding, vascular injury extravasation Expensive
Intramuscular (IM)	Depot storage if oil-based = slow release of drug Aqueous solution = rapid onset of action	Pain/hematoma at site of injection
Subcutaneous (SC)	Non-irritating drugs, small volumes Constant, even absorption Alternative to IV	Pain at site of injection Smaller volumes than IM May have tissue damage from multiple injections
Intrathecal	Direct into CSF Bypass BBB and blood-CSF barrier	Risk of infection
Inhalation	Immediate action in lungs Rapid delivery to blood No hepatic first-pass effect	Must be gas, vapour, or aerosol
Topical	Easy to administer Localized (limited systemic absorption)	Effects are mainly limited to site of application
Transdermal	Drug absorption through intact skin No hepatic first-pass effect	Irritation at site of application Delayed onset of action Hydrophilic drugs not easily absorbed
Others (intraperitoneal, intra-articular)	Local effect	Risk of infection

Pharmacokinetics

- study of "what the body does to a drug"
- **definition**: relationship between drug administration, time-course/rate of absorption and distribution, concentration changes in the body compartments, and the drug's removal from the body

Absorption

- **definition**: movement of the drug from the site of administration into plasma

Mechanisms of Drug Absorption
- most drugs are absorbed into the systemic circulation via passive diffusion
- other mechanisms include active transport, facilitated diffusion, and pinocytosis/phagocytosis

Factors Affecting the Rate and Extent of Drug Absorption
- $P_{o/w}$
- **local blood flow** at the site of administration (e.g. sublingual vessels facilitate rapid absorption of sublingual medications)
- **molecular size** (e.g. drugs with smaller molecular weight absorb faster)
- **pH and drug ionization**
  - drugs are usually weak acids (e.g. ASA) or weak bases (e.g. ketoconazole) and thus exist in ionized and non-ionized forms
  - non-ionized forms cross cell membranes much faster than ionized (charged) forms
  - the ratio of ionized to non-ionized forms is determined by body compartment pH and drug pKa (HH equation)
- **total surface area for absorption**
  - small intestinal villi are the primary site of absorption for most oral drugs

$P_{o/w}$
- Ratio of a drug's solubility in oil/lipid (e.g. cell membrane) as compared to water (e.g. extracellular fluid)
- A large $P_{o/w}$ (e.g. anesthetics) means that a drug is highly soluble in lipid and will cross cell membranes easily

Bioavailability (F)
- **definition**: proportion of dose that reaches systemic circulation in an unchanged state
- decreased by limited drug absorption or first-pass effect
- IV dose has 100% bioavailability (F = 1)

First-Pass Effect
- **definition**: drug metabolism by the liver and/or the gut before it reaches systemic circulation, resulting in reduced F
- occurs with PO administration of a drug: GI tract (absorption) → portal vein to liver (first-pass metabolism) → systemic circulation
- occurs less with PR administration because drug absorbed in colon bypasses the portal system

Examples of Drugs with High First-Pass Effect
- Levodopa
- Morphine
- Propranolol
- Lidocaine
- Organic nitrates

Efflux Pump
- Pgp is a protein found in various parts of the body that acts as a multidrug efflux pump involved in the transport of drugs out of cells
- for example, opposes intestinal absorption (e.g. dabigatran etexilate) and also enhances renal elimination of certain drugs (e.g. digoxin, etoposide, paclitaxel, tacrolimus, cyclosporine)
- some drugs (e.g. macrolide antibiotics) inhibit Pgp function, leading to increased serum levels of drugs transported by Pgp; Pgp inducers (e.g. St. John's wort) do the opposite
- some tumours overexpress Pgp leading to multidrug resistance to chemotherapeutic agents

Examples of Drugs with Low First-Pass Effect
- Diazepam
- Digoxin
- Phenytoin
- Warfarin

Distribution

- **definition**: movement of drugs between different body compartments and to the site of action
- major body fluid compartments include plasma, interstitial fluid, intracellular fluid, transcellular fluid (e.g. CSF, peritoneal, pleural)
- tissue compartments include fat, brain

Factors Affecting the Rate and Extent of Drug Distribution
- physiochemical properties of the drug (e.g. $P_{o/w}$ and pK_a)
- pH of fluid
- plasma protein binding
- binding within compartments (i.e. depots)
- regional blood flow

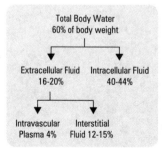

Figure 1. Distribution of total body water (TBW)

Multiple drugs and endogenous substances can compete for the same protein binding sites. For example, ASA displaces highly protein-bound acidic drugs such as phenytoin, thus increasing risk of toxicity, and sulfonamide displaces bilirubin, which could potentially lead to jaundice and kernicterus in neonates

Special consideration must be given in dosing patients in hypoalbuminemic states (e.g. liver failure or nephrotic syndrome) to prevent drug toxicity. Highly protein-bound drugs (e.g. warfarin, digoxin, diazepam, furosemide, amitriptyline) will exert a greater effect in these patients than in healthy individuals because of higher levels of free drug

Main Factors Governing Penetration of BBB
- Small molecular size (<500 Da)
- High lipid solubility
- Active transport mechanisms
(e.g. Pgp efflux pump)

Volume of Distribution
- V_d: the apparent volume of fluid into which a drug distributes
- maximum actual V_d (anatomic fluid volume accessible to drug) = TBW (TBW~40 L for average adult)
    - a calculated value (V_d) = amount of drug in body ÷ plasma drug concentration
    - a theoretical value that does not correspond to an anatomical space (i.e. can exceed TBW)
    - small V_d corresponds to a drug that concentrates in plasma and/or binds plasma proteins to a high degree
    - large V_d corresponds to a drug that distributes into tissues (fat, muscle, etc.); most is not in blood (measured) space, and it therefore "appears" to distribute in a large volume
    - V_d of plasma protein bound drugs can be altered by liver and kidney disease
- example: amiodarone distributes into TBW (actual V_d = 40 L), but it also concentrates in fat tissues giving instead an apparent V_d of 400 L; therefore, to achieve a given plasma concentration of amiodarone, we dose as though the drug distributes into 400 L of body fluid

Plasma Protein Binding
- drug molecules in the blood exist in an equilibrium of two forms:
    1. bound to plasma protein: acidic drugs bind to albumin, basic drugs bind to α1-acid glycoprotein
    2. free or unbound: can leave the circulation to distribute into tissues and exert an effect, subject to metabolism and elimination
- bound fraction is determined by drug concentration, binding affinity, and plasma protein concentration (number of binding sites)
- reduced number of binding sites (e.g. hypoalbuminemia) or saturation of binding sites (e.g. competition/displacement) may result in increased concentration of free drug, which is often metabolized with no harmful effects, although toxicity is possible

Depots
- a body compartment in which drug molecules tend to be stored and released slowly over a long period of time
- fat is a depot for very lipid soluble drugs (e.g. diazepam)
- some oil-based medications are injected IM for slow release (e.g. depot medroxyprogesterone acetate q3mo; depot risperidone q2wk)

Barriers (relative)
- body structures that limit or prevent diffusion of drug molecules, such as the placenta or BBB (a barrier composed of tight junctions between capillary endothelial cells and astrocytes)
- many of these barriers result, in part, from the activity of multidrug efflux pumps (e.g. Pgp), which serve as a natural defense mechanism against drugs and xenobiotics
- need to consider dosing route if drugs are meant to cross these barriers

Metabolism (Biotransformation)

- **definition**: chemical transformation of a drug *in vivo* to enhance elimination
- sites of biotransformation include liver (main), GI tract, lung, plasma, kidney
- as a result of the process of biotransformation:
    - an inactive prodrug may be **activated** (e.g. tamoxifen to endoxifen; codeine to morphine)
    - a drug may be **changed** to another active metabolite (e.g. diazepam to oxazepam)
    - a drug may be **changed** to a toxic metabolite (e.g. meperidine to normeperidine)
    - a drug may be **inactivated** (most drugs)

Drug Metabolizing Pathways
- **phase I (P450) reactions**
    - minor molecular changes introduce or unmask polar groups on a parent compound to increase water solubility (e.g. oxidation-reduction, hydrolysis, hydroxylation); the change in $P_{o/w}$ is typically minimal compared to phase II, and often phase I places a polar 'handle' on a lipophilic drug to allow for phase II
    - mediated by CYPs found in the endoplasmic reticulum
    - product of the reaction can be excreted or undergo further phase II reactions
- **phase II (conjugation) reactions**
    - conjugation with large polar endogenous substrates (e.g. glucuronidation, glutathione conjugation, sulfation)
    - dramatically increases water solubility and renal elimination
    - can result in biologically active metabolites (e.g. glucuronides of morphine)
    - can occur independently of phase I reactions

Factors Affecting Drug Biotransformation
- **genetic polymorphisms** of metabolizing enzymes
  - individual genotypes may determine rate of drug metabolism (e.g. poor, intermediate, extensive, or ultrarapid metabolizers)
  - may lead to toxicity or ineffectiveness of a drug at a normal dose
    - tamoxifen and codeine are prodrugs activated by CYP2D6 (nonfunctional alleles reduce effectiveness, whereas overactive/duplicated alleles impart "ultrarapid metabolizer" phenotype)
    - warfarin is metabolized by CYP2C9 (nonfunctional alleles lead to greater effect and lower dose requirements)
- **enzyme inhibition** may sometimes be due to other drugs
  - CYP inhibition leads to an increased concentration and bioavailability of the substrate drug (e.g. erythromycin [CYP3A4 inhibitor] can predispose patients to simvastatin toxicity [metabolized by CYP3A4])
- **enzyme induction**
  - certain medications enhance gene transcription leading to an increase in the activity of a metabolizing enzyme
  - a drug may induce its own metabolism (e.g. carbamazepine) or that of other drugs (e.g. phenobarbital can induce the metabolism of OCPs) by inducing the CYP system
- **liver dysfunction** (e.g. hepatitis, alcoholic liver, biliary cirrhosis, or hepatocellular carcinoma) may decrease drug metabolism but this may not be clinically significant due to the liver's reserve capacity
- **renal disease** often results in decreased drug clearance
- **extremes of age** (neonates or elderly) have reduced biotransformation capacity, and doses should be adjusted accordingly
- **nutrition**: insufficient protein and fatty acid intake decreases CYP biotransformation, and vitamin/mineral deficiencies may also impact other metabolizing enzymes
- **alcohol**: while acute alcohol ingestion inhibits CYP2E1, chronic consumption can induce CYP2E1 and increase risk of hepatocellular damage from acetaminophen by increasing the generation of acetaminophen's toxic metabolite
- **smoking** can induce CYP1A2, thus increasing the metabolism of some drugs (e.g. theophylline, antipsychotic)

Elimination

- **definition**: removal of drug from the body

Routes of Drug Elimination
- **kidney** (main organ of elimination): two mechanisms
  1. **glomerular filtration**
     - a passive process, so that only the free drug fraction can be eliminated
     - drug filtration rate depends on GFR, degree of protein binding of drug, and size of drug
  2. **tubular secretion**
     - an active process that is saturable allowing both protein-bound and free drug fractions to be excreted
     - distinct transport mechanisms for weak acids (e.g. penicillin, salicylic acid, probenecid, chlorothiazide) and weak bases (e.g. quinine, quaternary ammonium compounds such as choline)
     - drugs may competitively block mutual secretion if both use the same secretion system (e.g. probenecid can reduce the excretion of penicillin)
- **tubular reabsorption**: drugs can be passively reabsorbed back to the systemic circulation, countering elimination mechanisms
- **renal function** (assessed using serum Cr levels) decreases with age and is affected by many disease states such as diabetes
- **stool**: some drugs and metabolites are actively excreted in the bile or directly into the GI tract
  - enterohepatic reabsorption counteracts stool elimination, and can prolong the drug's duration in the body
  - some glucuronic acid conjugates that are excreted in bile may be hydrolyzed in the intestines by bacteria back to their original form and can be systemically reabsorbed
- **lungs**: elimination of anesthetic gases and vapours by exhalation
- **saliva**: saliva concentrations of some drugs parallel their plasma levels (e.g. rifampin)

Cytochrome P450 System
The CYPs are a superfamily of heme proteins that are grouped into families and subfamilies according to their amino acid sequence. These proteins are responsible for the metabolism of drugs, chemicals, and other substances

Nomenclature: CYP3A4
"CYP" = cytochrome P450 protein
1st number = family
letter = subfamily
2nd number = isoform

The CYP1, CYP2, and CYP3 families metabolize most drugs in humans. The most important isoforms are CYP3A4 and CYP2D6; therefore, anticipate drug interactions if prescribing drugs using these enzymes

Examples of CYP Substrates, Inhibitors and Inducers
http://www.medicine.iupui.edu/CLINPHARM/ddis/main-table

The Cockcroft-Gault Equation can Estimate CrCl in Adults 20 yr of Age and Older
- For males
CrCl (mL/min) =
$$\frac{[(140 - \text{age in yr}) \times \text{Weight (kg)}] \times 1.2}{\text{serum Cr } (\mu\text{mol/L})}$$
- For females, multiply above equation x 0.85

***Only applies when renal function is at steady state

Avoid toxicity from drug or metabolite accumulation by adjusting a drug's dosage according to the elimination characteristics of the patient

Principles of Pharmacokinetics
V_d = amount of drug in the body/ plasma drug concentration

Cl = rate of elimination of drug/plasma drug concentration

Half-life (t1/2) = $0.7 \times V_d / Cl$

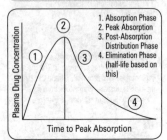

1. Absorption Phase
2. Peak Absorption
3. Post-Absorption Distribution Phase
4. Elimination Phase (half-life based on this)

Figure 2. Time course of drug action

For most drugs it takes 5 half-lives to reach steady state with repeated dosing or to eliminate a drug once dosing is stopped

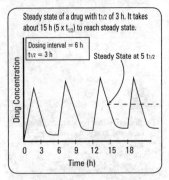

Steady state of a drug with t1/2 of 3 h. It takes about 15 h (5 x $t_{1/2}$) to reach steady state.

Dosing interval = 6 h
t1/2 = 3 h
Steady State at 5 t1/2

Figure 3. Steady state of a drug displaying first-order kinetics

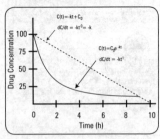

$C(t) = -kt + C_0$
$dC/dt = -kt^0 = -k$

$C(t) = C_0 e^{-kt}$
$dC/dt = -kt^1$

Figure 4. First and zero order kinetics
In first order kinetics (solid line), a constant fraction of the drug is eliminated per unit time; in zero order kinetics (dashed line), a constant amount of the drug is eliminated per unit time

Pharmacokinetic Calculation

- **definition**: the quantitative description of the rates of the various steps of drug disposition (i.e. how drugs move through the body)
- the pharmacokinetic principles of ADME (absorption, distribution, metabolism, and elimination) can be graphically represented on a concentration vs. time graph

Time Course of Drug Action
- many kinetic parameters are measured using IV dosing, such that absorption is immediate and distribution for most drugs is rapid; thus elimination is the main process being measured
- the concentration axis is converted to a log10 concentration to allow for easier mathematical calculations
- drugs such as warfarin can exhibit hysteresis (for a single drug concentration, there may be two different response levels)

Half-Life
- **definition**: time taken for the serum drug level to fall 50% during elimination
- drugs with first order kinetics require five half-lives to reach steady state with repeated dosing or for complete drug elimination once dosing is stopped

# of Half-Lives	1	2	3	3.3	4	5
% of Steady State Concentration	50	75	87.5	90	93.8	96.9

Steady State
- drug concentration remains constant when amount of drug entering the system is eliminated from the system
- drug levels in therapeutic drug monitoring are of greatest utility when the steady state has been reached
- special situations
    - use a loading dose for drugs with a long half-life and when there is clinical need to rapidly achieve therapeutic levels (e.g. amiodarone, digoxin, phenytoin)
    - use continuous infusion for drugs with a very short half-life and when there is need for a long-term effect and multiple or frequently repeated doses are too inconvenient (e.g. nitroprusside, insulin, unfractionated heparin)

Clearance
- a quantitative measurement of the body fluid volume from which a substance is removed per unit time
- Cl = rate of elimination of drug ÷ plasma drug concentration
- must consider Cl from a specific part of the body and total body Cl

Elimination Kinetics
- first-order kinetics (most common type)
    - constant fraction of drug eliminated per unit time
    - some drugs can follow first-order kinetics until elimination is saturated (usually at large doses) at which point the Cl decreases
    - becomes linear relationship when plotted on a log (concentration) vs. time graph
- zero-order kinetics (less common, associated with overdose, e.g. alcohol)
    - drug is eliminated at a constant rate regardless of concentration; concept of half-life does not apply
    - the concentration axis is converted to a log (concentration) to allow for easier mathematical calculations

Table 2. Loading vs. Maintenance Dosing

Loading Dose	Maintenance Dose
Use when you need an IMMEDIATE effect	After a loading dose OR beginning with maintenance doses
Often parenteral medication	Steady-state levels achieved after ~5 half-lives
Rationale: give large dose of medication to "fill up" the volume of distribution	Can be given as either a continuous infusion (relatively rare, short half-life drug) OR much more commonly as intermittent doses

Pharmacodynamics

- study of "what the drug does to the body"

Dose-Response Relationship

- graded dose-response relationships: relates dose to intensity of effect

Efficacy
- the maximum biological response produced by a drug
- measured by Emax (the maximal response that a drug can elicit in a RCT or under optimal circumstances)

Potency
- measured by EC50 (the concentration of a drug needed to produce 50% of Emax)
- a drug that reaches its EC50 at a lower dose is more potent

Efficacy vs. Potency
- Efficacy measures the maximal effect of a drug
- Potency measures the concentration of a drug needed to produce a certain effect

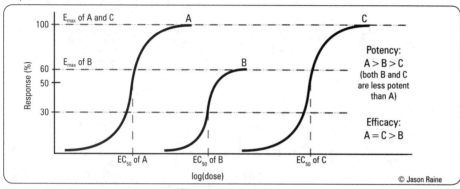

Figure 5. Log(dose)-response curve illustrating efficacy and potency

Effects of Drugs on Receptors

Agonists
- drugs that mimic the effects of the endogenous ligand and evoke a response when bound to the receptor
  - **affinity**: the ability of the agonist to bind to the receptor (e.g. the β2-agonist salbutamol has greater affinity for β2-receptors than β1-receptors)
  - **efficacy**: the ability to recapitulate endogenous response via the receptor interaction (e.g. binding of salbutamol to β2-receptors results in smooth muscle relaxation)
- **full agonists**: can elicit a maximal effect at a receptor
- **partial agonists**: can only elicit a partial effect, no matter the concentration at the receptor (i.e. reduced efficacy compared to full agonists)

Antagonists
- drugs that block the action of an agonist or of an endogenous ligand
- **chemical antagonism**: direct chemical interaction between agonist and antagonist prevents agonist-receptor binding (e.g. chelating agents for removal of heavy metals)
- **functional antagonism**: two agonists that act independently at different receptors and have opposite physiological effects (e.g. acetylcholine at the muscarinic receptor compared to epinephrine at the adrenergic receptor)
- **reversible and irreversible competitive antagonism**
  - drugs that exert no direct effect upon binding to a given receptor
  - reversible competitive antagonists reversibly bind to the same receptor as the agonist, thus displacing it (e.g. naloxone is an antagonist to morphine or heroin)
  - irreversible antagonists form a covalent bond with the receptor, thus irreversibly blocking substrates from binding (e.g. phenoxybenzamine forms a covalent bond with adrenergic receptors preventing adrenaline and NE from binding)
- **non-competitive antagonism**
  - antagonist binds to an alternate site near the agonist site, producing allosteric effects that change the ability of the agonist to bind (e.g. organophosphates irreversibly bind acetylcholinesterase)

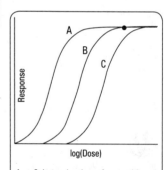

A → C increasing dose of competitive antagonist
At each dose of antagonist, increasing the concentration of agonist can overcome the inhibition

Figure 6. The log(dose)-response curve for competitive reversible antagonism

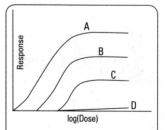

A → D increasing dose of irreversible antagonist. With co-administration of antagonist, increasing dose of agonist does not completely overcome antagonism, as seen in B. Eventually with high enough antagonism concentrations, no amount of agonist can elicit a response, as seen in D

Figure 7. The log(dose)-response curve for irreversible antagonism

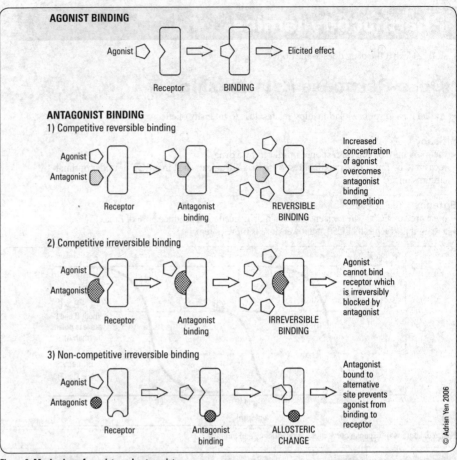

Figure 8. Mechanism of agonists and antagonists

Effectiveness and Safety

Effectiveness
- ED_{50} (effective dose): the dose of a drug needed to cause a therapeutic effect in 50% of a test population of subjects

Safety
- LD_{50} (lethal dose): the dose of a drug needed to cause death in 50% of a test population of subjects
- TD_{50} (toxic dose): the dose needed to cause a harmful effect in 50% of a test population of subjects

Therapeutic Indices

Therapeutic Index: TD_{50}/ED_{50}
- reflects the "margin of safety" for a drug – the likelihood of a therapeutic dose to cause serious toxicity or death
- the larger the TI, the safer a drug (e.g. warfarin has a narrow TI and requires drug monitoring)
- factors that can change the TI
  - presence of interacting drugs
  - changes in drug ADME

Certain Safety Factor: TD_1/ED_{99}
- >1 translates to a dose effective in at least 99% of the population and toxic in less than 1% of the population

The two most clinically relevant properties of any drug are effectiveness and safety

Drugs with a narrow TI have a high likelihood of causing toxicity and need close therapeutic monitoring

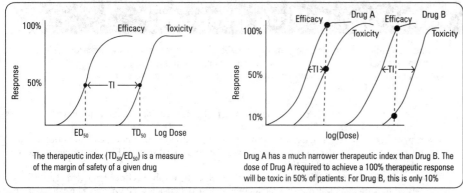

Figure 9. ED$_{50}$, TD$_{50}$, and the therapeutic index

Therapeutic Drug Monitoring

- **definition**: using serum drug concentration data to optimize drug therapy (e.g. dose adjustment, monitor compliance)
  - serum drug samples are usually taken when the drug has reached steady state (after approximately 5 half-lives)
- TDM is often used for drugs that have: narrow TIs, unpredictable dose-response relationships, significant consequences associated with therapeutic failure or toxicity, and wide inter-patient PK variability

Adverse Drug Reactions

Table 3. Characteristics of Type A-E Adverse Drug Reactions

Classification	Definition	Characteristics
A (Augmented)	Dose related	Predictable extension of drug's pharmacologic effect (e.g. β-blockers causing bradycardia) >80% of all ADRs
B (Bizarre)	Non-dose related	Reactions unrelated to the known pharmacological actions of the drug Examples include: drug hypersensitivity syndromes, immunologic reactions (penicillin hypersensitivity), and idiosyncratic reactions (malignant hyperthermia)
C (Chronic)	Dose and time related	Related to cumulative doses Effects are well-known and can be anticipated (e.g. atypical femoral fracture from bisphosphonates)
D (Delayed)	Time related	Occurs some time after use of drug (e.g. carcinogen) May also be dose-related
E (End of use)	Withdrawal	Occurs after cessation of drug use (e.g. opiate withdrawal)

Examples of drugs whose levels need to be monitored include warfarin (via INR levels), digoxin, lithium, anti-epileptics (e.g. phenytoin, carbamazepine)

Approach to Suspected Adverse Drug Reactions

- history and physical exam: signs and symptoms of reaction (e.g. rash, fever, hepatitis, anaphylaxis), timing, risk factors, detailed medication history including all drugs and timing, de-challenge (response when drug is removed), and re-challenge (response when drug is given again)
- differentiate between drug therapy vs. disease pathophysiology
- treatment: stop the drug, supportive care, symptomatic relief
- resources: check recent literature, Health Canada, and FDA; contact the pharmaceutical company; call Poison Control (1-888-268-9017) if overdose or poisoning suspected; check with Motherisk (www.motherisk.org) in cases involving pregnant or breastfeeding women
- report all suspected ADRs that are: 1) unexpected, 2) serious, or 3) reactions to recently marketed drugs (on the market <5 yr) regardless of nature or severity
  - Canadian Adverse Drug Reaction Monitoring Program available for online reporting

Sample of Clinically Relevant Adverse Drug Reactions

Classification	Drug(s)	ADR
A	β-blockers	Bradycardia
A	ACEIs	Cough
A	NSAIDs	GI bleeding
A	Opiates	GI upset, constipation, urinary retention, respiratory depression
A	Acetaminophen	Hepatotoxicity
A	Vancomycin	Red Man syndrome
A	Aminoglycosides	Ototoxicity and nephrotoxicity
B	Sulfa Drugs	Stevens-Johnson syndrome, Toxic epidermal necrolysis
B	Penicillins	Rash
B	Valproic acid, Chinese herbs	Hepatotoxicity

Variability in Drug Response

- recommended patient dosing is based on clinical research and represents mean values for a select population, but each person may be unique in their dosing requirements
- possible causes of individual variability in drug response include problems with:
  - intake: patient adherence
  - PK
    - absorption: vomiting, diarrhea, or steatorrhea; first pass effect increased due to enzyme induction or decreased due to liver disease
    - drug interactions (e.g. calcium carbonate complexes with iron, thyroxine, and fluoroquinolones)
    - distribution: very high or low percentage body fat; intact or disrupted BBB; patient is elderly or a neonate, or has liver dysfunction
    - biotransformation and elimination: certain genetic polymorphisms or enzyme deficiencies related to drug metabolism (e.g. acetylcholinesterase deficiency, CYP polymorphism); kidney or liver dysfunction
  - PD: genetic variability in drug response (e.g. immune-mediated reactions); diseases that affect drug PD; drug tolerance or cross-tolerance

Drug Interactions

Examples of Clinically Relevant Drug Interactions

Interaction	Potential Effect
Warfarin plus ciprofloxacin, clarithromycin, erythromycin, metronidazole or trimethoprim-sulfamethoxazole	Increased effect of warfarin
Oral contraceptive pills plus rifampin, antibiotics	Decreased effectiveness of oral contraception
Sildenafil plus nitrates	Hypotension
SSRI plus St. John's wort, naratriptan, rizatriptan, sumatriptan, zolmitriptan	Serotonin syndrome
SSRI plus selegiline or non-selective MAO-I	Serotonin syndrome
Some **HMG-CoA reductase inhibitors** plus niacin, gemfibrozil, erythromycin or itraconazole	Possible rhabdomyolysis

- concomitant prescriptions: one drug alters the effect of another by changing its PK and/or PD
- PK interactions involve changes in drug concentration
  - absorption: alterations in gastrointestinal pH, gastric emptying, intestinal motility, gut mucosal function
  - biotransformation: alterations in drug metabolizing enzymes
  - excretion: alterations in renal elimination
- PD interactions are due to two drugs that exert similar effects (additive) or opposing effects (subtractive)
- drug interactions can also involve herbal medications (e.g. St. John's wort) and food (e.g. grapefruit)

Autonomic Pharmacology

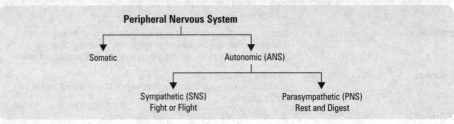

Peripheral Nervous System

Somatic

Autonomic (ANS)

Sympathetic (SNS)
Fight or Flight

Parasympathetic (PNS)
Rest and Digest

Figure 10. Subdivisions of the peripheral nervous system

- most organs are innervated by both sympathetic and parasympathetic nerves, which have opposing effects (see Neurology, N8)
- ACh and NE are the main neurotransmitters of the autonomic NS
- ACh binds to cholinergic receptors, which include nicotinic and muscarinic receptors
- NE binds to adrenergic receptors, which principally include $\beta1$, $\beta2$, $\alpha1$, and $\alpha2$
- ACh action is terminated by metabolism in the synaptic cleft by acetylcholinesterase and in the plasma by pseudocholinesterase
- acetylcholinesterase inhibitors (pyridostigmine, donepezil, galantamine, rivastigmine) can be used to increase ACh levels in conditions such as myasthenia gravis or Alzheimer's disease
- NE action is terminated by reuptake at the presynaptic membrane, diffusion from the synaptic cleft, and degradation at monoamine oxidase (MAO) and catechol-O-methyl transferase (COMT)

Parasympathetic Nervous System

- blood vessels, adrenals, sweat glands, spleen capsule, and adrenal medulla do NOT have parasympathetic innervation
- parasympathetic pre-ganglionic fibres originate in the lower brainstem from cranial nerves III, VII, IX, X, and in the sacral spinal cord at levels S2-S4 and connect with post-ganglionic fibres via nicotinic receptors in ganglionic cells located near or within the target organ
- post-ganglionic fibres connect with effector tissues via:
  - M_1 muscarinic receptors located in the CNS
  - M_2 muscarinic receptors located in smooth muscle, cardiac muscle, and glandular epithelium

Sympathetic Nervous System

- sympathetic pre-ganglionic fibres originate in the spinal cord at spinal levels T1-L2/L3
- pre-ganglionic fibres connect with post-ganglionic fibres via nicotinic receptors located in one of two groups of ganglia
    1. paravertebral ganglia (i.e. the sympathetic trunk) that lie in a chain close to the vertebral column
    2. pre-vertebral ganglia (i.e. celiac and mesenteric ganglia) that lie within the abdomen
- post-ganglionic fibres connect with effector tissues via:
    - β1 receptors in cardiac tissue
    - β2 receptors in smooth muscle of bronchi and GI tract
    - α1 receptors in vascular smooth muscle
    - α2 receptors in vascular smooth muscle
    - M3 muscarinic receptors located in sweat glands

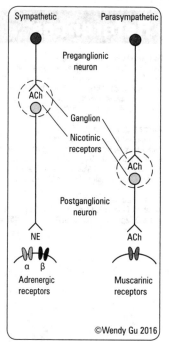

Figure 11. Autonomic nervous system efferent tracts

Table 4. Direct Effects of Autonomic Innervation on the Cardiorespiratory System

Organ	Sympathetic NS		Parasympathetic NS	
	Receptor	Action	Receptor	Action
Heart				
1. Sinoatrial	β1	Increased HR	M	Decreased conduction
2. Atrioventricular node	β1	Increased conduction	M	Decreased conduction
3. Atria	β1	Increased contractility	M	Decreased conduction
4. Ventricles	β1	Increased contractility	M	Decreased HR
Blood Vessels				
1. Skin, splanchnic	α1, β2	Constriction	M	Dilatation
2. Skeletal muscle	α	Constriction	M	Dilatation
3. Coronary	β2 (large muscles)	Dilatation	M	Dilatation
	α1, β2	Constriction	M	Dilatation
	β2	Dilatation	M	Dilatation
Lungs				
1. Bronchiolar smooth muscle	β2	Relaxation	M	Constriction
2. Bronchiolar glands	α1, β2	Increased secretion	M	Stimulation

Common Drug Endings

Table 5. Common Drug Endings

Ending	Category	Example
-afil	5-PDE inhibitor	sildenafil
-ane	Inhaled general anesthetic	halothane
-azepam	Benzodiazepine	lorazepam
-azole	Antifungal	ketoconazole
-caine	Local anesthetic	lidocaine
-olol	β-blocker	propranolol
-prazole	Proton pump inhibitor	omeprazole
-pril	ACE inhibitor	captopril
-sartan	ARB	candesartan
-statin	HMG-CoA inhibitor	atorvastatin
-terol	β2 agonist	albuterol
-tidine	H2 antagonist	cimetidine
-tropin	Pituitary hormone	somatotropin
-vir	Antiviral	acyclovir
-zosin	α1 antagonist	prazosin

Note: Some medications are exceptions to the rule, e.g. methimazole (antithyroid)

References

Principles of Clinical Pharmacology
Hardman JG, Limbird LR. Goodman and Gilman's the pharmacological basis of therapeutics, 9th ed. New York: McGraw-Hill, 1996.
Hardy B, Bedard M. Compendium of pharmaceuticals and specialties. Chapter: Serum drug concentration monitoring. Ottawa: Canadian Pharmacists Association, 2002.
Kalant H, Grant DM, Mitchell J. Principles of medical pharmacology, 7th ed. Toronto: Elsevier Canada, 2007.
Katzung BG. Basic and clinical pharmacology, 8th ed. New York: McGraw-Hill, 2001.
Rang H, Dale M, Ritter J. Pharmacology, 4th ed. Edinburgh: Churchill Livingstone, 1999.

Adverse Drug Reactions
Baker GR, Norton PG, Flintoft V, et al. The Canadian adverse events study: the incidence of adverse events among hospital patients in Canada. CMAJ 2004;170:1678-1686.
Lewis T. Using the NO TEARS tool for medication review. BMJ 2004;329:434.
MedEffect Canada. Canada vigilance adverse reaction online database. Ottawa: Health Canada. 1964. Available from: http://www.hc-sc.gc.ca/dhp-mps/medeff/databasdon/index_e.html.
Pirmohamed M, James S, Meakin S, et al. Adverse drug reactions as cause of admission to hospital: prospective analysis of 18820 patients. BMJ 2004;329:315.
Samoy LJ, Zed PJ, Wilbur K, et al. Drug-related hospitalizations in a tertiary care internal medicine service of a Canadian hospital: a prospective study. Pharmacotherapy 2006;26:1578-1586.

Drug Interactions
Ament PW, Bertolino JG, Liszewski JL. Clinically significant drug interactions. Am Fam Physician 2000;61:1745-1754.
Indiana University, Division of Clinical Pharmacology. P450 drug interaction table. Indiana University, 2009. Available from: http://www.medicine.iupui.edu/clinpharm/DDIs/table.aspx.

D

Dermatology

Danny Mansour, Cristina Olteanu, and Venus Valbuena, chapter editors
Narayan Chattergoon and Desmond She, associate editors
Arnav Agarwal and Quynh Huynh, EBM editors
Dr. David Adam and Dr. Jensen Yeung, staff editors

Acronyms 2

Introduction to Skin 2
Skin Anatomy
Skin Function

Definitions 3
Primary Morphological Lesions
Secondary Morphological Lesions
Other Morphological Lesions
Patterns and Distribution

Differential Diagnoses of Common
    Presentations. 5

Common Skin Lesions. 5
Cysts
Fibrous Lesions
Hyperkeratotic Lesions
Keloids
Pigmented Lesions
Vascular Lesions
Lipoma

Acneiform Eruptions 11
Acne Vulgaris/Common Acne
Perioral Dermatitis
Rosacea

Dermatitis (Eczema) 13
Asteatotic Dermatitis
Atopic Dermatitis
Contact Dermatitis
Dyshidrotic Dermatitis
Nummular Dermatitis
Seborrheic Dermatitis
Stasis Dermatitis
Lichen Simplex Chronicus

Papulosquamous Diseases 16
Lichen Planus
Pityriasis Rosea
Psoriasis

Vesiculobullous Diseases 19
Bullous Pemphigoid
Pemphigus Vulgaris
Dermatitis Herpetiformis
Porphyria Cutanea Tarda

Drug Eruptions. 21
Exanthematous
Urticarial
Pustular
Bullous
Other

Heritable Disorders 23
Ichthyosis Vulgaris
Neurofibromatosis (Type I; von
    Recklinghausen's Disease)
Vitiligo

Infections 25
Bacterial Infections
Dermatophytoses
Parasitic Infections
Viral Infections
Yeast Infections
Sexually Transmitted Infections

Pre-Malignant Skin Conditions. 33
Actinic Keratosis (Solar Keratosis)
Leukoplakia

Malignant Skin Tumours. 34
Non-Melanoma Skin Cancers
Malignant Melanoma
Other Cutaneous Cancers

Diseases of Hair Density 37
Hair Growth
Non-Scarring (Non-Cicatricial) Alopecia
Scarring (Cicatricial) Alopecia

Nails and Disorders of the Nail Apparatus 39

Skin Manifestations of Systemic Disease 40

Pediatric Exanthems P55

Miscellaneous Lesions 41
Angioedema and Urticaria
Erythema Nodosum
Pruritus
Wounds and Ulcers
Sunscreens and Preventative Therapy
Topical Steroids
Dermatologic Therapies

References 46

Acronyms

β-hCG	β-human chorionic gonadotropin	Fe	iron	MTP	metatarsal phalangeal	SLE	systemic lupus erythematosus
AAFP	American Academy of Family Physicians	FTA-ABS	fluorescent treponemal antibody-absorption	NB-UVB	narrow band ultraviolet wavelength B	SPF	sun protection factor
AD	atopic dermatitis	GAS	group A β-hemolytic *Streptococcus*	NCN	neocellular nevus	SSRI	selective serotonin reuptake inhibitor
AK	actinic keratosis	GVHD	graft-versus-host disease	Nd: Yag	neodymium-doped yttrium aluminum garnet	SSSS	staphylococcal scalded skin syndrome
ASO	anti-streptolysin O	HHV	human herpes virus	NMN	nevomelanocytic nevus	STI	sexually transmitted infection
BCC	basal cell carcinoma	HPA	hypothalamic-pituitary-adrenal	NMSC	nonmelanoma skin cancers	TB	tuberculosis
BSA	body surface area	HPV	human papillomavirus	NSAID	nonsteroidal anti-inflammatory drug	TEN	toxic epidermal necrolysis
BUN	blood urea nitrogen	HRT	hormone replacement therapy	OCP	oral contraceptive pill	TMP/SMX	trimethoprim-sulfamethoxazole
CBC	complete blood count	HSV	herpes simplex virus	OTC	over-the-counter	TSH	thyroid stimulating hormone
CMV	cytomegalovirus	HZV	herpes zoster virus	PABA	para-aminobenzoic acid	UC	ulcerative colitis
CNS	central nervous system	IFN	interferon	PASI	Psoriasis Area and Severity Index	URTI	upper respiratory tract infection
Cr	creatinine	IVIg	intravenous immunoglobulin	PPD	purified protein derivative	UV	ultraviolet
CXR	chest x-ray	LFT	liver function test	PUVA	psoralens and UVA	UVA	ultraviolet A
DLE	discoid lupus erythematosus	MAOI	monoamine oxidase inhibitor	RA	rheumatoid arthritis	UVB	ultraviolet B
DM	diabetes mellitus	MM	malignant melanoma	SCC	squamous cell carcinoma	UVC	ultraviolet C
DVT	deep vein thrombosis	MMR	measles/mumps/rubella	SHBG	sex hormone-binding globulin	VDRL	venereal disease research laboratory
EM	erythema multiforme	MRSA	methicillin-resistant *Staphylococcus aureus*	SJS	Stevens-Johnson syndrome	VZV	varicella zoster virus

Introduction to Skin

Skin Anatomy

Layers of the Epidermis
"Californians Like Getting Sun Burns"
OR
"Canadians Like Good Sushi Boxes"

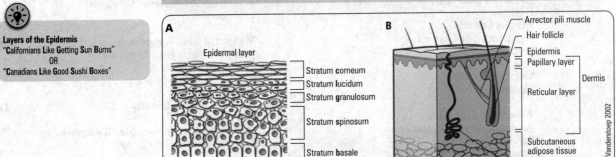

Figure 1. Histologic layers of the skin. Epidermal layer is detailed in A

© Ken Vanderstoep 2002

Skin
- divided anatomically into epidermis, dermis, and subcutaneous tissue
- **epidermis**
  - avascular: receives its nutrition from the dermal capillaries
  - derived from keratinocytes with the youngest presenting at the stratum basale
  - cells progress from stratum basale to stratum corneum in about 4 wk
    - stratum basale (germinativum): mitotic figures that give rise to keratinocytes
    - stratum spinosum (prickle cells): junctions in this layer (tonofilaments) give the epidermis its strength
    - stratum granulosum: flat cells containing basophilic granules which characterize skin
    - stratum lucidum: transparent layers of packed dead cells
    - stratum corneum: flat scales of the water-resistant protein keratin
  - cells of the epidermis
    - keratinocytes: located in all layers of the epidermis, except the stratum corneum; connected to each other by desmosomes
    - melanocytes: located in the stratum basale; keratinocyte to melanocyte ratio in the basal layer is 10:1; melanocyte number is equal among races; produce melanosomes containing melanin, which are transferred to keratinocytes
    - Langerhans cells: dendritic cells which are important for immune surveillance
    - Merkel cells: located in the basal layer; involved in touch sensation
- **dermis:** comprised of connective tissue divided into two regions
  - papillary: contains numerous capillaries that supply nutrients to the dermis and epidermis
  - reticular: provides a strong structure for skin; consists of collagen bundles woven together along with elastic fibres, fibroblasts, and macrophages
  - cells of dermis
    - fibroblasts: produces collagen, elastin, and ground substance
    - mast cells: releases histamines which mediate type I hypersensitivity
  - other components of dermis include: blood vessels, nerves, pilosebaceous units, and sweat glands
- **subcutaneous tissue** (hypodermis)
  - consists primarily of adipose cells, larger calibre vessels, nerves and fascia

Epidermal Appendages
- epidermal in origin, can extend into the dermis; includes hair, nails, and cutaneous glands
- pilosebaceous unit = hair + hair follicle + sebaceous gland + arrector pili muscle

Cutaneous Glands
- **sebaceous gland:** part of pilosebaceous unit, produces sebum which is secreted into the hair follicle via the sebaceous duct, where it covers the skin surface (protective function)
    - sebum has some antifungal properties
    - these glands cover entire skin surface and are absent only in non-hair bearing areas (e.g. palms, soles, lips)
- **apocrine sweat gland:** apocrine duct empties into hair follicle above sebaceous gland
    - found in axillae and perineum
    - likely a vestigial structure, functions in other species to produce scent (e.g. pheromones)
- **eccrine sweat gland:** not part of pilosebaceous unit
    - found over entire skin surface except lips, nail beds, and glans penis
    - important in temperature regulation via secretion of sweat to cool skin surface

Skin Function

- **protection**
    - due to continuous recycling and avascularity of epidermis
    - barrier to UV radiation (melanin), mechanical/chemical insults (sensory/mechanoreceptors), pathogens (immune cells), and dehydration (lipid rich barrier)
- **thermal regulation**
    - insulation to maintain body temperature in cool environments via peripheral vasoconstriction, hair, and subcutaneous adipose tissue
    - dissipation of heat in warm environments via increased activity of sweat glands and increased blood flow within dermal vascular networks
- **sensation**
    - touch, pain, and temperature sensation
- **metabolic function**
    - vitamin D synthesis
    - energy storage (mainly in the form of triglycerides)

Definitions

Primary Morphological Lesions

Definition
- an initial lesion that has not been altered by trauma or manipulation, and has not regressed

Table 1. Types of Primary Morphological Lesions

Profile	<1 cm Diameter	≥1 cm Diameter
Flat lesion	Macule (e.g. freckle)	Patch (e.g. vitiligo)
Raised superficial lesion	Papule (e.g. wart)	Plaque (e.g. psoriasis)
Deep palpable (dermal or subcutaneous)	Nodule (e.g. dermatofibroma)	Tumour (e.g. lipoma)
Elevated fluid-filled lesions	Vesicle (e.g. HSV)	Bulla (e.g. bullous pemphigoid)

> **Describe a Lesion with SCALDA**
> **S**ize and **S**urface area
> **C**olour (e.g. hyperpigmented, hypopigmented, erythematous)
> **A**rrangement (e.g. solitary, linear, reticulated, grouped, herpetiform)
> **L**esion morphology
> **D**istribution (e.g. dermatomal, intertriginous, symmetrical/asymmetrical, follicular)
> **A**lways check hair, nails, mucous membranes and intertriginous areas

Secondary Morphological Lesions

Definition
- develop during the evolutionary process of skin disease, or created by manipulation, or due to complication of primary lesion (e.g. rubbing, scratching, infection)
- **crust:** dried fluid (serum, blood, or purulent exudate) originating from a lesion (e.g. impetigo)
- **scale:** excess keratin (e.g. seborrheic dermatitis)
- **lichenification:** thickening of the skin and accentuation of normal skin markings (e.g. chronic atopic dermatitis)
- **fissure:** a linear slit-like cleavage of the skin
- **excoriation:** a scratch mark
- **erosion:** a disruption of the skin involving the epidermis alone; heals without scarring
- **ulcer:** a disruption of the skin that extends into the dermis or deeper; may heal with scarring
- **xerosis:** pathologic dryness of skin (xeroderma), conjunctiva (xerophthalmia), or mucous membranes (xerostomia)
- **atrophy:** histological decrease in size or number of cells or tissues, resulting in thinning or depression of the skin

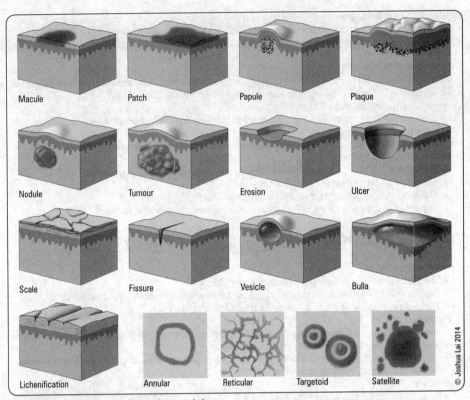

Figure 2. Examples of primary and secondary morphology

Other Morphological Lesions

- **cyst:** an epithelial-lined collection containing semi-solid or fluid material
- **pustule:** an elevated lesion containing purulent fluid (white, grey, yellow, green)
- **scar:** replacement fibrosis of dermis and subcutaneous tissue (hypertrophic or atrophic)
- **wheal:** a special form of papule or plaque that is transient (<24 h) and blanchable often with a halo and central clearing, formed by edema in the dermis (e.g. urticaria)
- **comedone**: a special collection of sebum and keratin
  - open comedo (blackhead)
  - closed comedo (not a pustule; rather a minute dome-shaped, skin-coloured papule)
- **petechiae:** pinpoint extravasation of blood into dermis resulting in hemorrhagic lesions; non-blanchable, <3 mm in size
- **purpura:** larger than petechia, 3 mm-1 cm in size
- **ecchymosis:** larger than purpura, >1 cm in size (i.e. a "bruise")
- **telangiectasia:** dilated superficial blood vessels; often blanchable, reticulated, and of small calibre, can be associated with benign or malignant entities

Patterns and Distribution

- **acral:** relating to the hands and feet (e.g. perniosis, secondary syphilis)
- **annular:** ring-shaped (e.g. granuloma annulare)
- **follicular:** involving hair follicles (e.g. folliculitis)
- **guttate:** lesions following a "drop-like" pattern (e.g. guttate psoriasis)
- **Koebner phenomenon:** i.e. isomorphic response, appearance of lesions at an injury site (e.g. lichen planus, psoriasis, vitiligo)
- **morbilliform:** literally means "measles-like", an eruption composed of macules and papules with truncal predominance
- **reticular:** lesions following a net-like pattern (e.g. livedo reticularis)
- **satellite:** small lesions scattered around the periphery of a larger lesion (e.g. candida diaper dermatitis)
- **serpiginous:** lesions following a snake-like pattern (e.g. cutaneous larva migrans)
- **target/targetoid:** concentric ring lesions, like a dartboard (e.g. erythema multiforme)
- **other descriptive terms:** discrete, clustered, linear, confluent, dermatitic, indurated (i.e. hard or firm)

Differential Diagnoses of Common Presentations

Table 2. Differential Diagnosis of Common Presenting Problems

Lesion	Infectious	Inflammatory	Drug/Toxin	Miscellaneous
Brown Macule		Post-inflammatory hyper-pigmentation	UV radiation, actinic/solar lentigo, freckle (ephelide)	Congenital: café-au-lait spots, congenital nevus, epidermal/junctional nevus Neoplasia: lentigo maligna, MM, pigmented BCC Other: melasma/chloasma ("mask of pregnancy")
Discrete Red Papule	Folliculitis Furuncle Scabies	Acne vulgaris Rosacea Psoriasis Urticaria	Bites/stings	Autoimmune: lichen planus; see *Papulosquamous Diseases*, D16 Vascular: hemangioma, pyogenic granuloma Other: dermatofibroma, miliaria rubra
Red Scales	Pityriasis rosea Secondary syphilis Tinea	Dermatitis (atopic, contact, nummular, seborrheic) Discoid lupus Psoriasis	Gold	Autoimmune: lichen planus; see *Papulosquamous Diseases*, D16 Neoplastic: mycosis fungoides
Vesicle	Cat scratch disease Impetigo Viral: HSV, HZV, VZV, Molluscum, Coxsackie Scabies	Acute contact dermatitis Dyshidrotic eczema		Other: dermatitis herpetiformis, porphyria cutanea tarda
Bulla	Bullous impetigo	Acute dermatitis EM, SJS, TEN, SLE	Fixed drug eruption	Autoimmune: bullous pemphigoid, pemphigus vulgaris Other: dermatitis herpetiformis, porphyria cutanea tarda
Pustule	Candida Dermatophyte Impetigo Sepsis Varicella	Acne vulgaris Rosacea Dyshidrotic dermatitis Pustular folliculitis Pustular psoriasis Hidradenitis suppurativa	Acute generalized exanthematous pustulosis (usually secondary to drug reaction)	
Oral Ulcer	Aspergillosis CMV Coxsackie Cryptococcosis HSV/HZV HIV, TB, Syphilis	Allergic stomatitis EM/SJS/TEN Lichen planus Seronegative arthropathies, SLE Recurrent aphthous stomatitis Behçet's disease	Chemotherapy Radiation therapy	Autoimmune: pemphigus vulgaris Congenital: XXY Hematologic: sickle cell disease Neoplasia: BCC, SCC
Skin Ulcer	Plague Syphilis TB Tularemia	RA, SLE, vasculitis UC (pyoderma gangrenosum)		Autoimmune: necrobiosis lipoidica diabeticorum (e.g. DM) Congenital: XXY Hematologic: sickle cell disease Neoplasia: SCC Vascular: arterial, neurotrophic, pressure, venous, aphthous, leukoplakia, traumatic

Common Skin Lesions

Cysts

Table 3. Cysts

	Clinical Presentation	Pathophysiology	Epidemiology	Clinical Course	Management
Epidermal Cyst	Round, yellow/flesh-coloured, slow growing, mobile, firm, fluctuant, nodule or tumour	Epithelial cells displaced into dermis, epidermal lining becomes filled with keratin and lipid-rich debris May be post-traumatic, rarely syndromic	Most common cutaneous cyst in youth – middle age	Central punctum may rupture (foul, cheesy odour, creamy colour) and produce inflammatory reaction Increase in size and number over time, especially in pregnancy	Excise completely before it becomes infected
Pilar Cyst (Trichilemmal)	Multiple, hard, variable sized nodules under the scalp, lacks central punctum	Thick-walled cyst lined with stratified squamous epithelium and filled with dense keratin Idiopathic Post-trauma, often familial	2nd most common cutaneous cyst F>M	Rupture causes pain and inflammation	Excision
Dermoid Cyst	Firm nodule most commonly found at lateral third of eyebrow or midline under nose	Rare, congenital hamartomas, which arise from inclusion of epidermis along embryonal cleft closure lines, creating a thick-walled cyst filled with dense keratin	Rare	If nasal midline, risk of extension into CNS	Excision
Ganglion Cyst	Usually solitary, rubbery, translucent; a clear gelatinous viscous fluid may be extruded	Cystic lesion that originates from joint or tendon sheath, called a digital mucous cyst when found on fingertip Associated with osteoarthritis	Older age	Stable	Incision and expression of contents Laser ablation and electrodessication
Milium	1-2 mm superficial, white to yellow subepidermal papules occurring on eyelids, cheeks, and forehead	Small epidermoid cyst, primarily arising from pluripotential cells in epidermal or adnexal epithelium Can be secondary to blistering, ulceration, trauma, topical corticosteroid atrophy, or cosmetic procedures	Any age 40-50% of infants	In newborns, spontaneously resolves in first 4 wk of life	Incision and expression of contents Laser ablation and electrodessication Multiple facial milia respond to topical retinoid therapy

Common Skin Lesions

Fibrous Lesions

DERMATOFIBROMA

Clinical Presentation
- button-like, firm dermal papule or nodule, skin-coloured to red-brown colouring
- majority are asymptomatic but may be pruritic and/or tender
- site: legs > arms > trunk
- dimple sign (Fitzpatrick's sign): lateral compression causes dimpling of the lesion

Pathophysiology
- benign tumour due to fibroblast proliferation in the dermis

Etiology
- unknown; may be associated with history of minor trauma (e.g. shaving or insect bites)
- eruptive dermatofibromata can be associated with SLE

Epidemiology
- adults, F>M

Differential Diagnosis
- dermatofibrosarcoma protuberans, malignant melanoma, Kaposi's sarcoma, blue nevus

Investigations
- biopsy if diagnosis is uncertain

Management
- no treatment required
- excision or cryosurgery if bothersome

SKIN TAGS

Clinical Presentation
- small (1-10 mm), soft, skin-coloured or darker pedunculated papule, often polypoid
- sites: eyelids, neck, axillae, inframammary, and groin

Pathophysiology
- benign outgrowth of skin

Epidemiology
- middle-aged and elderly, F>M, obese, can increase in size and number during pregnancy

Differential Diagnosis
- pedunculated seborrheic keratosis, compound or dermal melanocytic nevus, neurofibroma, fibroepithelioma of Pinkus (rare variant of BCC)

Management
- excision, electrodessication, cryosurgery

Hyperkeratotic Lesions

SEBORRHEIC KERATOSIS

Clinical Presentation
- known as 'wisdom spots', 'age spots', or 'barnacles of life'
- well-demarcated waxy papule/plaque with classic "stuck on" appearance
- rarely pruritic
- over time lesions appear more warty, greasy and pigmented
- sites: face, trunk, upper extremities (may occur at any site except palms or soles)

Pathophysiology
- very common benign epithelial tumour due to proliferation of keratinocytes and melanocytes

Epidemiology
- unusual <30 yr old
- M>F
- autosomal dominant inheritance
- Leser-Trelat: sudden appearance of SK that can be associated with malignancy, commonly gastric adenocarcinomas

Skin Phototypes (Fitzpatrick)

Phototype	Colour of Skin	Skin's Response to Sun Exposure (without SPF protection)
I	White	Always burns, never tans
II	White	Always burns, little tan
III	White	Slight burn, slow tan
IV	Pale brown	Slight burn, faster tan
V	Brown	Rarely burns, dark tan
VI	Dark brown or black	Never burns, dark tan

Skin tags are also known as...
- Acrochordons
- Fibroepithelial polyps
- Soft fibromas
- Pedunculated lipofibromas
- Cutaneous papillomas

Differential Diagnosis
- malignant melanoma (lentigo maligna, nodular melanoma), melanocytic nevi, pigmented BCC, solar lentigo, spreading pigmented AK

Investigations
- biopsy only if diagnosis uncertain

Management
- none required, for cosmetic purposes only
- cryotherapy, curettage

ACTINIC KERATOSIS (SOLAR KERATOSIS)
- see *Pre-Malignant Skin Conditions*, D33

KERATOACANTHOMA
- see *Malignant Skin Tumours*, D35

CORNS (HELOMATA)

Clinical Presentation
- firm papule with a central, translucent, cone-shaped, hard keratin core
- painful with direct pressure
- sites: most commonly on dorsolateral fifth toe and dorsal aspects of other toes

Pathophysiology
- localized hyperkeratosis induced by pressure on hands and feet

Epidemiology
- F>M, can be caused by chronic microtrauma

Differential Diagnosis
- tinea pedis, plantar warts

Management
- relieve pressure with padding or alternate footwear, orthotics
- paring, curettage

Corns vs. Warts vs. Calluses
- **Corns** have a whitish yellow central translucent keratinous core; painful with direct pressure
- **Warts** bleed with paring and have a black speckled central appearance due to thrombosed capillaries; plantar warts destroy dermatoglyphics (epidermal ridges)
- **Calluses** have layers of yellowish keratin revealed with paring; there are no thrombosed capillaries or interruption of epidermal ridges

Keloids

Clinical Presentation
- firm, shiny, skin-coloured or red-bluish papules/nodules that most often arise from cutaneous injury (e.g. piercing, surgical scar, acne), but may appear spontaneously
- extends beyond the margins of the original injury, and may continue to expand in size for years with claw-like extensions
- can be pruritic and painful
- sites: earlobes, shoulders, sternum, scapular area, angle of mandible

Pathophysiology
- excessive deposition of randomly organized collagen fibres following trauma to skin

Epidemiology
- most common in black patients, followed by those of Asian descent (predilection for darker skin)
- M=F, all age groups

Management
- intralesional corticosteroid injections
- cryotherapy
- silicone compression

Keloids vs. Hypertrophic Scars
- **Keloids:** extend beyond margins of original injury with claw-like extensions
- **Hypertrophic scars:** confined to original margins of injury

Pigmented Lesions

CONGENITAL NEVOMELANOCYTIC NEVI (CNMN)

Clinical Presentation
- sharply demarcated pigmented papule or plaque with regular borders ± coarse hairs
- classified by size: small (<1.5 cm), medium (M1: 1.5-10 cm, M2: >10-20 cm), large (L1: >20-30 cm, L2 >30-40 cm), giant (G1: >40-60 cm, G2: >60 cm)
- may be surrounded by smaller satellite nevi

Pathophysiology
- nevomelanocytes in epidermis (clusters) and dermis (strands)

Epidemiology
- present at birth or develops in early infancy to childhood
- malignant transformation is rare (1-5%) and more correlated with size of the lesion
- neurocutaneous melanosis can occur in giant CNMN (melanocytes in the central nervous system)

Management
- surgical excision if suspicious, due to increased risk of melanoma
- MRI if suspicious for neurological involvement

OTHER CONGENITAL PIGMENTED LESIONS

Table 4. Comparison of Other Congenital Pigmented Lesions

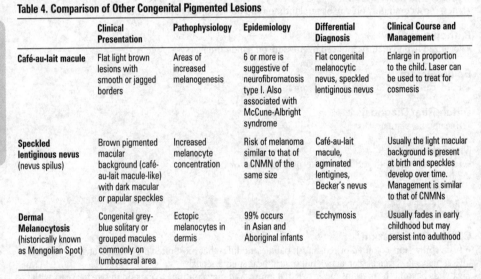

	Clinical Presentation	Pathophysiology	Epidemiology	Differential Diagnosis	Clinical Course and Management
Café-au-lait macule	Flat light brown lesions with smooth or jagged borders	Areas of increased melanogenesis	6 or more is suggestive of neurofibromatosis type I. Also associated with McCune-Albright syndrome	Flat congenital melanocytic nevus, speckled lentiginous nevus	Enlarge in proportion to the child. Laser can be used to treat for cosmesis
Speckled lentiginous nevus (nevus spilus)	Brown pigmented macular background (café-au-lait macule-like) with dark macular or papular speckles	Increased melanocyte concentration	Risk of melanoma similar to that of a CNMN of the same size	Café-au-lait macule, agminated lentigines, Becker's nevus	Usually the light macular background is present at birth and speckles develop over time. Management is similar to that of CNMNs
Dermal Melanocytosis (historically known as Mongolian Spot)	Congenital grey-blue solitary or grouped macules commonly on lumbosacral area	Ectopic melanocytes in dermis	99% occurs in Asian and Aboriginal infants	Ecchymosis	Usually fades in early childhood but may persist into adulthood

ACQUIRED NEVOMELANOCYTIC NEVI

Clinical Presentation
- common mole: well circumscribed, round, uniformly pigmented macules/papules <1.5 cm
- average number of moles per person: 18-40
- 3 stages of evolution: junctional NMN, compound NMN, and dermal NMN

Table 5. Evolution of Acquired Nevomelanocytic Nevi

Type	Age of Onset	Clinical Presentation	Histology
Junctional	Childhood Majority progress to compound nevus	Flat, irregularly bordered, uniformly tan-dark brown, sharply demarcated smooth macule	Melanocytes at dermal-epidermal junction above basement membrane
Compound	Any age	Domed, regularly bordered, smooth, round, tan-dark brown papule Face, trunk, extremities, scalp NOT found on palms or soles	Melanocytes at dermal-epidermal junction; migration into dermis
Dermal	Adults	Soft, dome-shaped, skin-coloured to tan/brown papules or nodules, often with telangiectasia Sites: face, neck	Melanocytes exclusively in dermis

Management
- new or changing pigmented lesions should be evaluated for atypical features which could indicate a melanoma
- excisional biopsy can be considered if the lesion demonstrates asymmetry, varied colours, irregular borders, pruritus or persistent bleeding

OTHER ACQUIRED PIGMENTED LESIONS

Table 6. Comparison of Other Acquired Pigmented Lesions

	Clinical Presentation	Pathophysiology	Epidemiology	Differential Diagnosis	Clinical Course and Management
Atypical nevus (Dysplastic Nevus)	Variegated macule/papule with irregular distinct melanocytes in the basal layer. Risk factors: family history	Hyperplasia and proliferation of melanocytes extending beyond dermal compartment of the nevus. Often with region of adjacent nests	>5 atypical nevi increases risk for melanoma. Numerous dysplastic nevi may be part of Familial Atypical Mole and Melanoma syndrome	Melanoma	Follow with colour photographs for changes. Excisional biopsy if lesion changing or highly atypical
Ephelides (Freckles)	Small (<5 mm) well-demarcated light brown macules. Sites: sun-exposed skin	Increased melanin within basal layer keratinocytes secondary to sun exposure	Skin phototypes I-II	Junctional nevi, Juvenile lentigines	Multiply and darken with sun exposure, fade in winter. No treatment required. Sunscreen may prevent the appearance of new freckles
Solar Lentigo (Liver Spot)	Well-demarcated brown/black irregular macules. Sites: sun-exposed skin	Benign melanocytic proliferation in dermal-epidermal junction due to chronic sun exposure	Most common in Caucasians >40 yr. Skin phototypes I-III	Lentigo maligna, seborrheic keratosis, pigmented solar keratosis	Laser therapy, shave excisions, cryotherapy
Becker's Nevus	Hairy, light brown macule/patch with a papular verrucous surface. Sites: trunk and shoulders, onset in teen years	Pigmented hamartoma with increased melanin in basal cells	M>F. Often becomes noticeable at puberty	Hairy congenital melanocytic nevus	Hair growth follows onset of pigmentation. Cosmetic management (usually too large to remove)
Melasma	Dark, usually symmetrical, skin discolouration on sun-exposed areas of face (forehead, upper lip, cheeks, chin)	Increase in number and activity of melanocytes. Associated with estrogen and progesterone	F>M. Common in pregnancy and women taking OCP or HRT. Risk factors: sun exposure, dark skin tone. Can occur with mild endocrine disturbances, antiepileptic medications and other photosensitizing drugs	Post-inflammatory hyperpigmentation, Riehl melanosis	Often fades over several months after stopping hormone treatment or delivering baby. Treatment: hydroquinone, azelaic acid, retinoic acid, topical steroid, combination creams, destructive modalities (chemical peels, laser treatment), camouflage make-up, sunscreen, sun avoidance

Vascular Lesions

Table 7. Vascular Tumours Compared to Vascular Malformations

	Vascular Tumours	Vascular Malformations
Definition	Endothelial hyperplasia	Congenital malformation with normal endothelial turnover
Presence at Birth	Usually postnatal	100% at birth (not always obvious)
M:F	1:3-5	1:1
Natural History	Phases: Proliferating, Involuting, Involuted	Proportionate growth (can expand)

HEMANGIOMAS

Clinical Presentation
- red or blue subcutaneous mass that is soft/compressible, blanches with pressure; feels like a "bag of worms" when palpated

Pathophysiology
- benign vascular tumour
- includes: cavernous hemangioma, capillary/infantile hemangioma, spider hemangioma

A spider angioma will blanch when the tip of a paperclip is applied to the centre of the lesion

Table 8. Vascular Tumours

	Clinical Presentation	Pathophysiology	Epidemiology	Clinical Course	Management
Hemangioma of infancy	Hot, firm red to blue plaques or tumours	Benign vascular proliferation of endothelial lining	Appears shortly after birth; rarely may be congenital	Appears shortly after birth, increases in size over months, then regresses 50% of lesions resolve spontaneously by 5 yr	10% require treatment due to functional impairment (visual compromise, airway obstruction, high output cardiac failure) or cosmesis Consider treatment if not gone by school age; propranolol; systemic corticosteroids; laser treatment; surgery
Spider Angioma (Campbell Telangiectasia)	Central red arteriole with slender branches, faintly pulsatile, blanchable	Can be associated with hyperestrogenic state (e.g. in hepatocellular disease, pregnancy, OCP) but often is not		Increase in number over time	Reassurance Electrodesiccation or laser surgery if patient wishes
Cherry Angioma (Campbell De Morgan Spot)	Bright red to deep maroon, dome-shaped vascular papules, 1-5 mm Site: trunk Less friable compared to pyogenic granulomas	Benign vascular neoplasm	>30 yr old	Lesions do not fade in time Lesions bleed infrequently	Usually no treatment needed Laser or electrocautery for small lesions Excision of large lesions if necessary
Pyogenic Granuloma	Bright red, dome-shaped sessile or pedunculated friable nodule Sites: fingers, lips, mouth, trunk, toes DDx: glomus tumour, nodular MM, SCC, nodular BCC	Rapidly developing hemangioma Proliferation of capillaries with erosion of epidermis and neutrophilia	<30 yr old		Surgical excision with histologic examination Electrocautery; laser; cryotherapy

VASCULAR MALFORMATIONS

Pyogenic granuloma is a misnomer: it is neither pyogenic nor granulomatous

Table 9. Vascular Malformations

Type	Clinical Presentation	Pathophysiology	Management
Nevus Flammeus (Port-wine stain)	Red to blue macule present at birth that follows a dermatomal distribution, rarely crosses midline Most common site: nape of neck Never spontaneously regresses but grows in proportion to the child	Congenital vascular malformation of dermal capillaries; rarely associated with Sturge-Weber syndrome (V1, V2 distribution)	Laser or make-up
Nevus Simplex (salmon patch)	Pink-red irregular patches Midline macule on glabella known as "Angel Kiss"; on nuchal region known as "Stork Bites" Present in 1/3 of newborns Majority regress spontaneously	Congenital dilation of dermal capillaries	No treatment required

Venous Lake: benign blue or violaceous papular lesion occurring on the face, lips, and ears due to dilation of a venule. Distinguished from malignant pigmented lesions through diascopy, as compression blanches the lesion

Lipoma

Clinical Presentation
- single or multiple non-tender subcutaneous tumours that are soft and mobile
- occurs most frequently on the trunk, and extremities but can be anywhere on the body

Pathophysiology
- adipocytes enclosed in a fibrous capsule

Epidemiology
- often solitary or few in number, if multiple can be associated with rare syndromes

Differential Diagnosis
- angiolipoma, liposarcoma

Investigations
- biopsy only if atypical features (painful, rapid growth, firm)

Management
- reassurance
- excision or liposuction only if desired for cosmetic purposes

Acneiform Eruptions

Acne Vulgaris/Common Acne

Clinical Presentation
- a common inflammatory pilosebaceous disease categorized with respect to severity
  - Type I: comedonal, sparse, no scarring
  - Type II: comedonal, papular, moderate ± little scarring
  - Type III: comedonal, papular, and pustular, with scarring
  - Type IV: nodulocystic acne, risk of severe scarring
- sites of predilection: face, neck, upper chest, and back

Pathophysiology
- hyperkeratinization at the follicular ostia (opening) blocks the secretion of sebum leading to the formation of microcomedones
- androgens promote excess sebum production
- *Propionibacterium* acnes metabolize sebum to free fatty acids and produces pro-inflammatory mediators

Epidemiology
- age of onset in puberty (10-17 yr in females, 14-19 yr in males)
- in prepubertal children consider underlying hormonal abnormality (e.g. late onset congenital adrenal hyperplasia)
- more severe in males than in females
- incidence decreases in adulthood
- genetic predisposition: majority of individuals with cystic acne have parent(s) with history of severe acne

Differential Diagnosis
- folliculitis, keratosis pilaris (upper arms, face, thighs), perioral dermatitis, rosacea

Table 10. Management of Acne

Compound/Drug Class	Product Names	Notes
MILD ACNE: Topical Therapies OTC		
Benzoyl peroxide (BPO)	Solugel, Benzac, Desquam, Fostex	Helps prevent *P. acnes* resistance, is a bactericidal agent (targets *P. acnes*) and is comedolytic
Salicylic acid	Akurza® Cream, DermalZone	Used when patients cannot tolerate a topical retinoid due to skin irritation
MILD ACNE: Prescription Topical Therapies		
Antimicrobials	Clindamycin (Dalacin T), Erythromycin	High rate of resistance when used as monotherapy
Retinoids	Vitamin A Acid (Tretinoin, Stieva-A, Retin A) Adapalene (Differin)	Backbone of topical acne therapy All regimens should include a retinoid unless patient cannot tolerate
Combination products	Clindoxyl (Clindamycin and BPO) Benzaclin (Clindamycin and BPO) Tactuo (Adapalene and BPO) Stievamycine (Tretinoin and Erythromycin) Benzamycine (BPO and Erythromycin)	Allows for greater adherence and efficacy Combines different mechanisms of action to increase efficacy and maximize tolerability
MODERATE ACNE		
Tetracycline/Minocycline/Doxycycline	Sumycin/Minocin/Vibramycin	Use caution with regard to drug interactions: do not use with isotretinoin Sun sensitivity Antibiotics require 3 mo of use before assessing efficacy
Cyproterone acetate-ethinyl estradiol	Diane-35®	After 35 yr of age, estrogen/progesterone should only be considered in exceptional circumstances, carefully weighing the risk/benefit ratio with physician guidance
Spironolactone (source ADA)	Aldactone	May cause hyperkalemia at higher doses Black box warning for breast cancer
SEVERE ACNE		
Isotretinoin	Accutane®, Clarus®, Epuris®	See Table 27 for full side effect profile Most adverse effects are temporary and will resolve when the drug is discontinued Baseline lipid profile (risk of hypertriglyceridemia), LFTs and β-hCG before treatment May transiently exacerbate acne before patient sees improvement Refractory cases may require multiple courses of isotretinoin

Treatment of Acne Scars
- Tretinoin creams
- Microdermabrasion for superficial scars
- Injectable fillers (collagen, hyaluronic acid)
- Fraxel laser

Acne Myths Debunked
- Eating greasy food and chocolate does not cause or worsen acne
- Blackheads (comedones) are black because of oxidized fatty acids, not dirt
- Acne is not caused by poor hygiene; on the contrary, excessive washing of face can be an aggravator

Antibiotics are used in inflammatory skin conditions since they also have anti-inflammatory properties (e.g. macrolides in acne). Topical antibiotics may also be used to treat secondary bacterial superinfections (e.g. impetigo)

Acne Exacerbating Factors
- Systemic medications: lithium, phenytoin, steroids, halogens, androgens, iodides, bromides, danazol
- Topical agents: steroids, tars, ointments, oily cosmetics
- Mechanical pressure or occlusion, such as leaning face on hands
- Emotional stress

A combination of topical retinoids and topical erythromycin or clindamycin is more effective than either agent used alone

Intralesional Injections
Intralesional corticosteroid injections are effective in the treatment of individual acne nodules

Isotretinoin and Pregnancy
- Use of Isotretinoin during pregnancy is associated with spontaneous abortion and major birth defects such as facial dysmorphism and cognitive impairment
- Pregnancy should be ruled out before starting isotretinoin
- Ideally, patients should use 2 forms of contraception while on isotretinoin

Important Controversies Associated with Isotretinoin Therapy for Acne
Am J Clin Dermatol 2013;14:71-76
Study: Review on isotretinoin and (1) depression and suicide, (2) inflammatory bowel disease (IBD), (3) pregnancy prevention programs.
Conclusions
1. The evidence on whether isotretinoin causes depression and suicide is inconsistent; however, numerous controlled studies have shown an improvement in anxiety and depression scores in those taking isotretinoin.
2. There is no association between IBD and isotretinoin use. Only one study showed a significantly increased risk of UC. When considering using isotretinoin in a patient with IBD or with a strong family history, consider involving a gastroenterologist.

Perioral Dermatitis

Clinical Presentation
- discrete erythematous micropapules that often become confluent, forming inflammatory plaques on perioral, perinasal, and periorbital skin
- commonly symmetrical, rim of sparing around vermillion border of lips

Epidemiology
- 15-40 yr old, occasionally in younger children
- predominantly females

Differential Diagnosis
- contact dermatitis, rosacea, acne vulgaris

Management
- avoid all topical steroids
- topical: metronidazole 0.75% gel or 0.75-1% cream to affected area bid
- systemic: tetracycline family antibiotic (utilized for its anti-inflammatory properties)
- occasional use of a non-steroidal anti-inflammatory cream (i.e. tacrolimus or pimecrolimus)

Rosacea

Clinical Presentation
- dome-shaped inflammatory papules ± pustules
- flushing, non-transient erythema, and telangiectasia
- distribution: typically on central face including forehead, nose, cheeks, and chin; rarely on scalp, neck, and upper body
- characterized by remissions and exacerbations
- exacerbating factors: heat, cold, wind, sun, stress, drinking hot liquids, alcohol, caffeine, spices
- all forms of rosacea can progress from mild to moderate to severe
- rarely in longstanding rosacea, signs of thickening, induration and lymphedema in the skin can develop
- phyma: a distinct swelling caused by lymphedema and hypertrophy of subcutaneous tissue, particularly affecting the nose (rhinophyma)
- ocular manifestations: blepharoconjunctivitis, keratitis, iritis

Pathophysiology
- unknown

Epidemiology
- although found in all skin types, highest prevalence in fair-skinned people
- 30-50 yr old; F>M

Differential Diagnosis
- acne vulgaris, seborrheic dermatitis, perioral dermatitis, contact dermatitis

Management
- trigger avoidance and daily sunscreen use for long-term management
- avoid topical corticosteroids
- telangiectasia: treated by physical ablation; electrical hyfrecators, vascular lasers, and intense pulsed light therapies
- phymas: treated by physical ablation or removal; paring, electrosurgery, cryotherapy, laser therapy (CO_2, argon, Nd:YAG)

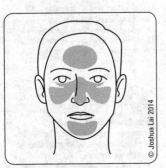

Figure 3. Rosacea distribution

Rosacea can be differentiated from acne by the absence of comedones, a predilection for the central face and symptoms of flushing

Guidelines for the Diagnosis of Rosacea
J Drugs Dermatol 2012;11(6):725-730
Presence of one or more of the following primary features:
• Flushing (transient erythema)
• Nontransient erythema
• Papules and pustules
• Telangiectasia
May include one or more of the following secondary features:
• Burning or stinging
• Dry appearance
• Edema
• Phymatous changes
• Ocular manifestations
• Peripheral location

Table 11. Specific Rosacea Treatments

1st Line	2nd Line	3rd Line
Oral tetracyclines (250-500 mg PO bid)	Topical clindamycin	Oral retinoids
Topical metronidazole	Topical erythromycin 2% solution	Topical sulfur
Oral erythromycin (250-500 mg PO bid)	Topical benzoyl peroxide	
Topical azelaic acid	Oral metronidazole	
	Ampicillin	

Dermatitis (Eczema)

Definition
- inflammation of the skin

Clinical Presentation
- poorly demarcated erythematous patches or plaques
- symptoms include pruritus and pain
- acute dermatitis: papules, vesicles
- subacute dermatitis: scaling, crusting, excoriations
- chronic dermatitis: lichenification, xerosis, fissuring

Asteatotic Dermatitis

Clinical Presentation
- diffuse, mild pruritic dermatitis secondary to dry skin
- very common in elderly, especially in the winter (i.e. "winter itch") but starts in the fall
- shins predominate, looks like a "dried river bed"

Management
- skin rehydration with moisturizing routine ± mild corticosteroid creams

Atopic Dermatitis

Clinical Presentation
- subacute and chronic eczematous reaction associated with prolonged severe pruritus
- distribution depends on age
- inflammation, lichenification, excoriations are secondary to relentless scratching
- atopic palms: hyperlinearity of the palms (associated with ichthyosis vulgaris)
- associated with: keratosis pilaris (hyperkeratosis of hair follicles, "chicken skin"), xerosis, occupational hand dryness

Epidemiology
- frequently affects infants, children, and young adults
- almost 15% of children in developed countries under the age of 5 are affected
- associated with personal or family history of atopy (asthma, hay fever), anaphylaxis, eosinophilia
- polygenic inheritance: one parent >60% chance for child; two parents >80% chance for child
- the earlier the onset, the more severe and persistent the disease
- long-term condition with 1/3 of patients continuing to show signs of AD into adulthood

Pathophysiology
- a T-cell driven process with epidermal barrier dysfunction

Investigations
- clinical diagnosis
- consider: skin biopsy, immunoglobulin serum levels (often elevated serum IgE level), patch testing, and skin prick tests

Management
- goal: reduce signs and symptoms, prevent or reduce recurrences/flares
- better outcome (e.g. less flare-ups, modified course of disease) if diagnosis made early and treatment plan individualized
- avoid triggers of AD
- **non-pharmacologic therapy**
  - moisturizers
    - apply liberally and reapply frequently with goal of minimizing xerosis
    - include in treatment of mild to severe disease as well as in maintenance therapy
  - bathing practices
    - bathe in plain warm water for a short period of time once daily followed by lightly but not completely drying the skin with a towel; immediately apply topical agents or moisturizers after this
    - use fragrance-free hypoallergenic non-soap cleansers
- **pharmacologic therapy**
  - topical corticosteroids
    - effective in reducing acute and chronic symptoms as well as prevention of flares
    - choice of steroid potency depends on age, body site, short vs. long-term use
    - apply 1 adult fingertip unit (0.5 g) to an area the size of 2 adult palms bid for acute flares, and 1-2x/wk for maintenance therapy
    - local side effects: skin atrophy, purpura, telangiectasia, striae, hypertrichosis, and acneiform eruption are all very rarely seen

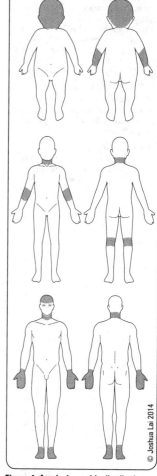

Figure 4. Atopic dermatitis distribution
The typical distribution of atopic dermatitis in infants <6 mo (top), children >18 mo (middle) and adults (bottom)

Triggers for Atopic Dermatitis
- Irritants (detergents, solvents, clothing, water hardness)
- Contact allergens
- Environmental aeroallergens (e.g. dust mites)
- Inappropriate bathing habits (e.g. long hot showers)
- Sweating
- Microbes (e.g. S. aureus)
- Stress

The Diagnostic Value of Atopy Patch Testing and Prick Testing in Atopic Dermatitis: Facts and Controversies
Clin Dermatol 2010;28:38-44
Study: Systematic review.
Conclusions
Use of the atopy patch test (APT) is controversial
• There is no gold standard for aeroallgergen provocation, so APT is used without comparison to another method.
• APT findings are not consistent among children with atopic dermatitis.

APT may be valuable
• May provide diagnostic information and may aid clinical decision making regarding the use of IgE-mediated sensitizations.

Future research is needed
• Need standardized provocation and avoidance testing to determine the clinical relevance of obtaining a positive APT result.

- topical calcineurin inhibitors
  - tacrolimus 0.03%, 0.1% (Protopic®) and pimecrolimus 1% (Elidel®)
  - use as steroid-sparing agents in the long-term
  - advantages over long-term corticosteroid use: rapid, sustained effect in controlling pruritus; no skin atrophy; safe for the face and neck
  - apply 2x/d for acute flares, and 2-3x/wk to recurrent sites to prevent relapses
  - local side effects: stinging, burning, allergic contact dermatitis
  - U.S. black box warning of malignancy risk: rare cases of skin cancer and lymphoma reported; no causal relationship established

Complications
- infections
  - treatment of infections
    - topical mupirocin or fusidic acid (Canada only, not available in US)
    - oral antibiotics (e.g. cloxacillin, cephalexin) for widespread *S. aureus* infections

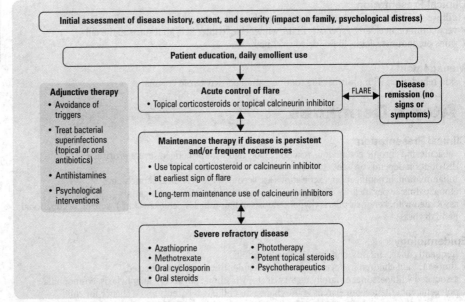

Figure 5. Atopic dermatitis treatment algorithm
Adapted from: Ellis C, et al. ICCAD II Faculty. International Consensus Conference on Atopic Dermatitis II (ICCAD II): clinical update and current treatment strategies. *Br J Dermatol* 2003;148(Suppl 63):3-10

Contact Dermatitis

Clinical Presentation
- cutaneous inflammation caused by an external agent(s)

Table 12. Contact Dermatitis

	Irritant Contact Dermatitis	Allergic Contact Dermatitis
Mechanism of Reaction	Toxic injury to skin; non-immune mechanism	Cell-mediated delayed (Type IV) hypersensitivity reaction (see Rheumatology, RH2)
Type of Reaction	Erythema, dryness, fine scale, burning. Acute: quick reaction, sharp margins (e.g. from acid/alkali exposure). Cumulative insult: slow to appear, poorly defined margins (e.g. from soap), more common	Erythema with a papulovesicular eruption, swelling, pruritus
Frequency	Majority; will occur in anyone given sufficient concentration of irritants	Minority; patient acquires susceptibility to allergen that persists indefinitely
Distribution	Hands are the most common site	Areas exposed to allergen
Examples	Soaps, weak alkali, detergents, organic solvents, alcohol, oils	Many allergens are irritants, so may coincide with irritant dermatitis
Management	Avoidance of irritants. Wet compresses with Burow's solution. Barrier moisturizers. Topical/oral steroids	Patch testing to determine specific allergen. Avoid allergen and its cross-reactants. Wet compresses soaked in Burow's solution (drying agent). Steroid cream (e.g. hydrocortisone 1%, betamethasone valerate 0.05% or 0.1% cream; bid). Systemic steroids prn (prednisone 1 mg/kg, taper over 2 wk)

Dyshidrotic Dermatitis

Clinical Presentation
- "tapioca pudding" papulovesicular dermatitis of hands and feet that coalesce into plaques, followed by painful fissuring
- acute stage often very pruritic
- secondary infections common
- lesions heal with desquamation and may lead to chronic lichenification
- sites: palms and soles ± dorsal surfaces of hands and feet

Pathophysiology
- NOT caused by hyperhidrosis (excessive sweating)
- emotional stress may precipitate flares

Management
- topical: high potency corticosteroid with plastic cling wrap occlusion to increase penetration
- intralesional triamcinolone injection
- systemic:
  - prednisone in severe cases
  - antibiotics for secondary *S. aureus* infection

Nummular Dermatitis

Clinical Presentation
- annular, coin-shaped, pruritic, dry, scaly, erythematous plaques, can become lichenified
- often associated with atopic and dyshidrotic dermatitis
- secondary infection common

Pathophysiology
- little is known, but it is often accompanied by xerosis, which results from a dysfunction of the epidermal lipid barrier; this in turn can allow permeation of environmental agents, which can induce an allergic or irritant response

Management
- moisturization
- mid to high potency corticosteroid ointment bid

Seborrheic Dermatitis

Clinical Presentation
- greasy, erythematous, yellow, scaling, minimally elevated papules and plaques in areas rich in sebaceous glands, can look moist and superficially eroded in flexural regions
- infants: "cradle cap"
- children: may be generalized with flexural and scalp involvement
- adults: diffuse involvement of scalp margin with yellow to white flakes, pruritus, and underlying erythema
- sites: scalp, eyebrows, eyelashes, beard, glabella, post-auricular, over sternum, trunk, body folds, genitalia

Pathophysiology
- possible etiologic association with *Malassezia* spp. (yeast)

Epidemiology
- common in infants and adolescents
- increased incidence and severity in immunocompromised patients
- in adults, can cause dandruff (pityriasis sicca)

Management
- face: ketoconazole (Nizoral®) cream daily or bid + mild steroid cream daily or bid
- scalp: salicylic acid in olive oil or Derma-Smoothe FS® lotion (peanut oil, mineral oil, fluocinolone acetonide 0.01%) to remove dense scales, 2% ketoconazole shampoo (Nizoral®), ciclopirox (Stieprox®) shampoo, selenium sulfide (e.g. Selsun®) or zinc pyrithione (e.g. Head and Shoulders®) shampoo, steroid lotion (e.g. betamethasone valerate 0.1% lotion bid)

Stasis Dermatitis

Clinical Presentation
- erythematous, scaly, pruritic plaques in lower legs, particularly the medial ankle
- brown hemosiderin deposition, woody fibrosis, atrophy blanche, and lipodermatosclerosis in late stages
- usually bilateral, accompanied by swelling, oozing, crusting, may have accompanying varicosities

Pathophysiology
- chronic venous insufficiency leads to venous stasis
- surrounding soft tissue inflammation and fibrosis results

Investigations
- Doppler and colour-coded Duplex sonography if suspicious for DVT
- culture for MRSA if there is crusting

Management
- compression stockings
- rest and elevate legs (above the level of the heart)
- moisturizer to treat xerosis
- mid-high potency topical corticosteroids to control inflammation

Complications
- ulceration (common at medial malleolus), secondary bacterial infections

Lichen Simplex Chronicus

Clinical Presentation
- well-defined plaque(s) of lichenified skin with increased skin markings ± excoriations
- common sites: neck, scalp, lower extremities, urogenital area
- often seen in patients with atopy

Pathophysiology
- skin hyperexcitable to itch, continued rubbing/scratching of skin results
- eventually lichenification occurs

Investigations
- if patient has generalized pruritus, rule out systemic cause: CBC with differential count, transaminases, bilirubin, renal and thyroid function tests
- CXR if lymphoma suspected

Management
- antipruritics (e.g. antihistamines, topical or intralesional glucocorticoids, Unna boot)

Papulosquamous Diseases

Lichen Planus

The 6 Ps of Lichen Planus
Purple
Pruritic
Polygonal
Peripheral
Papules
Penis (i.e. mucosa)

Clinical Presentation
- acute or chronic inflammation of mucous membranes or skin, especially on flexural surfaces
- morphology: pruritic, well-demarcated, violaceous, polygonal, flat-topped papules
- common sites: wrists, ankles, mucous membranes in 60% (mouth, vulva, glans), nails, scalp
- distribution: symmetrical and bilateral
- Wickham's striae: reticulate white-grey lines over surface; pathognomonic but may not be present
- mucous membrane lesions: lacy, whitish reticular network, milky-white plaques/papules; increased risk of SCC in erosions and ulcers
- nails: longitudinal ridging; dystrophic; pterygium formation
- scalp: scarring alopecia with perifollicular hyperkeratosis
- spontaneously resolves but may last for weeks, months or years (mouth and skin lesions)
- rarely associated with hepatitis C
- Koebner phenomenon

Pathophysiology
- autoimmune, antigen unknown
- lymphocyte activation leads to keratinocyte apoptosis

Epidemiology
- 1%
- 30-60 yr old, F>M

Investigations
- biopsy
- hepatitis C serology if patient has risk factors

Management
- topical or intralesional corticosteroids
- short courses of oral prednisone (rarely)
- phototherapy for generalized or resistant cases
- oral retinoids for erosive lichen planus in mouth
- systemic immunosuppressants (e.g. azathioprine, methotrexate, cyclosporine)

Pityriasis Rosea

Clinical Presentation
- acute, self-limiting eruption characterized by red, oval plaques/patches with central scale that does not extend to edge of lesion
- long axis of lesions follows skin tension lines (i.e. Langer's Lines) parallel to ribs producing "Christmas tree" pattern on back
- varied degree of pruritus
- most start with a "herald" patch which precedes other lesions by 1-2 wk
- common sites: trunk, proximal aspects of arms and legs

Etiology
- suspected HHV-7 or HHV-6 reactivation

Investigations
- none required

Management
- none required; clears spontaneously in 6-12 wk
- symptomatic: topical glucocorticoids if pruritic, cool compresses, emollients

Psoriasis

Classification

1. plaque psoriasis   2. guttate psoriasis   3. erythrodermic psoriasis
4. pustular psoriasis   5. inverse psoriasis

Pathophysiology
- not fully understood, genetic and immunologic factors
- shortened keratinocyte cell cycle leads to Th1- and Th17-mediated inflammatory response

Epidemiology
- 1.5-2%, M=F
- all ages: peaks of onset: 20-30 and 50-60
- polygenic inheritance: 8% with 1 affected parent, 41% with both parents affected
- risk factors: smoking, obesity, alcohol, drugs, infections

Differential Diagnosis
- AD, mycosis fungoides (cutaneous T-cell lymphoma), seborrheic dermatitis, tinea, nummular dermatitis, lichen planus

Investigations
- biopsy (if atypical presentation, rarely needed)

1. PLAQUE PSORIASIS

Clinical Presentation
- chronic and recurrent disease characterized by well-circumscribed erythematous papules/plaques with silvery-white scales
- often worse in winter (lack of sun and humidity)
- Auspitz sign: bleeds from minute points when scale is removed
- common sites: scalp, extensor surfaces of elbows and knees, trunk (especially buttocks), nails, pressure areas

PSORIASIS: Presentation and Pathophysiology
Pink papules/Plaques/Pinpoint bleeding (Auspitz sign)/Physical injury (Koebner phenomenon)
Silver scale/Sharp margins
Nail findings: pitting/onycholysis/Oil spots/ subungual hyperkeratosis/red lunula/
Itching (sometimes)
Immunologic with Th 1 and Th 17 helper cells being actively involved in the pathogenesis

PSORIASIS: Triggers
- Physical trauma (Koebner phenomenon)
- Infections (acute streptococcal infection precipitates guttate psoriasis)
- Stress (can be a major factor in flares)
- Drugs (rebound from stopping systemic glucocorticoids, lithium, antimalarial drugs, interferon)
- Smoking and heavy alcohol consumption

Mechanism of Biologics
"-mab" = monoclonal antibody
"-cept" = receptor

Topical Treatments for Chronic Plaque Psoriasis
Cochrane DB Syst Rev 2013;3:CD005028
Study: Systematic review of randomised trials comparing active topical treatments against placebo or against vitamin D analogues (used alone or in combination) in people with chronic plaque psoriasis.
Patients: 34,808 participants, including 26 trials of scalp psoriasis and 6 trials of inverse psoriasis, facial psoriasis, or both.
Intervention: Vitamin D analogues, corticosteroids, dithranol, tazarotene, coal tar.
Primary Outcomes: Investigator assessment of overall global improvement. Total severity scores. Psoriasis area and severity index. Patient assessment of overall global improvement.
Results: Corticosteroids perform at least as well as vitamin D analogues, and they are associated with a lower incidence of local adverse events. A combination of corticosteroids and vitamin D were better than either vitamin D or corticosteroids alone.

Calcipotriol is a Vitamin D Derivative
Dovobet® = calcipotriene combined
with betamethasone dipropionate and is
considered to be one of the most potent
topical psoriatic therapies

Management

- principles of management depends on severity of disease, as defined by BSA affected or less commonly Psoriasis Area and Severity Index (PASI)
- mild (<5% BSA)
  - topical steroids, topical vitamin D3 analogues, or a combinations of the two are first line
  - topical retinoid ± topical steroid combination, anthralin, and tar are also effective but tend to have more side effects than first line therapies
  - emollients potentiate the effect of topical therapies
  - phototherapy or systemic treatment may be necessary if the lesions are scattered or if it involves sites that are difficult to treat such as palms, soles, scalp, genitals
- moderate (5-10% BSA) to severe (>10% BSA)
  - goal of treatment is to attain symptom control that is adequate from patient's perspective
  - phototherapy if accessible
  - systemic or biological therapy based on patient's treatment history and comorbidities
  - topical steroid ± topical vitamin D3 analogue as adjunct therapy

Table 13. Topical Treatment of Psoriasis

Treatment	Mechanism	Comments
Emollients	Reduce fissure formation	Petrolatum is effective
Salicylic acid 1-12%	Remove scales	
Tar (LCD: liquor carbonis detergens)	Inhibits DNA synthesis, increases cell turnover	Poor long-term compliance
Topical Corticosteroids	Reduce scaling and thickness	Use appropriate potency steroid in different areas for degree of psoriasis
Vitamin D3 analogues: Calcipotriene / calcipotriol (Dovonex®, Silkis®)	Binds to skin 1,25-dihydroxyvitamin D3 to inhibit keratinocyte proliferation	Can be used on face and skin folds
Betamethasone + calcipotriene (Dovobet®)	Combined corticosteroid and vitamin D3 analogue. See above mechanisms	Not to be used on face and folds
Tazarotene (Tazorac®) (gel/cream)	Retinoid derivative, decreased scaling	Use on nails

Table 14. Systemic Treatment of Psoriasis

Treatment	Considerations	Adverse Effects
Acitretin	More effective when used in combination with phototherapy	Alopecia, cheilitis, teratogenicity, hepatotoxicity, photosensitivity, epistaxis, xerosis, hypertriglyceridemia
Cyclosporine	Used for intermittent control rather than continuouslyAvoid using for >1 yr	Renal toxicity, hypertension, hypertriglyceridemia, immunosuppression, lymphoma
Methotrexate	Has been used for over 50 yr	Bone marrow toxicity, hepatic cirrhosis, teratogenicity
Apremilast (Otezla®)	Extremely safe	GI upset, headache, weight loss
PUVA	Highly effective in achieving remission Avoid >200 sessions in lifetime	Pruritus, burning, cataracts, skin cancer
UVB and "Narrow band" UVB (311-312 nm)	Much less carcinogenic than PUVA	Rare burning

Table 15. Biologics Approved in Canada

Treatment	Route	Dosing Schedule	Effectiveness	Action
Etanercept (Enbrel®)*	SC	50 mg twice weekly for 3 mo, then 50 mg weekly	+++	Anti-TNF
Adalimumab (Humira®)*	SC	80 mg x 1, then 40 mg at wk 1 and every 2 wk thereafter	++++	Anti-TNF
Infliximab (Remicade®)*	IV	5 mg/kg at wk 0, 2, 6 and every 8 wk thereafter	+++++	Anti-TNF
Ustekinumab (Stelara®)	SC	45 mg or 90 mg at wk 0, 4 and every 12 wk thereafter	++++	Anti-IL 12/23
Secukinumab (Cosentyx®)	SC	300 mg at week 0, 1, 2, 3, 4 and every 4 wk thereafter	+++++	Anti-IL 17A

*Can also be used to treat psoriatic arthritis

- biologics under study for treatment of psoriasis: secukinumab, brodalumab, ixekizumab, tildrakizumab, guselkumab

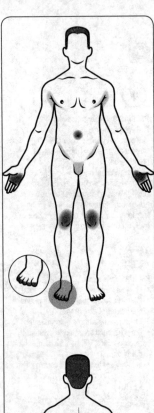

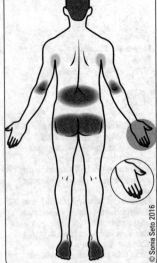

© Sonia Seto 2016

Figure 6. Psoriasis distribution

2. GUTTATE PSORIASIS ("DROP-LIKE")

Clinical Presentation
- discrete, scattered salmon-pink small scaling papules
- sites: diffuse, usually on trunk and legs, sparing palms and soles
- often antecedent streptococcal pharyngitis

Management
- UVB phototherapy, sunlight, lubricants
- penicillin V or erythromycin if Group A β-hemolytic *Streptococcus* on throat culture

3. ERYTHRODERMIC PSORIASIS

Clinical Presentation
- generalized erythema (> 90% of body surface area) with fine desquamative scale on surface
- associated signs and symptoms: arthralgia, pruritus, dehydration, electrolyte imbalance
- aggravating factors: lithium, β-blockers, NSAIDs, antimalarials, phototoxic reaction, infection

Management
- IV fluids, monitor fluids and electrolytes, may require hospitalization
- treat underlying aggravating condition, sun avoidance
- cyclosporine, acitretin, UV, biologics

4. PUSTULAR PSORIASIS

Clinical Presentation
- sudden onset of erythematous macules and papules which evolve rapidly into pustules, can be painful
- may be generalized or localized to palms/soles
- patient usually has a history of psoriasis; may occur with sudden withdrawal from steroid therapy

Management
- methotrexate, cyclosporine, acitretin, biologics

5. INVERSE PSORIASIS

Clinical Presentation
- erythematous plaques on flexural surfaces such as axillae, inframammary folds, gluteal fold, inguinal folds
- lesions may be macerated

Management
- low potency topical corticosteroids
- topical vitamin D derivatives such as calcipotriene or calcitriol
- topical calcineurin inhibitors such as tacrolimus or pimecrolimus

6. PSORIATIC ARTHRITIS
- 5-30% of patients with psoriasis can also be suffering from psoriatic arthritis
- psoriatic patients with nail or scalp involvement are at a higher risk for developing psoriatic arthritis
- see Rheumatology, RH23

Vesiculobullous Diseases

Bullous Pemphigoid

Clinical Presentation
- chronic autoimmune bullous eruption characterized by pruritis, pruritic, tense, subepidermal bullae on an erythematous or normal skin base
- can present as urticarial plaques without bullae
- common sites: flexor aspect of forearms, axillae, medial thighs, groin, abdomen, mouth in 33%

Pathophysiology
- IgG produced against dermal-epidermal basement membrane proteins (hemidesmosomes) leads to subepidermal bullae

Epidemiology
- mean age of onset: 60-80 yr old, F=M

Investigations
- immunofluorescence shows linear deposition of IgG and C3 along the basement membrane
- anti-basement membrane antibody (IgG) (pemphigoid antibody detectable in serum)

Prognosis
- heals without scarring, usually chronic
- rarely fatal

Management
- prednisone 0.5-1 mg/kg/day until clear, then taper ± steroid-sparing agents (e.g. azathioprine, methotrexate)
- topical potent steroids (clobetasol) may be as effective as systemic steroids in limited disease
- tetracycline ± nicotinamide is effective for some cases
- immunosuppressants such as azathioprine, mycophenolate mofetil, cyclosporine
- IVIg and plasmapheresis for refractory cases

Pemphigus Vulgaris

Clinical Presentation
- autoimmune blistering disease characterized by flaccid, non-pruritic intraepidermal bullae/vesicles on an erythematous or normal skin base
- may present with erosions and secondary bacterial infection
- sites: mouth (90%), scalp, face, chest, axillae, groin, umbilicus
- Nikolsky's sign: epidermal detachment with shear stress
- Asboe-Hansen sign: pressure applied to bulla causes it to extend laterally

Pathophysiology
- IgG against epidermal desmoglein-1 and -3 lead to loss of intercellular adhesion in the epidermis

Epidemiology
- 40-60 yr old, M=F, higher prevalence in Jewish, Mediterranean, Asian populations
- paraneoplastic pemphigus may be associated with thymoma, myasthenia gravis, malignancy, and use of D-penicillamine

Investigations
- immunofluorescence: shows IgG and C3 deposition intraepidermally
- circulating serum anti-desmoglein IgG antibodies

Prognosis
- lesions heal with hyperpigmentation but do not scar
- may be fatal unless treated with immunosuppressive agents

Management
- prednisone 1-2 mg/kg until no new blisters, then 1-1.5 mg/kg until clear, then taper ± steroid-sparing agents (e.g. azathioprine, methotrexate, gold, cyclophosphamide, cyclosporine, IVIg, mycophenolate mofetil, rituximab)

Dermatitis Herpetiformis

Clinical Presentation
- grouped papules/vesicles/urticarial wheals on an erythematous base, associated with intense pruritus, burning, stinging, excoriations
- lesions grouped, bilaterally symmetrical
- common sites: extensor surfaces of elbows/knees, sacrum, buttocks, scalp

Pathophysiology
- transglutaminase IgA deposits in the skin alone or in immune complexes leading to eosinophil and neutrophil infiltration
- 90% have HLA B8, DR3, DQWZ
- 90-100% associated with an often subclinical gluten-sensitive enteropathy (i.e. celiac disease)
- 30% have thyroid disease; increased risk of intestinal lymphoma in untreated comorbid celiac disease; iron/folate deficiency is common

Epidemiology
- 20-60 yr old, M:F = 2:1

Investigations
- biopsy
- immunofluorescence shows IgA deposits in perilesional skin

Pemphigus Vulgaris vs. Bullous Pemphigoid
Vulgari**S** = **S**uperficial, intraepidermal, flaccid lesions
Pemphigoi**D** = **D**eeper, tense lesions at the dermal-epidermal junction

Pemphigus Foliaceus
An autoimmune intraepidermal blistering disease that is more superficial than pemphigus vulgaris due to antibodies against desmoglein-1, a transmembrane adhesion molecule. Appears as crusted patches, erosions and/or flaccid bullae that usually start on the trunk. Localized disease can be managed with topical steroids. Active widespread disease is treated like pemphigus vulgaris

Management
- dapsone (sulfapyridine if contraindicated or poorly tolerated)
- gluten-free diet for life – this can reduce risk of lymphoma

Porphyria Cutanea Tarda

Clinical Presentation
- skin fragility followed by formation of tense vesicles/bullae and erosions on photoexposed skin
- gradual healing to scars, milia
- periorbital violaceous discolouration, diffuse hypermelanosis, facial hypertrichosis
- common sites: light-exposed areas subjected to trauma, dorsum of hands and feet, nose, and upper trunk

Pathophysiology
- uroporphyrinogen decarboxylase deficiency leads to excess heme precursors
- can be associated with hemochromatosis, alcohol abuse, DM, drugs (estrogen therapy, NSAIDs), HIV, hepatitis C, increased iron indices

Epidemiology
- 30-40 yr old, M>F

Investigations
- urine + 5% HCl shows orange-red fluorescence under Wood's lamp (UV rays)
- 24 h urine for uroporphyrins (elevated)
- stool contains elevated coproporphyrins
- immunofluorescence shows IgE at dermal-epidermal junctions

Management
- discontinue aggravating substances (alcohol, estrogen therapy)
- phlebotomy to decrease body iron load
- low dose hydroxychloroquine

Drug Eruptions

Exanthematous

EXANTHEMATOUS DRUG REACTION

Clinical Presentation
- morphology: erythematous macules and papules ± scale
- spread: symmetrical, trunk to extremities
- time course: 7-14 d after drug initiation, fades 7-14 d after withdrawal

Epidemiology
- most common cutaneous drug reaction; increased in presence of infections
- common causative agents: penicillin, sulfonamides, phenytoin

Management
- weigh risks and benefits of drug discontinuation
- antihistamines, emollients, topical steroids

Diagnosis of a Drug Reaction
Classification by Naranjo et. al has 4 criteria:
1. Temporal relationship between drug exposure and reaction
2. Recognized response to suspected drug
3. Improvement after drug withdrawal
4. Recurrence of reaction on re-challenge with the drug
Definite drug reaction requires all 4 criteria to be met
Probable drug reaction requires #1-3 to be met
Possible drug reaction requires only #1

DRUG INDUCED HYPERSENSITIVITY SYNDROME (DIHS) / DRUG REACTION WITH EOSINOPHILIA AND SYSTEMIC SYMPTOMS (DRESS)

Clinical Presentation
- morphology: morbilliform rash involving face, trunk, arms; can have facial edema
- systemic features: fever, malaise, cervical lymphadenopathy, internal organ involvement (e.g. hepatitis, arthralgia, nephritis, pneumonitis, lymphadenopathy, hematologic abnormalities, thyroid abnormalities)
- spread: starts with face or periorbitally and spreads caudally; no mucosal involvement
- time course: onset 1-6 weeks after first exposure to drug, persists weeks after withdrawal of drug

Epidemiology
- rare: incidence varies considerably depending on drug
- common causative agents: anticonvulsants (e.g. phenytoin, phenobarbital, carbamazepine, lamotrigine), sulfonamides, and allopurinol
- 10% mortality if severe, undiagnosed, and untreated

Management
- discontinue offending drug ± prednisone 0.5mg/kg per day, consider cyclosporine in severe cases
- may progress to generalized exfoliative dermatitis/erythroderma if drug is not discontinued

Drug Hypersensitivity Syndrome Triad
- Fever
- Exanthematous eruption
- Internal organ involvement

Urticarial

DRUG INDUCED URTICARIA AND ANGIOEDEMA

Clinical Presentation
- morphology: wheals lasting <24hrs, angioedema (face and mucous membranes)
- systemic features: may be associated with systemic anaphylaxis (bronchospasm, laryngeal edema, shock)
- time course: hours to days after exposure depending on the mechanism

Epidemiology
- second most common cutaneous drug reaction
- common causative agents: penicillins, ACEI, analgesics/anti-inflammatories, radiographic contrast media

Management
- discontinue offending drug, antihistamines, steroids, epinephrine if anaphylactic

SERUM SICKNESS-LIKE REACTION

Clinical Presentation
- morphology: symmetrical cutaneous eruption (usually urticarial)
- systemic features: malaise, low grade fever, arthralgia, lymphadenopathy
- time course: appears 1-3 wks after drug initiation, resolve 2-3 wks after withdrawal

Epidemiology
- more prevalent in kids 0.02-0.2%
- common causative agents: cefaclor in kids; bupropion in adults

Management
- discontinue offending drug ± topical/oral corticosteroids

Pustular

ACUTE GENERALIZED EXANTHEMATOUS PUSTULOSIS (AGEP)

Clinical Presentation
- morphology: erythematous edema and sterile pustules prominent in intertriginous areas
- systemic features: high fever, leukocytosis with neutrophilia
- spread: starts in face and intertriginous areas and spread to trunk and extremities
- time course: appears 1 wk after drug initiation, resolve 2 wks after withdrawal

Epidemiology
- rare: 1-5/million
- common causative agents: aminopenicillins, cephalosporins, clindamycin, calcium channel blockers

Management
- discontinue offending drug and systemic corticosteroids

Bullous

STEVEN-JOHNSON SYNDROME (SJS)/TOXIC EPIDERMAL NECROLYSIS (TEN)

Clinical Presentation
- morphology: prodromal rash (morbilliform/targetoid lesions ± purpura, or diffuse erythema), confluence of flaccid blisters, positive Nikolsky sign (epidermal detachment with shear stress), full thickness epidermal loss; dusky tender skin, bullae, desquamation/skin sloughing, atypical targets
- classification: BSA with epidermal detachment: <10% in SJS, 10-30% in SJS/TEN overlap, and >30% in TEN
- spread: face and extremities; may generalize; scalp, palms, soles relatively spared; erosion of mucous membranes (lips, oral mucosa, conjunctiva, GU mucosa)
- systemic features: fever (higher in TEN), cytopenias, renal tubular necrosis/AKI, tracheal erosion, infection, contractures, corneal scarring, phimosis, vaginal synechiae
- time course: appears 1-3 wk after drug initiation; progression <4 d; epidermal regrowth in 3 wk
- can have constitutional symptoms: malaise, fever, hypotension, tachycardia

Epidemiology
- SJS: 1.2-6/million; TEN: 0.4-1.2/million
- risk factors: SLE, HIV/AIDS, HLA-B1502 (associated with carbamazepine), HLA-B5801 (associated with allopurinol)
- common causative agents: drugs (allopurinol, anti-epileptics, sulfonamides, NSAIDs, cephalosporins) responsible in 50% of SJS and 80% of TEN; viral or mycoplasma infections;
- prognosis: 5% mortality in SJS, 30% in TEN due to fluid loss and infection

SCORTEN Score for TEN Prognosis
One point for each of: age ≥40, malignancy, body surface area detached ≥10%, tachycardia ≥120 bpm, serum urea >10 mmol/L, serum glucose >14 mmol/L, serum bicarbonate <20 mmol/L

Used to determine appropriate clinical setting: score 0-1 can be treated in non-specialized wards; score ≥2 should be transferred to intensive care or burn unit

Score at admission is predictive of survival: 94% for 0-1, 87% for 2, 53% for 3, 25% for 4, and 17% for ≥5

Differential Diagnosis
- Scarlet fever, phototoxic eruption, GVHD, SSSS, exfoliative dermatitis, AGEP, paraneoplastic pemphigus

Management
- discontinue offending drug
- admit to intermediate/intensive care/burn unit
- supportive care: IV fluids, electrolyte replacement, nutritional support, pain control, wound care, sterile handling, monitor for and treat infection
- IVIg or cyclosporine

Other

FIXED DRUG ERUPTION

Clinical Presentation
- morphology: sharply demarcated erythematous oval patches on the skin or mucous membranes
- spread: commonly face, mucosa, genitalia, acral; recurs in same location upon subsequent exposure to the drug (fixed location)

Epidemiology
- common causative agents: antimicrobials (tetracycline, sulfonamides), anti-inflammatories, psychoactive agents (barbiturates), phenolphthalein

Management
- discontinue offending drug ± prednisone 1mg/kg/d x 2 wk for generalized lesions ± potent topical corticosteroids for non-eroded lesions or antimicrobial ointment for eroded lesions

PHOTOSENSITIVITY REACTION

Clinical Presentation
- phototoxic reaction: "exaggerated sunburn" (erythema, edema, vesicles, bullae) confined to sun-exposed areas
- photoallergic reaction: pruritic eczematous eruption with papules, vesicles, scaling, and crusting that may spread to areas not exposed to light

Pathophysiology
- phototoxic reaction: direct tissue injury
- photoallergic reaction: type IV delayed hypersensitivity

Epidemiology
- common causative agents: chlorpromazine, doxycycline, thiazide diuretics, procainamide

Management
- sun protection ± topical/oral corticosteroids

Heritable Disorders

Ichthyosis Vulgaris

Clinical Presentation
- xerosis with fine scaling as well as large adherent scales ("fish-scales")
- affects arms, legs, palms, soles, back, forehead, and cheeks; spares flexural creases
- improves in summer, with humidity, and as the child grows into adulthood

Pathophysiology
- genetic deficiency in filaggrin protein leads to abnormal retention of keratinocytes (hyperkeratosis)
- scaling without inflammation

Epidemiology
- 1:300 incidence
- autosomal dominant inheritance
- associated with AD and keratosis pilaris

Investigations
- electron microscopy: keratohyalin granules

Management
- immersion in bath and oils followed by an emollient cream, humectant cream, or creams/oil containing urea or α- or β-hydroxy acids
- intermittent systemic retinoids for severe cases

Intravenous Immunoglobulin in the Treatment of Stevens-Johnson Syndrome and Toxic Epidermal Necrolysis: A Meta-Analysis with Meta-Regression of Observational Studies
Int J Dermatol 2015;54(1):108-15
Study: Systematic review of 17 articles (retrospective cohort studies were most common, no RCTs).
Patients: Individuals with a diagnosis of SJS/TEN treated with IVIg.
Intervention: Various doses and regimens of IVIg.
Outcomes: Time to disease cessation, time to healing.
Results: Eleven of 14 TEN studies reported positive results, while three studies did not observe a statistically significant improvement. Two of three SJS studies reported positive results, with one study observing no significant difference in mortality, or speed of healing.
Conclusion: IVIg appears to have a positive impact on TEN/SJS but results cannot be statistically analyzed as a whole due to variability and inconsistency in data presented from each study. However, it is considered the gold standard treatment.

Neurofibromatosis (Type I; von Recklinghausen's Disease)

Clinical Presentation
- diagnostic criteria includes 2 or more of the following
    1. more than 5 café-au-lait patches >1.5 cm in an adult or more than 5 café-au-lait macules >0.5 cm in a child under 5 yr
    2. axillary or inguinal freckling
    3. iris hamartomas (Lisch nodules)
    4. optic gliomas
    5. neurofibromas
    6. distinctive bony lesion (sphenoid wing dysplasia or thinning of long bone cortex)
    7. first degree relative with neurofibromatosis type 1
- associated with pheochromocytoma, astrocytoma, bilateral acoustic neuromas, bone cysts, scoliosis, precocious puberty, developmental delay, and renal artery stenosis
- skin lesions less prominent in neurofibromatosis Type II (see Pediatrics, P84)

Pathophysiology
- autosomal dominant disorder with excessive and abnormal proliferation of neural crest elements (Schwann cells, melanocytes), high incidence of spontaneous mutation
- linked to absence of neurofibromin (a tumour suppressor gene)

Epidemiology
- incidence 1:3,000

Investigations
- Wood's lamp examination to detect café-au-lait macules in patients with pale skin

Management
- refer to orthopedics, ophthalmology, plastics, and psychology for relevant management
- follow-up annually for brain tumours such as astrocytoma
- excise suspicious or painful lesions
- see Pediatrics, P84

Vitiligo

Clinical Presentation
- primary pigmentary disorder characterized by depigmentation
- acquired destruction of melanocytes characterized by sharply marginated white patches
- associated with streaks of depigmented hair, chorioretinitis
- sites: extensor surfaces and periorificial areas (mouth, eyes, anus, genitalia)
- Koebner phenomenon, may be precipitated by trauma

Pathophysiology
- acquired autoimmune destruction of melanocytes

Epidemiology
- 1% incidence, polygenic
- 30% with positive family history

Investigations
- rule out associated autoimmune diseases: thyroid disease, pernicious anemia, Addison's disease, Type I DM
- Wood's lamp to detect lesions: illuminates UV light onto skin to detect amelanosis (porcelain white discolouration)

Management
- sun avoidance and protection
- topical calcineurin inhibitor (e.g. tacrolimus, pimecrolimus) or topical corticosteroids
- PUVA or Narrow band UVB
- make-up
- "bleaching" normal pigmented areas (i.e. monobenzyl ether of hydroquinone 20%) if widespread loss of pigmentation

Interventions for Vitiligo
Cochrane Database Syst Rev. 2015;2:CD003263.
Study: Systematic review of 96 randomized controlled trials with 4,512 participants with vitiligo.
Intervention: Topical treatments, light therapies, oral treatments, surgical methods.
Outcome Measures: Quality of life, >75% repigmentation, adverse effects
Results: Some evidence of therapies for vitiligo but further research required due to differences in design and outcome measures. Evidence exists to support use of combination therapies to be more effective than single agent. Narrowband UVB light, alone or in combination, show better results. Use of topical corticosteroids reported most adverse effects.

Infections

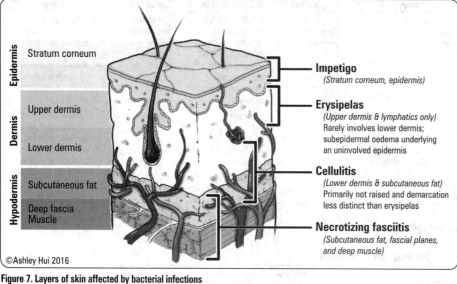

Figure 7. Layers of skin affected by bacterial infections

Location Matters!

e.g. Group A Strep Infections
- Impetigo → just below stratum corneum
- Erysipelas → epidermis and upper dermis only
- Cellulitis → primarily lower dermis and subcutis (primarily not raised, and demarcation less distinct than erysipelas)
- Necrotizing fasciitis → deep fascia and muscle

Bacterial Infections

EPIDERMIS

IMPETIGO

Clinical Presentation
- acute purulent infection which appears vesicular; progresses to golden yellow "honey-crusted" lesions surrounded by erythema
- can present with bullae
- common sites: face, arms, legs, and buttocks

Etiology
- GAS, *S.aureus*, or both

Epidemiology
- preschool and young adults living in crowded conditions, poor hygiene, neglected minor trauma

Differential Diagnosis
- infected eczema, HSV, VZV

Investigations
- Gram stain and culture of lesion fluid or biopsy

Management
- remove crusts, use saline compresses, and topical antiseptic soaks bid
- topical antibacterials such as 2% mupirocin or fusidic acid (Canada only) tid; continue for 7-10 d after resolution
- systemic antibiotics such as cloxacillin or cephalexin for 7-10 d

DERMIS

Table 16. Comparison of Erysipelas and Cellulitis

	Clinical Presentation	Etiology	Complications	Differential Diagnosis	Investigations	Management
Erysipelas	Involves upper dermis Confluent, erythematous, sharp raised edge, warm plaque, well demarcated Very painful ("St. Anthony's fire") Sites: face and legs Systemic symptoms: fever, chills, headache, weakness (if present, sign of more serious infection)	GAS	Scarlet fever, streptococcal gangrene, fat necrosis, coagulopathy Spreads via lymphatics	DVT (less red, less hot, smoother), superficial phlebitis, contact dermatitis, photosensitivity reaction, stasis dermatitis, panniculitis, vasculitis	Clinical diagnosis: rarely do skin/blood culture If suspect necrotizing fasciitis: do immediate biopsy and frozen section, histopathology	1st line: penicillin, cloxacillin or cefazolin 2nd line: clindamycin or cephalexin If allergic to penicillin, use erythromycin
Cellulitis	Involves lower dermis/subcutaneous fat Unilateral erythematous flat lesion, often with vesicles poorly demarcated, not uniformly raised Tender Sites: commonly on legs Systemic symptoms (uncommon): fever, leukocytosis, lymphadenopathy	GAS, S. aureus (large sized wounds), H. influenzae (periorbital), Pasteurella multocida (dog/cat bite)	Uncommon	Same as erysipelas	Same as erysipelas	1st line: cloxacillin or cefazolin/cephalexin 2nd line: erythromycin or clindamycin Children: cefuroxime If DM (foot infections): TMP/SMX and metronidazole

COMMON HAIR FOLLICLE INFECTIONS

Table 17. Comparison of Superficial Folliculitis, Furuncles, and Carbuncles

	Clinical Presentation	Etiology	Management
Superficial Folliculitis	Superficial infection of the hair follicle (versus pseudofolliculitis: inflammation of follicle due to friction, irritation, or occlusion) Acute lesion consists of a dome-shaped pustule at the mouth of hair follicle Pustule ruptures to form a small crust Sites: primarily scalp, shoulders, anterior chest, upper back, other hair-bearing areas	Normal non-pathogenic bacteria (Staphylococcus – most common; Pseudomonas – hot tub) Pityrosporum	Antiseptic (Hibiclens®) Topical antibacterial (fusidic acid, mupirocin, erythromycin or clindamycin) Oral cloxacillin for 7-10 d
Furuncles (Boils)	Red, hot, tender, inflammatory nodules with central yellowish point, which forms over summit and ruptures Involves subcutaneous tissue that arises from a hair follicle Sites: hair-bearing skin (thigh, neck, face, axillae, perineum, buttocks)	S. aureus	Incise and drain large furuncles to relieve pressure and pain If afebrile: hot wet packs, topical antibiotic If febrile/cellulitis: culture blood and aspirate pustules (Gram stain and C&S) Cloxacillin for 1-2 wk (especially for lesions near external auditory canal/nose, with surrounding cellulitis, and not responsive to topical therapy)
Carbuncles	Deep-seated abscess formed by multiple coalescing furuncles Usually in areas of thicker skin Occasionally ulcerates Lesions drain through multiple openings to the surface Systemic symptoms may be associated	S. aureus	Same as for furuncles

Dermatophytoses

Clinical Presentation
- infection of skin, hair, and nails caused by dermatophytes (fungi that live within the epidermal keratin or hair follicle and do not penetrate into deeper structures)

Pathophysiology
- digestion of keratin by dermatophytes results in scaly skin, broken hairs, crumbling nails/onycholysis

Etiology
- *Trichophyton, Microsporum, Epidermophyton* species (*Pityrosporum* is a superficial yeast and not a dermatophyte)

Investigations
- skin scrapings, hair, and/or nail clippings analyzed with potassium hydroxide (KOH) prep to look for hyphae and mycelia

Management
- topicals as first line agents for tinea corporis/cruris and tinea pedis (interdigital type): clotrimazole, or terbinafine or ciclopirox olamine cream applied bid
- oral therapy is indicated for onychomycosis or tinea capitis: terbinafine (Lamisil® – liver toxicity, CYP2D6 inhibitor) or itraconazole (Sporanox® – CYP3A4 inhibitor, liver toxicity)

Table 18. Different Manifestations of Dermatophyte Infection

	Clinical Presentation	Differential Diagnosis	Investigations	Management
Tinea Capitis	Round, scaly patches of alopecia, possibly with broken off hairs; pruritic Sites: scalp, eyelashes, and eyebrows; involving hair shafts and follicles Kerion (boggy, elevated, purulent inflamed nodule/plaque) may form secondary to infection by bacteria and result in scarring May have occipital lymphadenopathy Affects children (mainly black), immunocompromised adults Very contagious and may be transmitted from barber, hats, theatre seats, pets	Alopecia areata, psoriasis, seborrheic dermatitis, trichotillomania	Wood's light examination of hair: green fluorescence only for Microsporum infection Culture of scales/hair shaft Microscopic examination of KOH preparation of scales or hair shafts	Terbinafine (Lamisil®) x 4 wk NB: oral agents are required to penetrate the hair root where dermatophyte resides Adjunctive antifungal shampoos or lotions may be helpful, and may prevent spread (e.g. selenium sulfide, ketoconozole, ciclopirox)
Tinea Corporis (Ringworm)	Pruritic, scaly, round/oval plaque with active erythematous margin, and central clearing Site: trunk, limbs, face	Granuloma annulare, pityriasis rosea, psoriasis, seborrheic dermatitis	Microscopic examinations of KOH prep of scales shows hyphae Culture of scales	Topicals: 1% clotrimazole, 2% ketoconazole 2% miconazole, terbinafine or ciclopirox olamine cream bid for 2-4 wk Oral terbinafine, or itraconazole, or fluconazole, or ketoconazole if extensive
Tinea Cruris ("Jock Itch")	Scaly patch/plaque with a well-defined, curved border and central clearing Pruritic, erythematous, dry/macerated Site: medial thigh	Candidiasis (involvement of scrotum and satellite lesions), contact dermatitis, erythrasma	Same as for tinea corporis	Same as for tinea corporis
Tinea Pedis (Athlete's Foot)	Pruritic scaling and/or maceration of the web spaces, and powdery scaling of soles Acute infection: interdigital (esp. 4th web space) red/white scales, vesicles, bullae, often with maceration Secondary bacterial infection may occur Chronic: non-pruritic, pink, scaling keratosis on soles and sides of feet May present as flare-up of chronic tinea pedis Predisposing factors: heat, humidity, occlusive footwear	AD, contact dermatitis, dyshidrotic dermatitis, erythrasma, intertrigo, inverse psoriasis	Same as for tinea corporis	Same as for tinea corporis
Tinea Manuum	Primary fungal infection of the hand is rare; usually associated with tinea pedis Acute: blisters at edge of red areas on hands Chronic: single dry scaly patch	AD, contact dermatitis, granuloma annulare, psoriasis	Same as for tinea corporis	Same as for tinea corporis
Tinea Unguium (Onychomycosis)	Crumbling, distally dystrophic nails; yellowish, opaque with subungual hyperkeratotic debris Toenail infections usually precede fingernail infections *T. rubrum* (90% of all toenail infections)	Psoriasis, lichen planus, contact dermatitis, traumatic onychodystrophies, bacterial infections	Microscopic examinations of KOH prep of scales from subungual scraping shows hyphae Culture of subungual scraping or nail clippings on Sabouraud's agar PAS stain of nail clipping by pathology	Terbinafine (Lamisil®) (6 wk for fingernails, 12 wk for toenails) Itraconazole (Sporanox®) 7 d on, 3 wk off (2 pulses for fingernails, 3 pulses for toenails) Topical: ciclopirox (Penlac®); nail lacquer (often ineffective), Efinaconazole (Jublia®) (48 weeks)

Parasitic Infections

SCABIES

Clinical Presentation
- characterized by superficial burrows, intense pruritus (especially nocturnal), and secondary infection
- primary lesion: superficial linear burrows; inflammatory papules and nodules in the axilla and groin
- secondary lesion: small urticarial crusted papules, eczematous plaques, excoriations
- common sites: axillae, groin, buttocks, hands/feet (especially web spaces), sparing of head and neck (except in infants)

Pathophysiology
- scabies mite remains alive 2-3 d on clothing/sheets
- incubation of 1 mo, then pruritus begins
- re-infection followed by hypersensitivity in 24 h

Etiology
- *Sarcoptes scabiei* (a mite)
- risk factors: sexual promiscuity, crowding, poverty, nosocomial, immunocompromised

Differential Diagnosis
- asteatotic eczema, dermatitis herpetiformis, lichen simplex chronicus (neurodermatitis)

Investigations
- microscopic examination of root and content of burrow and mineral oil mount for mite, eggs, feces
- skin biopsy may sometimes show scabies mite

Management
- bathe, then apply permethrin 5% cream (i.e. Nix®) from neck down to soles of feet (must be left on for 8-14 h and requires second treatment 7 d after first treatment)
- change underwear and linens; wash twice with detergent in hot water cycle then machine dry
- treat family and close contacts
- pruritus may persist for 2-3 wk after effective treatment due to prolonged hypersensitivity reaction
- mid potency topical steroids and antihistamines for symptom management

LICE (PEDICULOSIS)

Clinical Presentation
- intensely pruritic, red excoriations, morbilliform rash, caused by louse (a parasite)
- scalp lice: nits (i.e. louse eggs) on hairs; red, excoriated skin with secondary bacterial infection, lymphadenopathy
- pubic lice: nits on hairs; excoriations
- body lice: nits and lice in seams of clothing; excoriations and secondary infection mainly on shoulders, belt-line and buttocks

Etiology
- *Phthirus pubis* (pubic), *Pediculus humanus capitis* (scalp), *Pediculus humanus humanus* (body): attaches to body hair and feeds
- can transmit infectious agents such as *Bartonella quintana* and *Rickettsia prowazekii*

Differential Diagnosis
- bacterial infection of scalp, seborrheic dermatitis

Diagnosis
- lice visible on inspection of affected area or clothing seams

Management
- permethrin 1% (Nix® cream rinse) (ovicidal) or permethrin 1% (RC & Cor®, Kwellada-P® shampoo)
- comb hair with fine-toothed comb using dilute vinegar solution to remove nits
- repeat in 7 d after first treatment
- shave hair if feasible, change clothing and linens; wash with detergent in hot water cycle then machine dry

BED BUGS (HEMIPTERA)

Clinical Presentation
- burning wheals, turning to firm papules, often in groups of three – "breakfast, lunch and dinner" – in areas with easy access (face, neck, arms, legs, hands)

Etiology
- caused by *Cimex lectularius*, a small insect that feeds mainly at night (hide in crevices in walls and furniture during the day)

Differential Diagnosis
- dermatitis herpetiformis, drug eruptions, ecthyma, other insect bites, scabies

Investigations
- none required, but lesional biopsy can confirm insect bite reaction

Management
- professional fumigation
- topical steroids and oral H1-antagonists for symptomatic relief
- definitive treatment is removal of clutter in home and application of insecticides to walls and furniture

Viral Infections

HERPES SIMPLEX

Clinical Presentation
- herpetiform (i.e. grouped) vesicles on an erythematous base on skin or mucous membranes
- transmitted via contact with erupted vesicles or via asymptomatic viral shedding
- **primary**
  - children and young adults
  - usually asymptomatic; may have high fever, regional lymphadenopathy, malaise
  - followed by antibody formation and latency of virus in dorsal nerve root ganglion
- **secondary**
  - recurrent form seen in adults; much more common than primary
  - prodrome: tingling, pruritus, pain
  - triggers for recurrence: fever, excess sun exposure, physical trauma, menstruation, emotional stress, URTI
- **complications:** dendritic corneal ulcer, EM, herpes simplex encephalitis (infants at risk), HSV infection on AD causing Kaposi's varicelliform eruption (eczema herpeticum)
- two biologically and immunologically different subtypes: HSV-1 and HSV-2
  - HSV-1
    - typically "cold sores" (grouped vesicles at the mucocutaneous junction which quickly burst)
    - recurrent on face, lips and hard palate, but NOT on soft, non-keratinized mucous membranes (unlike aphthous ulcers)
  - HSV-2
    - usually sexually transmitted; incubation 2-20 d
    - gingivostomatitis: entire buccal mucosa involved with erythema and edema of gingiva
    - vulvovaginitis: edematous, erythematous, extremely tender, profuse vaginal discharge
    - urethritis: watery discharge in males
    - recurrent on vulva, vagina, penis for 5-7 d
    - differential diagnosis of genital ulcers: *Candida balanitis*, chancroid, syphilitic chancres

Both HSV-1 and HSV-2 can occur on face or genitalia

Investigations
- Tzanck smear with Giemsa stain shows multinucleated giant epithelial cells
- viral culture, electron microscopy, and direct fluorescence antibody test of specimen taken from the base of a relatively new lesion
- serologic testing for antibody for current or past infection if necessary

Management
- HSV-1
  - treat during prodrome to prevent vesicle formation
  - topical antiviral (Zovirax®/Xerese®) cream, apply 5-6x/d x 4-7 d for facial/genital lesions
  - oral antivirals (e.g. acyclovir, famciclovir, valacyclovir) are far more effective and have an easier dosing schedule than topicals
- HSV-2
  - rupture vesicle with sterile needle if you wish to culture it
  - wet dressing with aluminum subacetate solution, Burow's compression, or betadine solution
  - 1st episode: acyclovir 200 mg PO 5x/d x 10 d
    - maintenance: acyclovir 400 mg PO bid
  - famciclovir and valacyclovir may be substituted and have better enteric absorption and less frequent dosing
  - in case of herpes genitalis, look for and treat any other sexually-transmitted infections STIs
  - for active lesions in pregnancy, see Obstetrics, OB29

Erythema Multiforme
Etiology: most often HSV or mycoplasma pneumoniae, rarely drugs
Morphology: macules/papules with central vesicles; classic bull's-eye pattern of concentric light and dark rings (typical target lesions)
Management: symptomatic treatment (oral antihistamines, oral antacids); corticosteroids in severely ill (controversial); prophylactic oral acyclovir for 6-12 mo for HSV-associated EM with frequent recurrences

HERPES ZOSTER (SHINGLES)

Clinical Presentation
- unilateral dermatomal eruption occurring 3-5 d after pain and paresthesia of that dermatome
- vesicles, bullae, and pustules on an erythematous, edematous base
- lesions may become eroded/ulcerated and last days to weeks
- pain can be pre-herpetic, synchronous with rash, or post-herpetic
- severe post-herpetic neuralgia often occurs in elderly
- Hutchinson's sign: shingles on the tip of the nose signifies ocular involvement. Shingles in this area involves the nasociliary branch of the ophthalmic branch of the trigeminal nerve (V1)
- distribution: thoracic (50%), trigeminal (10-20%), cervical (10-20%); disseminated in HIV

Herpes zoster typically involves a single dermatome; lesions rarely cross the midline

Etiology
- caused by reactivation of VZV
- risk factors: immunosuppression, old age, occasionally associated with hematologic malignancy

Differential Diagnosis
- before thoracic skin lesions occur, must consider other causes of chest pain
- contact dermatitis, localized bacterial infection, zosteriform HSV (more pathogenic for the eyes than VZV)

Investigations
- none required, but can do Tzanck test, direct fluorescence antibody test, or viral culture to rule out HSV

Management
- compress with normal saline, Burow's, or betadine solution
- analgesics (NSAIDs, amitriptyline)
- famciclovir, valacyclovir, or acyclovir for 7 d; must initiate within 72 h to be of benefit
- gabapentin 300-600 mg PO tid for post-herpetic neuralgia

MOLLUSCUM CONTAGIOSUM

Clinical Presentation
- discrete dome-shaped and umbilicated pearly, white papules caused by DNA Pox virus (Molluscum contagiosum virus)
- common sites: eyelids, beard (likely spread by shaving), neck, axillae, trunk, perineum, buttocks

Etiology
- virus is spread via direct contact, auto-inoculation, sexual contact
- common in children and sexually active young adults (giant molluscum and severe cases can be seen in the setting of HIV)
- virus is self-limited and can take 1-2 yr to resolve

Investigations
- none required, however can biopsy to confirm diagnosis

Management
- topical cantharidin (a vesicant)
- cryotherapy
- curettage
- topical retinoids
- Aldara® (imiquimod): immune modulator that produces a cytokine inflammation

WARTS (VERRUCA VULGARIS) (HUMAN PAPILLOMAVIRUS INFECTIONS)

Table 19. Different Manifestations of HPV Infection

	Definition and Clinical Features	Differential Diagnosis	Distribution	HPV Type
Verruca Vulgaris (Common Warts)	Hyperkeratotic, elevated discrete epithelial growths with papillated surface caused by HPV Paring of surface reveals punctate, red-brown specks (thrombosed capillaries)	Molluscum contagiosum, seborrheic keratosis	Located at trauma sites: fingers, hands, knees of children and teens	At least 80 types are known
Verruca Plantaris (Plantar Warts) and **Verruca Palmaris** (Palmar Warts)	Hyperkeratotic, shiny, sharply marginated growths Paring of surface reveals red-brown specks (capillaries), interruption of epidermal ridges	May need to scrape ("pare") lesions to differentiate wart from callus and corn	Located at pressure sites: metatarsal heads, heels, toes	Commonly HPV 1, 2, 4, 10
Verruca Planae (Flat Warts)	Multiple discrete, skin coloured, flat topped papules grouped or in linear configuration Common in children	Syringoma, seborrheic keratosis, molluscum contagiosum, lichen planus	Sites: face, dorsa of hands, shins, knees	Commonly HPV 3, 10
Condyloma Acuminata (Genital Warts)	Skin-coloured pinhead papules to soft cauliflower like masses in clusters Often occurs in young adults, infants, children Can be asymptomatic, lasting months to years Highly contagious, transmitted sexually and non-sexually (e.g. Koebner phenomenon via scratching, shaving), and can spread without clinically apparent lesions Investigations: acetowhitening (subclinical lesions seen with 5% acetic acid x 5 min and hand lens) Complications: fairy-ring warts (satellite warts at periphery of treated area of original warts)	Condyloma lata (secondary syphilitic lesion, dark field strongly +ve), molluscum contagiosum	Sites: genitalia and perianal areas	Commonly HPV 6 and 11 HPV 16, 18, 31, 33 cause cervical dysplasia, SCC and invasive cancer

Treatment for Warts
- **first line therapies**
  - salicylic acid preparations (patches, solutions, creams, ointments), cryotherapy, topical cantharone
- **second line therapies**
  - topical imiquimod, topical 5-fluorouracil, topical tretinoin, podophyllotoxin
- **third line therapies**
  - curettage, cautery, surgery for non plantar warts, CO_2 laser, oral cimetidine (particularly children), intralesional bleomycin (plantar warts), trichloroacetic acid, diphencyprone
- other viruses associated with skin changes, such as measles, roseola, fifth disease, etc.
- see <u>Pediatrics</u>, *Pediatric Exanthems*, P55

Yeast Infections

CANDIDIASIS

Etiology
- many species of *Candida* (70-80% of infections are from *Candida albicans*)
- opportunistic infection in those with predisposing factors (e.g. trauma, malnutrition, immunodeficiency)

Candidal Paronychia
- clinical presentation: painful red swellings of periungual skin
- management: topical agents not as effective; oral antifungals recommended

Candidal Intertrigo
- clinical presentation
  - macerated/eroded erythematous patches that may be covered with papules and pustules, located in intertriginous areas often under breast, groin, or interdigitally
  - peripheral "satellite" pustules
  - starts as non-infectious maceration from heat, moisture, and friction
- predisposing factors: obesity, DM, systemic antibiotics, immunosuppression, malignancy
- management: keep area dry, terbinafine, ciclopirox olamine, ketoconazole/clotrimazole cream bid until rash clears

Oral Terbinafine (Lamisil®) is not effective because it is not secreted by sweat glands

PITYRIASIS (TINEA) VERSICOLOR

Clinical Presentation
- asymptomatic superficial fungal infection with brown/white scaling macules
- affected skin darker than surrounding skin in winter, lighter in summer (does not tan)
- common sites: upper chest and back

Pathophysiology
- microbe produces azelaic acid → inflammatory reaction inhibiting melanin synthesis yielding variable pigmentation
- affinity for sebaceous glands; require fatty acids to survive

Etiology
- *Pityrosporum ovale* (*Malassezia furfur*)
- also associated with folliculitis and seborrheic dermatitis
- predisposing factors: summer, tropical climates, excessive sweating, Cushing's syndrome, prolonged corticosteroid use

Investigations
- clinical diagnosis but can perform microscopic examination, KOH prep of scales for hyphae and spores

Management
- ketoconazole shampoo or cream daily
- topical terbinafine or ciclopirox olamine bid
- systemic fluconazole or itraconazole for 7 d if extensive

Sexually Transmitted Infections

SYPHILIS

Clinical Presentation
- characterized initially by a painless ulcer (chancre)
- following inoculation, systemic infection with secondary and tertiary stages

Etiology
- *Treponema pallidum*
- transmitted sexually, congenitally, or rarely by transfusion

Natural History of Untreated Syphilis
- Inoculation
- Primary syphilis (10-90 d after infection)
- Secondary syphilis (simultaneous to primary syphilis or up to 6 mo after healing of primary lesion)
- Latent syphilis
- Tertiary syphilis (2-20 yr)

Latent Syphilis
70% of untreated patients will remain in this stage for the rest of their lives and are immune to new primary infection

Table 20. Stages of Syphilis

	Clinical Presentation	Investigations	Management
Primary Syphilis	Single red, indurated, painless chancre, that develops into painless ulcer with raised border and scanty serous exudate Chancre develops at site of inoculation after 3 wk of incubation and heals in 4-6 wk; chancre may also develop on lips or anus Regional non-tender lymphadenopathy appears <1 wk after onset of chancre DDx: chancroid (painful), HSV (multiple lesions)	CANNOT be based on clinical presentation alone VDRL negative – repeat weekly for 1 mo Fluorescent treponemal antibody-syphilis (FTA-ABS) test has greater sensitivity and may detect disease earlier in course Dark field examination – spirochete in chancre fluid or lymph node aspirate	Penicillin G, 2.4 million units IM, single dose
Secondary Syphilis	Presents 2-6 mo after primary infection (patient may not recall presence of primary chancre) Associated with generalized lymphadenopathy, splenomegaly, headache, chills, fever, arthralgias, myalgias, malaise, photophobia Lesions heal in 1-5 wk and may recur for 1 yr 3 types of lesions: 1. Macules and papules: flat top, scaling, non-pruritic, sharply defined, circular/annular rash (DDx: pityriasis rosea, tinea corporis, drug eruptions, lichen planus) 2. Condyloma lata: wart-like moist papules around genital/perianal region 3. Mucous patches: macerated patches mainly found in oral mucosa	VDRL positive FTA-ABS +ve; –ve after 1 yr following appearance of chancre Dark field +ve in all secondary	As for primary syphilis
Tertiary Syphilis	Extremely rare 3-7 yr after secondary Main skin lesion: 'Gumma' – a granulomatous non-tender nodule	As in primary syphilis, VDRL can be falsely negative	Treatment: penicillin G, 2.4 million units IM weekly x 3 wk

GONOCOCCEMIA

Clinical Presentation
- disseminated gonococcal infection
- hemorrhagic, tender, pustules on a purpuric/petechial background
- common sites: distal aspects of extremities
- associated with fever, arthritis, urethritis, proctitis, pharyngitis, and tenosynovitis
- neonatal conjunctivitis if infected via birth canal

Etiology
- *Neisseria gonorrhoeae*

Investigations
- requires high index of clinical suspicion plays because tests are often negative
- bacterial culture of blood, joint fluid, and skin lesions
- joint fluid cell count and Gram stain

Management
- notify Public Health authorities
- screen for other STIs
- cefixime 400 mg PO (drug of choice) or ceftriaxone 1 g IM

HSV
- see *Viral Infections*, D29

HPV
- see *Viral Infections*, D30

Pre-Malignant Skin Conditions

Actinic Keratosis (Solar Keratosis)

Clinical Presentation
- ill-defined, scaly erythematous papules or plaques on a background of sun-damaged skin (solar heliosis)
- sandpaper-like, gritty sensation felt on palpation, often easier to appreciate on palpation rather than inspection
- sites: areas of sun exposure (face, ears, scalp if bald, neck, sun-exposed limbs)

Pathophysiology
- UV radiation damage to keratinocytes from repeated sun exposure (especially UVB)
- risk of transformation of AK to SCC (~1/1,000), but higher likelihood if AK is persistent
- UV-induced p53 gene mutation
- risk factors: increased age, light skin/eyes/hair, immunosuppression, syndromes such as albinism or xeroderma pigmenotsum
- risk factors for malignancy: immunosuppression, history of skin cancer, persistence of the AK

Epidemiology
- common with increasing age, outdoor occupation, M>F
- skin phototypes I-III, rare in darker skin as melanin is protective

Differential Diagnosis
- SCC *in situ*, superficial BCC, seborrheic keratosis, cutaneous lupus erythematosus

Investigations
- biopsy lesions that are refractory to treatment

Management
- destructive: cryotherapy, electrodessication, and curettage
- topical pharmacotherapy (mechanism: destruction of rapidly growing cells or immune system modulation)
  - topical 5-Fluorouracil cream (for 2-4 wk), Imiquimod 5% (2 times per wk for 16 wk), Imiquimod 3.75% (daily for 2 wk then none for 2 wk then daily for 2 wk), Ingenol Mebutate gel 0.015% (daily for 3 d on the head and neck), Ingenol mebutate 0.05% gel (daily for 2 d on the body)
- photodynamic therapy
- excision

Types of AK
- Erythematous: typical AK lesion
- Hypertrophic: thicker, rough papule/plaque
- Cutaneous horn: firm hyperkeratotic outgrowth
- Actinic cheilitis: confluent AKs on the lip
- Pigmented: flat, tan-brown, scaly plaque
- Spreading pigmented
- Proliferative
- Conjunctival: pinguecula, pterygium

Leukoplakia

Clinical Presentation
- a morphologic term describing homogenous or speckled white plaques with sharply demarcated borders
- sites: oropharynx, most often floor of the mouth, soft palate, and ventral/lateral surfaces of the tongue

Pathophysiology
- precancerous or premalignant condition
- oral form is strongly associated with tobacco use and alcohol consumption

Epidemiology
- 1-5% prevalence in adult population after 30 yr of age; peak at age 50
- M>F, fair-skinned
- most common oral mucosal premalignant lesion

Differential Diagnosis
- lichen planus, oral hairy leukoplakia

Investigations
- biopsy is mandatory because it is premalignant

Management
- low risk sites on buccal/labial mucosal or hard palate: eliminate carcinogenic habits, follow-up
- moderate/dysplastic lesions: excision, cryotherapy

Malignant Skin Tumours

Non-Melanoma Skin Cancers

BASAL CELL CARCINOMA

Subtypes
- noduloulcerative (typical)
  - skin-coloured papule/nodule with rolled, translucent ("pearly") telangiectatic border, and depressed/eroded/ulcerated centre
- pigmented variant
  - flecks of pigment in translucent lesion with surface telangiectasia
  - may mimic malignant melanoma
- superficial variant
  - flat, tan to red-brown plaque, often with scaly, pearly border and fine telangiectasia at margin
  - least aggressive subtype
- sclerosing (morpheaform) variant
  - flesh/yellowish-coloured, shiny papule/plaque with indistinct borders, indurated

Pathophysiology
- malignant proliferation of basal keratinocytes of the epidermis
  - low grade cutaneous malignancy, locally aggressive (primarily tangential growth), rarely metastatic
  - usually due to UVB light exposure, therefore >80% on face
  - may also occur in previous scars, radiation, trauma, arsenic exposure, or genetic predisposition (Gorlin syndrome)

Epidemiology
- most common malignancy in humans
- 75% of all malignant skin tumours >40 yr, increased prevalence in the elderly
- M>F, skin phototypes I and II, chronic cumulative sun exposure, ionizing radiation, immunosuppression, arsenic exposure

Differential Diagnosis
- benign: sebaceous hyperplasia, intradermal melanocytic nevus, dermatofibroma
- malignant: nodular malignant melanoma, SCC

Management
- imiquimod 5% cream (Aldara®) or cryotherapy is indicated for superficial BCCs on the trunk
- fluorouracil and photodynamic therapy can also be used for superficial BCC
- shave excision + electrodessication and curettage for most types of BCCs, not including morpheaform
- Mohs surgery: microscopically controlled, minimally invasive, stepwise excision for lesions on the face or in areas that are difficult to reconstruct
- radiotherapy used in advanced cases of BCC where surgical intervention is not an option
- vismodegib is approved for metastatic BCC
- life-long follow up every 6 mo to 1 yr
- 95% cure rate if lesion <2 cm in diameter or if treated early

SQUAMOUS CELL CARCINOMA

Clinical Presentation
- indurated, pink/red/skin-coloured papule/plaque/nodule with surface scale/crust ± ulceration
- more rapid enlargement than BCC
- exophytic (grows outward), may present as a cutaneous horn
- sites: face, ears, scalp, forearms, dorsum of hands

Pathophysiology
- malignant neoplasm of keratinocytes (primarily vertical growth)
- predisposing factors include: UV radiation, PUVA, ionizing radiation therapy/exposure, chemical carcinogens (such as arsenic, tar, and nitrogen mustards), HPV 16, 18, immunosuppression
- may occur in previous scar (SCC more commonly than BCC)

Epidemiology
- second most common type of cutaneous neoplasm
- primarily on sun-exposed skin in the elderly, M>F, skin phototypes I and II, chronic sun exposure
- in organ transplant recipients SCC is most common cutaneous malignancy, with increased mortality as compared to non-immunocompromised population

Differential Diagnosis
- benign: nummular eczema, psoriasis, irritated seborrheic keratosis
- malignant: keratoacanthoma, Bowen's disease, BCC

Workup/Investigations of BCC and other NMSCs
- **History:** duration, growth rate, family/personal Hx of skin cancer, prior therapy to the particular lesion
- **Physical:** location, size, whether circumscribed, tethering to deep structures, full skin exam, lymph node exam
- **Biopsy:** if shallow lesion, can do shave biopsy; otherwise punch or excisional biopsy may be more appropriate

Surgical Margins
- **Smaller lesions:** electrodessication and curettage with 2-3 mm margin of normal skin
- **Deep infiltrative lesions:** surgical excision with 3-5 mm margins beyond visible and palpable tumour border, which may require skin graft or flap; or Mohs surgery, which conserves tissue and does not require margin control

Management
- surgical excision with primary closure, skin flaps or grafting
- Mohs surgery
- lifelong follow-up (more aggressive treatment than BCC)

Prognosis
- good prognostic factors: early treatment, negative margins, and small size of lesion
- SCCs that arise from AK metastasize less frequently (~1%) than other SCCs arising de novo in old burns (2-5% of cases)
- overall control is 75% over 5 yr, 5-10% metastasize
- metastasis rates are higher if diameter > 2 cm, depth > 4 mm, recurrent, involvement of bone/muscle/nerve, location on scalp/ears/nose/lips, immunosuppressed, caused by arsenic ingestion, or tumour arose from scar/chronic ulcer/burn/genital tract/sinus tract

BOWEN'S DISEASE (SQUAMOUS CELL CARCINOMA *IN SITU*)

Clinical Presentation
- sharply demarcated erythematous patch/thin plaque with scale and/or crusting
- often 1-3 cm in diameter and found on the skin and mucous membranes
- evolves to SCC in 10-20% of cutaneous lesions and >20% of mucosal lesions

Management
- same as for BCC
- biopsy required for diagnosis
- topical 5-fluorouracil (Efudex®) or imiquimod (Aldara®) used if extensive and as a tool to identify margins of poorly defined tumours
- cryosurgery
- shave excision with electrodessication and curettage

KERATOACANTHOMA

Clinical Presentation
- rapidly growing, firm, dome-shaped, erythematous or skin-coloured nodule with central keratin-filled crater, resembling an erupting volcano
- may spontaneously regress within a year, leaving a scar
- sites: sun-exposed skin

Pathophysiology
- epithelial neoplasm with atypical keratinocytes in epidermis
- low grade variant of SCC

Etiology
- HPV, UV radiation, chemical carcinogens (tar, mineral oil)

Epidemiology
- >50 yr, rare <20 yr

Differential Diagnosis
- treat as SCC until proven otherwise
- hypertrophic solar keratosis, verruca vulgaris

Management
- surgical excision or saucerization (shave biopsy) followed by electrodesiccation of the base, treated similarly to SCC

Malignant Melanoma

Clinical Presentation
- malignant characteristics of a mole: "ABCDE" mnemonic
- sites: skin, mucous membranes, eyes, CNS

Clinical Subtypes of Malignant Melanoma
- lentigo maligna
  - malignant melanoma in situ (normal and malignant melanocytes confined to the epidermis)
  - 2-6 cm, tan/brown/black uniformly flat macule or patch with irregular borders
  - lesion grows radially and produces complex colours
  - often seen in the elderly
  - 10% evolve to lentigo maligna melanoma

Does this Patient have a Mole or Melanoma?

ABCDE checklist
Asymmetry
Border (irregular and/or indistinct)
Colour (varied)
Diameter (increasing or >6 mm)
Enlargement, elevation, evolution (i.e. change in colour, size, or shape)

Sensitivity 92% (CI 82-96%)
Specificity 100% (CI 54-100%)

JAMA 1998;279:696-701

- **lentigo maligna melanoma** (15% of all melanomas)
  - malignant melanocytes invading into the dermis
  - associated with pre-existing solar lentigo, not pre-existing nevi
  - flat, brown, stain-like, gradually enlarging with loss of skin surface markings
  - with time, colour changes from uniform brown to dark brown with black and blue
  - found on all skin surfaces, especially those often exposed to sun, such as the face and hands
- **superficial spreading melanoma** (60-70% of all melanomas)
  - atypical melanocytes initially spread laterally in epidermis then invade the dermis
  - irregular, indurated, enlarging plaques with red/white/blue discolouration, focal papules or nodules
  - ulcerate and bleed with growth
- **nodular melanoma** (30% of all melanomas)
  - atypical melanocytes that initially grow vertically with little lateral spread
  - uniformly ulcerated, blue-black, and sharply delineated plaque or nodule
  - rapidly fatal
  - may be pink or have no colour at all, this is called an amelanotic melanoma
  - "EFG" Elevated, Firm, Growing
- **acrolentiginous melanoma** (5% of all melanomas)
  - ill-defined dark brown, blue-black macule
  - palmar, plantar, subungual skin
  - melanomas on mucous membranes have poor prognosis

Pathophysiology
- malignant neoplasm of pigment forming cells (melanocytes and nevus cells)

Epidemiology
- incidence 1/75 (Canada) 1/50 (US)
- risk factors: numerous moles, fair skin, red hair, positive personal/family history, 1 large congenital nevus (>20 cm), familial dysplastic nevus syndrome, any dysplastic nevi, immunosuppression, > 50 common nevi, and sun exposure with sunburns, tanning beds
- most common sites: back (M), calves (F)
- worse prognosis if: male, on scalp, hands, feet, late lesion, no pre-existing nevus present

Differential Diagnosis
- benign: nevi, solar lentigo, seborrheic keratosis
- malignant: pigmented BCC

Management
- excisional biopsy preferable, otherwise incisional biopsy
- remove full depth of dermis and extend beyond edges of lesion only after histologic diagnosis
- beware of lesions that regress – tumour is usually deeper than anticipated
- high dose IFN for stage II (regional), chemotherapy (cis-platinum, BCG) and high dose IFN for stage III (distant) disease
- newer chemotherapeutic, gene therapies, and vaccines starting to be used in metastatic melanoma
- radiotherapy may be used as adjunctive treatment

Table 21. American Joint Committee on Cancer Staging System Based on Breslow's Thickness of Invasion

Tumour Depth	Stage	Approximate 5 Yr Survival
T1 <1.0 mm	Stage I T1a – T2a	5-yr survival 90%
T2 1.01-2.0 mm	Stage II T2b – T4b	5-yr survival 70%
T3 2.01-4.0 mm	Stage III any nodes	5-yr survival 45%
T4 >4.0 mm	Stage IV any mets	5-yr survival 10%

a = no ulceration; b = ulceration

Other Cutaneous Cancers

CUTANEOUS T-CELL LYMPHOMA

Clinical Presentation
- **Mycosis fungoides** (limited superficial type)
  - characterized by erythematous patches/plaques/nodules/tumours, which may be pruritic and poikilodermic (atrophy, telangiectasia, hyperpigmentation, hypopigmentation)
  - common sites include: trunk, buttocks, proximal limbs
  - mildly symptomatic, usually excellent prognosis for early disease
- **Sézary syndrome** (widespread systemic type)
  - rare variant characterized by erythroderma, lymphadenopathy, WBC >20 x 10^9/L with Sézary cells
  - associated with intense pruritus, alopecia, palmoplantar hyperkeratosis, and systemic symptoms (fatigue, fever)
  - often fatal

Risk Factors for Melanoma

no SPF is a SIN
Sun exposure
Pigment traits (blue eyes, fair/red hair, pale complexion)
Freckling
Skin reaction to sunlight (increased incidence of sunburn)
Immunosuppressive states (e.g. renal transplantation)
Nevi (dysplastic nevi; increased number of benign melanocytic nevi)

Node Dissection for Lesions
>1 mm thick OR <1 mm and ulcerated OR >1 mitoses/mm2 (Stage IB or higher melanoma patients should be offered a sentinel lymph node biopsy)
- Assess sentinel node at time of wide excision

Pathophysiology
- clonal proliferation of skin-homing CD4 T-cells

Epidemiology
- >50 yr old, M:F 2:1

Differential Diagnosis
- tinea corporis, nummular dermatitis, psoriasis, DLE, Bowen's disease

Investigations
- skin biopsy (histology, "lymphocyte antigen cell" markers, TcR gene arrangement)
- blood smear looking for Sézary cells or flow cytometry (e.g. CD4:CD8 >10 is Sézary)
- imaging (for systemic involvement)

Management
- **Mycosis fungoides**
  - depends on stage of disease
  - topical steroids and/or PUVA, narrow band UVB (NBUVB, 311-313mm)
- **Sézary syndrome**
  - oral retinoids and IFN
  - extra-corporeal photopheresis
  - may need radiotherapy for total skin electron beam radiation
  - may maintain on UV therapy
  - other chemotherapy agents

Diseases of Hair Density

Hair Growth

- hair grows in a cyclic pattern that is defined in 3 stages (most scalp hairs are in anagen phase)
  1. growth stage = anagen phase
  2. transitional stage = catagen stage
  3. resting stage = telogen phase
- total duration of the growth stage reflects the type and location of hair: eyebrow, eyelash, and axillary hairs have a short growth stage in relation to the resting stage
- growth of the hair follicles is also based on the hormonal response to testosterone and DHT; this response is genetically controlled

Non-Scarring (Non-Cicatricial) Alopecia

ANDROGENETIC ALOPECIA

Clinical Presentation
- male- or female-pattern alopecia
- males: fronto-temporal areas progressing to vertex, entire scalp may be bald
- females: widening of central part, "Christmas tree" pattern

Pathophysiology
- action of testosterone on hair follicles

Epidemiology
- males: early 20s-30s
- females: 40s-50s

Management
- minoxidil (Rogaine®) solution or foam to reduce rate of loss/partial restoration
- females: spironolactone (anti-androgenic effects), cyproterone acetate (Diane-35®)
- males: finasteride (Propecia®) (5-α-reductase inhibitor) 1 mg/d
- hair transplant

PHYSICAL
- trichotillomania: impulse-control disorder characterized by compulsive hair pulling with irregular patches of hair loss, and with remaining hairs broken at varying lengths
- traumatic (e.g. tight "corn-row" braiding of hair, wearing tight pony tails, tight tying of turbans)

Hair Loss

TOP HAT
Telogen effluvium, tinea capitis
Out of Fe, Zn
Physical: trichotillomania, "corn-row" braiding
Hormonal: hypothyroidism, androgenic
Autoimmune: SLE, alopecia areata
Toxins: heavy metals, anticoagulants, chemotherapy, vitamin A, SSRIs

DDx of Non-Scarring (Non-Cicatricial) Alopecia
- **Autoimmune**
  - Alopecia areata
- **Endocrine**
  - Hypothyroidism
  - Androgens
- **Micronutrient deficiencies**
  - Iron
  - Zinc
- **Toxins**
  - Heavy metals
  - Anticoagulants
  - Chemotherapy
  - Vitamin A
- **Trauma to the hair follicle**
  - Trichotillomania
  - 'Corn-row' braiding
- **Other**
  - Syphilis
  - Severe illness
  - Childbirth

TELOGEN EFFLUVIUM

Clinical Presentation
- uniform decrease in hair density secondary to hairs leaving the growth (anagen) stage and entering the resting (telogen) stage of the cycle

Pathophysiology
- variety of precipitating factors
- hair loss typically occurs 2-4 mo after exposure to precipitant
- regrowth occurs within a few months but may not be complete

ANAGEN EFFLUVIUM

Clinical Presentation
- hair loss due to insult to hair follicle impairing its mitotic activity (growth stage)

Pathophysiology
- precipitated by chemotherapeutic agents (most common), other meds (bismuth, levodopa, colchicine, cyclosporine), exposure to chemicals (thallium, boron, arsenic)
- dose-dependent effect
- hair loss 7-14 d after single pulse of chemotherapy; most clinically apparent after 1-2 mo
- reversible effect; follicles resume normal mitotic activity few weeks after agent stopped

ALOPECIA AREATA

Clinical Presentation
- autoimmune disorder characterized by patches of complete hair loss often localized to scalp but can affect eyebrows, beard, eyelashes, etc.
- may be associated with dystrophic nail changes – fine stippling, pitting
- "exclamation mark" pattern (hairs fractured and have tapered shafts, i.e. looks like "!")
- may be associated with pernicious anemia, vitiligo, thyroid disease, Addison's disease
- spontaneous regrowth may occur within months of first attack (worse prognosis if young at age of onset and extensive loss)
- frequent recurrence often precipitated by emotional distress

Management
- generally unsatisfactory
- intralesional triamcinolone acetonide (corticosteroids) can be used for isolated patches
- UV or PUVA therapy
- immunomodulatory (diphencyprone)

Scarring (Cicatricial) Alopecia

Clinical Presentation
- irreversible loss of hair follicles with fibrosis

Etiology
- physical: radiation, burns
- infections: fungal, bacterial, TB, leprosy, viral (HZV)
- inflammatory
  - lichen planus (lichen planopilaris)
  - DLE (note that SLE can cause an alopecia unrelated to DLE lesions which are non-scarring)
  - morphea: "coup de sabre" with involvement of centre of scalp
  - central centrifugal cicatricial alopecia (CCCA): seen in up to 40% of black women, starting at central scalp; one of most commonly diagnosed scarring alopecias, may be associated with hair care practices in this population

Investigations
- biopsy from active border

Management
- infections: treat underlying infection
- inflammatory: topical/intralesional steroids, anti-inflammatory antibiotics, antimalarials

---

Precipitants of Telogen Effluvium
"SEND" hair follicles out of anagen and into telogen
Stress and **S**calp disease (surgery)
Endocrine (hypothyroidism, post-partum)
Nutritional (iron and protein deficiency)
Drugs (citretin, heparin, lithium, IFN, β-blockers, valproic acid, SSRIs)

Non-scarring alopecia: intact hair follicles on exam → biopsy not required (but may be helpful)
Scarring alopecia: absent hair follicles on exam → biopsy required

Alopecia Areata Subtypes

Alopecia totalis: loss of all scalp hair and eyebrows

Alopecia universalis: loss of all body hair

DDx of Scarring (Cicatricial) Alopecia

Developmental/Hereditary Disorders
- Aplasia cutis congenita
- Epidermal nevi
- Romberg's syndrome
- Generalized follicular hamartoma

Primary Causes
- Group 1: Lymphocytic
  - DLE
  - Lichen planopilaris
  - Central centrifugal cicatricial alopecia
  - Classic pseudopelade
- Group 2: Neutrophilic
  - Folliculitis decalvans
  - Dissecting scalp cellulitis
- Group 3: Mixed
  - Acne keloidalis nuchae

Secondary Causes
- Infectious agents
  - Bacterial (e.g. post-cellulitis)
  - Fungal (e.g. kerion tinea capitis)
- Neoplasms (e.g. BCC, SCC, lymphomas, and metastatic tumours)
- Physical agents
  - Mechanical trauma
  - Burns
  - Radiotherapy
  - Caustic chemicals

Nails and Disorders of the Nail Apparatus

Table 22. Nail Changes in Systemic and Dermatological Conditions

Nail Abnormality	Definition/Etiology	Associated Disease
NAIL PLATE CHANGES		
Clubbing	Proximal nail plate has greater than 180° angle to nail fold, watch-glass nails, bulbous digits	Cyanotic heart disease, bacterial endocarditis, pulmonary disorders, GI disorders, etc.
Koilonychia	Spoon shaped nails	Iron deficiency, malnutrition, DM
Onycholysis	Separation of nail plate from nail bed	Psoriasis, dermatophytes, thyroid disease
Onychogryphosis	Hypertrophy of the nail plate producing a curved, clawlike deformity	Poor circulation, chronic inflammation, tinea
Onychohemia	Subungual hematoma	Trauma to nail bed
Onychomycosis	Fungal infection of nail (e.g. dermatophyte, yeast, mould)	HIV, DM, peripheral arterial disease
Onychocryptosis	Ingrown toenail often hallux with congenital malalignment, painful inflammation, granulation tissue	Tight fitting shoes, excessive nail clipping
SURFACE CHANGES		
V-shaped nicking	Distal margin has v-shaped loss of the nail plate	Darier's disease (keratosis follicularis)
Pterygium inversus unguium	Distal nail plate does not separate from underlying nail bed	Scleroderma
Pitting	Punctate depressions that migrate distally with growth	Psoriasis (random pattern), alopecia areata (geometric, gridshaped arrangement), eczema
Transverse ridging	Transverse depressions often more in central portion of nail plate	Serious acute illness slows nail growth (when present in all nails = Beau's lines), eczema, chronic paronychia, trauma
Transverse white lines	Bands of white discolouration	Poisons, hypoalbuminemia (Muehrcke's lines)
COLOUR CHANGES		
Yellow		Tinea, jaundice, tetracycline, pityriasis rubra pilaris, yellow nail syndrome, psoriasis, tobacco use
Green		*Pseudomonas*
Black		Melanoma, hematoma
Brown		Nicotine use, psoriasis, poisons, longitudinal melanonychia (ethnic)
Splinter hemorrhages	Extravasation of blood from longitudinal vessels of nail bed, blood attaches to overlying nail plate and moves distally as it grows	Trauma, bacterial endocarditis, blood dyscrasias, psoriasis
Oil spots	Brown-yellow discolouration	Psoriasis
NAIL FOLD CHANGES		
Herpetic whitlow	HSV infection of distal phalanx	HSV infection
Paronychia	Local inflammation of the nail fold around the nail bed	Acute: painful infection Chronic: constant wetting (e.g. dishwashing, thumbsucking)
Nail fold telangiectasias	Cuticular hemorrhages, roughness, capillary changes	Scleroderma, SLE, dermatomyositis

Skin Manifestations of Systemic Disease

Table 23. Skin Manifestations of Internal Conditions

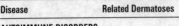

Disease	Related Dermatoses
AUTOIMMUNE DISORDERS	
Behçet's disease	Painful aphthous ulcers in oral cavity ± genital mucous membranes, erythema nodosum, acneiform papules
Buerger's disease	Superficial migratory thrombophlebitis, pallor, cyanosis, gangrene, ulcerations, digital resorptions
Dermatomyositis	Periorbital and extensor violaceous erythema, heliotrope with edema, Gottron's papules (violaceous flat-topped papules with atrophy), periungual erythema, telangiectasia, calcinosis cutis
Polyarteritis nodosa	Subcutaneous nodules, stellate purpura, erythema, gangrene, splinter hemorrhages, livedo reticularis, ulceration
Reactive arthritis	Keratoderma blennorrhagica (on feet), balanitis circinata (on male penis)
Rheumatic fever	Petechiae, urticaria, erythema nodosum, rheumatic nodules, evanescent rash
Scleroderma	Raynaud's, nonpitting edema, waxy/shiny/tense atrophic skin (morphea), ulcers, cutaneous calcification, periungual telangiectasia, acrosclerosis, salt-and-pepper pigmentation
SLE	Malar erythema, discoid rash (erythematous papules or plaques with keratotic scale, follicular plugging, atrophic scarring on face, hands, and arms), hemorrhagic bullae, palpable purpura, urticarial purpura, patchy/diffuse alopecia, mucosal ulcers, photosensitivity
Crohn's disease/UC	Pyoderma gangrenosum, erythema nodosum, Sweet's syndrome
ENDOCRINE DISORDERS	
Addison's disease	Generalized hyperpigmentation or limited to skin folds, buccal mucosa, and scars
Cushing's syndrome	Moon facies, purple striae, acne, hyperpigmentation, hirsutism, atrophic skin with telangiectasia
DM	Infections (e.g. boils, carbuncles, *Candidiasis*, *S. aureus*, dermatophytoses, tinea pedis and cruris, infectious eczematoid dermatitis), pruritus, eruptive xanthomas, necrobiosis lipoidica diabeticorum, granuloma annulare, diabetic foot, diabetic bullae, acanthosis nigricans, calciphylaxis
Hyperthyroidism	Moist, warm skin, seborrhea, acne, nail atrophy, hyperpigmentation, toxic alopecia, pretibial myxedema, acropachy, onycholysis
Hypothyroidism	Cool, dry, scaly, thickened, hyperpigmented skin; toxic alopecia with dry, coarse hair, brittle nails, myxedema, loss of lateral 1/3 eyebrows
HIV-RELATED	
Infections	Viral (e.g. HSV, HZV, HPV, CMV, molluscum contagiosum, oral hairy leukoplakia), bacterial (impetigo, acneiform folliculitis, dental caries, cellulitis, bacillary epithelioid angiomatosis, syphilis), fungal (candidiasis, histoplasmosis, cryptococcus, blastomycosis)
Inflammatory dermatoses	Seborrhea, psoriasis, pityriasis rosea, vasculitis
Malignancies	Kaposi's sarcoma, lymphoma, BCC, SCC, MM
MALIGNANCY	

Adenocarcinoma
  Gastrointestinal
  Cervix/anus/rectum
	
	Peutz-Jeghers: pigmented macules on lips/oral mucosa
	Paget's disease: eroding scaling plaques of perineum

Carcinoma
  Breast
  GI
  Thyroid
  Breast/lung/ovary
	
	Paget's disease, eczematous and crusting lesions of the skin of the nipple and usually areola of the breast
	Palmoplantar keratoderma: thickened skin of palms/soles
	Sipple's syndrome: multiple mucosal neuromas
	Dermatomyositis: heliotrope erythema of eyelids and violaceous plaques over knuckles

Lymphoma/leukemia
  Hodgkin's
  Acute leukemia
	
	Ataxia Telangiectasia: telangiectasia on pinna, bulbar conjunctiva
	Ichthyosis: generalized scaling especially on extremities, Sweet's syndrome
	Bloom's syndrome: butterfly erythema on face, associated with short stature

Multiple myeloma	Amyloidosis: large, smooth tongue with waxy papules on eyelids, nasolabial folds and lips, as well as facial petechiae
OTHERS	
Liver disease	Pruritus, hyperpigmentation, spider nevi, palmar erythema, white nails (Terry's nails), porphyria cutanea tarda, xanthomas, hair loss, jaundice
Renal disease	Pruritus, pigmentation, half and half nails, perforating dermatosis, calciphylaxis
Pruritic urticarial papules and plaques of pregnancy	Erythematous papules or urticarial plaques in distribution of striae distensae: buttocks, thighs, upper inner arms and lower back
Cryoglobulinemia	Palpable purpura in cold-exposed areas, Raynaud's, cold urticaria, acral hemorrhagic necrosis, bleeding disorders, associated with hepatitis C infection

Raynaud's Phenomenon DDx

COLD HAND
Cryoglobulins/**C**ryofibrinogens
Obstruction/**O**ccupational
Lupus erythematosus, other connective tissue disease
DM/**D**rugs
Hematologic problems (polycythemia, leukemia, etc)
Arterial problems (atherosclerosis)
Neurologic problems (vascular tone)
Disease of unknown origin (idiopathic)

Acanthosis Nigricans
An asymptomatic dark thickened velvety hyperpigmentation of flexural skin most commonly around the neck. Associated with DM, obesity, and other endocrine disorders and malignancy. It is a cutaneous marker of tissue insulin resistance

Pediatric Exanthems

• see Pediatrics, P55

Miscellaneous Lesions

Angioedema and Urticaria

Angioedema
- deeper swelling of the skin involving subcutaneous tissues; often involves the eyes, lips, and tongue
- may or may not accompany urticaria
- hereditary or acquired forms
- hereditary angioedema (does not occur with urticaria)
  - onset in childhood; 80% have positive family history
  - recurrent attacks; 25% die from laryngeal edema
  - triggers: minor trauma, emotional upset, temperature changes
- types of acquired angioedema
  - acute allergic angioedema (allergens include food, drugs, contrast media, insect venom, latex)
  - non-allergic drug reaction (drugs include ACEI)
  - acquired C1 inhibitor deficiency
- treatment
  - prophylaxis with danazol or stanozolol for hereditary angioedema
  - epinephrine pen to temporize until patient reaches hospital in acute attack

Urticaria
- also known as "hives"
- transient, red, pruritic well-demarcated wheals
- each individual lesion lasts less than 24 h
- second most common type of drug reaction
- results from release of histamine from mast cells in dermis
- can also result after physical contact with allergen

Table 24. Classification of Urticaria

Type	Etiology
Acute Urticaria >2/3 of cases Attacks last <6 wk Individual lesions last <24 h	Drugs: especially ASA, NSAIDs Foods: nuts, shellfish, eggs, fruit Idiopathic (vast majority) Infection Insect stings (bees, wasps, hornets) Percutaneous absorption: cosmetics, work exposures Stress Systemic diseases: SLE, endocrinopathy, neoplasm

Chronic Urticaria
<1/3 of cases
Attacks last >6 wk
Individual lesion lasts <24 h
	IgE-dependent: trigger associated
	  Idiopathic (90% of chronic urticaria patients)
	  Aeroallergens
	  Drugs (antibiotics, hormones, local anesthetics)
	  Foods and additives
	  Insect stings
	  Parasitic infections
	  Physical contact (animal saliva, plant resins, latex, metals, lotions, soap)
	Direct mast cell release
	  Opiates, muscle relaxants, radio-contrast agents
	Complement-mediated
	  Serum sickness, transfusion reactions
	  Infections, viral/bacterial (>80% of urticaria in pediatric patients)
	  Urticarial vasculitis
	Arachidonic acid metabolism
	  ASA, NSAIDs
	Physical
	  Dermatographism (friction, rubbing skin), cold (ice cube, cold water), cholinergic (hot shower, exercise), solar, pressure (shoulder strap, buttocks), aquagenic (exposure to water), adrenergic (stress), heat
	Other
	  Mastocytosis, urticaria pigmentosa

Urticarial Vasculitis
Individual lesions last >24 h
Often painful, less likely pruritic, heals with bruise type lesions
Requires biopsy
	Idiopathic
	Infections
	  Hepatitis
	Autoimmune diseases
	  SLE
	Drug hypersensitivity
	  Cimetidine and diltiazem

DDx for Urticaria

DAM HIVES
Drugs and foods
Allergic
Malignancy
Hereditary
Infection
Vasculitis
Emotions
Stings

Approach to Urticaria
- Thorough Hx and P/E
- **Acute:** no immediate investigations needed; consider referral for allergy testing
- **Chronic:** further investigations required: CBC and differential, urinalysis, ESR, TSH, LFTs to help identify underlying cause
- **Vasculitic:** biopsy of lesion and referral to dermatology

Wheal
- Typically erythematous flat-topped, palpable lesions varying in size with circumscribed dermal edema
- Individual lesion lasts <24 h
- Associated with mast cell release of histamine
- May be pruritic

Mastocytosis (Urticaria Pigmentosa)
Rare disease due to excessive infiltration of the skin by mast cells. It manifests as many reddish-brown elevated plaques and macules. Friction to a lesion produces a wheal surrounded by intense erythema (Darier's sign), due to mast cell degranulation; this occurs within minutes

Erythema Nodosum

Clinical Presentation
- acute or chronic inflammation of subcutaneous fat (panniculitis)
- round, red, tender, poorly demarcated nodules
- sites: asymmetrically arranged on extensor lower legs, knees, arms, (typically shins)
- associated with arthralgia, fever, malaise

Etiology
- 40% are idiopathic
- drugs: sulfonamides, OCPs (also pregnancy), analgesics, trans retinoic acid
- infections: GAS, TB, histoplasmosis, *Yersinia*
- inflammation: sarcoidosis, Crohn's > UC
- malignancy: acute leukemia, Hodgkin's lymphoma

Epidemiology
- 15-30 yr old, F:M = 3:1
- lesions last for days and spontaneously resolve in 6 wk

Investigations
- chest x-ray (to rule out chest infection and sarcoidosis)
- throat culture, ASO titre, PPD skin test

Management
- symptomatic: bed rest, compressive bandages, wet dressings
- NSAIDs, intralesional steroids
- treat underlying cause

Pruritus

Clinical Presentation
- a sensation provoking a desire to scratch, with or without skin lesions
- lesions may arise from the underlying disease, or from excoriation causing crusts, lichenified plaques, or wheals

Etiology
- dermatologic – generalized
  - asteatotic dermatitis ("winter itch" due to dry skin)
  - pruritus of senescent skin (may not have dry skin, any time of year)
  - infestations: scabies, lice
  - drug eruptions: ASA, antidepressants, opiates
  - psychogenic states
- dermatologic – local
  - atopic and contact dermatitis, lichen planus, urticaria, insect bites, dermatitis herpetiformis
  - infection: varicella, candidiasis
  - lichen simplex chronicus
  - prurigo nodularis
- systemic disease – usually generalized
  - hepatic: obstructive biliary disease, cholestatic liver disease of pregnancy
  - renal: chronic renal failure, uremia secondary to hemodialysis
  - hematologic: Hodgkin's lymphoma, multiple myeloma, leukemia, polycythemia vera, hemochromatosis, Fe deficiency anemia, cutaneous T-cell lymphoma
  - neoplastic: lung, breast, gastric (internal solid tumours), non-Hodgkin's lymphoma
  - endocrine: carcinoid, DM, hypothyroid/thyrotoxicosis
  - infectious: HIV, trichinosis, echinococcosis, hepatitis C
  - psychiatric: depression, psychosis
  - neurologic: post-herpetic neuralgia, multiple sclerosis

Investigations
- blood work: CBC, ESR, Cr/BUN, LFT, TSH, fasting blood sugar, stool culture and serology for parasites

Management
- treat underlying cause
- cool water compresses to relieve pruritus
- bath oil and emollient ointment (especially if xerosis is present)
- topical corticosteroid and antipruritics (e.g. menthol, camphor, phenol, mirtazapine, capsaicin)
- systemic antihistamines: H1 blockers are most effective, most useful for urticaria
- phototherapy with UVB or PUVA
- doxepin, amitriptyline
- immunosuppressive agents if severe: steroids and steroid-sparing

DDx of Erythema Nodosum

NODOSUMM
NO cause (idiopathic) in 40%
Drugs (sulfonamides, OCP, etc.)
Other infections (GAS+)
Sarcoidosis
UC and Crohn's
Malignancy (leukemia, Hodgkin's lymphoma)
Many Infections

DDx of Pruritus

SCRATCHED
Scabies
Cholestasis
Renal
Autoimmune
Tumours
Crazies (psychiatric)
Hematology (polycythemia, lymphoma)
Endocrine (thyroid, parathyroid, Fe)
Drugs, Dry skin

Consider biopsy of any nonhealing wound to rule out cancer

Wounds and Ulcers

- see Plastic Surgery, PL8, PL15

Sunscreens and Preventative Therapy

Sunburn
- erythema 2-6 h post UV exposure often associated with edema, pain and blistering with subsequent desquamation of the dermis, and hyperpigmentation
- chronic UVA and UVB exposure leads to photoaging, immunosuppression, photocarcinogenesis
- prevention: avoid peak UVR (10 am-4 pm), wear appropriate clothing, wide-brimmed hat, sunglasses, and broad-spectrum sunscreen
- clothing with UV protection expressed as UV protection factor (UPF) is analogous to SPF of sunscreen

SPF = burn time with cream/burn time without cream

Sunscreens
- under ideal conditions an SPF of 10 means that a person who normally burns in 20 min will burn in 200 min following the application of the sunscreen
- topical chemical: absorbs UV light
  - requires application at least 15-30 min prior to exposure, should be reapplied every 2 h (more often if sweating, swimming)
  - UVB absorbers: PABA, salicylates, cinnamates, benzylidene camphor derivatives
  - UVA absorbers: benzophenones, anthranilates, dibenzoylmethanes, benzylidene camphor derivatives
- topical physical: reflects and scatters UV light
  - titanium dioxide, zinc oxide, kaolin, talc, ferric chloride, and melanin
    - all are effective against the UVA and UVB spectrum
  - less risk of sensitization than chemical sunscreens and waterproof, but may cause folliculitis or miliaria
- some sunscreen ingredients may cause contact or photocontact allergic reactions, but are uncommon

UV Radiation

UVA (320-400 nm): Aging
- Penetrates skin more effectively than UVB or UVC
- Responsible for tanning, burning, wrinkling, photoallergy and premature skin aging
- Penetrates clouds, glass and is reflected off water, snow and cement

UVB (290-320 nm): Burning
- Absorbed by the outer dermis
- Is mainly responsible for burning and premature skin aging
- Primarily responsible for BCC, SCC
- Does not penetrate glass and is substantially absorbed by ozone

UVC (200-290 nm)
- Is filtered by ozone layer

Management
- sunburn: if significant blistering present, consider treatment in hospital; otherwise, symptomatic treatment (cool wet compresses, oral anti-inflammatory, topical corticosteroids)
- antioxidants, both oral and topical are being studied for their abilities to protect the skin; topical agents are limited by their ability to penetrate the skin

Topical Steroids

Table 25. Potency Ranking of Topical Steroids

Relative Potency	Relative Strength	Generic Names	Trade Names	Usage
Weak	x1	hydrocortisone – 2.5% (1% available over-the-counter)	Emo Cort®	Intertriginous areas, children, face, thin skin
Moderate	x3	hydrocortisone 17-valerate – 0.2% desonide mometasone furoate	Westcort® Tridesilon® Elocom®	Arm, leg, trunk
Potent	x6	betamethasone – 0.1% 17-valerate – 0.1% amcinonide	Betnovate® Celestoderm – V® Cyclocort®	Body
Very Potent	x9	betamethasone dipropionate – 0.05% fluocinonide – 0.05% halcinonide	Diprosone® Lidex, Topsyn gel® Lyderm® Halog®	Palms and soles
Extremely Potent	x12	clobetasol propionate – 0.05% (most potent) betamethasone dipropionate ointment halobetasol propionate – 0.05%	Dermovate® Diprolene® Ultravate®	Palms and soles

Body Site:
Relative Percutaneous Absorption
Forearm	1.0
Plantar foot	0.14
Palm	0.83
Back	1.7
Scalp	3.7
Forehead	6.0
Cheeks	13.0
Scrotum	42.0

Calculation of strength of steroid compared to hydrocortisone on forearm: relative strength of steroid x relative percutaneous absorption

Surface Area
30 g covers full adult body once. Children have a greater surface area/volume ratio and there are consequently greater side effects

Side Effects of Topical Steroids
- Local: atrophy, perioral dermatitis, steroid acne, rosacea, contact dermatitis, tachyphylaxis (tolerance), telangectasis, striae, hypertrichosis, hypopigmentation
- Systemic: suppression of HPA axis

Dermatologic Therapies

Topical Vehicles
- Ointment (water in oil): hydrate, greasy
- Cream (oil in water): hydrate, variable
- Lotion (powder in water): drying, cosmesis
- Solutions (water, alcohol, propylene glycol)
- Gel (solution that melts on contact with skin, alcohol): drying

Table 26. Common Topical Therapies

Drug Name	Dosing Schedule	Indications	Comments
Calcipotriol (Dovonex®)	0.005% cream, ointment, scalp solution, apply bid. For maintenance therapy apply OD	Psoriasis	Burning, itching, skin irritation, worsening of psoriasis. Avoid face, mucous membranes, eyes; wash hands after application. Maximum weekly dosage of cream by age: 2-5 yr – 25 g/wk; 6-10 yr – 50 g/wk; 11-14 yr – 75 g/wk; >14 yr – 100 g/wk. Inactivated by light (do not apply before phototherapy)
Imiquimod (Aldara®)	5% cream applied 3x/wk. Apply at bedtime, leave on 6-10 h, then wash off with mild soap and water. Max duration 16 wk	Genital warts, Cutaneous warts, AK, Superficial BCC	Avoid natural/artificial UV exposure. Local skin and application site reactions. Erythema, ulceration, edema, flu-like symptoms. Works best for warts on mucosal surfaces. May induce inflammation and erosion
Permethrin (Kwellada® P Lotion and Nix® Dermal Cream)	1% or 5% cream, applied once overnight to all skin areas from neck down, repeated one week later	Scabies (Kwellada-P Lotion, Nix® Dermal Cream), Pediculosis (Kwellada-P Crème Rinse®, Nix Crème Rinse®)	Do not use in children <2 yr. Hypersensitivity to drug, or known sensitivity to chrysanthemums. Local reactions only (resolve rapidly); including burning, pruritus. Low toxicity, excellent results. Consider second application after 7 d
Pimecrolimus (Elidel®)	1% cream bid. Use for as long as lesions persist and discontinue upon resolution of symptoms	AD (mild to moderate)	Burning. Lacks adverse effects of steroids. May be used on all skin surfaces including head, neck, and intertriginous areas. Expensive
Tacrolimus Topical (Protopic®)	0.03% (children) or 0.1% (adults) ointment bid. Continue for duration of disease PLUS 1 wk after clearing	AD (mild to moderate)	Burning. Lacks adverse effects of steroids. May be used on all skin surfaces including head, neck, and intertriginous areas. Expensive

Table 27. Common Oral Therapies

Drug Name	Dosing Schedule	Indications	Comments
Acitretin (Soriatane®)	25-50 mg PO OD; maximum 75 mg/d	Severe psoriasis, Other disorders of hyperkeratinization (ichthyosis, Darier's disease)	Monitoring strategies: Monitor lipids, LFTs at baseline and q1-2wk until stable. Contraindications: Women of childbearing potential unless strict contraceptive requirements are met. Drug interactions: Other systemic retinoids, methotrexate, tetracyclines, certain contraceptives. May be combined with PUVA phototherapy (known as re-PUVA)
Antivirals	famciclovir (Famvir®) 250 mg PO tid x 7-10 d (for 1st episode of genital herpes) 125 mg PO bid x 5 d (for recurrent genital herpes)	Chickenpox, Herpes zoster, Genital herpes, Acute and prophylactic to reduce transmission in infected patients, Herpes labialis	Side effects: Headache, nausea, diarrhea, abdominal pain. Reduce dose if impaired renal function
	valacyclovir (Valtrex®) 1000 mg PO bid x 7-10 d (for 1st episode of genital herpes) 500 mg PO bid x 5 d (for recurrent genital herpes)		Side effects: Dizziness, depression, abdominal pain. Reduce dose if impaired renal function. Drug interactions: cimetidine
Cyclosporine (Neoral®)	2.5-4 mg/kg/d PO divided bid. Max 4 mg/kg/d. After 4 wk may increase by 0.5 mg/kg/d q2wks. Concomitant dose of magnesium may protect the kidneys	Psoriasis. May also be effective in: Lichen planus, EM, Recalcitrant urticaria, Recalcitrant AD	Monitoring strategies: Blood pressure, renal function. Contraindications: Abnormal renal function, uncontrolled hypertension, malignancy (except NMSC), uncontrolled infection, immunodeficiency (excluding autoimmune disease), hypersensitivity to drug. Long-term effects preclude use of cyclosporine for >2 yr; discontinue earlier if possible. May consider rotating therapy with other drugs to minimize adverse effects of each drug
Dapsone	50-100-150 mg PO OD tapering to 25-50 mg PO OD to as low as 50 mg 2x/wk	Dermatitis herpetiformis, neutrophilic dermatoses	Monitoring strategies: Obtain G6PD levels before initiating; in the initial two wk obtain methemoglobin levels and follow the blood counts carefully for the first few months. Side effects: Neuropathy. Hemolysis (Vitamin C and E supplementation can help prevent this). Drug interactions: Substrate of CYP2C8/9 (minor), 2C19 (minor), 2E1 (minor), 3A4 (major). Often a dramatic response within hours

Table 27. Common Oral Therapies (continued)

Drug Name	Dosing Schedule	Indications	Comments
Isotretinoin (Accutane®)	0.5-1 mg/kg/d given OD, to achieve a total dose of 120 mg/kg (20-24 wk)	Severe nodular and/or inflammatory acne Acne conglobata Recalcitrant acne Widespread comedonal acne	Monitoring strategies Baseline lipid profile and LFTs before treatment, β-hCG Contraindications Teratogenic – in sexually active females, 2 forms of reliable contraception necessary Generally regarded as unsafe in lactation Side effects Night blindness, decreased tolerance to contact lenses, dry mucous membranes May transiently exacerbate acne, dry skin Depression, myalgia Drug interactions Do not use at the same time as tetracycline or minocycline – both may cause pseudotumour cerebri Discontinue vitamin A supplements Drug may be discontinued at 16-20 wk when nodule count has dropped by >70%; a second course may be initiated after 2 mo prn Refractory cases may require >3 courses
Itraconazole (Sporanox®)	100-400 mg PO OD, depending on infection Tinea corporis/cruris/versicolor: 200 mg PO OD x 7 d Tinea pedis: 200 mg PO bid x 7 d Toenails: 200 mg PO bid x 7 d once per month, repeated 3x Fingernail involvement only: 200 mg bid PO x 7 d once per month, repeated 2x	Onychomycosis Tinea corporis, cruris, pedis, versicolor, capitis	Contraindications CHF Side effects Serious hepatotoxicity Drug Interactions Inhibits CYP3A4 Increases concentration of some drugs metabolized by this enzyme (i.e. statins, diabetic drugs) Give capsules with food, capsules must be swallowed whole
Ivermectin (Mectizan®, Stromectol®)	200-250 μg/kg PO qweekly x 2 Take once as directed; repeat one wk later	Onchocerciasis (USA only) Not licensed for use in Canada Also effective for: scabies	No significant serious side effects Efficacious
Methotrexate (Trexall®)	10-25 mg qwk, PO, IM, or IV Max: 30 mg/wk To minimize side effects, administer with folic acid supplementation: 1-5 mg OD	Psoriasis AD Lymphomatoid papulosis May also be effective in: cutaneous sarcoidosis	Monitoring strategies Baseline renal, liver, and hematological studies Contraindications Pregnancy, lactation, alcohol abuse, liver dysfunction, immunodeficiency syndrome, blood dyscrasias, hypersensitivity to drug Restricted to severe, recalcitrant or disabling psoriasis not adequately responsive to other forms of therapy May be combined with cyclosporine to allow lower doses of both drugs
Minocycline (Minocin®)	50-100 mg PO bid Taper to 50 mg PO OD as acne lessens	Acne vulgaris Rosacea	Contraindications Caution if impaired renal or liver function Drug interactions Do not use with isotretinoin (Accutane®) Side effects Extensive; affects multiple organ systems including CNS, teeth, eyes, bones, renal, and skin (photosensitivity and blue pigmentation) Drug-induced lupus (check p-ANCA) Alternative to tetracycline
OCPs (TriCyclen®, Diane 35®, Alesse®)	1 pill PO once daily	Hormonal acne (chin, jawline) Acne associated with polycystic ovarian syndrome or other endocrine abnormalities	All combined OCPs are helpful in acne but those listed on the left have undergone RCTs Contraindications Smoking, HTN, migraines with aura, pregnancy Routine gynecological health maintenance should be up to date
Spironolactone	50-100 mg PO OD alone or with OCPs	Hormonal acne (chin, jawline) Acne with endocrine abnormality	Contraindications Pregnancy Side effects Menstrual irregularities at higher doses if not on OCPs Breast tenderness, mild diuresis common Risk of hyperkalemia – counsel patients to reduce intake of potassium rich foods such as bananas
Terbinafine (Lamisil®)	250 mg PO OD x 2 wk Fingernails x 6 wk Toenails x 12 wk Confirm diagnosis prior to treatment	Onychomycosis Tinea corporis, cruris, pedis, capitis	Contraindications Pregnancy, chronic or active liver disease Drug interactions Potent inhibitor of CYP2D6; use with caution when also taking β-blockers, certain anti-arrhythmic agents, MAOI type B, and/or antipsychotics Drug concentrates rapidly in skin, hair, and nails at levels associated with fungicidal activity
Tetracycline	250-500 mg PO bid to tid Taken 1 h before or 2 h after a meal	Acne vulgaris Rosacea Bullous pemphigoid	Contraindications Severe renal or hepatic dysfunction

References

Aoyama H, Tanaka M, Hara M, et al. Nummular eczema: An addition of senile xerosis and unique cutaneous reactivities to environmental aeroallergens. Dermatology 1999;199(2):135-139.

Bolognia JL, Jorizzo JL, Rapini RP (editors). Textbook of dermatology. Vol. 1 and 2. Toronto: Mosby, 2003.

Cribier B, Caille A, Heid E. Erythema nodosum and associated diseases. Int J Dermatol 1998;37:667-672.

Cummings SR, Tripp MK, Herrmann NB. Approaches to the prevention and control of skin cancer. Cancer Metast Rev 1997;16:309-327.

deShazo RD, Kemp SF. Allergic reactions to drugs and biologic agents. JAMA 1997;278:1895-1906.

Ellis C, Luger T, Abeck D, et al. International Consensus Conference on Atopic Dermatitis II (ICCAD II): clinical update and current treatment strategies. Br J Dermatol 2003;148(suppl 63):3-10.

Faergemann J, Baron R. Epidemiology, clinical presentation, and diagnosis of onychomycosis. Br J Dermatol 2003;149(suppl 65):1-4.

Fitzpatrick JE, Aeling JL. Dermatology secrets. 2nd ed. Philadelphia: Hanley & Belfus, 2001.

Friedmann PS. Assessment of urticaria and angio-oedema. Clin Exp Allergy 1999;2(suppl 3):109-112.

Goldsmith L, Katz S, Gilchrest B, et al. Fitzpatrick's Dermatology in General Medicine, 8th edition. New York: McGraw Hill, 2012.

Goodheart H. Goodheart's photoguide to common skin disorders: diagnosis and management, 3rd ed. Philadelphia: Lippincott, Williams and Wilkins, 2008.

Gordon ML, Hecker MS. Care of the skin at midlife: diagnosis of pigmented lesions. Geriatrics 1997;52:56-67.

Johnson RA, Suurmond D, Wolff K (editors). Color atlas and synopsis of clinical dermatology, 5th ed. New York: McGraw Hill, 2005.

Krafchik BR. Treatment of atopic dermatitis. J Cutan Med Surg 1999;3(suppl 2):16-23.

Lebwohl MG, Heymann WR, Berth-Jones J, et al. (editors). Treatment of skin disease: comprehensive therapeutic strategies, 2nd ed. Philadelphia: Mosby, 2006.

Mastrolorenzo A, Urbano FG, Salimbeni L, et al. Atypical molluscum contagiosum in an HIV-infected patient. Int J Dermatol 1998;27:378-380.

Ozkaya E. Adult-onset atopic dermatitis. J Am Acad Dermatol 2005;52(4):579-582.

Paller AS, Mancini AJ. Hurwitz clinical pediatric dermatology: a textbook of skin disorders of childhood and adolescence, 3rd ed. China: Elsevier, 2006.

Price VH. Treatment of hair loss. NEJM 1999;341:964-973.

Roujeau JC. Stevens-Johnson syndrome and toxic epidermal necrolysis are severe variants of the same disease which differs from erythema multiforme. J Dermatol 1997;24:726-729.

Sivamani RK, Goodarzi H, Garcia MS, et al. Biologic therapies in the treatment of psoriasis: a comprehensive evidence-based basic science and clinical review and a practical guide to tuberculosis monitoring. Clin Rev Allerg Immu 2013;44:121-140.

Sterry W, Paus W, Burgdorf W (editors). Thieme clinical companions: dermatology, 5th ed. New York: Thieme, 2005.

Ting PT, Banankin B. Can you identify this condition? Melasma. Can Fam Physician 2005;51:353-355.

Walsh SRA, Shear NH. Psoriasis and the new biologic agents: interrupting a T-AP dance. CMAJ 2004;170:1933-1941.

Whited JD, Grichnik JM. The rational clinical examination. Does this patient have a mole or a melanoma? JAMA 1998;279:696-701.

Wilkin J, Dahl M, Detmar M, et al. Standard classification of rosacea: report of the National Rosacea Society Expert Committee on the classification and staging of rosacea. J Am Acad Dermatol 2002;46:584-587.

Wolff K, Johnson RA. Fitzpatrick's colour atlas and synopsis of clinical dermatology, 6th ed and 7th ed. New York: McGraw Hill, 2009.

ER Emergency Medicine

Devon Alton, Ali El Hamouly, Jonah Himelfarb, and Hamza Sami, chapter editors
Narayan Chattergoon and Desmond She, associate editors
Arnav Agarwal and Quynh Huynh, EBM editors
Dr. Mark Freedman, Dr. Kevin Skarratt, and Dr. Fernando Teixeira, staff editors

Acronyms

AAA	abdominal aortic aneurysm	DIC	disseminated intravascular coagulation
ABG	arterial blood gas		
ACS	acute coronary syndrome	DKA	diabetic ketoacidosis
AED	automatic external defibrillator	DRE	digital rectal exam
AFib	atrial fibrillation	DT	delirium tremens
AG	anion gap	DVT	deep vein thrombosis
ARDS	acute respiratory distress syndrome	ED	emergency department
AVN	avascular necrosis	EM	erythema multiforme
AVPU	alert, voice, pain, unresponsive	ETT	endotracheal tube
AXR	abdominal X-ray	FAST	focused abdominal sonogram for trauma
Bi-PAP	bilevel positive airway pressure		
BSA	body surface area	FFP	fresh frozen plasma
CAS	Children's Aid Society	GERD	gastroesophageal reflux disease
CPAP	continuous positive airway pressure	GCS	Glasgow Coma Scale
CPP	cerebral perfusion pressure	HI	head injury
CSF	cerebrospinal fluid	IBD	inflammatory bowel disease
CVA	costovertebral angle	IBS	irritable bowel syndrome
CXR	chest X-ray	ICP	intracranial pressure
D&C	dilatation and curettage	ICS	intercostal space
DGI	disseminated gonococcal infection	JVP	jugular venous pressure

LBBB	left bundle branch block
LOC	level of consciousness
LP	lumbar puncture
LVH	left ventricular hypertrophy
MAP	mean arterial pressure
MDI	metered dose inhaler
MVC	motor vehicle collision
NG	nasogastric
NS	normal saline
OD	once daily
PE	pulmonary embolism
PID	pelvic inflammatory disease
PNS	parasympathetic nervous system
POG	plasma osmolar gap
pRBC	packed red blood cells
RBBB	right bundle branch block
ROM	range of motion
RPS	rapid primary survey
RSI	rapid sequence induction
rt-PA	recombinant tissue plasminogen activator

SAH	subarachnoid hemorrhage
SCI	spinal cord injury
SJS	Stevens-Johnson syndrome
SNS	sympathetic nervous system
SOB	shortness of breath
SSSS	staphylococcal scalded skin syndrome
STEMI	ST elevation myocardial infarction
TBI	traumatic brain injury
TCA	tricyclic antidepressant
TEN	toxic epidermal necrolysis
TSS	toxic shock syndrome
U/A	urinalysis
U/S	ultrasound
UTox	urine toxicology screen
VBG	venous blood gas
VFib	ventricular fibrillation
VTach	ventricular tachycardia
VTE	venous thromboembolism

Patient Assessment/Management

1. Rapid Primary Survey

Approach to the Critically Ill Patient
1. Rapid Primary Survey (RPS)
2. Resuscitation (often concurrent with RPS)
3. Detailed Secondary Survey
4. Definitive Care

- **A**irway maintenance with C-spine control
- **B**reathing and ventilation
- **C**irculation (pulses, hemorrhage control)
- **D**isability (neurological status)
- **E**xposure (complete) and **E**nvironment (temperature control)
  - continually reassessed during secondary survey
  - changes in hemodynamic and/or neurological status necessitates a return to the primary survey beginning with airway assessment
- **IMPORTANT**: Always watch for signs of shock while doing primary survey

A. AIRWAY
- first priority is to secure airway
- assume a cervical injury in every trauma patient and immobilize with collar
- assess ability to breathe and speak
- can change rapidly, therefore reassess frequently
- assess for facial fractures/edema/burns (impending airway collapse)

Signs of Airway Obstruction
- Agitation, confusion, "universal choking sign"
- Respiratory distress
- Failure to speak, dysphonia, stridor
- Cyanosis

Airway Management
- anatomic optimization to allow for oxygenation and ventilation

1. Basic Airway Management
- protect the C-spine
- head-tilt (if C-spine injury not suspected) or jaw thrust to open the airway
- sweep and suction to clear mouth of foreign material

2. Temporizing Measures
- nasopharyngeal airway (if gag reflex present, i.e. conscious)
- oropharyngeal airway (if gag reflex absent, i.e. unconscious)
- "rescue" airway devices (e.g. laryngeal mask airway, Combitube®)
- transtracheal jet ventilation through cricothyroid membrane (last resort)

Medications that can be Delivered via ETT

NAVEL
Naloxone (Narcan®)
Atropine
Ventolin® (salbutamol)
Epinephrine
Lidocaine

3. Definitive Airway Management
- ETT intubation with in-line stabilization of C-spine
  - orotracheal ± RSI preferred
  - nasotracheal may be better tolerated in conscious patient
    - relatively contraindicated with basal skull fracture
  - does not provide 100% protection against aspiration
- surgical airway (if unable to intubate using oral/nasal route and unable to ventilate)
- cricothyroidotomy

Contraindications to Intubation
- supraglottic/glottic pathology that would preclude successful intubation

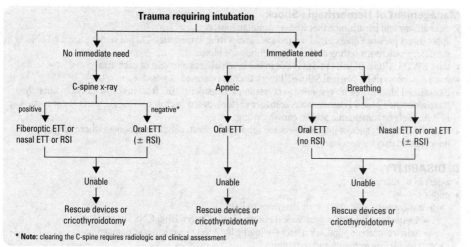

Figure 1. Approach to endotracheal intubation in an injured patient

Indications for Intubation
- Unable to protect airway (e.g. GCS <8; airway trauma)
- Inadequate oxygenation with spontaneous respiration (O_2 saturation <90% with 100% O_2, or rising pCO_2)
- Anticipatory: in trauma, overdose, CHF, asthma, COPD, and smoke inhalation injury
- Anticipated transfer of critically ill patients

Rescue Techniques in Intubation
- Bougie (used like a guidewire)
- Glidescope®
- Lighted stylet (use light through skin to determine if ETT in correct place)
- Fiberoptic intubation – indirect visualization using fiberoptic cable

B. BREATHING
- **Look**
  - mental status (anxiety, agitation, decreased LOC), colour, chest movement (bilateral vs. asymmetrical), respiratory rate/effort, nasal flaring
- **Listen**
  - auscultate for signs of obstruction (e.g. stridor), breath sounds, symmetry of air entry, air escaping
- **Feel**
  - tracheal shift, chest wall for crepitus, flail segments, sucking chest wounds, subcutaneous emphysema

Noisy breathing is obstructed breathing until proven otherwise

Breathing Assessment
- objective measures of respiratory function: rate, oximetry, ABG, A-a gradient

Management of Breathing
- nasal prongs → simple face mask → non-rebreather mask → CPAP/BiPAP (in order of increasing FiO_2)
- Bag-Valve mask and CPAP to supplement inadequate ventilation

C. CIRCULATION

Definition of Shock
- inadequate organ and tissue perfusion with oxygenated blood (brain, kidney, extremities)

Shock in a trauma patient is hemorrhagic until proven otherwise

Table 1. Major Types of Shock

Hypovolemic	Cardiogenic	Distributive (vasodilation)	Obstructive
Hemorrhage (external and internal)	Myocardial ischemia	Septic	Cardiac tamponade
Severe burns	Dysrhythmias	Anaphylactic	Tension pneumothorax
High output fistulas	CHF	Neurogenic (spinal cord injury)	PE
Dehydration (diarrhea, DKA)	Cardiomyopathies		Aortic stenosis
	Cardiac valve problems		Constrictive pericarditis

Medications that can be Delivered via ETT

NAVEL
Naloxone (Narcan®)
Atropine **Causes of Shock**

SHOCKED
Septic, spinal/neurogenic,
Hemorrhagic
Obstructive (e.g. tension pneumothorax, cardiac tamponade, PE)
Cardiogenic (e.g. blunt myocardial injury, dysrhythmia, MI)
anaphylacti**K**
Endocrine (e.g. Addison's, myxedema, coma)
Drugs
Ventolin® (salbutamol)
Epinephrine
Lidocaine

Clinical Evaluation
- early: tachypnea, tachycardia, narrow pulse pressure, reduced capillary refill, cool extremities, and reduced central venous pressure
- late: hypotension and altered mental status, reduced urine output

Table 2. Estimation of Degree of Hemorrhagic Shock

Class	I	II	III	IV
Blood loss	<750 cc	750-1,500 cc	1,500-2,000 cc	>2,000 cc
% of blood volume	<15%	15-30%	30-40%	>40%
Pulse	<100	>100	>120	>140
Blood pressure	Normal	Normal	Decreased	Decreased
Respiratory rate	20	30	35	>45
Capillary refill	Normal	Decreased	Decreased	Decreased
Urinary output	30 cc/h	20 cc/h	10 cc/h	None
Fluid replacement	Crystalloid	Crystalloid	Crystalloid + blood	Crystalloid + blood

Estimated Systolic Blood Pressure Based on Position of Most Distal Palpable Pulse

	sBP (mmHg)
Radial	>80
Femoral	>70
Carotid	>60

3:1 Rule
Since only 30% of infused isotonic crystalloids remains in intravascular space, you must give 3x estimated blood loss

Management of Hemorrhagic Shock
- clear airway and breathing either first or simultaneously
- apply direct pressure on external wounds while elevating extremities. Do not remove impaled objects in the emergency room setting as they may tamponade bleeds
- start TWO LARGE BORE (14-16G) IVs in the brachial/cephalic vein of each arm
- run 1-2 L bolus of IV Normal Saline/Ringer's Lactate (warmed, if possible)
- if continual bleeding or no response to crystalloids, consider pRBC transfusion, ideally crossmatched. If crossmatched blood is unavailable, consider O- for women of childbearing age and O+ for men. Use FFP, platelets or tranexamic acid in early bleeding
- consider common sites of internal bleeding (abdomen, chest, pelvis, long bones) where surgical intervention may be necessary

D. DISABILITY
- assess LOC using GCS
- pupils
  - assess equality, size, symmetry, reactivity to light
    - inequality/sluggish suggests local eye problem or lateralizing CNS lesion
    - relative afferent pupillary defect (swinging light test) – optic nerve damage
  - extraocular movements and nystagmus
  - fundoscopy (papilledema, hemorrhages)
  - reactive pupils + decreased LOC: metabolic or structural cause
  - non-reactive pupils + decreased LOC: structural cause (especially if asymmetric)

Fluid Resuscitation
- Give bolus until HR decreases, urine output increases, and patient stabilizes
  - Maintenance: 4:2:1 rule
  - 0-10 kg: 4 cc/kg/h
  - 10-20 kg: 2 cc/kg/h
  - Remaining weight: 1 cc/kg/h
  - Replace ongoing losses and deficits (assume 10% of body weight)

Glasgow Coma Scale
- for use in trauma patients with decreased LOC; good indicator of severity of injury and neurosurgical prognosis
- most useful if repeated; change in GCS with time is more relevant than the absolute number
- less meaningful for metabolic coma
- patient with deteriorating GCS needs immediate attention
- prognosis based on best post-resuscitation GCS
- reported as a 3 part score: Eyes + Verbal + Motor = Total
- if patient intubated, GCS score reported out of 10 + T (T = tubed, i.e. no verbal component)

Table 3. Glasgow Coma Scale

Eyes Open		Best Verbal Response		Best Motor Response	
Spontaneously	4	Answers questions appropriately	5	Obeys commands	6
To voice	3	Confused, disoriented	4	Localizes to pain	5
To pain	2	Inappropriate words	3	Withdraws from pain	4
No response	1	Incomprehensible sounds	2	Decorticate (flexion)	3
		No verbal response	1	Decerebrate (extension)	2
				No response	1

13-15 = mild injury, 9-12 = moderate injury, ≤8 = severe injury   See Table 36, ER57 for modified GCS for infants and children

Unilateral, Dilated, Non-Reactive Pupil, Think
- Focal mass lesion
- Epidural hematoma
- Subdural hematoma

E. EXPOSURE/ENVIRONMENT
- expose patient completely and assess entire body for injury; log roll to examine back
- DRE
- keep patient warm with a blanket ± radiant heaters; avoid hypothermia
- warm IV fluids/blood
- keep providers safe (contamination, combative patient)

2. Resuscitation

- done concurrently with primary survey
- attend to ABCs
- manage life-threatening problems as they are identified
- vital signs q5-15 min
- ECG, BP, and O₂ monitors
- Foley catheter and NG tube if indicated
- tests and investigations: CBC, electrolytes, BUN, Cr, glucose, amylase, INR/PTT, β-hCG, toxicology screen, cross and type

Contraindications to Foley Insertion
- Blood at urethral meatus
- Scrotal hematoma
- High-riding prostate on DRE

NG Tube Contraindications
- Significant mid-face trauma
- Basal skull fracture

Table 4. 2010 AHA CPR Guidelines

Step/Action	Adult: >8 yr	Child: 1-8 yr	Infant: <1 yr
Airway	Head tilt-chin lift		
Breaths	2 breaths at 1 second/breath – stop once see chest rise		
Foreign-Body Airway Obstruction	Abdominal thrust		Back slaps and chest thrusts
Compressions			
Compression landmarks	In the centre of the chest, between nipples		Just below nipple line
Compression method: push hard and fast, and allow for complete recoil	2 hands: heel of 1 hand with second hand on top	2 hands: heel of 1 hand with second on top, or 1 hand: heel of 1 hand only	2 fingers, or thumbs
Compression depth	2-2.4 inches	About 1/3 to 1/2 the depth of the chest	
Compression rate	100-120/min with complete chest wall recoil between compressions		
Compression-ventilation ratio	30 compressions to 2 ventilations		
Compression-only CPR	Hands-only CPR is preferred if the bystander is not trained or does not feel confident in their ability to provide conventional CPR or if the bystander is trained but chooses to use compressions only		
Defibrillation	Immediate defibrillation for all rescuers responding to a sudden witnessed collapse Compressions (5 cycles/2 min) before AED is considered if unwitnessed arrest Manual defibrillators are preferred for children and infants but can use adult dose AED if a manual defibrillator is not available		

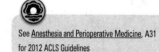

See Anesthesia and Perioperative Medicine, A31 for 2012 ACLS Guidelines

3. Secondary Survey

- done after primary survey once patient is hemodynamically and neurologically stabilized
- identifies major injuries or areas of concern
- full physical exam and x-rays (C-spine, chest, pelvis – required in blunt trauma, consider T-spine and L-spine)

HISTORY

- "**SAMPLE**": **S**igns and symptoms, **A**llergies, **M**edications, **P**ast medical history, **L**ast meal, **E**vents related to injury

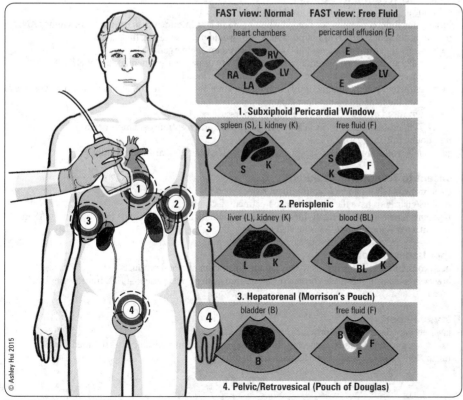

Figure 2. Four areas of a FAST

PHYSICAL EXAM

Head and Neck
- palpation of facial bones, scalp

Chest
- inspect for: 1. midline trachea and 2. flail segment: ≥2 rib fractures in ≥2 places; if present look for associated hemothorax, pneumothorax, and contusions
- auscultate lung fields
- palpate for subcutaneous emphysema

Abdomen
- assess for peritonitis, abdominal distention, and evidence of intra-abdominal bleeding
- DRE for GI bleed, high riding prostate and anal tone

Musculoskeletal
- examine all extremities for swelling, deformity, contusions, tenderness, ROM
- check for pulses (using Doppler probe) and sensation in all injured limbs
- log roll and palpate thoracic and lumbar spines
- palpate iliac crests and pubic symphysis and assess pelvic stability (lateral, AP, vertical)

Neurological
- GCS
- full cranial nerve exam
- alterations of rate and rhythm of breathing are signs of structural or metabolic abnormalities with progressive deterioration in breathing indicating a failing CNS
- assess spinal cord integrity
- conscious patient: assess distal sensation and motor function
- unconscious patient: response to painful or noxious stimulus applied to extremities

INITIAL IMAGING
- non-contrast CT head/face/C-spine (rule out fractures and bleeds)
- chest x-ray
- FAST (see Figure 2) or CT abdomen/pelvis (if stable)
- pelvis x-ray

Signs of Increased ICP
- Deteriorating LOC (hallmark)
- Deteriorating respiratory pattern
- Cushing reflex (high BP, low heart rate, irregular respirations)
- Lateralizing CNS signs (e.g. cranial nerve palsies, hemiparesis)
- Seizures
- Papilledema (occurs late)
- N/V and headache

Non-contrast head CT is the best imaging modality for intracranial injury

Ethical Considerations

Consent to Treatment: Adults
- see Ethical, Legal, and Organizational Medicine, ELOM6
- Emergency Rule: consent is not needed when a patient is at imminent risk from a serious injury AND obtaining consent is either: a) not possible, OR b) would increase risk to the patient
  - assumes that most people would want to be saved in an emergency
- any capable and informed patient can refuse treatment or part of treatment, even if it is life-saving
- exceptions to the Emergency Rule - treatment cannot be initiated if
  - a competent patient has previously refused the same or similar treatment and there is no evidence to suggest the patient's wishes have changed
  - an advanced directive is available (e.g. do not resuscitate order)
  - NOTE: refusal of help in a suicide situation is NOT an exception; care must be given
- if in doubt, initiate treatment
- care can be withdrawn if necessary at a later time or if wishes are clarified by family

Consent to Treatment: Children
- treat immediately if patient is at imminent risk
- parents/guardians have the right to make treatment decisions
- if parents refuse treatment that is life-saving or will potentially alter the child's quality of life, CAS must be contacted – consent of CAS is needed to treat

Other Issues of Consent
- need consent for HIV testing, as well as for administration of blood products
- however, if delay in substitute consent for blood transfusions puts patient at risk, transfusions can be given

Duty to Report
- law may vary depending on province and/or state
- examples: gunshot wounds, suspected child abuse, various communicable diseases, medical unsuitability to drive, risk of substantial harm to others

Jehovah's Witnesses
- Capable adults have the right to refuse medical treatment
- May refuse whole blood, pRBCs, platelets, and plasma even if life-saving
- Should be questioned directly about the use of albumin, immunoglobulins, hemophilic preparations
- Do not allow autologous transfusion unless there is uninterrupted extra corporeal circulation
- Usually ask for the highest possible quality of care without the use of the above interventions (e.g. crystalloids for volume expansion, attempts at bloodless surgery)
- Patient will generally sign hospital forms releasing medical staff from liability
- Most legal cases involve children of Jehovah's Witnesses; if life-saving treatment is refused, contact CAS

Traumatology

- epidemiology
  - leading cause of death in patients <45 yr
  - 4th highest cause of death in North America
  - causes more deaths in children/adolescents than all diseases combined
- trimodal distribution of death
  - minutes: lethal injuries, death usually at the scene
  - early: death within 4-6 h – "golden hour" (decreased mortality with trauma care)
  - days-weeks: death from multiple organ dysfunction, sepsis, etc.
- injuries fall into two categories
  - blunt (most common): MVC, pedestrian-automobile impact, motorcycle collision, fall, assault, sports
  - penetrating (increasing in incidence): gunshot wound, stabbing, impalement

Always completely expose and count the number of wounds

Considerations for Traumatic Injury

- important to know the mechanism of injury in order to anticipate traumatic injuries
- always look for an underlying cause (alcohol, medications, illicit substances, seizure, suicide attempt, medical problem)
- always inquire about HI, loss of consciousness, amnesia, vomiting, headache, and seizure activity

Cardiac Box: sternal notch, nipples, and xiphoid process; injuries inside this area should increase suspicion of cardiac injury

Table 5. Mechanisms and Considerations of Traumatic Injuries

Mechanism of Injury	Special Considerations	Associated Injuries
MVC	Vehicle(s) involved: weight, size, speed, damage Location of patient in vehicle Use and type of seatbelt Ejection of patient from vehicle Entrapment of patient under vehicle Airbag deployment Helmet use in motorcycle collision	Head-on collision: head/facial, thoracic (aortic), lower extremity Lateral/T-bone collision: head, C-spine, thoracic, abdominal, pelvic, and lower extremity Rear-end collision: hyper-extension of C-spine (whiplash injury) Rollover
Pedestrian-Automobile Impact	High morbidity and mortality Vehicle speed is an important factor Site of impact on car	Children at increased risk of being run over (multisystem injuries) Adults tend to be struck in lower legs (lower extremity injuries), impacted against car (truncal injuries), and thrown to ground (HI)
Falls	1 storey = 12 ft = 3.6 m Distance of fall: 50% mortality at 4 storeys and 95% mortality at 7 storeys Landing position (vertical vs. horizontal)	Vertical: lower extremity, pelvic, and spine fractures; HI Horizontal: facial, upper extremity, and rib fractures; abdominal, thoracic, and HI

High Risk Injuries
- MVC at high speed, resulting in ejection from vehicle
- Motorcycle collisions
- Vehicle vs. pedestrian crashes
- Fall from height >12 ft (3.6 m)

Vehicle vs. Pedestrian Crash
In adults look for triad of injuries (Waddle's triad)
- Tibia-fibula or femur fracture
- Truncal injury
- Craniofacial injury

Head Trauma

- see Neurosurgery, NS29
- 60% of MVC-related deaths are due to HI

Specific Injuries
- fractures
  - Dx: non-contrast head CT and physical exam
  - A. skull fractures
  - vault fractures
    - linear, non-depressed
      - most common
      - typically occur over temporal bone, in area of middle meningeal artery (commonest cause of epidural hematoma)
    - depressed
      - open (associated overlying scalp laceration and torn dura, skull fracture disrupting paranasal sinuses or middle ear) vs. closed
  - basal skull
    - typically occur through floor of anterior cranial fossa (longitudinal more common than transverse)
    - clinical diagnosis superior as poorly visualized on CT
  - B. facial fractures (see Plastic Surgery, PL29)
  - neuronal injury
  - beware of open fracture or sinus fractures (risk of infection)
  - severe facial fractures may pose risk to airway from profuse bleeding

Signs of Basal Skull Fracture
- Battle's sign (bruised mastoid process)
- Hemotympanum
- Raccoon eyes (periorbital bruising)
- CSF rhinorrhea/otorrhea

- **scalp laceration**
  - can be a source of significant bleeding
  - achieve hemostasis, inspect and palpate for skull bone defects ± CT head (rule-out skull fracture)
- **neuronal injury**
  - A. diffuse
    - mild TBI = concussion
      - transient alteration in mental status that may involve loss of consciousness
        - hallmarks of concussion: confusion and amnesia, which may occur immediately after the trauma or minutes later
        - loss of consciousness (if present) must be less than 30 min, initial GCS must be between 13-15, and post-traumatic amnesia must be less than 24 h
    - diffuse axonal injury
      - mild: coma 6-24 h, possibly lasting deficit
      - moderate: coma >24 h, little or no signs of brainstem dysfunction
      - severe: coma >24 h, frequent signs of brainstem dysfunction
  - B. focal injuries
    - contusions
    - intracranial hemorrhage (epidural, subdural, intracerebral)

ASSESSMENT OF BRAIN INJURY

History
- pre-hospital status
- mechanism of injury

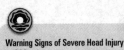

Physical Exam
- assume C-spine injury until ruled out
- vital signs
  - shock (not likely due to isolated brain injury, except in infants)
  - Cushing's response to increasing ICP (bradycardia, HTN, irregular respirations)
- severity of injury determined by
  1. LOC
     - GCS ≤8 intubate, any change in score of 3 or more = serious injury
     - mild TBI = 13-15, moderate = 9-12, severe = 3-8
  2. pupils: size, anisocoria >1 mm (in patient with altered LOC), response to light
  3. lateralizing signs (motor/sensory)
     - may become more subtle with increasing severity of injury
- reassess frequently

Investigations
- labs: CBC, electrolytes, PT/PTT or INR/PTT, glucose, toxicology screen
- CT scan (non-contrast) to exclude intracranial hemorrhage/hematoma
- C-spine imaging, often with CT head and neck to exclude intracranial hemorrhage/hematoma

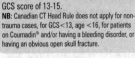

Management
- goal in ED: reduce secondary injury by avoiding hypoxia, ischemia, decreased CPP, seizure
- general
  - ABCs
  - ensure oxygen delivery to brain through intubation and prevent hypercarbia
  - maintain BP (sBP >90)
  - treat other injuries
- early neurosurgical consultation for acute and subsequent patient management
  - medical management
    - seizure treatment/prophylaxis
      - benzodiazepines, phenytoin, phenobarbital
      - steroids are of no proven value
    - treat suspected raised ICP, consider if HI with signs of increased ICP:
      - intubate
      - calm (sedate) if risk for high airway pressures or agitation
      - paralyze if agitated
      - hyperventilate (100% O_2) to a pCO_2 of 30-35 mmHg
      - elevate head of bed to 20°
      - adequate BP to ensure good cerebral perfusion
      - diurese with mannitol 1g/kg infused rapidly (contraindicated in shock/renal failure)

Disposition
- neurosurgical ICU admission for severe HI
- in hemodynamically unstable patient with other injuries, prioritize most life-threatening injuries and maintain cerebral perfusion
- for minor HI not requiring admission, provide 24 h HI protocol to competent caregiver, follow-up with neurology as even seemingly minor HI may cause lasting deficits

Mild Traumatic Brain Injury

Epidemiology
- TBI results in 1.7 million deaths, hospitalizations, and ED visits each year (US)
- 75% are estimated to be mild TBI; remainder are moderate or severe (see <u>Neurosurgery</u>, NS29)
- highest rates in children 0-4 yr, adolescents 15-19 yr, and elderly >65 yr

Clinical Features
- somatic: headache, sleep disturbance, N/V, blurred vision
- cognitive dysfunction: attentional impairment, reduced processing speed, drowsiness, amnesia
- emotion and behaviour: impulsivity, irritability, depression
- severe concussion: may precipitate seizure, bradycardia, hypotension, sluggish pupils

Etiology
- falls, MVC, struck by an object, assault, sports

Investigations
- neurological exam
- concussion recognition tool (see thinkfirst.ca)
- imaging – CT as per Canadian CT Head Rules, or MRI if worsening symptoms despite normal CT

Treatment
- close observation and follow-up; for patients at risk of intracranial complications, give appropriate discharge instructions to patient and family; watch for changes to clinical features above, and if change, return to ED
- hospitalization with normal CT (GCS <15, seizures, bleeding diathesis), or with abnormal CT
- early rehabilitation to maximize outcomes
- pharmacological management of pain, depression, headache
- follow Return to Play guidelines

Prognosis
- most recover with minimal treatment
  - athletes with previous concussion are at increased risk of cumulative brain injury
- repeat TBI can lead to life-threatening cerebral edema or permanent impairment

Spine and Spinal Cord Trauma

- assume cord injury with significant falls (>12 ft), deceleration injuries, blunt trauma to head, neck, or back
- spinal immobilization (cervical collar, spine board during patient transport only) must be maintained until spinal injury has been ruled out (Figure 3)
- vertebral injuries may be present without spinal cord injury; normal neurologic exam does not exclude spinal injury
- cord may be injured despite normal C-spine x-ray (SCIWORA = spinal cord injury without radiologic abnormality)
- injuries can include: complete/incomplete transection, cord edema, spinal shock

History
- mechanism of injury, previous deficits, SAMPLE
- neck pain, paralysis/weakness, paresthesia

Physical Exam
- ABCs
- abdominal: ecchymosis, tenderness
- neurological: complete exam, including mental status
- spine: maintain neutral position, palpate C-spine; log roll, then palpate T-spine and L-spine, assess rectal tone
  - when palpating, assess for tenderness, muscle spasm, bony deformities, step-off, and spinous process malalignment
- extremities: check capillary refill, suspect thoracolumbar injury with calcaneal fractures

Investigations
- bloodwork: CBC, electrolytes, Cr, glucose, coagulation profile, cross and type, toxicology screen
- imaging
  - full C-spine x-ray series for trauma (AP, lateral, odontoid)
- thoracolumbar x-rays
  - AP and lateral views

Extent of retrograde amnesia correlates with severity of injury

Every Patient with One or More of the Following Signs or Symptoms should be Placed in a C-Spine Collar
- Midline tenderness
- Neurological symptoms or signs
- Significant distracting injuries
- HI
- Intoxication
- Dangerous mechanism
- History of altered LOC

Of the investigations, the lateral C-spine x-ray is the single most important film; 95% of radiologically visible abnormalities are found on this film

Cauda Equina Syndrome can occur with any spinal cord injury below T10 vertebrae. Look for incontinence, anterior thigh pain, quadriceps weakness, abnormal sacral sensation, decreased rectal tone, and variable reflexes

The Canadian C-Spine Rule vs. the NEXUS Low-Risk Criteria in Patients with Trauma
NEJM 2003;349:2510-2518
Purpose: To compare the clinical performance of the Canadian C-Spine Rule (CCR) and the National Emergency X-Radiography Utilization Study (NEXUS) Low-Risk Criteria (NLC).
Study: Trauma patients (n=8,283) in stable condition were prospectively evaluated by both the CCR and NLC by 394 physicians before radiography. 2% of these patients had a C-spine injury.
Results: Compared to the NLC, the CCR was more sensitive (99.4 vs. 90.7%) and more specific (45.1 vs. 36.8%) after exclusion of indeterminate cases. The number of missed patients would be 1 for the CCR and 16 for the NLC. The ROM was not evaluated in some CCR cases likely because physicians were not comfortable with the procedure and this may slightly lower the sensitivity or specificity of the CCR in practice.
Summary: The CCR is superior to the NLC in alert and stable patients with trauma. The use of the CCR can result in lower radiography rates.

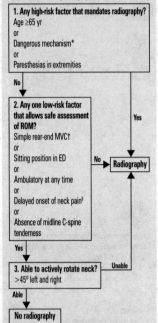

The Canadian C-Spine Rule
JAMA 2001;286:1841-1848

For Alert (GCS Score = 15) and Stable Trauma Patients where C-Spine Injury is a Concern

1. Any high-risk factor that mandates radiography?
Age ≥65 yr
or
Dangerous mechanism*
or
Paresthesias in extremities

↓ No

2. Any one low-risk factor that allows safe assessment of ROM?
Simple rear-end MVC†
or
Sitting position in ED
or
Ambulatory at any time
or
Delayed onset of neck pain§
or
Absence of midline C-spine tenderness

→ No → **Radiography**
↑ Yes

↓ Yes

3. Able to actively rotate neck?
>45° left and right

→ Unable ↑ (to Radiography)

↓ Able

No radiography

*Dangerous Mechanism:
• Fall from ≥1 meter/5 stairs
• Axial load to head (e.g. diving)
• MVC high speed (>100 km/h), rollover, ejection
• Motorized recreational vehicles
• Bicycle collision

†Simple rear-end MVC excludes:
• Pushed into oncoming traffic
• Hit by bus/large truck
• Rollover
• Hit by high-speed vehicle

§Delayed: not immediate onset of neck pain

- indications
  - patients with C-spine injury
  - unconscious patients (with appropriate mechanism of injury)
  - patients with neurological symptoms or findings
  - patients with deformities that are palpable when patient is log rolled
  - patients with back pain
  - patients with bilateral calcaneal fractures (due to fall from height)
    - concurrent burst fractures of the lumbar or thoracic spine in 10% (T11-L2)
  - consider CT (for subtle bony injuries), MRI (for soft tissue injuries) if appropriate

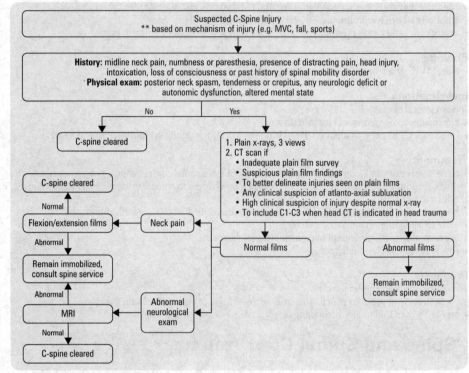

Figure 3. Approach to clearing the C-spine

Can Clear C-Spine if
- oriented to person, place, time, and event
- no evidence of intoxication
- no posterior midline cervical tenderness
- no focal neurological deficits
- no painful distracting injuries (e.g. long bone fracture)

Management of Cord Injury
- immobilize
- evaluate ABCs
- treat neurogenic shock (maintain sBP >100 mmHg)
- insert NG and Foley catheter
- high dose steroids: methylprednisolone 30 mg/kg bolus, then 5.4 mg/kg/h drip, start within 6-8 h of injury (controversial and recently has less support)
- complete imaging of spine and consult spine service if available
- continually reassess high cord injuries as edema can travel up cord
- if cervical cord lesion, watch for respiratory insufficiency
  - low cervical transection (C5-T1) produces abdominal breathing (phrenic innervation of diaphragm still intact but loss of innervation of intercostals and other accessory muscles of breathing)
  - high cervical cord injury (above C4) may require intubation and ventilation
- treatment: warm blanket, Trendelenburg position (occasionally), volume infusion, consider vasopressors

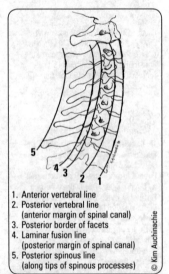

1. Anterior vertebral line
2. Posterior vertebral line (anterior margin of spinal canal)
3. Posterior border of facets
4. Laminar fusion line (posterior margin of spinal canal)
5. Posterior spinous line (along tips of spinous processes)

© Kim Auchinachie

Figure 4. Lines of contour on a lateral C-spine x-ray

Prevertebral soft tissue swelling is only 49% sensitive for injury

Approach to C-Spine X-Rays
- 3-view C-spine series is the screening modality of choice
  1. lateral C1-T1 ± swimmer's view
     - lateral view is best, identifies 90-95% of injuries
  2. odontoid view (open mouth or oblique submental view)
     - examine the dens for fractures
       - if unable to rule out fracture, repeat view or consider CT or plain film tomography
     - examine lateral aspects of C1 and spacing relative to C2

3. AP view
- alignment of spinous processes in the midline
- spacing of spinous processes should be equal
- check vertebral bodies and facet dislocations

Table 6. Interpretation of Lateral View: The ABCS

A	Adequacy and Alignment
	Must see C1 to C7-T1 junction; if not, downward traction of shoulders, swimmer's view, bilateral supine obliques, or CT scan needed
	Lines of contour in children <8 yr of age, can see physiologic subluxation of C2 on C3, and C3 on C4, but the spino-laminal line is maintained
	Fanning of spinous processes suggests posterior ligamentous disruption
	Widening of facet joints
	Check atlanto-occipital joint
	Line extending inferiorly from clivus should transect odontoid
	Atlanto-axial articulation, widening of predental space (normal: <3 mm in adults, <5 mm in children) indicates injury of C1 or C2
B	**Bones**
	Height, width, and shape of each vertebral body
	Pedicles, facets, and laminae should appear as one – doubling suggests rotation
C	**Cartilage**
	Intervertebral disc spaces – wedging anteriorly or posteriorly suggests vertebral compression
S	**Soft Tissues**
	Widening of retropharyngeal (normal: <7 mm at C1-4, may be wide in children <2 yr on expiration) or retrotracheal spaces (normal: <22 mm at C6-T1, <14 mm in children <5 yr)

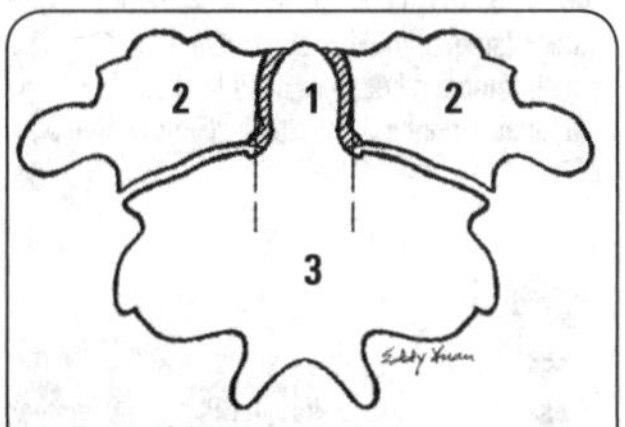

1. Dens of C2
2. C1 lateral mass
3. C2

To clear the x-ray ensure that:
A. The dens is centred between the lateral masses of C1
B. C1 and C2 are aligned laterally
C. The lateral masses of C1 are symmetrical in size

© Eddy Xuan

Figure 5. C-spine x-ray; odontoid view

Sequelae of C-Spine Fractures
- see Neurosurgery, NS32
- acute phase of SCI
  - spinal shock: absence of all voluntary and reflex activity below level of injury
    - decreased reflexes, no sensation, flaccid paralysis below level of injury, lasting days to months
  - neurogenic shock: loss of vasomotor tone, SNS tone
    - watch for: hypotension (lacking SNS), bradycardia (unopposed PNS), poikilothermia (lacking SNS so no shunting of blood from extremities to core)
    - occurs within 30 min of SCI at level T6 or above, lasting up to 6 wk
    - provide airway support, fluids, atropine (for bradycardia), vasopressors for BP support
- chronic phase of SCI
  - autonomic dysreflexia: in patients with an SCI at level T6 or above
    - signs and symptoms: pounding headache, nasal congestion, feeling of apprehension or anxiety, visual changes, dangerously increased sBP and dBP
    - common triggers
      - GU causes: bladder distention, urinary tract infection, and kidney stones
      - GI causes: fecal impaction or bowel distension
    - treatment: monitoring and controlling BP, prior to addressing causative issue

Supine Oblique Views
- Rarely used
- Better visualization of posterior element fractures (lamina, pedicle, facet joint)
- Good to assess patency of neural foramina
- Can be used to visualize the C7-T1 junction

20% of C-spine fractures are accompanied by other spinal fractures, so ensure thoracic and lumbar spine x-rays are normal before proceeding to OR

Chest Trauma

- two types: those found and managed in 1° survey and those found and managed in 2° survey

Table 7. Life-Threatening Chest Injuries Found in 1° Survey

	Physical Exam	Investigations	Management
Airway Obstruction	Anxiety, stridor, hoarseness, altered mental status Apnea, cyanosis	Do not wait for ABG to intubate	Definitive airway management Intubate early Remove foreign body if visible with laryngoscope prior to intubation
Tension Pneumothorax Clinical diagnosis One-way valve causing accumulation of air in pleural space	Respiratory distress, tachycardia, distended neck veins, cyanosis, asymmetry of chest wall motion Tracheal deviation away from pneumothorax Percussion hyperresonance Unilateral absence of breath sounds	Non-radiographic diagnosis	Needle thoracostomy – large bore needle, 2nd ICS mid clavicular line, followed by chest tube in 5th ICS, anterior axillary line

Trauma to the chest accounts for 50% of trauma deaths

80% of all chest injuries can be managed non-surgically with simple measures such as intubation, chest tubes, and pain control

Table 7. Life-Threatening Chest Injuries Found in 1° Survey (continued)

	Physical Exam	Investigations	Management
Open Pneumothorax Air entering chest from wound rather than trachea	Gunshot or other wound (hole >2/3 tracheal diameter) ± exit wound Unequal breath sounds	ABG: decreased pO₂	Air-tight dressing sealed on 3 sides Chest tube Surgery
Massive Hemothorax >1,500 cc blood loss in chest cavity	Pallor, flat neck veins, shock Unilateral dullness Absent breath sounds, hypotension	Usually only able to do supine CXR – entire lung appears radioopaque as blood spreads out over posterior thoracic cavity	Restore blood volume Chest tube Thoracotomy if: >1,500 cc total blood loss ≥200 cc/h continued drainage
Flail Chest Free-floating segment of chest wall due to >2 rib fractures, each at 2 sites Underlying lung contusion (cause of morbidity and mortality)	Paradoxical movement of flail segment Palpable crepitus of ribs Decreased air entry on affected side	ABG: decreased pO₂, increased pCO₂ CXR: rib fractures, lung contusion	O₂ + fluid therapy + pain control Judicious fluid therapy in absence of systemic hypotension Positive pressure ventilation ± intubation and ventilation
Cardiac Tamponade Clinical diagnosis Pericardial fluid accumulation impairing ventricular function	Penetrating wound (usually) Beck's triad: hypotension, distended neck veins, muffled heart sounds Tachycardia, tachypnea Pulsus paradoxus Kussmaul's sign (increased JVP with inspiration)	Echocardiogram FAST	IV fluids Pericardiocentesis Open thoracotomy

Table 8. Potentially Life-Threatening Chest Injuries Found in 2° Survey

	Physical Exam	Investigations	Management
Pulmonary Contusion	Blunt trauma to chest Interstitial edema impairs compliance and gas exchange	CXR: areas of opacification of lung within 6 h of trauma	Maintain adequate ventilation Monitor with ABG, pulse oximeter, and ECG Chest physiotherapy Positive pressure ventilation if severe
Ruptured Diaphragm	Blunt trauma to chest or abdomen (e.g. high lap belt in MVC)	CXR: abnormality of diaphragm/lower lung fields/NG tube placement CT scan and endoscopy: sometimes helpful for diagnosis	Laparotomy for diaphragm repair and associated intra-abdominal injuries
Esophageal Injury	Usually penetrating trauma (pain out of proportion to degree of injury)	CXR: mediastinal air (not always) Esophagram (Gastrograffin®) Flexible esophagoscopy	Early repair (within 24 h) improves outcome but all require repair
Aortic Tear 90% tear at subclavian (near ligamentum arteriosum), most die at scene Salvageable if diagnosis made rapidly	Sudden high speed deceleration (e.g. MVC, fall, airplane crash), complaints of chest pain, dyspnea, hoarseness (frequently absent) Decreased femoral pulses, differential arm BP (arch tear)	CXR, CT scan, transesophageal echo, aortography (gold standard)	Thoracotomy (may treat other severe injuries first)
Blunt Myocardial Injury (rare)	Blunt trauma to chest (usually in setting of multi-system trauma and therefore difficult to diagnose) Physical exam: overlying injury, e.g. fractures, chest wall contusion	ECG: dysrhythmias, ST changes Patients with a normal ECG and normal hemodynamics never get dysrhythmias	O₂ Antidysrhythmic agents Analgesia

Other Potentially Life-Threatening Injuries Related to the Chest

Penetrating Neck Trauma
- includes all penetrating trauma to the three zones of the neck
- management: injuries deep to platysma require further evaluation by angiography, contrast CT, or surgery
- do not explore penetrating neck wounds except in the OR

3-way Seal for Open Pneumothorax (i.e. sucking chest wound)
Allows air to escape during the expiratory phase (so that you do not get a tension pneumothorax) but seals itself to allow adequate breaths during the inspiratory phase

Pulsus Paradoxus: a drop in BP of >10 mmHg with inspiration. Recall that BP normally drops with inspiration, but what's "paradoxical" about this is that it drops more than it should

Ruptured diaphragm is more often diagnosed on the left side, as liver conceals right side defect

Aortic Tear

ABC WHITE
X-ray features of **A**ortic tear
Depressed left mainstem **B**ronchus pleural **C**ap
Wide mediastinum (most consistent)
Hemothorax
Indistinct aortic knuckle
Tracheal deviation to right side
Esophagus (NG tube) deviated to right
(Note: present in 85% of cases, but cannot rule out)

Airway Injuries

- always maintain a high index of suspicion
- larynx
  - history: strangulation, direct blow, blunt trauma, any penetrating injury involving platysma
  - triad: hoarseness, subcutaneous emphysema, palpable fracture
  - other symptoms: hemoptysis, dyspnea, dysphonia
  - investigations: CXR, CT scan, arteriography (if penetrating)
  - management
    - airway: manage early because of edema
    - C-spine may also be injured, consider mechanism of injury
    - surgical: tracheotomy vs. repair
- trachea/bronchus
  - frequently missed
  - history: deceleration, penetration, increased intra-thoracic pressure, complaints of dyspnea, hemoptysis
  - examination: subcutaneous air, Hamman's sign (crunching sound synchronous with heart beat)
  - CXR: mediastinal air, persistent pneumothorax or persistent air leak after chest tube inserted for pneumothorax
  - management: surgical repair if >1/3 circumference

Abdominal Trauma

- two mechanisms
  - blunt: usually causes solid organ injury (spleen = most common, liver = 2nd)
  - penetrating: usually causes hollow organ injury or liver injury (most common)

BLUNT TRAUMA
- results in two types of hemorrhage: intra-abdominal and retroperitoneal
- adopt high clinical suspicion of bleeding in multi-system trauma

History
- mechanism of injury, SAMPLE history

Physical Exam
- often unreliable in multi-system trauma, wide spectrum of presentations
  - slow blood loss not immediately apparent
  - tachycardia, tachypnea, oliguria, febrile, hypotension
  - other injuries may mask symptoms
  - serial examinations are required
- abdomen
  - inspect: contusions, abrasions, seat-belt sign, distention
  - auscultate: bruits, bowel sounds
  - palpate: tenderness, rebound tenderness, rigidity, guarding
  - DRE: rectal tone, blood, bone fragments, prostate location
  - placement of NG, Foley catheter should be considered part of the abdominal exam
- other systems to assess: cardiovascular, respiratory (possibility of diaphragm rupture), genitourinary, pelvis, back/neurological

Investigations
- labs: CBC, electrolytes, coagulation, cross and type, glucose, Cr, CK, lipase, amylase, liver enzymes, ABG, blood EtOH, β-hCG, U/A, toxicology screen

If Penetrating Neck Trauma Present, DON'T:
- Clamp structures (can damage nerves)
- Probe
- Insert NG tube (leads to bleeding)
- Remove weapon/impaled object

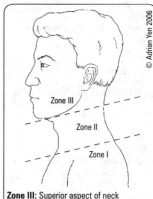

Zone III: Superior aspect of neck
Zone II: Midportion of neck (cricoid to the angle of mandible)
Zone I: Base of neck (thoracic inlet to cricoid cartilage)

Figure 6. Zones of the neck in trauma

Seatbelt Injuries May Cause
- Retroperitoneal duodenal trauma
- Intraperitoneal bowel transection
- Mesenteric injury
- L-spine injury

Indications for Foley and NG Tube in Abdominal Trauma
Foley catheter: unconscious or patient with multiple injuries who cannot void spontaneously
NG tube: used to decompress the stomach and proximal small bowel Contraindications: facial fractures or basal skull fractures suspected

Table 9. Imaging in Abdominal Trauma

Imaging	Strengths	Limitations
X-Ray	Chest (looking for free air under diaphragm, diaphragmatic hernia, air-fluid levels), pelvis, cervical, thoracic, lumbar spines	Soft tissue not well visualized
CT Scan	Most specific test	Radiation exposure 20x more than x-ray Cannot use if hemodynamic instability
Diagnostic Peritoneal Lavage (rarely used)	Most sensitive test Tests for intra-peritoneal bleed	Cannot test for retroperitoneal bleed or diaphragmatic rupture Cannot distinguish lethal from trivial bleed Results can take up to 1 h
Ultrasound: FAST	Identifies presence/absence of free fluid in peritoneal cavity RAPID exam: less than 5 min Can also examine pericardium and pleural cavities	NOT used to identify specific organ injuries If patient has ascites, FAST will be falsely positive

Criteria for Positive Lavage
- >10 cc gross blood
- Bile, bacteria, foreign material
- RBC count >100,000 x 10^6/L
- WBC >500 x 10^6/L,
- Amylase >175 IU

- imaging must be done if
  - equivocal abdominal examination, altered sensorium, or distracting injuries (e.g. head trauma, spinal cord injury resulting in abdominal anesthesia)
  - unexplained shock/hypotension
  - patients have multiple traumas and must undergo general anesthesia for orthopedic, neurosurgical, or other injuries
  - fractures of lower ribs, pelvis, spine
  - positive FAST

Laparotomy is Mandatory if Penetrating Trauma and:
- Shock
- Peritonitis
- Evisceration
- Free air in abdomen
- Blood in NG tube, Foley catheter, or on DRE

Management
- general: ABCs, fluid resuscitation, and stabilization
- surgical: watchful waiting vs. laparotomy
- solid organ injuries: decision based on hemodynamic stability, not the specific injuries
- hemodynamically unstable or persistently high transfusion requirements: laparotomy
- hollow organ injuries: laparotomy
- even if low suspicion of injury: admit and observe for 24 h

PENETRATING TRAUMA
- high risk of gastrointestinal perforation and sepsis
- history: size of blade, calibre/distance from gun, route of entry
- local wound exploration under direct vision may determine lack of peritoneal penetration (not reliable in inexperienced hands) with the following exceptions:
- thoracoabdominal region (may cause pneumothorax)
- back or flanks (muscles too thick)

"Rule of Thirds" for Stab Wounds
- 1/3 do not penetrate peritoneal cavity
- 1/3 penetrate but are harmless
- 1/3 cause injury requiring surgery

Management
- general: ABCs, fluid resuscitation, and stabilization
- gunshot wounds always require laparotomy

Genitourinary Tract Injuries

- see Urology, U32

Etiology
- blunt trauma: often associated with pelvic fractures
  - upper tract
    - renal
      - contusions (minor injury – parenchymal ecchymoses with intact renal capsule)
      - parenchymal tears/laceration: non-communicating (hematoma) vs. communicating (urine extravasation, hematuria)
    - ureter: rare, at uretero-pelvic junction
  - lower tract
    - bladder
      - extraperitoneal rupture of bladder from pelvic fracture fragments
      - intraperitoneal rupture of bladder from trauma and full bladder
    - urethra
      - posterior urethral injuries: MVCs, falls, pelvic fractures
      - anterior urethral injuries: blunt trauma to perineum, straddle injuries/direct strikes
  - external genitalia
- penetrating trauma
  - damage to: kidney, bladder, ureter (rare), external genitalia
- acceleration/deceleration injury
  - renal pedicle injury: high mortality rate (laceration and thrombosis of renal artery, renal vein, and their branches)
- iatrogenic
  - ureter and urethra (from instrumentation)

Gross hematuria suggests bladder injury

History
- mechanism of injury
- hematuria (microscopic or gross), blood on underwear
- dysuria, urinary retention
- history of hypotension

Physical Exam
- abdominal pain, flank pain, CVA tenderness, upper quadrant mass, perineal lacerations
- DRE: sphincter tone, position of prostate, presence of blood
- scrotum: ecchymoses, lacerations, testicular disruption, hematomas
- bimanual exam, speculum exam
- extraperitoneal bladder rupture: pelvic instability, suprapubic tenderness from mass of urine or extravasated blood
- intraperitoneal bladder rupture: acute abdomen
- urethral injury: perineal ecchymosis, scrotal hematoma, blood at penile meatus, high riding prostate, pelvic fractures

Investigations
- urethra: retrograde urethrography
- bladder: U/A, CT scan, urethrogram ± retrograde cystoscopy ± cystogram (distended bladder + post-void)
- ureter: retrograde ureterogram
- renal: CT scan (best, if hemodynamically stable), intravenous pyelogram

> In the case of gross hematuria, the GU system is investigated from distal to proximal (i.e. urethrogram, cystogram, etc.)

Management
- urology consult
- renal
  - minor injuries: conservative management
    - bedrest, hydration, analgesia, antibiotics
  - major injuries: admit
    - conservative management with frequent reassessments, serial U/A ± re-imaging
    - surgical repair (exploration, nephrectomy): hemodynamically unstable or continuing to bleed >48 h, major urine extravasation, renal pedicle injury, all penetrating wounds and major lacerations, infections, renal artery thrombosis
- ureter
  - ureterouretostomy
- bladder
  - extraperitoneal
    - minor rupture: Foley drainage x 10-14 d
    - major rupture: surgical repair
  - intraperitoneal
    - drain abdomen and surgical repair
- urethra
  - anterior: conservative, if cannot void, Foley or suprapubic cystostomy and antibiotics
  - posterior: suprapubic cystostomy (avoid catheterization) ± surgical repair

Orthopedic Injuries

- see Orthopedics (see *Shoulder* OR10, *Knee* OR31, *Wrist* OR20, *Ankle* OR27)

Goals of ED Treatment
- diagnose potentially life/limb threatening injuries
- reduce and immobilize fractures (cast/splint) as appropriate
- provide adequate pain relief
- arrange proper follow-up if necessary

History
- use SAMPLE
- mechanism of injury may be very important

> **Description of Fractures**
>
> **SOLARTAT**
> Site
> Open vs. closed
> Length
> Articular
> Rotation
> Translation
> Alignment/Angulation
> Type e.g. Salter-Harris, etc.

Physical Exam
- look (inspection): "SEADS" swelling, erythema, atrophy, deformity, and skin changes (e.g. bruises)
- feel (palpation): all joints/bones for local tenderness, swelling, warmth, crepitus, joint effusions, and subtle deformity
- move: joints affected plus those above and below injury – active ROM preferred to passive
- neurovascular status: distal to injury (before and after reduction)

LIFE- AND LIMB-THREATENING INJURIES

Table 10. Life- and Limb-Threatening Orthopedic Injuries

Life-Threatening Injuries (usually blood loss)	Limb-Threatening Injuries (usually interruption of blood supply)
Major pelvic fractures	Fracture/dislocation of ankle (talar AVN)
Traumatic amputations	Crush injuries
Massive long bone injuries and associated fat emboli syndrome	Compartment syndrome
	Open fractures
Vascular injury proximal to knee/elbow	Dislocations of knee/hip
	Fractures above knee/elbow

Open Fractures
- communication between fracture site and external surface of skin – increased risk of osteomyelitis
- remove gross debris, irrigate, cover with sterile dressing – formal irrigation and debridement often done in the OR
- control bleeding with pressure (no clamping)
- splint
- antibiotics (1st generation cephalosporin and aminoglycoside) and tetanus prophylaxis
- standard of care is to secure definitive surgical management within 6 h, time to surgery may vary from case-to-case

> **When Dealing with an Open Fracture, Remember "STAND"**
> Splint
> Tetanus prophylaxis
> Antibiotics
> Neurovascular status (before and after)
> Dressings (to cover wound)

Vascular injury/compartment syndrome is suggested by **"The 6 Ps"**
Pulse discrepancies
Pallor
Paresthesia/hypoesthesia
Paralysis
Pain (especially when refractory to usual analgesics)
Polar (cold)

Vascular Injuries
- realign limb/apply longitudinal traction and reassess pulses (e.g. Doppler probe)
- surgical consult
- direct pressure if external bleeding

Compartment Syndrome
- when the intracompartmental pressure within an anatomical area (e.g. forearm or lower leg) exceeds the capillary perfusion pressure, eventually leading to muscle/nerve necrosis
- clinical diagnosis: maintain a high index of suspicion
  - pain out of proportion to the injury
  - pain worse with passive stretch
  - tense compartment
  - look for "the 6 Ps" (note: radial pulse pressure is 120/80 mmHg while capillary perfusion pressure is 30 mmHg, seeing any of the 6ps indicates advanced compartment syndrome, therefore do not wait for these signs to diagnose and treat)
- requires prompt decompression: remove constrictive casts, dressings; emergent fasciotomy may be needed

UPPER EXTREMITY INJURIES
- anterior shoulder dislocation
  - axillary nerve (lateral aspect of shoulder) and musculocutaneous nerve (extensor aspect of forearm) at risk
  - seen on lateral view: humeral head anterior to glenoid
  - reduce (traction, scapular manipulation), immobilize in internal rotation, repeat x-ray, out-patient follow-up with orthopedics
  - with forceful injury, look for fracture
- Colles' fracture
  - distal radius fracture with dorsal displacement from "Fall on Outstretched Hand" (FOOSH)
  - AP film: shortening, radial deviation, radial displacement
  - lateral film: dorsal displacement, volar angulation
  - reduce, immobilize with splint, out-patient follow-up with orthopedics or immediate orthopedic referral if complicated fracture
  - if involvement of articular surface, emergent orthopedic referral
- scaphoid fracture
  - tenderness in anatomical snuff box, pain on scaphoid tubercle, pain on axial loading of thumb
  - negative x-ray: thumb spica splint, repeat x-ray in 1 wk ± CT scan/bone scan
  - positive x-ray: thumb spica splint x 6-8 wk, repeat x-ray in 2 wk
  - risk of AVN of scaphoid if not immobilized
  - outpatient orthopedics follow-up

LOWER EXTREMITY INJURIES
- ankle and foot fractures
  - see Ottawa Ankle and Foot Rules
- knee injuries
  - see Ottawa Knee Rules
- avulsion of the base of 5th metatarsal
  - occurs with inversion injury
  - supportive tensor or below knee walking cast for 3 wk
- calcaneal fracture
  - associated with fall from height
  - associated injuries may involve ankles, knees, hips, pelvis, lumbar spine

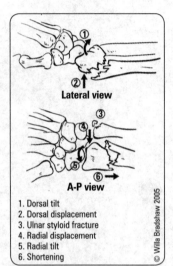

Lateral view

A-P view

1. Dorsal tilt
2. Dorsal displacement
3. Ulnar styloid fracture
4. Radial displacement
5. Radial tilt
6. Shortening

© Willa Bradshaw 2005

Figure 7. Colles' fracture

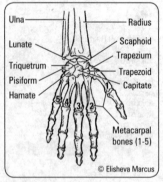

Ulna — Radius
Lunate — Scaphoid
— Trapezium
Triquetrum — Trapezoid
Pisiform — Capitate
Hamate
Metacarpal bones (1-5)

© Elisheva Marcus

Figure 8. Carpal bones

A knee x-ray examination is required only for acute injury patients with one or more of:
- Age 55 yr or older
- Tenderness at head of fibula
- Isolated tenderness of patella
- Inability to flex to 90°
- Inability to bear weight both immediately and in the ED (four steps)

Figure 9. Ottawa knee rules
Adapted from: Stiell IG, et al. *JAMA* 1997;278:2075-2079

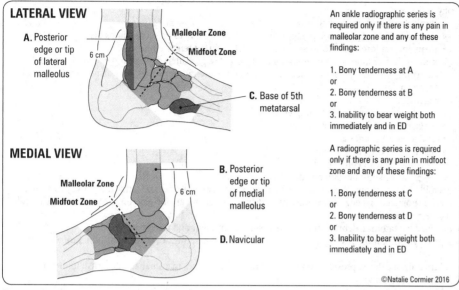

LATERAL VIEW

A. Posterior edge or tip of lateral malleolus

6 cm

Malleolar Zone

Midfoot Zone

C. Base of 5th metatarsal

MEDIAL VIEW

Malleolar Zone

Midfoot Zone

6 cm

B. Posterior edge or tip of medial malleolus

D. Navicular

An ankle radiographic series is required only if there is any pain in malleolar zone and any of these findings:

1. Bony tenderness at A
or
2. Bony tenderness at B
or
3. Inability to bear weight both immediately and in ED

A radiographic series is required only if there is any pain in midfoot zone and any of these findings:

1. Bony tenderness at C
or
2. Bony tenderness at D
or
3. Inability to bear weight both immediately and in ED

©Natalie Cormier 2016

Figure 10. Ottawa ankle and foot rules
Adapted from: Stiell IG, et al. *JAMA* 1994;271:827-832

Wound Management

Goals of ED Treatment
- identify injuries and stop any active bleeding – direct pressure
- manage pain
- wound examination and exploration (history and physical)
- cleansing ± antibiotic and tetanus prophylaxis
- closure and dressing

Tetanus Prophylaxis
- both tetanus toxoid (Td) and immunoglobulin (TIG) are safe in pregnancy

Table 11. Guidelines for Tetanus Prophylaxis for Wounds

	Clean, minor wounds		All other wounds*	
Vaccination History	Tdap or Td[†]	TIG	Tdap or Td[†]	TIG
Unknown or fewer than 3 doses	Yes	No	Yes	Yes
3 or more doses	No§	No	No¶	No

*Such as, but not limited to, wounds contaminated with dirt, feces, soil, and saliva; puncture wounds; avulsions; and wounds resulting from missiles, crushing, burns, and frostbite.
†Tdap is preferred to Td for adults who have never received Tdap. Single antigen tetanus toxoid (TT) is no longer available in the United States.
§Yes, if more than ten years since the last tetanus toxoid-containing vaccine dose.
¶Yes, if more than five years since the last tetanus toxoid-containing vaccine dose.
Source: *MMWR* 1991;40(No. RR-10):1-28.

Bruises
- non-palpable = ecchymosis
- palpable collection (not swelling) = hematoma following blunt trauma
- assess for coagulopathy (e.g. liver disease), anticoagulant use

Abrasions
- partial to full thickness break in skin
- management
  - clean thoroughly with brush to prevent foreign body impregnation ± local anesthetic antiseptic ointment (Polysporin® or Vaseline®) for 7 d for facial and complex abrasions
  - tetanus prophylaxis

Lacerations
- see Plastic Surgery, PL8
- consider every structure deep to a laceration injured until proven otherwise
- in hand injury patients, include the following in history: handedness, occupation, mechanism of injury, previous history of injury

Acute Treatment of Contusions

RICE
Rest
Ice
Compression
Elevation

High Risk Factors for Infection
Wound Factors
- Puncture wounds
- Crush injuries
- Wounds >12 h old
- Hand or foot wounds
- Immunocompromised

Patient Factors
- Age >50 yr
- Prosthetic joints or valves (risk of endocarditis)

Suture Use and Duration

Suture to:	Close with Nylon or Other Non-absorbable Suture	Approx. Duration (days)
Face	6-0	5
Not Joint	4-0	7
Joint	3-0	10
Scalp	4-0	7
Mucous Membrane	absorbable (vicryl)	N/A

N.B. Patients on steroid therapy may need sutures for longer periods of time

- physical exam
  - think about underlying anatomy
  - examine tendon function actively against resistance and neurovascular status distally
  - clean and explore under local anesthetic; look for partial tendon injuries
  - x-ray or U/S wounds if a foreign body is suspected (e.g. shattered glass) and not found when exploring wound (remember: not all foreign bodies are radioopaque), or if suspect intra-articular involvement
- management
  - disinfect skin/use sterile techniques
  - irrigate copiously with normal saline
  - analgesia ± anesthesia
  - maximum dose of lidocaine
    - 7 mg/kg with epinephrine
    - 5 mg/kg without epinephrine
- in children, topical anesthetics such as LET (lidocaine, epinephrine, and tetracaine), and in selected cases a short-acting benzodiazepine (midazolam or other agents) for sedation and amnesia are useful
- secure hemostasis
- evacuate hematomas, debride non-viable tissue, remove hair and foreign bodies
- ± prophylactic antibiotics (consider for animal/human bites, intra-oral lesion, or puncture wounds to the foot)
- suture unless: delayed presentation (>6-8 h), puncture wound, mammalian bite, crush injury, or retained foreign body
- take into account patient and wound factors when considering suturing
- advise patient when to have sutures removed
- cellulitis and necrotizing fasciitis (see Plastic Surgery, PL15)

Early wound irrigation and debridement are the most important factors in decreasing infection risk

Where **NOT** to use local anesthetic with epinephrine:
Ears, Nose, Fingers, Toes, and Penis

Alternatives to Sutures
- Tissue glue
- Steristrips®
- Staples

Approach to Common ED Presentations

Abdominal Pain

Table 12. Selected Differential Diagnosis of Abdominal Pain

	Emergent	Usually Less Emergent
GI	Perforated viscus, bowel obstruction, ischemic bowel, appendicitis, strangulated hernia, IBD flare, esophageal rupture, peptic ulcer disease	Diverticulitis, gastroenteritis, GERD, esophagitis, gastritis, IBS
Hepatobiliary	Hepatic/splenic injury, pancreatitis, cholangitis, spontaneous bacterial peritonitis	Biliary colic, cholecystitis, hepatitis
Genital	Female: Ovarian torsion, PID, ectopic pregnancy Male: Testicular torsion	Female: tubo-ovarian abscess, ovarian cyst, salpingitis, endometriosis Male: epididymitis, prostatitis
Urinary	Pyelonephritis	Renal colic, cystitis
CVS	MI, aortic dissection, AAA	Pericarditis
Respirology	PE, empyema	Pneumonia
Metabolic	DKA, sickle cell crisis, toxin, Addisonian crisis	Lead poisoning, porphyria
Other	Significant trauma, acute angle closure glaucoma	Abdominal wall injury, herpes zoster, psychiatric, abscess, hernia, mesenteric adenitis

Be vigilant: very young, elderly, alcoholics, immunosuppressed patients often present atypically
Old age, pregnancy (T3), and chronic corticosteroid use can blunt peritoneal findings, so have an increased level of suspicion for an intra-abdominal process in these individuals

Unstable patients should not be sent for imaging

- differential can be focused anatomically by location of pain: RUQ, LUQ, RLQ, LLQ, epigastric, periumbilical, diffuse

History
- pain: OPQRST
- review symptoms from GU, gynecological, GI, respiratory, and CV systems
- abdominal trauma/surgeries most recent colonoscopy

Physical Exam
- vitals, abdominal (including DRE, CVA tenderness), pelvic/genital, respiratory, and cardiac exams as indicated by history

Investigations
- ABCs, do not delay management and consultation if patient unstable
- CBC, electrolytes, glucose, BUN/Cr, U/A ± liver enzymes, LFTs, lipase, β-hCG, ECG, troponins, ± VBG/lactate
- AXR: look for calcifications, free air, gas pattern, air fluid levels
- CXR upright: look for pneumoperitoneum (free air under diaphragm), lung disease
- U/S: biliary tract, ectopic pregnancy, AAA, free fluid
- CT: trauma, AAA, pancreatitis, nephro-/urolithiasis, appendicitis, and diverticulitis

If elevated AST and ALT
Think hepatocellular injury
AST > ALT: alcohol-related
ALT > AST: viral, drug, toxin

If elevated ALP and GGT
Think biliary tree obstruction

Management
- NPO, IV, NG tube, analgesics, consider antibiotics and anti-emetics
- growing evidence that small amounts of opioid analgesics improve diagnostic accuracy of physical exam of surgical abdomen
- consult as necessary: general surgery, vascular surgery, gynecology, etc.

Disposition
- admission: surgical abdomen, workup of significant abnormal findings, need for IV antibiotics or pain control
- discharge: patients with a negative lab and imaging workup who improve clinically during their stay; instruct the patient to return if severe pain, fever, or persistent vomiting develops

Acute Pelvic Pain

Etiology
- gynecological
  - second most common gynecological complaint (after vaginal bleeding)
  - ovaries: ruptured ovarian cysts (most common cause of pelvic pain), ovarian abscess, ovarian torsion (rare, 50% will have ovarian mass)
  - fallopian tubes: salpingitis, tubal abscess, hydrosalpinx
  - uterus: leiomyomas (uterine fibroids) – especially with torsion of a pedunculated fibroid or in a pregnant patient (degeneration), PID, endometriosis
  - other: ectopic pregnancy (ruptured/expanding/leaking), spontaneous abortion (threatened or incomplete), endometriosis and dysmenorrhea, sexual or physical abuse
- non-gynecological (see causes of lower abdominal pain above)

History and Physical Exam
- pain: OPQRST
- associated symptoms: vaginal bleeding, discharge, dyspareunia, bowel or bladder symptoms
- pregnancy and sexual history
- vitals
- gynecological exam: assess for cervical motion tenderness/"chandelier sign" (suggests PID)
- abdominal exam

Investigations
- β-hCG for all women of childbearing age
- CBC and differential, electrolytes, glucose, Cr, BUN, G&S, PTT/INR
- vaginal and cervical swabs for C&S during physical exam
- pelvic and abdominal U/S: evaluate adnexa, thickness of endometrium, pregnancy, free fluid or masses in the pelvis
- Doppler flow studies for ovarian torsion

Management
- general: analgesia, determine if admission and consults are needed
- specific
  - ovarian cysts
    - unruptured or ruptured and hemodynamically stable: analgesia and follow-up
    - ruptured with significant hemoperitoneum: may require surgery
  - ovarian torsion: surgical detorsion or removal of ovary
  - uncomplicated leiomyomas, endometriosis, and secondary dysmenorrhea can usually be treated on an outpatient basis, discharge with gynecology follow-up
  - PID: requires broad spectrum antibiotics

Disposition
- referral: gynecological or obstetrical causes requiring surgical intervention, requiring admission, or oncological in nature
- admission: patients requiring surgery, IV antibiotics/pain management
- discharge: negative workup and resolving symptoms; give clear instructions for appropriate follow-up

Altered Level of Consciousness

Definitions
- altered mental status: collective, non-specific term referring to change in cognitive function, behaviour, or attentiveness, including:
  - delirium (see Psychiatry, PS19)
  - dementia (see Psychiatry, PS20)
  - lethargy: state of decreased awareness and alertness (patient may appear wakeful)
  - stupor: unresponsiveness but rousable
  - coma: a sleep-like state, not rousable to consciousness

Analgesia in Patients with Acute Abdominal Pain
Cochrane DB Syst Rev 2011;1:CD005660
Study: systematic review of all RCTs of adult patients with acute abdominal pain (AAP) comparing use of opioid analgesia during initial evaluation with placebo. Included in the review: 8 RCTs.
Population: patients age >14 with non traumatic AAP <1 week duration.
Intervention: six trials used morphine, one trial used Tramadol, one study Papaveretum as analgesia.
Main Outcome Measure: diagnostic accuracy.
Results: there were no significant differences in the physical examination among the groups or when comparing by drug. There were no significant differences in rate of 'incorrect diagnosis' among the groups.
Conclusion: the use of analgesia for acute abdominal pain does not increase risk of diagnostic error and does not mask clinical findings.

Gynecological Causes of Pelvic Pain
- Ovarian cyst
- Dysmenorrhea
- Mittelschmerz
- Endometriosis
- Ovarian torsion
- Uterine fibroids/neoplasm
- Adnexal neoplasm
- PID + cervicitis

U/S is the preferred imaging modality in the assessment of acute pelvic pain

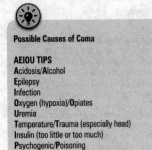

Possible Causes of Coma

AEIOU TIPS
Acidosis/Alcohol
Epilepsy
Infection
Oxygen (hypoxia)/Opiates
Uremia
Temperature/Trauma (especially head)
Insulin (too little or too much)
Psychogenic/Poisoning
Stroke

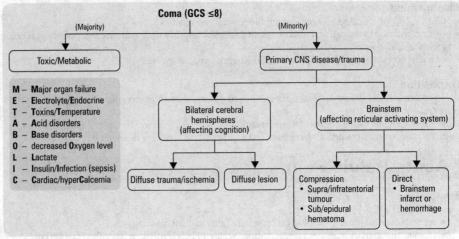

Figure 11. Etiology of coma

MANAGEMENT OF ALTERED LOC

In general, intubate if GCS <8; but ability to protect airway is primary consideration

History
- obtain collateral from family, friends, police, paramedics, old chart, MedicAlert® bracelet, etc.
- onset and progression
  - antecedent trauma, seizure activity, fever
  - abrupt onset suggests CNS hemorrhage/ischemia or cardiac cause
  - progression over hours to days suggests progressive CNS lesion or toxic/metabolic cause
- determine patient's baseline LOC
- past medical history (e.g. similar episode, depression, overdose)

Physical Exam
- ABCs, vitals including temperature; cardiac, respiratory, abdominal exams
- complete neurological exam; in particular, examination of the eyes ("PEARL" pupils equal and reactive to light)
  - use the GCS to evaluate LOC (see *Initial Patient Assessment/Management*, ER2)

Investigations
- blood work
  - rapid blood sugar, CBC, electrolytes, Cr, BUN, LFTs, glucose, serum osmolality, VBG, PT/PTT/INR, troponins
  - serum EtOH, acetaminophen, and salicylate levels
- imaging
  - CXR, CT head
- other tests
  - ECG, U/A, UTox

Diagnosis
- administer appropriate universal antidotes
  - thiamine 100 mg IV if history of EtOH or patient looks malnourished
  - one ampule D50W IV if low blood sugar on finger-prick
  - naloxone 0.4-2 mg IV or IM if opiate overdose suspected
- distinguish between structural and toxic-metabolic coma
  - structural coma
    - pupils, extraocular movements, and motor findings, if present, are usually asymmetric
    - look for focal or lateralizing abnormalities
  - toxic-metabolic coma
    - dysfunction at lower levels of the brainstem (e.g. caloric unresponsiveness)
    - respiratory depression in association with an intact upper brainstem (e.g. equal and reactive pupils; see exceptions in Table 13)
    - extraocular movements and motor findings are symmetric or absent
- essential to re-examine frequently because status can change rapidly
- diagnosis may become apparent only with the passage of time
  - delayed deficit after head trauma suggestive of epidural hematoma (characteristic "lucid interval")

Table 13. Toxic-Metabolic Causes of Fixed Pupils

Dilated	Dilated to Normal	Constricted
Anoxia Anticholinergic agents (e.g. atropine, TCAs) Methanol (rare) Cocaine Opioid withdrawal Amphetamines Hallucinogens	Hypothermia Barbiturates Antipsychotics	Cholinergic agents (e.g. organophosphates) Opiates (e.g. heroin), except meperidine

Disposition
- admission: if ongoing decreased LOC, admit to service based on tentative diagnosis, or transfer patient if appropriate level of care not available
- discharge: readily reversible alteration of LOC; ensure adequate follow-up care available

Chest Pain

Table 14. Differential Diagnosis for Chest Pain

	Emergent	Usually Less Emergent
CVS	MI, unstable angina, aortic dissection, cardiac tamponade, arrhythmia	Stable angina, pericarditis, myocarditis
Respirology	PE, pneumothorax	Pneumonia, pleural effusion, malignancy
GI	Esophageal rupture, pneumomediastinum	Peptic ulcer disease, esophagitis, GERD, esophageal spasm, pancreatitis, cholecystitis
MSK		Rib fracture, costochondritis
Other		Herpes zoster, psychiatric/panic attack

History and Physical Exam
- OPQRST, previous episodes and change in pattern
- cardiac risk factors (HTN, DM, dyslipidemia, smoking, FHx)
- vitals, cardiac, respiratory, peripheral vascular, abdominal exams

Investigations
- CBC, electrolytes, Cr, BUN, glucose, PTT/INR
- ECG: always compare with previous; may be normal in up to 50% of PE and acute MI
- CXR: compare with previous

Management and Disposition
- ABCs, O_2, cardiac monitors, IV access
- treat underlying cause and involve consultants as necessary
- consider further observation/monitoring if unclear diagnosis or risk of dysrhythmia
- discharge: patients with a low probability of life-threatening illness due to resolving symptoms and negative workup; arrange follow-up and instruct to return if SOB or increased chest pain develops

Life-Threatening Causes of Chest Pain

PET MAP
PE
Esophageal rupture
Tamponade
MI/angina
Aortic dissection
Pneumothorax

Imaging is necessary for all suspected aortic dissections, regardless of BP

Angina Characteristics
1. Retrosternal location
2. Provoked by exertion
3. Relieved by rest or nitroglycerin

Risk for CAD
3/3 = "typical angina" - high risk
2/3 = intermediate risk for women >50 yr, all men
1/3 = Intermediate risk in men >40 yr, women >60 yr

ACS more likely to be atypical in females, diabetics, and >80 yr. Anginal equivalents include dyspnea, diaphoresis, fatigue, non-retrosternal pain

Signs of PE on CXR
Westermark's sign: abrupt tapering of a vessel on chest film
Hampton's hump: a wedge-shaped infiltrate that abuts the pleura
Effusion, atelectasis, or infiltrates 50% normal

It is important to look for reciprocal changes in STEMI in order to differentiate from pericarditis (diffuse elevations)

Tracheal deviation is away from tension or towards non-tension pneumothorax

Addition of Clopidogrel to Aspirin® and Fibrinolytic Therapy for Myocardial Infarction with ST-Segment Elevation
NEJM 2005;352:1179-1191
Purpose: To assess the benefit of adding clopidogrel to Aspirin® and fibrinolytic therapy in ST-elevation MI.
Study Characteristics: Double-blind, RCT, following intention-to-treat analysis, with 3,491 patients and clinical follow-up at 30 d.
Participants: Individuals presenting within 12 h of onset of ST-elevation MI (mean age 57, 80.3% male, 50.3% smokers, 9.1% previous MI). Those presenting after 12 h, age >75, or with previous CABG, were excluded.
Intervention: Clopidogrel (300 mg loading dose followed by 75 mg OD until day of angiogram) or placebo, in addition to Aspirin®, a fibrinolytic agent, and heparin when appropriate.
Primary Outcome: Composite of occluded infarct-related artery on angiography (thrombosis in MI flow grade 0 or 1), or death or recurrent MI prior to angiography.
Results: Rates of primary end point were 21.7% in the placebo group and 15.0% in the clopidogrel group (95% CI 24-47%). Among the individual components of the primary end point, clopidogrel had a significant effect on the rate of an occluded infarct-related artery and the rate of recurrent MI, but no effect on the rate of death from any cause. At 30 d clinical follow-up, there was no difference in rate of death from cardiovascular causes, a significant reduction in the odds of recurrent MI, and a non-significant reduction in recurrent ischemia with need for urgent revascularization. The rates of major bleeding and intracranial hemorrhage were similar between the two groups.
Conclusion: Addition of clopidogrel improves the patency rate of infarct-related arteries and reduces ischemic complications, both of which are associated with improved long-term survival after MI. The trial was not powered to detect a survival benefit, and none was seen.

Table 15. Comparison of Chest Pain Diagnoses

	Classic History	Classic Findings	Diagnostic Investigations	Management and Disposition
Acute Coronary Syndrome	New or worsening pattern of retrosternal squeezing/pressure pain, radiation to arm/neck, dyspnea, worsened by exercise, relieved by rest N/V; syncope	New or worsened murmur, hypotension, diaphoresis, pulmonary edema	ECG: ischemia (15-lead if hypotensive, AV node involvement or inferior MI), serial troponin I (sensitive 6-8 h after onset), CK-MB, CXR	ABCs, aspirin, anticoagulation and emergent cardiology consult to consider percutaneous intervention or thrombolytic
Pulmonary Embolism	Pleuritic chest pain (75%), dyspnea; risk factors for venous thromboembolism	Tachycardia, hypoxemia; evidence of DVT	Wells' criteria: D-dimer, CT pulmonary angiogram*, V/Q scan; leg Doppler, CXR	ABCs, anticoagulation; consider airway management and thrombolysis if respiratory failure
Acute Pericarditis	Viral prodrome, anterior precordial pain, pleuritic, relieved by sitting up and leaning forward	Triphasic friction rub	ECG: sinus tachycardia, diffuse ST elevation, PR depression in II, III, avF and V4-6; reciprocal PR elevation and ST depression in aVR ±V1; echocardiography	ABCs, rule out MI, high dose NSAIDs +/- colchicine; consult if chronic/recurrent or non-viral cause (e.g. SLE, renal failure, requires surgery)
Pneumothorax	Trauma or spontaneous pleuritic chest pain often in tall, thin, young male athlete	Hemithorax with decreased/absent breath sounds, hyper-resonance; deviated trachea and hemodynamic compromise	Clinical diagnosis CXR: PA, lateral, expiratory views – lung edge, loss of lung markings, tracheal shift; deep sulcus sign on supine view	ABCs, if unstable, needle to 2nd ICS at MCL; urgent surgical consult / thoracostomy 4th ICS and chest tube
Aortic Dissection	Sudden severe tearing retrosternal or midscapular pain ± focal pain/neurologic loss in extremities in context of HTN	HTN; systolic BP difference >20 mmHg or pulse deficit between arms; aortic regurgitant murmur	CT angio; CXR - wide mediastinum, left pleural effusion, indistinct aortic knob, >4 mm separation of intimal calcification from aortic shadow, 20% normal	ABCs, reduce BP and HR; classify type A (ascending aorta, urgent surgery) vs. B (not ascending aorta, medical) on CT angio and urgent consult
Cardiac Tamponade	Dyspnea, cold extremities, ±chest pain; often a recent cardiac intervention or symptoms of malignancy, connective tissue disease	Beck's triad - hypotension, elevated JVP, muffled heart sounds; tachycardia, pulsus paradoxus >10 mmHg	Clinical diagnosis CXR: may show cardiomegaly, evidence of trauma	ABCs, cardiac surgery or cardiology consult, pericardiocentesis if unstable, treat underlying cause
Esophageal Rupture	Sudden onset severe pain after endoscopy, forceful vomiting, labour, or convulsion, or in context of corrosive injury or cancer	Subcutaneous emphysema, findings consistent with sepsis	CXR: pleural effusion (75%), pneumomediastinum; CT or water soluble contrast esophagogram	ABCs, early antibiotics, resuscitation, thoracics consult, NPO, consider chest tube
Esophagitis or GERD	Frequent heartburn, acid reflux, dysphagia, relief with antacids	Oral thrush or ulcers (rare)	None acutely	ABCs, PPI, avoid EtOH, tobacco, trigger foods
Herpes Zoster	Abnormal skin sensation – itching/tingling/pain – preceding rash by 1-5 d	None if early; maculopapular rash developing into vesicles and pustules that crust	Clinical diagnosis; direct immunofluorescence assay	ABCs, anti-virals, analgesia ±steroids, dressing; r/o ocular involvement/refer if necessary
MSK	History of injury	Reproduction of symptoms with movement or palpation (not specific – present in 25% of MI)	MSK injury or fracture on X-rays	ABCs, NSAIDs, rest, orthopedics consultation for fractures
Anxiety	Symptoms of anxiety, depression, history of psychiatric disorder; may coexist with physical disease	Tachycardia, diaphoresis, tremor	Diagnosis of exclusion	ABCs, arrange social supports, rule out suicidality and consider psychiatry consult

Table 16. Common Life-Threatening ECG Changes

Pathology	ECG Findings
Dysrhythmia	
a) Torsades de pointes	Ventricular complexes in upward-pointing and downward-pointing continuum (250-350 bpm)
b) Ventricular tachycardia	6 or more consecutive premature ventricular beats (150-250 bpm)
c) Ventricular flutter	Smooth sine wave pattern of similar amplitude (250-350 bpm)
d) Ventricular fibrillation	Erratic ECG tracing, no identifiable waves
Conduction	
a) 2nd degree heart block (Mobitz Type II)	PR interval stable, some QRSs dropped
	Total AV dissociation, but stable P-P and R-R intervals
b) 3rd degree heart block	Prolonged QRS complex (>0.12 s)
	RSR' in V5 or V6
	Monophasic I and V6
c) Left bundle branch block	May see ST elevation
	Difficult to interpret, new LBBB is considered STEMI equivalent
Ischemia	
a) STEMI	ST elevation in leads associated with injured area of heart and reciprocal lead changes (depression)
Metabolic	
a) Hyperkalemia	Tall T waves
b) Hypokalemia	P wave flattening
	QRS complex widening and flattening
	U waves appear
	Flattened T waves
Digitalis Toxicity	Gradual downward curve of ST
	At risk for AV blocks and ventricular irritability
Syndromes	
a) Brugada	RBBB with ST elevation in V1, V2, and V3
	Susceptible to deadly dysrhythmias, including VFib
b) Wellens	Marked T wave inversion in V2 and V3
	Left anterior descending coronary stenosis
c) Long QT syndrome	QT interval longer than ½ of cardiac cycle
	Predisposed to ventricular dysrhythmias

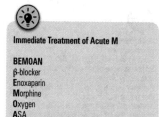

Immediate Treatment of Acute M

BEMOAN
β-blocker
Enoxaparin
Morphine
Oxygen
ASA
Nitroglycerin

Headache

- see Neurology, N44

Etiology
- **the common**
  - common migraine (without aura)/classic migraine (with aura)
    - common: unilateral, throbbing, aggravated by activity, moderate/severe, N/V, photo-/phonophobia
    - classic: varied aura symptoms, e.g. flashing lights, pins and needles (paresthesia), loss of vision, dysarthria
    - abortive treatment: fluids, NSAIDs, antiemetics, antiepileptic drugs, vasoactive medications
    - family doctor to consider prophylactic treatment
  - tension/muscular headache
    - mild-moderate headache with gradual onset lasting minutes to days
    - bilateral-frontal or nuchal-occipital
    - increased with stress, sleep deprivation
    - treatment: modify stressor(s), local measures, NSAIDs, tricyclic antidepressants
- **the deadly**
  - subarachnoid hemorrhage (SAH) (see Neurosurgery, NS17)
    - sudden onset, "worst headache of life" maximum intensity within minutes
    - increased pain with exertion, N/V, meningeal signs
    - diagnosis
      - new generation CT 100% sensitive within 6h of onset (hyperattentuating signal around Circle of Willis)
      - LP if suspected SAH and normal CT after 6h
    - management: urgent neurosurgery consult
  - increased ICP
    - worse in morning, when supine or bending down, with cough or valsalva
    - physical exam: neurological deficits, cranial nerve palsies, papilledema
    - diagnosis: CT head
    - management: consult neurosurgery

Common Therapeutic Approach to Severe Migraine
- 1L bolus of NS
- prochlorperazine 10 mg IV
- diphenhydramine 25 mg IV
- ketorolac 30 mg IV
- dexamethasone 10 mg IV
- Other options include haloperidol, metoclopramide, ergotamine, sumatriptan, analgesics

Ottawa SAH Rule
JAMA 2013;310(12): 1248-1255
- Use for alert patients older than 15 yr with new severe non-traumatic headache reaching maximum intensity within 1 h
- Not for patients with new neurologic deficits, previous aneurysms, SAH, brain tumours, or history of recurrent headaches (≥3 episodes over the course of ≥6 mo)
- Investigate if ≥1 high-risk variables present:
- Age ≥40 yr
- Neck pain or stiffness
- Witnessed loss of consciousness
- Onset during exertion
- Thunderclap headache (instantly peaking pain)
- Limited neck flexion on examination
Subarachnoid hemorrhage can be predicted with 100% sensitivity using this rule.

Meningitis
- Do not delay IV antibiotics for LP
- Deliver first dose of dexamethasone with or before first dose of antibiotic therapy

Which Patients can Safely Undergo Lumbar Puncture Without Screening CT?
Arch Intern Med 1999;159(22):2681-2685
Study: a prospective study to identify patients who can safely undergo LP without CT.
Population: 113 patients, age >18 yr, needing urgent LP as determined by ED physician.
Intervention: all patients were examined before CT by staff physicians. Physician examiners involved in the study then recorded the presence or absence of 10 clinical findings and answered 8 questions regarding the patient's past medical history and recorded their perceived likelihood that LP would be contraindicated.
Main Outcome Measure: results of non-contrast CTs interpreted by staff radiologist.
Results: 2.7% of patients had lesions on CT that contra-indicated LP. Overall, clinical impression had the highest predictive value in identifying patients with contraindications to LP (+LR 18.8). When used in aggregate- altered mentation, focal neurological examination and papilledema were three statistically significant identified predictors of new intracranial lesions(-LR 0). When used alone these predictors were inadequate.
Conclusion: given the low prevalence of lesions that contraindicate LP, screening CT solely to establish the safety of LP provides minimal extra information. Physicians can rely on their clinical judgement and the three predictors.

Parenteral Dexamethasone for Preventing Recurrence of Acute Severe Migraine Headache
BMJ 2008;336(7657):1359
A meta-analysis of 7 RCTs examined the effectiveness of parenteral corticosteroids use after administration of standard abortive therapy. The primary outcome was recurrence of migraine within 72 hours of treatment. All trials compared single dose parenteral dexamethasone with placebo. Results showed dexamethasone and placebo provided similar acute pain reduction (weighted mean difference 0.37, 95 CI -0.2, 0.94). Dexamethasone was, however, more effective than placebo in reducing recurrence rates (RR 0.74, 95 CI 0.6-0.9). Conclusion: when added to standard abortive therapy for migraine headaches, single dose of parenteral dexamethasone is associated with 26% RRR in recurrent headaches (NNT=9).

CT Head within 6 h is 100% Sensitive for Diagnosis of Subarachnoid Hemorrhage (SAH)
BMJ 2012;343(d4277)
Study: a prospective multicentre cohort study was conducted in 11 tertiary care emergency departments across Canada to measure the sensitivity of CT head in the evaluation of ED patients for SAH.
Population: neurologically intact adults who presented with new onset non-traumatic headache reaching maximum intensity in less than one hour who had head CT as part of their diagnostic workup to rule out SAH.
Design: patients were deemed positive for SAH if there was subarachnoid blood on CT, xanthochromia in the CSF or red blood cells in the final tube of CSF collected. Some patients with normal results on CT received LPs at the discretion of the treating physician. Unless patients had a negative result on LP or a definitive cause for the headache identified through neuroimaging patients were followed for six months to ascertain their outcome.
Main Outcome Measure: Results of CT interpreted by staff radiologist.
Results: Overall sensitivity of CT for detecting subarachnoid hemorrhage was 92.9%, specificity 100%. Subgroup analysis revealed 100% sensitivity for patients scanned within 6 h of headache onset.
Conclusion: CT is extremely sensitive in identifying subarachnoid hemorrhage when it is carried out within 6 h of headache

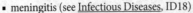

- meningitis (see Infectious Diseases, ID18)
    - flu-like symptoms (fever, N/V, malaise), meningeal signs, petechial rash
    - altered LOC and confusion
    - rule out increased ICP; if CT head or normal mental status, no neurological signs and no papilledema, then do LP for diagnosis
    - treatment: early empiric antibiotics ± acyclovir, steroid therapy
- temporal arteritis (causes significant morbidity, blindness) (see Ophthalmology, OP35)
    - vasculitis of large and mid-sized arteries, gender 3:1 F:M, most commonly age >70 yr
    - headache, scalp tenderness, jaw claudication, arthralgia, myalgia, fever, malaise or weight loss
    - temporal artery tender on palpation, relative afferent pupillary defect (RAPD), optic disc edema on fundoscopy
    - labs: elevated ESR, CRP
    - temporal artery biopsy is gold standard for diagnosis
    - associated with polymyalgia rheumatica
    - treatment: high-dose steroids immediately if suspected, no need to hold treatment until pathology results

Disposition
- admission: if underlying diagnosis is critical or emergent, if there are abnormal neurological findings, if patient is elderly or immunocompromised (atypical presentation), or if pain is refractory to oral medications
- discharge: assess for risk of narcotic misuse; most patients can be discharged with appropriate analgesia and follow-up with their family physician; instruct patients to return for fever, vomiting, neurologic changes, or increasing pain

Joint and Back Pain

JOINT PAIN (see Rheumatology, RH3)
- rule out life threatening causes: septic joint (see Orthopedics, OR10)

History and Physical Exam
- associated symptoms: fever, constitutional symptoms, skin lesions, conjunctivitis, urethritis
- patterns of joint involvement: polyarticular vs. monoarticular, symmetric vs. asymmetric
- inflammatory symptoms: prolonged morning stiffness, stiffness and pain ease through the day, mid-day fatigue, soft tissue swelling
- non-inflammatory symptoms: stiffness short lived after inactivity, short duration stiffness in the morning, pain increases with activity
- assess ROM, presence of joint effusion, warmth
- assess for localized joint pain, erythema, warmth, swelling with pain on active ROM, inability to bear weight, fever; may indicate presence of septic joint

Investigations
- blood work: CBC, ESR, CRP, WBC, INR/PTT, blood cultures, urate
- joint x-ray ± contralateral joint for comparison
- bedside U/S to identify effusion
- test joint aspirate for: WBC, protein, glucose, Gram stain, crystals

Management
- septic joint: IV antibiotics ± joint decompression and drainage
    - antibiotics can be started empirically if septic arthritis cannot be ruled out
- crystalline synovitis: NSAIDs at high dose, colchicine within first 24 h, corticosteroids
    - do not use allopurinol, as it may worsen acute attack
- acute polyarthritis: NSAIDs, analgesics (acetaminophen ± opioids), local or systemic corticosteroids
- osteoarthritis: NSAIDs, acetaminophen
- soft tissue pain: allow healing with enforced rest ± immobilization
    - non-pharmacologic treatment: local heat or cold, electrical stimulation, massage
    - pharmacologic: oral analgesics, NSAIDs, muscle relaxants, corticosteroid injections, topical agents

BACK PAIN (see Family Medicine, FM38)
- rule out vascular emergencies: aortic dissection, AAA, PE, MI, retroperitoneal bleed
- rule out spinal emergencies using red flags (see sidebar): osteomyelitis, cauda equina, epidural abscess or hematoma
- evaluate risk for fracture (osteoporosis, age), infection (IV drug user, recent spinal intervention, immunosuppression), cancer, vascular causes (cardiac risk factors)
- typical benign back pain is moderate, dull, aching, worse with movement or cough
- palpate spine for bony tenderness; precordial, respiratory, abdominal and neurological exams guided by history
- reserve imaging for suspicion of emergencies, metastases, and patients at high risk of fracture, infection, cancer, or vascular causes

Management
- treat underlying cause
- lumbosacral strain and disc herniation: analgesia and continue daily activities as much as tolerated; discuss red flags and organize follow-up
- spinal infection: early IV antibiotics and ID consultation
- cauda equina: dexamethasone, early neurosurgical consultation

Hospitalization is required for joint pain in the presence of
- Significant, concomitant internal organ involvement
- Signs of bacteremia, including vesiculopustular skin lesions, Roth spots, shaking chills, or splinter hemorrhages
- Systemic vasculitis
- Severe pain
- Severe constitutional symptoms
- Purulent synovial fluid in one or more joints
- Immunosuppression

Seizures

- see Neurology, N18

Definition
- paroxysmal alteration of behaviour and/or EEG changes resulting from abnormal, excessive activity of neurons
- status epilepticus: continuous or intermittent seizure activity for greater than 5 min without regaining consciousness (life threatening)

Categories
- generalized seizure (consciousness always lost): tonic/clonic, absence, myoclonic, atonic
- partial seizure (focal): simple partial, complex partial
- causes: primary seizure disorder, structural (trauma, intracranial hemorrhage, infection, increased ICP), metabolic disturbance (hypo-/hyperglycemia, hypo-/hypernatremia, hypocalcemia, hypomagnesemia, toxins/drugs)
- differential diagnosis: syncope, pseudoseizures, migraines, movement disorders, narcolepsy/cataplexy, myoclonus

Red Flags for Back Pain
Bowel or bladder dysfunction
Anesthesia (saddle)
Constitutional symptoms
K - Chronic disease, Constant pain
Paresthesia
Age >50 and mild trauma
IV drug use/infection
Neuromotor deficits

History
- from patient and bystander: flaccid and unconscious, often with deep rapid breathing
- preceding aura, rapid onset, loss of bladder/bowel control, tongue-biting (sides of the tongue)
- length of seizure and post-ictal symptoms

Physical Exam
- injuries to head and spine and bony prominences (e.g. elbows), tongue laceration, aspiration, urinary incontinence

Table 17. Concurrent Investigation and Management of Status Epilepticus

Timing	Steps

Immediate	Protect airway with positioning; intubate if airway compromised or elevated ICP
	Monitor: vital signs, ECG, oximetry; bedside blood glucose
	Establish IV access
	   Benzodiazepine - IV lorazepam 0.1 mg/kg up to 4 mg/dose at 2 mg/min preferred over IV diazepam 0.15 mg/kg up to 10 mg/dose at 5 mg/min; repeat at 5 min if ineffective
	   Fluid resuscitation
	   Give 50 mL 50% glucose (preceded by thiamine 100 mg IM in adults)
	Obtain blood samples for glucose, CBC, electrolytes, Ca²⁺, Mg²⁺, toxins, and antiepileptic drug levels; consider prolactin, β-hCG
	Vasopressor support if sBP <90 or MAP <70 mmHg

Urgent	Establish second IV line, urinary catheter If status persists, phenytoin 20 mg/kg IV at 25-50 mg/min in adults; may give additional 10 mg/kg IV 10 minutes after loading infusion If seizure resolves, antiepileptic drug still required to prevent recurrence EEG monitoring to evaluate for non-convulsive status epilepticus

Refractory	If status persists after maximum doses above, consult ICU and start one or more of:
	   Phenobarbital 20 mg/kg IV at 50 mg/min
	   Midazolam 0.2 mg/kg IV loading dose and 0.05-0.5 mg/kg/h
	   Propofol 2-5 mg/kg IV loading dose then 2-10 mg/kg/h

Post-Seizure	Investigate underlying cause: consider CT, LP, MRI, intracranial pressure monitoring

Note: All interventions should be done as soon as possible
Adapted from Brophy et al. Guidelines for the Evaluation and Management of Status Epilepticus. *Neurocrit Care* 2012;17:3-23

Minimum Workup in an Adult with 1st Time Seizure
CBC and differential
Electrolytes including Ca²⁺, Mg²⁺, PO₄³⁻
Head CT

If administering phenytoin, patient must be on a cardiac monitor as dysrhythmias and/or hypotension may occur

If IV access is not feasible, midazolam 0.2 mg/kg IM up to 10 mg can be used for initial control of seizure in adults

Disposition
- decision to admit or discharge should be based on the underlying disease process identified
  - if a patient has returned to baseline function and is neurologically intact, then consider discharge with outpatient follow-up
- first-time seizure patients being discharged should be referred to a neurologist for follow-up
- admitted patients should generally have a neurology consult
- patient should not drive until medically cleared (local regulations vary)
  - complete notification form to appropriate authority regarding ability to drive
- warn regarding other safety concerns (e.g. no swimming, bathing children alone, etc.)

Shortness of Breath

- see Respirology, R3 and Cardiology and Cardiac Surgery, C5

Table 18. Differential Diagnosis for Dyspnea

	High Mortality/Morbidity	Usually Less Emergent
Respiratory	Airway obstruction (Foreign body, epiglottitis, abscess, anaphylaxis) Pneumo/hemothorax Gas exchange –Pulmonary edema, PE, pneumonia, AECOPD	Chronic obstructive, interstitial or restrictive lung disease Pleural effusion
Cardiac	CHF, MI, valvular disease, tamponade, arrhythmia	Chronic CHF, Angina
Metabolic	Metabolic acidosis NYD, carbon monoxide inhalation	Anemia, Hemoglobinopathy
Neuromuscular	Myasthenia gravis, diaphragmatic paralysis	CNS lesion, primary muscle weakness
Other		Anxiety, deconditioning

History and Physical Exam
- acute SOB is often due to a relatively limited number of conditions; associated symptoms and signs are key to the appropriate diagnosis
  - substernal chest pain with cardiac ischemia
  - fever, cough, and sputum with respiratory infections
  - urticaria with anaphylaxis
  - wheezing with acute bronchospasm
  - environmental or occupational exposures
- dyspnea may be the sole complaint and the physical exam may reveal few abnormalities (e.g. PE, pneumothorax)
- vitals including pulse oximetry
  - wheeze and stridor (airway) vs. crackles (parenchymal), JVP, and murmurs

Investigations
- blood work
  - CBC and differential (hematocrit to exclude anemia), electrolytes, consider VBG
  - serial cardiac enzymes and ECG if considering cardiac source
  - Wells scores to consider appropriateness of d-dimer
- imaging
  - CXR (hyperinflation and bullous disease suggestive of obstructive lung disease, or changes in interstitial markings consistent with inflammation, infection, or interstitial fluid)
  - CT chest usually is not indicated in the initial evaluation of patients with dyspnea, but can be valuable in patients with interstitial lung disease, occult emphysema, or chronic thromboembolic disease (i.e. PE)

Management of Life-Threatening Dyspnea NYD
- see *Primary and Secondary Surveys*, ER2-3
- treat underlying cause

Disposition
- the history and physical exam lead to accurate diagnoses in patients with dyspnea in approximately two-thirds of cases; the decision to admit or discharge should be based on the underlying disease process identified
  - consider intubation in CO_2 retainers (e.g. COPD)
- if discharging, organize follow-up and educate regarding signs to return to hospital

Syncope

5 Types of Syncope
- Vasomotor
- Cardiac
- CNS
- Metabolic
- Psychogenic

Definition
- sudden, transient loss of consciousness and postural tone with spontaneous recovery
- usually caused by generalized cerebral or reticular activating system hypoperfusion

Etiology
- cardiogenic: dysrhythmia, outflow obstruction (e.g. PE, pulmonary HTN), MI, valvular disease
- non-cardiogenic: peripheral vascular (hypovolemia), vasovagal, cerebrovascular disorders, CNS, metabolic disturbances (e.g. EtOH intoxication)

History
- gather details from witnesses, and clarify patient's experience (e.g. dizziness, ataxia, or true syncope)
  - two key historical features: prodrome and situation
- distinguish between syncope and seizure (see Neurology, N19)
  - some patients may have myoclonic jerks with syncope – NOT a seizure
    - signs and symptoms during presyncope, syncope, and postsyncope
    - past medical history, drugs
    - think anatomically in differential; pump (heart), blood, vessels, brain
- syncope is cardiogenic until proven otherwise if
  - there is sudden loss of consciousness with no warning or prodrome
  - syncope is accompanied by chest pain

Physical Exam
- postural BP and HR
- cardiovascular, respiratory, and neurological exam
- examine for signs of trauma caused by syncopal episode

Investigations
- ECG (tachycardia, bradycardia, blocks, Wolff-Parkinson White, long QT interval, Brugada Syndrome, RV strain), bedside glucose
- blood work: CBC, electrolytes, BUN/Cr, ABGs, troponin, Ca^{2+}, Mg^{2+}, β-hCG, D-dimer
- consider toxicology screen

Management
- ABCs, IV, O_2, monitor
- cardiogenic syncope: admit to medicine/cardiology
- low risk syncope: discharge with follow-up as indicated by cause (non-cardiogenic syncope may still be admitted)

Disposition
- decision to admit is based on etiology
- most patients will be discharged
- on discharge, instruct patient to follow up with family physician
  - educate about avoiding orthostatic or situational syncope
  - evaluate the patient for fitness to drive or work
  - patients with recurrent syncope should avoid high-risk activities (e.g. driving)

Causes of Syncope by System

HEAD, HEART, VeSSELS
Hypoxia/Hypoglycemia
Epilepsy
Anxiety
Dysfunctional brainstem
Heart attack
Embolism (PE)
Aortic obstruction
Rhythm disturbance
Tachycardia
Vasovagal
Situational
Subclavian steal
ENT (glossopharyngeal neuralgia)
Low systemic vascular resistance
Sensitive carotid sinus

San Francisco Syncope Rule: High risk of adverse outcomes in syncope patients if:

CHESS
CHF: Hx of CHF
Hct: Low
ECG: Abnormal
SOB: Hx of dyspnea
SBP: sBP <90 at triage

Sexual Assault

Epidemiology
- 1 in 4 women and 1 in 10 men will be sexually assaulted in their lifetime; only 7% are reported

General Approach
- ABCs, treat acute, serious injuries; physician priority is to treat medical issues and provide clearance
- ensure patient is not left alone and provide ongoing emotional support
- obtain consent for medical exam and treatment, collection of evidence, disclosure to police (notify police as soon as consent obtained)
- Sexual Assault Kit (document injuries, collect evidence) if <72 h since assault
- label samples immediately and pass directly to police
- offer community crisis resources (e.g. shelter, hotline)
- do not report unless victim requests or if <16 yr old (legally required)

History
- ensure privacy for the patient – others should be asked to leave
- questions to ask: who, when, where did penetration occur, what happened, any weapons, or physical assault?
- post-assault activities (urination, defecation, change of clothes, shower, douche, etc.)
- gynecologic history
  - gravidity, parity, last menstrual period
  - contraception use
  - last voluntary intercourse (sperm motile 6-12 h in vagina, 5 d in cervix)
- medical history: acute injury/illness, chronic diseases, psychiatric history, medications, allergies, etc.

Physical Exam
- never re-traumatize a patient with the examination
- general examination
  - mental status
  - sexual maturity
  - patient should remove clothes and place in paper bag
  - document abrasions, bruises, lacerations, torn frenulum/broken teeth (indicates oral penetration)

Interprofessional teams are key; many centres or regions have sexual assault teams who specialize in the assessment and treatment of sexual assault victims, leaving emergency physicians responsible only for significant injuries and medical clearance

- pelvic exam and specimen collection
  - ideally before urination or defecation
  - examine for seminal stains, hymen, signs of trauma
  - collect moistened swabs of dried seminal stains
  - pubic hair combings and cuttings
  - speculum exam
    - lubricate with water only
    - vaginal lacerations, foreign bodies
    - Pap smear, oral/cervical/rectal culture for gonorrhea and chlamydia
    - posterior fornix secretions if present or aspiration of saline irrigation
    - immediate wet smear for motile sperm
    - air-dried slides for immotile sperm, acid phosphatase, ABO group
- fingernail scrapings and saliva sample from victim

Investigations
- VDRL: repeat in 3 mo if negative
- serum β-hCG
- blood for ABO group, Rh type, baseline serology (e.g. hepatitis, HIV)

Management
- involve local/regional sexual assault team
- medical
  - suture lacerations, tetanus prophylaxis
  - gynecology consult for foreign body, complex lacerations
  - assumed positive for gonorrhea and chlamydia
    - management: azithromycin 1 g PO x 1 dose (alt: doxycycline 100 mg PO bid x 7 d) and cefixime 800 mg PO x 1 dose (alt: ceftriaxone 250 mg IM x 1 dose)
  - may start prophylaxis for hepatitis B and HIV
  - pre and post counselling for HIV testing
  - pregnancy prophylaxis offered
    - levonorgestrel 0.75 mg PO STAT, repeat within 12 h (Plan B*)
- psychological
  - high incidence of psychological sequelae
  - have victim change and shower after exam completed

Disposition
- discharge if injuries/social situation permit
- follow-up with physician in rape crisis centre within 24 h
- best if patient does not leave ED alone

DOMESTIC VIOLENCE
- women are usually the victims, but male victimization also occurs
- identify the problem (need high index of suspicion)
  - suggestive injuries (bruises, sprains, abrasions, occasionally fractures, burns, or other injuries; often inconsistent with history provided)
  - somatic symptoms (chronic and vague complaints)
  - psychosocial symptoms
  - clinician impression (your 'gut feeling', e.g. overbearing partner that won't leave patient's side)
- if disclosed, be supportive and assess danger
- patient must consent to follow-up investigation/reporting (unless for children)

Management
- treat injuries and document findings
- ask about sexual assault and children at home (encourage notification of police)
- safety plan with good follow-up with family doctor/social worker

Medical Emergencies

Anaphylaxis and Allergic Reactions

Etiology
- anaphylaxis is an exaggerated immune mediated hypersensitivity reaction that leads to systemic histamine release, increased vascular permeability, and vasodilation; regardless of the etiology, the presentation and management of anaphylactic reactions are the same
- allergic (re-exposure to allergen)
- non-allergic (e.g. exercise induced)

Risk of Sexually Transmitted Disease after Sexual Assault
- Gonorrhea: 6-18%
- Chlamydia: 4-17%
- Syphilis: 0.5-3%
- HIV: <1%

How do you get a patient who is accompanied by her partner alone without arousing suspicion?
Order an x-ray

Most Common Triggers for Anaphylaxis
- Foods (nuts, shellfish, etc.)
- Stings
- Drugs (penicillin, NSAIDs, ACEI)
- Radiographic contrast media
- Blood products
- Latex

Diagnostic Criteria

- anaphylaxis is highly likely with any of
  1. acute onset of an illness (min to hrs) with involvement of the skin, mucosal tissue and at least one of
     - respiratory compromise (e.g. dyspnea, wheeze, stridor, hypoxemia)
     - hypotension/end-organ dysfunction (e.g. hypotonia, collapse, syncope, incontinence)
  2. two or more of the following after exposure to a LIKELY allergen for that patient (min to hrs)
     - involvement of the skin-mucosal tissue
     - respiratory compromise
     - hypotension or associated symptoms
     - persistent gastrointestinal symptoms (e.g. crampy abdominal pain, vomiting)
  3. hypotension after exposure to a KNOWN allergen for that patient (min to hrs)
     - management is also appropriate in cases which do not fulfill criteria, but who have had previous episodes of anaphylaxis
     - life-threatening differentials for anaphylaxis include asthma and septic shock
     - angioedema may mimic anaphylaxis but tends not to improve with standard anaphylaxis treatment

Anaphylaxis should be suspected if airway, breathing, or especially circulation compromise is present after exposure to a known allergen

Hypotension is defined as systolic BP >30% decrease from baseline or
- Adults: <90 mmHg
- ≥11 yr: <90 mmHg
- 1-10 yr: <70 mmHg + 2 x age
- 1 mo-1 yr: <70 mmHg

Management

- moderate reaction: generalized urticaria, angioedema, wheezing, tachycardia
  - epinephrine (1:1000) 0.3-0.5 mg IM
  - antihistamines: diphenhydramine (Benadryl®) 25-50 mg IM
  - salbutamol (Ventolin®) 1 cc via MDI
- severe reaction/evolution: severe wheezing, laryngeal/pulmonary edema, shock
  - –ABCs, may need ETT due to airway edema
  - epinephrine (1:1000) 0.1-0.3 mg IV (or via ETT if no IV access) to start, repeat as needed
  - antihistamines: diphenhydramine (Benadryl®) 50 mg IV (~1 mg/kg)
  - steroids: hydrocortisone (Solucortef®) 100 mg IV (~1.5 mg/kg) or methylprednisolone (Solumedrol®) 1 mg/kg IV q6h x 24 h
  - large volumes of crystalloid may be required

Early epinephrine is lifesaving and there are no absolute contraindications

Pediatric Dosing
- Epinephrine: 0.01 mg/kg IM up to 0.5mg q5-15min
- Initial crystalloid bolus: 20 mL/kg, reassess
- Epinephrine infusion: 0.1-1 μg/kg/min up to 10 μg/min
- Diphenhydramine: 1 mg/kg up to 50 mg IM/IV q4-6h
- Ranitidine: 1 mg/kg up to 50 mg PO/IV
- Methylprednisolone: 1 mg/kg up to 125 mg IV

Disposition

- monitor for 4-6 h in ED (minimum) and arrange follow-up with family physician in 24-48 h
- can have second phase (biphasic) reaction up to 48 h later, patient may need to be supervised
- educate patient on avoidance of allergens
- medications
  - H₁ antagonist (cetirizine 10 mg PO OD or Benadryl® 50 mg PO q4-6h x3d)
  - H₂ antagonist (ranitidine 150 mg PO OD x3d)
  - corticosteroid (prednisone 50 mg PO OD) x5d to prevent secondary reaction

Asthma

- see Respirology, R7
- chronic inflammatory airway disease with episodes of bronchospasm and inflammation resulting in reversible airflow obstruction

Beware of the silent chest in asthma exacerbations. This is a medical emergency and may require emergency intubation

History and Physical

- find cause of asthma exacerbation (viral, environmental, etc.)
- history of asthma control; severity of exacerbations (ICU, intubation history)
- signs of respiratory distress
- vitals, specifically O₂

Investigations

- peak flow meter
- ± ABG if in severe respiratory distress
- CXR if diagnosis in doubt to rule out pneumonia, pneumothorax, etc.

Table 19. Asthma Assessment and Management

Classifications	History and Physical Exam	Management
Respiratory Arrest Imminent	Exhausted, confused, diaphoretic, cyanotic Silent chest, ineffective respiratory effort Decreased HR, RR >30, pCO_2 >45 mmHg O_2 sat <90% despite supplemental O_2	100% O_2, cardiac monitor, IV access Intubate (consider induction with ketamine) Short acting β-agonist (Ventolin): nebulizer 5 mg continually Short-acting Anticholinergic (Atrovent): nebulizer 0.5 mg x 3 IV steroids: methylprednisolone 125 mg
Severe Asthma	Agitated, diaphoretic, laboured respirations Speaking in words No relief from β-agonist O_2 sat <90%, FEV_1 <50%	Anticipate need for intubation Similar to above management Magnesium sulphate 2 g IV O_2 to achieve O_2 sat >92%
Moderate Asthma	SOB at rest, cough, congestion, chest tightness Speaking in phrases Inadequate relief from β-agonist FEV_1 50-80%	O_2 to achieve O_2 sat >92% Short-acting β-agonist (Ventolin): MDI or nebulizer q5min Short-acting Anticholinergic (Atrovent): MDI or nebs x 3 Steroids: prednisone 40-60 mg PO
Mild Asthma	Exertional SOB/cough with some nocturnal symptoms Difficulty finishing sentences FEV_1 >80%	β-agonist Monitor FEV_1 Consider steroids (MDI or PO)

Elements of Well-Controlled Asthma
Can Respir J 2010;17(1):15-24
- Daytime symptoms <4x/wk
- Nocturnal symptoms <1x/wk
- No limitation in activity
- No absence from work/school
- Rescue inhaler use <4x/wk
- FEV_1 <90% personal best
- PEF <10-15% diurnal variation
- Mild infrequent exacerbations

Disposition
- discharge safe in patients with FEV1 or PEF > 60% predicted, and may be safe if FEV1 or PEF 40-60% predicted based on patient's risk factors for recurrence of severe attack
  - risk factors for recurrence: frequent ED visits, frequent hospitalizations, recent steroid use, recent exacerbation, poor medication compliance, prolonged use of high dose beta-agonists
- β-agonist MDI with aerochamber 2-4 puffs q2-4h until symptoms controlled, then prn
- initiate inhaled corticosteroids with aerochamber if not already prescribed
- if moderate to severe attack, administer prednisone 30-60 mg/d for 7 d with no taper
- counsel on medication adherence and educate on use of aerochamber
  - follow-up with primary care physician or asthma specialist

Cardiac Dysrhythmias

- see Cardiology and Cardiac Surgery, C16

Bradydysrhythmias and AV Conduction Blocks
- AV conduction blocks
  - 1st degree: prolonged PR interval (>200 msec), no treatment required
  - 2nd degree
    - Mobitz I: gradual prolongation of PR interval then dropped QRS complex, usually benign
    - Mobitz II: PR interval constant with dropped QRS complex, can progress to 3rd degree AV block
  - 3rd degree: P wave unrelated to QRS complex, PP and RR intervals constant
    - atropine and transcutaneous pacemaker (atropine with caution)
    - if transcutaneous pacemaker fails consider dopamine, epinephrine IV
  - long-term treatment for Mobitz II and 3rd degree block – internal pacemaker
- sinus bradycardia (rate <60 bpm)
  - can be normal (especially in athletes)
  - causes: vagal stimulation, vomiting, myocardial infarction/ischemia, increased ICP, sick sinus node, hypothyroidism, drugs (e.g. β-blockers, CCBs)
  - treat if symptomatic (hypotension, chest pain)
    - acute: atropine ± transcutaneous pacing
    - sick sinus: transcutaneous pacing
    - drug induced: discontinue/reduce offending drug, consider antidotes

Supraventricular Tachydysrhythmias (narrow QRS)
- sinus tachycardia (rate >100 bpm)
  - causes: increased sympathetic tone, drugs, fever, hypotension, anemia, thyrotoxicosis, MI, PE, emotional, pain, etc.
  - search for and treat underlying cause, consider β-blocker if symptomatic
- regular rhythm (i.e. not sinus tachycardia)
  - vagal maneuvers (carotid massage, Valsalva), adenosine 6 mg IV push, if no conversion give 12 mg, can repeat 12 mg dose once
  - rhythm converts: probable re-entry tachycardia (AVNRT more common than AVRT)
    - monitor for recurrence
    - treat recurrence with adenosine or longer acting medications

If the patient with tachydysrhythmia is unstable, perform immediate synchronized cardioversion

- rhythm does not convert: atrial flutter, ectopic atrial tachycardia, junctional tachycardia
  - rate control (diltiazem, β-blockers) and consult cardiology
- irregular rhythm
  - probable AFib, atrial flutter, or multifocal atrial tachycardia
  - rate control (diltiazem, β-blockers)

Atrial Fibrillation

- most common sustained dysrhythmia; no organized P waves (atrial rate >300/min), irregularly irregular heart rate, narrow QRS (typically)
- etiology: HTN, CAD, thyrotoxicosis, EtOH (holiday heart), valvular disease, pericarditis, cardiomyopathy, sick sinus syndrome
- treatment principles: stroke prevention, treat symptoms, identify/treat underlying cause
- decreases cardiac output by 20-30% (due to loss of organized atrial contractions)
- acute management
  - if unstable: immediate synchronized cardioversion
  - if onset of AFib is >48 h: rate control, anticoagulate 3 wk prior to and 4 wk after cardioversion, or do transesophageal echocardiogram to rule out clot
  - if onset <48 h or already anticoagulated: may cardiovert
    - electrical cardioversion: synchronized direct current (DC) cardioversion
    - chemical cardioversion: procainamide, flecainide, propafenone
- long-term management: rate or rhythm control, consider anticoagulation (CHADS2 score, see Cardiology and Cardiac Surgery, C20)

Ventricular Tachydysrhythmias (wide QRS)

- VTach (rate usually 140-200 bpm)
  - definition: 3 or more consecutive ventricular beats at >100 bpm
  - etiology: CAD with MI is most common cause
  - treatment: sustained VTach (>30 s) is an emergency
    - hemodynamic compromise: synchronized DC cardioversion
    - no hemodynamic compromise: synchronized DC cardioversion, amiodarone, procainamide
- VFib: call a code blue, follow ACLS for pulseless arrest
- Torsades de pointes
  - looks like VTach but QRS 'rotates around baseline' with changing axis and amplitude (twisted ribbon)
  - etiology: prolonged QT due to drugs (e.g. quinidine, TCAs, erythromycin, quinolones), electrolyte imbalance (hypokalemia, hypomagnesemia), congenital
  - treatment
    - IV Mg^{2+}, temporary overdrive pacing, isoproterenol
    - correct cause of prolonged QT

Acute Exacerbation of COPD (AECOPD)

- for chronic management of COPD see Respirology, R9
- progressive development of irreversible airway obstruction, typically caused by smoking

History and Physical Exam

- cardinal symptoms of AECOPD: increased dyspnea, increased coughing frequency or severity, increased sputum volume or purulence
- triggers: virus, pneumonia, urinary tract infection, PE, CHF, MI, drugs
- characterize previous episodes and hospitalizations, smoking history
- vital signs, level of consciousness, signs of respiratory distress, respiratory exam

Investigations

- CBC, electrolytes, ABG, CXR, ECG
- PFTs are NOT useful in managing acute exacerbations

Management

- oxygen: keep O_2 sat 88-92% (be aware when giving O_2 to chronic hypercapnic/CO_2 retainers but do not withhold O_2 if hypoxic)
- bronchodilators: short-acting β-agonist (Salbutamol 4-8 puffs via MDI with spacer q15min x3 prn) ± short-acting anticholinergic (Ipratropium 4-8 puffs via MDI q15min x3 prn)
- steroids: prednisone 40-60 mg PO for 7-14 d, or methylprednisolone 125 mg IV bid-qid if severe exacerbation, or unable to take PO
- antibiotics: TMP-SMX, cephalosporins, respiratory quinolones (given if all 3 cardinal symptoms present or 2 cardinal symptoms with increased sputum purulence or mechanical ventilation)
- ventilation: apply NIPPV (CPAP or BiPAP) if severe distress or signs of fatigue, arterial pH <7.35, or hypercapnic
- if life-threatening, ICU admission for intubation and ventilation (chance of ventilation dependency)

Disposition

- no guidelines for admission - based on clinical judgement and comorbidities
- lower threshold to admit if comorbid illness (diabetes, CHF, CAD, alcohol abuse)
- if discharging, use antibiotics, tapering steroids, up to 4-6 puffs qid of ipratropium and salbutamol and organize follow-up

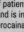

If patient has Wolff-Parkinson-White and is in AFib use amiodarone or procainamide; avoid AV nodal blocking agents (adenosine, digoxin, diltiazem, verapamil, β-blockers), as this can increase conduction through bypass tract, leading to cardiac arrest

Causes of Atrial Fibrillation

C ("sea") PIRATES
CHF, Cardiomyopathy
Pulmonary embolism
Ischemic heart disease
Rheumatic or valvular disease
Anemia
Thyroid
EtOH, Elevated blood pressure
Sick Sinus, Stress - surgery, sepsis

Physical Exam Findings in COPD
- Wheeze
- Maximum laryngeal height ≤4 cm
- Forced expiratory time ≥6 s
- Decreased breath sounds
- Decreased cardiac dullness

Need to Rule Out with COPD Exacerbation
- Pneumothorax
- CHF exacerbation
- Acute MI
- Pneumonia and other infectious causes
- PE

Acute Decompensated Heart Failure (ADHF)

- for chronic management of CHF see <u>Cardiology and Cardiac Surgery</u>, C36

Etiology
- Causes of CHF: decreased myocardial contractility (ischemia, infarction, cardiomyopathy, myocarditis), pressure overload states (HTN, valve abnormalities, congenital heart disease), restricted cardiac output (myocardial infiltrative disease, cardiac tamponade)
- Precipitants of acute decompensation of CHF
  - cardiac (ischemia, infarction, arrhythmia - Afib)
  - medications (beta-blockers, CCBs, NSAIDs, steroids, non-compliance)
  - dietary (increased sodium and/or water intake)
  - high output (anemia, infection, pregnancy, hyperthyroid)
  - other (renal failure, hypertensive crisis, iatrogenic fluid overload - blood transfusions or IV fluids)

Presentation
- left-sided heart failure
  - dyspnea, SOBOE, orthopnea, PND, nocturia, fatigue, altered mental status, presyncope/syncope, angina, systemic hypotension
  - hypoxia, decreased air entry to lungs, crackles, S3 or S4, pulmonary edema (on CXR), pleural effusion (usually right-sided)
- right-sided heart failure
  - dependent bilateral pitting edema, JVP elevation and positive AJR, ascites, hepatomegaly
- patients often present with a combination of right-sided and left-sided symptoms

Investigations
- blood work: CBC, electrolytes, AST, ALT, bilirubin, Cr, BUN, cardiac enzymes, brain natriuretic peptide
- CXR: most useful test (see sidebar)
- ECG: look for MI, ischemia (ST elevation/depression, T-wave inversion), LVH, atrial enlargement, conduction abnormalities
- ABG: if severe or refractory to treatment
  - hypoxemia, hypercapnia and acidosis are signs of severe CHF
- echocardiogram: not usually used in emergency evaluation, previous results may aid in diagnosis
- rule out serious differentials such as PE, pneumothorax, pneumonia/empyema, AECOPD

Management
- ABCs, may require intubation if severe hypoxia
- sit upright, cardiac monitoring, and continuous pulse oximetry
- saline lock IV, Foley catheter (to follow effectiveness of diuresis)
- 100% O₂ by mask
  - if poor response, may require BiPAP or intubation
- drugs
  - diuretic (if volume overloaded): Furosemide 40-80 mg IV
  - vasodilators (if sBP > 100): Nitroglycerin 0.3 mg SL q5min prn ± topical Nitrodur patch (0.4-0.8 mg/h)
    - if not responding or signs of ischemia (angina): Nitroglycerine 10-20 µg/min IV, titrate to response
    - if severe or refractory hypertension: Nitroprusside 0.5 µg/kg/min, titrate to response
  - inotropes/vasopressors (if sBP < 90)
    - without signs of shock: Dobutamine 2.5 µg/kg/min IV, titrate up to sBP > 90 mmHg
    - with signs of shock: Dopamine 5-10 µg/kg/min IV, titrate up to sBP > 90 mmHg
- treat precipitating factor - e.g. rate control (beta-blocker, CCB) or rhythm-control (electrical or chemical cardioversion) if new Afib
- cardiology or medicine consult

Venous Thromboembolism (VTE)

- see <u>Respirology</u>, R20

Risk Factors
- Virchow's triad: alterations in blood flow (venous stasis), injury to endothelium, hypercoagulable state (including pregnancy, use of OCP, malignancy)
- clinical risk factors (see sidebar)

DEEP VEIN THROMBOSIS (DVT)

Presentation
- calf pain, unilateral leg swelling/erythema/edema, palpable cord along the deep venous system on exam; can be asymptomatic
- clinical signs/symptoms are unreliable for diagnosis and exclusion of DVT; investigation often needed

---

Precipitants of CHF Exacerbation

FAILURE
Forgot medication
Arrhythmia (Dysrhythmia)/**A**nemia
Ischemia/Infarction/Infection
Lifestyle (e.g. high salt intake)
Upregulation of cardiac output
(pregnancy, hyperthyroidism)
Renal failure
Embolism (pulmonary)

CHF on CXR
- Pulmonary vascular redistribution
- Perihilar infiltrates
- Interstitial edema, Kerley B lines
- Alveolar edema, bilateral infiltrates
- May see cardiomegaly, pleural effusions
- Peribronchial cuffing
- Fissural thickening (fluid in fissure)

Acute Treatment of CHF

LMNOP
Lasix (furosemide)
Morphine
Nitroglycerin
Oxygen
Position (sit upright), **P**ressure (BiPAP)

Hospital Management Required if
- Acute MI
- Pulmonary edema or severe respiratory distress
- Severe complicating medical illness (e.g. pneumonia)
- Anasarca
- Symptomatic hypotension or syncope
- Refractory to outpatient therapy
- Thromboembolic complications requiring interventions
- Clinically significant dysrhythmias
- Inadequate social support for safe outpatient management
- Persistent hypoxia requiring supplemental oxygen

Risk Factors for VTE

THROMBOSIS
Trauma, travel
Hypercoagulable, HRT
Recreational drugs (IVDU)
Old (age >60 yr)
Malignancy
Birth control pill
Obesity, obstetrics
Surgery, smoking
Immobilization
Sickness (CHF, MI, nephrotic syndrome, vasculitis)

Investigations

- use Wells' criteria for DVT to guide investigations (Figure 12)
- D-dimer is only useful at ruling out a DVT if it is negative in low to moderate risk patients (highly sensitive)
  - high risk of false positives in: elderly, infection, recent surgery, trauma, hemorrhage, late in pregnancy, liver disease, cancer
- U/S has high sensitivity & specificity for proximal clot but only 73% sensitivity for calf DVT (may need to repeat in 1 wk)
  - if positive – treat for DVT regardless of risk
  - if negative and low risk – rule out DVT
  - if negative and moderate to high risk – repeat U/S in 5-7 days to rule out DVT

Management

- LMWH unless patient also has renal failure
  - dalteparin 200 IU/kg SC q24h or enoxaparin 1.5 mg/kg SC q24h
- warfarin started at same time as LMWH (5 mg PO OD initially followed by dosing based on INR)
- LMWH discontinued when INR has been therapeutic (2-3) for 2 consecutive days
- rivaroxaban can be used in acute management of symptomatic DVT
  - 15 mg PO bid for first 21 d; 20 mg PO daily for remaining treatment (taken with food at approximately the same time each day)
- consider thrombolysis if extensive DVT causing limb compromise
- IVC filter or surgical thrombectomy considered if anticoagulation is contraindicated
- duration of anticoagulation: 3 months if transient coagulopathy; 6 months if unprovoked DVT; life-long if ongoing coagulopathy

PULMONARY EMBOLISM (PE)

Presentation

- dyspnea, pleuritic chest pain, hemoptysis, tachypnea, cyanosis, hypoxia, fever
- clinical signs/symptoms are unreliable for diagnosis and exclusion of DVT; investigation often needed

Investigations

- use Wells' criteria for PE to guide investigations (Figures 13-14)
- PERC score alone can rule out PE in low risk patients (as determined by Wells' criteria) unless patient is pregnant
- ECG and CXR are useful to rule out other causes (e.g. ACS, pneumonia, pericarditis) or to support diagnosis of PE
  - ECG changes in PE: sinus tachycardia, right ventricular strain (S1Q3T3), T wave inversions in anterior and inferior leads
  - CXR findings in PE: Hampton's hump (triangular density extending from pleura) or Westermark's sign
- D-dimer is only useful at ruling out a PE if it is negative in low to moderate risk patients (highly sensitive)
  - if positive D-dimer or high-probability patient, then pursue CT angiography or V/Q scan
- CT angiography has high sensitivity and specificity for PE, may also suggest other etiology
- V/Q scan useful in pregnancy, when CT angiography not available, or IV contrast contraindicated

Management of PE

- treatment of PE with anticoagulation and duration of treatment is the same as for DVT (see above)
- consider thrombolysis if extensive PE causing hemodynamic compromise or cardiogenic shock
- catheter-directed thrombolysis or surgical thrombectomy rarely considered in massive PE or contraindication to anticoagulation
- often can be treated as outpatient, may require analgesia for chest pain (narcotic or NSAID)
- admit if hemodynamically unstable, require supplemental O₂, major comorbidities, lack of sufficient social supports, unable to ambulate, need invasive therapy
  - referral to medicine for coagulopathy and malignancy workup

Wells' Criteria for DVT

Active cancer	+1
Paralysis, paresis or recent immobilization of leg	+1
Recently bedridden x 3 d or major surgery within 4 wks	+1
Local tenderness	+1
Entire leg swollen	+1
Calf swelling 3cm > asymptomatic leg	+1
Unilateral pitting edema	+1
Collateral superficial veins	+1
Alternative dx more likely	-2

0: Low probability
1-2: Moderate probability
>3: High probability

Wells' Criteria for PE

Previous Hx of DVT/PE	+1.5
HR >100	+1.5
Recent immobility or surgery	+1.5
Clinical signs of DVT	+3
Alternate Dx less likely than PE	+3
Hemoptysis	+1
Cancer	+1

< 2: Low probability
2-6: Intermediate probability
>6: High probability

PERC Score
- Age >50 yr
- HR >100 bpm
- O₂ sat on RA <94%
- Prior history DVT/PE
- Recent trauma or surgery
- Hemoptysis
- Exogenous estrogen
- Clinical signs suggesting DVT

Score 1 for each question; a score 0/8 means patient has <1.6% chance having a PE and avoids further investigation. Caution using the PERC score in pregnant women as the original study excluded pregnant women

D-dimer is only useful if it is negative; negative predictive value >99%

50% of patients with symptomatic proximal DVT will develop PE, often within days to weeks of the event

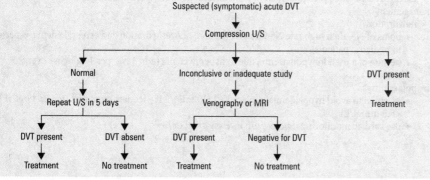

Figure 12. Approach to suspected DVT

Clinical Criteria to Prevent Unnecessary Diagnostic Testing in Emergency Department Patients with Suspected Pulmonary Embolism
J Thromb Haemost 2004;2:1247-1255
Purpose: To develop PE rule-out criteria (PERC) that can be used at the bedside, and prevents overtesting for PE, which includes the D-dimer test that frequently results in false positives.
Study: 21 variables were collected prospectively from 3,148 ER patients evaluated for possible PE to develop rule-out criteria. The application of the developed rules was investigated in 1,427 low-risk patients and 382 very low-risk patients.
Results: Eight variables were included in a block rule (age <50 yr, pulse <100 bpm, SaO2 >94%, no unilateral leg swelling, no hemoptysis, no recent trauma or surgery, no prior PE or DVT, no hormone use) and a negative score was used to rule-out PE. In low-risk and very low-risk patients, the rule had a sensitivity of 96 and 100%, respectively and a specificity of 27 and 15%, respectively.
Summary: D-dimer testing for PE may not be favourable if all eight factors in the PERC are negative.

Oral Rivaroxaban for the Treatment of Symptomatic Pulmonary Embolism
NEJM 2012;366:1287-1297
Background: Evidence supporting rivaroxaban as effective therapy in DVT may also apply to simplify treatment of PE.
Methods: A randomized, open-label, event-driven, non-inferiority trial involving 4,832 patients with acute symptomatic PE with or without DVT, was undertaken to compare rivaroxaban (15 mg twice daily for 3 wk, followed by 20 mg once daily) with standard therapy of enoxaparin followed by an adjusted-dose vitamin K antagonist.
Results: Rivaroxaban was non-inferior to standard therapy (non-inferiority margin, 2.0; p=0.003) for preventing recurrent VTE (HR: 1.12; 95% CI 0.75-1.68). Major bleeding occurred less in the rivaroxaban group (hazard ratio, 0.49; 95% CI 0.31-0.79; p=0.003). Rates of other adverse events were similar in the two groups.
Conclusions: A fixed-dose regimen of rivaroxaban alone was non-inferior to standard therapy for the initial and long-term treatment of PE.

Oral Rivaroxaban for the Treatment of Symptomatic Venous Thromboembolism
NEJM 2010;363:2499-2510
Background: Rivaroxaban, an oral factor Xa inhibitor, hypothesized to provide a simple, fixed-dose regimen for treating acute DVT and for continued treatment, without the need for laboratory monitoring.
Methods: An open-label, randomized, event-driven, non-inferiority study compared oral rivaroxaban alone (15 mg twice daily for 3 wk, followed by 20 mg once daily) with subcutaneous enoxaparin followed by vitamin K antagonist in patients with acute, symptomatic DVT (sample size: 3,449 patients). In parallel, a double-blind, randomized, event-driven superiority study was conducted to compare rivaroxaban alone (20 mg once daily) versus placebo in patients who had received treatment for VTE (sample size: 602 patients in intervention vs 594 in placebo group).
Results: Rivaroxaban had non-inferior efficacy with respect to recurrent VTE (HR: 0.68 95%CI: 0.44-1.04). Similar bleeding prevalence were reported in each group. In the parallel continued-treatment study, rivaroxaban had superior efficacy with respect to preventing VTE (HR: 0.18 95%CI 0.09-0.39). Four patients in the rivaroxaban group had nonfatal major bleeding vs. none in the placebo group (p=0.11).
Conclusions: Rivaroxaban offers a single-drug approach to treatment of VTE that may improve the benefit-to-risk profile of anticoagulation.

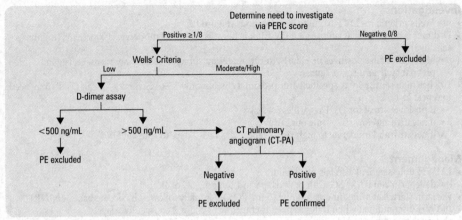

Figure 13. Approach to suspected PE

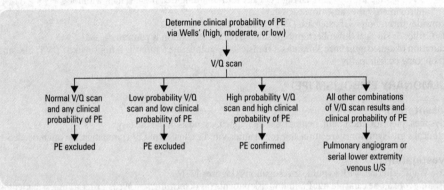

Figure 14. V/Q-based algorithm for suspected PE

Diabetic Emergencies

- see Endocrinology, E11

Diabetic Ketoacidosis
- triad of hyperglycemia, ketosis, and acidosis due to severe insulin deficiency and counter-regulatory hormone excess
- clinical presentation
  - often young, Type 1 DM patients, (may rarely be first presentation of undiagnosed Type 2 DM) with symptoms evolving within a day
  - early signs and symptoms: polyuria, polydipsia, malaise, nocturia, weight loss
  - late signs and symptoms
    - GI: anorexia, nausea, vomiting, abdominal pain
    - neurological: fatigue, drowsiness, stupor, coma
    - respiratory: Kussmaul's respiration, dyspnea (often due to acidosis), fruity ketotic breath
- investigations
  - blood work: CBC, electrolytes, Ca^{2+}, Mg^{2+}, PO_4^{3-}, Cr, BUN, glucose, ketones, osmolality, AST/ALT/ALP, amylase, troponin
  - urine: glucose and ketones
  - ABG
  - ECG (MI is possible precipitant; electrolyte disturbances may predispose to dysrhythmia)
- management
  - rehydration
    - bolus of NS, then high rate NS infusion (beware of overhydration and cerebral edema, especially in pediatric patients)
    - beware of a pseudohyponatremia due to hyperglycemia (add 3 Na^+ per 10 glucose over 5.5 mmol/L)
  - potassium
    - essential to avoid hypokalemia: replace KCl (20 mEq/L if adequate renal function and initial K^+ <5.5 mmol/L)
    - use cardiac monitoring if potassium levels normal or low

- insulin
  - critical, as this is the only way to turn off gluconeogenesis/ketosis
  - do not give insulin if K^+ <3.3 mmol/L
  - initial bolus of 5-10 U short-acting/regular insulin (or 0.2 U/kg) IV in adults (controversial – may just start with infusion)
  - followed by continuous infusion at 5-10 U (or 0.1 U/kg) per hour
  - once the blood glucose < 14 mmol/L, patient should receive their regular insulin SC injection and the infusion stopped in 1 hour
  - add D5W to IV fluids when blood glucose <15 mmol/L to prevent hypoglycemia
- bicarbonate is not given unless patient is at risk of death or shock (typically pH <7.0)

Hyperosmolar Hyperglycemic State
- state of extreme hyperglycemia (44-133.2 mmol/L) due to relative insulin deficiency, counter-regulatory hormones excess, gluconeogenesis, and dehydration (due to osmotic diuresis)
- clinical presentation
  - often older, Type 2 DM patients with more co-morbid illnesses and larger fluid losses with symptoms evolving over days to weeks, less GI symptoms and more neurological deficits than DKA including: mental disturbances, coma, delirium, seizures
  - polyuria, N/V
- investigations
  - blood work: CBC, electrolytes, Ca^{2+}, Mg^{2+}, PO_4^{3-}, Cr, BUN, glucose, ketones, osmolality
  - urine: glucose and ketones
  - ABG
  - find underlying cause: ECG, CXR, blood and urine C&S
- management
  - rehydration with IV NS (total water deficit estimated at average 100 cc/kg body weight)
  - O_2 and cardiac monitoring, frequent electrolyte and glucose monitoring
  - insulin is controversial
  - identify and treat precipitant if present (the 5 Is)

Hypoglycemia
- characterized by Whipple's triad: low plasma glucose, symptoms suggestive of hypoglycemia, prompt resolution of symptoms with glucose
- clinical presentation
  - neuroglycopenic symptoms: headaches, confusion, seizures, coma
  - autonomic symptoms: diaphoresis, nausea, hunger, tachycardia, palpitations
- history and physical exam
  - last meal, known DM, prior similar episodes, drug therapy, and compliance
  - liver/renal/endocrine/neoplastic disease
  - depression, alcohol or drug use
- management
  - IV access and rapid blood glucose measurement
  - D50W 50 mL IV push, glucose PO if mental status permits
  - if IV access not possible, glucagon 1-2 mg IM, repeat x 1 in 10-20 min
  - O_2, cardiac, frequent blood glucose monitoring
  - thiamine 100 mg IM
  - full meal as soon as mental status permits
  - if episode due to long-acting insulin, or sulfonylureas, watch for prolonged hypoglycemia due to long t1/2 (may require admission for monitoring)
  - search for cause (most often due to exogenous insulin, alcohol, or sulfonylureas)

4 Criteria for DKA Dx
- Hyperglycemia
- Metabolic acidosis
- Hyperketonemia
- Ketonuria

Signs and Symptoms of DKA
D: Diuresis, dehydration, drowsy, delirium, dizziness
K: Kusmaul's breathing, ketotic breath
A: Abdominal pain, anorexia

Precipitating Factors in DKA

The 5 Is
Infection
Ischemia
Infarction
Intoxication
Insulin missed

Causes of Hypoglycemia
Most common: excessive insulin use in setting of poor PO intake
Common: alcohol intoxication, sepsis, liver disease, oral anti-hyperglycemics
Rare: insulinomas, hypopituitarism, adrenal insufficiency, med side effects

Cerebral edema may occur if hyperosmolality is treated too aggressively

Electrolyte Disturbances

- see Nephrology, NP7 and Endocrinology, E36

Table 20. Electrolyte Disturbances

Electrolyte Disturbance	Common Causes	Symptoms	Treatment	Special Considerations
Hypernatremia Inadequate H_2O intake (elderly/disabled) or inappropriate excretion of H_2O (diuretics, Li, and DI)		Lethargy, weakness, irritability, and edema; seizures and coma occur with severe elevations of Na^+ levels (>158 mmol/L)	Salt restrict and give free water	No more than 12 mmol/L in 24 h drop in Na^+ (0.5 mmol/L/h) due to risk of cerebral edema, seizures, death
Hyponatremia	Hypovolemic (GI, renal, skin, blood fluid loss), euvolemic (SIADH/stress, adrenal insufficiency, hypothyroid, diet/intake), hypervolemic (CHF, cirrhosis, nephrotic syndrome)	Neurologic symptoms 2° to cerebral edema, headache, decreased LOC, depressed reflexes; chronic milder than acute	Water restrict/NPO; Seizure/Coma: 100cc 3% NaCl; Treat hypovolemia with RL and hypervolemia with furosemide	Limit total rise to 8 mmol/L in 24 h (0.5 mmol/L/h maximum) as patients are at risk of central pontine myelinolysis
Hyperkalemia	Rhabdomyolysis, insulin deficiency, metabolic acidosis (e.g. acute renal failure, missed dialysis)	Nausea, palpitations, muscle stiffness, areflexia	Protect heart: calcium gluconate Shift K^+ into cells: D50W + Insulin, $NaHCO_3$, salbutamol Remove K^+: Fluids+furosemide, dialysis	High risk of dysrhythmia - ECG: peaked/narrow T wave, decreased P wave, prolonged PR interval, widening of QRS, AV block, VFib
Hypokalemia	Metabolic alkalosis (e.g. diarrhea), insulin, diuretics, anorexia, salbutamol	N/V, fatigue, muscle cramps, constipation	K-Dur®, K^+ sparing diuretics, IV solutions with 20-40 mEq/L KCl over 3-4 h	ECG: U waves most important, flattened/inverted T waves, prolonged QT, depressed ST May need to restore Mg^{2+}
Hypercalcemia	Hyper-PTH and malignancy account for ~90% of cases	Multisystem including CVS, GI (groans), renal (stones), rheumatological, MSK (bones), psychiatric (moans)	Isotonic saline (+ furosemide if hypervolemic) Bisphosphonates, dialysis, chelation (EDTA or oral PO_4^{3-})	Patients with more severe or symptomatic hypercalcemia are usually dehydrated and require saline hydration as initial therapy
Hypocalcemia	Iatrogenic, low Mg^{2+}, liver dysfunction, 1° hypo-PTH	Laryngospasm, hyperreflexia, paresthesia, tetany, Chvostek's and Trousseau's sign	Acute (ionized Ca^{2+} <0.7 mM) requires immediate treatment: IV calcium gluconate 1-2 g in 10-20 min followed by slow infusion	Prolonged QT interval can arise, leading to dysrhythmia as can upper airway obstruction

Hypertensive Emergencies

HELLP Syndrome (seen only in preeclampsia/eclampsia)
Hemolytic anemia
Elevated **L**iver enzymes
Low **P**latelet count

Hypertensive Emergency (Hypertensive Crisis)
- definition: severe elevation of BP with evidence of end-organ damage (CNS, retinal, CVS, renal, GI)
- etiology
  - essential HTN, emotional exertion, pain, use of sympathomimetic drugs (cocaine, amphetamine, etc.), MAOI use with ingestion of tyramine-containing food (cheese, red wine, etc.), pheochromocytoma, pregnancy
- clinical presentation

Table 21. Signs and Symptoms of Hypertensive Emergencies

	CNS	Retinal	Renal	Cardiovascular	Gastrointestinal
Complication	Stroke/TIA, headache, altered mental status, seizures, hemorrhage	Vision change, hemorrhage, exudates, papilledema	Nocturia, elevated Cr, proteinuria, hematuria, oliguria	Ischemia/angina, infarction, dissection (back pain), CHF	N/V, abdominal pain, elevated liver enzymes

- investigations
  - blood work: CBC, electrolytes, BUN, Cr
  - urinalysis
  - peripheral blood smear: to detect microangiopathic hemolytic anemia
  - CXR: if SOB or chest pain
  - ECG, troponins, CK: if chest pain
  - CT head: if neurological findings or severe headache
  - toxicology screen if sympathomimetic overdose suspected
- management

Catecholamine-Induced Hypertensive Emergencies
Avoid use of non-selective β-blockers as they inhibit β-mediated vasodilation and leave α-adrenergic vasoconstriction unopposed

  - in general, the strategy for management is to gradually and progressively reduce BP in 24-48 h
  - lower BP by 25% over the initial 60 min by initiating antihypertensive therapy (usually nitroprusside and labetalol)
  - if preeclampsia, immediately consult OB/GYN (see Obstetrics, OB24)
  - establish arterial line; transfer to ICU for further reduction in BP under monitored setting
  - in case of ischemic stroke: do no rapidly reduce BP, maintain BP > 150/100 for 5 d
  - in case of aortic dissection: rapid reduction of sBP to 110-120 STAT (do not resuscitate with IV fluids)
  - in case of excessive catecholamines: avoid β-blockers (except labetalol)
  - in case of ACS: address ischemia initially, then BP

Hypertensive Urgency
- definition: severely elevated BP (usually sBP >180, dBP >110) with no evidence of end-organ damage
- most commonly due to non-adherence with medications
- treatment: initiate/adjust antihypertensive therapy, monitor in ED (up to 6 h) and discharge with follow up for 48-72 h
- goal: differentiate hypertensive emergencies from hypertensive urgencies

With CNS manifestations of severe HTN, it is often difficult to differentiate causal relationships (i.e. HTN could be secondary to a cerebral event with an associated Cushing reflex)

Table 22. Commonly Used Agents for the Treatment of Hypertensive Crisis

Drug	Dosage	Onset of Action	Duration of Action	Adverse Effects*	Special Indications
VASODILATORS					
Sodium Nitroprusside (vascular smooth muscle dilator) 1st line	0.25-10 μg/kg/min	Immediate	3-5 min	N/V, muscle twitching, sweating, cyanide intoxication, coronary steal syndrome	Most hypertensive emergencies (especially CHF, aortic dissection) Use in combination with β-blockers (e.g. esmolol) in aortic dissection Caution with high ICP and azotemia
Nicardipine (CCB)	2 mg IV bolus, then 4 mg/kg/h IV	15-30 min	40 min	Tachycardia, headache, flushing, local phlebitis (e.g. encephalopathy, RF, eclampsia, sympathetic crisis)	Most hypertensive emergencies Caution with acute CHF
Fenoldopam Mesylate (dopamine receptor antagonist)	0.05-0.1 μm/kg/min IV	<5 min	8-10 min	Tachycardia, headache, nausea, flushing (e.g. acute RF)	Most hypertensive emergencies Caution with glaucoma
Enalapril (ACEI)	0.625-1.25 mg IV q6h	15-30 min	12-24 h	Theoretical fall in pressure in high renin states not seen in studies	Acute LV failure Avoid in acute MI, pregnancy, acute RF
Nitroglycerin	5-20 μg/min IV	1-2 min	3-5 min	Hypotension, bradycardia, headache, lightheadedness, dizziness	MI/pulmonary edema
Hydralazine	5-10 mg IV/IM q20min (max 20 mg)	5-20 min	2-6 h	Dizziness, drowsiness, headache, tachycardia, Na+ retention	Eclampsia
ADRENERGIC INHIBITORS					
Labetalol	20 mg IV bolus q10min or 0.5-2 mg/min	5-10 min	3-6 h	Vomiting, scalp tingling, burning in throat, dizziness, nausea, heart block, orthostatic hypotension	Most hypertensive emergencies (especially eclampsia) Avoid in acute CHF, heart block >1st degree
Esmolol	250-500 μg/kg/min 1 min, then 50 μg/kg/min for 4 min; repeat	1-2 min	10-20 min	Hypotension, nausea, bronchospasm	Aortic dissection, acute MI SVT dysrhythmias, perioperative HTN Avoid in acute CHF, heart block >1st degree
Phentolamine	5-15 mg q5-15min	1-2 min	3-10 min	Tachycardia, headache, flushing	Catecholamine excess (e.g. pheochromocytoma)

*Hypotension may occur with all of these agents

Acute Coronary Syndrome

- see Cardiology and Cardiac Surgery, C27
- definition: new onset of chest pain, or acute worsening of previous chest pain, or chest pain at rest with:
  - negative cardiac biomarkers and no ECG changes = Unstable angina (UA)
  - positive cardiac biomarkers (elevated troponin) and no ECG changes = NSTEMI
  - positive cardiac biomarkers (elevated troponin) and ST segment elevation on ECG = STEMI
- investigations
  - ECG STAT (as soon as ACS is suspected on history), troponin (2-6 hours after symptom onset), CXR (to rule out other causes)
- management
  - stabilize: ABCs, oxygen, IV access, cardiac monitors, oximetry
  - ASA 162-325 mg chewed and swallowed
  - nitroglycerin 0.3 mg SL q5min x 3; IV only if persistent pain, CHF, or hypertensive
    - contraindications: hypotension, phosphodiesterase inhibitor use, right ventricular infarctions (⅓ of all inferior MIs)

- anticoagulation: choice of anticoagulation (unfractionated heparin, LMWH, or fondaparinux) and additional antiplatelet therapy (clopidogrel, ticagrelor, or prasugrel) depends on STEMI vs. NSTEMI and reperfusion strategy
- early cardiology consult for reperfusion therapy
  - UA/NSTEMI: early coronary angiography recommended if high TIMI risk score
  - STEMI: primary percutaneous coronary intervention (within 90 min) preferred; thrombolytics if unavailable within 120 min of medical contact, symptoms <12 hr and no contraindications
- atorvastatin 80 mg to stabilize plaques
- β-blocker if no signs of CHF, hemodynamic compromise, bradycardia or severe reactive airway disease
- ACEI initiated within 24 hours

Sepsis

- see Infectious Diseases, ID21 and Respirology, R33
- definitions
  - SIRS: Two or more of: 1) T < 36 or > 38; 2) Pulse > 90 bpm; 3) RR > 20 breaths per min (or $PaCO_2$ < 30 mmHg); 4) WBC > 12 x 10 cells/L^9, or < 4 x 10 cells/L^9, or > 10% bands
  - sepsis: SIRS in response to infection
  - severe sepsis: sepsis and signs of organ dysfunction (altered mental status, lung injury, renal failure, coagulopathy, decreased urine output, lactic acidosis, liver failure)
  - septic shock: severe sepsis and hypotension (sBP <90) unresponsive to IV crystalloid fluid bolus
- management
  - early recognition of sepsis and investigations to locate source of infection
  - identify severe sepsis with lactate or evidence of tissue hypoperfusion
  - treatment priorities
    - ABCs, monitors, lines
    - aggressive fluid resuscitation; consider ventilatory and inotropic support
    - cultures, then early empiric appropriate antibiotics - consider broad spectrum and atypical coverage
    - source control - e.g. remove infected Foley or surgery for ischemic gut
    - monitor adequate resuscitation with vital signs, inferior vena cava on U/S, and serial lactates

Stroke and TIA

- see Neurology, N48
- definitions
  - stroke: sudden loss of brain function due to ischemia (80%) or hemorrhage (20%) with persistence of symptoms >24 hr or neuroimaging evidence
  - TIA: transient episode of neurologic dysfunction from focal ischemia without acute infarction typically lasting <1 h, but defined as <24 h
- clinical presentation

7 Causes of Emboli from the Heart
- AFib
- MI
- Endocarditis
- Valvular disease
- Dilated cardiomyopathy
- Left heart myxoma
- Prosthetic valves

Table 23. Signs and Symptoms of Stroke

	General	Language/ Throat	Vision	Coordination	Motor	Sensation	Reflex
Signs/ Symptoms	Decreased LOC, changed mental status, confusion, neglect	Dysarthria, aphasia, swallowing difficulty	Diplopia, eye deviation, asymmetric pupils, visual field defect	Ataxia, intention tremor, lack of coordination	Increased tone, loss of power, spasticity	Loss of sensation	Hyper-reflexia, clonus

- patients with hemorrhagic stroke can present with sudden onset thunderclap headache that is usually described as "worst headache of life"
- stroke mimics: seizure, migraine, hypoglycemia, Todd's paresis, peripheral nerve injury, Bell's palsy, tumour, syncope

Differentiation of UMN Disease vs. LMN Disease

Category	UMN Disease	LMN Disease
Muscular deficit	Muscle groups	Individual muscles
Reflexes	Increased	Decreased/absent
Tone	Increased	Decreased
Fasciculations	Absent	Present
Atrophy	Absent/minimal	Present
Babinski	Present Upgoing	Present Downgoing

Table 24. Stroke Syndromes

Region of Stroke	Stroke Syndrome
Anterior Cerebral Artery	Primarily frontal lobe function affected Altered mental status, impaired judgment, contralateral lower extremity weakness and hypoesthesia, gait apraxia
Middle Cerebral Artery	Contralateral hemiparesis (arm and face weakness > leg weakness) and hypoesthesia, ipsilateral hemianopsia, gaze preference to side of lesion ± agnosia, receptive/expressive aphasia
Posterior Cerebral Artery	Affects vision and thought Homonymous hemianopsia, cortical blindness, visual agnosia, altered mental status, impaired memory
Vertebrobasilar Artery	Wide variety of cranial nerve, cerebellar, and brainstem deficits: vertigo, nystagmus, diplopia, visual field deficits, dysphagia, dysarthria, facial hypoesthesia, syncope, ataxia Loss of pain and temperature sensation in ipsilateral face and contralateral body

Investigations
- CBC, electrolytes, blood glucose, coagulation studies ± cardiac biomarkers ± toxicology screen
- non-contrast CT head: look for hemorrhage, ischemia
- ECG ± echocardiogram: rule out AFib, acute MI as source of emboli
- other imaging: carotid Dopplers, CTA, MRA as appropriate

Management
- ABCs; intubation with RSI if GCS ≤8, rapidly decreasing GCS, or inadequate airway protection reflexes
- thrombolysis: immediate assessment for eligibility; need acute onset, <4.5 h from drug administration time AND compatible physical findings AND normal CT with no bleed
- elevating head of bed if risk of elevated ICP, aspiration, or worsening cardiopulmonary status
- NPO, IV ± cardiac monitoring
  - judge fluid rate carefully to avoid overhydration (cerebral edema) as well as underhydration (underperfusion of the ischemic penumbra)
- BP control: only treat severe HTN (sBP >200, dBP >120, mean arterial BP >140) or HTN associated with hemorrhagic stroke transformation, cardiac ischemia, aortic dissection, or renal damage; use IV nitroprusside or labetalol
- glycemic control: keep fasting glucose <6.5 in acute phase (5 d)
- cerebral edema control: hyperventilation, mannitol to decrease ICP if necessary
- consult neurosurgery, neurology, medicine as indicated

Medications
- acute ischemic stroke: thrombolytics (rt-PA, e.g. alteplase) if within 4.5 h of symptom onset with no evidence of hemorrhage on CT scan
- antiplatelet agents: prevent recurrent stroke or stroke after TIAs, e.g. Aspirin® (1st line); clopidogrel, Aggrenox® (2nd line)
- anticoagulation: DVT prophylaxis if immobile; treat AFib if present
- follow-up for consideration of carotid endarterectomy, cardiovascular risk optimization

If patient presents within 4.5 h of onset of disabling neurological deficits greater than 60 min with no signs of resolution, they may be a candidate for thrombolysis. Do brief assessment and order stat CT head

Absolute Exclusion Criteria for tPA
- Suspected subarachnoid hemorrhage
- Previous intracranial hemorrhage
- Cerebral infarct or severe HI within the past 3 mo
- Recent LP or arterial puncture at non-compressible site
- Brain tumour
- Metastatic cancer diagnosis
- BP >185 mmHg systolic, or >110 mmHg diastolic
- Bleeding diathesis
- Prolonged PT > 15 s or INR >1.7
- Platelet count <100,000
- Blood glucose <2.8 or >22 mmol/L
- Intracranial hemorrhage on CT or large volume infarct
- Previously ADL dependent (clinical judgment)
- Seizure at onset causing postictal impairments

Relative Exclusion Criteria for tPA
- Only minor or rapidly improving symptoms
- Very severe symptoms (NIHSS > 22) or coma
- Major surgery within the past 14 d
- GI or urinary hemorrhage within the past 21 d

Otolaryngological Presentations and Emergencies

- see Otolaryngology, OT6
- ear associated symptoms: otalgia, aural fullness, otorrhea, hearing loss, tinnitus, vertigo, pruritis, fever
- risk factors: Q-tip use, hearing aids, headphones, occupational noise exposure

Dizziness and Vertigo
- distinguish four types of dizziness: vertigo ("room spinning"), lightheadedness ("disconnected from environment"), presyncope ("almost blacking out"), dysequilibrium ("unstable, off-balance")
- broad differential and diverse management (see Family Medicine, FM25; Otolaryngology, OT6)
- consider medication adverse effects

Otalgia (see Otolaryngology, OT6)
- differential diagnosis
  - infections: acute otitis externa, acute otitis media, otitis media with effusion, mastoiditis, myringitis, malignant otitis in diabetics, herpes simplex/zoster, auricular cellulitis, external canal abscess, dental disease
  - others: trauma, temporomandibular joint dysfunction, neoplasm, foreign body, cerumen impactions, trigeminal neuralgia, granulomatosis with polyangiitis
- observe for otorrhea, palpation of outer ear/mastoid, otoscope to see bulging erythematous tympanic membrane, perforation
- C&S of ear canal discharge, if present
- CT head if suspicion of mastoiditis, malignant otitis externa
- antibiotics/antifungals/antivirals for respective infections

Hearing Loss (see Otolaryngology, OT7)
- differentiate conductive versus sensorineural hearing loss
- rule out sudden sensorineural hearing loss (SNHL), a medical emergency requiring high dose steroids and urgent referral
- in elderly, unilateral tinnitus or SNHL is acoustic neuroma until proven otherwise
- consider audiogram and referral or follow-up with family physician

Epistaxis

- see Otolaryngology, OT26
- 90% of nosebleeds stem from the anterior nasal septum (at Kiesselbach's plexus located in Little's area)
- can be life-threatening

Etiology
- most commonly caused by trauma (digital, blunt, foreign bodies)
- other causes: barometric changes, nasal dryness, chemicals (cocaine, Otrivin®), or systemic disease (coagulopathies, HTN, etc.)

Investigations
- blood work: CBC, PT/PTT (as indicated)
- imaging: X-ray, CT as needed

Treatment
- aim is to localize bleeding and achieve hemostasis
- first-aid: ABCs, clear clots by blowing nose or suctioning, lean forward, pinch cartilaginous portion of nose for 20 min twice
- assess blood loss: vitals, IV NS, cross match 2 units pRBC if significant
- if first aid measures fail twice, proceed to packing
- apply an anterior pack
  - clear nose of any clots
  - apply topical anesthesia/vasoconstrictors (lidocaine with epinephrine, cocaine, or soaked pledgets)
  - insert either a traditional Vaseline® gauze pack or a commercial nasal tampon or balloon
  - if bleeding stops, arrange follow-up in 48-72 h for reassessment and pack removal
  - if packing both nares, prophylactic anti-staphylococcal antibiotics to prevent sinusitis or toxic shock syndrome
  - if bleeding is controlled with anterior pressure, cautery with silver nitrate can be performed if the site of bleeding is identified (one side of septum only because if both are cauterized this can lead to septal perforation)
- if suspect posterior bleed or anterior packing does not provide hemostasis, consult ENT for posterior packing and further evaluation
  - posterior packing requires monitoring because can cause significant vagal response and posterior bleeding source can lead to significant blood loss, therefore usually requires admission

Disposition
- discharge: discharged upon stabilization and appropriate follow-up; educate patients about prevention (e.g. humidifiers, saline spray, topical ointments, avoiding irritants, managing HTN)
- admission: severe cases of refractory bleeding, and most cases of posterior packing

Gynecologic/Urologic Emergencies

Vaginal Bleeding

- see Gynecology, GY10 and Obstetrics, OB13

Etiology
- pregnant patient
  - 1st/2nd trimester pregnancy: ectopic pregnancy, abortion (threatened, incomplete, complete, missed, inevitable, septic), molar pregnancy, implantation bleeding, friable cervix (most common cause)
  - 2nd/3rd trimester pregnancy: placenta previa, placental abruption, premature rupture of membranes, preterm labour
  - other: trauma, bleeding cervical polyp, passing of mucous plug
- postpartum
  - postpartum hemorrhage, uterine inversion, retained placental tissue, endometritis
- non-pregnant patients
  - dysfunctional uterine bleeding, uterine fibroids, pelvic tumours, trauma, endometriosis, PID, exogenous hormones

History
- characterize bleeding (frequency, duration, number of pads/tampons, cyclicity)
- pain, if present (OPQRSTU)
- menstrual history, sexual history, STI history, syncope/pre-syncope
- details of pregnancy, including gush of fluid and fetal movement (>20 wk)

Physical Exam
- ABC (especially noting postural BP/HR and mucous membrane)
- abdominal examination (peritoneal signs, tenderness, distension, mass)
- speculum examination (NOT IF 2nd/3rd trimester bleeding; perform only when placenta previa is ruled out with U/S)
  - look for active bleeding, trauma/anomaly, and cervical dilatation
  - use sterile speculum if pregnant
- bimanual examination (cervical tenderness, size of uterus, cervical length/dilatation)
- sterile gloves if pregnant

Thrombocytopenic patients – use resorbable packs to avoid risk of re-bleeding caused by pulling out the removable pack

Complications of Nasal Packing
- Hypoxemia
- Toxic-shock syndrome
- Aspiration
- Pharyngeal fibrosis/stenosis
- Alar/septal necrosis

Vaginal bleeding can be life-threatening Always start with ABCs and ensure your patient is stable

Investigations
- β-hCG test for all patients with childbearing potential
- CBC, blood and Rh type, quantitative β-hCG, PTT, INR
- type and cross if significant blood loss
- transvaginal U/S (rule out ectopic pregnancy and spontaneous abortion)
- abdominal U/S (rule out placenta previa and fetal demise)
- postpartum
  - U/S for retained products
  - β-hCG if concerned about retained tissue

Management
- ABCs
- pulse oximeter and cardiac monitors if unstable
- Rh immune globulin (Rhogam®) for vaginal bleeding in pregnancy and Rh-negative mother
- 1st/2nd trimester pregnancy
  - ectopic pregnancy: definitive treatment with surgery or methotrexate
  - intrauterine pregnancy, no concerns of coexistent ectopic: discharge patient with obstetrics follow-up
  - U/S indeterminate or β-hCG >1,000-2,000 IU: further workup and/or gynecology consult
  - abortions: if complete, discharge if stable; for all others, acquire gynecology consult
- 2nd/3rd trimester pregnancy
  - placenta previa or placental abruption: obstetrics consult for possible admission
- postpartum
  - manage ABCs: start 2 large bore IV rapid infusion, type and cross 4 units of blood, consult OB/GYN immediately
- non-pregnant
  - dysfunctional uterine bleeding (prolonged or heavy flow ± breakthrough bleeding and without ovulation, a diagnosis of exclusion)
    - <35-40 yr of age: Provera® 10 mg PO OD x 10 d, warn patient of a withdrawal bleed, discharge if stable
    - if unstable, admit for IV hormonal therapy, possible D&C
    - >35-40 yr of age: uterine sampling necessary prior to initiation of hormonal treatment to rule out endometrial cancer, U/S for any masses felt on exam
    - tranexamic acid (Cyklokapron®) to stabilize clots
  - structural abnormalities: fibroids or uterine tumours may require excision for diagnosis/treatment, U/S for workup of other pelvic masses, Pap smear/biopsy for cervical lesions

Disposition
- decision to admit or discharge should be based on the stability of the patient, as well as the nature of the underlying cause; consult gynecology for admitted patients
- if patient can be safely discharged, ensure follow-up with family physician or gynecologist
- instruct patient to return to ED for increased bleeding, presyncope

Need β-hCG ≥1,200 to see intrauterine changes on transvaginal U/S

An ectopic pregnancy can be ruled out by confirming an intrauterine pregnancy by bedside U/S unless the patient is using IVF due to the high risk of heterotopic pregnancy

Vaginal bleeding (and its underlying causes) can be a very distressing event for patients; ensure appropriate support is provided

Pregnant Patient in the ED

Table 25. Complications of Pregnancy

Trimester	Fetal	Maternal

First 1-12 wk	Pregnancy failure
	    Spontaneous abortion
	    Fetal demise
	    Gestational trophoblastic disease
		Ectopic pregnancy
		Anemia
		Hyperemesis gravidarum
		UTI/pyelonephritis

Second 13-27 wk	Disorders of fetal growth
	    IUGR
	    Oligo/polyhydramnios
		Gestational DM
		Rh incompatibility
		UTI/pyelonephritis

Third 28-41 wk	Vasa previa	Preterm labour/PPROM Preeclampsia/eclampsia Placenta previa Placental abruption Uterine rupture DVT

Nephrolithiasis (Renal Colic)

- see Urology, U17

Epidemiology and Risk Factors
- 10% of population (twice as common in males)
- recurrence 50% at 5 yr
- peak incidence 30-50 yr of age
- 75% of stones <5 mm pass spontaneously within 2 wk, larger stones may require consultation

Clinical Features
- urinary obstruction → upstream distention of ureter or collecting system → severe colicky pain
- may complain of pain at flank, groin, testes, or tip of penis
- writhing, never comfortable, N/V, hematuria (90% microscopic), diaphoresis, tachycardia, tachypnea
- occasionally symptoms of trigonal irritation (frequency, urgency)
- fever, chills, rigors in secondary pyelonephritis
- peritoneal findings/anterior abdominal tenderness usually absent

Differential Diagnosis of Renal Colic
- acute ureteric obstruction
- acute abdomen: biliary, bowel, pancreas, AAA
- urogynecological: ectopic pregnancy, torsion/rupture of ovarian cyst, testicular torsion
- pyelonephritis (fever, chills, pyuria, vomiting)
- radiculitis (L1): herpes zoster, nerve root compression

Investigations
- screening
- CBC: elevated WBC in presence of fever suggests infection
- electrolytes, Cr, BUN to assess renal function
- U/A: R&M (WBCs, RBCs, crystals), C&S
- imaging
- non-contrast spiral CT is the study of choice
- abdominal U/S may demonstrate stone or hydronephrosis (consider in females of childbearing age)
- AXR will identify large radiopaque stones (calcium, struvite, and cystine stones) but may miss smaller stones, uric acid stones, or stones overlying bony structures; consider as an initial investigation in patients who have a history of radioopaque stones and similar episodes of acute flank pain (CT necessary if film is negative)
- strain all urine stone analysis

Management
- analgesics: NSAIDs (usually ketorolac [Toradol®], preferable over opioids), antiemetics, IV fluids
- urology consult may be indicated, especially if stone >5 mm, or if patient has signs of obstruction or infection
- α-blocker (e.g. tamsulosin) may be helpful to increase stone passage in select cases

Disposition
- most patients can be discharged
- ensure patient is stable, has adequate analgesia, and is able to tolerate oral medications
- may advise hydration and limitation of protein, sodium, oxalate, and alcohol intake

---

Ophthalmologic Emergencies

- see Ophthalmology, OP5

History and Physical Exam
- patient may complain of pain, tearing, itching, redness, photophobia, foreign body sensation, trauma
- mechanism of foreign body insertion – if high velocity injury suspected (welding, metal grinding, metal striking metal), must obtain orbital X-rays, U/S, or CT scan to exclude presence of intraocular metallic foreign body
- visual acuity in both eyes, pupils, extraocular structures, fundoscopy, tonometry, slit lamp exam

Management of Ophthalmologic Foreign Body
- copious irrigation with saline for any foreign body
- remove foreign body under slit lamp exam with cotton swab or sterile needle
- antibiotic drops qid until healed
- patching may not improve healing or comfort – do not patch contact lens wearers
- limit use of topical anesthetic to examination only
- consider tetanus prophylaxis
- ophthalmology consult if globe penetration suspected

Kidney Stones
- 80% Calcium oxalate
- 10% Struvite
- 10% Uric acid

Obstruction + Infection
= Urological Emergency
Urgent urology consult

Indications for Admission to Hospital
- Intractable pain
- Fever (suggests infection) or other evidence of pyelonephritis
- Single kidney with ureteral obstruction
- Bilateral obstructing stones
- Intractable vomiting
- Compromised renal function

Visual acuity is the "vital sign" of the eyes and should ALWAYS be assessed and documented in both eyes when a patient presents to the ER with an ophthalmologic complaint

Table 26. Differential Diagnosis of Red Eye in the Emergency Department

Symptom	Possible Serious Etiology
Light sensitivity	Iritis, keratitis, abrasion, ulcer
Unilateral	Above + herpes simplex, acute angle closure glaucoma
Significant pain	Above + scleritis
White spot on cornea	Corneal ulcer
Non-reactive pupil	Acute glaucoma, iritis
Copious discharge	Gonococcal conjunctivitis
Blurred vision	All of the above

Contraindications to Pupil Dilation
- Shallow anterior chamber
- Iris-supported lens implant
- Potential neurological abnormality requiring pupillary evaluation
- Caution with CV disease – mydriatics can cause tachycardia

Table 27. Select Ophthalmologic Emergencies

Condition	Signs and Symptoms	Management
Acute Angle Closure Glaucoma	Unilateral red, painful eye Decreased visual acuity, halos around lights Fixed, mid-dilated pupil N/V Marked increase in IOP (>40 mmHg) Shallow anterior chamber ± cells	Ophthalmology consult for laser iridotomy Topical β-blockers, adrenergics, and cholinergics Systemic carbonic anhydrase inhibitors and hyperosmotic agents
Chemical Burn	Known exposure to acids or alkali (worse) Pain, decreased visual acuity Vascularization or defects of cornea Iris and lens damage	Irrigate at site of accident IV NS drip in ED with eyelid retracted Swab fornices Cycloplegic drops Topical antibiotics and patching
Orbital Cellulitis	Red, painful eye, decreased visual acuity Headache, fever Lid erythema, edema, and difficulty opening eye Conjunctival injection and chemosis Proptosis, opthalmoplegia ± RAPD	Admission, ophthalmology consult Blood cultures, orbital CT IV antibiotics (ceftriaxone+ vancomycin) Drainage of abscess
Retinal Artery Occlusion	Sudden, painless, monocular vision loss RAPD Cherry red spot and retinal pallor on fundoscopy	Restore blood flow <2 h Massage globe Decrease IOP (topical β-blockers, inhaled O_2/CO_2 mix, IV Diamox®, IV mannitol, drain aqueous fluid)
Retinal Detachment	Flashes of light, floaters, and curtains of blackness/peripheral vision loss Painless Loss of red reflex, decreased IOP Detached areas are grey ± RAPD	Ophthalmology consult for scleral buckle/pneumatic retinoplexy

Other Ophthalmologic Emergencies
Infectious: Red eye, endophthalmitis, hypopyon
Trauma: Globe rupture, orbital blow-out fractures, corneal injuries, eyelid laceration, hyphema, lens dislocation, retrobulbar hemorrhage
Painful vision loss: Acute iritis, corneal abrasion, globe rupture, lens dislocation, retrobulbar hemorrhage, optic neuritis, temporal arteritis, endophthalmitis, keratitis
Painless vision loss: Central retinal vein occlusion, amaurosis fugax, occipital stroke

Dermatologic Emergencies

Rash Characteristics
A. Diffuse Rashes
- Staphylococcal Scalded Skin Syndrome (SSSS)
    - caused by an exotoxin from infecting strain of coagulase-positive *S. aureus*
    - mostly occurs in children
    - prodrome: fever, irritability, malaise, and skin tenderness
    - sudden onset of diffuse erythema: skin is red, warm, and very tender
    - flaccid bullae that are difficult to see, then desquamate in large sheets
    - Nikolsky's sign: gentle lateral stroking of skin causes epidermis to separate
- Toxic Epidermal Necrolysis (TEN): >30% of BSA
    - see <u>Dermatology</u>, D22
    - caused by drugs (e.g. phenytoin, sulfas, penicillins, and NSAIDs), bone marrow transplantation, and blood product transfusions
    - usually occurs in adults
    - diffuse erythema followed by necrosis
    - severe mucous membrane blistering
    - entire epidermis desquamation
    - high mortality (>50%)
- Toxic Shock Syndrome (TSS)
    - see <u>Infectious Diseases</u>, ID23
    - caused by superantigen from *S. aureus* or GAS activating T-cell and cytokines
    - patient often presents with onset of shock and multi-organ failure, fever
    - diffuse erythematous macular rash
    - at least 3 organ systems involved: CNS, respiratory, GI, muscular, mucous membranes, renal, liver, hematologic, and skin (necrotizing fasciitis, gangrene)

- vesicobullous lesions
- Erythema Multiforme (EM)
  - see Dermatology, D29
  - immunologic reaction to herpes simplex
  - viral prodrome 1-14 d before rash
  - "target lesion": central grey bulla or wheal surrounded by concentric rings of erythema and normal skin
- Stevens-Johnson Syndrome (SJS): <10% of BSA
  - see Dermatology, D22
  - related to drugs such as antiepileptics and biologic agents (e.g. infliximab)
  - EM with constitutional symptoms and mucous membrane involvement (milder mucous membrane involvement than TEN)

B. Discrete Lesions
- pyoderma gangrenosum
  - often associated with immunocompromised patients (HIV, leukemia, or lymphoma) with Gram-negative sepsis
  - often occurs in arms, hands, feet, or perineal region
  - usually begins as painless macule/vesicle pustule/bulla on red/blue base sloughing, leaving a gangrenous ulcer
- disseminated gonococcal infection
  - see Dermatology, D32
  - fever, skin lesions (pustules/vesicles on erythematous base ~5 mm in diameter), arthritis (joint swelling and tenderness), and septic arthritis (in larger joints, such as knees, ankles, and elbows)
  - most commonly in gonococcus positive women during menstruation or pregnancy
  - skin lesions usually appear in extremities and resolve quickly (<7 d)
- meningococcemia
  - flu-like symptoms of headache, myalgia, N/V
  - petechial, macular, or maculopapular lesions with grey vesicular centres
  - usually a few millimeters in size, but may become confluent and hemorrhagic
  - usually appear in extremities, but may appear anywhere
  - look for signs of meningeal irritation: Brudzinski, Kernig, nuchal rigidity, jolt accentuation

Thorough dermatologic examinations are required; examination of asymptomatic skin may identify more lesions; ensure adequate draping during dermatologic examinations

History and Physical Exam
- determine onset, course, and location of skin lesions
- fever, joint pain
- associated symptoms: CNS, respiratory, GU, GI, renal, liver, mucous membranes
- medication history
- vitals

Investigations
- immediate consultation if patient unstable
- CBC, electrolytes, Cr, AST, ALT, ALP, blood culture, skin biopsy, serum immunoglobulin levels (serum IgE)

Management
- general: judicious IV fluids and electrolyte control, consider vasopressors if hypotensive, prevention of infection
- determine if admission and consult needed: dermatology or infectious diseases
- specific management is determined by etiology
  - SSSS, TSS, DGI, and meningococcemia
    - IV antibiotics
  - EM, SJS, and TEN
    - stop precipitating medication
    - fluids
    - symptomatic treatment: antihistamines, antacids, topical corticosteroids, systemic corticosteroids (controversial), prophylactic oral acyclovir, consider IVIG
    - TEN: debride necrotic tissue

Disposition
- most cases will require urgent care and hospitalization
- TEN: early transfer to burn centre improves outcome

Environmental Injuries

Heat Exhaustion and Heat Stroke

- predisposing factors: young persons who overexert themselves, older adults who cannot dissipate heat at rest (e.g. using anticholinergic drugs such as antihistamines or TCAs), and patients with schizophrenia who are using anticholinergic or antiepileptic medications

Heat Exhaustion
- clinical features relate to loss of circulating volume caused by exposure to heat stress
- "water depletion": heat exhaustion occurs if lost fluid not adequately replaced
- "salt depletion": heat exhaustion occurs when losses replaced with hypotonic fluid

Heat exhaustion may closely resemble heat stroke; heat exhaustion may eventually progress to heat stroke, so if diagnosis is uncertain treat as heat stroke

Heat Stroke
- life-threatening emergency resulting from failure of normal compensatory heat-shedding mechanisms
- divided into classical and exertional subtypes
- if patient does not respond relatively quickly to cooling treatments, consider other possible etiologies of hyperpyrexia (e.g. meningitis, thyroid storm, anticholinergic poisoning, delirium tremens, other infections)

Table 28. Heat Exhaustion vs. Heat Stroke

	Heat Exhaustion	Classical Heat Stroke	Exertional Heat Stroke
Clinical Features	Non-specific malaise, headache, fatigue Body temp <40.5°C (usually normal) No coma or seizures Dehydration (HR, orthostatic hypotension)	Occurs in setting of high ambient temperatures (e.g. heat wave, poor ventilation) Often patients are older, poor, and sedentary or immobile Dry, hot skin Temp usually >40.5°C Altered mental status, seizures, delirium, or coma May have elevated AST, ALT	Occurs with high endogenous heat production (e.g. exercise) that overwhelms homeostatic mechanisms Patients often younger, more active Skin often diaphoretic Other features as for classical heat stroke, but may also have DIC, acute renal failure, rhabdomyolysis, marked lactic acidosis
Treatment	Rest in a cool environment IV NS if orthostatic hypotension; otherwise replace losses slowly PO	Cool body temperature with water mist (e.g. spray bottle) and standing fans Ice water immersion also effective; monitor body temperature closely to avoid hypothermic overshoot Secure airway because of seizure and aspiration risk Give fluid resuscitation if still hypotensive after above therapy Avoid β-agonists (e.g. epinephrine), peripheral vasoconstriction, and antipyretics (e.g. ASA)	

Hypothermia and Cold Injuries

HYPOTHERMIA
- predisposing factors: extremes of age, lack of housing, drug overdose, EtOH ingestion, trauma (incapacitating), cold water immersion, outdoor sports
- treatment based on re-warming and supporting cardiorespiratory function
- complications: coagulopathy, acidosis, ventricular dysrhythmias (VFib), asystole, volume and electrolyte depletion
- labs: CBC, electrolytes, ABG, serum glucose, Cr/BUN, Mg^{2+}, Ca^{2+}, amylase, coagulation profile
- imaging: CXR (aspiration pneumonia, pulmonary edema are common)
- monitors: ECG, rectal thermometer, Foley catheter, NG tube, monitor metabolic status frequently

Afterdrop Phenomenon
Warming of extremities causes vasodilation and movement of cool pooled blood from extremities to core, resulting in a drop in core temperature leading to cardiac arrest

Table 29. Classification of Hypothermia

Class	Temp	Symptoms/Signs
Mild	32-34.9°C	Tachypnea, tachycardia, ataxia, dysarthria, shivering
Moderate	28-31.9°C	Loss of shivering, dysrhythmias, Osborne (J) waves on ECG, decreased LOC, combative behaviour, muscle rigidity, dilated pupils
Severe	<28°C	Coma, hypotension, acidemia, VFib, asystole, flaccidity, apnea

Re-warming Options
- gentle fluid and electrolyte replacement in all (due to cold diuresis)
- **passive external re-warming**
  - suitable for most stable patients with core temperature >32.2°C
  - involves covering patient with insulating blanket; body generates heat and re-warms through metabolic process, shivering

- **active external re-warming**
  - involves use of warming blankets
  - beware of "afterdrop" phenomenon
  - safer when done in conjunction with active core re-warming
- **active core re-warming**
  - generally for patients with core temperature <32.2°C, and/or with cardiovascular instability
  - avoids "afterdrop" seen with AER alone
  - re-warm core by using
    - warmed humidified oxygen, IV fluids
    - peritoneal dialysis with warm fluids
    - stric/colonic/pleural irrigation with warm fluids
    - external circulation (cardiopulmonary bypass machine) is most effective and fastest

Approach to Cardiac Arrest in the Hypothermic Patient
- do all procedures gently or may precipitate VFib
- check pulse and rhythm for at least 1 min; may have profound bradycardia
- **if any pulse at all (even very slow) do NOT do CPR**
- if in VFib try to defibrillate up to maximum 3 shocks if core temperature <30°C
- intubate if required, ventilate with warmed, humidified O₂
- medications (vasopressors, antidysrhythmics) may not be effective at low temperatures
  - controversial; may try one dose
- focus of treatment is re-warming

FROSTBITE

Classification
- ice crystals form between cells
- classified according to depth – similar to burns (1st to 3rd degree)
- 1st degree
  - symptoms: initial paresthesia, pruritus
  - signs: erythema, edema, hyperemia, no blisters
- 2nd degree
  - symptoms: numbness
  - signs: blistering (clear), erythema, edema
- 3rd degree
  - symptoms: pain, burning, throbbing (on thawing); may be painless if severe
  - signs: hemorrhagic blisters, skin necrosis, edema, no movement

Management
- treat for hypothermia: O₂, IV fluids, maintenance of body warmth
- remove wet and constrictive clothing
- immerse in 40-42°C agitated water for 10-30 min (very painful; administer adequate analgesia)
- clean injured area and leave it open to air
- consider aspiration/debridement of blisters (controversial)
- debride skin
- tetanus prophylaxis
- consider penicillin G as frost bite injury has high risk of infection
- surgical intervention may be required to release restrictive eschars
- never allow a thawed area to re-chill/freeze

Burns

- see Plastic Surgery, PL17

Clinical Presentation/Physical Exam Findings
- burn size
  - rule of nines; does not include 1st degree burns
- burn depth
  - superficial (1st degree): epidermis only (e.g. sunburn), painful and tender to palpation
  - superficial partial thickness (2nd degree): extends to epidermis and superficial dermis, blister formation occurs, very painful
  - deep partial thickness (2nd degree): involves hair follicles, sebaceous glands; skin is blistered, exposed dermis is white to yellow, absent sensation
  - full thickness (3rd degree): epidermis and all dermal layers; skin is pale, insensate, and charred or leathery
  - deep (4th degree): involvement of fat, muscle, even bone

Management
- remove noxious agent/stop burning process
- establish airway if needed (indicated with burns >40% BSA or smoke inhalation injury)
- resuscitation for 2nd and 3rd degree burns (after initiation of 2 large bore IVs)

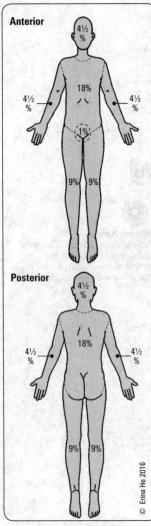

Anterior

Posterior

© Erina He 2016

Figure 15. Rule of 9s for total BSA

- fluid boluses if unstable
  - Parkland Formula: Ringer's lactate 4 cc/kg/%BSA burned; give half in first 8 h, half in next 16 h; maintenance fluids are also required if patient cannot tolerate PO hydration
  - urine output is best measure of resuscitation, should be 40-50 cc/h or 0.5 cc/kg/h; avoid diuretics
- pain relief: continuous morphine infusion with breakthrough bolus
- investigations: CBC, electrolytes, U/A, CXR, ECG, ABG, carboxyhemoglobin
- burn wound care: prevent infection, clean/debride with mild soap and water, sterile dressings
- escharotomy or fasciotomy for circumferential burns (chest, extremities)
- topical antibiotics, systemic antibiotics infrequently indicated
- tetanus prophylaxis if burn is deeper than superficial dermis

Use palm of the patient's hand to estimate 1% of BSA affected

Disposition
- admit
  - 2nd degree burns >10% BSA, or any significant 3rd degree burns
  - 2nd degree burns on face, hands, feet, perineum, or across major joints
  - electrical, chemical burns, and inhalation injury
  - burn victims with underlying medical problems or immunosuppressed patients

Burn Causes
- Thermal (flame, scald)
- Chemical
- Radiation (UV, medical/therapeutic)
- Electrical

Inhalation Injury

Etiology
- CO or cyanide poisoning
- direct thermal injury: limited to upper airway
- smoke causes bronchospasm and edema from particulate matter and toxic inhalants (tissue asphyxiates, pulmonary irritants, systemic toxins)

History and Physical Exam
- risk factors: closed space fires, period of unconsciousness, noxious chemicals involved
- cherry red skin (unreliable, usually post-mortem finding)
- singed nasal hairs, soot on oral/nasal membranes, sooty sputum
- hoarseness, stridor, dyspnea
- decreased LOC, confusion
- PO_2 normal but O_2 saturation low suggests CO poisoning

Investigations
- measure carboxyhemoglobin levels, co-oximetry
- ABG
- CXR ± bronchoscopy

Management
- CO poisoning: 100% O_2 ± hyperbaric O_2 (controversial)
- direct thermal injury: humidified oxygen, early intubation, pulmonary toilet, bronchodilators, and mucolytics (N-acetylcysteine)

Intubate early if you suspect inhalation injury, as airway can become obstructed due to edema

Bites

MAMMALIAN BITES
- see Plastic Surgery, PL10

History
- time and circumstances of bite, symptoms, allergies, tetanus immunization status, comorbid conditions, rabies risks, HIV/hepatitis risk (human bite)
- high morbidity associated with clenched fist injuries, "fight bites"

Physical Exam
- assess type of wound: abrasion, laceration, puncture, crush injury
- assess for direct tissue damage: skin, bone, tendon, neurovascular status

Investigations
- if bony injury or infection suspected, check for fracture and gas in tissue with x-rays
- get skull films in children with scalp bite wounds ± CT to rule out cranial perforation
- ultrasound may be helpful for identifying abscess formation as well as locating radiolucent foreign bodies in infected wounds

Initial Management
- wound cleansing and copious irrigation as soon as possible
- irrigate/debride puncture wounds if feasible, but not if sealed or very small openings; avoid hydrodissection along tissue planes
- debridement is important in crush injuries to reduce infection and optimize cosmetic and functional repair

- culture wound if signs of infection (erythema, necrosis, or pus); obtain anaerobic cultures if wound foul smelling, necrotizing, or abscess; notify lab that sample is from bite wound
- suturing
  - vascular structures (i.e. face and scalp) are less likely to become infected, therefore consider suturing
  - allow avascular structures (i.e. pretibial regions, hands, and feet) to heal by secondary intention
  - tetanus immunization if >10 yr or incomplete primary series

Prophylactic Antibiotics
- types of infections resulting from bites: cellulitis, lymphangitis, abscesses, tenosynovitis, osteomyelitis, septic arthritis, sepsis, endocarditis, meningitis
- a 3-5 d course of antibiotics is recommended for all bite wounds to the hand and should be considered in other bites if any high-risk factors present (efficacy not proven)
- dog and cat bites (pathogens: *Pasteurella multocida, S. aureus, S. viridans*)
  - 10-50% of cat bites, 5% of dog bites become infected
  - 1st line: amoxicillin + clavulanic acid
- human bites (pathogens: *Eikenella corrodens, S. aureus, S. viridans*, oral anaerobes)
  - 1st line: amoxicillin + clavulanic acid
- rabies (see Infectious Diseases, ID20)
  - reservoirs: warm-blooded animals except rodents, lagomorphs (e.g. rabbits)
  - post-exposure vaccine is effective; treatment depends on local prevalence

INSECT BITES
- bee stings
  - 5 types of reactions to stings (local, large local, systemic, toxic, unusual)
  - history and physical exam key to diagnosis; no lab test will confirm
  - investigations: CBC, electrolytes, BUN, Cr, glucose, ABGs, ECG
  - ABC management, epinephrine 0.1 mg IV over 5 min if shock, antihistamines, cimetidine 300 mg IV/IM/PO, steroids, β-agonists for SOB/wheezing 3 mg in 5 mL NS via nebulizer, local site management
- West Nile virus (see Infectious Diseases, ID24)

Near Drowning

- most common in children <4 yr and teenagers
- causes lung damage, hypoxemia, and may lead to hypoxic encephalopathy
- must also assess for shock, C-spine injuries, hypothermia, and scuba-related injuries (barotrauma, air emboli, lung re-expansion injury)
- complications: volume shifts, electrolyte abnormalities, hemolysis, rhabdomyolysis, renal, DIC

Physical Exam
- ABCs, vitals: watch closely for hypotension
- respiratory: rales (ARDS, pulmonary edema), decreased breath sounds (pneumothorax)
- CVS: murmurs, dysrhythmias, JVP (CHF, pneumothorax)
- H&N: assess for C-spine injuries
- neurological: GCS or AVPU, pupils, focal deficits

Investigations
- labs: CBC, electrolytes, ABGs, Cr, BUN, INR, PTT, U/A (drug screen, myoglobin)
- imaging: CXR (pulmonary edema, pneumothorax) ± C-spine imaging
- ECG

Management
- ABCs, treat for trauma, shock, hypothermia
- cardiac and O_2 monitors, IV access
- intensive respiratory care
  - ventilator assistance if decreased respirations, pCO_2 >50 mmHg, or pO_2 <60 mmHg on maximum O_2
  - may require intubation for airway protection, ventilation, pulmonary toilet
  - high flow O_2/CPAP/BiPAP may be adequate but some may need mechanical ventilation with positive end-expiratory pressure
- dysrhythmias: usually respond to corrections of hypoxemia, hypothermia, and acidosis
- vomiting: very common, NG suction to avoid aspiration
- convulsions: usually respond to O_2; if not, diazepam 5-10 mg IV slowly
- bronchospasm: bronchodilators
- bacterial pneumonia: prophylactic antibiotics not necessary unless contaminated water or hot tub (*Pseudomonas*)
- always initiate CPR in drowning-induced cardiac arrest even if patient hypothermic; continue CPR until patient is fully rewarmed

Disposition
- non-significant submersion: discharge after short observation
- significant submersion (even if asymptomatic): long period of observation (24 h) as pulmonary edema may appear late
- CNS symptoms or hypoxemia: admit
- severe hypoxemia, decreased LOC: ICU

> "Secondary drowning" where the onset of symptoms, as a result of pulmonary edema or infection, can be insidious, developing over hours, or possibly even days, must be anticipated in the near drowning patient

Toxicology

"ABCD₃EFG" of Toxicology

- basic axiom of care is symptomatic and supportive treatment
- address underlying problem only once patient is stable

A	Airway (consider stabilizing the C-spine)
B	Breathing
C	Circulation
D1	Drugs
	• ACLS as necessary to resuscitate the patient
	• universal antidotes
D2	Draw bloods
D3	Decontamination (decrease absorption)
E	Expose (look for specific toxidromes)/Examine the patient
F	Full vitals, ECG monitor, Foley, X-rays
G	Give specific antidotes and treatments

- reassess
- call Poison Information Centre
- obtain corroborative history from family, bystanders

Principles of Toxicology
4 principles to consider with all ingestions:
- Resuscitation (ABCD₃EFG)
- Screening (toxidrome? clinical clues?)
- Decrease absorption of drug
- Increase elimination of drug

D1 – Universal Antidotes

- treatments that will not harm patients and may be essential

Dextrose (glucose)
- give to any patient presenting with altered LOC
- measure blood glucose prior to glucose administration if possible
- adults: 0.5-1.0 g/kg (1-2 mL/kg) IV of D50W
- children: 0.25 g/kg (2-4 mL/kg) IV of D25W

Universal Antidotes

DONT
Dextrose
Oxygen
Naloxone
Thiamine (must give BEFORE dextrose)

Oxygen
- do not deprive a hypoxic patient of oxygen no matter what the antecedent medical history (i.e. even COPD with CO_2 retention)
- if depression of hypoxic drive, intubate and ventilate
- exception: paraquat or diquat (herbicides) inhalation or ingestion (oxygen radicals increase morbidity)

Naloxone (central μ-receptor competitive antagonist, shorter t1/2 than naltrexone)
- antidote for opioids: administration is both diagnostic and therapeutic (1 min onset of action)
- used for the undifferentiated comatose patient
- loading dose
  - adults
    - response to naloxone can be drastic, so stepwise delivery of initial 2 mg bolus is recommended
    - draw up 2 mg to deliver IV/IM/SL/SC or via ETT (ETT dose = 2-2.5x IV dose)
      - 1st dose 0.4 mg
      - if no response, deliver second dose 0.6 mg
      - if still no response, deliver remaining 1 mg
  - child
    - 0.01 mg/kg initial bolus IV/IO/ETT
    - 0.1 mg/kg if no response and opioid still suspected to max of 10 mg
  - maintenance dose
    - may be required because half-life of naloxone (30-80 min) is much shorter than many opioids
    - hourly infusion rate at 2/3 of initial dose that allowed patient to be roused

> Administration of naloxone can cause opioid withdrawal in chronic users:
> **Minor** withdrawal may present as lacrimation, rhinorrhea, diaphoresis, yawning, piloerection, HTN, and tachycardia
> **Severe** withdrawal may present as hot and cold flashes, arthralgias, myalgias, N/V, and abdominal cramps

Thiamine (Vitamin B1)
- 100 mg IV/IM with IV/PO glucose to all patients
- given to prevent/treat Wernicke's encephalopathy
- a necessary cofactor for glucose metabolism (may worsen Wernicke's encephalopathy if glucose given before thiamine), but do not delay glucose if thiamine unavailable
- must assume all undifferentiated comatose patients are at risk

Populations at Risk for Thiamine Deficiency
- Alcoholics
- Anorexics
- Hyperemesis of pregnancy
- Malnutrition states

D2 – Draw Bloods

- essential tests
  - CBC, electrolytes, BUN/Cr, glucose, INR/PTT, osmolality
  - ABGs, measure O_2 sat
  - ASA, acetaminophen, EtOH levels
- potentially useful tests
  - drug levels – this is NOT a serum drug screen
  - Ca^{2+}, Mg^{2+}, PO_4^{3-}
  - protein, albumin, lactate, ketones, liver enzymes, CK – depending on drug and clinical presentation

Serum Drug Levels

- treat the patient, not the drug level
- negative toxicology screen does not rule out a toxic ingestion – signifies only that the specific drugs tested were not detectable in the specimen
- specific drugs available on general screen vary by institution; check before ordering
- urine screens also available (qualitative only)

Urine drug screen is costly and generally not helpful in the ED management of the poisoned patient

Table 30. Toxic Gaps (see Nephrology, NP16)

METABOLIC ACIDOSIS

Increased AG: "MUDPILES CAT" (* = toxic)
Methanol*
Uremia
Diabetic ketoacidosis/Starvation ketoacidosis
Phenformin*/Paraldehyde*
Isoniazid, Iron, Ibuprofen
Lactate (anything that causes seizures or shock)
Ethylene glycol*
Salicylates*
Cyanide, CO*
Alcoholic ketoacidosis
Toluene, theophylline*

Increased POG: "MAE DIE" (if it ends in "-ol", it will likely increase the POG)
Methanol
Acetone
Ethanol
Diuretics (glycerol, mannitol, sorbitol)
Isopropanol
Ethylene glycol

Note: normal POG does not rule out toxic alcohol; only an elevated gap is helpful

Decreased AG
Electrolyte imbalance (increased $Na^+/K^+/Mg^{2+}$)
Hypoalbuminemia (50% fall in albumin ~5.5 mmol/L decrease in the AG)
Lithium, bromine elevation
Paraproteins (multiple myeloma)

Increased O_2 saturation gap
Carboxyhemoglobin
Methemoglobin
Sulfmethemoglobin

Normal AG
High K^+: pyelonephritis, obstructive nephropathy, renal tubular acidosis IV, TPN
Low K^+: small bowel losses, acetazolamide, renal tubular acidosis I, II

Anion Gap
= $Na^+ - Cl^- - HCO_3^-$
Normal AG ≤12 mM/L

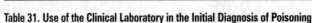

Table 31. Use of the Clinical Laboratory in the Initial Diagnosis of Poisoning

Test	Finding	Selected Causes
ABG	Hypoventilation (pCO₂) Hyperventilation (pCO₂)	CNS depressants (opioids, sedative-hypnotic agents, phenothiazines, EtOH) Salicylates, CO, other asphyxiants
Electrolytes	AG metabolic acidosis Hyperkalemia Hypokalemia	"MUDPILES CAT": see Table 30 Digitalis glycosides, fluoride, potassium Theophylline, caffeine, β-adrenergic agents, soluble barium salts, diuretics, insulin
Glucose	Hypoglycemia	Oral hypoglycemic agents, insulin, EtOH, ASA
Osmolality and Osmolar Gap	Elevated osmolar gap	"MAE DIE": see Table 30
ECG	Wide QRS complex Prolonged QT interval Atrioventricular block	TCAs, quinidine, other class Ia and Ic antidysrhythmic agents Terfenadine, astemizole, antipsychotics Ca^{2+} antagonists, digitalis glycosides, phenylpropanolamine
Abdominal X-Ray	Radioopaque pills or objects	"CHIPES": Calcium, Chloral hydrate, CCl₄, Heavy metals, Iron, Potassium, Enteric coated Salicylates, and some foreign bodies
Serum Acetaminophen	Elevated level (>140 mg/L or 1,000 μmol/L 4 h after ingestion)	May be only sign of acetaminophen poisoning

D3 – Decontamination and Enhanced Elimination

Ocular Decontamination
- saline irrigation to neutralize pH; alkali exposure requires ophthalmology consult

Dermal Decontamination (Wear Protective Gear)
- remove clothing, brush off toxic agents, irrigate all external surfaces

Gastrointestinal Decontamination
- single dose activated charcoal
  - adsorption of drug/toxin to activated charcoal prevents availability
  - contraindications: caustics, small bowel obstruction, perforation
  - dose: 10 g/g drug ingested or 1g/kg body weight
  - odourless, tasteless, prepared as slurry with H_2O
- whole bowel irrigation
  - 500 mL/h (child) to 2,000 mL/h (adult) of polyethylene glycol solution by mouth until clear effluent per rectum
  - start slow (500 mL in an adult) and aim to increase rate hourly as tolerated
  - indications
    - awake, alert, can be nursed upright OR intubated and airway protected
    - delayed release product
    - drug/toxin not bound to charcoal
    - drug packages (if any evidence of breakage emergency surgery)
    - recent toxin ingestion
- contraindications
  - evidence of ileus, perforation, or obstruction
- surgical removal in extreme cases
  - indicated for drugs that are toxic, form concretions, or cannot be removed by conventional means
- no evidence for the routine use of cathartics (i.e. ipecac)

Urine Alkalinization
- may be used for: ASA, methotrexate, phenobarbital, chlorpropamide
- weakly acidic substances can be trapped in alkali urine (pH >7.5) to increase elimination

Multidose Activated Charcoal
- may be used for: carbamazepine, phenobarbital, quinine, theophylline
- for toxins which undergo enterohepatic recirculation
- removes drug that has already been absorbed by drawing it back into GI tract
- various regimens: 12.5 g (1/4 bottle) PO q1h or 25 g (1/2 bottle) PO q2h until non-toxic

Hemodialysis
- indications/criteria for hemodialysis
  - toxins that have high water solubility, low protein binding, low molecular weight, adequate concentration gradient, small volume of distribution, or rapid plasma equilibration
  - removal of toxin will lead to clinical improvement
  - advantage is shown over other modes of therapy
  - predicted that drug or metabolite will have toxic effects
  - impairment of normal routes of elimination (cardiac, renal, or hepatic)
  - clinical deterioration despite maximal medical support
- useful for the following toxins

- methanol
- ethylene glycol
- salicylates
- lithium
- phenobarbital
- chloral hydrate (trichloroethanol)

- others include theophylline, carbamazepine, valproate, methotrexate

E – Expose and Examine the Patient

- vital signs (including temperature), skin (needle tracks, colour), mucous membranes, pupils, odours, and CNS
- head-to-toe survey including
  - C-spine
  - signs of trauma, seizures (incontinence, "tongue biting", etc.), infection (meningismus), or chronic alcohol/drug abuse (track marks, nasal septum erosion)
- mental status

Table 32. Specific Toxidromes

Toxidrome	Overdose Signs and Symptoms		Examples of Drugs
Anticholinergic	Hyperthermia	"Hot as a hare"	Antidepressants (e.g. TCAs)
	Dilated pupils	"Blind as a bat"	Cyclobenzaprine (Flexeril®)
	Dry skin	"Dry as a bone"	Carbamazepine
	Vasodilation	"Red as a beet"	Antihistamines (e.g. diphenhydramine)
	Agitation/hallucinations	"Mad as a hatter"	Antiparkinsonians
	Ileus	"The bowel and bladder	Antipsychotics
	Urinary retention	lose their tone and the	Antispasmodics
	Tachycardia	heart goes on alone"	Belladonna alkaloids (e.g. atropine)
Cholinergic	"DUMBELS"		Natural plants: mushrooms, trumpet flower
	Diaphoresis, **D**iarrhea, **D**ecreased BP		Anticholinesterases: physostigmine
	Urination		Insecticides (organophosphates, carbamates)
	Miosis		Nerve gases
	Bronchospasm, **B**ronchorrhea, **B**radycardia		
	Emesis, **E**xcitation of skeletal muscle		
	Lacrimation		
	Salivation, **S**eizures		
Extrapyramidal	Dysphonia, dysphagia		Major tranquilizers
	Rigidity and tremor		Antipsychotics
	Motor restlessness, crawling sensation (akathisia)		
	Constant movements (dyskinesia)		
	Dystonia (muscle spasms, laryngospasm, trismus, oculogyric crisis, torticollis)		
Hemoglobin Derangements	Increased respiratory rate		CO poisoning (carboxyhemoglobin)
	Decreased LOC		Drug ingestion (methemoglobin, sulfmethemoglobin)
	Seizures		
	Cyanosis unresponsive to O_2		
	Lactic acidosis		
Opioid, Sedative/ Hypnotic, EtOH	Hypothermia		EtOH
	Hypotension		Benzodiazepines
	Respiratory depression		Opioids (morphine, heroin, fentanyl, etc.)
	Dilated or constricted pupils (pinpoint in opioid)		Barbiturates
	CNS depression		Gamma hydroxybutyrate
Sympathomimetic	Increased temperature		Amphetamines, caffeine, cocaine, LSD, phencyclidine
	CNS excitation (including seizures)		Ephedrine and other decongestants
	Tachycardia, HTN		Thyroid hormone
	N/V		Sedative or EtOH withdrawal
	Diaphoresis		
	Dilated pupils		
Serotonin Syndrome	Mental status changes, autonomic hyperactivity, neuromuscular abnormalities, hyperthermia, diarrhea, HTN		MAOI, TCA, SSRI, opiate analgesics Cough medicine, weight reduction medications

Note: ASA poisoning and hypoglycemia mimic sympathomimetic toxidrome

F – Full Vitals, ECG Monitor, Foley, X-Rays

G – Give Specific Antidotes and Treatments

Urine Alkalinization Treatment for ASA Overdose
- urine pH >7.5
- fluid resuscitate first, then 3 amps $NaHCO_3$/L of D5W at 1.5x maintenance
- add 20-40 mEq/L KCl if patient is able to urinate

Table 33. Protocol for Warfarin Overdose

INR	Management: Consider Prothrombin Complex Concentrate (Octaplex®, Beriplex®) for any elevated INR, AND either life-threatening bleeding, or a plan for the patient to undergo a surgical procedure within the next 6 h
<5.0	Cessation of warfarin administration, observation, serial INR/PT
5.1–9.0	If no risk factors for bleeding, hold warfarin x 1-2 d and reduce maintenance dose OR Vitamin K 1-2 mg PO if patient at increased risk of bleeding
9.1–20.0	Hold warfarin, vitamin K 2-4 mg PO, serial INR/PT, additional vitamin K if necessary
>20.0	Hold warfarin, vitamin K 10 mg IV over 10 min, increase vitamin K dosing (q4h) if needed

Table 34. Specific Antidotes and Treatments for Common Toxins*

Toxin	Treatment	Considerations
Acetaminophen	Decontaminate (activated charcoal) N-acetylcysteine	Often clinically silent; evidence of liver/renal damage delayed >24 h Toxic dose >200 mg/kg (>7.5 g adult) Monitor drug level 4 h post-ingestion; also liver enzymes, INR, PTT, BUN, Cr Hypoglycemia, metabolic acidosis, encephalopathy poor prognosis
Acute Dystonic Reaction	Benztropine: 1-2 mg IM/IV then 2 mg PO x 3 d OR Diphenhydramine 1-2 mg/kg IV, then 25 mg PO qid x 3 d	Benztropine (Cogentin®) has euphoric effect and potential for abuse
Anticholinergics	Decontaminate (activated charcoal) Supportive care	Special antidotes available; consult Poison Information Centre
ASA	Decontaminate (activated charcoal) Alkalinize urine; want urine pH >7.5	Monitor serum pH and drug levels closely Monitor K^+ level; may require supplement for urine alkalinization Hemodialysis may be needed if intractable metabolic acidosis, very high levels, or end-organ damage (i.e. unable to diurese)
Benzodiazepines	Decontaminate (activated charcoal) Flumazenil Supportive care	
β-blockers	Decontaminate (activated charcoal) Consider high dose insulin euglycemia therapy Some dialyzable, some use intralipids	Consult Poison Information Centre
Calcium Channel Blockers	Decontaminate (activated charcoal) $CaCl_2$ 1-4 g of 10% solution IV if hypotensive Other: high dose insulin euglycemia inotropes or intralipids	Order ECG, electrolytes (especially Ca^{2+}, Mg^{2+}, Na^+, K^+)
Cocaine	Decontaminate (activated charcoal) if oral Aggressive supportive care	Beta-blockers are contraindicated in acute cocaine toxicity Intralipid for life-threatening symptoms
CO Poisoning	See Inhalation Injury, ER47 Supportive care 100% O_2	
Cyanide	Hydroxocobalamin	
Digoxin	Decontaminate (activated charcoal) Digoxin-specific Ab fragments 10-20 vials IV if acute; 3-6 if chronic 1 vial (40 mg) neutralizes 0.5 mg of toxin	Use for life-threatening dysrhythmias unresponsive to conventional therapy, 6 h serum digoxin >12 nmol/L, initial K^+ >5 mmol/L, ingestion >10 mg (adult)/>4 mg (child) Common dysrhythmias include VFib, VTach, and conduction blocks
Ethanol	Thiamine 100 mg IM/IV Manage airway and circulatory support	Hypoglycemia very common in children Mouthwash = 70% EtOH; perfumes and colognes = 40-60% EtOH Order serum EtOH level and glucose level; treat glucose level appropriately
Ethylene Glycol/ Methanol	Fomepizole (4-methylpyrazole) 15 mg/kg IV load over 30 min, then 10 mg/kg q12h OR Ethanol (10%) 10 mL/kg over 30 min, then 1.5 mL/h	CBC, electrolytes, glucose, ethanol level Consider hemodialysis
Heparin	Protamine sulfate 25-50 mg IV	For unfractionated heparin overdose only
Insulin IM/SC/ Oral Hypoglycemic	Glucose IV/PO/NG tube Glucagon: 1-2 mg IM (if no access to glucose)	Glyburide carries highest risk of hypoglycemia among oral agents Consider octreotide for oral hypoglycemics (50-100 μg SC q6h) in these cases; consult local Poison Information Centre
MDMA	Decontaminate (activated charcoal), supportive care	Monitor CK; treat rhabdomyolysis with high flow fluids: aggressive external cooling for hyperthermia
Opioids	See Universal Antidotes, ER49	
TCAs	Decontaminate (activated charcoal) Aggressive supportive care $NaHCO_3$ bolus for wide QRS/seizures	Flumazenil antidote contraindicated in combined TCA and benzodiazepine overdose Also consider cardiac and hypotension support, seizure control Intralipid therapy (consult local Poison Information Centre)

* Call local Poison Information Centre for specific doses and treatment recommendations

Alcohol Related Emergencies

- see Psychiatry, PS23

Acute Intoxication
- slurred speech, CNS depression, disinhibition, lack of coordination
- nystagmus, diplopia, dysarthria, ataxia may progress to coma
- hypotension (peripheral vasodilation)
- if obtunded, rule out
  - head trauma/intracranial hemorrhage
  - associated depressants/street drugs, toxic alcohols
    - may also contribute to respiratory/cardiac depression
  - hypoglycemia (screen with bedside glucometer)
  - hepatic encephalopathy: confusion, altered LOC, coma
    - precipitating factors: GI bleed, infection, sedation, electrolyte abnormalities, protein meal
  - Wernicke's encephalopathy (ataxia, ophthalmoplegia, delirium)
  - post-ictal state, basilar stroke

Withdrawal
- beware of withdrawal signs
- treatment
  - diazepam 10-20 mg IV/PO or lorazepam 2-4 mg IV/PO q1h until calm
    - frequency of dosing may have to be increased depending on clinical response
  - may use CIWA protocol and give benzodiazepines as above until CIWA <10
  - thiamine 100 mg IM/IV then 50-100 mg/d
  - magnesium sulfate 4 g IV over 1-2 h (if hypomagnesemic)
  - admit patients with DT or multiple seizures

Table 35. Alcohol Withdrawal Signs

Time Since Last Drink	Syndrome	Description
6-8 h	Mild withdrawal	Generalized tremor, anxiety, agitation, but no delirium Autonomic hyperactivity (sinus tachycardia), insomnia, N/V
1-2 d	Alcoholic hallucinations	Visual (most common), auditory, and tactile hallucinations Vitals often normal
8 h-2 d	Withdrawal seizures	Typically brief generalized tonic-clonic seizures May have several within a few hours CT head if focal seizures have occurred
3-5 d	DT	5% of untreated withdrawal patients Severely confused state, fluctuating LOC Agitation, insomnia, hallucinations/delusions, tremor Tachycardia, hyperpyrexia, diaphoresis High mortality rate

Cardiovascular Complications
- HTN
- cardiomyopathy: SOB, edema
- dysrhythmias ("holiday heart")
- AFib (most common), atrial flutter, SVT, VTach (especially Torsades if hypomagnesemic/hypokalemic)

Metabolic Abnormalities
- alcoholic ketoacidosis
  - AG metabolic acidosis, urine ketones, low glucose, and normal osmolality
  - history of chronic alcohol intake with abrupt decrease/cessation
  - malnourished, abdominal pain with N/V
  - treatment: dextrose, thiamine (100 mg IM/IV prior to dextrose), volume repletion (with NS)
  - generally resolves in 12-24 h
- other alcohols
  - ethylene glycol CNS, CVS, renal findings
  - methanol
    - early: lethargy, confusion
    - late: headache, visual changes, N/V, abdominal pain, tachypnea
  - both ethylene glycol and methanol produce severe metabolic acidosis with anion gap (as the alcohol is metabolized) and osmolar gap (initially after ingestion but before metabolism)
  - EtOH co-ingestion is protective

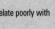

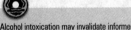
Alcohol levels correlate poorly with intoxication

Alcohol intoxication may invalidate informed consent

Common Deficiencies
- Thiamine
- Niacin
- Folate
- Glycogen
- Magnesium
- Potassium

CIWA Withdrawal Symptoms
- N/V
- Tremor
- Paroxysmal sweats
- Anxiety
- Agitation
- Visual disturbances
- Tactile disturbances
- Auditory disturbances
- Headache
- Disorientation

10 symptoms each scored out of 7 except orientation is out of 4

- treatment
  - urgent hemodialysis required
  - fomepizole 15 mg/kg IV bolus OR EtOH 10% IV bolus and infusion to achieve blood level of 22 mmol/L (EtOH loading may be done PO)
  - consider folic acid for methanol, and pyridoxine and thiamine for ethylene glycol – both help reduce conversion to active metabolites
- other abnormalities associated with alcohol: hypomagnesemia, hypophosphatemia, hypocalcemia, hypoglycemia, hypokalemia

Gastrointestinal Abnormalities
- gastritis
  - common cause of abdominal pain and GI bleed in chronic alcohol users
- pancreatitis
  - serum amylase very unreliable in patients with chronic pancreatitis, may need serum lipase
  - hemorrhagic form (15%) associated with increased mortality
  - fluid resuscitation very important
- hepatitis
  - AST/ALT ratio >2 suggests alcohol as the cause as well as elevated GGT with acute ingestion
- peritonitis/spontaneous bacterial peritonitis
  - leukocytosis, fever, generalized abdominal pain/tenderness
  - occasionally accompanies cirrhosis
  - paracentesis for diagnosis (common pathogens: *E. coli*, *Klebsiella*, *Streptococcus*)
- GI bleeds
  - most commonly gastritis or ulcers, even if patient known to have varices
  - consider Mallory-Weiss tear secondary to retching
  - often complicated by underlying coagulopathies
  - minor: treat with antacids
  - severe or recurrent: endoscopy

Disposition
- before patient leaves ED ensure stable vital signs, can walk unassisted, and fully oriented
- offer social services to find shelter or detox program
- ensure patient can obtain any medications prescribed and can complete any necessary follow-up

Approach to the Overdose Patient

History
- age, weight, underlying medical problems, medications
- substance and how much
- time and symptoms since exposure determines prognosis and need for decontamination
- route
- intention, suicidality

Physical Exam
- focus on: ABCs, LOC/GCS, vitals, pupils

Suspect Overdose when
- Altered LOC/coma
- Young patient with life-threatening dysrhythmia
- Trauma patient
- Bizarre or puzzling clinical presentation

Disposition from the Emergency Department

- methanol, ethylene glycol
  - delayed onset, admit and watch clinical and biochemical markers
- TCAs
  - prolonged/delayed cardiotoxicity warrants admission to monitored (ICU) bed
  - if asymptomatic and no clinical signs of intoxication: 6 h ED observation adequate with proper decontamination and no ECG abnormalities
  - sinus tachycardia alone (most common finding) with history of overdose warrants observation in ED
- hydrocarbons/smoke inhalation
  - pneumonitis may lag 6-8 h
  - consider observation for repeated clinical and radiographic examination
- ASA, acetaminophen
  - if borderline level, get second level 2-4 h after first
  - for ASA, must have at least 2 levels going down before discharge (3 levels minimum)
- oral hypoglycemics
  - admit all patients for minimum 24 h if hypoglycemic and 12 h after last octreotide dose
  - observe asymptomatic patient for at least 8 h

Psychiatric Consultation
- once patient medically cleared, arrange psychiatric intervention if required
- beware – suicidal ideation may not be expressed

Psychiatric Emergencies

Approach to Common Psychiatric Presentations

- see Psychiatry, PS4
- before seeing patient, ensure your own safety; have security/police available if necessary

History
- safety
  - assess suicidality: suicidal ideation (SI), intent, plan, lethal means, and past attempts
  - assess homicidality: homicidal ideation (HI), access to weapons, intended victim, and history of violence
  - driving and children
  - command hallucinations
- identify current stressors and coping strategies
- mood symptoms: manic, depressive
- anxiety: panic attacks, generalized anxiety, phobias, obsessive-compulsive disorder, post-traumatic stress disorder
- psychotic symptoms: delusions, hallucinations, disorganized speech, disorganized or catatonic behaviour, negative symptoms (affective flattening, alogia, avolition)
- substance use history: most recent use, amount, previous withdrawal reactions
- past psychiatric history, medications, adherence with medications
- medical history: obtain collateral if available

Physical Exam
- complete physical exam focusing on: vitals, neurological exam, signs of head trauma, signs of drug toxicity, signs of metabolic disorder
- mental status exam: general appearance, behaviour, cooperation, speech, mood and affect, thought content and form, perceptual disturbances, cognition (including MMSE if indicated), judgment, insight, reliability

Investigations
- investigations vary with age, established psychiatric diagnosis vs. first presentation, history and physical suggestive of organic cause
- as indicated: blood glucose, urine and serum toxicology screen, pregnancy test, electrolytes, TSH, AST/ALT, bilirubin, serum Cr, BUN, and osmolality
- blood levels of psychiatric medications
- CT head if suspect neurological etiology
- LP if indicated

Key Functions of Emergency Psychiatric Assessment
- Is the patient medically stable?
- Rule out medical cause
- Is psychiatric consult needed?
- Are there safety issues (SI, HI)?
- Is patient certifiable? (must demonstrate risk [present/past test] and apparent mental illness [future test])

Psychiatric Review of Systems

MOAPS
Mood
Organic
Anxiety
Psychosis
Safety
intoxication

Acute Psychosis

Differential Diagnosis
- primary psychotic disorder (e.g. schizophrenia)
- secondary to medical condition (e.g. delirium)
- drugs: substance intoxication or withdrawal, medications (e.g. steroids, anticholinergics)
- infectious (CNS)
- metabolic (hypoglycemic, hepatic, renal, thyroid)
- structural (hemorrhage, neoplasm)

Management
- violence prevention
  - remain calm, empathic, and reassuring
  - ensure safety of staff and patients, have extra staff and/or security on hand
  - patients demonstrating escalating agitation or overt violent behaviour may require physical restraint and/or chemical tranquilization
- treat agitation: whenever possible, offer medication to patients as opposed to administering with force (helps calm and engage patient)
  - benzodiazepines: lorazepam 2 mg PO/IM/SL
  - antipsychotics: olanzapine 5 mg PO, haloperidol 5 mg PO/IM
- treat underlying medical condition
- psychiatry or Crisis Intervention Team consult

Suicidal Patient

Epidemiology
- attempted suicide F>M, completed suicide M>F
- second leading cause of death in people <24 yr

Management
- ensure patient safety: close observation, remove potentially dangerous objects from person and room
- assess thoughts (ideation), means, action (preparatory, practice attempts), previous attempts
- admit if there is evidence of intent and organized plan, access to lethal means, psychiatric disorder, intoxication (suicidal ideation may resolve with few days of abstinence)
- patient may require certification if unwilling to stay voluntarily
- do not start long-term medications in the ED
- psychiatry or Crisis Intervention Team consult

See Psychiatry, Common Forms, PS50 for certification (involuntary assessment/admission) considerations

High Risk Patients

SAD PERSONS
Sex = male
Age >45 yr old
Depression
Previous attempts
Ethanol use
Rational thinking loss
Suicide in family
Organized plan
No spouse, no support system
Serious illness

Common Pediatric ED Presentations

Modified Glasgow Coma Score

Table 36. Modified GCS

Modified GCS for Infants

Eye Opening	Verbal Response	Motor Response
4 – spontaneously	5 – coos, babbles	6 – normal, spontaneous movement
3 – to speech	4 – irritable cry	5 – withdraws to touch
2 – to pain	3 – cries to pain	4 – withdraws to pain
1 – no response	2 – moans to pain	3 – decorticate flexion
	1 – no response	2 – decerebrate extension
		1 – no response

Modified GCS for Children <4 years

Eye Opening	Verbal Response	Motor Response
4 – spontaneously	5 – oriented, social, speaks, interacts	6 – normal, spontaneous movement
3 – to speech	4 – confused speech, disoriented, consolable	5 – localizes to pain
2 – to pain	3 – inappropriate words, not consolable/aware	4 – withdraws to pain
1 – no response	2 – incomprehensible, agitated, restless, not aware	3 – decorticate flexion
	1 – no response	2 – decerebrate extension
		1 – no response

Any trauma or suspected trauma patient <1 yr of age with a large, boggy scalp hematoma requires U/S or CT

Respiratory Distress

- see Pediatrics, P84

History and Physical Exam
- infants not able to feed, older children not able to speak in full sentences
- anxious, irritable, lethargic – may indicate hypoxia
- tachypnea >60 (>40 if preschool age, >30 if school age), retractions, tracheal tug
  - see Pediatrics, P3 for age specific vital signs
- pulsus paradoxus
- wheezing, grunting, vomiting

Table 37. Stridorous Upper Airway Diseases: Diagnosis

Feature	Croup	Bacterial Tracheitis	Epiglottitis[1]
Age Range (yr)	0.5-4	5-10	2-8
Prodrome	Days	Hours to days	Minutes to hours
Temperature	Low grade	High	High
Radiography	Steeple sign	Exudates in trachea	Thumb sign
Etiology	Parainfluenza	S. aureus/GAS	H. influenzae type b
Barky Cough	Yes	Yes	No
Drooling	Yes	No	Yes
Appear Toxic	No	Yes	Yes
Intubation/ICU	No	Yes	Yes
Antibiotics	No	Yes	Yes
NOTE	Oral exam	Oral exam	No oral exam, consult ENT

[1]Now rare with Hib vaccine in common use

Management
- croup (usually laryngotracheitis caused by parainfluenza viruses)
  - humidified O₂ should not be given (no evidence for efficacy)
  - racemic epinephrine q1h x 3 doses, observe for 'rebound effects'
  - nebulized 1:1000 epinephrine (racemic has limited availability)
  - dexamethasone x 1 dose
  - consider bacterial tracheitis/epiglottitis if unresponsive to croup therapy
- bacterial tracheitis
  - start croup therapy, but may have poor response
  - usually require intubation, ENT consult, ICU
  - start antibiotics (e.g. cloxacillin), pending C&S
- epiglottitis
  - 4 D's: drooling, dyspnea, dysphagia, dysphonia + tripod sitting
  - do not examine oropharynx or agitate patient
  - immediate anesthesia, ENT call – intubate
  - then IV fluids, antibiotics, blood cultures
- asthma
  - supplemental O₂ if saturation <90% or PaO₂ <60%
  - bronchodilator therapy: salbutamol (Ventolin®) 0.15 mg/kg by masks q20min x 3
  - add 250-500 µg ipratropium (Atrovent®) to first 3 doses salbutamol
  - give corticosteroid therapy as soon as possible after arrival (prednisolone 2 mg/kg, dexamethasone 0.3 mg/kg)
  - if critically ill, not responding to inhaled bronchodilators or steroids: give IV bolus, then infusion of MgSO₄
  - IV β2-agonists if critically ill and not responding to above

Febrile Infant and Febrile Seizures

FEBRILE INFANT
- see Pediatrics, P51
- for fever >38°C without obvious focus
  - <28 d
    - admit
    - full septic workup (CBC and differential, blood C&S, urine C&S, LP ± stool C&S, CXR if indicated)
    - treat empirically with broad spectrum IV antibiotics
  - 28-90 d
    - as above unless infant meets Rochester criteria, investigate as indicated by history and physical
  - >90 d
    - toxic: admit, treat, full septic workup
    - non-toxic and no focus: investigate as indicated by history and physical

FEBRILE SEIZURES
- see Pediatrics, P82

Etiology
- children aged 6 mo-6 yr with fever or history of recent fever
- typical vs. atypical febrile seizures
- normal neurological exam afterward
- no evidence of intracranial infection or history of previous non-febrile seizures
- often positive family history of febrile seizures
- relatively well-looking after seizure

Investigations and Management
- if it is a febrile seizure: treat fever and look for source of fever
- if not a febrile seizure: treat seizure and look for source of seizure
  - note: may also have fever but may not meet criteria for febrile seizure
- ± EEG (especially if first seizure), head U/S (if fontanelle open)

Rochester Criteria for Febrile Infants Age 28-90 Days Old
- Non-toxic looking
- Previously well (>37 wk gestational age, home with mother, no hyperbilirubinemia, no prior antibiotics or hospitalizations, no chronic/underlying illness)
- No skin, soft tissue, bone, joint, or ear infection on physical exam
- WBC 5,000-15,000, bands <1,500, urine <10 WBC/HPF, stool <5 WBC/HPF

Table 38. Typical vs. Atypical Febrile Seizures

Characteristic	Typical	Atypical
Duration	<15 min	>15 min
Type of Seizure	Generalized	Focal features
Frequency	1 in 24 h	>1 in 24 h

Abdominal Pain

- see Pediatrics, P37

History
- nature of pain, associated fever
- associated GI, GU symptoms
- anorexia, decreased fluid intake

Physical Exam
- HEENT, respiratory, abdominal exam including DRE, testicular/genital exam

Table 39. Differential Diagnosis of Abdominal Pain in Infants/Children/Adolescents

Medical	Surgical
Colic	Malrotation with volvulus
UTI	Hirschsprung's disease
Constipation	Necrotizing enterocolitis
Gastroenteritis	Incarcerated hernia
Sepsis	Intussusception
Henoch-Schönlein purpura	Duodenal atresia
IBD	Appendicitis
Hemolytic uremic syndrome	Cholecystitis
Pneumonia	Pancreatitis
Strep throat	Testicular torsion
Sickle cell disease crisis	Ectopic pregnancy
DKA	Trauma
Functional	Pyloric stenosis

*Remember to keep an index of suspicion for child abuse

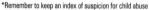

Red Flags for Abdominal Pain
- Significant weight loss or growth retardation (need growth chart)
- Fever
- Joint pain with objective physical findings
- Rash
- Rectal bleeding
- Rebound tenderness and radiation of pain to back, shoulders, or legs
- Pain wakes from sleep
- Severe diarrhea and encopresis
- Trauma or suspected trauma patient <1 yr of age with a large, boggy scalp hematoma requires U/S or CT

Common Infections

- see Pediatrics, P51

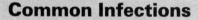

Table 40. Antibiotic Treatment of Pediatric Bacterial Infections

Infection	Pathogens	Treatment
MENINGITIS SEPSIS		
Neonatal	GBS, E. coli, Listeria, Gram-negative bacilli	ampicillin + cefotaxime
1-3 mo	Same pathogens as above and below	ampicillin + cefotaxime + vancomycin
>3 mo	S. pneumoniae, H. influenzae type b (>5 yr), meningococcus	ceftriaxone + vancomycin
OTITIS MEDIA		
1st line	S. pneumoniae, H. influenzae type b, M. catarrhalis	amoxicillin 80-90 mg/kg per day
2nd line		clarithromycin 15 mg/kg/d bid (for penicillin allergy)
Treatment failure		90 mg/kg/d amoxicillin and 6.4 mg/kg/d clavulanate divided into bid dosage
STREP PHARYNGITIS		
	Group A β-hemolytic Streptococcus	penicillin/amoxicillin or erythromycin (penicillin allergy)
UTI		
	E. coli, Proteus, H. influenzae, Pseudomonas, S. saprophyticus, Enterococcus, GBS	Oral: cephalexin (older children) IV: ampicillin and aminoglycoside
PNEUMONIA		
1-3 mo	Viral, S. pneumoniae, C. trachomatis, B. pertussis, S. aureus, H. influenzae	cefuroxime ± macrolide (erythromycin) OR ampicillin ± macrolide
3 mo-5 yr	Viral, S. pneumoniae, S. aureus, H. influenzae, Mycoplasma pneumoniae	ampicillin/amoxicillin or cefuroxime
>5 yr	As above	ampicillin/amoxicillin + macrolide or cefuroxime + macrolide

Child Abuse and Neglect

- see Pediatrics, P14
- obligation to report any suspected/known case of child abuse or neglect to CAS yourself (do not delegate)
- document injuries
- consider skeletal survey x-rays (especially in non-ambulatory child), ophthalmology consult, CT head
- injury patterns associated with child abuse
  - HI: torn frenulum, dental injuries, bilateral black eyes, traumatic hair loss, diffuse severe CNS injury, retinal hemorrhage
  - Shaken Baby Syndrome: diffuse brain injury, subdural/SAH, retinal hemorrhage, minimal/no evidence of external trauma, associated bony fractures
  - skin injuries: bites, bruises/burns in shape of an object, glove/stocking distribution of burns, bruises of various ages, bruises in protected areas
  - bone injuries: rib fractures without major trauma, femur fractures age <1 yr, spiral fractures of long bones in non-ambulatory children, metaphyseal fractures in infants, multiple fractures of various ages, complex/multiple skull fractures
  - GU/GI injuries: chronic abdominal/perineal pain, injury to genitals/rectum, STI/pregnancy, recurrent vomiting or diarrhea

Presentation of Neglect
- Failure to thrive, developmental delay
- Inadequate or dirty clothing, poor hygiene
- Child exhibits poor attachment to parents

Procedures that may Require Sedation
- Setting fractures
- Reducing dislocations
- Draining abscesses
- Exploring wounds/ulcers/superficial infections
- Endoscopic examination
- Reduce patient anxiety/agitation for imaging/procedures

Common Medications

Table 41. Commonly Used Medications

Drug	Dosing Schedule	Indications	Comments
Acetaminophen	325-650 mg PO q4-6h prn	Pain control	Max 4 g daily
Activated charcoal	30-100 g PO in 250 mL H_2O	Poisoning/overdose	
ASA	325-650 mg PO q4h max 4g/d stroke/MI risk: 81-325 mg PO OD 160 mg chewed	Pain control Cardiac prevention ACS	
β-blockers (metoprolol)	5 mg slow IV q5min x 3 if no contraindications	Acute MI	
Diazepam	anxiety: 2-10 mg PO tid/qid alcohol withdrawal: 10-20 mg PO/IV q1h titrated to signs/symptoms	Anxiety Alcohol withdrawal	
Enoxaparin	1 mg/kg SC bid	Acute MI	
Epinephrine	anaphylaxis: 0.1-0.5 mg IM; can repeat q10-15min	Anaphylaxis	Max 1 mg/dose
Fentanyl	0.5-1.0 μg/kg IV	Procedural sedation	Very short acting narcotic (complication=apnea)
Flumazenil	0.3 mg IV bolus q5min x 3 doses	Reversal of procedural sedation	Benzodiazepine antagonist Can cause seizures/status epilepticus in chronic benzodiazepine users
Furosemide (Lasix®)	CHF: 40-80 mg IV HTN: 10-40 mg PO bid	CHF HTN	Monitor for electrolyte imbalances
Glucose	0.5-1.0 g/kg (1-2 mL/kg) IV of D50W	Hypoglycemia/DKA	
Haloperidol	2.5-5.0 mg PO/IM initial effective dose 6-20 mg/d	Psychosis	Monitor with Parkinson's; results in CNS depression
Ibuprofen	200-800 mg PO tid prn max 1,200 mg/d	Mild to moderate acute pain Analgesic and anti-inflammatory properties	
Insulin	bolus 5-10 U (0.2 U/kg) then 5-10 U (0.1 U/kg) per h	Hyperglycemia	Monitor blood glucose levels Consider K^+ replacement, also measure blood glucose levels before administration
Ipratropium bromide	2-3 puffs inhaled tid-qid, max 12 puffs/d	Asthma	Contraindicated with peanut/soy allergy Caution with narrow-angle glaucoma
Lidocaine with epi	max 7 mg/kg SC	Local anesthetic	Not to be used in fingers, nose, toes, penis, ears
Lidocaine w/o epi	max 5 mg/kg SC	Local anesthetic	
Lorazepam	anxiety: 0.5-2 mg PO/IM/IV q6-8h status epilepticus: 4 mg IV repeat up to q5min	Anxiety Status epilepticus	
Midazolam	50 μg/kg IV	Procedural sedation	Short acting benzodiazepine (complication=apnea when used with narcotic) Fentanyl and midazolam often used together for procedural sedation

Table 41. Commonly Used Medications (continued)

Drug	Dosing Schedule	Indications	Comments
Morphine	15-30 mg PO q8-12h 0.1-0.2 mg/kg max 15 mg IV q4h	Mild to moderate acute/chronic pain Prescribed in combination with NSAIDs or acetaminophen	GI and constipation side effects DO NOT CRUSH, CUT, or CHEW
Naloxone	0.5-2 mg or 0.01-0.02 mg/kg initial bolus IV/IM/SL/SC or via ETT (2-2.5x IV dose), increase dose by 2 mg until response/max 10 mg	Comatose patient Opioid overdose Reversal in procedural sedation	
Nitroglycerin	acute angina: 0.3-0.6 mg SL q5min, OR 5 μg/min IV increasing by 5-20 μg/min q3-5min	Angina Acute MI	Not to be used with other antihypertensives Not in right ventricular MI
Percocet 10/325®	1-2 tabs PO q6h prn	Moderate pain control	Oxycodone + acetaminophen Max 4 g acetaminophen daily
Phenytoin	Status epilepticus: see Table 17	Status epilepticus	Begin maintenance dose 12 h after loading dose Continuous ECG, BP monitoring mandatory
Polysporin®	Apply to affected area bid-tid	Superficial infections	
Propofol	0.25-1 mg/kg IV	Procedural sedation	Short acting Anesthetic/sedative (complication=apnea, decreased BP)
Salbutamol	2 puffs inhaled q4-6h max 12 puffs/d	Asthma	Caution with cardiac abnormalities
Thiamine	100 mg IV/IM initially, then 50-100 mg IM/IV/PO OD x 3d	To treat/prevent Wernicke's encephalopathy	Caution use in pregnancy
Tylenol #3®	1-2 tabs PO q4-6h prn	Pain control	Max 4 g acetaminophen daily

References

American College of Emergency Physicians. Clinical policy for the initial approach to patients presenting with altered mental status. Ann Emerg Med 1999;33:251-280.

Andreoli TE, Carpenter CJ, Griggs RC, et al. Cecil essentials of medicine, 8th ed. Saunders, 2010.

Bachmann LM, Kolb E, Koller MT, et al. Accuracy of Ottawa ankle rules to exclude fractures of the ankle and mid-foot: systematic review. BMJ 2003;326:417.

Barash PG, Cullen BF, Stoelting RK. Clinical anesthesia, 5th ed. Philadelphia: Lippincott, 2005.

Chu P. Blunt abdominal trauma: current concepts. Curr Orthopaed 2003;17:254-259.

Dargan P, Wallace C, Jones AL. An evidence based flowchart to guide the management of acute salicylate (Aspirin®) overdose. Emerg Med J 2002;19;206-209.

The EINSTEIN-PE Investigators. Oral rivaroxaban for the treatment of symptomatic pulmonary embolism. NEJM 2012;366:1287-1297.

The EINSTEIN-PE Investigators. Oral rivaroxaban for the treatment of symptomatic venous thromboembolism. NEJM 2010;363:2499-2510.

Elliott WJ. Hypertensive emergencies. Crit Care Clin 2001;17:435-451.

Frampton A. Reporting of gunshot wounds by doctors in emergency departments: A duty or a right? Some legal and ethical issues surrounding breaking patient confidentiality. Emerg Med J 2005;22;84-86.

Kalant H, Roschlau WH. Principles of medical pharmacology, 7th ed. New York: Oxford University Press, 2006.

Keim S. Emergency medicine on call. McGraw Hill, 2004.

Kline JA, Mitchell AM, Kabrhel C, et al. Clinical criteria to prevent unnecessary diagnostic testing in emergency department patients with suspected pulmonary embolism. J Thromb Haemost 2004;2:1247-1255.

Marx J, Hockberger R, Walls R (editors). Rosen's emergency medicine: concepts and clinical practice, 8th ed. Mosby, 2013.

Munro P. Management of eclampsia in the accident and emergency department. Emerg Med J 2000;7:7-11.

Perry JJ, Stiell IG, Sivilotti MA, et al. Clinical decision rules to rule out subarachnoid hemorrhage for acute headache. JAMA 2013;310(12):1248-1255.

Perry JJ, Stiell IG, Sivilotti MA, et al. Sensitivity of computed tomography performed within six hours of onset of headache for diagnosis of subarachnoid haemorrhage: prospective cohort study. BMJ 2011;343:d4277.

Righini M, Van Es J, Den Exter PL, et al. Age adjusted d dimer cutoff levels to rule out pulmonary embolism: The ADJUST-PE Study. JAMA 2014;311(11):1117-1124.

Roberts JR, Hedges JR. Clinical procedures in emergency medicine, 5th ed. WB Saunders, 2009.

Sabatine MS, Cannon CP, Gibson M, et al. Addition of clopidogrel to Aspirin® and fibrinolytic therapy for myocardial infarction with ST-segment elevation. NEJM 2005;352:1179-1189.

Schulman S, Kearon C, Kakkar AK, et al. Extended use of dabigatran, warfarin, or placebo in venous thromboembolism. NEJM 2013;368:709-718.

Soar J, Pumphrey R, Cant A, et al. Emergency treatment of anaphylactic reactions: guideline for healthcare providers. Resuscitation 2008;77:157-169.

Stiell IG, Wells GA, Vandemheen KL, et al. The Canadian CT head rule for patients with minor head injury. Lancet 2001;357:1391-1396.

Stiell IG, Wells GA, Vandemheen KL, et al. The Canadian C-spine rule for radiography in alert and stable trauma patients. JAMA 2001;286:1841-1848.

Tintinalli JE, Kelen GE. Emergency medicine: a comprehensive study guide, 7th ed. McGraw-Hill, 2004.

Varon J, Marik P. The diagnosis and management of hypertensive crises. Chest 2000;118:214-227.

Vidt DG. Emergency room management of hypertensive urgencies and emergencies. J Clin Hypertens 2004;6:520-525.

Warden CR, Zibulewsky J, Mace S, et al. Evaluation and management of febrile seizures in the out-of-hospital and emergency department settings. Ann Emerg Med 2003;41;215-222.

Wells PS, Anderson DR, Rodger M, et al. Derivation of a simple clinical model to categorize patients probability of pulmonary embolism: increasing the models utility with the simpliRED d-dimer. J Thromb Haemost 2000;83:416-420.

Wells PS, Anderson DR, Rodger M, et al. Excluding pulmonary embolism at the beside without diagnostic imaging: management of patients with suspected pulmonary embolism presenting to the emergency department by using a simple clinical model. Ann Int Med 2000;135:98-107.

E | Endocrinology

Raghad Al-Saqqar, Cecilia Alvarez-Veronesi and Sumedha Arya, chapter editors
Claudia Frankfurter and Inna Gong, associate editors
Brittany Prevost and Robert Vanner, EBM editors
Dr. Alice Cheng and Dr. Adam Millar, staff editors

Acronyms

[ ]	concentration	DM	diabetes mellitus	hs-CRP	highly sensitive C-reactive protein	PTU	propylthiouracil
Ab	antibody	DXM	dexamethasone	HVA	homovanillic acid	RAIU	radioactive iodine uptake
ACR	albumin-creatinine ratio	ECF	extracellular fluid	ICF	intracellular fluid	RAAS	renin-angiotensin-aldosterone system
ACTH	adrenocorticotropic hormone	EtOH	ethanol	IDL	intermediate density lipoprotein	RH	releasing hormone
ADH	antidiuretic hormone	FFA	free fatty acids	IFG	impaired fasting glucose	SHBG	sex hormone binding globulin
AG	anion gap	FNA	fine needle aspiration	IGT	impaired glucose tolerance	T2DM	type 2 diabetes mellitus
AVP	arginine vasopressin	FPG	fasting plasma glucose	LCAT	lecithin-cholesterol acyltransferase	T_3	triiodothyronine
BG	blood glucose	FSH	follicle stimulating hormone	LDL	low density lipoprotein	T_4	thyroxine
BMD	bone mineral density	GFR	glomerular filtration rate	LH	luteinizing hormone	TBG	thyroid binding globulin
BMI	body mass index	GH	growth hormone	LP	lipoprotein	TC	total cholesterol
CAD	coronary artery disease	GHRH	growth hormone releasing hormone	MEN	multiple endocrine neoplasia	TG	triglycerides
CAH	congenital adrenal hyperplasia	GnRH	gonadotropin releasing hormone	MMI	methimazole	TgAb	thyroglobulin antibodies
CHO	carbohydrates	Hb	hemoglobin	MTC	medullary thyroid cancer	TPOAb	anti-thyroid peroxidase antibodies
CK	creatine kinase	hCG	human chorionic gonadotropin	NS	normal saline	TRAb	TSH receptor antibodies
CMV	cytomegalovirus	HDL	high density lipoprotein	OGTT	oral glucose tolerance test	TRH	thyrotropin releasing hormone
CrCl	creatinine clearance	HHS	hyperosmolar hyperglycemic state	PAD	peripheral arterial disease	TSH	thyroid stimulating hormone
CRH	corticotropin releasing hormone	HLA	human leukocyte antigen	PCOS	polycystic ovarian syndrome	TSI	thyroid stimulating immunoglobulin
CVD	cardiovascular disease	HMG-CoA	3-hydroxy-3-methylglutaryl-coenzyme A	POMC	pro-opiomelanocorticotropin	VLDL	very low density lipoprotein
DDAVP	desmopressin (1-deamino-8-D-arginine vasopressin)	HPA	hypothalamic pituitary adrenal	PRL	prolactin	VMA	vanillylmandelic acid
DHEA	dehydroepiandrosterone			PTH	parathyroid hormone	WC	waist circumference
DI	diabetes insipidus						
DKA	diabetic ketoacidosis						

Basic Anatomy Review

Major Endocrine Organs

GENERAL FUNCTION OF ORGANS

The Hypothalamic-Pituitary Axis
Information about cortical inputs, automatic function, environmental cues (light, temperature) and peripheral hormonal feedback is synthesized at the coordinating centre of the endocrine system, the hypothalamus. The hypothalamus then sends signals to the pituitary to release hormones that affect the thyroid, adrenals, gonads, growth, milk production, and water balance

Anatomy ⟷ Function
Hypothalamic hormones: small peptides, non-binding protein → rapid degradation
High [ ] in pituitary-portal blood system
Low [ ] in peripheral circulation
Proximity of axis preserves the pulsatile output signals from the hypothalamic neurons

Thyroid
Thyroid hormone is critical to 1) brain and somatic development in fetus and infants, 2) metabolic activity in adults, and 3) function of virtually every organ system

Adrenal
Each gland (6-8 g) has 1) a cortex with 3 layers that act like independent organs (zona glomerulosa → aldosterone, fasciculata → cortisol, reticularis → androgen and estrogen precursors), and 2) a medulla that acts like a sympathetic ganglion to store/synthesize adrenaline and noradrenaline

Gonads
Bifunctional: sex steroid synthesis and gamete production
Sex steroids control sexuality and affect metabolic and brain functions

Parathyroid
Synthesize and secrete PTH, a principle regulator of ECF Ca^{2+}, regulated by $[Ca^{2+}]$, $[Mg^{2+}]$, $1,25(OH)_2D$ (active metabolite of vit D), and phosphate

Pancreas
Endocrine islet β-cells produce insulin: oppose glucose production (glycogenolysis, gluconeogenesis), increase glucose uptake into muscle and fat. Glucagon, epinephrine, cortisol, and GH are the counterregulatory hormones

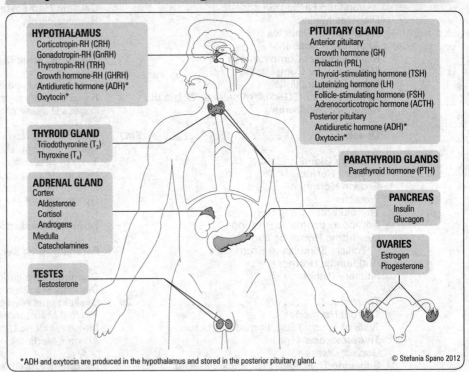

Figure 1. Endocrine system

Dyslipidemias

Definition
- metabolic disorders characterized by elevations of fasting plasma LDL-cholesterol, and/or triglycerides (TG), and/or low HDL-cholesterol

Overview of Lipid Transport

- lipoproteins are spherical complexes that consist of a lipid core surrounded by a shell of water-soluble cholesterol, apoproteins, and phospholipids
- lipoproteins transport lipids within the body
- apolipoproteins serve as enzyme co-factors, promote clearance of the particle by interacting with cellular receptors, and stabilize the lipoprotein micelle

Table 1. Lipoproteins

Lipoprotein	Apolipoproteins	Function
Exogenous Pathway		
Chylomicron	B-48, C, E, A-I, A-II, A-IV	Transports dietary TG from gut to adipose tissue and muscle
Endogenous Pathway		
VLDL	B-100, C, E	Transports hepatic synthesized TG from liver to adipose tissue and muscle
IDL	B-100, E	Product of hydrolysis of TG in VLDL by lipoprotein lipase resulting in depletion of TG core Enriched in cholesterol esters
LDL	B-100	Formed by further removal of residual TG from IDL core by hepatic lipase resulting in greater enriched particles with cholesterol esters Transports cholesterol from liver to peripheral tissues (gonads, adrenals)
HDL	A-I, A-II, C, E	Transports cholesterol from peripheral tissues to liver Acts as a reservoir for apolipoproteins

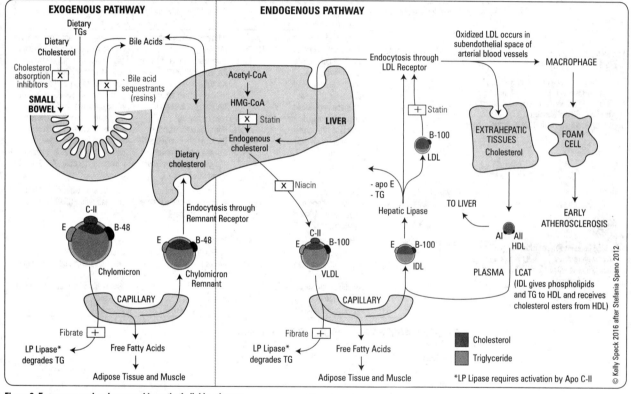

Figure 2. Exogenous and endogenous biosynthetic lipid pathways

Hypertriglyceridemia (Elevated Triglycerides)

PRIMARY HYPERTRIGLYCERIDEMIA

Table 2. Primary Hypertriglyceridemias

Hypertriglyceridemia	Etiology/ Pathophysiology	Labs	Clinical Presentation	Treatment
Familial Lipoprotein Lipase Deficiency	Autosomal recessive deficiency of lipoprotein lipase or its cofactor	↑ TG ↑ Chylomicrons Moderate ↑ in VLDL	Presents at infancy Recurrent abdominal pain Hepatosplenomegaly Splenic infarct Anemia, granulocytopenia, thrombocytopenia 2° to hypersplenism Pancreatitis Lipemia retinalis Eruptive xanthomata	Decrease dietary fat intake to <10% of total calories Decrease dietary simple carbohydrates Cook with medium chain fatty acids Abstain from EtOH Gene therapy (Glybera)
Familial Hypertriglyceridemia	Autosomal dominant for inactivating mutations of the LP lipase gene Several genetic defects resulting in ↑ hepatic VLDL synthesis or ↓ removal of VLDL	↑ TG ↑ VLDL	Possible premature CAD Develop syndrome of obesity, hypertriglyceridemia, hyperinsulinemia, and hyperuricemia in early adulthood	Decrease dietary simple carbohydrates and fat intake Abstain from EtOH Fibrates or niacin

SECONDARY HYPERTRIGLYCERIDEMIA

Hypertriglyceridemia and Pancreatitis
Serum triglyceride levels >10 mmol/L
increases the risk of developing pancreatitis
(even some reports of TG >5 mmol/L)

Etiology
- endocrine: obesity/metabolic syndrome, hypothyroidism (more for high LDL, not TG), acromegaly, Cushing's syndrome, DM
- renal: chronic renal failure, polyclonal and monoclonal hypergammaglobulinemia
- hepatic: chronic liver disease, hepatitis, glycogen storage disease
- drugs: alcohol, corticosteroids, estrogen, hydrochlorothiazide, retinoic acid, β-blockers without intrinsic sympathomimetic action (ISA), anti-retroviral drugs, atypical antipsychotics, oral contraceptive pills
- other: pregnancy

Hypercholesterolemia

PRIMARY HYPERCHOLESTEROLEMIA

Table 3. Primary Hypercholesterolemias

Hypercholesterolemia	Etiology/Pathophysiology	Labs	Clinical Presentation	Treatment
Familial Hypercholesterolemia	1/500 in U.S. population. Autosomal codominant with high penetrance. More prevalent in French Canadian, Dutch Afrikanner, Christian Lebanese populations. Most commonly due to defects in the normal LDL receptor on cell membranes	↑ LDL ↑ TC	Tendinous xanthomatosis (Achilles, patellar, and extensor tendons of hand). Arcus cornealis. Xanthelasmata. Heterozygotes: premature CAD, 50% risk of MI in men by age 30. Homozygotes: manifest CAD and other vascular disease early in childhood and can be fatal (<20 yr) if untreated	Heterozygotes: improvement of LDL with statins, often in combination with ezetimibe or bile acid sequestrants or PCSK9 inhibitor. Homozygotes: partial control with portacaval shunt or LDL apheresis in conjunction with niacin; large dose statin is modestly effective; potential liver transplant; consider lomitapide (inhibitor of the microsomal TG transfer protein) and mipomersen (inhibits ApoB gene)
Polygenic Hypercholesterolemia	Most common. Few mild inherited defects in cholesterol metabolism	↑ TC ↑ LDL	Asymptomatic until vascular disease develops. No xanthomata	Statins, ezetimibe, niacin, bile acid sequesterant, PCSK9 inhibitor
Familial Combined Hyperlipidemia	In many cases, over-population of VLDL and associated ↑ LDL 2° to excess hepatic synthesis of apolipoprotein B. Autosomal dominant	↑ TC + G ↑ VLDL ↑ LDL	Xanthelasma. CAD and other vascular disease	Weight reduction. Decrease simple carbohydrates, fat, cholesterol, and EtOH in diet. Statins. Niacin, fibrates, ezetimibe, PCSK9 inhibitor

FH and Cardiovascular Risk Calculators
- Risk calculators such as Framingham and SCORE do not apply to patients with familial hypercholesterolemia
- Consider all adults with FH as "high risk"

Familial Combined Hyperlipidemia
- A common disorder (1-2% of the population)
- Contributes to 1/3 to 1/2 of familial coronary artery disease

SECONDARY HYPERCHOLESTEROLEMIA

Etiology
- endocrine: hypothyroidism
- renal: nephrotic syndrome
- immunologic: monoclonal gammopathy
- hepatic: cholestatic liver disease (e.g. primary biliary cirrhosis)
- nutritional: diet, anorexia nervosa
- drugs: cyclosporin, anabolic steroids, carbamazepine

Low High-Density Lipoprotein

PRIMARY CAUSES

Table 4. Primary Low HDL Cholesterol Levels

Disorder	Etiology/Pathophysiology	Clinical Presentation	Treatment
Familial Hypoalphalipoproteinemia or Familial HDL Deficiency	Autosomal dominant inheritance of a mutation in the ABCA1 or the APOA1 gene	Premature atherosclerosis. Cerebrovascular disease. Premature atherosclerosis. Xanthomas	Reduce the risk of atherosclerosis with lifestyle changes, management of concomitant hypercholesterolemia, hypertriglyceridemia, and metabolic syndrome if present
Tangier Disease	Autosomal recessive inheritance of mutations in the ABCA1 gene. Impaired HDL-mediated cholesterol efflux from macrophages and impaired intracellular lipid trafficking	Mild hypertriglyceridemia. Neuropathy. Enlarged, orange-coloured tonsils. Premature atherosclerosis. Splenomegaly. Hepatomegaly. Corneal clouding. Type 2 DM	Reduce the risk of atherosclerosis with lifestyle changes, management of concomitant hypercholesterolemia, hypertriglyceridemia, and metabolic syndrome if present

SECONDARY CAUSES

Etiology
- endocrine: obesity/metabolic syndrome, DM
- drugs: β-blockers, benzodiazepines, anabolic steroids
- other: acute infections, inflammatory conditions

Dyslipidemia and the Risk for Coronary Artery Disease

- increased LDL is a major risk factor for atherosclerosis and CAD as LDL is the major atherogenic lipid particle
- increased HDL is associated with decreased cardiovascular disease and mortality
- moderate hypertriglyceridemia (triglyceride level 2.3-9 mmol/L) is an independent risk factor for CAD, especially in people with DM and in post-menopausal women
- treatment of hypertriglyceridemia has not been shown to reduce CAD risk

Screening
- screen men over age 40, women over age 50 or post-menopausal
- if following risk factors present, screen at any age
  - DM
  - current cigarette smoking or COPD
  - HTN (sBP >140, dBP >90)
  - obesity (BMI >27 kg/m²)
  - family history of premature CAD
  - clinical signs of hyperlipidemia (xanthelasma, xanthoma, arcus cornealis)
  - evidence of atherosclerosis
  - inflammatory disease (rheumatoid arthritis, SLE, psoriatic arthritis, ankylosing spondylitis, inflammatory bowel disease)
  - HIV infection on highly active anti-retroviral therapy (HAART)
  - chronic kidney disease (estimated GFR <60 mL/min/1.73 m²)
  - erectile dysfunction
- screen children with a family history of hypercholesterolemia or chylomicronemia

Factors Affecting Risk Assessment
- metabolic syndrome
- apolipoprotein B (apo B)
  - each atherogenic particle (VLDL, IDL, LDL, and lipoprotein A) contains one molecule of apo B
  - serum [apo B] reflects the total number of particles and may be useful in assessing cardiovascular risk and adequacy of treatment in high risk patients and those with metabolic syndrome
- C-reactive protein (hs-CRP) levels
  - highly sensitive acute phase reactant
  - may be clinically useful in identifying those at a higher risk of cardiovascular disease than predicted by the global risk assessment

Treatment of Dyslipidemias

Approach to Treatment
For clinical guidelines see *Can J Cardiol* 2012;29:151-167
- estimate 10 yr risk of CAD using Framingham model
- establish treatment targets according to level of risk

Table 5. Target Lipids by Risk Group

Level of Risk	Definition (10 Yr Risk of CAD)	Initiate Treatment if:	Primary Target LDL-C	Alternate
High	Risk ≥20%, or Clinical atherosclerosis Abdominal aortic aneurysm DM >15 yr duration and age older than 30 yr DM with age older than 40 yr Microvascular disease High risk kidney disease High risk HTN	Consider treatment in all patients	≤2 mmol/L or ≥50% ↓ in LDL	apo B ≤0.80 g/L or non-HDL-C ≤2.6 mmol/L
Moderate	Risk 10 -19%	LDL >3.5 mmol/L For LDL-C<3.5 consider if: apo B ≥1.2 g/L or non-HDL-C ≥4.3 mmol/L	≤2 mmol/L or ≥50% ↓ in LDL	apo B <0.80 g/L or non-HDL-C ≤2.6 mmol/L
Low	Risk <10%	LDL ≥5.0 mmol/L Familial hypercholesterolemia	≥50% ↓ in LDL	

Treatment Effect
Each 1.0 mmol/L decrease in LDL corresponds to 20-25% relative risk reduction in cardiovascular disease

6% Rule
If the dose of a statin is doubled there is approximately a 6% increase in the LDL lowering efficacy

For Statin Follow-Up
- Liver enzymes and lipid profile: liver enzymes measured at the beginning of treatment then once after therapy initiated. Lipids (once stabilized) measured annually. Order both if patient complains of jaundice, RUQ pain, dark urine
- CK at baseline and if patient complains of myalgia
- D/C statin if CK >10x upper limit of normal or patient has persistent myalgia

A Report of the American College of Cardiology/ American Heart Association Task Force on Practice Guidelines
Circulation 2013;00:000-000.
Purpose: To examine the evidence supporting specific end-point LDL targets in statin therapy
Study: Systematic review, searching 1995-2009 inclusive identified 19 RCTs.
Results: None of the trials examined demonstrated better cardiovascular outcomes for a particular target LDL. Moreover, many trials showed best outcomes from maximum tolerated dose of statin, irrespective of the treated LDL level.
Conclusion: Based on systematic review, the ACC/ AHA is no longer recommending a "Treat to Target" approach for statin therapy. Primary prevention in patients with increased risk should be treated with moderate to high intensity statin therapy without tracking LDL targets. Similarly, patients needing secondary prevention should receive high intensity statin therapy without attention to LDL targets.

Simvastatin to Lower CAD Risk – The Heart Protection Study (HPS)
Lancet 2002;360:7-22
Study: Randomized, double-blind, placebo-controlled trial (median follow-up 5.0 yr).
Patients: 20,536 patients with coronary disease, other occlusive arterial disease or DM (aged 40-80 yr) who had a total cholesterol level of ≥3.5 mmol/L.
Intervention: Simvastatin 40 mg/d or placebo.
Main Outcomes: Mortality, fatal or non-fatal vascular events.
Results: The use of simvastatin significantly decreased total mortality (12.9 vs. 14.7, p=0.0003) and the first event rate of any cardiovascular event by 25% (p<0.0001).
Conclusion: Treatment with simvastatin improved survival and cardiovascular outcomes in high-risk CAD patients.

Table 6. Treatment of Hypercholesterolemia and Hypertriglyceridemia

Treatment of Hypercholesterolemia	Treatment of Hypertriglyceridemia

Conservative: 4-6 mo trial unless high risk group, in which case medical treatment should start immediately
  Diet
    Decrease fat: <30% calories
    Decrease saturated fat: <10% calories
    Decrease cholesterol: <200 mg/d
    Increase fibre: >30 g/d
  Decrease alcohol intake to ≤1-2 drinks/d
  Smoking cessation
  Aerobic exercise: ≥150 min/wk in bouts of ≥10 min
  Weight loss: target BMI <25
Medical
  HMG-CoA reductase inhibitors, ezetimibe, bile acid sequestrants, niacin (see *Common Medications*, E49)
	Conservative: 4-6 mo trial
	  Diet
	    Decrease fat and simple carbohydrates
	    Increase omega-3 polyunsaturated fatty acid
	  Control blood sugars
	  Decrease alcohol intake to ≤1-2 drinks/d
	  Smoking cessation
	  Aerobic exercise: ≥150 min/wk in bouts of ≥10 min
	  Weight loss: target BMI <25
	Medical: fibrates, niacin (see *Common Medications*, E49)
	Indications:
	  Failed conservative measures
	  TG >10 mmol/L (885 mg/dL) to prevent pancreatitis
	  Combined hyperlipidemia

Disorders of Glucose Metabolism

Overview of Glucose Regulation

Glucose Related Emergencies
- DKA
- HHS
- Hypoglycemia

Three Year Efficacy of Complex Insulin Regimens in Type 2 DM: 4T Trial
NEJM 2009;361:1736-1747
Study: Randomized unblinded trial with 3 yr of follow-up.
Population: 708 patients with type 2 DM, not on insulin or thiazolidinedione therapy on maximal metformin and sulfonylurea therapy.
Intervention: Thrice-daily prandial insulin aspart, versus twice-daily biphasic insulin aspart, versus once-daily basal insulin detemir. Sulfonylurea therapy was replaced with a secondary insulin regime specific to each arm if there was persistent hyperglycemia.
Primary Outcome: Three yr hemoglobin HbA1c.
Results: Significant difference in rates of patient withdrawal from the study: 5.1% biphasic, 11.7% prandial, 8.5% basal regimens (p=0.04). There were no significant differences in median HbA1c levels between all three arms from yr 1-3. A smaller proportion of patients reached HbA1c <6.5% or <7.0% in the biphasic arm. The basal arm had least weight gain and least weight circumference increase, but highest rate of secondary insulin requirement. The basal arm had fewest severe hypoglycemic events per patient yr, while the biphasic had the most serious adverse effects.
Conclusion: Basal insulin regime provides the best glycemic control over a 3 yr study; with better HbA1c control, fewer hypoglycemic events, and less weight gain.

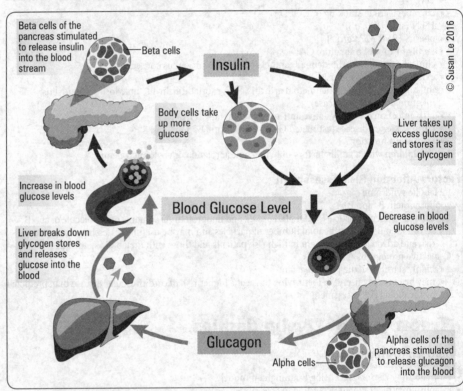

Figure 3. Blood glucose regulation

Pre-Diabetes (Impaired Glucose Tolerance/ Impaired Fasting Glucose)

- 1-5% per yr go on to develop DM
- 50-80% revert to normal glucose tolerance
- weight loss may improve glucose tolerance
- increased risk of developing macrovascular complications (IGT >IFG)
- lifestyle modifications decrease progression to DM by 58%

Diagnostic Criteria (CDA Guidelines)
- impaired fasting glucose (IFG): fasting plasma glucose (FPG) 6.1-6.9 mmol/L
- impaired glucose tolerance (IGT): 2h 75 g oral glucose tolerance test (OGTT) 7.8-11.0 mmol/L
- HbA1c: 6.0-6.4%

Diabetes Mellitus

Definition
- syndrome of disordered metabolism and inappropriate hyperglycemia secondary to an absolute/relative deficiency of insulin, or a reduction in biological effectiveness of insulin, or both

Diagnostic Criteria (CDA Guidelines)
- any one of the following is diagnostic
- FPG ≥7.0 mmol/L (fasting = no caloric intake for at least 8 h) OR
- 2h 75 g OGTT ≥11.1 mmol/L OR
- random PG ≥11.1 mmol/L OR
- HbA1c ≥6.5% (not for diagnosis of suspected Type 1 DM, children, adolescents, or pregnant women)
- in the presence of hyperglycemia symptoms (polyuria, polydipsia, polyphagia, weight loss, blurry vision,), a confirmatory test is not required
- in the absence of hyperglycemic symptoms, a repeat confirmatory test is required to make the diagnosis of diabetes

Etiology and Pathophysiology

Table 7. Etiologic Classification of Diabetes Mellitus

I. Type 1 DM (immune-mediated β cell destruction, usually leading to absolute insulin deficiency)

II. Type 2 DM (ranges from predominantly insulin resistance with relative insulin deficiency to a predominantly insulin secretory defect with insulin resistance 2o to β cell dysfunction)

III. Other Specific Causes of DM
- a. Genetic defects of β cell function (e.g. MODY – Maturity-Onset Diabetes of the Young) or insulin action
- b. Diseases of the exocrine pancreas:
  Pancreatitis, pancreatectomy, neoplasia, cystic fibrosis, hemochromatosis ("bronze diabetes")
- c. Endocrinopathies:
  Acromegaly, Cushing's syndrome, glucagonoma, pheochromocytoma, hyperthyroidism
- d. Drug-induced:
  Glucocorticoids, thyroid hormone, β-adrenergic agonists, thiazides, phenytoin, clozapine
- e. Infections:
  Congenital rubella, CMV, coxsackie
- f. Genetic syndromes associated with DM:
  Down's syndrome, Klinefelter's syndrome, Turner's syndrome

IV. Gestational Diabetes Mellitus (see Obstetrics, OB26)

Table 8. Comparison of Type 1 and Type 2 Diabetes Mellitus

	Type 1	Type 2
Onset	Usually <30 yr of age	Usually >40 yr of age Increasing incidence in pediatric population 2° to obesity
Epidemiology	More common in Caucasians Less common in Asians, Hispanics, Aboriginals, and Blacks Accounts for 5-10% of all DM	More common in Blacks, Hispanics, Aboriginals, and Asians Accounts for >90% of all DM
Etiology	Autoimmune	Complex and multifactorial
Genetics	Monozygotic twin concordance is 30-40% Associated with HLA class II DR3 and DR4, with either allele present in up to 95% of type 1 DM Certain DQ alleles also confer a risk	Greater heritability than type 1 DM Monozygotic twin concordance is 70-90% Polygenic Non-HLA associated
Pathophysiology	Synergistic effects of genetic, immune, and environmental factors that cause β cell destruction resulting in impaired insulin secretion Autoimmune process is believed to be triggered by environmental factors (e.g. viruses, bovine milk protein, urea compounds) Pancreatic cells are infiltrated with lymphocytes resulting in islet cell destruction 80% of β cell mass is destroyed before features of DM present	Impaired insulin secretion, peripheral insulin resistance (likely due to receptor and post receptor abnormality), and excess hepatic glucose production

Effects of Intensive Treatment of Type 1 DM on the Development and Progression of Long-Term Complications: The DCCT Study
NEJM 1993;329:977-986.
Study: Multicentre RCT, with 6.5 yr of mean follow-up
Patients: 1,441 patients (aged 13-39 yr) with type 1 DM with no cardiovascular history or severe diabetic complications
Intervention: Intensive therapy (3 or more daily insulin injections or treatment with an insulin pump with dose adjustments as needed, BG monitoring minimum qid, monthly visits, strict BG targets) vs. Conventional therapy (1 or 2 insulin injections per day with no dose adjustments, daily BG monitoring, visits q3 months).
Outcomes: Primary outcome was development or progression of retinopathy. Secondary outcomes were development or progression of renal, neurological, cardiovascular, and neuropsychological outcomes
Results: Intensive treatment of Type 1 DM significantly reduced the risk for the development and progression of retinopathy in the primary- and secondary-intervention cohorts, respectively. Intensive therapy also reduced the occurrence of microalbuminuria, albuminuria, and clinical neuropathy. The chief adverse event associated with intensive therapy was an increase in the occurrence of severe hypoglycemia.
Conclusions: Intensive treatment of Type 1 DM significantly reduces the development and progression of diabetic retinopathy, nephropathy, and neuropathy in patients with Type 1 DM.

Blood Glucose Control in Type 2 DM – UKPDS 33
Lancet 1998;352:837-853
Study: RCT (mean follow-up 10 yr).
Patients: 3,867 patients with newly diagnosed type 2 DM (mean age 53 yr, 61% men, 81% white, mean fasting plasma glucose [FPG] 6.1-15.0 mmol/L). Exclusions included severe cardiovascular disease, renal disease, retinopathy, and others.
Intervention: Intensive treatment with a sulfonylurea or insulin (target FPG <6 mmol/L) vs. conventional treatment with diet alone (target FPG <15 mmol/L without hyperglycemic symptoms).
Main Outcomes: DM-related endpoints (MI, angina, heart failure, stroke, renal failure, amputation, retinopathy, blindness, death from hyperglycemia or hypoglycemia), DM-related death, and all-cause mortality.
Results: Patients allocated to intensive treatment had lower median HbA1c levels (p<0.001).

Outcome	RRR % (p value)
DM-related endpoint	12 (0.029)
DM-related death	10 (0.34)
All-cause mortality	6 (0.44)

Patients allocated to intensive therapy had more hypoglycemic episodes and greater weight gain.
Conclusion: Intensive blood glucose control reduces microvascular, but not macrovascular complications in type 2 DM.

Targeting Intensive Glycemic Control vs. Targeting Conventional Glycemic Control for Type 2 DM
Cochrane DB Syst Rev 2011;6:CD008143
Study: Systematic review of randomized clinical trials of glycemic control in adults with type 2 DM.
Patients: Twenty trials randomized 16,106 patients with type 2 DM to intensive control and 13,880 patients with type 2 DM to conventional glycemic control.
Intervention: Intensive glycemic control (HbA1c ≤6.5%) versus conventional glycemic control (determined by local guidelines).
Primary Outcomes: All-cause mortality, compositive macrovascular (death from cardiovascular cause, nonfatal MI, nonfatal stroke) and microvascular events (nephropathy, retinopathy).
Results: There was no significant difference between targeting intensive and conventional glycemic control for all-cause mortality or cardiovascular mortality. Targeting intensive glycemic control reduced the risk of amputation, the composite risk of microvascular disease, retinopathy, retinal photocoagulation, and nephropathy. The risks of both mild and severe hypoglycemia were increased with targeting intensive glycemic control.
Conclusions: Intensive glycemic control did not reduce all-cause mortality and cardiovascular mortality compared to conventional glycemic control. Intensive glycemic control reduced the risk of microvascular complications while increasing the risk of hypoglycemia. Intensive glycemic control may also reduce the risk of non-fatal MI in trials exclusively dealing with glycemic control in usual care settings.

Canadian Diabetes Guidelines 2013

	Target
HbA1c	<7.0%
Fasting plasma glucose	4-7 mmol/L (72-126 mg/dL)
2h post-prandial glucose	5-10 mmol/L (90-180 mg/dL) 5-8 mmol/L (90-144 md/dL) if not meeting target A1c and can be safely achieved
Lipids	As per high risk group if age >40 or age >30 if DM duration >15 yr
Blood pressure	<130/80

Cardiovascular Effects of Intensive Lifestyle Intervention in Type 2 DM: The Look AHEAD Trial
NEJM 2013;369:145-154
Study: RCT, with 9.6 yr of median follow-up.
Population: 5,145 overweight or obese patients with type 2 DM.
Intervention: Intensive lifestyle intervention promoting weight loss through decreased caloric intake and increased physical activity (intervention) or DM support and education (control).
Primary Outcome: First occurrence of death from cardiovascular (CV) causes, non-fatal MI, non-fatal stroke, or hospitalization for angina.
Results: Although the intensive lifestyle intervention produced greater weight loss and reductions in glycated hemoglobin, the intervention did not significantly reduce the risk of CV morbidity or mortality.
Conclusions: An intensive lifestyle intervention focusing on weight loss did not significantly reduce the rate of cardiovascular events in overweight or obese adults with type 2 DM.

Table 8. Comparison of Type 1 and Type 2 Diabetes Mellitus (continued)

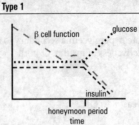

	Type 1	Type 2
Natural History	After initial presentation, honeymoon period often occurs where glycemic control can be achieved with little or no insulin treatment as residual cells are still able to produce insulin. Once these cells are destroyed, there is complete insulin deficiency	Early on, glucose tolerance remains normal despite insulin resistance as β cells compensate with increased insulin production. As insulin resistance and compensatory hyperinsulinism continue, the β cells are unable to maintain the hyperinsulinemic state which results in glucose intolerance and DM
Circulating Autoantibodies	Islet cell Ab present in up to 60-85%. Most common islet cell Ab is against glutamic acid decarboxylase (GAD). Up to 60% have Ab against insulin	<10%
Risk Factors	Personal history of other autoimmune diseases including Graves', myasthenia gravis, autoimmune thyroid disease, celiac disease, and pernicious anemia. Family history of autoimmune diseases	Age >40 yr. Schizophrenia. Abdominal obesity/overweight. Fatty liver. First-degree relative with DM. Hyperuricemia. Race/ethnicity (Black, Aboriginal, Hispanic, Asian-American, Pacific Islander). Hx of IGT or IFG. HTN. Dyslipidemia. Medications e.g. 2nd generation antipsychotics. PCOS. Hx of gestational DM or macrosomic baby (>9 lb or 4 kg)
Body Habitus	Normal to thin	Typically overweight with increased central obesity
Treatment	Insulin	Lifestyle modification. Non-insulin antihyperglycemic agents - unless contraindicated, metformin should be the initial antihyperglycemic agent of choice. Additional agents to be selected on the basis of clinically relevant issues, such as glucose lowering effectiveness, risk of hypoglycemia, and effect on body weight. Insulin therapy
Acute Complication	Diabetic ketoacidosis (DKA) in severe cases	Hyperosmolar hyperglycemic state (HHS). DKA in severe cases
Screening	Subclinical prodrome can be detected in first and second-degree relatives of those with type 1 DM by the presence of pancreatic islet autoantibodies	Screen individuals with risk factors

Treatment of Diabetes

Glycemic Targets
- HbA1c reflects glycemic control over 3 mo and is a measure of patient's long-term glycemic control
- therapy in most individuals with type 1 or type 2 DM (especially younger patients) should be targeted to achieve a HbA1c ≤7.0% in order to reduce the risk of microvascular and if implemented early in the course of disease, macrovascular complications
- more intensive glucose control, HbA1c <6.5%, may be targeted in type 2 DM in patients with a shorter duration of DM with no evidence of significant CVD and longer life expectancy, to further reduce risk of nephropathy and retinopathy, provided this does not result in a significant increase in hypoglycemia
- less stringent HbA1c targets (7.1-8.5%) may be more appropriate in type 1 and type 2 patients with limited life expectancy, higher level of functional dependency, a history of recurrent severe hypoglycemia, multiple comorbidities, extensive CAD, or a failure to attain HbA1c <7.0% despite intensified basal and bolus insulin therapy
- there may be harm associated with strategy to target HbA1c <6.0% (see *ACCORD trial*, E9)

Diet
- daily carbohydrate intake 45-60% of energy, protein 15-20% of energy, and fat <35% of energy
- intake of saturated fats <7% and polyunsaturated fats <10% of total calories each
- limit sodium, alcohol, and caffeine intake
- type 1: carbohydrate counting is used to titrate insulin regimen
- type 2: weight reduction

Lifestyle
- regular physical exercise to improve insulin sensitivity, lower lipid concentrations and control blood pressure
- smoking cessation

Medical Treatment: Non-insulin Antihyperglycemic Agents (Type 2 DM)
- initiate non-insulin antihyperglycemic therapy within 2-3 mo if lifestyle management does not result in glycemic control
- if initial HbA1c >8.5% at the time of diagnosis, initiate pharmacologic therapy with metformin immediately and consider combination of therapies or insulin immediately
- continue to add additional pharmacologic therapy in a timely fashion to achieve target HbA1C within 3-6 months of diagnosis
- see *Common Medications*, E49 for details on antihyperglycemic agents

Medical Treatment: Insulin (Figure 5)
- used for type 1 DM at onset, may be used in type 2 DM at any point in treatment
- routes of administration: subcutaneous injections, continuous subcutaneous insulin infusion pump, IV infusion (regular insulin only)
- bolus insulins: short-acting (Insulin regular), rapid-acting analogue (Insulin aspart, Insulin glulisine, Insulin lispro)
- basal insulins: intermediate-acting (Insulin NPH), long-acting analogue (Insulin detemir, glargine)
- premixed insulins (combination of basal and bolus insulins) available but not used regularly
- estimated total daily insulin requirement: 0.5-0.7 units/kg (often start with 0.3-0.5 units/kg/d)

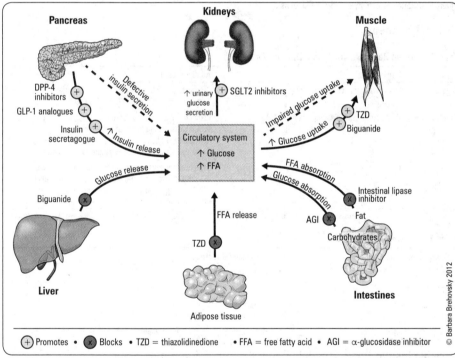

Figure 4. Antihyperglycemic agents

Table 9. Available Insulin Formulations

Insulin Type (trade name)	Onset	Peak	Duration
PRANDIAL (BOLUS) INSULINS			
Rapid-acting insulin analogues			
Insulin aspart (NovoRapid®)	10-15 min	1-1.5 h	3-5 h
Insulin lispro (Humalog®, Humalog 200 units/mL)	10-15 min	1-2 h	3.5-4.75 h
Insulin glulisine (Apidra®)	10-15 min	1-1.5 h	3-5 h
Short-acting insulins	30 min	2-3 h	6.5 h
Humulin R®			
Novolin Toronto®			
BASAL INSULINS			
Intermediate-acting	1-3 h	5-8 h	Up to 18 h
Humulin N®			
Novolin NPH®			
Long-acting basal insulin analogues	90 min	Not applicable	Up to 24 h (glargine 24 h, detemir 16-24 h)
Insulin detemir (Levemir®)			
Insulin glargine 100 units/mL (Lantus®)			
Insulin glargine 300 units/mL (Toujeo)			

DPP-IV Inhibitors
- Antihyperglycemic agents (e.g. sitagliptin, saxagliptin, linagliptin) that inhibit DPP-IV, which is an enzyme that degrades endogenous incretin hormones like GLP-1
- Incretin hormones stimulate glucose-dependent insulin secretion and inhibit glucagon release from the pancreas

GLP-1 Analogues (Incretins)
- Human glucagon-like peptide-1 analogues: exenatide, liraglutide
- These activate GLP-1 causing increased insulin secretion, decreased inappropriate glucagon secretion, increased B-cell growth/replication, slowed gastric emptying, and decreased food intake
- Associated with weight loss
- Subcutaneous formulation

Effects of Intensive Glucose Lowering in Type 2 DM: The ACCORD Trial
NEJM 2008;358:2545-2559
Study: Multicentre RCT.
Patients: 10,251 patients (mean age 62.2) with type 2 DM, and cardiovascular risk factors.
Intervention: Intensive therapy targeting a HbA1c level of less than 6.0% or standard therapy targeting 7.0-7.9%.
Outcomes: First occurrence of nonfatal MI, nonfatal stroke, or death from CV causes.
Results: The intensive therapy arm was stopped early (3.5 yr vs. 5.6 yr planned) due to evidence of increased mortality. There was no difference in primary outcome for either study arm. There was a significant increase in all-cause mortality, CV mortality, nonfatal MI, and CHF in the intensive therapy group. There were increased rates of all hypoglycemic events, any nonhypoglycemic serious adverse events, fluid retention, and weight gain >10 kg, but lower systolic and diastolic blood pressure in the intensive therapy group. There was an increased incidence of elevated ALT (>3x upper limit) and ACE drug use in the standard therapy group.
Conclusions: Intensive glucose lowering therapy in type 2 DM does not improve clinic outcomes and actually increases the risk of mortality with more adverse events compared to standard therapy. Additional research is required to discern the cause.

Effects of Intensive Blood Pressure Control in Type 2 DM: The ACCORD Trial
NEJM 2010;362:1575-1585
Study: RCT, unblinded with 4.7 yr of mean follow-up.
Population: 4,733 patients with type 2 DM, risk factors for cardiovascular (CV) disease, systolic blood pressure (sBP) between 130-180 mmHg.
Intervention: sBP control less than 120 mmHg (intensive) or 140 mmHg (standard).
Primary Outcomes: Major CV event (composite nonfatal MI, nonfatal stroke, or CV-related death).
Results: Mean number of medications at 1 yr for intensive therapy was 3.4 (95% CI 3.4-3.5) versus 2.1 (95% CI 2.1-2.2) for standard therapy. There was a significant increase in all serious adverse events in the intensive treatment arm (3.3% vs. 1.27%, p=<0.001); especially bradycardia or arrhythmia (0.5% vs. 0.13%, p=0.02) and hyperkalemia (0.4% vs. 0.04%, p=0.01). There was no significant difference in primary outcomes in the two study arms, or all-cause mortality. There was a significant reduction in any stroke (0.32%/yr vs. 0.53%/yr, p=0.01) and nonfatal stroke incidences (0.30%/yr vs. 0.47%/yr, p=0.03) in the intensive therapy arm.
Conclusions: Intensive BP lowering to less than 120 mmHg vs. 140 mmHg in patients with type 2 DM and CV risk factors does not reduce major CV event risk reduction except for stroke events.

Effects of Combination Lipid Therapy in Type 2 DM: the ACCORD Trial
NEJM 2010;362:1563-1574
Study: RCT, double-blinded trial with 4.7 yr of mean follow-up.
Population: 5,518 patients with type 2 DM.
Intervention: Statin with or without fibrate therapy.
Primary Outcome: Major cardiovascular (CV) event (composite nonfatal MI, nonfatal stroke, or CV-related death).
Results: No significant differences in primary outcome between the two arms. No difference in all MI, all stroke, or all-cause mortality between study arms.
Conclusions: The addition of fibrate therapy to statin therapy in patients with type 2 DM does not reduce major CV event risk.

Effects of a Mediterranean Diet in Preventing Cardiovascular Events in Type 2 DM: The PREDIMED Trial
NEJM 2013;368:1279-1290
Study: RCT, with 4.8 yr of median follow-up.
Population: 7,447 patients with type 2 DM or other high cardiovascular risk factors.
Intervention: Mediterranean diet supplemented with extra-virgin olive oil, Mediterranean diet supplemented with mixed nuts, or control diet with advice to reduce dietary fat.
Primary Outcome: Major cardiovascular (CV) event (MI, stroke, or death from CV causes).
Results: Both Mediterranean diets were associated with a reduced incidence of major CV events compared to the control diet.
Conclusions: A Mediterranean diet with extra-virgin olive oil or nuts reduces rates of MI, stroke, and CV death in those at high risk for CV disease.

Treatment of DKA/HHS
- Fluids
- Insulin
- Potassium
- Search for and treat precipitant

Conversion Chart for Percentage HbA1c to Average Blood Sugar Control

Average blood sugar level (mmol/L)		Hemoglobin A1c (% HbA1c)
17		12%
16	Inadequate Control	11%
14		10%
12		9%
10	Suboptimal	8%
8		7%
6	Optimal	6%

Conversion chart adapted from Nathan DM, et al. The clinical information value of a glycosylated hemoglobin assay. *NEJM* 1984;310:341-346

The 8 Is Precipitating DKA
Infection
Ischemia or Infarction
Iatrogenic (glucocorticoids)
Intoxication
Insulin missed
Initial presentation
Intra-abdominal process (e.g. pancreatitis, cholecystitis)
Intraoperative/perioperative stress

Table 9. Available Insulin Formulations (continued)

Insulin Type (trade name)	Onset	Peak	Duration
PRE-MIXED INSULINS			
Premixed regular insulin – NPH Humulin 30/70® Novolin 30/70®	A single vial or cartridge contains a fixed ratio of insulin (% of rapid acting or short-acting insulin to % of intermediate-acting insulin)		
Premixed insulin analogues Biphasic insulin aspart (NovoMix 30®) Insulin lispro/lispro protamine (Humalog Mix25® and Mix50®)			

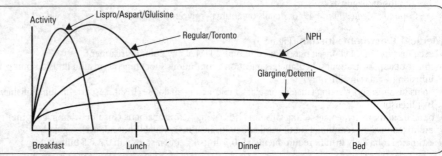

Figure 5. Duration of activity of different insulins

Insulin Regimens

Table 10. Insulin Regimens for Type 2 DM and Type 1 DM

	Regimen	Administration
Type 2 DM	Non-insulin antihyperglycemic agent + basal insulin	Start with 10 units of basal insulin at bedtime Titrate up by 1 unit until FPG <7.0 mmol/L
Type 1 DM	Basal-bolus (multiple daily injections (MDI))	Estimated total insulin requirement is 0.5-0.7 U/kg 40% is given as basal insulin at bedtime 20% is given as bolus insulin before breakfast, lunch, and dinner Continue metformin but discontinue secretagogue
	Premixed	Estimated total insulin requirement is 0.5-0.7 U/kg 2/3 dose is given as pre-mixed insulin before breakfast 1/3 dose is given as pre-mixed insulin before dinner Continue metformin but discontinue secretagogue

*Bolus insulin: Aspart, Glulisine, Lispro; *Basal insulin: Gargine, Detemir, NPH; *Pre-mixed insulin: Humulin 30/70, Novolin 30/70, Novomix 30, Humalog Mix25, Humalog Mix50

Table 11. Titrating Insulin Doses

Hyperglycemic Reading	Insulin Correction
High AM sugar	Increase bedtime basal insulin
High lunch sugar	Increase AM rapid/regular insulin
High supper sugar	Increase lunch rapid/regular insulin, or Increase AM basal insulin
High bedtime sugar	Increase supper rapid/regular insulin

Variable Insulin Dose Schedule ("Supplemental/Correction Scale")
- for patients on Basal-Bolus regimen: patient takes usual doses of basal insulin but varies doses of bolus insulin based on BG reading at time of dose
- use baseline bolus insulin dose when within BG target range; add or subtract units when above or below target
- when used in hospital (including perioperative management of DM), patient should also receive basal insulin to prevent fluctuations in blood sugar levels or long periods of hyperglycemia
- construction of a supplemental sliding scale for a patient on anti-hyperglycemics
- Correction Factor (CF) = 100/Total Daily Dose of insulin (TDD)
  - BG <4: call MD and give 15 g carbohydrates
  - BG between 4 to 8: no additional insulin
  - BG between 8 to (8 + CF): give one additional unit
  - BG between (8 + CF) to (8 + 2CF): give two additional units
  - BG between (8 + 2CF) to (8 + 3CF): give three additional units

Insulin Pump Therapy: Continuous Subcutaneous Insulin Infusion (CSII)
- external battery-operated device provides continuous basal dose of rapid-acting insulin analogue (aspart, glulisine, or lispro) through small subcutaneous catheter
- at meals, patient programs pump to deliver insulin bolus
- provides improved quality of life and flexibility
- risk of DKA if pump is inadvertently disconnected
- coverage available for insulin pumps for individuals with Type 1 DM varies by province

Acute Complications

All Ketonemia is not DKA
Consider starvation or alcohol ketosis

Table 12. Acute Complications of Diabetes Mellitus: Hyperglycemic Comatose States

	Diabetic Ketoacidosis (DKA)	Hyperosmolar Hyperglycemic State (HHS)
Pathophysiology	• Usually occurs in type 1 DM • Insulin deficiency with ↑ counterregulatory hormones (glucagon, cortisol, catecholamines, GH) • Can occur with lack of insulin (non-adherence, inadequate dosage, 1st presentation) or increased stress (surgery, infection, exercise) • Unopposed hepatic glucose production → hyperglycemia → osmotic diuresis → dehydration and electrolyte disturbance → ↓ Na^+ (water shift to ECF causing pseudohyponatremia) • Fat mobilization → ↑ FFA → ketoacids → metabolic acidosis • Severe hyperglycemia exceeds the renal threshold for glucose and ketone reabsorption → glucosuria and ketonuria • Total body K^+ depletion but serum K^+ may be normal or elevated, 2° to shift from ICF to ECF due to lack of insulin, ↑ plasma osmolality • Total body PO_4^{3-} depletion	• Occurs in type 2 DM • Often precipitated by sepsis, stroke, MI, CHF, renal failure, trauma, drugs (glucocorticoids, immunosuppressants, phenytoin, diuretics), dialysis, recent surgery, burns • Partial or relative insulin deficiency decreases glucose utilization in muscle, fat, and liver while inducing hyperglucagonemia and hepatic glucose production • Presence of a small amount of insulin prevents the development of ketosis by inhibiting lipolysis • Characterized by hyperglycemia, hyperosmolality, and dehydration without ketosis • More severe dehydration compared to DKA due to more gradual onset and ↑ duration of metabolic decompensation plus impaired fluid intake which is common in bedridden or elderly • Volume contraction → renal insufficiency → ↑ hyperglycemia, ↑ osmolality → shift of fluid from neurons to ECF → mental obtundation and coma
Clinical Features	• Polyuria, polydipsia, polyphagia with marked fatigue, N/V • Dehydration (orthostatic changes) • LOC may be ↓ with ketoacidosis or with high serum osmolality (osm >330 mmol/L) • Abdominal pain • Fruity smelling breath • Kussmaul's respiration	• Onset is insidious → preceded by weakness, polyuria, polydipsia • History of decreased fluid intake • History of ingesting large amounts of glucose containing fluids • Dehydration (orthostatic changes) • ↓ LOC → lethargy, confusion, comatose due to high serum osmolality • Kussmaul's respiration is absent unless the underlying precipitant has also caused a metabolic acidosis
Serum	• ↑ BG (typically 11-55 mmol/L, ↓ Na^+ (2° to hyperglycemia → for every ↑ in BG by 10 mmol/L) there is a ↓ in Na^+ by 3 mmol/L) • Normal or ↑ K^+, ↓ HCO_3^-, ↑ BUN, ↑ Cr, ketonemia, ↓ PO_4^{3-} • ↑ osmolality	• ↑ BG (typically 44.4-133.2 mmol/L) • In mild dehydration, may have hyponatremia (spurious 2° to hyperglycemia → for every ↑ in BG by 10 mmol/L there is a ↓ in Na+ by 3 mmol/L) – if dehydration progresses, may get hypernatremia • Ketosis usually absent or mild if starvation occurs • ↑ osmolality
ABG	• Metabolic acidosis with ↑ AG, possible 2° respiratory alkalosis • If severe vomiting/dehydration there may be a metabolic alkalosis	• Metabolic acidosis absent unless underlying precipitant leads to acidosis (e.g. lactic acidosis in MI)
Urine	• +ve for glucose and ketones	• -ve for ketones unless there is starvation ketosis • Glycosuria

Treatment	• ABCs are first priority
	• Monitor degree of ketoacidosis with AG, not BG or serum ketone level
	• Rehydration
	   – 1 L/h NS in first 2 h
	   – after 1st 2 L, 300-400 mL/h NS. Switch to 0.45% NaCl once euvolemic (continue NS if corrected sodium is falling faster than 3 mosm/kg water/h)
	   – once BG reaches 13.9 mmol/L then switch to D5W to maintain BG in the range of 12-14 mmol/L
	• Insulin therapy
	   – critical to resolve acidosis, not hyperglycemia
	   – do not use with hypokalemia (see below), until serum K^+ is corrected to >3.3 mmol/L
	   – use only regular insulin (R)
	   – maintain on 0.1 U/kg/h insulin R infusion
	   – check serum glucose hourly
	• K^+ replacement
	   – with insulin administration, hypokalemia may develop
	   – if serum K^+ <3.3 mmol/L, hold insulin and give 40 mEq/L K^+ replacement
	   – when K^+ 3.5-5.0 mmol/L add KCL 20-40 mEq/L IV fluid to keep K^+ in the range of 3.5-5 mEq/L
	• HCO_3^-
	   – if pH <7.0 or if hypotension, arrhythmia, or coma is present with a pH of <7.1 give HCO_3^- in 0.45% NaCl
	   – do not give if pH >7.1 (risk of metabolic alkalosis)
	   – can give in case of life-threatening hyperkalemia
	• ± mannitol (for cerebral edema)
		• Same resuscitation and emergency measures as DKA
		• Rehydration
		   – IV fluids: 1 L/h NS initially
		   – evaluate corrected serum Na^+
		   – if corrected serum Na^+ high or normal, switch to 0.45% NaCl (4-14 mL/kg/h)
		   – if corrected serum Na^+ low, maintain NS (4-14 mL/kg/h)
		   – when serum BG reaches 13.9 mmol/L switch to D5W
		• K^+ replacement
		   – less severe K^+ depletion compared to DKA
		   – if serum K^+ <3.3 mmol/L, hold insulin and give 40 mEq/L K^+ replacement
		   – if K^+ is 3.3-5.0, give KCl 20-30 mEq/L IV fluid
		   – if serum K^+ ≥5.5 mmol/L, check K^+ every 2 h
		• Search for precipitating event
		• Insulin therapy
		   – use only regular insulin (R)
		   – initially load 0.1 U/kg body weight insulin R bolus
		   – maintenance 0.1 U/kg/h insulin R infusion or IM
		   – check serum glucose hourly
		   – in general lower insulin requirement compared to DKA

Prognosis	• 2-5% mortality in developed countries • Serious morbidity from sepsis, hypokalemia, respiratory complications, thromboembolic complications, and cerebral edema (the latter in children)	• Overall mortality approaches 50% primarily because of the older patient population and underlying etiology/precipitant

Average fluid loss runs at 3-6 L in DKA, and 8-10 L in HHS

Laboratory Testing: Ketones
The nitroprusside test for ketones identifies acetone and acetoacetate but does NOT detect β-hydroxybutyrate (BHB), the ketone most frequently in excess. This has two clinical consequences:
- Be wary of a patient with a clinical picture of DKA but negative serum or urinary ketones. These could be false negatives because of the presence of BHB
- As DKA is treated, BHB is converted to acetone and acetoacetate. Serum or urinary ketones may therefore rise, falsely suggesting that the patient is worsening when in fact they are improving

Empagliflozin, Cardiovascular Outcomes, and Mortality in Type 2 Diabetes
NEJM 2015;373:2117-2128
Purpose: To examine whether Empagliflozin (an SGLT2 inhibitor) has any effect on cardiovascular risk in patients with Type 2 DM.
Study: Multi-centre RCT comparing Empagliflozin to placebo control; 7020 patients (test N=4687, placebo N=2333), median observation 3.1 yr.
Outcome: Death from cardiovascular causes, nonfatal MI, or nonfatal stroke.
Results: Both groups concurrently received the standard treatment for T2 DM. The Empagliflozin group had significantly lower rates of death from cardiovascular causes than control (3.7% vs. 5.9%; 38% decreased relative risk). The test group also had lower all-cause mortality (5.7% and 8.3%, respectively; 32% decreased relative risk).
Conclusion: Adding Empagliflozin to standard treatment for Type 2 DM reduced death from macrovascular complications and all-cause mortality when compared to placebo.

Management of Diabetic Retinopathy: A Systematic Review
JAMA 2007;298:902-916
Purpose: To review the best evidence for primary and secondary interventions in the management of diabetic retinopathy (DR), including diabetic macular edema.
Study Selection: English-language RCTs with more than 12 mo of follow-up and meta-analyses were included.
Results: Forty-four studies (including 3 meta-analyses) met the inclusion criteria. Tight glycemic and blood pressure control reduces the incidence and progression of DR. Pan-retinal laser photocoagulation reduces the risk of moderate and severe visual loss by 50% in patients with severe nonproliferative and proliferative retinopathy. Focal laser photocoagulation reduces the risk of moderate visual loss by 50-70% in eyes with macular edema. Early vitrectomy improves visual recovery in patients with proliferative retinopathy and severe vitreous hemorrhage. Intravitreal injections of steroids may be considered in eyes with persistent loss of vision when conventional treatment has failed.
Conclusions: Tight glycemic and blood pressure control remains the cornerstone in the primary prevention of DR. Pan-retinal and focal retinal laser photocoagulation reduces the risk of visual loss in patients with severe DR and macular edema, respectively. There is currently insufficient evidence to recommend routine use of other treatments.

Macrovascular Complications

- increased risk of CAD, ischemic stroke, and peripheral arterial disease secondary to accelerated atherosclerosis
- CAD (see Cardiology and Cardiac Surgery, C32)
    - risk of MI is 3-5x higher in those with DM compared to age-matched controls
    - CAD is the leading cause of death in type 2 DM
    - most patients with DM are considered "high risk" under the risk stratification for CAD (see *Dyslipidemias*, E5)
- ischemic stroke (see Neurology, N50)
    - risk of stroke is approximately 2.5x higher in those with DM
    - level of glycemia is both a risk factor for stroke and a predictor of a poorer outcome in patients who suffer a stroke
    - HbA1c level is a significant and independent predictor of the risk of stroke
- peripheral arterial disease (see Vascular Surgery, VS2)
    - manifested by intermittent claudication in lower extremities, intestinal angina, foot ulceration
    - risk of foot gangrene is 30x higher in those with DM compared to age-matched controls
    - risk of lower extremity amputation is 15x higher in those with DM
- treatment
    - tight blood pressure control (<130/80 mmHg); especially for stroke prevention
    - tight glycemic control in early DM without established CVD (refer to ACCORD, VADT, ADVANCE, DCCT, EDIC, UKPDS extension studies)
    - tight low density lipoprotein (LDL) cholesterol control (LDL ≤2.0 mmol/L)
    - ACEI or angiotensin receptor blocker in high-risk patients
    - smoking cessation

Microvascular Complications

DIABETIC RETINOPATHY (see Ophthalmology, OP33 for a more detailed description)

Epidemiology
- type 1 DM: 25% affected at 5 yr, 100% at 20 yr
- type 2 DM: 25% affected at diagnosis, 60% at 20 yr
- leading cause of blindness in North America between the ages of 20-74
- most important factor is disease duration

Clinical Features
- nonproliferative
- preproliferative
- proliferative

Treatment and Prevention

- tight glycemic control (delays onset, decreases progression), tight lipid control, manage HTN, smoking cessation
- ophthalmological treatments available – see Ophthalmology, OP33 for more details
- annual follow-up visits with an optometrist or ophthalmologist examination through dilated pupils whether symptomatic or not (immediate referral after diagnosis of type 2 DM; 5 yr after diagnosis of type 1 DM)
- interval for follow-up should be tailored to severity of retinopathy

DIABETIC NEPHROPATHY (see Nephrology, NP31 for a more detailed description)

Epidemiology
- DM-induced renal failure is the most common cause of renal failure in North America
- 20-40% of persons with type 1 DM (after 5-10 yr) and 4-20% with type 2 DM have progressive nephropathy

Screening
- serum creatinine
- random urine test for albumin to creatinine ratio (ACR) plus urine dipstick test for all type 2 DM patients at diagnosis, then annually, and for postpubertal type 1 DM patients with ≥5yr duration of DM

Treatment and Prevention
- appropriate glycemic control
- appropriate blood pressure control (<130/80 mmHg)
- use either ACEI or ARB (often used first line for their CVD protection)
- limit use of nephrotoxic drugs and dyes

DIABETIC NEUROPATHY

Epidemiology
- approximately 50% of patients within 10 yr of onset of type 1 DM and type 2 DM

Pathophysiology
- can have peripheral sensory neuropathy, motor neuropathy, or autonomic neuropathy
- mechanism poorly understood
- acute cranial nerve palsies and diabetic amyotrophy are thought to be due to ischemic infarction of peripheral nerve
- the more common motor and sensory neuropathies are thought to be related to metabolic or osmotic toxicity secondary to increased sorbitol and/or decreased myoinositol (possible mechanisms include accumulation of advanced glycation endproducts [AGE], oxidative stress, protein kinase C, nerve growth factor deficiency)

Screening
- 128 Hz tuning fork or 10 g monofilament at diagnosis and annually in people with type 2 DM and after 5 yr duration of type 1 DM

Clinical Features

Table 13. Clinical Presentation of Diabetic Neuropathies

Peripheral Sensory Neuropathy	Motor Neuropathy	Autonomic Neuropathy
Paresthesias (tingling, itching), neuropathic pain, radicular pain, numbness, decreased tactile sensation	Less common than sensory neuropathy Delayed motor nerve conduction and muscle weakness/atrophy	Postural hypotension, tachycardia, decreased cardiovascular response to Valsalva maneuver
Bilateral and symmetric with decreased perception of vibration and pain/temperature; especially true in the lower extremities but may also be present in the hands	May involve one nerve trunk (mononeuropathy) or more (mononeuritis multiplex) Some of the motor neuropathies spontaneously resolve after 6-8 wk	Gastroparesis and alternating diarrhea and constipation Urinary retention and erectile dysfunction
Decreased ankle reflex	Reversible CN palsies: III (ptosis/ophthalmoplegia, pupil sparing), VI (inability to laterally deviate eye), and VII (Bell's palsy)	
Symptoms may first occur in entrapment syndromes e.g. carpal tunnel	Diabetic amyotrophy: refers to pain, weakness, and wasting of hip flexors or extensors	
May result in neuropathic ulceration of foot		

Treatment and Management
- tight glycemic control
- for neuropathic pain syndromes: tricyclic antidepressants (e.g. amitriptyline), pregabalin, duloxetine, anti-epileptics (e.g. carbamazepine, gabapentin), and capsaicin
- foot care education
- Jobst® fitted stocking and tilting of head of bed may decrease symptoms of orthostatic hypotension
- treat gastroparesis with domperidone and/or metoclopramide (dopamine antagonists), erythromycin (stimulates motilin receptors)
- medical, mechanical, and surgical treatment for erectile dysfunction (see Urology, U30)

Other Complications

Dermatologic
- diabetic dermopathy: atrophic brown spots commonly in pretibial region known as "shin spots", secondary to increased glycosylation of tissue proteins or vasculopathy
- eruptive xanthomas secondary to increased triglycerides
- necrobiosis lipoidica diabeticorum: rare complication characterized by thinning skin over the shins allowing visualization of subcutaneous vessels

Bone and Joint Disease
- juvenile cheiroarthropathy: chronic stiffness of hand caused by contracture of skin over joints secondary to glycosylated collagen and other connective tissue proteins
- Dupuytren's contracture
- bone demineralization: bone density 10-20% below normal
- adhesive capsulitis ("frozen shoulder")

Cataracts
- subcapsular and senile cataracts secondary to glycosylated lens protein or increased sorbitol causing osmotic change and fibrosis

Infections
- see Infectious Diseases, ID15

Effect of a Multifactorial Intervention on Mortality in Type 2 DM: The Steno-2 Study
NEJM 2008;358:580-591
Study: Single centre RCT.
Patients: People (n=160) with type 2 DM and persistent microalbuminuria.
Intervention: Random assignment to receive either conventional multifactorial treatment or intensified, target-driven therapy involving a combination of medications and focused behaviour modification. Targets included an HbA1c level of <6.5%, a fasting serum total cholesterol level of <4.5 mmol/L, a fasting serum triglyceride level of <1.7 mmol/L, a sBP of <130 mmHg, and a dBP of <80 mmHg. Patients were treated with blockers of the renin–angiotensin system because of their microalbuminuria, regardless of blood pressure, and received low-dose Aspirin® as primary prevention.
Outcomes: The primary end point was the time to death from any cause. Other endpoints examined were death from CV causes and various CV events along with diabetic neuropathy, nephropathy, and retinopathy.
Results: Twenty-four patients in the intensive-therapy group died, as compared with 40 in the conventional-therapy group (hazard ratio, 0.54; 95% confidence interval [CI] 0.32-0.89; p=0.02). Intensive therapy was associated with a lower risk of death from CV causes (hazard ratio, 0.43; 95% CI 0.19-0.94; p=0.04) and of CV events (hazard ratio, 0.41; 95% CI 0.25-0.67; p<0.001). One patient in the intensive-therapy group had progression to end-stage renal disease, as compared with six patients in the conventional-therapy group (p=0.04). Fewer patients in the intensive-therapy group required retinal photocoagulation (relative risk, 0.45; 95% CI 0.23-0.86; p=0.02).
Conclusions: In at-risk patients with type 2 DM, intensive intervention with multiple drug combinations and behaviour modification had sustained beneficial effects with respect to vascular complications and on rates of death from any cause and from CV causes.

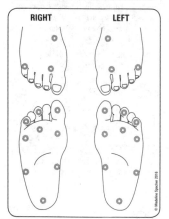

Figure 6. Monofilament testing for diabetic neuropathy

Effects of Treatments for Symptoms of Painful Diabetic Neuropathy: Systematic Review
BMJ 2007;335:87
Purpose: To evaluate the effects of treatments for the symptoms of painful diabetic neuropathy.
Study Selection: RCTs comparing topically applied and orally administered drugs with a placebo in adults with painful diabetic neuropathy.
Results: 25 included reports compared anticonvulsants (n=1,270), antidepressants (94), opioids (329), ion channel blockers (173), NMDA antagonist (14), duloxetine (805), capsaicin (277), and isosorbide dinitrate spray (22) with placebo. The odds ratios in terms of 50% pain relief were 5.33 (95% CI 1.77-16.02) for traditional anticonvulsants, 3.25 (95% CI 2.27-4.66) for newer generation anticonvulsants, and 22.24 (95% CI 5.83-84.75) for tricyclic antidepressants. The odds ratios in terms of withdrawals related to adverse events were 1.51 (95% CI 0.33-6.96) for traditional anticonvulsants, 2.98 (95% CI 1.75-5.07) for newer generation anticonvulsants, and 2.32 (95% CI 0.59-9.69) for tricyclic antidepressants.
Conclusion: Anticonvulsants and antidepressants are still the most commonly used options to manage diabetic neuropathy. Tricyclic antidepressants and traditional anticonvulsants are better for short-term pain relief than newer anticonvulsants. Evidence of the long-term effects of antidepressants and anticonvulsants is lacking. Further studies are needed on opioids, NMDA antagonists, and ion channel blockers.

Other Players in Glucose Homeostasis
These hormones act to increase blood glucose levels
• Glucagon
• Epinephrine
• Cortisol
• Growth hormone

C-Peptide
A short peptide released into the circulation when proinsulin is cleaved to insulin

Use C-peptide Levels to Distinguish between Exogenous and Endogenous Source of Hyperinsulinemia
Increased = endogenous
Decreased or normal = exogenous

Treatment of Acute Hypoglycemic Episode (Blood Glucose <4.0 mmol/L) in the Awake Patient (e.g. able to self-treat)

1) Eat 15 g of carbohydrates (CHO) (e.g. 3 packets sugar dissolved in water; 3/4 cup of juice)
↓
2) Wait 15 min
↓
3) Retest Blood Glucose (BG)
↓
4) Repeat steps 1-3 until BG >5 mmol/L
↓
5) Eat next scheduled meal. If next meal is >1 h away, eat snack including 15 g of CHO and protein

Hypoglycemia Unawareness (Type 1 DM >>> Type 2 DM)

Patient remains asymptomatic until severely hypoglycemic levels are reached

Causes:
• Decreased glucagon/epinephrine response
• History of repeated hypoglycemia or low HbA1c
• Autonomic neuropathy
• Not safe to drive

Suggest that patient obtain a Medic-Alert bracelet if at risk for hypoglycemia, especially with hypoglycemia unawareness

Hypoglycemia (BG <4.0 mmol/L or 72 mg/dL)

Etiology and Pathophysiology
• hypoglycemia occurs most frequently in people with DM receiving insulin or certain antihyperglycemic therapies (insulin secretagogues)
• in people without DM, care must be taken to distinguish fasting from post-prandial hypoglycemia as each invokes separate differential diagnoses

Table 14. Common Causes of Hypoglycemia

Fasting		Post-Prandial (Nonfasting, Reactive)
Hyperinsulinism	**Without Hyperinsulinism**	
Exogenous insulin	Severe hepatic dysfunction	Alimentary
Sulfonylurea or meglitinide reaction	Chronic renal insufficiency	Functional
Autoimmune hypoglycemia (autoantibodies to insulin or insulin receptor)	Hypocortisolism	Noninsulinoma pancreatogenous hypoglycemic syndrome
	Alcohol use	Occult DM
Pentamidine	Non-pancreatic tumours	Leucine sensitivity
Pancreatic β cell tumour – insulinoma	Inborn error of carbohydrate metabolism, glycogen storage disease, gluconeogenic enzyme deficiency	Hereditary fructose intolerance
		Galactosemia
		Newborn infant of diabetic mother

Clinical Features
• Whipple's triad
  1. serum glucose <2.5 mmol/L in males and <2.2 mmol/L in females
  2. neuroglycopenic symptoms
  3. rapid relief provided by administration of glucose
• adrenergic symptoms (typically occur first; caused by autonomic nervous system activity)
  ▪ palpitations, sweating, anxiety, tremor, tachycardia
• neuroglycopenic symptoms (caused by decreased activity of CNS)
  ▪ dizziness, headache, clouding of vision, mental dullness, fatigue, confusion, seizures, coma

Investigations
• electrolytes, creatinine, LFTs, drugs/toxins, cortisol
• if concerned about possible insulinoma
  ▪ blood work to be drawn when patient is hypoglycemic (e.g. during hospitalized 72-h fast) for glucose, serum ketones, insulin, pro-insulin, C-peptide, insulin antibodies

Treatment
• for fasting hypoglycemia, must treat underlying cause
• for post-prandial (reactive) hypoglycemia, frequent small feeds
• see Emergency Medicine, ER35
• treatment of hypoglycemic episode in the unconscious patient or patient NPO
  ▪ D50W 50 mL (1 ample) IV or 1 mg glucagon SC (if no IV available)
  ▪ may need ongoing glucose infusion once BG >5 mmol/L

Metabolic Syndrome

• several definitions exist
• postulated syndrome related to insulin resistance associated with hyperglycemia, hyperinsulinemia, HTN, central obesity, and dyslipidemia
• obesity aggravates extent of insulin resistance
• complications include DM, atherosclerosis, CAD, MI, and stroke
• women with PCOS are at increased risk for developing insulin resistance, hyperlipidemia, and metabolic syndrome
• not to be confused with syndrome X related to angina pectoris with normal coronary arteries (Prinzmetal angina)

Obesity

• see Family Medicine, FM7

Pituitary Gland

Pituitary Hormones

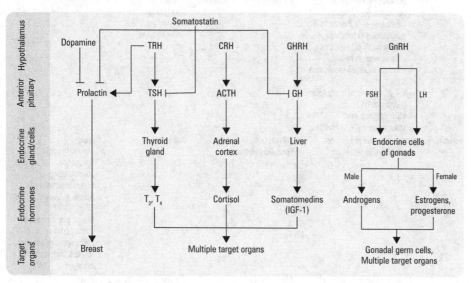

Figure 7. Hypothalamic-pituitary hormonal axes
CRH = corticotropin-releasing hormone; GHRH = growth hormone-releasing hormone; GnRH = gonadotropin-releasing hormone; PRH = prolactin-releasing hormone; TRH = thyrotropin-releasing hormone

Hypothalamic Control of Pituitary
- trophic and inhibitory factors control the release of pituitary hormones
- most hormones are primarily under trophic stimulation except prolactin which is primarily under inhibitory control by dopamine, as well as GH and TSH which are inhibited by somatostatin
- transection of the pituitary stalk (i.e. dissociation of hypothalamus and pituitary) leads to pituitary hypersecretion of prolactin and hyposecretion of all remaining hormones

Anterior Pituitary Hormones
- growth hormone (GH), luteinizing hormone (LH), follicle stimulating hormone (FSH), thyroid stimulating hormone (TSH), adrenocorticotropic hormone (ACTH), and prolactin (PRL)

Posterior Pituitary (Hypothalamic) Hormones
- antidiuretic hormone (ADH) and oxytocin
- peptides synthesized in the supraoptic and paraventricular nuclei of the hypothalamus
- although ADH and oxytocin are produced in the hypothalamus these hormones are stored and released from the posterior pituitary

Table 15. The Physiology and Action of Pituitary Hormones

Hormone	Function	Physiology	Inhibitory Stimulus	Secretory Stimulus
ACTH	Stimulates growth of adrenal cortex and secretion of its hormones	Polypeptide Pulsatile and diurnal variation (highest in AM, lowest at midnight)	Dexamethasone Cortisol	CRH Metyrapone Insulin-induced hypoglycemia Vasopressin Fever, pain, stress
GH	Needed for linear growth IGF-1 stimulates growth of bone and cartilage	Polypeptide Acts indirectly through serum factors synthesized in the liver: IGF-1 (somatomedin-C) Serum GH undetectable for most of the day and suppressed after meals high in glucose Sustained rise during sleep	Glucose challenge Glucocorticoids Hypothyroidism Somatostatin Dopamine D2 receptor agonists IGF-1 (long-loop) Tonically by dopamine	GHRH Insulin-induced hypoglycemia Exercise REM sleep Arginine, clonidine, propranolol, L-dopa

Table 15. The Physiology and Action of Pituitary Hormones (continued)

Hormone	Function	Physiology	Inhibitory Stimulus	Secretory Stimulus
LH/FSH	Stimulate gonads via cAMP Ovary: LH: production of androgens (thecal cells) which are converted to estrogens (granulosa cells); induces luteinization in follicles FSH: growth of granulosa cells in ovarian follicle; controls estrogen production Testes: LH: production of testosterone (Leydig cells) FSH: production of spermatozoa (Sertoli cells)	Polypeptide Glycoproteins (similar α subunit as TSH and hCG) Secreted in pulsatile fashion	Estrogen Progesterone Testosterone Inhibin Continuous (i.e. non-pulsatile) GnRH infusion	Pulsatile GnRH
Prolactin	Promotes milk production Inhibits GnRH secretion	Polypeptide Episodic secretion	Dopamine	Sleep Stress, hypoglycemia Pregnancy, breastfeeding Mid-menstrual cycle Sexual activity TRH Drugs: psychotropics, antihypertensives, dopamine antagonists, opiates, high dose estrogen
TSH	Stimulates growth of thyroid and secretion of T_3 and T_4 via cAMP	Glycoprotein	Circulating thyroid hormones (T_3, T_4) Opiates, dopamine	TRH Epinephrine Prostaglandins
ADH	Acts at renal collecting ducts on V2 receptors to cause insertion of aquaporin channels and increases water reabsorption thereby concentrating urine	Octapeptide Secreted by posterior pituitary Osmoreceptors in hypothalamus detect serum osmolality Contracted plasma volume detected by baroreceptors is a more potent stimulus than ↑ osmolality	↓ serum osmolality	Hypovolemia or ↓ effective circulatory volume ↑ serum osmolality Stress, pain, fever, paraneoplastic Lung or brain pathology
Oxytocin	Causes uterine contraction Breast milk secretion	Nonapeptide Secreted by posterior pituitary	EtOH	Suckling Distention of female genital tract during labour via stretch receptors

Growth Hormone

GH DEFICIENCY

- cause of short stature in children (see Pediatrics, P26)
- controversial significance in adults; often not clinically apparent, may present as fatigue

GH EXCESS

Risks Associated with GH Excess
- Cardiac disease (e.g. CAD, cardiomegaly, cardiomyopathy) in 1/3 of patients, with a doubling of risk of death from cardiac disease
- HTN in 1/3 of patients
- Risk of cancer (particularly GI) increased 2-fold to 3-fold

Etiology
- GH secreting pituitary adenoma, carcinoid or pancreatic islet tumours secreting ectopic GHRH resulting in excess GH

Pathophysiology
- normally GH is a catabolic hormone that acts to increase blood glucose levels
- in growth hormone excess states, secretion remains pulsatile but there is loss of hypoglycemic stimulation, glucose suppression, and the nocturnal surge
- proliferation of bone, cartilage, soft tissues, organomegaly
- insulin resistance and IGT

Clinical Features
- in children (before epiphyseal fusion) leads to gigantism
- in adults (after epiphyiseal fusion) leads to acromegaly
- enlargement of hands and feet, coarsening of facial features, thickening of calvarium, prognathism, thickening of skin, increased sebum production, sweating, acne, sebaceous cysts, fibromata mollusca, acanthosis nigricans, arthralgia, carpal tunnel syndrome, degenerative osteoarthritis, barrel chest, thyromegaly, renal calculi, HTN, cardiomyopathy, obstructive sleep apnea, colonic polyps, erectile dysfunction, menstrual irregularities, and DM

Investigations
- elevated serum insulin-like growth factor-1 (IGF-1) is usually the first line diagnostic test
- glucose suppression test is the most specific test (75 g of glucose PO suppresses GH levels in healthy individuals but not in patients with acromegaly)
- CT, MRI, or skull x-rays may show cortical thickening, enlargement of the frontal sinuses, and enlargement and erosion of the sella turcica
- MRI of the sella turcica is needed to look for a tumour

Treatment
- surgery, octreotide (somatostatin analogue), dopamine agonist (bromocriptine/cabergoline), growth hormone receptor antagonist (pegvisomant), radiation

Prolactin

HYPERPROLACTINEMIA

Etiology
- pregnancy and breastfeeding
- prolactinoma: most common pituitary adenoma (prolactin-secreting tumours may be induced by estrogens and grow during pregnancy)
- pituitary masses with pituitary stalk compression causing reduced dopamine inhibition of prolactin release
- primary hypothyroidism (increased TRH)
- decreased clearance due to chronic renal failure or severe liver disease (prolactin is metabolized by both the kidney and liver)
- medications with anti-dopaminergic properties are a common cause of high prolactin levels: antipsychotics (common), antidepressants, antihypertensives, anti-migraine agents (triptans/ergotamines), bowel motility agents (metoclopramide/domperidone), H_2-blockers (ranitidine)
- macroprolactinemia (high molecular weight prolactin also known as big big prolactin)

Approach to Nipple Discharge
- Differentiate between galactorrhea (fat droplets present) versus breast discharge (usually unilateral, may be bloody or serous)
- If galactorrhea, determine if physiologic (e.g. pregnancy, lactation, stress) versus pathologic
- If abnormal breast discharge, must rule out a breast malignancy

Clinical Features
- galactorrhea (secretion of breast milk in women and, in rare cases, men), infertility, hypogonadism, amenorrhea, erectile dysfunction

Investigations
- serum PRL, TSH, liver enzyme tests, creatinine, macroprolactin level in select cases
- MRI of the sella turcica in select cases

Treatment
- long-acting dopamine agonist: bromocriptine, cabergoline, or quinagolide
- surgery ± radiation (rare)
- prolactin-secreting tumours are often slow-growing and sometimes require no treatment
- if medication-induced, consider stopping medication if possible
- in certain cases if microprolactinoma and not planning on becoming pregnant, may consider OCP

Thyroid Stimulating Hormone

- see *Thyroid*, E20

Adrenocorticotropic Hormone

- see *Adrenal Cortex*, E29

Luteinizing Hormone and Follicle Stimulating Hormone

HYPOGONADOTROPIC HYPOGONADISM

Etiology
- primary/congenital: Kallmann syndrome, CHARGE syndrome, GnRH insensitivity
- secondary: CNS or pituitary tumours, pituitary apoplexy, brain/pituitary radiation, drugs (GnRH agonists/antagonists, glucocorti-coids, narcotics, chemotherapy, drugs causing hyperprolactinemia), functional deficiency due to another cause (hyperprolactinemia, chronic systemic illnesses, eating disorders, hypothyroidism, DM, Cushing's disease), systemic diseases (hemochromatosis, sarcoido-sis, histiocytosis)

Clinical Features
- hypogonadism, amenorrhea, erectile dysfunction (see Urology, U30), loss of body hair, fine skin, testicular atrophy, failure of pubertal development

Treatment
- combined FSH/LH hormone therapy, hCG, rFSH, or pulsatile GnRH analogue if fertility desired
- symptomatic treatment with estrogen/testosterone

HYPERGONADOTROPIC HYPOGONADISM

- hypogonadism due to impaired response of the gonads to FSH and LH

Etiology
- congenital:
  - chromosomal abnormalities (Turner's syndrome, Klinefelter syndrome, XX gonadal dysgenesis)
  - enzyme defects (17α-hydroxylase deficiency, 17, 20-lyase deficiency)
  - gonadotropin resistance (Leydig cell hypoplasia, FSH Insensitivty, pseudohypoparathyroidism type 1A)

- acquired:
  - gonadal toxins (chemotherapy, radiation)
  - drugs (glucocorticoids, antiandrogens, opioids, alcohol)
  - infections (STIs, Mumps)
  - gonadal failure in adults (androgen decline and testicular failure in men, premature ovarian failure and menopause in women)

Clinical Features
- hypogonadism, amenorrhea, erectile dysfunction (see Urology, U30), loss of body hair, fine skin, testicular atrophy, failure of pubertal development, low libido, infertility

Treatment
- hormone replacement therapy consisting of androgen (for males) and estrogen (for females) administration

Antidiuretic Hormone

DIABETES INSIPIDUS

Definition
- disorder of ineffective ADH (decreased production or peripheral resistance) resulting in passage of large volumes of dilute urine

Etiology and Pathophysiology
- central DI: insufficient ADH due to pituitary surgery, tumours, idiopathic/autoimmune, stalk lesion, hydrocephalus, histiocytosis X, trauma, familial central DI
- nephrogenic DI: collecting tubules in kidneys resistant to ADH due to drugs (e.g. lithium), hypercalcemia, hypokalemia, chronic renal disease, hereditary nephrogenic DI
- psychogenic polydipsia and osmotic diuresis must be ruled out

Diagnosing Subtypes of DI with DDAVP Response
Concentrated urine = Central
No effect = Nephrogenic

Clinical Features
- passage of large volumes of dilute urine, polydipsia, and dehydration; hypernatremia can develop with inadequate water consumption or secondary to an impaired thirst mechanism

Diagnostic Criteria
- fluid deprivation will differentiate true DI (high urine output persists, urine osmolality < plasma osmolality) from psychogenic DI (psychogenic polydipsia)
- response to exogenous ADH (DDAVP) will distinguish central from nephrogenic DI

Treatment
- DDAVP/vasopressin for central DI
- chlorpropamide, clofibrate, thiazides, NSAIDs, or carbamazepine as second line or for partial DI
- nephrogenic DI treated with solute restriction NSAIDs and thiazide diuretics; DDAVP (if partial)

SYNDROME OF INAPPROPRIATE ADH SECRETION

Diagnostic Criteria
- hyponatremia with corresponding plasma hypo-osmolality, urine sodium concentration above 40 mEq/L, urine less than maximally diluted (>100 mOsm/kg), euvolemia (edema absent), and absence of adrenal, renal, or thyroid insufficiency

Etiology and Pathophysiology
- stress (pain, nausea, post-surgical)
- malignancy (lung, pancreas, lymphoma)
- CNS disease (inflammatory, hemorrhage, tumour, Guillain-Barré syndrome)
- respiratory disease (TB, pneumonia, empyema)
- drugs (SSRIs, vincristine, chlorpropamide, cyclophosphamide, carbamazepine, nicotine, morphine, DDAVP, oxytocin)

Clinical Features
- symptoms of hyponatremia: headaches, nausea, vomiting, muscle cramps, tremors, cerebral edema If severe (confusion, mood swings, hallucinations, seizures, coma)

Treatment
- treat underlying cause, fluid restriction (800-1000 mL/day), vasopressin receptor antagonists (e.g. tolvaptan, conivaptan), and demeclocycline (antibiotic with anti-ADH properties, rarely-used) fludrocortisone, furosemide

Pituitary Pathology

PITUITARY ADENOMA (see Neurosurgery, NS13)

Clinical Features
- local mass effects
  - visual field defects (bitemporal hemianopsia due to compression of the optic chiasm), diploplia (due to oculomotor nerve palsies), headaches; increased ICP is rare
- hypofunction
  - hypopituitarism
- hyperfunction
  - PRL (galactorrhea), GH (acromegaly in adults, gigantism in children), ACTH (Cushing's disease = Cushing's syndrome caused by a pituitary tumour)
  - tumours secreting LH, FSH, and TSH are rare

Investigations
- radiological evaluation (MRI is imaging procedure of choice)
- formal visual field testing
- hypothalamic-pituitary hormonal function

HYPOPITUITARISM

Etiology (The Eight Is)
- Invasive
  - pituitary tumours, craniopharyngioma, cysts (Rathke's cleft, arachnoid, or dermoid), metastases
- Infarction/hemorrhage
  - Sheehan's syndrome (pituitary infarction due to excessive post-partum blood loss and hypovolemic shock)
  - pituitary apoplexy (acute hemorrhage/infarction of a pituitary tumour; presents with sudden loss of pituitary hormones, severe headache, and altered level of consciousness; can be fatal if not recognized and treated early)
- Infiltrative/inflammatory
  - sarcoidosis, hemochromatosis, histiocytosis
- Infectious
  - syphilis, TB, fungal (histoplasmosis), parasitic (toxoplasmosis)
- Injury
  - severe head trauma
- Immunologic
  - autoimmune destruction
- Iatrogenic
  - following surgery or radiation
- Idiopathic
  - familial forms, congenital midline defects

Clinical Features
- symptoms depend on which hormone is deficient:
  - ACTH: fatigue, weight loss, hypoglycemia, anemia, hyponatremia, failure to thrive and delayed puberty in children
  - GH: short stature in children
  - TSH: tiredness, cold intolerance, constipation, weight gain, hair loss
  - LH and FSH: oligo- or amenorrhea, infertility, decreased facial/body hair and muscle mass in men, delayed puberty
  - Prolactin: inability to breastfeed
  - ADH: symptoms of diabetes insipidus (extreme thirst, polydipsia, hypernatremia)
  - Oxytocin: usually asymptomatic- only needed during labour and breastfeeding

SIADH vs. Cerebral Salt Wasting (CSW)
CSW can occur in cases of subarachnoid hemorrhage. Na+ is excreted by malfunctioning renal tubules, mimicking findings of SIADH; hallmark is hypovolemia

Presentations of Pituitary Lesions
- Mass effect (visual field deficits, diplopia, ptosis, headaches, CSF leak)
- Hyperfunction
- Hypofunction

Important Deficiencies to Recognize are:
- Adrenal insufficiency
- Hypothyroidism
Concurrent adrenal insufficiency and hypothyroidism should be treated with glucocorticoids first and then with thyroid hormone to avoid adrenal crisis

The Pituitary Hormones
Order they are usually lost with compression by a mass:
"Go Look For The Adenoma Please"
GH, LH, FSH, TSH, ACTH, PRL + posterior pituitary hormones: ADH and oxytocin

Investigations
- triple bolus test
  - stimulates release of all anterior pituitary hormones in normal individuals
  - rapid sequence of IV infusion of insulin, GnRH, and TRH
  - insulin (usual dose 0.1 unit/kg of human regular insulin) → hypoglycemia → increased GH and ACTH/cortisol
  - GnRH (100 μg IV push) → increased LH and FSH
  - TRH (200 μg IV push over 120 s) → increased TSH and PRL (no longer available in Canada)
  - GnRH and TRH stimulation tests are very limited in their utility; the insulin tolerance test is the only truly useful test in the triple bolus assessment

Thyroid

Thyroid Hormones

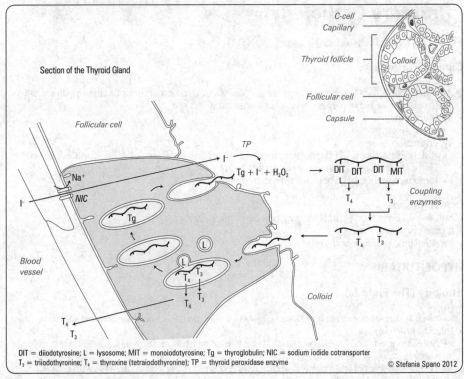

Section of the Thyroid Gland

DIT = diiodotyrosine; L = lysosome; MIT = monoiodotyrosine; Tg = thyroglobulin; NIC = sodium iodide cotransporter
T_3 = triiodothyronine; T_4 = thyroxine (tetraiodothyronine); TP = thyroid peroxidase enzyme

© Stefania Spano 2012

Figure 8. Thyroid hormone synthesis

Synthetic Function of Thyroid Gland
- the synthesis of thyroid hormones T_4 (thyroxine) and T_3 (triiodothyronine) by the thyroid gland involves trapping and oxidation of iodide, iodination of thyroglobulin, digestion of thyroglobulin, and release of T_3 and T_4
- free T_4 (0.03%) and free T_3 (0.3%) represent the hormonally active fraction of thyroid hormones
  - the remaining fraction is bound to thyroxine binding globulin (TBG) and albumin and is biologically inactive
- T_3 is more biologically active (3-8x more potent), but T_4 has a longer half-life
- 85% of T_4 is converted to T_3 or reverse T_3 (RT3) in the periphery by deiodinases
- RT3 is metabolically inactive but produced in times of stress to decrease metabolic activity
- most of the plasma T_3 pool is derived from the peripheral conversion of T_4
- calcitonin, a peptide hormone, is also produced in the thyroid, by the parafollicular cells or C cells
  - it functions by inhibiting osteoclast activity and increasing renal calcium excretion

Role of Thyroid Hormones
- thyroid hormones act primarily through modifying gene transcription by binding to nuclear receptors
- action of these hormones is diffuse, effecting nearly every organ system
- they increase the basal metabolic rate including: increased Na^+/K^+ATPase activity, increased O_2 consumption, increased respiration, heat generation, and increased cardiovascular activity
- also play crucial role during fetal life in both neurological and somatic development

Patterns of Hormone Levels

	TSH	T_3, T_4
1° Hyper	↓	↑
2° Hyper	↑	↑
1° Hypo	↑	↓
2° Hypo	↓	↓

Regulation of Thyroid Function

- extrathyroid
  - stimulation of thyroid by TSH, epinephrine, prostaglandins (cAMP stimulators)
  - T_3 negatively feeds back on anterior pituitary to inhibit TSH and on hypothalamus to inhibit TRH
- intrathyroid (autoregulation)
  - synthesis (Wolff-Chaikoff effect, Jod-Basedow effect)
  - there is varying thyroid sensitivity to TSH in response to iodide availability
  - increased ratio of T_3 to T_4 in iodide deficiency
  - increased activity of peripheral 5' deiodinase in hypothyroidism increases T_3 production despite low T_4 levels

Thyroid Assessment
- Serum thyroid hormones (TSH, T_3, T_4)
- Antibodies (TRAb, TgAb and TPOAb)
- Thyroglobulin (to monitor thyroid cancer)
- Thyroid ultrasound
- Nuclear uptake and scan (for hyperthyroidism)
- Biopsy (FNA)

Tests of Thyroid Function and Structure

TSH

- sensitive TSH (sTSH) is the best test for assessing thyroid function
- hyperthyroidism
  - primary: TSH is low because of negative feedback from increased levels of circulating T_3 and T_4
  - secondary: increased TSH results in increased T_3 and T_4
- hypothyroidism
  - primary: increased TSH (most sensitive test) because of less negative feedback from T_3 and T_4
  - secondary: TSH is low or normal with variable response to TRH depending on the site of the lesion (pituitary or hypothalamic)

Free T_3 and Free T_4

- standard assessment of thyroid function measures TSH and if necessary free T_4. Free T_3 should only be measured in the small subset of patients with hyperthyroidism and suspected T3 toxicosis. TSH would be suppressed, free T_4 normal, and free T_3 elevated

Thyroid Autoantibodies

- thyroglobulin antibodies (TgAb), anti-thyroid peroxidase antibodies (TPOAb), and TSH receptor antibodies (TRAb) of the blocking variety are increased in Hashimoto's disease; normal variant in 10-20% of individuals
- TRAb of the stimulating variety are also referred to as thyroid stimulating immunoglobulins (TSI) and cause Graves' disease. However, both TRAb receptor blocking and stimulating antibodies are seen in patients with Graves' disease

Plasma Thyroglobulin

- used to monitor for residual thyroid tissue post-thyroidectomy, e.g. tumour marker for thyroid cancer recurrence
- normal or elevated levels may suggest persistent, recurrent, or metastatic disease

Serum Calcitonin

- not routinely done to investigate thyroid nodules
- ordered if suspicion of medullary thyroid carcinoma or family history of MEN IIa or IIb syndromes
  - used to monitor for residual or recurrent medullary thyroid cancer

Thyroid Imaging/Scans

- normal gland size 15-20 g (estimated by palpation)
- thyroid U/S
  - to measure size of gland, solid vs. cystic nodule, facilitate fine needle aspirate biopsy (FNAB)
- radioisotope thyroid scan (Technetium-99)
- test of structure: order if there is a thyroid nodule and patient is hyperthyroid with low TSH
  - differentiates between hot (functioning → excess thyroid hormone production) and cold (non-functioning) nodules
    - hot nodule → very low chance malignancy; treat hyperthyroidism
    - cold nodule → ~5% chance malignancy; further workup required (U/S and FNAB)
- radioactive iodine uptake (RAIU)
  - test of function: order if patient is thyrotoxic
  - RAIU measures the turnover of iodine by thyroid gland *in vivo*
  - if ↑ uptake (i.e. incorporated), gland is overactive (hyperthyroid)
  - if ↓ uptake (i.e. not incorporated), gland is leaking thyroid hormone (e.g. thyroiditis), exogenous thyroid hormone use, or excess iodine intake (e.g. amiodarone or contrast dye, which has high iodine content)
- see Figure 9, *Approach to the Evaluation of a Thyroid Nodule*, E28 for further information regarding the utility of these scans

Thyroid Biopsy

- fine needle aspiration (FNA) for cytology
  - differentiates between benign and malignant disease
  - best done under U/S guidance
  - accuracy decreased if nodule is greater than 50% cystic, or if nodule located posteriorly in the gland

Does this Patient have a Goitre?
From The Rational Clinical Examination
JAMA 2009; http://www.jamaevidence.com/content/3480618
Study: Systematic review of articles assessing the accuracy and precision of the clinical exam in the diagnosis of a goitre.
Results: Clinical diagnosis was based on degree of lateral prominence, visibility, and palpability of the thyroid gland. No evidence exists to support the superiority of any one method.
The combined results of 4 studies detail the predictive utility of assessing grades of thyroid gland weight:

Weight	Reference	LR+	95% CI
0-20 g	normal	0.15	(0.10-0.21)
20-40 g	1-2x	1.9	(1.1-3.0)
>40 g	>2x	25.0	(2.6-175)

Alternatively, defining a goitre as mass larger than the distal phalanx of the thumb has been shown to have an LR+ of 3.0 (95% CI 2.5-3.5) and LR- of 0.30 (95% CI 0.24-0.37) in children, and an LR+ of 4.7 (95% CI 3.6-6.0) and LR- of 0.08 (95% CI 0.02-0.27) for the presence of a goitre.
Conclusions: Use of weight of thyroid tissue is an appropriate method of diagnosing a goitre, while comparing the size of thyroid mass to the distal phalanx of the thumb may be a useful alternative.

Caution with Amiodarone

Amiodarone-Induced Hypothyroidism (AIH):
AIH occurs more often in iodine-sufficient areas, and is more common in populations with a higher prevalence of autoimmune thyroid disease, such as women and the elderly. AIH can also occur in patients without pre-existing thyroid dysfunction.

Amiodarone-Induced Thyrotoxicosis (AIT):
AIT occurs more often in iodine-deficient areas. It may occur in patients with pre-existing thyroid deficiencies, as an iodine load on an already dysfunctional thyroid may result in excessive thyroid hormone synthesis and release. AIT may also occur in patients without thyroid abnormalities through a cytotoxic mechanism that results in leakage of thyroid hormone into the systemic circulation.

Signs and Symptoms of HYPERthyroidism

Tremor
Heart rate up
Yawning (fatigued)
Restlessness
Oligomenorrhea/amenorrhea
Intolerance to heat
Diarrhea
Irritability
Sweating
Muscle wasting/weight loss

Common Etiologies

Thyrotoxicosis	Hypothyroidism
Graves' Disease	Hashimoto's
Toxic Nodular Goitre	Congenital
Toxic Nodule	Iatrogenic (thionamides, radioactive iodine, or surgery)
Thyroiditis	Hypothyroid phase of thyroiditis

Table 16. Summary of Diagnostic Testing in Hyperthyroidism and Hypothyroidism

	Hyperthyroidism	Hypothyroidism
TSH	Decreased in 1° hyperthyroidism Increased in 2° hyperthyroidism	Increased in 1° hypothyroidism Decreased in 2° hypothyroidism
Free T4	Increased in 1° hyperthyroidism Increased in 2° hyperthyroidism	Decreased in 1° hypothyroidism Decreased in 2° hypothyroidism
Antibodies	Graves': thyroid stimulating Ig (TSI)	Hashimoto's: antithyroid peroxidase (TPOAb, TgAb)

RAIU	Increased uptake
	  Graves'
	  Toxic multinodular goitre
	  Toxic adenoma
		Decreased uptake
		  Subacute thyroiditis
		  Recent iodine load
		  Exogenous thyroid hormone	

Radioisotope Thyroid Scan	Graves': homogenous diffuse uptake Multinodular goitre: heterogeneous uptake Toxic adenoma: single intense area of uptake with suppression elsewhere	

Thyrotoxicosis

Definition
• clinical, physiological, and biochemical findings in response to elevated thyroid hormone

Epidemiology
• 1% of general population have hyperthyroidism
• F:M = 5:1

Etiology and Pathophysiology

Table 17. Differential Diagnosis of Thyrotoxicosis

Disorder	TSH	Free T4/T3	Thyroid Antibodies	RAIU	Other
HYPERTHYROIDISM					
Graves' Disease	Decreased	Increased	TSI	Increased	Homogenous uptake on scan
Toxic Nodular Goitre	Decreased	Increased	None	Increased	Heterogeneous uptake on scan
Toxic Nodule	Decreased	Increased	None	Increased	Intense uptake in hot nodule on scan with no uptake in the rest of the gland
THYROIDITIS					
Subacute, Silent, Postpartum	Decreased	Increased	Up to 50% of cases	Decreased (increases once entering hypothyroid phase, when TSH rises)	In classical subacute painful thyroiditis, ESR increased
EXTRATHYROIDAL SOURCES OF THYROID HORMONE					
Endogenous (struma ovariae, ovarian teratoma, metastatic follicular carcinoma)	Decreased	Increased	None	Decreased	
Exogenous (drugs)	Decreased	Increased (T4 would be decreased if taking T3)	None	Decreased	
EXCESSIVE THYROID STIMULATION					
Pituitary thyrotrophoma	Increased	Increased	None	Increased	
Pituitary thyroid hormone receptor resistance	Increased	Increased	None	Increased	
Increased hCG (e.g. pregnancy)	Decreased	Increased	None	Increased DO NOT DO THIS TEST IN PREGNANCY	

Clinical Features

Table 18. Clinical Features of Thyrotoxicosis

General	Fatigue, heat intolerance, irritability, fine tremor
CVS	Tachycardia, atrial fibrillation, palpitations Elderly patients may have only cardiovascular symptoms, commonly new onset atrial fibrillation
GI	Weight loss with increased appetite, thirst, increased frequency of bowel movements (hyperdefecation)
Neurology	Proximal muscle weakness, hypokalemic periodic paralysis (more common in Asians)
GU	Oligomenorrhea, amenorrhea, decreased fertility
Dermatology	Fine hair, skin moist and warm, vitiligo, soft nails with onycholysis (Plummer's nails), palmar erythema, pruritis Graves' disease: clubbing (acropachy), pretibial myxedema (rare)
MSK	Decreased bone mass, proximal muscle weakness
Hematology	Graves' disease: leukopenia, lymphocytosis, splenomegaly, lymphadenopathy (occasionally)
Eye	Graves' disease: lid lag, retraction, proptosis, diplopia, decreased acuity, puffiness, conjuctival injection

Treatment

- thionamides: propylthiouracil (PTU) or methimazole (MMI); MMI recommended (except in first trimester pregnancy)
- β-blockers for symptom control
- radioactive iodine thyroid ablation for Graves' disease
- surgery in the form of hemi, sub-total, or complete thyroidectomy

Graves' Disease

Definition

- an autoimmune disorder characterized by autoantibodies to the TSH receptor that leads to hyperthyroidism

Epidemiology

- most common cause of thyrotoxicosis
- occurs at any age with peak in 3rd and 4th decade
- F:M = 7:1, 1.5-2% of U.S. women
- familial predisposition: 15% of patients have a close family member with Graves' disease and 50% have family members with positive circulating antibodies
- association with HLA B8 and DR3
- may be associated with other inherited autoimmune disorders (e.g. pernicious anemia, Hashimoto's disease)

Etiology and Pathophysiology

- autoimmune disorder due to a defect in T-suppressor cells
- B lymphocytes produce TSI that binds and stimulates the TSH receptor and stimulates the thyroid gland
- immune response can be triggered by postpartum state, iodine excess, lithium therapy, viral or bacterial infections, glucocorticoid withdrawal
- ophthalmopathy (thyroid associated orbitopathy) is a result of increased tissue volume due to inflammation and accumulation of glycosaminoglycans, stimulated by TSI, that increase osmotic pressure within the orbit; this leads to fluid accumulation and displacement of the eyeball forward
- dermopathy may be related to cutaneous glycosaminoglycan deposition

Clinical Features

- signs and symptoms of thyrotoxicosis
- diffuse thyroid goitre ± thyroid bruit secondary to increased blood flow through the gland
- ophthalmopathy: proptosis, diplopia, conjunctival injection, corneal abrasions, periorbital puffiness, lid lag, decreased visual acuity (plus signs of hyperthyroidism: lid retraction, characteristic stare)
- dermopathy (rare): pretibial myxedema (thickening of dermis that manifests as *non-pitting* edema)
- acropachy: clubbing and thickening of distal phalanges

Investigations

- low TSH
- increased free T4 (and/or increased T3)
- positive for TSI (specific but not sensitive for Graves' disease)
- increased radioactive iodine (I-131) uptake
- homogeneous uptake on thyroid scan (only do this test in the presence of nodule)

Graves' Ophthalmopathy

NO SPECS (in order of changes usually)
No signs
Only signs: lid lag, lid retraction
Soft tissue: periorbital puffiness, conjuctival injection, chemosis
Proptosis/exophthalmos
Extraocular (diplopia)
Corneal abrasions (since unable to close eyes)
Sight loss

Treatment

- thionamides: propylthiouracil (PTU) or methimazole (MMI)
  - PTU and MMI inhibit thyroid hormone synthesis by inhibiting peroxidase-catalyzed reactions, thereby inhibiting organification of iodide, blocking the coupling of iodotyrosines
  - PTU also inhibits peripheral deiodination of T_4 to T_3
  - continue treatment until remission occurs (20-40% of patients achieve spontaneous remission at 6-18 mo of treatment)
  - small goitre and recent onset are good indicators for long-term remission with medical therapy
  - major side effects: hepatitis, agranulocytosis, and fever/arthralgias
  - minor side effects: rash
  - iodinated contrast agents: sodium ipodate and iopanoic acid can inhibit conversion of T_4 to T_3 and are especially effective in combination with MMI
  - MMI preferred vs. PTU due to longer duration of action (once daily for most), more rapid efficacy, and lower incidence of side effects
  - in pregnancy: use PTU during first trimester and MMI during second and third trimester. MMI is contraindicated in the first trimester due to risk of aplasia cutis; MMI is preferred in the second and third trimester due to the potential risk of hepatotoxicity with PTU in the second and third trimesters
- symptomatic treatment with β-blockers
- thyroid ablation with radioactive ^{131}I if PTU or MMI trial does not produce disease remission
  - high incidence of hypothyroidism after ^{131}I requiring lifelong thyroid hormone replacement
  - contraindicated in pregnancy
  - may worsen ophthalmopathy
- subtotal or total thyroidectomy (indicated for large goitres, suspicious nodule for Ca, if patient is intolerant to thionamides and refusing RAI ablation)
  - risks include hypoparathyroidism and vocal cord palsy
- ophthalmopathy/orbitopathy
  - smoking cessation is important
  - prevent drying of eyes
  - high dose prednisone in severe cases
  - orbital radiation, surgical decompression

Prognosis

- course involves remission and exacerbation unless gland is destroyed by radioactive iodine or surgery
- lifetime follow-up needed
- risk of relapse is 37%, 21%, 6% in thionamides, radioiodine ablation, and surgery groups, respectively

Subacute Thyroiditis (Thyrotoxic Phase)

Definition

- acute inflammatory disorder of the thyroid gland characterized by an initial thyrotoxic state followed by hypothyroidism eventually followed by euthyroidism in most cases
- two subtypes: painful ("De Quervain's") and painless ("Silent")

Etiology and Pathophysiology

- acute inflammation of the thyroid gland characterized by giant cells and lymphocytes
- disruption of thyroid follicles by inflammatory process results in the release of stored hormone rather than excessive production of new thyroid hormone
- painful = viral (usually preceded by URTI), De Quervain's (granulomatous thyroiditis)
- painless = postpartum, auto-immune, lymphocytic
  - occurs in 5-10% of postpartum mothers and is symptomatic in 1/3 of patients

Clinical Features

- painful (thyroid, ears, jaw, and occiput) or painless
- fever and malaise may be present, especially in De Quervain's
- postpartum: thyrotoxicosis 2-3 mo postpartum with a subsequent hypothyroid phase at 4-8 mo postpartum
- may be mistakenly diagnosed as postpartum depression

Laboratory Investigations

- initial elevated free T_4, T_3, low TSH, RAIU markedly reduced
- marked elevation of ESR in painful variety only
- as disease progresses values consistent with hypothyroidism may appear

Treatment

- painful – high dose NSAIDs, prednisone may be required for severe pain, fever, or malaise
- iodinated contrast agents (e.g. iopanoic acid, ipodate) to inhibit peripheral conversion of T_4 to T_3
- β-adrenergic blockade is usually effective in reversing most of the hypermetabolic and cardiac symptoms in both subtypes
- if symptomatically hypothyroid, may treat short-term with thyroxine

Prognosis

- full recovery in most cases, but permanent hypothyroidism in 10% of painless thyroiditis
- postpartum: most resolve spontaneously without need for supplementation, however may recur with subsequent pregnancies

Other Medications Used in the Treatment of Graves'

Glucocorticoids have been useful in the treatment of severe Graves' hyperthyroidism and thyroid storm, by inhibiting the conversion of peripheral T_4 to T_3

Lithium is also used to treat Graves' hyperthyroidism. It acts by blocking thyroid hormone release, but its toxicity has limited its use in practice

Caution with Thionamides
These drugs are effective in controlling hyperthyroidism and induce permanent remission in 20-30% of patients with Graves' disease. They inhibit thyroid hormone synthesis. They are most often employed to achieve a euthyroid state before definitive treatment. Adverse effects include teratogenicity, agranulocytosis, hepatotoxicity, and ANCA-positive vasculitis

Radioiodine Therapy for Graves' Disease and the Effect on Ophthalmopathy: A Systematic Review
Clin Endocrinol 2008;69:943-950
Purpose: To assess whether radioiodine therapy (RAI) for Graves' disease (GD) is associated with increased risk of ophthalmopathy compared with antithyroid drugs (ATDs) or surgery. To assess the efficacy of glucocorticoid prophylaxis in the prevention of occurrence or progression of Graves' ophthalmopathy (GO), when used with RAI.
Study Selection: RTCs regardless of language or publication status.
Results: RAI was associated with an increased risk of GO compared with ATD (Relative Risk (RR) 4.23, 95% confidence interval (CI 2.04-8.77) but compared with thyroidectomy, there was no statistically significant increased risk (RR 1.59, 95% CI 0.89-2.81). The risk of severe GO was also increased with RAI compared with ATD (RR 4.35, 95% CI 1.28-14.73). Prednisolone prophylaxis for RAI was highly effective in preventing the progression of GO in patients with pre-existing GO (RR 0.03; 95% CI 0.00-0.24). The use of adjunctive ATD with RAI was not associated with any significant benefit on the course of GO.
Conclusions: RAI therapy for GD is associated with a small but definite increased risk of development or worsening of GO compared with ATDs. Steroid prophylaxis is beneficial for patients with pre-existing GO.

Toxic Adenoma/Toxic Multinodular Goitre

Etiology and Pathophysiology
- autonomous thyroid hormone production from a functioning adenoma that is hypersecreting T_3 and T_4
- may be singular (toxic adenoma) or multiple (toxic multinodular goitre [Plummer's disease])

Clinical Features
- goitre with adenomatous changes
- tachycardia, heart failure, arrhythmia, weight loss, nervousness, weakness, tremor, and sweats
- seen most frequently in elderly people, often with presentation of atrial fibrillation

Investigations
- low TSH, high T_3 and T_4
- thyroid scan with increased RAIU in nodule(s) and suppression of the remainder of the gland

Treatment
- initiate therapy with PTU or MMI to attain euthyroid state
- use high dose radioactive iodine (I-131) to ablate hyperfunctioning nodules
- β-blockers often necessary for symptomatic treatment prior to definitive therapy
- surgical excision may also be used as 1st line treatment

Thyrotoxic Crisis/Thyroid Storm

Definition
- acute exacerbation of all of the symptoms of thyrotoxicosis presenting in a life-threatening state secondary to uncontrolled hyperthyroidism – medical emergency!
- rare, but serious with mortality rate between 10-30%

Etiology and Pathophysiology
- often precipitated by infection, trauma, or surgery in a hyperthyroid patient

Differential Diagnosis
- sepsis, pheochromocytoma, malignant hyperthermia, drug overdose, neuroleptic malignant syndrome

Clinical Features
- hyperthyroidism
- extreme hyperthermia (≥40°C), tachycardia, vomiting, diarrhea, vascular collapse, hepatic failure with jaundice, and confusion
- tachyarrhythmia, CHF, shock
- mental status changes ranging from delirium to coma

Laboratory Investigations
- increased free T_3 and T_4, undetectable TSH
- ± anemia, leukocytosis, hyperglycemia, hypercalcemia, elevated LFTs

General Measures
- fluids, electrolytes, and vasopressor agents should be used as indicated
- a cooling blanket and acetaminophen can be used to treat the pyrexia
- propranolol or other β-blockers that additionally decrease peripheral conversion of $T_3 \to T_4$ can be used, but should be used with caution in CHF patients as it may worsen condition

Specific Measures
- PTU is the anti-thyroid drug of choice and is used in high doses
- Give iodide, which acutely inhibits the release of thyroid hormone, one hour after the first dose of PTU is given
  - Sodium iodide 1 g IV drip over 12h q12h
    OR
  - Lugol's solution 2-3 drops q8h
    OR
  - Potassium iodide (SSKI) 5 drops q8h
- dexamethasone 2-4 mg IV q6h for the first 24-48 hours lowers body temperature and inhibits peripheral conversion of $T_3 \to T_4$

Prognosis
- probably <20% mortality rate if rapidly recognized and treated

Hypothyroidism

Definition
- clinical syndrome caused by cellular responses to insufficient thyroid hormone production

Epidemiology
- 2-3% of general population
- F:M = 10:1
- 10-20% of women over age 50 have subclinical hypothyroidism (normal T4, TSH mildly elevated)
- iodine deficiency most common cause worldwide, but not in North America

Etiology and Pathophysiology
- primary hypothyroidism (90%)
  - inadequate thyroid hormone production secondary to intrinsic thyroid defect
  - iatrogenic: post-ablative (^{131}I or surgical thyroidectomy)
  - autoimmune: Hashimoto's thyroiditis, chronic thyroiditis, idiopathic, burnt out Graves'
  - hypothyroid phase of subacute thyroiditis
  - drugs: goitrogens (iodine), PTU, MMI, lithium
  - infiltrative disease (progressive systemic sclerosis, amyloid)
  - iodine deficiency
  - congenital (1/4,000 births)
  - neoplasia
- secondary hypothyroidism: pituitary hypothyroidism
  - insufficiency of pituitary TSH
- tertiary hypothyroidism: hypothalamic hypothyroidism
  - decreased TRH from hypothalamus (rare)
- peripheral tissue resistance to thyroid hormone (Refetoff syndrome)

Table 19. Interpretation of Serum TSH and Free T₄ in Hypothyroidism

	Serum TSH	Free T₄
Overt Primary Hypothyroidism	Increased	Decreased
Subclinical Primary Hypothyroidism	Increased	Normal
Secondary Hypothyroidism	Decreased or not appropriately elevated	Decreased

Clinical Features

Table 20. Clinical Features of Hypothyroidism

General	Fatigue, cold intolerance, slowing of mental and physical performance, hoarseness, macroglossia
CVS	Pericardial effusion, bradycardia, hypotension, worsening CHF + angina, hypercholesterolemia, hyperhomocysteinemia, myxedema heart
Respiratory	Decreased exercise capacity, hypoventilation secondary to weak muscles, decreased pulmonary responses to hypoxia, sleep apnea due to macroglossia
GI	Weight gain despite poor appetite, constipation
Neurology	Paresthesia, slow speech, muscle cramps, delay in relaxation phase of deep tendon reflexes ("hung reflexes"), carpal tunnel syndrome, asymptomatic increase in CK, seizures
GU	Menorrhagia, amenorrhea, impotence
Dermatology	Puffiness of face, periorbital edema, cool and pale, dry and rough skin, hair dry and coarse, eyebrows thinned (lateral 1/3), discolouration (carotenemia)
Hematology	Anemia: 10% pernicious due to presence of anti-parietal cell antibodies with Hashimoto's thyroiditis

Treatment
- L-thyroxine (dose range: 0.05-0.2 mg PO OD ~1.6 µg/kg/d)
- elderly patients and those with CAD: start at 0.025 mg daily and increase gradually every 6 wk (start low, go slow)
- after initiating L-thyroxine, TSH needs to be evaluated in 6 wk; dose is adjusted until TSH returns to normal reference range
- once maintenance dose achieved, follow-up TSH with patient annually
- secondary/tertiary hypothyroidism
  - monitor via measurement of free T₄ (TSH is unreliable in this setting)

CONGENITAL HYPOTHYROIDISM
- see Pediatrics, P28

Thyroid Hormone Replacement for Subclinical Hypothyroidism
Cochrane DB Syst Rev 2007;3:CD003419
Purpose: To assess the effects of thyroid hormone replacement for subclinical hypothyroidism.
Study Selection: RCTs comparing thyroid hormone replacement with placebo in adults with subclinical hypothyroidism. Minimum duration of follow-up was one month.
Results: No trial assessed (cardiovascular) mortality or morbidity. Seven studies evaluated symptoms, mood, and quality of life with no statistically significant improvement. One study showed a statistically significant improvement in cognitive function. Six studies assessed serum lipids, there was a trend for reduction in some parameters following levothyroxine replacement. Some echocardiographic parameters improved after levothyroxine replacement therapy, like myocardial relaxation. Only four studies reported adverse events with no statistically significant differences between groups.
Conclusions: In current RCTs, levothyroxine replacement therapy for subclinical hypothyroidism did not result in improved survival or decreased cardiovascular morbidity. Data on health-related quality of life and symptoms did not demonstrate significant differences between intervention groups. Some evidence indicates that levothyroxine replacement improves some parameters of lipid profiles and left ventricular function.

Signs and Symptoms of Hypothyroidism

HIS FIRM CAP
Hypoventilation
Intolerance to cold
Slow HR
Fatigue
Impotence
Renal impairment
Menorrhagia/amenorrhea
Constipation
Anemia
Paresthesia

Hashimoto's Thyroiditis

- most common form of primary hypothyroidism in North America
- chronic autoimmune thyroiditis characterized by both cellular and humoral factors in the destruction of thyroid tissue
- two major forms: goitrous and atrophic; both forms share same pathophysiology but differ in the extent of lymphocytic infiltration, fibrosis, and thyroid follicular cell hyperplasia
- goitrous variant usually presents with a rubbery goitre and euthyroidism, then hypothyroidism becomes evident
    - associated with fibrosis
- atrophic variant patients are hypothyroid from the start
    - associated with thyroid lymphoma

Etiology and Pathophysiology
- defect in clone of T-suppressors leads to cell-mediated destruction of thyroid follicles
- B lymphocytes produce antibodies against thyroid components including thyroglobulin, thyroid peroxidase, TSH receptor, Na^+/I^- symporter

Risk Factors
- female gender (F:M = 7:1)
- genetic susceptibility: increased frequency in patients with Down's syndrome, Turner's syndrome, certain HLA alleles, cytotoxic T-lymphocyte-associated protein 4 (CTLA-4)
- family Hx or personal Hx of other autoimmune diseases
- cigarette smoking
- high iodine intake
- stress and infection

Investigations
- high TSH, low T_4 (not necessary to measure T_3 as it will be low as well)
- presence of anti-thyroid peroxidase (TPOAb) and thyroglobulin antibodies (TgAb) in serum

Treatment
- if hypothyroid, replace with L-thyroxine (analog of T_4)

Myxedema Coma

Definition
- severe hypothyroidism complicated by trauma, sepsis, cold exposure, MI, inadvertent administration of hypnotics or narcotics, and other stressful events – medical emergency!
- rare, high level of mortality when it occurs (up to 40%, despite therapy)

Clinical Features
- hallmark symptoms of decreased mental status and hypothermia; hyponatremia, hypotension, hypoglycemia, bradycardia, hypoventilation, and generalized edema often present

Investigations
- decreased T_4, increased TSH, decreased glucose
- check ACTH and cortisol for evidence of adrenal insufficiency

Treatment
- aggressive treatment required
- ABCs: ICU admission
- corticosteroids (for risk of concomitant adrenal insufficiency): hydrocortisone 100 mg q8h
- L-thyroxine 0.2-0.5 mg IV loading dose, then 0.1 mg IV OD until oral therapy tolerated; also consider T_3 therapy
- supportive measures: mechanical ventilation, vasopressor drugs, passive rewarming, IV dextrose, fluids if necessary (risk of overload)
- monitor for arrhythmia

Sick Euthyroid Syndrome

Definition
- changes in circulating thyroid hormones amongst patients with serious illness, trauma, or stress
- not due to intrinsic thyroid or pituitary disease
- initially low free T_3 may be followed by low TSH and if severe illness low free T_4
- with recovery of illness, TSH may overshoot and become transiently high

Pathophysiology
- abnormalities include alterations in
  - peripheral transport and metabolism of thyroid hormone
  - regulation of TSH secretion
  - thyroid function itself
- may be protective during illness by reducing tissue catabolism

Labs
- initially decreased free T_3 followed by decreased TSH and finally decreased free T_4

Treatment
- treat the underlying disease; thyroid hormone replacement worsens outcomes
- thyroid function tests normalize once patient is well (initially with a transient increase in TSH)

Non-Toxic Goitre

Definition
- generalized enlargement of the thyroid gland in a euthyroid individual that does not result from inflammatory or neoplastic processes

Pathophysiology
- the appearance of a goitre is more likely during adolescence, pregnancy, and lactation because of increased thyroid hormone requirements
  - early stages: goitre is usually diffuse
  - later stages: multinodular non-toxic goitre with nodule, cyst formation and areas of ischemia, hemorrhage, and fibrosis

Etiology
- iodine deficiency or excess
- goitrogens: brassica vegetables (e.g. turnip, cassava)
- drugs: iodine, lithium, para-aminosalicylic acid
- any disorder of hormone synthesis with compensatory growth
- peripheral resistance to thyroid hormone

Treatment
- remove goitrogens
- radioiodine therapy (need very high doses given low iodine uptake, used as last resort)
- suppression with L-thyroxine (rarely done)
- surgery may be necessary for severe compressive symptoms

Complications
- compression of neck structures causing stridor, dysphagia, pain, and hoarseness
- multinodular goitre may become autonomous leading to toxic multinodular goitre and hyperthyroidism

Thyroid Nodules

Definition
- clearly defined discrete mass, separated from the thyroid parenchyma
- palpable nodules are found in approximately 5% of women and 1% of men

Etiology
- benign tumours (e.g. colloid nodule, follicular adenoma)
- thyroid malignancy
- hyperplastic area in a multinodular goitre
- cyst: true thyroid cyst, area of cystic degeneration in a multinodular goitre

Investigations

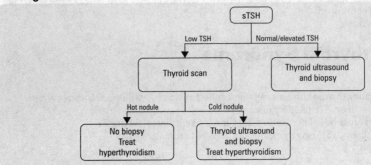

Figure 9. Approach to the evaluation of a thyroid nodule
Adapted from Dr. J Goguen, University of Toronto, MMMD 2013

Thyroid Malignancies

- see Otolaryngology, OT34

Adrenal Cortex

Adrenocorticotropic Hormone

- a polypeptide (cleaved from prohormone POMC), secreted in a pulsatile fashion from the anterior pituitary with diurnal variability (peak: 0200-0400; trough: 1800-2400)
- secretion regulated by corticotropin-releasing hormone (CRH) and arginine vasopressin (AVP)
- stimulates growth of adrenal cortex and release of glucocorticoids, androgens and, to a limited extent, mineralocorticoids
- some melanocyte stimulating activity

Adrenocortical Hormones

Aldosterone

- a mineralocorticoid which regulates extracellular fluid (ECF) volume through Na^+ (and Cl^-) retention and K^+ (and H^+) excretion (stimulates distal tubule Na^+/K^+ ATPase)
- regulated by the renin-angiotensin-aldosterone system (Figure 12)
- negative feedback to juxtaglomerular apparatus (JGA) by long loop (aldosterone ↑ volume expansion) and short loop (angiotensin II ↑ peripheral vasoconstriction)

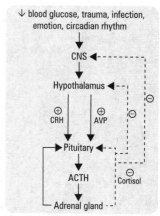

Figure 10. Regulation of CRH-ACTH-adrenal gland axis

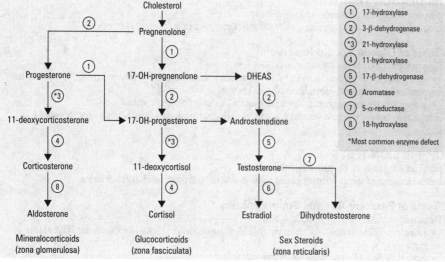

Figure 11. Pathways of major steroid synthesis in the adrenal gland and their enzymes

Enzyme legend:
1. 17-hydroxylase
2. 3-β-dehydrogenase
*3. 21-hydroxylase
4. 11-hydroxylase
5. 17-β-dehydrogenase
6. Aromatase
7. 5-α-reductase
8. 18-hydroxylase

*Most common enzyme defect

Mineralocorticoids (zona glomerulosa)
Glucocorticoids (zona fasciculata)
Sex Steroids (zona reticularis)

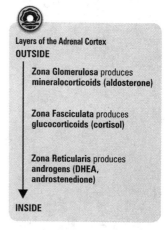

Layers of the Adrenal Cortex
OUTSIDE

Zona Glomerulosa produces mineralocorticoids (aldosterone)

Zona Fasciculata produces glucocorticoids (cortisol)

Zona Reticularis produces androgens (DHEA, androstenedione)

INSIDE

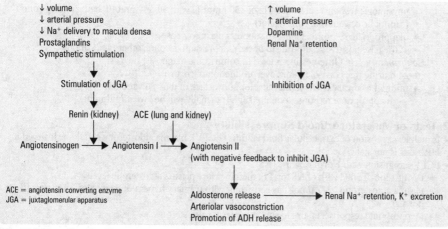

ACE = angiotensin converting enzyme
JGA = juxtaglomerular apparatus

Figure 12. Renin-angiotensin-aldosterone axis (see Nephrology, NP4)

Cortisol
- a glucocorticoid, regulated by the HPA axis
- involved in regulation of metabolism; counteracts the effects of insulin
- support blood pressure, vasomotor tone
- also involved in regulation of behaviour and immunosuppression

Table 21. Physiological Effects of Glucocorticoids

Stimulatory Effects	Inhibitory Effects
Stimulate hepatic glucose production (gluconeogenesis)	Inhibit bone formation; stimulate bone resorption
Increase insulin resistance in peripheral tissues	Inhibit fibroblasts, causing collagen and connective tissue loss
Increase protein catabolism	Suppress inflammation; impair cell-mediated immunity
Stimulate leukocytosis and lymphopenia	Inhibit growth hormone axis
Increase cardiac output, vascular tone, Na^+ retention	Inhibit reproductive axis
Increase PTH release, urine calcium excretion	Inhibit vitamin D3 and inhibit calcium uptake

Androgens
- sex steroids regulated by ACTH; primarily responsible for adrenarche (growth of axillary and pubic hair)
- principal adrenal androgens are dihydroepiandrosterone (DHEA), androstenedione, and 11-hydroxyandrostenedione
- proportion of total androgens (adrenal to gonadal) increases in old age

Adrenocortical Functional Workup

STIMULATION TEST
- purpose: diagnosis of hormone deficiencies
- method: measure target hormone after stimulation with tropic (pituitary) hormone

1. Tests of Glucocorticoid Reserve
- Cosyntropin (ACTH analogue) Stimulation Test
  - give 1 μg or 250 μg cosyntropin IV, then measure plasma cortisol levels at time 0, 30, and 60 min
  - physiologic response: stimulated plasma cortisol of >500 nmol/L
  - inappropriate response: inability to stimulate increased plasma cortisol
- insulin tolerance is the gold standard test used to diagnose adrenal insufficiency (see *Pituitary Gland*, E15)

SUPPRESSION TESTS
- purpose: diagnosis of hormone hypersecretion
- method: measure target hormone after suppression of its tropic (pituitary) hormone

1. Tests of Pituitary-Adrenal Suppressibility
- Dexamethasone (DXM) Suppression Test
  - principle: DXM suppresses pituitary ACTH, plasma cortisol should be lowered if HPA axis is normal
  - *Screening Test*: Overnight DXM Suppression Test
    - oral administration of 1 mg DXM at midnight measure plasma cortisol levels the following day at 8 am
    - physiologic response: plasma cortisol <50 nmol/L, with 50-140 nmol/L being a "grey zone" (cannot be certain if normal or not)
    - inappropriate response: failure to suppress plasma cortisol
    - <20% false positive results due to obesity, depression, alcohol, other medications
  - *Confirmatory Test*: Other testing is used to confirm the diagnosis, such as:
    - 24 h urine free cortisol (shows overproduction of cortisol)
    - midnight salivary cortisol (if available), shows lack of diurnal variation
      - inappropriate response: remains high (normally will be low at midnight)

2. Tests of Mineralocorticoid Suppressibility
- principle: expansion of extracellular fluid volume (ECFV); plasma aldosterone should be lowered if HPA axis is normal
- ECFV Expansion with Normal Saline (NS)
  - IV infusion of 500 mL/h of NS for 4 h, then measure plasma aldosterone levels
  - plasma aldosterone >277 pmol/L is consistent with primary hyperaldosteronsim, <140 pmol/L is normal
  - inappropriate response: failure to suppress plasma aldosterone

Mineralocorticoid Excess Syndromes

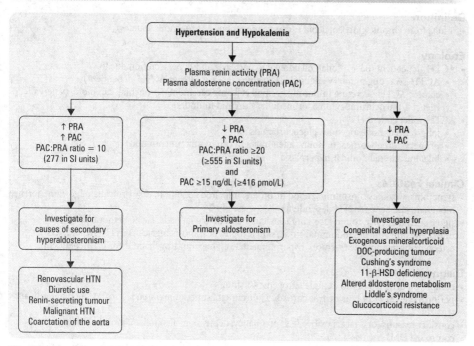

Figure 13. Approach to mineralocorticoid excess syndromes

Definition
- primary hyperaldosteronism (PH): excess aldosterone production (intra-adrenal cause)
- secondary hyperaldosteronism (SH): aldosterone production in response to excess RAAS (extra-adrenal cause)

Etiology
- primary hyperaldosteronism
  - aldosterone-producing adrenal adenoma (Conn's syndrome)
  - bilateral or idiopathic adrenal hyperplasia
  - glucocorticoid-remediable aldosteronism
  - aldosterone-producing adrenocortical carcinoma
  - unilateral adrenal hyperplasia
- secondary hyperaldosteronism

Clinical Features
- HTN
- hypokalemia (may have mild hypernatremia), metabolic alkalosis
- normal K^+, low Na^+ in SH (low effective circulating volume leads to ADH release) edema
- increased cardiovascular risk: LV hypertrophy, atrial fibrillation, stroke, MI
- fatigue, weakness, paresthesia, headache; severe cases with tetany, intermittent paralysis

Diagnosis
- investigate plasma aldosterone to renin ratio in patients with HTN and hypokalemia
- confirmatory testing for PH: aldosterone suppression test (demonstrate inappropriate aldosterone secretion with ECF volume expansion)
- imaging: CT adrenal glands

Table 22. Diagnostic Tests in Hyperaldosteronism

Test	Primary Hyperaldosteronism	Secondary Hyperaldosteronism
Plasma aldosterone to renin ratio (PAC/PRA)	Elevated (↑ aldo, ↓ renin)	Normal (↑ aldo, ↑ renin)
Salt loading test A) Oral test B) IV saline test	↑ urine aldosterone ↑ plasma aldosterone	Not performed if normal PAC/PRA

Treatment
- inhibit action of aldosterone: spironolactone, eplerenone, triamterene, amiloride (act on sodium channels)
- surgical excision of adrenal adenoma
- secondary hyperaldosteronism: treat underlying cause

Cushing's Syndrome

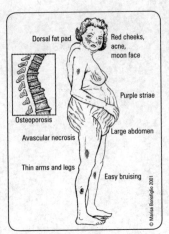

Figure 14. Clinical features of Cushing's syndrome

Labels on figure:
Dorsal fat pad
Red cheeks, acne, moon face
Purple striae
Osteoporosis
Avascular necrosis
Large abdomen
Thin arms and legs
Easy bruising
© Marisa Bonofiglio 2001

Definition
- results from chronic glucocorticoid excess (endogenous or exogenous sources)

Etiology
- ACTH-dependent (85%) – bilateral adrenal hyperplasia and hypersecretion due to:
  - ACTH-secreting pituitary adenoma (Cushing's disease; 80% of ACTH-dependent)
  - ectopic ACTH-secreting tumour (e.g. small cell lung carcinoma, bronchial, carcinoid, pancreatic islet cell, pheochromocytoma, or medullary thyroid tumours)
- ACTH-independent (15%)
  - long-term use of exogenous glucocorticoids
  - primary adrenocortical tumours: adenoma and carcinoma (uncommon)
  - bilateral adrenal nodular hyperplasia

Clinical Features
- symptoms: weakness, insomnia, mood disorders, impaired cognition, easy bruising, oligo-/amenorrhea, hirsutism, and acne (ACTH dependent)
- signs: central obesity, round face, supraclavicular and dorsal fat pads, facial plethora, proximal muscle wasting, purple abdominal striae, skin atrophy, acanthosis nigricans, HTN, hyperglycemia, osteoporosis, pathologic fractures, hyperpigmentation, hyperandrogenism if ACTH-dependent

Diagnosis
- complete a drug history to exclude iatrogenic Cushing's
- perform one of: 1) 24 h urine free cortisol, 2) dexamethasone suppression test, or 3) late night salivary cortisol
- consider reasons for a false positive (e.g. pregnancy, depression, alcoholism, morbid obesity, poorly controlled DM)
- confirm with one of the remaining tests if necessary (do not rely on random cortisol, insulin tolerance, loperamide, or urinary 17-ketosteroid tests)

Treatment
- adrenal
  - adenoma: unilateral adrenalectomy (curative) with glucocorticoid supplementation post-operatively
  - carcinoma: adjunctive chemotherapy often not useful (frequent metastases, poor prognosis)
  - medical treatment: mitotane, ketoconazole to reduce cortisol
- pituitary
  - trans-sphenoidal resection, with glucocorticoid supplement post-operatively
- ectopic ACTH tumour (paraneoplastic syndrome): usually bronchogenic cancer (poor prognosis)
  - surgical resection, if possible; chemotherapy/radiation for primary tumour
  - medical treatment with mitotane or ketoconazole to reduce cortisol synthesis. Often required when surgery is delayed, contraindicated, or unsuccessful

Congenital Adrenal Hyperplasia

- see <u>Pediatrics</u>, P29

Hyperandrogenism

Definition
- state of having excessive secretion of androgens (DHEA, DHEA sulfate, testosterone)

Etiology and Pathophysiology

Table 23. Etiology of Hyperandrogenism

Constitutional/Familial	Family history, predisposing ethnic background Premature adrenarche
Medications Androgen-Mediated	Anabolic steroids, ACTH, androgens, progestational agents
Ovarian	PCOS Ovarian hyperthecosis Theca cell tumours Pregnancy: placental sulfatase/aromatase deficiency
Adrenal	Congenital adrenal hyperplasia (CAH, late-onset CAH) Tumours (adenoma, carcinoma)
Pituitary	Cushing's disease – high ACTH Hyperprolactinemia

Adrenal Cortex

Clinical Features
Females
- hirsutism
  - male pattern growth of androgen-dependent terminal body hair in women: back, chest, upper abdomen, face, linea alba
  - Ferriman-Gallwey scoring system is used to quantify severity of hirsutism
- virilization
  - masculinization: hirsutism, temporal balding, clitoral enlargement, deepening of voice, acne
  - increase in musculature
- defeminization
  - loss of female secondary sex characteristics (i.e. amenorrhea, ↓ breast size, infertility)

Males
- minimal effects on hair, muscle mass, etc.
- inhibition of gonadotropin secretion may cause reduction in: testicular size, testicular testosterone production, and spermatogenesis

Conditions that do NOT Represent True Hirsutism
- Androgen-independent hair (e.g. lanugo hair)
- Drug-induced hypertrichosis (e.g. phenytoin, diazoxide, cyclosporine, minoxidil)
- Topical steroid use

Investigations
- testosterone, DHEA-S as a measure of adrenal androgen production
- LH/FSH (commonly in PCOS >2.5)
- 17-OH progesterone, elevated in CAH due to 21-OH deficiency; check on day 3 of menstrual cycle with a progesterone level
- for virilization: CT/MRI of adrenals and ovaries (identify tumours)
- if PCOS, check blood glucose, lipids, 75 g OGTT

Treatment
- discontinue causative medications
- antiandrogens, e.g. spironolactone
- oral contraceptives (increase sex hormone binding globulin, which binds androgens>estrogens; reduce ovarian production of androgens)
- surgical resection of tumour
- low dose glucocorticoid ± mineralocorticoid if CAH suspected
- treat specific causative disorders, e.g. tumours, Cushing's, etc.
- cosmetic therapy (laser, electrolysis)

Adrenocortical Insufficiency

Definition
- state of inadequate cortisol and/or aldosterone production by the adrenal glands

Etiology

PRIMARY (ADDISON'S DISEASE)

Table 24. Etiology of Primary Adrenocortical Insufficiency

Autoimmune (70-90%)	Isolated adrenal insufficiency Polyglandular autoimmune syndrome type I and II Antibodies often directed against adrenal enzymes and 3 cortical zones
Infection	TB (7-20%) (most common in developing world) Fungal: histoplasmosis, paracoccidioidomycosis HIV, CMV Syphilis African trypanosomiasis
Infiltrative	Metastatic cancer (lung>stomach>esophagus>colon>breast); lymphoma Sarcoidosis, amyloidosis, hemochromatosis
Vascular	Bilateral adrenal hemorrhage (risk increased by heparin and warfarin) Sepsis (meningococcal, *Pseudomonas*) Coagulopathy in adults or Waterhouse-Friderichsen syndrome in children Thrombosis, embolism, adrenal infarction
Drugs	Inhibit cortisol: ketoconazole, etomidate, megestrol acetate Increase cortisol metabolism: rifampin, phenytoin, barbiturates
Others	Adrenoleukodystrophy Congenital adrenal hypoplasia (impaired steroidogenesis) Familial glucocorticoid deficiency or resistance

SECONDARY ADRENOCORTICAL INSUFFICIENCY
- inadequate pituitary ACTH secretion
- multiple etiologies (see *Hypopituitarism*, E19), including withdrawal of exogenous steroids

Clinical Features

Table 25. Clinical Features of Primary and Secondary Adrenal Insufficiency (AI)

	Primary AI (Addison's or Acute AI)	Secondary AI
Skin and Mucosa	Dark (palmar crease, extensor surface)	Pale
Potassium	High	Normal
Sodium	Low	Normal or Low
Metabolic Acidosis	Present	Absent
Associated Diseases	Primary hypothyroidism, type 1 DM, vitiligo, neurological deficits	Central hypogonadism or hypothyroidism, growth hormone deficiency, DI, headaches, visual abnormalities
Associated Symptoms	Weakness, fatigue, weight loss, hypotension, salt craving, postural dizziness, myalgia, arthralgia GI: N/V, abdominal pain, diarrhea	Same except: No salt craving GI less common
Diagnostic Test	Insulin tolerance test Cosyntropin Stimulation Test High morning plasma ACTH	Insulin tolerance test Cosyntropin Stimulation Test Low morning plasma ACTH

Adapted from: Salvatori R. *JAMA* 2005;294:2481-2488

Treatment
- acute condition – can be life-threatening
  - IV NS in large volumes (2-3 L); add D5W if hypoglycemic from adrenal insufficiency
  - hydrocortisone 50-100 mg IV q6-8h for 24h, then gradual tapering
  - identify and correct precipitating factors
- maintenance
  - hydrocortisone 15-20 mg total daily dose, in 2-3 divided doses, highest dose in the AM
  - Florinef® (fludrocortisone, synthetic mineralocorticoid) 0.05-0.2 mg PO daily if mineralocorticoid deficient increase dose of steroids 2-3 fold for a few days during moderate-severe illness (e.g. with vomiting, fever)
  - major stress (e.g. surgery, trauma) requires 150-300 hydrocortisone IV daily divided into 3 doses
  - medical alert bracelet and instructions for emergency hydrocortisone/dexamethasone IM/SC injection

Adrenal Medulla

Catecholamine Metabolism

ABC of Adrenaline

Adrenaline activates
β-receptors, increasing
Cyclic AMP

- catecholamines are synthesized from tyrosine in postganglionic sympathetic nerves (norepinephrine) and chromaffin cells of adrenal medulla (epinephrine)
- broken down into metanephrines and other metabolites (VMA, HVA) and excreted in urine

Pheochromocytoma

Definition
- rare catecholamine secreting tumour derived from chromaffin cells of the sympathetic system

Epidemiology
- most commonly a single tumour of adrenal medulla
- rare cause of HTN (<0.2% of all hypertensives)

Etiology and Pathophysiology
- most cases sporadic (80%)
- familial: associated with multiple endocrine neoplasia II (MEN IIA and IIB) (50% penetrance; i.e. 50% of people with the mutation get pheochromocytoma), von Hippel-Lindau (10-20% penetrance), paraganglioma (20% penetrance), or neurofibromatosis type 1 (0.1-5.7% penetrance)
- tumours, via unknown mechanism, able to synthesize and release excessive catecholamines

Clinical Features
- 50% suffer from paroxysmal HTN; the rest have sustained HTN
- classic triad (not found in most patients): episodic "pounding" headache, palpitations/tachycardia, diaphoresis
- other symptoms: tremor, anxiety, chest or abdominal pain, N/V, visual blurring, weight loss, polyuria, polydipsia
- other signs: orthostatic hypotension, papilledema, hyperglycemia, dilated cardiomyopathy
- symptoms may be triggered by stress, exertion, anesthesia, abdominal pressure, certain foods (especially tyramine containing foods)

Investigations
- urine catecholamines
  - increased catecholamine metabolites (metanephrines) and free catecholamines
  - plasma metanephrines if available (most sensitive)
    - cut-off values will depend on assay used
- CT abdomen
  - if negative, whole body CT and meta-iodo-benzoguanidine (MIBG) scintigraphy, Octreoscan, or MRI

Treatment
- surgical removal of tumour (curative) with careful pre- and post-operative ICU monitoring
- adequate pre-operative preparation
  - α-blockade for BP control: doxazosin or calcium channel blockers (10-21 d pre-operative), IV phentolamine (perioperative, if required)
  - β-blockade for HR control once α blocked for a few days
  - metyrosine (catecholamine synthesis inhibitor) + phenoxybenzamine or prazosin
  - volume restoration with vigorous salt-loading and fluids
- rescreen urine 1-3 mo post-operatively
- screen urine in first degree relatives; genetic testing in patients <50 yr old

Disorders of Multiple Endocrine Glands

Multiple Endocrine Neoplasm

- neoplastic syndromes involving multiple endocrine glands
- tumours of neuroectodermal origin
- autosomal dominant inheritance with variable penetrance
- genetic screening for RET proto-oncogene on chromosome 10 has long-term benefit in MEN II
  - early cure and prevention of medullary thyroid cancer

MEN I – Wermer's Syndrome Affects
the 3 Ps

Pituitary
Parathyroid
Pancreas

Table 26. MEN Classification

Type	Tissues Involved	Clinical Manifestations
MEN I (chromosome 11)		
Wermer's Syndrome	Pituitary (15-42%) Anterior pituitary adenoma	Headache, visual field defects, often non-secreting but may secrete GH (acromegaly) and PRL (galactorrhea, erectile dysfunction, decreased libido, amenorrhea)
	Parathyroid (≥95%) Primary hyperparathyroidism from hyperplasia	
	Entero-pancreatic endocrine (30-80%) Pancreatic islet cell tumours	Nephrolithiasis, bone abnormalities, MSK complaints, symptoms of hypercalcemia
	Gastrinoma	Epigastric pain (peptic ulcers and esophagitis)
	Insulinomas	Hypoglycemia
	Vasoactive intestinal peptide (VIP)-omas	Secretory diarrhea
	Glucagonoma	Rash, anorexia, anemia, diarrhea, glossitis
	Carcinoid syndrome	Flushing, diarrhea, bronchospasm
MEN II (chromosome 10)		
1. IIa Sipple's Syndrome	Thyroid (>90%) Medullary thyroid cancer (MTC)	Physical signs are variable and often subtle
	Adrenal medulla (40-50%) Pheochromocytoma (40-50%)	Neck mass or thyroid nodule; non-tender, anterior lymph nodes
	Parathyroid (10-20%) 1° parathyroid hyperplasia	HTN, palpitations, headache, sweating
	Skin	Symptoms of hypercalcemia
	Cutaneous lichen amyloidosis	Scaly skin rash

Table 26. MEN Classification (continued)

Type	Tissues Involved	Clinical Manifestations
2. Familial Medullary Thyroid Ca (a variant of IIa)	Thyroid MTC (≥95%)	MTC without other clinical manifestations of MEN IIa or IIb

3. IIb	Thyroid
	  MTC
	Adrenal medulla
	  Pheochromocytoma (≥50%)
	Neurons
	  Mucosal neuroma, intestinal ganglioneuromas (100%)
	MSK (100%)
		MTC: most common component, more aggressive and earlier onset than MEN IIa
		HTN, palpitations, headache, sweating
		
		Chronic constipation; megacolon
		
		Marfanoid habitus (no aortic abnormalities)

Investigations
- MEN I
  - laboratory
    - may consider genetic screening for MEN-1 mutation in index patients
      - if a mutation is identified, screen family members who are at risk
    - gastrinoma: elevated serum gastrin level (>200 ng/mL) after IV injection of secretin
    - insulinoma: reduced fasting blood glucose (hypoglycemia) with elevated insulin and C-peptide levels
    - glucagonoma: elevated blood glucose and glucagon levels
    - pituitary tumours: assess GH, IGF-1, and prolactin levels (for over-production), TSH, free T_4, 8 AM cortisol, LH, FSH, bioavailable testosterone or estradiol (for underproduction due to mass effect of tumour)
    - hyperparathyroidism: serum Ca^{2+} and albumin, PTH levels; bone density scan (DEXA)
  - imaging
    - MRI for pituitary tumours, gastrinoma, insulinoma
- MEN II
  - laboratory
    - genetic screening for RET mutations in all index patients
      - if a mutation is identified screen family members who are at risk
    - calcitonin levels (MTC); urine catecholamines and metanephrines (pheochromocytoma); serum Ca^{2+}, albumin, and PTH levels (hyperparathyroidism)
    - pentagastrin ± calcium stimulation test if calcitonin level is within reference range
    - FNA for thyroid nodules-cytology
  - imaging
    - CT or MRI of adrenal glands, metaiodobenzylguanidine (MIBG) scan for pheochromocytoma
    - octreoscan and/or radionuclide scanning for determining the extent of metastasis

Treatment
- MEN I
  - medical
    - proton pump inhibitor (PPI) for acid hypersecretion in gastrinoma
    - cabergoline or other dopamine agonists to suppress prolactin secretion
    - somatostatin for symptomatic carcinoid tumours
  - surgery for hyperparathyroidism, insulinoma, glucagonoma, pituitary tumours (if medical treatment fails for the latter)
    - trans-sphenoidal approach with prn external radiation
- MEN II
  - surgery for MEN IIa with pre-operative medical therapy
    - prostaglandin inhibitors to alleviate diarrhea associated with thyroid cancer
    - α-blocker for at least 10-21 d for pheochromocytoma pre-operatively
    - hydration, calcitonin, IV bisphosphonates for hypercalcemia

Calcium Homeostasis

- normal total serum Ca^{2+}: 2.2-2.6 mmol/L
- ionic/free Ca^{2+} levels: 1.15-1.31 mmol/L
- serum Ca^{2+} is about 40% protein bound (mostly albumin), 50% ionized, and 10% complexed with PO_4^{3-} and citrate
- regulated mainly by two factors: parathyroid hormone (PTH) and vitamin D
- actions mainly on three organs: GI tract, bone, and kidney

Table 27. Major Regulators in Calcium Homeostasis

Major Regulators	Source	Regulation	Net Effect
PTH	Parathyroid glands	Stimulated by low serum Ca^{2+} and high serum PO_4^{3-}; inhibited by chronic low serum Mg^{2+}, high serum Ca^{2+}, and calcitriol	↑ Ca^{2+} ↑ Cacitriol ↓ PO_4^{3-}
Calcitriol (1,25-(OH)₂D₃)	Dietary intake Synthesized from cholesterol: UV on skin makes cholecalciferol (vitD3) liver makes calcidiol (25-(OH)D₃) kidneys make calcitriol	Renal calcitriol production is stimulated by low serum PO_4^{3-} and PTH; inhibited by high serum PO_4^{3-} and calcitriol in negative feedback	↑ Ca^{2+} ↑ PO_4^{3-}
Calcitonin	Thyroid C cells	Stimulated by pentagastrin (GI hormone) and high serum Ca^{2+}; inhibited by low serum Ca^{2+}	↓ Ca^{2+} (in pharmacologic doses) ↓ PO_4^{3-}
Mg^{2+}	Major intracellular divalent cation	See Magnesium, NP15	Cofactor for PTH secretion
PO_4^{3-}	Intracellular anion found in all tissues	See Phosphate, NP14	↓ Ca^{2+}

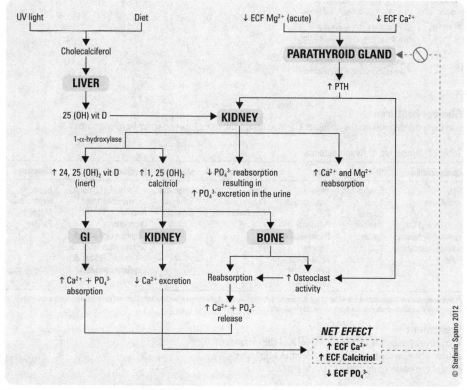

Figure 15. Parathyroid hormone (PTH) regulation

© Stefania Spano 2012

Primary Hyperparathyroidism Increased PTH secretion commonly due to parathyroid adenoma, lithium therapy; less often parathyroid carcinoma or parathyroid hyperplasia

Secondary Hyperparathyroidism Partial resistance to PTH action leads to parathyroid gland hyperplasia and increased PTH secretion, often in patients with renal failure and osteomalacia (due to low or low normal serum calcium levels)

Tertiary Hyperparathyroidism Irreversible clonal outgrowth of parathyroid glands, usually in long-standing inadequately treated chronic renal failure on dialysis

Primary Hyperparathyroidism is the most common cause of hypercalcemia in healthy outpatients. Most commonly related to a solitary adenoma or less commonly multiple gland hyperplasia. Surgical excision acts as definitive treatment and is recommended for patients who are symptomatic. For mild asymptomatic disease medical surveillance may be appropriate with annual serum calcium, creatinine, and bone mineral density (BMD)

For asymptomatic patients surgery is recommended for those who meet ≥1 of the following criteria:
- Serum calcium concentration more than 0.25 mmol/L (1.0 mg/dL) above the upper limit of normal
- Creatinine clearance <60 mL/min
- BMD T-score <-2.5 at hip, spine, or distal radius, and/or previous fragility fracture
- Age <50 yr

Pseudohypercalcemia: increased protein binding leading to an elevation in serum total Ca^{2+} without a rise in the ionized/free form, e.g. hyperalbuminemia from severe dehydration

Hypercalcemia

Definition
- total corrected serum Ca^{2+} >2.6 mmol/L OR ionized Ca^{2+} >1.35 mmol/L

Approach to Hypercalcemia
1. Is the patient hypercalcemic? (correct for albumin – see sidebar)
2. Is the PTH high/normal or low?
3. If PTH is low, is phosphate high/normal or low? If phosphate is high/normal is the level of vitamin D metabolites high or low?

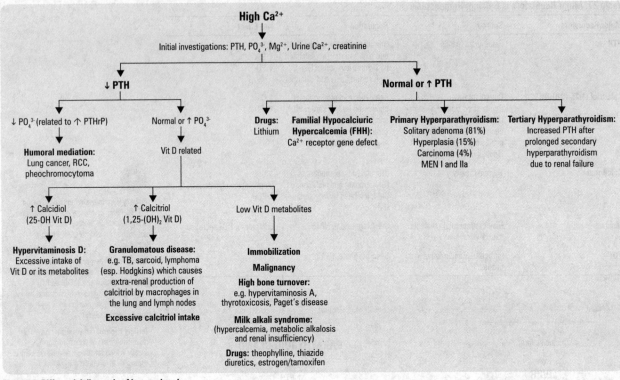

Figure 16. Differential diagnosis of hypercalcemia

Corrected Ca²⁺ (mmol/L) = measured Ca²⁺ + 0.02 (40 – albumin)

For every decrease in albumin by 10, increase in Ca²⁺ by 0.2

Benign (less likely malignant):
Ca²⁺ <2.75 mmol/L

Pathologic (more likely malignant):
Ca²⁺ >3.25 mmol/L

The symptoms and signs of hypercalcemia include:
"Bones, stones, groans, and psychiatric overtones"

The most common cause of **hypercalcemia in hospital** is **malignancy-associated hypercalcemia**
• Usually occurs in the later stages of disease
• Most commonly seen in lung, renal, breast, ovarian, and squamous tumours, as well as lymphoma and multiple myeloma

Mechanisms:
• Secretion of parathyroid hormone-related protein (PTHrP) which mimics PTH action by preventing renal calcium excretion and activating osteoclast-induced bone resorption
• Cytokines in multiple myeloma
• Calcitriol production by lymphoma
• Osteolytic bone metastases direct effect
• Excess PTH in parathyroid cancer

Clinical Features
• symptoms depend on the absolute Ca²⁺ value and the rate of its rise (may be asymptomatic)

Table 28. Symptoms of Hypercalcemia

Cardiovascular	GI	Renal	Rheumatological	MSK	Psychiatric	Neurologic
HTN	Constipation	Polyuria	Gout	Weakness	>3 mmol/L (12 mg/dL)	Hypotonia
Arrhythmia	Anorexia	(Nephrogenic	Pseudogout	Bone pain	Increased alertness	Hyporeflexia
Short QT	Nausea	DI)	Chondrocalcinosis	**(bones)**	Anxiety	Myopathy
Deposition of Ca²⁺	Vomiting	Polydipsia			Depression	Paresis
on valves, coronary	**(groans)**	**Nephrolithiasis**			Cognitive dysfunction	
arteries, myocardial	PUD	**(stones)**			Organic brain syndromes	
fibres	pancreatitis	Renal failure			>4 mmol/L (16 mg/dL)	
		(irreversible)			**Psychosis (moans)**	
		Dehydration				

** **Hypercalcemic crisis (usually >4 mmol/L or 16 mg/dL):** primary symptoms include oliguria/anuria and mental status changes including somnolence and eventually coma → this is a medical emergency and should be treated immediately!

Treatment
• treatment depends on the Ca²⁺ level and the symptoms
• treat acute, symptomatic hypercalcemia aggressively
• treat the underlying cause of the hypercalcemia

Table 29. Treatment of Acute Hypercalcemia/Hypercalcemic Crisis

Increase Urinary Ca²⁺ Excretion	Isotonic saline (4-5 L) over 24 h ± loop diuretic (e.g. furosemide) but only if hypervolemic (urine output >200mL/h)
	Calcitonin:
	  4 IU/kg IM/SC q12h
	  8 IU/kg IM/SC q6h
	  Only works for 48 h
	  Rapid onset within 4-6 h

Diminish Bone Resorption	Bisphosphonates (treatment of choice)
	  Inhibits osteoclastic bone resorption and promotes renal excretion of calcium
	  Acts rapidly but often transient response (decreased by 0.3-0.5 mmol/L beginning within 4-6 h) max effect usually in 7 d
	  Combination of calcitonin and steroids may prolong reduction in calcium
	  Tachyphylaxis may occur
	  Indicated in malignancy-related hypercalcemia (IV pamidronate or zoledronic acid used)
	  Mithramycin (rarely used) – effective when patient cannot tolerate large fluid load
	  Dangerous – hematotoxic and hepatotoxic

Decrease GI Ca²⁺ Absorption	Corticosteroids in hypervitaminosis D and hematologic malignancies
	  Anti-tumour effects → decreased calcitriol production by the activated mononuclear cells in lung and lymph node
	  Slow to act (5-10 d); need high dose

Dialysis	Treatment of last resort Indication: severe malignancy-associated hypercalcemia and renal insufficiency or heart failure

Hypocalcemia

Definition
- total corrected serum Ca^{2+} <2.2 mmol/L

Table 30. Clinical Features of Hypocalcemia

Acute Hypocalcemia	Chronic Hypocalcemia
Paresthesia Laryngospasm (with stridor) Hyperreflexia Tetany Chvostek's sign (tap CN VII) Trousseau's sign (carpal spasm) ECG changes Delirium Psychiatric Sx: emotional instability, anxiety, and depression	CNS: lethargy, seizures, psychosis, basal ganglia calcification, Parkinson's, dystonia, hemiballismus, papilledema, pseudotumour cerebri CVS: prolonged QT interval → Torsades de pointes (ventricular tachycardia) GI: steatorrhea ENDO: impaired insulin release SKIN: dry, scaling, alopecia, brittle and transversely fissured nails, candidiasis, abnormal dentition OCULAR: cataracts MSK: generalized muscle weakness and wasting

Approach to Hypocalcemia
1. Is the patient hypocalcemic?
2. Is the PTH high or low?
3. If PTH is high, is phosphate low or normal?
4. Is the Mg^{2+} level low?

Approach to Treatment
- correct underlying disorder
- mild/asymptomatic (ionized Ca^{2+} >0.8 mmol/L)
  - treat by increasing dietary Ca^{2+} by 1000 mg/d
  - calcitriol 0.25 µg/d (especially in renal failure)
- acute/symptomatic hypocalcemia (ionized Ca^{2+} <0.7 mmol/L)
  - immediate treatment required
  - IV calcium gluconate 1-2 g over 10-20 min followed by slow infusion if necessary
  - goal is to raise Ca^{2+} to low normal range (2.0-2.1 mmol/L) to prevent symptoms but allow maximum stimulation of PTH secretion
- if PTH recovery not expected, requires long-term therapy with calcitriol and calcium
- **do not correct hypocalcemia if asymptomatic and suspected to be transient**

Differential Diagnosis of Hypercalcemia
- Primary hyperparathyroidism
- Malignancy: hematologic, humoral, skeletal metastases (>90% from 1 or 2)
- Renal disease: tertiary hyperparathyroidism
- Drugs: calcium carbonate, milk alkali syndrome, thiazide, lithium, theophylline, vitamin A/D intoxication
- Familial hypocalciuric hypercalcemia
- Granulomatous disease: sarcoidosis, TB, Hodgkin's lymphoma
- Thyroid disease: thyrotoxicosis
- Adrenal disease: adrenal insufficiency, pheochromocytoma
- Immobilization

Watch Out for:
- Volume depletion via diuresis
- Arrhythmias

Acute Management of Hypercalcemia/ Hypercalcemic Crisis
- Volume expansion (e.g. NS IV 300-500 cc/h): initial therapy
- Calcitonin: transient, partial response
- Bisphosphonate: treatment of choice
- Corticosteroid: most useful in vitamin D toxicity, granulomatous disease, some malignancies
- Saline diuresis + loop diuretic (for volume overload): temporary measure

Hypomagnesmia can impair PTH secretion and action

Differential Diagnosis of Tetany
- Hypocalcemia
- Metabolic alkalosis (with hyperventilation)
- Hypokalemia
- Hypomagnesemia

Signs and Symptoms of Acute Hypocalcemia
- Paresthesias: perioral, hands, and feet
- Chvostek's sign: percussion of the facial nerve just anterior to the external auditory meatus elicits ipsilateral spasm of the orbicularis oculi or orbicularis oris muscles
- Trousseau's sign: inflation of a blood pressure cuff above systolic pressure for 3 min elicits carpal spasm and paresthesia

Transient hypoparathyroidism (resulting in hypocalcemia) common after subtotal thyroidectomy (permanent in <3% of surgeries)

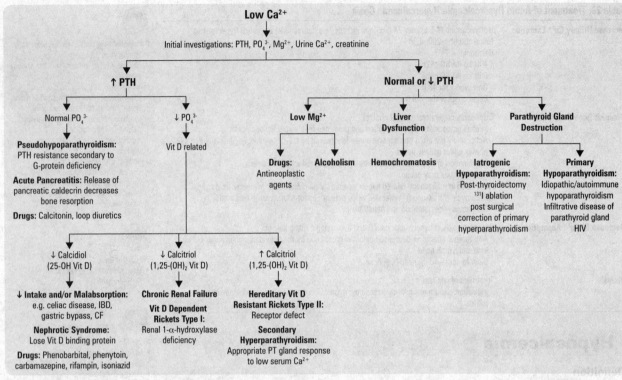

Figure 17. Etiology and clinical approach to hypocalcemia

Metabolic Bone Disease

Osteoporosis

Online Clinical Tools
CAROC
www.osteoporosis.ca/multimedia/pdf/
CAROC.pdf
FRAX
www.shef.ac.uk/FRAX/tool.aspx

Definition
- a condition characterized by decreased bone mass and microarchitectural deterioration of bone tissue with a consequent increase in bone fragility and susceptibility to fracture
- bone mineral density (BMD) ≥2.5 standard deviations below the peak bone mass for young adults (i.e. T-score ≤–2.5)
- osteopenia: BMD with T-score between -1.0 and -2.5

ETIOLOGY AND PATHOPHYSIOLOGY

Primary Osteoporosis (95% of osteoporosis in women and 80% in men)
- primary type 1: most common in post-menopausal women, due to decline in estrogen, worsens with age
- primary type 2: occurs after age 75, seen in females and males at 2:1 ratio, possibly due to zinc deficiency

Secondary Osteoporosis

Corticosteroid Therapy is a Common Cause of Secondary Osteoporosis
Individuals receiving ≥7.5 mg of prednisone daily for over 3 mo should be assessed for bone-sparing therapy
Mechanism: increased resorption + decreased formation + increased urinary calcium loss + decreased intestinal calcium absorption + decreased sex steroid production

- gastrointestinal diseases
  - gastrectomy
  - malabsorption (e.g. celiac disease)
  - chronic liver disease
- bone marrow disorders
  - multiple myeloma
  - lymphoma
  - leukemia
- endocrinopathies
  - Cushing's syndrome
  - hyperparathyroidism
  - hyperthyroidism
  - premature menopause
  - DM
  - hypogonadism
- malignancy
  - secondary to chemotherapy
  - myeloma
- drugs
  - corticosteroid therapy
  - phenytoin
  - chronic heparin therapy
  - androgen deprivation therapy
  - aromatase inhibitors
- other
  - rheumatologic disorders
    - rheumatoid arthritis
    - SLE
    - ankylosing spondylitis
  - renal disease
  - poor nutrition
  - immobilization
- COPD (due to disease, tobacco, and glucocorticoid use)

Clinical Features
- commonly asymptomatic
- height loss due to collapsed vertebrae
- fractures: most commonly in hip, vertebrae, humerus, and wrist
  - fragility fractures: fracture with fall from standing height
  - Dowager's hump: collapse fracture of vertebral bodies in mid-dorsal region
  - x-ray: vertebral compression and crush fractures, wedge fractures, "codfishing" sign (weakening of subchondral plates and expansion of intervertebral discs)
- pain, especially backache, associated with fractures

Approach to Osteoporosis
1. assess risk factors for osteoporosis on history and physical
2. decide if patient requires BMD testing with dual-energy x-ray absorptiometry (DEXA): men and women ≥65 yr or younger if presence of risk factors
3. Initial investigations
   - all patients with osteoporosis: calcium corrected for albumin, CBC, creatinine, ALP, TSH
   - also consider serum and urine protein electrophoresis, celiac workup, and 24 h urinary Ca²⁺ excretion to rule out additional secondary causes
   - **25-OH-Vitamin D level should only be measured after 3-4 mo of adequate supplementation and should not be repeated if an optimal level ≥75 nmol/L is achieved**
   - lateral thoracic and lumbar x-ray if clinical evidence of vertebral fracture
4. Assess 10-yr fracture risk by combining BMD result and risk factors (only if ≥50 yr)
   1) WHO Fracture Risk Assessment Tool (FRAX)
   2) Canadian Association of Radiologists and Osteoporosis Canada Risk Assessment Tool (CAROC)
      - approach to management guided by 10-yr risk stratification into low, medium, high risk
5. For all patients being assessed for osteoporosis, encourage appropriate lifestyle changes (see Table 33)

Table 31. Indications for BMD Testing

Older Adults (age ≥50 yr)	Younger Adults (age <50 yr)
All women and men age ≥65 yr	Fragility fracture
Menopausal women, and men aged 50-64 yr with clinical risk factors for fracture:	Prolonged use of glucocorticoids
Fragility fracture after age 40	Use of other high-risk medications
Prolonged glucocorticoid use	(aromatase inhibitors, androgen
Other high-risk medication use (aromatase inhibitors, androgen deprivation therapy)	deprivation therapy, anticonvulsants)
Parental hip fracture	Hypogonadism or premature menopause
Vertebral fracture or osteopenia identified on x-ray	Malabsorption syndrome
Current smoking	Primary hyperparathyroidism
High alcohol intake	Other disorders strongly associated with
Low body weight (<60 kg) or major weight loss (>10% of weight at age 25 yr)	rapid bone loss and/or fracture
Rheumatoid arthritis	
Other disorders strongly associated with osteoporosis: primary hyperparathyroidism, type 1 DM, osteogenesis imperfecta, uncontrolled hyperthyroidism, hypogonadism or premature menopause (<45 yr), Cushing's disease, chronic malnutrition or malabsorption, chronic liver disease, COPD and chronic inflammatory conditions (e.g. inflammatory bowel disease)	

Table 32. Osteoporisis Risk Stratification

Low Risk	
10-yr fracture risk <10%	Unlikely to benefit from pharmacotherapy; encourage lifestyle changes Reassess risk in 5 yr

Medium Risk	
10-yr fracture risk 10-20%	Discuss patient preference for management and consider additional risk factors Factors that warrant consideration for pharmacological therapy: Additional vertebral fracture(s) identified on vertebral fracture assessment (VFA) or lateral spine x-ray Previous wrist fracture in individuals ≥65 or with T-score ≤-2.5 Lumbar spine T-score much lower than femoral neck T-score Rapid bone loss Men receiving androgen-deprivation therapy for prostate cancer Women receiving aromatase-inhibitor therapy for breast cancer Long-term or repeated systemic glucocorticoid use (oral or parenteral) that does not meet the conventional criteria for recent prolonged systemic glucocorticoid use Recurrent falls (defined as falling 2 or more times in the past 12 mo) Other disorders strongly associated with osteoporosis Repeat BMD and reassess risk every 1-3 yr initially

High Risk	
10-yr fracture risk >20%; OR Prior fragility fracture of hip or spine; OR More than one fragility fracture	Start pharmacotherapy

Calcium Plus Vitamin D Supplementation and Risk of Fractures. Osteoporosis
Int 2015;27:367-376
Purpose: To review trials of Vitamin D and Calcium therapy for reducing fracture risk in osteoporosis.
Study: Systematic review searching 2011-2015, inclusive, identified 8 RCTs totalling 30,970 participants. RCTs reviewed included healthy adults and ambulatory older adults with medical conditions (excluding cancer). Vitamin D and Calcium combination therapy was compared to placebo.
Results: Analysis of RCT data revealed that calcium plus vitamin D supplementation produced a statistically significant reduction in risk of total fractures (0.85; CI:0.73–0.98) and in hip fractures (0.70;CI:0.56–0.87). Subgroup analysis was significant for community dwelling or institutionalized patients.
Conclusions: Systematic analysis suggests that Vitamin D and Calcium therapy significantly decreases fracture risk. This study did not specifically look at individuals with osteoporosis. However, it still supports that Vitamin D and Calcium should continue to be used as preventative treatment for individuals at increased risk of fractures.

Clinical Signs of Fractures or Osteoporosis
- Height loss >3 cm (Sn 92%)
- Weight <51 kg
- Kyphosis (Sp 92%)
- Tooth count <20 (Sp 92%)
- Grip strength
- Armspan-height difference >5 cm (Sp 76%)
- Wall-occiput distance >0 cm (Sp 87%)
- Rib-pelvis distance ≤2 finger breadth (Sn 88%)

Alendronate for the Primary and Secondary Prevention of Osteoporotic Fractures in Postmenopausal Women
Cochrane DB Syst Rev 2008;1:CD001155

Etidronate for the Primary and Secondary Prevention of Osteoporotic Fractures in Postmenopausal Women
Cochrane Database Syst Rev 2008;(1):CD003376

Risedronate for the Primary and Secondary Prevention of Osteoporotic Fractures in Postmenopausal Women
Cochrane Database Syst Rev 2008;(1):CD004523

Purpose: To assess the efficacy of three bisphosponates in the primary and secondary prevention of osteoporotic fractures in postmenopausal women.
Study Selection: Women receiving at least one yr of bisphosphonates for postmenopausal osteoporosis were compared to those receiving placebo or concurrent calcium/vitamin D or both. The outcome was fracture incidence.
Results: Levels of evidence: http://www.cochranemsk.org/review/writing/%RRR and %ARR for 5 yr fracture incidence reduction.

Aledronate (10 mg/d)
1° Prevention – Vertebral 45% RRR, 2% ARR (Gold)
1° Prevention – Hip   Not significant
1° Prevention – Wrist   Not significant
2° Prevention – Vertebral 45% RRR, 6% ARR (Gold)
2° Prevention – Hip   53% RRR, 1% ARR (Gold)
2° Prevention – Wrist   50% RRR, 2% ARR (Gold)

Etidronate (400 mg/d)
1° Prevention – Vertebral Not significant
1° Prevention – Hip   Not significant
1° Prevention – Wrist   Not significant
2° Prevention – Vertebral 47% RRR, 5% ARR (Silver)
2° Prevention – Hip   No benefit
2° Prevention – Wrist   No benefit

Risedronate (5 mg/d)
1° Prevention – Vertebral Not significant
1° Prevention – Hip   Not significant
1° Prevention – Wrist   Not significant
2° Prevention – Vertebral 39% RRR, 5% ARR (Gold)
2° Prevention – Hip   26% RRR, 1% ARR (Silver)
2° Prevention – Wrist   Not significant

Before prescribing Calcitonin, remember to ask about fish allergies

Factors Necessary for Mineralization
- Quantitatively and qualitatively normal osteoid formation
- Normal concentration of calcium and phosphate in ECF
- Adequate bioactivity of ALP
- Normal pH at site of calcification
- Absence of inhibitors of calcification

Treatment of Osteoporosis

Table 33. Treatment of Osteoporosis in Women and Men

Treatment for Both Men and Women	
Lifestyle	Diet: Elemental calcium 1000-1200 mg/d; Vit D 1000 IU/d Exercise: 3x30 min weight-bearing exercises/wk Cessation of smoking, reduce caffeine intake Stop/avoid osteoporosis-inducing medications
Drug Therapy	
Bisphosphonate: inhibitors of osteoclast binding	1st line in prevention of hip, nonvertebral, and vertebral # (Grade A): alendronate, risedronate, zoledronic acid 2nd line (Grade B): etidronate
RANKL Inhibitors	Denosumab: 1st line in prevention of hip, nonvertebral, vertebral # (Grade A)
Parathyroid Hormone	YES fragility #: 18-24 mo duration
Calcitonin (2nd line) osteoclast receptor binding	YES fragility #: Calcitonin 200 IU nasally OD with Calcitriol 0.25 μg bid
Treatment Specific to Post-Menopausal Women	
SERM (selective estrogen-receptor modulator): agonistic effect on bone but antagonistic effect on uterus and breast	Raloxifene: 1st line in prevention of vertebral # (Grade A) +ve: prevents osteoporotic # (Grade A to B evidence), improves lipid profile, decreased breast ca risk -ve: increased risk of DVT/PE, stroke mortality, hot flashes, leg cramps
HRT: combined estrogen + progesterone (see Gynecology, GY34)	1st line in prevention of hip, nonvertebral, and vertebral # (Grade A) For most women, risks > benefits Combined estrogen/progestin prevents hip, vertebral, total # Increased risks of breast cancer, cardiovascular events, and DVT/PE

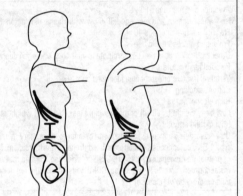

Figure 18. Physical examination test

Osteomalacia and Rickets

- **rickets:** osteopenia with disordered calcification leading to a higher proportion of osteoid (unmineralized) tissue prior to epiphyseal closure (in childhood)
- **osteomalacia**: osteopenia with disordered calcification leading to a higher proportion of osteoid (unmineralized) tissue after epiphyseal closure (in adulthood)

Etiology and Pathophysiology

Vitamin D Deficiency
- deficient uptake or absorption
  - nutritional deficiency
  - malabsorption: post-gastrectomy, small bowel disease (e.g. Celiac sprue), pancreatic insufficiency

- defective 25-hydroxylation
  - liver disease
  - anticonvulsant therapy (phenytoin, carbamazepine, phenobarbital)
- loss of vitamin D binding protein
  - nephrotic syndrome
- defective 1-α-25 hydroxylation
  - hypoparathyroidism
- renal failure
- pathophysiology: leads to secondary hyperparathyroidism and hypophosphatemia

Mineralization Defect
- abnormal matrix
  - osteogenesis imperfecta
  - fibrogenesis imperfecta
  - axial osteomalacia
- enzyme deficiency
  - hypophosphatasia (inadequate ALP bioactivity)
- presence of calcification inhibitors
  - bisphosphonates, aluminum, high dose fluoride, anticonvulsants

Table 34. Clinical Presentations of Rickets and Osteomalacia

Rickets	Osteomalacia
Skeletal pain and deformities, bow legged	Not as dramatic
Fracture susceptibility	Diffuse skeletal pain
Weakness and hypotonia	Bone tenderness
Disturbed growth	Fractures
Ricketic rosary (prominent costochondral junctions)	Gait disturbances (waddling)
Harrison's groove (indentation of lower ribs)	Proximal muscle weakness
Hypocalcemia	Hypotonia

Investigations

Table 35. Laboratory Findings in Osteomalacia and Rickets

Disorder	Serum Phosphate	Serum Calcium	Serum ALP	Other Features
Vitamin D deficiency	Decreased	Decreased to normal	Increased	Decreased calcitriol
Hypophosphatemia	Decreased	Normal	Decreased to normal	
Proximal RTA	Decreased	Normal	Normal	Associated with hyperchloremic metabolic acidosis
Conditions associated with abnormal matrix formation	Normal	Normal	Normal	

- radiologic findings
  - pseudofractures, fissures, narrow radiolucent lines – thought to be healed stress fractures or the result of erosion by arterial pulsation
  - loss of distinctness of vertebral body trabeculae; concavity of the vertebral bodies
  - changes due to secondary hyperparathyroidism: subperiosteal resorption of the phalanges, bone cysts, resorption of the distal ends of long bones
  - others: bowing of tibia, coxa profundus hip deformity
- bone biopsy: usually not necessary but considered the gold standard for diagnosis

Treatment
- definitive treatment depends on the underlying cause
- vitamin D supplementation
- PO_4^{3-} supplements if low serum PO_4^{3-}, Ca^{2+} supplements for isolated calcium deficiency
- bicarbonate if chronic metabolic acidosis

Renal Osteodystrophy

- changes to mineral metabolism and bone structure secondary to chronic kidney disease
- represents a mixture of four types of bone disease:
  - osteomalacia: low bone turnover combined with increased unmineralized bone (osteoid)
  - adynamic bone disease: low bone turnover due to excessive suppression of parathyroid gland
  - osteitis fibrosa cystica: increased bone turnover due to secondary hyperparathyroidism
  - mixed uremic osteodystrophy: both high and low bone turnover, characterized by marrow fibrosis and increased osteoid
- metastatic calcification secondary to hyperphosphatemia may occur

Pathophysiology
- metabolic bone disease secondary to chronic renal failure
- combination of hyperphosphatemia (inhibits 1,25(OH)$_2$-Vit D synthesis) and loss of renal mass (reduced 1-α-hydroxylase)

KDIGO 2012 Clinical Practice Guideline for the Evaluation and Management of Chronic Kidney Disease
Kidney Inter Suppl 2013;3:1-150

Recommendations for Metabolic Bone Disease in CKD

Screening
- Regular bone mineral density screening of patients with eGFR < 45 is not recommended
- No consensus regarding optimal intervals for screening PO_4^{3-} and Ca^{2+} levels
- Screening Vitamin D and PTH is not recommended

Management
- Best fracture prevention strategy is fall risk assessment and fall prevention measures (see Geriatric Medicine, GM5)
- No clear evidence that manipulation of Ca^{2+}, Vitamin D, PO_4^{3-}, or PTH results in improved outcomes

Clinical Features
- soft tissue calcifications, necrotic skin lesions if vessels involved
- osteodystrophy, generalized bone pain and fractures
- pruritus
- neuromuscular irritability and tetany may occur
- radiologic features of osteitis fibrosa cystica, osteomalacia, osteosclerosis, osteoporosis

Investigations
- serum Ca^{2+} corrected for albumin, PO_4^{3-}, PTH, ALP, ± imaging (x-ray, BMD), ± bone biopsy

Treatment
- prevention
- maintenance of normal serum Ca^{2+} and PO_4^{3-} by restricting PO_4^{3-} intake to 1 g OD
- Ca^{2+} supplements; PO_4^{3-} binding agents (calcium carbonate, aluminum hydroxide)
- vitamin D with close monitoring to avoid hypercalcemia and metastatic calcification

Paget's Disease of Bone

Definition
- a metabolic disease characterized by excessive bone destruction and repair

Epidemiology
- a common disease: 5% of the population, 10% of population >80 yr old
- consider Paget's disease of bone in older adults with ↑ ALP but normal GGT

Etiology and Pathophysiology
- postulated to be related to a slowly progressing viral infection of osteoclasts, possibly paramyxovirus
- strong familial incidence
- initiated by increased osteoclastic activity leading to increased bone resorption; osteoblastic activity increases in response to produce new bone that is structurally abnormal and fragile

Differential Diagnosis
- primary bone lesions
  - osteogenic sarcoma
  - multiple myeloma
  - fibrous dysplasia
- secondary bone lesions
  - osteitis fibrosa cystica
  - metastases

Clinical Features
- usually asymptomatic (routine x-ray finding or elevated ALP)
- severe bone pain (e.g. pelvis, femur, tibia) is often the presenting complaint
- skeletal deformities: bowed tibias, kyphosis, frequent fractures
- skull involvement: headaches, increased hat size, deafness
- increased warmth over involved bones due to increased vascularity
- high output CHF
- hypercalcemia with immobilization
- osteosarcoma

Investigations
- laboratory
  - ↑↑ serum ALP (unless burnt out), Ca^{2+} normal or ↑, PO_4^{3-} normal
  - urinary hydroxyproline ↑ (indicates resorption)
- imaging
  - bone scan to evaluate the extent of disease
  - confirmation on x-ray required to establish the diagnosis
  - skeletal survey: involved bones are denser and expanded with cortical thickening
    - initial lesion may be destructive and radiolucent
    - multiple fissure fractures in long bones

Complications
- local
  - fractures; osteoarthritis
  - cranial nerve compression and palsies (e.g. deafness), spinal cord compression
  - osteosarcoma/sarcomatous change in 1-3%
    - indicated by marked bone pain, new lytic lesions and suddenly increased ALP
- systemic
  - hypercalcemia and nephrolithiasis
  - high output CHF due to increased vascularity

Bones Most Often Affected in Paget's Disease (in decreasing order)
- Pelvis
- Femur
- Skull
- Tibia
- Vertebrae
- Clavicle
- Humerus

Comparison of a Single Infusion of Zoledronic Acid with Risedronate for Paget's Disease
NEJM 2005;353:898-908
Study: Two identical, randomized, double-blind, actively controlled trials (combined for analysis).
Patients: 357 men and women who were older than 30 yr of age and had radiologically confirmed Paget's disease. All but 4 patients had alkaline phosphatase levels that were more than twice the upper limit of normal.
Intervention: One 15-min infusion of 5 mg of zoledronic acid compared with 60 d of oral risedronate (30 mg/d) with follow up at 6 mo.
Primary Outcome: Rate of therapeutic response at 6 mo, defined as a normalization of alkaline phosphatase levels or a reduction of at least 75% in the total alkaline phosphatase excess.
Results: At 6 mo, 96% of patients receiving zoledronic acid had a therapeutic response (169 of 176), as compared with 74.3% of patients receiving risedronate (127 of 171, p<0.001). Alkaline phosphatase levels normalized in 88.6% of patients in the zoledronic acid group and 57.9% of patients in the risedronate group (p<0.001). Zoledronic acid was associated with a shorter median time to a first therapeutic response (64 vs. 89 d, p<0.001). Quality of life increased significantly from baseline at both 3 and 6 mo in the zoledronic acid group and differed significantly from those in the risedronate group at 3 mo. Pain scores improved in both groups. During post-trial follow-up (median, 190 d), 21 of 82 patients in the risedronate group had a loss of therapeutic response, as compared with 1 of 113 patients in the zoledronic acid group (p<0.001).
Conclusions: A single infusion of zoledronic acid produces more rapid, more complete, and more sustained responses in Paget's disease than does daily treatment with risedronate.

Treatment
- symptomatic therapy (pain management)
- weight-bearing exercise
- adequate calcium and vitamin D intake to prevent development of secondary hyperparathyroidism
- treat medically if ALP >3x normal
  - bisphosphonates, e.g. alendronate 40 mg PO OD x 6 mo OR risedronate 30 mg PO OD x 3 mo OR zoledronic acid 5 mg IV per yr
  - calcitonin 50-100 U/d SC
- surgery for fractures, deformity, degenerative changes

Male Reproductive Endocrinology

Androgen Regulation

- negative feedback may occur by androgens directly or after conversion to estrogen
- testosterone (from Leydig cells) primarily involved in negative feedback on LH and GnRH, whereas inhibin (from Sertoli cells) suppresses FSH secretion

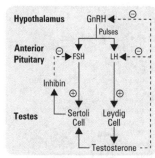

Figure 19. Hypothalamo-pituitary-gonadal axis

Tests of Testicular Function

- testicular size (lower limit = 4 cm x 2.5 cm)
- LH, FSH, total, bioavailable, and/or free testosterone
- human chorionic gonadotropin (hCG) stimulation test
  - assesses ability of Leydig cell to respond to gonadotropin
- semen analysis
  - semen volume, sperm concentration, morphology, and motility are the most commonly used parameters
- testicular biopsy
  - indicated with normal FSH and azoospermia/oligospermia

Hypogonadism and Infertility

- see Urology, U34
- deficiency in gametogenesis or testosterone production

Etiology
- causes include primary (testicular failure), secondary (hypothalamic-pituitary failure), and idiopathic
- primary hypogonadism is more common than secondary

Two Distinct Features of Primary Hypogonadism
- The decrease in sperm count is affected to a greater extent than the decrease in serum testosterone level
- Likely to be associated with gynecomastia

Table 36. Classification and Features of Hypogonadism

Two Features of Secondary Hypogonadism
- Associated with an equivalent decrease in sperm count and serum testosterone
- Less likely to be associated with gynecomastia

	Hypergonadotropic Hypogonadism (Primary Hypogonadism)	Hypogonadotropic Hypogonadism (Secondary Hypogonadism)
Definition	Primary testicular failure ↑ LH and FSH, ↑ FSH:LH ratio ↓ testosterone and sperm count	Hypothalamic-pituitary axis failure ↓ LH + FSH (LH sometimes inappropriately normal) ↓ testosterone and sperm count

Etiology	Congenital
	  Chromosomal defects (Klinefelter's, Noonan)
	  Cryptorchidism
	  Disorders of sexual development (DSD)
	  Bilateral anorchia (vanishing testicle syndrome)
	  Myotonic dystrophy
	  Mutation of FSH or LH receptor gene
	  Disorders of androgen synthesis
	Germ cell defects
	  Sertoli cell only syndrome
	  Leydig cell aplasia/failure
	Infection/Inflammation
	  Orchitis – TB, lymphoma, mumps, leprosy
	  Genital tract infection
	Physical factors
	  Trauma, heat, irradiation, testicular torsion, varicocele
	Drugs
	  Marijuana, alcohol, chemotherapy, ketoconazole, glucocorticoid, spironolactone
		Congenital
		  Kallman's syndrome
		  Prader-Willi syndrome
		  Abnormal subunit of LH or FSH
		Infection
		  Tuberculosis, meningitis
		Endocrine
		  Adrenal androgen excess
		  Cushing's syndrome
		  Hypo or hyperthyroidism
		  Hypothalamic-pituitary disease (tumour, hyperprolactinemia, hypopituitarism)
		Drugs
		  Alcohol, marijuana, spironolactone, ketoconazole, GnRH agonists, androgen/estrogen/progestin use, chronic narcotic use
		Chronic illness
		  Cirrhosis, chronic renal failure, AIDS
		  Sarcoidosis, Langerhan's cell histiocytosis hemochromatosis
		Critical illness
		  Surgery, MI, head trauma
		Obesity
		Idiopathic

Diagnosis	Testicular size and consistency (soft/firm) Sperm count LH, FSH, total, and/or bioavailable testosterone hCG stimulation (mainly used in pediatrics) Karyotype	Testicular size and consistency (soft/firm) Sperm count LH, FSH, total, and/or bioavailable testosterone Prolactin levels MRI of hypothalamic-pituitary region

Treatment
- testosterone replacement (improve libido, muscle mass, strength, body hair growth, bone mass)
  - IM injection, transdermal testosterone patch/gel, oral
  - side effects: acne, fluid retention, erythrocytosis, sleep apnea, benign prostatic hypertrophy, uncertain effects on cardiac events/mortality in older men
  - contraindicated if history of metastatic prostate cancer, breast cancer, severe LUTS associated with BPH, uncontrolled or poorly controlled CHF, PSA>4, hematocrit >50%
- GnRH agonist to restore fertility, if hypothalamic dysfunction with intact pituitary
  - administered SC in pulsatile fashion using an external pump
- hCG ± recombinant follicular stimulating hormone (rFSH) can be used to restore fertility in cases of either hypothalamic or pituitary lesions
- testicular sperm extraction (TESE) or microscopic sperm extraction (MICROTESE) – only if testicular tissues are not functioning

Other Causes of Male Infertility
- hereditary disorders: Kartagener syndrome (primary ciliary dyskinesia), cystic fibrosis
- anatomy: hypospadias, retrograde ejaculation
- obstruction: vasal occlusion, vasal aplasia, vasectomy, seminal vesicle disease
- sexual dysfunction: erectile dysfunction, premature ejaculation, infrequent coitus
- surgery: TURP, radical prostatectomy, orchiectomy

DEFECTS IN ANDROGEN ACTION

Etiology
- complete androgen insensitivity (CAIS)
- partial androgen insensitivity (PAIS)
- 5-α-reductase deficiency
- mixed gonadal dysgenesis
- defects in testosterone synthesis
- infertile male syndrome
- undervirilized fertile male syndrome

Clinical Features
- depends on age of onset

Table 37. Effects of Testosterone Deficiency

First Trimester *in utero*	Incomplete virilization of external genitalia (ambiguous genitalia) Incomplete development of Wolffian ducts to form male internal genitalia (male pseudohermaphrodism)
Third Trimester *in utero*	Micropenis Cryptorchidism (failure of normal testicular descent)
Prepuberty	Incomplete pubertal maturation (high pitch voice, sparse pubic + axillary hair, absence of facial hair) Eunuchoidal body habitus (greater growth of extremity long bones relative to axial bones) Poor muscle development, reduced peak bone mass
Postpuberty	Decrease in energy, mood, and libido Fine wrinkles in corners of mouth and eyes Decrease in pubic/axillary hair, hematocrit, muscle mass, strength, and BMD

Adapted from: UpToDate, 2010; *Cecil's Essentials of Medicine*

Treatment
- appropriate gender assignment in the newborn
- hormone replacement or supplementation
- psychological support
- gonadectomy for cryptorchidism (due to increased risk for testicular cancer)
- reduction mammoplasty for gynecomastia

Erectile Dysfunction

- see Urology, U30

Gynecomastia

Definition
- true gynecomastia refers to benign proliferation of the glandular component of the male breast, resulting in the formation of a concentric, rubbery, firm mass extending from the nipple(s)
- pseudogynecomastia or lipomastia refers to enlargement of soft adipose tissue, especially seen in obese individuals

Etiology

Physiologic
- puberty
- elderly (involutional)
- neonatal (maternal hormone)

Pathologic
- endocrinopathies: primary or secondary hypogonadism, hyperthyroidism, extreme hyperprolactinemia, adrenal disease
- tumours: pituitary, adrenal, testicular, breast, ectopic production of hCG
- chronic diseases: cirrhosis, renal, malnutrition (with refeeding)
- drugs: estrogens and estrogen agonists, spironolactone, ketoconazole, cimetidine, digoxin, chemotherapy, marijuana, alcohol
- congenital/genetic: Klinefelter's syndrome, androgen insensitivity
- other: idiopathic (majority of gynecomastia is classified as idiopathic), familial

Pathophysiology
- hormonal imbalance due to increased estrogen activity (increased production, or increased availability of estrogen precursors for peripheral conversion to estrogen) or decreased androgen activity (decreased androgen production, binding of androgen to sex hormone binding globulin (SHBG), or androgen receptor blockage)

History
- recent change in breast characteristics
- trauma to testicles
- mumps
- alcohol and/or drug use
- FHx
- sexual dysfunction

Physical Exam
- signs of feminization
- breast
  - rule out red flags suggesting breast cancer: unilateral, eccentric, hard or fixed mass, skin dimpling or retraction, and nipple discharge or crusting
  - gynecomastia occurs concentrically around nipple, is not fixed to underlying tissue
- genito-urinary exam
- stigmata of liver or thyroid disease

Investigations
- laboratory: serum TSH, PRL, LH, FSH, testosterone, estradiol, LFTs, creatinine, hCG (if hCG is elevated need to locate the primary tumour)
- CXR and CT of chest/abdomen/pelvis (to locate neoplasm)
- testicular U/S to rule out testicular mass
- MRI of hypothalamic-pituitary region if pituitary adenoma suspected

Treatment
- initial observation for most men with gynecomastia
- medical
  - correct the underlying disorder, discontinue responsible drug
  - androgens for hypogonadism
  - anti-estrogens: tamoxifen has most evidence for benefit
  - aromatase inhibitors: less evidence of benefit as compared to anti-estrogens
- surgical
  - usually required for macromastia, gynecomastia present for >1 yr (fibrosis is unresponsive to medication), or failed medical treatment and for cosmetic purposes

Female Reproductive Endocrinology

- see Gynecology, GY23

Pubertal Gyencomastia
- This benign condition peaks between 13-14 years of age and spontaneously regresses in 90% of cases within 2yr
- Waiting is often the best approach

Causes of Gynecomastia

DOC TECH
Drugs
Other
Congenital
Tumour
Endocrine
CHronic disease

Occurrence of Gynecomastia

3 Peaks	% Affected
Infancy	60-90
Puberty	4-69
Ages 50-80	24-65

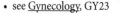

Paraneoplastic Syndrome

- clinical syndromes involving non-metastatic systemic effects that accompany malignant disease
- triggered by antibodies against neoplasm cross-reacting with normal tissue or by production of a physiologically active substance by the neoplasm
- commonly present with cancers of lung, breast, ovaries, or lymphatic system

Table 38. Clinical Presentation

Syndrome Class	Symptoms/Syndrome	Associated Malignancies	Mechanism
Endocrine	Cushing's syndrome	Small-cell lung cancer Pancreatic carcinoma Neural tumours Thymoma	Ectopic ACTH and ACTH-like substance secretion
	SIADH	Small-cell lung cancerCNS malignancies	Antidiuretic hormone secretion
	Hypercalcemia	Lung cancer Breast carcinoma Renal cell carcinoma Multiple myeloma Ovarian carcinoma	PTH-related protein, TGF-α, TNF secretion
	Hypoglycemia	Hepatocellular carcinomaFibrosarcoma	Insulin or insulin-like substance secretion
	Carcinoid	Pancreatic carcinomaGastric carcinoma	Serotonin, bradykinin secretion
Neurologic	Lambert-Eaton myasthenic syndrome (LEMS) Muscle weakness in limbs	Small-cell lung cancer	Ab interferes with ACh release
	Myasthenia gravis Fluctuating muscle weakness and fatiguability	Thymoma	Ab interferes with ACh release
	Paraneoplastic limbic encephalitis Depression, seizures, short-term memory loss	Small-cell lung cancer	Unknown
Renal	Hypokalemic nephropathy	Small-cell lung cancer	Ectopic ACTH and ACTH-like substance secretion
	Nephrotic syndrome	Lymphoma Melanomas	Immunocomplex sedimentation in nephrons
GI	Watery diarrhea	Medullary thyroid carcinomas	Prostaglandin secretion
Hematologic	Erythrocytosis	Renal cell carcinoma Hepatocellular carcinoma	EPO production
Rheumatologic	SLE	Lymphomas Lung cancer Breast carcinoma Gonadal carcinoma	Anti-nuclear Ab production
	Scleroderma	Breast carcinoma Lung cancer Uterine cancer	Anti-nuclear Ab production

Investigations

- CBC, electrolytes, creatinine, LFTs, ALP, ESR, CRP, serum/urine electrophoresis
- serum autoantibodies, lumbar puncture
- imaging: skeletal survey, CT, MRI, PET scan
- ± endoscopy

Treatment

- treat underlying tumour: surgery, radiation, chemotherapy
- treat immune-mediated disorder: IVIg, steroids, immunosuppressive drugs, plasmapheresis (reserved for patients with identifiable antibodies in serum)

Common Medications

Diabetes Medications

Drug Class	Mechanism of Action	Generic Drug Name	Canada Name	US Name (if different)	Dosing	Indications	Contraindications	Side Effects	Comments
Biguanide	Sensitizes peripheral tissues to insulin → increases glucose uptake. Decreases hepatic glucose production by simulation of hepatic AMP-activated protein kinase (AMPK)	metformin	Glucophage® Glumetza®		500 mg OD titrated to 2000 mg/d maximum	Useful in obese type 2 DM. Improves both fasting and postprandial hyperglycemia. Also ↓ TG	ABSOLUTE: Moderate to severe liver dysfunction. Moderate renal dysfunction GFR <30 mL/min. Cardiac dysfunction	GI upset (abdo discomfort, bloating, diarrhea). Lactic acidosis. Anorexia	↓ HbA1c 1.0-1.5%. Weight neutral
Insulin Secretagogue	Stimulates insulin release from β cells by causing K+ channel closure → depolarization → Ca2+ mediated insulin release. Use in nonobese type 2 DM	sulfonylureas: glyburide	Diabeta® Euglucon®	Micronase® Glynase PreTab®	2.5-5.0 mg/d titrated to >5 mg bid Max: 20 mg/d		ABSOLUTE: Moderate to severe liver dysfunction. RELATIVE (glyburide and glimepiride): Adjust dose in mild to moderate kidney dysfunction and avoid in severe kidney dysfunction. Avoid glyburide in the elderly. INTERACTIONS: Do not combine with a non-sulfonylurea insulin secretagogue or preprandial insulin	Hypoglycemia. Weight gain	↓ HbA1c 0.8%. Glicazide lowest incidence of hypoglycemia
		gliclazide	Diamicron® Diamicron® MR		40-160 mg bid 30-120 mg OD				
		glimepiride	Amaryl®		1-8 mg OD				
		non-sulfonylureas: repaglinide	GlucoNorm®		0.5-4 mg tid	Short t½ of 1 h causes brief but rapid ↑ in insulin, therefore effective for post-prandial control	ABSOLUTE: Severe liver dysfunction. INTERACTIONS: Do not combine with a non-sulfonylurea or pre-prandial insulin	Hypoglycemia. Weight gain	↓ HbA1c 0.7% for repaglinide and 0.5-1.0% for nateglinide
		nateglinide	Starlix®		60-120 mg tid				
Insulin Sensitizers (thiazolidinedione)	Sensitizes peripheral tissues to insulin → increases glucose uptake. Decreases FFA release from adipose. Binds to nuclear receptor PPAR-γ	rosiglitazone	Avandia®		2-8 mg OD	Rosiglitazone – indicated only in patients with type 2 DM for whom all other oral antidiabetic agents, in monotherapy or in combination, do not result in adequate glycemic control or are inappropriate due to contraindications or intolerance	ABSOLUTE: NYHA > class II CHF. INTERACTIONS: Do not combine with insulin	Peripheral edema. CHF. Anemia. Fluid retention and CHF. Increased risk of cardiac events with rosiglitazone (requires written informed consent when prescribing). Increased risk of bladder cancer with pioglitazone. Fractures	↓ HbA1c 0.8%
		pioglitazone	Actos®		15-45 mg OD				
α-Glucosidase Inhibitor	↓ carbohydrate GI absorption by inhibiting brush border α-glucosidase	acarbose	Glucobay®		25 mg OD titrated to 100 mg tid	↓ postprandial hyperglycemia	ABSOLUTE: Inflammatory bowel disease. Severe liver dysfunction	Flatulence. Abdominal cramps. Diarrhea	↓ HbA1c 0.6%. Not recommended as initial therapy in patients with A1c >8.5%
Dipeptidyl Peptidase-IV (DPP-IV) Inhibitor	Inhibits degradation of endogenous antihyperglycemic incretin hormones. Incretin hormones stimulate insulin secretion, inhibit glucagon release, and delay gastric emptying	sitagliptin	Januvia®		100 mg OD		ABSOLUTE (sitagliptin): Type 1 DM. DKA. RELATIVE (sitagliptin and saxagliptin): Use with dose reduction in kidney dysfunction	Nasopharyngitis. URTI. Headache. Pancreatitis. Stevens Johnson syndrome	↓ HbA1c 0.7%. Weight neutral
		saxagliptin	Onglyza™		2.5-5 mg OD				
		linagliptin	Trajenta®		5 mg OD				

Diabetes Medications (continued)

Drug Class	Mechanism of Action	Generic Drug Name	Canada Name	US Name (if different)	Dosing	Indications	Contraindications	Side Effects	Comments
Glucagon-Like Peptide (GLP)-1 Analogue	Binds to GLP-1 receptor to promote insulin release Insulinotropic effect suppressed as plasma glucose <4 mmol/L Slows gastric emptying, suppresses inappropriately elevated glucagon levels Causes β-cell regeneration and differentiation in vitro	Exenatide	Byetta®		5-10 µg SC bid 1 h before meals		ABSOLUTE: Type 1 DM DKA Acute pancreatitis Hx RELATIVE: Gastroparesis ESRD Personal or family history of medually thyroid cancer	N/V, diarrhea Dizziness, headache Muscle weakness Anti-exentide antibodies Pancreatitis	↓ HbA1c 1.0%
		Liraglutide	Victoza®		0.6-1.8 mg OD SC				
Sodium-glucose linked transporter 2 (SGLT2) Inhibitor	Enhances urinary glucose excretion by inhibiting glucose reabsorption in the proximal renal tubule	Canagliflozin	Invokana®		100 mg OD before first meal of the day		ABSOLUTE: Severe renal impairment ESRD Patients on dialysis	UTI, genital infections Hypotension caution with concomitant loop diuretic use Caution with renal dysfunction Hyperlipidemia (raises LDL and HDL) Dapagliflozin not to be used in patients with active or history of bladder cancer Rare diabetic ketoacidosis (may occur with no hyperglycemia)	↓ HbA1c 0.7-1.0% Negligible risk of hypoglycemia as monotherapy Cause weight loss
		Dapagliflozin	Forxiga®		5 mg OD in the morning with or without food				
		Empagliflozin	Jardiance®		10 mg OD in the morning with or without food				

For insulin formulations see Table 9, E9

Dyslipidemia Medications

Drug Class	Mechanism of Action	Generic Drug Name	Canada Name	US Name (if different)	Dosing	Indications	Contraindications	Side Effects
HMG-CoA Reductase Inhibitor (statins)	Inhibits cholesterol biosynthesis, ↓ LDL synthesis, ↑ LDL clearance, modest ↑ HDL, limited ↓ VLDL	atorvastatin fluvastatin lovastatin pravastatin rosuvastatin simvastatin	Lipitor® Lescol® Mevacor® Pravachol® Crestor® Zocor®		10-80 mg/d 20-80 mg/d 20-80 mg/d 10-40 mg/d 5-40 mg/d 10-80 mg/d	1st line monotherapy Used for ↑ LDL, ↑ TG	Active liver disease Persistent ↑ in AST, ALT unexplained	GI symptoms Rash, pruritus ↑ liver enzymes Myositis (↑ risk if combined with fibrates) Rhabdomyolysis
Fibrates	Upregulate lipoprotein lipase + apo A1, ↓ VLDL, ↓ TG, modest ↓ LDL, modest ↑ HDL	bezafibrate fenofibrate gemfibrozil	Bezalip® Lipidil® Lopid®		400 mg/d 48-200 mg/d 600-1200 mg/d	Used for ↑ TG, hyperchylomicronemia	Hepatic disease Renal disease	GI upset Skin rashes ↑ risk of gallstone formation ↑ risk of rhabdomyolysis when combined with statins
Niacin	Inhibits secretion of hepatic VLDL via lipoprotein lipase (LPL) pathway → decreased VLDL and LDL; decreased clearance of HDL	nicotinic acid	Niaspan® generic niacin	Niacor®	0.5-2 g/d 1-3 g/d	Used for ↑ LDL, ↑ VLDL	Hypersensitivity Hepatic dysfunction Active PUD Hyperuricemia	Generalized flushing Abnormal liver enzymes Pruritus IGT Watch glucose control with overt DM
Bile Acid Sequestrants	Resins that bind bile acids in intestinal lumen and prevent absorption thereby ↓ LDL	cholestyramine	Questran®		2-24 g/d	Used for ↑ LDL Use as adjunct with statins or fibrates	Complete biliary obstruction Pregnancy, lactation TG >3.5 mmol/L GI motility disorder	Constipation Nausea Flatulence Bloating Rise in TG
		colestipol	Colestid®		5-30 g/d			
Cholesterol Absorption Inhibitors	Inhibits cholesterol absorption at the small intestine brush border	ezetimibe	Ezetrol®	Zetia®	10 mg/d	Used for ↑ LDL, apo B	Hypersensitivity Hepatic dysfunction Do not combine with fibrates or bile acid resins	Fatigue Pharyngitis Sinusitis Abdominal pain Diarrhea Arthralgia

Thyroid Medications

Drug Class	Mechanism of Action	Generic Drug Name	Canada Name	US Name (if different)	Dosing	Indications	Contraindications	Side Effects
Antithyroid Agent (thionamides)	Decreases thyroid hormone production by inhibiting iodine and peroxidase from interacting with thyroglobulin to form T_4 and T_3 PTU also interferes with conversion of T_4 to T_3	propylthiouracil (PTU)	Propyl-Thyracil®		Start 100 mg PO tid, then adjust accordingly Thyroid storm: start 200-300 PO qid, then adjust accordingly	Hyperthyroidism	Hypersensitivity Relative: renal failure, liver disease PTU recommended in 1st trimester, MMI during 2nd and 3rd trimester Lactation: safe with PTU <300 mg/day and MMI <20-30 mg/d	N/V Rash Drug-induced hepatitis Agranulocytosis Hepatitis with PTU Cholestasis with MMI
		methimazole (MMI)	Tapazole®		Start 5-20 mg PO OD, then adjust accordingly Up to 60 mg OD may be required			
Thyroid Hormone	Synthetic form of thyroxine (T_4)	levothyroxine l-thyroxine	Synthroid® Eltroxin®	Levoxyl®	0.05-2.0 mg/d, usually 1.6x weight (kg) is dose in micrograms In elderly patients start at 0.025 mg/d	Hypothyroidism	Recent MI, thyrotoxicosis	If wrong dosing: symptoms of hypothyroidism or hyperthyroidism Skin rash from dye in pill
Antithyroid Agent Radiopharmaceutical	Radioactive isotope of iodine that is incorporated into the thyroid gland irradiating the area and destroying local glandular tissue	sodium iodide I-131	Iodotope®		Dose corrected for 24 h radioactive iodine uptake Hyperthyroidism 4-12 mCi Thyroid Ca 50-150 mCi	Hyperthyroidism Thyroid malignancy	Hypersensitivity Concurrent antithyroid medication Pregnancy, lactation	N/V Bone marrow suppression Sialadenitis Thyroiditis

Metabolic Bone Disease Medications

Drug Class	Mechanism of Action	Generic Drug Name	Canada Name	US Name (if different)	Dosing	Indications	Contraindications	Side Effects
Bisphosphonates	Inhibits osteoclast-mediated bone resorption	alendronate	Fosamax®		Osteoporosis: 5-10 mg OD 70 mg once weekly Paget's: 40 mg OD for 6 mo	Prevention of postmenopausal osteoporosis Treatment of osteoporosis Glucocorticoid-induced osteoporosis Paget's disease	Esophageal stricture or achalasia (oral) Unable to stand or sit upright for >30 min (oral) Hypersensitivity Hypocalcemia Renal insufficiency	GI MSK pain Headache Osteonecrosis of the jaw
		risedronate	Actonel®		Osteoporosis: 5 mg OD 35 mg once weekly 150 mg once monthly Paget's: 30 mg OD for 2 mo	Treatment and prevention of postmenopausal osteoporosis Treatment and prevention of glucocorticoid-induced osteoporosis Paget's disease		
		etidronate	Didronel®		Paget's: 5-10 mg /kg OD x 6 mo	Symptomatic Paget's disease Prevention and treatment of heterotopic ossification after total hip replacement or spinal cord injury		
		ibandronate	Boniva®		2.5 mg OD or 150 mg once monthly	Treatment and prevention of postmenopausal osteoporosis (US only)		
		pamidronate	Aredia®		Hypercalcemia of malignancy 60-90 mg IV over 2-24 h Wait at least 7 d before considering retreatment	Hypercalcemia of malignancy Paget's disease Osteolytic bone metastases of breast cancer Osteolytic lesions of multiple myeloma		
		zoledronate	Zometa® Aclasta®		5 mg IV once yearly IV	Treatment of osteoporosis Hypercalcemia of malignancy Treatment and prevention of skeletal complications related to cancer		

Metabolic Bone Disease Medications (continued)

Drug Class	Mechanism of Action	Generic Drug Name	Canada Name	US Name (if different)	Dosing	Indications	Contraindications	Side Effects
Selective Estrogen Receptor Modulators	Decreases resorption of bone through binding to estrogen receptors	raloxifene	Evista®		60 mg OD	Treatment and prevention of postmenopausal osteoporosis (2nd line)	Lactation Pregnancy Active or past history of DVT, PE, or retinal vein thrombosis	Hot flashes Leg cramps Increased risk of fatal stroke, venous thromboembolism
Calcitonin	Inhibits osteoclast-mediated bone resorption	calcitonin	Miacalcin®		One spray (200 IU) per d, alternating nostrils	Treatment of postmenopausal osteoporosis, greater than 5 yr postmenopause	Clinical allergy to salmon-calcitonin	Rhinitis Epistaxis Sinusitis Nasal dryness
Anti-RANKL Monoclonal Ab	Inhibits RANKL (osteoclast differentiating factor) → inhibits osteoclast formation and decreases bone resorption	denosumab	Prolia™ Xgeva™		60 mg SC q6mo	Treatment of postmenopausal women at high risk of fracture Prevent skeletal-related events in patients with bone metastasis from solid tumours	Hypocalcemia	Fatigue/headache Dermatitis/rash Hypophosphatemia/Hypocalcemia Hypercholesterolemia GI discomfort
PTH	Stimulates new bone formation by preferential stimulation of osteoblastic activity over osteoclastic activity	teriparatide	Forteo®		20 µg SC OD x 18-24 mo	Treatment of postmenopausal women with osteoporosis who are at high risk for fracture Treatment of men with primary or hypogonadal osteoporosis who are at high risk for fracture	Paget's disease Prior external beam or implant radiation therapy involving the skeleton Bone metastases Metabolic bone diseases other than osteoporosis	Orthostatic hypotension Hypercalcemia Dizziness Leg cramps
Calcium	Inhibits PTH secretion				1200 mg/d (including diet) Divided in 3 doses	Osteopenia Osteoporosis Prevention of metabolic bone disease	Caution with renal stones	Vomiting Constipation Dry mouth
Vitamin D	Regulation of calcium and phosphate homeostasis	cholecalciferol (vitamin D3)			800 -2000 IU/d	Osteopenia Osteoporosis Prevention of metabolic bone disease	Caution in patients on digoxin (risk of hypercalcemia which may precipitate arrhythmia)	Hypercalcemia Headache N/V Constipation
		ergocalciferol (vitamin D2)	Drisdol® Ergol®		50,000 IU/wk	Osteoporosis in patients with liver dysfunction, refractory rickets, hypoparathyroidism	Hypercalcemia Malabsorption syndrome Decreased renal function	
		calcitriol (1,25(OH)₂-D)	Rocaltrol®		Start 0.25 µg/d Titrate up by 0.25 µg/d at 4-8 wk intervals to 0.5-1 µg/d	Hypocalcemia and osteodystrophy in patients with chronic renal failure on dialysis	Hypercalcemia Vitamin D toxicity	
			Calcijex®		Start 0.25 µg/d Titrate up by 0.25 µg/d at 2-4 wk intervals to 0.5-2 µg/d	Hypoparathyroidism		

Adrenal Medications

Drug Class	Mineralocorticoid Activity	Generic Drug Name	Potency Relative to Cortisol	Equivalent Dose (mg)	Duration of Action (t₁/₂ in h)	Dosing	Comments
Hydrocortisone	Yes	Cortef Solu-Cortef	1.0	20	8	Adrenal Crisis: 50-100 mg IV bolus, then 50-100 mg q8h (continuous infusion x 24-48 h) PO once stable (50 mg q6h x 48 h, then taper over 14 d) Chronic AI: 15-20 mg PO OD (2/3 AM, 1/3 PM)	In high doses, mineralocorticoid side effects may emerge (salt + water retention, ECF volume expansion, HTN, low K⁺ metabolic alkalosis)
Cortisone Acetate	Yes	Cortisone Acetate	0.8	25	oral = 8 IM = 18+	Adrenal Crisis: 75-300 mg/d PO/IM divided q12-24h Chronic AI: 25 mg/d	Pro-drug which is converted to active form as hydrocortisone High doses can result in mineralocorticoid side effects (see above)
Prednisone	No	Prednisone	4	5	16-36	Adrenal Crisis: 15-60 mg/d PO qd or divided bid/qid Chronic AI: 5 mg daily	Pro-drug which is converted to active form as prednisolone
Dexamethasone	No	Dexamethasone	30	0.7	36-54	Adrenal Crisis: 4 mg IV, repeat q2-6h if necessary	Used for undiagnosed adrenal insufficiency (does not interfere with measurement of serum cortisol levels)

Landmark Endocrinology Trials

Trial	Reference	Results
DIABETES		
ACCORD	*NEJM* 2008; 358:2560-72	Compared with standard therapy the use of intensive therapy to target normal HbA1c levels (<6%) for 3.5 yr increased mortality and did not significantly reduce major cardiovascular events
ADVANCE	*NEJM* 2008; 358:2545-59	Intensive glucose control that lowered the HbA1c value to 6.5% reduced the incidence of nephropathy but did not significantly reduce major macrovascular events, death from cardiovascular events, or death from any cause; hypoglycemia was more common in the intensive control group
BARI-2D	*NEJM* 2009; 360:2503-15	In patients with both type 2 DM and CAD no significant difference was found in the rates of death and major cardiovascular events in patients undergoing prompt revascularization and those undergoing medical therapy or between strategies of insulin sensitization and insulin
DCCT	*NEJM* 1993; 329:977-86	Intensive blood glucose control delayed the onset and reduced the progression of microvascular complications (retinopathy, nephropathy, and neuropathy) in type 1 DM
EDIC	*NEJM* 2005; 353:2644-53	Compared with conventional therapy intensive DM therapy early on without macrovascular disease (goal HbA1c <6.05%) has long-term beneficial effects on the risk of cardiovascular disease in patients with type 1 DM
Look AHEAD	*NEJM* 2013; 369:145-54	Moderate weight loss (<7% BW) and increased exercise are not associated with reduction in CVD and its complications among overweight or obese patients with type 2 DM
NAVIGATOR	*NEJM* 2010; 362:1463-90	In patients with impaired glucose tolerance, nateglinide did not reduce progression to DM or risk of cardiovascular events while valsartan only reduced progression to DM
PREDIMED	*NEJM* 2013; 368:1279-90	A Mediterranean diet with extra-virgin olive oil or nuts reduces rates of MI, CVA, or CV death in those at high risk for CV disease (outcome was driven by reduction in rates of CVA)
Steno-2	*NEJM* 2008; 358:580-91	In at-risk patients with type 2 DM intensive intervention with multiple drug combinations and behaviour modification had sustained significant beneficial effects with respect to vascular complications and mortality; multifactorial intervention is critical in the management of type 2 DM
UKPDS	*Lancet* 1998; 352:837-53	Intensive blood glucose control reduces microvascular but not macrovascular complications in type 2 DM
UKPDS Extension	*NEJM* 2008; 359:1577-89	Continued risk reduction in microvascular risk and emergent risk reductions for MI and death from any cause 10 yr post UKPDS trial follow up in type 2 DM
VADT	*NEJM* 2009; 360:1-11	In patients with longstanding poorly controlled type 2 DM intensive glucose control had no significant effect on the rates of major cardiovascular events, death, or microvascular complications; adverse events, predominantly hypoglycemia, were more common in the intensive control group
LIPIDS		
4S	*Lancet* 1994; 344:1383-89	In patients with angina or previous MI and high total cholesterol simvastatin reduced: all-cause mortality, fatal and nonfatal coronary events, and need for coronary artery bypass surgery or angioplasty
FIELD	*Lancet* 2005; 366:1849-61	In patients with type 2 DM not previously on statin therapy fenofibrate did not significantly reduce the risk of the primary outcome of coronary events; it did reduce non-fatal MI and revascularizations
HPS	*Lancet* 2002; 360:7-22	In high-risk patients with various cholesterol values simvastatin reduced all-cause mortality, coronary deaths, and major vascular events
Jupiter	*NEJM* 2008; 359:2195-207	Rosuvastatin significantly reduced the incidence of major cardiovascular events in patients with elevated high-sensitivity CRP levels and no hyperlipidemia
TNT	*NEJM* 2005; 352:1425-35	Lipid-lowering therapy with atorvastatin 80 mg/d in patients with stable CHD provides clinical benefit beyond atorvastatin 10 mg/d

References

Agus AZ. Etiology of hypercalcemia. Rose BD (editor). Waltham: UpToDate. 2010.

Agus AZ. Overview of metabolic bone disease. Rose BD (editor). Waltham: UpToDate. 2002.

American Diabetes Association. Management of dyslipidemia in adults with diabetes (position statement). Diabetes Care 2002;25:S74-77.

Anderson TJ, Gregoire J, Hegele RA, et al. 2012 Update of the Canadian Cardiovascular Society guidelines for the diagnosis and treatment of dyslipidemia for the prevention of cardiovascular disease in the adult. Can J Cardiol 2012;29:151-167.

Arnold A. Classification and pathogenesis of the multiple endocrine neoplasia syndromes. Rose BD (editor). Waltham: UpToDate. 2002.

Braunwald E, Fauci AS, Kasper DL, et al. Harrison's principles of internal medicine, vol 2. New York: McGraw Hill, 2001. Chapter: DM; p2109-2135.

Burman KD. Overview of thyroiditis. Rose BD (editor). Waltham: UpToDate. 2002.

Canadian Diabetes Association Clinical Practice Guidelines Expert Committee. Canadian Diabetes Association 2013 clinical practice guidelines for the prevention and management of diabetes in Canada. Can J Diabetes 2013;37(S1):S1-S212.

Canadian Task Force on Preventive Health Care. Prevention of osteoporosis and osteoporotic fractures in post-menopausal women. CMAJ 2004;170:1665-1667.

Cheng A, Fantus IG. Oral antihyperglycemic therapy for type 2 DM. CMAJ 2005;172:213-226.

Collins R, Armitage J, Parish S, et al. MRC/BHF heart protection study of cholesterol lowering with simvastatin in 20,536 high risk individuals: a randomized placebo-controlled trial. Lancet 2002;360:7-22.

Dayan CM. Interpretation of thyroid function tests. Lancet 2001;357:619-624.

Dawson-Hughes B, Gold DT, Rodbard HW, et al. Physician's guide to prevention and treatment of osteoporosis. Washington: National Osteoporosis Foundation, 2003.

Estruch R, Ros E, Salas-Salvado J, et al. Primary prevention of cardiovascular disease with a Mediterranean diet. NEJM 2013;368:1279-1290.

Fodor JG, Frohlich JJ, Genest JJG, et al. Recommendations for the management and treatment of dyslipidemia. CMAJ 2000;162:1441-1447.

Genest J, Frohlich JJ, Fodor JG, et al. Recommendations of the management of dyslipidemia and the prevention of cardiovascular disease: 2003 update. CMAJ 2003;168(9):921-4.

Greenspan FS, Garber DG. Basic and clinical endocrinology. New York: Lange Medical Books/McGraw Hill, 2001. 100-163, 201-272, 623-761.

Harper W, Clement M, Goldenberg R, et al. Pharmacologic management of type 2 diabetes. Canadian Journal of Diabetes 2013;37(Suppl 1):S61-8.

Hemmingssen B, Lund SS, Gluud C, et al. Targeting intensive glycaemic control versus targeting conventional glycaemic control for type 2 DM. Cochrane DB Syst Rev 6 2011;CD008143.

Hirsch IB, Paauw DS, Brunzell J. Inpatient management of adults with diabetes. Diabetes Care 1995;18:870-878.

KDIGO CKD Work Group. KDIGO 2012 clinical practice guideline for the evaluation and management of chronic kidney disease. Kidney Intern Suppl 2013;3:1-150.

Kitabachi AE, Umpierrez GE, Murphy MB, et al. Management of hyperglycemic crises in patients with diabetes. Diabetes Care 2001;24:131-152.

Kronenberg HM, Larsen PR, Melmed S, et al. Williams textbook of endocrinology, 9th ed. Philadelphia: WB Saunders, 1998.

NIH Consensus Development Panel on Osteoporosis Prevention, Diagnosis and Therapy. Osteoporosis prevention, diagnosis, and therapy. JAMA 2001;285:785-795.

Orth DN. Evaluation of the response to ACTH in adrenal insufficiency. Rose BD (editor). Waltham: UpToDate. 2002.

Rosen HN, Rosenblatt M. Overview of the management of osteoporosis in women. Rose BD (editor). Waltham: UpToDate. 2002.

Ross DS. Disorders that cause hypothyroidism. Rose BD (editor). Waltham: UpToDate. 2002.

Ryan EA. Pregnancy in diabetes. Med Clin of N Amer 1998;82:823-845.

Schilcher J, Michaelsson K, Aspenberg P. Bisphosphonate use and atypical fractures of the femoral shaft. NEJM 2011;364:1728-1737.

Stone NJ, Robinson J, Lichtenstein AH et al. A report of the American College of Cardiology/American Heart Association task force on practice guidelines. Circulation 2013;00:000-000.

The Scandinavian Simvastatin Survival Study Group. Randomized trial of cholesterol lowering in 4444 patients with coronary heart disease: the Scandinavian Simvastatin Survival Study (4S). Lancet 1994;344:1383-1389.

Tsui E, Barnie A, Ross S, et al. Intensive insulin therapy with insulin lispro: a randomized trial of continuous subcutaneous insulin infusion versus multiple daily insulin injection. Diabetes Care 2001;24:1722-1727.

United Kingdom Prospective Diabetes Study (UKPDS) Group. Intensive blood-glucose control with sulfonylureas or insulin compared with conventional treatment and risk of complications in patients with type 2 diabetes. Lancet 1998;352:837-853.

Weaver CM, Alexander DD, Boushey CJ et al. Calcium plus vitamin D supplementation and risk of fractures. Osteoporosis Int 2015;27:367-376.

Wing RR, Bolin P, Brancati F, et al. Cardiovascular effects of intensive lifestyle intervention in type 2 diabetes. NEJM 2013;369:145-154.

Young WF, Kaplan NM. Diagnosis and treatment of pheochromocytoma in adults. Rose BD (editor). Waltham: UpToDate. 2002.

Zinman B, Wanner C, Lachin JM et al. Empagliflozin, cardiovascular outcomes, and mortality in Type 2 Diabetes. NEJM 2015;373:2117-2128.

FM Family Medicine

Julianne Bagg, Tina Hu, Lisa Saldanha, and **Roland Wong**, chapter editors
Narayan Chattergoon and **Desmond She**, associate editors
Arnav Agarwal and **Quynh Huynh**, EBM editors
Dr. Ruby Alvi and **Dr. Azadeh Moaveni**, staff editors

Acronyms

AAA	abdominal aortic aneurysm	FBG	fasting blood glucose	MAOI	monoamine oxidase inhibitor	PUFA	polyunsaturated fatty acids
ACR	albumin:creatinine ratio	FOBT	fecal occult blood test	MMSE	mini mental status examination	PVD	peripheral vascular disease
AIN	anal intraepithelial neoplasia	FRS	Framingham Risk Score	MOCA	Montreal cognitive assessment	RA	rheumatoid arthritis
AMC	another medical condition	GAD	generalized anxiety disorder	MSM	men who have sex with men	RCT	randomized controlled trial
AKI	acute kidney injury	GERD	gastroesophageal reflux disease	MUFA	monounsaturated fatty acids	SAH	subarachnoid hemorrhage
BMI	body mass index	GTT	drops	NPH	human insulin isophane	SDRI	serotonin dopamine reuptake inhibitor
ABG	arterial blood gas	HAART	highly active anti-retroviral therapy	NTD	neural tube defects	SERM	selective estrogen receptor modulator
AR	absolute reduction	HDL-C	high density lipoprotein cholesterol	NTG	nitroglycerin	SIDS	sudden infant death syndrome
BPPV	benign paroxysmal positional vertigo	HNPCC	hereditary non polyposis colon cancer	O&P	ova and parasites	SLE	systemic lupus erythematosis
CA	cancer	HSIL	high-grade squamous	OA	osteoarthritis	SNRI	serotonin norepinephrine
CABG	coronary artery bypass graft		intraepithelial lesion	OCD	obsessive compulsive disorder		reuptake inhibitor
CAD	coronary artery disease	HPV	human papillomavirus	OCP	oral contraceptive pill	SOB	shortness of breath
CHEP	Canadian Hypertension Education	HRT	hormone replacement therapy	OCPD	obsessive compulsive personality disorder	SSRI	selective serotonin reuptake inhibitor
	Program	IBD	inflammatory bowel disease	OD	once a day	TIA	transient ischemic attack
CVD	cardiovascular disease	IBS	irritable bowel syndrome	OGCT	oral glucose challenge test	TC	total cholesterol
CBT	cognitive behavioural therapy	ICS	inhaled corticosteroids	OGTT	oral glucose tolerance test	TCA	tricyclic antidepressant
CF	cystic fibrosis	IFG	impaired fasting glucose	OTC	over the counter	TG	triglyceride
CHF	congestive heart failure	IGT	impaired glucose tolerance	PCOS	polycystic ovarian syndrome	TM	tympanic membrane
CPAP	continuous positive airway pressure	IHD	ischemic heart disease	PFT	pulmonary function test	TMJ	temporomandibular joint
CRC	colorectal cancer	INH	isoniazid	PHE	periodic health examination	TUIP	transurethral incision of the prostate
DHP	dihydropyridine	IPT	interpersonal therapy	PID	pelvic inflammatory disease	TURP	transurethral resection of the prostate
DMPA	depot medroxyprogesterone	IVP	intravenous pyelogram	PMS	premenstrual syndrome	UC	ulcerative colitis
DRE	digital rectal exam	KUB	kidneys, ureter, bladder x-ray	PND	paroxysmal nocturnal dyspnea	URTI	upper respiratory tract infection
DS	double strength	LDL-C	low density lipoprotein cholesterol	PPI	proton pump inhibitor	UTI	urinary tract infection
ED	emergency department	LSIL	low-grade squamous intraepithelial lesion	PPD	purified protein derivative	VAIN	vaginal intraepithelial neoplasia
ER	extended release	LV	left ventricle	PSA	prostate specific antigen	VIN	vulvar intraepithelial neoplasia
F/U	follow-up	LVH	left ventricle hypertrophy	PTSD	post-traumatic stress disorder	VBI	vertebrobasilar insufficiency
FAP	familial adenomatous polyposis	MDI	metered dose inhaler	PUD	peptic ulcer disease	WSIB	Workplace Safety and Insurance Board

Four Principles of Family Medicine

College of Family Physicians of Canada Guidelines
1. The family physician is a skilled clinician
   - diagnoses and manages diseases common to the population served
   - recognizes importance of early diagnosis of serious life-threatening illnesses
2. Family medicine is a community-based discipline
   - provides information and access to community services
   - responds/adapts to changing needs and circumstances of the community
3. The family physician is a resource to a defined practice population
   - serves as a health resource
   - advocates for public policy to promote health
4. The patient-physician relationship is central to the role of the family physician
   - commits to the person, not just the disease
   - promotes continuity of patient care

Periodic Health Examination

Adult Periodic Health Exam
Male and female evidence-based preventive care checklist forms are available online at http://www.cfpc.ca

- Canadian Task Force on Preventive Health Care established in 1976, first published in 1979
- mandate: to develop and disseminate clinical practice guidelines for primary and preventive care
- recommendations are based on systematic analysis of scientific evidence
   - most notable recommendation is the abolition of the annual physical exam; replaced by the PHE

Purpose of the Periodic Health Examination

- **primary prevention:** identify risk factors for common diseases; counsel patients to promote healthy behaviour
- **secondary prevention:** presymptomatic detection of disease to allow early treatment and to prevent disease progression
- update clinical data
- enhance patient-physician relationship

Classification of Recommendations (GRADE, 2011)

Strength of Recommendation
- **strong:** high level of confidence that desirable effects outweigh undesirable effects (strong recommendation for an intervention) or that the undesirable effects outweigh desirable effects (strong recommendation against an intervention)
   - implies that most individuals will be best served by the recommended course of action

- **weak:** desirable effects probably outweigh the undesirable effects (weak recommendation for an intervention) or undesirable effects probably outweigh the desirable effects (weak recommendation against an intervention); uncertainty exists
  - implies that most people would want the recommended course of action but that many would not
  - different choices will be appropriate for different individuals, patients require support in reaching a management decision consistent with his/her values and preferences

Quality of Evidence
- high: high level of confidence that true effect lies close to the estimate of the effect
- moderate: true effect likely to be close to the estimate of the effect, but there is a possibility that it is substantially different
- low or very low: true effect may be substantially different from the estimate of the effect

Table 1. Periodic Health Exam

	General Population	Special Population

DISCUSSION	Dental hygiene (community fluoridation, brushing, flossing) (A)
	Noise control and hearing protection (A)
	Screen for poverty
	Smokers: counsel on smoking cessation, provide:
	  Nicotine replacement therapy (A)
	  Referral to smoking cessation program (B)
	Dietary advice on leafy green vegetables and fruits (B)
	Seat belt use (B)
	Injury prevention (bicycle helmets, smoke detectors) (B)
	Moderate physical activity (B)
	Avoid sun exposure and wear protective clothing (B)
	Problem drinking screening and counselling (B)
	Counselling to protect against STIs (B)
	Nutritional counselling and dietary advice on fat and cholesterol (B)
	Dietary advice on calcium and vitamin D requirements (B)
		Pediatrics: Home visits for high risk families (A), Inquiry into developmental milestones (B)
		
		Adolescents: Counsel on sexual activity and contraceptive methods (B), Counsel to prevent smoking initiation (B)
		
		Perimenopausal Women (>50): Assess for risk factors for: osteoporosis and fracture (A), Counsel on osteoporosis, Counsel on risks/benefits of hormone replacement therapy (B)
		
		Adults >65: Follow-up on caregiver concern of cognitive impairment (A), Multidisciplinary post-fall assessment (A)

PHYSICAL	Blood pressure measurement, using techniques described in CHEP guidelines (strong recommendation; moderate quality evidence) BMI measurement in obese adults (B)	**Pediatrics:** Repeated examinations of hips, eyes and hearing (especially in first year of life) (A), Serial height, weight and head circumference (B), Visual acuity testing after age 2 (B) **Adults >65:** Visual acuity (Snellen sight chart) (B), Hearing impairment (inquiry, whispered voice test, audioscope) (B) **First-Degree Relative with Melanoma:** Full body skin exam (B)
TESTS	See recommendations below for age and gender specific screening for diabetes, dyslipidemia, hypertension and cancer screening (colon, prostate, cervical, lung, and breast)	**Pediatrics:** Routine hemoglobin for high risk infants (B), Blood lead screening of high risk infants (B) **TB High Risk Groups:** Mantoux skin testing (A) **STI High Risk Groups:** Voluntary HIV antibody screening (A) Gonorrhea screening (A) Chlamydia screening in women (B) Syphillis screen (A) **Syphilis Risk Group:** VDRL test (A)
THERAPY	Folic acid supplementation to women of child-bearing age (A) Pharmacologic treatment of HTN (Refer to CHEP Guidelines) (A) Varicella vaccine for children age 1-12 and susceptible adolescents/adults (A) Rubella vaccine for all non-pregnant women of child-bearing age unless there is proof of immunity via immunization records or serology (B) Tetanus vaccine: routine booster q10yr if had 1° series (A) Pertussis vaccine: adults <65 should receive one booster given as Tdap– Adacel® or Boostrix® (A) Herpes zoster vaccine for adults ≥60	**Pediatrics:** Routine immunizations (A), Hepatitis B, HPV and Meningococcal immunizations are offered in schools in most Canadian provinces **Influenza High Risk Groups:** Outreach strategies for vaccination (A), annual immunization (B), now recommended for all **TB High Risk Groups** INH prophylaxis for household contacts or skin test converters (B) INH prophylaxis for high risk sub-groups (B) **Immunocompromised/Age≥65/COPD/Asthma/CHF/ Asplenia/Liver Disease/Renal Failure/DM:** Pneumococcalvaccine (Pneumovax®) (A)

Classification of recommendation in brackets. See sidebar on FM2 for classification details. See www.canadiantaskforce.ca – for up-to-date guidelines
Reference: Canadian Task Force on Preventive Health Care, 2014

Choosing Wisely Canada
http://www.choosingwiselycanada.org/
A campaign to help clinicians and patients engage in conversations about unnecessary tests and treatments and make smart and effective choices to ensure high quality care

Folic Acid Supplementation in Pregnancy (Joint SOGC-Motherisk Clinical Guideline)
- To prevent neural tube defects in all women capable of becoming pregnant
- Low risk women (no personal health risks, planned pregnancy): 0.4-1.0 mg daily folic acid supplementation for at least 2-3 mo before conception and throughout pregnancy and postpartum period
- High risk women (health risks including epilepsy, insulin dependent diabetes, BMI >35, family history of NTD, high risk ethnic group): at least 3 mo prior to conception until 10-12 wk post conception: daily supplementation with multivitamins with 5 mg folic acid
- From wk 12 post-conception until postpartum period (4-6 wks or as long as breastfeeding continues): 0.4-1.0 mg of folic acid supplementation is sufficient
- Women with additional lifestyle issues (poor compliance with medications, no consistent birth control, taking possible teratogenic substances): higher folic acid dose of 5 mg and counselling about prevention of birth defects

Breast Cancer Screening Guidelines

2011 Recommendations on Screening for Breast Cancer in Average-Risk Women (The Canadian Task Force on Preventive Health Care)
- average-risk women: women age 40-74 with no personal history of breast cancer, history of breast cancer in 1st degree relatives, known mutations of the *BRCA1/BRCA2* genes or previous exposures of the chest wall to radiation

Mammography
- age 40-49: routine screening with mammography not recommended (weak recommendation - moderate quality evidence)
- age 50-74: routine screening q2-3yr (age 50-69: weak recommendation; moderate quality evidence, age 70-74: weak recommendation; low quality evidence)
- age 75+: screen if benefits outweigh harm, must take overall health into account

Magnetic Resonance Imaging
- no routine screening with MRI scans (weak recommendation - low quality evidence)

Clinical Breast Examination
- no routine CBE alone or in conjunction with mammography to screen for breast cancer (weak recommendation - low quality evidence)

Breast Self-Examination

- recommend not advising women to routinely practice breast self-examination
- for more information on benign breast lesions and breast cancer, see General Surgery, GS55

Lung Cancer Screening Guidelines

2016 Canadian Task Force on Preventative Health Care
- apply to adults aged 18 and older who are not suspected of having lung cancer
- annual screening with low dose CT for adults aged 55-74 with at least a 30 pack-year smoking history who currently smoke or quit less than 15 years ago, up to three consecutive times

Colorectal Cancer Screening Guidelines

- recommendations for average risk individuals (asymptomatic, no family history of UC, polyps, or CRC)
- average risk testing should begin at age 50, but assessment for risk factors should begin earlier to identify high-risk individuals
  - Canadian Task Force on Preventative Health Care (2016)
    - FOBT (either high sensitivity FOBT or FIT - fecal immunochemical testing) q2yr OR flexible sigmoidoscopy q10yr
    - no colonoscopy as a screening test
    - no screening after age 75 is recommended for average risk patients, but it may be assessed on an individual basis for ages 76-85

- for more information on colorectal neoplasms, see General Surgery, GS33

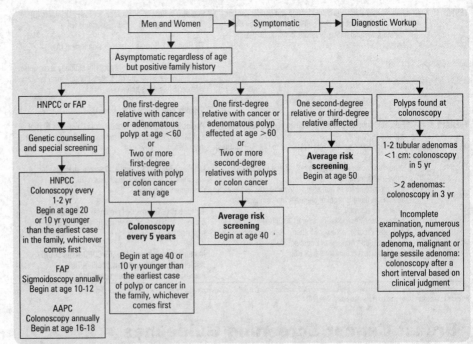

Figure 1. Approach to higher risk screening
AAPC = attenuated adenomatous polyposis; FAP = familial adenomatous polyposis; HNPCC = hereditary nonpolyposis colorectal cancer; 1st degree relatives: parents, siblings, children; 2nd degree relatives: grandparents, aunts, uncles; 3rd degree relatives: great grandparents or cousins. Figure printed with permission from Can J Gastroenterol 2004;18:93-99. Also see: Colorectal Screening for Cancer Prevention in Asymptomatic Patients, March 2013. Available from http://www.bcguidelines.ca/pdf/colorectal_screening.pdf

Cervical Cancer Screening

- either conventional Papanicolaou (Pap) smear or liquid based cytology testing
- endocervical and exocervical cell sampling (aim is to sample the transitional zone)
- best identifies squamous cell abnormalities, less reliable for glandular abnormalities
  - false positives 5-10%, false negatives 10-40% (for single test)
  - false negative rate 50% for existing cervical cancer
- cervical cancer screening guidelines differ by provincial jurisdiction (see The Society of Obstetricians and Gynaecologists of Canada guidelines)

- **Canadian Task Force for Preventative Care Guidelines**
  - screen all women age ≥25 q3yr (age 25-29: weak recommendation; moderate quality evidence, age 30-69: strong recommendation; high quality evidence)
  - women age ≥70: if 3 normal tests in a row and no abnormal tests in last 10 yr, can discontinue screening (weak recommendation; low quality evidence)
- **Ontario guidelines**
  - screen all women age ≥21 who are or have ever been sexually active (includes intercourse or digital/oral activity with partner of either gender)
  - if cytology is normal, can screen every 3 yr
  - women age ≥70: if 3 successive negative Pap tests in last 10 yr, can discontinue screening
  - women who are not sexually active by age 21 should delay cervical cancer screening until sexually active
- pregnant women and women who have sex with women should follow the routine cervical screening regimen
- women who have had a hysterectomy
  - total: discontinue screening if hysterectomy was for benign disease and no history of cervical dysplasia or HPV infection, continue to swab vaginal vault if history of uterine malignancy/dysplasia
  - subtotal: continue screening according to guidelines
- exceptions to guidelines
  - immunocompromised (transplant, steroids, diethylstilbestrol exposure, HIV)
  - previously unscreened patients
- for more information on cervical cancer (see Gynecology, GY43)

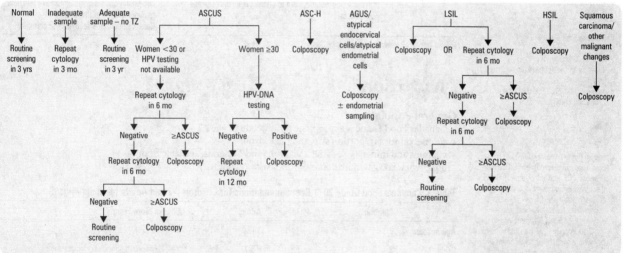

Figure 2. Decision making chart for cervical cancer screening (not applicable for adolescents)
AGUS = atypical glandular cells of unknown significance; ASCUS = abnormal squamous cells of unknown significance; ASC-H = abnormal squamous cells cannot rule out HSIL; HSIL = high grade squamous intraepithelial lesion; LSIL = low grade squamous intraepithelial lesion; TZ = transitional zone
Adapted from: Ontario Cervical Screening Cytology Guidelines. May 2012

Prostate Cancer Screening

- Canadian Task Force for Preventative Care Guidelines
  - screening for prostate cancer with the prostate specific antigen test is not recommended for any age group (age <55: strong recommendation; low quality evidence, age 55-69: weak recommendation; moderate quality evidence, age >70: strong recommendation; low quality evidence)

Prostate Cancer Mortality at 11 Years of Follow-Up
NEJM 2012;366:981-990
Study: Updated "ERSPC" study – multicentre randomized trial of screening for prostate cancer using PSA.
Patients: 162,388 men, ages 55-69 from 8 different European countries.
Intervention: PSA-based screening.
Main Outcome: Mortality from prostate cancer.
Results: After median follow up of 11 yr, the RRR of death from prostate cancer was 21%. The ARR was 1.07 deaths/1,000 men. NNT=1,055 – therefore to prevent one death from prostate cancer at 11 yr follow up, 1,055 men would need to be screened.

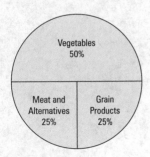

Figure 3. Plate layout

Handy Serving Size Comparisons
- 3 oz meat, fish, poultry → palm of hand
- 1 cup dairy (milk/yogurt) → size of fist
- Bread/grains → one slice, palm of hand
- ½ cup rice/pasta → one hand cupped
- 1 cup of fruit/vegetables → two cupped hands
- 1 oz cheese → full length of thumb
- 1 tsp oil/butter → tip of thumb
- Nuts/chips/snacks → palm covered

Energy Content of Food
- Carbohydrates 4 kcal/g
- Protein 4 kcal/g
- Fat 9 kcal/g
- Ethanol 7 kcal/g

Calculating Total Daily Energy Expenditure (TDEE)
- Roughly 35 kcal/kg/d
- Varies by age, weight, sex, and activity level
- Average 2000-2100 kcal/d for women, 2700-2900 kcal/d for men

Canadian Cancer Society (CCS) Recommendations for Vitamin D Use
- Based on CCS research on Vitamin D and the prevention of colorectal, breast and prostate cancer
- In consultation with their healthcare provider, the Society is recommending that:
  - Adults living in Canada should consider taking Vitamin D supplementation of 1,000 international units (IU) a day during the fall and winter
  - Adults at higher risk of having lower Vitamin D levels should consider taking Vitamin D supplementation of 1,000 IU/d all year round. This includes people: who are older, with dark skin, who do not go outside often, and who wear clothing that covers most of their skin
  - Babies who are exclusively breast-fed: 400 IU/d

Health Promotion and Counselling

- health promotion is the most effective preventive strategy
- there are several effective ways to promote healthy behavioural change, such as discussions appropriate to a patient's present stage of change
- for more information about motivational interviewing, see www.motivationalinterviewing.org

Motivational Strategies for Behavioural Change

Table 2. Motivational Strategies for Behavioural Change

Patient's Stage of Change	Physician's Aim	Physician's Plan
Pre-Contemplation	Encourage patient to consider the possibility of change Assess readiness for change Increase patient's awareness of the problem and its risks	Raise issue in a sensitive manner Offer (not impose) a neutral exchange of information to avoid resistance
Contemplation	Understand patient's ambivalence and encourage change Build confidence and gain commitment to change	Offer opportunity to discuss pros and cons of change using reflective listening
Preparation	Explore options and choose course most appropriate to patient Identify high-risk situations and develop strategies to prevent relapse Continue to strengthen confidence and commitment	Offer realistic options for change and opportunity to discuss inevitable difficulties
Action	Help patients design rewards for success Develop strategies to prevent relapse Support and reinforce convictions towards long-term change	Offer positive reinforcement and explore ways of coping with obstacles Encourage self-rewards to positively reinforce change
Maintenance	Help patient maintain motivation Review identified high-risk situations and strategies for preventing relapse	Discuss progress and signs of impending relapse
Relapse	Help patient view relapse as a learning experience Provide support appropriate to present level of readiness post-relapse	Offer a non-judgmental discussion about circumstances surrounding relapse and how to avoid relapse in the future Reassess patient's readiness to change

Adapted from: Hunt P. Motivating Change. *Nursing Standard* 2001;16:45-52, 54-55

Nutrition

General Population
- Canada's Food Guide is appropriate for individuals age ≥2
- counsel on variety, portion size, and plate layout
- vitamins and minerals: see CDC-Vitamins and Minerals, available from http://www.cdc.gov/nutrition/everyone/basics/vitamins/

Table 3. Canada's Food Guide 2011 Recommendations for Children >2 and Adults (# of servings/d)

	Children			Teens	Adults		Choose More From
Age in Years	2-3	4-8	9-13	14-18	19-50	51+	
Grain Products	3	4	6	F:6 M:7	F:6-7 M:8	F:6 M:7	Whole grain and enriched grain products
Vegetables and Fruit	4	5	6	F:7 M:8	F:7-8 M:8-10	F:7 M:7	Dark green vegetables, orange vegetables and fruit
Milk and Alternatives	2	2	3-4	F:3-4 M:3-4	F:2 M:2	F:3 M:3	Lower-fat dairy products
Meat and Alternatives	1	1	1-2	F:2 M:3	F:2 M:3	F:2 M:3	Lean meat, poultry, fish, peas, beans, lentils

Cardiovascular Disease Prevention

Table 4. Dietary Guidelines for Reducing Risk of Cardiovascular Disease

	Recommendations	Effects
Fat, Carbohydrates, Protein	Overall fat intake: 26-27% of total energy Saturated fat: 5-6% of total energy Trans fat: reduce intake, replace with MUFA or PUFA Carbohydrates: 55-59% of total energy Protein: 15-18% of total energy	Lower LDL
Omega-3 Fatty Acid Rich Foods	≥2 servings/wk of fish (especially oily fish like salmon)	Decreased sudden death, death from CAD Lower TG
Salt	≤2,400 mg/d	Lower BP Combining decreased sodium intake with the DASH diet (see below) achieves even greater BP-lowering effects
Alcohol	≤3 drinks/d for men, max 15/wk ≤2 drink/d for women, max 10/wk	Decreased risk of hypertriglyceridemia, HTN, osteoporosis, certain cancers
Dietary Approaches	DASH diet (Dietary Approaches to Stop Hypertension), recommended by the American Heart Association (AHA) Diet: high in vegetables/fruits, low-fat dairy, whole grains, poultry, fish, and nuts; Low in sweets, sugar-sweetened beverages, red meats Macronutrients: low in saturated/total fat and cholesterol; high in potassium, magnesium, calcium, protein, and fibre Mediterranean diet (fruits, vegetables, whole grains, legumes, nuts, olive oil, and herbs)	Lower BP, lower LDL

MUFA = monounsaturated fatty acids; PUFA = polyunsaturated fatty acids
Eckel RH, et al. 2013 AHA/ACC Guideline on Lifestyle Management to Reduce Cardiovascular Risk: A Report of the American College of Cardiology/American Heart Association Task Force on Practice Guidelines. *Circulation* 2013.
Dietary approaches to stop hypertension (DASH), available from: http://www.nhlbi.nih.gov/health/public/heart/hbp/dash/dash_brief.pdf
Lichtenstein AH, et al. Diet and lifestyle recommendations revision 2006: a scientific statement from the American Heart Association Nutrition Committee. *Circulation* 2006;114:82-96

Obesity

- see Canadian Task force on Preventive Health Care recommendations (*CMAJ* February 2015) at: canadiantaskforce.ca/ctfphc-guidelines/2015-obesity-adults/
- body mass index (BMI) = weight (kg)/height (m)^2 = weight (lbs)/height (in)^2 x 703; BMI is a poor predictor of obesity
- waist circumference (WC) = flexible tape placed on horizontal plane at iliac crest, normal depends on ethnic background
- increased WC for BMI 25-35 increases the risk of cardiovascular disease and type 2 diabetes

Table 5. Classification of Weight by BMI, Waist Circumference, and Associated Disease Risks in Adults

	BMI (kg/m²)	Obesity Class	Men ≤102 cm (40 in) Women ≤88 cm (35 in)	Men >102 cm (40 in) Women >88 cm (35 in)
Underweight	<18.5			
Normal	18.5-24.9			
Overweight	25.0-29.9		Increased	High
Obesity Class I	30.0-34.9	I	High	Very High
Obesity Class II	35.0-39.9	II	Very High	Very High
Obesity Class III (Extreme Obesity)	40.0 +	III	Extremely High	Extremely High

From: Classification of Overweight and Obesity by BMI, Waist Circumference, and Associated Disease Risks, National Institute of Health, National Heart Lung and Blood Institute, Obesity Education Initiative, http://www.nhlbi.nih.gov/health/public/heart/obesity/lose_wt/bmi_dis.htm

Epidemiology

- 16% (4 million) of people ≥18 yr old are obese, 32% (8 million) are overweight in Canada, according to StatsCan (2007)
- obesity rate in people of Aboriginal origin is 1.6 times higher than the national average
- proportion of children aged 6-11 who are overweight has more than doubled in the last 25 yr; percentage of overweight adolescents has tripled
- overweight and obesity rates in children are directly proportional to screen time (see *Exercise*, FM10)
- only 10-15% of population consume <30% fat daily
- obese persons generally consume more energy-dense food which tends to be highly processed, micronutrient poor, and high in fats, sugars, or starch

Osteoporosis Canada Recommendations for Calcium and Vitamin D Daily Requirements
- Vitamin D: 800-1,000 IU for individuals age <50 yr, 800-2,000 IU for individuals ≥50 yr
- Calcium: 1,000 mg daily from all sources for individuals 19-50 yr and pregnant/lactating women; 1,200 mg daily for individuals >50 yr (recommended to obtain calcium from nutrition whenever possible vs. supplementation)

Effectiveness of behavioural and pharmacologic treatment for overweight and obesity in adults. *CMAJ* Open 2014;2:E306–17.
Study: Review of 68 RCTs comparing the interventions: diet, exercise, diet and exercise, lifestyle, orlistat or metformin to control groups: no intervention, usual care, placebo or minimal interventions (e.g. newsletter or single information session on healthy living).
Population: overweight and obese adults >18 yr.
Outcome measure: weight 12 mo post intervention and secondary health outcomes: total cholesterol, LDL, fasting blood glucose, incidence of DM-2, systolic and diastolic BP.
Results:
1. Intervention participants had a greater mean weight loss, greater reduction in waist circumference and greater reduction in BMI. There was no significant difference between behavioural and pharmacologic intervention for any weight outcome.
2. For cholesterol and fasting glucose- the reduction was greater for participants in pharmacologic plus behavioural intervention as opposed to those using behavioural interventions alone.
3. A diagnosis of new onset type 2 DM was less likely to occur in intervention participants compared with the control group.
Conclusion: Behavioural and pharmacological interventions for overweight and obesity in adults leads to clinically significant results.

Losing Weight
- Aim for caloric intake 500-1000 kcal/d less than total daily energy expenditure (TDEE)
- 3500 kcal energy expended/ lb of fat burned
- Results in 1-2 lb (0.5-1 kg) weight loss per wk
- Achieved by combination of increased activity and/or decreased caloric intake

Low BMI Associations
- Osteoporosis
- Eating disorders
- Under-nutrition
- Pregnancy complications

Adverse Medical Consequences of Obesity
- Type 2 DM
- CAD
- Stroke
- HTN
- Gallbladder disease
- Non-alcoholic steatohepatitis
- Complications of pregnancy
- Dyslipidemia
- Osteoarthritis
- Sleep apnea
- Certain cancers
- CHF
- Low back pain
- Increased total mortality

Pharmacotherapy for Obesity
- Orlistat: gastrointestinal lipase inhibitor, reduces fat absorption by 30% by inhibition of pancreatic lipase
- Orlistat is associated with several adverse effects and not approved for clinical use longer than 2 yr
- Orlistat should be avoided in people with inflammatory or chronic bowel disease

"The Latest Evidence on Fad Diets…"
Comparison of the Atkins, Ornish, Weight Watchers, and Zone Diets for Weight Loss and Heart Disease Risk Reduction
JAMA 2005;293:43-53
Purpose: To assess the effectiveness and adherence rates of four popular diets for weight loss and reduction of cardiac risk factors.
Study Characteristics: Single centre RCT at academic medical centre in Boston, MA; 160 participants were randomized to either Atkins (carbohydrate restriction), Zone (macronutrient balanced and low glycemic load), Weight Watchers (low calorie/portion size), or Ornish (fat restriction) diet groups for a period of 18 mo.
Participants: Adults age 22-72 with known HTN, dyslipidemia, or fasting hyperglycemia.
Results: Assuming that participants who discontinued the study remained at baseline, the mean weight loss at 1 yr (and self selected dietary adherence rates per self report) were 2.1 kg for Atkins (53% of participants completed, p=0.009), 3.2 kg for the Zone (65% of participants completed, p=0.002), 3.0 kg for Weight Watchers (65% completed, p<0.001), 3.3 kg for Ornish (50% completed, p=0.007). Each diet significantly reduced the LDL/HDL ratio by ~10% (p<0.05), with no significant effects on blood pressure or glucose. Amount of weight loss was associated with adherence level (r = 0.60; p<0.001) but not with diet type (r = 0.07; p=0.40). Weight loss for each diet was significantly associated with reduction in levels of total/HDL cholesterol (r=0.36), C-reactive protein (r=0.37), and insulin (r=0.39), with no significant difference between diets.
Conclusion: Each popular diet was associated with modest weight loss and reduction of several cardiac risk factors. Adherence level, and not diet type, was the most important predictor of weight loss and cardiac risk factor reduction.

Hyperlipidemia Signs
- Atheromata: plaques in blood vessel walls
- Xanthelasmata: a sharply demarcated yellowish deposit of cholesterol underneath the skin, usually on or around the eyelid
- Tendinous xanthoma: lipid deposit in tendon (especially Achilles)
- Eruptive xanthoma: hypertriglyceridemia induced reddish yellow, pruritic, and painful papular or nodular rash
- Lipemia retinalis: thin atheromata seen in the retinal blood vessels
- Corneal arcus (arcus senilis): lipid deposit in cornea

Screening Recommendations
- the CANRISK or FINRISC scores can be used to assess the risk for type 2 diabetes in overweight and obese patients
- BMI risk assessment should be done every 3-5 yr in people at high risk of developing diabetes within 10 yr

Management
Behavioural/ Lifestyle
- weight loss of >5% is clinically significant for reducing many cardiovascular risk factors (e.g. elevated blood pressure, glucose and lipids)
- efficacious behavioural interventions are greater than 12 months duration, include diet and/or exercise and/or lifestyle components, and include group and individual sessions
- structured behavioural and lifestyle interventions should be offered or arranged for overweight individuals BMI >25
- strong recommendation for those with increased risk of Type 2 DM
- BMI >35 + risk factors or BMI >40 are candidates for bariatric surgery failing behavioural modification

Pharmacologic
- the task force recommends against pharmacologic intervention to manage patients who are overweight and obese, although some patients may prefer medications and be good candidates for pharmacologic treatment
- high benefit of behavioural modification alone, NNH (number needed to harm) 10 (mostly GI side effects) for pharmacotherapy

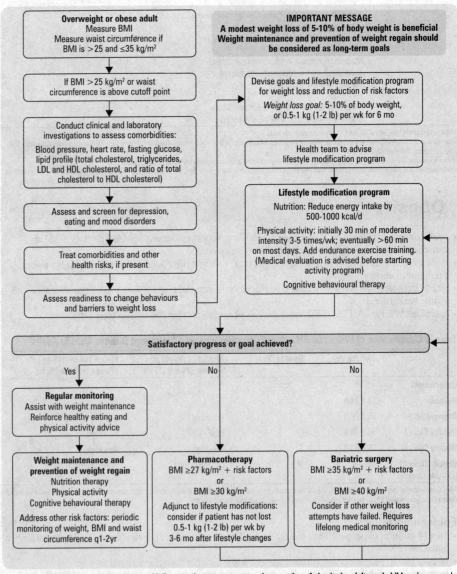

Figure 4. 2006 Canadian clinical practice guidelines on the management and prevention of obesity in adults and children (summary)
Adapted from: *CMAJ* 2007;176:S1-S13

Dyslipidemia

- see Endocrinology, E2
- defined as abnormal elevation of plasma cholesterol or triglyceride levels

Assessment

- measure fasting serum TC, LDL-C, HDL-C, and TG
- screen with full fasting lipid profile q1-3yr in males >40 yr and females >50 yr or who are menopausal, or at any age for adults with additional dyslipidemia risk factors (see sidebar)
- screen for secondary causes: hypothyroidism, chronic kidney disease, DM, nephrotic syndrome, liver disease
- risk category
  - estimate using the model for 10 yr CAD risk developed from the Framingham data (Framingham Risk Score – FRS)
    - FRS calculated based on the following factors: gender, age, HDL-C, total cholesterol, sBP, smoking, DM
    - family history of CVD <55 male relative or <65 in female relative doubles FRS
    - to be completed for men age 40-75, and women age 50-75 q3-5yr
    - cardiovascular age calculated as patient's age ± the difference between his or her estimated remaining life expectancy
      - used to increase adherence to therapy and reaffirm positive effect of following therapy
  - treatment decisions focus on LDL-C level and/or FRS risk; the alternate primary targets are apolipoprotein B (apo B) and non-HDL-C (not used widely yet)
  - if moderate risk and LDL-C <3.5, treatment decision thresholds shifted to apo B >1.2g/L or non-HDL C >4.3 mmol/L
  - other targets include: TC:HDL-C ratio, apo B:apo AI ratio, hs-CRP (used more for risk stratification of CAD), non-HDL-C, and serum TG levels

To calculate Framingham Risk Score, go to http://www.framinghamheartstudy.org/risk-functions/cardiovascular-disease/10-year-risk.php#

Risk Factors for Screening for Dyslipidemia
- First Nations or of South Asian ancestry
- Current cigarette smoking
- Diabetes
- Arterial Hypertension
- Family history of premature CVD
- Family history of hyperlipidemia
- Erectile dysfunction
- Chronic kidney disease
- Inflammatory disease (lupus, rheumatoid arthritis, psoriatic arthritis, IBD)
- HIV infection
- Chronic obstructive pulmonary disease
- Clinical evidence of atherosclerosis or abdominal aneurysm
- Clinical manifestation of hyperlipidemia
- Obesity (BMI >27)

Table 6. Target Lipid Values for Primary Prevention of CAD (2012 Canadian Cholesterol Guidelines)

Risk Category	Initiate Treatment if	Primary Targets LDL-C	Alternate
High (FRS ≥20%) Also: AAA, history of DM (>40 yrs, DM for 15 yr and age >30, microvascular complications), CAD, PVD, atherosclerosis, CKD, or Male with HTN plus one of: smoking, EKG abnormality, LVH, Fam hx of premature death, age >55 yr, TC/ HDL-C >6, microalbuminuria	Consider treatment in all patients	≤2 mmol/L or ≥50% decrease in LDL-C	apo B <0.80 g/L non HDL-C ≤2.6mmol/L
Moderate (FRS 10-19%)	LDL-C ≥3.5 mmol/L For LDL-C <3.5 consider if: apo B ≥1.2 g/L or non-HDL-C ≥4.3 mmol/L	≤2 mmol/L or ≥50% decrease in LDL-C	apo B ≤ 0.80 g/L non HDL-C ≤2.6mmol/L
Low (FRS <10%)	LDL-C ≥5.0 mmol/L Familial hypercholesterolemia	≥50% decrease in LDL-C	

Anderson TJ, et al. 2012 Update of the Canadian Cardiovascular Society Guidelines for the Diagnosis and Treatment of Dyslipidemia and Prevention of Cardiovascular Disease in the Adult. *Can J Cardiol* 2013; 29:151-167

Non-fasting Lipids vs. Fasting Lipids
Non-fasting (TC and non-HDL cholesterol) can be used for Framingham Risk Assessment and hold same prognostic value as fasting lipids In fasted vs. non-fasted samples, Non-HDL and TC varies by 2%, LDL-C by 10% and TG by 20%
Recently, non- fasting LDL-C has the same prognostic value as fasting LDL-C
Ontario Association of Medical Laboratories Guidelines for Lipid Testing in Adults (2013): http://www.oaml.com/documents/elineforAdultLipidTestingFinal2013_000.pdf

Management

- intensity and type of treatment is guided by "risk category" assigned (see Table 6)
1. health behaviours (can decrease LDL-C by up to 10%)
   - smoking cessation: probably the most important for preventing CAD
   - dietary modification: reduce saturated fat, red meat, refined sugar, alcohol; consume nuts, fruits/vegetables, poultry, fish
   - physical activity: at least 150 min of moderate to vigorous intensity aerobic exercise per wk
   - employ consistent lifestyle modifications for at least 3 mo before considering drug therapy; high risk patients should start treatment immediately with concurrent health behaviour interventions
2. pharmacologic therapy (can decrease LDL-C by up to 40%)
   - for a comparison of dyslipidemia medications, see Endocrinology, E50
   - 1st line monotherapy: statins (HMG-CoA reductase inhibitors)
     - risks: myopathy and hepatotoxicity
     - if severe side effects: ezetimibe (cholesterol absorption inhibitor) can be used for 19% reduction in LDL-C
     - post-ACS, cholesterol absorption inhibitors (e.g. ezetimibe) in addition to simvastatin reduced mortality, attained lipid targets <1.8, and improved outcomes in high risk individuals
     - lower evidence for other agents: bile acid sequestrants, nicotinic acid, fibrates, psyllium
   - monitoring
     - ALT, CK, Cr at baseline then 6 wk later for signs of transaminitis or myositis; tolerate rise in CK up to 10 times upper limit of normal vs. 2-3 times if symptomatic, or serum creatinine rise of ≤25%
     - no routine repeated measures of ALT and CK necessary in asymptomatic patients using statin therapy
     - if adequate response is achieved, evaluate fasting lipids q6-12mo

LDL cannot be calculated when TG ≥4.5 mmol/L

Safety of Statins: An Update
Therapeutic Advances in Drug Safety 2012;3:133-144
Trials have shown that statin therapy slightly increases the incidence of diabetes; however, the absolute risk is small. Relative to the reduction in coronary events, the clinical significance is not great enough to recommend against their use.

Use with caution when prescribing combined statin and fibrate therapy as there has been concern regarding the safety of certain combinations (potential increased risk of myopathy and rhabdomyolysis)

Isolated Hypertriglyceridemia

• does not increase your cardiovascular risk
• normal HDL-C and TC, elevated TG
• mild ≥2.2 mmol/L (≥200 mg/dL); marked ≥5.6 mmol/L (≥500 mg/dL)
• principal therapy is lifestyle modification
  ▪ weight loss, exercise, avoidance of smoking and alcohol, effective blood glucose control in diabetics, increased omega-3 fatty acid intake
  ▪ severe hypertriglyceridemia (typically >10 mmol/L) is associated with an increased risk of acute pancreatitis
• drug therapy (used to prevent pancreatitis, NOT cardiovascular disease!)
  ▪ nicotinic acid
  ▪ fibrates

Exercise

Epidemiology
• 25% of the population exercises regularly, 50% occasionally, 25% are sedentary

Management
• assess current level of fitness, motivation, and access to exercise
• encourage warm up and cool down periods to allow transition between rest and activity and to avoid injuries
• exercise with caution for patients with CAD, DM (risk of hypoglycemia), exercise-induced asthma
• patients with known CAD should have cardiac assessment prior to commencing exercise
• benefits of exercise
  ▪ reduces risk of premature death, heart disease, stroke, HTN, certain types of cancer, type 2 DM, osteoporosis, and overweight/obesity
  ▪ leads to improved fitness, strength, and mental health (morale and self-esteem)

Table 7. Canadian Physical Activity and Sedentary Behaviour Guidelines (2012 CSEP Guidelines)

Age Category	Physical Activity Guidelines	Example Activities	Sedentary Behaviour Guidelines
Infant (<1y)	Active several times daily	Interactive floor-based play including tummy time, reaching for toys, crawling	Minimize time spent sedentary, including sitting and being restrained (stroller, etc.) Screen time not recommended for infants <1y, limit to <1h/d ages 2-4
Toddler (1-2)	Accumulate 180 min of physical activity at any intensity spread throughout the day	Moving around the home Climbing stairs Exploring environment Brisk walking, running Dancing	apo B <0.80 g/L non HDL-C ≤2.6mmol/L
Preschool (2-4)			apo B ≤ 0.80 g/L non HDL-C ≤2.6mmol/L
Children (5-11)	Accumulate 60 min of moderate to vigorous intensity physical activity daily	Moderate: bike riding, playground Vigorous: running, swimming	Minimize time spent being sedentary Limited recreational screen time no more than 2 h per day Limit sedentary (motorized) transport, sitting, and time spent indoors
Youth (12-17)	Accumulate 60 min of moderate to vigorous intensity physical activity daily Vigorous intensity activities at least 3 d per wk Activities that strengthen muscle and bone at least 3 d per wk	Moderate: skating, bike riding Vigorous: running, roller blading	
Adults (18-64)	Accumulate 150 min of moderate to vigorous intensity aerobic physical activity per wk, in bouts of 10 m or more. It is beneficial to add muscle and bone strengthening activities using major muscle groups, at least 2 d per wk	Moderate: brisk walking, bike riding Vigorous: jogging, cross country skiing	No specific guidelines
Older Adults (65 and older)		Moderate: brisk walking, bike riding Vigorous: cross country skiing, swimming Those with poor mobility should perform physical activities to enhance balance and prevent falls	

Smoking Cessation

Epidemiology
- smoking is the single most preventable cause of premature illness and death
- 70% of smokers see a physician each year
- 2012 Canadian data from the Canadian Tobacco Use Monitoring Survey (CTUMS) on population age ≥15
  - 16% are current smokers (lowest since 1965)
  - highest prevalence in age group 20-24 (20%)
  - 11% of youth age 15-19 smoke (decreased from 25% in 2000): more males smoke than females; number of cigarettes consumed per day also decreasing

Management
- general approach
  - identify tobacco users; elicit smoking habits, previous quit attempts and results
  - CAN-ADAPTT 2012 guidelines
    - tobacco use status should be updated for all patients regularly (Grade 1A)
    - health care providers should clearly advise patients to quit (Grade 1C)
    - health care providers should also monitor the patient's mental health status/other addictions while quitting smoking. Medication dosage should be monitored and adjusted as necessary (Grade 1A)
  - every smoker should be offered treatment
    - combining counselling and smoking cessation medication is more effective than either alone (Grade 1A)
  - make patient aware of withdrawal symptoms
    - low mood, insomnia, irritability, anxiety, difficulty concentrating, restlessness, decreased heart rate, increased appetite
  - ≥4 counselling sessions >10 min each with 6-12 mo follow-up yields better results
  - 14% abstinent with counselling vs. 10% without counselling
  - approach depends on patient's stage of change (see *Motivational Strategies for Behavioural Change*, FM6)
- willing to quit
  - provision of social support, community resources (self-help, group, helpline, web-based strategies)
  - pregnant patients: counselling is recommended as 1st line treatment (Grade 1A). Nicotine replacement therapy (NRT) should be made available to pregnant women who are unable to quit using non-pharmacologic methods; intermittent NRT use (lozenges, gum) is preferred over continuous dosing of the patch (Grade 1C). Use buproprion (no evidence of fetal or reproductive harm) only if benefits > risks; consult Motherisk. Varenicline has not been studied in pregnancy and should not be used in pregnant women
- pharmacologic therapy
  1. Nicotine Replacement Therapy
     - 19.7% abstinent at 12 mo with NRT vs. 11.5% for placebo
     - no difference in achieving abstinence for different forms of NRT
     - reduces cravings and withdrawal symptoms without other harmful substances that are contained in cigarettes
     - use with caution: immediately post-MI, serious/worsening angina, serious arrhythmia
     - advise NO smoking while using NRT
  2. Antidepressants (note: mode of action appears to be independent of antidepressant effect)
     - Bupropion SR (Zyban®)
     - 21% abstinent at 12 mo vs. 8% for placebo
     - no advantage for NRT vs. bupropion (similarly effective)
  3. Varenicline (Champix®)
     - partial nicotinic receptor agonist (to reduce cravings) and partial competitive nicotinic receptor antagonist (to reduce the response to smoked nicotine)
     - more effective than bupropion (23% abstinent from 9-52 wk with varenicline vs. 16% for bupropion vs. 9% with placebo)
     - significant side effects may lower patient compliance

Table 8. Types of Nicotine Replacement Therapy

Type	Dosage	Comment	Side Effects
Nicotine Gum (OTC)	2 mg if <25 cig/d 4 mg if >25 cig/d 1 piece q1-2h for 1-3 mo (max 24 pieces/d)	Chew until "peppery" taste then "park" between gum and cheek to facilitate absorption Continue to chew-park intermittently for 30 min	Mouth soreness Hiccups Dyspepsia Jaw ache Most are transient
Nicotine Patch (OTC)	Use for 8 wk 21 mg/d x 4 wk 14 mg/d x 2 wk 7 mg/d x 2 wk	Start with lower dose if <10 cig/d Change patch q24h and alternate sides	Skin irritation Insomnia Palpitations Anxiety
Nicotine Inhaler (OTC)	6-16 cartridges/d for up to 12 wk	Nicotine inhaled through mouth, absorbed in mouth and throat not in lungs	Local irritation Coughing
Nicotine Nasal Spray (Rx)		Newer form of NRT	Local irritation, coughing

Physician Advice for Smoking Cessation
Cochrane DB Syst Rev 2013;5:CD000165
This systematic review of 17 trials compared brief advice by the physician versus no advice.
Conclusions: Simple advice can increase cessation rates by 1-3%. More intensive advice and providing follow-up support may further increase the quit rates.

The 5 A's for Patients Willing to Quit
Ask if the patient smokes
Advise patients to quit
Assess willingness to quit
Assist in quit attempt
Arrange follow-up

The 2-3 Pattern of Smoking Cessation
- Onset of withdrawal is 2-3 h after last cigarette
- Peak withdrawal is at 2-3 d
- Expect improvement of withdrawal symptoms at 2-3 wk
- Resolution of withdrawal at 2-3 mo
- Highest relapse rate within 2-3 mo

Assist Patient in Developing Quit Plan

STAR
Set quit date
Tell family and friends (for support)
Anticipate challenges (e.g. withdrawal)
Remove tobacco-related products (e.g. ashtrays/lighters)

Antidepressants for Smoking Cessation
Cochrane DB Syst Rev 2014;1:CD000031
This systematic review of 90 randomized trials compared antidepressant medication to placebo or alternative pharmacotherapy for smoking cessation and where follow-up was longer than 6 mo.
Conclusions: The antidepressants bupropion and nortriptyline can aid smoking cessation and have a similar efficacy to NRT. Bupropion is less effective than varenicline. Neither SSRIs (e.g. fluoxetine) nor MAOIs aid smoking cessation.

Nicotine Replacement Therapy for Smoking Cessation
Cochrane DB Syst Rev 2012;11:CD000146
This systematic review of 132 randomized trials compared NRT to placebo or no treatment or compared different NRT doses.
Conclusions: All commercially available forms of NRT (gum, transdermal patch, nasal spray, inhaler, and sublingual tablets/lozenges) are effective as part of a strategy to promote smoking cessation. They increase the rate of quitting by 50-70% regardless of setting and independent on the level of additional support provided to the smoker. Compared to a single form of NRT, combining a nicotine patch with a rapid delivery form of NRT may be more effective.

Nicotine Partial Receptor Agonists for Smoking Cessation
Cochrane DB Syst Rev 2012;4:CD006103
Conclusions: Cytisine increases the chances of quitting, although absolute quit rates were modest in two recent trials. Varenicline at standard dose increased the chances of successful long-term smoking cessation between two- and threefold compared with pharmacologically unassisted quit attempts. Lower dose regimens also conferred benefits for cessation, while reducing the incidence of adverse events. More participants quit successfully with varenicline than with bupropion.

Table 9. Pharmacologic Treatments for Smoking Cessation

Drug	Mechanism	Dosage	Prescribing*	Contraindications
Bupropion	Inhibits re-uptake of dopamine and/or norepinephrine. Side effects: insomnia, dry mouth	1. 150 mg qAM x 3 d 2. Then 150 mg bid x 7-12 wk 3. For maintenance consider 150 mg bid for up to 6 mo	1. Decide on a quit date 2. Continue to smoke for first 1-2 wk of treatment and then completely stop (therapeutic levels reached in 1 wk)	Seizure disorder Eating disorder MAOI use in past 14 d Simultaneous use of bupropion (Wellbutrin®) for depression
Varenicline	Partial nicotinic receptor agonist, and partial nicotinic receptor competitive antagonist. Side effects: N/V, constipation, headache, dream disorder, insomnia, increased risk of psychosis, depression, suicidal ideation	1. 0.5 mg qAM x 3 d 2. Then 0.5 mg bid x 4 d 3. Continue 1 mg bid x 12 wk ± additional 12 wk as maintenance	1. Decide on a quit date 2. Continue to smoke for first wk of treatment and then completely stop	Caution with pre-existing psychiatric condition

*Bupropion and Verenicline may be used in combination with nicotine replacement therapy

- unwilling to quit
  - motivational intervention (5 Rs)
  1. **R**elevance to patient
     - relevant to patient's disease status or risk, family or social situation (e.g. having children in the home), health concerns, age, gender
  2. **R**isks of smoking
     - short-term: SOB, asthma exacerbation, impotence, infertility, pregnancy complications, heartburn, URTI
     - long-term: MI, stroke, COPD, lung CA, other cancers
     - environmental: higher risk in spouse/children for lung CA, SIDS, asthma, respiratory infections
  3. **R**ewards: benefits
     - improved health, save money, food tastes better, good example to children
  4. **R**oadblocks: obstacles
     - fear of withdrawal, weight gain, failure, lack of support
  5. **R**epetition
     - reassure unsuccessful patients that most people try many times before successfully quitting (average number of attempts before success is 7)
- recent quitter
  - highest relapse rate within 3 mo of quitting
    - minimal practice: congratulate on success, encourage ongoing abstinence, review benefits and problems
    - prescriptive interventions: address problem of weight gain, negative mood, withdrawal, lack of support

Alcohol

- see <u>Psychiatry</u>, PS23

Definition
- diagnostic categories occur along a continuum

Epidemiology
- 10-15% of patients in family practice are problem drinkers
- 20-50% of hospital admissions, 10% of premature deaths, 30% of suicides, and 50% of fatal traffic accidents in Canada are alcohol-related
- more likely to miss diagnosis in women or elderly, patients with high socioeconomic status

Assessment
- screen for alcohol dependence with CAGE questionnaire
  - if CAGE positive, explore with further questions for alcohol abuse/dependence
- assess drinking profile
  - setting, time, place, occasion, with whom
  - impact on: family, work, social
  - quantity-frequency history
    - how many drinks per day?
    - how many days per week?
    - maximum number of drinks on any one day in the past month?

Standard Drink Equivalents
One standard drink = 14 g of pure alcohol
- Beer (5% alcohol) = 12 oz
- Wine (12-17% alcohol) = 5 oz
- Fortified wine = 3 oz
- Hard liquor (40%) = 1.5 oz

CAGE Questionnaire
C Have you ever felt the need to **CUT** down on your drinking?
A Have you ever felt **ANNOYED** at criticism of your drinking?
G Have you ever felt **GUILTY** about your drinking?
E Have you ever had a drink first thing in the morning to steady your nerves or get rid of a hangover?
(EYE OPENER)
≥2 for men or ≥1 for women suggests possibility of problem drinking (sensitivity 85%, specificity 89%)

- if identified positive for alcohol problem
  - screen for other drug use
  - identify medical/psychiatric complications
  - ask about drinking and driving
  - ask about past recovery attempts and current readiness for change

Investigations
- GGT and MCV for baseline and follow-up monitoring
- AST, ALT (usually AST:ALT approaches 2:1 in an alcoholic)
- CBC (anemia, thrombocytopenia), INR (decreased clotting factor production by liver)

Management
- intervention should be consistent with patient's motivation for change
- individualized counselling and regular follow-up is crucial
- 10% of patients in alcohol withdrawal will have seizures or delirium tremens
- Alcoholics Anonymous/12-step program
  - outpatient/day programs for those with chronic, resistant problems
  - family treatment (Al-Anon, Alateen, screen for spouse/child abuse)
- in-patient program if
  - dangerous or highly unstable home environment
  - severe medical/psychiatric problem
  - addiction to drug that may require in-patient detoxification
  - refractory to other treatment programs
- pharmacologic
  - diazepam for withdrawal
  - disulfiram (Antabuse®): impairs metabolism of alcohol by blocking conversion of acetaldehyde to acetic acid, leading to flushing, headache, N/V, hypotension if alcohol is ingested (available in U.S., but no longer available in Canada)
  - naltrexone: competitive opioid antagonist that reduces cravings and pleasurable effects of drinking
  - may trigger withdrawal in opioid-dependent patients
  - acamprosate: glutamate receptor modulator that also reduces craving
- see Psychiatry, PS23

Prognosis
- relapse is common and should not be viewed as failure
- monitor regularly for signs of relapse
- 25-30% of abusers exhibit spontaneous improvement over 1 yr
- 60-70% of individuals with jobs and families have an improved quality of life 1 yr post-treatment

Common Presenting Problems

Abdominal Pain

- see Gastroenterology, G11 and General Surgery, GS4

Epidemiology
- 20% of individuals have experienced abdominal pain within the last 6-12 mo
- 90% resolve in 2-3 wk
- only 10% are referred to specialists, of those <10% admitted to hospital

Etiology
- most common diagnosis in family medicine at 28% is "nonspecific abdominal pain," which has no identifiable cause and is usually self-limited
- GI disorders (e.g. PUD, pancreatitis, IBD, appendicitis, gastroenteritis, IBS, diverticular disease, biliary tract disease)
- urinary tract disorders (e.g. UTI, renal calculi)
- gynecological disorders (e.g. PID, ectopic pregnancy, endometriosis)
- cardiovascular disorders (e.g. CAD, AAA, ischemic bowel)
- other: DKA, porphyria, hypercalcemia, medications (e.g. NSAIDs), alcohol, toxic ingestion, foreign body, psychogenic

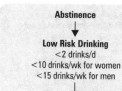

Some Adverse Medical Consequences of Problem Drinking
- GI: gastritis, dyspepsia, pancreatitis, liver disease, bleeds, diarrhea, oral/esophageal cancer
- Cardiac: HTN, alcoholic cardiomyopathy
- Neurologic: Wernicke-Korsakoff syndrome, peripheral neuropathy
- Hematologic: anemia, coagulopathies
- Other: trauma, insomnia, family violence, anxiety/depression, social/family dysfunction, sexual dysfunction, fetal damage

Abstinence → **Low Risk Drinking** <2 drinks/d, <10 drinks/wk for women, <15 drinks/wk for men → **At Risk Drinking** Consumption above low-risk level but no alcohol-related physical or social problems → **Alcohol Use Disorder** Physical or social problems, Continued use despite consequences, Inability to fulfill life roles, Legal problems, No evidence of dependence → **Alcohol Use Disorder**

Figure 5. Continuum of alcohol use

If pain precedes nausea/vomiting, cause of abdominal pain is more likely to be surgical

In patient age >50, keep a high index of suspicion for AAA – its presentation may mimic renal colic or diverticulitis

Pathophysiology
- type of pain
  - somatic pain: sharp, localized pain
  - visceral pain: dull, generalized pain
- location of pain
  - epigastric (foregut): distal esophagus, stomach, proximal duodenum, biliary tree, pancreas, liver
    - RUQ: biliary, hepatic, colonic, pulmonary, renal
    - LUQ: cardiac, gastric, pancreatic, renal, vascular
  - periumbilical (midgut): distal duodenum to proximal 2/3 of transverse colon,
  - hypogastric (hindgut): distal 1/3 of transverse colon to rectosigmoid region,
    - RLQ: colonic, appendix, gynecologic, renal
    - LLQ: colonic, gynecologic, renal
  - any location: aneurysm, dissection, ischemia, zoster, muscle strain, hernia, bowel obstruction, ischemia, peritonitis, porphyria, DKA

Investigations
- guided by findings on history and physical
- possible blood work: CBC, electrolytes, BUN, Cr, amylase, lipase, AST, ALT, ALP, bilirubin, glucose, INR/PTT, tox screen, β-hCG
- imaging
  - CXR (for free air under the diaphragm) in setting of perforation in surgical abdomen
  - abdominal x-ray, KUB (consider: gas pattern, free air, kidney stones, constipation)
  - ultrasound (renal stones, gallbladder disease, gynecological problems, liver disease, pancreatitis, diverticular disease, appendicitis)
  - CT scan (AAA, appendicitis), non-contrast helical CT-Scan (first choice for renal stones)
- other tests
  - urinalysis
  - endoscopy (for peptic ulcers, gastritis, tumours, etc.)
  - *H. pylori* testing (urea breath test, serology, biopsy)

Allergic Rhinitis

- see <u>Otolaryngology</u>, OT23

Definition
- inflammation of the nasal mucosa that is triggered by an allergic reaction
- classification
  - seasonal
    - symptoms during a specific time of the year
    - common allergens: trees, grass and weed pollens, airborne moulds
  - perennial
    - symptoms throughout the year with variation in severity
    - common allergens: dust mites, animal dander, moulds
- persistent allergic rhinitis may lead to chronic rhinosinusitis

Rhinitis Medicamentosa
Rebound nasal congestion. Occurs with prolonged use (>5-7 d) of vasoconstrictive intranasal medications. Patient may become dependent, requiring more frequent dosing to achieve the same decongestant effect

Etiology
- increased IgE levels to certain allergens → excessive degranulation of mast cells → release of inflammatory mediators (e.g. histamine) and cytokines → local inflammatory reaction

Epidemiology
- affects approximately 40% of children and 20-30% of adults
- prevalence has increased in developed countries, particularly in the past two decades
- associated with asthma, eczema, sinusitis, and otitis media

Assessment
- identify allergens
- take an environmental/occupational history
- ask about related conditions (e.g. atopic dermatitis, asthma, sinusitis, and family history)

Management
- conservative
  - minimize exposure to allergens
    - most important aspect of management, often sufficient (may take months)
  - maintain hygiene, saline nasal rinses
- pharmacologic agents
  - oral antihistamines – first line therapy for mild symptoms
    - e.g. cetirizine (Reactine®), fexofenadine (Allegra®), loratadine (Claritin®)
  - intranasal corticosteroids for moderate/severe or persistent symptoms (>1 mo of consistent use to see results)
  - intranasal decongestants (use must be limited to <5 d to avoid rhinitis medicamentosa)

- allergy skin testing
    - for patients with chronic rhinitis
    - symptoms not controlled by allergen avoidance, pharmacological therapy
    - may identify allergens to include in immunotherapy treatment
- immunotherapy (allergy shots)
    - reserved for severe cases unresponsive to pharmacologic agents
    - consists of periodic (usually weekly) subcutaneous injections of custom prepared solutions of one or more antigens to which the patient is allergic

Amenorrhea

- see Gynecology, GY10

Anxiety

- see Psychiatry, PS13

Epidemiology
- 25-30% of patients in primary care settings have psychiatric disorders
- many are undiagnosed or untreated; hence the need for good screening
- high rate of coexistence of anxiety disorders and depression

Screening
- screening tools such as the GAD-7 tool
- screening questions
    - Do you tend to be an anxious or nervous person?
    - Have you felt unusually worried about things recently?
    - Has this worrying affected your life? How?

Assessment
- associated symptoms
- risk factors
    - family history of anxiety or depression, past history of anxiety, stressful life event, social isolation, female, comorbid psychiatric diagnosis (e.g. depression)
- assess substance abuse, comorbid depression, stressful life events, trauma, suicidal ideation/self-harm
- to differentiate anxiety disorders, consider symptoms (panic attacks, specific situations/stressors, excessive worry about common concerns, repetitive thoughts and/or behaviours to neutralize the anxiety) and their duration
- Generalized Anxiety Disorder 7–item (GAD – 7) scale to assess level of anxiety

Symptoms of GAD

AND I C REST
Anxious, nervous, or worried
No control over the worry
Duration >6 mo
Irritability
Concentration impairment
Restlessness
Energy decreased
Sleep impairment
Tension in muscles
Can Fam Physician 2005;51:1340-1342

Differential Diagnosis of Anxiety Disorders
- Panic disorder
- GAD
- Social Anxiety Disorder (previously Social Phobia)
- Agoraphobia
- Specific phobia
- Selective Mutism
- Separation Anxiety Disorder
- Other: GMC, AMC, mood disorder, psychotic disorder, OCD, PTSD

Rule Out
- Cardiac (post MI, arrhythmias)
- Endocrine (hyperthyroidism, diabetes, pheochromocytoma)
- Respiratory (asthma, COPD)
- Somatoform disorders
- Psychotic disorders
- Mood disorders (depression, bipolar)
- Personality disorder (OCPD)
- Drugs (amphetamines, thyroid preparations, caffeine, OTC for colds/decongestants, alcohol/benzodiazepine withdrawal)

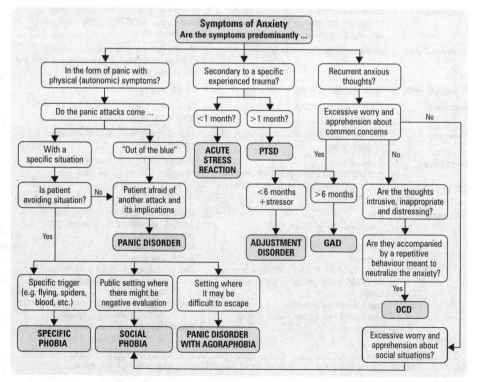

Figure 6. Differentiating anxiety disorders
Adapted from: Evans M, Bradwejn J, Dunn L. Anxiety Review Panel. Guidelines for the treatment of anxiety disorders in primary care. Toronto: Queen's Printer of Ontario, 2000.41

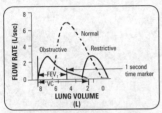

Figure 7. Expiratory flow volume curves (obstructive, normal, and restrictive disease)

See Respirology, R8 Adapted from: Weinberger SE. Principles of pulmonary medicine, 5th ed. With permission from *Elsevier.* ©2008

Signs of Poorly Controlled Asthma
- β2 agonist use >4x/wk
- Asthma-related absence from work/school
- Exercise induced asthma
- Night-time symptoms >1x/wk

What Colour is Your Inhaler?

Name	Body/Cap Colour
β₂-Agonists	
Salbutamol – Ventolin®	light blue/navy
Salmeterol – Serevent®	teal/light teal
Terbutaline – Bricanyl®	blue/white
ICS	
Fluticasone – Flovent®	orange/peach
Budesonide – Pulmicort®	white/brown
Combined Long-Acting β₂-Agonist + ICS	
Fluticasone/Salmeterol – Advair®	purple discus
Budesonide/Formoterol – Symbicort®	red/white
Ipratropium/Albuterol – Combivent®	clear/orange
Anticholinergics	
Ipratropium – Atrovent®	clear/green
Tiotropium – Spiriva®	white/turquoise

More About Inhalers
- Aerosols (puffers=MDI, MDI + spacer) MDIs should be used with spacers to:
  - Reduce side effects
  - Improve amount inhaled
  - Increase efficiency of use
- Dry Powder Inhalers (discus, turbuhaler, and diskhaler) require deep and fast breathing (may not be ideal for children)
- Nebulizers can be used to convert liquid medications into a fine mist: recommended for use if contraindications to MDIs

Differential Diagnosis of Wheezing
- Allergies, anaphylaxis
- Asthma, reactive airway disease
- GERD
- Infections (bronchitis, pneumonia)
- Obstructive Sleep Apnea
- COPD
- Less common: congestive heart disease, foreign body, malignancy, cystic fibrosis, vocal cord dysfunction

When prescribing salbutamol, watch out for signs of **hypokalemia**: lethargy, irritability, paresthesias, myalgias, weakness, palpitations, N/V, polyuria

Management
- patient education: emphasize prevalence, good recovery rate of anxiety conditions
- lifestyle advice: decrease caffeine and alcohol intake, exercise, relaxation techniques, mindfulness strategies
- self-help materials, community resources (e.g. support groups)
- CBT: cognitive interventions, exposure therapy, etc.
- treat any underlying medical and/or comorbid conditions
- provide support to family and caregivers
- for pharmacotherapy, see Psychiatry, PS48

Asthma/COPD

- see Respirology, R7

Definition
- asthma
  - chronic, reversible airway inflammation characterized by periodic attacks of wheezing, SOB, chest tightness, and coughing
  - airways hyper-responsive to triggers/antigens leading to acute obstructive symptoms by bronchoconstriction, mucous plugs and increased inflammation
  - cannot be diagnosed at first presentation; called reactive airway disease until recurrent presentations
  - pulmonary function tests (PFTs) can be done from age 6 or when child able to follow instructions to do PFTs
  - peak flow meters are useful in the office and at home for monitoring
- chronic obstructive pulmonary disease (COPD)
  - group of chronic, progressive, non-reversible lung diseases characterized by limited airflow with variable degrees of air sac enlargement and lung tissue destruction
  - emphysema and chronic bronchitis are the most common forms

Table 10. Differentiating COPD from Asthma

	COPD	Asthma
Age of Onset	Usually in 6th decade	Any age (but 50% of cases diagnosed in children age <10)
Role of Smoking	>10 pack yr	Not causal, known trigger
Reversibility of Airflow Obstruction	Airflow obstruction is chronic and persistent	Airflow obstruction is episodic and usually reversible with therapy
Evolution	Slow, progressive worsening (with periodic exacerbations)	Stable, episodic, less than 50% will outgrow
History of Allergy	Infrequent	Over 50% patients
Precipitators	Environmental irritants (air pollution, cigarette smoking, α-1 antitrypsin deficiency, viral infection, occupational exposure (firefighters, dusty jobs)	Environmental irritants (dust, pollen), animal fur, cold air, exercise, URTIs, cigarette smoke, use of β-blockers/ASA
Symptoms/Signs	Chronic cough, sputum, and/or dyspnea	Wheeze (hallmark symptom), dyspnea, chest tightness, cough which is worse in cold, at night, and in early AM, prolonged expiration
Diffusion Capacity	Decreased (more so in pure emphysema)	Normal (for pure asthma)
Hypoxemia	Chronic in advanced stages	Not usually present Episodic with severe attacks
Spirometry	May have improvement with bronchodilators but not universally seen	Marked improvement with bronchodilators or steroids
Chest X-Ray	Often normal Increased bronchial markings (chronic bronchitis) and chronic hyperinflation (emphysema) often co-exist, bullae	Often normal or episodic hyperinflation Hyperinflation during asthma attack
Management	**Mild** Step 1: SABA prn (salbutamol) Step 2: SABA prn + LAAC (i.e. tiotropium) or + LABA (e.g. salmeterol) **Moderate** Step 3: SABA prn + LAAC + low-dose combined ICS/LABA; consider inhaled vs. oral steroids **Severe** Step 4: ± theophylline Pneumococcal vaccination, annual influenza immunization	Ongoing patient education, and environmental control SABA taken prn as rescue medication + maintenance meds Maintenance medications Step 1: Low-dose ICS Step 2: Medium/high-dose ICS or low-dose ICS plus either LABA, LT modifier, or long-acting theophylline Step 3: Medium/high-dose ICS plus either LABA, LT modifier, or long-acting theophylline Step 4: As above plus immunotherapy ± oral glucocorticosteroids + pneumococcal vaccination, annual influenza immunization

ICS = inhaled corticosteroids; LAAC = long-acting anticholinergic; LABA = long-acting β-agonist; LT modifier = leukotriene modifier; SABA = short-acting β-agonist

Benign Prostatic Hyperplasia

- see Urology, U7

Definition
- hyperplasia of the stroma and epithelium in the periurethral transition zone

History and Physical
- include current/past health, surgeries, trauma, current and OTC meds
- specific urinary symptoms
- physical exam must include DRE for size, symmetry, nodularity, and texture of prostate (prostate is symmetrically enlarged, smooth, and rubbery in BPH)

Investigations
- urinalysis to exclude UTI and for microscopic hematuria (common sign)
- serum PSA: protein produced by prostatic tissue
  - values
    - <4.0 ng/mL: normal, but must take into account patient's age and velocity of PSA increase
    - 4-10 ng/mL: consider measuring free/total PSA
    - >10 ng/mL: high likelihood of prostate pathology
  - PSA testing is inappropriate in men with a life expectancy less than 10 yr or patients with prostatitis, UTI
  - increased PSA in a younger man is more often due to cancer than other causes
  - abnormal DRE or PSA should trigger further assessment
  - discuss test with men at increased risk of prostate cancer (FHx, African ancestry) or who are concerned about development of prostate cancer
  - decision to test PSA in an asymptomatic man should involve discussion about the risks and possible benefits
- other tests
  - Cr, BUN
  - post-void residual volume by ultrasound
  - urodynamic studies, renal ultrasound
  - patient voiding diary
- tests NOT recommended as part of routine initial evaluation include:
  - cystoscopy
  - cytology
  - prostate ultrasound or biopsy
  - IVP
  - urodynamic studies

Table 11. Symptoms and Complications of BPH

Obstructive Symptoms	Irritative Symptoms	Late Complications
Hesitancy (difficulty starting urine flow)	Urgency	Hydronephrosis
Diminution in size and force of urinary stream	Frequency	Loss of renal concentrating ability
Stream interruption (double voiding)	Nocturia	Systemic acidosis
Urinary retention (bladder does not feel completely empty)	Urge incontinence	Renal failure
Post-void dribbling	Dysuria	
Overflow incontinence		
Nocturia		

Differential Diagnosis
- Prostate cancer
- Urethral obstruction
- Bladder neck obstruction
- Neurogenic bladder
- Overactive bladder
- Cystitis
- Prostatitis

Management
- referral to urologist if moderate/severe symptoms
- conservative: for patients with mild symptoms or moderate/severe symptoms considered by the patient to be non-bothersome
  - fluid restriction (avoid alcohol and caffeine)
  - avoidance/monitoring of certain medications (e.g. antihistamines, diuretics, antidepressants, decongestants)
  - pelvic floor/Kegel exercises
  - bladder retraining (scheduled voiding)
- pharmacological: for moderate/severe symptoms
  - α-receptor antagonists (e.g. terazosin [Hytrin®], doxazosin [Cardura®], tamsulosin [Flomax®], alfuzosin [Xatral®])
  - relaxation of smooth muscle around the prostate and bladder neck
  - 5-α reductase inhibitor (e.g. finasteride [Proscar®])
  - only for patients with demonstrated prostatic enlargement due to BPH
  - inhibits enzyme responsible for conversion of testosterone into dihydrotestosterone (DHT) thus reducing growth of prostate
  - phytotherapy (e.g. saw palmetto berry extract, *Pygeum africanum*)
  - more studies required before this can be recommended as standard therapy
  - considered safe

- surgical
  - TURP (transurethral resection of the prostate), TUIP (transurethral incision of the prostate, for prostates <30 g)
  - absolute indications: failed medical therapy, intractable urinary retention, benign prostatic obstruction leading to renal insufficiency
  - complications: impotence, incontinence, ejaculatory difficulties (retrograde ejaculation), decreased libido

Bronchitis (Acute)

Definition
- acute infection of the tracheobronchial tree causing inflammation leading to bronchial edema and mucus formation

Epidemiology
- 5th most common diagnosis in family medicine, most common is URTI

Etiology
- 80% viral: rhinovirus, coronavirus, adenovirus, influenza, parainfluenza, respiratory syncytial virus (RSV)
- 20% bacterial: *M. pneumoniae, C. pneumoniae, S. pneumoniae*

Investigations
- acute bronchitis is typically a clinical diagnosis
- sputum culture/Gram stain is not useful
- CXR if suspect pneumonia (cough >3 wk, abnormal vital signs, localized chest findings) or CHF
- PFT with methacholine challenge if suspect asthma

Management
- primary prevention: frequent hand washing, smoking cessation, avoid irritant exposure
- symptomatic relief: rest, fluids (3-4 L/d when febrile), humidity, analgesics and antitussives as required
- bronchodilators may offer improvement of symptoms (e.g. salbutamol)
- current literature does not support routine antibiotic treatment for the management of acute bronchitis because it is most likely to be caused by a viral infection
  - antibiotics may be useful if elderly, comorbidities, suspected pneumonia, or if the patient is toxic (see *Antimicrobial Quick Reference*, FM49)
  - antibiotics in children show no benefit

Chest Pain

- see Cardiology and Cardiac Surgery, C4 and Emergency Medicine, ER21

Differential Diagnosis

Table 12. Differential Diagnosis of Chest Pain

Cardiac	Pulmonary	GI	MSK/Neuro	Psychologic
Angina*	Hemothorax*	Cholecystitis	Arthritis	Anxiety
Aortic dissection*	Lung CA	Esophageal spasm	Costochondritis	Depression
Endocarditis	PE*	GERD	Herpes zoster	Panic
MI*	Pneumonia	Hepatitis	Intercostal strain	
Myocarditis	Pneumothorax*	Perforated viscus*	Rib fractures	
Pericarditis*	Pulmonary HTN	PUD	Trauma	

*Emergent

Investigations
- ECG, CXR, and others if indicated (cardiac enzymes, d-dimers, liver function tests [LFTs], etc.)
- refer to ED if suspect serious etiology (e.g. aortic dissection, MI)

Management of Common Causes of Chest Pain
- angina/ischemic heart disease
  - nitroglycerin (NTG): wait 5 min between sprays and if no effect after 3 sprays, send to ED
- myocardial infarction
  - ASA (160-325 mg, chewed stat), clopidogrel (Plavix®), LMWH (enoxaparin), morphine, oxygen, NTG
  - ± reperfusion therapy with fibrinolytics (e.g. tPA, RPA, TNK, or SK) if within 12h (ideally <30 min) or percutaneous intervention (cath lab) if <90 min
  - start β-blocker (e.g. metoprolol starting dose 25 mg PO q6h or bid, titrating to HR goal of 55-60 bpm)
- endocarditis: antibiotic choice is based on whether patient has a native or prosthetic heart valve as well as culture and sensitivity results
- GERD: antacids, H_2-blockers, PPIs, patient education
- costochondritis: NSAIDs

Treatment of Stable Ischemic Heart Disease
- see Cardiology and Cardiac Surgery, C27

Differential Diagnosis of Bronchitis
- URTI
- Asthma
- Acute exacerbation of chronic bronchitis
- Sinusitis
- Pneumonia
- Bronchiolitis
- Pertussis
- Environmental/occupational exposures
- Post-nasal drip
- Others: GERD, CHF, cancer, aspiration syndromes, CF, foreign body

How to Tell if Viral or Bacterial?
Bacterial infections tend to give a higher fever, excessive amounts of purulent sputum production, and may be associated with concomitant COPD

Risk Factors for CAD

Major
- Smoking
- Diabetes
- HTN
- Hyperlipidemia
- Family history of early CAD in first degree relative (males <55 yr, females <65 yr)
- Untreated obstructive sleep apnea
- Chronic kidney disease

Minor
- Obesity
- Sedentary lifestyle
- Age

Red Flags
- Severe pain
- Pain for >20 min
- New onset pain at rest
- Severe SOB
- Loss of consciousness
- Hypotension
- Tachycardia
- Bradycardia
- Cyanosis

Ruling out Coronary Artery Disease in Primary Care
CMAJ 2010;182(12):1295-1300
Components of the prediction rule used to determine the presence or absence of CAD in patients with chest pain in primary care:
- Age/sex (female ≥65, male ≥55): 1 pt
- Known clinical vascular disease (coronary artery disease, occlusive vascular disease, or cerebrovascular disease): 1 pt
- Pain worse during exercise: 1 pt
- Pain not reproducible by palpation: 1 pt
- Patient assumes pain is of cardiac origin: 1 pt
Positive result: 3-5 pts; negative result: ≤2 pts
(sensitivity: 87.1%, specificity: 80%)

Common Cold (Acute Rhinitis)

- see Infectious Diseases, *Pneumonia and Influenza*, ID7

Definition
- viral URTI with inflammation

Epidemiology
- most common diagnosis in family medicine, peaks in winter months
- incidence: adults = 2-4/yr, children = 6-10/yr
- organisms
  - mainly rhinoviruses (30-35% of all colds)
  - others: coronavirus, adenovirus, RSV, influenza, parainfluenza, coxsackie virus
- incubation: 1-5 d
- transmission: person-person contact via secretions on skin/objects and by aerosol droplets

Risk Factors
- psychological stress, excessive fatigue, allergic nasopharyngeal disorders, smoking, sick contacts

Clinical Features
- symptoms
  - local: nasal congestion, clear to mucopurulent secretions, sneezing, sore throat, conjunctivitis, cough
  - general: malaise, headache, myalgias, mild fever
- signs
  - erythematous nasal/oropharyngeal mucosa, enlarged lymph nodes
  - normal chest exam
- complications
  - secondary bacterial infection: otitis media, sinusitis, bronchitis, pneumonia
  - asthma/COPD exacerbation

Differential Diagnosis
- allergic rhinitis, pharyngitis, influenza, laryngitis, croup, sinusitis, bacterial infections

Management
- patient education
  - symptoms peak at 1-3 d and usually subside within 1 wk
  - cough may persist for days to weeks after other symptoms disappear
  - no antibiotics indicated because of viral etiology
  - secondary bacterial infection can present within 3-10 d after onset of cold symptoms
- prevention
  - frequent hand washing, avoidance of hand to mucous membrane contact, use of surface disinfectant
  - yearly influenza vaccination
- symptomatic relief
  - rest, hydration, gargling warm salt water, steam, nasal irrigation (spray/pot)
  - analgesics and antipyretics: acetaminophen, ASA (not in children because of risk of Reye's syndrome)
  - cough suppression: dextromethorphan or codeine if necessary (children under 6 yr of age should not use any cough/cold medications)
  - decongestants, antihistamines
- patients with reactive airway disease will require increased use of bronchodilators and inhaled steroids

Concussion/Mild Traumatic Brain Injury

- see Neurosurgery, NS29, and Emergency Medicine, ER9
- a useful tool for the assessment of individuals and athletes with concussion is the Sport Concussion Assessment Tool, 3rd edition (SCAT3), *Br J Sports Med* 2013 47: 259

Contraception

- see Gynecology, GY16

EMERGENCY CONTRACEPTION
- hormonal EC (Yuzpe® or Plan B®, usually 2 doses taken 12 h apart) or post-coital copper IUD insertion
- hormonal EC is effective if taken within 72 h of unprotected intercourse (reduces chance of pregnancy by 75-85%), most effective if taken within 24 h, does not affect an established pregnancy
- copper IUDs inserted within 5 d of unprotected intercourse are significantly more effective than hormonal EC (reduces chance of pregnancy by ~99%)
- pregnancy test should be performed if no menstrual bleeding within 21 d of either treatment
- advance provision of hormonal EC increases the use of EC without decreasing the use of regular contraception
- pharmacists across Canada can dispense Plan B® OTC

MI in Elderly Women
Elderly women can often present with dizziness, back pain, lightheadedness, or weakness, in the absence of chest pain

MI in Diabetics
May present with dyspnea, syncope, and fatigue in the absence of chest pain

Influenza vs. Colds: A Guide to Symptoms

Features	Flu	Cold
Onset of illness	Sudden	Slow
Fever	High fever	None
Exhaustion level	Severe	Mild
Cough	Dry severe or hacking	±
Throat	Fine	Sore
Nose	Dry and clear	Runny
Head	Achy	Headache-free
Appetite	Decreased	Normal
Muscles	Achy	Fine
Chills	Yes	No

Echinacea for Preventing and Treating the Common Cold
Cochrane DB Syst Rev 2014;2:CD000530
This systematic review of 24 trials assessed the effect of Echinacea in preventing and treating common colds. Trials compared preparations containing Echinacea with placebo, no treatment, or an alternative common cold treatment.
Conclusions: Echinacea products have not been shown to provide benefits for treating colds, although, it is possible there is a weak benefit from some Echinacea products. Individual prophylaxis trials consistently show positive (if non-significant) trends, although potential effects are of questionable clinical relevance.

Differential Diagnosis

Common Causes
- Upper airway cough syndrome (post-nasal drip)
- Asthma/COPD
- GERD
- Non-asthmatic eosinophilic bronchitis

Other Causes
- ACEI
- Aspiration
- Bronchiectasis
- Cystic fibrosis
- Chronic interstitial lung disease
- CHF
- Lung/laryngeal cancer
- Pertussis
- Psychogenic
- Restrictive lung disease
- TB, atypical mycobacterium, and other chronic lung infections

Dementia Quick Screen = Mini Cog + Animal naming
- 3 simple tests, takes about 2 min
- Use when suspect mild cognitive impairment or when patient is at high risk
- Mini Cog = 3-word recall + clock drawing
  - Clock Drawing – including numbers and hands so time shows 10 min past 11 (normal = correct number/hand placing, or only minor spacing problems)
  - 0 word recall = impairment, 1-2 words and clock drawing abnormal = impairment, 3- word recall = normal.
- Naming animals in 1 min (normal = >15 in one min)
- Interpretation: If all 3 results within normal range, cognitive impairment unlikely
- Return for further evaluation if:
  - <15 animals named
  - 0-1 words recalled
  - Clock Drawing Abnormal

Cough

History and Physical
- duration (chronic - 8 wk), onset, frequency, quality (dry vs. productive), sputum characteristics, provoking/relieving factors, recent changes
- associated symptoms: fever, dyspnea, hemoptysis, wheezing, chest pain, orthopnea, PND, rhinitis, reflux, post-nasal drip
- constitutional symptoms: fever, chills, fatigue, night sweats
- risk factors: smoking, occupation, exposure, family history of lung CA or other CA, TB status, recent travel
- medications (e.g. ACEI, β-blockers), allergies
- PMH: lung (asthma, COPD, CF), heart (CHF, MI, arrhythmias), chronic illness, GI (reflux)
- vitals including O_2 saturation, respiratory exam, HEENT and precordial exam

Investigations
- guided by findings on history and physical
  - consider throat swab, CXR, PFTs, upper GI series, sputum culture test for acid-fast bacilli (if TB is suspected)

Dementia (Major Neurocognitive Disorder)

- see <u>Psychiatry</u>, PS20

Epidemiology
- 15% of Canadians 65 and older are living with dementia; risk for dementia doubles every 5 years after age 65
- prevalence of depression in dementia is 20-60%; major depression decreases as dementia severity increases; vascular and mixed dementias have a higher prevalence of depression
- differential diagnosis: Alzheimer's dementia, vascular dementia, Lewy-Body dementia, frontotemporal dementia

Investigations
- history, physical exam, MMSE, MOCA (best screening test), dementia quick screen (see sidebar)
- investigations are completed to exclude reversible causes of dementia and should be selected based on the clinical circumstances
- CBC, liver enzymes, TSH, renal function tests, serum electrolytes, serum calcium, serum glucose, vitamin B_{12}, folate, VDRL, HIV, head CT

Management
- treat and prevent reversible causes
- provide orientation cues (e.g. calendars, clocks) and optimize vision and hearing
- family education, counselling, and support (respite programs, group homes)
- pharmacologic therapy: NMDA receptor antagonists and cholinesterase inhibitors slow rate of cognitive decline; low-dose neuroleptics and antidepressants can be used to treat behavioural and emotional symptoms
- 20% of patients develop clinical depression, most commonly seen in vascular dementia

Depression

- see <u>Psychiatry</u>, PS10

Etiology
- often presents as non-specific complaints (e.g. sleep disturbance, chronic fatigue, pain)
- depression is a clinical diagnosis and tests are done in order to rule out other causes of symptoms
- 2/3 of patients may not receive appropriate treatment for their depression
- early diagnosis and treatment improve outcomes

Screening Questions
- Canadian Task Force on Preventive Health Care (2103) recommends not routinely screening for depression
- high-yield screening questions are:
  - "Are you depressed?" (high specificity and sensitivity)
  - "Have you lost interest or pleasure in the things you usually like to do?" (anhedonia)
  - "Do you have problems sleeping?"
- PHQ9 tool is useful to screen, diagnose and monitor depression; use Geriatric Depression Scale (GDS) for the geriatric population

Assessment

- risk factors: see Psychiatry, PS10
- personal or family history of depression
- medications and potential substance abuse problems
- high risk for suicide/homicide
  - fill out Form 1 (in Ontario): application by physician to hospitalize a patient against his/her will for psychiatric assessment (up to 72 h)
- functional impairment (e.g. work, relationships)
- at least 5 out of 9 criteria including at least one of anhedonia or depressed mood ≥2 wk for actual diagnosis to be met (see sidebar)
- validated depression rating scales: Beck's depression inventory, Zung's self-rating depression scale, Children's depression inventory, Geriatric Depression Scale, Personal Health Questionnaire Depression Scale (PHQ-9)
- routine medical workup (physical exam, CBC, TSH, ferritin, folate, B12, electrolytes, urinalysis, glucose, etc.)

Treatment

- goal: full remission of symptoms and return to baseline psychosocial function
- phases of treatment
  - acute phase (8-12 wk): relieve symptoms and improve quality of life
  - maintenance phase (6-12 mo after symptom resolution): prevent relapse/recurrence, must stress importance of continuing medication treatment for full duration to patients
- treatment options are pharmacotherapy psychotherapy, or a combination of both
- combination therapy is synergistic and most effective
- treatment of youth (age 10-21)
  - for mild depression, a period of active support and monitoring before initiating treatment is recommended
  - fluoxetine is first line among SSRIs (most evidence)
    - monitor closely for adverse effects such as suicidal ideation and behaviour
  - psychotherapy
    - CBT or interpersonal therapy (IPT) alone can be used for mild depression
    - psychotherapy plus medication is recommended for moderate to severe depression
  - treatment should continue for at least 6 months
    - ongoing management should include assessment in key domains (school, home, social setting)
    - reassessment and referral recommended if no improvement after 6-8 wk of treatment
- for adolescents with moderate/severe depression and coexisting psychosis and/or substance abuse, consider referral

Table 13. Common Medications

Class	Examples	Action	Side Effects	Notes
SSRI	paroxetine (Paxil®) fluoxetine (Prozac®) sertraline (Zoloft®) citalopram (Celexa®) fluvoxamine (Luvox®) escitalopram (Cipralex®)	Block serotonin reuptake	Sexual dysfunction (impotence, decreased libido, delayed ejaculation, anorgasmia), headache, GI upset, weight loss, tremors, insomnia, fatigue, increase QT interval (baseline ECG is suggested)	First line therapy for youth is fluoxetine; paroxetine is not recommended for youth (controversial)
SNRI	venlafaxine (Effexor®) duloxetine (Cymbalta®)	Block serotonin and NE reuptake	Insomnia, tremors, tachycardia, sweating	
SDRI	bupropion (Wellbutrin®)	Block dopamine and NE reuptake	Headache, insomnia, nightmares, seizures, less sexual dysfunction than SSRIs	Often chosen for lack of sexual side effects, can be used for augmentation of anti-depressant effects with other classes of medication
TCA	amitriptyline (Elavil®)	Block serotonin and NE reuptake	Sexual dysfunction, weight gain, tremors, tachycardia, sweating	Narrow therapeutic window, lethal in overdose

Prognosis

- up to 40% resolve spontaneously within 6-12 mo
- risks of recurrence: 50% after 1 episode; 70% after 2 episodes; 90% after 3 episodes

Diabetes Mellitus

- see Endocrinology, E7
- see 2013 Clinical Practice Guidelines from Canadian Diabetes Association (updated in 2016), available from: http://guidelines.diabetes.ca/fullguidelines

Definition

- metabolic disorder characterized by the presence of hyperglycemia due to defection insulin secretion, defective insulin action or both

Must Ask About/Rule Out
- Suicidal/homicidal ideation
- Psychosis
- Substance use/abuse/withdrawal
- Anxiety
- Bipolar/manic/hypomanic episodes
- Bereavement
- Intimate partner violence
- Post-partum depression
- Organic cause

Differential Diagnosis
- Other psychiatric disorders (e.g. anxiety, personality, bipolar, adjustment disorder, schizoaffective, seasonal affective disorder, substance abuse/withdrawal)
- Cancer (50% of patients with tumours, especially of brain, lung, and pancreas, develop symptoms of depression before the diagnosis of cancer is made)
- Chronic fatigue syndrome
- Early dementia
- Endocrine (e.g. hyper/hypothyroidism, DM, adrenal disorders)
- Infections (mononucleosis)
- Liver failure, renal failure
- Medication side effects (β-blockers, benzodiazepines, glucocorticoids, interferon)
- Menopause
- Neurological (Parkinson's, MS)
- Vitamin deficiency (pernicious anemia, pellagra)

Criteria for Depression (≥5/9 with at least one of anhedonia or depressed mood for ≥2 wk)

M-SIGECAPS
M Depressed **M**ood
S Increased/decreased **S**leep
I Decreased **I**nterest
G **G**uilt
E Decreased **E**nergy
C Decreased **C**oncentration
A Increased/decreased **A**ppetite and weight
P **P**sychomotor agitation/retardation
S **S**uicidal ideation

Combined Pharmacotherapy and Psychological Treatment for Depression: A Systematic Review
Arch Gen Psychiatry 2004;61:714-719
Study: Systematic review of randomized clinical trials.
Patients: 16 trials comprising 1,842 patients.
Intervention: Antidepressant treatment alone vs. combination of psychological intervention and antidepressant therapy.
Main Outcomes: Efficacy of and adherence to therapy.
Results: Overall, combined therapy was significantly more effective than antidepressant therapy alone (OR 1.86; 95% CI 1.38-2.52), however there was no difference in the rate of dropouts and non-responders in either treatment arm. In studies lasting >12 wk, combined therapy showed a reduction in dropouts compared to non-responders (OR 0.59; 95% CI 0.39-0.88).

Classification
- type 1: primarily a result of pancreatic β-cell destruction
- type 2: characterized by insulin resistance
- GDM: glucose intolerance with onset or first recognition during pregnancy

Epidemiology
- major health concern, affecting up to 10% of Canadians
- incidence of type 2 DM is rising due to increasing obesity, sedentary lifestyle, and age of the population
- leading cause of new-onset blindness and renal dysfunction
- Canadian adults with DM are twice as likely to die prematurely, compared to persons without DM

Risk Factors
- type 1 DM
  - personal or family history of autoimmune disease
- type 2 DM
  - first degree relative with DM
  - age ≥40 yr
  - obesity (especially abdominal), HTN, hyperlipidemia, CAD, vascular disease
  - prior GDM, macrosomic baby (>4 kg)
  - PCOS
  - history of IGT or IFG
  - presence of complications associated with DM
  - presence of associated diseases: PCOS, acanthosis nigricans, psychiatric disorders, HIV
  - medications: glucocorticoids, atypical antipsychotics, HAART
- both
  - member of a high risk population (e.g. Aboriginal, Hispanic, Asian, or African descent)

Diagnosis
- persistent hyperglycemia is the hallmark of all forms of DM

Long-Term Complications of DM
- Microvascular: nephropathy, retinopathy, neuropathy
- Macrovascular: CAD, CVD, PVD

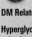

DM Related Symptoms

Hyperglycemia: polyphagia, polydipsia, polyuria, weight change, blurry vision, yeast infections

Diabetic Ketoacidosis (DKA): fruity breath, anorexia, N/V, fatigue, abdominal pain, Kussmaul breathing, dehydration

Hypoglycemia: hunger, anxiety, tremors, palpitations, sweating, headache, fatigue, confusion, seizures, coma

Table 14. Diagnosis of Prediabetes and Diabetes

Condition	Diagnostic Criteria
DM	One of the following on 2 occasions: Random BG ≥11.1 mmol/L (200 mg/dL) with symptoms of DM (fatigue, polyuria, polydipsia, unexplained weight loss) OR Fasting BG ≥7.0 mmol/L (126 mg/dL) OR BG 2 h post 75 g OGTT ≥11.1 mmol/L (200 mg/dL) OR HbA1c ≥6.5% (in adults) **If asymptomatic (and meet any of the above criteria) a repeat test must be done to confirm the diagnosis. If symptomatic (fatigue, polyuria, polydipsia, unexplained weight loss), the diagnosis is made with one test.
Impaired Fasting Glucose (IFG)	Fasting BG = 6.1-6.9 mmol/L (110-124 mg/dL)
Impaired Glucose Tolerance (IGT)	BG 2 h post 75 g OGTT = 7.8-11.0 mmol/L (141-198 mg/dL)
Prediabetes	HbA1C = 6.0-6.4%

Screening
- type 2 DM
  - FBG in everyone ≥40 q3yr, or at high risk using the CANRISK calculator
  - more frequent and/or earlier testing if presence of ≥1 risk factor (see above)
- GDM (see Obstetrics, OB26)
  - all pregnant women between 24-28 wk gestation

Goals of Therapy

Table 15. Goals of Therapy in Diabetes

General	Avoid complications (e.g. ketoacidosis, hyperglycemia, infection) Prevent long-term complications (microvascular and macrovascular) Minimize negative sequelae associated with therapies (e.g. hypoglycemia, weight gain)
Fasting or Preprandial BG	Ideal: 4-7 mmol/L (72-126 mg/dL) Suboptimal: 7.1-10 mmol/L (128-180 mg/dL); action may be required Inadequate: >10.0 mmol/L (180 mg/dL); action required Frail Elderly: target is 5-12 mmol/L
HbA1c	≤7% or ≤6.5% in some type 2 DM patients at risk for nephropathy Suboptimal: 7-8.4% Inadequate: >8.4% Frail elderly, advanced co-morbidities, recurrent severe hypoglycemia or hypoglycemia unawareness: target is 7.1-8.5%
2 h Postprandial BG	5-10 mmol/L (90-180 mg/dL) if HbA1c target met 5-8 mmol/L (90-144 mg/dL) if HbA1c target not met Frail elderly: use clinical judgment
Blood Pressure	<130/80 in adults (DM and HTN guidelines)
Lipids	LDL <2.0 mmol/L (36 mg/dL)

Assessment and Monitoring

Table 16. Assessment and Monitoring

	Initial Assessment	q2-4mo	Annually
History	Symptoms of hyperglycemia, ketoacidosis, hypoglycemia Past medical history Functional inquiry Family history Risk factors Medications Sexual function Lifestyle	DM-directed history Screen for awareness and frequency of hypoglycemia and DKA Glucose monitoring Use of insulin and oral agents Smoking cessation	DM-directed history Screen for awareness and frequency of hypoglycemia and DKA Glucose monitoring Use of insulin and oral agents Sexual function Lifestyle counselling Screen for depression
Physical Exam	General: Ht, Wt, BMI, BP, WC Head and neck: fundoscopy, thyroid exam Cardiovascular exam: signs of PVD, pulses, bruits Abdominal exam (e.g. for organomegaly) Hand/foot/skin exam Neurological exam	Wt, BP, BMI, WC	Foot exam for sensation (using a 10 g monofilament), ulcers or infection Remainder of exam as per PHE
Investigations	FBG, HbA1c, fasting lipids, Cr, microalbumin:creatinine ratio Baseline ECG; repeat testing q2yrs for those at high risk	HbA1c q3mo FBG as needed	Fasting lipid profile Annual random ACR and eGFR

Management	Nutritional and physical education
	Consider referral to DM education program if available
	Monitoring BG: explain methods and frequency
	Medication counselling: oral hypoglycemics and/or insulin, method of administration, dosage adjustments
	Pneumococcal vaccination
	Ophthalmology consult
	  type 1 DM within 5 yr
	  type 2 DM at diagnosis
		Assess progress towards long-term complications
		Adjust treatment plan if necessary
			Calibrate home glucose monitor
			Arrange retinopathy screening
			Influenza vaccination annually

Calculate Total Insulin Required
type 1 DM: 0.5-0.7 units/kg/d
type 2 DM: 0.3 units/kg/d

Dietary Advice for Treatment of Type 2 DM in Adults
Cochrane DB Syst Rev 2007;3:CD004097
A meta-analysis of 36 RCTs in which dietary advice was the main intervention for adults with T2DM demonstrated no data available for efficacy of dietary changes. Exercise improved HbA1c at 6 and 12-mo timepoints.

Nonpharmacologic Management
- diet
  - all diabetics should see a registered dietician for nutrition counselling
  - can reduce HbA1c by 1-2%
  - moderate weight loss (5%) improves glycemic control and CVD risk factors
  - decrease combined saturated fats and trans-fatty acids to <10% of calories
  - avoid simple sugars, choose low glycemic-index foods, ensure regularity in timing and spacing of meals
- physical activity and exercise
  - at least 150 min of aerobic exercise per wk, plus 2 sessions per wk of resistance exercise is recommended
  - encourage 30-45 min of moderate exercise 4-7 d/wk
  - promote cardiovascular fitness: increases insulin sensitivity, lowers BP, and improves lipid profile
  - if insulin treated, may require alterations of diet, insulin regimen, injection sites, and self-monitoring

Self-Monitoring of Blood Glucose
- type 1 DM: 3 or more self-tests/d is associated with a 1% reduction in HbA1c
- type 2 DM: recommendations vary based on treatment regimen (e.g. insulin dependent requires more frequent monitoring – refer to 2013 Canadian Practice Guidelines)
- if FBG >14 mmol/L, perform ketone testing to rule out DKA
- if bedtime level is <7 mmol/L, have bedtime snack to reduce risk of nocturnal hypoglycemia

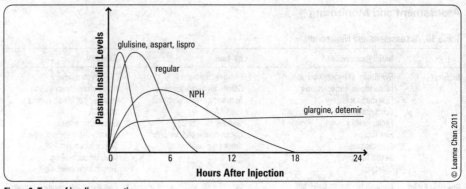

Figure 8. Types of insulin preparation

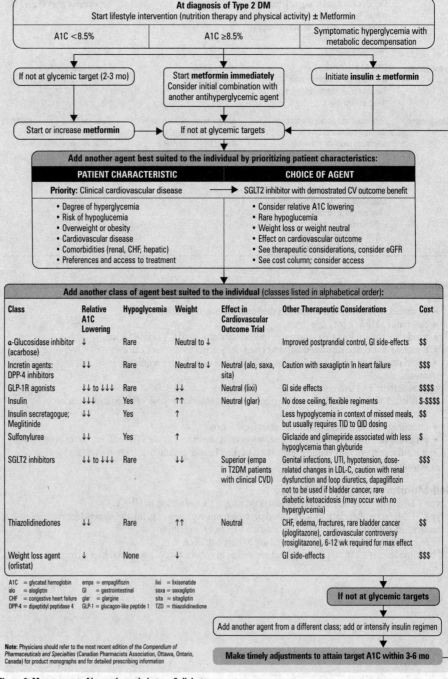

Figure 9. Management of hyperglycemia in type 2 diabetes
With permission of: Canadian Diabetes Association Clinical Practice Guidelines Expert Committee. Pharmacologic Management of Type 2 Diabetes. *Can J Diabetes* 2013;37:S61-S68

Hypoglycemic Agents (Type 2 DM)
- oral
  - biguanide: metformin (Glucophage®)
  - thiazolidinedione: troglitazone (Rezulin®), rosiglitazone (Avandia®)
  - α-glucosidase inhibitor: acarbose (Precose®)
  - nonsulfonylureas: nateglinide (Starlix®), repaglinide (Gluconorm®)
  - sulfonylureas: glyburide (DiaBeta®), glimepiride (Amaryl®), gliclazide (Diamicron®)
  - DPP-4 inhibitor: sitagliptin (Januvia®)
- injectable
  - GLP-1 analogue: liraglutide (Victoza®)

Other Medications Used in DM
- ACEI or ARB in those with any of
  - clinical macrovascular disease
  - age ≥55 years
  - age <55 and microvascular complications
- statin in those with any of
  - clinical macrovascular disease
  - age ≥40 years
  - age <40 and any of the following:
  - diabetes duration >15 years and age >30 years
  - microvascular complications
  - other cardiovascular risk factors
- low dose ASA (81-325 mg)
  - for secondary prevention in people with established CVD (NOT to be used routinely for primary prevention)

Rosiglitazone Revisited: An Updated Meta-Analysis of Risk for Myocardial Infarction and Cardiovascular Mortality
Arch Intern Med 2010;170:1191-1201
Eleven years after the introduction of rosiglitazone, the totality of randomized clinical trials continue to demonstrate increased risk for MI although not for CV or all-cause mortality. The current findings suggest an unfavourable benefit to risk ratio for rosiglitazone.

Dizziness

- see Otolaryngology, OT6

Epidemiology
- 70% see general practitioners initially; 4% referred to specialists
- frequency proportional to age; commonest complaint of ambulatory patients age >75

Differential Diagnosis

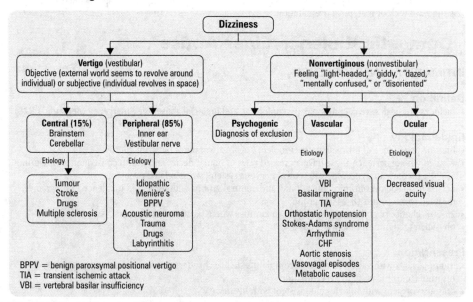

Figure 10. Differential diagnosis of dizziness

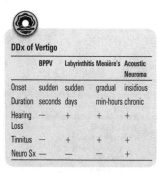

History
- clarify type of dizziness: vertigo, pre-syncope, disequilibrium, light-headedness
- duration
- exacerbations
  - worse with head movement or eye closure (vestibular)
  - no change with head movement and eye closure (nonvestibular)
  - worse with exercise (cardiac/pulmonary causes)

- associated symptoms
  - neurologic (central)
    - transient diplopia, dysphagia, dysarthria, ataxia (TIA, VBI, migraine)
    - persistent headache, alterations in level of consciousness, sensory and/or motor deficits (CNS)
  - audiologic (peripheral)
    - hearing loss, tinnitus, otalgia, aural fullness
  - others
    - N/V (peripheral vestibular disorders)
    - SOB, palpitations (hyperventilation, cardiac problem)
- general medical history
  - HTN, DM, heart disease, fainting spells, seizures, cerebrovascular disease, migraines
  - ototoxic drugs: aminoglycosides (gentamicin, streptomycin, tobramycin), erythromycin, ASA, antimalarials
  - hypotension (secondary to diuresis): furosemide, caffeine, alcohol
  - depression/anxiety: can present with light-headedness

Physical Exam/Investigations
- syncopal
  - cardiac (orthostatic changes in vitals), peripheral vascular, and neurologic exams
  - blood work, ECG, 24 h Holter, treadmill stress test, loop ECG, tilt table testing, carotid, and vertebral doppler, EEG
- vertiginous
  - ENT and neurologic exams
  - Dix-Hallpike, consider audiometry and MRI if indicated
- non-syncopal, non-vertiginous
  - assess gait, vision and test for neuropathy
  - cardiac and neurologic exams
  - 3-min hyperventilation trial (patient is coached to hyperventilate until patient becomes dizzy to identify if symptoms are reproducible and confirm that hyperventilation is the etiology of the symptoms), ECG, EEG
  - Romberg test: test for disequilibrium (patient sways towards the side of vestibular dysfunction)

Treatment
- guided by history, physical exam, and investigations
- include education, lifestyle modification, physical maneuvers (e.g. Epley for BPPV), symptomatic management (e.g. antiemetics), pharmacotherapy, and surgery
- refer when significant central disease is suspected, when vertigo of peripheral origin is persistent (lasting >2-4 wk), or if atypical presentation

Domestic Violence/Elder Abuse

INTIMATE PARTNER VIOLENCE

Definition
- includes physical, sexual, emotional, psychological, and financial abuse (see Emergency Medicine, ER28)

Epidemiology
- lifetime prevalence of intimate partner violence against women is between 25-30%
- women who experience abuse have increased rates of injury, death, and health consequences including 50-70% increase in gynecological, central nervous system, stress-related problems
- occurs in all socioeconomic, educational, and cultural groups with increased incidence in pregnancy, disabled women, and 18-24 age group
- 25-50% chance of child abuse or neglect in families where partner abuse occurs
- physician recognition rates as low as 5%

Presentation
- multiple visits with vague, ill-defined complaints such as: headaches, gastrointestinal symptoms, insomnia, chronic pain, hyperventilation
- may also present with injuries inconsistent with history

Management
- screen ALL patients
  - always have a high index of suspicion
  - asking about abuse is the strongest predictor of disclosure
  - several screening tools (see sidebar) exist to identify victims of partner violence
  - make sure to determine the victim's level of immediate and long-term danger and ask if there are weapons in the house
- ensure patient safety
  - victim most at risk for homicide when attempting to leave home or following separation

Dix-Hallpike Test
- Have the patient seated with legs extended and head at 45° rotation
- Rapidly shift patient to supine position with head fully supported in slight extension (for 45 s)
- Observe for rotatory nystagmus and ask about sensation of vertigo

Screening Instruments for Domestic Violence
A) Woman Abuse Screening Tool (WAST)-SHORT
1. In general how would you describe your relationship?
   a. A lot of tension
   b. Some tension
   c. No tension
2. Do you and your partner work out arguments with . . .?
   a. Great difficulty
   b. Some difficulty
   c. No difficulty
Endorsing either question 1 ("a lot of tension") or question 2 ("great difficulty") makes intimate partner violence exposure likely
B) HITS
How often does your partner:
1. Physically hurt you?
2. Insult you?
3. Threaten you with harm?
4. Scream or curse at you?
Each question on HITS to be answered on a 5 point scale ranging from 1 (= never) to 5 (= frequently)
A total score of 10.5 is significant

- provide community resources
  - safety planning includes ensuring that there is access to an exit in the home, establishing a safe place to go and having money, clothes, keys, medications, important documents, and other emergency items prepared should the patient need to leave quickly
  - shelter or helpline number with legal advocacy and counselling services
  - involve social workers or domestic violence advocates
- appointment for follow-up to assess whether condition is better or worse
- reassure patient she/he is not to blame and that the assault is a crime
  - goal is to convey the message that "As your doctor, I am concerned for your safety" and "Your partner has a problem that he/she needs help with" and "I want to help you"
  - reporting suspected or known child abuse is mandatory
  - spousal abuse is a criminal act, but not reportable without the woman's/man's permission
- DOCUMENT all evidence of abuse-related visits for medico-legal purposes

ELDER ABUSE

- see Geriatric Medicine, GM4

Dyspepsia

- see Gastroenterology, G10

Definition and Clinical Features
- defined as epigastric pain or discomfort
- can be associated with fullness, belching, bloating, heartburn, food intolerance, N/V

Epidemiology
- annual incidence 1-2%, prevalence 20-40%

Etiology
- common: functional, PUD, GERD, gastritis
- others: cholelithiasis, irritable bowel syndrome, esophageal or gastric cancer, pancreatitis, pancreatic cancer, Zollinger-Ellison syndrome, and abdominal angina

History
- symptoms may not be useful in finding cause
- associated with eating, anorexia, N/V, alcohol, NSAID use
- red flags: vomiting, bleeding/ anemia, abdominal mass, dysphagia (VBAD)

Investigations and Management
- for new onset dyspepsia, test for *H. pylori* using the urea breath test or serology
- upper endoscopy (preferred), upper GI series (not in patients with alarm symptoms)
- lifestyle modifications: decreased caffine and alcohol intake, avoid citrus food , avoid supine position right after meals, smoking cessation
- pharmacologic treatment
- gastric acid suppression: H₂ blockers, PPI's; both are effective for PUD and GERD
- prokinetics: e.g. Metoclopramide; effective for functional dyspepsia
- *H. pylori* eradication
- do not keep patients on PPI without at least 1 trial off the medication per year (http://www.choosingwiselycanada.org/in-action/toolkits/bye-bye-ppi/)
- for non-responders, gastroscopy should be considered

Dyspnea

- see Respirology, R3 and Emergency Medicine, ER26

Definition
- uncomfortable, abnormal awareness of breathing

History and Physical Exam
- history
  - cough, sputum, hemoptysis, wheezing, chest pain, palpitations, dizziness, edema, SOB
  - asthma, allergy, eczema, ASA/NSAID sensitivity, nasal polyps
  - constitutional symptoms
  - smoking, recreational drugs, medications
  - occupational exposure, environmental exposure (e.g. pets, allergens, smoke)
  - travel and birth place
  - FHx of atopy
  - previous CXR or PFTs
- physical exam: vitals, respiratory, precordial, HEENT, signs of anemia/liver failure/heart failure

How to Document Abuse
- Take photographs (with permission) of known or suspected injuries
- Use an injury location chart or "body map" when documenting physical findings
- Document any investigations ordered (e.g. x-ray)
- Write legibly or use a computer
- Record the patient's own words in quotation marks
- Avoid phrases that imply doubt about the patient's reliability (e.g. "patient claims that...")
- Record the patient's demeanor (e.g. upset, agitated)
- Record the time of day the patient is examined and how much time has elapsed since the abuse occurred

Dyspepsia Red Flags
- Weight Loss
- Dysphagia
- Persistent vomiting
- GI bleeding (hematemesis, hematochezia, melena)
- Onset age >50

***H. pylori* Eradication**
Take the following 10 day treatment
1) PPI 1 tablet 2x/d for 10 d and
2) Amoxicillin 1 g twice a day for 5 d (day 1-5)
Followed by
3) Clarithromycin 500 mg 2x/d (day 6-10) and
4) Metronidazole 500 mg 2x/d (day 6-10)

DDx of Dyspnea

Pulmonary
- COPD
- Asthma
- Restrictive lung disease
- Pneumothorax
- Congenital lung disease
- PE

Cardiac
- CHF
- CAD
- MI (recent or past)
- Cardiomyopathy
- Valve dysfunction
- Pericarditis
- Arrhythmia
- Hypertrophy

Mixed/Other
- Deconditioning
- Trauma
- Pain
- Neuromuscular
- Metabolic condition
- Functional: anxiety, panic attack, hyperventilation

UTI Clinical Decision Aid
- Dysuria
- +Leukocytes
- +Nitrites

If 2 or more criteria MET, then treat without culture, otherwise culture required prior to treatment
Arch Intern Med 2007;67:2201-2206

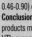

Risk Factors for Complicated UTI
- Male
- Pregnancy
- Recent urinary tract instrumentation
- Functional or anatomic abnormality of the urinary tract
- Chronic renal disease
- DM
- Immunosuppression
- Indwelling catheter

Cranberries for Preventing Urinary Tract Infections
Cochrane DB Syst Rev 2008;1:CD001321
Study: Meta-analysis of 10 RCTs (n=1,049).
Patients: All populations.
Intervention: Cranberry juice vs. placebo, juice or water was evaluated in seven studies, and cranberry tablets vs. placebo in four studies.
Main Outcome: UTIs – symptomatic and asymptomatic.
Results: Cranberry products significantly reduced the incidence of UTIs at 12 mo (RR 0.65, 95% CI 0.46-0.90) compared with placebo/control.
Conclusion: There is some evidence that cranberry products may decrease the number of symptomatic UTIs over a 12 mo period, particularly for women with recurrent UTIs.

Prevention of UTIs
- Maintain good hydration (especially with cranberry juice) (recommendation level I)
- Wipe urethra from front to back to avoid contamination of the urethra with feces from the rectum
- Avoid feminine hygiene sprays and scented douches
- Empty bladder immediately before and after intercourse

Investigations
- CXR, ECG
- PFTs, ABG acutely if indicated

Management
- ABCs: send to ED if in severe respiratory distress
- depends on cause

Dysuria

- see Urology, U10

Definition
- the sensation of pain, burning, or discomfort on urination

Epidemiology
- in adulthood, more common in women than men
- approximately 25% of women report one episode of acute dysuria per year
- most common in women age 25-54 and in those who are sexually active
- in men, dysuria becomes more prevalent with increasing age

Etiology
- infectious
  - most common cause
  - presents as cystitis, urethritis, pyelonephritis, vaginitis, cervicitis, epididymo-orchitis, or prostatitis
- non-infectious
  - hormonal conditions (hypoestrogenism), obstruction (BPH, urethral strictures), allergic reactions, radiation, drugs/chemicals, foreign bodies, trauma, neoplasm, kidney stones, inflammatory diseases, endometriosis, psychogenic

Table 17. Etiology, Signs and Symptoms of Common Causes of Dysuria

Infection	Etiology	Signs and Symptoms
UTI/Cystitis	KEEPS bacteria (*Klebsiella, E. coli, Enterobacter, Proteus mirabilis, Pseudomonas, S. saprophyticus*)	Internal dysuria throughout micturition, frequency, urgency, incontinence, hematuria, nocturia, back pain, suprapubic discomfort, low grade fever (rare)
Urethritis	*C. trachomatis, N. gonorrhoeae, Trichomonas, Candida*, herpes	Initial dysuria, urethral/vaginal discharge, history of STI
Vaginitis	*Candida, Gardnerella, Trichomonas, C. trachomatis,* atrophic, herpes, lichen sclerosis	External dysuria/pain, vaginal discharge, irritation, dyspareunia, abnormal vaginal bleeding
Prostatitis	*E. coli, C. trachomatis, S. saprophyticus, Proteus mirabilis, Enterobacter, Klebsiella, Pseudomonas*	Dysuria, fever, chills, urgency, frequency, tender prostate, rectal pain
Pyelonephritis	*E. coli, S. saprophyticus, Proteus mirabilis, Enterobacter, Klebsiella, Pseudomonas*	Internal dysuria, fever, chills, flank pain radiating to groin, CVA tenderness, N/V

Investigations
- no investigations necessary when history and physical consistent with uncomplicated UTI – treat empirically (urinalysis can be performed when indicated by dipstick or microscopy)
- urinalysis/dipstick: positive for nitrites and leukocytes
- urine R&M: pyuria, bacteriuria, hematuria
- urine C&S
- CBC and differential if suspecting pyelonephritis
- if vaginal/urethral discharge present: wet mount, Gram stain, KOH test, vaginal pH, culture for yeast and trichomonas, endocervical/urethral swab or urine PCR for *N. gonorrhoeae* and *C. trachomatis*
- radiologic studies and other diagnostic tests if atypical presentation
- see Pediatrics, P62 for UTI in children

Management
- UTI/cystitis
  - pregnant women with bacteriuria (2-7%) must be treated even if asymptomatic, due to increased risk of pyelonephritis, preterm labour, low birth weight and perinatal mortality; need to follow with monthly urine cultures and retreat if still infected
  - patients with recurrent UTIs (>3/yr) should be considered for prophylactic antibiotics
  - if complicated UTI, patients require longer courses of broader spectrum antibiotics
- urethritis
  - when swab or PCR is positive for chlamydia or gonorrhea must report to Public Health
  - all patients should return 4-7 d after completion of therapy for clinical evaluation

Epistaxis

- see <u>Otolaryngology</u>, OT26

Erectile Dysfunction

- see <u>Urology</u>, U30

Definition
- consistent or recurrent inability to attain and/or maintain penile erection sufficient for sexual performance of ≥3 mo duration

Epidemiology
- ~20% of men age 40; ~50% of men age 70

Etiology
- organic: vascular (90%) (arterial insufficiency, atherosclerosis), endocrine (low testosterone, DM), anatomic (structural abnormality, e.g. Peyronie's), neurologic (post-operative, DM), medications (clonidine, antihypertensives, psychotropics)
- psychogenic (10%)

Table 18. Differentiation Between Organic and Psychogenic ED

Characteristic	Organic	Psychogenic
Onset	Gradual	Acute
Circumstances	Global	Situational
Course	Constant	Varying
Non-Coital Erection	Poor	Rigid
Morning Erection	Absent	Present
Psychosexual Problem	Secondary	Long history
Partner Problem	Secondary	At onset
Anxiety and Fear	Secondary	Primary

Walsh: Campbell's Urology, 8th ed. Table 46-4

History
- comprehensive sexual, medical, and psychosocial history
- time course
  - last satisfactory erection
  - gradual or sudden onset
  - attempts at sexual activity
- quantify
  - presence of morning or night time erections
  - stiffness (scale of 1-10)
  - ability to initiate and maintain an erection with sexual stimulation
  - erection stiffness during sex (scale of 1-10)
- qualify
  - partner or situation specific
  - loss of erection before penetration or climax
  - degree of concentration required to maintain an erection
  - percentage of sexual attempts satisfactory to patient and/or his partner
  - significant bends in penis or pain with erection
  - difficulty with specific positions
  - impact on quality of life and relationship

Investigations
- hypothalamic-pituitary-gonadal axis evaluation: testosterone (free + total), prolactin, LH
- risk factor evaluation: fasting glucose, HbA1c, lipid profile
- others: TSH, CBC, urinalysis
- specialized testing
  - psychological and/or psychiatric consultation
  - in-depth psychosexual and relationship evaluation
  - nocturnal penile tumescence and rigidity (NPTR) assessment
  - vascular diagnostics (e.g. doppler studies, angiography)

DDx of Erectile Dysfunction

PENIS
Psychogenic
Endocrine (type 2 DM, testosterone)
Neurogenic (type 2 DM, post-operative)
Insufficiency of blood (atherosclerosis)
Substances

The Effect of Lifestyle Modification and Cardiovascular Risk Factor Reduction on Erectile Dysfunction
Arch Intern Med 2011;171:1797-1803
Study: Meta-analysis of 6 RCTs.
Population: 740 male participants.
Intervention: Lifestyle modification and pharmacotherapy targeting CAD risk factors.
Main Outcome Measure: International Index of Erectile Dysfunction (IIEF-5) score.
Results: Lifestyle modifications and pharmacotherapy for cardiovascular risk factors had a statistically significant association with improved sexual function (weighted mean difference 2.66; 95% CI 1.86-3.47). Lifestyle modification without use of statins was also statistically significantly associated with improved sexual function (weighted mean difference 2.40; 95% CI 1.19-3.61).
Conclusion: Lifestyle modification alone or combined with pharmacotherapy can improve sexual function.

Reasons for Referral to Urology
- Significant penile anatomic disease
- Younger patient with a history of pelvic or perineal trauma
- Cases requiring vascular or neuro- surgical intervention
- Complicated endocrinopathies
- Complicated psychiatric or psychosocial problems
- Patient or physician desire for further evaluation

Management

Table 19. Management of Erectile Dysfunction

Nonpharmacologic	Pharmacologic	Surgical
Lifestyle changes (alcohol, smoking, exercise)	Oral agents	Implants
	Suppository	Vascular repair
Relationship/sexual counselling	Male urethral suppository for erection (MUSE)	Realignment
Vacuum devices	Injections	

- pharmacologic treatment
  - phosphodiesterase type 5 inhibitors
  - α-adrenergic blockers (e.g. yohimbine)
  - serotonin antagonist and reuptake inhibitor (e.g. trazodone)
  - testosterone – currently only indicated in patients presenting with hypogonadism and testosterone deficiency (note: breast/prostate cancer are absolute contraindications)

Table 20. Phosphodiesterase Type 5 Inhibitors

Examples	Dosing (1 dose/d)	Specifics	Side Effects	Contraindications
sildenafil (Viagra®)	25-100 mg/dose	Take 0.5-4 h prior to intercourse May last 24 h	Flushing, headache, indigestion	Not to be used in patients taking nitrates
tadalafil (Cialis®)	5-20 mg/dose	Effects may last 36 h	As above	As above
vardenafil (Levitra®)	2.5-20 mg/dose	Take 1 h prior to intercourse	As above	As above

Fatigue

Fatigue Red Flags
- Fever
- Weight loss
- Night sweats
- Neurological deficits
- Ill-appearing

Epidemiology
- 25% of office visits to family physicians
  - peaks in ages 20-40
  - F:M = 3-4:1
- 50% have associated psychological complaints/problems, especially if <6 mo duration

Differential Diagnosis

Table 21. Differential Diagnosis of Fatigue: PS VINDICATE

P	**Psychogenic**	**Depression, life stresses,** anxiety disorder, chronic fatigue syndrome, fibromyalgia
	Physiologic	**Pregnancy, caregiving demands (young children, elderly)**
S	Sleep disturbance	**Obstructive sleep apnea, sleep disorder,** poor sleep hygiene, BPH, shift work, pain
	Sedentary	Unhealthy/sedentary lifestyle
V	Vascular	Stroke
I	**Infectious**	Viral (e.g. mononucleosis, hepatitis, HIV), bacterial (e.g. TB), fungal, parasitic
N	**Neoplastic**	Any malignancy
	Nutrition	**Anemia** (Fe^{2+} deficiency, B_{12} deficiency)
	Neurogenic	Myasthenia gravis, multiple sclerosis, Parkinson's disease
D	**Drugs**	β-blockers, antihistamines, anticholinergics, benzodiazepines, antiepileptics, antidepressants
I	Idiopathic	
C	Chronic illnesses	CHF, lung diseases (e.g. COPD, sarcoidosis), renal failure, chronic liver disease
A	Autoimmune	SLE, RA, mixed connective tissue disease, polymyalgia rheumatica
T	Toxin	**Substance abuse** (e.g. alcohol), heavy metal
E	Endocrine	**Hypothyroidism, DM,** Cushing's syndrome, adrenal insufficiency, pregnancy

Common causes are in **bold**

Investigations
- psychosocial causes are common, so usually minimal investigation is warranted
- physical causes of fatigue usually have associated symptoms/signs that can be elicited from a focused history and physical exam
- investigations should be guided by history and physical exam and may include
  - CBC and differential, electrolytes, BUN, Cr, ESR, glucose, TSH, ferritin, vitamin B_{12}, serum protein electrophoresis, Bence-Jones protein, albumin, AST, ALT, ALP, bilirubin, calcium, phosphate, ANA, β-hCG
  - urinalysis, CXR, ECG
  - additional tests: serologies (Lyme disease, hepatitis B and C screen, HIV, ANA) and Mantoux skin tests

Treatment
- treat underlying cause
- if etiology cannot be identified (1/3 of patients)
  - reassurance and follow-up, especially with fatigue of psychogenic etiology
  - quick follow-up for reassurance
  - supportive counselling, behavioural, or group therapy
  - encourage patient to stay physically active to maximize function
  - review all medications, OTC, and herbal remedies for drug-drug interactions and side effects
  - prognosis: after 1 yr, 40% are no longer fatigued

CHRONIC FATIGUE SYNDROME

Definition (CDC 2006) – must meet both criteria
1. new or definite onset of unexplained, clinically evaluated, persistent or relapsing chronic fatigue, not relieved by rest, which results in occupational, educational, social, or personal dysfunction
2. concurrent presence of ≥4 of the following symptoms for a minimum of 6 mo
   - impairment of short-term memory or concentration, severe enough to cause significant decline in function
   - sore throat
   - tender cervical or axillary lymph nodes
   - muscle pain
   - multi-joint pain with no swelling or redness
   - new headache
   - unrefreshing sleep
   - post-exertion malaise lasting >24 h
- exclusion criteria: medical conditions that may explain the fatigue, certain psychiatric disorders (depression with psychotic or melancholic features, schizophrenia, eating disorders), substance abuse, severe obesity (BMI >45)

Epidemiology
- F>M, Caucasians > other groups, majority in their 30s
- found in <5% of patients presenting with fatigue

Etiology
- unknown, likely multifactorial
- may include infectious agents, immunological factors, neurohormonal factors, and/or nutritional deficiency

Investigations
- no specific diagnostic laboratory tests

Treatment
- promote sleep hygiene
- provide support and reassurance that most patients improve over time
- non-pharmacological
  - regular physical activity, optimal diet, psychotherapy (e.g. CBT), family therapy, support groups
- pharmacological
  - to relieve symptoms: e.g. antidepressants, anxiolytics, NSAIDs, antimicrobials, antiallergy therapy, antihypotensive therapy

> **Exercise Therapy for Chronic Fatigue**
> Cochrane Depression, Anxiety, and Neurosis Group
> *Cochrane DB Syst Rev* 2004;Issue 3
> **Purpose:** To determine the effectiveness of exercise therapy for Chronic Fatigue Syndrome (CFS).
> **Methods:** Systematic review of 5 RCTs with 336 patients of all ages with a clinical diagnosis of CFS.
> **Interventions:** Exercise therapy alone was compared with treatment as usual (or relaxation and flexibility), pharmacotherapy (fluoxetine), or exercise therapy combined with either pharmacotherapy or patient education.
> **Results:** At 12 wk, patients undergoing exercise therapy were less fatigued than controls (SMD -0.77; 95% CI -1.26 to -0.28). Physical functioning was also significantly improved, but there were more dropouts with exercise therapy. Compared with fluoxetine, patients receiving exercise therapy were less fatigued (WMD -1.24; 95% CI -5.3-2.83). Patients receiving combination therapy with exercise therapy and either fluoxetine or patient education, did better than those on monotherapy.
> **Conclusions:** Patients may benefit from exercise therapy. Combination therapy with either fluoxetine or education may offer additional benefit. Further high quality trials are needed.

Fever

- see Pediatrics, P51

Definition
- oral temperature >37.2°C (AM), 37.7°C (PM)
- fever in children under 2 must be a rectal temperature for accuracy
- TM not accurate for measurement until child is >5 yr

Table 22. Differential Diagnosis of Fever

Infection	Cancer	Medications		Other
Bacterial	Leukemia	Allopurinol	Nifidepine	Irritable Bowel Syndrome
Viral	Lymphoma	Captopril	Phenytoin	Collagen Vascular Disease
TB	Other Malignancies	Cimetidine	Diuretics	DVT
		Heparin	Barbiturates	
		INH	Antihistamines	
		Meperidine		

History
- fever
  - peak temperature, thermometer, route, duration
  - time of day
  - response to antipyretics
- systemic symptoms
  - weight loss, fatigue, rash, arthralgia, night sweats
- symptoms of possible source
  - UTI/pyelonephritis: dysuria, foul-smelling urine, incontinence, frequency, hematuria, flank pain
  - pneumonia: cough, pleuritic chest pain
  - URTI: cough, coryza, ear pain
  - meningitis: headache, confusion, stiff neck, rash
  - osteomyelitis: bone pain
  - skin: purulent discharge
  - PID: discharge, dyspareunia, lower abdominal pain
  - gastroenteritis: abdominal pain, diarrhea, blood per rectum, vomit
  - medications
  - PE/DVT: swollen legs, pain in calf, SOB, pleuritic chest pain
  - history of cancer/family history of cancer
- infectious contacts
  - travel history, camping, day care, contact with TB, foodborne, animals

Possible Investigations
- CBC and differential, blood culture, urine culture, urinalysis
- stool O&P, Gram stain, culture
- CXR, Mantoux skin test, sputum culture
- LP

Management
- increase fluid intake
- general: sponge bath, light clothing
- acetaminophen/ibuprofen as needed
- treat underlying cause

Headache

- see Neurology, N44

Primary Headaches

Migraine Screen

POUND
Pulsatile quality
Over 4-72 h
Unilateral
Nausea and vomiting
Disabling intensity
if ≥4 present then a diagnosis is likely
(+LR = 24)

Table 23. Primary Headaches

	Migraine	Tension-Type	Cluster	Caffeine Withdrawal
Epidemiology	12% of adults F>M 20% with aura 80% without aura	38% of adults, can be episodic or chronic	<0.1% of adults, M>>F	~50% of people drinking >2.5 cups/d
Duration	5-72 h	May occur as isolated incident or daily, duration is variable	<3 h at same time of day	Begins 12-24 h after last caffeine intake, can last ~1 wk
Pain	Classically unilateral and pulsatile, but 40% are bilateral, moderate-severe intensity, N/V, photo-/phonophobia	Mild to moderate pain, bilateral, fronto-occipital or generalized pain, band-like pain, ± contracted neck/scalp muscles, associated with little disability	Sudden, unilateral, severe, usually centred around eye, frequently awakens patient. Associated conjunctival injection and tearing. "Suicide" headache	Severe, throbbing, associated with drowsiness, anxiety, muscle stiffness, nausea, waves of hot or cold sensations
Triggers	Numerous (e.g. food, sleep disturbance, stress, hormonal, fatigue, weather, high altitude). Aggravated by physical activity	Stressful events, NOT aggravated by physical activity	Often alcohol	Discontinuing caffeine
Treatment of Acute Headache	1st line: acetaminophen, NSAIDs, ASA ± caffeine 2nd line: NSAIDs 3rd line: 5-HT agonists ± antiemetic	Rest and relaxation NSAIDs or acetaminophen	Sumatriptan Dihydroergotamine High-flow O₂ Intranasal lidocaine	Caffeine Acetaminophen or ASA ± caffeine
Prophylactic Therapy	1st line: β-blockers 2nd line: TCAs 3rd line: anticonvulsants	Rest and relaxation, physical activity, biofeedback	Lithium carbonate, prednisone, methysergide	Cut down on caffeine

Secondary Headaches
- caused by underlying organic disease
- account for <10% of all headaches, may be life-threatening

Etiology
- aneurysm
- medication overuse headache
- space-occupying lesion
- systemic infection (meningitis, encephalitis)
- stroke
- subarachnoid hemorrhage
- systemic disorders (thyroid disease, HTN, pheochromocytoma, etc.)
- temporal arteritis
- traumatic head injuries
- TMJ or C-spine pathology
- serious ophthalmological and otolaryngological causes of headache

Investigations
- indicated only when red flags are present and may include:
  - CBC for suspected systemic or intracranial infection
  - ESR for suspected temporal arteritis
  - neuroimaging (CT or MRI) to rule out intracranial pathology
  - CSF analysis for suspected intracranial hemorrhage, infection

Management
- based on underlying disorder
- analgesics may provide symptomatic relief

Hearing Impairment

- see Otolaryngology, OT7

Definition
- hearing impairment: a raised hearing threshold measured as decibels of hearing loss relative to the normal population at specific frequencies
- hearing disability: hearing impairment that interferes with performing daily tasks

Epidemiology
- prevalence increases with age (6% of 35-44 yr old, 43% of 65-84 yr old)
- 90% of age-related hearing loss (presbycusis) is sensorineural
- hearing loss detectable by audiology is present in greater than 1/3 of people >65 yr
- associated with significant physical, functional, and mental health consequences

Classification
- conductive (external sound does not reach the middle ear)
- sensorineural involving the inner ear, cochlea, or auditory nerve
- mixed

Assessment
- infants
  - universal newborn hearing screening program
- elderly
  - presbycusis is characterized by the progressive, symmetric loss of high-frequency hearing
    - tinnitus, vertigo, and disequilibrium may be present
    - can cause low self-esteem, isolation, and depression
  - whispered-voice test
    - whisper 6 test words 6 in-2 ft away from the patient's ear out of the visual field, ask patient to repeat the words (with non-test ear distraction)
  - tuning fork test (to distinguish conductive from sensorineural hearing loss)
    - Rinne and Weber (not for general screening)
  - formal audiologic assessment
    - pure tone, air, and bone conduction testing
    - speech audiometry
    - impedance audiometry

Management
- counsel about noise control and hearing protection programs (Grade A evidence)
- investigations in patients with unexplained sensorineural hearing loss
  - blood sugar, CBC+ differential, TSH, syphilis testing
- referral
  - refer patients with hearing loss for a complete audiological examination
  - unclear etiology of hearing loss: referral to ENT
  - **sudden hearing loss: urgent referral** as treatment success is related to early treatment
- patients with progressive asymmetric sensorineural hearing loss should have an MRI/CT scan to exclude vestibular schwannoma (acoustic neuroma)
- hearing amplification (e.g. hearing aids), assistive listening devices, and cochlear implants can dramatically improve quality of life

---

Headache Red Flags

SNOOP
Systemic symptoms of illness
- fever
- anticoagulation
- pregnancy
- cancer

Neurologic signs/symptoms
- impaired mental status
- neck stiffness
- seizures
- focal neurological deficits

Onset
- sudden and severe
- new headache after age 50

Other associated conditions
- following head trauma
- awakens patient from sleep
- jaw claudication
- scalp tenderness
- worse with exercise, sexual activity or Valsalva

Prior headache history
- different pattern
- rapidly progressing in severity/frequency

Acupuncture for Migraine Prophylaxis
Cochrane DB Syst Rev 2009;4:CD001218
Study: Meta-analysis of 22 RCTs.
Population: 4,419 participants with diagnosed migraine.
Intervention: Preventive treatment with acupuncture, sham acupuncture, no prophylactic treatment/routine care only, other interventions.
Main Outcome Measure: Proportion of responders in 3-4 mo.
Other Outcomes: Frequency of migraine attacks, number of migraine days, headache frequency.
Results: Patients receiving acupuncture had higher response rates and fewer headaches after 3-4 mo than those with no prophylactic treatment or routine care only. There was no statistically significant difference between "true" vs. "sham" acupuncture.
Conclusion: Acupuncture is a viable prophylactic treatment option for migraine attacks. Selecting specific points for acupuncture is not as important as believed by practitioners.

Does this Patient have Hearing Impairment?
JAMA 2006;295:416-428
Purpose: To evaluate bedside clinical maneuvers used to evaluate the presence of hearing impairment.
Study: Evidence-based review of studies examining the accuracy or precision of screening questions and tests. 24 studies were included in this analysis.
Conclusions: Elderly patients who admit to having hearing impairment should be offered audiometry, while those who do not should undergo a whispered-voice test. Those who hear the whispered voice require no further testing, while those who do not require audiometry. The Weber and Rinne tests are not useful in screening for hearing impairment.

Hypertension

Hypertension Guidelines are reviewed and updated annually, for up-to-date recommendations, please see www.hypertension.ca/chep

Epidemiology
- 22% of Canadian adults suffer from HTN (prevalence is 52% in the 60-70 age group)
- lifetime risk of developing hypertension is approximately 90%
- 64% of Canadians who have HTN are treated and controlled, while 17% are unaware that they have HTN
- 3rd leading risk factor associated with death
  - risk factor for CAD, CHF, cerebrovascular disease, renal failure, peripheral vascular disease

Definitions
- HTN
  - BP ≥140/90 mmHg, unless DM (≥130/80 mmHg), or age ≥80 yr (≥150/90 mmHg)
- isolated systolic HTN
  - sBP ≥140 and dBP <90
  - associated with progressive reduction in vascular compliance
  - usually begins in 5th decade
- hypertensive urgency
  - sBP >210 or dBP >120 with minimal or no target-organ damage
- hypertensive emergency
  - severe HTN + acute target-organ damage
  - accelerated HTN
    - significant recent increase in BP over previous hypertensive levels associated with evidence of vascular damage on fundoscopy, but without papilledema
  - malignant HTN
    - sufficient elevation in BP to cause papilledema and other manifestations of vascular damage (retinal hemorrhages, bulging discs, mental status changes, increasing creatinine)
- white coat hypertension
  - high clinic BP with normal home BP and 24 ambulatory BP, caused by anxiety in clinic
- masked hypertension
  - normal clinic BP with high BP in home and/or ambulatory setting, often provoked by anxiety, job stress, exercise

Etiology
- essential (primary) HTN (>90%)
  - undetermined cause
- secondary HTN (10%)

Predisposing Factors
- family history
- obesity (especially abdominal)
- alcohol consumption
- stress
- sedentary lifestyle
- smoking
- male
- age >30
- excessive salt intake/fatty diet
- African American ancestry
- dyslipidemia

Table 24. Causes of Secondary HTN

	Common Cause	
Renal	Renovascular HTN Renal parenchymal disease, glomerulonephritis, pyelonephritis, polycystic kidney	
Endocrine	1° hyperaldosteronism Pheochromocytoma Cushing's syndrome Hyperthyroidism/hyperparathyroidism Hypercalcemia of any cause	
Vascular	Coarctation of the aorta Renal artery stenosis	
Drug-Induced	Estrogens/OCP Steroids NSAIDs MAOIs Lithium Decongestants Cocaine Amphetamines Alcohol	

Investigations
- for all patients with HTN
  - electrolytes, Cr, fasting glucose and/or HbA1c, lipid profile, 12-lead ECG, urinalysis
  - self-measurement of BP at home is encouraged (recommended devices listed at www.hypertension.ca)
- for specific patient subgroups
  - DM or chronic kidney disease: urinary protein excretion
  - if suspected renovascular HTN: renal ultrasound, captopril renal scan (if GFR >60 mL/min), MRA/CTA (if normal renal function)

Symptoms of HTN are usually NOT PRESENT (this is why it is called the "silent killer")
May have occipital headache upon awakening or organ-specific complaints if advanced disease

Renovascular HTN Suspected if Patient Presenting with 2 or more of:
- Sudden onset or worsening of HTN and age >55 or <30 yr
- Presence of abdominal bruit
- HTN resistant to 3 or more drugs
- Rise in Cr of 30% or more associated with use of an ACEI or ARB
- Other atherosclerotic vascular disease, particularly in patients who smoke or have dyslipidemia
- Recurrent pulmonary edema associated with hypertensive surges

Suspect Hyperaldosteronism when
- HTN refractory to treatment with 3 or more drugs
- Spontaneous hypokalemia
- Profound diuretic-induced hypokalemia (<3.0 mmol/L)
- Incidental adrenal adenomas

Hypertensive Emergencies
- **Malignant HTN**
- **Cerebrovascular**
  Hypertensive encephalopathy
  CVA
  Intracerebral hemorrhage
  SAH
- **Cardiac**
  Acute aortic dissection
  Acute refractory LV failure
  Myocardial infarction/ischemia
  Acute pulmonary edema
- **Renal Failure**

- if suspected endocrine cause: plasma aldosterone, plasma renin
  - measured from morning samples taken from patients in sitting position after resting 15 min
  - discontinue aldosterone antagonists, ARBs, β-blockers, and clonidine prior to testing
- if suspected pheochromocytoma: 24 h urine for metanephrines and creatinine
- echocardiography for left ventricular dysfunction assessment if indicated

Diagnosis

- all Canadian adults should have BP assessed at all appropriate clinical visits, oscillometric preferred to manual

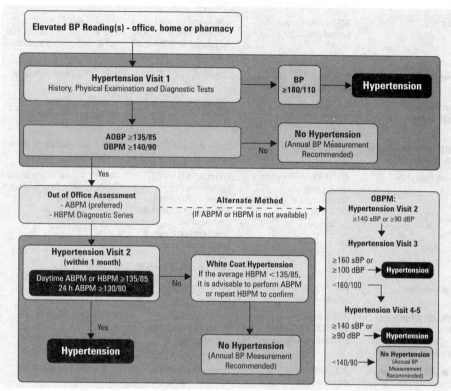

Figure 11. Assessment of patients with hypertension   Adapted from: CHEP 2015 Guidelines

Treatment

- treat to target BP: <140/90 mmHg, <130/80 mmHg if DM, sBP<150 in very elderly (>80 yrs)
- optimum management of hypertension requires assessment of overall cardiac risk
- lifestyle modification (in all HTN patients)
  - may be sufficient in patients with stage 1 HTN (140-159/90-99)
  - diet
    - follow Canada's Guide to Healthy Eating (see *Nutrition*, FM6) and **D**ietary **A**pproaches to **S**top **H**ypertension (**DASH**) (reduced cholesterol and saturated fats)
    - limit daily sodium intake to 65-100 mmol (1.5-2.3 g)
    - potassium/magnesium/calcium supplementations are NOT recommended for HTN
  - moderate intensity dynamic exercise: 30-60 min, 4-7 x/wk; higher intensity exercise is no more effective
  - smoking cessation
  - stress management
  - low-risk alcohol consumption (see *Alcohol*, FM12)
  - achieve and maintain a healthy BMI (18.5-24.9 kg/m²) and waist circumference (<102 cm for men, <88 cm for women); use multidisciplinary approach to weight loss
  - individualized cognitive behavioural interventions for stress management
- pharmacological
  - indications regardless of age (caution with elderly patients)
    - dBP ≥90 mmHg with target organ damage or independent cardiovascular risk factors
    - dBP ≥100 mmHg or sBP ≥160 mmHg without target organ damage or cardiovascular risk factors
    - sBP ≥140 with target organ damage
  - first line antihypertensives: thiazide/thiazide-like diuretic, ACEI (for non-African patients), ARB, long-acting CCB, β-blocker (if age <60)
  - if partial response to standard dose monotherapy, add another first-line drug
  - caution with combination of non-DHP CCB and β-blocker
  - combination of ACEI and ARB is <u>not</u> recommended
  - be cautious of hypokalemia in patients treated with thiazide/thiazide-like diuretic monotherapy
  - if still not controlled or adverse effects, can add other classes of anti-hypertensives
- focus on adherence to health behaviour modification and pharmacotherapy; should be assessed at each visit

Impact of Health Behaviour on Blood Pressure

Intervention	Systolic BP (mmHg)	Diastolic BP (mmHg)
Diet and weight control	-6.0	-4.8
Reduced salt/ sodium intake	-5.4	-2.8
Reduced alcohol intake (heavy drinkers)	-3.4	-3.4
DASH diet	-11.4	-5.5
Physical activity	-3.1	-1.8
Relaxation therapies	-3.7	-3.5

CHEP (Canadian Hypertension Education Program) Guidelines 2014. Available from: http://www.hypertension.ca/en/chep

β-blocker
Not recommended as first line for patients of age ≥60

ACEI
Not recommended as monotherapy in people of African descent

How to Combine Antihypertensive Medications (in general)

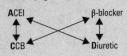

Table 25. Pharmacologic Treatment of Hypertension in Patients with Unique Conditions

Condition or Risk Factor	Recommended Drugs	Alternative Drugs	Not Recommended/Notes
Isolated Diastolic HTN	Thiazide diuretic, β-blocker, ACEI, ARB, or long-acting CCB (consider ASA and statin in select patients)	Combinations of first-line drugs	β-blocker monotherapy (age >60) or combination of ACEI with an ARB
Isolated Systolic HTN	Thiazide diuretic, ARB, or long acting dihydropyridine CCB	Combinations of first-line drugs	Same as above
CAD	ACEI or ARB; β-blocker for patients with stable angina	Long acting CCB, when combination therapy for high risk patients, ACEI/DHP CCB is preferred	Short-acting CCB (nifedipine) or ACEI + ARB is not recommended dBP 60 mmHg may exacerbate MI
Prior MI	β-blocker + ACEI (ARB if cannot tolerate ACEI)	Long-acting CCB	ACEI + ARB combination is not recommended
Left Ventricular Hypertrophy	ACEI, ARB, thiazide, or long-acting CCB	Combination of additional agents	Hydralazine and minoxidil can increase LVH, thus not recommended
Cerebrovascular Disease (stroke/TIA)	ACEI + diuretic	Combination of additional agents	ACEI + ARB combination after a stroke is not recommended
Heart Failure	ACEI (ARB if ACEI intolerant) and β-blocker Spironolactone in patients with NYHA class II-IV	ARB in addition to ACEI Hydralazine/isosorbide dinitrate combination if ARB or ACEI not tolerated/contraindicated Thiazide or loop diuretic is recommended as additive therapy DHP CCB can also be used	Non-DHP CCB not recommended Carefully monitor for side effects if using ACEI + ARB
Dyslipidemias	Does not affect initial treatment recommendations	Combination of additional agents	
DM with Albuminuria (ACR >2.0 mg/mmol in men and >2.8 mg/mmol in women)	ACEI or ARB (DHP CCB > HCTZ for combination therapy with ACEI)	Add thiazide diuretic, cardioselective β-blocker, long acting CCB	If serum Cr >150 μmol/L, a loop diuretic should be considered instead of low-dose thiazide diuretic
DM without Albuminuria (criteria listed above)	ACEI, ARB, DHP CCB, or thiazide diuretic	Combination of first-line drugs or, first-line agents not tolerated, cardioselective β-blocker or non-DHP CCB	ACEI + ARB combination not recommended
Non-Diabetic Chronic Kidney Disease with Proteinuria (urinary protein >500 mg/24 h or ACR >30 mg/mmol)	ACEI (ARB if ACEI intolerant), diuretic as additive therapy	Thiazide for additive antihypertensive therapy, loop diuretic for volume overload	ACEI + ARB combination is not recommended
Renovascular Disease	Same as HTN without other indications		Caution in using ACEI or ARB – monitor for AKI Renal angioplasty and stenting offer no benefits over optimal medical therapy alone
Asthma	K+-sparing + thiazide diuretic for patients on salbutamol		β-blocker, unless specific indications like angina or post-MI
Gout			Thiazide, but asymptomatic hyperuricemia is not a contraindication
Smoking	Low dose thiazide ACEI		β-blocker
Pregnancy	Methyldopa Hydralazine	Labetolol Nifedipine	ACEI
Elderly (>60 yr)	As for uncomplicated isolated diastolic HTN, except for use of β-blocker		β-blocker not recommended as first line treatment
Emergency	BP >169/90 = labetolol, nifedipine		
If >3 Cardiovascular Risk Factors or Established Atherosclerotic Disease	Statin (age >40), low-dose ASA (age >50)		Caution with use of ASA in patients with uncontrolled BP

Adapted from: McAlister FA, Zarnke KB, Campbell NRC, et al. The 2001 Canadian recommendations for the management of hypertension: Part two – Therapy. *Can J Cardiol* 2002;18:625-641 and The 2012 Canadian Hypertension Education Program Recommendations

Follow-Up
- assess and encourage adherence to pharmacological and non-pharmacological therapy at every visit
- lifestyle modification q3-6mo
- pharmacological
  - q1-2mo until BP under target for 2 consecutive visits
  - more often for symptomatic HTN, severe HTN, antihypertensive drug intolerance, target organ damage
  - q3-6mo once at target BP
- referral is indicated for cases of refractory HTN, suspected secondary cause or worsening renal failure
- hospitalization is indicated for malignant HTN

Joint Pain

- see Rheumatology, RH3

Table 26. Differential Diagnosis of Joint Pain

Non-Articular		Articular		
Localized	Generalized	Inflammatory	Degenerative	Other
Bursitis	Fibromyalgia	Seropositive	Primary	Neoplastic
Tendonitis	Polymyalgia rheumatica	RA	Familial Heberden's node	Drug-induced
Capsulitis	Myofascial pain syndrome	Systemic lupus erythematosus	Osteoarthritis	Endocrine (hyperthyroid, hypothyroid, hyperparathyroid)
		Scleroderma	Regional hip or knee	
		Polymyositis/Dermatomyositis		
		Sjögren's syndrome		
		Seronegative	Secondary	
		Ankylosing spondylitis	Metabolic	
		Inflammatory bowel disease	Hemophiliac	
		Psoriatic arthritis	Neuropathic	
		Reactive arthritis	Traumatic	
		Crystal		
		Gout		
		Pseudogout		
		Hydroxyapatite		
		Infectious/septic		
		Gonococcal		
		Non-gonococcal		
		Systemic vasculitis disease		

History
- number of joints involved: monoarticular, oligoarticular, polyarticular
- pattern of joints involved: symmetrical vs. asymmetrical, large vs. small joints, axial skeleton
- onset: acute vs. chronic (>6 wk)
- trauma, infection, medications (steroids, diuretics)
- morning stiffness (duration) vs. worse at end of day
- FHx of arthritis
- comorbidities: DM (carpal tunnel syndrome), renal insufficiency (gout), psoriasis (psoriatic arthritis), myeloma (low back pain), osteoporosis (fracture), obesity (OA)
- constitutional symptoms (neoplasm)

Physical Exam
- vitals
- specific joint exams
- systemic features (skin, nails, eyes, hands)

Investigations (Guided by the History and Physical Exam)
- general: CBC and differential, electrolytes, Cr
- acute phase reactants: ESR, CRP, ferritin, albumin, fibrinogen
- complement (C3, C4)
- urinalysis to detect disease complications (proteinuria, active sediment)
- serology (ANA, anti-dsDNA, HLA-B27, anti-Jo-1, anti-Sm, anti-La, anti-Ro, RhF, and anti-CCP, etc.)
- synovial fluid analysis (cell count + differential, culture, Gram stain, microscopy)
- tissue cultures
- radiology (plain film, CT, MRI, U/S, bone densitometry, angiography, bone scan)

Treatment
- patient education including lifestyle modifications
- physiotherapy, occupational therapy
- manage pain (acetaminophen, NSAIDs)
- treat specific causes (e.g. antibiotics, DMARDs etc., see Rheumatology, RH26)

Signs and Symptoms of Inflammatory Arthritis

WARM(S) Joints
Worse with rest, better with activity
Awakening in the latter half of the night
Redness around joint
Morning stiffness (>30 min)
Soft tissue swelling, erythema

Systemic Features
- Fever (SLE, infection)
- Rash (SLE, psoriatic arthritis)
- Nail abnormalities (psoriatic, reactive arthritis)
- Uveitis (psoriatic, reactive arthritis, ankylosing spondylitis)
- Myalgias (fibromyalgia, myopathy)
- Weakness (polymyositis, neuropathy)
- GI symptoms (scleroderma, IBD)
- GU symptoms (reactive arthritis, gonococcemia)

Common Presenting Problems

Low Back Pain

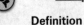

• see Orthopedics, OR25

Definition
• acute: <6 wk
• subacute: 6-12 wk
• chronic: >12 wk

Epidemiology
• 5th most common reason for visiting a physician
• lifetime prevalence: 90%
• peak prevalence: age 45-60
• largest WSIB category
• most common cause of chronic disability for individuals <45 yr old
• 90% resolve in 6 wk, <5% become chronic

Etiology
• source of pain can be local, radicular, referred, or related to a psychiatric illness
• 98% are mechanical causes
  ▪ pain is worse with movement, better with rest
  ▪ sprain (ligament), strain (muscle), facet joint degeneration, disc degeneration/herniation, spinal stenosis (e.g. spondylosis), spondylolisthesis, compression fracture, pregnancy
• 2% are non-mechanical causes
  ▪ surgical emergencies
    ◆ cauda equina syndrome (areflexia, lower extremity weakness, decreased anal tone, saddle anesthesia, fecal incontinence, urinary retention), AAA (pulsatile abdominal mass)
  ▪ medical conditions
    ◆ neoplastic (primary, metastatic, multiple myeloma)
    ◆ infectious (osteomyelitis, TB)
    ◆ metabolic (osteoporosis, osteomalacia, Paget's disease)
    ◆ rheumatologic (ankylosing spondylitis, polymyalgia rheumatica)
    ◆ referred pain (perforated ulcer, pancreatitis, pyelonephritis, ectopic pregnancy, herpes zoster)

Physical Exam
• inspection: curvature, posture, gait
• palpation: bony deformities/tenderness, paraspinal muscle bulk/tenderness, trigger points
  ▪ percussion of spine to elicit pain due to fracture or infection
• ROM and peripheral pulses
• neurologic exam for L4/L5/S1 helps determine level of spinal involvement (power, reflexes, sensation)
• special tests
  ▪ straight leg raise (positive if pain at <70 degrees and aggravated by ankle dorsiflexion), positive test is indicative of sciatica
  ▪ crossed straight leg raise (raising of uninvolved leg elicits pain in leg with sciatica), more specific than straight leg raise
  ▪ femoral stretch test (patient prone, knee flexed, examiner extends hip) to diagnose L4 radiculopathy

Investigations
• plain films not recommended in initial evaluation
• if infection/cancer suspected: CBC, ESR
• if neurologic deficits worsening or infection/cancer suspected: consider CT or MRI

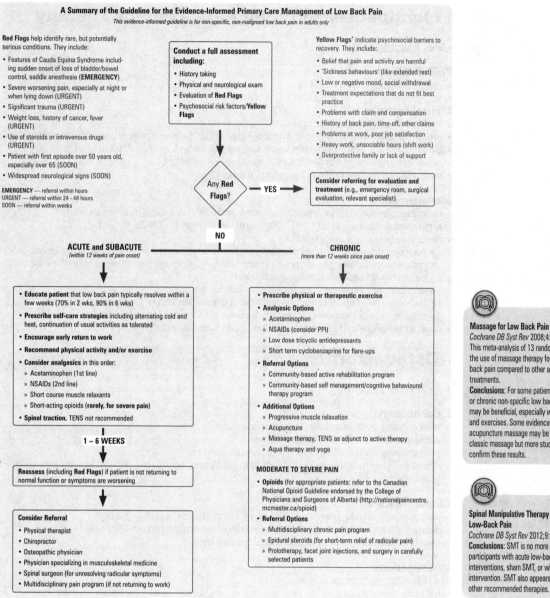

Figure 12. Low back pain treatment
Reprinted with permission from: Kendall NAS, et al. Guide to Assessing Psycho-Social Yellow Flags in Acute Low Back Pain. ACC & NZGG, Wellington, NZ. (2004 ed.); Toward Optimized Practice. Guideline for the evidence-informed primary care management of low back pain, 2nd ed. 2007. Available from: www.topalbertadoctors.org

Table 27. Approach to Non-Traumatic Low Back Pain

	Back Dominant (Pain greatest above gluteal fold)		Leg Dominant (Pain greatest below gluteal fold)	
History	**Pattern 1** Worse with flexion Constant/intermittent	**Pattern 2** Worse with extension Never worse with flexion Always intermittent	**Pattern 3** Pain changes with back movement/position Currently/previously constant	**Pattern 4** Worse with activity Improves with rest and posture change Intermittent/short duration
Physical Exam	Normal neuro exam Fast responder Improves with extension Slow responder No change or worsens with extension	Normal neuro exam ± improves with flexion Worse with extension	Leg pain can improve but not disappear Positive straight leg raise ± conduction loss Fast responder Improves with specific back position Slow responder Not better with position changes	No irritative findings ± conduction loss
Likely Pathology	Arising from intervertebral discs or adjacent ligaments	Posterior joint complex (associated ligaments and capsular structures)	Sciatica	Neurogenic claudication
Initial Management	Scheduled extension Lumbar roll Night lumbar roll Medication as required	Scheduled flexion Limited extension Night lumbar roll Medication as required	Prone extension Supine "Z" lie Lumbar roll Night lumbar roll Medication as required	Abdominal exercises Night lumbar roll Sustained flexion Pelvic tilt Medication as required

Adapted from: American Academy of Orthopaedic Surgeons. Acute care: nontraumatic low back pain. *Orthopaedic Knowledge Update: Spine 2* 2001;153-166

Menopause/Hormone Replacement Therapy

- see <u>Gynecology</u>, GY34

Epidemiology
- mean age of menopause = 51.4 yr

Clinical Features
- associated with estrogen deprivation
- urogenital tract: atrophy, vaginal dryness/itching, urinary frequency/urgency/incontinence, bleeding
- blood vessels and heart: vasomotor instability (e.g. hot flashes), increased risk of heart disease
- bones: bone loss, joint/muscle/back pain, fractures, loss of height
- brain: depression, irritability, mood swings, memory loss

Management
- encourage physical exercise, smoking cessation, and a balanced diet with adequate intake/supplementation of calcium (1,200-1,500 mg/d) and vitamin D (800-2,000 IU/d)
- hormone replacement therapy (HRT)
  - prescribe for moderate to severe symptoms for no longer than 5 yr; routine use is not recommended
  - regimens: cyclic estrogen-progestin, continuous estrogen-progestin, estrogen only (if no uterus), estrogen patch/gel/cream/ring/vaginal tablet
  - decreases risk of osteoporotic fractures, colorectal cancer
  - increases risk of breast cancer, coronary heart disease, stroke, DVT, and PE
  - initiation of HRT requires a thorough discussion of short- and long-term benefits and risks
- consider venlafaxine, SSRIs, or gabapentin to ease vasomotor instability

Osteoarthritis

- see <u>Rheumatology</u>, RH5

Epidemiology
- most common form of arthritis seen in primary care
- prevalence is 10-12% and increases with age
- results in long-term disability in 2-3% of patients with OA
- almost everyone over the age of 65 shows signs of OA on x-ray, but only 33% of these individuals will be symptomatic

Clinical Features
- joint pain with activity, improved with rest, morning stiffness or gelling <30 min
- deformity, bony enlargement, crepitus, limitation of movement, peri-articular muscle atrophy
- usually affects distal joints of hands, spine, hips, and knees

Investigations
- no laboratory tests for the diagnosis of OA
- hallmark radiographic features: joint space narrowing, subchondral sclerosis, subchondral cysts, osteophytes

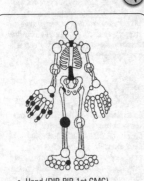

- Hand (DIP, PIP, 1st CMC)
- Hip
- Knee
- 1st MTP
- L-spine (L4-L5, L5-S1)
- C-spine
- Uncommon: ankle, shoulder, elbow, MCP, rest of wrist

© Linda Colati

Figure 13. Common sites of involvement in OA

Management
- goals: relieve pain, preserve joint motion and function, prevent further injury
- conservative
  - patient education, weight loss, low-impact exercise (OT/PT), assistive devices (e.g. canes, orthotics, raised toilet seats)
- pharmacological
  - consider comorbidities such as PUD, HTN, IHD, hepatic disease, and renal disease
  - medications do not alter natural course of OA
  - 1st line: acetaminophen up to 4 g/d (OA is not an inflammatory disorder)
  - 2nd line: NSAIDs in the lowest effective dose for the shortest duration of time, along with gastroprotection; COX-2 selective inhibitors (celecoxib/Celebrex®, Meloxicam/Mobicox®) are recommended if long-term treatment or if high risk for serious GI problems
  - combination analgesics (e.g. acetaminophen and codeine)
  - intra-articular hyaluronic acid injections
  - intra-articular corticosteroid injections (no more than 3-4x/yr) may be helpful in acute flares (benefits last 4-6 wk, can be up to 6 mo)
  - topical NSAID (diclofenac/Pennsaid®)
  - capsaicin cream (Zostrix®)
  - oral glucosamine
- surgery
  - consider if persistent significant pain and functional impairment despite optimal pharmacotherapy (e.g. debridement, osteotomy, total joint arthroplasty)

Glucosamine Therapy for Treating Osteoarthritis
Cochrane DB Syst Rev 2005;2:CD002946
This meta-analysis of 25 single- and double-blinded randomized controlled trials with 4,963 patients compared glucosamine treatment, administered by any route, against placebo or another treatment.
Conclusions: Glucosamine can decrease pain and functional impairment resulting from OA and is not associated with any side effects compared to placebo. Differences in the effectiveness of Rotta and non-Rotta preparations highlight variability between glucosamine preparations and patients should be made aware of this.

Osteoporosis

- see <u>Endocrinology</u>, E40

- for current guidelines and tools see www.osteoporosis.ca
- age-related disease characterized by decreased bone mass and increased susceptibility to fractures
- affects 1 in 4 Canadian women and 1 in 8 Canadian men

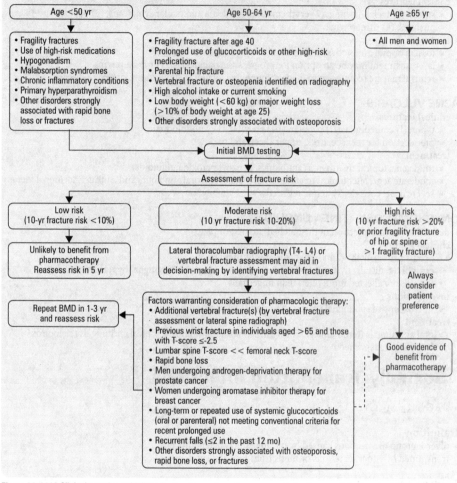

Figure 14. 2010 Clinical practice guidelines for the diagnosis and management of osteoporosis in Canada (integrated management model). Adapted from: *CMAJ* 2010;182:1864-1873

Management
- see <u>Endocrinology</u>, E42

Palliative and End-of-Life Care

- see <u>Geriatric Medicine</u>, GM12

Rash

ATOPIC DERMATITIS
- **clinical features**
  - affects all ages but is more common in children
  - pruritus is the most common symptom; scratching worsens the rash creating a vicious cycle
- **treatment**
  - goals: limit itching, repair skin
  - moisturizers, emollients, topical corticosteroids; oral corticosteroids and topical calcineurin inhibitors may be used

---

Disorders Strongly Associated with Osteoporosis Include
Primary hyperparathyroidism, type 1 DM, osteogenesis imperfecta, uncontrolled hyperthyroidism, hypogonadism or premature menopause (<45 yr), Cushing's disease, chronic malnutrition or malabsorption, chronic liver disease, COPD, and chronic inflammatory conditions (e.g. IBD)

10 Yr Fracture Risk Assessment
FRAX (WHO Fracture Risk Assessment Tool) and CAROC (Canadian Association of Radiologists and Osteoporosis Canada) have been validated in the Canadian Population FRAX and CAROC are available online from: https://www.osteoporosis.ca/health-care-professionals/clinical-tools-and-resources/

How much Calcium do we Need?

Age	
4-8	1,000 mg
9-18	1,300 mg
19-50	1,200 mg
>50	1,200 mg
Pregnant and lactating women 19-50	1,000 mg

Calcium Content of Common Foods
- 1 cup milk = 300 mg
- ¾ cup yogurt = 332 mg
- ½ can salmon with bones = 240 mg
- ½ cup cooked broccoli = 33 mg
- 1 medium orange = 50 mg

Vitamin D Content in Food
- Milk fortified with vitamin D_3 contains 100 IUs per 250 mL glass
- Foods such as margarine, eggs, chicken livers, salmon, sardines, herring, mackerel, swordfish, and fish oils (halibut and cod liver oils) all contain small amounts; supplementation is necessary to obtain adequate levels as dietary intake has minimal impact
- Most multivitamins provide 400 IUs of vitamin D_3

SEBORRHEIC DERMATITIS
- clinical features
  - affects all ages but is most common in infants within the first 3 mo of life (e.g. pityriasis capitis or "cradle cap") and adults age 30-60 yr
  - affects the scalp, central face, and anterior chest; often presents as scalp scaling (dandruff) in adolescents and adults
  - may cause mild to marked erythema of the nasolabial fold, often with greasy scaling
- treatment
  - topical antifungals, topical low-potency steroids; topical calcineurin inhibitors may be used

ROSACEA
- clinical features
  - stages: (1) facial flushing, (2) erythema and/or edema and ocular symptoms, (3) papules and pustules, (4) rhinophyma
- treatment
  - topical or oral antibiotics, oral retinoids
  - laser treatment may be an option for progressive telangiectasias or rhinophyma
  - referral may be required to manage rhinophyma, ocular complications, or severe disease

ACNE VULGARIS
- clinical features
  - types: (I) comedonal, (II) papular, (III) pustular, (IV) nodulocystic
  - predilection for the face, neck, upper chest, and back
- treatment
  - mild acne: topical treatments (antibiotics, benzoyl peroxide, retinoids)
  - moderate acne: after topical treatments have failed, add oral antibiotics and consider hormonal therapy
  - severe acne: consider systemic retinoids

ONYCHOMYCOSIS (TINEA UNGUIUM)
- **definition:** fungal infection of the nail bed, matrix, or plate
- clinical features
  - occurs primarily in adults, most commonly after age 60
  - crumbling, distally dystrophic nails; yellowish, opaque with subungual hyperkeratotic debris
  - toenails are affected more often than fingernails
- investigations
  - microscopy of subungual scrapings under KOH preparation, culture
- treatment
  - oral antifungals (terbinafine/Lamisil®, itraconazole/Sporanox®), topical antifungals (ciclopirox/Loprox®) are less effective

Sexually Transmitted Infections

- see Gynecology, GY27

Definition
- diverse group of infections caused by multiple microbial pathogens
- transmitted by either secretions or fluids from mucosal surfaces

Epidemiology
- high incidence rates worldwide
- Canadian prevalence in clinical practice
  - common: chlamydia (most common), gonorrhea (2nd most common), HPV, genital herpes (increasing incidence of chlamydia and gonorrhea)
  - less common: hepatitis B, HIV, and syphilis (increasing in incidence), trichomoniasis
  - rare: chancroid, granuloma inguinale, lymphogranuloma venereum
- non-sexually transmitted genital tract infections: vulvovaginal candidiasis (VVC), bacterial vaginosis (BV)
- three most common infections associated with vaginal discharge in adult women are BV, VVC, and trichomoniasis

History
- sexual history
  - age of first intercourse, sexual orientation, sexual activity (oral, anal, and/or vaginal intercourse), sexual activity during travel
  - total number of partners in the past year/month/week and duration of involvement with each
- STI history
  - STI awareness, contraception, previous STIs and testing (including Pap tests), partner communication regarding STIs
  - local symptoms such as burning, itching, discharge, sores, vesicles, testicular pain, dysuria, abdominal pain
  - systemic symptoms such as fever, lymphadenopathy, arthralgia

When an STI is detected in a child, evaluation for sexual abuse is mandatory

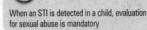

STI Risk Factors
- Sexually active males and females <25 yr old
- Unprotected sex, sexual contact with a known case of STI, previous STI
- New sexual partner or >2 sexual partners in the past 12 mo
- Street involved, homeless, and/or substance abuse

Sexual History
5 P's
Partners (numbers, gender)
Practices (vaginal, oral, anal insertive/receptive)
Protection
Past history of STIs
Pregnancy prevention

Investigations/Screening
- individuals at increased risk, even those who are asymptomatic, should be screened for chlamydia, gonorrhea, hepatitis B, HIV, and syphilis
- Pap test if none performed in the preceding 12 mo

Management
- primary prevention is vastly more effective than treating STIs and their sequelae
- offer hepatitis B vaccine if not immune
- offer Gardasil® to women over 9 years of age (can be offered to men as well but not covered by OHIP)
- discuss STI risk factors (e.g. decreasing the number of sexual partners)
- direct advice to ALWAYS use condoms or to abstain from intercourse
- condoms are not 100% effective against HPV or HSV
- an STI patient is not considered treated until the management of his/her partner(s) is ensured (contact tracing by Public Health)
- patients diagnosed with bacterial STI or trichomonal infection should abstain from sexual activity until treatment completion and for 7 d after treatment for both partners, or until test of cure completed
- mandatory reporting: chlamydia, gonorrhea, hepatitis B, HIV, syphilis

Efficacy of Human Papillomavirus Vaccines – A Systematic Quantitative Review
Int J Gynecol Cancer 2009;19:1166-1176
Study: Systematic review of 6 randomized placebo-controlled double-blind trials.
Patients: 47,236 women between ages 9-26.
Intervention: Vaccination with HPV L1 virus-like particle in either quadrivalent (HPV 6, 11, 16, 18), bivalent (HPV 16, 18), or univalent (HPV 16) form vs. placebo.
Main Outcome: Prevention of cytologically and/or histologically proven lesions (including LSIL, HSIL, VIN, VAIN, AIN, adenocarcinoma in situ of the cervix, or cancer of the cervix associated with HPV infection).
Results: Bivalent and quadrivalent vaccines reduced the rate of lesions in the cervix, vulva, vagina, and anogenital region with efficacy of 93% and 62%, respectively.

Table 28. Diagnosis and Treatment of Common STIs

	Signs and Symptoms	Investigations	Treatment	Complications
Gonococcal Urethritis/ Cervicitis (*Neisseria gonorrhoeae*)	M: urethral discharge, unexplained pyuria, dysuria, irritation, testicular swelling, Sx of epididymitis F: mucopurulent endocervical discharge, vaginal bleeding, dysuria, pelvic pain, dyspaurenia M and F: often asymptomatic, can involve rectal symptoms in cases of unprotected anal sex	M: urethral swab for Gram stain and culture F: urine PCR, endocervical swab for Gram stain and culture, vaginal swab for wet mount (to rule out trichomonas) M and F: urine PCR, rectal/pharyngeal swabs if indicated	Ceftriaxone 250 mg IM single dose* If risk factors for treatment failure (e.g. pregnancy, pharyngeal/rectal infection, potentially reduced susceptibility) Test of cure: culture 4 d post-treatment (preferred) or urine PCR 2 wk post treatment (alternative) If no risk factors, rescreen 6-12 months post treatment	M: urethral strictures, epididymitis, infertility F: PID, infertility, ectopic pregnancy, perinatal infection, chronic pelvic pain M and F: Arthritis, increased risk of acquiring and transmitting HIV
Non-Gonococcal Urethritis/Cervicitis (Usually *Chlamydia trachomatis***)	~70% asymptomatic If symptoms appear (usually 2-6 wk after infection) then similar to gonococcal symptoms (see above)	Same as above	Azithromycin 1 g PO single dose + gonococcal urethritis/cervicitis Rx* Same follow-up as above	Same as above
Human Papillomavirus (genital warts, cervical dysplasia)	Most are asymptomatic M: cauliflower lesions (condylomata acuminata) on skin/mucosa of penile or anal area F: cauliflower lesions and/or pre-neoplastic/neoplastic lesions on cervix/vagina/vulva	None needed if simple condylomata Potential biopsy of suspicious lesions F: screening for cervical dysplasia through regular Pap smears	For condylomata: cryotherapy, electrocautery, laser excision, topical therapy (patient-applied or office-based) For cervical dysplasia: colposcopy and possible excision, dependent on grade of lesion	M and F: anal cancer MSM and F who have receptive anal sex: rectal cancer F: cervical/vaginal/vulvar cancer
Genital Herpes (HSV-1 and -2)	1° episode: painful vesiculocerative genital lesions ± fever, tender lymphadenopathy, protracted course Recurrent episodes: less extensive lesions, shorter course may have "trigger factors"	Swab of vesicular content for culture, type-specific serologic testing for HSV-1 vs. HSV-2 antibodies and to determine 1° vs. recurrent episode	1° Episode Acyclovir 200 mg PO 5x/d x 5-10 d or Famciclovir 250 mg PO tid x 5 d or Valacyclovir 1,000 mg PO bid x 10 d Recurrent Episode Acyclovir 200 mg PO 5x/d x 5d or 800 mg PO tid x 2 d or Famciclovir 125 mg PO bid x 5 d or Valacyclovir 500 mg PO bid x 3 d or 1,000 mg PO OD x 3 d	Genital pain, urethritis, cervicitis, aseptic meningitis, increased risk of acquiring and transmitting HIV
Infectious Syphilis (*Treponema pallidum*)	1°: chancre (painless sore), regional lymphadenopathy 2°: rash and flu-like symptoms, meningitis, H/A, uveitis, retinitis, condyloma lata, mucus lesions, alopecia Latent Phase: asymptomatic 3°: neurologic, cardiovascular, and tissue complications	Specimen collection from 1° and 2° lesions, screen high risk individuals with serologic syphilis testing (VDRL), universal screening of pregnant women	Benzathine penicillin G IM (dose depends on stage and patient population. Check Public Health Canada guidelines) Notify partners (last 3-12 mo) Continuous follow-up and testing until patients are seronegative	Chronic neurologic and cardiovascular sequelae, increased risk of acquiring and transmitting HIV

F = females; M = males
*N.B. if urethritis/cervicitis is suspected, always treat for both gonococcal and non-gonococcal types (i.e. ceftriaxone AND azithromycin)
**Most common reportable STI in Canada

Sinusitis

- see <u>Otolaryngology</u>, OT24

Etiology
- viral etiology is more common
- viral: rhinovirus, influenza, parainfluenza
- bacterial: *S. pneumoniae, H. influenzae, M. catarrhalis*

Management of Acute Sinusitis
- may provide symptom relief: oral analgesics (acetaminophen, NSAIDs), nasal saline rinse, short-term use of topical or oral decongestants
- do not prescribe antihistamines
- intra-nasal corticosteroids if diagnosed with mild to moderate acute bacterial sinusitis
- antibiotics and intra-nasal corticosteroids if diagnosed with severe acute bacterial sinusitis
- ENT referral if: anatomic defect (e.g. deviated septum, polyp, adenoid hypertrophy), failure of second-line therapy, ≥4 episodes/yr, development of complications (e.g. mucocele, orbital extension, meningitis, intra-cranial abscess, venous sinus thrombosis)

Red Flags for Urgent Referral
- Altered mental status
- Headache
- Systemic toxicity
- Swelling of the orbit or change in visual acuity or EOM
- Hard neurological findings
- Signs of meningeal irritation
- Suspected intra-cranial complications (meningitis, intra-cranial abscess, cavernous sinus thrombosis)
- Involvement of associated structures (periorbital cellulitis, Pott's puffy tumour)

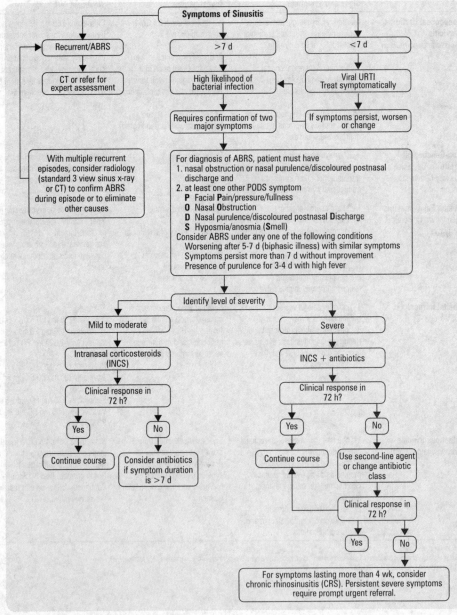

Figure 15. Diagnosis and management of sinusitis
ABRS = acute bacterial rhinosinusitis
Adapted from: Desrosiers M, et al. *Allergy Asthma Clin Immunol* 2011;7:doi:10.1186/1710-1492-7-2

Sleep Disorders

- see Respirology, R31 and Neurology, N46

Definition
- most often characterized by one of three complaints
  - insomnia
    - difficulty falling asleep, difficulty maintaining sleep, early-morning wakening, non-refreshing sleep
  - parasomnias
    - night terrors, nightmares, restless leg syndrome, somnambulism (performing complex behaviour during sleep with eyes open but without memory of event)
  - excessive daytime sleepiness

Epidemiology
- 1/3 of patients in primary care setting have occasional sleep problems, 10% have chronic sleep problems

Etiology
- primary sleep disorders
  - primary insomnia, narcolepsy, obstructive sleep apnea, restless leg syndrome, periodic limb movements of sleep
- secondary causes
  - medical: COPD, asthma, CHF, hyperthyroidism, chronic pain, BPH, menopause, GERD, PUD, pregnancy, neurological disorders
  - drugs: alcohol, caffeine, nicotine, nicotine replacement therapy, β-agonists, antidepressants, steroids
  - psychiatric: mood and anxiety disorders
  - lifestyle factors: shift work, jet-lag

Investigations
- complete sleep diary every morning for 1-2 wk
  - record bedtime, sleep latency, total sleep time, awakenings, quality of sleep
- rule out specific medical problems (e.g. CBC and differential, TSH)
- refer for sleep study, nocturnal polysomnogram, or daytime multiple sleep latency test if suspicion of sleep apnea or periodic leg movements of sleep

Treatment of Specific Problems
- **Primary insomnia**
  - majority of cases
  - person reacts to insomnia with fear or anxiety around bedtime or with a change in sleep hygiene, which can progress to a chronic disorder (psychophysiological insomnia)
  - treat any suspected medical or psychiatric cause
  - behaviour-based treatment
  - sleep hygiene: avoid alcohol, caffeine, nicotine; comfortable sleep environment; regular sleep schedule; no napping
  - exercise regularly, avoid heavy exercise within 3 h of bedtime
  - relaxation therapy: deep breathing, meditation, biofeedback
  - stimulus control therapy: re-association of bed/bedroom with sleep, re-establishment of a consistent sleep-wake schedule, reduce activities that cue staying awake
    - sleep restriction therapy: total time in bed should closely match the total sleep time of the patient (improves sleep efficacy)
    - CBT: address inappropriate beliefs and attitudes that perpetuate dysfunctional sleep
  - pharmacologic treatment
    - short-acting benzodiazepines (e.g. lorazepam, oxazepam, temazepam) at the lowest effective dose should be used <7 consecutive nights to break cycle of chronic insomnia or to manage an exacerbation of previously controlled primary insomnia
    - non-benzodiazepines: zoplicone (Imovane®), zolpidem (Sublinox®), melatonin, low dose anti-depressants with sedating properties (amitriptyline, trazodone, mirtazapine)
    - follow-up every 2-4 wk initially (to reinforce behavioural interventions and renew/consider pharmacotherapy) then every 3 mo; if no progress or limited improvement, consider referral to sleep medicine program
- **Snoring**
  - results from soft tissue vibration at the back of the nose and throat due to turbulent airflow through narrowed air passages
  - physical exam: obesity, nasal polyps, septal deviation, hypertrophy of the nasal turbinates, enlarged uvula and tonsils
  - investigations (only if severely symptomatic): nocturnal polysomnography and airway assessment (CT/MRI)
  - treatment
    - sleep on side (position therapy), weight loss
    - nasal dilators (noninvasive external dilator made with elastic adhesive backing applied over nasal bridge), tongue-retaining devices, mandibular advancement devices
  - at risk of developing obstructive sleep apnea

- **Obstructive Sleep Apnea (OSA)**
  - apnea (no breathing for ≥10 s) resulting from upper airway obstruction due to collapse of the base of the tongue, soft palate with uvula, and epiglottis; respiratory effort is present
  - leads to a distinctive snorting, choking, awakening type pattern as the body rouses itself to open the airway (resuscitative breath)
  - apneic episodes can last from 20 s-3 min and occur 100-600 episodes/night
  - diagnosis is based on nocturnal polysomnography: >15 apneic/hypopneic episodes per hour of sleep with arousal recorded
  - consequences
    - daytime somnolence, non-restorative sleep
    - poor social and work performance
    - mood changes: anxiety, irritability, depression
    - sexual dysfunction: poor libido, impotence
    - morning headache (due to hypercapnia)
    - HTN (2x increased risk), CAD (3x increased risk), stroke (4x increased risk), arrhythmias
    - OSA is an independent risk factor for CAD
    - pulmonary HTN, right ventricular dysfunction, cor pulmonale (due to chronic hypoxemia)
    - memory loss, decreased concentration, confusion
  - investigations
    - valuate BP, inspect nose and oropharynx (enlarged adenoids or tonsils)
    - blood gas not helpful, TSH if clinically indicated
    - nocturnal polysomnography
  - treatment
    - modifiable factors: avoid sleeping supine; weight loss; avoid alcohol, sedatives, opioids; inhaled steroids if nasal swelling present; dental appliances to modify mandibular position
    - primary treatment of OSA is CPAP: maintains patent airway in 95% of OSA cases
    - surgery: somnoplasty, uvulopalatopharyngoplasty (UPPP), tonsillectomy, and adenoidectomy (in children)
    - report patient to Ministry of Transportation if OSA is not controlled by CPAP

Sore Throat (Pharyngitis)

Definition
- inflammation of the oropharynx
- may be caused by a wide range of infectious organisms, most of which produce a self-limited infection with no significant sequelae

Etiology
- viral: adenovirus, rhinovirus, influenza virus, RSV, EBV, coxsackie virus, herpes simplex virus, CMV, HIV
- bacterial: Group A β-Hemolytic *Streptococcus* (GABHS), Group C and Group β-Hemolytic *Streptococcus*, *Neisseria gonorrhoeae*, *Chlamydia pneumoniae*, *Mycoplasma pneumoniae*, *Corynebacterium diphtheriae*

Epidemiology
- viral
  - most common cause (90% in adults is viral), occurs year round
- bacterial
  - GABHS (Group A β-Hemolytic Streptococcal Infections)
    - most common bacterial cause
    - occurs most often in winter months
    - 5-15% of adult cases and up to 50% of all pediatric cases of acute pharyngitis
    - most prevalent between 5-17 yr old

Clinical Features
- viral
  - pharyngitis, conjunctivitis, rhinorrhea, hoarseness, cough
  - nonspecific flu-like symptoms such as fever, malaise, and myalgia
  - often mimics bacterial infection
  - common viral infections
    - EBV (infectious mononucleosis)
      - pharyngitis, tonsillar exudate, fever, lymphadenopathy, fatigue, rash
    - coxsackie virus (hand, foot, and mouth disease)
      - primarily late summer, early fall
      - sudden onset of fever, pharyngitis, headache, abdominal pain, and vomiting
      - appearance of small vesicles that rupture and ulcerate on soft palate, tonsils, pharynx
      - ulcers are pale grey and several mm in diameter, have surrounding erythema, and may appear on hands and feet
    - herpes simplex virus
      - like coxsackie virus but ulcers are fewer and larger
      - pharyngitis, tonsillar exudate, fever, lymphadenopathy, fatigue, rash

- bacterial
  - symptoms: pharyngitis, fever, malaise, headache, abdominal pain, absence of cough
  - signs: fever, tonsillar or pharyngeal erythema/exudate, swollen/tender anterior cervical nodes, halitosis
  - complications: rheumatic fever, glomerulonephritis, suppurative complications (abscess, sinusitis, otitis media, cervical adenitis, pneumonia), meningitis, impetigo

Investigations
- suspected GABHS
  - see Table 29 for approach to diagnosis and management of GABHS
  - gold standard for diagnosis is throat culture
  - rapid test for streptococcal antigen: high specificity (95%) but low sensitivity (50-90%)
  - suspected EBV (infectious mononucleosis)
    - peripheral blood smear, heterophile antibody test (i.e. the latex agglutination assay or "monospot")

Table 29. Modified Centor Score: Approach to Diagnosis and Management of GABHS

	POINTS
Cough absent?	1
History of fever >38°C?	1
Tonsillar exudate?	1
Swollen, tender anterior nodes?	1
Age 3-14	1
Age 15-44	0
Age >45	−1

In communities with moderate levels of strep infection (10-20% of sore throats):

Score	0	1	2	3	4 or more
Chance patient has strep	1-2.5%	5-10%	11-17%	28-35%	51-53%
Suggested action	NO culture or antibiotic		Culture all, treat with antibiotics only if culture is positive		Culture all, treat with antibiotics on clinical grounds[1], discontinue antibiotics if culture comes back negative

[1]Clinical grounds include a high fever or other indicators that the patient is clinically unwell and is presenting early in the course of the illness
Limitations: *This score is not applicable to patients <3 yr of age
    *If an outbreak or epidemic of illness caused by GABHS is occuring in any community, the score is invalid and should not be used
Adapted from: Centor RM, et al. Med Decis Making 1981;1:239-46; McIssac WI, et al. CMAJ 1998;158:75-83

Management
- viral pharyngitis
  - antibiotics not indicated
  - symptomatic therapy: acetaminophen/NSAIDs for fever and muscle aches, decongestants
- GABHS
  - antibiotic treatment decreases severity and duration of symptoms, risk of transmission (after 24 h of treatment), and risk of rheumatic fever and suppurative complications
  - incidence of glomerulonephritis is not decreased with antibiotic treatment
  - no increased incidence of rheumatic fever with 48 h delay in antibiotic treatment; if possible, delay antibiotic treatment until culture confirms diagnosis
  - routine F/U and/or post-treatment throat cultures are not required for most patients
  - F/U throat culture only recommended for: patients with history of rheumatic fever, patients of family member(s) with history of acute rheumatic fever, suspected streptococcal carrier
- infectious mononucleosis (EBV)
  - self-limiting course; antibiotics are not indicated
  - symptomatic treatment: acetaminophen/NSAIDs for fever, pharyngitis, malaise
  - avoid heavy physical activity and contact sports for at least one month or until splenomegaly resolves because of risk of splenic rupture
  - if acute airway obstruction, give corticosteroids and consult ENT

Complementary and Alternative Medicine

Most Common Uses of CAM
- Back/neck problems
- Gynecological problems
- Anxiety
- Headaches
- Digestive problems
- Chronic fatigue syndromes

Epidemiology
- 50-75% of Canadians report some use of CAM over their lifetime, and only half will disclose this use to their physician
- use is highest in Western provinces and lowest in Atlantic provinces
- more likely to be used by younger patients and those with higher education and income
- examples: chiropractic, acupuncture, massage, naturopathy, homeopathy, traditional Chinese medicine, craniosacral therapy, osteopathy

Herbal Products
- over 50% of Canadians use natural health products (NHPs)
- most commonly used include echinacea, ginseng, ginkgo, garlic, St. John's wort, and soy
- relatively few herbal products have been shown to be effective in clinical trials
- many patients believe herbal products are inherently safe and are unaware of potential side effects and interactions with conventional medicines
- all NHPs must be regulated under The Natural Health Products Regulations as of January 1, 2004, including herbal remedies, homeopathic medicines, vitamins, minerals, traditional medicines, probiotics, amino acids, and essential fatty acids (e.g. omega-3)
- always ask patients whether they are taking any herbal product, herbal supplement, or other natural remedy. Further questions may include:
  - Are you taking any prescription or non-prescription medications for the same purpose as the herbal product?
  - Are you allergic to any plant products?
  - Are you pregnant or breastfeeding?
- information resources: National Center for CAM (www.nccam.nih.gov), Health Canada website

Table 30. Common Herbal Products

Common Name	Reported Uses	Possible Adverse Effects	Possible Drug Interactions
Black Cohosh	Menopausal symptoms, PMS, labour induction, arthritis	Hepatitis, liver failure, headaches, GI discomfort, heaviness in legs, weight problems	None reported
Chamomile	Mild sedative, anxiolytic, GI complaints, common cold	Allergic/contact dermatitis, anaphylaxis	Anxiolytics, sedatives
Echinacea	Common cold, flu, wound treatment, UTI, cancer	Hypersensitivity, hepatotoxicity with prolonged use, avoid use if immunosuppressed	Potentiates warfarin
Evening Primrose	Dysmenorrhea, menopausal sx, inflammation, allergies, eczema, arthritis, MS	Headache, restlessness, nausea, diarrhea, may decrease seizure threshold	Anticoagulants, antiplatelets
Feverfew	Migraine prevention, RA, anti-inflammatory	Anxiety, upset stomach, skin rash, miscarriage	Anticoagulants, antiplatelets
Flaxseed Oil	Laxative, menopausal symptoms, source of omega-3 fatty acids	Diarrhea	Do not take with other medications as fibre content can bind drugs
Garlic	Elevated lipids, HTN, hyperglycemia, antimicrobial	GI irritation, contact dermatitis, may increase post-operative bleeding	Anticoagulants, potentiates antihypertensives
Ginger	Nausea, motion sickness, dyspepsia, anti-inflammatory	Heartburn, not to be used for morning sickness	None known
Ginkgo Biloba	Increases peripheral circulation (AD, dementia, intermittent claudication), premenstrual syndrome, vertigo	Headache, cramping, bleeding, mild digestive problems; reports of intracranial hemorrhage	Anticoagulants, thiazide diuretics, MAO inhibitors
Ginseng	Energy enhancer, decreases stress, adjunct support for chemotherapy/radiation	HTN, nervousness, insomnia, breakthrough bleeding, palpitations	Stimulant medications, antihypertensives, hormonal therapies
Glucosamine (Chondroitin)	Osteoarthritis	GI distress, headache, drowsiness, palpitations	Caution if shellfish allergy
Saw Palmetto	BPH, adjunct to finasteride	Mild GI distress	α-adrenergics, finasteride
St. John's Wort	Mild to moderate depression	Photosensitivity, increased liver enzymes, drowsiness, dizziness, nausea, headache	CNS depressants, contraindicated with indinavir
Valerian Root	Sedative, anxiolytic, muscle relaxant, PMS	Drowsiness, headache, digestive problems, paradoxical insomnia	CNS depressants, antihistamines

Zink T, Chaffin J. Herbal "health" products: What family physicians need to know. *American Family Physician* 1998;58:1133-1140; NIH National Center for Complementary and Alternative Medicine website (http://nccam.nih.gov/)

Primary Care Models

Table 31. Primary Care Models (Adapted from www.healthforceontario.ca)

	Characteristics
Comprehensive Care Model	FPs/GPs in solo practice with limited after-hours availability Payment model: fee-for-service
Family Health Team	Groups of health care professionals (e.g. FPs, GPs, RNs, NPs, dieticians, social workers) Wider range of services (e.g. rehabilitation, palliative care), with increased after-hours availability Receives provincial funding for allied health Patient enrolment is strongly encouraged Payment model: paid annually per patient rostered depending on demographic category (blended capitation model)
Family Health Group	Group of ≥3 FPs, can utilize nurse-staffed, telephone health advisory services to provide around the clock primary care coverage Physicians commit to enroll patients Payment model: blended capitation model i.e. age- and sex-adjusted base rate remuneration plus bonuses and incentives
Family Health Network	Group of ≥3 FPs, can utilize nurse practitioners, with telephone health advisory services to provide around the clock primary care coverage Payment model: salary-based
Family Health Organization	Same as FHT but usually larger in scale in terms of personnel Physicians commit to enrol patients Must sign governance and Family Health Organization agreements to join Payment model: blended capitation model i.e. age- and sex-adjusted base rate remuneration plus bonuses and incentives

Antimicrobial Quick Reference

Condition	Microorganisms	Antimicrobial
RESPIRATORY/ENT		
Acute Rhinitis (common cold)	Rhinovirus, coronavirus, influenza, RSV, parainflunenza, adenovirus	None
Pharyngitis (sore throat)	Rhinovirus, adenovirus, influenza, parainfluenza, coxsackievirus, coronavirus	None
Strep Pharyngitis	Group A β-Hemolytic *Streptococcus*	*Children:* <u>1st line:</u> penicillin V 40 mg/kg/d PO div bid-tid (max 750 mg/d) x 10 d (use adult dose if >27 kg) amoxicillin 40 mg/kg/d PO div bid-tid x 10 d <u>2nd line:</u> erythromycin estolate 40 mg/kg/d PO div bid-tid x 10 d <u>3rd line:</u> cephalexin 25-50 mg/kg/d PO div qid x 10 d cefprozil 15 mg/kg/d PO div bid x 10 d *Adults:* <u>1st line:</u> penicillin V 300 mg PO tid or 600 mg bid x 10 d <u>2nd line:</u> erythromycin 250 mg PO qid x 10 d <u>3rd line:</u> cephalexin 250 mg PO qid x 10 d cefadroxil 500 mg PO bid x 10 d
Sinusitis	S. pneumoniae H. influenzae M. catarrhalis S. aureus	*Children:* <u>1st line:</u> amoxicillin 80 mg/kg/d PO div bid-tid x 5-10 d (max 3 g/d) x 10-14 d <u>2nd line:</u> amoxicillin/clavulanate 40-80 mg/kg/d div bid (max 3 g/d) x 10-14 d cefprozil 30 mg/kg/d PO div bid x 10-14 d <u>3rd line:</u> cefuroxime-AX 30-40 mg/kg/d PO div bid x 10-14 d clarithromycin 15 mg/kg/d PO div bid x 10-14 d *Adults:* <u>1st line:</u> amoxicillin 500 mg PO tid x 5-10 d <u>2nd line:</u> amoxicillin/clavulanate 500 or 875 mg PO bid x 5-10 d cefuroxime-AX 250-500 mg PO bid x 5-10 d <u>3rd line:</u> levofloxacin 500 mg PO OD x 5-10 d moxifloxacin 400 mg PO OD x 5-10 d

Condition	Microorganisms	Antimicrobial
RESPIRATORY/ENT		
Acute Otitis Media	*S. pneumoniae* *H. influenzae* *M. catarrhalis* Group A *Strep* *S. aureus*	*Children:* Treat if under age 6 mo If age 6-24 mo, watchful waiting appropriate if parents can observe child for 48-72 h with appropriate medical follow-up If age >24 mo, treat if worsens after 48-72 h 10 d course if age <24 mo, 5 d course if age >24 mo <u>1st line</u>: amoxicillin 80 mg/kg/d PO div bid-tid (max 3 g/d) <u>2nd line</u>: amoxicillin/clavulanate 40-80 mg/kg/d PO div bid (max 3 g/d) cefprozil 30 mg/kg/d PO div bid <u>3rd line</u>: cefuroxime-AX 30-40 mg/kg/d PO div bid clarithromycin 15 mg/kg/d PO div bid Chronic TM perforation or ventilation tubes: Ciprodex® otic suspension 4 drops bid x 5 d *Adults:* <u>1st line</u>: amoxicillin 500 mg PO tid x 7-10 d <u>2nd line</u>: amoxicillin/clavulanate 500 mg PO tid or 875 mg PO bid x 7-10 d cefprozil 250-500 mg PO bid x 7-10 d Chronic TM perforation or ventilation tubes: Ciprodex® otic suspension 4 drops bid x 5 d
Otitis Externa	*P. aeruginosa* Coliforms *S. aureus*	Cortisporin® otic solution 4 drops tid or qid (3 drops tid or qid for children) TM defect: Ciprodex® otic suspension 4 drops bid x 5 d Necrotizing (i.e. bone involvement): ciprofloxacin 750 mg PO bid x 4-8 wk
Bronchitis	*H. influenzae,* parainfluenza, coronavirus, rhinovirus, RSV	None
Community Acquired Pneumonia: Outpatient without Comorbidity	*S. pneumoniae* *M. pneumoniae* *C. pneumoniae*	<u>1st line</u>: amoxicillin 1,000 mg PO tid x 7-14 d (for patients over age 50 where mycoplasma infection is less likely) erythromycin 500 mg PO qid x 7-14 d clarithromycin 500 mg PO bid or 1,000 mg (ER) PO OD x 7-14 d azithromycin 500 mg PO on 1st d then 250 mg PO OD x 4 d or 500 mg PO OD x 3 d <u>2nd line</u>: doxycycline 100 mg PO on 1st d then 100 mg PO OD x 7-14 d
Community Acquired Pneumonia: Outpatient with Comorbidity	*S. pneumoniae* *M. pneumoniae* *C. pneumoniae* *H. influenzae*	**ANYONE of the β-lactam agents below:** amoxicillin 1,000 mg PO tid x 7-14 d amoxicillin/clavulanate 500 mg PO tid or 875 mg PO bid x 7-14 d cefuroxime-AX 500 mg PO bid x 7-14 d cefprozil 500 mg PO bid x 7-14 d **PLUS ONE of the following:** clarithromycin 500 mg PO bid or 1,000 mg (ER) PO OD x 7-14 d azithromycin 500 mg PO OD on 1st d then 250 mg PO OD x 4 d doxycycline 100 mg PO bid on 1st d then 100 mg PO OD x 7-14 d **OR ANY ONE of the following:** levofloxacin 750 mg PO OD x 7-14 d moxifloxacin 400 mg PO OD x 7-14 d
Dental Infections/ Periapical and Periodontal Abscesses	Oral Flora	penicillin V potassium 500 mg PO qid x 7-10 d clindamycin 300 mg PO qid or 600 mg bid x 7-10 d
GASTROENTEROLOGY		
Diarrhea – Enteritis	Enterotoxigenic *E. coli* (ETEC) *Campylobacter* *Salmonella* *Shigella* Viruses Protozoa	<u>Mild to moderate</u> (i.e. <3 BM/d, no blood, no fever): OTC loperamide 4 mg PO STAT then 2 mg PO after each loose stool (max 8 doses/d) OTC bismuth subsalicylate (Pepto Bismol®) 2 tabs or 30 mL repeat q30min prn (max 8 doses/d) (prevention: 2 tabs or 30 mL qid with meals and in the evening) <u>Moderate to severe</u> (i.e. >3 BM/d, blood, fever): ofloxacin 400 mg PO single dose or 300 mg PO bid x 3 d (prevention: 300 mg PO OD) norfloxacin 800 mg PO single dose or 400 mg PO bid x 1-3 d (prevention: 400 mg PO OD) ciprofloxacin 750 mg PO single dose or 500 mg PO bid x 1-3 d (prevention: 500 mg PO OD) levofloxacin 500 mg PO OD x 1-3 d (prevention: 500 mg PO OD) azithromycin 1,000 mg PO single dose or 500 mg PO OD x 1-3 d (children: 10 mg/kg/d x 3 d) *Azithromycin:* Recommended primarily for Thailand, India, Nepal, and Indonesia where *Campylobacter* resistance to quinolones is high Considered drug of choice for children because of safety, tolerability, and ease of administration
Diarrhea – Post Abx (common with clindamycin)	*C. difficile*	<u>Mild to moderate</u> (WBC <5 x 10⁹/L and Cr <1.5 x baseline): metronidazole 500 mg PO tid or 250 mg PO qid x 10 d (children: 15-30 mg/kg/d PO div tid-qid max 4 g/d) <u>Severe</u> (WBC ≥15 x 10⁹/L and Cr ≥1.5 x baseline): vancomycin 125 mg PO qid x 10-14 d (children: 40 mg/kg/d PO div tid-qid x 10-14 d max 2 g/d)
Peptic Ulcer Disease (non-NSAID related)	*H. pylori*	<u>1st line</u>: (PPI PO bid + amoxicillin 1,000 mg PO bid + clarithromycin 500 mg PO bid x 7 d [e.g. HP-PAC: lansoprazole 30 mg PO bid + amoxicillin 1,000 mg PO bid + clarithromycin 500 mg PO bid x 7 d]) (PPI PO bid + metronidazole 500 mg PO bid + clarithromycin 500 mg or 250 mg PO bid x 7 d) <u>2nd line</u>: (PPI PO bid + metronidazole 500 mg PO bid + amoxicillin 1,000 mg PO bid x 7 d) (PPI PO bid + bismuth subsalicylate 2 tabs or 30 mL qid + metronidazole 250 mg PO qid + tetracycline 500 mg PO qid x 7-14 d) PPI: lansoprazole 30 mg or omeprazole 20 mg or pantoprazole 40 mg or rabeprazole 20 mg

Condition	Microorganisms	Antimicrobial
DERMATOLOGIC		
Head and Pubic Lice (crabs)	*Pediculosis humanus capitis* *Phthirus pubis*	permethrin cream 1%: apply as liquid onto washed hair for 10 min, then rinse; repeat in 1 wk
Vulvovaginal Candidiasis	*Candida*	Treat only if patient is symptomatic fluconazole 150 mg PO single dose miconazole 2% cream (Monistat 7®): one applicator (5 g) intravaginally qhs x 7 d multiple other OTC azole treatments
Bacterial Vaginosis	Overgrowth of: *G. vaginalis* *M. hominis* Anaerobes	If patient is asymptomatic, treatment is unnecessary unless high-risk pregnancy, prior IUD insertion, gynecologic surgery, induced abortion, or upper tract instrumentation <u>1st line:</u> metronidazole 500 mg PO bid x 7 d metronidazole 0.75% gel: one applicator (5 g) intravaginally qhs x 5 d clindamycin 2% cream: one applicator (5 g) intravaginally qhs x 7 d <u>2nd line:</u> metronidazole 2 g PO single dose clindamycin 300 mg PO bid x 7 d
Herpes	Herpes simplex virus	<u>1° episode:</u> acyclovir 400 mg PO tid x 5-7 d famciclovir 250 mg PO tid x 5-7 d valacyclovir 500-1,000 mg PO bid x 5-7 d <u>Recurrent Episode:</u> acyclovir 400 mg PO tid x 5 d or 800 mg PO bid x 5 d or 800 mg PO tid x 2 d famciclovir 125 mg PO bid x 5 d valacyclovir 500 mg PO bid x 3 d or 1,000 mg PO OD x 3 d <u>Pregnancy:</u> 1° episode: acyclovir 200 mg PO 5x/d x 5-10 d Prior infection within previous yr: acyclovir 200 mg PO qid at 36 wk valacyclovir 500 mg PO bid at 36 wk
Gonorrhea/Chlamydia	*N. gonorrhoeae* *C. trachomatis*	ceftriaxone 250 mg IM x 1 dose + azithromycin 1 g PO single dose or doxycycline 100 mg PO bid x 7 d
Mastitis	*S. aureus* *S. pyogenes*	cloxacillin 500 mg PO qid x 7 d cephalexin 500 mg PO qid x 7 d
Tinea Cruris/Pedis (jock itch/athlete's foot)	Trichophyton	clotrimazole 1% cream bid ketoconazole 2% cream bid
Uncomplicated Cellulitis	*S. aureus* Group A *Streptococcus*	*Children:* <u>1st line:</u> cephalexin 50-100 mg/kg/d div qid x 10-14 d <u>2nd line:</u> cloxacillin 50 mg/kg/d div qid x 10-14 d clindamycin 25 mg/kg/d x 10-14 d *Adults:* <u>1st line:</u> cephalexin 500 mg PO qid x 10-14 d <u>2nd line:</u> cloxacillin 500 mg PO qid x 10-14 d clindamycin 300 mg PO x 10-14 d

References

Comprehensive Family Medicine Resources
The Hub -Family Medicine. Department of Family and Community Medicine, The University of Toronto. Available from: http://thehub.utoronto.ca/family/
Ponka D, Kirlew M. Top 10 Differential Diagnosis in Primary Care. 2006. Available from http://www.familymedicine.uottawa.ca/assets/documents/underGrad/Top10_Differential_Diagnosis_In_Primary_Care.pdf

Abuse
Fogarty CT, Burge S, McCord E. Communicating with patients about intimate partner violence: screening and interviewing approaches. Fam Med 2002;34:369-375.
National Center on Elder Abuse at the American Public Human Services Association. National elder abuse incidence study. Available from: http://www.aoa.gov/eldfam/Elder_Rights/Elder_Abuse/AbuseReport_Full.pdf
Wathen CN, MacMillan HL. Interventions for violence against women. JAMA 2003;289:589-599.

Breast Cancer Screening Guidelines
CTFPHC Breast Cancer Screening Guidelines, 2011. Available from: http://canadiantaskforce.ca/guidelines/2011-breast-cancer/

Colorectal Cancer Screening Guidelines
Colorectal Screening for Cancer Prevention in Asymptomatic Patients, March 2013. Available from: http://www.bcguidelines.ca/pdf/colorectal_screening.pdf

Diabetes
Canadian Diabetes Association 2013 Clinical Practice Guidelines. Available from: http://guidelines.diabetes.ca/Browse.aspx.
Moore H, Summerbell C, Hooper L, et al. Dietary advice for treatment of type 2 diabetes mellitus in adults. Cochrane DB Syst Rev 2007;Issue 3.
Norris SL, Zhang X, Avenell A, et al. Long-term non-pharmacological weight loss interventions for adults with pre-diabetes. Cochrane DB Syst Rev 2005;Issue 2.
Saenz A, Fernandez-Esteban I, Mataix A, et al. Metformin monotherapy for type 2 diabetes mellitus. Cochrane DB Syst Rev 2005;Issue 3.

Diet, Exercise, and Obesity
Calle E, Thun MJ, Petrelli JM, et al. Body-mass index and mortality in a prospective cohort of US adults. NEJM 1999;341:1097-1105.
Canada's Food Guide to Healthy Eating. Health Canada. Last updated 2011.
Canadian Cancer Society Vitamin D Guidelines. Available from: http://www.cancer.ca/en/prevention-and-screening/live-well/vitamin-d/.
Canadian Task Force For Preventive Health Care 2015 Obesity Guidelines from: canadiantaskforce.ca/ctfphc-guidelines/2015-obesity-adults/.
Canadian Task Force on Preventive Health Care.. Recommendations for prevention of weight gain and use of behavioural and pharmacologic interventions to manage overweight and obesity in adults in primary care. CMAJ 2015. DOI: 10.1503/cmaj.140887
Canadian Society for Exercise Physiology (CSEP) Physical Activity Guidelines. Available from: http://www.csep.ca/english/view.asp?x=949.
Clinical Guidelines on the Identification, Evaluation, and Treatment of Overweight and Obesity in Adults, NIH 1998.
Lau D, Douketis JD, Morrison KM, et al. 2006 Canadian clinical practice guidelines on the management and prevention of obesity in adults and children. CMAJ 2007;176:S1-13.
National Institute of Health, National Heart Lung and Blood Institute, Obesity Education Initiative. Classification of overweight and obesity by BMI, waist circumference, and associated disease risks. Available from: http://www.nhlbi.nih.gov/health/public/heart/obesity/lose_wt/bmi_dis.htm.
Dansinger ML, Gleason JA, Griffith JL, et al. Comparison of the Atkins, Ornish, Weight Watchers, and Zone diets for weight loss and heart disease risk reduction. JAMA 2005;293:43-53.
Health Canada. Canada's physical activity guide to healthy active living. Available from: http://www.hc-sc.gc.ca/hppb/paguide/main.html.
Krauss RM, Eckel RH, Howard B, et al. AHA dietary guidelines: revision 2000: A statement for healthcare professionals from the nutrition committee of the American Heart Association. Stroke 2000;31:2751-2766.
Litchenstein AH, Appel LJ, Brands M, et al. Diet and lifestyle recommendations revision 2006: a scientific statement from the American Heart Association Nutrition Committee. Circulation 2006;114:82-96.
Osteoporosis Canada Nutrition Guidelines. Available from: http://www.osteoporosis.ca/osteoporosis-and-you/nutrition/

Dyslipidemia, Hypertension, and Heart Disease
Anderson TJ, Grégoire J, Hegele RA, et al. 2012 Update of the Canadian Cardiovascular Society for the diagnosis and treatment of dyslipidemia for the prevention of cardiovascular disease in the adult. Canadian Journal of Cardiology 2013;29;151-167.
Canadian Health Measures Survey, Cycle 2, CHHS, CHMS, Statistics Canada, 2012. Available from: http://www.hypertension.ca/en/professional/chep/diagnosis-measurement/assessment-of-hypertensive-patients.
Canadian Hypertension Education Program. 2009 Canadian hypertension education program recommendations: an annual update. Can Fam Phys 2009;55:697-700.
Canadian Hypertension Education Program. 2010 Canadian hypertension education program recommendations for the management of hypertension. Can J Cardiol 2010;26:241-258.
CHEP (Canadian Hypertension Education Program) Guidelines 2014. Available from: http://www.hypertension.ca/en/chep.
Elmer PJ, Obarzanek E, Vollmer WM, et al. Effects of comprehensive lifestyle modification on diet, weight, physical fitness, and blood pressure control: 18-month results of a randomized trial. Ann Intern Med 2006;144:485-495.
Eckel RH, Jakicic JM, Ard JD, et al. 2013 AHA/ACC Guideline on Lifestyle Management to Reduce Cardiovascular Risk: A Report of the American College of Cardiology/American Heart Association Task Force on Practice Guidelines. Circulation 2013.
Graham DJ, Staffa JA, Shatin D, et al. Incidence of hospitalized rhabdomyolysis in patients treated with lipid-lowering drugs. JAMA 2004;292:2585-2590.
Genest J, McPherson R, Frohlich J, et al. 2009 Canadian Cardiovascular Society/Canadian guidelines for the diagnosis and treatment of dyslipidemia and prevention of cardiovascular disease in the adult – 2009 recommendations. Can J Cardiol 2009;25:567-579.
Manson JE, Hsia J, Johnson KC, et al. Estrogen plus progestin and the risk of coronary heart disease. NEJM 2003;349:523-534.
McPherson R, Frohlich J, Fodor G, et al. Canadian Cardiovascular Society position statement – Recommendations for the diagnosis and treatment of dyslipidemia and prevention of cardiovascular disease. Can J Cardiol 2006;22:913-27.
Ontario Drug Therapy Guidelines for Stable Ischemic Heart Disease in Primary Care. Ontario Program for Optimal Therapeutics. Toronto: Queen's Printer of Ontario, 2000:10.
Onusko E. Diagnosing secondary hypertension. Am Fam Phys 2003;67:67-74.
Pandor A, Ara RM, Tumur I, et al. Ezetimibe monotherapy for cholesterol lowering in 2,722 people: systematic review and meta-analysis of randomized controlled trials. 2009;265(5):568-580
Recommendations for the management of dyslipidemia and the prevention of cardiovascular disease: Summary of the 2003 update. CMAJ 2003;169:921-924.
Anderson TJ, Gregoire J, Hegele R et al. 2012 Update of the Canadian Cardiovascular Society Guidelines for the Diagnosis and Treatment of Dyslipidemia and Prevention of Cardiovascular Disease in the Adult. Can J Cardiol 2013;29:151-167
Peirson L, Douketis J, Cliska D et al. Treatment for overweight and obesity in adult population: a systematic review and meta-analysis. CMAJ 2014;E306-17.

Periodic Health Examination
Grades of Recommendation, Assessment, Development, and Evaluation (GRADE) Working Group, 2011. Available from: http://www.gradeworkinggroup.org/publications/JCE_series.htm.
Canadian Task Force on Preventative Health Care Guidelines. Available from: canadiantaskforce.ca
Towards Optimized Care Guidelines. Available from: http://www.topalbertadoctors.org/cpgs/

Smoking and Alcohol
Cahill K, Stevens S, Perera R, et al. Pharmacological interventions for smoking cessation: an overview and network meta-analysis. Cochrane Database of Systematic Reviews 2013, Issue 5.
Cahill K, Stead LF, Lancaster T. Nicotine receptor partial agonists for smoking cessation. Cochrane Database of Systematic Reviews 2012, Issue 4.
CAN-ADAPTT. Canadian Smoking Cessation Clinical Practice Guideline. Toronto, Canada: Canadian Action Network for the Advancement, Dissemination and Adoption of Practice-informed Tobacco Treatment, Centre for Addiction and Mental Health, 2011.
Health Canada. Canadian tobacco use monitoring survey (CTUMS): annual results 2012. Available from: http://www.hc-sc.gc.ca/hc-ps/tobac-tabac/research-recherche/stat/ctums-esutc_2012-eng.php#tab1.
Hughes JR, Stead LF, Hartmann-Boyce J, et al. Antidepressants for smoking cessation. Cochrane Database of Systematic Reviews 2014, Issue 1.
Ontario Medical Association. OMA position paper: rethinking stop-smoking medications. Available from: https://www.oma.org/Resources/Documents/e2008RethinkingStop-Smoking/Medications.pdf.
Shroeder SA. What to do with a patient who smoked. JAMA 2005;294:482-487.
Stead LF, Perera R, Bullen C, et al. Nicotine replacement therapy for smoking cessation. Cochrane DB Syst Rev 2008;Issue 1.
Stead LF, Buitrago D, Preciado N, et al. Physician advice for smoking cessation. Cochrane DB Syst Rev 2008;Issue 2.
Moyer A, Finney JW. Brief interventions for alcohol misuse. CMAJ 2015.

Other
American Psychiatric Association. Diagnostic and statistical manual of mental disorders, 5th ed. Arlington, VA: American Psychiatric Publishing, 2013.
American Psychiatric Association. Treating Major Depressive Disorder: A Quick Reference Guide, 2010. Available from: http://ajp.psychiatryonline.org/content.aspx?bookid=28&sectionid=1663150.
Arlinger S. Negative consequences of uncorrected hearing loss: a review. Int J Audiol 2003;42 Suppl 2:2S17.
Bagai A, Thavendiranathan P, Detsky AS. Does this patient have hearing impairment? JAMA 2006;295:416-428.
Beck E, Sieber WJ, Trejo R. Management of cluster headaches. Am Fam Phys 2005;71:717724.

Bent S, Nallamothu BK, Simel DL, et al. Does this woman have an acute uncomplicated urinary tract infection? JAMA 2002;287:2701-2710.

Brcic V, Ebderdt C, Kaczorowski J. Development of a tool to identify poverty in a family practice setting: a pilot study. Int J Family Med 2011;2011:812182.

British Columbia Medical Association and British Columbia Ministry of Health Services. Osteoarthritis in peripheral joints: diagnosis and treatment. Guidelines & Protocol, Advisory Committee, 2008.

Brown JP, Josse RG. 2002 Clinical practice guidelines for the diagnosis and management of osteoporosis in Canada. CMAJ 2002;167:S1-34.

Burge SK, Schneider FD. Alcohol-related problems: recognition and intervention. Am Fam Phys 1999;59:361-370.

Butt P, Gliksman L, Beirness D, et al. Alcohol and health in Canada: A summary of evidence and guidelines for low-risk drinking. Ottawa, ON: Canadian Centre on Substance Abuse, 2011.

Canadian Paediatric Society. Use of selective serotonin reuptake inhibitor medications for the treatment of child and adolescent mental illness (2013). Available from: https://onlinereview.cps.ca/papers/use-of-SSRIs-for-child-adolescent-mental-illness/print_ready.pdf

Canadian Task Force on Preventive Health Care. The Canadian guide to clinical preventive health care. Ottawa: Minister of Supply and Services Canada. Available from: http://www.ctfphc.org.

Canadian Task Force on Preventive Health Care. Recommendations on screening for breast cancer in average-risk women aged 40-74 years. CMAJ 2011;183:1991-2001.

Canadian Task Force on Preventive Health Care. Recommendations on screening for depression in adults. CMAJ 2013;185(9):775-782.

Canadian Guidelines on Sexually Transmitted Infections. Section 2 - Primary Care and Sexually Transmitted Infections. Available from: http://www.phac-aspc.gc.ca/std-mts/sti-its/cgsti-ldcits/section-2-eng.php#a8.

Cartwright SL, Knudson MP. Evaluation of Acute Abdominal Pain in Adults. Am Fam Phys 2008;77(7):971-978.

Centor RM, Witherspoon JM, Dalton HP, et al. The diagnosis of strep throat in adults in the emergency room. Med Decis Making 1981;1:239-246.

Cheung AM, Feig DS, Kapral M, et al. Prevention of osteoporosis and osteoporotic fractures in post-menopausal women: recommendation statement from the Canadian Task Force on Preventive Health Care. CMAJ 2004;170:1665-1667.

Clark MS, Jansen KL, Cloy JA. Treatment of childhood and adolescent depression. Am Fam Phys 2012;86(5):442-448.

Comuz J, Guessous I, Farrat B. Fatigue: a practical approach to diagnosis in primary care. CMAJ 2006;174:765-767.

Derby CA, Mohr BA, Goldstein I, et al. Modifiable risk factors and erectile dysfunction: can lifestyle changes modify risk? Urology 2000;56:302-306.

Desrosiers M, Evans GA, Keith PK, et al. Canadian clinical practice guidelines for acute and chronic rhinosinusitis. Allergy, Asthma & Clin Immunol 2011;7:doi:10.1186/1710-1492-7-2.

Domino FJ. The 5-minute clinical consult, 18th ed. Lippincott Williams & Wilkins, 2009.

Ebell MH. Evidence-based diagnosis: a handbook of clinical prediction rules. Springer, 2001.

Ebell MH. Treating adult women with suspected UTI. Am Fam Phys 2006;73:293-296.

Edmonds M, McGuire H, Price J. Exercise therapy for chronic fatigue syndrome. Cochrane DB Syst Rev 2004;Issue 3.

Evans M (editor). Mosby's family practice sourcebook: an evidence based approach to care, 4th ed. Elsevier Canada, 2006: 343-345.

Evans M, Bradwejn J, Dunn L. Guidelines for the treatment of anxiety disorders in primary care. Toronto: Queen's Printer of Ontario, 2002.

Fauci AS, Braunwald E, Kasper D, et al. Harrison's principles of internal medicine, 17th ed. McGraw-Hill Professional, 2008.

Furlan AD, van Tulder MW, Cherkin DC, et al. Acupuncture and dry-needling for low back pain. Cochrane DB Syst Rev 2005;Issue 1.

Furlan AD, Imamura M, Dryden T, et al. Massage for low-back pain. Cochrane DB Syst Rev 2008;Issue 4.

Gilbert DN, Moellering RC, Eliopoulos GM. The Sanford guide to antimicrobial therapy, 43rd ed. Sperryville: Antimicrobial Therapy, 2013.

Guidelines for Adolescent Depression in Primary Care (GLAD-PC). Guidelines on identification, assessment and initial management, 2007. Available from: http://pediatrics.aappublications.org/content/120/5/e1299.full.

Gupta BP, Murad MH, Clifton MM, et al. The effect of lifestyle modification and cardiovascular risk factor reduction on erectile dysfunction. Arch Intern Med 2011;171:1797-1803.

Health Canada. An advisory committee statement: National Advisory Committee on Immunization: prevention of pertussis in adolescents and adults. Canada Communicable Disease Report 2003;29:ACS5-6.

Health Canada. Natural health products directorate 2004. Available from: http://www.hc-sc.gc.ca/hpfb-dgpsa/nhpd-dpsn/.

Holbrook AM (Chair: Ontario Musculoskeletal Therapy Review Panel). Ontario treatment guidelines for osteoarthritis, rheumatoid arthritis, and acute, musculoskeletal injury. Toronto; Queen's Printer of Ontario, 2000:13-24.

Hueston WJ, Mainous AG. Acute bronchitis. Am Fam Phys 1998;57:1270-1279.

Hui D. Approach to internal medicine. A resource book for clinical practice, 3rd ed. Springer New York, 2012.

Hunt P. Motivating change. Nursing Standard 2001;16:45-55.

Jepson RG, Craig JC. Cranberries for preventing urinary tract infections. Cochrane DB Syst Rev 2008;Issue 1

Leddin DJ, Enns R, Hilsden R, et al. Canadian Association of Gastroenterology position statement on screening individuals at average risk of developing colorectal cancer, 2010. Can J Gastroenterol 2010;24:12.

Linde K, Allais G, Brinkhaus B, et al. Acupuncture for migraine prophylaxis. Cochrane DB Syst Rev 2009;Issue 4.

Linde K, Barrett B, Wolkart K, et al. Echinacea for preventing and treating the common cold. Cochrane DB Syst Rev 2006;Issue 1.

Linde K, Mulrow CD, Berner M, et al. St John's wort for depression. Cochrane DB Syst Rev 2005;Issue 2.

Linde K, Berner MM, Kriston L. St John's wort for major depression. Cochrane Database of Systematic Reviews 2008, Issue 4.

Low DE, Desrosiers M, McSherry J, et al. A practical guide for the diagnosis and treatment of acute sinusitis. CMAJ 1997;156:1S.

Marshall IIR. Zinc for the common cold. Cochrane DB Syst Rev 2006;Issue 3.

McIsaac WJ, White D, Tannenbaum D, et al. A clinical score to reduce unnecessary antibiotic use in patients with sore throat. CMAJ 1998;158:75-83.

McIsaac WJ, Moineddin R, Ross S. Validation of a decision aid to assist physicians in reducing unnecessary antibiotic drug use for acute cystitis. Arch Intern Med 167:2201-2206.

Montgomery L, Scoville C. What is the best way to evaluate acute diarrhea? J Fam Pract 2002;51.

Murphy J, Kennedy EB, Dunn S, et al. Cervical screening: a guideline for clinical practice in Ontario. JOGC 2012;34:453-458.

National Institute of Health. Herbs at a glance: black cohosh. National Center for Complementary and Alternative Medicine, 2008. Available from: http://nccam.nih.gov/health/blackcohosh/ataglance.htm.

Nash SD, Cruickshanks KJ, Klein R, et al. The prevalence of hearing impairment and associated risk factors: the Beaver Dam Offspring Study. Arch Otolaryngol Head Neck Surg. 2011;137(5):432.

Osteoporosis Canada. Calcium requirements. 2009. Available from: http://www.osteoporosis.ca/index.php/ci_id/5535/la_id/1.htm.

Pandor A, Ara RM, Tumur I, et al. Ezetimibe monotherapy for cholesterol lowering in 2,722 people: systematic review and meta-analysis of randomized controlled trials. 2009;265(5):568-580

Papaioannou A, Morin S, Cheung AM, et al. 2010 Clinical practice guidelines for the diagnosis and management of osteoporosis in Canada: summary. CMAJ 2010;182:1864-1873.

Pampallona S, Bollini P, Tibaldi G, et al. Combined pharmacotherapy and psychological treatment for depression: a systematic review. Arch Gen Psychiatry 2004;61:714-9.

ParticipACTION. Available from: http://www.participaction.com.

Ponka D, Kirlew M. Top ten differential diagnoses in family medicine: Generalized abdominal pain. Canadian Family Physician 2007;53(9):1509.

Public Health Canada. Canadian Guidelines on Sexually Transmitted Infections. Section 5, Management and treatment of specific infections, Syphilis. Available from: http://www.phac-aspc.gc.ca/std-mts/sti-its/cgsti-ldcits/section-5-10-eng.php.

Public Health Ontario. Testing and treatment of gonorrhea in Ontario, 2013. Available from: http://www.publichealthontario.ca/en/eRepository/Guidelines_Gonorrhea_Ontario_Guide_2013.pdf.

Rambout L, Hopkins L, Hutton B, et al. Prophylactic vaccination against human papillomavirus infection and disease in women: a systematic review of randomized controlled trials. CMAJ 2007;177:469-479.

Richie AM, Francis ML. Diagnostic approach to polyarticular joint pain. Am Fam Phys 2003;68(6):1151-1160.

Ridker PM, Danielson E, Fonseca FA, et al. Rosuvastatin to prevent vascular events in men and women with elevated c-reactive protein. NEJM 2008;359:2195-2207.

Roelofs PD, Deyo RA, Koes BW, et al. Non-steroidal anti-inflammatory drugs for low back pain. Cochrane DB Syst Rev 2008;Issue 1.

Sabatine MS. Pocket medicine: the Massachusetts General Hospital handbook of internal medicine, 4th ed. Lippincott Williams & Wilkins, Philadelphia 2011.

Schiller LR. Chronic diarrhea. Curr Treat Options Gastroenterol 2005;8:259-266.

Smith-Bindman R, Aubin C, Bailitz J, et al. Ultrasound versus Computed Tomography for Suspected Nephrolithiasis. 2014;371:1100-1110

Society of Obstetricians and Gynecologists of Canada. Canadian Consensus Guidelines on Human Papillomavirus. JOGC 2007;29(8, suppl 3):S29

Spinar J, Spinarova L, Vitovec J. IMProved Reduction of Outcomes: Vytorin Efficacy International Trial (studie IMPROVE-IT). Vnitr Lek. 2014; 60(12):1095-101

Sport Concussion Assessment Tool, 3rd edition (SCAT3), Br J Sports Med 2013;47:259.

Swinson RP, Antony MM, Bleau P, et al. Clinical practice guidelines: management of anxiety disorders. Can J Psychiatry 2006;51:Supplement 2.

Taylor RB. Family medicine: principles and practice, 6th ed. New York: Springer-Verlag, 2003.

Toward Optimized Practice Program. Guideline for assessment to diagnosis of adult insomnia. 2006 (2010 update).

Toward Optimized Practice Program. Guideline for the diagnosis and management of adult primary insomnia. 2006 (2010 update).

Toward Optimized Practice Program. Guideline for the diagnosis and management of community acquired pneumonia: adult. 2002 (2008 update).

Toward Optimized Practice Program. Guideline for the diagnosis and management of acute otitis media. 1999 (2008 update).

Toward Optimized Practice Program. Guideline for the diagnosis and management of acute pharyngitis. 1999 (2008 update).

Toward Optimized Practice Program. Guideline for the management of acute bronchitis. 2000 (2008 update).

Toward Optimized Practice Program. Guideline for the treatment of Helicobacter pylori infection in adults. 2000 (2009 update).

Toward Optimized Practice Program. Guideline for the management of low back pain. 2009 (2011 update).

Toward Optimized Practice Program. Use of PSA and the early diagnosis of prostate cancer. 2006 (2009 update).

Towheed TE, Maxwell L, Anastassiades T, et al. Glucosamine therapy for treating osteoarthritis. Cochrane DB Syst Rev 2005;Issue 2.

Weber PC. Evaluation of hearing loss in adults. Rose BD (editor). Waltham: UpToDate. 2013.

Wong T, Latham-Carmanico C. Canadian guidelines on sexually transmitted infections. Ottawa; Public Health Agency of Canada 2006 (reviewed 2008).

Wren BG. The benefits of oestrogen following menopause: why hormone replacement therapy should be offered to postmenopausal women. Med J Aust 2009;190:321-325.

Yueh B, Collins MP, Souza PE, et al. Screening for auditory impairment: Which hearing aid tests? A randomized clinical trail. Department of Veterns Affairs, Seattle, WA 2001

Zink T, Chaffin J. Herbal "health"products: what family physicians need to know. Am Fam Phys 1998;58:1133-1140

Notes

G Gastroenterology

Rory Blackler, Michael Tjong, and Gary Tran, chapter editors
Claudia Frankfurter and Inna Gong, associate editors
Brittany Prevost and Robert Vanner, EBM editors
Dr. Maria Cino, Dr. Gabor Kandel, and Dr. Piero Tartaro, staff editors

Acronyms

ALF	acute liver failure	EVL	endoscopic variceal ligation	IBD	inflammatory bowel disease	PBC	primary biliary cirrhosis
BE	Barrett's esophagus	FAP	familial adenomatous polyposis	IBS	irritable bowel syndrome	PN	parenteral nutrition
BT	biologic therapy	GE	gastroesophageal	ICP	Intracranial pressure	PPI	proton pump inhibitor
CCK	cholecystokinin	GERD	gastroesophageal reflux disease	INH	isoniazid	PSC	primary sclerosing cholangitis
CD	Crohn's disease	GI	gastrointestinal	LES	lower esophageal sphincter	PTC	percutaneous transhepatic
DM	diabetes mellitus	HAV	hepatitis A virus	MRCP	magnetic resonance		cholangiography
DPG	deamidated gliadin peptides	HBV	hepatitis B virus		cholangiopancreatography	PUD	peptic ulcer disease
DES	diffuse esophageal spasm	HCC	hepatocellular carcinoma	MS	multiple sclerosis	SBP	spontaneous bacterial peritonitis
EIM	extraintestinal manifestation	HCV	hepatitis C virus	NAC	N-acetylcysteine	TIPS	transjugular intrahepatic
EN	enteral nutrition	HNPCC	hereditary non-polyposis colorectal	NAFLD	non-alcoholic fatty liver disease		portosystemic shunt
ERCP	endoscopic retrograde		cancer	NERD	non-erosive reflux disease	TPN	total parenteral nutrition
	cholangiopancreatography	HRS	hepatorenal syndrome	NMS	neuroleptic malignant syndrome	TTG	tissue transglutaminase
EUS	endoscopic ultrasound	HVPG	hepatic venous pressure gradient	OGD	oesophagogastroduodenoscopy	UC	ulcerative colitis

Anatomy Review

Overview of Gastrointestinal Tract

- the gastrointestinal tract runs from mouth to anus ("gum to bum")

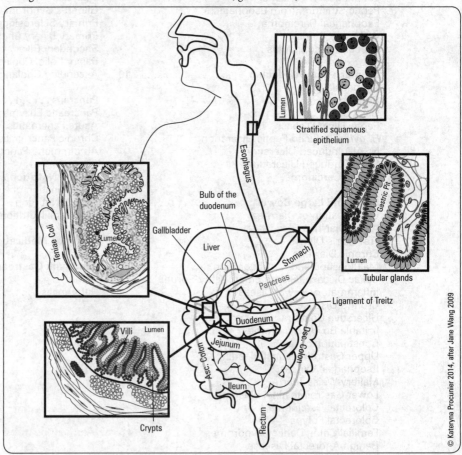

Figure 1. Overview of gastrointestinal tract

© Kateryna Procunier 2014, after Jane Wang 2009

Table 1. Summary of Gastrointestinal Tract Structure and Function

Organ	Function	Blood Supply	Innervation	Histology and Structural Features
Esophagus	Muscular tube approximately 25 cm long with a diameter of 2 cm Extends from pharynx to the stomach	Arterial: left gastric artery and left inferior phrenic artery Venous: Left gastric vein → portal venous system Esophageal veins → azygos vein → IVC (systemic)	Parasympathetic innervation via anterior and posterior gastric nerves (vagal trunks) Sympathetic innervation via thoracic trunks of the greater splanchnic nerves	Mucosa: stratified squamous epithelium Submucosa: connective tissue, lymphocytes, plasma cells, nerve cells Muscularis propria (muscularis externa): inner circular, outer longitudinal muscle Upper 1/3: striated muscle Middle 1/3: transition zone Lower 1/3: smooth muscle
Stomach	Delivers food to intestine for digestion and absorption Secretes acid, probably to reduce enteric infections/pneumonia; facilitate digestion of protein/iron/B12 Secretes intrinsic factor to facilitate B12 absorption Minor contribution to initial protein digestion via pepsin	Lesser curvature Right and left gastric arteries (from celiac trunk) Greater curvature Right and left gastro-omental (gastroepiploic) arteries (from gastroduodenal and splenic arteries respectively) Fundus: short and posterior gastric arteries (from the splenic artery)	Parasympathetic innervation via vagus nerve Sympathetic innervation via celiac plexus (from T6-T9)	5 parts Cardia Fundus Body Antrum Pylorus
Duodenum	Modulates enteral pH via secretin → decreased gastric acid secretion, increased bicarbonate secretion Secretes CCK to stimulate bile secretion Site of iron absorption	Branches of celiac artery and superior mesenteric artery	Parasympathetic innervation via vagus nerve Sympathetic innervation via greater and lesser splanchnic nerves	4 parts Superior (5 cm) Descending (7-10 cm) Horizontal (6-8 cm) Ascending (5 cm) 1st part is intraperitoneal; rest is retroperitoneal
Jejunum	Absorption of sodium, water, and nutrients (protein, carbohydrates, fat, folic acid, and vitamin A, B, C, D, E, K)	Superior mesenteric artery	Parasympathetic innervation via fibres of the posterior vagal trunk Sympathetic innervation via fibres of T8-T10	Deep red colour 2-4 cm in thickness Thick and heavy wall Plicae circulares are large, tall, and closely packed Has long vasa recta Scant fat in mesentery Scant Peyer's patches
Ileum	Absorption of sodium, water, nutrients, soluble vitamins (only site of vitamin B12 absorption), and bile salts (entero-hepatic circulation)	Superior mesenteric artery	Same as jejunum	When compared to jejunum Paler pink colour 2-3 cm in thickness Thin and light walls Plicae circulares are small and sparse Contains more mesenteric fat Many Peyer's patches
Large Bowel	Absorption of water (5-10% of total water) Bacteria: further digestion of chyme and metabolism of undigested CHO to short chain fatty acids Formation and storage of feces	Branches of superior and inferior mesenteric arteries Rectal blood supply: sigmoid, right pudendal, and rectal arteries	Parasympathetic innervation via vagus nerve Sympathetic innervation via greater and lesser splanchnic nerves	Consists of cecum, colon (ascending, transverse, descending, and sigmoid), rectum and anal canal Features include teniae coli, haustra, and omental appendices
Liver	Glucose homeostasis Plasma protein synthesis Lipid and lipoprotein synthesis Bile acid synthesis and secretion Vitamin A, D, E, K, B12 storage Biotransformation, detoxification Excretion of compounds	2 sources Portal vein (75-80%) Hepatic artery (20-25%)	Parasympathetic innervation via fibres of the anterior and posterior vagal trunks Sympathetic innervation via fibres of the celiac plexus	Largest internal organ Composed of 4 lobes (left, right, caudate, quadrate), and divided into 8 segments
Biliary Tract	Gallbladder functions to store and release bile that is produced in the liver Bile is used to emulsify fat and is composed of cholesterol, lecithin, bile acids, and bilirubin CCK stimulates gallbladder emptying while trypsin and chymotrypsin inhibit bile release	Cystic artery	Parasympathetic innervation via vagus nerve Sympathetic and visceral innervation via celiac nerve plexus Somatic afferent fibres via right phrenic nerve	Consists of the hepatic ducts (intrahepatic, left, right and common), gallbladder, cystic duct, common bile duct, and ampulla of Vater
Pancreas	Endocrine function: islets of Langerhans produce glucagon, insulin, and somatostatin (from the α, β, and δ cells, respectively) Exocrine function: digestive enzymes are produced including amylase, lipase, trypsin, chymotrypsin, and carboxypeptidase	Anterior superior pancreaticoduodenal artery (from the celiac trunk) Anterior inferior pancreaticoduodenal artery (from the superior mesenteric artery) Dorsal pancreatic artery (from the splenic artery) Pancreatic veins drain into the portal, splenic, and superior mesenteric veins	Parasympathetic innervation via vagus nerve Sympathetic innervation via abdominopelvic splanchnic nerves	4 parts of pancreas: head (includes uncinate process), neck, body, and tail (Major) pancreatic duct connecting to common bile duct prior to ampulla of Vater Accessory pancreatic duct connected directly to duodenum

Visualizing the GI Tract

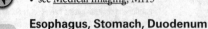

- see <u>Medical Imaging</u>, MI15

Esophagus, Stomach, Duodenum
- OGD: best visualization of mucosa; also allows for therapeutic intervention (e.g. banding varices, thermal therapy/clipping/injecting bleeding ulcers, and dilatation e.g. treatment of esophageal strictures)
  - consider barium swallow first if dysphagia, decreased level of consciousness (increases risk of aspiration), inability to cooperate (increases risk of pharyngeal trauma during intubation), possibility of fistulas
  - endotracheal intubation first if massive upper GI bleed, acidemia, or inability to protect airway

Small Bowel
- most difficult to visualize, especially if mucosal detail is needed
- CT enterography more accurate than small bowel follow through, but both have low sensitivity
- MRI small bowel imaging increasingly available, especially useful if radiation exposure is an issue (e.g. young patient, multiple radiological images already done)
  - note: MRI enteroclysis: luminal contrast administered by nasojejunal tube to dilate the small bowel – disliked by both radiologist and patient, but may improve sensitivity
- "double balloon" enteroscopy (enteroscope with proximal and distal balloons to propel endoscope into jejunum from mouth or into jejunum/ileum or into ileus from anus) may be most sensitive but currently available only in selected centres; technically demanding
- wireless endoscopy capsule (26 x 11 mm capsule is swallowed, transmits images to a computer; contraindicated in bowel obstruction) is also accurate in diagnosis but unable to provide any therapeutic intervention

Colon and Terminal Ileum
- colonoscopy, with biopsy if required; contraindicated in perforation, acute diverticulitis, and severe colitis (increased risk of perforation)
- CT colonography ("virtual colonoscopy") more accurate in diagnosing diverticulosis, extrinsic pressure on colon (e.g. ovarian cancer compressing sigmoid colon), and fistulae; increasing evidence for use in colorectal cancer screening, especially for assessment of right side of colon in cases where colonoscopy is less sensitive. Most often used when optical endoscopic colonoscopy is a risk (e.g. frail elderly) or unsuccessful (e.g. stricture).
- most often used when optical endoscopic colonoscopy is a risk (e.g. frail elderly) or unsuccessful (e.g. stricture)

Pancreatic/Biliary Duct
- MRCP almost as sensitive as ERCP in determining if bile duct obstruction present, but less accurate in determining cause of obstruction (tumour, stone, stricture)
- ERCP if therapeutic intervention likely to be required: strong suspicion of stone, obstruction requiring stenting, or if tissue sampling required

Differential Diagnosis of Common Complaints

- see <u>General Surgery</u>, *Acute Abdominal Pain*, GS4

Table 2. Differential Diagnosis of Common Presenting Complaints

CHRONIC/ RECURRENT ABDOMINAL PAIN	Inflammatory	Neoplastic/ Vascular	Toxin	Other
	PUD Biliary colic IBD Chronic pancreatitis	Recurrent bowel obstruction Mesenteric ischemia Sickle cell anemia	Lead poisoning	Mittleschmertz Endometriosis Porphyria IBS Radiculopathy Abdominal wall pain syndrome
ACUTE DIARRHEA	Inflammatory		Non-Inflammatory	
*Causes of bloody diarrhea	**Bacterial** *Shigella** *Salmonella** *Campylobacter** *Yersinia** *E. coli* (EHEC 0157:H7)*	**Protozoal** *E. histolytica** (amoebiasis) Strongyloides **Others** NSAIDs IBD* Ischemic*	**Bacterial** *S. aureus* *C. perfringens* *B. cereus* *E. coli* (ETEC, EPEC) *Salmonella enteritidis* *Vibrio cholera* **Protozoal** *Giardia lamblia*	**Viral** Rotavirus Norwalk CMV **Drugs** Antibiotics Colchicine Laxatives Antacids (magnesium)

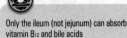

Retroperitoneal Structures
Suprarenal glands (adrenal glands)
Aorta/IVC
Duodenum (second to fourth segments)
Pancreas (tail is intraperitoneal)
Ureters
Colon (only the ascending and descending branches)
Kidneys
Esophagus
Rectum

Only the ileum (not jejunum) can absorb vitamin B$_{12}$ and bile acids

Acute Upper Abdominal Pain
Remember to rule out thoracic sources, e.g. myocardial infarction, pneumonia, dissecting aneurysm

Obscure But Treatable Causes of Abdominal Pain
- Acute Intermittent Porphyria
- Hereditary Angioedema
- Familial Mediterranean Fever
- Vasculitis (e.g. polyarteritis nodosa)

Inflammatory Diarrhea: Occurs when there is damage to the mucosal lining or brush border, which leads to a passive loss of protein-rich fluids and a decreased ability to absorb these lost fluids. Diarrhea may be profuse or very small in volume. Often associated with abdominal pain ± fever and chills
Non-Inflammatory Diarrhea: No damage to the mucosal lining. N/V may be present. Fever, chills, blood in the stool, severe abdominal pain or tenderness are not present

Table 2. Differential Diagnosis of Common Presenting Complaints (continued)

CHRONIC DIARRHEA

*Causes of bloody diarrhea

	Organic				Functional
	Inflammatory	Secretory	Steatorrhea	Osmotic	
	IBD* Infectious (TB, CMV, HSV) Ischemic* bowel Radiation colitis Neoplasia C. difficile rarely causes bleeding	Stimulant laxatives Post-ileal resection/ cholecystectomy (bile salts) Bacterial toxins Vasculitis Neoplasia* (colon ca, carcinoid, VIPoma) Addison's disease Congenital syndromes	Giardia lamblia Celiac sprue Chronic pancreatitis Chronic cholestasis	Osmotic laxatives Lactose intolerance Chewing gum (sorbitol, mannitol)	IBS Constipation (overflow diarrhea) Anal sphincter dysfunction

IBD Is a common cause of bloody diarrhea but can be diagnosed only If mimickers are excluded. Chiefly, infection, ischemia and medication side-effects

CONSTIPATION: if no associated rectal bleeding/weight loss, etc., usually no cause found (and dysmotility assumed)

Colorectal cancer Stricture Extrinsic compression Anal disease Rectocele	Medications (narcotics, antidepressants, calcium channel blockers) Metabolic (DM, thyroid, hypercalcemia)	Neurologic (Parkinson's, MS, stroke) Collagen vascular disease (scleroderma, dermatomyositis)

NAUSEA/VOMITING

	With Abdominal Pain		Without Abdominal Pain	
	Relieved by Vomiting	Not Relieved by Vomiting	Headache/Dizziness	No Other Symptoms
	Gastric outlet obstruction Small bowel obstruction GERD (regurgitation more common)	Gallbladder disease Pancreatitis Myocardial infarction Hepatitis Infectious Gastroenteritis	Cerebral tumour Migraine Vestibular disease Increased ICP	Drugs Uremia Pregnancy Metabolic (e.g. hypercalcemia) Gastroparesis (e.g. DM) Ketoacidosis

Commonly Forgotten Causes of Vomiting
- Drugs
- Uremia
- CNS Disease
- Pregnancy
- Marijuana (cannabinoid hyperemesis)

DYSPEPSIA

Common		Uncommon	Rare
Functional dyspepsia Drug side effect Peptic ulcer GERD (esophagitis)		Angina Crohn's disease Cancer (stomach, pancreas, liver) Gallstones Aerophagia	Giardia lamblia Malabsorption (celiac sprue) Pancreatitis

UPPER GI BLEED

Common		Uncommon	Rare
Ulcers (H. pylori, ASA, NSAIDs) Esophageal varices Mallory-Weiss tears Erosive esophagitis Erosive gastritis		Tumours Arteriovenous malformation Dieulafoy's lesion (arterial) Gastric antral vascular ectasia (GAVE) Portal hypertensive gastropathy	Aorto-enteric fistulas Hemobilia

LOWER GI BLEED

Common		Uncommon	Rare
Diverticulosis Ischemia Angiodysplasia (elderly) Infectious Anorectal (hemorrhoids, fissure, ulcer)		Upper GI bleed (brisk) Post-polypectomy Radiation colitis IBD	Intussusception Vasculitides Stercoral ulcer Coagulopathies

DYSPHAGIA

Mechanical (Solids)		Motility (Solids and Liquids)	Other
Peptic stricture/cancer Eosinophilic esophagitis Extrinsic compression Schatzki ring/esophageal web Zenker's diverticulum		Achalasia Diffuse esophageal spasm Scleroderma	Foreign body Eosinophilic esophagitis

Difference Between Dysphagia and Odynophagia
- **Dysphagia**: Difficulty swallowing due to mechanical obstruction or dysmotility of the esophagus or pharynx
- **Odynophagia**: Pain when swallowing due to ulceration or Inflammation (e.g. eosinophilic esophagitis) in the esophagus pharynx

ODYNOPHAGIA

Infection	Inflammation/Ulceration	Drugs	Other
Candida Herpes CMV (common in those who are immunosuppressed)	Caustic damage Eosinophilic esophagitis	Quinidine Iron Vitamin C Antibiotics (e.g. tetracycline) Bisphosphonates	Radiation

ABDOMINAL DISTENTION

Fluid (Ascites)		Flatulence	Feces	Other
Portal HTN	**Normal Portal Pressure**			
Cirrhosis Cardiac failure Hepatic vein thrombosis	Cancer (especially ovarian) Pancreatitis TB	Functional bowel disease (e.g. IBS) Fibre Lactose intolerance Chewing gum (e.g. sorbitol, mannitol)	Constipation Colonic obstruction Dysmotility	Pregnancy (fetus) Obesity (fat) Blood Large tumours (fatal growth)

Differential Diagnosis of Abdominal Distention

6 Fs
Fat
Feces
Fetus
Flatus
Fluid
Fatal Growth

Bowel Ischemia
The splenic flexure and rectosigmoid junction are watershed areas and are susceptible to ischemia. History and symptoms include acute onset crampy left abdominal pain, absence of abdominal tenderness on exam, rectal bleeding, and risk factors for embolization, atherosclerosis and atrial fibrillation

Table 2. Differential Diagnosis of Common Presenting Complaints (continued)

JAUNDICE (UNCONJUGATED BILIRUBIN)	Overproduction	Decreased Hepatic Intake	Decreased Conjugation
	Hemolysis Ineffective erythropoiesis (e.g. megaloblastic anemias)	Gilbert's syndrome Drugs (e.g. rifampin)	Drug inhibition (e.g. chloramphenicol) Crigler-Najjar syndromes type I and II Gilbert's syndrome Neonatal jaundice
JAUNDICE (CONJUGATED BILIRUBIN)	Common		Uncommon
	Hepatocellular disease Drugs Cirrhosis (any cause) Inflammation (hepatitis, any cause) Infiltrative (e.g. hemochromatosis) Familial disorders (e.g. Rotor syndrome, Dubin-Johnson syndrome, cholestasis of pregnancy) PBC PSC Sepsis Post-operative/TPN		Intraductal obstruction Gallstones Biliary stricture Parasites Malignancy (cholangiocarcinoma) Sclerosing cholangitis **Extraductal obstruction** Malignancy (e.g. pancreatic cancer, lymphoma) Metastases in peri-portal nodes **Inflammation (e.g. pancreatitis)**

Esophagus

Gastroesophageal Reflux Disease

Dyspepsia = postprandial fullness, early satiety, epigastric pain, or burning

Definition
- condition in which the stomach contents (most characteristically acid) moves backwards from the stomach into the esophagus

Etiology
- inappropriate transient relaxations of LES – most common cause
- low basal LES tone (especially in scleroderma)
- contributing factors include: delayed esophageal clearance, delayed gastric emptying, obesity, pregnancy, acid hypersecretion (rare) from Zollinger-Ellison syndrome (gastrin-secreting tumour)
- hiatus hernia worsens reflux, does not cause it (see General Surgery, GS13)

Foods/Substances that Aggravate GERD Symptoms (but not the underlying disease)
- EtOH
- Caffeine
- Tobacco
- Fatty/fried foods
- Chocolate
- Peppermint
- Spicy foods
- Citrus fruit juices

Clinical Features
- "heartburn" (pyrosis) and acid regurgitation (together are 80% sensitive and specific for reflux) ± sour regurgitation; less sensitive and less specific: water brash, sensation of a lump in the throat (globus sensation), and frequent belching
- non-esophageal symptoms are increasingly recognized of being poor predictors of reflux

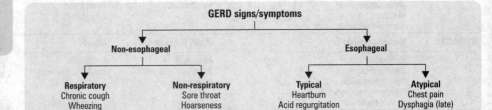

Figure 2. Signs and symptoms of GERD

Investigations
- usually, a clinical diagnosis is sufficient based on symptom history and relief following a trial of pharmacotherapy (PPI: symptom relief 80% sensitive for reflux)
- gastroscopy indications (*Ann Intern Med* 2012;157:808-816)
  - absolute indications
    - heartburn accompanied by red-flags (bleeding, weight loss, etc.)
    - persistent reflux symptoms or prior severe erosive esophagitis after therapeutic trial of 4-8 wk of PPI 2x daily
    - history suggests esophageal stricture especially dysphagia
    - high risk for Barrett's (male, age >50, obese, white, tobacco use, long history of symptoms)
- repeat endoscopy after 6-8 wks of PPI therapy indicated if: severe esophagitis because it can mask Barrett's esophagus or symptoms
- esophageal manometry (study of esophageal motility)
  - done to diagnose abnormal peristalsis and/or decreased LES tone, but cannot detect presence of reflux; indicated before surgical fundoplication to ensure intact esophageal function

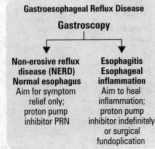

Gastroesophageal Reflux Disease

Gastroscopy

Non-erosive reflux disease (NERD)
Normal esophagus
Aim for symptom relief only; proton pump inhibitor PRN

Esophagitis
Esophageal inflammation
Aim to heal inflammation; proton pump inhibitor indefinitely or surgical fundoplication

Figure 3. Classification and gastroscopic findings of GERD

- surgical fundoplication (wrapping of gastric fundus around the lower end of the esophagus) more likely to alleviate symptoms if lower esophageal pressure is diminished; less likely to be successful if abnormal peristalsis
- 24 h pH monitoring: most accurate test for reflux, but not required or performed in most cases
  - most useful if PPIs do not improve symptoms

Treatment
- PPIs are the most effective therapy and usually need to be continued as maintenance therapy
- on-demand: antacids ($Mg(OH)_2$, $Al(OH)_3$, alginate), H_2-blockers, or PPIs can be used for NERD
- diet helps symptoms, not the disease; avoid alcohol, coffee, spices, tomatoes, and citrus juices
- only beneficial lifestyle changes are weight loss (if obese) and elevating the head of bed (if nocturnal symptoms)
- symptoms may recur if therapy is discontinued

Complications
- esophageal stricture disease – scarring can lead to dysphagia (solids)
- ulcer
- bleeding
- Barrett's esophagus and esophageal adenocarcinoma – gastroscopy is recommended for patients with chronic GERD or symptoms suggestive of complicated disease (e.g. anorexia, weight loss, bleeding, dysphagia)

Barrett's Esophagus

Definition
- metaplasia of normal squamous esophageal epithelium to abnormal columnar epithelium containing-type intestinal mucosa (intestinal metaplasia)

Etiology
- thought to be acquired via long-standing GERD and consequent damage to squamous epithelium

Epidemiology
- in North America and Western Europe, 0.5-2.0% of adults are thought to have Barrett's esophagus
- up to 10% of GERD patients will have already developed BE by the time they seek medical attention
- more common in males, age >50, Caucasians, smokers, overweight, hiatus hernia, and long history of reflux symptoms

Pathophysiology
- endoscopy shows erythematous epithelium in distal esophagus; diagnosis of BE relies on biopsy demonstrating the presence of specialized intestinal epithelium of any length within the esophagus
- BE predisposes first to premalignant changes characterized as low or high-grade dysplasia, which then progresses to adenocarcinoma

Significance
- rate of malignant transformation is approximately 0.12% per yr for all BE patients prior to dysplasia
- risk of malignant transformation in high-grade dysplasia is significantly higher; studies have reported a 32-59% transformation rate over 5-8 yr of surveillance
- increased gastric acid secretion is more frequently associated with Barrett's esophagus as opposed to reflux alone

Treatment
- acid suppressive therapy with high-dose PPI indefinitely (or surgical fundoplication)
- endoscopy every 3 yr if no dysplasia
- high grade dysplasia: regular and frequent surveillance with intensive biopsy, endoscopic ablation/resection, or esophagectomy produce similar outcomes; however, evidence increasingly favouring endoscopic ablation with mucosal resection or radiofrequency ablation
- if low grade dysplasia, both surveillance and endoscopic ablation/resection are satisfactory options

Esophageal damage from reflux is most severe at first gastroscopy, therefore gastroscopy is necessary only once for patients with NERD

Up to 25% of patients with Barrett's esophagus do not report symptoms of GERD

Should Patients with Barrett's Esophagus Undergo Periodic Upper GI Endoscopy for Esophageal Cancer Screening?
Impact of Endoscopic Surveillance on Mortality From Barrett's Esophagus - Associated Esophageal Adenocarcinomas
Gastroenterology 2013;145:312-319
There is no question that Barrett's esophagus (BE) increases the incidence of esophageal adenocarcinoma, which can be recognized early on with a safe procedure, endoscopy. Indeed, because early cancer is often asymptomatic and curable, most clinicians recommend period upper endoscopy. Yet Corley et al. found no difference in endoscopy rates in BE patients who died of esophageal adenocarcinoma compared to BE patients who died of other diseases. Perhaps this result is due to statistics, but as the accompanying editorial emphasizes (Gastroenterology 2013; 145:273-6) at the very least this finding should question the value of a screening program. In fact, there are multiple other lines of evidence indicating that endoscopic surveillance is of marginal benefit at most. Possible explanations for this disappointing finding include: most esophageal adenocarcinomas may not arise from BE, esophageal carcinoma is too rare a cause of death in BE, morbidity from esophageal cancer treatments, or that endoscopic screening is just not that effective in the real world. The situation is analogous to the disappointing value of serum PSA screening for prostate cancer. Therefore, adoption of screening programs require more than theoretical calculations.

Dysphagia

Remember:
Dysphagia = Difficulty in swallowing
Odynophagia = Pain on swallowing

Definition
- difficulty swallowing

Key Questions in Dysphagia
- Difficulty in starting swallowing?
- Associated symptoms? (regurgitation, change in voice pitch, weight loss)
- Solids, liquids, or both?
- Intermittent or progressive?
- History of heartburn?
- Change in eating habits/diet?

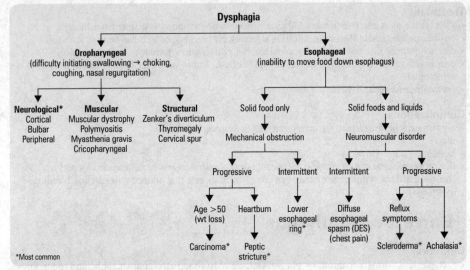

Figure 4. Approach to dysphagia (eosinophilic esophagitis omitted)

Esophageal Motor Disorders

Clinical Features
- dysphagia with solids and liquids
- chest pain (in some disorders)

Diagnosis
- motility study (esophageal manometry)
- barium swallow sometimes helpful

Causes
- idiopathic
- achalasia (painless)
- scleroderma (painless)
- DM
- DES: rare and can be difficult to diagnose due to intermittent presentation

Table 3. Esophageal Motor Disorders

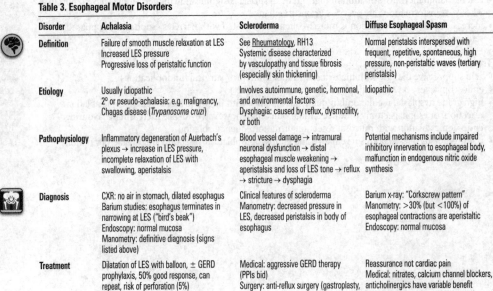

Disorder	Achalasia	Scleroderma	Diffuse Esophageal Spasm
Definition	Failure of smooth muscle relaxation at LES Increased LES pressure Progressive loss of peristaltic function	See Rheumatology, RH13 Systemic disease characterized by vasculopathy and tissue fibrosis (especially skin thickening)	Normal peristalsis interspersed with frequent, repetitive, spontaneous, high pressure, non-peristaltic waves (tertiary peristalsis)
Etiology	Usually idiopathic 2° or pseudo-achalasia: e.g. malignancy, Chagas disease (Trypanosoma cruzi)	Involves autoimmune, genetic, hormonal, and environmental factors Dysphagia: caused by reflux, dysmotility, or both	Idiopathic
Pathophysiology	Inflammatory degeneration of Auerbach's plexus → increase in LES pressure, incomplete relaxation of LES with swallowing, aperistalsis	Blood vessel damage → intramural neuronal dysfunction → distal esophageal muscle weakening → aperistalsis and loss of LES tone → reflux → stricture → dysphagia	Potential mechanisms include impaired inhibitory innervation to esophageal body, malfunction in endogenous nitric oxide synthesis
Diagnosis	CXR: no air in stomach, dilated esophagus Barium studies: esophagus terminates in narrowing at LES ("bird's beak") Endoscopy: normal mucosa Manometry: definitive diagnosis (signs listed above)	Clinical features of scleroderma Manometry: decreased pressure in LES, decreased peristalsis in body of esophagus	Barium x-ray: "Corkscrew pattern" Manometry: >30% (but <100%) of esophageal contractions are aperistaltic Endoscopy: normal mucosa
Treatment	Dilatation of LES with balloon, ± GERD prophylaxis, 50% good response, can repeat, risk of perforation (5%) Injection of botulinum toxin into LES (temporary) POEM (perioral endoscopicmyotomy)	Medical: aggressive GERD therapy (PPIs bid) Surgery: anti-reflux surgery (gastroplasty, last resort)	Reassurance not cardiac pain Medical: nitrates, calcium channel blockers, anticholinergics have variable benefit Surgical: long esophageal myotomy if unresponsive to above treatment (rarely helpful); balloon dilatation

Esophageal Diverticula

Definition
- outpouchings of one or more layers of the esophageal tract

Clinical Features
- commonly associated with motility disorders
- dysphagia, regurgitation, retrosternal pain, intermittent vomiting, may be asymptomatic

Classification
- classified according to location
  - pharyngoesophageal (Zenker's) diverticulum
    - most frequent form of esophageal diverticulum
    - posterior pharyngeal outpouching most often on the left side, above cricopharyngeal muscle and below the inferior pharyngeal constrictor muscle
    - symptoms: dysphagia, regurgitation of undigested food, halitosis
    - treatment: endoscopic or surgical myotomy of cricopharyngeal muscle ± surgical excision of sac
  - mid-esophageal diverticulum
    - secondary to mediastinal inflammation ("traction" diverticulae), motor disorders
    - usually asymptomatic; no treatment required
  - just proximal to LES (pulsatile type)
    - usually associated with motor disorders
    - usually asymptomatic, no treatment required

Peptic Stricture (from Esophagitis)

- presents as dysphagia alongside a long history of reflux symptoms, but reflux symptoms may disappear as stricture develops
- diagnosed with endoscopy or barium study if endoscopy contraindicated or unavailable

Treatment
- endoscopic dilatation and indefinite PPI

Esophageal Carcinoma

- see General Surgery, GS15

Webs and Rings

- web = partial occlusion (upper esophagus)
- ring = circumferential narrowing (lower esophagus)

Clinical Features
- asymptomatic with lumen diameter >12 mm, provided peristalsis is normal
- dysphagia with large food boluses
- Schatzki ring
  - mucosal ring at squamo-columnar junction above a hiatus hernia
  - causes intermittent dysphagia with solids
  - treatment involves disrupting ring with endoscopic bougie

Plummer-Vinson Syndrome Triad
- Iron deficiency anemia
- Dysphagia
- Esophageal webs
- rare (prevalence <1 in 1,000,000) but good prognosis when treated with iron and esophageal dilatation

Infectious Esophagitis

Definition
- severe mucosal inflammation and ulceration as a result of a viral or a fungal infection

Risk Factors
- DM
- chemotherapeutic agents
- immunocompromised states

Clinical Features
- characteristically odynophagia, less often dysphagia
- diagnosis is via endoscopic visualization and biopsy

Appearance
- Candida (most common): whitish-yellow plaques without visible ulceration or inflammation
- Herpes (second most common), CMV: focal ulcers

Eosinophilic Esophagitis
- Eosinophils infiltrate the epithelium of the esophagus
- Causes odynophagia, dysphagia, common cause of bolus food impaction
- Usually primary, but can be part of the spectrum of eosinophilic gastroenteritis, secondary to drugs, parasites etc.
- Often associated with allergies
- Most characteristically occurs in young men
- Diagnosis established by endoscopic biopsy, suggested by mucosal rings seen in the esophageal mucosa at endoscopy
- Treatment: (a)diet, (b)swallow corticosteroid nasal spray (fluticasone), (c)swallow viscous corticosteroid (budesonide mixed with sucralose

Investigations
- diagnosis via endoscopic visualization and biopsy

Treatment
- Candida: nystatin swish and swallow, ketoconazole, fluconazole
- Herpes: often self-limiting; acyclovir, valacyclovir, famciclovir
- CMV: IV gancyclovir, famciclovir, or oral valganciclovir

Stomach and Duodenum

Dyspepsia

The most common cause of dyspepsia is functional (idiopathic) dyspepsia

Definition
- one or more of the following symptoms: postprandial fullness, early satiation, epigastric pain or burning (Rome III criteria)
- multiple causes: esophagitis, GERD, peptic ulcer, stomach cancer, drugs, but overall functional disease is most common

History and Physical Exam
- history: most important are age, associated symptoms (such as weight loss and vomiting), and drugs (especially NSAIDs)
- physical exam: adenopathy, abdominal mass/organomegaly, Carnett's sign (if pain is due to abdominal wall muscle problem then the pain will increase during muscle contraction, such as during a sit-up)

Red Flags of Dyspepsia
(raise suspicion of gastric malignancy):
- Unintended weight loss
- Persistent vomiting
- Progressive dysphagia
- Odynophagia
- Unexplained anemia or iron deficiency
- Hematemesis
- Jaundice
- Palpable abdominal mass or lymphadenopathy
- Family history of upper GI cancer
- Previous gastric surgery

Investigations
- laboratory: usual (CBC, liver enzymes, glucose, Cr, etc.), amylase, albumin, calcium, protein electrophoresis, TSH, *H. pylori* serology
- consider trial of empiric anti-secretory drug therapy, non-invasive testing for *H. pylori* infection, endoscopy; barium radiography is outdated

Stomach

Table 4. Cells of the Gastric Mucosa

Cell Type	Secretory Product	Important Notes
Parietal Cells	Gastric acid (HCl)	
Intrinsic Factor	Stimulated by histamine, ACh, gastrin	
Chief Cells	Pepsinogen	Stimulated by vagal input and local acid
G-Cells	Gastrin	Stimulates H^+ production from parietal cells
Superficial Epithelial Cells	Mucus, HCO_3^-	Protect gastric mucosa
Neuroendocrine Cells	Multiple (e.g. somatostatin, inhibits cell secretion)	Involved in neural, hormonal, and paracrine pathways

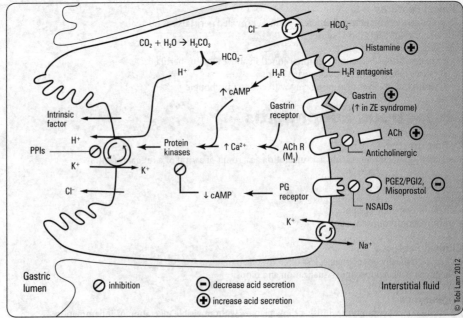

Figure 5. Stimulation of H^+ secretion from the parietal cell

Gastritis

Definition
- defined histologically: inflammation of the stomach mucosa

Etiology
- some causative agents may play a role in more than one type of gastritis and an individual patient may have histopathological evidence of more than one type of gastritis

Table 5. Updated Sydney Classification of Gastritis

Type	Common Etiology
Acute Gastritis	
Hemorrhagic/erosive gastritis	Alcohol, Aspirin®/NSAID, shock/physiological stress (seen in ICU patients)
Helicobacter gastritis	*H. pylori**
Chronic Gastritis	
Non-atrophic	*H. pylori*
Atrophic	*H. pylori*, dietary, environmental factors (multi-focal), autoimmunity
Chemical	NSAID, bile
Radiation	Radiation injury
Lymphocytic	Celiac disease, drug
Eosinophilic	Food allergies
Non-infectious granulomatous	Crohn's disease, sarcoidosis
Other infectious gastritides	Bacteria, viruses, fungi, parasite, TB, syphilis

Clinical Features
- non-erosive gastritis is asymptomatic (except in certain rare causes like Crohn's disease), does not cause pain; difficult to diagnose clinically or endoscopically – requires biopsy for diagnosis
- erosive gastritis can cause bleeding (pain only if progresses to ulcers – rare); can be seen endoscopically

Treatment
- determined by etiology (see *H. pylori*, G13, *NSAID*, G13 and *Stress-Induced Ulceration*, G14)
- non-pharmacological: avoidance of mucosal irritants such as alcohol, NSAIDs, and foods that trigger symptoms

Peptic Ulcer Disease

Definition
- focal defects in the mucosa that penetrate the muscularis mucosal layer results in scarring (defects superficial to the muscularis mucosa are erosions and do not cause scarring)
- peptic ulcer disease includes defects located in the stomach (gastric ulcers) and duodenum (duodenal ulcers)

Etiology

Table 6. Etiology of Peptic Ulcer Disease

	Duodenal	Gastric
H. pylori Infection	90%	60%
NSAIDs	7%	35%
Physiologic Stress-Induced	<3%	<5%
Zollinger-Ellison Syndrome	<1%	<1%
Idiopathic	15%	10%

- NSAID negative, *H. pylori* negative ulcers becoming more commonly recognized
- others: CMV, ischemic, idiopathic
- alcohol: damages gastric mucosa but rarely causes ulcers
- peptic ulcer associated with cigarette smoking, cirrhosis of liver, COPD, and chronic renal failure

Cigarette Smoking and PUD
- Increased risk of ulcer
- Increased risk of complications
- Increased chance of death from ulcer
- Impairs healing

Clinical Features
- dyspepsia: most common presenting symptom
  - only 5% of patients with dyspepsia have ulcers, while most have functional disease
- may present with complications
  - bleeding 10% (severe if from gastroduodenal artery), perforation 2% (usually anterior ulcers), gastric outlet obstruction 2%
  - posterior inflammation (penetration) 2%; may also cause pancreatitis

Stomach and Duodenum

- duodenal ulcers: 6 classical features, but history alone cannot distinguish from functional dyspepsia
  - epigastric pain; may localize to tip of xiphoid
  - burning
  - develops 1-3 h after meals
  - relieved by eating and antacids
  - interrupts sleep
  - periodicity (tends to occur in clusters over wk with subsequent periods of remission)
- gastric ulcers: more atypical symptoms; a biopsy is necessary to exclude malignancy

Investigations
- endoscopy (most accurate)
- upper GI series
- *H. pylori* tests (see Table 7)
- fasting serum gastrin measurement if Zollinger-Ellison syndrome suspected (but most common cause of elevated serum gastrin level is atrophic gastritis)

Gastric vs. Duodenal Ulcers
Gastric ulcers must always be biopsied to rule out malignancies; duodenal ulcers are rarely malignant

Treatment
- specific management depends on etiology; (see *H. pylori*, G13, *NSAID-Induced Ulceration*, G13 and *Stress-Induced Ulceration*, G14)
- eradicate *H. pylori* if present; chief advantage of triple therapy over PPI is to lower ulcer recurrence rate
- stop NSAIDs if possible
- start PPI: inhibits parietal cell H^+/K^+-ATPase pump which secretes acid
- heals most ulcers, even if NSAIDs are continued
- other medications (e.g. histamine H2-antagonists) less effective
- discontinue cigarette smoking
- no diet modifications required but some people have fewer symptoms if they avoid caffeine, alcohol, and spices

Approach to PUD
- Stop NSAIDs
- Acid neutralization
- *H. pylori* eradication
- Quit smoking

Management of Bleeding Peptic Ulcers
- OGD to explore upper GI tract
- IV pantoprazole continuous drip
- establish risk of rebleeding/continuous bleed (since most ulcers stop bleeding spontaneously)
  - clinical risk factors: increased age (>60), bleeding diathesis, history of PUD, comorbid disease, hemodynamically unstable
  - endoscopic signs of recurrent bleeding (active bleeding, visible vessel, clot, red spot) more predictive than clinical risk factors
    - if high risk, consider ICU admission

Bleeding Peptic Ulcers
Risk Factors for Increased Mortality
- Co-existent illness
- Hemodynamic instability
- Age >60 yr
- Transfusion required

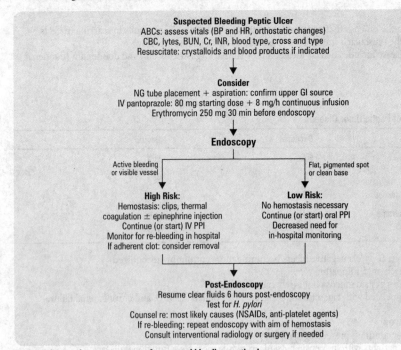

Figure 6. Approach to management of suspected bleeding peptic ulcer
Adapted from: Gralnek I, Barkun A, Bardou M. Management of acute bleeding from a peptic ulcer. *NEJM* 2008;359:928-937

H. pylori-Induced Peptic Ulceration

Pathophysiology
- *H. pylori*: Gram-negative flagellated rod that resides within the gastric mucosa, causing persistent infection and inflammation
- acid secreted by parietal cells (stimulated by vagal acetylcholine, gastrin, histamine) necessary for most ulcers
- theories of how *H. pylori* causes ulcers: none satisfactory, but pattern of colonization correlates with outcome
- gastritis only in antrum (15% of patients), high gastric acid, associated with duodenal ulcer, may progress to gastric metaplasia of duodenum where ulcer forms
- gastritis throughout stomach ("pangastritis" – 85% of patients), low gastric acid, associated with stomach ulcer and cancer

Epidemiology
- *H. pylori* is found in about 20% of all Canadians
- highest prevalence in those raised during 1930s
- infection most commonly acquired in childhood, presumably by fecal-oral route
- high prevalence in developing countries, low socioeconomic status (poor sanitation and overcrowding)

Outcome
- gastritis (non-erosive) in 100% of patients but asymptomatic
- peptic ulcer in 15% of patients
- gastric carcinoma and mucosal associated lymphomatous tissue [MALT] lymphoma in 0.5% of patients
- most are asymptomatic but still worthwhile eradicating to lower future risk of peptic ulcer/gastric malignancy and prevent spread to others (mostly children <5 yr of age)

Diagnosis

Table 7. Diagnosis of H. pylori Infection

Test	Sensitivity	Specificity	Comments
Non-invasive Tests			
Urea breath test	90-100%	89-100%	Affected by PPI therapy (false negatives)
Serology	88-99%	89-95%	Can remain positive after treatment
Invasive Tests (require endoscopy)			
Histology	93-99%	95-99%	Gold standard; affected by PPI therapy (false negatives)
Rapid urease test (on biopsy)	89-98%	93-100%	Rapid
Microbiology culture	98%	95-100%	Research only

Treatment: *H. pylori* Eradication
- triple therapy for 7-14 d (Hp-Pac®): PPI bid (e.g. lansoprazole 30 mg bid) + amoxicillin 1 g bid + clarithromycin 500 mg bid
- becoming less successful as prevalence of *H. pylori* clarithromycin-resistance increases
- quadruple therapy for 10-14 d now recommended: PPI bid + bismuth 525 mg qid + tetracycline 500 mg qid + metronidazole 250 mg qid
- levofloxacin can replace metronidazole or tetracycline
- sequential therapy
- days 1-5: PPI bid + amoxicillin 1 g bid
- days 6-10: PPI bid + clarithromycin 500 mg bid + tinidazole (generally substitute with metronidazole as tinidazole not available in Canada) 500 mg bid
- 5-15% of cases are resistant to all known therapies

NSAID-Induced Ulceration

- NSAID use causes gastric mucosal petechiae in virtually all, erosions in most, ulcers in some (25%)
- erosions bleed, but usually only ulcers cause significant clinical problems
- most NSAID ulcers are clinically silent: dyspepsia is as common in patients with ulcers as in patients without ulcers; NSAID-induced ulcers characteristically present with complications (bleeding, perforation, obstruction)
- NSAIDs more commonly cause gastric ulcers than duodenal ulcers
- may exacerbate underlying duodenal ulcer disease

Pathophysiology
- direct: erosions/petechiae – are due to local (direct) effect of drug on gastric mucosa
- indirect: systemic NSAID effect (intravenous NSAID causes ulcers, but not erosions), inhibits mucosal cyclooxygenase, leading to decreased synthesis of protective prostaglandins, thus leading to ulcers

Risk Factors for NSAID-induced Peptic Ulcer
- previous peptic ulcers/UGIB
- age (≥65 yr)
- high dose of NSAID/multiple NSAIDs being taken
- concomitant corticosteroid use
- concomitant cardiovascular disease/other significant diseases

Treatment
- prophylactic cytoprotective therapy with a PPI is recommended if any of the above risk factors exist concomitantly with ASA/NSAID use
- lower NSAID dose or stop all together and replace with acetaminophen
- combine NSAID with PPI or misoprostol (less effective) in one tablet
- enteric coating of Aspirin® (ECASA) provides minor benefit since this decreases incidence of erosion, not incidence of ulceration

If at high risk for development of ulcers, prophylaxis with PPI indicated

Stress-Induced Ulceration

Definition
- ulceration or erosion in the upper GI tract of ill patients, usually in ICU (stress is physiological, not psychiatric)
- lesions most commonly in fundus of stomach

Pathophysiology
- unclear: likely involves ischemia; may be caused by CNS disease, acid hypersecretion, Cushing ulcers
- mechanical ventilation is the most important risk factor

Curling's and Cushing's Ulcers
- **Curling's ulcer**: acute peptic ulcer of the duodenum resulting as a complication from severe burns when reduced plasma volume leads to ischemia and cell necrosis (sloughing) of the gastric mucosa (think BURN from a CURLing iron)
- **Cushing's ulcer**: peptic ulcer produced by elevated intracranial pressure (may be due to stimulation of vagal nuclei secondary to elevated ICP which leads to increased secretion of gastric acid)

Risk Factors
- mechanical ventilation
- anti-coagulation
- multi-organ failure
- septicemia
- severe surgery/trauma
- CNS injury ("Cushing's ulcers")
- burns involving more than 35% of body surface

Clinical Features
- UGIB (see *Upper Gastrointestinal Bleeding*, G25)
- painless

Treatment
- prophylaxis with gastric acid suppressants decreases risk of UGIB; PPI most potent but may increase risk of pneumonia; H2 blockers less potent but less likely to cause pneumonia
- treatment same as for bleeding peptic ulcer but often less successful

Gastric Carcinoma

- see General Surgery, GS19

Small and Large Bowel

Classification of Diarrhea

Stool Osmotic Gap
Stool osmolality is normally about 290 mOsm/kg and can be approximated by the calculated stool osmolality
$(2 \times [Na^+]_{stool} + [K^+]_{stool})$
In osmotic diarrhea, measured stool osmolality > calculated stool osmolality
In secretory diarrhea measured stool osmolality = calculated stool osmolality
Stool osmolarity Is always the same as serum

Definition
- clinically: diarrhea defined as stools that are looser and/or more frequent than normal (i.e. ≥3x per day); physiologically: 24 h stool weight >200 g (less useful clinically)

Classification
- acute vs. chronic
- small volume (tablespoons of stool; typical of colonic diseases) vs. large volume (>1/2 cup stool; typical of small bowel diseases)
- watery: secretory (diarrhea persists with fasting) vs. osmotic (diarrhea stops with fasting)
- steatorrhea
- inflammatory
- functional

Acute Diarrhea

Definition
- passage of frequent unformed stools for <14 d

Etiology
- most commonly due to infections
- most infections are self-limiting and resolve within 7 d

Risk Factors
- food (seafood, chicken, turkey, eggs, beef)
- medications: antibiotics, laxatives
- others: high risk sexual activity, infectious outbreaks, family history (IBD)

Table 8. Classification of Acute Diarrhea

	Inflammatory	Non-Inflammatory
Definition	Disruption of intestinal mucosa	Intestinal mucosa intact
Site	Usually colon	Usually small intestine
Mechanism	Organisms and cytotoxins invade mucosa, killing mucosal cells, and further perpetuating the diarrhea	Stimulation of intestinal water secretion and inhibition of water absorption (i.e. secretory problem)
Sigmoidoscopy	Usually abnormal mucosa seen	Usually normal
Symptoms	Bloody (not always) Small volume, high frequency Often lower abdominal cramping with urgency ± tenesmus May have fever ± shock	Watery, little or no blood Large volume Upper/periumbilical pain/cramp ± shock
Investigations	Fecal WBC and RBC positive	Fecal WBC negative
Etiology	See *Differential Diagnosis of Presenting Complaints*, G4	See *Differential Diagnosis of Presenting Complaints*, G4
Differential Diagnosis	Acute presentation of idiopathic inflammatory bowel disease	Acute presentation of non-inflammatory chronic diarrhea (e.g. celiac disease)
Significance	Higher yield with stool C&S Can progress to life-threatening megacolon, perforation, hemorrhage Antibiotics may benefit	Lower yield with stool C&S Chief life-threatening problem is electrolyte disturbances/ fluid depletion Antibiotics unlikely to be helpful

Investigations
- stool cultures/microscopy (C&S/O&P) are required only if diarrhea is inflammatory, severe, or for epidemiological purposes (day care worker, nursing home resident, community outbreaks, e.g. Walkerton, etc.)
  - C&S only tests *Campylobacter, Salmonella, Shigella, E. coli*
    - other organisms must be ordered separately
- flexible sigmoidoscopy (without bowel preparation): useful if inflammatory diarrhea suspected
  - biopsies are the most useful method of distinguishing idiopathic IBD (Crohn's disease and ulcerative colitis) from infectious colitis or acute self-limited colitis
- *C. difficile* toxin: indicated when recent/remote antibiotic use, hospitalization, nursing home, or recent chemotherapy

Treatment
- fluid and electrolyte replacement orally in most cases, intravenous if severe extremes of age/coma
- anti-diarrheals
  - antimotility agents: diphenoxylate, loperamide (Imodium®); contraindicated in mucosal inflammation
    - side effects: abdominal cramps, toxic megacolon
  - absorbants: kaolin/pectin (Kaopectate®), methylcellulose, activated attapulgite
    - act by absorbing intestinal toxins/micro-organisms, or by coating intestinal mucosa
    - much less effective than antimotility agents
  - modifiers of fluid transport: bismuth subsalicylate (Pepto-Bismol®) may be helpful (but should not be used in the presence of bloody diarrhea or fever)
- antibiotics: rarely indicated
  - risks
    - prolonged excretion of enteric pathogen (especially *Salmonella*)
    - drug side effects (including *C. difficile* infection)
    - development of resistant strains
    - renal failure/hemolysis (enterohemorrhagic *E. coli* O157:H7)

Useful Questions in Acute Diarrhea

Those Fads Wilt
Travel
Homosexual contacts
Outbreaks
Seafood
Extra-intestinal signs of IBD
Family history
Antibiotics
Diet
Steatorrhea
Weight loss
Immunosuppressed
Laxatives
Tumour history

Infectious Causes of Inflammatory Diarrhea

Your Stool Smells Extremely Crappy
Yersinia
Shigella
Salmonella
E. coli (EHEC 0157:H7), *E. histolytica*
Campylobacter, *C. difficile*

Finally: A Role for Bacteriotherapy
Duodenal Infusion of Donor Feces for Recurrent
Clostridium difficile
NEJM 2013; 368:407-15
For centuries, out-of-the-box thinkers have speculated that the colonic bacteria all of us have, but which differs among individuals, play a role in disease. More recently, the colonic microbiome has become the hottest area of research in gastroenterology. The best documented medical indication for manipulating the colonic bacteria is recurrent *C. difficile* infection. In this randomized study of this disease, infusion of donor feces via a nasoduodenal tube resolved diarrhea in 81% of patients, without side-effects, compared to 31% given the standard treatment of oral vancomycin, and 23% of patients given oral vancomycin plus bowel lavage. It takes little prescience to predict an onslaught of future studies investigating the therapeutic potential of altering the human microbiome.

- indications for antimicrobial agents in acute diarrhea
  - septicemia
  - prolonged fever with fecal blood or leukocytes
  - clearly indicated: *Shigella, V. cholerae, C. difficile*, traveller's diarrhea (enterotoxigenic *E. coli* [ETEC]), *Giardia, Entamoeba histolytica, Cyclospora*
  - situational: *Salmonella, Campylobacter, Yersinia*, non-enterotoxigenic *E. coli*
  - *Salmonella*: always treat *Salmonella typhi* (typhoid or enteric fever); treat other *Salmonella* only if there is underlying immunodeficiency, hemolytic anemia, extremes of age, aneurysms, prosthetic valve grafts/joints, sickle cell disease

Traveller's Diarrhea

- see Infectious Diseases, ID13

Chronic Diarrhea

Definition
- passage of frequent unformed stool for >4 wk (persistent diarrhea as 14-30 d)
- approach is similar to that of acute diarrhea except that the majority of cases are non-infectious

Etiology/Classification
- see *Differential Diagnosis of Common Presenting Complaints*, G4

Investigations
- guided by history
- stool analysis for: *C. difficile* toxin, C&S, O&P ± fecal fat, WBC
- blood for: CBC, electrolytes, CRP, TSH, celiac serology (IgA anti-tTG; ask for serum protein electrophoresis or immunoglobulin quantitation to rule out IgA deficiency which has an increased frequency in celiac disease)
- colonoscopy and ileoscopy with biopsy
- upper GI endoscopy with duodenal biopsy
- wireless small bowel endoscopy capsule (low yield)
- trial of lactose free diet
  - caveat: may delay diagnosis of IBD and celiac disease

Maldigestion and Malabsorption

Definition
- maldigestion: inability to break down large molecules in the lumen of the intestine into their component small molecules
- malabsorption: inability to transport molecules across the intestinal mucosa into circulation
- malassimilation: encompasses both maldigestion and malabsorption

Etiology
- maldigestion
  - inadequate mixing of food with enzymes (e.g. post-gastrectomy)
  - pancreatic exocrine deficiency
  - primary diseases of the pancreas (e.g. cystic fibrosis, pancreatitis, cancer)
  - bile salt deficiency
    - terminal ileal disease (impaired recycling), bacterial overgrowth (deconjugation of bile salts), rarely liver disease (cholestatic, e.g. primary biliary cirrhosis)
  - specific enzyme deficiencies (e.g. lactase)
- malabsorption
  - inadequate absorptive surface
    - infections/infestations (e.g. Whipple's disease, Giardia)
    - immunologic or allergic injury (e.g. celiac disease)
    - infiltration (e.g. lymphoma, amyloidosis)
    - fibrosis (e.g. systemic sclerosis, radiation enteritis)
    - bowel resection (length, site, location, presence/absence of ileocecal valve are important)
    - extensive ileal Crohn's disease
  - drug-induced
    - cholestyramine, ethanol, neomycin, tetracycline, and other antibiotics
  - endocrine
    - DM (complex pathogenesis)

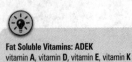

Clinical Features
- symptoms usually vague unless disease is severe
- weight loss, diarrhea, steatorrhea, weakness, fatigue
- manifestations of malabsorption/deficiency

Table 9. Absorption of Nutrients and Fat Soluble Vitamins

Deficiency	Absorption	Clinical Disease and/or Features	Investigations
Iron	Duodenum, upper jejunum	Hypochromic, microcytic anemia, glossitis, koilonychia (spoon nails), pica	↓ Hb, ↓ serum Fe, ↓ serum ferritin
Calcium	Duodenum, upper jejunum (binds to Ca^{2+} binding-protein in cells; levels increased by Vit D)	Metabolic bone disease, may get tetany and paresthesias if serum calcium falls (see Endocrinology, E36)	↓ serum Ca^{2+}, ↓ serum Mg^{2+}, and ↑ ALP. Evaluate for ↓ bone mineralization radiographically (DEXA)
Folic Acid	Jejunum	Megaloblastic anemia, glossitis, ↓ red cell folate (may see ↑ folic acid with bacterial overgrowth)	↓ serum folic acid
Vitamin B12	B12 ingested and bound to R proteins mainly from salivary glands; stomach secretes intrinsic factor (IF) in acidic medium; in basic medium, proteases from the pancreas cleave R protein and B12-IF complex forms, protecting B12 from further protease attack; B12 absorbed in ileum and binds to transcobalamin (TC)	Subacute combined degeneration of the spinal cord, peripheral/optic neuropathy, dementia, megaloblastic anemia, glossitis	Differentiate causes by nuclear Schilling test (when available). Positive anti-intrinsic factor antibodies and atrophic gastritis point toward pernicious anemia (see Hematology, H24)
Carbohydrate	Complex polysaccharides hydrolyzed to oligosaccharides, and disaccharides by salivary and pancreatic enzymes. Monosaccharides absorbed in duodenum/jejunum	Generalized malnutrition, weight loss, flatus, and diarrhea	Hydrogen breath test. Trial of carbohydrate-restricted diet. D-xylose test
Protein	Digestion at stomach, brush border, and inside cell. Absorption occurs primarily in the jejunum	General malnutrition and weight loss, amenorrhea, and ↓ libido if severe	↓ serum albumin (low sensitivity)
Fat	Lipase, colipase, phospholipase A (pancreatic enzymes), and bile salts needed for digestion. Products of lipolysis form micelles which solubilize fat and aid in absorption. Fatty acids diffuse into cell cytoplasm	Generalized malnutrition, weight loss, and diarrhea. Foul-smelling feces + gas. Steatorrhea	Small bowel biopsy. MRCP, ERCP, pancreatic function tests (not routinely available). Quantitative stool fat test (72 h). May start with qualitative stool fat test (Sudan stain of stool). C-triolein breath test (not routinely available)
Vitamin A	Dietary sources (e.g. milk, eggs, liver, carrots, sweet potatoes)	Night blindness. Dry skin. Keratomalacia	
Vitamin D	Skin (via UV light) or diet (e.g. eggs, fish oil, fortified milk)	Osteomalacia in adults. Ricketts in children	
Vitamin E	Dietary sources (e.g. vegetable oils, nuts, leafy green vegetables)	Retinopathy, neurological problems	
Vitamin K	Synthesized by intestinal flora. ↑ risk of deficiency after prolonged use of broad spectrum antibiotics and/or starvation	Prolonged INR may cause bleeding	

* Calcium malabsorption more commonly causes decreased bone density rather than hypocalcemia because serum calcium levels are protected by leaching calcium from the bone

Investigations
- transglutaminase (tTG) antibody serology/immunoglobulin quantitation and abdominal imaging are most useful because celiac disease and chronic pancreatitis are the two most common causes of steatorrhea
- 72 h stool collection (weight, fat content) documents steatorrhea (gold standard)
- fecal elastase (not routinely available) to screen for pancreatic insufficiency and/or consider empiric trial of pancreatic enzymes based on clinical context
- serum carotene (precursor to vitamin A), folate, Ca^{2+}, Mg^{2+}, vitamin B12, albumin, ferritin, serum iron solution, INR/PTT
- stool fat globules on fecal smear stained with Sudan (rarely used)
- other tests specific for etiology (e.g. CT scan/MRI to visualize pancreas)

Treatment
- dependent on underlying etiology

Celiac Disease (Gluten Enteropathy/Sprue)

Definition
- abnormal small intestine mucosa due to intestinal reaction to gluten, a protein found in cereal grains

Etiology
- only autoimmune disease in which antigen (various gliadin peptides) is recognized
- associated with other autoimmune diseases, especially Sjögren's, thyroid disease
- gluten, a protein in cereal grains, is broken down to gliadin, which is the toxic factor
- HLA-DQ2 (chromosome 6) found in 80-90% of patients compared with 20% in general population; celiac also associated with HLA-DQ8 (note: up to 40% of Caucasians carry the HLA alleles, but will never develop celiac disease)

Epidemiology
- more common in women
- family history: 10-15% of first-degree relatives
- may present any time from infancy (when cereals introduced) to elderly
- peak presentation in infancy

Clinical Features
- classic presentation: diarrhea, weight loss, anemia, symptoms of vitamin/mineral deficiency, failure to thrive; more common current presentation: bloating, gas, iron deficiency
- improves with gluten-free diet, deteriorates when gluten reintroduced
- disease is usually most severe in proximal bowel
    - thus iron, calcium, and folic acid deficiency (proximal absorption) more common than vitamin B_{12} deficiency (absorbed in ileum)
- gluten enteropathy may be associated with dermatitis herpetiformis skin eruption, epilepsy, myopathy, depression, paranoia, infertility, bone fractures/metabolic bone disease

Investigations
- serological tests
    - serum anti-tTG antibody, IgA, is 90-98% sensitive, 94-97% specific
    - IgA deficient patients have false-negative anti-tTG
        - therefore, measure serum IgA concomitantly (via serum quantitative protein electrophoresis)
        - incorporate serum testing tTG and/or DGP IgG in IgA deficiencies
- small bowel mucosal biopsy (usually duodenum) is diagnostic with increased intraepithelial lymphocytes (earliest pathologic finding)
    - crypt hyperplasia
    - villous atrophy
    - note: villous atrophy also seen in small bowel overgrowth, Crohn's, lymphoma, Giardia, HIV
- improvement with a gluten-free diet, but should not be started before serological tests and biopsy
- consider CT enterography to visualize small bowel to rule out lymphoma
- evidence of malabsorption (localized or generalized)
    - steatorrhea
    - low levels of ferritin/iron saturation, Ca^{2+}, Fe, albumin, cholesterol, carotene, B_{12} absorption
- fecal fat >7%

Treatment
- dietary counselling
    - gluten free diet; avoid barley, rye, wheat (as these grains are related and also have toxic factor, similar to gliadin)
    - oats allowed if not contaminated by other grains (grown in soil without cross-contamination)
    - rice and corn flour are acceptable
    - iron, folate supplementation (with supplementation of other vitamins as needed)
- if poor response to diet change, consider
    - alternate diagnosis
    - non-adherence to gluten-free diet
    - concurrent disease (e.g. microscopic colitis, pancreatic insufficiency)
    - development of intestinal (enteropathy-associated T-cell) lymphoma (abdominal pain, weight loss, palpable mass)
    - development of diffuse intestinal ulceration, characterized by aberrant intraepithelial T-cell population (precursor to lymphoma)

Prognosis
- associated with increased risk of lymphoma, carcinoma (e.g. small bowel and colon; slight increase compared with general population), autoimmune diseases
- risk of lymphoma may be lowered by dietary gluten restriction

Gluten Found in BROW
Barley
Rye
Oats (controversial)
Wheat

Inflammatory Bowel Disease

Definition
- Crohn's disease (CD), ulcerative colitis (UC), indeterminate colitis or IBD-unclassified (IBDU)

Pathophysiology
- poorly understood
- most likely a sustained response of the immune system, perhaps to enteric flora
- lack of appropriate down-regulation of immune responsiveness after an infection in a genetically predisposed individual

Genetics
- increased risk of both UC and CD in relatives of patients with either disease, especially siblings, early onset disease
    - familial risk greater if proband has CD rather than UC
- likely polygenomic pattern: 9 gene loci are associated
- CARD15/NOD2 gene mutation associated with CD (relative risk in heterozygote is 3, in homozygote is 40), especially Ashkenazi Jews, early onset disease, ileal involvement, fistulizing and stenotic disease
    - CARD15 gene product modulates NFκB, which is required for the innate immune response to microbial pathogens, best expressed in monocytes-macrophages

Clinical Features

Table 10. Clinical Differentiation of Ulcerative Colitis from Crohn's Disease

	Crohn's Disease	Ulcerative Colitis
Location	Any part of GI tract Small bowel + colon: 50% Small bowel only: 30% Colon only: 20%	Isolated to large bowel Always involves rectum, may progress proximally
Rectal Bleeding	Uncommon	Very common (90%)
Diarrhea	Less prevalent, non-bloody	Frequent, mucous, bloody, small volume stools
Abdominal Pain	Post-prandial/colicky	Less common
Fever	Common	Uncommon
Urgency/Tenesmus	Uncommon (unless rectum involved)	Common
Palpable Mass	Frequent (25%), RLQ	Rare (if present, often related to cecum full of stool)
Recurrence After Surgery	Common	None post-colectomy
Endoscopic Features	Ulcers (aphthous, stellate, linear), patchy lesions, pseudopolyps, cobblestoning	Continuous diffuse inflammation, erythema, friability, loss of normal vascular pattern, pseudopolyps
Histologic Features	Transmural distribution with skip lesions Focal inflammation ± noncaseating granulomas, deep fissuring + aphthous ulcerations, strictures Glands intact	Mucosal distribution, continuous disease (no skip lesions) Architectural distortion, gland disruption, crypt abscess Granulomas absent
Radiologic Features	Cobblestone mucosa Frequent strictures and fistulae AXR: bowel wall thickening "string sign"	Lack of haustra Strictures rare; need to rule out complicating cancer
Complications	Strictures, fistulae, perianal disease	Toxic megacolon
Colon Cancer Risk	Increased if >30% of colon involved	Increased except in proctitis

Table 11. Extraintestinal Manifestations (EIM) of IBD

System	Crohn's Disease	Ulcerative Colitis
Dermatologic		
Erythema nodosum	15%	10%
Pyoderma gangrenosum	10%	Less common
Perianal skin tags	75-80%	Rare
Oral mucosal lesions	Common	Rare
Psoriasis	Statistically associated in 5-10% of those with IBD but not an EIM	
Stomatitis		
Rheumatologic		
Peripheral arthritis	15-20% of those with IBD (CD>UC)	
Ankylosing spondylitis	10% of those with IBD (CD>UC)	
Sacroiliitis	Occurs equally in CD and UC	
Ocular (~10% of IBD)		
Uveitis (vision threatening)		
Episcleritis (benign)	3-4% of IBD patients (CD>UC)	
Hepatobiliary		
Cholelithiasis	15-35% of patients with ileal Crohn's	
PSC	1-5% of IBD cases involving colon	
Fatty liver		
Gallstones		
Urologic		
Calculi	Most common in CD, especially following ileal resection	
Ureteric obstruction		
Fistulae	Characteristic of Crohn's	
Others		
Thromboembolism		
Vasculitis		
Osteoporosis		
Vitamin deficiencies (B12, Vit ADEK)		
Cardiopulmonary disorders		
Pancreatitis (rare)		
Phlebitis		

Crohn's Disease

Definition
- chronic transmural inflammatory disorder potentially affecting the entire gut from mouth to perianal region ("gum to bum")

Epidemiology
- incidence 1-6/100,000; prevalence 10-100/100,000
- bimodal: onset before 30 yr, second smaller peak age 60; M=F
- incidence of Crohn's increasing (relative to UC) especially in young females
- more common in Caucasians, Ashkenazi Jews
  - risk in Asians increases with move to Western countries
- smoking incidence in Crohn's patients is higher than general population

Pathology
- most common location: ileum + ascending colon
- linear ulcers leading to mucosal islands and "cobblestone" appearance
- granulomas are found in 50% of surgical specimens, 15% of mucosal biopsies

Clinical Features
- natural history unpredictable; young age, perianal disease, and need for corticosteroids have been associated with poor prognosis, but associations are not strong enough to guide clinical decisions
- most often presents as recurrent episodes of abdominal cramps, non-bloody diarrhea, and weight loss
- ileitis may present with post-prandial pain, vomiting, RLQ mass; mimics acute appendicitis
- extra-intestinal manifestations are more common with colonic involvement
- fistulae, fissures, abscesses are common
- deep fissures with risk of perforation into contiguous viscera (leads to fistulae and abscesses)
- enteric fistulae may communicate with skin, bladder, vagina, and other parts of bowel

Investigations
- colonoscopy with biopsy to visualize (less often gastroscopy)
- CT/MR enterography to visualize small bowel
- CRP elevated in most new cases, useful to monitor treatment response (especially acutely in UC)
- bacterial cultures, O&P, *C. difficile* toxin to exclude other causes of inflammatory diarrhea

Management (see Figure 7)

Table 12. Management of Crohn's Disease

Management	Notes
Lifestyle/Diet	Smoking cessation Fluids only during acute exacerbation Enteral diets may aid in remission only for Crohn's ileitis, not colitis No evidence for any non-enteral diet changing the natural history of Crohn's disease, but may affect symptoms Those with extensive small bowel involvement or extensive resection require electrolyte, mineral, and vitamin supplements (vit D, Ca^{2+}, Mg^{2+}, zinc, Fe, B_{12})
Antidiarrheal Agents*	Loperamide (Imodium®) > diphenoxylate (Lomotil®) > codeine (cheap but addictive) All work by decreasing small bowel motility, used only for symptom relief CAUTION if colitis is severe (risk of precipitating toxic megacolon), therefore avoid during flare-ups

5-ASA**	Efficacy controversial: Is currently used for mild ileitis
	Sulfasalazine (Salazopyrin®): 5-ASA bound to sulfapyridine
	    Hydrolysis by intestinal bacteria releases 5-ASA (active component)
	    Dose-dependent efficacy
	Mesalamine (Pentasa®): coated 5-ASA releases 5-ASA in the ileum and colon when inflammation is mild

Antibiotics	e.g. metronidazole (20 mg/kg/d, bid or tid dosing) or ciprofloxacin Best described for perianal Crohn's, although characteristically relapse when discontinued
Corticosteroids	Prednisone: starting dose 40 mg OD for acute exacerbations; IV methylprednisolone if severe No proven role for steroids in maintaining remissions; masks intra-abdominal sepsis
Immunosuppressives	6-mercaptopurine (6-MP), azathioprine (Imuran®); methotrexate (used less often) More often used to maintain remission than to treat active inflammation Most commonly used as steroid-sparing agents i.e. to lower risk of relapse as corticosteroids are withdrawn May require >3 mo to have beneficial effect; usually continued for several years May help to heal fistulae, decrease disease activity Increases efficacy of biologicals plus lowers chances of biological dosing efficacy (tolerance) so often given in combination with biologics Side effects: vomiting, pancreatitis, bone marrow suppression, increased risk of malignancy (i.e. lymphoma)
Biologics	Infliximab IV (Remicade®) or adalimumab SC (Humira®): both = antibody to TNF-α Proven effective for treatment of fistulae and patients with medically refractory CD First-line immunosuppressive therapy with inflixmab + azathioprine more effective than using either alone

Surgical/ Experimental	Surgical treatment (see General Surgery, GS28)
	Surgery generally reserved for complications such as fistulae, obstruction, abscess, perforation, bleeding, and for medically refractory disease
	    If <50% or <200 cm of functional small intestine, risk of short bowel syndrome
	At least 50% clinical recurrence within 5 yr; 85% within 15 yr; endoscopic recurrence rate even higher
	40% likelihood of second bowel resection, 30% likelihood of third bowel resection
	Complications of ileal resection
	    <100 cm resected → watery diarrhea or cholorrhea (impaired bile salt absorption)
	        Treatment: cholestyramine or anti-diarrheals e.g. loperamide
	    >100 cm resected → steatorrhea (reduced mucosal surface area, bile salt deficiency)
	        Treatment: fat restriction, medium chain triglycerides

*Cholestyramine: a bile-salt binding resin; for watery diarrhea with <100 cm of terminal ileum diseased or resected; however, non-specific anti-diarrheals are more convenient and often more potent

** 5-ASA use in Crohn's is controversial; however, initial trial for mild ileitis only is warranted (induction and maintenance if clinical response)

Prognosis
- highly variable course
- 10% disabled by the disease eventually, spontaneous remission also described
- increased mortality, especially with more proximal disease, greatest in the first 4-5 yr
- complications include
  - intestinal obstruction/perforation
  - fistula formation
  - malignancy (lower risk compared to UC)
- surveillance colonoscopy same as ulcerative colitis (see *Ulcerative Colitis*) if more than 1/3 of colon involved

Ulcerative Colitis

Definition
- inflammatory disease affecting colonic mucosa anywhere from rectum (always involved) to cecum

Epidemiology
- incidence 2-10/100,000; prevalence 35-100/100,000 (more common than Crohn's)
- 2/3 onset by age 30 (with second peak after 50); M=F
- small hereditary contribution (15% of cases have 1st degree relative with disease)
- risk is less in smokers
- inflammation limited to rectum or left colon is more common than pancolitis

Traditional Medical Management of Crohn's

	Induction of Remission	Maintenance
5-ASA*	?	?
Steroids	+	
Immunosuppressive	+	+
Antibiotics	+	
MTX	+	+
Infliximab	+	+

*5-ASA use in Crohn's is controversial. However, initial trial for mild ileitis only is warranted (induction and maintenance if clinical response)

Note: Starting with immunosupressives plus immunomodulators ("bottom-up approach") increasingly being used (*Lancet* 2008;371;660-667). Combination of azathioprine and infliximab has the highest remission rate yet described with medical treatment (*NEJM* 2010;362;1383-1395). Characteristically more than 1 yr between onset of symptoms and diagnosis of Crohn's disease.

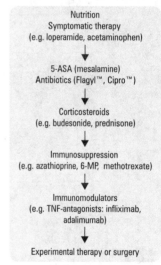

Nutrition
Symptomatic therapy
(e.g. loperamide, acetaminophen)
↓
5-ASA (mesalamine)
Antibiotics (Flagyl™, Cipro™)
↓
Corticosteroids
(e.g. budesonide, prednisone)
↓
Immunosuppression
(e.g. azathioprine, 6-MP, methotrexate)
↓
Immunomodulators
(e.g. TNF-antagonists: infliximab, adalimumab)
↓
Experimental therapy or surgery

Figure 7. Traditional graded approach to induction therapy in Crohn's disease
Note: immunosuppressants and immunomodulators are increasingly used initially ("top-down management strategy")

Pathology
- disease can involve any portion of lower bowel ranging from rectum only (proctitis) to entire colon (pancolitis)
- inflammation is diffuse, continuous and confined to mucosa

Clinical Features
- rectal bleeding is the hallmark feature; diarrhea present if more than the rectum is involved
  - can also have abdominal cramps/pain, especially with defecation
- severity of colonic inflammation correlates with symptoms (stool volume, amount of blood in stool)
- tenesmus, urgency, incontinence
- systemic symptoms: fever, anorexia, weight loss, fatigue in severe cases
- extra-intestinal manifestations (see Table 11)
- characteristic exacerbations and remissions; 5% of cases are fulminant

Investigations
- sigmoidoscopy with mucosal biopsy (to exclude self-limited colitis) without bowel prep often sufficient for diagnosis
- colonoscopy helpful to determine extent of disease; contraindicated in severe exacerbation
- CT colonography (formerly barium enema) if colonoscopy cannot be done; contraindicated in severe disease
- stool culture, microscopy, *C. difficile* toxin assay necessary to exclude infection
- no single confirmatory test

Treatment
- mainstays of treatment: 5-ASA (mesalamine) derivatives (only in mild to moderate disease) and corticosteroids, with azathioprine used in steroid-dependent or resistant cases
- diet of little value in decreasing inflammation but may alleviate symptoms
- anti-diarrheal medications generally not indicated in UC
  - 5-ASA
    - topical (suppository or enema): effective for distal disease (rectum to splenic flexure) if inflammation is mild, preferable to corticosteroids
    - oral: effective for mild to moderate, but not severe colitis (e.g. sulfasalazine 3-4 g/d, mesalamine 4 g/d)
    - commonly used in maintaining remission (decreases yearly relapse rate from 60% to 15%)
    - may decrease rate of colorectal cancer
- corticosteroids
  - to remit acute disease, especially if severe or first attack; may need maximum dose IV steroids initially (e.g. methylprednisolone 30 mg IV q12h)
  - limited role as maintenance therapy for mild to moderate disease
  - use suppositories for proctitis
  - use enemas and topical steroids (e.g. hydrocortisone foam, budesonide enemas) for inflammation distal to splenic flexure
- immunosuppressants (steroid-sparing)
  - in hospitalized patients with severe UC – add IV infliximab if no response to IV methylprednisolone within 3 days; then colectomy if inadequate response
  - biologics (infliximab, adalimumab, golimumab, vedolizumab) can also be used for outpatients with moderate-severe disease, particularly those that are steroid-unresponsive or steroid-dependent
  - azathioprine and 6-mercaptopurine: too slow to rapidly resolve acute relapse
    - most commonly used to maintain remission as corticosteroids withdrawn
    - given with biologics: increase efficacy of biologics and decrease likelihood of tolerance to biologics (~ 10% chance/yr)
- surgical treatment curative
  - aim for cure with colectomy; bowel continuity can be restored with ileal pouch-anal anastamosis (IPAA)
  - indications: failure of adequate medical therapy, toxic megacolon, uncontrollable bleeding, pre-cancerous changes detected either by endoscopy or endoscopic biopsies (dysplasia), inability to taper corticosteroids, overt malignancy

Complications
- similar to CD, except
  - more liver problems (especially PSC in men)
  - greater risk of colorectal cancer
    - risk increases with duration and extent of disease (5% at 10 yr, 15% at 20 yr for pancolitis; overall relative risk is 8%)
    - risk also increases with active mucosal inflammation and sclerosing cholangitis
    - thus, regular colonoscopy and biopsy in pancolitis of ≥8 yr is indicated
  - toxic megacolon (transverse colon diameter >6 cm on abdominal x-ray) with immediate danger of perforation (see General Surgery, GS37)

In UC, non-bloody diarrhea is frequently the initial presentation; eventually progressing to bloody diarrhea

Medical Management of Ulcerative Colitis

	Induction of Remission	Maintenance
5-ASA	+	+
Steroids	+	
Immunosuppressive	±	+

When Considering Complications of IBD, Think:

ULCERATIVE COLITIS
Urinary calculi
Liver problems
Cholelithiasis
Epithelial problems
Retardation of growth/sexual maturation
Arthralgias
Thrombophlebitis
Iatrogenic complications
Vitamin deficiencies
Eyes
Colorectal cancer
Obstruction
Leakage (perforation)
Iron deficiency
Toxic megacolon
Inanition (wasting)
Strictures

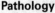

Prognosis
- chronic relapsing pattern in most patients
- 10-15% chronic continuous pattern
- >1 attack in almost all patients
- more colonic involvement in the 1st yr correlates with increased severity of attacks and increased colectomy rate
  - colectomy rate = 1% for all patients after the 1st yr; 20-25% eventually undergo colectomy
- normal life expectancy
- if proctitis only, usually benign course
- stool calprotectin increasingly recognized as a marker of bowel mucosal inflammation, reported especially to be useful in monitoring the activity of inflammatory bowel disease, but still accuracy is still controversial

Irritable Bowel Syndrome

Definition
- a form of functional bowel disease; more than just a label for GI symptoms unexplained after normal investigations

Epidemiology
- 20% of North Americans
- onset of symptoms usually in young adulthood
- F>M

Pathophysiology
- associated with either abnormal perception of intestinal activity or abnormal intestinal motility
- abnormal motility: multiple abnormalities described; unclear if associations or if causative
- psychological: stress may increase IBS symptoms but probably does not cause IBS
- types of IBS: IBS with diarrhea, IBS with constipation, IBS-mixed type (both diarrhea and constipation), and IBS untyped (insufficient abnormality in stool consistency to meet other types)

Diagnosis

Table 13. Rome III Criteria for Diagnosing Irritable Bowel Syndrome

IBS Rome III Criteria

≥12 wk in the past 12 mo of abdominal discomfort plus pain that has 2 out of 3 features
  Relieved with defecation
  Associated with a change in frequency of stool
  Associated with a change in consistency of stool

The following are supportive, but not essential to the diagnosis:
  Abnormal stool frequency (>3/d or <3/wk)
  Abnormal stool form (lumpy/hard/loose/watery) >1/4 of defecations
  Abnormal stool passage (straining, urgency, feeling of incomplete evacuation) >1/4 of defecations
  Passage of mucus >1/4 of defecations
  Bloating

Diagnosis of IBS Less Likely in Presence of "Red Flag" Features

Weight loss	Anemia
Fever	Blood or pus in stool
Nocturnal defecation	Abnormal gross findings on flexible sigmoidoscopy

Normal Physical Exam

Investigations
- if history consistent with Rome III criteria, no alarm symptoms, and no family history of IBD or colorectal cancer, limited investigations required
- aim is to rule out diseases which mimic IBS, particularly celiac disease and IBD
- investigations can be limited to CBC, inflammatory markers (ESR, CRP) and celiac serology
- if available, fecal calprotectin is likely more reliable test to rule out IBD
- consider TSH, stool cultures depending on clinical circumstances
- consider colonoscopy (e.g. if alarming features present, family history of IBD or age > 50)

IBS Mimickers
- Enteric infections e.g. *Giardia*
- Lactose intolerance/other disaccharidase deficiency
- Crohn's disease
- Celiac sprue
- Drug-induced diarrhea
- Diet-induced (excess tea, coffee, colas)

Treatment
- reassurance, explanation, support, aim for realistic goals
- relaxation therapy, biofeedback, hypnosis, stress reduction, probably exercise
- low FODMAP diet for pain, bloating gas, irregular bowel movements
- no therapeutic agent consistently effective, pain most difficult to control, no drug changes natural history so the drug should be "wanted, since it is not needed"

Rifaximin Therapy for Patients with Irritable Bowel Syndrome Without Constipation
NEJM 2011;364:22-32
Purpose: Previous evidence suggests that gut flora may play an important role in the pathophysiology of IBS. This study evaluated rifaximin, a minimally absorbed antibiotic, in treating IBS without constipation.
Methods: Two phase 3, double-blind, placebo-controlled trials (TARGET 1 and TARGET 2). 1,260 patients who had IBS without constipation were randomly assigned to rifaximin (550 mg dose) or placebo, 3 times daily for 2 wk, with a follow-up of 10 wk. The primary endpoint was adequate self-reported relief of global IBS symptoms.
Results: Significantly more patients in the rifaximin group had adequate self-reported relief of global IBS symptoms compared to the placebo group during the first 4 wk after treatment (40.8% vs. 31.2% respectively). Also, more patients in the rifaximin group had adequate relief of bloating compared to the placebo group (39.5% vs. 28.7% respectively).
Conclusions: Rifaximin therapy for 2 wk provided significant relief of symptoms, bloating, abdominal pain, and stool consistency associated with IBS without constipation.

- symptom-guided treatment
  - pain predominant
    - antispasmodic medication before meals (e.g. hyoscine, pinaverium, trimebutine - low level evidence)
    - increase dietary fibre (bran or psyllium)
    - tricyclic antidepressants (TCA), selective serotonin reuptake inhibitors (SSRI - moderate level of evidence)
  - IBS with diarrhea (IBS-D)
    - increase dietary fibre (bran or psyllium) to increase stool consistency but worsens abdominal gas
    - loperamide (Imodium*)
    - diphenoxylate (Lomotil*)
    - cholestyramine
  - IBS with constipation (IBS-C)
    - increase fibre in diet
    - linaclotide
    - osmotic or other laxatives (help more with the constipation than the pain)
  - mixed (alternating constipation and diarrhea) (IBS-M)

Prognosis
- 80% improve over time
- most have intermittent episodes
- normal life expectancy

Constipation

Definition
- passage of infrequent or hard stools with straining (stool water <50 mL/d); bowel frequency <3x/wk

Epidemiology
- increasing prevalence with age; F>M
- rare in Africa and India where stool weight is 3-4x greater than in Western countries

Etiology
- most common: idiopathic attributed to colon dysmotility but this is difficult to measure
- organic causes
  - medication side effects (narcotics, antidepressants) are the most common
  - intestinal obstruction, left sided colon cancer (consider in older patients), and fecal impaction
  - metabolic
    - DM
    - hypothyroidism
    - hypercalcemia, hypokalemia, uremia
  - neurological
    - intestinal pseudo-obstruction
    - Parkinson's disease
    - MS
  - collagen vascular disease (e.g. scleroderma)
  - painful anal conditions (e.g. fissures

Causes of Constipation

DOPED
Drugs
Obstruction
Pain
Endocrine dysfunction
Depression

Clinical Presentation
- overlaps with IBS
- stool firm, difficult to expel, passed with straining, abdominal pain relieved by defecation, flatulence, overflow diarrhea, tenesmus, abdominal distension, infrequent BMs (<3/wk)

Investigations
- underlying disease rarely found if constipation is the only presenting symptom
  - only test indicated in this situation is a CBC (2013 recommendation of American Gastroenterology Association), but also consider TSH, calcium, and glucose, X-ray of abdomen
- colon visualization if concomitant symptoms such as rectal bleeding, weight loss, or anemia (colonoscopy, CT colonography)
- if refractory to treatment, consider classification based on colon transit time; can measure colonic transit time with radio-opaque markers that are ingested and followed with a series of plain film abdominal x-rays (normal: 70 h)
  1. normal = misperception of normal defecation (IBS)
  2. prolonged throughout = "colonic inertia" (infrequent bowel movements with gas/bloating, tends to occur in youth)
  3. outlet obstruction = inability to coordinate pelvic floor muscles to empty rectum, straining, stool in rectum on digital exam, tends to occur in old age
- combination of 1 and 3 common

Treatment (in order of Increasing Potency)
- dietary fibre
  - useful if mild or moderate constipation, but not if severe
  - aim for 30 g daily, increase dose slowly
- surface-acting (soften and lubricate)
  - docusate salts, mineral oils
- osmotic agents (effective in 2-3 d)
  - lactulose, sorbitol, magnesium salts (e.g. magnesium hydroxide, i.e. milk of magnesia), lactitol (β-galactosido-sorbitol), polyethylene glycol 3350
- cathartics/stimulants (effective in 24 h)
  - castor oil, senna (avoid prolonged use to prevent melanosis coli), bisacodyl
- enemas and suppositories (e.g. saline enema, phosphate enema, glycerin suppository, bisacodyl suppository)
- prokinetic agents (prucalopride)
- linaclotide (increases water secretion into the intestinal lumen)

Upper Gastrointestinal Bleeding

Definition
- bleeding proximal to the ligament of Treitz, see *Gastrointestinal Tract*, G2 (75% of GI bleeds)
  - ligament of Treitz: suspensory ligament where fourth portion of the duodenum transitions to jejunum

Etiology
- above the GE junction
  - epistaxis
  - esophageal varices (10-30%)
  - esophagitis
  - esophageal cancer
  - Mallory-Weiss tear (10%)
- stomach
  - gastric ulcer (20%) (see *Peptic Ulcer Disease*, G11)
  - erosive gastritis (e.g. from EtOH or post-surgery) (20%)
  - gastric cancer
  - gastric antral vascular ectasia (rare, associated with cirrhosis and CTD)
  - Dieulafoy's lesion (very rare)
- duodenum
  - ulcer in bulb (25%)
  - aortoenteric fistula: usually only if previous aortic graft (see sidebar)
- coagulopathy (drugs, renal disease, liver disease)
- vascular malformation (Dieulafoy's lesion, AVM)

Clinical Features
- in order of decreasing severity of the bleed: hematochezia (brisk upper GI bleed) > hematemesis > coffee ground emesis > melena > occult blood in stool

Treatment
- stabilize patient (1-2 large bore IVs, IV fluids, monitor)
- send blood for CBC, cross and type, platelets, PT, PTT, electrolytes, BUN, Cr, LFTs
- keep NPO
- consider NG tube to determine upper vs. lower GI bleeding in some cases
- IV PPI: decrease risk of rebleed if endoscopic predictors of rebleeding seen (see prognosis section)
  - given to stabilize clot, not to accelerate ulcer healing
  - if given before endoscopy, decreases need for endoscopic therapeutic intervention
- for variceal bleeds, octreotide 50 μg loading dose followed by constant infusion of 50 μg/h
- consider IV erythromycin (or metoclopramide) to accelerate gastric emptying prior to gastroscopy to remove clots from stomach
- endoscopy (OGD): establish bleeding site + treat lesion
  - if bleeding peptic ulcer: most commonly used method of controlling bleeding is injection of epinephrine around bleeding point + thermal hemostasis (bipolar electrocoagulation or heater probe); less often thermal hemostasis may be used alone, but injection alone not recommended
  - endoclips
  - hemospray

Prognosis
- 80% stop spontaneously
- peptic ulcer bleeding: low mortality (2%) unless rebleeding occurs (25% of patients, 10% mortality)
- endoscopic predictors of rebleeding (Forrest classification): spurt or ooze, visible vessel, fibrin clot
- can send home if clinically stable, bleed is minor, no comorbidities, endoscopy shows clean ulcer with no high risk predictors of rebleeding
- H2-antagonists should not be used since they impact minimally on rebleeding rates and need for surgery
- esophageal varices have a high rebleeding rate (55%) and mortality (29%)

Always ask about NSAID/Aspirin® or anticoagulant therapy in GI bleed

Aortoenteric Fistula is a rare and lethal cause of GI bleed, most common in patients with a history of aortic graft surgery. Therefore, perform emergency endoscopy if suspected, emergency surgery if diagnosed. Note: The window of opportunity is narrow. Suspect if history of aortic graft, abdominal pain associated with bleeding

Transfusion Strategies for Acute Upper Gastrointestinal Bleeding
NEJM 2013;368:11-21
Study: Prospective, unblinded, RCT, follow-up up to 45 d.
Populations: 921 patients with hematemesis, bloody nasogastric aspirate, melena, or both. Exclusion criteria included massive bleed, ACS, stroke/TIA or transfusion within previous 90 d; recent trauma/surgery; lower GI bleed.
Intervention: Patients randomized to restrictive (<70 g/L) or liberal (<90 g/L) transfusion.
Outcome: Mortality, further bleeding, adverse events.
Results: Fewer patients in the restrictive group required transfusion (51% vs. 15%; p<0.001). The hazard ratio for death for restrictive compared to liberal transfusion was 0.55; 95% CI 0.33-0.92; p=0.02. Further bleeding occurred in 10% vs. 16% (p=0.01) of patients, while adverse effects occurred in 40% vs. 48% (p=0.02) of patients in the restrictive and liberal strategies, respectively. The restrictive strategy had a better survival rate in patients with bleeding associated with cirrhosis Child-Pugh class A or B (HR: 0.30; 95% CI 0.11-0.85), but not in cirrhosis Child-Pugh class C (HR: 1.04; 95% CI 0.45-2.37) or a peptic ulcer (HR: 0.70; 95% CI 0.26-1.25).
Conclusions: Transfusing patients with an acute upper GI bleed at hemoglobin of <70 g/L rather than 90 g/L is associated with fewer transfusions, better survival, and fewer adverse events.

Forrest Prognostic Classification of Bleeding Peptic Ulcers

Forrest Class	Type of Lesion	Risk of Rebleed (%)
I	Arterial bleeding (oozing/spurting)	55-100
IIa	Visible vessel	43
IIb	Sentinel clot	22
IIc	Hematin covered flat spot	10
III	No stigmata of hemorrhage	5

Lancet 1974;2:394-397

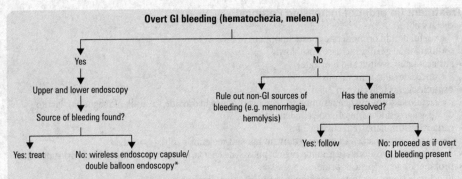

Figure 8. Approach to iron deficiency anemia

Esophageal Varices

Etiology
- almost always due to portal hypertension

Clinical Features
- characteristically massive upper GI bleeding

Prognosis
- risk of bleeding: 30% in 1st yr
- risk of rebleeding: 50-70% (20% mortality at 6 wk)

Investigations
- endoscopy

Management

If varices isolated to stomach, think of splenic vein thrombosis

Gastric varices best treated by endoscopic injection of cyanoacetate ("crazy glue")

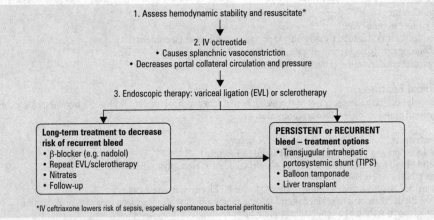

Figure 9. Management of bleeding esophageal varices
Not depicted: Intravenous ceftriaxone (lowers risk of sepsis, especially spontaneous bacterial peritonitis)

Mallory-Weiss Tear

Definition
- longitudinal laceration in gastric mucosa on lesser curvature near GE junction (20% straddle junction, 5% in distal esophagus)

Etiology
- due to rapid increases in gastric pressure from retching/vomiting against a closed glottis
- hiatus hernia usually present

Clinical Features
- hematemesis ± melena, classically following an episode of retching without blood
- can lead to fatal hematemesis

Management
- 90% stop spontaneously
- if persistent: endoscopy with epinephrine injection ± clips or surgical repair

Lower Gastrointestinal Bleeding

Definition
• bleed distal to ligament of Treitz

Etiology
• if blood per rectum with hemodynamic instability, rule out upper GI source
• diverticular (60% from right colon)
• vascular
  ▪ angiodysplasia (small vascular malformations of the gut)
  ▪ anorectal (hemorrhoids, fissures)
• neoplasm
  ▪ cancer
  ▪ polyps
• inflammation
  ▪ colitis (ulcerative, infectious, radiation, ischemic)
• post-polypectomy

Lower GI Bleed

CHAND
Colitis (radiation, infectious, ischemic, IBD [UC > CD])
Hemorrhoids/fissure
Angiodysplasia
Neoplastic
Diverticular disease

Clinical Features
• hematochezia (see Figure 10)
• anemia
• occult blood in stool
• rarely melena

Treatment
• treat underlying cause

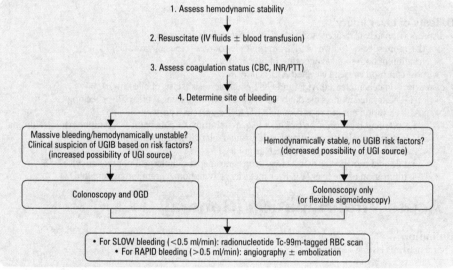

1. Assess hemodynamic stability

2. Resuscitate (IV fluids ± blood transfusion)

3. Assess coagulation status (CBC, INR/PTT)

4. Determine site of bleeding

| Massive bleeding/hemodynamically unstable? Clinical suspicion of UGIB based on risk factors? (increased possibility of UGI source) | Hemodynamically stable, no UGIB risk factors? (decreased possibility of UGI source) |
| Colonoscopy and OGD | Colonoscopy only (or flexible sigmoidoscopy) |

• For SLOW bleeding (<0.5 ml/min): radionucleotide Tc-99m-tagged RBC scan
• For RAPID bleeding (>0.5 ml/min): angiography ± embolization

Always exclude upper GI lesion before localizing the site of the bleeding to the lower GI tract

Figure 10. Approach to hematochezia

Colorectal Carcinoma

• see General Surgery, GS34

Colorectal Polyps

• see General Surgery, GS33

Familial Colon Cancer Syndromes

• see General Surgery, GS33

Benign Anorectal Disease

• see General Surgery, GS38

Liver

Investigations of Hepatobiliary Disease

A. Tests of Liver Function

Table 14. Liver Function Tests

Test	What Do Levels Correlate With?	Increased by	How to Interpret
Prothrombin Time (PT or INR)	Hepatic protein synthesis All coagulation factors except VIII	Hepatocellular dysfunction Vitamin K deficiency (due to malnutrition, malabsorption, etc.)	PT/INR will promptly correct if vitamin K is administered, so increased PT/INR in absence of vitamin K deficiency is a reliable marker of hepatocellular dysfunction
Serum Albumin	Hepatic protein synthesis (and other causes listed in next column)	Hepatocellular dysfunction Malnutrition Renal or GI losses Significant inflammation Malignancy	Rule out potential causes other than hepatocellular dysfunction
Serum Direct Bilirubin*	Hepatic excretion from hepatocyte to biliary system	Liver dysfunction	Conjugation is preserved even in end stage liver failure, thus increased direct bilirubin indicates liver dysfunction

*Serum Bilirubin
• canaliculus breakdown product of hemoglobin; metabolized in the reticuloendothelial system of liver, transported through biliary system, excreted via gut
• direct bilirubin = conjugated; indirect = unconjugated bilirubin

B. Tests of Liver Injury
- disproportionately increased AST or ALT = hepatocellular damage
  - ALT more specific to liver; AST from multiple sources (especially muscle)
  - elevation of both highly suggestive of liver injury
  - most common cause of elevated ALT is fatty liver
- disproportionately increased ALP (and GGT) = cholestasis (stasis of bile flow)
  - if ALP is elevated alone, rule out bone disease by fractionating ALP and/or checking GGT
  - if ALP elevation out of proportion to ALT/AST elevation, consider
    1. obstruction of common bile duct (e.g. extraluminal = pancreatic Ca, lymphoma; intraluminal = stones, cholangiocarcinoma, sclerosing cholangitis, helminths)
    2. destruction of microscopic ducts (e.g. PBC)
    3. bile acid transporter defects (e.g. drugs, intrahepatic cholestasis of pregnancy)
    4. infiltration of the liver (e.g. liver metastases, lymphoma, granulomas, amyloid)

Acute Viral Hepatitis (General)

Definition
- viral hepatitis lasting <6 mo

Clinical Features
- most are subclinical
- flu-like prodrome may precede jaundice by 1-2 wk
  - nausea/vomiting, anorexia, headaches, fatigue, myalgia, low-grade fever, arthralgia and urticaria (especially HBV)
- only some progress to icteric (clinical jaundice) phase, lasting days to weeks
  - pale stools and dark urine 1-5 d prior to icteric phase
  - hepatomegaly and RUQ pain
  - splenomegaly and cervical lymphadenopathy (10-20% of cases)

Investigations
- AST and ALT (>10-20x normal in hepatocellular necrosis)
- ALP minimally elevated
- viral serology, particularly the IgM antibody directed to the virus

Treatment
- supportive (hydration, diet)
- usually resolves spontaneously, but if severe HBV infection, treatment with entecavir should be considered; in anicteric hepatitis C, anti-viral treatment should be considered (see hepatitis C)
- indications for hospitalization: encephalopathy, coagulopathy, severe vomiting, hypoglycemia

Prognosis
- poor prognostic indicators: comorbidities, persistently high bilirubin (>340 mmol; 20 mg/dL), increased INR, decreased albumin, hypoglycemia

All clotting factors except factor VIII and von Willebrand factor are exclusively synthesized in the liver. Factor VIII is also produced in the endothelium. In cirrhosis, risk of bleeding does not correlate closely with elevations in INR/PTT since so many of the proteins in the coagulation cascade are affected

ALT > AST = most causes of hepatitis
AST > ALT = alcoholic liver disease or other causes of hepatitis (i.e. non-alcoholic liver disease) that have progressed to advanced cirrhosis

Serum Transaminases >1000 due to
• Viral hepatitis
• Drugs/toxins
• Autoimmune hepatitis
• Hepatic ischemia
• Less often, common bile duct stone

Alcoholic hepatitis: history of recent alcohol, RUQ abdominal pain, AST/ALT>2, AST usually <300, low grade fever, mildly elevated WBC

Major Sources of ALP
• Hepatobiliary tree
• Bone
• Placenta

Complications
- cholestasis (most commonly associated with HAV infection)
- hepatocellular necrosis: AST, ALT >10-20x normal, ALP and bilirubin minimally increased, increased cholestasis

Hepatitis A Virus

- RNA virus
- fecal-oral transmission; incubation period 4-6 wk
- diagnosed by elevated transaminases, positive anti-HAV IgM
- in children: characteristically asymptomatic
- in adults: fatigue, nausea, arthralgia, fever, jaundice
- can cause acute liver failure and subsequent death (<1-5%)
- can relapse (rarely), but never becomes chronic

Hepatitis B Virus

Table 15. Hepatitis B Serology

	HBsAg	Anti-HBs	HBeAg	Anti-HBe	Anti-HBc	Liver Enzymes
Acute HBV	+	–	+	–	IgM	
Chronic (e-Ag positive) HBV (generally high HBV DNA)	+	–	+	–	IgG	ALT, AST elevated
Chronic (e-Ag negative) HBV (generally low HBV DNA)	+	–	–	+	IgG	ALT, AST normal
Resolved infection	–	±	–	±	IgG	
Immunization	–	+	–	–	–	

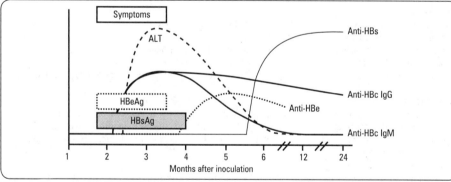

Figure 11. Time course of acute hepatitis B infection

Epidemiology
- 4 phases of chronic hepatitis B: not all carriers will go through all 4 phases, but all carriers will have positive HBsAg
  1. **immune tolerance**: extremely high HBV-DNA (>20,000 IU/mL), HBeAg positive, but normal ALT/AST; due to little immune control and minimal immune-mediated liver damage; characteristic of perinatal infection (or 'incubation period' in adult with newly-acquired HBV)
  2. **immune clearance** (or immunoactive): HBV-DNA levels (>20,000 IU/mL), HBeAg positive; due to immune attack on the virus and immune-mediated liver damage; characterized by progressive disease without treatment and increasing liver fibrosis (sometimes progressing to cirrhosis and/or hepatocellular carcinoma); likely to benefit from treatment
  3. **immune control**: lower HBV-DNA (<20,000 IU/mL), HBeAg negative, anti-HBe positive, ALT/AST normal; due to immune control without immune-mediated liver damage; risk of reactivation to phase 2 (clinically resembles acute hepatitis B), especially with immunosuppression e.g. corticosteroids or chemotherapy
  4. **immune escape** ("core or precore mutant"): elevated HBV-DNA (>2,000 IU/mL), HBeAg negative because of pre-core or core promoter gene mutation, anti-HBe positive, ALT/AST high; characterized by progressive disease without treatment and increasing liver fibrosis (sometimes progressing to cirrhosis and/or hepatocellular carcinoma); likely to benefit from treatment

DDx for Hepatitis
- Viral infection
- Alcohol
- Drugs
- Immune-mediated
- Toxins

Causes of Elevated Serum Transaminases in Chronic Hepatitis B
- Ongoing immune-mediated liver injury without immune control of HBV (HBeAg positive)
- Immune escape (anti-HBe positive)
- Reactivation, seroconversion (conversion from anti-HBe to HBeAg)
- Hepatitis D
- Heptocellular carcinoma
- Other liver insult (fatty liver, alcohol, drugs, hepatitis A)

Risk Factors for Progression
- EtOH
- HIV coinfection
- Old age at diagnosis

In acute hepatitis B, HDV coinfection increases severity of hepatitis but does not increase risk of progression to chronic hepatitis. However in the context of chronic hepatitis B, superinfection with HDV increases progression to cirrhosis

Without treatment, 8-20% of those with ongoing immunoactive chronic hepatitis can develop cirrhosis within 5 yr. In contrast, those in the immune tolerant phase (with extremely high HBV-DNA levels) are at minimal risk for liver fibrosis as they do not have immune-mediated liver injury

Risk of hepatocellular carcinoma in HBV increases with increasing age, which is likely a surrogate for increasing liver fibrosis/cirrhosis, and serum HBV-DNA
Risk of hepatocellular carcinoma in HCV increases only after cirrhosis develops

HCV (and HBV) treatment lowers the risk of hepatocellular carcinoma

DDx for Hepatomegaly
- Congestive (right heart failure, Budd-Chiari syndrome)
- Infiltrative
  - Malignant (primary, secondary, lymphoproliferative, leukemia)
  - Benign (fatty liver, cysts, hemochromatosis, extramedullary hematopoiesis, amyloid)
- Proliferative
  - Infectious (viral, tuberculosis, abscess, echinococcus)
  - Inflammatory (granulomas [sarcoid], histiocytosis X)

From Description to Cure in One Generation
Ledipasvir and Sofosbuvir for Untreated HCV Genotype 1 Infection
NEJM 2014;370;1889-1898.
If you ever need an example to demonstrate the miraculous advances of modern medicine, consider using chronic hepatitis C. It inflicts about 6 per 1000 of Canadians and is the commonest reason for liver transplant in most studies. Yet until 1989, when the virus was first cloned, this condition was so poorly understood that it was labelled as what it wasn't - it was called hepatitis non-A, non-B because there was insufficient evidence to even appreciate that it was one disease, let alone an infection. Today it can be cured by taking a safe drug regimen for 6 to 24 weeks, depending on the virus strain, previous treatments, and the degree of liver damage. This recent study showed that sofosbuvir (nucleoside polymerase inhibitor) and ledispavir (NS5A inhibitor) led to a 99% cure rate in genotype 1 (the most common) infection with only minimal side-effects. These antiviral drugs are designer drugs: specifically tailored in the laboratory to combat pathogenic features of the hepatitis C virus.

Treatment of Hepatitis C: A Systematic Review
JAMA 2014;312(6):631-40.
Purpose: To evaluate the evidence for the safety, efficacy and tolerability of interferon and non-interferon based, oral therapies in the treatment of Hepatitis C virus (HCV).
Study: Literature review of phase 2, 3, and 4 studies published from January 1, 2009 – May 30, 2014, with data graded according to Oxford Centre for Evidence-Based Medicine criteria.
Population: 19, 063 adult patients infected with HCV genotype 1, 2, or 3 with or without HIV coinfection.
Outcome: Sustained virologic response (SVR) of undetectable plasma HCV RNA at 12 or 24 weeks post-therapy.
Results: Achievement of SVR was more difficult in HCV genotype 1 patients. Treatment of HCV genotype 1 patients with sofosvubir with pegylated interferon and ribavirin yielded high rates of SVR (89-90%) and shorter duration of therapy. HCV genotype 2 or 3 patients treated with sofosbuvir and ribavirin alone achieved SVR of 82-93% and 80-95% for genotype 2 at 12 weeks and genotype 3 at 24 weeks, respectively. Patients with HCV and HIV coinfection with compensated cirrhosis should be treated in the same manner as HCV-monoinfected patients.
Conclusions: High SVR rates can be achieved for HCV patients with or without HIV coinfection using shorter durations of non-interferon therapies. HCV genotype 1 patients are likely to benefit from co-treatment with interferon and non-interferon therapies.

Treatment
- counselling: 40% of men and 10% of women with perinatal infection without treatment will die from HBV-related complications
- prolonged immune-mediated damage leads to higher risk of liver fibrosis
- hepatocellular carcinoma screening with ultrasound q6mo, especially if high serum HBV-DNA levels, cirrhosis, men, (age >40 in Asian men, >50 in Asian women, and >20 in African descent)
- consider pharmacological therapy if
  1. HBeAg positive + HBV-DNA >20, 000 IU/mL + elevated ALT ; or
  2. HBeAg negative + HBV-DNA >2,000 IU/mL + elevated ALT ± stage ≥2 fibrosis on liver biopsy
  3. treat to prevent flare when placed on immunosuppressive therapy such as prednisone, chemotherapy, biologics, etc.
- treatment goal: reduce serum HBV-DNA to undetectable level
- treatment options: interferon, tenofovir, entacavir, lamivudine
- vaccinate against HAV if serology negative (to prevent further liver damage)
- follow blood and sexual precautions

Hepatitis D

- defective RNA virus requiring HBsAg for entry into hepatocyte, therefore infects only patients with HBV; causes more aggressive disease than hepatitis B virus alone
- coinfection: acquire HDV and HBV at the same time
- HDV can present as ALF and/or accelerate progression to cirrhosis
- treatment: low-dose interferon (20% response) and liver transplant for end-stage disease

Hepatitis C Virus

- RNA virus (7 genotypes; genotype 1 is most common in North America)
- blood-borne transmission; sexual transmission is "inefficient"
- major risk factor: injection drug use
- other risk factors: blood transfusion received before 1992 (or received in developing world), tattoos, intranasal cocaine use
- clinical manifestation develops 6-8 wk after exposure
  - symptoms mild and vague (fatigue, malaise, nausea) therefore not commonly diagnosed in acute stage

Diagnosis
- suspected on basis of elevated ALT/AST and positive serum anti-HCV
- diagnosis established by detectable HCV-RNA in serum
- virus genotype correlates with response to treatment but not prognosis
  - serum HCV-RNA inversely correlates with response to treatment
- normal transaminases can have underlying cirrhosis on biopsy, but otherwise excellent prognosis

Treatment
- blood-borne precautions; vaccinate for hepatitis A and B if serology negative; avoid alcohol
- clearest indication for treatment is in subgroup likely to develop clinically significant liver disease
- persistently elevated transaminases, liver biopsy shows fibrosis/cirrhosis and at least moderately severe necrosis/inflammation
- treatment depends on genotype
- oral interferon-free regimens (e.g. sofosbuvir/ledipasvir, ombitasvir/paritaprevir/ritonavir+dasabuvir, or elbasvir/grazoprevir) are now becoming the standard of care with >90% success rate without significant side-effects including those who failed previous interferon-based treatment

Prognosis
- 80% of acute hepatitis C become chronic (of these 20% evolve to cirrhosis)
- risk of hepatocellular carcinoma increases if cirrhotic
- can cause cryoglobulinemia; associated with membranoproliferative glomerulonephritis, lymphoma

Table 16. Characteristics of the Viral Hepatitides

	HAV	HBV	HCV	HDV	HEV	CMV	EBV	Yellow Fever
Virus Family	*Picornaviridae*	*Hepadnaviridae*	*Flaviviridae*	*Deltaviridae*	*Caliciviridae*	*Herpesviridae*	*Herpesviridae*	*Flavivirus*
Genome	RNA	DNA	RNA	RNA	RNA	DNA	RNA	RNA
Envelope	No	Yes	Yes	Yes	No	Yes	Yes	Yes
Transmission	Fecal-oral	Parenteral/sexual or equivalent Vertical	Parenteral/sexual (transfusion, IVDU, sexual [<HBV]) 40% have no known risk factors	Non-parenteral (close contact in endemic areas) Parenteral (blood products, IVDU)- sexual transmission is inefficient	Fecal-oral (endemic: Africa, Asia, central America, India, Pakistan)	Close contacts, most body fluids	Saliva-oral	Vector (mosquito)
Incubation	4-6 wk	6 wk-6 mo	2-26 wk	3-13 wk	2-8 wk	20-60 d	30-50 d	3-6 d
Onset	Usually abrupt	Usually insidious	Insidious	Usually abrupt	Usually abrupt	Variable	Variable	Usually abrupt
Communicability	2-3 wk in late incubation to early clinical phase Acute hepatitis in most adults, 10% of children	HBsAg+ state highly communicable Increased during third trimester or early post-partum	Communicable prior to overt symptoms and throughout chronic illness	Infectious only in presence of HBV (HBsAg required for replication)	Unknown	Variable – dormant or persistent	Communicable highest during year after primary infection but never zero	Variable, vector-dependent
Chronicity	None, although can relapse	5% adults, 90% infants	80%, 20% of which develop cirrhosis	5%	None	Common; latent	Common; latent	Infection confers lifelong immunity
Serology	Anti-HAV (IgM)	See Table 15	HCV-RNA Anti-HCV (IgG/IgM)	HBsAg Anti-HDV (IgG/IgM)	Anti-HEV (IgG/IgM)	Anti- CMV (IgM/IgG)	Monospot; anti-EBV IgM/IgG, EBV DNA quantitation	Anti-YF (IgM/IgG)
Immunity	Yes	Yes	?	Yes	?	?	?	Yes
Vaccine	Havrix, 2 doses q6mo, combined with Twinrix at 0, 7, and 21 d	Recombivax HBTM, age 11-15, 2 doses q6mo	No	No	No	No	No	YF-VAX, 1 dose booster q10yr
Management	General hygiene Treat close contacts (anti-HAV Ig) Prophylaxis for high-risk groups (HAV vaccine ± HAV Ig) unless immune	Prevention: HBV vaccine and/or hepatitis B Ig (HBIG) for needlestick, sexual contact, infants of infected mothers unless already immune Rx: oral antivirals vs interferon if indications met	Prevention: no vaccine Rx: IFN + ribavirin ± protease inhibitor; although all oral anti-viral (IFN-free) therapy now available is highly efficacious	Prevention: HBV vaccine	Prevention: general hygiene, no vaccine	In high risk transplant patients: CMV IG and anti-virals (ganciclovir, valganciclovir)	Supportive treatment post infection	Prevention Supportive treatment post infection
Acute Mortality	0.1-0.3%	0.5-2%	1%	2-20% coinfection with HBV, 30% superinfection Predisposes HBV carriers to more severe hepatitis and faster progression to cirrhosis	1-2% overall, 10-20% in pregnancy	Rare in immunocompetent adults	Rare	20-60% in developing countries
Oncogenicity	No	Yes	Yes	?	No	No	Yes	No
Complications	Can cause acute liver failure and subsequent death (<1-5%)	Hepatocellular carcinoma secondary to cirrhosis, serum sickness-like syndrome, glomerulonephritis, cryoglobulinemia, polyarteritis nodosa, porphyria cutanea tarda	Hepatocellular carcinoma in 2-5% of cirrhosis per yr, cryoglobulinemia, B-cell non-Hodgkin lymphoma	Leukocytoclastic vasculitis, membranous glomerulonephropathy	Mild, except in third trimester (10-20% fulminant liver failure)	5% of newborns with multiple handicaps Immunocomprimised patients at risk of CMV-induced hepatitis, retinitis, colitis, esophagitis, pneumonitis	Associated with Burkitt's lymphoma and nasopharyngeal carcinoma (rare in Western world)	Can cause a recurrent toxic phase with liver damage, GI bleeding, and high mortality rates

Autoimmune Chronic Active Hepatitis

- diagnosis of exclusion: rule out viruses, drugs, metabolic, or genetic causes
- can be severe: 40% mortality at 6 mo without treatment
- extrahepatic manifestations
  - sicca, Raynaud's, thyroiditis, Sjögren's, arthralgias
  - hypergammaglobulinemia
    - anti-smooth muscle antibody elevation is most characteristic; also elevations in
    - anti-LKM elevation (liver kidney microsome), especially in children
      - less specific: elevated ANA, RF
    - can have false positive viral serology (especially anti-HCV)
    - biopsy – periportal (zone 1) and interface inflammation and necrosis
- treatment: corticosteroids (80% respond) ± azathioprine (without this, most will relapse as corticosteroids are withdrawn)

Drug-Induced Liver Disease

Table 17. Classification of Hepatotoxins

	Direct	Indirect
Example	Acetaminophen, CCl4	Phenytoin, INH
Dose-Dependence	Usual	Unusual
Latent Period	Hours-days	Weeks-months
Host Factors	Not important	Very important
Predictable	Yes	No (idiosyncratic)

Hy's Law: drug-induced hepatocellular jaundice indicates a mortality of at least 10%

Specific Drugs
- acetaminophen
    - metabolized by hepatic cytochrome P450 system
    - can cause ALF (transaminases >1,000 U/L followed by jaundice and encephalopathy)
    - requires 10-15 g in healthy, 4-6 g in alcoholics/anticonvulsant users
    - mechanism: high acetaminophen dose saturates glucuronidation and sulfation elimination pathways → reactive metabolite is formed → covalently binds to hepatocyte membrane
    - presentation
        - first 24 h: N/V (usually within 4-12 h of overdose)
        - 24-48 h: asymptomatic, but ongoing hepatic necrosis resulting in increased transaminases
        - >48 h: continued hepatic necrosis possibly complicated with ALF or resolution
        - note: potential delay in presentation in sustained-release products
    - blood levels of acetaminophen correlate with the severity of hepatic injury, particularly if time of ingestion known
    - therapy
        - gastric lavage/emesis (if <2 h after ingestion)
        - oral activated charcoal
        - N-acetylcysteine (NAC, Mucomyst®) can be given PO or IV (most effective within 8-10 h of ingestion, but should be given no matter when time of ingestion)
            – promotes hepatic glutathione regeneration
        - no recorded fatal outcomes if NAC given before increase in transaminases
- chlorpromazine: cholestasis in 1% after 4 wk; often with fever, rash, jaundice, pruritus, and eosinophilia
- INH (isoniazid)
    - 20% develop elevated transaminases but <1% develop clinically significant disease
    - susceptibility to injury increases with age
- methotrexate
    - causes fibrosis/cirrhosis; increased risk in the presence of obesity, DM, alcoholism (i.e. with underlying risk for pre-existing fatty liver)
    - scarring develops without symptoms or changes in liver enzymes, therefore biopsy may be needed in long-term treatment
- amiodarone: can cause same histology and clinical outcome as alcoholic hepatitis
- others: azoles, statins, methyldopa, phenytoin, propylthiouracil (PTU), rifampin, sulfonamides, tetracyclines
- herbs: chaparral, Chinese herbs (e.g. germander, comfrey, bush tea)

Wilson's Disease

Definition
- autosomal recessive defect in copper metabolism (gene ATP7B)

Etiology
- decreased biliary excretion of copper plus decreased incorporation of copper into ceruloplasmin

Clinical Manifestations of Wilson's Disease

ABCD
Asterixis
Basal ganglia degeneration: suspect if parkinsonian features in the young
Ceruloplasmin decreases
Cirrhosis
Corneal deposits (Kayser-Fleischer ring)
Copper
Dementia

Clinical Features
- liver: acute hepatitis, acute liver failure, chronic active hepatitis, cirrhosis, low risk of hepatocellular carcinoma
- eyes: Kayser-Fleischer rings (copper deposits in Descemet's membrane); more common in patients with CNS involvement, present in 50% if only liver involvement
- CNS: basal ganglia (wing flapping tremor, Parkinsonism), cerebellum (dysarthria, dysphagia, incoordination, ataxia), cerebrum (psychosis, affective disorder)
- kidneys: Fanconi's syndrome (proximal tubule transport defects) and stones
- blood: intravascular hemolysis; may be initial presentation in fulminant hepatitis
- joints: arthritis, bone demineralization, calcifications

Investigations
- suspect if increased liver enzymes with clinical manifestations at young age (<30); especially combination of liver disease with dystonia, psychiatric symptoms

- screening tests
    1. reduced serum ceruloplasmin (<50% of normal)
    2. Kayser-Fleischer rings (usually require slit-lamp examination)
    3. increased urinary copper excretion
- gold standard
    1. increased copper on liver biopsy by quantitative assay
    2. genetic analysis imperfect as many mutations in ATP7B are possible

Treatment
- 4 drugs available
    1. penicillamine chelates copper, poorly tolerated
    2. trientine chelates copper
    3. zinc impairs copper excretion in stool and decreases copper absorption from gut
    4. tetrathiomolybdate preferred if neurological involvement
- screen relatives
- liver transplant in severe cases

Hemochromatosis

Definition
- excessive iron storage causing multiorgan system dysfunction (liver, in particular) with total body stores of iron increased to 20-40 g (normal 1 g)

Etiology
- primary (hereditary) hemochromatosis
    - hepcidin deficiency results in ongoing gut absorption of iron despite adequate iron stores
- secondary hemochromatosis
    - parenteral iron overload (e.g. transfusions)
    - chronic hemolytic anemia: thalassemia, pyruvate kinase deficiency
    - excessive iron intake

Epidemiology
- hereditary hemochromatosis most common in Northern European descent
- primarily due to common recessive gene (HFE, 5%); 1/400 patients are homozygotes

Clinical Features
- usually presents with trivial elevation in serum transaminases
- liver: cirrhosis (30%), HCC (200x increased risk) – most common cause of death (1/3 of patients)
- pancreas: DM, chronic pancreatitis
- skin: bronze or grey (due to melanin, not iron)
- heart: dilated cardiomyopathy
- pituitary: hypogonadotropic hypogonadism (impotence, decreased libido, amenorrhea)
- joints: arthralgia (any joint, but especially MCP joints), chondrocalcinosis

Hemochromatosis Clinical Features ABCD
- Arthralgia
- Bronze skin
- Cardiomyopathy, cirrhosis of liver
- Diabetes (pancreatic damage)
- Hypogonadism (anterior pituitary damage)

Investigations
- screening for individuals with clinical features and/or family history (1/4 chance of sibling having the disease)
    - transferrin saturation (free Fe^{2+}/TIBC) >45%
    - serum ferritin >400 ng/mL
    - HFE gene analysis: 90% of primary hemochromatosis involves C282Y allele, while H63D and S65C alleles also commonly involved and screened
- liver biopsy (generally used to detect cirrhosis or if potential for other causes of liver disease)
    - markers of advanced fibrosis: if any of the following are present at the time of diagnosis → age >40, elevated liver enzymes, or ferritin >1000
    - considered if compound heterozygote and potential other cause of liver injury (e.g. fatty liver, etc.)
    - if C282Y/C282Y and no markers of advanced fibrosis, then biopsy generally not needed
- HCC screening if cirrhosis

Ferritin may never normalize if other causes of high ferritin present (e.g. fatty liver from metabolic syndrome or alcohol)

Gene mutation not 100% penetrant, so not all with homozygous gene defect have clinically significant iron overload

Treatment
- phlebotomy: weekly or q2wk then lifelong maintenance phlebotomies q2-6mo
- deferoxamine if phlebotomy contraindicated (e.g. cardiomyopathy, anemia)
- primary hemochromatosis responds well to phlebotomy
- secondary hemochromatosis usually requires chelation therapy (administration of agents that bind and sequester iron, and then excreted)

Prognosis
- normal life expectancy if treated before the development of cirrhosis or DM

Alcoholic Liver Disease

Standard Drink Equivalent
1 standard drink= 14 g EtOH
= 12 oz beer (5% alcohol)
= 5 oz wine (12-17%)
= 3 oz fortified wine (17-22%)
= 1.5 oz liquor (40%)
Tip: percentage alcohol multiplied by oz in 1 standard drink roughly equals 60

Definition
- fatty liver (all alcoholics): always reversible if alcohol stopped
- alcoholic hepatitis (35% of alcoholics): usually reversible if alcohol stopped
- cirrhosis (10-15% of alcoholics): potentially irreversible

Pathophysiology
- several mechanisms, poorly understood
- ethanol oxidation to acetaldehyde
  - reduces NAD^+ to NADH; increased NADH decreases ATP supply to liver, impairing lipolysis so fatty acids and triglycerides accumulate in liver
  - binds to hepatocytes evoking an immune reaction
- ethanol increases gut permeability leading to increased bacterial translocation
- alcohol metabolism causes
  - relative hypoxia in liver zone III (near central veins; poorly oxygenated) > zone I (around portal tracts, where oxygenated blood enters)
  - necrosis and hepatic vein sclerosis
- histology of alcoholic hepatitis
  - ballooned (swollen) hepatocytes often containing Mallory bodies, characteristically surrounded by neutrophils
  - large fat globules
  - fibrosis: space of Disse and perivenular

Biopsy + Histology of Alcoholic Hepatitis (triad)
- Hepatocyte necrosis with surrounding inflammation in zone III
- Mallory bodies (intracellular eosinophilic aggregates of cytokeratins)
- Chicken-wire fibrosis (network of intralobular connective tissue surrounding cells and venules)

Clinical Features
- >2-3 standard drinks/d in females and >3-6 standard drinks/d in men for >10 yr leads to cirrhosis, but only in about 10-20% of those who consume this amount daily on a continuous basis; cirrhosis risk increases with amount of alcohol consumed above threshold
- clinical findings do not accurately predict type of liver involvement
- fatty liver
  - mildly tender hepatomegaly; jaundice rare
  - mildly increased transaminases <5x normal
- alcoholic hepatitis
  - variable severity: mild to fatal liver failure
  - mild: stops drinking because feels unwell, resumes when feeling better (if assessed, findings of hepatitis, potentially mild jaundice, and mildly elevated INR)
  - severe: stops drinking but feels unwell, low grade fever, RUQ discomfort, increased white blood cell count – mimics RLL pneumonia and cholecystitis

GI Complications of Alcohol Abuse
- Esophagus
  - Mallory-Weiss tear
  - Esophageal varices (secondary to portal hypertension)
- Stomach
  - Alcoholic gastritis
- Pancreas
  - Acute pancreatitis
  - Chronic pancreatitis
- Liver
  - Alcoholic hepatitis
  - Fatty liver
  - Cirrhosis
  - Hepatic encephalopathy
  - Portal hypertension
  - Ascites
  - HCC

Investigations
- blood tests are non-specific, but in general
  - AST:ALT >2:1 (both usually <300)
  - if ALT>AST, usually cirrhosis has developd (assuming alcohol in the cause of the liver disease)
  - CBC: increased MCV, increased WBC

Treatment
- alcohol cessation (see Psychiatry, PS23)
  - Alcoholics Anonymous, disulfiram, naltrexone, acamprosate
- multivitamin supplements (especially thiamine)
- caution with drugs metabolized by the liver
- prednisone and pentoxifylline less used since most definitive trial did not show efficacy

Prognosis
- Maddrey's discriminant function (based on PT and bilirubin) and MELD predict mortality and guide treatment
- fatty liver: complete resolution with cessation of alcohol intake
- alcoholic hepatitis mortality
  - immediate: 30%-60% in the first 6 mo if severe
  - with continued alcohol: 70% in 5 yr
  - with cessation: 30% in 5 yr

Non-Alcoholic Fatty Liver Disease

Definition
- spectrum of disorders characterized by macrovesicular hepatic steatosis, sometimes with inflammation and/or fibrosis
- most common cause of liver disease in North America

Etiology
- pathogenesis not well elucidated; insulin resistance implicated as key mechanism, leading to hepatic steatosis
- histological changes indistinguishable from those of alcoholic hepatitis despite negligible history of alcohol consumption

Risk Factors
- likely a component of the metabolic syndrome along with type 2 DM, HTN, hypertriglyceridemia
- rapid weight loss or weight gain

Clinical Features
- often asymptomatic
- may present with fatigue, malaise, and vague RUQ discomfort
- elevated serum triglyceride/cholesterol levels and insulin resistance

Investigations
- elevated serum AST, ALT ± ALP; AST/ALT <1
- presents as echogenic liver texture on ultrasound
- liver biopsy diagnostic, but often necessary only for prognosis

Treatment
- mainstay is gradual weight loss (0.5-1 kg/wk) as rapid weight loss can worsen liver disease
  - ideally, aim to lose at least 7-10% of body weight
- some evidence for vitamin E (800 U daily) if there is hepatic inflammation
- some evidence for benefits of coffee drinking (3 cups per day) and vitamin D

Prognosis
- most die from cardiovascular or cerebrovascular disease
- better prognosis than alcoholic hepatitis
  - <25% progress to cirrhosis over a 7-10 yr period
- risk of progression increases if inflammation or scarring occurs alongside fat infiltration (non-alcoholic steatohepatitis)
- other clinical indicators of unfavourable prognosis: DM, age, metabolic syndrome

Acute Liver Failure (formerly Fulminant Hepatic Failure)

Definition
- severe decline in liver function characterized by coagulation abnormality (INR>1.5) and encephalopathy
- in setting of previously normal liver
- rapid (<26 wk duration)

Etiology
- drugs (especially acetaminophen), hepatitis B (measure anti-HBc, IgM fraction because sometimes HBV-DNA and even HBsAg rapidly becomes negative), hepatitis A, hepatitis C (rare), ischemic, idiopathic

Treatment
- correct hypoglycemia, monitor level of consciousness, prevent GI bleeding with PPI, monitor for infection and multiorgan failure (usually requires ICU)
- consider liver biopsy before INR becomes too high
- chief value of biopsy is to exclude chronic disease, less helpful for prognosis
- liver transplant (King's College criteria can be used as prognostic indicator): consider early, especially if time from jaundice to encephalopathy >7 d (e.g. not extremely rapid), age <10 or >40, cause is drug or unknown, bilirubin >300 μmol/L, INR >3.5, creatinine >200 μmol/L

Cirrhosis

Definition
- liver damage characterized by diffuse distortion of the basic architecture and replacement with scar tissue and formation of regenerative nodules
- Stage 1 cirrhosis is compensated and asymptomatic, can last for 10-20 yr with almost normal life expectancy
- Stage 2 cirrhosis is decompensation, typically development of ascites (most common), variceal bleeding, encephalopathy, characteristically presents abruptly even though histologically the liver fibrosis is gradually progressive

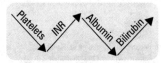

Figure 12. Progression of liver dysfunction based on liver function tests – the "W"

Etiology
- fatty liver (alcoholic or non-alcoholic fatty liver disease)
- chronic viral hepatitis (B, B+D, C; not A or E)

- autoimmune hepatitis
- hemochromatosis
- primary biliary cirrhosis
- chronic hepatic congestion
    - cardiac cirrhosis (chronic right heart failure, constrictive pericarditis)
    - hepatic vein thrombosis (Budd-Chiari)
- cryptogenic (i.e. no identifiable cause, although many of these patients may represent "burnt-out NASH")
- rare: Wilson's disease, Gaucher's disease, α1-antitrypsin deficiency

Investigations
- definitive diagnosis is histologic (liver biopsy)
- other tests may be suggestive
    - blood work: fall in platelet count <150 is the earliest finding, followed many years later with rise in INR, fall in albumin, rise in bilirubin, fall in glucose level (pre-terminal event)
    - FibroTest: combination of various clinical and biochemical markers that can predict degree of fibrosis
    - imaging
        - U/S is the primary imaging modality but only finds advanced cirrhosis
        - CT to look for varices, nodular liver texture, splenomegaly, ascites
        - Ultrasound elastography (FibroScan): non-invasive tool using elastography (variable availability)
- gastroscopy: varices or portal gastropathy

MELD-Na (Model for End Stage Liver Disease)
- Predicts 3 mo survival and used to stratify patients on transplant list
- Based on creatinine, INR, total bilirubin, and serum sodium concentration

Treatment
- treat underlying disorder
- decrease insults (e.g. alcohol cessation, hepatotoxic drugs, immunize for Hep A and B if non-immune)
- follow patient for complications (esophageal varices, ascites, HCC defines stage 2 cirrhosis)
- prognosis: Child-Pugh Score and MELD score
- liver transplantation for end-stage disease if no alcohol for >6 mo; use MELD score

Table 18. Child-Pugh Score and Interpretation

Classification	1	2	3
Serum bilirubin (μmol/L)	<34	34-51	>51
Serum albumin (g/L)	>35	28-35	<28
INR	<1.7	1.7-2.3	>2.3
Presence of ascites	Absent	Controllable	Refractory
Encephalopathy	Absent	Minimal	Severe

Interpretation			
Points	Class	Life Expectancy	Perioperative Mortality
5-6	A	15-50 yr	10%
7-9	B	Candidate for transplant	30%
10-15	C	1-3 mo	82%

Score: 5-6 (Child's A), 7-9 (Child's B), 10-15 (Child's C)
*Note: Child's classification is rarely used for shunting (TIPS or other surgical shunts), but is still useful to quantitate the severity of cirrhosis

Cirrhosis Complications

VARICES
Varices
Ascites/Anemia
Renal failure (hepatorenal syndrome)
Infection
Coagulopathy
Encephalopathy
Sepsis

Complications
- hematologic changes in cirrhosis
    - pancytopenia from hypersplenism: platelets first, then WBC, then hemoglobin
    - decreased clotting factors resulting in elevated INR
    - relationship of INR to bleeding tendency is controversial; some patients may be hypocoagulable, others may be hypercoagulable
- variceal bleeds
    - half of patients with cirrhosis have gastroesophageal varices and one-third of these develop hemorrhage with an overall mortality of >30%
    - hepatic venous pressure gradient (HVPG) ≥10 mmHg is the strongest predictor of variceal development
    - treatment: resuscitation, antibiotic prophylaxis, vasoactive drugs (e.g. octreotide IV) combined with endoscopic band ligation or sclerotherapy, TIPS
- renal failure in cirrhosis
    - classifications
        - pre-renal (usually due to over-diuresis)
        - acute tubular necrosis
        - HRS
            - Type I: sudden and acute renal failure (rapid doubling of creatinine over 2 wk)
            - Type II: gradual increase in creatinine with worsening liver function (creatinine doubling over years)

Usual causes of death in cirrhosis: renal failure (hepatorenal syndrome), sepsis, GI bleed, or HCC

Hepatorenal Syndrome vs. Pre-Renal Failure – Difficult to Differentiate
- Similar blood and urine findings
- Urine sodium: very low in hepatorenal; low in pre-renal
- Intravenous fluid challenge: giving volume expanders improves pre-renal failure, but not hepatorenal syndrome

- HRS can occur at any time in severe liver disease, especially after
  - overdiuresis or dehydration, such as diarrhea, vomiting, etc.
  - GI bleed
  - sepsis
- treatment for hepatorenal syndrome (generally unsuccessful at improving long-term survival)
  - for type I HRS: octreotide + midodrine + albumin (increases renal blood flow by increasing systemic vascular resistance)
  - definitive treatment is liver transplant
- hepatopulmonary syndrome
  - majority of cases due to cirrhosis, though can be due to other chronic liver diseases, such as non-cirrhotic portal HTN
  - thought to arise from ventilation-perfusion mismatch, intrapulmonary shunting and limitation of oxygen diffusion, failure of damaged liver to clear circulating pulmonary vasodilators vs. production of a vasodilating substance by the liver
  - clinical features
    - hyperdynamic circulation with cardiac output >7 L/min at rest and decreased pulmonary + systemic resistance (intrapulmonary shunting)
    - dyspnea, platypnea (increase in dyspnea in upright position, improved by recumbency), and orthodeoxia (desaturation in the upright position, improved by recumbency)
    - diagnosis via contrast-enhanced echocardiography: inject air bubbles into peripheral vein; air bubbles appear in left ventricle after third heartbeat (normal = no air bubbles; in ventricular septal defect, air bubbles seen <3 heart beats)
    - only proven treatment is liver transplantation

Hepatopulmonary Syndrome Clinical Triad
- Liver disease
- Increased alveolar-arterial gradient while breathing room air
- Evidence for intrapulmonary vascular abnormalities

Fibrosis may regress and disappear if cause of liver injury is treated or resolves

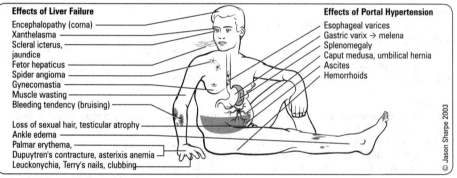

Effects of Liver Failure
Encephalopathy (coma)
Xanthelasma
Scleral icterus, jaundice
Fetor hepaticus
Spider angioma
Gynecomastia
Muscle wasting
Bleeding tendency (bruising)
Loss of sexual hair, testicular atrophy
Ankle edema
Palmar erythema,
Dupuytren's contracture, asterixis anemia
Leuckonychia, Terry's nails, clubbing

Effects of Portal Hypertension
Esophageal varices
Gastric varix → melena
Splenomegaly
Caput medusa, umbilical hernia
Ascites
Hemorrhoids

© Jason Sharpe 2003

Figure 13. Clinical features of liver disease

Hepatocellular Carcinoma

- see General Surgery, GS44

Liver Transplantation

- see General Surgery, GS45

Portal Hypertension

Definition
- pressure gradient between hepatic vein pressure and wedged hepatic vein pressure (corrected sinusoidal pressure) >5 mmHg

Pathophysiology
- 3 sites of increased resistance (remember pressure = flow x resistance)
  - pre-sinusoidal (e.g. portal vein thrombosis, schistosomiasis, sarcoidosis)
  - sinusoidal (e.g. cirrhosis, alcoholic hepatitis)
  - post-sinusoidal (e.g. right-sided heart failure, hepatic vein thrombosis, veno-occlusive disease, constrictive pericarditis)

Complications
- GI bleeding from varices in esophagus, less commonly in stomach, even less frequently from portal hypertensive gastropathy
- ascites
- hepatic encephalopathy
- thrombocytopenia
- renal dysfunction
- sepsis
- arterial hypoxemia

Portal Hypertension

Signs
- Esophageal varices
- Melena
- Splenomegaly
- Ascites
- Hemorrhoids

Management
- β-blockers
- Nitrates
- Shunts (e.g. TIPS)

Treatment
- non-selective β-blockers (propanolol, nadolol) decrease risk of bleeding from varices
- TIPS: to decrease portal venous pressure
  - radiologically inserted stent between portal and hepatic vein via transjugular vein catheterization and percutaneous puncture of portal vein
  - can be used to stop acute bleeding or prevent rebleeding or treat ascites
  - shunt usually remains open for <1 yr
  - complications: hepatic encephalopathy, deterioration of hepatic function
  - contraindicated with severe liver dysfunction
  - most commonly used as a "bridge" to liver transplant
- other surgically created shunts: portacaval, distal spleno-renal (Warren shunt) - all used only rarely in the modern era

Hepatic Encephalopathy

Definition
- spectrum of potentially reversible neuropsychiatric syndromes secondary to liver disease diagnosed after ruling out other causes for symptoms (e.g. structural/metabolic)

Pathophysiology
- portosystemic shunt around hepatocytes and decreased hepatocellular function increase level of systemic toxins (believed to be ammonia from gut, mercaptans, fatty acids, amino acids) which go to the brain

Precipitating Factors for Hepatic Encephalopathy

Hepatics
Hemorrhage in GI tract/**H**ypokalemia
Excess dietary protein
Paracentesis
Alkalosis/**A**Anemia
Trauma
Infection
Colon surgery
Sedatives

Precipitating Factors
- nitrogen load (GI bleed, protein load from food intake, renal failure, constipation)
- drugs (narcotics, CNS depressants)
- electrolyte disturbance (hypokalemia, alkalosis, hypoxia, hypovolemia)
- infection (spontaneous bacterial peritonitis)
- deterioration in hepatic function or superimposed liver disease

Stages
- I: apathy, restlessness, reversal of sleep-wake cycle, slowed intellect, impaired computational abilities, impaired handwriting
- II: asterixis, lethargy, drowsiness, disorientation
- III: stupor (rousable), hyperactive reflexes, extensor plantar response (upgoing Babinski)
- IV: coma (response to painful stimuli only)

Investigations
- clinical diagnosis: supported by laboratory findings and exclusion of other neuropsychiatric diseases
- rule out
  - non-liver-related neuropsychiatric disease in a patient with liver problems (e.g. alcohol withdrawal or intoxication, sedatives, subdural hematoma, metabolic encephalopathy)
  - causes of metabolic encephalopathy (e.g. renal failure, respiratory failure, severe hyponatremia, hypoglycemia)
- characteristic EEG findings: diffuse (non-focal), slow, high amplitude waves
- serum ammonia levels increased, but not often necessary to measure in routine clinical use

Treatment
- treat underlying precipitating factors
- decrease generation of nitrogenous compounds
  - routine protein restriction is no longer recommended given patients generally have concurrent malnutrition and muscle wasting; however, vegetable protein is better tolerated than animal protein
  - lactulose: titrated to achieve 2-3 soft stools/d
    - prevents diffusion of NH3 (ammonia) from the colon into blood by lowering pH and forming non-diffusible NH4 (ammonium)
    - serves as a substrate for incorporation of ammonia by bacteria, promotes growth in bowel lumen of bacteria which produce minimal ammonia
    - also acts as a laxative to eliminate nitrogen-producing bacteria from colon
- oral rifaximin for both acute treatment and maintenance therapy has high level evidence for efficacy
- best acute treatment in comatose patient is lactulose enemas
- other antibiotics that may be used include metronidazole and vancomycin

Ascites

Definition
- accumulation of excess fluid in the peritoneal cavity

Etiology

Table 19. Serum-Ascites Albumin Gradient as an Indicator of the Causes of Ascites

Serum [Alb] – Ascitic [Alb] >11 g/L (1.1 g/dL) Portal Hypertension Related	Serum [Alb] – Ascitic [Alb] <11 g/L (1.1 g/dL) Non-Portal Hypertension Related
Cirrhosis/severe hepatitis	Peritoneal carcinomatosis
Chronic hepatic congestion (right heart failure, Budd-Chiari)	TB
Massive liver metastases	Pancreatic disease
Myxedema	Serositis
	Nephrotic syndrome*

* In nephrotic syndrome: decreased serum [Alb] to begin with therefore gradient not helpful

Pathophysiology
- key factor in pathogenesis is increased sodium (and water) retention by the kidney for reasons not fully understood. Theories include:
  - underfill hypothesis: first step in ascites formation is increased portal pressure and low oncotic pressure (e.g. low serum albumin) driving water out of the splanchnic portal circulation into abdominal cavity; the resulting decreased circulating volume causes secondary sodium retention by the kidney
  - overfill hypothesis: cirrhosis directly causes increased sodium retention by the kidney in the absence of hypovolemia and ascites arises secondarily
  - peripheral arterial vasodilation theory (most popular): as portal HTN develops in cirrhosis, production of local mediators such as nitric oxide lead to splanchnic arterial vasodilation which ultimately results in reduction of effective arterial volume and compensatory sodium and fluid retention by the kidneys (i.e. circulation volume is increased, as per overflow hypothesis, but relatively underfilled, as per underfill hypothesis)

Diagnosis
- abdominal ultrasound
- physical exam (clinically detectable when >500 mL)
  - bulging flanks, shifting dullness, fluid-wave test positive
  - most sensitive symptom: ankle swelling

Investigations
- diagnostic paracentesis
  - 1st aliquot: cell count and differential
  - 2nd aliquot: chemistry (especially albumin, but also total protein; amylase if pancreatitis; TG and chylomicrons if turbid and suspect chylous ascites)
  - 3rd aliquot: C&S, Gram stain
  - 4th aliquot: cytology (usually positive in peritoneal carcinomatosis)

Treatment
- non-refractory ascites
  - Na^+ restriction (daily sodium intake <2 g)
  - diuretics: spironolactone, furosemide
  - aim for weight loss 0.5-1 kg/d, more if concomitant peripheral edema (which is mobilized quicker than ascitic fluid); overly rapid weight loss increases risk of renal failure
  - if target weight loss is not achieved and there are no complications, increase dose to achieve target while monitoring for complications
- refractory ascites (diuretics are inadequate or not tolerated)
  - therapeutic paracentesis with intravenous albumin
  - TIPS in an appropriate patient (no contraindications) with potential transplant-free survival advantage
  - liver transplantation should be considered in every case, since development of ascites in patients with cirrhosis is associated with 50% 2 yr mortality

Secondary bacterial peritonitis (as opposed to primary bacterial peritonitis) usually results from a perforated viscus or surgical manipulation

Serum Ascites Albumin Gradient (SAAG) = serum albumin – ascites albumin
- >11 g/L portal HTN
  - ascitic fluid total protein >25 g/L, suggests cardiac portal hypertension
  - ascitic fluid total protein <25 g/L, suggests cirrhosis portal hypertension
- <11 g/L unrelated to portal HTN

Complication: Primary/Spontaneous Bacterial Peritonitis
- primary/spontaneous bacterial peritonitis (SBP)
  - complicates ascites, but does not cause it (occurs in 10% of cirrhotic ascites); higher risk in patients with GI bleed
  - 1/3 of patients are asymptomatic, thus do not hesitate to do a diagnostic paracentesis in ascites even if no clinical indication of infection
  - fever, chills, abdominal pain, ileus, hypotension, worsening encephalopathy, acute kidney injury
  - Gram-negatives compose 70% of pathogens: *E. coli* (most common), *Streptococcus*, *Klebsiella*
- diagnosis
  - absolute neutrophil count in peritoneal fluid >0.25x10^9 cells/L (250 cells/mm³)
  - Gram stain positive in only 10-50% of patients
  - culture positive in <80% of patients (not needed for diagnosis)
- prophylaxis: consider in patients with
  - cirrhosis or GI bleed: ceftriaxone IV daily or norfloxacin bid x 7 d
  - previous episode of SBP: long-term prophylaxis with daily norfloxacin or TMP-SMX
- treatment
  - IV antibiotics (cefotaxime 2 g IV q8h or ceftriaxone 2g IV daily is the treatment of choice for 5 d; modify if response inadequate or culture shows resistant organisms)
  - IV albumin (1.5 g/kg at time of diagnosis and 1 g/kg on day 3) decreases mortality by lowering risk of acute renal failure

Biliary Tract

Jaundice

- see Table 2 and Figures 15 and 16

Signs and Symptoms
- dark urine, pale stools: suggests that bilirubin elevation is from direct fraction
- pruritus: suggests chronic disease, cholestasis
- abdominal pain: suggests biliary tract obstruction from stone or pancreatic tumour (obstructive jaundice)
- painless jaundice in the elderly: think of pancreatic cancer, although most patients with pancreatic cancer have pain
- kernicterus: rarely seen in adults due to maturation of blood brain barrier

Investigations
- blood work: CBC, bilirubin (direct and total), liver enzymes (AST, ALT, ALP, GGT), liver function tests (INR/PT, PTT, albumin), amylase
- U/S or CT for evidence of bile duct obstruction (e.g. bile duct dilation)
- direct bile duct visualization
- magnetic resonance cholangiopancreatography (MRCP): non-invasive
- endoscopic ultrasound (EUS): sensitive for stones and pancreatic tumours
- endoscopic retrograde cholangiopancreatography (ERCP): invasive, most accurate, allows for therapeutic intervention
- percutaneous transhepatic cholangiography (PTC): if ERCP fails (endoscopic access not possible)

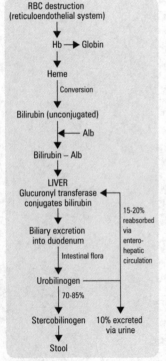

Figure 15. Production and excretion of bilirubin

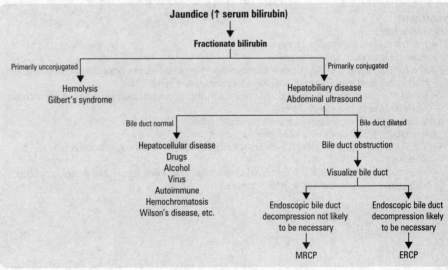

Figure 14. Approach to jaundice

Gilbert's Syndrome

Definition
- mild decrease in glucuronyltransferase activity leading to defective conjugation of bilirubin
- an abnormality of bilirubin metabolism with no clinical relevance

Etiology/Epidemiology
- some patients have decreased hepatobiliary uptake
- affects 7% of population, especially males
- autosomal dominant, 70% due to a mutation in the UGT gene

Clinical Features
- presents in teens-20s, often an incidental finding
- only manifestation is intermittent jaundice with increased serum unconjugated bilirubin developing most characteristically while fasting, or at times of acute illness; no other clinical implications

Treatment
- none indicated (entirely benign)

Gilbert's Syndrome vs. Crigler-Najjar Syndrome
Gilbert's Syndrome: mild decrease in glucuronyltransferase activity
Crigler-Najjar Syndrome: complete deficiency of glucuronyltransferase

Primary Sclerosing Cholangitis

Definition
- narrowing of biliary tree (intra and/or extrahepatic bile ducts) from scarring

Etiology
- primary/idiopathic (most common)
  - associated with IBD, more commonly UC, in up to 70% of patients (usually male)
  - one of the most common indications for liver transplant
- secondary (less common)
  - long-term choledocholithiasis
  - cholangiocarcinoma
  - surgical/traumatic injury (iatrogenic)
  - contiguous inflammatory process
  - post-ERCP
  - associated with HIV/AIDS ("HIV cholangiopathy")
  - IgG4-related disease

Signs and Symptoms
- often insidious, may present with fatigue and pruritus
- may present with signs of episodic bacterial cholangitis secondary to biliary obstruction

Investigations
- increased ALP (hallmark), less often increased bilirubin
- mildly increased AST, usually <300 U/L
- p-ANCA (30-80%), elevated IgM (40-50%)
- MRCP and ERCP shows narrowing and dilatations of bile ducts that may result in "beading", both intrahepatic and extrahepatic bile ducts
  - if intrahepatic narrowing only, do anti-mitochondrial antibody to rule out PBC

Complications
- repeated bouts of cholangitis may lead to complete biliary obstruction with resultant secondary biliary cirrhosis and hepatic failure
- increased incidence of cholangiocarcinoma (10-15%): difficult to diagnose and treat

Treatment
- image bile duct (MRCP) at least annually for early detection of cholangiocarcinoma (controversial)
- endoscopic sphincterotomy, biliary stent in selected cases of dominant CBD stricture
- antibiotics for cholangitis
- suppurative cholangitis requires emergency drainage of pus in CBD
- liver transplantation appears to be the best treatment for advanced sclerosing cholangitis (nearly 90% 1-yr survival; mean follow-up from time of diagnosis to need for transplant is 10 yr)
- ursodiol: previously recommended, but studies suggest that at least in high doses it increases mortality

Prognosis
- unfavourable regardless of treatment
- mean survival after diagnosis remains 4-10 yr

Primary Biliary Cholangitis (formerly cirrhosis)

Definition
- chronic inflammation and fibrous obliteration of intrahepatic bile ductules

Etiology/Epidemiology
- likely autoimmune (associated with Sjögren's syndrome, scleroderma, CREST syndrome, RA, thyroiditis)
- affects mainly middle-aged women (M:F = 1:9)

MRCP/ERCP
- Absence of narrowing in PBC
- Narrowing of intra and extrahepatic ducts in PSC

Signs and Symptoms
- often asymptomatic
- initial symptoms: pruritus, fatigue
- chronic: jaundice and melanosis (darkening skin) and other signs of cholestasis
- end-stage: hepatocellular failure, portal HTN, ascites
- high incidence of osteoporosis

Investigations
- increased ALP, GGT; bilirubin rises in later stage
- positive anti-mitochondrial antibodies (AMA; 95% specificity and sensitivity)
- increased serum cholesterol (mild increase in LDL, larger increase in HDL)
  - may have: xanthelasmas, xanthomas
- liver biopsy confirms diagnosis and stages severity
- normal bile duct on MRCP rules out bile duct obstruction which can mimic PBC
- recently described "overlap" syndromes with autoimmune cholangitis, autoimmune hepatitis, sclerosing cholangitis

Treatment
- treat with ursodiol (less frequently colchicine, methotrexate)
- cholestyramine (for pruritus and hypercholesterolemia)
- calcium and vitamin D for low bone density; bisphosphonates if osteoporosis severe
- monitor for thyroid disease
- liver transplant if disease severe, progressive

Prognosis
- can be fatal, although not all asymptomatic patients show progression

Table 20. Primary Sclerosing Cholangitis vs. Primary Biliary Cholangitis

	Primary Sclerosing Cholangitis	Primary Biliary Cholangitis
Predominant Gender	Male	Female
Associated Comorbidities	IBD, especially UC	Other autoimmune disorders (Sjögren's, CREST, RA)
Affected Ducts	Both intra- and extra-hepatic	Intrahepatic only
Investigations	ERCP/MRCP (narrowing and dilatations of ducts visualized)	Anti-mitochondrial antibodies, IgM, increased lipids, liver biopsy (absence of duct narrowing on ERCP)

Secondary Biliary Cirrhosis

Definition
- cirrhosis from prolonged partial or total obstruction of major bile ducts

Etiology
- acquired: post-operative strictures, chronic pancreatitis, sclerosing cholangitis, stone in bile duct
- congenital: CF, congenital biliary atresia, choledochal cysts

Investigations
- cholangiography and liver biopsy

Treatment
- treat obstruction, give antibiotics for cholangitis prophylaxis

Biliary Colic, Cholecystitis

- see <u>General Surgery</u>, GS47

Ascending Cholangitis

- see <u>General Surgery</u>, GS49

Definition
- infection of the biliary tree

Etiology
- stasis in the biliary tract due to obstruction or stricture (usually from previous cholecystectomy)
- infection originates in the duodenum or spreads hematogenously from the portal vein
- bacteria
  - *E. coli, Klebsiella, Enterobacter, Enterococcus*
  - co-infection with *Bacteroides* and Clostridia can occur

Charcot's Triad
- RUQ pain
- Fever
- Jaundice

Signs and Symptoms
- Charcot's triad: fever, RUQ pain, jaundice (50-70%)
- Reynolds' Pentad in patients with suppurative cholangitis: fever, RUQ pain, jaundice, hypotension, altered mental status

Reynolds Pentad
- Charcot's triad
- Hypotension
- Altered mental status

Investigations
- increased WBC
- usually increased ALP and bilirubin, ALT variably elevated
- blood culture
- abdominal U/S: CBD dilation, stones

Treatment
- most important is drainage, ideally via ERCP, but if not possible technically by percutaneous biliary or least often by surgical routes
- antibiotic therapy: broad spectrum to cover Gram-negatives, *Enterococcus*, and anaerobes (especially if CBD manipulation); no clear consensus on antibiotic choice but consider:
  - ampicillin + sulbactam or piperacillin/tazobactam
  - metronidazole + 3rd generation cephalosporin (e.g. ceftriaxone) or fluoroquinolone (e.g. ciprofloxacin or levofloxacin)
  - carbapenem monotherapy (e.g. imipenem or meropenem)

Prognosis
- good with effective drainage and antibiotics in mild to moderate cases
- high mortality (~50%) in patients with Reynolds Pentad

Pancreas

Pancreatic Enzyme Abnormalities

Causes of Increased Serum Amylase
- pancreatic disease
  - pancreatitis, pancreatic duct obstruction (e.g. ampullary cancer), pseudocyst, abscess, ascites, trauma, cancer
- non-pancreatic abdominal disease
  - biliary tract disease, bowel obstruction/ischemia, perforated or penetrating ulcer, ruptured ectopic pregnancy, aneurysm, chronic liver disease, peritonitis
- non-abdominal disease
  - cancer (lung, ovary, esophagus, etc.), salivary gland lesions, bulimia, renal transplant/insufficiency, burns, ketoacidosis
  - macroamylasemia

Pancreatic Enzymes

TALC
Trypsin
Amylase
Lipase
Chymotrypsin

Causes of Increased Serum Lipase
- pancreatic disease: same as above
- non-pancreatic abdominal disease (mild elevations only): same as above
- non-abdominal disease
  - macrolipasemia
  - renal failure

When serum amylase >5x normal, the cause is almost always pancreatitis or renal disease

Acute Pancreatitis

Etiology (most common are alcohol and gallstones)

When thinking about the causes of acute pancreatitis remember: **I GET SMASHED**, but vast majority due to gallstones or ethanol

Idiopathic: thought to be hypertensive sphincter or microlithiasis
Gallstones (45%)
Ethanol (35%)
Tumours: pancreas, ampulla, choledochocele
Scorpion stings
Microbiological
- bacterial: *Mycoplasma, Campylobacter*, TB, *M. avium intracellulare, Legionella*, leptospirosis
- viral: mumps, rubella, varicella, viral hepatitis, CMV, EBV, HIV, Coxsackie virus, echovirus, adenovirus
- parasites: ascariasis, clonorchiasis, echinococcosis
Autoimmune: SLE, polyarteritis nodosa (PAN), Crohn's disease
Surgery/trauma
- manipulation of sphincter of Oddi (e.g. ERCP), post-cardiac surgery, blunt trauma to abdomen, penetrating peptic ulcer
Hyperlipidemia (TG >11.3 mmol/L; >1000 mg/dL), **H**ypercalcemia, **H**ypothermia
Emboli or ischemia
Drugs/toxins
- azathioprine, mercaptopurine, furosemide, estrogens, methyldopa, H₂-blockers, valproic acid, antibiotics, acetaminophen, salicylates, methanol, organophosphates, steroids (controversial)

Pathophysiology
- activation of proteolytic enzymes within pancreatic cells, starting with trypsin, leading to local and systemic inflammatory response
- in gallstone pancreatitis, this is due to mechanical obstruction of the pancreatic duct by stones
- in ethanol-related pancreatitis, pathogenesis is unknown
- in rare genetic diseases, mutations prevent the physiological breakdown of trypsin required normally to stop proteolysis (e.g. mutant trypsin in hereditary pancreatitis or mutation in SPINK 1 gene which normally inhibits activated trypsin); may be model for ethanol-related pancreatitis

Gallstones only cause acute pancreatitis (not chronic pancreatitis)

Pathology
- mild (interstitial)
  - peri-pancreatic fat necrosis
  - interstitial edema
- severe (necrotic)
  - extensive peri-pancreatic and intra-pancreatic fat necrosis
  - parenchymal necrosis and hemorrhage → infection in 60%
  - release of toxic factors into systemic circulation and peritoneal space (causes multi-organ failure)
- severity of clinical features may not always correlate with pathology
- 3 phases
  - local inflammation + necrosis → hypovolemia
  - systemic inflammation in multiple organs, especially in lungs, usually after IV fluids given → pulmonary edema
  - local complications 2 wk after presentation → pancreatic sepsis/abscess

Signs and Symptoms
- pain: epigastric, noncolicky, constant
- can radiate to back
- may improve when leaning forward (Inglefinger's sign)
- tender rigid abdomen; guarding
- N/V
- abdominal distention from paralytic ileus
- fever: chemical, not due to infection
- jaundice: compression or obstruction of bile duct
- Cullen's/Grey-Turner's signs
- tetany: transient hypocalcemia
- hypovolemic shock: can lead to renal failure
- acute respiratory distress syndrome
- coma

Cullen's Sign
Periumbilical ecchymosis

Grey-Turner's Sign
Flank ecchymosis

Investigations
- increased serum pancreatic enzymes: amylase, lipase (more specific)
- ALT >150 specific for biliary cause
- increased WBC, glucose, low calcium
- imaging: CT most useful for diagnosis and prognosis
  - x-ray: "sentinel loop" (dilated proximal jejunum), calcification, and "colon cut-off sign" (colonic spasm)
  - U/S: useful for evaluating biliary tree (67% sensitivity, 100% specificity)
  - CT scan with IV contrast: useful for diagnosis and prognosis because contrast seen only in viable pancreatic tissue, non-viable areas can be biopsied percutaneously to differentiate sterile from infected necrosis
  - ERCP or MRCP if cause uncertain, assess for duct stone, pancreatic or ampullary tumour, pancreas divisum

Increased Amylase
- Sensitive, not specific

Increased Lipase
- Higher sensitivity and specificity
- Stays elevated longer

Classification
- interstitial edematous vs. necrotizing
- mild, moderate, severe

Prognosis
- usually a benign, self-limiting course, single or recurrent
- occasionally severe leading to
  - shock
  - pulmonary edema
  - multi-organ dysfunction syndrome
  - GI ulceration due to stress
  - death
  - numerous scales to describe severity: probably most useful is proportion of pancreas not taking up contrast on CT done 48 hours after presentation (necrotic pancreas does not take up the contrast dye)
  - presence of organ failure, particularly organ failure that persists > 48 hours, is associated with worse outcomes

Table 21. Collections in pancreatitis (Revised 2012 Atlanta Classification)

	Liquid	Solid
Acute	Acute peripancreatic fluid collection (APFC)	Acute necrotic collection (ANC)
Chronic	Pancreatic pseudocyst	Walled-off necrosis (WON)

All of these collections are classified as infected or not infected

Treatment
- goals (only supportive therapy available)
  1. hemodynamic stability
  2. analgesia
  3. oxygen
  4. stop progression of damage (difficult)
  5. treat local and systemic complications
- antibiotics controversial except in documented infection (use cephalosporins, imipenem)
- aspirate necrotic areas of pancreas to diagnose infection; drain if infected
- IV fluids (crystalloid or colloid)
  - beware third spacing of fluid, monitor urine output carefully
- NG suction (lets pancreas rest) if vomiting, stomach very dilated
- endoscopic sphincterotomy if severe gallstone pancreatitis (i.e. cholangitis or ongoing obstruction)
- nutritional support: nasojejunal feeding tube or TPN if cannot tolerate enteric feeds
  - recent evidence supports nasogastric enteral (or oral if feasible) feeds
- no benefit: glucagon, atropine, aprotinin, H₂-blockers, peritoneal lavage
- follow clinically and CT/ultrasound to exclude complications
- chief role of invasive intervention is to excise necrotic tissue (necrosectomy) in the case of infected pancreatic necrosis (try to delay for >2 wk to allow demarcation between viable and necrotic tissue), better done endoscopically or radiologically than surgically if technically possible

Late Complications
- pseudocysts: follow if asymptomatic, drain if symptomatic or growing
  - drain: choice of endoscopic, percutaneous under radiological guidance, or surgical
- infected necrosis/abscesses: antibiotics + percutaneous drainage, endoscopic vs. surgical
- bleeding: (1) gastric varices if splenic vein thrombosis, (2) pseudoaneurysm of vessels in areas of necrosis, especially splenic artery, (3) duodenal ulcer related to compression of duodenum by enlarged pancreas
- splenic and portal vein thrombosis: no effective therapy described, anticoagulation not proven, hazardous
- rare: DM, pancreatic duct damage

Chronic Pancreatitis

Definition
- irreversible damage to pancreas characterized by
  1. pancreatic cell loss (from necrosis)
  2. inflammation
  3. fibrosis

Etiology/Pathophysiology
- alcohol (most common)
  - causes a larger proportion (>90%) of chronic pancreatitis than acute pancreatitis
  - changes composition of pancreatic juice (e.g. increases viscosity)

When to call the surgeon in acute pancreatitis? Endoscopic Transgastric vs Surgical Necrosectomy for Infected Necrotizing Pancreatitis: A Randomized Trial
JAMA 2012; 307:1053-61
Once it was recognized that severe acute (necrotizing) pancreatitis had a terrible prognosis because of an exuberant inflammatory response leading to multiorgan failure, pancreatectomy was attempted. However, contrary to the expected favourable results, clinical experience has shown that surgical pancreatectomy is usually not helpful, perhaps because once the inflammatory cascade starts, it persists as a self-perpetuating cycle. The problems caused by acute pancreatitis can be thought of a widespread burn initiated by inflammation in the pancreas, but having little do with ongoing problems within the pancreas itself. Studies suggest that the only compelling indication for surgery is infected necrotizing pancreatitis not responding to antibiotics. As predicted, without removal of such infected pancreatic tissue, death is likely from sepsis.
In this recent randomized trial, transgastric necrosectomy, an endoscopic technique that also removes infected necrotic pancreatic tissue, reduced both a composite end-point of major pancreatitis complications (especially new onset organ failure) and the pro-inflammatory response (as measured by serum IL-6 levels) to a greater extent than surgical necrosectomy. Of course, not all necrotic collections are in areas amenable to endoscopic intervention, and the advice of an experienced surgeon should always be welcomed in severe acute pancreatitis, but the role of surgery in this previously considered surgical disease is rapidly diminishing.

Prophylactic Antibiotics Cannot Reduce Infected Pancreatic Necrosis and Mortality in Acute Necrotizing Pancreatitis: Evidence from a Meta-Analysis of Randomized Controlled Trials
Am J Gastroenterol 2008;103:104-110
Purpose: To review the effectiveness of IV antibiotics on pancreatic necrosis.
Study Selection: RCTs comparing antibiotics with placebo or no treatment.
Results: Seven trials (n=467) were included. Antibiotics were not statistically superior to controls in reduction of infected necrosis and mortality.
Conclusion: Prophylactic antibiotics cannot reduce infected pancreatic necrosis and mortality in patients with acute necrotizing pancreatitis.
Note: In practice the temptation to give antibiotics for pancreatitis is mainly in the setting of a sick patient with fever and suggestive pancreatic necrosis on CT scan. It is difficult to determine whether pancreatic necrosis has become infected without aspiration biopsy (see Curr *Gastroenterol Rep* 2009;11:104-110).

Symptoms of Chronic Pancreatitis
- Abdominal pain
- Diabetes
- Steatorrhea

Etiology = Almost Always Alcohol

Treatment
- Alcohol abstinence
- Pancreatic enzyme replacement
- Analgesics
- Pancreatic resection if ductular blockage

- decreases pancreatic secretion of pancreatic stone protein (lithostathine) which normally solubilizes calcium salts
  - precipitation of calcium within pancreatic duct results in duct and gland destruction
- toxic effect on acinar and duct cells – directly or via increasing free radicals
- acinar cell injury leads to cytokine release, which stimulates pancreatic stellate cells to form collagen (leading to fibrosis)
- varying degrees of ductular dilatation, strictures, protein plugs, calcification
- no satisfactory theory to explain why only a minority of alcoholics develop pancreatitis
- unusual causes
- CF
  - severe protein-calorie malnutrition
  - hereditary
  - idiopathic

Signs and Symptoms
- early stages
  - recurrent attacks of severe abdominal pain (upper abdomen and back)
  - chronic painless pancreatitis: 10%
- late stages: occurs in 15% of patients
  - malabsorption syndrome when >90% of function is lost, steatorrhea
  - diabetes, calcification, jaundice, weight loss, pseudocyst, ascites, GI bleed

Investigations
- laboratory
  - increase in serum glucose
  - increase in serum ALP, less commonly bilirubin (jaundice)
  - serum amylase and lipase usually normal
  - stool elastase is low in steatorrhea
- AXR: pancreatic calcifications
- U/S or CT: calcification, dilated pancreatic ducts, pseudocyst
- MRCP or ERCP: abnormalities of pancreatic ducts-narrowing and dilatation
- EUS: abnormalities of pancreatic parenchyma and pancreatic ducts, most sensitive test
- 72-h fecal fat test: measures exocrine function
- secretin test: gold standard, measures exocrine function but difficult to perform, unpleasant for patient, expensive
- fecal pancreatic enzyme measurement (elastase-1, chymotrypsin): available only in selected centres

Treatment
- most common problem is pain, difficult to control
- general management
  - total abstinence from alcohol
  - enzyme replacement may help pain by resting pancreas via negative feedback
  - analgesics
  - celiac ganglion blocks
  - time: pain decreases with time as pancreas "burns out"
- endoscopy: sphincterotomy, stent if duct dilated, remove stones from pancreatic duct
- surgery: drain pancreatic duct (pancreaticojejunostomy) if duct dilated (more effective than endoscopy); resect pancreas if duct contracted
- steatorrhea
  - pancreatic enzyme replacement
  - restrict fat, increase carbohydrate and protein (may also decrease pain)
  - neither endoscopy nor surgery can improve pancreatic function

Autoimmune Pancreatitis

- most commonly presents as a mimicker of pancreatic cancer (pancreatic mass detected because of jaundice ± abdominal pain)

Investigations
- histology: lymphocyte and plasma cell infiltration of pancreas
- imaging: focal or diffuse enlargement of pancreas on CT or MRI, sausage shaped, low density rim around pancreas
- serology: increased serum IgG4
- other organ involvement: sialadenitis, retroperitoneal fibrosis, biliary duct narrowing, nephritis

Treatment
- responds to prednisone

Clinical Nutrition

Determination of Nutritional Status

- corrected weight loss (expressed as body mass index [kg/m²]) is most important parameter in assessing need for nutritional support
- Subjective Global Assessment: simple bedside tool to assess nutritional status, to help identify those who will benefit from nutritional support

Investigations
- plasma proteins: albumin, pre-albumin (shorter half life than albumin), transferrin
- decrease may indicate decreased nutritional status or disease state
- thyroid-binding globulin, retinol-binding protein (may be too sensitive)
- anthropometry (e.g. triceps skinfold thickness), grip strength less often used

Table 22. Areas of Absorption of Nutrients

	Fe	CHO	Proteins, Lipids Na⁺, H₂O	Bile Acids	Vit B₁₂
Duodenum	+++	+++	+++	+	
Jejunum	+	+	++	+	+
Ileum	+	+	++	+++	+++

Enteral Nutrition

Definition
- enteral nutrition (tube feeding) is a way of providing food through a tube placed in the stomach or the small intestine
- choice of tubes: nasogastric (NG), nasojejunal (NJ), percutaneous endoscopic gastrostomy ("G-tube" or "PEG tube"), percutaneous endoscopic jejunostomy (J-tube) or tubes can be placed radiologically, surgically

Indications
- oral feeding inadequate or contraindicated

Feeds
- polymeric feeds contain whole protein, carbohydrate, fat as a liquid, with or without fibre
- elemental feeds contain protein as amino acids, carbohydrate as simple sugars, fat content low (therefore high osmolarity)
- specific diets: low carbohydrate/high fat solution for ventilated patients (carbohydrate has a high respiratory quotient so minimizes carbon dioxide production), high energy, low electrolyte solutions for dialysis patients

Relative Contraindications
- non-functioning gut (e.g. intestinal obstruction, enteroenteral or enterocutaneous fistulae)
- uncontrolled diarrhea
- GI bleeding

Complications
- aspiration
- diarrhea
- refeeding syndrome (rare): carbohydrate can stimulate excessive insulin release, leading to cellular uptake and low serum levels of phosphate, magnesium, potassium
- overfeeding syndrome (rare): hypertonic dehydration, hyperglycemia, hypercapnea, azotemia (from excess protein)

Enteral Nutrition Advantages over Parenteral Nutrition
- fewer serious complications (especially sepsis)
- nutritional requirements for enterally administered nutrition better understood
- can supply gut-specific fuels such as glutamine and short chain fatty acids
- nutrients in the intestinal lumen prevent atrophy of the gut and pancreas
- prevents gallstones by stimulating gallbladder motility
- much less expensive

Most Common Indications for Artificial Nutrition Support
- Preexisting nutritional deprivation
- Anticipated or actual inadequate energy intake by mouth
- Significant multiorgan system disease

Whenever possible, enteral nutrition is ALWAYS preferable over parenteral nutrition

Hypomagnesemia may be an initial sign of short bowel syndrome in patients who have undergone surgical bowel resection

Enteral vs. Parenteral Nutrition for Acute Pancreatitis
Cochrane DB of Syst Rev 2010;1:CD002837
Purpose: Compare EN vs. TPN on mortality, morbidity, and hospital stay in patients with pancreatitis.
Study Selection: RCTs of TPN vs. EN in pancreatitis.
Results: Eight trials (n=348) were included. Enteral nutrition decreases RR of death (0.50), multiple organ failure (0.55), infection (0.39), and other local complications (0.70). It also decreased hospital stay by 2.37 d.
Conclusion: EN reduces mortality, organ failure, infections, and length of hospital stay in patients with pancreatitis.

Parenteral Nutrition

Definition
- parenteral nutrition (PN) is the practice of feeding a person intravenously, bypassing the usual process of eating and digestion

Indications
- short-term (<1 mo)
  - whenever GI tract not functioning
  - only situations where PN has been well shown to increase survival are after bone marrow transplant and in short bowel syndrome, some evidence for benefit in gastric cancer, but often used in ICU, perioperatively, and in difficult to control sepsis
  - pre-operative: only useful in severely malnourished (e.g. loss of >15% of pre-morbid weight, serum albumin <28 g/L or <2.8 g/dL), and only if given for ≥2 wk
  - renal failure: PN shown to increase rate of recovery; no increase in survival
  - liver disease: branched chain amino acids may shorten duration of encephalopathy; no increase in survival
  - IBD: PN closes fistulae and heals acute exacerbations of mucosal inflammation, but effect is transient (EN is equally effective)
  - some evidence for efficacy, but convincing data not available for
    - radiation/chemotherapy-induced enteritis
    - AIDS with wasting diarrhea
    - severe acute pancreatitis
- long-term (>1 mo): can be given at home
  - severe untreatable small bowel disease (e.g. radiation enteritis, extensive CD, high output fistulae)
  - following surgical resection of >70% of small bowel (e.g. small bowel infarction)
  - severe motility diseases (e.g. scleroderma affecting bowel)

Relative Contraindications
- functional GI tract for enteral nutrition
- active infection; at least until appropriate antibiotic coverage
- inadequate venous access; triple-lumen central venous lines usually prevent this problem
- unreliable patient or clinical setting

Complications of PN
- sepsis: most serious of the common complications
- mechanical pneumothorax from insertion of central line, catheter migration and thrombosis, air embolus
- metabolic: CHF, hyperglycemia, gallstones, cholestasis

Common Medications

Table 23. Common Drugs Prescribed in Gastroenterology

Class	Generic Drug Name	Trade Name	Dosing	Mechanism of Action	Indications	Contraindications	Side Effects
Proton Pump Inhibitors (H$^+$/K$^+$-ATPase inhibitors)	omeprazole	Losec®/ Prilosec®	20 mg PO OD	Inhibits gastric enzymes H$^+$/K$^+$-ATPase (proton pump)	Duodenal ulcer, gastric ulcer, NSAID-associated gastric and duodenal ulcers, reflux esophagitis, symptomatic GERD, dyspepsia, Zollinger-Ellison syndrome, eradication of H. pylori (combined with antibiotics)	Hypersensitivity to drug	Dizziness, headache, flatulence, abdominal pain, nausea, rash, increased risk of osteoporotic fracture (secondary to impaired calcium absorption)
	lansoprazole or dexlansoprazole	Prevacid® Dexilant®	Oral therapy: lansoprazole 15-30 mg OD (before breakfast), dexlansoprazole 30-60mg OD (does not need to be taken before breakfast)	Same as above	Same as above	Same as above	Same as above
	pantoprazole	Pantoloc® Protonix®	40 mg PO ODfor UGIB: 80 mg IV bolus then 8 mg/h infusion	Same as above	Same as above and UGIB	Same as above	Same as above
	rabeprazole	Pariet®/ Aciphex®	40 mg PO OD	Same as above	Same as above	Same as above	Same as above
	esomeprazole	Nexium®	20-40 mg PO OD	Same as above	Same as above	Same as above	Same as above
Histamine H2-Receptor Antagonists	ranitidine	Zantac®	300 mg PO OD or 150 mg bid IV therapy: 50 mg q8h (but tachyphylaxis aproblem)	Inhibits gastric histamine H2-receptors	Duodenal ulcer, gastric ulcer, NSAID-associated gastric and duodenal ulcers, ulcer prophylaxis, reflux esophagitis, symptomatic GERD; not useful for acute GI bleeds	Hypersensitivity to drug	Confusion, dizziness, headache, arrhythmias, constipation, nausea, agranulocytosis, pancytopenia, depression
	famotidine	Pepcid®	Oral therapy: duodenal/gastric ulcers: 40 mg qhs GERD: 20 mg bid IV therapy: 20 mg bid	Same as above	Same as above	Same as above	Same as above
Stool Softener	docusate sodium	Colace®	100-400 mg PO OD, divided in 1-4 doses	Promotes incorporation of water into stool	Relief of constipation	Presence of abdominal pain, fever, N/V	Throat irritation, abdominal cramps, rashes
Osmotic Laxatives	lactulose	Lactulose/ Constulose®	Constipation: 15-30 mL PO OD to bid Encephalopathy: 15-30 mL bid to qid	Poorly absorbed in GI tract and is broken down by colonic bacteria into lactic acid in the colon, increases osmotic colonic contents, increases stool volume	Chronic constipation, prevention, and treatment of portal-systemic encephalopathy	Patients who require a low galactose diet	Flatulence, intestinal cramps, nausea, diarrhea if excessive dosage
	PEG3350	Lax-a-day®/ Golytely®	Constipation: 17 g powder dissolved in 4-8 oz liquid PO OD	Osmotic agent causes water retention in stool and promotes frequency of stool	Relief of constipation Colonoscopy prep	Hypersensitivity to drug	Abdominal distension, pain, anal pain, thirst, nausea, rigor, tonic-clonic seizures (rare)
	magnesium hydroxide	Milk of Magnesia/ Pedia-Lax®	Constipation (adult): 400 mg/5 mL: 30-60 mL PO qhs	Osmotic retention of fluid which distends the colon and increases peristaltic activity	Relief of constipation	Patients with myasthenia gravis or other neuromuscular disease Renal impairment	Abdominal pain, vomiting, diarrhea
Stimulant Laxatives	senna	Senokot®	Tablets: 1-4 PO qhs Syrup: 10-15 mL PO qhs	Induce peristalsis in lower colon	Constipation	Patients with acute abdomen	Abdominal cramps, discolouration of breast milk, urine, feces, melanosis coli and atonic colon from prolonged use (controversial)
	bisacodyl	Bisacodyl®	5-30 mg PO OD (start at 10 mg for bowel preparation)	Enteric nerve stimulation and local contact-induced secretory effects Colonic movements	Constipation Preparation of bowel for procedure	GI obstruction Gastroenteritis	Abdominal colic, abdominal discomfort, proctitis (with suppository use), diarrhea
	metoclopramide	Maxeran®	See anti-emetics	See anti-emetics	See anti-emetics	See anti-emetics	See anti-emetics
Bulk Laxatives	psyllium	Metamucil®	2-6 tabs (1 tab = 0.52 g) PO od-tid prn	Increases stool bulk → water retention in stool	Constipation	Hypersensitivity to drug GI obstruction	GI obstruction, diarrhea, constipation, abdominal cramps
Antidiarrheal Agents	loperamide	Imodium®	Acute diarrhea: 4 mg PO initially, followed by 2 mg after each unformed stool	Acts as antidiarrheal viacholinergic, noncholinergic, opiate, and nonopiate receptor-medicated mechanisms; decreases activity of myenteric plexus	Adjunctive therapy for acute non-specific diarrhea, chronic diarrhea associated with IBD and for reducing the volume of discharge for ileostomies, colostomies, and other intestinal resections	Children <2 yr, known hypersensitivity to drug, acute dysentery characterized by blood in stools and fever, acute ulcerative colitis or pseudomembranous colitis associated with broad-spectrum antibiotics	Abdominal pain or discomfort, drowsiness or dizziness, tiredness, dry mouth, nausea and vomiting, hypersensitivity reaction
	diphenoxylate/ atropine	Lomotil®	5 mg PO tid to qid	Inhibits GI propulsion via direct action on smooth muscle, resulting in a decrease in peristaltic action and increase in transit time	Adjunctive therapy for diarrhea, as above	Hypersensitivity to diphenoxylate or atropine, jaundice, pseudomembranous enterocolitis, diarrhea caused by enterotoxin producing bacteria	Dizziness, drowsiness, insomnia, headache, N/V, cramps, allergic reaction

Table 23. Common Drugs Prescribed in Gastroenterology (continued)

Class	Generic Drug Name	Trade Name	Dosing	Mechanism of Action	Indications	Contraindications	Side Effects
Anti-Emetics	dimenhydrinate	Gravol®	25-50 mg PO/IV/IM q4-6h prn	Competitive H1 receptor antagonist in GI tract, blood vessels, and respiratory tract. Blocks chemoreceptor trigger zone. Diminishes vestibular simulation and disrupts labyrinthine function through central anticholinergic action	Motion sickness, radiation sickness, postoperative vomiting, and drug-induced N/V	Hypersensitivity to drug	Xerostomia, sedation
	prochlorperazine	Stemetil®	5-10 mg PO/IV/IM bid-tid prn	D1, D2 receptor antagonist in chemoreceptor trigger zone and α adrenergic and anti-cholinergic effects Depresses reticular activating system (RAS) affecting emesis	Post-operative N/V, antipsychotic, anxiety	Hypersensitivity to drug	Dystonia, EPS, seizure, neuroleptic malignant syndrome (NMS) (rarely)
	metoclopramide	Maxeran®	10 mg IV/IM q2-3h prn, 10-15 mg PO qid (30 min before meals and qhs)	Dopamine and 5-HT receptor antagonist in chemoreceptor trigger zone. Enhances response to ACh in upper GI tract, enhancing motility and gastric emptying. Increases LES tone	GERD, diabetic gastroparesis, post-operative and chemotherapy induced N/V, migraines, constipation	Hypersensitivity to drug, GI obstruction, perforation, hemorrhage, pheochromocytoma, seizures, and EPS	Restlessness, drowsiness, dizziness, fatigue, EPS, some rare serious side effects include NMS, agranulocytosis
	ondansetron	Zofran®	Depends on procedure, generally 8-16 mg PO	Selective 5HT3 receptor antagonist in central chemoreceptor trigger zone and peripherally on vagus nerve	N/V caused by cancer chemotherapy and radiation therapy; multiple off label uses, including gastroenteritis N/V	Morphine, hypersensitivity to drug	Constipation, diarrhea, increased liver enzymes, headache, fatigue, malaise, cardiac dysrhythmia
	granisetron	Kytril®	1 mg PO bid (for nausea from chemotherapy/ radiation)	Same as above	N/V caused by cancer chemotherapy and radiation therapy	Same as above	Constipation, prolonged QT interval (rarely)
IBD Agents	mesalamine	Pentasa® Salofalk® Asacol® Mesasal®	CD: 1 g PO tid/qid Active UC: 1 g PO qid Maintenance UC: 1.6 g PO divided doses daily also as suppositories and enemas	5-ASA: Blocks arachidonic acid metabolism to prostaglandins and leukotrienes	IBD	Hypersensitivity to mesalamine salicylates; Asacol contains phthalate, potential urogenital teratogenicity for male fetus	Abdominal pain, constipation, arthralgia, headache
	sulfasalazine	Salazopyrin®	3-4 g/d PO in divided doses	Compound composed of 5-ASA bound to sulfapyridine, hydrolysis by intestinal bacteria releases 5-ASA, the active component	Colonic disease	Hypersensitivity to sulfasalazine, sulfa drugs, salicylates; intestinal or urinary obstruction, porphyria	Rash, loss of appetite, N/V, headache, oligospermia (reversible)
						Hypersensitivity to sulfasalazine, sulfa drugs, salicylates; intestinal or urinary obstruction, porphyria	Rash, loss of appetite, N/V, headache, oligospermia (reversible)
	prednisone		20-40 mg PO OD for acute exacerbation	Anti-inflammatory	Mod-severe CD and UC		Complications of steroid therapy
Immuno-suppressive Agents	6-mercaptopurine (6-MP)	Purinethol®	CD: 1.5 mg/kg/d PO	Immunosuppressive	IBD: active inflammation and to maintain remission	Hypersensitivity to mercaptopurine, prior resistance to mercaptopurine or thioguanine, history of treatment with alkylating agents, hypersensitivity to azathioprine, pregnancy	Pancreatitis, bone marrow suppression, increased risk of cancer
	azathioprine	Azasan® Imuran®	IBD: 2-3 mg/kg/d PO	Same as above	Same as above	Same as above	Same as above
Biologics	infliximab	Remicade®	5-10 mg/kg IV over 2 h	Monoclonal antibody to TNFα	Medically refractory CD	Heart failure, moderate to severe, doses >5 mg/kg	Reported cases of reactivated TB, PCP, lymphoma, other infections Other TNFα share similar serious side-effects
	adalimumab	Humira®	CD induction: four 40 mg SC on day 1, then 80 mg 2 wks later (day 15) CD maintenance: 40 mg every other wk beginning day 29	Monoclonal antibody to TNFα	Medically refractory CD or poor response to infliximab	Hypersensitivity to adalimumab Severe infection Moderate-to-severe heart failure	Headaches, skin rashes, upper respiratory tract infection
	golimumab	Simponi®	RA: 2 mg/kg at wks 0, 4 and then every 8 wks thereafter (use with methotrexate) UC induction: 200 mg SC at wk 0, then 100 mg at wk 2 UC maintenance: 50 mg every 4 wk	Monoclonal antibody to TNFα	Active ankylosing spondylitis Psoriatic arthritis Moderate-to-severe active RA (combined with methotrexate) UC: medically refractory UC	Hypersensitivity to golimumab or latex Severe infection Moderate-to-severe heart failure	
	vedolizumab	Entyvio®	CD/UC: 300 mg at 0, 2, 6 wks and then every 8 wks thereafter	Monoclonal antibody to α4β7 integrin	Medically refractory CD/UC, including other TNFα inhibitors and corticosteroids	Hypersensitivity to vedolizumab	Infections, liver injury, and progressive multifocal leukoencephalopathy

Landmark Gastroenterology Trials

Trial	Reference	Results
MELD score as a predictor of death in chronic liver disease	*Gastroenterology* 2003;124:91-6	MELD score can be applied for allocation of donor livers as it accurately predicts 3 mo mortality in patients with chronic liver failure
Infliximab, azathioprine, or combination for Crohn's disease	*NEJM* 2010; 362:1383-95	In moderate-severe Crohn's disease, infliximab + azathioprine was more likely to result in corticosteroid-free remission than infliximab monotherapy. Infliximab monotherapy was more effective than azathioprine monotherapy. Similar results have been reported for ulcerative colitis (Gastroenterology 2014; 146:392-400)
Enteral versus parenteral nutrition for acute pancreatitis	*Cochrane DB Syst Rev* 2010; 1: CD002837	For acute pancreatitis, no trial was convincing alone, but in aggregate, enteral feeds via nasogastric tube is preferable to either no feeding or parenteral nutrition
Rifaximin treatment in hepatic encephalopathy	*NEJM* 2010; 362:1071-81	The most convincing of several articles establishing this non-absorbable antibiotic as the treatment of choice for hepatic encephalopathy for maintaining remission from hepatic encephalopathy and reducing hospitalization associated with the disease
Adenoma detection rate and risk of colorectal cancer and death	*NEJM* 2014; 370:1298-1306	A high miss rate for colorectal cancers has been suggested, chiefly in the right colon. This study demonstrates a method of assessing the competence of endoscopists in detecting cancers using adenoma detection rate (the proportion of colonoscopic exams in which a physician detects one or more adenomas) as a surrogate marker. Adenoma detection rate was associated with lower risk of interval colorectal cancer and has launched quality assurance programs for screening colonoscopies
Prednisolone or pentoxifylline for alcoholic hepatitis	*NEJM* 2015; 372:1619-28	For alcoholic hepatitis, prednisolone improved survival when the Maddrey's discriminant function > 32, but the benefit did not reach statistical significance and pentoxifylline was of no advantage at all. Other studies had shown some benefit with pentoxifylline, but this study was the most definitive

References

Atlas
Kandel G. Division of Gastroenterology, St. Michael's Hospital, Toronto.
Olscamp G. Division of Gastroenterology, St. Michael's Hospital, Toronto.
Saibil F. Division of Gastroenterology, Sunnybrook and Women's College Health Sciences Centre, Toronto.
Haber G. Division of Gastroenterology, Lennox Hall Hospital, New York.

Esophageal and Gastric Disease
Devault KR, Castell DO. Guidelines for the diagnoses and treatment of gastroesophageal reflux disease. Arch Intern Med 1995;115:2165-2173.
DiPalma JA. Management of severe gastroesophageal reflux disease. J Clin Gastroenterol 2001;32:19-26.
Sharma P, Sarin SK. Improved survival with the patients with variceal bleed. Int J Hepatol 2011: Epub 2011Jul 7.
Verbeek RE, van Oijen MG, ten Kate FJ, et al. Surveillance and follow-up strategies in patients with high-grade dysplasia in Barrett's esophagus: a Dutch population-based study. Am J Gastroenterol 2012;107:534-542.
Wang KK, Sampliner RE. Updated guidelines 2008 for the diagnosis, surveillance and therapy of Barrett's esophagus. Am J Gastroenterol 2008;103:788-797.
Wilcox CM, Karowe MW. Esophageal infections: etiology, diagnosis, and management. Gastroenterol 1994;2:188-206.

Stomach and Duodenum
American Gastroenterological Association position statement: evaluation of dyspepsia. Gastroenterol 1998;114:579-581.
Howden CW, Hunt RH. Guidelines for the management of helicobacter pylori infection. Am J Gastroenterol 1998;93:2330-2338.
Hunt RH, Fallone CA, Thomson ABR. Canadian helicobacter pylori consensus conference update: infection in adults. J Gastroenterol 1999;13:213-216.
Laine L, Peterson WL. Bleeding peptic ulcer. NEJM 1994;331:717-727.
Lanza FL. A guideline for the treatment and prevention of NSAID-induced ulcer. Am J Gastroenterol 1998;93:2037-2046.
McColl KE. Clinical practice helicobacter pylori infection. NEJM 2010;362:1597-601.
Peek RM, Blaser MJ. Pathophysiology of helicobacter pylori-induced gastritis and peptic ulcer disease. Am J Med 1997;102:200-207.
Salcedo JA, Al-Kawas F. Treatment of helicobacter pylori infection. Arch Intern Med 1998;158:842-851.
Schmid CH, Whitling G, Cory D, et al. Omeprazole plus antibiotics in the eradication of Helicobacter pylori infection: a meta-regression analysis of randomized, controlled trials. Am J Ther 1999;6:25-36.
Soll AH. Practice parameters: committee of the American College of Gastroenterology: medical treatment of peptic ulcer disease. JAMA 1996;275:622-629.
Thijs JC, van Zwet AA, Thijs WJ, et al. Diagnostic tests for helicobacter pylori: a prospective evaluation of their accuracy, without selecting a single test as the gold standard. Am J Gastroenterol 1996;91:2125-2129.

Small and Large Bowel
Aranda-Michel J, Giannella R. Acute diarrhea: a practical review. Am J Med 1999;670-676.
Colorectal cancer screening: recommendation statement from the Canadian task force on preventative health care. CMAJ 2001;165:206-208.
Donowitz M, Kokke FT, Saidi R. Evaluation of patients with chronic diarrhea. NEJM 1995;332:725-729.
Drossma DA. The functional gastrointestinal disorders and the Rome III process. Gastroenterol 2006;130:1377-1390.
Forrest JA, Finlayson ND, Shearman DJ. Endoscopy in gastrointestinal bleeding. Lancet 1974;2:394-397.
Ghosh S, Shand A. Ulcerative colitis. BMJ 2000;320:1119-1123.
Hanauer SB. Drug therapy: inflammatory bowel disease. NEJM 1996;334:841-848.
Hatchette TF, Farina D. Infectious diarrhea: when to test and when to treat. CMAJ 2011;183:339-344.
Horwitz BJ, Fisher RS. Current concepts: the irritable bowel syndrome. NEJM 2001;344:1846-1850.
Jennings JSR, Howdle PD. Celiac disease. Curr Opin Gastroen 2001;17:118-126.
Laine L, Sahota A, Shah A. Does capsule endoscopy improve outcomes in obscure gastrointestinal bleeding? Randomized trial vs. dedicated small bowel radiography. Gastroenterol 2010;138:1673-1680.
Pimentel M, Lembo A, Chey WD, et al. Rifaximin therapy for patients with irritable bowel syndrome without constipation. NEJM 2011;364:22-32.
Rubio-Tapia A, Hill ID, Kelly CP, et al. ACG clinical guidelines: Diagnosis and management of celiac disease. Am J Gastroenterol 2013; 108: 656-676.

Liver and Biliary Tract
Angulo P. Primary biliary cirrhosis and primary sclerosing cholangitis. Clin Liv Dis 1999;3:529-570.
Andreoli T, Carpenter C, Griggs R, et al. (editors). Cecil essentials of medicine, 5th ed. Philadephia: WB Saunders Company, 2001.
Custis K. Common biliary tract disorders. Clin Fam Pract 2000;2:141-154.
Diehl AM. Alcoholic liver disease. Clin Liv Dis 1998;2:103-118.
Feldman M, Friedman LS, Sleisenger MH (editors). Gastrointestinal and liver disease: pathophysiology, diagnosis, management, 7th ed., vol. 2. Philadelphia: WB Saunders Company, 2004.
Haubrich WS, Schaffner F, Berk JE (editors). Bockus gastroenterology, 5th ed., vol 4. Chapter 74: Pregnancy-related hepatic and gastrointestinal disorders. Philadelphia: WB Saunders Company, 1995. 1448-1458.
Haubrich WS, Schaffner F, Berk JE (editors). Bockus gastroenterology, 5th ed., vol 4. Chapter 184: Pregnancy and the gastrointestinal tract. Philadelphia: WB Saunders Company, 1995. 3446-3452.
Kohli A, Shaffer A, Sherman A, and Kottilil S. Treatment of hepatitis C: a systematic review. JAMA 2014; 312: 631-640.
Malik AH. Acute and chronic viral hepatitis. Clin Fam Pract 2000;2:35-57.
Reynolds T. Ascites. Clin Liv Dis 2000;4:151-168.
Sandowski SA. Cirrhosis. Clin Fam Pract 2000;2:59-77.
Sherman M. Chronic viral hepatitis and chronic liver disease. Can J Diag 2001;18:81-90.
Sternlieb I. Wilson's disease. Clin Liv Dis 2000;4:229-239.
Williams JW, Simel DL. Does this patient have ascites? JAMA 1992;267:2645-2648.
Yapp TR. Hemochromatosis. Clin Liv Dis 2000;4:211-228.
Yu AS, Hu KQ. Management of ascites. Clin Liv Dis 2001;5:541-568.

Pancreas
Beckingham IJ, Bornman PC. ABC of diseases of liver, pancreas, and biliary system. Acute pancreatitis. BMJ 2001;322:595-598.
Beckingham IJ, Bornman PC. ABC of diseases of liver, pancreas, and biliary system. Chronic pancreatitis. BMJ 2001;322:660-663.
Steer ML. Chronic pancreatitis. NEJM 1995;332:1482-1490.
Sternby B, O'Brien JF, Zinsmeister AR, et al. What is the best biochemical test to diagnose acute pancreatitis? A prospective clinical study. Mayo Clin Proc 1996;71:1138-1144.
Whytcomb DC. Acute pancreatitis. NEJM 2006;354:2142-2150.

Rational Clinical Examination
Grover SA, Barkun AN, Sackett DL. Does this patient have splenomegaly? JAMA 1993;270:2218-2221.
Kitchens JM. Does this patient have an alcohol problem? JAMA 1994;272:1782-1787.
Naylor CD. Physical exam of the liver. JAMA 1994;271:1859-1865.
Williams JW, Simel DL. Does this patient have ascites? How to divine fluid in the abdomen. JAMA 1992;267:2645-2648.

Notes

General Surgery and Thoracic Surgery

Nishaan Brar, Shaidah Deghan, and Eric Walser, chapter editors
Dhruvin Hirpara and Sneha Raju, associate editors
Valerie Lemieux and Simran Mundi, EBM editors
Dr. Abdollah Behzadi and Dr. Alice Wei, staff editors

Acronyms

5-FU	5-fluorouracil	DRE	digital rectal exam
AAA	abdominal aortic aneurysm	EBL	estimated blood loss
ABG	arterial blood gas	ERCP	endoscopic retrograde cholangiopancreatography
ABI	ankle brachial index		
ALND	axillary lymph node dissection	EUA	examination under anesthesia
APR	abdominoperineal resection	EUS	endoscopic ultrasound
ARDS	acute respiratory distress syndrome	FAP	familial adenomatous polyposis
ATN	acute tubular necrosis	FAST	focused abdominal sonography for trauma
BRBPR	bright red blood per rectum		
BCS	breast conserving surgery	FNA	fine needle aspiration
CBD	common bile duct	FOBT	fecal occult blood test
CF	cystic fibrosis	GERD	gastroesophageal reflux disease
CHF	congestive heart failure	GI	gastrointestinal
CRC	colorectal cancer	GIST	gastrointestinal stromal tumour
CVA	costovertebral angle	GU	genitourinary
CVP	central venous pressure	HDGC	hereditary diffuse gastric carcinoma
DCIS	ductal carcinoma in situ	HIDA	hepatobiliary imino-diacetic acid
DIC	disseminated intravascular coagulation	HNPCC	hereditary nonpolyposis colorectal cancer
DPL	diagnostic peritoneal lavage		

I&D	incision and drainage	PPI	proton pump inhibitor
IPAH	idiopathic pulmonary arterial hypertension	PTC	percutaneous transhepatic cholangiography
IPF	idiopathic pulmonary fibrosis	PUD	peptic ulcer disease
LAR	low anterior resection	SBO	small bowel obstruction
LBO	large bowel obstruction	SCC	squamous cell carcinoma
LCIS	lobular carcinoma in situ	SIADH	syndrome of inappropriate anti-diuretic hormone
LES	lower esophageal sphincter		
LGIB	lower gastrointestinal bleed	SMA	superior mesenteric artery
LVRS	lung volume reduction surgery	SMV	superior mesenteric vein
MALT	mucosa-associated lymphoid tissue	SNLB	sentinel lymph node biopsy
MEN	multiple endocrine neoplasia	TED	thromboembolic deterrent
MIBG	metaiodobenzylguanidine	TEE	transesophageal echocardiogram
MIS	minimally invasive surgery	TTE	transthoracic echocardiogram
MRCP	magnetic resonance cholangiopancreatography	UGIB	upper gastrointestinal bleed
NGT	nasogastric tube	VATS	video-assisted thorascopic surgery
OGD	oesophagogastroduodenoscopy	VIP	vasoactive intestinal peptide
POD	post-operative day		

Basic Anatomy Review

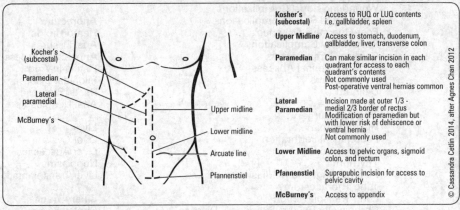

Kosher's (subcostal)	Access to RUQ or LUQ contents i.e. gallbladder, spleen
Upper Midline	Access to stomach, duodenum, gallbladder, liver, transverse colon
Paramedian	Can make similar incision in each quadrant for access to each quadrant's contents. Not commonly used. Post-operative ventral hernias common
Lateral Paramedian	Incision made at outer 1/3 - medial 2/3 border of rectus. Modification of paramedian but with lower risk of dehiscence or ventral hernia. Not commonly used
Lower Midline	Access to pelvic organs, sigmoid colon, and rectum
Pfannenstiel	Suprapubic incision for access to pelvic cavity
McBurney's	Access to appendix

© Cassandra Cetlin 2014, after Agnes Chan 2012

Figure 1. Abdominal incisions

Lateral Abdominal Wall Layers and their Continuous Spermatic and Scrotal Structures (superficial to deep)

1. skin (epidermis, dermis, subcutaneous fat)
2. superficial fascia
   - Camper's fascia (fatty) → Dartos fascia
   - Scarpa's fascia (membranous) → Colles' superficial perineal fascia
3. muscle (see Figure 2 and Figure 3)
   - external oblique → inguinal ligament → external spermatic fascia and fascia lata
   - internal oblique → cremasteric muscle/fascia
   - transversus abdominis → posterior inguinal wall
4. transversalis fascia → internal spermatic fascia
5. preperitoneal fat
6. peritoneum → tunica vaginalis

Midline Abdominal Wall Layers (superficial to deep)

1. skin
2. superficial fascia
3. rectus abdominis muscle: in rectus sheath, divided by linea alba
   - above arcuate line (midway between symphysis pubis and umbilicus)
     - anterior rectus sheath = external oblique aponeurosis and anterior leaf of internal oblique aponeurosis
     - posterior rectus sheath = posterior leaf of internal oblique aponeurosis and transversus abdominis aponeurosis
   - below arcuate line
     - aponeuroses of external oblique, internal oblique, transversus abdominis all pass in front of rectus abdominis
4. arteries: superior epigastric (branch of internal thoracic), inferior epigastric (branch of external iliac); both arteries anastomose and lie behind the rectus muscle (superficial to posterior rectus sheath above arcuate line)
5. transversalis fascia
6. peritoneum

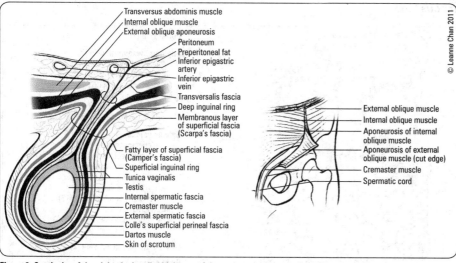

Figure 2. Continuity of the abdominal wall with layers of the scrotum and spermatic cord

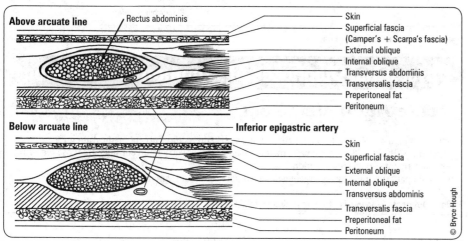

Figure 3. Midline cross-section of abdominal wall

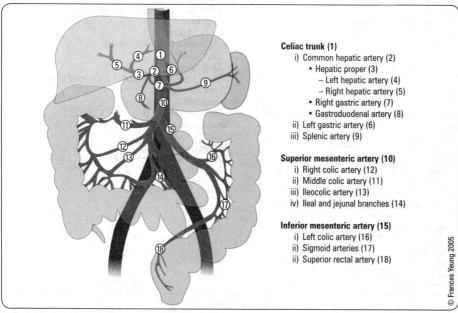

Figure 4. Blood supply to the GI tract

Venous Flow

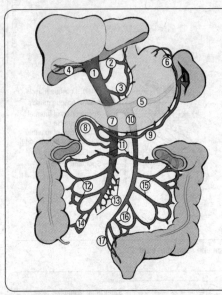

Organ	Arteries
Liver	Left and right hepatic (branches of hepatic proper)
Spleen	Splenic
Gallbladder	Cystic (branch of right hepatic artery)
Stomach	1. Lesser curvature: right and left gastric 2. Greater curvature: right (branch of gastroduodenal) and left (branch of splenic) gastroepiploic 3. Fundus: short gastrics (branch of splenic)
Duodenum	1. Gastroduodenal 2. Pancreaticoduodenals (superior branch of gastroduodenal, inferior branch of superior mesenteric)
Pancreas	1. Pancreatic branches of splenic 2. Pancreaticoduodenals
Small intestine	Superior mesenteric branches: jejunal, ileal, ileocolic
Large intestine	1. Superior mesenteric branches: right colic, middle colic 2. Inferior mesenteric branches: left colic, sigmoid, superior rectal

Portal vein (1)

Superior mesenteric vein (7)
  i) Ileal and jejunal veins (13)
  ii) Ileocolic vein (14)
  iii) Right colic vein (12)
  iv) Middle colic vein (11)
  v) Pancreaticoduodenal vein (8)
  vi) Right gastroepiploic vein (9)

Splenic vein (5)
  i) Inferior mesenteric vein (10) (superior rectal vein until crossing common iliac vessels)
    • Left colic veins (15)
    • Sigmoid veins (16)
    • Superior rectal veins (17)
  ii) Pancreatic veins
  iii) Left gastroepiploic vein
  iv) Short gastric veins (6)

Left gastric (coronary) vein (2)

Right gastric vein (3)

Cystic vein (4)

Paraumbilical vein

© Carly Vanderlee 2011

Figure 5. Venous drainage of the GI tract

Differential Diagnoses of Common Presentations

Acute Abdominal Pain

- acute abdomen = severe abdominal pain of acute onset and requires urgent medical attention
- in patients with acute abdominal pain, the first diagnoses that you should consider are those requiring potential urgent surgical intervention
- two main patterns constituting urgent general surgery referrals are peritonitis and obstruction

Table 1. Differential Diagnosis of Acute Abdominal Pain

RUQ	RLQ

Hepatobiliary
  Biliary colic
  Cholecystitis
  Cholangitis
  CBD obstruction (stone, tumour)
  Hepatitis
  Budd-Chiari
  Hepatic abscess/mass
  Right subphrenic abscess
Gastrointestinal
  Pancreatitis
  Presentation of gastric, duodenal, or pancreatic pathology
  Hepatic flexure pathology (CRC, subcostal incisional hernia)
Genitourinary
  Nephrolithiasis
  Pyelonephritis
  Renal: mass, ischemia, trauma
Cardiopulmonary
  RLL pneumonia
  Effusion/empyema
  CHF (causing hepatic congestion and R pleural effusion)
  MI
  Pericarditis
  Pleuritis
Miscellaneous
  Herpes zoster
  Trauma
  Costochondritis
	Gastrointestinal
	  Appendicitis
	  Crohn's disease
	  Tuberculosis of the ileocecal junction
	  Cecal tumour
	  Intussusception
	  Mesenteric lymphadenitis (Yersinia)
	  Cecal diverticulitis
	  Cecal volvulus
	  Hernia: femoral, inguinal obstruction, Amyand's (and resulting cecal distention)
	Gynecological
	  See 'suprapubic'
	Genitourinary
	  See 'suprapubic'
	Extraperitoneal
	  Abdominal wall hematoma/abscess
	  Psoas abscess

In all patients presenting with an acute abdomen, order the following:
KEY TESTS FOR SPECIFIC DIAGNOSIS
- ALP, ALT, AST, bilirubin
- Lipase/ amylase
- Urinalysis
- β-hCG (in women of childbearing age)
- Troponins
- Lactate

KEY TESTS FOR OR PREPARATION
- CBC, electrolytes, creatinine, glucose
- INR/PTT
- CXR (if history of cardiac or pulmonary disease)
- ECG if clinically indicated by history or if >69 years and no risk factors

Types of Peritonitis
- Primary peritonitis: spontaneous without clear etiology
- Secondary peritonitis: due to a perforated viscus
- Tertiary peritonitis: recurrent secondary peritonitis more often with resistant organisms

Localization of Pain
Most digestive tract pain is perceived in the midline because of bilaterally symmetric innervation; kidney, ureter, ovary, or somatically innervated structures are more likely to cause lateralized pain

Referred Pain
- Biliary colic: to right shoulder or scapula
- Renal colic: to groin
- Appendicitis: periumbilical to right lower quadrant (RLQ)
- Pancreatitis: to back
- Ruptured aortic aneurysm: to back or flank
- Perforated ulcer: to RLQ (right paracolic gutter)
- Hip pain: to groin

Table 1. Differential Diagnosis of Acute Abdominal Pain (continued)

LUQ	LLQ

Pancreatic
  Pancreatitis (acute vs. chronic)
  Pancreatic pseudocyst
  Pancreatic tumours
Gastrointestinal
  Gastritis
  PUD
  Splenic flexure pathology
  (e.g. CRC, ischemia)
Splenic
  Splenic infarct/abscess
  Splenomegaly
  Splenic rupture
  Splenic artery aneurysm
Cardiopulmonary (see RUQ and Epigastric)
Genitourinary (see RUQ)
	Gastrointestinal
	  Diverticulitis
	  Diverticulosis
	  Colon/sigmoid/rectal cancer
	  Fecal impaction
	  Proctitis (ulcerative colitis, infectious;
	  i.e. *gonococcus* or *Chlamydia*)
	  Sigmoid volvulus
	  Hernia
	Gynecological
	  See 'suprapubic'
	Genitourinary
	  See 'suprapubic'
	Extraperitoneal
	  Abdominal wall hematoma/abscess
	  Psoas abscess
	
	See <u>Gynecology</u>, <u>Urology</u>,
	and <u>Respirology</u> for further details regarding respective RLQ and suprapubic pain

EPIGASTRIC	SUPRAPUBIC	DIFFUSE

Cardiac
  Aortic dissection/ruptured
  AAA
  MI
  Pericarditis
Gastrointestinal
  Gastritis
  GERD/esophagitis
  PUD
  Pancreatitis
  Mallory-Weiss tear
	Gastrointestinal (see RLQ/LLQ)
	  Acute appendicitis
	  IBD
	Gynecological
	  Ectopic pregnancy
	  PID
	  Endometriosis
	  Threatened/incomplete
	  abortion
	  Hydrosalpinx/salpingitis
	  Ovarian torsion
	  Hemorrhagic fibroid
	  Tubo-ovarian abscess
	  Gynecological tumours
	Genitourinary
	  Cystitis (infectious,
	  hemorrhagic)
	  Hydroureter/urinary colic
	  Epididymitis
	  Testicular torsion
	  Acute urinary retention
	Extraperitoneal
	  Rectus sheath hematoma
		Gastrointestinal
		  Peritonitis
		  Early appendicitis, perforated appendicitis
		  Mesenteric ischemia
		  Gastroenteritis/colitis
		  Constipation
		  Bowel obstruction
		  Pancreatitis
		  Inflammatory bowel disease
		  Irritable bowel syndrome
		  Ogilvie's syndrome
		Cardiovascular/Hematological
		  Aortic dissection/ruptured AAA
		  Sickle cell crisis
		Genitourinary/Gynecological
		  Perforated ectopic pregnancy
		  PID
		  Acute urinary retention
		Endocrinological
		  Carcinoid syndrome
		  Diabetic ketoacidosis
		  Addisonian crisis
		  Hypercalcemia
		Other
		  Lead poisoning
		  Tertiary syphilis

> **Most Common Presentations of Surgical Pain**
> - Sudden onset with rigid abdomen = perforated viscus
> - Pain out of proportion to physical findings = ischemic bowel
> - Vague pain that subsequently localizes = appendicitis or other intra-abdominal process that irritates the parietal peritoneum
> - Waves of colicky pain = bowel obstruction

Abdominal Mass

Table 2. Differential Diagnosis of Abdominal Mass

Right Upper Quadrant (RUQ)	Upper Midline	Left Upper Quadrant (LUQ)
Gallbladder: cholecystitis, cholangiocarcinoma, peri-ampullary malignancy, cholelithiasis **Biliary tract**: Klatskin tumour **Liver**: hepatomegaly, hepatitis, abscess, tumour (hepatocellular carcinoma, metastatic tumour, etc.)	**Pancreas**: pancreatic adenocarcinoma, other pancreatic neoplasm, pseudocyst **Abdominal aorta**: AAA (pulsatile) **GI**: gastric tumour (adenocarcinoma, gastrointestinal stromal tumour, carcinoid tumour), MALT lymphoma	**Spleen**: splenomegaly, tumour, abscess, subcapsular splenic hemorrhage, can also present as RLQ mass if extreme splenomegaly **Stomach**: tumour

Right Lower Quadrant (RLQ)	Lower Midline	Left Lower Quadrant (LLQ)
Intestine: stool, tumour (CRC), mesenteric adenitis, appendicitis, appendiceal phlegmon or other abscess, typhlitis, intussusception, Crohn's inflammation **Ovary**: ectopic pregnancy, cyst (physiological vs. pathological), tumour (serous, mucinous, struma ovarii, germ cell, Krukenberg) **Fallopian tube**: ectopic pregnancy, tubo-ovarian abscess, hydrosalpinx, tumour	**Uterus**: pregnancy, leiomyoma (fibroid), uterine cancer, pyometra, hematometra **GU**: bladder distention, tumour	**Intestine**: stool, tumour, abscess (see RLQ) **Ovary**: see RLQ **Fallopian tube**: see RLQ

> Pancreatitis can look like a surgical abdomen, but is rarely an indication for immediate surgical intervention

Gastrointestinal Bleeding

- see <u>Gastroenterology</u>, G25 and G27

Indications for Surgery
- failure of medical management
- exsanguinating hemorrhage: hemodynamic instability despite vigorous resuscitation
- recurrent hemorrhage after initial stabilization procedures with up to two attempts of endoscopic hemostasis
- prolonged bleeding with transfusion requirement >3 units
- bleeding at rate >1 unit/8 h

Surgical Management of GI Bleeding
- UGIB
    - bleeding from a source proximal to the ligament of Treitz
    - often presents with hematemesis and melena unless very brisk (then can present with hematochezia)
    - initial management with endoscopy; if fails, then consider surgery
    - PUD accounts for approximately 55% of severe UGIB
- LGIB
    - bleeding from a source distal to the ligament of Treitz
    - often presents with BRBPR unless proximal to transverse colon
        - may occasionally present with melena
    - initial management with colonoscopy to detect and potentially stop source of bleeding
    - 75% of patients will spontaneously stop bleeding, however if bleeding continues barium enema should NOT be performed
    - angiography or RBC scan to determine source as indicated
    - surgery indicated if bleeding is persistent - aimed at resection of area containing source of bleeding
    - obscure bleed may require blind total colectomy if the source is not found

Table 3. Differential Diagnosis of GI Bleeding

Anatomical Source	Etiology	
Hematological	Excess anticoagulation (coumadin, heparin, etc.) Excess antiplatelet (clopidogrel, ASA)	DIC Congenital bleeding disorders
Nose	Epistaxis	
Esophagus	Esophageal varices Mallory-Weiss tear Esophagitis	Aorto-esophageal fistula (generally post endovascular aortic repair)* Esophageal cancer
Stomach	Gastritis Gastric varices Dieulafoy's lesion	Gastric ulcer Gastric cancer*
Duodenum	Duodenal ulcer Perforated duodenal ulcer*	Duodenal cancer*
Jejunum	Tumours* Polyps Ulcers	
Ileum and Ileocecal Junction	Meckel's diverticulum (rare surgical management) Small bowel obstruction	Crohn's disease* Tuberculosis of ileocecal junction
Large Intestine	Colorectal cancer* Mesenteric thrombosis/ischemic bowel* Ulcerative colitis* (subtotal colectomy if failure of medical management) Angiodysplasia Diverticulosis (*if bleeding is persistent)	Crohn's disease (less frequently presents with bleeding)* Pancolitis (infectious, chemotherapy, or radiation induced) Bleeding post-gastrointestinal anastomosis
Sigmoid	Diverticulosis (*if bleeding is persistent) Sigmoid cancer* Bleeding post-polypectomy	Polyps (*if not amenable to colonoscopic polypectomy) Inflammatory bowel disease (IBD)
Rectum and Anus	Hemorrhoids Fissures Rectal cancer* Anal varices	Polyps (*if not amenable to colonoscopic polypectomy) Crohn's or ulcerative colitis* Solitary rectal ulcer syndrome

*Managed surgically in most cases

Jaundice

- see <u>Gastroenterology</u>, G40

Indications for Urgent Operation

IHOP
Ischemia
Hemorrhage
Obstruction
Perforation

Overt bleeding: obvious hematochezia or melena per rectum visible to naked eye
Occult bleeding: bleeding per rectum is not obvious to naked eye (e.g. positive guaiac test)
Obscure bleeding: overt bleeding with no identifiable source after colonoscopy and endoscopy

Transfusion Strategies for Acute Upper Gastrointestinal Bleeding
NEJM 2013;368:11-21
Recent study by Villanueva et al., demonstrates that a restrictive transfusion strategy (transfusion with hemoglobin below 70 g/L) significantly improves outcomes in patients with acute UGIB, compared to a liberal transfusion strategy (transfusion with hemoglobin below 90 g/L). Refer to study for details.

Biochemical Signs for Differentiating Jaundice
Hepatocellular: Elevated bilirubin + elevated ALT/AST
Cholestatic: Elevated bilirubin + elevated ALP/GGT ± duct dilatation upon biliary U/S
Hemolysis: ↓ haptoglobin ↑ LDH

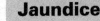

Note: cholestatic jaundice is often surgical

Pre-Operative Preparations

Considerations

- informed consent (see <u>Ethical, Legal, and Organizational Medicine</u>, ELOM6)
- screening questionnaire to determine risk factors e.g. age, exercise capacity, medication use, allergies
- consider pre-operative anesthesia, medicine consult as indicated to optimize patient status
- NPO according to guidelines (see <u>Anesthesia and Perioperative Medicine</u>, A4)
- IV – balanced crystalloid at maintenance rate (4:2:1 rule → roughly 100-125 cc/h): normal saline or Ringer's lactate; bolus to catch up on estimated losses including losses from bowel prep
    - appropriate use of fluids perioperatively decreases risk of cardiorespiratory complications
- patient's regular medications included with the exception of hypoglycemic agents, diuretics and ACEI
- patients on steroids may require stress dose coverage, anticoagulation/ antiplatelet medication must be managed to decrease surgical bleeding but not put patient at risk for increased thrombotic events (e.g. switching from warfarin to LMWH)
- prophylactic antibiotics depending on wound class (within 1 h prior to incision): usually cefazolin (Ancef®) ± metronidazole (Flagyl®)
- consider bowel prep: cleans out bowel and decreases bacterial population
    - oral cathartic (e.g. fleet Phosphosoda®) starting previous day
    - in selected cases, current evidence does not support routine use
- consider VTE prophylaxis for all inpatient surgery (LMWH or heparin)
- do not hold anticoagulation prior to surgery unless epidural is expected
- smoking cessation and weight loss pre-operative can significantly decrease post-operative complications
- infection: delay elective surgery until infection controlled including respiratory infection particularly in asthma patients

Investigations

- see <u>Anesthesia and Perioperative Medicine</u>, A4
- routine pre-operative laboratory investigations for elective procedures should be selective
    - only ASA class and surgical risk have been found to independently predict post-operative adverse effects
- blood components: group and screen or cross and type depending on procedure
- CBC, electrolytes, creatinine
- INR/PT, PTT
- CXR (PA and lateral) for patients with history of cardiac or pulmonary disease
- ECG as indicated by history or if >69 yr and no risk factors
- β-hCG testing in all women of reproductive age

Drains

- NGT
    - indications: gastric decompression, analysis of gastric contents, irrigation/dilution of gastric contents, feeding, if necessary
    - contraindications: suspected basal skull fracture, obstruction of nasal passages due to trauma
- Foley catheter with urometer
    - indications: to accurately monitor urine output, decompression of bladder, relieve obstruction, rapidly expanding suprapubic mass
    - contraindications: suspected urethral injury, difficult insertion of catheter

Surgical Complications

- general principles in preventing complications during the post-operative period include
    - frequent examination of the patient (daily or more) and their wound
    - removal of surgical tubes as soon as possible (e.g. Foley catheters and surgical drains)
    - early ambulation
    - monitor fluid balance and electrolytes
    - analgesia - enough to adequately address pain, but not excessive
    - skillful nursing care

Post-Operative Fever

- fever does not necessarily imply infection particularly in the first 24-48 h post-operative
- fever may not be present or is blunted if patient is receiving chemotherapy, glucocorticoids, or immunosuppression
- timing of fever may help identify cause
    - hours after surgery – POD #1 (immediate)
        - inflammatory reaction in response to trauma from surgery; unlikely to be infectious
        - reaction to blood products received during surgery
        - malignant hyperthermia

Bilirubin Levels

	Prehepatic	Intrahepatic	Posthepatic
Serum Bilirubin			
Indirect	↑	↑	N
Direct	N	↑	↑
Urine			
Urobilinogen	↑	↑	–
Bilirubin	–	+	+
Fecal			
Urobilinogen	↑	↑	–

In patients with liver disease and an acute abdomen, spontaneous bacterial peritonitis must be ruled out

Surgical Emergencies: Take an AMPLE History
Allergies
Medications
Past medical/surgical history (including anesthesia and bleeding disorders)
Last meal
Events (HPI)

Best Practice in General Surgery (BPIGS)
http://www.bpigs.ca/
BPIGS is a University of Toronto initiative with the goal of standardizing care in general surgery. This link contains EBM based guidelines which have been implemented by consensus within all Toronto teaching hospitals. This is a highly recommended source for the most up-to-date pre-operative and general treatment guidelines

Drain Size
Measured by the unit French:
French = diameter (mm) x 3

Pre and Post-Operative Orders

ADDAVIDS
Admit to ward X under Dr. Y
Diagnosis
Diet
Activity
Vitals (q4h from ED and post-operative is standard)
IV, Investigations, Ins and Outs
Drugs, Dressings, Drains
Special procedures

5 Ws of Post-Operative Fever
Wind POD #1-2 (pulmonary – atelectasis, pneumonia)
Water POD #3-5 (urine – UTI)
Wound POD #5-8 (wound infection - if earlier think streptococcal or clostridial infection)
Walk POD #8+ (thrombosis – DVT/PE)
Wonder drugs POD #1+ (drug)

Drugs – 7 As
Analgesia
Anti-emetic
Anticoagulation
Antibiotics
Anxiolytics
Anticonstipation
All other patient meds (home meds, stress
dose steroids, and β-blockers)

**Approach to the Critically Ill Surgical/
Trauma Patient**

ABC, I'M FINE
ABC
IV: 2 large bore IVs with NS, wide open
Monitors: O₂ sat, ECG, BP
Foley catheter to measure urine output
Investigations: blood work
NGT if indicated
"Ex" rays (abdomen 3 views, CXR), other
imaging – only when stable

- POD #1-2 (acute)
  - atelectasis (most common cause of fever on POD #1)
  - early wound infection (especially *Clostridium*, Group A *Streptococcus* – feel for crepitus and look for "dishwater" drainage)
  - aspiration pneumonitis
  - other: Addisonian crisis, thyroid storm, transfusion reaction
- POD #3-7 (subacute): likely infectious
  - UTI, surgical site infection, IV site/line infection, septic thrombophlebitis, leakage at bowel anastomosis (tachycardia, hypotension, oliguria, abdominal pain)
- POD #8+ (delayed)
  - intra-abdominal abscess, DVT/PE (can be anytime post-operative, most commonly POD #8-10), drug fever
  - other: cholecystitis, peri-rectal abscess, URTI, infected seroma/biloma/hematoma, parotitis, C. difficile colitis, endocarditis

Treatment
- treat primary cause
- antipyrexia (e.g. acetaminophen)

Wound/Incisional Complications

WOUND CARE (see Plastic Surgery, PL8)

- can shower POD #2-3 after epithelialization of wound
- dressings can be removed POD #2 and left uncovered if dry
- examine wound if wet dressing, signs of infection (fever, tachycardia, pain)
- skin sutures and staples can be removed POD #7-10
  - exceptions: incision crosses crease (groin), closed under tension, in extremities (hand) or patient factors (elderly, corticosteroid use, immunosuppressed) removed POD #14, earlier if signs of infection
- negative pressure dressings consist of foam and suction, promote granulation
  - ideal for large (grafted sites) or non-healing wounds (irradiated skin, ulcer)

DRAINS
- drains may be placed selectively at the time of surgery to prevent fluid accumulation (blood, pus, serum, bile, urine)
  - can be used to assess quantity of third space fluid accumulation post-operatively
- potential route of infection; to decrease risk of wound infection bring out through separate incision (vs. operative wound) and remove as soon as possible
- types of drains
  - open (e.g. Penrose), higher risk of infection
  - closed: 1) Gravity drainage (e.g. Foley catheter); 2) Underwater-seal drainage system (e.g. chest tube); 3) Suction drainage (e.g. Jackson-Pratt)
  - sump (e.g. NGT)
- monitor drain outputs daily
- drains should be removed once drainage is minimal (usually <30-50 cc/24 h)
- drains do not guarantee that the patient will not form a collection of fluid
- ridged drains can erode through internal structures, and excessive suction can cause necrosis
- evidence does not support routine post-operative drainage of abdominal cavity

SURGICAL SITE INFECTION

Etiology
- *S. aureus, E. coli, Enterococcus, Streptococcus* spp., *Clostridium* spp.

Risk Factors

Table 4. Procedures and Their Impact on Surgical Site Infection

Classification	Clean	Clean-Contaminated	Contaminated	Dirty/Infected
Definition	Incision under sterile conditions; nontraumatic; no entrance of hollow organ	Incision under sterile conditions; ENTRANCE of hollow viscus; no evidence of active infection; minimal contamination	Incision under sterile conditions; MAJOR contamination of wound during procedure (i.e. gross spillage of stool, infection in biliary, respiratory, or GU systems)	Established infection present before wound is made in skin
Example	Wound created to repair hernia	Routine cholecystectomy; colon resection	Bowel obstruction with enterotomy and spillage of contents; necrotic bowel resection; fresh traumatic wounds	Appendiceal abscess; traumatic wound with contaminated devitalized tissue; perforated viscus
Infection Rate	<2%	3-4%	7-10%	30-40%
Wound Closure	Primary closure	Primary closure	Often secondary closure	Secondary closure

- patient characteristics
  - age, DM, steroids, immunosuppression, obesity, burn, malnutrition, patient with other infections, traumatic wound, radiation, chemotherapy
- other factors
  - prolonged pre-operative hospitalization, reduced blood flow, break in sterile technique, multiplantibiotics, hematoma, seroma, foreign bodies (drains, sutures, grafts), skin preparation, hypoxemia, hypothermia

Prophylaxis
- pre-operative antibiotics for most surgeries (cefazolin ± metronidazole or if β-lactam allergy, clindamycin ± gentamycin)
  - within 1 h pre-incision; can redose at 1-2 half-lives (~q4-8h) in the OR
  - not required for low risk elective cholecystectomy, hemorrhoidectomy, fistulotomy, sphincterotomy for fissure
  - some evidence suggests role in breast surgery
    - reserve post-operative antibiotics for treatment of suspected or documented intra-abdominal infection, hair removal should not be performed unless necessary; if so, clipping superior to shaving chlorhexidine-alcohol wash of surgical site
- normothermia (maintain patient temperature 36-38°C during OR)
- hyperoxygenation (consider FiO_2 of 80% in OR)
- consider delayed primary closure of incision for contaminated wounds

Clinical Presentation
- typically fever POD #5-8 (*Streptococcus* and *Clostridium* can present in 24 h)
- pain, blanchable wound erythema, induration, purulent discharge, warmth
- complications: fistula, sinus tracts, sepsis, abscess, suppressed wound healing, superinfection, spreading infection to myonecrosis or fascial necrosis (necrotizing fasciitis), wound dehiscence, evisceration, hernia

Treatment
- examination of the wound: inspect, compress adjacent areas, swab drainage for C&S and Gram stain
- re-open affected part of incision, drain, pack, heal by secondary intention in most cases
- for deeper infections, debride necrotic and non-viable tissue
- antibiotics and demarcation of erythema only if cellulitis or immunodeficiency

WOUND HEMORRHAGE/HEMATOMA
- secondary to inadequate surgical control of hemostasis

Risk Factors
- anticoagulant therapy, coagulopathies, thrombocytopenia, DIC, severe liver disease, myeloproliferative disorders, severe arterial HTN, severe cough
- more common with transverse incisions through muscle, due to cutting of muscle

Clinical Features
- pain, swelling, discolouration of wound edges, leakage
- rapidly expanding neck hematoma can compromise airway and is a surgical emergency: consider having a suture kit at bedside in all neck surgery in the event of having to open the wound emergently

Treatment
- pressure dressing
- open drainage ± wound packing (large hematoma only)
- if significant bleeding, may need to re-operate to find source (often do not find a discrete source)

SEROMA
- fluid collection other than pus or blood
- secondary to transection of lymph vessels
- delays healing
- increased infection risk

Treatment
- consider pressure dressing ± needle drainage
- if significant may need to re-operate

WOUND DEHISCENCE
- disruption of fascial layer, abdominal contents contained by skin only
- 95% caused by intact suture tearing through fascia

Clinical Features
- typically POD #1-3; most common presentation sign is serosanguinous drainage from wound ± evisceration
- palpation of wound edge: should normally feel a "healing ridge" from abdominal wall closure (raised area of tissue under incision)

Systemic Prophylactic Antibiotics Recommendations
Updated Recommendations for Control of Surgical Site Infections
Ann Surg 2011;253:1082-93
- Choice of routine prophylactic antibiotic depends on the pathogen and patient allergies.
- Vancomycin and fluoroquinolones should be administered 1-2 h prior to incision; all other antibiotics should be administered 30 min prior to incision.
- Short-acting antibiotics should be redosed ~3 h after incision.
- Antibiotic administration >24 h after surgery does not appear to add benefits.
- Antibiotics should no longer be routinely administered in three doses.
- The majority of antibiotics are renally excreted hence renal function must be considered in antibiotic administration.
- Obese patients need higher antibiotic doses to achieve therapeutic concentrations.
- Drug half-life and length of operation need to be considered in antibiotic administration.

Pre-Operative Skin Antiseptics for Preventing Surgical Wound Infections After Clean Surgery
Cochrane DB Syst Rev 2015;4:CD003949
Purpose: To determine if pre-operative skin antisepsis prior to clean surgery prevents surgical-site infection (SSI) and compare the effectiveness of other antiseptics.
Methods: Systematic review of randomized-controlled trials (RCTs) part of the Cochrane Wounds Group Specialised Register and the Chochrane Central Register of Controlled Trials (CENTRAL). Main outcome was SSI. Secondary outcomes included quality of life, mortality, and resource use.
Results: 13 RCTs (n=2,623 patients) were included that made 11 total comparisons between skin antiseptics. A single study found that 0.5% chlorhexidine solution in methylated spirits was significantly superior in preventing SSIs after clean surgery compared to alcohol based povidone iodine solution. No other statistically significant differences were found.
Conclusions: Further research is warranted to determine the effectiveness of one antiseptic over the others at preventing SSI post clean surgery.

Systemic Review and Meta-Analysis of Randomized Clinical Trials Comparing Primary vs. Delayed Primary Skin Closure in Contaminated and Dirty Abdominal Incisions
JAMA Surg 2013;148:779-786
Purpose: To compare rates of surgical site infection (SSI) with delayed primary closure (DPC) vs. primary skin closure (PC).
Results/Conclusions: 8 RCTs with 623 patients. Most common diagnosis was appendicitis (77.4%). Although there was significant heterogeneity between studies, DPC (2-5 d time to first review) was found to significantly reduce the chance of SSI (OR 0.65, 95% CI 0.40-0.93). Although current trials are poorly designed, DPC may be a simple and cost-effective way of reducing the rates of SSIs following abdominal surgery with contaminated or dirty wounds.

Risk Factors
- local: technical failure of closure, increased intra-abdominal pressure (e.g. COPD, ileus, bowel obstruction), hematoma, infection, poor blood supply, radiation, patient not fully paralyzed while closing, transverse incision
- systemic: smoking, malnutrition (hypoalbuminemia, vitamin C deficiency), connective tissue diseases, immunosuppression, pulmonary disease, ascites, poor nutrition, steroids, chemotherapy, obesity, other (e.g. age, sepsis, uremia)
- DM alone is not a risk factor

Treatment
- place moist dressing over wound with binder around abdomen and transfer to OR
- may consider conservative management with debridement of fascial and/or skin margins
- evisceration, also known as 'burst abdomen', is a surgical emergency): take patient for operative re-closure.

Urinary and Renal Complications

URINARY RETENTION
- may occur after any operation with general anesthesia or spinal anesthesia
- more likely in older males with history of benign prostatic hyperplasia, patients on anticholinergics

Clinical Presentation
- abdominal discomfort, palpable bladder, overflow incontinence, post-void residual urine volume >100 mL

Treatment
- Foley catheter to rest bladder, then trial of voiding

OLIGURIA/ANURIA (see Nephrology, NP18)

Etiology
- prerenal vs. renal vs. postrenal
- most common post-operative cause is prerenal ± ischemic ATN
  - external fluid loss: hemorrhage, dehydration, diarrhea
  - internal fluid loss: third-spacing due to bowel obstruction, pancreatitis

Clinical Presentation
- urine output <0.5 cc/kg/h, increasing Cr, increasing BUN

Treatment
- according to underlying cause; fluid deficit is treated with crystalloid (NS or RL)

Post-Operative Dyspnea

- see *Respiratory Complications* next and *Cardiac Complications*, GS12

Etiology
- respiratory: atelectasis, pneumonia, pulmonary embolus (PE), ARDS, asthma, pleural effusion
- cardiac: MI, arrhythmia, CHF
- inadequate pain control

Respiratory Complications

ATELECTASIS
- comprises 90% of post-operative pulmonary complications

Clinical Features
- low-grade fever on POD #1, tachycardia, crackles, decreased breath sounds, bronchial breathing, tachypnea

Risk Factors
- COPD, smoking, obesity, elderly persons
- upper abdominal/thoracic surgery, oversedation, significant post-operative pain, poor inspiratory effort

Treatment
- pre-operative prophylaxis
  - smoking cessation (best if >8 wk pre-operative)
- post-operative prophylaxis
  - incentive spirometry, deep breathing exercise, chest physiotherapy, intermittent positive-pressure breathing
  - selective NGT decompression after abdominal surgery
  - short-acting neuromuscular blocking agents
  - minimize use of respiratory depressive drugs, appropriate pain control, early ambulation

PNEUMONIA/PNEUMONITIS
- may be secondary to aspiration of gastric contents during anesthetic induction or extubation, causing a chemical pneumonitis

Risk Factors
- aspiration: general anesthetic, decreased LOC, GERD, full stomach, bowel/gastric outlet obstruction + non-functioning NGT, pregnancy, seizure disorder
- non-aspiration: atelectasis, immobility, pre-existing respiratory disease

Clinical Features
- productive cough, fever
- tachycardia, cyanosis, respiratory failure, decreased LOC
- CXR: pulmonary infiltrate

Treatment
- prophylaxis: see atelectasis prophylaxis, pre-operative NPO/NGT, rapid sequence anesthetic induction
- immediate removal of debris and fluid from airway
- consider endotracheal intubation and flexible bronchoscopic aspiration
- IV antibiotics to cover oral nosocomial aerobes and anaerobes (e.g. ceftriaxone, metronidazole)

PULMONARY EMBOLUS (See Respirology, R18)

Clinical Features
- unilateral leg swelling and pain (DVT as a source of PE), sudden onset shortness of breath, tachycardia, fever
- most commonly POD #8-10, but can occur anytime post-operatively, even after discharge
- diagnosis made by Chest CT scan usually

Treatment
- initial treatment IV heparin or therapeutic- dose LMWH, bridging to therapeutic anticoagulation is required for a minimum of 3 months; for patients with cancer, or other risk factors for hypercoagulability, the duration of anticoagulation may be longer
- Greenfield (IVC) filter if contraindications to anticoagulation
- prophylaxis: subcutaneous heparin (5,000 U bid) or LMWH, compression stockings (TED™ Hose), sequential compression devices

PULMONARY EDEMA

Etiology
- cardiogenic vs. noncardiogenic
- circulatory overload: excess volume replacement, LV failure, shift of fluid from peripheral to pulmonary vascular bed, negative airway pressure, alveolar injury due to toxins (e.g. ARDS)
  - more common with pre-existing cardiac disease
- negative pressure pulmonary edema due to inspiratory efforts against a closed glottis upon awakening from general anesthesia

New onset "asthma" and wheezing in the elderly is cardiogenic until proven otherwise

Clinical Features
- shortness of breath, crackles at lung bases, CXR abnormal

Treatment (LMNOP)
- Lasix
- Morphine (decreases symptoms of dyspnea, venodilator and afterload reduction)
- Nitrates (venodilator)
- Oxygen + non-invasive ventilation
- Position (sit patient up)

RESPIRATORY FAILURE

Clinical Features
- dyspnea, cyanosis, evidence of obstructive lung disease
- earliest manifestations – tachypnea and hypoxemia (RR >25, pO_2 <60)
- pulmonary edema, unexplained decrease in SaO_2

Treatment
- ABCs, O_2, ± positive pressure ventilation, intubation
- bronchodilators, diuretics to treat CHF
- adequate blood pressure to maintain pulmonary perfusion
- if these measures fail to keep PaO_2 >60, consider ARDS

Cardiac Complications

- abnormal ECGs common in post-operative period (compare to pre-operative ECG)
- common arrhythmias: supraventricular tachycardia, atrial fibrillation (secondary to fluid overload, PE, MI)

MYOCARDIAL INFARCTION
- see <u>Cardiology and Cardiac Surgery</u>, C27
- surgery increases risk of MI
- incidence
- 0.5% in previously asymptomatic men >50 yr old
- 40-fold increase in men >50 yr old with previous MI

Risk Factors
- pre-operative HTN, CHF
- previous MI (highest risk ≤6 mo, but risk never returns to baseline)
- increased age
- intra-operative hypotension
- operations >3 h
- angina

Clinical Features
- majority of cases on day of operation or POD #3-4 (shifting of third space fluid back into intravascular compartment)
- often silent without chest pain, may only present with new-onset CHF (dyspnea), arrhythmias, hypotension

Intra-Abdominal Abscess

Definition
- collection of pus walled-off from rest of peritoneal cavity by inflammatory adhesions and viscera

Etiology
- usually polymicrobial: Gram-negative bacteria, anaerobes
  - consider Gram-positives if coexisting cellulitis

Risk Factors
- emergency surgery, contaminated OR
- GI surgery with anastomoses
- poor healing risk factors (DM, poor nutrition, etc.)
- may occur POD #3 after laparotomy when third space fluid re-distribution occurs

Clinical Features
- persistent spiking fever, dull pain, weight loss
- mass difficult to palpate
- peritoneal signs if abscess perforation and secondary peritonitis
- leukocytosis or leukopenia (immunocompromised, elderly)
- co-existing effusion (pleural effusion with subphrenic abscess)
- common sites: pelvis, Morrison's pouch (space between kidney and liver), subphrenic, paracolic gutters, lesser sac, peri-appendiceal, post-surgical anastomosis, diverticular, psoas

Investigations
- CBC, blood cultures x2
- CT ± IV and water-soluble contrast
- DRE (pelvic abscess)

Treatment
- drain placement by interventional radiology (preferred), laparoscopy, open drainage
- subsequent antibiotic coverage; ceftriaxone + metronidazole or piperacilin-tazobactam (PepTazo)

Paralytic Ileus

- see *Bowel Obstruction*, GS23

Delirium

- see Psychiatry, PS19 and Neurology, N20

Thoracic Surgery

Hiatus Hernia

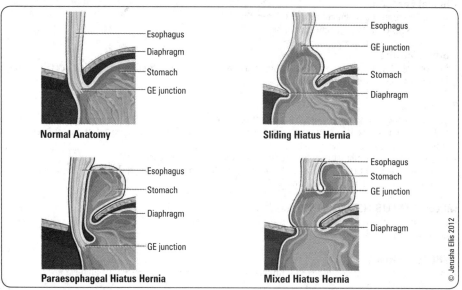

Figure 6. Types of hiatus hernia

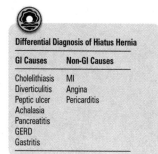

Differential Diagnosis of Hiatus Hernia

GI Causes	Non-GI Causes
Cholelithiasis	MI
Diverticulitis	Angina
Peptic ulcer	Pericarditis
Achalasia	
Pancreatitis	
GERD	
Gastritis	

SLIDING HIATUS HERNIA (TYPE I)
- see Figure 6
- herniation of both the stomach and the gastroesophageal (GE) junction into thorax
- 90% of esophageal hernias

Risk Factors
- age
- increased intra-abdominal pressure (e.g. obesity, pregnancy, coughing, heavy lifting)
- smoking

Clinical Features
- majority are asymptomatic
- hernias frequently associated with GERD due to decreased competence of LES

Complications
- most common complication is GERD
- other complications are rare and are related to reflux
- esophagitis (dysphagia, heartburn)
- consequences of esophagitis (peptic stricture, Barrett's esophagus, esophageal carcinoma)
- extra-esophageal complications (aspiration pneumonitis/pneumonia, asthma type bronchospasm, cough, laryngitis)

Investigations
- barium swallow, endoscopy (esophago-gastroscopy), or esophageal manometry (technique for measuring LES pressure)
- 24 h esophageal pH monitoring to quantify reflux
- endoscopy with biopsy to document type and extent of tissue damage and rule out esophagitis, Barrett's esophagus, and cancer

Treatment
- lifestyle modification
  - stop smoking, weight loss, elevate head of bed, no meals <3 h prior to sleeping, smaller and more frequent meals, avoid alcohol, coffee, mint, and fat
- medical
  - antacid, H_2-antagonist, PPI, prokinetic agent
- surgical (<15%)
  - if failure of medical therapy, complications of GERD such as esophageal stricture, severe nocturnal aspiration, Barrett's esophagus
  - anti-reflux procedure (usually laparoscopic) e.g. Nissen fundoplication
    - fundus of stomach is wrapped around the lower esophagus and sutured in place
    - 90% success rate

PARAESOPHAGEAL HIATUS HERNIA (TYPE II)
- see Figure 6
- herniation of all or part of the stomach through the esophageal hiatus into the thorax with an undisplaced GE junction
- least common esophageal hernia (<10%)

Clinical Features
- usually asymptomatic due to normal GE junction
- pressure sensation in lower chest, dysphagia

Complications
- hemorrhage, incarceration, strangulation (gastric volvulus), obstruction, gastric stasis ulcer (Cameron's lesion – causes Fe-deficiency anemia)

Treatment
- surgery to address symptoms or treat/prevent complications
- reduce hernia and excise hernia sac, repair defect at hiatus, and anti-reflux procedure (e.g. Nissen fundoplication)
- may consider suturing stomach to anterior abdominal wall (gastropexy)
- in very elderly patients at high surgical risk consider PEG (percutaneous endoscopic gastrostomy) to anchor the stomach in the abdomen

MIXED HIATUS HERNIA (TYPE III)
- see Figure 6
- combination of Types I and II

TYPE IV HERNIA
- herniation of stomach and other abdominal organs into thorax: colon, spleen, small bowel
- Fe-deficiency anemia is common

Esophageal Perforation

Etiology
- iatrogenic (most common)
  - endoscopic, dilatation, biopsy, intubation, operative, NGT placement (rare)
- barogenic
  - trauma
  - repeated, forceful vomiting (Boerhaave's syndrome)
  - other: convulsions, defecation, labour (rare)
- ingestion injury
  - foreign body, corrosive substance
- carcinoma

Clinical Features
- neck or chest pain
- fever, tachycardia, hypotension, dyspnea, respiratory compromise
- subcutaneous emphysema, pneumothorax, pleural effusion, and hematemesis,

Investigations
- CXR: pneumothorax, pneumomediastinum, pleural effusion, subdiaphragmatic air, widened mediastinum
- CT chest: neumomediastinum, pleural effusion, pneumothorax, contrast in the chest, subq emphysema
- Upper GI swallow study with water soluble contrast. If negative then perform with diluted barium: contrast extravasation

Boerhaave's syndrome: transmural esophageal perforation
Mallory-Weiss tear: non-transmural esophageal tear (partial thickness tear)
Both are associated with forceful emesis

6Ss of SCC
Smoking
Spirits (alcohol)
Seeds (betel nut)
Scalding (hot liquid)
Strictures
Sack (diverticula)

Treatment
- supportive if rupture is contained
  - NPO, fluid resuscitation, broad-spectrum antibiotics, possible percutaneous drainage of mediastinum or pleura
- surgical
  - <24 h
    - primary closure of a healthy esophagus or resection of diseased esophagus
  - >24 h or non-viable wound edges
    - diversion and exclusion followed by delayed reconstruction (i.e. esophagostomy proximally, close esophagus distally, gastrostomy/jejunostomy for decompression/feeding)

Complications
- sepsis, abscess, fistula, empyema, mediastinitis, death
- post-operative esophageal leak
- mortality 10-50% dependent on timing of diagnosis

Esophageal Carcinoma

Epidemiology
- M:F = 3:1
- onset 50-60 yr of age
- upper (20-33%), middle (33%), lower (33-50%)
- main types
  - most common worldwide: SCC in upper 2/3 of esophagus
  - most common in Western countries: adenocarcinoma in distal 1/3 of esophagus

Risk Factors
- geographic variation in incidence
- SCC
  - underlying esophageal disease such as strictures, diverticula, achalasia
  - smoking, alcohol, hot liquids
  - more common in patients from Asia
- adenocarcinoma
  - Barrett's esophagus (most important), smoking, obesity (increased reflux), GERD

Clinical Features
- progressive dysphagia (mechanical): first solids then liquids
- odynophagia then constant pain
- constitutional symptoms
- regurgitation and aspiration (aspiration pneumonia)
- hematemesis, anemia
- direct, hematogenous, or lymphatic spread
  - trachea (coughing), recurrent laryngeal nerves (hoarseness, vocal paralysis), aortic, liver, lung, bone, celiac and mediastinal nodes

Investigations and Staging
- barium swallow: shows narrowing – suggestive but not diagnostic
- endoscopic biopsy and assess resectability
- both SCC and adenocarcinoma use TNM staging system but have separate stage groupings according to histology
- endoscopic U/S (EUS)
  - visualize local disease
  - regional nodal involvement (number of nodes may be more important than location)
- bronchoscopy ± thoracoscopy
  - rule out airway invasion in tumours of the upper and mid esophagus
- full metastatic workup (CXR, bone scan, CT head, CT chest/abdomen/pelvis, LFTs, etc.)
- PET scan more sensitive than CT in detecting metastatic disease

Treatment
- if present with distant metastatic disease
  - treat with systemic therapy and treat symptoms (esophageal stent)
- if locally advanced (locally invasive disease or nodal disease on CT or EUS)
  - multimodal therapy
    - concurrent external beam radiation and chemotherapy (cisplatin and 5-FU)
    - possibility of curative esophagectomy after chemoradiation if disease responds well
  - if unable to tolerate multimodal therapy or if highly advanced disease, consider palliative resection, brachytherapy, or endoscopic dilatation/stenting/laser ablation for palliation

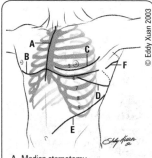

A. Median sternotomy
B. Transverse thoracotomy (clam shell)
C. Anterolateral thoracotomy
D. Lateral thoracotomy
E. Thoracoabdominal thoracotomy
F. Posterolateral thoracotomy

Figure 7. Typical thoracic surgery incisions

Perioperative Chemo(radio)therapy vs. Primary Surgery for Resectable Adenocarcinoma of the Stomach, Gastroesophageal Junction, and Lower Esophagus
Cochrane DB Syst Rev 2013;5:CD008107
Study: Review of RCTs to examine the effect of perioperative chemotherapy for gastroesophageal adenocarcinoma on survival and other clinically relevant outcomes.
Results/Conclusions: 14 RCTs, 2,422 participants.
1) Perioperative chemotherapy was associated with a significantly longer overall survival (HR 0.81, 95% CI 0.73 to 0.89), a relative survival increase of 19% and an absolute increase of 9%.
2) Tumours of the GE junction showed a more pronounced response to perioperative chemotherapy compared to other sites.
3) Combined chemoradiotherapy was more effective for tumours of the esophagus and GE junction compared to chemotherapy alone.
4) Perioperative chemotherapy was more effective in younger patients and is associated with longer disease-free survival, higher rates of R0 resection, and a more favourable tumour stage upon resection.
5) Resection with negative margins is a strong predictor of survival.

- if early stage (non-transmural and without evidence of nodal disease)
  - endoscopic mucosal resection can be considered for early mucosal cancer or high grade dysplasia
  - esophagectomy (transthoracic or trans-hiatal approach) and lymphadenectomy
    - anastomosis in chest or neck
    - stomach most often used for reconstruction; may also use colon
  - neoadjuvant chemotherapy and radiation are controversial
  - adjuvant chemotherapy ± radiation usually recommended for post-operative node-positive disease

Prognosis
- TNM status - usually poor because presentation is usually at advanced stage.

OTHER DISORDERS
- esophageal motor disorders (see Gastroenterology, G8)
- esophageal varices (see Gastroenterology, G26)
- Mallory-Weiss tear (see Gastroenterology, G26)

Thymoma

Epidemiology
- most common neoplasms in thymus including both thymoma and thymic carcinoma
- patients between 40 and 60 yr
- M > F

Risk Factors
- no known risk factors, strong association with myasthenia gravis and other paraneoplastic syndromes

Clinical Presentation
- frequently asymptomatic: incidental finding on imaging
- symptoms related to tumour size and location or myasthenia gravis: chest pain, SOB, cough, phrenic nerve palsy
- ddx includes lymphoma, other anterior mediastinal tumours (see Respirology, R21)

Investigations
- CT chest (and/or MRI)
- Germ cell tumour markers (β-hCG, alpha fetoprotein), thyroid function, PFTs

Treatment
- for patients with resectable disease
- surgical resection of thymus via median sternotomy or VATS depending on the size
- ± post-operative radiation based on Masaoka staging
- for non-surgical patients
- multimodal therapy including neoadjuvant or palliative chemotherapy and post-operative chemoradiotherapy if de-bulking procedure feasible

Prognosis
- depends upon stage of disease and resectability
- generally slow growing tumours and have good prognosis

Pleura, Lung, and Mediastinum

- see Respirology, R21

Tube Thoracostomy

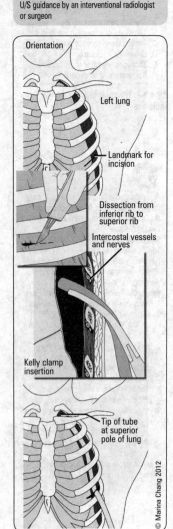
Tube thoracostomy can be completed under U/S guidance by an interventional radiologist or surgeon

Orientation
Left lung
Landmark for incision
Dissection from inferior rib to superior rib
Intercostal vessels and nerves
Kelly clamp insertion
Tip of tube at superior pole of lung
© Marina Chang 2012

Figure 8. Tube thoracostomy

Indications
- to drain abnormal large-volume air or fluid collections in the pleural space
  - hemothorax, pleural effusion, chylothorax, empyema
  - pneumothorax, if
    - large or progressive
    - patient is on mechanical ventilation
    - bronchopleural fistula
    - tension pneumothorax
- to treat symptomatic and/or recurrent pleural effusion
  - see Respirology, R22
  - for long-term drainage of malignant effusions use: 1. Tunneled pleural catheter; 2. Pleural drainage and chemical pleurodesis
  - via facilitation of pleurodesis (obliteration of the pleural space by instilling talc or doxycycline to cause fibrosis and adherence of parietal and visceral pleura)

Complications
- overall complications are rare (1-3%)
- malposition (most common complication), especially by inexperienced operators
  - tubes may dissect along the external chest wall, or may be placed below the diaphragm
- bleeding (anticoagulation is a relative contraindication)
- local infection, empyema
- perforation of lung parenchyma or vasculature
- risk of re-expansion pulmonary edema when large volumes of air or fluid are drawn off quickly (>1.0-1.5 L)

Lung Transplantation

Conditions Leading to Transplantation
- chronic acquired lung disease: COPD
- genetic: CF, emphysema due to α-1 antitrypsin deficiency
- idiopathic interstitial pneumonias: IPF, nonspecific interstitial pneumonitis
- HTN-related: IPAH, secondary pulmonary HTN, Eisenmenger's syndrome
- other: sarcoidosis, lymphangioleiomyomatosis, pulmonary Langerhans cell histiocytosis

Clinical Indications
- transplantation should be considered for patients with advanced lung disease refractory to maximal medical or surgical therapy
- patients who are symptomatic during activities of daily living and have limited expected survival over the next 2 yr

Criteria for Transplantation
- lung allocation score based on: 1) post-transplant survival measure, and 2) waiting list urgency measure
- transplant benefit = post-transplant survival (days) – waitlist survival (days)

Contraindications
- uncontrolled or untreatable pulmonary or extrapulmonary infection
- malignancy in the last 2 yr
- advanced cardiopulmonary disease
- significant chest wall/spinal deformity
- active cigarette smoking
- HIV infection, ongoing HBV or HCV infections

Post-Operative Complications
- primary graft dysfunction: main cause is ischemia-reperfusion injury, graded by PaO_2/FiO_2 ratio and CXR findings
- airway anastomotic complications (focal infection, bronchial necrosis and dehiscence, excess granulation tissue, tracheobronchomalacia, stenosis, fistula)
- chronic graft dysfunction: bronchiolitis obliterans syndrome
- infectious complications (bacterial, fungal, CMV, community-acquired respiratory viruses, mycobacteria)
- malignancy (non-melanoma skin cancer, post-transplant lymphoproliferative disease, colon, breast, Kaposi's sarcoma, bladder)

Prognosis
- median survival for all adult recipients: 5.4 yr
- 1 yr survival: COPD > IPF > IPAH
- 10 yr survival: CF, α-1 antitrypsin deficiency > IPAH > COPD, IPF

Chronic Obstructive Pulmonary Disease

- see Respirology, R9

Treatment
- indications for surgical management
  - dyspnea despite maximal medical therapy and pulmonary rehabilitation
  - CT showing hyperinflation and heterogeneously distributed emphysema predominant in the upper lung zone
  - may be used as a bridging procedure to lung transplantation
- contraindications
  - age >75, cigarette smoking within the prior 6 mo, higher risk of surgical mortality
  - homogeneously distributed emphysematous changes without areas of preserved lung tissue
  - diffusing capacity of lung for carbon monoxide <20% of predicted, $PaCO_2$ >60 mmHg, PaO_2 <45 mmHg
- surgical procedures
  - lung volume reduction surgery: wedge excision of emphysematous tissue
  - bilateral or unilateral, thoracotomy or VATS

Long-Term Survival Analysis of the Canadian Lung Volume Reduction Surgery Trial
Ann Thorac Surg 2013;96:1217-1222
Study: Retrospective observational study assessing the long-term survival of patients enrolled in the CLVRS at 8-10 yr follow-up.
Results/Conclusions: Compared with the best medical care group, patients in the LVRS group showed a 16-mo survival advantage and a 20% reduction in mortality. Although not statistically significant, LVRS may provide long-term benefits in the treatment of end-stage emphysema.

Complications of Treatment
- air leak: may require reintubation and mechanical ventilation
- arrhythmias, pneumonia

Prognosis
- total mortality at 2 yr same as with maximal medical therapy, but better exercise capacity and quality of life with LVRS

Stomach and Duodenum

Peptic Ulcer Disease

GASTRIC ULCERS
- see Gastroenterology, G11

Indications for Surgery
- refractory to medical management
- suspicion of malignancy (even if biopsy benign)
- complications of PUD: obstruction, perforation, bleeding (3x greater risk compared to duodenal ulcers)
- surgical treatment is increasingly rare due to *H. pylori* eradication and medical treatment

Procedures
- ligation of bleeding vessels
- distal gastrectomy with ulcer excision: Billroth II, Roux-en-Y gastrojejunostomy or Billroth I (rarely) reconstruction
- vagotomy and pyloroplasty only if acid hypersecretion (rare)
- wedge resection if possible or biopsy with primary repair

DUODENAL ULCERS
- see Gastroenterology, *Bleeding Peptic Ulcer*, G12, and *Peptic Ulcer Disease*, G11
- most within 2 cm of pylorus (duodenal bulb)

Indications for Surgery
- hemorrhage, rebleed in hospital, perforation, gastric outlet obstruction
- refractory to medical and endoscopic management

Procedures
- omental (Graham) patch: plication of ulcer supported by overlying omental patch
- oversewing of bleeding ulcer ± pyloroplasty
treat with *H. plyori* eradication protocol post operatively.

Complications of Gastric Surgery
- retained antrum
- fistula (gastrocolic/gastrojejunal)
- dumping syndrome, postvagotomy diarrhea, afferent loop syndrome (see *Complications of Gastric Surgery*, GS21)

Table 5. Complications of Duodenal Ulceration

Complication	Clinical Features	Management
Perforated Ulcer (typically on anterior surface)	Sudden onset of pain (possibly in RLQ due to track down right paracolic gutter) Acute abdomen: rigid, diffuse guarding Ileus Initial chemical peritonitis followed by bacterial peritonitis	Investigation CXR – free air under diaphragm (70% of patients) Treatment Oversew ulcer (plication) and omental (Graham) patch – most common treatment
Posterior Penetration	Elevated amylase/lipase if penetration into pancreas Constant mid-epigastric pain burrowing into back, unrelated to meals	
Hemorrhage (typically on posterior surface)	Gastroduodenal artery involvement	Resuscitation initially with crystalloids; blood transfusion if necessary Diagnostic and/or therapeutic endoscopy (laser, cautery, or injection); if recurs, may have second scope Consider interventional radiology: angiography with embolization/coiling Surgery if severe or recurrent bleeding, hemodynamically unstable, or failure of endoscopy and IR: oversewing of ulcer, pyloroplasty
Gastric Outlet Obstruction	Ulcer can lead to edema, fibrosis of pyloric channel, neoplasm N/V (undigested food, non-bilious), dilated stomach, crampy abdominal pain Succussion splash (splashing noise heard with stethoscope over the stomach when patient is shaken) Auscultate gas and fluid movement in obstructed organ	NGT decompression and correction of hypochloremic, hypokalemic metabolic alkalosis Medical management initially: high dose PPI therapy Surgical resection if obstruction does not resolve: either Billroth I, pyloroplasty, or gastrojejunostomy

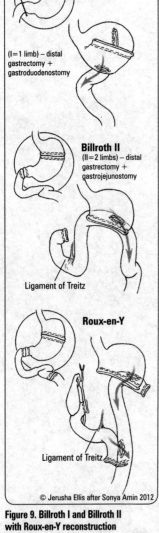

Billroth I

(I = 1 limb) – distal gastrectomy + gastroduodenostomy

Billroth II

(II = 2 limbs) – distal gastrectomy + gastrojejunostomy

Ligament of Treitz

Roux-en-Y

Ligament of Treitz

© Jerusha Ellis after Sonya Amin 2012

Figure 9. Billroth I and Billroth II with Roux-en-Y reconstruction (gastrojejunostomy)

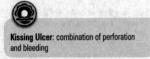

Kissing Ulcer: combination of perforation and bleeding

Gastric Carcinoma

Epidemiology
- 5th most common cancer in the world
- M:F = 3:2
- most common age group = 50-59 yr
- incidence has decreased by 2/3 in past 50 yr
- incidence of adenocarcinoma <10 (US) vs. 40 (Japan, Korea) per 100,000 (incidence highest in Asia, Latin America, and Caribbean)

Risk Factors
- compensatory epithelial cell proliferation via gastric atrophy from:
  - *H. pylori*, causing chronic atrophic gastritis
  - pernicious anemia associated with achlorhydria and chronic atrophic gastritis
  - previous partial gastrectomy (>10 yr post-gastrectomy)
- host-related factors
  - blood type A
  - hereditary nonpolyposis colorectal cancer (HNPCC), hereditary diffuse gastric carcinoma (HDGC)
  - gastric adenomatous polyps
  - hypertrophic gastropathy
  - genetic syndromes: hereditary diffuse gastric cancer E-cahedrin (CDH-1) gene
- environmental factors: smoking, alcohol, smoked food, nitrosamines

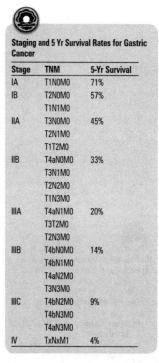

Signs of Metastatic Gastric Carcinoma
Virchow's node: left supraclavicular node
Blumer's shelf: mass in pouch of Douglas
Krukenberg tumour: metastases to ovary
Sister Mary Joseph node: umbilical metastases
Irish's node: left axillary nodes

Clinical Features
- clinical suspicion
  - ulcer fails to heal
  - lesion on greater curvature of stomach or cardia
- asymptomatic, insidious, or late onset of symptoms
  - postprandial abdominal fullness, vague epigastric pain
  - anorexia, weight loss
  - burping, N/V, dyspepsia, dysphagia
  - hepatomegaly, epigastric mass (25%)
  - hematemesis, fecal occult blood, melena, iron-deficiency anemia
- metastasis
  - peritoneum, ovarian, liver, lung, brain

Investigations
- OGD and biopsy; consider EUS to assess pre-operative T-stage and N-stage
- CT chest/abdomen/pelvis (for metastatic workup see Table 7)

Staging and 5 Yr Survival Rates for Gastric Cancer

Stage	TNM	5-Yr Survival
IA	T1N0M0	71%
IB	T2N0M0	57%
	T1N1M0	
IIA	T3N0M0	45%
	T2N1M0	
	T1T2M0	
IIB	T4aN0M0	33%
	T3N1M0	
	T2N2M0	
	T1N3M0	
IIIA	T4aN1M0	20%
	T3T2M0	
	T2N3M0	
IIIB	T4bN0M0	14%
	T4bN1M0	
	T4aN2M0	
	T3N3M0	
IIIC	T4bN2M0	9%
	T4bN3M0	
	T4aN3M0	
IV	TxNxM1	4%

Table 6. TNM Classification System for Staging of Gastric Carcinoma (AJCC/IUCC 2010)

Primary Tumour (T)		Regional Lymph Nodes (N)		Distant Metastasis (M)	
T0	No evidence of primary tumour	NX	Cannot be assessed	M0	No distant metastasis
Tis	Carcinoma *in situ*	N0	No regional node metastasis	M1	Distant metastasis
T1a	Invasion into lamina propria or muscularis mucosae	N1	Metastasis in 1-2 regional nodes		
T1b	Invasion into submucosa	N2	Metastasis in 3-6 regional nodes		
T2	Invasion into muscularis propria	N3a	Metastasis in 7-15 regional nodes		
T3	Penetration of subserosal connective tissue without tissue invasion of visceral peritoneum or adjacent structures	N3b	Metastasis in ≥16 regional nodes		
T4a	Invasion into serosa				
T4b	Invasion into adjacent structures				
N0	No regional node metastasis				
N1	Metastasis in 1-2 regional nodes				
N2	Metastasis in 3-6 regional nodes				
N3a	Metastasis in 7-15 regional nodes				
N3b	Metastasis in ≥16 regional nodes				

Treatment
- adenocarcinoma
  - proximal lesions
    - total gastrectomy and Roux-en-Y esophagojejunostomy
  - distal lesions
    - distal gastrectomy: wide margins, en bloc removal of omentum and lymph nodes with Roux-en-Y or Billroth II reconstruction
  - palliation
    - limited gastric resection or endoscopic stenting to decrease bleeding and relieve obstruction, enables the patient to eat
    - radiation therapy
  - studies are showing larger role for adjuvant/ neoadjuvant and palliative chemotherapy

- lymphoma
  - *H. pylori* eradication, chemotherapy ± radiation, surgery in limited cases (perforation, bleeding, obstruction)

Gastrointestinal Stromal Tumour

Epidemiology
- most common mesenchymal neoplasm of GI tract
- derived from interstitial cells of Cajal (cells associated with Auerbach's plexus that have autonomous pacemaker function which coordinate peristalsis throughout the GI tract)
- 75-80% associated with tyrosine kinase (c-KIT) mutations
- most common in stomach (50%) and proximal small intestine (25%), but can occur anywhere along GI tract
- typically present with vague abdominal mass, feeling of abdominal fullness, or with secondary symptoms of bleeding and anemia
- often discovered incidentally on CT, laparotomy, or endoscopy

Risk Factors
- Carney's triad: GISTs, paraganglioma, and pulmonary chondroma
- Type IA neurofibromatosis

Investigations
- pre-operative biopsy (endoscopic ultrasound): controversial, but useful for indeterminate lesions
  - not recommended if index of suspicion for GIST is high
  - percutaneous biopsy is NOT recommended due to high friability and risk of peritoneal spread

Treatment
- surgical resection if >2 cm; follow with serial endoscopy if <2 cm and resect if growing or symptomatic
- localized GIST
  - surgical resection with preservation of intact pseudocapsule
  - lymphadenectomy NOT required, as GISTs rarely metastasize to lymph nodes
  - consider adjuvant treatment with imatinib (Gleevec) or high-risk GIST (large, >4 cm with significant mitotic activity)
- advanced disease (i.e. metastases to liver and/or peritoneal cavity)
  - palliative intent chemotherapy with imatinib
  - metastectomy may be considered for liver limited disease

Prognosis
- risk of metastatic potential depends on
  - tumour size (worse if >10 cm)
  - mitotic activity (worse if >5 mitotic figures or 50/hpf)
  - degree of nuclear pleomorphism
  - location: with identical sizes, extra-gastric location has a higher risk of progression than GISTs in the stomach
- metastases to liver, omentum, peritoneum; nodal metastases rare

Bariatric Surgery

- weight reduction surgery for morbid obesity
- indications: BMI ≥40 without illness or BMI ≥35 with 1+ serious comorbidity (e.g. DM, CAD, sleep apnea, severe joint disease)

Surgical Options
- malabsorptive/restrictive
  - laparoscopic Roux-en-Y gastric bypass (most common – see Figure 9)
  - staple off small gastric pouch (restrictive) with Roux-en-Y limb to pouch (malabsorptive) with dumping syndrome physiology
  - most effective, higher complication rates
- restrictive
  - laparoscopic adjustable gastric banding
    - silicone band around fundus creates pouch, adjustable through port under skin
  - laparoscopic vertical sleeve gastrectomy
    - vertical stapled small gastric pouch
- malabsorptive
  - biliopancreatic diversion with duodenal switch
  - gastrectomy, enteroenterostomy, duodenal division closure and duodenoenterostomy

Bariatric (Weight Loss) Surgery for Obesity is Considered when Other Treatments have Failed
Cochrane DB Syst Rev 2009;2:CD003641
Benefits
- Greater weight loss in patients with BMI >30 at 2 yr.
- Reduction in comorbidities (type 2 DM, HTN, and medication use).
- Improvement in quality of life at 2 yr (physical function, physical role, general health, vitality, and emotional role).

Risks
- Complications: leaks, hernias, infection, pulmonary embolism, post-operative mortality.
- Side effects specific to type of procedure (i.e. vomiting, dumping syndrome, food intolerance).
- Cholecystitis occurs as a result of rapid weight loss.

Complications
- perioperative mortality ~1% (anastomotic leak with peritoneal signs, PE)
- obstruction at enteroenterostomy (see *Complications of Gastric Surgery*)
- staple line dehiscence
- dumping syndrome
- cholelithiasis due to rapid weight loss (20-30%)
- band abscess (if long-term)

Complications of Gastric Surgery

- most resolve within 1 yr

Alkaline Reflux Gastritis (see Figure 10A)
- duodenal contents (bilious) reflux into stomach causing gastritis ± esophagitis
- treatment
  - medical: H_2-blocker, metoclopramide, cholestyramine (bile acid sequestrant)
  - surgical: conversion of Billroth I or II to Roux-en-Y

Afferent Loop Syndrome (see Figure 10B)
- accumulation of bile and pancreatic secretions causes intermittent mechanical obstruction and distention of afferent limb
- clinical features
  - early postprandial distention, RUQ pain, nausea, bilious vomiting, anemia
- treatment: surgery (conversion to Roux-en-Y increases afferent loop drainage)

Dumping Syndrome (see Figure 10C)
- early – 15 min post-prandial
  - etiology
    - hyperosmotic chyme released into small bowel (fluid accumulation and jejunal distention)
  - clinical features
    - post-prandial symptoms
    - epigastric fullness or pain, emesis, nausea, diarrhea, palpitations, dizziness, tachycardia, diaphoresis
  - treatment
    - small multiple low carbohydrate, low fat, and high protein meals and avoidance of liquids with meals
    - last resort is interposition of antiperistaltic jejunal loop between stomach and small bowel to delay gastric emptying
- late – 3 h post-prandial
  - etiology: large glucose load leads to large insulin release and hypoglycemia
  - treatment: small snack 2 h after meals

Blind-Loop Syndrome (see Figure 10D)
- bacterial overgrowth of colonic Gram-negative bacteria in afferent limb
- clinical features
  - anemia/weakness, diarrhea, malnutrition, abdominal pain, and hypocalcemia
- treatment: broad-spectrum antibiotics, surgery (conversion to Billroth I)

Postvagotomy Diarrhea (see Figure 10E)
- up to 25%
- bile salts in colon inhibit water resorption
- treatment: medical (cholestyramine), surgical (reversed interposition jejunal segment)

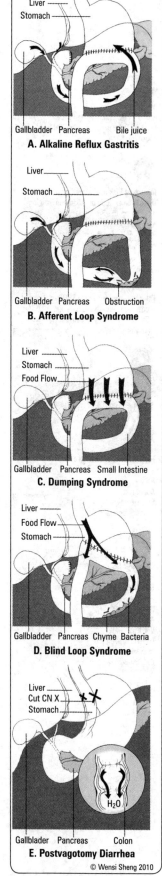

A. Alkaline Reflux Gastritis

B. Afferent Loop Syndrome

C. Dumping Syndrome

D. Blind Loop Syndrome

E. Postvagotomy Diarrhea

© Wensi Sheng 2010

Figure 10. Complications of gastric surgery

SMALL INTESTINE

Small Bowel Obstruction

Mechanical Small Bowel Obstruction

MUST DO
Rule out CRC in constipated patient
Send for TURP in patient with BPH (treat intra-abdominal HTN)

Increased Risk of Perforation with Distention as seen on Abdomen Imaging
- Small bowel ≥3 cm
- Distal colon ≥6 cm
- Proximal colon ≥9 cm
- Cecum ≥12 cm

Patients presenting with a SBO in setting of "virgin" abdomen should have surgery ASAP – EXCEPTION: malignant obstruction from history and imaging

In a non-virgin abdomen – adhesional SBOs resolve spontaneously with NGT decompression 70% of time

Top 3 Causes of SBO (in order)

ABC
Adhesions
Bulge (hernias)
Cancer (neoplasms)

Causes of SBO

SHAVING
Stricture
Hernia
Adhesions
Volvulus
Intussusception/IBD
Neoplasm
Gallstones

Etiology

Table 7. Common Causes of SBO

Intraluminal	Intramural	Extramural
Intussusception	Crohn's	Adhesions from previous surgeries (75% SBO)
Gallstones	Radiation stricture	Incarcerated hernia
Bezoars	Adenocarcinoma	Peritoneal carcinomatosis

Pathophysiology
- obstruction → gas & fluid (swallowed or GI secretions) accumulate proximal to site of obstruction and distal decompression → intestinal activity increases to overcome obstruction → colicky pain and diarrhea (initially)
- bowel wall edema and disruption of normal bowel absorptive function can lead to increased intraluminal fluid and transudative fluid loss into peritoneal cavity, electrolyte disturbances
- increase intramural pressure can lead to impaired microvascular perfusion leading to intestinal ischemia and necrosis (strangulated bowel obstruction)
- **three types**
  - partial SBO: only a portion of intestinal lumen is occluded, allows passage of some gas & fluid, low risk of strangulation
  - complete SBO: the lumen of the intestine is occluded, no passage of gas or stool, at higher risk of strangulation
  - closed-loop obstruction: segment of intestine is obstructed both proximally and distally (e.g. volvulus), leading to rapid rise in intraluminal pressure from gas and fluid that cannot escape, high risk of strangulation due to bowel wall ischemia

Risk Factors
- prior abdominal or pelvic surgery, abdominal wall or groin hernia, history of malignancy, prior radiation

Clinical Features
- 1) distinguish mechanical obstruction from ileus; 2) determine etiology of obstruction; 3) recognize partial from complete SBO; 4) differentiate simple from complicated (e.g. strangulated) obstruction
- **symptoms**: colicky abdominal pain, nausea/vomiting, obstipation
  - vomiting is more prominent with proximal than distal
  - more feculent vomitus suggest more established obstruction because of bacterial overgrowth
  - continue passage of gas and/or stool 6-12 h after onset of symptoms suggest partial than complete obstruction
- **signs**: abdominal distention (most prominent if obstruction at distal ileum), hyperactive proceeding to minimal bowel sound
- strangulated obstruction: abdominal pain disproportionate to physical exam findings suggest intestinal ischemia
  - may have tachycardia, localized abdominal tenderness, fever, marked leukocytosis, lactate acidosis

Investigations
- **radiological**
  - abdominal x-ray (3 views): triad of dilated small bowel (>3 cm in diameter), air-fluid levels on upright film, paucity of air in colon (high sensitivity, low specificity as ileus and LBO can present similarly)
  - CT: discrete transition zone with proximal bowel dilation, distal bowel decompression, and intraluminal contrast does not pass the transition zone
    - most importantly to r/o ischemic bowel/strangulation: pneumatosis intestinalis (free air in bowel wall) & thickened bowel wall, air in portal vein, free intraperitoneal fluids, differential wall enhancements (poor uptake of IV contrast into the wall of the affected bowel)
  - other
    - less used: upper GI series/small bowel series (if no cause apparent, i.e. no hernias, no previous surgeries)
    - may consider U/S or MRI in pregnant patients
- **laboratory**
  - may be normal early in disease course
  - creatinine, hematocrit to assess degree of dehydration
  - fluid, electrolyte abnormalities; metabolic alkalosis due to frequent emesis; amylase elevated
  - if strangulation: leukocytosis with left shift, , elevated lactate (late signs)

Treatment
- IV isotonic fluid resuscitation + urine output monitoring with catheter
  - SBO related vomiting and decrease PO intake leads to volume depletion
- NG tube in the stomach for gastric decompression; decrease nausea, distention, and risk of aspiration from vomiting
- **Partial SBO/Crohn's/Carcinomatosis**: conservative management with fluid resuscitation and NG tube decompression
  - 48 h of watchful waiting; if no improvement or develops complications, surgery
- **Complete SBO**, if no clinical features of strangulation, short course of conservative management with fluid resuscitation and NG tube decompression with frequent re-examination by surgical team
  - duration of observation varies from hours to a few days
  - if SBO fails to resolve, or if symptoms of strangulation develop then surgery

High risk for strangulation based on clinical symptoms: urgent surgery to prevent irreversible ischemia
- early post-operative SBO: if bowel function do not return within 3-5 d after surgery; usually partial, extended conservative therapy (2-3 wk) with bowel rest, fluids, and TPN is appropriate
  - surgery if presence of peritonitis or complete SBO demonstrated

Prognosis
- related to etiology; mortality: non-strangulating <1%, strangulating 8% (25% if >36 h), ischemic = up to 50%

Prevention
- open surgery has four fold increase in risk of SBO in 5 yr compared to laparoscopic surgery

Paralytic Ileus

Pathogenesis
- temporary, reversible impairment of intestinal motility; mostly frequently caused by:
  - abdominal operations, infections & inflammation, medications (opiates, anesthetics, psychotropics), and electrolyte abnormalities
  - passing gas is the most useful indicator
- **NOT** the same as intestinal pseudo-obstruction
  - chronic pseudo-obstruction refers to specific disorders that affect the smooth muscle and myenteric plexus, leading to **irreversible** intestinal dysmotility

Clinical Features
- symptoms and signs of intestinal obstruction without mechanical obstruction
  - bowel sounds are diminished or absent (in contrast to initial hyperactive bowel sounds in SBO)

Investigations
- routine post-operative ileus: expected, no investigation needed
- if ileus persists or occurs without abdominal surgery
  - review patient medications (especially opiates)
  - measure serum electrolyte to monitor for electrolyte abnormalities (including extended lytes like Mg, Ca^{2+}, PO_4)
  - CT scan to rule out abscess or peritoneal sepsis, or to exclude complete mechanical obstruction

Treatment
- most important: NPO + fluid resuscitation
- NGT decompression, correct causative abnormalities (e.g. sepsis, medications, electrolytes), consider TPN for prolonged ileus
- **post-operative**: gastric and small bowel motility returns by 24-48 h, colonic motility by 3-5 d
- current interest in novel therapies such as gum chewing and pharmacologic therapy (e.g. alvimopan, an opioid antagonists)

Intestinal Ischemia

Etiology
- acute
  - arterio-occlusive mesenteric ischemia (AOMI)
    - thrombotic, embolic, extrinsic compression (e.g. strangulating hernia)
  - non-occlusive mesenteric ischemia (NOMI)
    - mesenteric vasoconstriction secondary to systemic hypoperfusion (preserves supply to vital organs)
  - mesenteric venous thrombosis (MVT)
    - consider hypercoagulable state (i.e. rule out malignancy), DVT (prevents venous outflow)
- chronic: usually due to atherosclerotic disease – look for CVD risk factors
- can lead to occlusion in vessels that supplies the small intestine and the large intestine

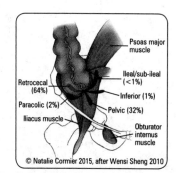

Figure 11. Appendix anatomy

Pain "out of keeping with physical findings" is the hallmark of early intestinal ischemia

An acute abdomen + metabolic acidosis is bowel ischemia until proven otherwise

Clinical Features
- acute: severe abdominal pain out of proportion to physical findings, vomiting, bloody diarrhea, bloating, minimal peritoneal signs early in course, hypotension, shock, sepsis
- chronic: postprandial pain (from mesenteric angina), fear of eating, weight loss
- common sites: SMA supplied territory, "watershed" areas of colon – splenic flexure, left colon, sigmoid colon

Investigations
- laboratory: leukocytosis (non-specific), lactic acidosis (late finding)
  - amylase, lactate, CK, ALP can be used to observe progress
  - hypercoagulability workup if suspect venous thrombosis
- AXR: portal venous gas, intestinal pneumatosis, free air if perforation
- contrast CT: thickened bowel wall, luminal dilatation, SMA or SMV thrombus, mesenteric/portal venous gas, pneumatosis
- CT angiography is the gold standard for acute arterial ischemia

Treatment
- fluid resuscitation, correct metabolic acidosis, NPO, NGT decompression of stomach, prophylactic broad-spectrum antibiotics, avoid vasoconstrictors and digitalis
- exploratory laparotomy
- angiogram, embolectomy/thrombectomy, bypass/graft, mesenteric endarterectomy, anticoagulation therapy, percutaneous transluminal angioplasty ± stent
- segmental resection of necrotic intestine
- assess extent of viability; if extent of bowel viability is uncertain, a second look laparotomy 12-24 h later is mandatory

Tumours of Small Intestine

Carcinoid Syndrome Symptoms

FDR
Flushing
Diarrhea
Right-sided heart failure

BENIGN TUMOURS
- 10x more common than malignant
- usually asymptomatic until large
- most common sites: terminal ileum, proximal jejunum
- polyps
  - adenomas
  - hamartomas
  - FAP (see *Familial Colon Cancer Syndromes*, GS33)
  - juvenile polyps
- other: leiomyomas, lipomas, hemangiomas

Table 8. Malignant Tumours of the Small Intestine

	Adenocarcinoma	Carcinoid	Lymphoma	Metastatic
Epidemiology	Usually 50-70 yr M>F	Increased incidence 50-60 yr	Highest incidence in 70s M>F Usually non-Hodgkin's lymphoma	Most common site of GI metastases in patients with metastatic melanoma
Risk Factors	Crohn's, FAP, history of CRC, HNPCC		Crohn's, celiac disease, autoimmune disease, immunosuppression, radiation therapy, nodular lymphoid hyperplasia	Melanoma, breast, lung, ovary, colon, cervical cancer
Clinical Features	Early metastasis to lymph nodes 80% metastatic at time of operation Abdominal pain (common)	N/V, anemia, GI bleeding, jaundice, weight loss (less common) Often slow-growing Usually asymptomatic, incidental finding Obstruction, bleeding, crampy abdominal pain, intussusception Carcinoid syndrome (<10%) Hot flashes, hypotension, diarrhea, bronchoconstriction, right heart failure Requires liver involvement: lesion secretes serotonin, kinins, and vasoactive peptides directly to systemic circulation (normally inactivated by liver)	Fatigue, weight loss, fever malabsorption, abdominal pain, anorexia, vomiting, constipation, mass Rarely – perforation, obstruction, bleeding, intussusception	Obstruction and bleeding
Investigations	CT abdomen/pelvis Endoscopy	Most found incidentally at surgery for obstruction or appendectomy Chest thorax/abdomen/pelvis Consider small bowel enteroclysis to look for primary Serum chromogranin A as a tumour marker Elevated 5-HIAA (breakdown product of serotonin) in urine or increased 5-HT in blood Radiolabelled octreotide or MIBG scans to search for metastases and locate tumour	CT abdomen/pelvis	CT abdomen/pelvis

Table 8. Malignant Tumours of the Small Intestine (continued)

	Adenocarcinoma	Carcinoid	Lymphoma	Metastatic
Treatment	Surgical resection ± chemotherapy	Surgical resection ± chemotherapy Carcinoid syndrome treated with steroids, histamine, octreotide Metastatic risk 2% if size <1 cm, 90% if >2 cm	Low grade: chemotherapy with cyclophosphamide High grade: surgical resection, radiation Palliative: somatostatin, doxorubicin	Palliation
Prognosis	5 yr survival 25% (if node positive)	5 yr survival 70%; 20% with liver metastases	5 yr survival 40%	Poor
Origin/Location	Usually in proximal small bowel, incidence decreases distally	Classified based on embryological origin (foregut, midgut, hindgut) Originate from gut enterochromaffin cell Appendix 46%, distal ileum 28%, rectum 17%	Usually distal ileum Proximal jejunum in patients with celiac disease	Hematogenous spread from breast, lung, kidney Direct extension from cervix, ovaries, colon
Staging System	TNM	TNM	Ann Arbor	

Short Gut Syndrome

Definition
- reduced surface area (length) of small bowel causing insufficient intestinal absorption leading to diarrhea, malnutrition, and dehydration

Risk Factors
- acute mesenteric ischemia: resection of large amount of bowel at once
- Crohn's disease: cumulative resections
- malignancies

Prognostic Factors
- residual small bowel length, residual colon length (reabsorption of water and electrolytes and some reabsorption of nutrients), condition of the remnant small bowel (healthier bowel facilitate better reabsorption), presence of ileocecal valve (delay transition into colon leading to more reabsorption)
- resection of ileum is less tolerated than resection of jejunum (ileum reabsorbs bile salt and vitamin B12)

Therapy
- medical
  - TPN: replenish lost fluid and electrolytes in diarrhea
  - HT2R antagonist or PPI to prevent gastric acid secretion
  - antimotility agent to prolong transit time in the small intestine
  - consider octreotide to decrease GI secretion & cholestyramine for bile acid absorption
- surgical: non-transplant
  - to slow transit time: small bowel segmental reversal, intestinal valve construction, or electrical pacing of small bowel
  - to increase intestinal length:
    - LILT (longitudinal intestinal lengthening and tailoring) procedure
    - STEP (serial transverse enteroplasty procedure) in dilated small bowels
- surgical: transplant
  - indication: life-threatening complication from intestinal failure or long-term TPN
    - liver failure, thrombosis of major central veins, recurrent catheter-related sepsis, recurrent severe dehydration

Abdominal Hernia

- see *Hiatus Hernia*, GS13

Definition
- defect in abdominal wall causing abnormal protrusion of intra-abdominal contents

Epidemiology
- M:F = 9:1
- lifetime risk of developing a hernia: males 20-25%, females 2%
- frequency of occurrence: 50% indirect inguinal, 25% direct inguinal, 8-10% incisional (ventral), 5% femoral, 3-8% umbilical
- most common surgical disease of males

Risk Factors
- activities which increase intra-abdominal pressure
  - obesity, chronic cough, asthma, COPD, pregnancy, constipation, bladder outlet obstruction, ascites, heavy lifting
- congenital abnormality (e.g. patent processus vaginalis, indirect inguinal hernia)
- previous hernia repair, especially if complicated by wound infection
- loss of tissue strength and elasticity (e.g. hiatus hernia, aging, repetitive stress)

Indirect Inguinal Hernias: Rule of 5s
5% lifetime incidence in males
5x more common than direct inguinal hernias
5-10x more common in males than females
Generally occur by 5th decade of life

Inguinal Hernias – MD's don't LIe
MD: Medial to the inferior epigastric a. = **D**irect inguinal hernia
LI: Lateral to the inferior epigastric a. = **I**ndirect inguinal hernia

Inguinal Canal Walls = MALT x 2
2M Roof	2 muscles (internal oblique, transversus abdominis)
2A Ant. wall	2 aponeuroses (external and internal oblique)
2L Floor	2 ligaments (inguinal and lacunar)
2 Ts Post. wall	2T (transversalis fascia, conjoint tendon)

Borders of Hesselbach's Triangle
- Lateral: inferior epigastric artery
- Inferior: inguinal ligament
- Medial: lateral margin of rectus sheath

Abdominal Hernia

Shouldice Technique vs. Other Open Techniques for Inguinal Hernia Repair
Cochrane DB Syst Rev 2012;4:CD001543
Purpose: To evaluate the efficacy and safety of the Shouldice technique to other non-laparoscopic techniques.
Results/Conclusions: 16 RCTs or quasi-randomized RCTs with 2,566 hernias (1,121 mesh; 1,608 non-mesh). The recurrence rate with Shouldice was higher than mesh (OR 3.80, 95% CI 1.99-7.26) but lower than non-mesh (OR 0.62, 95% CI 0.45-0.85). There was no difference in chronic pain or complications. In conclusion, with respect to recurrence rates, Shouldice herniorrhaphy is the best non-mesh technique, although inferior to mesh. However, it is also more time consuming and results in slightly longer post-operative hospital stays.

Watchful Waiting vs. Repair of Inguinal Hernia in Minimally Symptomatic Men: A Randomized Clinical Trial
JAMA 2006;295:285-292
Purpose: To compare pain and the physical component score (PCS) of the Short Form-36 Version 2 survey at 2 yr in men with minimally symptomatic inguinal hernias treated with watchful waiting or surgical repair.
Methods: RCT of 720 men (n=364 watchful waiting, n=356 surgical repair) followed up for 2-4.5 yr. Watchful-waiting patients were followed up at 6 mo and annually and watched for hernia symptoms; repair patients received standard open tension-free repair and were followed up at 3 and 6 mo and annually. The main outcome was pain and discomfort interfering with usual activities at 2 yr and change in PCS from baseline to 2 yr. Secondary outcomes were complications, patient-reported pain, functional status, activity levels, and satisfaction with care.
Results: Primary intention-to-treat outcomes were similar at 2 yr for watchful waiting vs. surgical repair: pain limiting activities (5.1% vs. 2.2%, respectively; p=0.06 [corrected]); PCS (improvement over baseline, 0.29 points vs. 0.13 points; p=0.79). Twenty-three percent of patients assigned to watchful waiting crossed over to receive surgical repair (increase in hernia-related pain was the most common reason offered); 17% assigned to receive repair crossed over to watchful waiting. Self-reported pain in watchful-waiting patients crossing over improved after repair. Occurrence of post-operative hernia-related complications was similar in patients who received repair as assigned and in watchful-waiting patients who crossed over. One watchful-waiting patient (0.3%) experienced acute hernia incarceration without strangulation within 2 yr; a second had acute incarceration with bowel obstruction at 4 yr, with a frequency of 1.8/1,000 patient/yr inclusive of patients followed up for as long as 4.5 yr.
Conclusion: Watchful waiting is an acceptable option for men with minimally symptomatic inguinal hernias. Delaying surgical repair until symptoms increase is safe because acute hernia incarcerations occur rarely.

Outcomes of Laparoscopic vs. Open Repair of Primary Ventral Hernias
JAMA Surg 2013;148:1043-1048
Purpose: To compare outcomes (surgical site infection (SSI), hernia recurrence and bulging) of patients undergoing laparoscopic ventral hernia repair (LVHR) versus open ventral hernia repair (OVHR).
Results/Conclusions: 79 patients with LVHR matched to 79 patients with OVHR with mesh with a median follow-up of 56 mo. LVHR was associated with fewer SSIs (7.6% vs. 34.1%) but more cases of bulging (21.5% vs. 1.3%) and port-site hernia (2.5% vs. 0.0%). No differences in recurrence were observed.

Clinical Features
- mass of variable size
- tenderness worse at end of day, relieved with supine position or with reduction
- abdominal fullness, vomiting, constipation
- transmits palpable impulse with coughing or straining

Investigations
- physical examination usually sufficient
- U/S ± CT (CT required for obturator hernias, internal abdominal hernias, and Spigelian and/or femoral hernias in obese patients)

Classification
- complete: hernia sac and contents protrude through defect
- incomplete: partial protrusion through the defect
- internal hernia: sac herniating into or involving intra-abdominal structure
- external hernia: sac protrudes completely through abdominal wall
- strangulated hernia: vascular supply of protruded viscus is compromised (ischemia)
  - requires **emergency** repair
- incarcerated hernia: irreducible hernia, not necessarily strangulated
- Richter's hernia: only part of bowel circumference (usually anti-mesenteric border) is incarcerated or strangulated so may not be obstructed
  - a strangulated Richter's hernia may self-reduce and thus be overlooked, leaving a gangrenous segment at risk of perforation in the absence of obstructive symptoms
- sliding hernia: part of wall of hernia sac formed by retroperitoneal structure (usually colon)

Anatomical Types
- groin
  - indirect and direct inguinal, femoral
  - pantaloon: combined direct and indirect hernias, peritoneum draped over inferior epigastric vessels
- epigastric: defect in linea alba above umbilicus
- incisional: ventral hernia at site of wound closure, may be secondary to wound infection
- other: Littre's (involving Meckel's), Amyand's (containing appendix), lumbar, obturator, peristomal, umbilical, Spigelian (ventral hernia through linea semilunaris)

Complications
- incarceration
- strangulation
  - small, new hernias more likely to strangulate
  - femoral >> indirect inguinal > direct inguinal
  - intense pain followed by tenderness
  - intestinal obstruction, gangrenous bowel, sepsis
  - surgical emergency
  - **DO NOT** attempt to manually reduce hernia if septic or if contents of hernial sac gangrenous
  - will cause closed loop SBO – and EMERGENCY

Treatment
- surgical treatment (herniorrhaphy) is only to prevent strangulation and evisceration, for symptomatic relief, for cosmesis; if asymptomatic can delay surgery
- repair may be done open or laparoscopic and may use mesh for tension-free closure
- most repairs are now done using tension free techniques – a plug in the hernial defect and a patch over it or patch alone
- observation is acceptable for small asymptomatic inguinal hernias

Post-Operative Complications
- recurrence (15-20%)
  - risk factors: recurrent hernia, age >50, smoking, BMI >25, poor pre-operative functional status (ASA ≥3 – see Anesthesia and Perioperative Medicine, A4), associated medical conditions: type 2 DM, hyperlipidemia, immunosuppression, any comorbid conditions increasing intra-abdominal pressure
  - less common with mesh/"tension-free" repair
- scrotal hematoma (3%)
  - painful scrotal swelling from compromised venous return of testes
  - deep bleeding: may enter retroperitoneal space and not be initially apparent
  - difficulty voiding
- nerve entrapment
  - ilioinguinal (causes numbness of inner thigh or lateral scrotum)
  - genital branch of genitofemoral (in spermatic cord)
- stenosis/occlusion of femoral vein
  - acute leg swelling
- ischemic colitis

Groin Hernias

Table 9. Groin Hernias

	Direct Inguinal	Indirect Inguinal	Femoral
Epidemiology	1% of all men	Most common hernia in men and women M>F	Affects mostly females
Etiology	Acquired weakness of transversalis fascia "Wear and tear" Increased intra-abdominal pressure	Congenital persistence of processus vaginalis in 20% of adults	Pregnancy – weakness of pelvic floor musculature Increased intra-abdominal pressure
Anatomy	Through Hesselbach's triangle **Medial** to inferior epigastric artery Usually does not descend into scrotal sac	Originates in deep inguinal ring Lateral to inferior epigastric artery Often descends into scrotal sac (or labia majora)	Into femoral canal, below inguinal ligament but may override it Medial to femoral vein within femoral canal
Treatment	Surgical repair	Surgical repair	Surgical repair
Prognosis	3-4% risk of recurrence	<1% risk of recurrence	

Table 10. Superficial Inguinal Ring vs. Deep Inguinal Ring*

Superficial Inguinal Ring	Deep Inguinal Ring
Opening in external abdominal aponeurosis; palpable superior and lateral to pubic tubercle	Opening in transversalis fascia: palpable superior to mid-inguinal ligament
Medial border: medial crus of external abdominal aponeurosis	Medial border: inferior epigastric vessels
Lateral border: lateral crus of external oblique aponeurosis	Superior-lateral border: internal oblique and transversus abdominis muscles
Roof: intercrural fibres	Inferior border: inguinal ligament

*see *Basic Anatomy Review*, Figure 2, GS3

Appendix

Appendicitis

Epidemiology
- 6% of population, M>F
- 80% between 5-35 yr of age

Pathogenesis
- luminal obstruction → bacterial overgrowth → inflammation/swelling → increased pressure → localized ischemia → gangrene/perforation → localized abscess (walled off by omentum) or peritonitis
- etiology
  - children or young adult: hyperplasia of lymphoid follicles, initiated by infection
  - adult: fibrosis/stricture, fecolith, obstructing neoplasm
  - other causes: parasites, foreign body

Clinical Features
- most reliable feature is progression of signs and symptoms
- low grade fever (38°C), rises if perforation
- abdominal pain then anorexia, N/V
- classic pattern: pain initially periumbilical; constant, dull, poorly localized, then well localized pain over McBurney's point
  - due to progression of disease from visceral irritation (causing referred pain from structures of the embryonic midgut, including the appendix) to irritation of parietal structures
  - McBurney's sign
- signs
  - inferior appendix: McBurney's sign (see sidebar), Rovsing's sign (palpation pressure to left abdomen causes McBurney's point tenderness). McBurney's sign is present whenever the opening of the appendix at the cecum is directly under McBurney's point; therefore McBurney's sign is present even when the appendix is in different locations
  - retrocecal appendix: psoas sign (pain on flexion of hip against resistance or passive hyperextension of hip)
  - pelvic appendix: obturator sign (flexion then external or internal rotation about right hip causes pain)
- complications
  - perforation (especially if >24 h duration)
  - abscess, phlegmon
  - sepsis

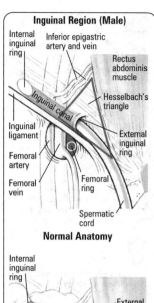

Inguinal Region (Male)

Normal Anatomy

Indirect Hernia

Direct Hernia

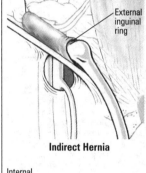
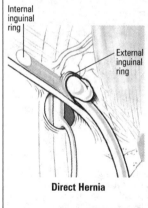
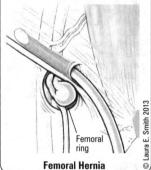

Femoral Hernia

© Laura E. Smith 2013

Figure 12. Schematic of inguinal (direct and indirect) and femoral hernias

McBurney's Sign
Tenderness 1/3 the distance from the ASIS to the umbilicus on the right side

Laparoscopic vs. Open Appendectomy
Cochrane DB Syst Rev 2010;10:CD001546
Laparoscopic Surgery
- Wound infection less likely
- Intra-abdominal abscesses 2x more likely
- Reduced pain on POD #1
- Reduced hospital stay by 1.1 d
- Sooner return to normal activity, work, and sport
- Costs outside hospital are reduced
Open Surgery
- Shorter duration of surgery
- Lower operation costs
Overview
Diagnostic laparoscopy and laparoscopic appendectomy appear to be advantageous over open appendectomy, particularly for young female patients and obese patients.

Effect of Delay to Operation on Outcomes in Adults with Acute Appendicitis
Arch Surg 2010;145:886-892
Purpose: To examine the effect of delay to appendectomy on morbidity and mortality among adults with appendicitis.
Method: Retrospective cohort study with the main exposure being time to operation, and main outcomes being 30 d overall morbidity and serious morbidity/mortality.
Results: Of 32,782 patients in the study, 75.2%, 15.1%, and 9.8% underwent surgeries within 6 h, 6-12 h, and >12 h of admission, respectively. Differences in operative duration and length of post-operative stay were statistically significant but not clinically meaningful. No significant differences were observed in adjusted overall morbidity or serious morbidity/mortality. Duration from surgical admission to anesthesia induction was not predictive in regression models for either outcomes.
Conclusions: Delay of appendectomy for acute appendicitis among adults does not adversely affect outcomes.

Antibiotics vs. Placebo for Prevention of Post-Operative Infection After Appendectomy
Cochrane DB Syst Rev 2005;3:CD001439
Purpose: To determine the effectiveness of antibiotics against post-operative infections after appendectomy.
Method: Meta-analysis of randomized controlled trials (RCTs) and controlled clinical trials (CCTs), on both adults and children, in which any antibiotic regime was compared to placebo in patients undergoing appendectomy for suspected appendicitis. The main outcomes of interest were wound infection, intra-abdominal abscess, length of hospital stay, and mortality.
Results: 45 studies (n=9,576) were included. Treatment with antibiotics decreased wound infection and abscess rates.
Conclusion: Various prophylactic antibiotic regimens are effective in preventing post-operative complications after appendectomy.

Crohn's 3 Major Patterns
- Ileocecal 40% (RLQ pain, fever, weight loss)
- Small intestine 30% (especially terminal ileum)
- Colon 25% (diarrhea)

Investigations
- laboratory
  - mild leukocytosis with left shift (may have normal WBC counts)
  - higher leukocyte count with perforation
  - β-hCG to rule out ectopic pregnancy
  - urinalysis
- imaging
  - U/S: may visualize appendix, but also helps rule out gynecological causes – overall accuracy 90-94%, can rule in but CANNOT rule out appendicitis (if >6 mm, SENS/SPEC/NPV/PPV 98%)
  - =CT scan: thick wall, appendicolith, inflammatory changes – overall accuracy 94-100%, optimal investigation

Treatment
- hydrate, correct electrolyte abnormalities
- appendectomy (gold standard)
  - laparoscopic vs. open (see sidebar)
  - complications: intra-abdominal abscess, appendiceal stump leak
  - perioperative antibiotics:
    - cefazolin + metronidazole if uncomplicated peri-operative dose is adequate
    - consider treatment with post-operative antibiotics for perforated appendicitis
- for patients who present with an abscess (palpable mass or phlegmon on imaging and often delayed diagnosis with symptoms for >4-5 d), consider radiologic drainage + antibiotics x 14 d ± interval appendectomy once inflammation has resolved =(controversial)
- recent research supports antibiotic only treatment as reasonable for uncomplicated appendicitis, with 10-20% recurrence rates
- colonoscopy in the elderly to rule out other etiology (neoplasm)

Prognosis
- mortality rate: 0.08% (non-perforated), 0.5% (perforated appendicitis)

Inflammatory Bowel Disease

- see Gastroenterology, G19

Principles of Surgical Management
- can alleviate symptoms, address complications, improve quality of life
- conserve bowel: resect as little as possible to avoid short gut syndrome
- perioperative management
  - optimize medical status: may require TPN (especially if >7 d NPO) and bowel rest
  - hold immunosuppressive therapy pre-operative, provide pre-operative stress dose of corticosteroid if patient had recent steroid therapy, taper steroids post-operative
  - VTE prophylaxis: LMWH or heparin (IBD patients at increased risk of thromboembolic events)

Crohn's Disease

- see Gastroenterology, G20

Treatment
- surgery is for symptom management, it is NOT curative, but over lifetime ~70% of Crohn's patients will have surgery
- indications for surgical management
  - failure of medical management
  - SBO (due to stricture/inflammation): indication in 50% of surgical cases
  - abscess, fistula (enterocolic, vesicular, vaginal, cutaneous abscess), quality of life, perforation, hemorrhage, chronic disability, failure to thrive (children), perianal disease
- surgical procedures
  - resection and anastomosis/stoma if active or subacute inflammation, perforation, fistula
    - resection margin only has to be free of gross disease (microscopic disease irrelevant to prognosis)
  - stricturoplasty – widens lumen in chronically scarred bowel: relieves obstruction without resecting bowel (contraindicated in acute inflammation)

Complications of Treatment
- short gut syndrome (diarrhea, steatorrhea, malnutrition)
- fistulas
- gallstones (if terminal ileum resected, decreased bile salt resorption → increased cholesterol precipitation)
- kidney stones (loss of calcium in diarrhea → increased oxalate absorption and hyperoxaluria → stones)

Prognosis
- recurrence rate at 10 yr: ileocolic (25-50%), small bowel (50%), colonic (40-50%)
- re-operation at 5 yr: primary resection (20%), bypass (50%), stricturoplasty (10% at 1 yr)
- 80-85% of patients who need surgery lead normal lives
- mortality: 15% at 30 yr

Findings in Crohn's
- "Cobblestoning" on mucosal surface due to edema and linear ulcerations
- "Skip lesions": normal mucosa in between
- "Creeping fat": mesentery infiltrated by fat
- Granulomas: 25-30%

Ulcerative Colitis

- see Gastroenterology, G21

Treatment
- indications for surgical management
  - failure of medical management (including inability to taper steroids)
  - complications: hemorrhage, obstruction, perforation, toxic megacolon (emergency), failure to thrive (children)
  - reduce cancer risk (1-2% risk per yr after 10 yr of disease)
- surgical procedures
  - proctocolectomy and ileal pouch-anal anastomosis (IPAA) ± rectal mucosectomy (operation of choice)
  - proctocolectomy with permanent end ileostomy (if not a candidate for ileoanal procedures)
  - colectomy and IPAA ± rectal mucosectomy
  - in emergency: total colectomy and ileostomy with Hartmann closure of the rectum, rectal preservation

Complications of Treatment
- early: bowel obstruction, transient urinary dysfunction, dehydration (high stoma output), anastomotic leak
- late: stricture, anal fistula/abscess, pouchitis, poor anorectal function, reduced fertility

Findings in Ulcerative Colitis
- Patients usually present with diarrhea (± blood in their stool)
- Associated symptoms include colicky abdominal pain, urgency, tenesmus, and incontinence
- Presence of extra-intestinal manifestations
- Endoscopically, there is loss of vascular markings, erythema, granularity of mucosa, petechiae, exudates, edema, erosions, and spontaneous bleeding
- Biopsy features included crypt abscesses, crypt branching, shortening and disarray, and crypt atrophy
- Inflammation is continuous and usually involves rectum

Prognosis
- mortality: 5% over 10 yr
- total proctocolectomy will eliminate risk of cancer
- perforation of the colon is the leading cause of death from ulcerative colitis

LARGE INTESTINE

Large Bowel Obstruction

Mechanical Large Bowel Obstruction

Etiology

Table 11. Common Causes of LBO

Intraluminal	Intramural	Extramural
Constipation	Adenocarcinoma	Volvulus
Foreign bodies	Diverticulitis	Adhesions
	IBD stricture	Hernias (sigmoid colon in a large groin hernia)
	Radiation stricture	

Top 3 Causes of LBO (in order)
- Cancer
- Diverticulitis
- Volvulus

Clinical Features (unique to LBO)
- open loop (10-20%)
  - incompetent ileocecal valve allows relief of colonic pressure as contents reflux into ileum, therefore clinical presentation similar to SBO
- closed loop (80-90%) (dangerous)
  - competent ileocecal valve, resulting in proximal and distal occlusions
  - massive colonic distention → increased pressure in cecum → bowel wall ischemia → necrosis → perforation

In a patient with clinical LBO consider impending perforation when:
- Cecum ≥12 cm in diameter
- Tenderness present over cecum

Treatment
- surgical correction of obstruction (usually requires resection + temporary diverting colostomy)
- volvulus requires sigmoidoscopic or endoscopic decompression followed by operative reduction if unsuccessful
  - if successful, consider interval sigmoid resection on same admission
- cecal volvulus can be a true volvulus or a cecal 'bascule' (cecum folds anteriorly to the ascending colon producing a flap valve occlusion to cecal emptying) – both need surgical treatment

Prognosis
- overall mortality: 10%
- cecal perforation + feculent peritonitis: 20% mortality

Table 12. Bowel Obstruction vs. Paralytic Ileus

	SBO	LBO	Paralytic Ileus
N/V	Early, may be bilious	Late, may be feculent	Present
Abdominal Pain	Colicky	Colicky	Minimal or absent
Abdominal Distention	+ (prox SBO), ++ (distal SBO)	++	+
Constipation	+	+	+
Bowel Sounds	Normal, increased Absent if secondary ileus (delayed presentation)	Normal, increased (borborygmi) Absent if secondary ileus (delayed presentation)	Decreased, absent
AXR Findings	Air-fluid levels "Ladder" pattern (plicae circularis) Proximal distention (>3 cm) + no colonic gas	Air-fluid levels "Picture frame" appearance Proximal distention + distal decompression No small bowel air if competent ileocecal valve Coffee bean sign (sigmoid volvulus)	Air throughout small bowel and colon

Functional LBO: Colonic Pseudo-Obstruction (Ogilvie's Syndrome)

Definition
- acute pseudo-obstruction
- distention of colon without mechanical obstruction in distal colon
- exact mechanism unknown, likely autonomic motor dysregulation → possibly sympathetic deprivation to colon, unopposed parasympathetic tone, and interruption of sacral parasympathetic tone to distal bowel

Associations
- most common: trauma, infection, cardiac (MI, CHF)
- disability (long-term debilitation, chronic disease, bed-bound nursing home patients, paraplegia), drugs (narcotic use, laxative abuse, polypharmacy), other (recent orthopedic or neurosurgery, post-partum, electrolyte abnormalities including hypokalemia, retroperitoneal hematoma, diffuse carcinomatosis)

Clinical Features
- most prominent is abdominal distention (acute or graduate over 3-7 days)
- abdominal pain, nausea and vomiting, constipation/diarrhea
- watch out for fever, leukocytosis, and presence of peritoneal signs

Investigations
- AXR: cecal dilatation – if diameter ≥12 cm, increased risk of perforation

Treatment
- treat underlying cause
- NPO, NGT
- decompression: rectal tube, colonoscopy, neostigmine (cholinergic drug), surgical decompression (ostomy/resection) uncommon
- surgery (extremely rare): if perforation, ischemia, or failure of conservative management

Prognosis
- most resolve with conservative management

Diverticular Disease

Definitions
- diverticulum: abnormal sac-like protrusion from the wall of a hollow organ
- diverticulosis: presence of multiple diverticula
- diverticulitis: inflammation of diverticula
- true (congenital) diverticuli: contain all layers of colonic wall, often right-sided
- false (acquired) diverticuli: contain mucosa and submucosa, often left-sided

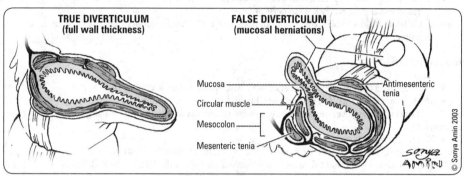

TRUE DIVERTICULUM
(full wall thickness)

FALSE DIVERTICULUM
(mucosal herniations)

Mucosa
Circular muscle
Mesocolon
Mesenteric tenia
Antimesenteric tenia

Figure 13. Diverticular disease – cross-sections of true and false diverticuli

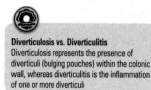

Diverticulosis vs. Diverticulitis
Diverticulosis represents the presence of diverticuli (bulging pouches) within the colonic wall, whereas diverticulitis is the inflammation of one or more diverticuli

Diverticulosis

Epidemiology
- 5-50% of Western population, lower incidence in non-Western countries, M=F
- prevalence is age dependent: <5% by age 40, 30% by age 60, 65% by age 85
- 95% involve sigmoid colon (site of highest pressure)

Pathogenesis
- risk factors
  - lifestyle: low-fibre diet (predispose to motility abnormalities and higher intraluminal pressure), inactivity, obesity
  - muscle wall weakness from aging and illness (e.g. Ehler-Danlos, Marfan's)
- high intraluminal pressures cause outpouching to occur at point of greatest weakness, most commonly where vasa recta penetrate the circular muscle layer, therefore increased risk of hemorrhage

Clinical Features
- uncomplicated diverticulosis: asymptomatic (70-80%)
- episodic abdominal pain (often LLQ), bloating, flatulence, constipation, diarrhea
- absence of fever/leukocytosis
- no physical exam findings or poorly localized LLQ tenderness
- complications
  - diverticulitis (15-25%): 25% of which are complicated (i.e. abscess, obstruction, perforation, fistula)
  - bleeding (5-15%): PAINLESS rectal bleeding, 30-50% of massive LGIB
  - diverticular colitis (rare): diarrhea, hematochezia, tenesmus, abdominal pain

Treatment
- uncomplicated diverticulosis: high fibre, education
- diverticular bleed
  - initially workup and treat as any LGIB
  - if hemorrhage does not stop, resect involved region

Diverticulitis

Epidemiology
- 95% left-sided in patients of Western countries, 75% right-sided in Asian populations

Pathogenesis
- erosion of the wall by increased intraluminal pressure or inspissated food particles → inflammation and focal necrosis → micro or macroscopic perforation
- usually mild inflammation with perforation walled off by pericolic fat and mesentery; abscess, fistula, or obstruction can ensue
- poor containment results in free perforation and peritonitis

Clinical Features

- depend on severity of inflammation and whether or not complications are present; hence ranges from asymptomatic to generalized peritonitis
- LLQ pain/tenderness (2/3 of patients) often for several days before admission
- constipation, diarrhea, N/V, urinary symptoms (with adjacent inflammation)
- complications (25% of cases)
    - abscess: palpable tender abdominal mass
    - fistula: colovesical (most common), coloenteric, colovaginal, colocutaneous
    - colonic obstruction: due to scarring from repeated inflammation
    - perforation: generalized peritonitis (feculent vs. purulent)
        - recurrent attacks rarely lead to peritonitis
- low-grade fever, mild leukocytosis common, occult or gross blood in stool rarely coexist with acute diverticulitis

Investigations

- AXR, upright CXR
    - localized diverticulitis (ileus, thickened wall, SBO, partial colonic obstruction)
    - free air may be seen in 30% with perforation and generalized peritonitis
- CT scan (test of choice): very useful for assessment of severity and prognosis; usually done with rectal contrast
    - 97% sensitive, 99% specific
    - increased soft tissue density within pericolic fat secondary to inflammation, diverticula secondary to inflammation, bowel wall thickening, soft tissue mass (pericolic fluid, abscesses), fistula
    - 10% of diverticulitis cannot be distinguished from carcinoma
- elective evaluation: establish extent of disease and rule out other diagnoses (polyps, malignancy) AFTER resolution of acute episode
    - colonoscopy or barium enema and flexible sigmoidoscopy

Treatment

- uncomplicated: conservative management
- outpatient: clear fluids only until improvement and antibiotics (e.g. cefazolin and metronidazole) 7-10 d to cover gram negative rods and anaerobes (e.g. *B. fragilis*)
- hospitalize: if severe presentation, inability to tolerate oral intake, significant comorbidities, fail to improve outpatient management
- treat with NPO, IVF, IV antibiotics (e.g. IV ceftriaxone + metronidazole)
- indications for surgery
    - unstable patient with peritonitis
    - Hinchey stage 3-4
    - after 1 attack if immunosuppressed
    - consider if recurrent episodes of diverticulitis (3 or more), recent trend is toward conservative management of recurrent mild/moderate attacks
    - complications: perforation, abscess, fistula, obstruction, hemorrhage, inability to rule out colon cancer on endoscopy, or failure of medical management
- surgical procedures
    - for unstable patient or complex cases: Hartmann procedure
        - colon resection + colostomy and rectal stump → colostomy reversal in 3-6 mo
    - for more stable patients with Hinchey stage III and IV acute diverticulitis, colonic resection, primary anastomosis + diverting loop ileostomy is becoming more common, with benefits for mortality and morbidity
    - laparoscopic peritoneal lavage with drain placement near the affected colon, in addition to IV antibiotics (NO resection) has been proposed for Hinchey stage III

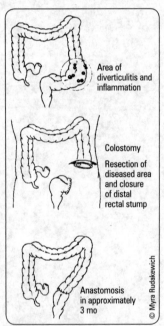

Area of diverticulitis and inflammation

Colostomy

Resection of diseased area and closure of distal rectal stump

Anastomosis in approximately 3 mo

© Myra Rudakewich

Figure 14. Hartmann procedure

Prognosis

- mortality rates: 6% for purulent peritonitis, 35% for feculent peritonitis
- recurrence rates: 13-30% after first attack, 30-50% after second attack

Table 13. Hinchey Staging and Treatment for Diverticulitis

Hinchey Stage	Description	Acute Treatment
1	Phlegmon/small pericolic abscess	Medical
2	Large abscess/fistula	Medical, abscess drainage ± resection with primary anastomosis
3	Purulent peritonitis (ruptured abscess)	Resection or Hartmann procedure
4	Feculent peritonitis	Hartmann procedure

Colorectal Neoplasms

Colorectal Polyps

Definition
- polyp: protuberance into the lumen of normally flat colonic mucosa
- sessile (flat) or pedunculated (on a stalk)

Epidemiology
- 30% of the population have polyps by age 50, 40% by age 60, 50% by age 70

Clinical Features
- 50% in the rectosigmoid region, 50% are multiple
- usually asymptomatic, do not typically bleed, tenesmus, intestinal obstruction, mucus
- usually detected during routine endoscopy or familial/high risk screening

Pathology
- non-neoplastic
  - hyperplastic: most common non-neoplastic polyp
  - mucosal polyps: small <5 mm, no clinical significance
  - inflammatory pseudopolyps: associated with IBD, no malignant potential
  - submucosal polyps: lymphoid aggregates, lipomas, leiomyomas, carcinoids
- neoplastic
  - lipomas, leiomyomas, carcinoids
  - hamartomas: juvenile polyps (large bowel), Peutz-Jegher syndrome (small bowel)
    - malignant risk due to associated adenomas (large bowel)
    - low malignant potential → most spontaneously regress or autoamputate
  - adenomas: premalignant, considered carcinoma in situ IF high grade dysplasia
  - some may contain invasive carcinoma ("malignant polyp" – 3-9%): invasion into submucosa
    - malignant potential: villous > tubulovillous > tubular

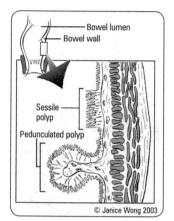

Figure 15. Sessile and pedunculated polyps

Table 14. Characteristics of Tubular vs. Villous Polyps

	Tubular	Villous
Incidence	Common (60-80%)	Less common (10%)
Size	Small (<2 cm)	Large (usually >2 cm)
Attachment	Pedunculated	Sessile
Malignant Potential	Lower	Higher
Distribution	Even	Left-sided predominance

Investigations
- colonoscopy is the gold standard for diagnosis and treatment of colonic polyps
- CT colonography: increasing in availability; patients still require bowel prep and will require colonoscopy if polyps are identified
- other: flexible sigmoidoscopy if polyps are detected, proceed to colonoscopy for examination of entire bowel and biopsy

Treatment
- indications: symptoms, malignancy or risk of malignancy (i.e. adenomatous polyps)
- endoscopic removal of entire growth
- indications for segmental resection for malignant polyps: 1) lymphovascular invasion; 2) tumour budding; 3) positive resection margin; 4) poorly differentiated cells; 5) evidence of regional or distant metastases on staging. Most of these cases are usually discussed at multi-disciplinary tumour boards
- follow-up endoscopy 1 yr later, then every 3-5 yr

Familial Colon Cancer Syndromes

FAMILIAL ADENOMATOUS POLYPOSIS

Pathogenesis
- autosomal dominant inheritance, mutation in adenomatous polyposis coli (APC) gene on chromosome 5q21

Clinical Features
- hundreds to thousands of colorectal adenomas usually by age 20 (by 40s in attenuated FAP)
- extracolonic manifestations
  - carcinoma of small bowel (i.e. polyps in colon), bile duct, pancreas, stomach, thyroid, adrenal, small bowel
  - congenital hypertrophy of retinal pigment epithelium presents early in life in 2/3 of patients; 97% sensitivity
  - virtually 100% lifetime risk of colon cancer (because of number of polyps)
- variants
  - Gardner's syndrome: FAP + extra-intestinal lesions (sebaceous cysts, osteomas, desmoid tumours)
  - Turcot syndrome: FAP + CNS tumours (childhood cerebellar medulloblastoma)

Investigations
- genetic testing (80-95% sensitive, 99-100% specific)
- if no polyposis found: annual flexible sigmoidoscopy from puberty to age 50, then routine screening
- if polyposis or APC gene mutation found: annual colonoscopy and consider surgery (see Figure 14); consider upper endoscopy to evaluate for periampullary tumours

Treatment
- surgery indicated by age 17-20
- total proctocolectomy with ileostomy or total colectomy with ileorectal anastomosis
- doxorubicin-based chemotherapy
- NSAIDs for intra-abdominal desmoids

HEREDITARY NON-POLYPOSIS COLORECTAL CANCER – LYNCH SYNDROME

Pathogenesis
- autosomal dominant inheritance, mutation in a DNA mismatch repair gene (MSH2, MSH6, MLH1) resulting in microsatellite genomic instability and subsequent mutations
- microsatellite instability account for approximately 15% of all colorectal cancers

Clinical Features
- early age of onset, right > left colon, synchronous and metachronous lesions
- mean age of cancer presentation is 44 yr, lifetime risk 70-80% (M>F)
  - HNPCC I: hereditary site-specific colon cancer
  - HNPCC II: cancer family syndrome – high rates of extracolonic tumours (endometrial, ovarian, hepatobiliary, small bowel)

Diagnosis
- Amsterdam Criteria
  - 3 or more relatives with verified Lynch syndrome associated cancers, and 1 must be 1st degree relative of the other 2
  - 2 or more generations involved
  - 1 case must be diagnosed before 50 yr old
  - FAP is excluded
- genetic testing (80% sensitive) – colonoscopy mandatory even if negative
  - refer for genetic screening individuals who fulfill EITHER the Amsterdam Criteria OR the revised Bethesda Criteria
- colonoscopy (starting age 20) annually
- surveillance for extracolonic lesions

Treatment
- total colectomy and ileorectal anastomosis with annual proctoscopy

Colorectal Carcinoma

Epidemiology
- 4th most common cancer (after lung, prostate, and breast), 2nd most common cause of cancer death

Risk Factors
- most patients have no specific risk factors
- age >50 (dominant risk factor in sporadic cases), mean age is 70
- genetic: FAP, HNPCC, family history of CRC
- colonic conditions
  - adenomatous polyps (especially if >1 cm, villous, multiple)
  - IBD (especially UC: risk is 1-2%/yr if UC >10 yr)
  - previous colorectal cancer (also gonadal or breast)
- diet (increased fat, red meat, decreased fibre) and smoking
- DM and acromegaly (insulin and IGF-1 are growth factors for colonic mucosal cells)

Referral Criteria for Genetic Screening for APC
- To confirm the diagnosis of FAP (in patients with ≥100 colorectal adenomas)
- To provide pre-symptomatic testing for individuals at risk for FAP (1st degree relatives who are ≥10 yr old)
- To confirm the diagnosis of attenuated FAP (in patients with ≥20 colorectal adenomas)

Revised Bethesda Criteria for HNPCC and Microsatellite Instability (MSI)
Tumours from individuals should be tested for MSI in the following situations:
- Colorectal cancer diagnosed in a patient who is <50 yr
- Presence of synchronous, metachronous colorectal, or other HNPCC-associated tumours, regardless of age
- Colorectal cancer with the MSI-H histology diagnosed in a patient who is <60 yr
- Colorectal cancer diagnosed in one or more first-degree relatives with an HNPCC-related tumour, with one of the cancers being diagnosed <50 yr
- Colorectal cancer diagnosed in two or more first- or second-degree relatives with HNPCC-related tumours, regardless of age

Elderly persons who present with iron-deficiency anemia should be investigated for colon cancer

Staging for CRC
I   T1,2 N0M0
II   T3,4 N0M0
III   TxN+M0
IV   TxNxM1

APR removes distal sigmoid colon, rectum, and anus; permanent end colostomy required
LAR removes distal sigmoid and rectum with anastomosis of distal colon to anus

Pathogenesis
- adenoma-carcinoma sequence; rarely arise de novo

Clinical Features
- often asymptomatic
- hematochezia/melena, abdominal pain, change in bowel habits
- others: weakness, anemia, weight loss, palpable mass, obstruction
- 20% patients have distant metastatic disease at time of presentation
- spread
  - direct extension, lymphatic, hematogenous (liver most common, lung, bone, brain; tumour of distal rectum → IVC → lungs)
  - peritoneal seeding: ovary, Blumer's shelf (pelvic cul-de-sac)

Table 15. Clinical Presentation of CRC

	Right Colon	Left Colon	Rectum
Frequency	25%	35%	30%
Pathology	Exophytic lesions with occult bleeding	Annular, invasive lesions	Ulcerating
Symptoms	Weight loss, weakness, rarely obstruction	Constipation ± overflow (alternating bowel patterns), abdominal pain, decreased stool calibre, rectal bleeding	Obstruction, tenesmus, rectal bleeding
Signs	Fe-deficiency anemia, RLQ mass (10%)	BRBPR, LBO	Palpable mass on DRE, BRBPR

Investigations
- colonoscopy (best), look for synchronous lesions (3-5% of patients); alternative: air contrast barium enema ("apple core" lesion) + sigmoidoscopy
- if a patient is FOBT +ve, or has microcytic anemia or has a change in bowel habits, do colonoscopy
- laboratory: CBC, urinalysis, liver enzymes, liver function tests, carcinogenic embryonic antigen (CEA) (pre-operative for baseline, >5 ng/mL have worse prognosis)
- staging: CT chest/abdomen/pelvis; bone scan, CT head only if lesions suspected
- rectal cancer: pelvic MRI or endorectal U/S to determine T and N stage

Table 16. TNM Classification System for Staging of Colorectal Carcinoma (AJCC/IUCC 2010)

Primary Tumour (T)		Regional Lymph Nodes (N)		Distant Metastasis (M)	
T0	No primary tumour found	N0	No regional node involvement	M0	No distant metastasis
Tis	Carcinoma *in situ*	N1	Metastasis in 1-3 regional nodes	M1	Distant metastasis
T1	Invasion into submucosa	N2	Metastasis in 4 or more regional nodes		
T2	Invasion into muscularis propria				
T3	Invasion through muscularis propria and into serosa				
T4	Invasion into adjacent structures or organs				

Treatment
- **colon cancer**
  - wide surgical resection of lesion and regional lymphatic drainage; usually colectomy with primary anastomosis
    - curative: wide resection of lesion (5 cm margins) with nodes (>12) and mesentery
    - metastatic lesions confined to the liver can be resected with curative intent
    - palliative: if distant spread, local control for hemorrhage or obstruction
    - care is taken to not spread tumour by unnecessary palpation
    - cancer-bearing portion of colon is removed according to vascular distribution of segment
  - adjuvant chemotherapy (5-FU or oral capecitabine with oxaliplatin) for stage III and is considered in select stage II patients
- **rectal cancer**
  - choice of operation depends on individual case; types of operations
    - low anterior resection of rectum (LAR): curative procedure of choice if adequate distal margins (~2cm); uses technique of total mesorectal excision
    - abdominoperineal resection of rectum (APR): if adequate distal margins cannot be obtained; involves the removal of distal sigmoid colon, rectum, and anus – permanent end colostomy required
    - transanal minimally invasive surgery (TAMIS)- local excision for select T1 lesions only
    - palliative procedures involve proximal diversion with an ostomy for obstruction and radiation for bleeding or pain
  - adjuvant therapy
    - combined neoadjuvant chemoradiation therapy followed by post-operative adjuvant chemotherapy for stages II and III

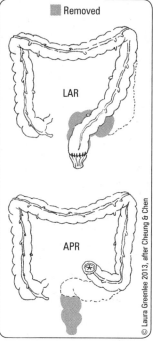

Figure 16. APR vs. LAR

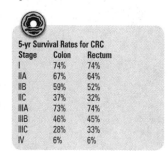

5-yr Survival Rates for CRC		
Stage	**Colon**	**Rectum**
I	74%	74%
IIA	67%	64%
IIB	59%	52%
IIC	37%	32%
IIIA	73%	74%
IIIB	46%	45%
IIIC	28%	33%
IV	6%	6%

Pre-Operative vs. Post-Operative Chemoradiotherapy for Locally Advanced Rectal Cancer: Results of the German CAO/ARO/AIO-94 Randomized Phase III Trial after a Median Follow-Up of 11 Yr
J Clin Oncol 2012;30:1926-1933
Background: The CAO/ARO/AIO-94 trial (published 2004) recommended pre-operative chemoradiotherapy (CRT) as standard treatment for locally advanced rectal cancer. However, no survival benefit was shown after median follow-up of 46 mo, and this study reports long-term effects.
Methods: Patients with stage II to III rectal cancer (n=799) were randomly assigned to pre-operative (n=404) or post-operative CRT (n=395) with fluorouracil (FU), radiation, and adjuvant FU chemotherapy, in addition to total mesorectal excision surgery. Follow-up was designed to assess long-term overall survival as the primary end point; and cumulative incidence of local and distant relapses and disease-free survival as secondary end points.
Results: 10 yr incidence of local relapse was significantly lower in the pre-operative CRT group than in the post-operative group (7.1% vs. 10.1%, p=0.048). Overall survival at 10 yr was similar at ~60% for patients treated with pre-operative or post-operative CRT (p=0.85). Disease-free survival rates at 10 yr was similar at ~68% for patients treated with pre-operative or post-operative CRT (p=0.54). No significant difference was detected for 10-yr incidence of distant metastases (pre-operative CRT 29.8% vs. post-operative CRT 29.6%, p=0.9).
Conclusion: There is long-term reduction in local recurrence of stage II to III rectal cancer with pre-operative chemotherapy, but no improvement in overall survival or distant recurrence of disease.

Follow-Up
- currently there are no data suggesting optimal follow-up
- combination of periodic CT chest/abdomen/pelvis, CEA, and colonoscopy is recommended
- CEA to monitor for initial response to treatment, and for surveillance (q6months)

Other Conditions of the Large Intestine

Angiodysplasia

Definition
- vascular anomaly: focal submucosal venous dilatation and tortuosity

Clinical Features
- most frequently in right colon of patients >60 yr old
- bleeding typically intermittent, rarely massive, not usually hypotensive (melena, anemia, guaiac positive stools)

Investigations
- colonoscopy: cherry red spots, branching pattern from central vessel
- angiography: early-filling vein, vascular tuft, delayed emptying vein; rarely active bleeding
- RBC technetium-99 scan
- barium enema is contraindicated (obscures other x-rays, i.e. angiogram)

Treatment
- none if asymptomatic
- cautery, right hemicolectomy, embolization, vasopressin infusion, sclerotherapy, band ligation, laser, octreotide, and rarely segmental resection if other treatments fail

Volvulus

Definition
- rotation of segment of bowel about its mesenteric axis
- sigmoid (65%), cecum (30%), transverse colon (3%), splenic flexure (2%)
- 5-10% of large bowel obstruction; 25% of intestinal obstruction during pregnancy

Risk Factors
- age (50% of patients >70 yr: stretching/elongation of bowel with age is a predisposing factor)
- high fibre diet (can cause elongated/redundant colon), chronic constipation, laxative abuse, pregnancy, bedridden, institutionalization (less frequent evacuation of bowels)
- congenital hypermobile cecum

Cecal Volvulus
AXR: Central cleft of "coffee bean" sign points to RLQ

Sigmoid Volvulus
AXR: Central cleft of "coffee bean" sign points to LLQ
Barium enema: "ace of spades" or "bird's beak" sign

Clinical Features
- symptoms due to bowel obstruction (see *Large Bowel Obstruction*, GS29) or intestinal ischemia (see *Intestinal Ischemia*, GS23)
- colicky abdominal pain, persistence of pain between spasms, abdominal distention, vomiting

Investigations
- AXR (classic findings): "omega", "bent inner-tube", "coffee-bean" signs
- barium/Gastrografin® enema: "ace of spades" (or "bird's beak") appearance due to funnel-like luminal tapering of lower segment towards volvulus
- sigmoidoscopy or colonoscopy as appropriate
- CT

Treatment
- initial supportive management (same as initial management for bowel obstruction (see *Large Bowel Obstruction*, GS29)
- cecum
  - nonsurgical
    - may attempt colonoscopic detorsion and decompression
  - surgical
    - right colectomy + ileotransverse colonic anastomosis
- sigmoid
  - nonsurgical
    - decompression by flexible sigmoidoscopy and insertion of rectal tube past obstruction
    - subsequent elective surgery recommended (50-70% recurrence)
- surgical: Hartmann procedure (if urgent)
    - indications: strangulation, perforation, or unsuccessful endoscopic decompression

Toxic Megacolon

Pathogenesis
- extension of inflammation into smooth muscle layer causing paralysis
- damage to myenteric plexus and electrolyte abnormalities are not consistently found

Etiology
- inflammatory bowel disease (ulcerative colitis > Crohn's disease)
- infectious colitis: bacterial (*C. difficile, Salmonella, Shigella, Campylobacter*), viral (cytomegalovirus), parasitic (*E. histolytica*)

Clinical Features
- infectious colitis usually presents for >1 wk before colonic dilatation
- diarrhea ± blood (but improvement of diarrhea may portend onset of megacolon)
- abdominal distention, tenderness, ± local/general peritoneal signs (suggest perforation)
- triggers: hypokalemia, constipating agents (opioids, antidepressants, loperamide, anticholinergics), barium enema, colonoscopy

Diagnostic Criteria
- must have both colitis and systemic manifestations for diagnosis
- radiologic evidence of dilated colon
- three of: fever, HR >120, WBC >10.5, anemia
- one of: fluid and electrolyte disturbances, hypotension, altered LOC

Investigations
- CBC (leukocytosis with left shift, anemia from bloody diarrhea), electrolytes, elevated CRP, ESR
- metabolic alkalosis (volume contraction and hypokalemia) and hypoalbuminemia are late findings
- AXR: dilated colon >6 cm (right > transverse > left), loss of haustra
- CT: useful to assess underlying disease

Treatment
- NPO, NGT, stop constipating agents, correct fluid and electrolyte abnormalities, transfusion
- serial AXRs
- broad-spectrum antibiotics (reduce sepsis, anticipate perforation)
- aggressive treatment of underlying disease (e.g. steroids in IBD, metronidazole for *C. difficile*)
- indications for surgery (50% improve on medical management)
- worsening or persisting toxicity or dilation after 48-72 h
- severe hemorrhage, perforation
- high lactate and WBC especially for *C. difficile*
- procedure: subtotal colectomy + end ileostomy (may be temporary, with second operation for re-anastomosis later)

Prognosis
- average 25-30% mortality

Use caution when giving antidiarrheal agents, especially with bloody diarrhea

Fistula

Definition
- abnormal communication between two epithelialized surfaces (e.g. enterocutaneous, colovesical, aortoenteric, entero-enteric)

Etiology
- foreign object erosion (e.g. gallstone, graft)
- inflammatory states (e.g. infection, IBD [especially Crohn's], diverticular disease)
- iatrogenic/surgery (e.g. post-operative anastomotic leak, radiation)
- congenital, trauma
- neoplastic

Why Fistulae Stay Open

FRIENDO
Foreign body
Radiation
Infection
Epithelialization
Neoplasm
Distal obstruction (most common)
Others: increased flow; steroids (may inhibit closure, usually will not maintain fistula)

Investigations
- U/S, CT scan, fistulogram
- measure amount of drainage from fistula

Treatment
- decrease secretion: octreotide/somatostatin/omeprazole
- surgical intervention: dependent upon etiology (for non-closing fistulas); uncertainty of diagnosis

Stomas

Definition
- an opening of the GI tract onto the surface of the abdomen wall
  - stomas can be constructed as either **end stomas**: the proximal end of the GI tract forms the stoma and the distal end of the GI tract is not part of the stoma, or **loop stomas**: a loop of the GI tract is brought up to the skin and the anti-mesenteric surface of the bowel is matured as a stoma. The proximal and distal GI tract remain in continuity

Ileostomy
- usually positioned in RLQ; ileum is brought through rectus abdominus muscles
- indications: after protocolectomy for ulcerative colitis, in some cases of Crohn's disease or familial polyposis
- conventional ileostomy: discharges small quantities of liquid material continuously, appliance (plastic bag attached to a sheet of protective material) required at all times
- continent ileostomy: reservoir is constructed from distal ileum, emptied by inserting catheter into stoma several times a day; rarely used, has mostly been replaced by ileal pouch anal anastomosis

Colostomy
- indications: to decompress an obstructed colon, to protect a distal anastomosis after resection, or to evacuate stool after distal colon or rectum is removed
- colostomies can be done by making an opening in a loop of colon (loop colostomy) or by dividing the colon and bringing out one end (end colostomy)
- most common permanent colostomy is a sigmoid colostomy – expels stool once per day, no appliance required
- chronic paracolostomy hernia is a common complication

Complications (10%)
- obstruction: herniation, stenosis (skin and abdominal wall), adhesive bands, volvulus
- peri-ileostomy abscess and fistula
- skin irritation
- prolapse or retraction
- diarrhea (excessive output)

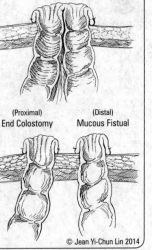

Colostomy/Ileostomy
- Connection of proximal limb of colon or ileum to abdominal wall skin

Mucous Fistula
- Connection of distal limb of colon to abdominal wall skin

Ileal Conduit
- Connection of bowel to ureter proximally and abdominal wall distally to drain urine

Loop Colostomy

(Proximal) End Colostomy   (Distal) Mucous Fistual

© Jean Yi-Chun Lin 2014

Figure 18. End vs. loop colostomy

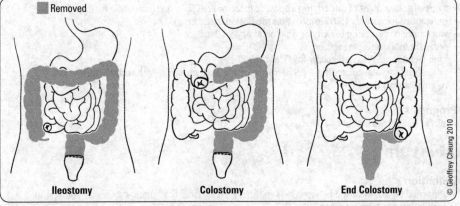

Removed

Ileostomy   Colostomy   End Colostomy

© Geoffrey Cheung 2010

Figure 17. Ostomies

Anorectum

Hemorrhoids

Etiology
- vascular and connective tissue complexes form a plexus of dilated veins (cushion)
- internal: superior hemorrhoidal veins, above dentate line, portal circulation
- external: inferior hemorrhoidal veins, below dentate line, systemic circulation

Risk Factors
- increased intra-abdominal pressure: chronic constipation, pregnancy, obesity, portal HTN, heavy lifting

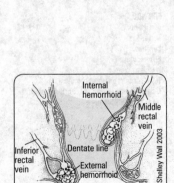

Internal hemorrhoid
Middle rectal vein
Inferior rectal vein
Dentate line
External hemorrhoid

© Shelley Wall 2003

Figure 19. Hemorrhoids

Clinical Features and Treatment

- internal hemorrhoids
  - engorged vascular cushions usually at 3, 7, 11 o'clock positions (patient in lithotomy position)
  - PAINLESS rectal bleeding, anemia, prolapse, mucus discharge, pruritus, burning pain, rectal fullness
    - **1st degree**: bleed but do not prolapse through the anus
      - treatment: high fibre/bulk diet, sitz baths, steroid cream, parmoxine (Anusol°), rubber band ligation, sclerotherapy, photocoagulation
    - **2nd degree**: bleed, prolapse with straining, spontaneous reduction
      - treatment: rubber band ligation, photocoagulation
    - **3rd degree**: bleed, prolapse, requires manual reduction
      - treatment: same as 2nd degree, but may require closed hemorrhoidectomy
    - **4th degree**: bleed, permanently prolapsed, cannot be manually reduced
      - treatment: closed hemorrhoidectomy
- external hemorrhoids
  - dilated venules usually mildly symptomatic
    - PAIN after bowel movement, associated with poor hygiene
    - medical treatment: dietary fibre, stool softeners, steroid cream (short course), parmoxine (Anusol°), avoid prolonged straining
  - thrombosed hemorrhoids are very painful
    - resolve within 2 wk, may leave excess skin = perianal skin tag
    - treatment: consider surgical decompression within first 48 h of thrombosis, otherwise medical treatment

Always rule out more serious causes (e.g. colon CA or anal canal cancer) in a person with hemorrhoids and rectal bleeding

Band ligation can be done as outpatient

External hemorrhoids will often recur

Table 17. Signs and Symptoms of Internal vs. External Hemorrhoids

Internal Hemorrhoids	External Hemorrhoids
Painless BRBPR	Sudden severe perianal pain
Rectal fullness or discomfort	Perianal mass
Mucus discharge	

Anal Fissures

Definition

- tear of anal canal below dentate line (very sensitive squamous epithelium)
- 90% posterior midline, 10% anterior midline
- if off midline: consider other possible causes such as IBD, STIs, TB, leukemia, or anal carcinoma
- repetitive injury cycle after first tear
  - sphincter spasm occurs preventing edges from healing and leads to further tearing
  - ischemia may ensue and contribute to chronicity

Etiology

- forceful dilation of anal canal: large, hard stools and irritant diarrheal stools
- tightening of anal canal secondary to nervousness/pain leads to further tearing
- others: habitual use of cathartics, childbirth

Clinical Features

- acute fissure
  - very painful bright red bleeding especially after bowel movement, sphincter spasm on limited DRE
  - treatment is conservative: stool softeners, bulking agent, sitz baths (heals 90%)
- chronic fissure (anal ulcer)
  - triad: fissure, sentinel skin tags, hypertrophied papillae
  - treatment
  - stool softeners, bulking agents, sitz baths
  - topical nitroglycerin or nifedipine: increases local blood flow, promoting healing and relieves sphincter spasm
  - lateral internal anal sphincterotomy (most effective): objective is to relieve sphincter spasm → increases blood flow and promotes healing; but 5% chance of fecal incontinence therefore not commonly done
  - alternative treatment
    - botulinum toxin: inhibits release of acetylcholine (ACh), reducing sphincter spasm

Anorectal Abscess

Definition
- infection in one or more of the anal spaces
- usually bacterial infection of blocked anal gland at the dentate line
- *E. coli, Proteus, Streptococci, Staphylococci, Bacteroides*, anaerobes

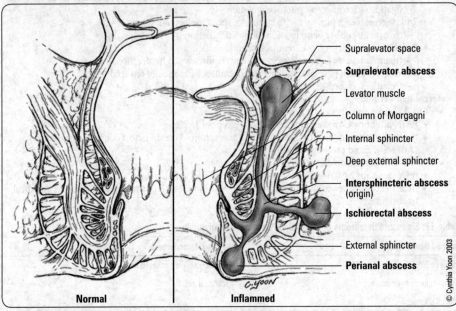

Figure 20. Different types of perianal abscesses

Clinical Features
- throbbing pain that may worsen with straining and ambulation
- abscess can spread vertically downward (perianal), vertically upward (supralevator), or horizontally (ischiorectal)
- tender perianal/rectal mass on exam

Treatment
- I&D
  - curative in 50% of cases
  - 50% develop anorectal fistulas
- may require antibiotics if diabetic, heart murmur, or cellulitis

Fistula-In-Ano

Definition
- anal fistula from rectum to perianal skin
- an inflammatory tract with internal os at dentate line, external os on skin

Etiology
- see *Fistula*, GS37
- same perirectal process as an anal abscess, therefore usually associated with an abscess
- other causes: post-operative, trauma, anal fissure, malignancy, radiation proctitis

Clinical Features
- intermittent or constant purulent discharge from perianal opening
- pain
- palpable cord-like tract

Treatment
- identification
  - internal opening
    - Goodsall's rule
      - fistulas originating anterior to a transverse line through the anus will have a straight course and exit anteriorly, whereas those originating posterior to the transverse line will begin in the midline and have a curved tract
  - fistulous tract
    - probing or fistulography under anesthesia

Recurrent perianal abscesses is associated with Crohn's disease

Antibiotics are not typically helpful in the treatment of perianal abscesses

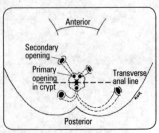

Figure 21. Goodsall's rule

- surgery
  - fistulotomy: unroof tract from external to internal opening, allow drainage, heals by secondary intention
  - low lying fistula (does not involve external sphincter) → primary fistulotomy
  - high lying fistula (involves external sphincter) → staged fistulotomy with Seton suture placed through tract
    - promotes drainage
    - promotes fibrosis and decreases incidence of incontinence
    - delineates anatomy
    - usually done to spare muscle cutting

Post-Operative
- sitz baths, irrigation, and packing to ensure healing proceeds from inside to outside

Complications
- recurrence
- rarely fecal incontinence

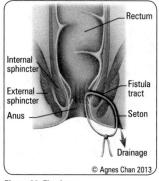

Figure 22. Fistulotomy

Pilonidal Disease

Definition
- chronic recurring abscess or chronic draining sinus in sacrococcygeal area

Epidemiology
- occurs most frequently in young men age 15-40 yr; rare in >50 yr

Etiology
- obstruction of the hair follicles in this area → formation of cysts, sinuses, or abscesses

Clinical Features
- asymptomatic until acutely infected, then pain/tenderness, purulent discharge, inspissated hair

Treatment
- acute abscess
  - I&D (often performed by primary care doctors)
  - wound packed open
  - 40% develop chronic pilonidal sinuses
- surgery
  - indication: failure of healing after I&D, recurrent disease, complex disease
  - pilonidal cystotomy: excision of sinus tract and cyst; wound closed by secondary intention, primary closure with tissue flap, or marsupialization (cyst edge sewn to surrounding tissue to leave sinus tract open)

Rectal Prolapse

Definition
- protrusion of some or all of rectal mucosa through external anal sphincter

Epidemiology
- extremes of ages: <5 yr old and >5th decade
- 85% women

Etiology
- lengthened attachment of rectum secondary to constant straining
- 2 types
  1. false/partial/mucosal: protrusion of mucosa only, radial furrows at junction with anal skin; most common type of rectal prolapse in childhood
  2. true/complete (most common): full thickness extrusion of rectal wall, concentric folds in:
     - first degree: prolapse includes mucocutaneous junction
     - second degree: without involvement of mucocutaneous junction
     - third degree (internal intussusception): prolapse is internal, concealed, or occult

Risk Factors
- gynecological surgery
- chronic neurologic/psychiatric disorders affecting motility

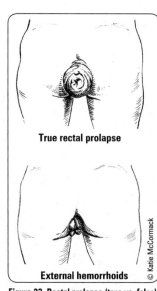

True rectal prolapse

External hemorrhoids

Figure 23. Rectal prolapse (true vs. false)

Clinical Features
- extrusion of mass with increased intra-abdominal pressure
  - straining, coughing, laughing, Valsalva
- difficulty in bowel regulation
  - tenesmus, constipation, fecal incontinence
- permanently extruded rectum with excoriation, ulceration, and constant soiling
- may be associated with urinary incontinence or uterine prolapse

Treatment
- Type I
  - conservative: gentle manual reduction of prolapsed area, especially in children
  - mucosectomy with excision of redundant mucosa, mostly in adults
- Type II
  - conservative: reduce if possible
  - surgery: abdominal, perineal, transsacral approaches

Anal Neoplasms

ANAL CANAL

Squamous Cell Carcinoma of Anal Canal (Above Dentate Line)
- most common tumour of anal canal (75%)
- anus prone to human papillomavirus (HPV) infection, therefore at risk for anal squamous intra-epithelial lesions (ASIL)
  - high grade squamous intra-epithelial lesion (HSIL) and low grade squamous intra-epithelial lesion (LSIL) terminology used
- clinical features: anal bleeding, pain, mass, ulceration, pruritus; 25% asymptomatic
- treatment: chemotherapy ± radiation ± surgery
- prognosis: 80% 5-yr survival

Malignant Melanoma of Anal Canal
- 3rd most common site for primary malignant melanoma after skin, eyes
- aggressive, distant metastases common at time of diagnosis
- treatment: wide excision or APR ± chemoradiation
- prognosis: <5% 5 yr survival

ANAL MARGIN
- clinical features and treatment as for skin tumours elsewhere
- squamous and basal cell carcinoma, Bowen's disease (SCC *in situ*), and Paget's disease

Liver

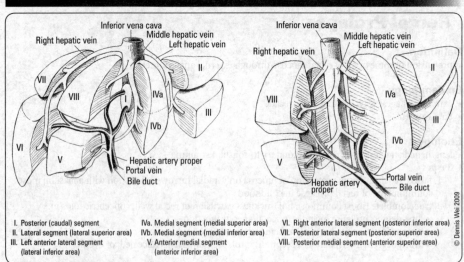

I. Posterior (caudal) segment
II. Lateral segment (lateral superior area)
III. Left anterior lateral segment (lateral inferior area)
IVa. Medial segment (medial superior area)
IVb. Medial segment (medial inferior area)
V. Anterior medial segment (anterior inferior area)
VI. Right anterior lateral segment (posterior inferior area)
VII. Posterior lateral segment (posterior superior area)
VIII. Posterior medial segment (anterior superior area)

Figure 24. Anatomy of liver

Liver Cysts

Table 18. Characteristics of Liver Cysts

	Simple Cysts	Polycystic Liver Disease	Choledochal Cysts	Hydatid (Cystic Echinococcosis)	Cystadenoma (Premalignant)/ Cystadenocarcinoma
Description	Contain clear fluid that do not communicate with the intrahepatic biliary tree Most common	Several cysts that replace much of the liver	Congenital malformations of pancreaticobiliary tree high risk of malignancy majority present before age 10	Infection with parasite *Echinococcus granulosus* associated with exposure to dogs, sheep, and cattle in Southern Europe, Middle East, Australasia, South America	Rare cystic tumours that occur in the liver parenchyma or the extrahepatic bile ducts Cystadenocarcinoma is an invasive carcinoma
Clinical Features	Usually asymptomatic may have multiple simple cysts	Progressive 50% associated with polycystic kidney disease	Recurrent abdominal pain Intermittent jaundice RUQ mass Cholangitis Pancreatitis	Asymptomatic mass chronic pain Hepatomegaly	Upper abdominal mass Abdominal pain Anorexia
Investigations	U/S: Used for diagnosis and follow-up CT: well demarcated lesion that does not enhance with contrast	U/S	U/S CT Transhepatic cholangiography LFTs	Anti-Echinococcus Ab (IgG) U/S CT: calcified mass Needle biopsy	Appear as complex cysts: internal septae, papillary projections, irregular lining Need histology for definite diagnosis
Treatment	Not required unless very large Monitor if >4 cm	Only if symptomatic partial liver resection drainage	Complete excision of cysts liver transplant if cyst involves intrahepatic bile ducts (Caroli's disease)	Albendazole (anti-helminthic) – cure up to 30% Surgical (risk of spillage into abdomen): Conservative: open endocystectomy or PAIR (Percutaneous Aspiration, Injection of protoscolicidal agent, Re-aspiration) Radical: partial hepatectomy or total pericystectomy	All complex, multiloculated cysts (except echinococcal) should be excised because of malignancy risk
Complications	Intracystic hemorrhage		Biliary cirrhosis, portal HTN, rupture, cholangiocarcinoma Abnormal pancreaticobiliary junction is associated with increased risk of malignancy	Inferior vena cava compression rupture can cause biliary colic, jaundice, cholangitis, pancreatitis, or anaphylactic reaction	Cystadenocarcinoma can invade adjacent tissues and metastasize

Liver Abscesses

Etiology
- types
- pyogenic (bacterial): most common etiology; most often polymicrobial – *E. coli*, *Klebsiella*, *Proteus*, *Strep. milleri*
- parasitic (amoebic): *Entamoeba histolytica*, *Echinococcal* cyst
- fungal: *Candida*
- sources: direct spread from biliary tract infection, portal spread from GI infection, systemic infection (e.g. endocarditis)

Clinical Features
- fever, malaise, chills, anorexia, weight loss, abdominal pain, nausea
- RUQ tenderness, hepatomegaly, jaundice

Investigations
- leukocytosis, anemia, elevated liver enzymes, echinoccocal serology
- U/S, CXR (right basilar atelectasis/effusion), CT, cyst aspiration with C&S, MRI

Treatment
- treat underlying cause
- bacterial abscesses generally will treat initially with antibiotics, and add surgical or percutaneous drainage and IV antibiotics for larger abscesses (initially ceftriaxone + metronidazole or piperacillin/ tazobactam)
- consider potential source of sepsis (e.g. biliary source, infected tumour)

Prognosis
- overall mortality 15% – higher rate if delay in diagnosis, multiple abscesses, malnutrition

Neoplasms

BENIGN LIVER NEOPLASMS

Hemangioma (cavernous)
- pathogenesis: most common benign hepatic tumour; results from malformation of angioblastic fetal tissue
- risk factors: F:M = 3:1
- clinical features
  - usually small and asymptomatic
  - consumptive coagulopathy if giant (in children)
- investigations
  - contrast CT (well-demarcated hypodense mass with peripheral enhancement on arterial phase with centripetal filling on delayed phases), U/S (homogenous hyperechoic mass), MRI
  - avoid biopsy: may result in hemorrhage
- treatment
  - usually none

Focal Nodular Hyperplasia
- pathogenesis: unclear, may be regenerative response to hyperperfusion from anomalous arteries at centre of nodule
- risk factors: female, age 20-50
- clinical features: asymptomatic, rarely grows or bleeds, no malignant potential
- investigations: central stellate scar on CT scan; MRI, biopsy may be required
- treatment: may be difficult to distinguish from adenoma/fibrolamellar HCC (malignant potential)
  - if confirmed to be FNH → no treatment required

Adenoma
- definition: benign glandular epithelial tumour
- risk factors: female, age 20-50, estrogen (OCP, pregnancy)
- clinical features: asymptomatic, 25% present with RUQ pain or mass, may present with bleeding
- investigations: CT (well-demarcated masses, often heterogeneous enhancement on arterial phase, isodense on venous phase without washout of contrast), U/S, MRI, biopsy often needed
- treatment
  - stop anabolic steroids or OCP
  - excise, especially if large (>5 cm), due to risk of transformation to hepatocellular carcinoma and spontaneous rupture/hemorrhage

MALIGNANT LIVER NEOPLASMS

Primary
- most comonlyhepatocellular carcinoma (HCC) and cholangiocarinomas
- others include angiosarcoma, hepatoblastoma, hemangioendothelioma, HCC
- epidemiology: 3rd leading cause of cancer death worldwide, 9th in United States; highest in Africa, China, Taiwan
- risk factors
  - chronic liver inflammation: cirrhosis from any cause, chronic hepatitis B (inherently oncogenic) and hepatitis C, hemochromatosis, α1-antitrypsin deficiency
  - medications: OCPs (3x increased risk), steroids
  - smoking, alcohol, Betel nuts
  - chemical carcinogens (aflatoxin, microcystin, vinyl chloride – associated with angiosarcoma)
- clinical features
  - RUQ discomfort, right shoulder pain
  - jaundice, weakness, weight loss, ± fever (if central tumour necrosis)
  - hepatomegaly, bruit, hepatic friction rub
  - ascites with blood (sudden intra-abdominal hemorrhage)
  - paraneoplastic syndromes – hypoglycemia, hypercalcemia, erythrocytosis, watery diarrhea
  - metastasis: lung, bone, brain, peritoneal seeding
- investigations
  - elevated ALP, bilirubin, and α-fetoprotein (80% of patients)
  - U/S (poorly-defined margins with internal echos), triphasic CT (enhancement on arterial phase and washout on portal venous phase), MRI
  - liver enzyme and liver function tests: AST, ALT, ALP, bilirubin, albumin, INR
- treatment
  - cirrhosis is a relative contraindication to tumour resection due to decreased hepatic reserve
  - surgical: resection (10% of patients have resectable tumours)
  - liver transplant; may use bridging therapy while awaiting transplant
    - **absolute contraindications**: extrahepatic disease, vascular invasion
    - **relative contraindications**: dependent on liver transplant protocol based on staging criteria followed by transplant centre

---

Differential Diagnosis of Metastatic Liver Mass

Some GU Cancers Produce Bumpy Lumps
Stomach
GenitoUrinary cancers (kidney, ovary, uterus)
Colon
Pancreas
Breast
Lung

Staging Criteria for Hepatocellular Carcinoma

Milan Criteria*	1 tumour ≤5 cm Up to 3 tumours each ≤3 cm
UCSF Criteria*	1 tumour ≤6.5 cm Up to 3 tumours each ≤4.5 cm, total diameter ≤8 cm
Toronto Criteria*	No tumour size of number restrictions No systemic symptoms Not poorly differentiated

*Each criteria assumes no extrahepatic and no macrovascular invasion

---

Child-Turcotte-Pugh Score (Prognosis of Chronic Liver Disease/Cirrhosis, Including Post-Operatively)

	1 Point	2 Points	3 Points
Albumin (g/L)	>35	28-35	<28
Ascites	Absent	Easily controlled	Poorly controlled
Bilirubin (μmol/L)	<34	34-51	>51
(mg/dL)	<2.0	2.0-3.0	>3.0
Coagulation (INR)	<1.7	1.7-2.3	>2.3
Hepatic Encephalopathy	None	Minimal (Grade I-II)	Advanced (Grade III-IV)

Points	Class	One Yr Survival	Two Yr Survival
5-6	A	100%	85%
7-9	B	81%	57%
10-15	C	45%	35%

- non-surgical: radiofrequency ablation, percutaneous ethanol injection, transcatheter arterial chemoembolization (TACE), chemotherapy (consider sorafenib for HCC; pre-operative chemotherapy for hepatoblastoma is standard of care), radiotherapy
- prognosis
  - median survival: 6-20 mo
  - 5 yr survival: all patients – 5%; patients undergoing complete resection – 11-40%

Secondary
- metastases to the liver are the most common malignant tumours found in the liver
- etiology
  - GI (colorectal most common), lung, breast, pancreas, ovary, uterus, kidney, gallbladder, prostate
- treatment
  - depends on the primary cancer site and prognosis. Often liver metastases are a manifestation of Stage IV disease, and chemotherapy is indicated
  - metastasectomy may be appropriate for some cancers
    - hepatic resection metastatic colorectal liver metastases is standard of care as part of multi-modality treatment that includes chemotherapy if complete resection of the primary cancer and metastases is possible
    - prognosis following liver resection for colorectal metastases is an overall survival of 30-60% at 5 yr

Liver Transplantation

Table 19. Conditions Leading to Transplantation

Parenchymal Disease	Cholestatic Disease	Inborn Errors	Tumours
Chronic hepatitis B or C*	Biliary atresia**	α1-antitrypsin deficiency	Hepatocellular carcinoma
Alcoholic cirrhosis	Primary biliary cirrhosis	Wilson's disease	
Acute liver failure	Sclerosing cholangitis	Hemochromatosis	
Budd-Chiari syndrome			
Congenital hepatic fibrosis			
CF			
Autoimmune hepatitis			
Cryptogenic cirrhosis			
Drug induced hepatotoxicity			
Non-alcoholic steatohepatitis			

*leading cause in adults; **leading cause in children

Clinical Indications
- early referral for transplant should be considered for all patients with progressive liver disease not responsive to medical therapy, especially:
  - decompensated cirrhosis (ascites, esophageal variceal hemorrhage, spontaneous hepatic encephalopathy, coagulopathy, progressive jaundice, severe fatigue)
  - unresectable primary liver cancers
  - fulminant hepatic failure
- end-stage liver disease with life expectancy <1 yr and if no other therapy is appropriate
  - suitable HCC not amenable to liver resection

Criteria for Transplantation
- Model for End-Stage Liver Disease (MELD): prognostic model to estimate 3 mo survival and disease severity if patient does not receive transplant; based on creatinine, bilirubin, INR; MELD scores from 6-40 used to prioritize liver allocation
- Child-Turcotte-Pugh Score: classification system to assess the prognosis and mortality of liver disease; patient must have ≥7 points (Class B)

Contraindications
- active alcohol/substance abuse
- extrahepatic malignancy within 5 yr
- advanced cardiopulmonary disease
- active uncontrolled infection

Post-Operative Complications
- primary non-function (graft failure): urgent re-transplantation is indicated
- acute and chronic rejection, ischemia-reperfusion injury
- vascular: hepatic artery or portal vein thrombosis, IVC obstruction
- biliary complications: fever, increasing bilirubin and ALP
- complications related to immunosuppression: HTN, renal disease, DM, obesity, hyperlipidemia, osteoporosis, malignancy, neurologic complications, infection (leading cause of mortality following transplant)

Prognosis
- patient survival at 1 yr: 85%
- graft survival at 1 yr: >80%, at 5 yr: 60-70%

Secondary liver metastases are common in many cancers, with some studies showing a prevalence of 40-50% amongst patients with extrahepatic cancers. They commonly arise from breast, lung, and colorectal cancers. For metastases secondary to colorectal cancer, surgical resection offers the greatest likelihood of cure

Living Liver Donors vs. Deceased Liver Donors
The right lobe of a living donor liver is transplanted into the recipient, whereas whole livers from deceased donors are transplanted orthotopically into the recipient

Which Matters Most: Number of Tumours, Size of the Largest Tumour, or Total Tumour Volume?
Liver Transplant 2011;17:S58-66
Purpose: To determine if the size and/or number of hepatocellular carcinoma (HCC) nodules predict disease recurrence and survival after liver transplantation.
Methods: Systematic review and meta-analysis.
Results: 74 studies were included for analysis. Patients beyond the Milan criteria had reduced overall and disease-free survivals and higher recurrence. Patients outside the UCSF criteria had reduced overall and disease-free survivals and higher recurrence. Patients outside the Milan criteria but within the UCSF criteria had reduced overall and disease-free survivals. Overall and disease-free survivals were reduced for patients with larger total tumour diameter, ≥10 cm vs. <10 cm and ≥9 cm vs. <9 cm, respectively. Similarly, patients with higher diameter of largest tumour nodule (≥3 cm vs. <3 cm) had reduced overall survival and higher recurrence. Overall and disease-free survivals were reduced and recurrence higher for patients with tumour size ≥5 cm vs. <5 cm. Mixed results were found regarding number of tumour nodules.
Conclusion: Tumour size and volume are important factors in survival after liver transplantation.

Living Donor Liver Transplantation vs. Deceased Donor Liver Transplantation for Hepatocellular Carcinoma: Comparable Survival and Recurrence
Liver Transplant 2012;18:315-322
Purpose: To compare the overall survival and hepatocellular carcinoma (HCC) recurrence rates after living donor liver transplantation (LDLT) versus deceased donor liver transplantation (DDLT) in a series of patients with HCC.
Methods: Study conducted between 1996 and 2009 at a single centre. 345 patients with HCC undergoing liver transplantation included.
Results: The overall survival rates at 1, 3, and 5 yr did not significantly differ between the LDLT and DDLT groups (p=0.62). Disease free survival at 1, 3, and 5 yr did not differ between the groups (p=0.82). The recurrence rates at 1, 3, and 5 yr also did not differ between the two group (p=0.54).
Conclusion: LDLT and DDLT lead to similar survival and recurrence rates.

Biliary Tract

Cholelithiasis

Definition
- the presence of gallstones

Pathogenesis
- imbalance of cholesterol and its solubilizing agents (bile salts and lecithin)
- excessive hepatic cholesterol secretion → bile salts and lecithin are "overloaded" → supersaturated cholesterol can precipitate and form gallstones
- North America: cholesterol stones (80%), pigment stones (20%)

Risk Factors
- cholesterol stones
  - obesity, age <50
  - estrogens: female, multiparity, OCPs
  - ethnicity: First Nations heritage (especially Pima Indians) > Caucasian > Black
  - terminal ileal resection or disease (e.g. Crohn's disease)
  - impaired gallbladder emptying: starvation, TPN, DM
  - rapid weight loss: rapid cholesterol mobilization and biliary stasis
- pigment stones (contain calcium bilirubinate)
  - cirrhosis
  - chronic hemolysis
  - biliary stasis (strictures, dilation, biliary infection)
  - protective factors: statins, vitamin C, coffee, exercise

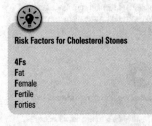

Risk Factors for Cholesterol Stones

4Fs
Fat
Female
Fertile
Forties

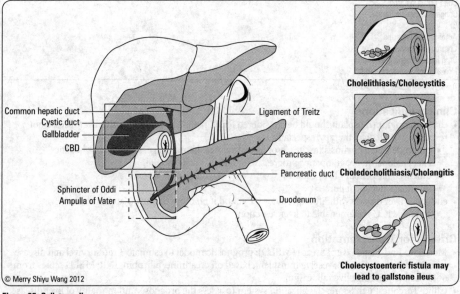

Cholelithiasis/Cholecystitis

Choledocholithiasis/Cholangitis

Cholecystoenteric fistula may lead to gallstone ileus

Figure 25. Gallstone disease

Clinical Presentation
- asymptomatic (80%)
  - most do NOT require treatment
  - consider cholecystectomy if: increased risk of malignancy (choledochal cysts, Caroli's disease, porcelain or calcified gallbladder), sickle cell disease, pediatric patient, bariatric surgery, immunosuppression
- biliary colic (10-25%)
- cholecystitis
- choledocholithiasis (8-15%)
- cholangitis
- gallstone pancreatitis (see *Acute Pancreatitis*, GS51)
- gallstone ileus (0.3-0.5%)
- other: empyema of the gallbladder, liver abscess, gallbladder perforation with bile peritonitis

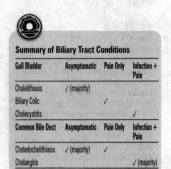

Summary of Biliary Tract Conditions

Gall Bladder	Asymptomatic	Pain Only	Infection + Pain
Cholelithiasis	✓ (majority)		
Biliary Colic		✓	
Cholecystitis			✓
Common Bile Duct	Asymptomatic	Pain Only	Infection + Pain
Choledocholithiasis	✓ (majority)	✓	
Cholangitis			✓ (majority)

Investigations

- Labs
  - CBC, LFTs, amylase, and lipase
- U/S: diagnostic procedure of choice
  - image for signs of inflammation, obstruction, localization of stones
  - 95% specific for detecting stones
  - signs: gallbladder wall thickening >4 mm, edema (double-wall sign), gallbladder sludge, pericholecystic fluid, sonographic Murphy's sign
- HIDA scan
  - used less commonly
  - radioisotope technetium-99 injected into a vein is excreted in high concentrations into bile, allowing visualization of the biliary tree
  - does not visualize stones; diagnosis by seeing occluded cystic duct or CBD

Choledhocholithiasis (suspected or confirmed)

- MRCP
  - visualization of ampullary region, biliary and pancreatic anatomy
  - non-invasive diagnostic test of choice
- ERCP
  - CBD stones in periampullary region
  - complications: retained stones, ERCP pancreatitis (1-2%), pancreatic or biliary sepsis

Percutanteous Transhepatic Cholangiography

- percutaneous approach to the proximal biliary tree (i.e. intra-hepatic biliary system) via the hepatic parenchyma
- useful for proximal bile duct obstruction or when ERCP fails or not available
- requires prophylactic antibiotics
- contraindications: coagulopathy, ascites, peri/intrahepatic sepsis, disease of right lower lung or pleura
- complications: bile peritonitis, chylothorax, pneumothorax, biliary sepsis, hemobilia

Biliary Colic

Pathogenesis

- gallstone transiently impacted in cystic duct, no infection

Clinical Features

- steady, severe dull pain in epigastrium or RUQ for minutes to hours (<6 h), crescendo-decrescendo pattern
- may present with chest pain
- N/V
- frequently occurs at night or after fatty meal, not after fasting
- can radiate to right shoulder or scapula
- no peritoneal findings, no systemic signs

Biliary colic is a **constant pain**, not colicky

Investigations

- normal blood work: CBC, electrolytes, LFTs, bilirubin, amylase
- U/S shows cholelithiasis, may show stone in cystic duct

2 Most Important Lab Tests for Biliary Pain
- Amylase
- Bilirubin

Treatment

- analgesia, rehydration during colic episode
- elective cholecystectomy (95% success)
  - complications: CBD injury (0.3-0.5%), hollow viscus injury, bile peritonitis, vessel injury
  - laparoscopic cholecystectomy is the standard of care, no benefit to delaying surgery
  - risk of open cholecystectomy higher in emergency situations

Biliary colic is treated with analgesia and elective cholecystectomy
Acute cholecystitis is treated with antibiotics and early cholecystectomy

Acute Cholecystitis

Pathogenesis

- inflammation of gallbladder resulting from sustained gallstone impaction in cystic duct or Hartmann's pouch
- no cholelithiasis in 5-10% (see *Acalculous Cholecystitis*, GS48)

Clinical Features

- often have history of biliary colic
- severe constant (<6hr) epigastric or RUQ pain, anorexia, N/V, low grade fever (<38.5°C)
- focal peritoneal findings: Murphy's sign, palpable, tender gallbladder (in 33%)
- Boas' sign: right subscapular pain

Early vs. Delayed Laparoscopic Cholecystectomy for Uncomplicated Biliary Colic
Cochrane DB Syst Rev 2013;6:CD007196
Study: To assess the benefits and harms of early vs. delayed laparoscopic cholecystectomy for patients with uncomplicated biliary colic due to gallstones.
Results: One trial with 75 participants, average age 43 yr. Early laparoscopic cholecystectomy (<24 h) vs. delayed (mean wait period 4.2 mo). The proportion of serious adverse events was lower in the early vs. delayed group (0% vs. 22.5%, respectively). There was a shorter hospital stay in the early group (MD -1.25 d, 95% CI -2.05 to -0.45) and a shorter operating time in the early group (MD -14.80 min, 95% CI -18.02 to -11.58). There was no difference in the proportion of patients requiring conversion to open cholecystectomy in the two groups.
Conclusion: Early laparoscopic cholecystectomy (<24 h of diagnosis of biliary colic) decreased morbidity during the waiting period for elective laparoscopic cholecystectomy, hospital stay, and operating time.

Mirizzi Syndrome
Extrinsic compression of the common hepatic duct by a gallstone in the cystic duct or Hartmann's pouch. Impacted gallstone may erode into the CHD or CBD, creating a cholecystohepatic or cholecystocholedochal fistula; Mirizzi syndrome has an association with gallbladder cancer

Rouviere's Sulcus
Fissure between right lobe and caudate process of liver; keeping dissection anterior to this landmark prevents bile duct injury

Critical View of Safety
Space between the gallbladder and liver clear of any structures other than the cystic artery

Laparoscopic vs. Open Cholecystectomy
Laparoscopic Cholecystectomy
• Shorter operating time
• Shorter length of stay
• Shorter sick leave
• Shorter time to return to daily activities
• Less post-operative pain
• Decreased use of post-operative analgesia
• Decreased reduction in pulmonary function*
• Fewer pulmonary complications
• Decreased acute phase response
• Less impairment in intestinal motility*
Open Cholecystectomy
• Lower conversion rates to open surgery (for mini-laparotomies)
*NOTE:
Pulmonary function = O₂ consumption, spirometric parameters, ABG, and acid-base balance
Intestinal motility = auscultating intestinal peristalsis, abdominal circumference measurement, and time interval to restitution of defecation

American Society of Gastrointestinal Endoscopy 2010 Predictors for Risk of CBD Stones
Very strong
• CBD stone on U/S
• Clinical ascending cholangitis
• Bilirubin >68 μmol/L
Strong
• CBD dilated >6 mm on U/S
• Bilirubin 31-68 μmol/L
Moderate
• Abnormal liver test (besides bilirubin)
• Age >55 yr
• Clinical gallstone pancreatitis

Investigations
• blood work: elevated WBC and left shift, mildly elevated bilirubin, AST, ALT, and ALP
• U/S: 98% sensitive, consider HIDA scan if U/S negative

Complications
• Mirizzi syndrome: extra-luminal compression of CBD/CHD due to large stone in cystic duct
• empyema of gallbladder: suppurative cholecystitis, pus in gallbladder + sick patient
• emphysematous cholecystitis: bacterial gas present in gallbladder lumen, wall, or pericholecystic space (risk in diabetic patient); organisms involved in secondary infection: *E. coli, Klebsiella, Enterococcus*
• gangrenous gallbladder (20%), perforation (2%): result in abscess formation or peritonitis
• cholecystoenteric fistula, from repeated attacks of cholecystitis, can lead to gallstone ileus

Treatment
• admit, hydrate, NPO, NGT (if persistent vomiting from associated ileus), analgesics once diagnosis is made
• antibiotics
  ▪ cefazolin if uncomplicated cholecystitis
• ERCP prior to surgery if US if CBD stones are present
  ▪ MRCP ± ERCP if CBD is markedly dilated or CBD stones suspected
• cholecystectomy
  ▪ early (within 72 h) vs. delayed (after 6 wk)
    ◆ equal morbidity and mortality
    ◆ early cholecystectomy preferred: shorter hospitalization and recovery time, no benefit to delaying surgery
    ◆ emergent OR indicated if high risk, e.g. emphysematous
  ▪ laparoscopic is standard of care (convert to open for complications or difficult case)
    ◆ laparoscopic: reduced risk of wound infections, shorter hospital stay, reduced post-operative pain, increased risk of bile duct injury
• intra-operative cholangiography (IOC)
  ▪ indications: clarify bile duct anatomy, history of biliary pancreatitis, small stones in gallbladder with a wide cystic duct (>15 mm), jaundice
• percutaneous cholecystostomy tube: critically ill or if general anesthetic contraindicated

Acalculous Cholecystitis

Definition
• acute or chronic cholecystitis in the absence of stones

Pathogenesis
• typically due to gallbladder ischemia, stasis

Risk Factors
• DM, immunosuppression, ICU admission, trauma patient, TPN, sepsis

Clinical Features
• see *Acute Cholecystitis*, GS47
• occurs in 20% of cases of acute cholecystitis

Investigations
• U/S: shows sludge in gallbladder, other U/S features of cholecystitis (see *Acute Cholecystitis*)
• CT or HIDA scan

Treatment
• broad-spectrum antibiotics, cholecystectomy
• if patient unstable → cholecystostomy

Choledocholithiasis

Definition
• stones in CBD

Clinical Features
• 50% asymptomatic
• often have history of biliary colic
• tenderness in RUQ or epigastrium
• acholic stool, dark urine, fluctuating jaundice
• primary vs. secondary stones
  ▪ primary: formed in bile duct, indicates bile duct pathology (e.g. benign biliary stricture, sclerosing cholangitis, choledochal cyst, CF)
  ▪ secondary: formed in gallbladder (85% of cases in U.S.)

Investigations
- CBC: usually normal; leukocytosis suggests cholangitis
- LFTs: increased AST, ALT early in disease, increased bilirubin (more sensitive), ALP, GGT later
- amylase/lipase: to rule out gallstone pancreatitis
- U/S: intra-/extra-hepatic duct dilatation; differential diagnosis is choledochal cyst
- MRCP (90% sensitive)

Complications
- cholangitis, pancreatitis, biliary stricture, and biliary cirrhosis

Treatment
- treat with ERCP for CBD stone extraction possibly followed by elective cholecystectomy in 25% of patients

Acute Cholangitis

Pathogenesis
- obstruction of CBD leading to biliary stasis, bacterial overgrowth, suppuration and biliary sepsis – may be life-threatening, especially in elderly

Etiology
- choledocholithiasis (60%), stricture, neoplasm (pancreatic or biliary), extrinsic compression (pancreatic pseudocyst or pancreatitis), instrumentation of bile ducts (PTC, ERCP), biliary stent
- organisms: *E. coli, Klebsiella, Pseudomonas, Enterococcus, B. fragilis, Proteus*

Charcot's Triad
Fever, RUQ pain, jaundice

Clinical Features
- Charcot's triad: fever, RUQ pain, jaundice
- Reynold's pentad: fever, RUQ pain, jaundice, shock, confusion
- may have N/V, abdominal distention, ileus, acholic stools, tea-coloured urine (elevated direct bilirubin)

Reynolds' Pentad
Fever, RUQ pain, jaundice, shock, confusion

Investigations
- CBC: elevated WBC + left shift
- may have positive blood cultures
- LFTs: obstructive picture (elevated ALP, GGT, and conjugated bilirubin, mild increase in AST, ALT)
- amylase/lipase: rule out pancreatitis
- U/S: intra-/extra-hepatic duct dilatation

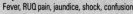

Common Bacteria in Biliary Tract

KEEPS
Klebsiella
Enterococcus
E. coli, Enterobacter
Proteus, Pseudomonas
Serratia

Treatment
- initial: NPO, fluid and electrolyte resuscitation, ± NGT, IV antibiotics (treats 80%)
- biliary decompression
  - ERCP + sphincterotomy: diagnostic and therapeutic
  - PTC with catheter drainage: if ERCP not available or unsuccessful
  - laparotomy with CBD exploration and T-tube placement if above fails
- all patients should also have a cholecystectomy, unless contraindicated

Prognosis
- suppurative cholangitis mortality rate: 50%

Gallstone Ileus

Pathogenesis
- repeated inflammation causing a cholecystoenteric fistula (usually duodenal) → large gallstone enters the gut and impacts near the ileocecal valve, causing a true bowel obstruction (note: ileus is a misnomer in this context)

Clinical Features
- crampy abdominal pain, N/V (see *Large Bowel Obstruction*, GS29)

Investigations
- AXR: dilated small intestine, air fluid levels, may reveal radiopaque gallstone, air in biliary tree (pneumobilia) (40%)
- CT: biliary tract air, obstruction, gallstone in intestine
- Rigler's triad: pneumobilia (air in biliary tree), small bowel obstruction (partial or complete), gallstone (usually in right iliac fossa)

Rigler's Triad of Gallstone Ileus
Pneumobilia
Small bowel obstruction
Gallstone

Bouveret's Syndrome
Gastric outlet/duodenal obstruction caused by a large gallstone passing through a cholecystogastric or cholecystoduodenal fistula

Treatment
- fluid resuscitation, NGT decompression
- surgery: enterolithotomy and removal of stone, inspect small and large bowel for additional proximal stones
- may close fistula surgically or manage expectantly (can resolve spontaneously)
- cholecystectomy is generally not performed

Carcinoma of the Gallbladder

Risk Factors
- chronic symptomatic gallstones (70% of cases), old age, female, gallbladder polyps, porcelain gallbladder, chronic infection (*Salmonella, Helicobacter*), abnormal pancreaticobiliary duct junction

Clinical Features
- majority are adenocarcinoma
- may be incidental finding on elective cholecystectomy (~1% of open cholecystectomies 0.1% in laparoscopic cholecystectomies)
- many patients are asymptomatic until late
- local: non-specific RUQ pain, ± palpable RUQ mass
- Courvoisier's gallbladder: an enlarged, often palpable gallbladder in a patient with carcinoma of the head of the pancreas; associated with jaundice due to obstruction of the CBD
- systemic: jaundice (50%) due to invasion of CBD or compression of CBD by pericholedochal nodes, weight loss, malaise, anorexia
- early local extension to liver, may extend to stomach, duodenum
- early metastasis common to liver, lung, bone

Investigations
- U/S: mural thickening, calcification, loss of interface between gallbladder and liver, fixed mass
- endoscopic U/S (EUS): good for distinguishing carcinomas from other diagnoses such as polyps, good for staging, allows sampling of bile for cytology
- abdominal CT: polypoid mass, mural thickening, liver invasion, nodal involvement, distant metastases
- MRI/MRCP: good for distinguishing benign and malignant polyps

Treatment
- if carcinoma of the gallbladder is suspected pre-operatively, an open cholecystectomy should be considered to avoid tumour seeding of the peritoneal cavity
- confined to mucosa (rare): cholecystectomy
- beyond mucosa: cholecystectomy, en bloc wedge resection of 3-5 cm underlying liver, dissection of hepatoduodenal lymph nodes

Prognosis
- poor 5 yr survival (10%) as gallbladder carcinoma is often detected late
- better outcomes when detected incidentally following cholecystectomy

Cholangiocarcinoma

Definition
- malignancy of extra- or intrahepatic bile ducts

Risk Factors
- age 50-70, gallstones, ulcerative colitis, primary sclerosing cholangitis, choledochal cyst, Clonorchis sinensis infection (liver fluke), chronic intrahepatic stones (hepatolithiasis)

Clinical Features
- majority are adenocarcinomas
- gradual signs of biliary obstruction: jaundice, pruritus, dark urine, pale stools
- anorexia, weight loss, RUQ pain, Courvoisier's sign (if CBD obstructed), hepatomegaly
- early metastases are uncommon, but commonly tumour grows into portal vein or hepatic artery
- Klatskin tumour: cholangiocarcinoma located at bifurcation of common hepatic duct

Investigations
- LFTs show obstructive picture
- U/S, CT: bile ducts usually dilated, but not necessarily
- ERCP or PTC: to determine resectability, for biopsies
- CXR, bone scan: for metastatic workup

Treatment
- if resectable: biliary drainage and wide excision margin
- intra-hepatic lesions: liver resection
    - upper third lesions: duct resection + Roux-en-Y hepaticojejunostomy, ± liver resection
    - middle third lesions (uncommon): duct resection + Roux-en-Y hepaticojejunostomy
    - lower third lesions: Whipple procedure
- unresectable lesions: stent or choledochojejunostomy (surgical bypass)
- chemotherapy ± radiotherapy
- role for transplantation in selected patients with Klatskins tumours

Prognosis
- overall 5 yr survival: 15%

Courvoisier's Sign
Palpable, nontender distended gallbladder due to CBD obstruction. Present in 33% of patients with pancreatic carcinoma. The distended gallbladder could not be due to acute cholecystitis or stone disease because the gallbladder would actually be scarred and smaller, not larger

Efficacy of Neoadjuvant Chemoradiation, Followed by Liver Transplantation, for Perihilar Cholangiocarcinoma at 12 US Centres
Gastroenterology 2012;143:88-98
Purpose: To determine the effectiveness of neoadjuvant chemoradiation and liver transplantation for unresectable perihilar cholangiocarcinoma and to determine the appropriateness of the United Network of Organ Sharing/Organ Procurement and Transplantation Network (UNOS/OPTN) criteria for model of end-stage liver disease (MELD) exception for patients with this disease.
Methods: Study conducted from 1993-2010 in 12 transplant centres. 287 patients included.
Results: Median follow-up was 2.5 yr. 43% of patients (n=122) died after a median of 1.2 yr from presentation, and of these, 60 died pretransplant. Post-transplant, 43 patients had recurrences and 62 died. Recurrence-free survival at 2, 5, and 10 yr were 78%, 65%, and 59%, respectively. Intention-to-treat survival rates at 2 and 5 yr were 68% and 53%, respectively. 25% of patients left the waiting list after a median of 4.6 mo. The waiting list drop-out rate increased by an average of 11.5% every 3 mo. Patients who received transplantation outside of the criteria for MELD exception or who had a malignancy within 5 yr had significantly worse recurrence-free survival compared to those who met the criteria (HR=2.98, 95% CI 1.79, 4.95). Recurrence-free survival at 5 yr was shorter for patients with tumours >3 cm vs. ≤3 cm (p<0.001).
Conclusions: Neoadjuvant chemoradiation and liver transplantation are effective treatments for unresectable perihilar cholangiocarcinoma. Furthermore, the UNOS/OPTN criteria for MELD exception appear to be appropriate.

Obstructive jaundice is the most common presenting symptom for cholangiocarcinoma

Ranson's Criteria
A. At admission
  1. Age >55 yr
  2. WBC >16 x 109/L
  3. Glucose >11 mmol/L
  4. LDH ≥350 IU/L
  5. AST >250 IU/L
B. During initial 48 h
  1. Hct drop >10%
  2. BUN rise >1.8 mmol/L
  3. Arterial PO_2 <60 mmHg
  4. Base deficit >4 mmol/L
  5. Calcium <2 mmol/L
  6. Fluid sequestration >6 L
C. Interpretation
  ≥2 = difficult course
  ≥3 = high mortality (≥15%)

Pancreas

Acute Pancreatitis

- see Gastroenterology, G44

GALLSTONE PANCREATITIS (35% of Acute Pancreatitis)

Pathogenesis
- obstruction of pancreatic duct by large or small gallstones and biliary sludge
- backup of pancreatic enzymes can cause autodigestion of the pancreas

Clinical Features (Pancreatitis of Any Etiology)
- pain (epigastric pain radiating to back), N/V, ileus, peritoneal signs, jaundice, fever
- Inglefinger's sign: pain worse when supine, better when sitting forward
- may have coexistent cholangitis or pancreatic necrosis
- Ranson's criteria for determining prognosis of acute pancreatitis (see sidebar)
- physical exam may show: tachypnea, tachycardia, hypotension, abdominal distention and tenderness, Cullen's sign, Grey Turner's sign

Investigations
- elevated amylase (higher than alcoholic pancreatitis), lipase, leukocytosis
- elevated ALT (>150 IU/L), AST strongly suggest gallstone etiology of pancreatitis
- U/S may show multiple stones (may have passed spontaneously), edematous pancreas
- CXR, AXR, CT (if severe to evaluate for complications)

Treatment
- supportive: e.g. NPO, hydration, analgesia, early enteric nutrition
- antibiotics for severe cases of necrotizing pancreatitis or signs of sepsis
- stone often passes spontaneously (~90%); usually no surgical management in uncomplicated acute pancreatitis
- cholecystectomy during same admission (25-60% recurrence if no surgery)
- may need urgent ERCP + sphincterotomy if CBD stone impacted or cholangitis
- **surgical indications** in acute pancreatitis (rare):
  - drain placement and debridement for necrotizing pancreatitis if refractory to medical management, if septic or in ICU without other sources of sepsis

Complications
- acute fluid collections
- pseudocyst (collection of pancreatic secretions >4 wk old surrounded by a defined wall of granulation tissue)
- abscess/infection, necrosis
- splenic/mesenteric/portal vessel thrombosis
- pancreatic ascites/pancreatic pleural effusion
- DM
- ARDS/sepsis/multiorgan failure
- coagulopathy/DIC
- severe hypocalcemia

Chronic Pancreatitis

- see Gastroenterology, G45

Surgical Treatment
- treatment is generally medical
- indications for surgery
  - failure of medical treatment
  - debilitating abdominal pain
  - pseudocyst complications: persistence, hemorrhage, infection, rupture
  - CBD obstruction (e.g. strictures), duodenal obstruction
  - pancreatic fistula, variceal hemorrhage secondary to splenic vein obstruction
  - rule out pancreatic cancer (present in 15% of chronic pancreatitis treated surgically)
  - anatomical abnormality causing recurrent pancreatitis
- pre-operative CT and/or ERCP are mandatory to delineate anatomy
- minimally invasive options
  - endoscopic pancreatic duct decompression: less effective than surgery
  - extracorporeal shockwave lithotripsy: if pancreatic duct stones
  - celiac plexus block: lasting benefit in 30% patients, less effective in those <45 yr or with prior pancreatic surgery

The hallmark of chronic pancreatitis is epigastric pain radiating to the back

- surgical options
  - drainage procedures: only effective if ductal system is dilated
    - Puestow procedure (lateral pancreaticojejunostomy): improves pain in 80% of patients
  - pancreatectomy: best option in absence of dilated duct
    - proximal disease: Whipple procedure (pancreaticoduodenectomy) – pain relief in 80%
    - distal disease: distal pancreatectomy ± Roux-en-Y pancreaticojejunostomy
    - total pancreatectomy: refractory disease
  - denervation of celiac ganglion and splanchnic nerves

PSEUDOCYST
- localized fluid collections rich in pancreatic enzymes, with a non-epithelialized wall consisting of fibrous and granulation tissue
- complication of chronic and/or acute pancreatitis
- often resolve spontaneously
- cyst wall must be mature prior to drainage (4-6 wk)
- pseudoaneurysm an absolute contraindication to endoscopic drainage, must embolize first

Treatment
- expectant management if asymptomatic
- endoscopic drainage
  - cystgastrostomy
  - cystduodenostomy
- percutaneous catheter drainage
- surgical drainage (gold standard)
  - cystgastrostomy
  - cystenterostomy
- resection
  - consider biopsy of cyst wall to rule out cystadenocarcinoma

Pancreatic Cancer

Epidemiology
- fourth most common cause of cancer-related mortality in both men and women in Canada
- M:F = 1.3:1, average age: 50-70

Risk Factors
- increased age
- smoking: 2-5x increased risk, most clearly established risk factor
- high fat/low fibre diets, heavy alcohol use
- obesity
- DM, chronic pancreatitis
- partial gastrectomy, cholecystectomy
- chemicals: betanaphthylamine, benzidine
- African descent

Clinical Features
- head of the pancreas (70%)
  - weight loss, obstructive jaundice, steatorrhea, vague constant mid-epigastric pain (often worse at night, may radiate to back)
  - painless jaundice, Courvoisier's sign
- body or tail of pancreas (30%)
  - tends to present later and usually inoperable
  - weight loss, vague mid-epigastric pain
  - <10% jaundiced
  - sudden onset DM

Investigations
- serum chemistry is non-specific, can have elevated ALP and high bilirubin
- CA 19-9 (most useful serum marker of pancreatic cancer)
- U/S, CT (also evaluates metastasis and resectability) ± ERCP, MRI, EUS

Pathology
- ductal adenocarcinoma: most common type (75-80%); exocrine pancreas
- intraductal papillary mucinous neoplasm (IPMN)
- other: pancreatic neuroendocrine tumours (non-functional, insulinoma, gastrinoma, VIPoma, glucagonoma, somatostatinoma), mucinous cystic neoplasm (MCN), acinar cell carcinoma
- see *Surgical Endocrinology*, GS60 for functional pancreatic neuroendocrine tumours

Trousseau's Sign
Spontaneous peripheral venous thrombosis, often associated with pancreatic and other cancers

Vague abdominal pain with weight loss ± jaundice in a patient over 50 yr old is pancreatic cancer until proven otherwise

Courvoisier's Sign
Palpable, nontender distended gallbladder due to CBD obstruction. Present in 33% of patients with pancreatic carcinoma. The distended gallbladder could not be due to acute cholecystitis or stone disease because the gallbladder would actually be scarred and smaller, not larger

Treatment
- resectable (10-20% of pancreatic cancer)
  - no involvement of liver, peritoneum, or vasculature (hepatic artery, SMA, SMV, portal vein, IVC, aorta), no distant metastasis
  - Whipple procedure (pancreaticoduodenectomy) for cure <5% mortality
  - distal pancreatectomy ± splenectomy, lymphadenectomy if carcinoma of midbody and tail of pancreas
- locally advanced, borderline resectable
  - tumours that abut the SMA, SMV, portal vein, hepatic artery, or celiac artery
- locally advanced, non-resectable (palliative → relieve pain, obstruction)
  - encasement of major vascular structures including arterie
  - most body/tail tumours are not resectable (due to late presentation)
  - relieve biliary/duodenal obstruction with endoscopic stenting or double bypass procedure (choledochoenterostomy + gastroenterostomy)
  - palliative chemotherapy (gemcitabine + nab-paclitaxel, FOLFIRNOX) ± radiotherapy

Prognosis
- most important prognostic indicators are lymph node status, margin status, size >3 cm, perineural invasion (invasion of tumour into microscopic nerves of pancreas)
- overall 5 yr survival for all patients with pancreas cancer is 1%; following surgical resection 5 yr survival is 20%
- median survival for unresectable disease: 3-6 mo if metastatic, 8-12 mo if locally advanced at presentation

Table 20. TNM Classification System for Exocrine and Endocrine Tumours of the Pancreas

Primary Tumour (T)		Regional Lymph Nodes (N)		Distant Metastasis (M)	
TX	Primary tumour cannot be assessed	NX	Regional lymph nodes cannot be assessed	M0	No distant metastasis
T0	No evidence of primary tumour	N0	No regional lymph node metastasis	M1	Distant metastasis
Tis	Carcinoma *in situ*	N1	Regional lymph node metastasis		
T1	Tumour limited to pancreas, <2 cm in greatest dimension				
T2	Tumour limited to pancreas, >2 cm in greatest dimension				
T3	Tumour extends beyond pancreas, no involvement of celiac axis or SMA				
T4	Tumour involves celiac axis or SMA (unresectable)				

Table 21. Staging and Treatment of Pancreatic Cancer

Stage	Classification	5 Yr Survival	Treatment
0	Tis, N0, M0		Surgical resection ± chemotherapy
IA	T1, N0, M0	14%	Same as above
IB	T2, N0, M0	12%	Same as above
IIA	T3, N0, M0	7%	Same as above
IIB	T1-3, N1, M0	5%	Same as above
III	T4, any N, M0	3%	Borderline resectable, trial of chemotherapy and radiation
IV	any T, any N, M1	1%	Non-resectable, palliative treatments

Steps of a Whipple Resection (Pancreaticoduodenectomy)
1. Assessment of metastatic disease (all peritoneal surfaces)
2. Mobilization of the duodenum and head of the pancreas
3. Identification of the superior mesenteric vein and mobilization of the pancreatic neck
4. Mobilization of the stomach; dissection of the hepatoduodenal ligament and cholecystectomy
5. Division of the stomach, proximal jejunum, and CBD
6. Transection of the pancreatic neck and dissection of the uncinate process from the retroperitoneum
7. Restoration of gastrointestinal continuity: construction of a pancreaticojejunostomy, hepaticojejunostomy, gastrojejunostomy using a neoduodenum

Removed
- CBD
- Gallbladder
- Duodenum
- Pancreatic head
- Distal stomach (sometimes)

Diagnostic Value of Serum Carbohydrate Antigen 19-9 in Pancreatic Cancer: A Meta-Analysis
Tumour Biol 2014 [Epub ahead of print]
Summary: 11 studies with 2,316 patients were included in the analysis. The sensitivity of CA19-9 in the diagnosis of pancreatic cancer was found to be 0.8 (95% CI 0.77-0.82) and the specificity also 80% (95% CI 0.77-0.82) with a diagnostic odds ratio of 14.79 (95% CI 8.55-25.59). Overall, CA19-9 plays an important role in the diagnosis of pancreatic cancer.

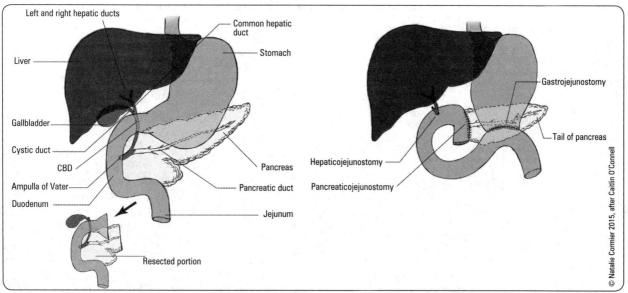

Figure 26. Schematic of Whipple resection, showing the resected components

© Natalie Cormier 2015, after Caitlin O'Connell

Spleen

Splenic Trauma

- typically from blunt trauma (especially in people with splenomegaly)
- most common intra-abdominal organ injury in blunt trauma
- may have Kehr's sign

Kehr's Sign
Left shoulder pain due to diaphragmatic irritation from splenic rupture, worsens with inspiration

Treatment
- non-operative
  - in stable patients: extended bed rest with serial hematocrit levels, close monitoring for 3-5 d; pediatric guidelines for days of bed rest is grade plus 1 (i.e. grade 3 splenic laceration requires 4 d of bed rest)
  - hemostatic control
  - splenic artery embolization if patient stable and one of: active contrast extravasation, splenic pseudoaneurysm, hemoperitoneum
- operative
  - splenorrhaphy (suture of spleen) ± splenic wrapping with hemostatic mesh – if patient hemodynamically stable, patient has stopped bleeding and laceration does not involve hilum
  - partial splenectomy, rarely performed due to risk of recurrent hemorrhage
  - total splenectomy if patient unstable or high-grade injury

Splenectomy

Indications
- splenic trauma (most common reason for splenectomy), hereditary spherocytosis, primary hypersplenism, chronic immune thrombocytopenic purpura (ITP), splenic vein thrombosis causing esophageal varices, splenic abscess, thrombotic thrombocytopenic purpura (TTP), sickle cell disease
- does not benefit all thrombocytopenic states (e.g. infection, most malignancies involving the bone marrow, drugs/toxins)
- probability of cure of ITP by splenectomy is 60-70%, may be predicted by response to IVIg

Indication of Splenectomy

SHIRTS
Splenic abscess/splenomegaly
Hereditary spherocytosis
Immune thrombocytopenic purpura
Rupture of spleen
Thrombotic thrombocytopenic purpura
Splenic vein thrombosis

Complications
- short-term
  - injury to surrounding structures (e.g. gastric wall, tail of pancreas)
  - post-operative thrombocytosis, leukocytosis
  - thrombosis of portal, splenic, or mesenteric veins
  - subphrenic abscess
- long-term
  - post-splenectomy sepsis (encapsulated organisms): 4% of splenectomized patients (highest risk in those <16 yr old)
    - 50% mortality
    - prophylaxis with vaccinations, ideally 2 wk pre- or post-operative (pneumococcal, *H. influenzae*, and meningococcus)
    - liberal use of penicillin especially in children <6 yr old
  - splenosis: intra-abdominal "seeding" of splenic tissue during removal

Breast

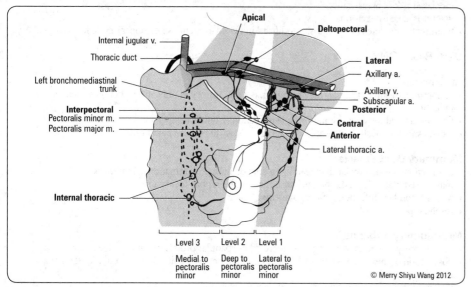

Figure 27. Anatomy of the breast

Labels in figure:
- Apical
- Deltopectoral
- Internal jugular v.
- Thoracic duct
- Lateral
- Axillary a.
- Axillary v.
- Subscapular a.
- Left bronchomediastinal trunk
- Posterior
- Interpectoral
- Pectoralis minor m.
- Pectoralis major m.
- Central
- Anterior
- Lateral thoracic a.
- Internal thoracic
- Level 3 / Medial to pectoralis minor
- Level 2 / Deep to pectoralis minor
- Level 1 / Lateral to pectoralis minor
- © Merry Shiyu Wang 2012

> **Levels of Axillary Lymph Nodes**
> **Level I:** lateral to pectoralis minor
> **Level II:** deep to pectoralis minor
> **Level III:** medial to pectoralis minor
> (higher level of nodal involvement = worse prognosis)

Benign Breast Lesions

Three Categories
1. nonproliferative
2. proliferative without atypia
3. atypical hyperplasia

NONPROLIFERATIVE LESIONS
- benign breast condition characterized by fibrous and cystic changes in the breast
- most common: breast cysts
- other lesions include papillary apocrine change, epithelial-related calcifications and mild hyperplasia of the usual type
- no increased risk of breast cancer
- age 30 to menopause (and after if HRT used)
- clinical features
  - breast pain, focal areas of nodularity or cysts often in the upper outer quadrant, frequently bilateral, mobile, varies with menstrual cycle, nipple discharge (straw-like, brown, or green)
- treatment
  - evaluation of breast mass (U/S, mammography as indicated) and reassurance
  - no strong evidence for avoidance of xanthine-containing products (coffee, tea, chocolate, cola)
  - analgesia (ibuprofen, ASA)
  - for severe symptoms: OCP, danazol, bromocriptine

> **DDx for Breast Mass**
> **Benign**
> - Fibrocystic changes
> - Fibroepithelial lesions (fibroadenoma most common; benign phyllodes also)
> - Fat necrosis
> - Papilloma/papillomatosis
> - Galactocele
> - Duct ectasia
> - Ductal/lobular hyperplasia
> - Sclerosing adenosis
> - Lipoma
> - Neurofibroma
> - Granulomatous mastitis (e.g. TB, granulomatosis with polyangiitis, sarcoidosis)
> - Abscess
> - Silicone implant
>
> **Malignant**
> - Breast cancer (likely invasive, DCIS rarely forms a breast mass)
> - Malignant phyllodes
> - Angiosarcoma (rare)

PROLIFERATIVE LESIONS – WITHOUT ATYPIA

Table 22. Proliferative Lesions - without Atypia

		Clinical Features	Diagnosis	Treatment	Risk of Breast Cancer
Fibroadenoma	Most common breast tumour in women <30 yr	Nodules: firm, rubbery, discrete, well-circumscribed, non-tender, mobile, hormone-dependent (unlike cysts), needle aspiration yields no fluid	Core or excisional biopsy some times required if concerned about malignancy U/S and FNA alone cannot differentiate fibroadenoma from Phyllodes tumour	Generally conservative: serial observation Consider excision if size 2-3 cm and growing on serial U/S (q6mo x 2 yr is usual follow-up), if symptomatic, formed after age 35, or patient preference or features on core biopsy suggestive of a Phyllodes tumour	Increased if complex, adjacent atypia or strong family history of breast cancer
Intraductal Papilloma	Solitary intraductal benign polyp	Can present as nipple discharge (most common cause of spontaneous, unilateral, bloody nipple discharge = pathologic nipple discharge), breast mass, nodule on U/S		Surgical excision of involved duct to ensure no atypia	Can harbour areas of atypia or DCIS
Usual Ductal Hyperplasia	Increased number of cells within the ductal space	Incidental finding on biopsy of mammographic abnormalities or breast masses		None required	Generally low risk, slightly increased if moderate or florid hyperplasia
Sclerosing Adenosis	Lobular lesion with increased fibrous tissue and glandular cells	Mass or mammographic abnormality		None required	Low risk

ATYPICAL HYPERPLASIA
- can involve ducts (ductal hyperplasia with atypia) or lobules (lobular hyperplasia with atypia)
- cells lose apical-basal orientation
- increased risk of breast cancer
- diagnosis: core or excisional biopsy
- treatment: complete resection, risk modification (avoid exogenous hormones), close follow-up

OTHER LESIONS

Fat Necrosis
- uncommon, result of trauma (may be minor, positive history in only 50%), after breast surgery (i.e. reduction)
- firm, ill-defined mass with skin or nipple retraction, ± tenderness
- regress spontaneously, but complete imaging ± biopsy to rule out carcinoma

Mammary Duct Ectasia
- obstruction of a subareolar duct leading to duct dilation, inflammation, and fibrosis
- may present with nipple discharge, bluish mass under nipple, local pain
- risk of secondary infection (abscess, mastitis)
- resolves spontaneously

Montgomery Tubercle
- Montgomery tubercles (or Morgagni tubercles) are papular projections at the edge of the areola
- obstruction of these glands can lead to inflammation or cystic collections (cyst of Montgomery i.e. retroareolar cyst)
- if signs of secondary infection, start treatment for mastitis
- resolves spontaneously in weeks to years

Abscess

- lactational (see Obstetrics, OB45) vs. periductal/subareolar
- unilateral localized pain, tenderness, erythema, subareolar mass, nipple discharge, nipple inversion
- rule out inflammatory carcinoma, as indicated
- treatment: initially broad-spectrum antibiotics and I&D, if persistent total duct excision (definitive)
- if mass does not resolve: U/S to assess for presence of abscess, core biopsy to exclude cancer, consider MRI

Breast Cancer

Epidemiology
- leading cancer diagnosis in women in NA, 2nd leading cause of cancer mortality in women
- 1 in 8 (12.9% life time risk) women in Canada will be diagnosed with breast cancer in their lifetime
- 1 in 30 women in Canada will die from breast cancer
- all age relative survival is 88%

Risk Factors

Gender followed by age are the two greatest risk factors for breast cancer

Any palpable dominant breast mass requires further investigation
- gender (99% female)
- age (80% >40 yr old)
- personal history of breast cancer and/or prior breast biopsy (regardless of pathology)
- family history of breast cancer (greater risk if relative was first degree and premenopausal)
- high breast density, nulliparity, first pregnancy >30 yr, menarche <12 yr, menopause >55 yr
- decreased risk with lactation, early menopause, early childbirth
- radiation exposure (e.g. mantle radiation for Hodgkin's disease)
- >5 yr HRT use, >10 yr OCP use
- BRCA1 and BRCA2 gene mutations
- alcohol use, obesity, sedentary lifestyle

Male breast cancer (<1%)
- most commonly invasive ductal carcinoma
- often diagnosed at later stages
- stage-for-stage similar prognosis to breast cancer in females
- consider genetic testing: most often hormone receptor positive

Investigations
- mammography
  - indications
    - screening guidelines (see Family Medicine, FM4)
  - findings indicative of higher risk of malignancy
    - mass that is poorly defined, spiculated border
    - microcalcifications
    - architectural distortion
    - interval mammographic changes
  - normal mammogram does not rule out suspicion of cancer based on clinical findings

- other radiographic studies
  - U/S: differentiate between cystic and solid
  - MRI: high sensitivity, low specificity
  - galactogram/ductogram (for nipple discharge): identifies lesions in ducts
  - metastatic workup indicated in Stage II-IV disease: bone scan, abdominal U/S, CXR (or CT chest/abdomen/pelvis), CT head (if specific neurological symptoms)

Diagnostic Procedures

- needle aspiration: for palpable cystic lesions; send fluid for cytology if blood or cyst does not completely resolve
- U/S or mammography guided core needle biopsy (most common)
- FNA: for palpable solid masses; need experienced practitioner for adequate sampling
- excisional biopsy: only performed as second choice to core needle biopsy; should not be done for diagnosis if possible

Diagnostic mammography is indicated in all patients, even in women <50 yr

Genetic Screening

- consider testing for BRCA1/2 if
  - patient diagnosed with breast AND ovarian cancer
  - strong family history of breast/ovarian cancer
  - family history of male breast cancer
  - young patient (<35 yr)
  - bilateral breast cancer in patients <50 yr

Phyllodes tumours are rare fibroepithelial breast tumours that can be benign or malignant that mostly affect women from 35-55 yr

Staging

- patients are assigned a clinical stage pre-operatively (cTNM); following surgery the pathologic stage is determined (pTNM)
- clinical
  - tumour size by palpation, mammogram, U/S and/or MRI
  - nodal involvement by palpation, imaging
  - metastasis by physical exam, CXR, and abdominal U/S (or CT chest/abdomen/pelvis), bone scan (usually done post-operative if node-positive disease)
- pathological
  - tumour size and type (see Pathology)
  - grade: modified Bloom and Richardson score (I to III) – histologic, nuclear, and mitotic grade
  - number of axillary nodes positive for malignancy out of total nodes resected, extranodal extension, sentinel lymph node biopsy (SLNB) positive/negative
  - tumour biology: estrogen receptor (ER), progesterone receptor (PR) and HER2/neu oncogene status
  - margins: for invasive breast cancer negative margin is sufficient, for DCIS prefer 2mm margin
  - lymphovascular invasion (LVI)
  - extensive in situ component (EIC): DCIS in surrounding tissue
  - involvement of dermal lymphatics (inflammatory) – automatically Stage IIIb

Table 23. Staging of Breast Cancer (American Joint Committee on Cancer)

Stage	Tumour	Nodes (regional) (clinical)	Metastasis	Survival (5 yr)
0	in situ	None	None	99%
I	<2 cm	None	None	94%
II A	<2 cm	Mobile ipsilateral	None	85%
II B	2-5 cm	None or mobile ipsilateral	None	70
	or >5 cm	None	None	
III A	Any size	Fixed ipsilateral or internal mammary	None	52%
III B	Skin/chest wall invasion	Any	None	48%
III C	Any size	Ipsilateral infraclavicular/internal mammary plus axillary nodes; ipsilateral supraclavicular node(s) ± axillary nodes	None	33%
IV	Any	Any	Distant	18%

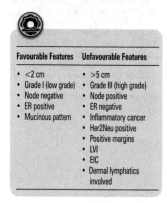

Favourable Features	Unfavourable Features
• <2 cm	• >5 cm
• Grade I (low grade)	• Grade III (high grade)
• Node negative	• Node positive
• ER positive	• ER negative
• Mucinous pattern	• Inflammatory cancer
	• Her2Neu positive
	• Positive margins
	• LVI
	• EIC
	• Dermal lymphatics involved

Pathology

NON-INVASIVE

Ductal Carcinoma in situ (DCIS)

- proliferation of malignant ductal epithelial cells completely contained within breast ducts, often multifocal
- 80% non-palpable, detected by screening mammogram
- risk of invasive ductal carcinoma in same breast up to 35% in 10 yr

Diagnosis of Breast Lesions: Fine-Needle Aspiration Cytology or Core Needle Biopsy? A Review
J Clin Pathol 2012;65:287-292
CNB
- High sensitivity (85%-100%) and specificity (86%-100%).
- High success rates for diagnosis of malignancy for palpable lesions (97%), non-palpable lesions (94%), and lesions <10 mm (90%).
- More accurate for histologic and immunohistochemistry examinations, and differentiation between in situ and invasive malignancies.
- Reliable for testing of ER, PR, and HER2 status and proliferation assessment.
- More painful procedure.

FNAC
- Variable sensitivity (35%-95%) and specificity (48%-100%).
- Quality correlates with skill of aspirator.
- Lower success rates for diagnosis of malignancy for palpable lesions (75-90%), non-palpable lesions (34-58%), and lesions <10 mm (50%).
- High rates of insufficient sampling for lesions >40 mm or calcified lesions.
- Quick to perform.
- Low technical costs.

Conclusions: FNAC is preferable for palpable, low malignancy-risk lesions. However, for potential malignancies, CNB is advantageous with respect to prognostication and prediction and is likely cost-effective in the long-term.

Analysis of Circulating Tumour DNA to Monitor Metastatic Breast Cancer
NEJM 2013;368:1199-1209
Study: The quantification of circulating tumour DNA, cancer antigen 15-3 (CA 15-3), and circulating tumour cells in 30 women with metastatic breast cancer receiving systemic therapy. The results were compared with radiographic imaging of tumours.
Results/Conclusions: Circulating tumour DNA was detected in 97% of women and showed greater correlation with changes in tumour burden than did CA 15-3 or circulating tumour cells, providing the earliest measure of treatment response in 53% of women. CA 15-3 and circulating tumour cells were detected in 78% and 87% of women, respectively. Circulating tumour DNA may therefore be an informative biomarker for metastatic breast cancer.

- treatment
  - lumpectomy with wide excision margins + radiation (5-10% risk of invasive cancer)
  - mastectomy if large area of disease, high grade, or multifocal (risk of invasive cancer reduced to 1%)
  - possibly tamoxifen as an adjuvant treatment
  - 99% 5 yr survival

Lobular Carcinoma *in situ* (LCIS)
- neoplastic cells completely contained within breast lobule
- no palpable mass, no mammographic findings, usually incidental finding on breast biopsy for another indication
- LCIS is a risk factor for invasive carcinoma (approximately 1%/yr)
- treatment
- if diagnosed on core biopsy, excisional biopsy necessary to rule out malignancy
- if diagnosed on excisional biopsy, wide excision not needed since LCIS if often multicentric and not managed as precursor lesion
- clinical follow-up and surveillance
- consider chemoprevention (e.g. tamoxifen)

INVASIVE

Invasive Ductal Carcinoma (most common 80%)
- originates from ductal epithelium and infiltrates supporting stroma
- characteristics: hard, scirrhous, infiltrating tentacles, gritty on cross-section

Invasive Lobular Carcinoma (8-15%)
- originates from lobular epithelium
- 20% bilateral (i.e. more often than infiltrating ductal carcinoma)
- does not form microcalcifications, harder to detect mammographically (may benefit from MRI)

Paget's Disease (1-3%)
- ductal carcinoma that invades nipple with scaling, eczematoid lesion

Inflammatory Carcinoma (1-4%)
- ductal carcinoma that invades dermal lymphatics
- most aggressive form of breast cancer
- clinical features: erythema, skin edema, warm, swollen, and tender breast ± lump
- peau d'orange indicates advanced disease (IIIb-IV)

Sarcomas: rare
- most commonly Phyllodes tumour, a variant of fibroadenoma with potential for malignancy
- can also be angiosarcomas – after previous radiation

Lymphoma: rare

Other
- papillary, medullary, mucinous, tubular cancers
- generally better prognosis

Treatment

Table 24. Breast Cancer Treatment by Stage

Stage	Primary Treatment Options	Adjuvant Systemic Therapy
0 (*in situ*)	BCS + radiotherapy BCS alone if margins >1 cm and low nuclear grade Mastectomy* ± SLNB	Consider post-operative tamoxifen for ER+, trastuzumab for HER2+
I	BCS + axillary node dissection + radiotherapy Mastectomy* + axillary node dissection/SLNB	May not be needed; discuss risks/benefits of chemotherapy and tamoxifen
II	BCS + axillary node dissection + radiotherapy Mastectomy* + axillary node dissection/SLNB	Chemotherapy for premenopausal women or postmenopausal and ER negative, followed by tamoxifen if ER+
III	Likely mastectomy + axillary node dissection + radiotherapy after chemotherapy (neoadjuvant)	Neoadjuvant therapy should be considered i.e. pre-operative especially if not resectable chemotherapy and/or hormone therapy. Adjuvant radiation and chemotherapy may also be appropriate (i.e. post-operative)
Inflammatory	Mastectomy + axillary node dissection + radiotherapy	Neoadjuvant therapy
IV	Surgery as appropriate for local control	Primary treatment is systemic therapy i.e. chemotherapy and/or hormone therapy

BCS = breast conserving surgery; SLNB = sentinel lymph node biopsy
*If no reason to select mastectomy, the choice between BCS + radiotherapy and mastectomy can be made according to patient's preference since choice of local treatment does not significantly affect survival if local control is achieved

PRIMARY SURGICAL TREATMENT

Breast Conservation Surgery (BCS)
- lumpectomy must be combined with radiation for survival equivalent to mastectomy
- contraindications include
    - high risk of local recurrence e.g. extensive malignant-type calcifications on mammogram, multifocal primary tumours
    - failure to obtain tumour-free margins after re-excision
    - not suitable for radiation therapy (pregnancy, previous radiation, collagen vascular disease)
    - large tumour size relative to breast

Breast conserving surgery can be offered to most women with stage I/II disease

Mastectomy
- radical mastectomy (rarely): removes all breast tissue, skin, pectoralis muscle, axillary nodes
- modified radical mastectomy (MRM): removes all breast tissue, skin, and axillary nodes
- simple mastectomy: removes all breast tissue and skin
- see Plastic Surgery, PL34 for breast reconstruction

There is no survival benefit of mastectomy over lumpectomy plus radiation for stage I and II disease

Sentinel Lymph Node Biopsy (SLNB)
- perform in women with clinically node-negative invasive breast cancer and those with extensive DCIS who are undergoing mastectomy
- patients with clinically suspicious nodes should U/S + FNA prior to decision to proceed with SLNB
- technetium-99 ± blue dye injected at tumour site prior to surgery to identify sentinel node(s)
- intra-operative frozen section evaluated can be considered
- proceed with ALND if >3 positive nodes, with 1-3 nodes whole breast radiation therapy may be alternative
- 5% false negative rate

Axillary Lymph Node Dissection (ALND)
- perform in all patients with pathologic confirmation of nodal involvement (including positive SLNB as above)
- risk of arm lymphedema (10-15%) especially if getting radiation therapy, decreased arm sensation, shoulder pain

ADJUVANT/NEOADJUVANT

Radiation
- indications
    - decrease risk of local recurrence; almost always used after BCS, sometimes after mastectomy
    - inoperable locally advanced cancer
    - axillary nodal radiation may be added if nodal involvement

Hormonal
- indications
    - ER positive plus node-positive or high-risk node-negative
    - SERM if premenopausal (e.g. tamoxifen) or aromatase inhibitors if postmenopausal (e.g. anastrozole); optimal duration 5-10 yr
    - ovarian ablation (e.g. goserelin/GnRH agonist, oophorectomy), progestins (e.g. megestrol acetate), androgens (e.g. fluoxymesterone) are other options
    - palliation for metastatic disease

Chemotherapy
- indications
    - ER negative plus node-positive or high-risk node-negative
    - ER positive and young age
    - stage I disease at high risk of recurrence (high grade, lymphovascular invasion)
    - palliation for metastatic disease
    - can consider oncotype DX (21 gene analysis) to provide recurrence score (low, intermediate, high)

FOLLOW-UP

Post-Treatment Follow-Up
- assessment and physical exam q3-6mo x 3 yr, q6-12mo x 2yr, and annually thereafter
- following BCS mammography q6-12mo; can reduce to annual once stable, no other routine imaging unless clinically indicated
- women who receive tamoxifen should have regular gynecologic follow-up (increased risk of endometrial cancer)
- psychosocial support and counselling
- delayed breast reconstruction if underwent a mastectomy

Local/Regional Recurrence
- recurrence in treated breast or ipsilateral axilla
- 1% per yr up to maximum of 15% risk of developing contralateral malignancy
- 5x increased risk of developing metastases

Metastasis
- bone > lungs > pleura > liver > brain
- treatment is palliative: hormone therapy, chemotherapy, radiation
- overall survival of metastatic breast cancer is 36-60 mo

Surgical Endocrinology

Thyroid and Parathyroid

- see Endocrinology, E20 and Otolaryngology, OT34

> **Hypertrophic Pyloric Stenosis**
> Non-bilious emesis in infant is the classic presentation

Thyroidectomy
- indications: thyroid cancer, symptomatic thyroid mass or goitre, medically refractory Graves' or hyperthyroidism
- contraindications: uncontrolled severe hyperthyroidism (i.e. Graves') due to risk of intra-operative or post-operative thyroid storm
- pre-operative workup: thyroid U/S for thyroid nodules, FNA for large nodules, U/S of the neck for lesions suspicious for papillary or medullary thyroid cancer, CT neck useful to rule out extension, vocal cord function
- complications: hypocalcemia secondary to hypoparathyroidism, recurrent/superior laryngeal nerve injury, neck hematoma, infection, thyrotoxic storm

Parathyroidectomy
- indications: symptomatic primary hyperparathyroidism due to effects of PTH on bone or kidneys, asymptomatic primary hyperparathyroidism with specific laboratory criteria (elevated serum Ca, marked hypercalciuria, Cr clearance <30% normal, bone density reduction with T score <2.5, <50 yr)
- contraindications: familial hypocalciuric hypercalcemia
- pre-operative workup: 99mTc sestamibi scanning, ± SPECT or CT, U/S
- complications: recurrent/superior laryngeal nerve injury, post-operative hypocalcemia, infection, bleeding

Adrenal Gland

- see Endocrinology, E29
- functional anatomy
  - cortex: glomerulosa (mineralocorticoids), fasciculata (glucocorticoids), reticularis (sex steroids)
  - medulla: catecholamines (epinephrine, norepinephrine)
- types of adrenal tumours: functional (e.g. Cushing's syndrome, Conn's syndrome) or non-functional

INCIDENTALOMA
- adrenal mass discovered by investigation of unrelated symptoms

Epidemiology
- benign adenoma (38%) > metastases to adrenal (22%) >> cyst, carcinoma, pheochromocytoma, neuroblastoma
- metastasis to adrenal gland from: lung > breast, colon, lymphoma, melanoma, kidney
- peak incidence of carcinoma: females age 50-60, risk decreases with increasing age and male gender

Investigations
- MRI, CT: size >6 cm is best predictor of primary adrenal carcinoma (92% are >6 cm)
- functional studies
  - pheochromocytoma: 24 h urine epinephrine, norepinephrine, metanephrine, normetanephrine, VMA (vanillylmandelic acid)
  - Cushing's: 24 h urine cortisol or 1 mg overnight dexamethasone suppression test
  - aldosteronoma: electrolytes, aldosterone:renin level, saline suppression test if appropriate
  - adrenal androgens: 17-OH progesterone, DHEAS
- FNA biopsy: if suspect metastasis to adrenal (must exclude pheochromocytoma first to prevent a hypertensive crisis)
  - indicated if history of cancer or patient is smoker
- iodocholesterol scintigraphy: may distinguish benign vs. malignant disease

Treatment
- functional tumour: resect
- non-functional tumour
  - >4 cm: resect
  - <4 cm: follow-up imaging in 6-12 mo, resect if >1 cm enlargement

Pancreas

INSULINOMA
- tumour that secretes insulin
- most common pancreatic endocrine neoplasm; 10% associated with MEN1 syndrome

Clinical Features
- Whipple's triad
- palpitations, trembling, diaphoresis, confusion, seizure, personality changes

Investigations
- blood work: decreased serum glucose and increased serum insulin and C-peptide
- U/S, CT: insulinomas evenly distributed throughout head, body, tail of pancreas

Treatment
- only 10% are malignant
- enucleation of solitary insulinomas may be done endoscopically
- tumours >2 cm located close to the pancreatic duct may require pancreatectomy or pancreaticoduodenectomy

GASTRINOMA
- tumour secreting gastrin; cause of Zollinger-Ellison syndrome

Clinical Features
- abdominal pain, PUD, severe esophagitis
- multiple ulcers in atypical locations refractory of antacid therapy

Investigations
- blood work: serum gastrin levels (usually >1,000 pg/mL), secretin stimulation test
- U/S, CT: 70-90% found in Passaro's triangle (head of pancreas medially, 2nd portion of duodenum inferiorly, and the confluence of the cystic and CBD superiorly)
- octreotide scintigraphy scan

Treatment
- 50% are malignant
- surgical resection of tumour dependent on location
- non-surgical treatment: chemotherapy, somatostatin analogues, interferon, chemoembolization
- if inoperable, vagotomy can be performed for symptomatic control

VASOACTIVE INTESTINAL PEPTIDE-SECRETING TUMOUR
- tumour secreting VIP; commonly located in the distal pancreas and most are malignant when diagnosed

Clinical Features
- severe watery diarrhea causing dehydration, weakness, electrolyte imbalance

Investigations
- blood work: serum VIP levels
- U/S, CT

Treatment
- somatostatin analogues
- surgical resection/palliative debulking

Whipple's Triad
- Symptomatic fasting hypoglycemia
- Serum glucose <50 mg/dL
- Relief of symptoms when glucose is administered

Rule of 2s for Meckel's Diverticulum
- **2%** of the population
- **2:1** male-to-female ratio
- Symptomatic in **2%** of cases
- Found within **2** feet (10-90 cm) of the ileocecal (IC) valve
- **2** inches in length
- **2** inches in diameter
- **2** types of tissue (gastric, pancreatic)
- Often present by **2** yr of age

Pediatric Surgery

Condition	Epidemiology and Risk Factors	Pathophysiology	Clinical Features and History	Physical Exam	Investigations	Treatment	Prognosis
Hydrocele (see Urology, U29)	1-2% of live births Present at birth, majority close spontaneous by 1 yr M:F = 6:1 Prematurity	**Communicating hydroceles:** processus vaginalis fails to close with small opening for fluid to move freely between peritoneal cavity through patent processus (if opening progresses to allow passage of intestine, it is a hernia) **Noncommunicating hydroceles:** fluid trapped in tunica vaginalis; in older children, may be secondary to testicular pathology (reactive hydrocele)	Painless scrotal mass Communicating hydroceles increase in size with standing or valsalva, may be absent in the morning and large in the evening	Transillumination suggests hydrocele Silk glove sign: gently palpating hydrocele sac over pubic tubercle feels like rubbing silk on silk	U/S if suspect pathology	Most resolve spontaneously by 1 yr Surgical repair if: Persistence >2 yr Pain Fluctuating in size which suggests communication Cosmetic reasons Infection	<2% recurrence
Hypertrophic Pyloric Stenosis	0.03-1.0% of live births Can present at 1-20 wk, most commonly at 6-8 wk M:F = 4:1 Early erythromycin exposure (<13 d old)	Acquired pyloric circular muscle hypertrophy results in gastric outlet obstruction Hypovolemia caused by emesis of gastric contents causes hypochloremic hypokalemic metabolic alkalosis Electrolyte exchange based volume retention in kidneys results in paradoxical aciduria	Projectile non-bilious vomiting Vomiting 30-60 min after feeds Hungry after vomiting Dehydration (variable severity)	Smooth oblong 1-2 cm mass palpable above umbilicus, "olive" visible left-to-right gastric contraction "waves" after feeding	Electrolytes (assess hypochloremia, dehydration) U/S shows pyloric length >14 mm, muscle thickness >4 mm Upper GI series necessary only when U/S unavailable or non-diagnostic will show "string sign"	Fluid resuscitate with normal saline, correct electrolyte and acid/base abnormalities with D5, 1/2NS + 20 mEq/L KCl at maintenance rate NGT decompression unnecessary Pyloromyotomy, open (Ramstedt vs. transumbilical or laparoscopic approach) Alternative therapies such as TPN/wait or atropine impractical due to long time course of effect	Pyloromyotomy curative
Congenital Diaphragmatic Hernias 3 types: Posterolateral (Bochdalek) Left-sided, 85% Right-sided, 13% Bilateral, rare, often fatal Anterior (Morgagni) Hiatus	1 in 2,000 to 5,000 live births Presents within hours of life although some cases of delayed presentation M=F >10% are associated with other congenital anomalies Prenatal diagnosis common	**Left-sided:** small bowel, large bowel, stomach, and solid viscera (spleen, left lobe of liver) herniate into thorax **Right-sided:** liver, large bowel herniate into thorax Pulmonary hypoplasia Pulmonary HTN	Early respiratory distress Cyanosis Scaphoid abdomen Prenatal diagnosis	Decreased air entry ± bowel sounds in the chest Displaced heart sounds	Prenatal US/MRI ABG CXR (bowel loops in hemithorax, shifted heart) Echocardiography Genetic consultation if warranted	Intubate Orogastric suction Period of respiratory stabilization due to associated pulmonary hypoplasia (may require ECMO) Surgical repair after stable by hernia reduction and closure of diaphragmatic defect – open vs. thoracoscopic vs. laparoscopic with or without prosthetic or muscular patch depending on size of defect	Better outcomes in later presentations Hearing deficit (40%) Associated GERD MSK defects – chest wall and scoliotic defects a potential complication of thoracotomy Long-term surveillance for potential recurrence Failure to thrive Chronic lung disease if severe hypoplasia
Meckel's Diverticulum Most common remnant of vitelline duct that connects yolk sac with primitive midgut	1-3% of population M:F = 3:1 Present most frequently during first 5 yr of life Symptomatic in 2% of cases	Failure of vitelline duct to regress 5-7 wk in utero; 50% contain heterotopic tissue (e.g. gastric mucosa, ectopic pancreas); other associated anomalies include omphalomesenteric fistula, umbilical sinus, umbilical cyst, fibrous band	BRBPR (heterotopic gastric mucosa in Meckel's causing mucosal ulceration and bleeding in adjacent small bowel mucosa) Abdominal sepsis (Meckel's diverticulitis ± perforation) Small bowel volvulus around fibrous band	Tenderness (lower abdomen) near umbilicus	AXR Meckel scan: scan for ectopic gastric mucosa with technetium Tc99m pertechnetate IV (sensitivity 85%, specificity 95%)	Stabilize, resection by laparotomy or laparoscopy ± incidental appendectomy	Resection curative

Condition	Epidemiology and Risk Factors	Pathophysiology	Clinical Features and History	Physical Exam	Investigations	Treatment	Prognosis
Malrotation	1:500 live births 1/3 present by 1 wk of age, 3/4 by 1 mo of age, 90% by 1 yr of age M:F = 1:1; higher incidence among patients with cardiac anomalies, heterotaxy syndromes	Failure of gut to normally rotate around SMA with associated abnormal intestinal attachments and anatomic positions Represent a spectrum of rotational abnormalities including complete non-rotation (which is not at high risk for volvulus)	Bilious emesis is THE cardinal sign, especially if abdomen nondistended If bilious emesis in ill child with distended abdomen, consider surgical exploration to rule out volvulus Rectal bleed (late/ominous signs) Intermittent symptoms	Bilious drainage from NGT Tachycardic, pale Diaphoretic Flat abdomen Tenderness	AXR: obstruction of proximal SBO, double-bubble sign, intestinal wall thickened Immediate UGI: dilated duodenum, duodenojejunal segment (Ligament of Treitz) right of midline and not fixed posteriorly over spinal column, "corkscrew" sign indicating volvulus U/S: "whirlpool" sign, abnormal SMA/SMV relationship indicates UGI to rule out rotational anomalies	IV antibiotics Fluid resuscitation EMERGENT LAPAROTOMY Ladd procedure: counterclockwise reduction of midgut volvulus, division of Ladd's bands, division of peritoneal attachments between cecum and abdominal wall that obstruct duodenum, broadening of the mesentery (open folded mesentery like a book and divide congenital adhesions), ± appendectomy Positioning the bowel into non-rotation (SBO in right abdomen, LBO in left abdomen)	Mortality related to length of bowel loss: 10% necrosis – 100% survival rate, 75% necrosis – 35% survival rate Recurrence 2-6%
Gastroschisis	1:2,000 live births Antenatal diagnosis common Increases with younger maternal age and associated with IUGR M:F = 1:1	Defect of abdominal wall, with free extrusion of intestine into amniotic cavity No specific environmental factor identified Defect in embryogenesis unclear	Not associated with genetic syndromes 10% with intestinal atresia Some cases associated with short bowel syndrome due to antenatal volvulus and necrosis of herniated bowel	Hollow viscera (stomach, small and large bowels) Defect lateral to cord (usually right) Bowel may be inflamed, thickened, matted, foreshortened Defect size variable	Prenatal U/S Elevated MS-AFP	NGT decompression IV fluids IV antibiotics Keep viscera moist and protected until surgical reduction with primary abdominal closure or staged closure with silo May have bowel dysmotility requiring motility medications	>90% survival rate
Omphalocele	1:5,000 live birth Antenatal diagnosis common Lower gestational age Increased maternal age M:F = 1.5:1	Defect of abdominal wall, with extrusion of sac covered viscera (amnion, Wharton's jelly, peritoneum) Duhamel's theory – failure of body wall morphogenesis	Associated with genetic syndromes 30-70% (e.g. Pentalogy of Cantrell, congenital heart disease, Beckwith-Wiedemann syndrome) Associated pulmonary hypoplasia	Hollow viscera (stomach, small and large bowels, often liver) Cord on the sac	Prenatal U/S Elevated MS-AFP	NGT decompression IV fluids, IV antibiotics Small defect (<2 cm): Primary closure Medium (2-4 cm) and large (>4 cm) defects: silver sulfadiazine coupled with compression dressing to allow epithelialization and gradual reduction, followed by future repair ±mesh	40-70% survival rate Higher survival rates most likely related to antenatal mortality of fetuses with giant omphaloceles
Umbilical Hernias	Incidence 2-14% Increases with prematurity Decreases with increasing age	Incomplete closure of peritoneal and fascial layers within umbilicus by 5 yr	Majority asymptomatic Majority spontaneously resolve by age 5 Incarceration prior to age 5 very rare Most symptoms occur in late adolescence or adulthood	Protrusion from umbilicus Different from less common abdominal wall hernias that do not spontaneously resolve (e.g. epigastric hernias) Most defects >1.5 cm in infancy will not close spontaneously	None if uncomplicated	Repair if not spontaneously closed by age 5 Earlier repair of large "proboscoid" hernias with extensive skin stretching may be warranted for cosmetic reasons Simple primary closure of fascial defect	Low risk of recurrence
Intestinal Atresia	Incidence 2-14% May be antenatally diagnosed by dilated bowel loops or "double-bubble" sign on x-ray for duodenal atresia Decreased with increasing age	Duodenal – failure of bowel to recanalize after endodermal epithelium proliferation (wk 8-10) Jejunal/ileal – acquired as a result of vascular disruption → ischemic necrosis → resorption of necrotic tissue → blind distal and proximal ends Colonic – mechanism unknown, thought to be similar to small bowel atresia	Gastric distension and vomiting (usually bilious) Duodenal – may be associated with other anomalies (tracheoesophageal fistula, cardiac, renal, and vertebral anomalies), 24-28% have Down syndrome Jejunal/ileal – within 2 d of birth, may be associated with CF Colonic – within 3 d of birth	Complete physical Special attention to abdominal exam Perineum and anus Include evaluation of respiratory distress and signs of volume depletion Congenital anomalies Jaundice	Contrast enema ± UGI with small bowel follow through (SBFT) Group and screen INR and PTT if for surgery	NPO NGT decompression Fluid resuscitate TPN Broad spectrum antibiotics Duodenal – duodenoduodenostomy or duodenojejunostomy Jejunal/ileal – primary anastomosis; or if atresia associated with short bowel then may create end stoma or defer surgery for bowel lengthening procedures Colonic – primary anastomosis	Long-term survival Duodenal – 86% Jejunal/ileal – 84% Colonic – 100%

Condition	Epidemiology and Risk Factors	Pathophysiology	Clinical Features and History	Physical Exam	Investigations	Treatment	Prognosis
Hirschsprung's Disease	1:5,000 births M:F = 3:1 to 4:1, approaches 1:1 when whole colon involved Can have aganglionosis of small bowel as well Familial Hirschsprung's in <5% of cases	Defect in migration of neurocrest cells to intestine resulting in aganglionic bowel that fails to peristalse and internal sphincter that fails to relax (internal anal sphincter achalasia) causing functional and partial mechanical obstruction, respectively; always starts in the rectum and variable involvement proximally; RET mutation	Failure to pass meconium spontaneously within 48 h of life is the classic history (95% pass meconium within 24h, 5% within 48h) Symptoms of bowel obstruction: abdominal distension, constipation, bilious emesis Enterocolitis/sepsis Failure to thrive	± abdominal distension Squirt/blast sign	Rectal biopsy (gold standard) – look for aganglionosis and neural hypertrophy AXR Contrast enema to find narrow rectum and transition zone Anal manometry unreliable in infants – classic finding is absence of rectoanal inhibitory reflex	Surgical resection of aganglionic intestinal segment and anastomosis of remaining intestine to anus Either in newborn period or staged if extensive aganglionosis	Most have normal/ near-normal anorectal function Complications: Fecal incontinence and constipation, post-operative enterocolitis (medical emergency if progresses to sepsis)
Cryptorchidism	2-5% of term males – most of these descend spontaneously by 6mo of age 1% of males do not spontaneously descend	Idiopathic Descent is mediated by descendin which is created in response to testosterone Descent usually begins at 28 wk	Palpable testicle within inguinal canal or testicle which can be milked down into scrotum (called retractile testis) Occasionally no palpable testis as it is intra-abdominal Consider other congenital abnormalities	Bi-annual testicular exam with palpation Distinguish truly undescended testis from retractile testis (which is "high" testis due to hyperactive cremasteric muscles)	Depends on age of presentation U/S or MRI if no palpable testis Older child: LH, FSH, MIS, hCG stimulation test for gonadotropin production Infant: U/S, FSH, LH, karyotype, MIS, 17-hydroxy-progesterone	hCG to stimulate testosterone production and descent Orchidopexy – especially if undescended by age 6 mo-2 yr	Orchidopexy Decreased risk of torsion and blunt trauma to testicle No effect on malignant potential of testicle Descent can preserve spermatogenesis if performed by 1 yr of age
Intussusception	Most common cause of bowel obstruction between 6-36 mo 26:100,000 newborns M:F = 3:2 Pathologic lead points: enlarged Peyer's patches due to viral infections of the GI tract, polyps, Meckel's diverticulum CF, lymphoma, IBD may increase risk	Idiopathic is most common Usually starts at ileocecal junction Telescoping of bowel into itself causing an obstruction and vascular compromise	Acute onset of abdominal pain which is classic episodic "colicky" pain Vomiting ± bilious Abdominal mass Currant-jelly stool suggests mucosal necrosis and sloughing	Abdominal exam Palpate for masses (especially sausage shaped upper abdominal mass) and tenderness Signs of bowel obstruction: distended abdomen Look for localized peritonitis which suggests transmural ischemia	AXR for signs of bowel obstruction or perforation U/S if suspect pathology	If peritonitis, then consider operative management Non-operative management involves reduction via air contrast enema Operative reduction can be done open or laparoscopically Resection of involved colon if failure to reduce or bowel appears compromised	10% recurrence rate If recurrent = more likely non-idiopathic If successfully reduced by enema in older children allow 2wk resolution of edema then perform SBFT to rule out pathologic lead points
Tracheoesophageal Fistula (TEF)	1:3,000-1:4,500	Associated anomalies in 50%: VACTERL association (see Pediatrics, P40)	Varies with type of fistula May have history of maternal polyhydramnios May present after several months (if no associated esophageal atresia) of non-bilious vomiting, coughing, cyanosis with feeds, respiratory distress, recurrent pneumonia, frothy bubbles of mucus in mouth and nose that return after suctioning		X-ray: anatomic abnormalities, NGT curled in pouch	Investigate for other congenital anomalies, early repair by surgical ligation to prevent lung damage and maintain nutrition and growth	Complications: pneumonia, sepsis, reactive airways disease Following repair: esophageal stenosis and strictures at repair site, GERD and poor swallowing (i.e. dysphagia, regurgitation)
Inguinal Hernias	5% of all term newborns 2x risk and more likely bilateral if pre-term M:F = 4:1 Low birth weight increases risk 1/5 inguinal hernias will become incarcerated if patient is <1 yr old Incarceration is more common in females Associated with other conditions: androgen insensitivity, connective tissue diseases	All infant hernias are indirect: descent of intra-abdominal contents through the internal inguinal ring through a patent tunica vaginalis	Most common presentation: painless intermittent mass in groin, may also note extension into scrotum (scrotal mass in absence of inguinal mass is a hydrocele) If incarcerated: tender, vomiting, firm mass, erythema then cyanosis of mass may be noted	Palpate for "bag of worms" suggests possible testicular varicocele Biannual testicular exam + palpation along inguinal canal to evaluate for any masses "Silk sign" – palpable thickening of cord Mass palpated at external inguinal ring and reducible through inguinal canal into abdomen Must always try reduction to confirm that hernia is not incarcerated	Physical exam is gold standard U/S only if physical exam uncertain (e.g. in small infants where exam can be difficult)	Manual reduction – to relieve acute symptoms Herniorraphy – definitive treatment by reduction of herniated contents and high ligation of sac for indirect hernias Laparoscopic or open techniques	Risk of recurrence after surgical reduction <3% but higher if repair done in premature infants or if hernia was incarcerated/ strangulated at repair

Skin Lesions

- see Dermatology, D5; Emergency Medicine, ER17; Plastic Surgery, PL5

Common Medications

All inguinal hernias of infancy and childhood require repair at the earliest convenience; emergent repair if incarcerated/strangulated

Antiemetics
- dimenhydrinate (Gravol®) 25-50 mg PO/IV/IM q4-6h prn
- prochlorperazine (Stemetil®) 5-10 mg PO/IV/IM bid-tid prn
- metoclopramide (Maxeran®) 10 mg IV/IM q2-3h prn, 10-15 mg PO qid (30 min before meals and qhs)
- ondansetron (Zofran®) 4-8 mg PO q8h prn
- granisetron (Kytril®) 1 mg PO bid (for nausea from chemotherapy/radiation)

Analgesics
- acetaminophen ± codeine (Tylenol® #3/plain) 1-2 tabs q4-6h PO/PR prn
- hydromorphone i-ii tabs PO q4h prn, 0.5-2 mg IV q3-4h prn
- ibuprofen 200-400 mg PO q4-6h prn
- morphine 2.5-10 mg IM/SC q4-6h prn + 1-2 mg IV q1h prn for breakthrough
- ketorolac (Toradol®) 30-60 mg IM/IV q6h prn
- Percocet® (acetaminophen/oxycodone, 325/5 mg) 1-2 tabs PO q4-6h prn

DVT Prophylaxis
- heparin 5,000 units SC bid, if cancer patient then heparin 5,000 units SC tid
- dalteparin (Fragmin®) 5,000 units SC daily
- enoxaparin (Lovenox®) 40 mg SC daily

Antidiarrheals
- loperamide (Imodium®) 4 mg PO initially, then 2 mg PO after each loose stool up to 16 mg/d
- diphenoxylate + atropine (Lomotil®) 2 tabs/10 mL PO qid

Laxatives
- sennosides (Senokot®) 1-2 tabs qhs
- docusate sodium (Colace®) 100 mg PO bid
- glycerine suppository 1 tab PR prn
- lactulose 15-30 mL PO qid prn
- milk of magnesia (MOM) 30-60 mL PO qid prn
- bisacodyl (Dulcolax®)10-15 mg PO prn

Sedatives
- zopiclone (Imovane®) 5-7.5 mg PO qhs prn
- lorazepam (Ativan®) 0.5-2 mg PO/SL qhs prn

Antibiotics
- cefazolin (Ancef®) 1 g IV/IM on call to OR or q8h – GP except *Enterococcus*, GN only *E. coli, Klebsiella,* and *Proteus*
- cefalexin (Keflex®) 250-500 mg PO qid – *Listeria*, GP except *Enterococcus*, GN only *E. coli, Klebsiella,* and *Proteus*
- ceftriaxone 1-2 g IM/IV q24h – broad coverage including *Pseudomonas*
- ampicillin 1-2 g IV q4-6h – *Listeria*, GP (*Enteroccus*) except *Streptococcus* and *E. coli*, oral anaerobes except *Bacteroides*
- gentamicin 3-5 mg/kg/d IM/IV divided q8h; monitor creatinine, gentamicin levels – GN including *Pseudomonas*
- ciprofloxacin 400 mg IV q12h, 500 mg PO bid – GN including *Pseudomonas*
- metronidazole (Flagyl®) 500 mg PO/IV bid (500 mg PO tid for *C. difficile*) – anaerobes
- clindamycin 600-900 mg IV q8h, 150-400 mg PO qid – GP except *Enterococcus*, anaerobes
- piperacillin/tazobactam 4.5 mg IV q6h – GP, GN, and anaerobes
- vancomycin 1g IV q12h – GP and MRSA
- sulfamethoxazole/trimethoprim DS (Septra®) PO bid – GP, GN including *Nocardia*

Over-the-Counter Medications
- Pepto-Bismol® (bismuth subsalicylate) 2 tabs or 30 mL PO q30min-1h up to 8 doses/d
  side effects: black stools, risk of Reye's syndrome in children
- Alka-Seltzer® (ASA + citrate + bicarbonate) 2 tabs in 4 oz water PO q4h prn, max 8 tabs
- Maalox® (aluminum hydroxide + magnesium hydroxide) 10-20 mL or 1-4 tabs PO prn
- Tums® (calcium carbonate) 1-3 g PO q2h prn
- Rolaids® (calcium carbonate and magnesium hydroxide) 2-4 tabs PO q1h prn, max 12 tabs/d

References

Alexander JW, Solomkin JS, Edwards MJ. Updated recommendations for control of surgical site infections. Ann Surg 2001;253:1082-1093.
Amato B, Moja L, Panico S, et al. Shouldice technique versus other open techniques for inguinal hernia repair. Cochrane DB Syst Rev 2012;4:CD001543.
Andersen BR, Kallehave FL, Andersen HK. Antibiotics versus placebo for prevention of post-operative infection after appendicectomy. Cochrane DB Syst Rev 2005;3:CD001439.
Andrén-Sandberg A. Diagnosis and management of gallbladder cancer. N Am J Med Sci. 2012;4:293-299.
Antimicrobial prophylaxis for surgery. Treat Guidel Med Lett 2009;7:47-52.
Applegate KE. Intussusception in children: evidence-based diagnosis and treatment. Pediatr Radiol 2009;39(Suppl 2):S140-143.
Aqzarian J, Miller JD, Kosa SD, et al. Long-term survival analysis of the Canadian lung volume reduction surgery trial. Ann Thorac Surg 2013;96:1217-1222.
Arnold DT, Reed JB, Burt K. Evaluation and management of the incidental adrenal mass. Proc (Bayl Univ Med Cent) 2003;16:7-12.
Bazarah BM, Peltekian KM, McAlister VC, et al. Utility of MELD and Child-Turcotte-Pugh scores and the Canadian waitlisting algorithm in predicting short-term survival after liver transplant. Clin Invest Med 2004;27:162-167.
Bhangu A, Singh P, Lundy J, et al. Systemic review and meta-analysis of randomized clinical trials comparing primary vs. delayed primary skin closure in contaminated and dirty abdominal incisions. JAMA Surg 2013;148:779-786.
Bland KI. The practice of general surgery, 1st ed. Toronto: WB Saunders, 2002.
Brandt ML. Pediatric hernias. Surg Clin N Am 2008;88:27-43,vii-viii.
Brunicardi FC, Andersen D, Billiar T, et al. Schwartz's principles of surgery, 9th ed. McGraw-Hill, 2010.
Canadian Task Force on Preventive Health Care. Colorectal cancer screening. CMAJ 2001;165:206-208.
Chandler CF, Lane JS, Fergusoan P, et al. Prospective evaluation of early versus delayed laparoscopic cholecystectomy for treatment of acute cholecystitis. Am J Surg 2000;66:896-900.
Cholongitas E, Burroughs AK. The evolution in the prioritization for liver transplantation. Ann Gastroenterol 2012;25:6-13.
Coha M, Cerutti E, Schellino MM, et al. Piedmont Intensive Care Units Network (PICUN). Continuous positive airway pressure for treatment of post-operative hypoxemia: a randomized controlled trial. JAMA 2005;293:589-595.
Colquitt JL, Picot J, Loveman E, et al. Surgery for obesity. Cochrane DB Syst Rev 2009;2:CD003641.
Darwish MS, Kim WR, Harnois DM, et al. Efficacy of neoadjuvant chemoradiation followed by liver transplantation, for perihilar cholangiocarcinoma at 12 US centers. Gastroenterology 2012;143:88-98.e3.
Dawson SJ, Tsui DW, Murtaza M, et al. Analysis of circulating tumor DNA to monitor metastatic breast cancer. NEJM 2013;368:1199-1209.
Dodson MK, Magann EF, Meeks GR. A randomized comparison of secondary closure and secondary intention in patients with superficial wound dehiscence. Obstet Gynecol 1992;80:321-324.
Darouiche RO, Wall MJ Jr, Itani KM, et al. Chlorhexidine-alcohol versus povidone-iodine for surgical-site antisepsis. NEJM 2010;362:18-26.
de Groen PC, Gores GJ, LaRusso NF, et al. Biliary tract cancers. NEJM 1999;341:1368-1378.
Doherty GM. Current surgical diagnosis and treatment, 12th ed. New York: McGraw-Hill, 2006.
Duncan CB, Riall TS. Evidence-based current surgical practice: calculous gallbladder disease. J Gastrointest Surg 2012;16:2011-2025.
Eagon JC, Miedema BW, Kelly KA. Postgastrectomy syndromes. Surg Clin N Am 1992;72:445.
Edell SL, Eisen MD. Current imaging modalities for the diagnosis of breast cancer. Delaware Med J 1999;71:377-382.
Ferzoco LB, Raptopoulos V, Silen W. Acute diverticulitis. NEJM 1998;338:1521-1526.
Fitzgibbons RJ Jr, Giobbie-Hurder A, Gibbs JO, et al. Watchful waiting vs. repair of inguinal hernia in minimally symptomatic men: a randomized clinical trial. JAMA 2006;295:285-292.
Gamme G, Birch DW, Karmali S. Minimally invasive splenectomy: an update and review. Can J Surg 2013;56:280-285.
García-Miguel FJ, Serrano-Aguilar PG, López-Bastida J. Preoperative assessment. Lancet 2003;362(9397):1749.
Germani G, Gurusamy K, Garcovich M, et al. Which matters most: number of tumors, size of the largest tumor, or total tumor volume? Liver Transplant 2011;Suppl2:S58-66.
Gibril F, Reynolds JC, Lubensky IA, et al. Ability of somatostatin receptor scintigraphy to identify patients with gastric carcinoids: a prospective study. J Nucl Med 2000;41:1646-1656.
Glasgow RE, Mulvihill SJ. Postgastrectomy syndromes. Probl Gen Surg 1997;14:132-152.
Goldhirsh A, Glick JH, Gelber RD, et al. Meeting highlights: International Consensus Panel on the treatment of primary breast cancer. J Clin Oncol 2001;19:3817-3827.
Graham DJ, McHenry CR. The adrenal incidentaloma: guidelines for evaluation and recommendations for management. Surg Onc Clin N Am1998;7:749-764.
Gurusamy KS, Koti R, Fusai G, et al. Early vs. delayed laparoscopic cholecystectomy for uncomplicated biliary colic. Cochrane DB Syst Rev 2013;6:CD007196.
Hilditch WG, Asbury AJ, Jack E, et al. Validation of a pre-anaesthetic screening questionnaire. Anaesthesia 2003;58:874-877.
Hong Z, Wu J, Smart G, et al. Survival analysis of liver transplant patients in Canada 1997-2002. Transplant Proc 2006;38(9):2951-2956.
Hutson JM, Balic A, Nation T, et al. Cryptorchidism. Semin Pediat Surg 2010;19:215-224.
Ingraham AM, Cohen ME, Bilimoria KY, et al. Effect of delay to operation on outcomes in adults with acute appendicitis. Arch Surg 2010;145:886-892.
Ivanovich JL, Read TE, Ciske DJ, et al. A practical approach to familial and hereditary colorectal cancer. Am J Med 1999;107:68-77.
Jannë PA, Mayer RJ. Chemoprevention of colorectal cancer. NEJM 2000;342:1960-198.
Jarrell BE, Carabasi RA. NMS Surgery, 5th ed. Philidelphia: Lippincott Williams & Wilkins, 2008.
Johnson CD. Upper abdominal pain: gallbladder. BMJ 2001;323:1170-1173.
Kanwal F, Dulai GS, Spiegel BMR, et al. A comparison of liver transplantation outcomes in the pre- vs. post-MELD eras. Aliment Pharm Ther 2005;21:169-177.
Kasper DL. Harrison's principles of internal medicine, 16th ed. 2005.
Kehlet H, Holte K. Review of post-operative ileus. Am J Surg 2001;182(Suppl):3S-10S.
Kemeny MM, Adak S, Gray B, et al. Combined-modality treatment for resectable metastatic colorectal carcinoma to the liver: surgical resection of hepatic metastases in combination with continuous infusion of chemotherapy – an intergroup study. J Clin Oncol 2002;20:1499-1505.
King JE, Dozois RR, Lindor NM, et al. Care of patients and their families with familial adenomatous polyposis. Mayo Clin Proc 2000;75:57-67.
Kittaneh M, Montero AJ, Gluck S. Molecular profiling for breast cancer: a comprehensive review. Biomark Cancer 2013;5:61-70.
Latif A. Gastric cancer update on diagnosis, staging and therapy. Postgrad Med 1997;102:231-236.
Lawrence PF. Essentials of general surgery. Philadelphia: Lippincott Williams & Wilkins, 2000.
Levine CD. Toxic megacolon: diagnosis and treatment challenges. AACN Clinical Issues 1999;10:492-499.
Li CI, Anderson BO, Daling JR, et al. Trends in incidence rates of invasive lobular and ductal breast carcinoma. JAMA 2003;289:1421-1424.
Liang MK, Berger RL, Li LT, et al. Outcomes of laparoscopic vs open repair of primary ventral hernias. JAMA Surg 2013;148:1043-1048.
Lickstein LH, Matthews JB. Elective surgical management of peptic ulcer disease. Probl Gen Surg 1997;14:37-53.
Maden AK, Aliabadi-Wahle S, Tesi D, et al. How early is early laparoscopic treatment of acute cholecystitis? Am J Surg 2002;183:232-236.
Mandel JS, Bond JH, Church TR, et al. Reducing mortality from colorectal cancer by screening for fecal occult blood. Minnesota Colon Cancer Control Study. NEJM 1993;328:1365-1371.
Mandel JS, Church TR, Bond JH, et al. The effect of fecal occult blood screening on the incidence of colorectal cancer. NEJM 2000;343:1603-1607.
Mamounas EP. NSABP breast cancer clinical trials: recent results and future directions. Clin Med Res 2003;1:309-326.
Martin RF, Rossi RL. The acute abdomen: an overview and algorithms. Surg Clin N Am 1997;77:1227-1243.
Mills P, Sever A, Weeks J, et al. Axillary ultrasound asessement in primary breast cancer: an audit of 653 cases. Breat J 2010:16(5):460.
Moore KL, Dalley AF, Agur AMR. Clinically oriented anatomy, 6th ed. Philadelphia: Lippincott Williams and Wilkins, 2010.
Paulson EK, Kalady MF, Pappas TN. Suspected appendicitis. NEJM 2003;348:236-242.
Penner RM, Majumdar SR. Diagnostic approach to abdominal pain in adults. Rose BD (editor). Waltham: UpToDate. 2013.
Polk H, Christmas B. Prophylactic antibiotics in surgery and surgical wound infections. Am Surgeon 2000;66:105-111.
Preoperative antibiotic prophylaxis. CDC. Available from: http://www.cdc.gov/ncidod/hip/SSI/SSI.pdf.
Ransohoff DF, Sandler RS. Screening for colorectal cancer. NEJM 2002;346:40-44.
Ravikumar R, Williams JG. The operative management of gallstone ileus. Ann R Coll Surg Engl 2010;92:279-281.
Ray BS, Neill CL. Abdominal visceral sensation in man. Ann Surg 1947;126:709-723.
Ronellenfitsch U, Schwarzbach M, Hofheinz R, et al. Perioperative chemo(radio)therapy versus primary surgery for resectable adenocarcinoma of the stomach, gastroesophageal junction, and lower esophagus. Cochrane DB Syst Rev 2013;5:CD008107.
Roy MA. Inflammatory bowel disease. Surg Clin N Am 1997;77:1419-1431.
Rubin BP, Heinrich MC, Corless CL. Gastrointestinal stromal tumour. Lancet 2007;369:1731-1741.
Rustgi AK. Hereditary gastrointestinal polyposis and nonpolyposis syndromes. NEJM 1994;331:1694-1702.
Sandhu L, Sandroussi C, Guba M, et al. Living donor liver transplantation versus deceased donor liver transplantation for hepatocellular carcinoma: comparable survival and recurrence. Liver Transplant 2012;18:315-322.
Sauerland S, Jaschinski T, Neugebauer EA. Laparoscopic versus open surgery for suspected appendicitis. Cochrane DB Syst Rev 2010;10:CD001546.
Sheth SG, LaMont JT. Toxic megacolon. Lancet 1998;351:509-513.
Simeone DM, Hassan A, Scheiman JM. Giant peptic ulcer: a surgical or medical disease? Surgery 1999;126:474-478.
Styblo TM, Wood WC. The management of ductal and lobular breast cancer. Surg Oncol 1999;8:67-75.
The Canadian Task Force on Preventive Health Care. Recommendations on screening for breast cancer in average-risk women aged 40-74 years. CMAJ 2011;183:1991-2001.
Tseng JF, Tamm EP, Lee JE, et al. Venous resection in pancreatic cancer surgery. Best Pract Res Clin Gastroenterol 2006;20:349-64.
Waki K. UNOS Liver Registry: ten year survivals. Clin Transplant 2006:29-39.
Way LW. Current surgical diagnosis and treatment, 11th ed. 2003.
Willems SM, van Deurzen CH, van Diest PJ. Diagnosis of breast lesions: fine-needle aspiration cytology or core needle biopsy? A review. J Clin Pathol 2012;65:287-92.
Yadav D, Agarwal N, Pitchumoni CS. A critical evaluation of laboratory tests in acute pancreatitis. Am J Gastroenterol 2002;97:1309-1318.

GM | Geriatric Medicine

Keith Lee and **Harry Zhou**, chapter editors
Claudia Frankfurter and **Inna Gong**, associate editors
Brittany Prevost and **Robert Vanner**, EBM editors
Dr. Vicky Chau and **Dr. Barry J. Goldlist**, staff editors

Acronyms

ACEI	angiotensin converting enzyme inhibitor	CVA	cerebrovascular accident	GCA	giant cell arteritis	NG	nasogastric
ADL	activities of daily living	DHPCCB	dihydropyridine calcium channel blocker	HR	heart rate	NSTEMI	non-ST elevation myocardial infarction
ARB	angiotensin receptor blocker			IBD	inflammatory bowel disease	PPI	proton pump inhibitor
BPH	benign prostatic hypertrophy	DM	diabetes mellitus	IBS	irritable bowel syndrome	PPS	palliative performance scale
CABG	coronary artery bypass graft	DNR	do not resuscitate	ICP	intracranial pressure	PTH	parathyroid hormone
CBT	cognitive behavioural therapy	ESAS	Edmonton symptom assessment scale	LOC	level of consciousness	RA	rheumatoid arthritis
CHF	congestive heart failure			MMSE	mini mental status examination	SLE	systemic lupus erythematosus
CO	cardiac output	FAP	familial adenomatous polyposis	NE	norepinephrine	UTI	urinary tract infection

Seniors in Canada and the U.S.

Health Status

Table 1. Causes of Mortality and Morbidity in Canadian and American Seniors

Mortality (Can[1]/U.S.[2])	Morbidity[1,2]	
1. Diseases of the heart and circulatory system (19.7/27.0%)	1. Hypertension	5. Ulcers
2. Malignant neoplasms (29.9/22.0%)	2. Arthritis	6. Stroke
3. Cerebrovascular disease (5.5/6.0%)	3. Heart disease	7. Asthma
4. Chronic lower respiratory disease (4.6/7.0%)	4. Diabetes	8. Allergies
5. Accidents (4.4%)		
6. Alzheimer's (2.6/5.0%)		

[1]Statistics Canada, 2011   [2]Minino AM, 2009

Physiology and Pathology of Aging

Definition
- major categories of impairment that appear with old age and affect the physical, mental, and social domains of the elderly, usually due to many predisposing and precipitating factors, rather than a single cause

Table 2. Changes Occurring Frequently with Aging

System	Physiological Changes	Pathological Changes
Neurologic	Decreased wakefulness, brain mass, cerebral blood flow, increased white matter changes	Increased insomnia, neurodegenerative disease, stroke, decreased reflex response
Special Senses	Decreased lacrimal gland secretion, lens transparency, dark adaptation, decreased sense of smell and taste	Increased glaucoma, cataracts, macular degeneration, presbycusis, presbyopia, tinnitus, vertigo, oral dryness
Cardiovascular	Increased sBP, dBP, decreased HR, CO. Decreased vessel elasticity, cardiac myocyte size and number, β-adrenergic responsiveness	Increased atherosclerosis, CAD, MI, CHF, hypertension, arrhythmias, orthostatic hypotension
Respiratory	Increased tracheal cartilage calcification, mucous gland hypertrophy. Decreased elastic recoil, mucociliary clearance, pulmonary function reserve	Increased COPD, pneumonia, pulmonary embolism
Gastrointestinal	Increased intestinal villous atrophy. Decreased esophageal peristalsis, gastric acid secretion, liver mass, hepatic blood flow, calcium and iron absorption	Increased cancer, diverticulitis, constipation, fecal incontinence, hemorrhoids, intestinal obstruction, malnutrition, weight loss
Renal and Urologic	Increased proteinuria, urinary frequency. Decreased renal mass, creatinine clearance, urine acidification, hydroxylation of vitamin D, bladder capacity	Increased urinary incontinence, nocturia, BPH, prostate cancer, pyelonephritis, nephrolithiasis, UTI
Reproductive	Decreased androgen, estrogen, sperm count, vaginal secretion. Decreased ovary, uterus, vagina, breast size	Increased breast and endometrial cancer, cystocele, rectocele, atrophic vaginitis
Endocrine	Increased NE, PTH, insulin, vasopressin. Decreased thyroid and adrenal corticosteroid secretion	Increased DM, hypothyroidism, stress response
Musculoskeletal	Increased calcium loss from bone. Decreased muscle mass, cartilage	Increased arthritis, bursitis, osteoporosis, muscle weakness with gait abnormalities, polymyalgia rheumatica
Integumentary	Atrophy of sebaceous and sweat glands. Decreased epidermal and dermal thickness, dermal vascularity, melanocytes, collagen synthesis	Increased lentigo, cherry hemangiomas, pruritus, seborrheic keratosis, herpes zoster, decubitus ulcers, skin cancer, easy bruising
Psychiatric	None	Increased depression, dementia, delirium, suicidality, anxiety, sleep disruption

Differential Diagnoses of Common Presentations

Constipation

- see Gastroenterology, G24

Definition
- less than 3 bowel movements in one wk and/or hard stools, straining, sense of blockade, needing manual maneuvers or incomplete evacuation on more than 25% of occasions for at least 12 wk (does not need to be consecutive)

Epidemiology
- chronic constipation increases with age (up to 1/3 of patients >65 yr experience constipation and 1/2 of patients >80)
- in the elderly, chronic constipation may present as fecal impaction

Pathophysiology
- impaired rectal sensation (increased rectal distention required to stimulate the urge to defecate)
- colorectal dysmotility

Treatment
- non-pharmacological
- increase fibre intake
- ensure adequate fluid intake
- discourage chronic laxative use
- engage in regular exercise
- review medication regime, reduce dosages or substitute
- pharmacologic
- see *Common Medications*, GM11

Common Causes of Constipation Include:
- Electrolyte abnormalities (hypokalemia, hypercalcemia)
- Endocrine (hypothyroidism, DM)
- GI (IBS, colon cancer)
- Neurologic (multiple sclerosis, Parkinson's disease)
- Psychiatric (depression, dementia)
- Other (dehydration, immobility)

Drugs Associated with Constipation Include:
- Analgesics (narcotics, NSAIDs)
- Anticholinergics
- Calcium channel blockers
- Diuretics
- Supplements (iron or calcium)

Am Fam Physician 2011;84:299-306

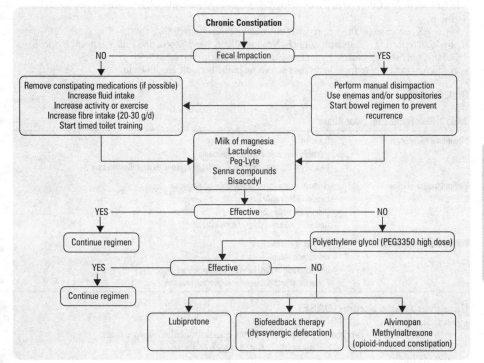

Treatment of Constipation in Older Adults
CMAJ 2013;185(8):663-70
Objectives: To discuss management of constipation in older adults.
Results/Conclusions: In older adults, the predominant symptom of constipation is more frequently straining than decreased stool frequency. RCTs support the use of osmotic agents to treat symptoms of constipation in older adults. In contrast evidence supporting the use of bulk agents, stool softeners stimulants and prokinetic agents is lacking, limited and inconsistent.

Figure 1. Treatment algorithm for the management of chronic constipation in the elderly
Adapted from: *Clin Interv Aging* 2010;5:163-171

Antipsychotics for Delirium
Cochrane DB Syst Rev 2009;CD005594
Objectives: To compare the efficacy and incidence of adverse effects of haloperidol with risperidone, olanzapine, and quetiapine in the treatment of delirium.
Selection Criteria: Types of studies included, unconfounded, randomized trials with concealed allocation of subjects.
Results: Three studies were included, comparing haloperidol with risperidone, olanzapine, and placebo in the management of delirium and in the incidence of adverse drug reactions. Decreases in delirium scores were not significantly different when comparing the effect of low dose haloperidol (<3.0 mg/d) with olanzapine and risperidone (odds ratio 0.63; 95% CI 10.29-1.38; p=0.25). High dose haloperidol (>4.5 mg/d) was associated with an increased incidence of extrapyramidal adverse effects compared with olanzapine. Low dose haloperidol decreased the severity and duration of delirium in post-operative patients, although not the incidence of delirium compared to placebo.
Conclusions: There is no evidence that haloperidol in low dosage has different efficacy in comparison with the atypical antipsychotics olanzapine and risperidone in the management of delirium or has a greater frequency of adverse drug effects than these drugs. High dose haloperidol was associated with a greater incidence of side effects. Low dose haloperidol may be effective in decreasing the degree and duration of delirium in post-operative patients, compared with placebo. However, all studies were small and should be repeated.

Elder Abuse Suspicion Index (EASI) Instructions
- Questions 1-5 are to be asked of the patient
- Question 6 is to be answered by the doctor
- A response of "yes" on one or more of questions 2-6 may establish concern
- Validated for use by family practitioners of cognitively intact seniors seen in ambulatory setting
1. Have you relied on people for any of the following: bathing, dressing, shopping, banking, or meals?
2. Has anyone prevented you from getting food, clothes, medication, glasses, hearing aids, or medical care, or from being with people you wanted to be with?
3. Have you been upset because someone talked to you in a way that made you feel shamed or threatened?
4. Has anyone tried to force you to sign papers or to use your money against your will?
5. Has anyone made you afraid, touched you in ways that you did not want, or hurt you physically?
6. Doctor: elder abuse may be associated with findings such as: poor eye contact, withdrawn nature, malnourishment, hygiene issues, cuts, bruises, inappropriate clothing, or medication compliance issues. Did you notice any of these today or in the last 12 mo?
NICE net. Elder Abuse Suspicion Index. 2006

Delirium, Dementia, and Depression

- see Psychiatry, PS19, PS20, PS10 and Neurology, N20

Definition
- all of the above may present with pathologic decrease in memory, language, or executive function

Differential Diagnosis
- delirium, dementia, or pseudodementia of depression (see Psychiatry)

Delirium Prevention in Elderly
- ensure optimal vision and hearing to support orientation (e.g. appropriate eye wear and hearing aids)
- provide adequate nutrition and hydration (up in chair to eat and drink whenever feasible)
- encourage regular mobilization to build and maintain strength, balance, and endurance
- avoid unnecessary medications and monitor for drug interactions
- avoid bladder catheterization if possible
- ensure adequate sleep

Elder Abuse

Definition
- includes physical abuse, sexual abuse, emotional/psychological abuse, financial abuse, abandonment, and neglect
- elder abuse is a criminal offence under the Criminal Code of Canada
- in the U.S., most states have criminal penalties for elder abuse

Epidemiology
- in Canada in 2013, almost 3000 seniors were victims of family violence. The perpetrators of family violence against seniors were identified to be their grown child (43% of cases) and their spouses (28% of the cases)
- in Canada in 2013, the rate of family-related homicides against seniors was 3.2 for every 1 million seniors
- in the U.S., estimates of the frequency of elder abuse range from 3-8%
- physician reporting is mandatory only in Newfoundland, Nova Scotia, and Prince Edward Island; in Ontario, only abuse occurring in nursing homes is mandatory to report
- insufficient evidence to include/exclude screening in the Periodic Health Exam

Risk Factors

Table 3. Risk Factors for Elder Abuse

Situational Factors	Isolation
	Unstable or unsafe living arrangements
	Lack of family, community or living facility resources for additional care
Victim Characteristics	Physical or emotional dependence on caregiver
	Lack of close family ties
	History of family violence
	Dementia or recent deterioration in health
Perpetrator Characteristics	Related to victim
	Living with victim
	Long duration of care for victim (mean 9.5 yr)
	Financial, marital, occupational or other stressors

Caregiver Abuse Screen (CASE)
- instructions
  - to be answered by caregivers, if answer "yes" to a question, further explore issue
  - the more "yes" responses, the more likely the presence of abuse
- screening tool
  - please answer the following questions as a helper/caregiver:
    1. Do you sometimes have trouble making _____ control his/her temper or aggression?
    2. Do you often feel you are being forced to act out of character/do things you feel badly about?
    3. Do you find it difficult to manage _____'s behaviour?
    4. Do you sometimes feel that you are forced to be rough with _____?
    5. Do you sometimes feel that you can't do what is really necessary or what should be done for _____?
    6. Do you often feel you have to reject/ignore _____?
    7. Do you often feel so tired and exhausted that you cannot meet _____'s needs?
    8. Do you often feel you have to yell at _____?

From: NICE. Case: Caregiver Abuse Screen. 2010. Reproduced with permission from NICE.

Management

- assess safety and determine capacity to make decisions about living arrangements
- establish need for hospitalization or alternate accommodation (e.g. immediate risk of physical harm by self or caregiver)
- involve multidisciplinary team (e.g. nurse, social worker, family members, and physicians including geriatrician, psychiatrist or family physician)
- educate and assist caregiver, contact local resources (e.g. legal aid, crisis support, PSW, caregiver support groups)
- interpret critical and lab findings that are key in exclusion, differentiation and diagnosis

Falls

Definition

- an event which results in a person coming to rest inadvertently on the ground or floor or other lower level

Epidemiology

- 30-40% of people >65 yr old and ~50% of people >80 yr old fall each year
  - equally common between men and women, but more likely to result in injury in women and death in men
  - 5% of falls lead to hospitalization
  - falls are the leading cause of death from injury in persons older than 65 yr
  - 25% associated with serious injuries (e.g. hip fracture, head injury, bruises, laceration)
  - between 25-75% do not recover to previous level of ADL function
  - mortality increases with age (171/100,000 in men >85 yr old) and type of injury (25% with hip fracture die within 6 mo)

Etiology

- multifactorial
  - extrinsic
  - environmental (e.g. home layout, lighting, stairs, overcrowding)
  - accidental, abuse
  - •side effects of medications and substance abuse (e.g. alcohol)
  - ace illness, exacerbation of chronic illness
- intrinsic
  - orthostatic/syncopal
  - age-related changes and diseases associated with aging: musculoskeletal (arthritis, muscle weakness), sensory (visual, proprioceptive, vestibular), cognitive (depression, dementia, delirium, anxiety), cardiovascular (CAD, arrhythmia, MI, low BP), neurologic (stroke, decreased LOC, gait disturbances/ataxia), metabolic (glucose, electrolytes)

Investigations

- directed by history and physical
- comprehensive geriatric assessment to identify all potential causes
- CBC, electrolytes, BUN, creatinine, glucose, Ca^{2+}, TSH, B_{12}, urinalysis, cardiac enzymes, ECG, CT head

Prevention

- multidisciplinary, multifactorial, health, and environmental risk factor screening and intervention programs in the community
- muscle strengthening, balance retraining, and group exercise programs (e.g. Tai Chi)
- home hazard assessment and modification (e.g. remove rugs, add shower bars, etc.)
- prescription of vitamin D 1000 IU daily
- tapering or gradually discontinuation of psychotropic medication
- postural hypotension, heart rate, and rhythm abnormalities management
- eyesight and footwear optimization

Red Flags for Elder Abuse
- Delay in seeking medical attention
- Disparity in histories
- Implausible or vague explanations
- Frequent emergency room visits for exacerbations of chronic disease despite plan for medical care and adequate resources
- Presentation of functionally impaired patient without designated caregiver
- Lab findings inconsistent with history

Key Physical Findings in the Elderly Patient Who Falls or Nearly Falls
I HATE FALLING
Inflammation of joints
Hypotension (orthostatic changes)
Auditory and visual abnormalities
Tremor
Equilibrium (balance) problem
Foot Problems
Arrhythmia, heart block or valvular disease
Leg-length discrepancy
Lack of conditioning (generalized weakness)
Illness
Nutrition
Gait disturbance
Am Fam Phys 2001;61:2159-2172

A history of falls within the past 1-2 yr is a predictor of motor vehicle crashes in the older population. These patients should be evaluated on their ability to drive and counselled about driving

Drugs That May Increase the Risk of Falling
- Sedative-hypnotic and anxiolytic drugs (especially long-acting benzodiazepines)
- Antidepressants (including MAOIs, SSRIs, TCAs)
- Antipsychotics and tranquilizers (phenothiazines and butyrophenones)
- Antihypertensive drugs
- Antiarrhythmics (Class IA)
- Diuretics
- Systemic corticosteroids
- NSAIDs
- Anticholinergic drugs
- Hypoglycemic agents
- Alcohol
Adapted from: *Am Fam Phys* 2001;61:2159-2172
Geriatrics At Your Fingertips, 13th ed. New York: *Am Geriat Soc*, 2011

Fall Prevention Tips
- Improve lighting, especially on stairs
- Caution while adjusting to new bifocal prescription (poor depth perception)
- Side rails in bathtubs
- Railings on steps
- Connect patient to lifeline button signaling systems
- Remove loose mats or carpets, telephone cords and other tripping hazards
- Recommend support hose for varicose veins and swelling of ankles
Essential Geriatrics: Managing 6 Conditions. *Patient Care Canada* 1997;8

Falls Prevention in Community-Dwelling Older Adults
JAMA 2013:309:1406-1407
Purpose: To identify interventions that led to decreased falls in community dwelling older patients.
Study Selection: Meta-analysis of RCTs testing interventions intended to reduce falls.
Results: 159 RCTs were assessed, yielding a population of 79 193 participants (30%M:70%F). The interventions tested included exercise programs, vitamin D supplementation, home assessment, and multi-factorial interventions. Primary outcomes were rate of falls and number of people who fell. Interventions that significantly reduced fall rates included exercise programs (group or home-based) and multi-factorial interventions. Vitamin D supplementation only significantly improved outcomes for patients with deficiency. Home assessment was only significant for patients with high fall risk.
Conclusions: Multiple interventions have been found to significantly decrease falls in patients living in the community. Assessment of fall risk may help to guide choice of interventions. It is noted that patients with dementia, Parkinson's disease, or stroke were not included in these studies.

Will My Patient Fall?
JAMA 2007;297:77-86
Purpose: To identify the prognostic value of risk factors for future falls among older patients.
Study Selection: Meta-analysis of prospective cohort studies of risk factors for falls.
Results: 18 studies were included. Clinically identifiable risk factors were identified across 6 domains: orthostatic hypotension, visual impairment, impairment of gait or balance, medication use, limitations in basic or instrumental activities of daily living, and cognitive impairment. The estimated pretest probability of falling at least once in any given yr for individuals 65 yr and older was 27% (95% CI 19-36%). Patients who have fallen in the past yr are more likely to fall again (LR2.3-2.8). Best predictors of future falls were disturbances in gait of balance (LR 1.7-2.4), while visual impairment, impaired cognition and medication were not reliable predictors.
Conclusions: Screening for risk of falling during the clinical examination begins with determining if the patient has fallen in the past yr. For patients who have not previously fallen, screening consists of an assessment of gait and balance. Patients who have fallen or who have a gait or balance problem are at higher risk of future falls.

Four Syndromes in Failure to Thrive

My Pa Can't Drive
Malnutrition
Physical impairment
Cognitive impairment
Depression

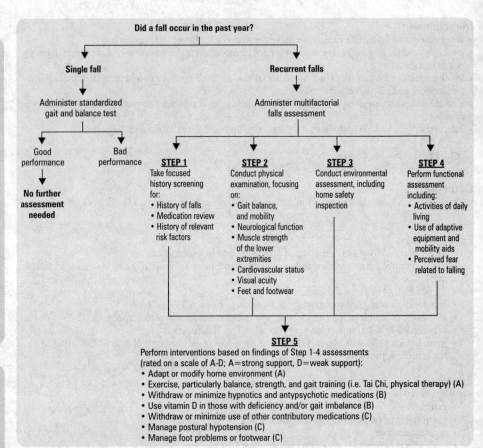

Figure 2. Approach to falls in the elderly
Adapted from: Davuluri S, Dharmarajan TS. Clinical Geriatrics 2013;21(10)

Frailty (Functional Decline/Failure to Thrive)

Definition
- frailty - clinical state of older adults with increased vulnerability to acute stressors resulted from functional decline
- functional decline - progressive limitation in the ability to carry out basic functional activities
- failure to thrive - a state of decline that may be characterized by weight loss, decreased appetite, poor nutrition, and inactivity

Etiology
- multifactorial - malnutrition, functional impairment, cognitive impairment, and depression

Table 4. Common Medical Conditions Associated with Failure to Thrive

Medical Condition	Cause of Failure to Thrive
Cancer	Metastases, malnutrition, cachexia
Chronic lung disease	Respiratory failure
Chronic renal insufficiency	Renal failure
Chronic steroid use	Steroid myopathy, diabetes, osteoporosis, vision loss
Cirrhosis, hepatitis	Hepatic failure
Depression, other psychiatric disorders	Major depression, psychosis, poor functional status, cognitive loss
Diabetes	Malabsorption, poor glucose homeostasis, end-organ damage
Gastrointestinal surgery	Malabsorption, malnutrition
Hip, long bone fracture	Functional impairment
Inflammatory bowel disease	Malabsorption, malnutrition
Myocardial infarction, congestive heart failure	Cardiac failure
Recurrent UTI, pneumonia	Chronic infection, functional impairment
Rheumatologic disease (GCA, RA, SLE)	Chronic inflammation
Stroke	Dysphagia, depression, cognitive loss, functional impairment
Tuberculosis, other systemic infections	Chronic infection

Adapted from: *Clin Geriatr Med* 1997;13:769-778

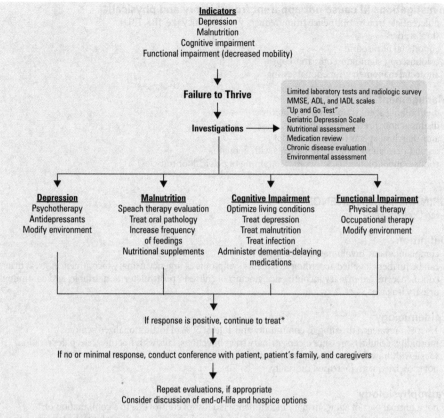

Figure 3. Failure to thrive in elderly patients
Adapted from: *American Family Physician* 2004;70: 343-350

A Global Clinical Measure of Fitness and Frailty in Elderly People
CMAJ 2005;173:489-495
The CHSA Clinical Frailty Scale – shown to predict death and need for institution
1. Very fit – robust, active, energetic, well motivated and fit; these people commonly exercise regularly and are in the most fit group for their age.
2. Well – without active disease, but less fit than people in category 1.
3. Well, with treated comorbid disease – its symptoms are well controlled compared with those in category 4.
4. Apparently vulnerable – although not frankly dependent, these people commonly complain of being "slowed up" or have disease symptoms.
5. Mildly frail – with limited dependence on others for instrumental activities of daily living.
6. Moderately frail – help is needed with both instrumental and non-instrumental activities of daily living.
7. Severely frail – completely dependent on others for the activities of daily living, or terminally ill.

Functional Assessment (ADLs and IADLs)

ADLs: ABCDE-TT	IADLs: SHAFT-TT
Ambulating	Shopping
Bathing	Housework
Continence	Accounting/Managing finances
Dressing	Food preparation
Eating	Transportation
Transferring	Telephone
Toileting	Taking medications

Can use formal assessment tools such as the Lawton-Brody Instrumental Activities of Daily Living Scale to assess functioning

Incontinence

FECAL INCONTINENCE

Definition
- involuntary passage or the inability to control the discharge of fecal matter through the rectum
- severity can range from unintentional flatus to the complete evacuation of bowel contents
- there are three subtypes
  1. passive incontinence: involuntary discharge of stool or gas without awareness
  2. urge incontinence: discharge of fecal matter in spite of active attempts to retain bowel contents
  3. fecal: leakage of stool following otherwise normal evacuation

Epidemiology
- second leading cause of nursing home placement
- US estimates show that 10-25% of hospitalized geriatric patients suffer from fecal incontinence

Etiology
- commonly multifactorial
  - structural abnormalities
  - trauma (e.g. prior vaginal delivery, surgery)
  - prolapse
  - tumour/trauma (e.g. brain, spinal cord, cauda equina)
  - overflow (e.g. encopresis, impaction)
- functional abnormalities
  - neurologic conditions – neuropathy, multiple sclerosis, stroke, dementia
- others
  - constipation with overflow may be a factor
  - psychosis (willful soiling)
  - age >80 yr: decreased external sphincter strength and weak anal squeeze, increased rectal compliance, decreased resting tone and internal sphincter, impaired anal sensation
  - medications (e.g. laxatives, anticholinergics, antidepressants, caffeine, muscle relaxants)

Transient Causes of Incontinence

DIAPERS
Delirium
Infection
Atrophic urethritis/vaginitis
Pharmaceuticals
Excessive urine output
Restricted mobility
Stool impaction

Investigations (if cause not apparent from history and physical)
- differentiate true incontinence from frequency and urgency (i.e. IBS, IBD)
- stool studies
- endorectal ultrasound
- colonoscopy, sigmoidoscopy, anoscopy
- anorectal manometry/functional testing

Management
- diet/bulking agent if stool is liquid or loose
- disimpaction, prevent impaction
- anti-diarrheal agents (e.g. loperamide)
- regular defecation program in patients with dementia
- counsel about biofeedback therapy (retraining of pelvic floor muscles)

URINARY INCONTINENCE
- see Urology, U5

Definition
- complaint of any involuntary loss of urine
- can be further classified according to patients symptoms as urgency urinary incontinence, stress urinary continence, mixed urinary incontinence, nocturnal enuresis, post-micturition dribble, and continuous urinary leakage

Epidemiology
- 15-30% prevalence dwelling in community and at least 50% of institutionalized seniors
- morbidity: cellulitis, pressure ulcers, urinary tract infections, falls with fractures, sleep deprivation, social withdrawal, depression, sexual dysfunction
- not associated with increased mortality

Pathophysiology
- not a normal part of aging, urinary incontinence is a loss of control due to a combination of:
- genitourinary pathology: increased post-void residual volume, increased involuntary bladder contractions (urge incontinence)
- age-related changes: decreased bladder capacity
- comorbid conditions and medications
- functional impairment
- in elderly women: decline in bladder outlet and urethral resistance pressure promoting stress incontinence
- in elderly men: prostatic enlargement can cause overflow and urge incontinence

Gait Disorders

- see Neurology, N10

Hazards of Hospitalization

Table 5. Recommendations for Sequelae of Hospitalization in Older Patients

Sequelae	Recommendations
Malnutrition	No dietary restrictions (except diabetes), assistance, dentures if necessary, sitting in a chair to eat
Urinary incontinence	Medication review, remove environmental barriers, discontinue use of catheter
Depression	Routine screening
Adverse drug event	Medication review
Confusion/delirium	Orientation, visual and hearing aids, volume repletion, noise reduction, early mobilization, medication review, remove restraints
Pressure ulcers	Low-resistance mattress, daily inspection, repositioning every 2 h
Infection	Early mobilization, remove unnecessary IV lines, catheters, NG tubes
Falls	Appropriate footwear, assistive devices, early mobilization, remove restraints, medication review
Hypotension/dehydration	Early recognition and repletion
Diminished aerobic capacity/loss of muscle strength/contractures	Early mobilization
Decreased respiratory function	Incentive spirometry, physiotherapy

Source: Asher, Richard AJ. Dangers of going to bed. British Medical Journal 2.4536 (1947): 967

Hypertension

- see Family Medicine, FM34

Definition
- blood pressure at which an otherwise healthy person would have increased risk of cardiovascular disease
- definition of high blood pressure has changed over time and differs between guidelines proposed by expert bodies
- target: <140/90 mm Hg for adults younger than 80. <130/80 mm Hg for individuals with DM. <150sBP for adults aged 80 or older

Epidemiology
- 60-80% of elderly (>65 yr old) have hypertension
  - 60% of these have isolated systolic HTN
  - the benefit of treating hypertension in the elderly is 2-4 times greater than that achieved in the treatment of younger patients with primary hypertension
  - systolic and pulse pressure are major predictors of outcome in the elderly patient
  - in older adults, base treatment on sBP

Management
- non-pharmacologic treatments are first-line, then thiazide or thiazide-like diuretic monotherapy is recommended in patients without comorbidities
- add ACEI/ARB if also atherosclerosis, DM, CHF or chronic kidney disease
- add β-blockers if also angina or CHF

Immobility

Complications
- cardiovascular: orthostatic hypotension, venous thrombosis, embolism
- respiratory: decreased ventilation, atelectasis, pneumonia
- gastrointestinal: anorexia, constipation, incontinence, dehydration, malnutrition
- genitourinary: infection, urinary retention, bladder calculi, incontinence
- musculoskeletal: atrophy, contractures, bone loss
- skin: pressure ulcers
- psychological: sensory deprivation, delirium, depression

Immunizations

- the following immunizations are recommended for people 65 yr of age and older
- tetanus: every 10 yr
- pneumococcus: every 5 yr
- influenza: every autumn
- herpes zoster: Zostivax®

Malnutrition

Definition
- involuntary weight loss of ≥5% baseline body weight or ≥5 kg
- hypoalbuminemia, hypocholesterolemia

Etiology
- nutritional
  - decreased assimilation: impaired transit, maldigestion, malabsorption
  - decreased intake: financial, psychiatric (depression), cognitive deficits, anorexia associated with chronic disease, functional deficits (e.g. difficulty shopping, preparing meals or feeding oneself due to functional impairment)
- stress: acute or chronic illness/infection, chronic inflammation, abdominal pain
- mechanical: dental problems, dysphagia
- age-related changes: appetite dysregulation, decreased thirst
- mixed: increased energy demands (e.g. hyperthyroidism), abnormal metabolism, protein-losing enteropathy

Clinical Features
- history
  - recent or chronic illness
    - depression, GI symptoms

Treatment of Hypertension in Patients 80 Years of Age or Older
NEJM 2008;358:1887-1898
Study: Randomized, double-blind, placebo-controlled, multicentre trial.
Subjects: 3,845 patients who were 80 yr of age or older and had a sustained systolic blood pressure of 160 mmHg were followed for a median 1.8 yr.
Intervention: Indapamide (sustained release, 1.5 mg) or matching placebo. The angiotensin-converting enzyme inhibitor perindopril (2 or 4 mg), or matching placebo, was added if necessary to achieve the target blood pressure of 150/80 mmHg.
Primary Outcome: Fatal or nonfatal stroke.
Results: Treatment was associated with a 30% reduction in the rate of fatal or nonfatal stroke (95% CI –1-51; p=0.06), 39% reduction in the rate of death from stroke (95% CI 1-62; p=0.05), 21% reduction in the rate of death from any cause (95% CI 4-35; p=0.02), 23% reduction in the rate of death from cardiovascular causes (95% C, –1-40; p=0.06), and 64% reduction in the rate of heart failure (95% CI 42-78; p<0.001). Fewer serious adverse events were reported in the treatment group (358 vs. 448 in the placebo group; p=0.001).
Conclusions: Antihypertensive treatment with indapamide (sustained release), with or without perindopril, in persons 80 yr of age or older reduces death from stroke, death from any cause, and the incidence of heart failure.

Etiology of Malnutrition in the Elderly

MEALS ON WHEELS
Medications
Emotional problems
Anorexia
Late-life paranoia
Swallowing disorders
Oral problems
Nosocomial infections
Wandering/dementia related activity
Hyperthyroid/Hypercalcemia/Hypoadrenalism
Enteric disorders
Eating problems
Low-salt/Low-fat diet
Stones

Remember to Calculate BMI
BMI outside 22-27 kg/m² is a health risk

Calculating Basic Caloric and Fluid Requirements
WHO daily energy estimates for adults >60 yr:
Female: 10.5 x (weight in kg) + 596
Male: 13.5 x (weight in kg) + 487
Maintenance fluid requirements for the elderly without cardiac or renal disease: 1500-2500 cc/24 h

- functional disability: impaired ADLs and IADLs
- social factors: economic barriers, dental problems and living situation (e.g. living alone)
- constitutional symptoms (e.g. recent weight loss)
- physical exam
  - BMI <23.5 in males, <22 in females should raise concern
  - temporal wasting, muscle wasting, presence of triceps skin fold
  - assess cognition

Investigations
- CBC, electrolytes, Ca^{2+}, Mg^{2+}, PO_4^{3-}, creatinine, LFTs (albumin, INR, bilirubin), B_{12}, folate, TSH, transferrin, lipid profile, urinalysis, ESR, CXR

Treatment
- direct treatment at underlying causes
- dietary modification: high calorie foods, oral nutritional supplementation

Osteoporosis

- see Endocrinology, E40

Presbycusis

- see Otolaryngology, OT19

Pressure Ulcers

- see Plastic Surgery, PL16

Risk Factors
- extrinsic factors: friction, pressure, shear force
- intrinsic factors: immobility, malnutrition, moisture, sensory loss

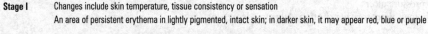

Risk Assessment and Prevention of Pressure Ulcers
Ann Intern Med 2015;162:359-369
The American College of Physicians (ACP) strongly recommends advanced static mattresses or advanced static overlays for patients who are at an increased risk of developing pressure ulcers. The ACP also recommends against using alternating air-mattresses or alternating-air overlays.

Table 6. Classification of Pressure Ulcers

Stage I	Changes include skin temperature, tissue consistency or sensation
	An area of persistent erythema in lightly pigmented, intact skin; in darker skin, it may appear red, blue or purple
Stage II	Partial thickness skin loss involving the epidermis, dermis or both
	The ulcer is superficial and presents as an abrasion, blister or shallow crater
Stage III	Full thickness skin loss involving damage or necrosis of subcutaneous tissue which may extend down to, but not through, underlying fascia
	Presents as a deep crater with or without undermining of adjacent tissue
Stage IV	Full thickness skin loss with extensive destruction, tissue necrosis or damage to muscle, bone or supporting structures
	May have associated undermining and/or sinus tracts

Prevention
- pressure reduction
  - frequent repositioning
  - pressure-reducing devices (static, dynamic)
- maintaining nutrition, encouraging mobility and managing incontinence

Pressure-Reducing Devices
Static devices distribute pressure over a greater surface area. Dynamic devices use alternating air currents to shift pressure to different body sites

Treatment
- optimize nutritional status
- minimize pressure on wound
- analgesia
- wound debridement (mechanical, enzymatic, autolytic) and dressing application
- maintain moist wound environment to enable re-epithelialization
- treatment of wound infections (topical gentamicin, silver sulfadiazine, mupirocin)
- swab wounds not demonstrating clinical improvement for C&S; biopsy chronic wounds to rule out malignancy
- stage IV ulcers typically warrant surgical debridement
- consider other treatment options
  - negative pressure wound therapy/vacuum-assisted closure (VAC)
  - biological agents: application of fibroblast growth factor, platelet-derived growth factor to wound
  - non-contact normothermic wound therapy
  - electrotherapy

Driving Competency

Reporting Requirements

- physician-reporting to the Ministry of Transportation is mandatory in all provinces and territories except in Quebec, Nova Scotia, and Alberta, where it is discretionary
- not an issue unique to geriatrics – any patient may suffer from a medical condition that impairs their ability to drive should be reported
- in the U.S., varies by state

Conditions that may Impair Driving

Table 7. Conditions that Impair Driving

Alcohol	Patients with history of impaired driving and those with high probability of future impaired driving should not drive until further assessed
	Alcohol dependence or abuse: if suspected, should be advised not to drive
	Alcohol withdrawal seizure: must complete a rehabilitation program and remain abstinent and seizure-free for 6 mo before driving
Blood Pressure Abnormalities	Hypertension: sustained BP >170/110 should be evaluated carefully
	Hypotension: if syncopal, discontinue until attacks are treated and preventable
Cardiovascular Disease	Suspected asymptomatic CAD or stable angina: no restrictions
	STEMI, NSTEMI with significant LV damage, coronary artery bypass surgery: no driving for one mo following hospital discharge
	NSTEMI with minor LV damage, unstable angina: no driving for 48 h if percutaneous coronary intervention (PCI) performed or 7 d if no PCI performed
Cerebrovascular Conditions	TIA: should not be allowed to drive until a medical assessment is completed
	Stroke: should not drive for at least one mo; may resume driving if functionally able; no clinically significant motor, cognitive, perceptual or vision deficits; no obvious risk of sudden recurrence; underlying cause appropriately treated; no post-stroke seizure
COPD	Mild/moderate impairment: no restrictions
	Moderate or severe impairment requiring supplemental oxygen: road test with supplemental oxygen
Cognitive Impairment/ Dementia	Moderate to severe dementia is a contraindication to driving; defined as the "inability to independently perform 2 or more IADLs or any basic ADL"
	Patients with mild dementia should be assessed; if indicated, refer to specialized driving testing centre; if deemed fit to drive, re-evaluate patient every 6-12 mo
	Poor performance on MMSE, clock drawing or Trails B suggests a need to investigate driving ability further
	MMSE score alone (whether normal or low) is insufficient to determine fitness to drive
Diabetes	Diet controlled or oral hypoglycemic agents: no restrictions in absence of diabetes complications that may impair ability to drive (e.g. retinopathy, nephropathy, neuropathy, cardiovascular or cerebrovascular disease)
	Insulin use: may drive if no complications (as above) and no severe hypoglycemic episode in the last 6 mo
Drugs	Be aware of: analgesics, anticholinergics, anticonvulsants, antidepressants, antipsychotics, opiates, sedatives, stimulants
	Degree of impairment varies: patients should be warned of the medication/withdrawal effect on driving
Hearing Loss	Effect of impaired hearing on ability to drive safely is controversial
	Acute labyrinthitis, positional vertigo with horizontal head movement, recurrent vertigo: advise not to drive until condition resolves
Musculoskeletal Disorders	Physician's role is to report etiology, prognosis and extent of disability (pain, range of motion, coordination, muscle strength)
Post-Operative	Outpatient, conscious sedation: no driving for 24 h
	Outpatient, general anesthesia: no driving for ≥24 h
Seizures	First, single, unprovoked: no driving for 3 mo until complete neurologic assessment, EEG, CT head
	Epilepsy: can drive if seizure-free on medication and physician has insight into patient compliance
Sleep Disorders	If patient is believed to be at risk due to a symptomatic sleep disorder but refuses investigation with a sleep study or refuses appropriate treatment, the patient should not drive
Visual Impairment	Visual acuity: contraindicated to drive if <20/50 with both eyes examined simultaneously
	Visual field: contraindicated to drive if <120° along horizontal meridian and 15° continuous above and below fixation with both eyes examined simultaneously

N.B. guidelines included refer specifically to private driving; please see CMA guidelines for commercial driving

Simplified Functional Approach to Driving Assessment
1. Unimpaired vision
2. Adequate cognition
3. Ability to maintain consciousness
4. Physical mobility (e.g. mobility of arms/ legs/neck)

Key Factors to Consider in Older Drivers
SAFEDRIVE
Safety record
Attention (e.g. concentration lapses, episodes of disorientation)
Family observations
Ethanol abuse
Drugs
Reaction time
Intellectual impairment
Vision/Visuospatial function
Executive functions (e.g. planning, decision-making, self-monitoring behaviours)
Geriatrics 1996;51:36-45

Systematic Review of Driving Risk and the Efficacy of Compensatory Strategies in Persons with Dementia
J Am Geriatr Soc 2007;55:878-884
Purpose: To determine whether persons with dementia are at greater driving risk and, if so, to estimate the magnitude of this risk and determine whether there are efficacious methods to compensate for or accommodate it.
Study Selection: Systematic review of the case-control studies of drivers with a diagnosis of dementia.
Results: Drivers with dementia universally exhibited poorer performance on road tests and simulator evaluations. The one study that used an objective measure of motor vehicle crashes found that the crash risk in persons with dementia was 2-2.5 times greater than matched controls. No studies were found that examined the efficacy of methods to compensate for or accommodate the decreased driving performance.
Conclusions: Drivers with dementia are poorer drivers than cognitively normal drivers, but studies have not consistently demonstrated higher crash rates. Clinicians and policy makers must take these findings into account when addressing issues pertinent to drivers with a diagnosis of dementia.

Health Care Institutions

Table 8. Classification of Health Care Services and Institutions

Institution/Service	Description
Community Support Services	Health care services offered at home for those who can live independently at home or under the care of family members including professional health care services, personal care and support (ADL assistance), homemaking (IADL assistance), community support services (e.g. transportation, meal delivery, day programs, caregiver relief, security checks, etc.)
Rehabilitation	Health care services offered in an institution to optimize patients' function, independence and quality of life
Residential	Divided into short (<60-90 d/yr) and long (indefinite) stay
a) Seniors Affordable Housing	Seniors who live independently and manage their own care but prefer to live near other seniors; usually has accessibility features and rent is adjusted based on income
b) Retirement/Nursing Home	Residents are fairly independent and require minimal support with ADLs and IADLs; often privately owned
c) Supportive Housing	Residents require minimal to moderate assistance with daily activities while living independently; often rental units in an apartment and may offer some physiotherapy and rehabilitation services
d) Long-term Care/Skilled Nursing Facility	Around the clock nursing care and on-call physician coverage; often offers occupational therapy, physiotherapy, respiratory therapy, and rehabilitation services; may be used short-term for caregiver respite or for supportive patient care to regain strength and confidence after leaving the hospital
e) Hospice	Free-standing facility or designated floor in a hospital or nursing home for care of terminally ill patients and their families; focus is on quality of life and often requires prognosis ≤3 mo

- names of community health care institutions, types of facilities, and services offered vary between geographical locations
- factors to consider when seeking services/institutions include level of care required, support networks, duration of stay, and cost

Palliative and End-of-Life Care

Principles and Quality of Life

- support, educate, and treat both patient and family
- address physical, psychological, social and spiritual needs
- focus on symptom management and comfort measures
- offer therapeutic environment and bereavement support
- ensure maintenance of human dignity

End-of-Life Care Discussions

When to Initiate End-of-Life Care Discussions
- recent hospitalization for serious illness
- severe progressive medical condition(s)
- death expected within 6-12 mo
- patient inquires about end-of-life care

Suggested Topics for Discussion
- goals of care (disease vs. symptom management)
- advance directives, power of attorney, public guardian and trustee
- treatment options and likelihood of success
- common medical interventions
  - mechanical ventilation
  - antibiotic therapy
  - feeding tubes
- resuscitation options and likelihood of success (Full Code vs. DNR status including preferences for CPR, intubation, ICU admission, artificial hydration)

Power of Attorney

- see Ethical, Legal, and Organizational Medicine, ELOM9

Guidance on the Management of Pain in Older People
Age and Aging 2013; 42:1-57
The three most common sites of pain in older adults are the back, leg/knee and hip. Acetaminophen should be considered first-line treatment for the management of both acute and persistent pain, particularly that which is of musculoskeletal origin. NSAIDs should be prescribed with caution and co-prescribed with a PPI.

Instructional Advance Directives

- see Ethical, Legal, and Organizational Medicine, ELOM9

Symptom Management

Assessment Tools
- **Edmonton Symptom Assessment System (ESAS):** a tool that asks patients to rate the intensity of symptoms from 0 to 10 and allows for tracking of the efficacy of interventions. Assesses: pain, tiredness, nausea, depression, anxiety, drowsiness, appetite, well-being, shortness of breath, and "other problems"
- **Palliative Performance Scale (PPS):** a tool that uses functional status to predict survival in terminally ill patients. Assesses 5 components: ambulation, activity and evidence of disease, self-care, intake and conscious level

Source: *J Palliat Care* 1991;7:6-9 and *Victoria Hospice Society* 2006;120-121

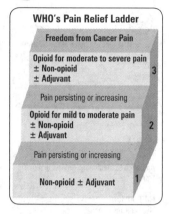

WHO's Pain Relief Ladder

Freedom from Cancer Pain

Opioid for moderate to severe pain
± Non-opioid
± Adjuvant   3

Pain persisting or increasing

Opioid for mild to moderate pain
± Non-opioid
± Adjuvant   2

Pain persisting or increasing

Non-opioid ± Adjuvant   1

Table 9. Management of Common End-of-Life Symptoms

Symptom	Non-Pharmacologic Management	Pharmacologic Management
Constipation	Rule out obstruction, impaction, anorectal disease; hydration and high fibre intake; increase mobility	Stop unnecessary opioids and medications with anticholinergic side effects; provide stool softener (e.g. docusate sodium), increase peristalsis (e.g. senna), alter water and electrolyte secretion (e.g. magnesium hydroxide, lactulose, peg3350)
Death Rattle/ Increased Pulmonary Secretions	Oral suctioning Discontinue unnecessary IV solutions	Scopolamine SC or transdermal
Dry mouth	Oral hygiene q2h, ice cubes, sugarless gum	Artificial saliva substitutes, bethanechol, pilocarpine 1% solution as mouth rinse
Dysphagia	Frequent small feeds, ideally seated, keep head of bed elevated for 30 min after eating, suction as necessary	Treat painful mucositis (diphenhydramine: lidocaine: Maalox® in a 1:2:8 mixture), candidiasis (fluconazole)
Dyspnea	Elevate head of bed, eliminate allergens, open window/use fan	Oxygen, bronchodilators, opioids (e.g. morphine, hydromorphone)
Hiccups	Dry sugar, breathing in paper bag	Chlorpromazine, haloperidol, metoclopramide, baclofen, marijuana
Nausea and Vomiting	Frequent and small meals, avoid offensive strong odours, treat constipation if present	Raised ICP: dexamethasone Anticipatory nausea, anxiety: lorazepam Vestibular disease, vertigo: dimenhydrinate Drug induced, hepatic or renal failure: prochlorperazine, haloperidol GERD: PPI or H2 antagonist Gastric stasis: metoclopramide Bowel obstruction: metoclopramide, dexamethasone, octreotide
Pain	Hot and cold compresses, music therapy, relaxation techniques, individualized program of physical activity designed to improve flexibility, strength and endurance, and cognitive behavioural therapy (CBT)	Nociceptive pain: non-opioids (NSAIDs, acetaminophen), weak opioids (codeine, hydrocodone, oxycodone), strong opioids (morphine, hydromorphone, oxycodone, fentanyl) Neuropathic pain: anticonvulsants (gabapentin, pregabalin), antidepressants (TCAs, SSRIs), steroids (dexamethasone) Bony pain: non-opioids, weak opioids, bisphosphonates, radiation therapy
Pruritus	Bathing with tepid water, avoid soap, bath oils; sodium bicarbonate for jaundice	Antihistamines, phenothiazines, topical corticosteroids, calamine lotion
Weakness	Modify environment and activities to decrease energy expenditure	Treat insomnia, anemia, depression; consider psychostimulants

Source: *J Am Geriatr Soc* 2002;50:S205-S224 and *On Continuing Practice* 1993;20:20-25 and *Am Fam Physician* 2009;79(12):1059-1065

Death Rattle
Noise caused by the oscillatory movement of mucous secretions in the upper airway with inspiration and expiration

Opioid Equivalent Doses
(to 10 mg of IV morphine)

Opioid	SC/IV dose	PO dose
Morphine	10 mg	20-30 mg
Codeine	Not recommended	180-240 mg
Oxycodone	Not recommended	10-15 mg
Hydromorphone	2 mg	4-6 mg

Fentanyl transdermal 25 μg/h = morphine 90 mg PO/24 h, however fentanyl takes 12-16 h to reach steady state
N.B. Dosing may need to be adjusted in the older adult population

Nociceptive Pain
Somatic: localized to bone/skin/joint/muscle; gnawing, dull pain
Visceral: not well localized; crampy pain, pressure

Neuropathic Pain
Burning, shooting, radiating pain; localized to dermatomal regions

Serum creatinine does not reflect creatinine clearance in the elderly

Instead, use:
$$CrCl = \frac{(weight\ in\ kg)(140 - age)(1.23)}{(serum\ creatinine\ in\ \mu mol/L)}$$
(mL/min)

Multiply by 0.85 for females

Geriatric Pharmacology

Pharmacokinetics

Table 10. Age-Associated Pharmacokinetics

Parameter	Age Effect	Implications
Absorption (less significant)	Increased gastric pH	Drug-drug and drug-food interactions are more likely to affect absorption
	Decreased splanchnic blood flow, GI absorptive surface and dermal vascularity; delayed gastric emptying	
Distribution	Increased total body fat and α1-glycoprotein	Lipophilic drugs have a larger volume of distribution
	Decreased lean body mass, total body water, and albumin	Decreased binding of acidic drugs, increased binding of basic drugs
Metabolism (less significant)	Decreased hepatic mass and hepatic blood flow; impaired phase I reactions (oxidative system)	Lower doses may be therapeutic
Elimination	Decreased renal blood flow, GFR, tubular secretion and renal mass	For every x% reduction in clearance, decrease the dose by x% and increase the interval by x%

Pharmacodynamics

Drug Sensitivity
- changes in pharmacokinetics as well as intrinsic sensitivity lead to altered drug responses
- increased sensitivity to warfarin, sedatives, antipsychotics, digoxin and narcotics
- decreased sensitivity to β-blockers in majority of elderly patients, though some may have increased sensitivity

Decreased Homeostasis
- poorer compensatory mechanisms leading to more adverse reactions (e.g. bleeding with NSAIDs/anticoagulants, altered mental status with anticholinergic/sympathomimetic/anti-Parkinsonian drugs)

Polypharmacy

Definition
- prescription, administration or use of five or more medications at the same time

Epidemiology
- in Canada, > 60% of elderly individuals reported using ≥5 medications
- hospitalized elderly are given an average of 10 medications during admission

Risk Factors for Non-Compliance
- risk of non-compliance correlates with medication factors, not age
  - number of medications: compliance with 1 medication is 80%, but drops to 25% with ≥6 medications
- increased dosing frequency, complicated container design, financial constraints, and cognitive impairment

Adverse Drug Reactions (ADRs)
- any noxious or unintended response to a drug that occurs at doses used for prophylaxis or therapy
- risk factors in the elderly
  - intrinsic: comorbidities, age-related changes in pharmacokinetics and pharmacodynamics
  - extrinsic: number of medications, multiple prescribers, unreliable drug history
- 90% of ADRs are from: ASA, analgesics, anticoagulants, antimicrobials, antineoplastics, digoxin, diuretics, hypoglycemics, and steroids

Preventing Polypharmacy
- consider drug: safer side effect profiles, convenient dosing schedules, convenient route, efficacy
- consider patient: other medications, clinical indications, medical comorbidities
- consider patient-drug interaction risk factors for ADRs
- review drug list regularly to eliminate medications with no clinical indication or with evidence of toxicity
- avoid treating an ADR with another medication

Inappropriate Prescribing in the Elderly

Epidemiology
- the estimated prevalence of potentially inappropriate prescribing ranges from 12-40%

Beers Criteria
- a list of medications to avoid in adults 65 yr and older due to safety concerns
- examples include long-acting benzodiazepines, strong anticholinergics, high-dose sedatives
- the elderly are also often under-treated (ACEI, ASA, β-blockers, thrombolytics, warfarin)

Beers Criteria
For full list of medications, consult the
following reference:
The American Geriatrics Society 2012 Beers
Criteria Update Expert Panel
J Am Geriatr Soc 2012;60(4):616-31
http://www.americangeriatrics.org

Common Medications

Table 11. Common Medications

Drug Name	Brand Name	Dosing Schedule	Indications	Contraindications	Side Effects	Mechanism of Action
Cognitive Enhancers						
donepezil	Aricept®	5-10 mg PO daily	Moderate to severe dementia of Alzheimer's type	Known hypersensitivity, caution in pulmonary disease, sick sinus syndrome, seizure disorder	N/V, diarrhea, anorexia, falls, hip fracture, increase need for pacemaker insertion	Reversible inhibition of acetylcholinesterase
galantamine	Reminyl®	8-12 mg PO bid	Mild to moderate dementia of Alzheimer's type	Known hypersensitivity, caution in sick sinus syndrome, seizure disorder, pulmonary disease, low body weight	N/V, diarrhea, anorexia, falls, hip fracture, increase need for pacemaker insertion	Reversible inhibition of acetylcholinesterase
rivastigmine	Exelon®	1.5 mg PO daily (starting) up to 6 mg PO bid	Mild to moderate dementia of Alzheimer's type	Known hypersensitivity, severe hepatic disease, caution in sick sinus syndrome, pulmonary disease, seizure disorder	N/V, diarrhea, anorexia, falls, hip fracture, increase need for pacemaker insertion	Acetylcholinesterase inhibition (reversible but very slow)
memantine	Ebixa®/Namenda® (Can)/(U.S.)	5 mg PO daily (starting) up to 10 mg PO bid	Mild to moderate dementia of Alzheimer's type	Known hypersensitivity, conditions that alkalinize urine, caution in cardiovascular conditions	Agitation, fatigue, dizziness, headache, hypertension, constipation	NMDA-receptor antagonist
Laxatives						
bran	All-Bran®	1 cup/d	Constipation		Bloating, flatus	Bulk-forming laxative
psyllium	Metamucil® Prodiem Plain®	1 tsp PO tid	Constipation, hypercholesterolemia	N/V, abdominal pain, obstruction	Bloating, flatus	Bulk-forming laxative
lactulose	Chronulac® Cephulac® Kristalose®	15-30 cc PO daily/bid	Constipation, hepatic encephalopathy, bowel evacuation following barium exam	Patients on low galactose diets Abdominal pain, N/V	Flatus, cramps, nausea, diarrhea	Hyperosmolar agent, lowers pH of colon to decrease blood ammonia levels
senna	Senokot®/Ex-lax® Glysennid®	1-2 tabs PO daily or 10-15 cc syrup PO daily	Constipation	Abdominal pain, N/V	Cramps, griping, dependence	Stimulant laxative
bisacodyl	Dulcolax®	5-15 mg PO (10 mg PR)	Constipation	Ileus, obstruction, abdominal pain, N/V, severe dehydration	Cramps, pain, diarrhea	Stimulant laxative
Parkinsonian Agents – see Neurology, N32						
Sleeping Medications						
zopiclone	Imovane®	3.75 mg PO qhs (initially)	Insomnia	Known hypersensitivity, caution in myasthenia gravis, severe hepatic disease Geriatrics: dose reduction (dose-related adverse events)	Bitter taste, palpitations, vomiting, anorexia, sialorrhea, confusion, agitation, anxiety, tremor, sweating, cognitive impairment, falls	Short-acting hypnotic (no tolerance effects)
temazepam	Restoril®	15 mg PO qhs	Short-term management of insomnia	Known hypersensitivity, myasthenia gravis, sleep apnea Geriatrics: dose reduction recommended	Drowsiness, dizziness, impaired coordination, hangover, lethargy, dependence, cognitive Impairment, falls	Benzodiazepine: generalized CNS depression mediated by GABA
lorazepam	Ativan®	0.5 mg PO qhs (initially)	Anxiety, insomnia	Known hypersensitivity, myasthenia gravis, narrow-angle glaucoma Geriatrics: dose reduction recommended	Dizziness, drowsiness, lethargy, dependence, cognitive impairment, falls	Benzodiazepine: generalized CNS depression mediated by GABA
melatonin	Good Neighbor Pharmacy Melatonin, Nature's Blend Melatonin	Immediate release 5mg PO qhs (initially), or extended release 2mg PO qhs	Insomnia	Known hypersensitivity, concurrent immunosuppressive treatment	Hypothermia, sedation, somnolence, fatigue	Mimics hormone produced by pineal gland, regulates sleep cycle

Note: Docusate has been shown to be ineffective for the prevention/treatment of constipation in the elderly

Landmark Geriatric Trials

Trial	Reference	Results
Optimal management of urinary tract infections in older people	*Clin Interv Aging* 2011; 6:173-180	UTIs are over diagnosed and over treated in older people. Asymptomatic bacteriuria is very common in later life and should not be screened for or treated
Delirium is a strong risk factor for dementia in the oldest-old: a population-based cohort study	*Brain* 2012; 135(9): 2809-16	First population study to show that delirium is a strong risk factor for dementia and cognitive decline in elderly patients
Donepezil and Memantine for Moderate-to-Severe Alzheimer's Disease	*NEJM* 2012; 366:893-903	Continued treatment with donepezil was associated with cognitive benefits over the course of 12 mo in patients with moderate or severe Alzheimer's disease
Early palliative care for metastatic lung cancer	*NEJM* 2010; 363:733-742	Among patients with metastatic non-small-cell lung cancer, early palliative care led to significant improvements in both quality of life and mood. As compared with patients receiving standard care, patients receiving early palliative care had less aggressive care at the end-of-life but longer survival
Hip protectors for fracture prevention	*NEJM* 2000; 343:1506-1513	The risk of hip fracture can be reduced in frail elderly adults by the use of an anatomically designed external hip protector
HYVET	*NEJM* 2008; 358:1887-1898	Antihypertensive treatment with indapamide (sustained release), with or without perindopril, in adults 80 yr or older is beneficial
PROFET	*Lancet* 1999; 353:93-97	Demonstrates that an interdisciplinary approach to elderly adults with a previous history of falls can significantly decrease the risk of further falls and limit functional impairment
Yale Delirium Prevention Trial	*NEJM* 1999; 340:669-676	A risk-factor intervention strategy can result in significant reductions in the number and duration of episodes of delirium in hospitalized older patients

References

Constipation
Gandell D, Straus SE, Bundookwala M, et al. Treatment of constipation in older people. CMAJ 2013; 185:663-70.
Higgins PDR, Johanson JF. Epidemiology of constipation in North America: a systematic review. Am J Gastroenterol 2004;99:750-759.
Jamshed N, Lee ZE, Olden KW. Diagnostic approach to chronic constipation in adults. Am Fam Physician 2011;84:299-306
Rao SSC. Diagnosis and management of fecal incontinence. American Journal of Gastroenerology 2004; 99(8): 1585-604.
Rao SSC, Go JT. Update on the management of constipation in the elderly: new treatment options. Clin Interv Aging 2010;5:163-171.Reuben DB, Herr KA, Pacala JT, et al. Geriatrics at your fingertips, 13th ed. New York: The American Geriatrics Society, 2011.

Delirium, Dementia, and Depression
British Geriatrics Society and Royal College of Physicians. Guidelines for prevention, diagnosis and management of delirium in older people. Concise guidance to good practice series. 2006;6:303-8.
Inouye SK, Westendorp RG, Saczynski JS. Delirium in elderly people. Lancet 2014;383(9920):911-22.
Young J, Murthy L, Westby M, et al. Diagnosis, prevention, and management of delirium: summary of NICE guidance. BMJ 2010;341:c3704.
Driving Competency
CMA. CMA Driver's guide: determining medical fitness to operate motor vehicles. Ottawa, 2012.
Grabowski DC, Campbell CM, Morrisey MA. Elderly licensure laws and motor vehicle fatalities. JAMA 2004;291:2840-2846.
Joseph, CB. Physician's guide to assessing and counselling older drivers. Second edition. J Med Libr Assoc 2013;101:230-231
Man-Son-Hing M, Marshall SC, Molnar FJ, et al. Systematic review of driving risk and the efficacy of compensatory strategies in persons with dementia. J Am Geriatr Soc 2007;55:878-884.
Wiseman EJ, Souder E. The older driver: a handy tool to assess competence behind the wheel. Geriatrics 1996;51:36-38, 41-42, 45.

Elder Abuse
Health Canada. The Canadian guide to clinical preventative health care. Ottawa: Canadian Task Force on Preventative Health Care, 2002.
Lachs MS, Pillemer KA. Elder abuse. NEJM 2015;373(20):1947-56.
NICE. Elder Abuse Suspicion Index, 2006. Available from: http://www.nicenet.ca/tools-easi-elder-abuse-suspicion-index.
Public Health Agency of Canada. Elder Abuse in Canada: A Gender-Based Analysis, 2009.
Takahashi PY, Okhravi HR, Lim LS, et al. Preventative health care in the elderly population: a guide for practicing physicians. Mayo Clin Proc 2004;79:416-27.
Wang XM, Brisbin S, Loo T, et al. Elder abuse: an approach to identification, assessment and intervention. CMAJ 2015;187(8):575-81.

Falls
Butt DA, Mamdani M, Austin PC, et al. The risk of falls on initiation of antihypertensive drugs in the elderly. Osteoporosis Int 2013;24:2649-2657.
Davuluri S, Dharmarajan TS. Falls: A complex, multifactorial syndrome with addressable risk factors. Consultant360 2013;21.
Ganz DA, Bao Y, Shekelle PE, et al. Will my patient fall? JAMA 2007;297:77-86.
Gillespie LD, Robertson MC, Gillespie WJ, et al. Interventions for preventing falls in older people living In the community. Cochrane DB Syst Rev 2012;9:CD007146.
Kiel DP, Rose BD, Wellesly MA. Overview of falls in the elderly. Rose BD (editor). Waltham: UpToDate, 2006.
Kwan E, Straus SE. Assessment and management of falls in older people. CMAJ 2014;186(16):610-621.
Milos V, Bondesson A, Magnusson M, et al. Fall risk-increasing drugs and falls: a cross-sectional study among elderly patients in primary care. BMC Geriatr 2014;14:40.
Moncada L. Management of falls in older persons: a prescription for prevention. Am Fam Physician 2011;84:1267-1276.
Phelan EA, Mahoney JE, Voit JC, et al. Assessment and management of fall risk in primary care settings. Med Clin North Am 2015;99(2):281-93.
Rao S. Prevention of falls in older patients. Am Fam Physician 2011;72:81-88.
Reuben DB, Herr KA, Pacala JT, et al. Geriatrics at your fingertips, 13th ed. New York: The American Geriatrics Society, 2011.
Tinetti ME, Baker DI, McAvay G, et al. A multifactorial intervention to reduce the risk of falling among elderly people living in the community. NEJM 1994;331:821-827.
Robertson MC, Gillespie LD. Fall prevention in community-dwelling older adults. JAMA 2013;309:1406-1407.

Frailty
Colon-Emeric CS, Whitson HE, Pavon J, et al. Functional decline in older adults. AAFP 2013;88(6):388-394.
Chan X, Mao G, Leng SX. Frailty syndrome: an overview. Clin Interv Aging 2014;9:433-441
Quinn TJ, McArthur K, Ellis G, et al. Functional assessment in older people. BMJ 2011;343:d4681.
Robertson RG, Montagnini M. Geriatric failure to thrive. Am Fam Phys 2004;70:343-348.
Rockwood K, Song X, MacKnight C, et al. A global clinical measure of fitness and frailty in elderly people. CMAJ 2005;173:489-495.
Sarkisian CA, Laches MS. "Failure to thrive" in older adults. Ann Intern Med 1996;124:1072-1078.
Verdery RB. Clinical evaluation of failure to thrive in older people. Clin Geriatr Med 1997;13:769-778.Geriatric Pharmacology
American Geriatrics Society 2012 Beers Criteria Update Expert Panel. American Geriatrics Society updated beers criteria for potentially inappropriate medication use in older adults.
Barry PJ, Gallagher P, Ryan C, et al. START (screening tool to alert doctors to the right treatment)-an evidence-based screening tool to detect prescribing omissions in elderly patients. Age Aging 2007;36:632-638.
Carlson JE. Perils of polypharmacy: 10 steps to prudent prescribing. Geriatrics 1996;51:26-35
Gallagher P, Ryan C, Byrne S, et al. STOPP (screening tool of older person's prescriptions) and START (screening tool to alert doctors to right treatment). consensus validation. Int J Clin Pharmacol Ther 2008;46(2):72-83.
JAGS 2012. Available from: http://www.americangeraitrics.org.
Fick DM, Cooper JW, Wade WE, et al. Updating the Beers Criteria for potentially inappropriate medication use in older adults. Arch Intern Med 2003;163:2716-2724.
Fordyce M. Geriatric pearls. Philadelphia: FA Davis, 1999.
Lewis T. Using the NO TEARS tool for medication review. BMJ 2004;329:434.
Reason B, Terner M, Moses McKeag A, et al. Impact of Polypharmacy on the health of Canadian Seniors. Fam Pract 2012;29:427-432.

Hazards of Hospitalization
Asher, Richard AJ. Dangers of going to bed. British Medical Journal 2.4536 (1947): 967.
Creditor MC. Hazards of Hospitalization of the Elderly. Ann Intern Med 1993;118:219-223.
Inouye SK, Bogardus ST Jr, Charpentier PA, et al. A multi-component intervention to prevent delirium in hospitalized older patients. NEJM 1999;340:669-676.
James PA, Oparil S, Carter BL, et al. 2014 Evidence-Based Guideline for the Management of High Blood Pressure in Adults. JAMA 2008;358:1887-1898.
Sager MA, Franke T, Inouye SK, et al. Functional outcomes of acute medical illness and hospitalization in older persons. Arch Internal Med 1996;156:645-652.
Wilson RS, Herbert LE, Scherr PA, et al. Cognitive decline after hospitalization in a community population of older persons. Neurology 2012;78:950-956.

Health Care Institutions
Government of Ontario. Reports on long-term care homes. Queen's Printer for Ontario, 2007.

Health Status
Heron M. Deaths: leading causes for 2004. National Vital Statistics Reports 2007;56:1-96
Minino AM. Death in the United Sates, 2009. NCHS Data Brief 2011;64:1-8.
Statistics Canada. Deaths, by selected grouped causes and sex, Canada, provinces and territories, annual. Ottawa, 2011.

Hypertension
Allen M, Kelly K, Fleming I. Hypertension in elderly patients: recommended systolic targets are not evidence based. CFP 2013;59:19-21.
Beckett NS, Peters R, Fletcher AE, et al. Treatment of hypertension in patients 80 years of age or older. NEJM 2008;358:1887-1898.
Reuben DB, Herr KA, Pacala JT, et al. Geriatrics at your fingertips, 13th ed. New York: The American Geriatrics Society, 2011.
Whelton PK, Appel LJ, Espeland MA, et al. The 2001 Canadian hypertension recommendations. Perspect in Cardiol 2002;38-46.

Immunizations
Rivetti D, Jefferson T, Thomas R, et al. Vaccines for preventing influenza in the elderly. Cochrane DB Syst Rev 2006;19:CD004876.

Malnutrition
Alibhai SMH, Greenwood C, Payett H. An approach to the management of unintentional weight loss in elderly people. CMAJ 2005;172(6):773-80.
Halsted CH. Harrison's principles of internal medicine, 16th ed. Kasper, DL. 2004. Chapter: Malnutrition and nutritional assessment. 411-415.

Palliative and End-of-Life Care
Abdulla A, Adams N, Bone M, et al. Guidance on the management of pain in older people. Age and Aging 2013; 42:1-57.
AGS Panel on Persistent Pain in Older Persons. The management of persistent pain in older persons. J Am Geriatr Soc 2002;50(Suppl6):S205-S224.
Bruera E, Kuehn N, Miller MJ, et al. The Edmonton Symptom Assessment System (ESAS): A simple method for the assessment of palliative care patients. J Pall Care 1991;7:6-9.
Knowles S. Symptom management in palliative care. On Continuing Practice 1993;20:20-5.
Medical care of the dying, 4th ed. Victoria: Victoria Hospice Society, 2006. Chapter: Palliative performance scale, version 2. 120-121.
The World Health Association. Cancer – The WHO's pain ladder. 2001. Available from: http://www.who.int/cancer/palliative/painladder/en/.
Clary P, Lawson P. Pharmacological Pearls for End-of-Life Care. Am Fam Physician. 2009;79(12):1059-1065.

Physiology and Pathology of Aging
Braunwald E, Fauci AS, Hauser SL, et al. Harrison's principles of internal medicine. New York: McGraw-Hill, 2004.

Pressure Ulcers
Berlowitz D. Pressure ulcers: staging; epidemiology; pathogenesis; clinical manifestations. Rose BD (editor). Waltham: UpToDate, 2006.
Qaseem A. Risk assessment and prevention of pressure ulcers: a clinical procedures guideline from the American College of Physicians. Ann Intern Med 2015; 162:359-369.

Notes

GY Gynecology

Katie Bies, Tahrin Mahmood, and **Tammy Ryan**, chapter editors
Dhruvin Hirpara and **Sneha Raju**, associate editors
Valerie Lemieux and **Simran Mundi**, EBM editors
Dr. Sari L. Kives, Dr. Ally Murji, and **Dr. Fay Weisberg**, staff editors

Acronyms

β-hCG	beta-human chorionic gonadotropin	GIFT	gamete intrafallopian transfer	JRA	juvenile rheumatoid arthritis	RPR	rapid plasma reagin
AFP	alpha-fetoprotein	GnRH	gonadotropin-releasing hormone	LDH	lactate dehydrogenase	SCC	squamous cell carcinoma
AIS	androgen insensitivity syndrome	GTD	gestational trophoblastic disease	LEEP	loop electrosurgical excision procedure	SERMs	selective estrogen receptor modifiers
ASCUS	atypical squamous cells of undetermined significance	GTN	gestational trophoblastic neoplasia	LH	luteinizing hormone	SHBG	sex hormone binding globulin
		HERS	heart and estrogen/progestin replacement study	LHRH	luteinizing hormone releasing hormone	SHG	sonohysterography
AUB	abnormal uterine bleeding			LMP	last menstrual period	SSRI	selective serotonin reuptake inhibitors
BMI	body mass index	HMG	human menopausal gonadotropin	LN	lymph node	STI	sexually transmitted infections
BSO	bilateral salpingo-oophorectomy	HPO	hypothalamic-pituitary-ovarian	LNMP	last normal menstrual period	TAH	total abdominal hysterectomy
BV	bacterial vaginosis	HPV	human papillomavirus	LSIL	low grade squamous intraepithelial lesion	TET	tubal embryo transfer
CAH	congenital adrenal hyperplasia	HRT	hormone replacement therapy	LVSI	lymphovascular space involvement	TH	total hysterectomy
CMV	cytomegalovirus	HSG	hysterosalpingography	MRKH	Mayer-Rokitansky-Küster-Hauser	TOT	tension-free obturator tape
D&C	dilatation and curettage	HSIL	high grade squamous intraepithelial lesion	NK	natural killer	TSH	thyroid stimulating hormone
DES	diethylstilbestrol	HSV	herpes simplex virus	OCP	oral contraceptive pill	TVT	tension-free vaginal tape
DHEA	dihydroepiandrosterone	IBD	inflammatory bowel disease	OGTT	oral glucose tolerance test	TZ	transformation zone
DMPA	depo -medroxyprogesterone acetate or Depo-Provera®	ICSI	intracytoplasmic sperm injection	PCOS	polycystic ovarian syndrome	VDRL	venereal disease research laboratory
		ITP	immune thrombocytopenic purpura	PCR	polymerase chain reaction	VIN	vulvar intraepithelial neoplasia
DUB	dysfunctional uterine bleeding	IUD	intrauterine device	PG	prostaglandin	VTE	venous thromboembolism
DVT	deep venous thrombosis	IUI	intrauterine insemination	PID	pelvic inflammatory disease	vWD	von Willebrand's disease
EPC	emergency postcoital contraception	IVDU	intravenous drug use	PMDD	premenstrual dysphoric disorder	W/D	withdrawal
FSH	follicle stimulating hormone	IVF	in vitro fertilization	PMN	polymorphonuclear neutrophils	WHI	Women's Health Initiative
GA	gestational age	IVM	in vitro maturation	PMS	premenstrual syndrome	ZIFT	zygote intrafallopian transfer

Basic Anatomy Review

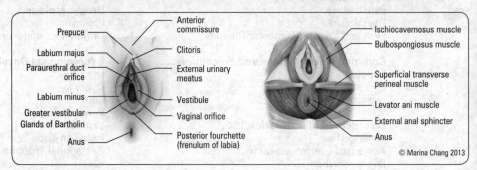

© Marina Chang 2013

Figure 1. Vulva and perineum

A. EXTERNAL GENITALIA
- referred to collectively as the vulva
- blood supply: internal pudendal artery
- sensory innervation: pudendal nerve
- lymphatic drainage: inguinal nodes

B. VAGINA
- muscular canal extending from cervix to vulva, anterior to rectum and posterior to bladder
- lined by rugated, stratified-squamous epithelium
- upper vagina separated by cervix into anterior, posterior, and lateral fornices
- blood supply: vaginal branch of internal pudendal artery with anastamoses from uterine, inferior vesical, and middle rectal arteries

C. UTERUS
- thick walled, muscular organ between bladder and rectum, consisting of two major parts:
  - uterine corpus
    - blood supply: uterine artery (branch of the internal iliac artery)
  - cervix
    - blood supply: cervical branch of uterine artery
- supported by the pelvic diaphragm, the pelvic organs, and 4 paired sets of ligaments
  - round ligaments: travel from anterior surface of uterus, through broad ligaments, and inguinal canals then terminate in the labia majora
    - function: anteversion
    - blood supply: Sampson's artery (branch of uterine artery running through round ligament)
  - uterosacral ligaments: arise from sacral fascia and insert into posterior inferior uterus
    - function: mechanical support for uterus and contain autonomic nerve fibres
  - cardinal ligaments: extend from lateral pelvic walls and insert into lateral cervix and vagina
    - function: mechanical support, prevent prolapse
  - broad ligaments: pass from lateral pelvic wall to sides of uterus; contain fallopian tube, round ligament, ovarian ligament, nerves, vessels, and lymphatics
- infundibulopelvic ligament: continuous tissue that connects ovary to pelvic wall
  - contains the ovarian artery, ovarian vein, ovarian plexus, and lymphatic vessels
- position of the uterus
  - anteverted (majority), retroverted, neutral

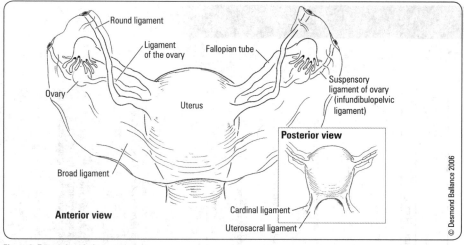

Figure 2. External genital organs

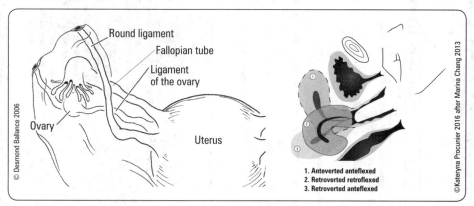

Figure 3. Positioning of uterus

Determination of uterine position by clinical exam
- If cervix faces anteriorly (under the urethra and less easily accessible), i.e. toward vaginal orifice, more likely RETROVERTED UTERUS
- If cervix faces posteriorly (easily accessible), i.e. toward sacrum or rectum, more likely ANTEVERTED UTERUS
- If uterus palpable on bimanual exam, more likely ANTEVERTED UTERUS

D. FALLOPIAN TUBES
- 8-14 cm muscular tubes extending laterally from the uterus to ovary
- interstitial, isthmic, ampullary, and infundibular segments; terminates at fimbriae
- mesosalpinx: peritoneal fold that attaches fallopian tube to broad ligament
- blood supply: uterine and ovarian arteries

"Water Under the Bridge"
The ureters run posterior to the uterine arteries

E. OVARIES
- consist of cortex with ova and medulla with blood supply
- supported by infundibulopelvic ligament (suspensory ligament of ovary)
- mesovarium: peritoneal fold that attaches ovary to broad ligament
- blood supply: ovarian arteries (branches off aorta), left ovarian vein (drains into left renal vein), right ovarian vein (drains into inferior vena cava)

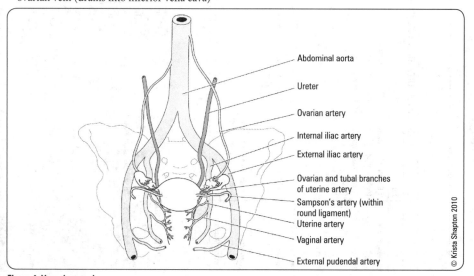

Figure 4. Vascular supply

Menstruation

Menstrual Cycle

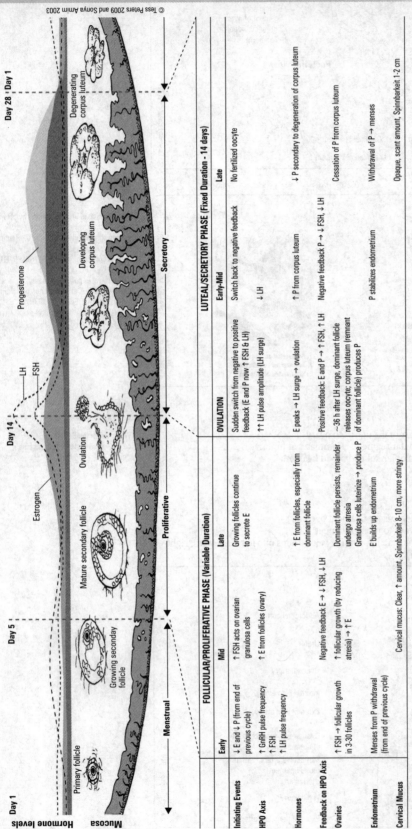

	FOLLICULAR/PROLIFERATIVE PHASE (Variable Duration)			LUTEAL/SECRETORY PHASE (Fixed Duration - 14 days)		
	Early	Mid	Late	OVULATION	Early-Mid	Late
Initiating Events	↓E and ↓P (from end of previous cycle)	↑FSH acts on ovarian granulosa cells; ↑E from follicles (ovary)	Growing follicles continue to secrete E	Sudden switch from negative to positive feedback (E and P now ↑FSH & LH); ↑↑LH pulse amplitude (LH surge)	Switch back to negative feedback; ↓LH	No fertilized oocyte
HPO Axis	↑GnRH pulse frequency; ↑FSH; ↑LH pulse frequency					
Hormones			↑E from follicles, especially from dominant follicle	E peaks → LH surge → ovulation	↑P from corpus luteum	↓P secondary to degeneration of corpus luteum
Feedback on HPO Axis		Negative feedback E → ↓FSH, ↓LH		Positive feedback: E and P → ↑↑FSH, ↑LH	Negative feedback P → ↓FSH, ↓LH	
Ovaries	↑FSH → follicular growth in 3-30 follicles	↑follicular growth (by reducing atresia) → ↑E	Dominant follicle persists, remainder undergo atresia; Granulosa cells luteinize → produce P	~36 h after LH surge, dominant follicle releases oocyte; corpus luteum (remnant of dominant follicle) produces P		Cessation of P from corpus luteum
Endometrium	Menses from P withdrawal (from end of previous cycle)		E builds up endometrium		P stabilizes endometrium	Withdrawal of P → menses
Cervical Mucus	Cervical mucus: Clear, ↑ amount, Spinnbarkeit 8-10 cm, more stringy			Opaque, scant amount, Spinnbarkeit 1-2 cm		

ESTROGEN

ESTROGEN is the main hormone in the follicular/proliferative phase and is stimulated by FSH. As the level increases it acts negatively on FSH. The majority of estrogen is secreted by the dominant follicle

Estrogen effects
- On the follicles in the ovaries
  - Reduces atresia
- On the endometrium
  - Proliferation of glandular and stromal tissue
- On all target tissues
  - Decreases E receptors

PROGESTERONE

PROGESTERONE is the main hormone in the luteal/secretory phase and is stimulated by LH. Increased progesterone acts negatively on LH and is secreted by the corpus luteum (remnant of dominant follicle)

Progesterone effects
- On the endometrium
  - Cessation of mitoses (stops building endometrium up)
  - "Organization" of glands (initiates secretions from glands)
  - Inhibits macrophages, interleukin-8, and enzymes from degrading endometrium
- On all target tissues
  - Decrease E receptors (the "anti-estrogen" effect)
  - Decrease P receptors

CHARACTERISTICS
- Menarche 10-15 yr
- Average 12.2 yr
- Entire cycle 28 ± 7 d with bleeding for 1-6 d
- 25-80 mL blood loss per cycle

E = estrogen; FSH = follicle-stimulating hormone; GnRH = gondatopin-releasing hormone; HPO = hypothalamic pituitar-ovarian; LH = luteinizing hormone; P = progesterone

Figure 5. Events of the normal menstrual cycle

Stages of Puberty

- see Pediatrics, P30
- adrenarche: increase in secretion of adrenal androgens; usually precedes gonadarche by 2 yr
- gonadarche: increased secretion of gonadal sex steroids; ~age 8 yr
- thelarche: breast development
- pubarche: pubic and axillary hair development
- menarche: onset of menses, usually following peak height velocity and/or 2 yr following breast budding

Premenstrual Syndrome

- synonyms: "ovarian cycle syndrome," "menstrual molimina" (moodiness)

Etiology

- multifactorial: not completely understood; genetics likely play a role
- CNS-mediated neurotransmitter interactions with sex steroids (progesterone, estrogen, and testosterone)
- serotonergic dysregulation – currently most plausible theory

Diagnostic Criteria for Premenstrual Syndrome
- at least one affective and one somatic symptom during the 5 d before menses in each of the three prior menstrual cycles
  - affective: depression, angry outbursts, irritability, anxiety, confusion, social withdrawal
  - somatic: breast tenderness, abdominal bloating, headache, swelling of extremities
- symptoms relieved within 4 d of onset of menses
- symptoms present in the absence of any pharmacologic therapy, drug or alcohol use
- symptoms occur reproducibly during 2 cycles of prospective recording
- patient suffers from identifiable dysfunction in social or economic performance

Treatment
- goal: symptom relief
- psychological support
- medications
  - NSAIDs for discomfort and pain
  - spironolactone for fluid retention: used during luteal phase
  - SSRIs: used during luteal phase x 14 d or continuously
  - OCP: primarily beneficial for physical/somatic symptoms
  - danazol: an androgen that inhibits the pituitary-ovarian axis
  - GnRH agonists if PMS is severe and unresponsive to treatment (may use prior to considering definitive treatment with BSO)
- mind/body approaches
  - regular aerobic exercise
  - cognitive behavioural therapy
  - relaxation, light therapy biofeedback, and guided imagery
- herbal remedies (variable evidence)
  - black cohosh, kava, ginkgo, agnus castus fruit extract
- BSO if symptoms severe

Premenstrual Dysphoric Disorder

Clinical Presentation
- irritability, depressed mood
- breast pain and bloating

Diagnostic Criteria for Premenstrual Dysphoric Disorder
- at least 5 of the following 11 symptoms during most menstrual cycles of the last year (with at least 1 of the first 4)
  - depressed mood or hopelessness
  - anxiety or tension
  - affective symptoms
  - anger or irritability
  - decreased interest in activities
  - difficulty concentrating
  - lethargy
  - change in appetite
  - hypersomnia or insomnia
  - feeling overwhelmed
  - physical symptoms: breast tenderness/swelling, headaches, joint/muscle pain, bloating, or weight gain
- symptoms interfere with social or occupational functioning
- symptoms must be discretely related to the menstrual cycle
- 1, 2 and 3 must be confirmed during at least 2 consecutive symptomatic menstrual cycles

Stages of Puberty

"Boobs, Pubes, Grow, Flow"
Thelarche, Pubarche, Growth spurt, Menarche

Tanner Stage

Thelarche
1. None
2. Breast bud
3. Further enlargement of areola and breasts with no separation of contours
4. 2° mound of areola and papilla
5. Areola recessed to general contour of breast – adult

Pubarche
1. None
2. Downy hair along labia only
3. Darker/coarse hair extends over pubis
4. Adult type covers smaller area, no thigh involvement
5. Adult hair in quantity and type; extends over thighs

Premenstrual Syndrome
Physiological and emotional disturbances that occur 1-2 wk prior to menses and last until a few days after onset of menses; common symptoms include depression, irritability, tearfulness, and mood swings

Differential Diagnoses of Common Presentations

Abnormal Uterine Bleeding

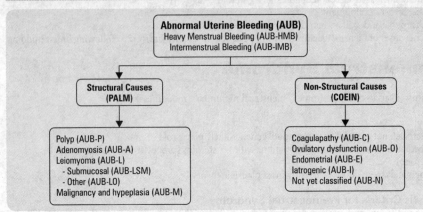

Figure 6. Differential diagnosis of abnormal uterine bleeding

Postmenopausal bleeding is endometrial cancer until proven otherwise

- see *Disorders of Menstruation*, GY11
- menstrual bleeding should be evaluated by ascertaining: frequency/regularity of menses, duration, volume of flow, affects on quality of life and timing (inter or premenstrual or breakthrough)
- classified as
  - regular: cycle to cycle variability of <20 d
  - irregular: cycle to cycle variability of ≥20 d
  - heavy menstrual bleeding: ≥80 cc of blood loss per cycle or ≥8 d of bleeding per cycle or bleeding that significantly affects quality of life
  - postmenopausal bleeding: any bleeding that presents >1 yr after menopause; must rule out endometrial cancer

Dysmenorrhea

- see *Disorders of Menstruation*, GY10
- primary/idiopathic
- secondary (acquired)
  - endometriosis
  - adenomyosis
  - uterine polyps
  - uterine anomalies (e.g. non-communicating uterine horn)
  - leiomyoma
  - intrauterine synechiae
  - ovarian cysts
  - cervical stenosis
  - imperforate hymen, transverse vaginal septum
  - pelvic inflammatory disease
  - IUD (copper)
  - foreign body

Pruritus

- see *Gynecological Infections*, GY25
- physiologic discharge and cervical mucus production
- non-physiologic
  - genital tract infection
  - vulvovaginitis: candidiasis, trichomoniasis, BV, polymicrobial superficial infection
  - chlamydia, gonorrhea
  - pyosalpinx, salpingitis
  - genital tract inflammation (non-infectious)
  - local: chemical irritants, douches, sprays, foreign body, trauma, atrophic vaginitis, desquamative inflammatory vaginitis, focal vulvitis
  - neoplasia: vulvar, vaginal, cervical, endometrial
  - systemic: toxic shock syndrome, Crohn's disease, collagen disease, dermatologic (e.g. lichen sclerosis)
  - IUD, OCP (secondary to progesterone)

Pelvic Pain

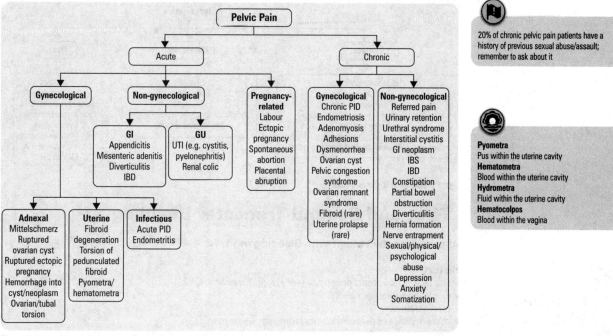

Figure 7. Approach to pelvic pain

20% of chronic pelvic pain patients have a history of previous sexual abuse/assault; remember to ask about it

Pyometra
Pus within the uterine cavity
Hematometra
Blood within the uterine cavity
Hydrometra
Fluid within the uterine cavity
Hematocolpos
Blood within the vagina

Pelvic Mass

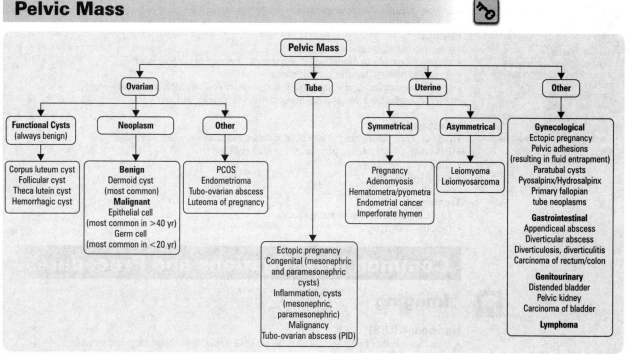

Figure 8. Differential diagnosis of pelvic mass

Dyspareunia

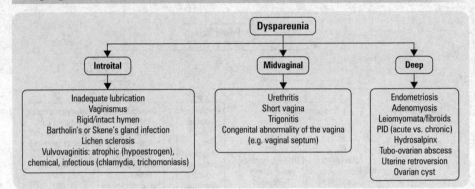

Figure 9. Approach to dyspareunia

First and Second Trimester Bleeding

Approach to the Patient with Bleeding in T1/T2

History
- risk factors for ectopic pregnancy (see *Ectopic Pregnancy*, GY21)
- previous spontaneous abortion
- recent trauma
- characteristics of the bleeding (including any tissue passed)
- characteristics of the pain (cramping pain suggests spontaneous abortion)
- history of coagulopathy
- gynecological/obstetric history
- fatigue, dizziness, syncopal episodes due to hypovolemia, fever (may be associated with septic abortion)

Physical
- vitals (including orthostatic changes)
- abdomen (symphysis fundal height, tenderness, presence of contractions)
- perineum (signs of trauma, genital lesions)
- speculum exam (cervical os open or closed, presence of active bleeding/clots/tissue)
- pelvic exam (uterine size, adnexal mass, uterine/adnexal tenderness)

Investigations
- β-hCG (lower than expected for GA in spontaneous abortion, ectopic pregnancy)
- U/S (confirm intrauterine pregnancy and fetal viability)
- CBC
- group and screen

Treatment
- IV resuscitation for hemorrhagic shock
- treat the underlying cause

Common Investigations and Procedures

Imaging

Ultrasound (U/S)
- transabdominal or transvaginal U/S is the imaging modality of choice for pelvic structures
- transvaginal U/S provides better resolution of uterus and adnexal structures
  - detects early pregnancy if β-hCG ≥1,500 (β-hCG must be ≥6,500 for transabdominal U/S)
- may be used to identify pelvic pathology
  - identify ectopic pregnancy, intrauterine pregnancy
  - assess uterine, adnexal, cul-de-sac, ovarian masses (e.g. solid or cystic)
  - determine endometrial thickness, locate/characterize fibroids
  - monitor follicles during assisted reproduction
  - assess endometrial lining in postmenopausal women

Endometrial Biopsy

- performed in the office using an endometrial suction curette (pipelle) guided through the cervix to aspirate fragments of endometrium
  - pre-treatment with misoprostol (Cytotec®) if nulliparous or postmenopausal
- more invasive procedure (D&C) may be done in the office or operating room ± hysteroscopy. This may be required if endometrial biopsy is not possible in the office setting
- indications
  - AUB/PMB
    - age > 40
    - risk factors for endometrial cancer
    - failure of medical treatment
    - significant intermenstrual bleeding
    - consider in women with infrequent menses suggesting anovulatory cycles

Hysterectomy

Indications
- uterine fibroids
- endometriosis, adenomyosis
- uterine prolapse
- pelvic pain
- AUB
- cancer (endometrium, ovaries, fallopian tubes, cervix)

Complications
- general anesthetic
- bleeding
- infection
- injury to other organs (ureter, bladder, rectum)
- loss of ovarian function (if ovaries removed, iatrogenic menopause)

Approaches
1. open (abdominal approach): uterus removed via transverse (pfannenstiel) or midline laparotomy
2. minimally Invasive Approaches
   - vaginal: uterus removed via vagina; uterus is separated from surrounding structures by vaginal route, no abdominal incisions
     - indications: mobile uterus, uterine size <12 wk
     - advantages : less pain, faster recovery time, allows for simultaneous repair of rectocele/cystocele/enterocele, improved aesthetics. This is the gold standard of the minimally invasive routes.
3. Robotic
   - similar advantages to laparoscopy
   - may be advantageous in high BMI patients
   - more costly

Table 1. Classification of Hysterectomy

Classification	Tissues Removed	Indications
Subtotal Hysterectomy	Uterus	Inaccessible cervix (e.g. adhesions) Patient choice/preference Severe endometriosis
Total Hysterectomy (extrafascial simple hysterectomy/type 1)	Uterus, cervix, uterine artery ligated at uterus	Uterine fibroids Endometriosis Adenomyosis Menorrhagia DUB
Total Hysterectomy (extrafasical simple hysterectomy/type 1) + Bilateral Salpingo-Oophorectomy	Uterus, cervix, uterine artery ligated at uterus, fallopian tubes, ovaries	Endometrial cancer Malignant adnexal masses Consider for endometriosis
Modified Radical Hysterectomy (type 2)	Uterus, cervix, proximal 1/3 parametria, uterine artery ligated medial to the ureter, mid point of uterosacral ligaments and upper 1-2 cm vagina	Cervical cancer (up to stage IBI)
Radical Hysterectomy (type 3)	Uterus, cervix, upper 1/3-1/2 vagina, entire parametria, uterine artery ligated at its origin from internal iliac artery, uterosacral ligament at most distal attachment (rectum)	Cervical cancer

Disorders of Menstruation

Amenorrhea

Differential Diagnosis of Amenorrhea

Table 2. Differential Diagnosis of Primary Amenorrhea

With Secondary Sexual Development		Without Secondary Sexual Development	
Normal breast and pelvic development	Normal breast, abnormal uterine development	High FSH (hypergonadotropic hypogonadism)	Low FSH (hypogonadotropic hypogonadism)

Hypothyroidism
Hyperprolactinemia
PCOS
Hypothalamic dysfunction
	Androgen insensitivity
	Anatomic abnormalities
	  Müllerian agenesis,
	  uterovaginal septum,
	  imperforate hymen
		Gonadal dysgenesis
		  Abnormal sex chromosome
		  (Turner's XO)
		  Normal sex chromosome
		  (46XX, 46XY)
			Constitutional delay (most common)
			Congenital abnormalities
			  Isolated GnRH deficiency
			  Pituitary failure (Kallman syndrome, head injury, pituitary adenoma, etc.)
			Acquired
			  Endocrine disorders (type 1 DM)
			  Pituitary tumours
			  Systemic disorders (IBD, JRA, chronic infections, etc.)

Table 3. Differential Diagnosis of Secondary Amenorrhea

With Hyperandrogenism	Without Hyperandrogenism

PCOS
Autonomous hyperandrogenism (androgen secretion independent of the HPO axis)
  Ovarian: tumour, hyperthecosis
  Adrenal androgen-secreting tumour
Late onset or mild congenital adrenal hyperplasia (rare)
	Hypergonadotropic hypogonadism (i.e. premature ovarian failure: high FSH, low estradiol)
	  Idiopathic
	  Autoimmune: type 1 DM, autoimmune thyroid disease, Addison's disease
	  Iatrogenic: cyclophosphamide drugs, radiation
	Hyperprolactinemia
	Endocrinopathies: most commonly hyper or hypothyroidism
	Hypogonadotropic hypogonadism (low FSH):
	  Pituitary compression or destruction: pituitary adenoma, craniopharyngioma, lymphocytic hypophysitis, infiltration (sarcoidosis), head injury, Sheehan's syndrome
	Functional hypothalamic amenorrhea (often related to stress excessive exercise and/or anorexia)

Functional hypothalamic amenorrhea is the most common cause of secondary amenorrhea

Investigations

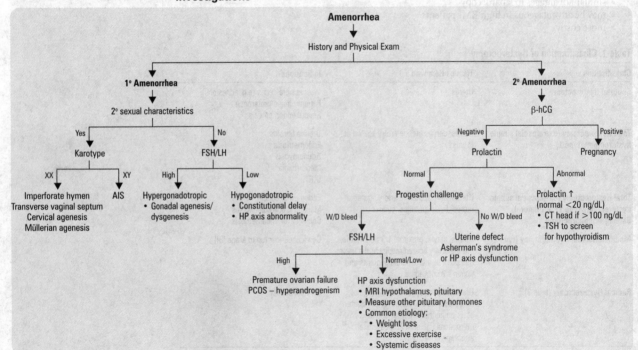

Figure 10. Diagnostic approach to amenorrhea

- β-hCG, hormonal workup (TSH, prolactin, FSH, LH, androgens, estradiol)
- progesterone challenge to assess estrogen status
  - medroxyprogesterone acetate (Provera®) 10 mg PO OD for 10-14 d
  - any uterine bleed within 2-7 d after completion of Provera® is considered to be a positive test/ withdrawal bleed
    - withdrawal bleed suggests presence of adequate estrogen to thicken the endometrium; thus withdrawal of progresterone results in bleeding
    - if no bleeding occurs, there may be inadequate estrogen (hypoestrogenism), excessive androgens, or progesterones (decidualization)
- karyotype: indicated if premature ovarian failure or absent puberty
- U/S to confirm normal anatomy, identify PCOS

Prolactinoma Symptoms
Galactorrhea, visual changes, headache

Treatment

Table 4. Management of Amenorrhea

Etiology	Management
1° AMENORRHEA	
Androgen insensitivity syndrome	Gonadal resection after puberty
	Psychological counselling
	Creation of neo-vagina
Anatomical	Surgical management
Imperforate hymen	
Transverse vaginal septum	
Cervical agenesis	
Müllerian dysgenesis (MRKH syndrome)	Psychological counselling
	Creation of neo-vagina with dilation
	Diagnostic study to confirm normal urinary system and spine
2° AMENORRHEA	
Uterine defect	Evaluation with hysterosalpingography or sonohysterography
Asherman's syndrome	Hysteroscopy: excision of synechiae
HP-axis dysfunction	**Identify modifiable underlying cause**
	Combined OCP to decrease risk of osteoporosis, maintain normal vaginal and breast development (NOT proven to work)
Premature ovarian failure	Screen for DM, hypothyroidism, hypoparathyroidism, hypocorticolism
	Hormonal therapy with estrogen + progestin to decrease risk of osteoporosis; can use OCP
Hyperprolactinemia	MRI/CT head to rule out lesion
	If no demonstrable lesions by MRI
	Bromocriptine, cabergoline if fertility desired
	Combined OCPs if no fertility desired
	Demonstrable lesions by MRI: surgical management
Polycystic ovarian syndrome	See *Polycystic Ovarian Syndrome*, GY24

Primary Amenorrhea
No menses by age 13 in absence of 2° sexual characteristics or no menses by age 15 with 2° sexual characteristics or no menses 2 yr after thelarche

Secondary Amenorrhea
No menses for >6 mo or 3 cycles after documented menarche

Oligomenorrhea
Episodic vaginal bleeding occurring at intervals >35 d

2° amenorrhea is pregnancy until proven otherwise

Abnormal Uterine Bleeding

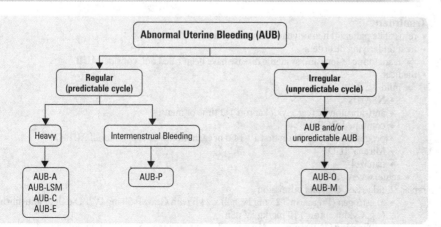

Figure 11. Diagnostic approach to abnormal uterine bleeding

Abnormal Uterine Bleeding
Change in frequency, duration, or amount of menstrual flow

Approach

- is it regular?
  - regular: cycle to cycle variability of <20 d – "Can you predict your menses within 20 days?"
  - irregular: cycle to cycle variability of ≥20 d
- is it heavy
  - ≥80 cc of blood loss per cycle or
  - ≥8 d of bleeding per cycle or
  - bleeding that significantly affects quality of life
- is it structural?
  - PALM
- is it non-structural?
  - COEIN

Table 5. AUB – Etiologies, Investigations, and Management

Etiology	Investigations	Management
STRUCTURAL		
Polyps (AUB-P)	Transvaginal Sonography Saline Infusion Sonohysterography MRI	Polypectomy (triage based on symptomatic, polyp size, histopathology and patient age)
Adenomyosis (AUB-A)	Transvaginal Sonography MRI	See *Adenomyosis*, GY15
Leiomyoma (AUB-L) Submucosal (AUB-Lsm) Other (AUB-Lo)	Transvaginal Sonography Saline Infusion Sonohysterography Diagnostic Hysteroscopy	See *Fibroids (Leiomyomata)*, GY15
Malignancy and Hyperplasia (AUB-M)	Transvaginal Sonography Endometrial Biopsy - consider biopsy in women >40 yr to exclude endometrial cancer	Dependent on diagnosis
NON-STRUCTURAL		
Coagulopathy (AUB-C)	CBC, coagulation profile (especially in adolescents), von Willebrand Factor, Ristocetin Cofactor, Factor VIII	Dependent on diagnosis (Hormonal modulation (e.g. OCP), Mirena IUD, endometrial ablation)
Ovulatory dysfunction (AUB-O)	Bloodwork: β-hCG, ferritin, prolactin, FSH, LH, serum androgens (free testosterone, DHEA), progesterone, 17-hydroxy progesterone, TSH, fT4 pelvic ultrasound	See *Infertility*, GY23
Endometrial (AUB-E)	Endometrial Biopsy	Tranexamic acid Hormonal modulation (eg. OCP) Mirena IUD endometrial ablation
Iatrogenic (AUB-I)	Transvaginal Sonography (rule out forgotten IUD) Review OCP/HRT use Review meds (especially neuroleptic use)	Remove offending agent
Not yet classified (AUB-N	—	—

*Ferrous gluconate 300 mg PO TID will raise Hb 10 points per wk

Abnormal Uterine Bleeding
Abnormal bleeding not attributable to organic (anatomic/systemic) disease
AUB is a diagnosis of exclusion
In the new nomenclature, AUB is referred to as AUB-O, AUB-E or AUB-C

AUB in women >40 yr requires an endometrial biopsy to rule out cancer even if known to have fibroids

Determine if patient is hemodynamically stable prior to any other task

Treatment

- resuscitate patient if hemodynamically unstable
- treat underlying disorders
  - if anatomic lesions and systemic disease have been ruled out, consider AUB
- medical
  - mild AUB
    - NSAIDs
    - anti-fibrinolytic (e.g. Cyklokapron®) at time of menses
    - combined OCP
    - progestins (Provera®) on first 10-14 d of each month or every 3 mo if AUB-O
    - Mirena® IUD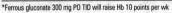
    - danazol
  - acute, severe AUB

replace fluid losses, consider admission
    - a) estrogen (Premarin®) 25 mg IV q4h x 24 h with Gravol® 50 mg IV/PO q4h or anti-fibrinolytic (e.g. Cyklokapron®) 10 mg/kg IV q8h
    - b) Tapering OCP regimen, 35μg pill TID x7d then taper to 1 pill/d for 3w with
    - Gravol® 50 mg IV/PO q4h
      - taper to 1 tab tid x 2 d → bid x 2 d → OD
    - after (a) or (b), maintain patient on monophasic OCP for next several months or consider alternativmedical treatment

- surgical
  - endometrial ablation
    - if finished childbearing
    - repeat procedure may be required if symptom reoccur especially if <40 yr
  - hysterectomy: definitive treatment

Dysmenorrhea

Etiology
- see *Differential Diagnoses of Common Presentations*, GY6

Table 6. Comparison of Primary and Secondary Dysmenorrhea

	Primary Dysmenorrhea	Secondary Dysmenorrhea
Features	Menstrual pain in absence of organic disease Begins 6 mo-2 yr after menarche (once ovulatory cycles established)	Menstrual pain due to organic disease Usually begins in women who are in their 20s, worsens with age May improve temporarily after childbirth
Signs and Symptoms	Colicky pain in abdomen, radiating to the lower back, labia, and inner thighs beginning hours before onset of bleeding and persisting for hours or days (48-72 h) Associated symptoms: N/V, altered bowel habits, headaches, fatigue (prostaglandin-associated)	Associated dyspareunia, abnormal bleeding, infertility
Diagnosis	Associated dyspareunia, abnormal bleeding, infertility Rule out underlying pelvic pathology and confirm cyclic nature of pain	Bimanual exam: uterine or adnexal tenderness, fixed uterine retroflexion, uterosacral nodularity, pelvic mass, or enlarged irregular uterus (findings are rare in women <20 yr) U/S, laparoscopy and hysteroscopy may be necessary to establish the diagnosis Screening for infections (vaginal and cervical cultures) may be required
Treatment	PG synthetase inhibitors (e.g. Anaprox®): should be started before onset of pain OCP: suppress ovulation/reduce menstrual flow	Treat underlying cause

Primary Dysmenorrhea
Menstrual pain in absence of organic disease

Secondary Dysmenorrhea
Menstrual pain due to organic disease

Endometriosis

Etiology
- not fully understood
- proposed mechanisms (combination likely involved)
  - retrograde menstruation (Sampson's theory)
  - immunologic theory: altered immunity may limit clearance of transplanted endometrial cells from pelvic cavity (may be due to decreased NK cell activity)
  - metaplasia of coelomic epithelium
  - extrapelvic disease may be due to aberrant vascular or lymphatic dissemination of cells
    - e.g. ovarian endometriosis may be due to direct lymphatic flow from uterus to ovaries

Epidemiology
- incidence: 15-30% of pre-menopausal women
- mean age at presentation: 25-30 yr
- regresses after menopause

Risk Factors
- family history (7-10x increased risk if affected 1st degree relative)
- obstructive anomalies of the genital tract (earlier onset) – resolve with treatment of anomaly
- nulliparity
- age >25 yr

Sites of Occurrence
- ovaries: 60% patients have ovarian involvement
- broad ligament, vesicoperitoneal fold
- peritoneal surface of the cul-de-sac, uterosacral ligaments
- rectosigmoid colon, appendix
- rarely may occur in sites outside abdomen/pelvis, including lungs

Endometriosis
The presence of endometrial tissue (glands and stroma) outside of the uterine cavity

Endometrioma
Endometriotic cyst encompassing the ovary

Differential Diagnoses
- Chronic PID, recurrent acute salpingitis
- Hemorrhagic corpus luteum
- Benign/malignant ovarian neoplasm
- Ectopic pregnancy

Classic Triad of Endometriosis
- Dysmenorrhea
- Dyspareunia (cul-de-sac, uterosacral ligament)
- Dyschezia (uterosacral ligament, cul-de-sac, rectosigmoid attachment)

A sharp, firm, and exquisitely tender "barb" on the uterosacral ligament is a classic feature of endometriosis

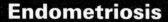

Clinical Features
- may be asymptomatic and can occur with one of 3 presentations
1. **pain**
   - menstrual symptoms
     - cyclic symptoms due to growth and bleeding of ectopic endometrium, usually precede menses (24-48 h) and continue throughout and after flow
     - secondary dysmenorrhea
     - sacral backache with menses
     - pain may eventually become chronic, worsening perimenstrually
     - deep dyspareunia
   - bowel and bladder symptoms
     - frequency, dysuria, hematuria
     - cyclic diarrhea/constipation, hematochezia, dyschezia (suggestive of deeply infiltrating disease)
2. **infertility**
   - 30-40% of patients with endometriosis will be infertile
   - 15-30% of those who are infertile will have endometriosis
3. **mass (endometrioma)**
   - ovarian mass can present with any of above symptoms or be asymptomatic
   - physical
   - tender nodularity of uterine ligaments and cul-de-sac felt on rectovaginal exam
   - fixed retroversion of uterus
   - firm, fixed adnexal mass (endometrioma)
   - physical findings not present in adolescent population

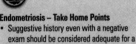

> **Endometriosis – Take Home Points**
> - Suggestive history even with a negative exam should be considered adequate for a presumptive diagnosis
> - Pelvic pain that is not primary dysmenorrhea should be considered endometriosis until proven otherwise
> - Medical management is the mainstay of endometriosis

Investigations
- definitive diagnosis requires
  - direct visualization of lesions typical of endometriosis at laparoscopy
  - biopsy and histologic exam of specimens (2 or more of: endometrial epithelium, glands, stroma, hemosiderin-laden macrophages)
- laparoscopy
  - mulberry spots: dark blue or brownish-black implants on the uterosacral ligaments, cul-de-sac, or anywhere in the pelvis
  - endometrioma: "chocolate" cysts on the ovaries
  - "powder-burn" lesions on the peritoneal surface
  - early white lesions and clear blebs
  - peritoneal "pockets"
- CA-125
  - may be elevated in patients with endometriosis but should NOT be used as a diagnostic test

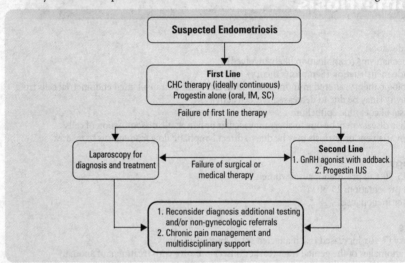

Figure 12. SOGC guidelines for treatment of endometriosis

Treatment
- **surgical** confirmation of disease is NOT required prior to starting medical management. Asymptomatic endometriosis does not require treatment. Management depends on certainty of the diagnosis, severity of symptoms, extent of disease, desire for future fertility, and impact to GI/GU systems (e.g. intestinal obstruction)
- medical
  - NSAIDs (e.g. naproxen sodium – Anaprox®)
  - 1st line
    - cyclic/continuous estrogen-progestin (OCP)
    - **progestin** (IM medroxyprogesterone (Depo-Provera®) or oral dienogest (Visanne®)
    - Mirena® IUS

- 2nd line
  - ◆ 2nd line: GnRH-a example: leuprolide (Lupron®): GnRH agonist (suppresses pituitary)
    - – side effects: hot flashes, vaginal dryness, reduced libido
    - – can use ≥12 mo with add-back progestin or estrogen
  - ◆ danazol (Danocrine®): weak androgen
    - – side effects: weight gain, fluid retention, acne, hirsutism, voice change
- surgical
  - ▪ conservative laparoscopy using laser, electrocautery ± laparotomy
    - ◆ ablation/resection of implants, lysis of adhesions, ovarian cystectomy of endometriomas
  - ▪ definitive: bilateral salpingo-oophorectomy ± hysterectomy
  - ▪ ± follow-up with medical treatment for pain control not shown to impact on preservation of fertility
  - ▪ best time to become pregnant is immediately after conservative surgery

Adenomyosis

- synonym: "endometriosis interna" (uterine wall may be diffusely involved)

Epidemiology
- 15% of females >35 yr old; found in 20-40% of hysterectomy specimens
- mean age at presentation: 40-50 yr old (older age group than seen in endometriosis)
- adenomyosis is a common histologic finding in asymptomatic patients

Adenomyosis
Extension of areas of endometrial glands and stroma into the myometrium

Clinical Features
- often asymptomatic
- menorrhagia, secondary dysmenorrhea, pelvic discomfort
- dyspareunia, dyschezia
- uterus symmetrically bulky, usually <14 cm, mobility not restricted, no associated adnexal pathology
- Halban sign: tender, softened uterus on premenstrual bimanual exam

Investigations
- clinical diagnosis
- U/S or MRI can be helpful
- endometrial sampling to rule out other pathology

Final diagnosis of adenomyosis is based on pathologic findings, but predictably identified on MRI

Treatment
- iron supplements as necessary
- analgesics, NSAIDs
- OCP, medroxyprogesterone (Depo-Provera®)
- GnRH agonists (e.g. leuprolide)
- Mirena® IUS
- low dose danazol 100-200 mg PO OD (trial x 4 mo)
- definitive: hysterectomy (no conservative surgical treatment)

Fibroids

Epidemiology
- diagnosed in approximately 40-50% of pre-menopausal women >35 yr
- more common in African Americans, where they are also larger and occur at earlier age
- common indication for major surgery in females
- minimal malignant potential (1:1,000)
- typically regress after menopause; enlarging fibroids in a postmenopausal woman should prompt consideration of malignancy

Pathogenesis
- estrogen stimulates monoclonal smooth muscle proliferation
- progesterone stimulates production of proteins that inhibit apoptosis
- degenerative changes (occur when tumour outgrows blood supply)
  - ▪ fibroids can degenerate, become calcified, have scarcomatous component or obtain parasitic blood supply

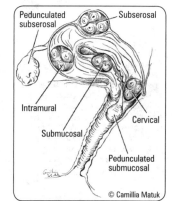

Figure 13. Possible anatomic locations of uterine leiomyomata

Clinical Features
- majority asymptomatic (60%), often discovered as incidental finding on pelvic exam or U/S
- abnormal uterine bleeding (30%): dysmenorrhea, menorrhagia
- pressure/bulk symptoms (20-50%)
  - ▪ pelvic pressure/heaviness
  - ▪ increased abdominal girth
  - ▪ urinary frequency and urgency
  - ▪ acute urinary retention (extremely rare but surgical emergency!)
  - ▪ constipation, bloating (rare)

Leiomyomata/Fibroids
Benign smooth muscle tumour of the uterus (most common gynecological tumour)

Ulipristal Acetate vs. Leuprolide Acetate for Uterine Fibroids
NEJM 2012;366:421-432
Study: Phase III, double-blind RCT of the efficacy and side-effect profile of ulipristal acetate versus those of leuprolide acetate for the treatment of symptomatic uterine fibroids before surgery.
Outcomes: Control of uterine bleeding at week 13 was the primary outcome. Secondary outcomes included bleeding pattern, amenorrhea, changes in fibroid/uterine volume, and global pain score.
Patients: 307 premenopausal women with symptomatic fibroids and excessive uterine bleeding were randomly assigned to oral ulipristal acetate (5 mg or 10 mg) or intramuscular injections of leuprolide acetate.
Results: Control of uterine bleeding at week 13 was not significantly different between the treatment groups. All three treatments reduced uterine volume, although this decrease was significantly greater in the leuprolide group (47% reduction) than in the ulipristal groups (20-22%). 40% of the leuprolide group reported moderate-to-severe hot flashes, but only 11% (5 mg) and 10% (10 mg) of the ulipristal groups did.
Conclusions: Oral ulipristal acetate (5 mg or 10 mg) is noninferior to intramuscular leuprolide acetate for control of uterine bleeding due to fibroids, and it had a better side-effect profile.

- acute pelvic pain
  - fibroid degeneration
  - fibroid torsion (pedunculated subserosal)
- infertility, recurrent pregnancy loss
- pregnancy complications (potential enlargement and increased pain, obstructed labour, difficult C-section)

Investigations
- bimanual exam: uterus asymmetrically enlarged, usually mobile
- CBC: anemia
- U/S: to confirm diagnosis and assess location of fibroids
- sonohysterogram: useful for differentiating endometrial polyps from submucosal fibroids, or if intracavitary growth
- endometrial biopsy to rule out uterine cancer for abnormal uterine bleeding (especially if age >40 yr)
- occasionally MRI is used for pre-operative planning (e.g. before myomectomy)

Treatment
- only if symptomatic, rapidly enlarging, menorrhagia, menometrorrhagia, or intracavitary
- treat anemia if present
- conservative approach (watch and wait) if
  - symptoms absent or minimal
  - fibroids <6-8 cm or stable in size
  - not submucosal (submucosal fibroids are more likely to be symptomatic)
  - currently pregnant due to increased risk of bleeding (follow-up U/S if symptoms progress)
- medical approach to treat AUB-L
  - antiprostaglandins (ibuprofen, other NSAIDs)
  - tranexamic acid (Cyklokapron®)
  - OCP/Depo-Provera®
  - GnRH agonist: leuprolide (Lupron®), danazol (Danocrine®)
    - ◆ short-term use only (6 mo)
    - ◆ often used pre-myomectomy or pre-hysterectomy to reduce fibroid size
    - ◆ reduced bleeding
  - ulipristal acetate: a partial progesterone receptor agonist
- interventional radiology approach
  - uterine artery embolization (occludes both uterine arteries) → shrinks fibroids by 50% at 6 mo; improves heavy bleeding in 90% of patients within 1-2 mo; not an option in women considering childbearing
- surgical approach
  - myomectomy (hysteroscopic, transabdominal, or laparoscopic): preserves fertility
  - hysteroscopic resection of fibroid and endometrial ablation for AUB-Lsm
  - hysterectomy (see *Hysterectomy*, GY9)
  - note: avoid operating on fibroids during pregnancy (due to → vascularity and potential pregnancy loss); expectant management usually best

Contraception

- see Family Medicine, FM19

Table 7. Classification of Contraceptive Methods

Type	Effectiveness (Perfect Use, Typical Use)
Physiological	
Withdrawal/coitus interruptus	77%
Rhythm method/calendar/mucus/symptothermal	98%, 76%
Lactational amenorrhea	98% (first 6 mo postpartum)
Chance – no method used	10%
Abstinence of all sexual activity	100%
Barrier Methods	
Condom alone	98%, 85%
Spermicide alone	82%, 71%
Sponge – Parous	80%, 68%
– Nulliparous	91%, 84%
Diaphragm with spermicide	94%, 84%
Female condom	95%, 79%
Cervical cap – Parous	74%, 68%
– Nulliparous	91%, 84%

Table 7. Classification of Contraceptive Methods (continued)

Type	Effectiveness (Perfect Use, Typical Use)
Hormonal	
OCP	99.7%, 92%
Nuva Ring®	99.7%, 92%
Transdermal (Ortho Evra®)	99.7%, 92%
Depo-Provera®	99.7%, 97%
Progestin-only pill (Micronor®)	90-99%
Mirena® IUS	99.9%
Jaydess® IUS	99.9%
Copper IUD	99.3%
Surgical	
Tubal ligation	99.65%
Vasectomy	99.9%
Emergency Postcoital Contraception (EPC)	
Yuzpe® method	98% (within 24 h), decreases by 30% at 72 h
"Plan B" levonorgestrel only	98% (within 24 h), decreases by 70% at 72 h
Postcoital IUD	99.9%
Ella	98% (within 120 h)

Effectiveness: percentage of women reporting no pregnancy after 1 yr of use

Hormonal Methods

Combined Oral Contraceptive Pills
- most contain low dose ethinyl estradiol (20-35 μg) plus progestin (norethinedrone, norgestrel, levonorgestrel, desogestrel, norgestimate, drospirenone)
- failure rate (0.3% to 8%) depending on compliance
- monophasic or triphasic formulations (varying amount of progestin throughout cycle)

Transdermal (Ortho Evra®)
- continuous release of 6 mg norelgestromin and 0.60 mg ethinyl estradiol into bloodstream
- applied to lower abdomen, back, upper arm, buttocks, NOT breast
- worn for 3 consecutive weeks (changed every wk) with 1 wk off to allow for menstruation
- as effective as OCP in preventing pregnancy (>99% with perfect use)
- may be less effective in women >90 kg
- may not be covered by drug plans

Contraceptive Ring (Nuva Ring®)
- thin flexible plastic ring; releases etonogestrel 120 μg/d and estradiol 15 μg/d
- works for 3 wk then removed for 1 wk to allow for menstruation
- as effective as OCP in preventing pregnancy (98%)
- side effects: vaginal infections/irritation, vaginal discharge
- may have better cycle control; i.e. decreased breakthrough bleeding

Starting Hormonal Contraceptives
- thorough history and physical exam, including blood pressure and breast exam
- can start at any time during cycle but ideal if within 5 d of LMP
- follow-up visit 6 wk after hormonal contraceptives prescribed
- pelvic exam not required as STI screening can be done by urine and pap smear screening does not start until >21 yr

Oral Contraceptives and the Risk of Venous Thromboembolism: An Update (2010)
J Obstet Gyn Canada 2010;32:1192-1197
Rates of Venous Thromboembolism
(VTE: DVT and PE) expressed in women/yr
Non-users of reproductive age   4-5/10,000
OCP users*   9-10/10,000
Pregnancy   29/10,000
Immediate post-partum   300-400/10,000
*Risk is highest in the first months of use and in medication switch and if stop and restart.
Effect of Ethinyl Estradiol Dose
ALL OCPs with ≤35 μg ethinyl estradiol carry a lower risk of VTE compared with oral contraceptives with 50 μg.
Effect of Progestin Type
Drospirenone: third generation progestin, e.g. Yasmin® and Yaz®
Levonorgestrel: second generation progestin, e.g. Alesse®
Two high quality research studies found comparable VTE rates with drospirenone-containing OCPs and other approved products.
1. Dinger et al., *Contraception* 2007;75:344-354
2. Seeger et al., *Obstet Gynecol* 2007;110:587-593
Two reports with significant methodological flaws found increased VTE risk. Results and conclusions may have been distorted by residual confounding.
1. Lidegaard et al., *BMJ* 2009;339:b2890
2. Van Hylckama Vlieg et al., *BMJ* 2009;339:b2921
Conclusion
- Occurrence of serious risks, such as VTE, is rare with all contemporary OCPs.
- Individualized risk assessment is mandatory.
- For most healthy women of reproductive age, the benefits of OCPs will outweigh the risks.

Thrombotic Stroke and Myocardial Infarction with Hormonal Contraception
NEJM 2012;366:2257-2266
Study: 15 yr Danish historical cohort study. Non-pregnant women 15-49 yr of age with no history of cardiovascular disease or cancer.
Results: Total of 1,626,158 women, thrombotic stroke rate 21.4/100,000 person yr, MI rate 10.1/100,000 person yr. Oral contraceptives with ethinyl estradiol at a dose of 30-40 μg according to progestin type and risk of thrombotic stroke and MI (RR [CI]): norethindrone 2.2 (1.5-3.2) and 2.3 (1.3-3.9); levonorgestrel 1.7 (1.4-2.0) and 2.0 (1.6-2.5); norgestimate 1.5 (1.2-1.9) and 1.3 (0.9-1.9); desogestrel 2.2 (1.8-2.7) and 2.1 (1.5-2.8); gestodene 1.8 (1.6-2.0) and 1.9 (1.6-2.3); and drospirenone 1.6 (1.2-2.2) and 1.7 (1.0-2.6). With ethinyl estradiol at a dose of 20 μg, risks according to progestin type were: desogestrel 1.5 (1.3-1.9) and 1.6 (1.1-2.1); gestodene 1.7 (1.4-2.1) and 1.2 (0.8-1.9) and drospirenone 0.9 (0.2-3.5) and 0.0.
Conclusions: Although the absolute risk of thrombotic stroke and MI with hormonal contraception is low, it is increased by a factor of 0.9-1.7 with oral contraceptives that contain ethinyl estradiol at a dose of 20 μg and by a factor of 1.3-2.3 with ethinyl estradiol doses of 30-40 μg, with relatively small differences in risk according to progestin type.

Table 8. Combined Estrogen and Progestin Contraceptive Methods

Mechanism of Action	Advantages	Side Effects	Contraindications
Ovulatory suppression through inhibition of LH and FSH Decidualization of endometrium Thickening of cervical mucus resulting in decreased sperm penetration	Highly effective Reversible Cycle regulation Decreased dysmenorrhea and menorrhagia (less anemia) Decreased benign breast disease and ovarian cyst development Decreased risk of ovarian and endometrial cancer Increased cervical mucus which may lower risk of STIs Decreased PMS symptoms Improved acne Osteoporosis protection (possibly)	**Estrogen-related** Nausea Breast changes (tenderness, enlargement) Fluid retention/bloating/edema Weight gain (rare) Migraine, headaches Thromboembolic events Liver adenoma (rare) Breakthrough bleeding (low estradiol levels) **Progestin-related** Amenorrhea/breakthrough bleeding Headaches Breast tenderness Increased appetite Decreased libido Mood changes HTN Acne/oily skin* Hirsutism* * Androgenic side effects may be minimized by prescribing formulations containing desogestrel, norgestimate, drospirenone, or cyproterone acetate	**Absolute** Known/suspected pregnancy Undiagnosed abnormal vaginal bleeding Prior thromboembolic events, thromboembolic disorders (Factor V Leiden mutation; protein C or S, or antithrombin III deficiency), active thrombophlebitis Cerebrovascular or coronary artery disease Estrogen-dependent tumours (breast, uterus) Impaired liver function associated with acute liver disease Congenital hypertriglyceridemia Smoker age >35 yr Migraines with focal neurological symptoms (excluding aura) Uncontrolled HTN **Relative** Migraines (non-focal with aura <1 h) DM complicated by vascular disease SLE Controlled HTN Hyperlipidemia Sickle cell anemia Gallbladder disease **Drug Interactions/Risks** Rifampin, phenobarbital, phenytoin, griseofulvin, primidone, and St. John's wort can decrease efficacy, requiring use of back-up method No evidence of fetal abnormalities if conceived on OCP No evidence that OCP is harmful to nursing infant but may decrease milk production; not recommended until 6 wk postpartum in BF and non BF moms, ideally 3 mo postpartum if BF

Reference: World Health Organization Guidelines for Oral Contraceptive Pill Use

Irregular breakthrough bleeding often occurs in the first few months after starting OCP; usually resolves after three cycles

Missed Combined OCPs
Miss 1 pill in <24 h
- Take 1 pill ASAP, and the next pill at the usual time

Miss ≥1 pill in a row in first wk
- Take 1 pill ASAP, and continue taking one pill daily until the end of the pack
- Use back-up contraception for 7 d; EPC may be necessary

Miss <3 pills in 2nd or 3rd wk of cycle
- Take 1 pill ASAP, and continue taking one pill daily until the end of the pack
- Do not take placebo (28-d packs) or do not take a hormone free interval (21-d packs)
- Start the next pack immediately after finishing the previous one
- No need for back-up contraception

Miss ≥3 pills during the 2nd or 3rd wk
- Take 1 pill ASAP, and continue taking one pill daily until the end of the pack
- Don't take placebo (28-d packs) or do not take a hormone free interval (21-d packs)
- Start the next pack immediately after finishing the previous one
- Use back-up contraception for 7 d; EPC may be necessary

SOGC Committee Opinion on Missed Hormonal Contraceptives: New Recommendations. *JOGC* 2008;30:1050-1062. http://www.sogc.org/guidelines/documents/gui219ECO0811.pdf

Table 9. Selected Examples of OCPs

Type	Active Compounds (estriol and progestin derivative)	Advantages	Disadvantages
Alesse®	20 μg ethinyl estradiol and 0.5 mg levonorgestrel	Low dose (20 μg) OCP Less estrogen side effects	Low-dose pills can often result in breakthrough bleeding If this persists for longer than 3 mo, patient should be switched to an OCP with higher estrogen content
Tri-cyclen®	35 μg ethinyl estradiol and 0.180/0.215/0.250 mg norgestimate Triphasic oral contraceptive (graduated levels of progesterone)	Low androgenic activity can help with acne	Triphasic OCPs not ideal for continuous use >3 weeks in a row (unlike monophasic formulation)
Yasmin® and Yaz®	Yasmin®: 30 μg ethinyl estradiol + 3 mg drospirenone (a new progestin) Yaz®: 20 μg ethinyl estradiol + 3 mg drospirenone – 24/4-d pill (4 d pill free interval) Drospirenone has antimineralocorticoid activity and antiandrogenic effects	Decreased perception of cyclic weight gain/bloating Fewer PMS symptoms Improved acne	Hyperkalemia (rare, contraindicated in renal and adrenal insufficiency) Check potassium if patient also on ACEI, ARB, K⁺-sparing diuretic, heparin Continue use of spironolactone

PROGESTIN-ONLY METHOD

Table 10. Progestin Only Contraceptive Methods

Indications	Mechanism of Action	Side Effects	Contraindications
Suitable for postpartum women (does not affect breast milk supply) Women with contraindications to combined OCP (e.g. thromboembolic or myocardial disease) Women intolerant of estrogenic side effects of combined OCPs	Progestin prevents LH surge Thickening of cervical mucus Decrease tubal motility Endometrial decidualization Ovulation suppression – oral progestins (not IM) do not consistently suppress compared to combined OCPs	Irregular menstrual bleeding Weight gain Headache Breast tenderness Mood changes Functional ovarian cysts Acne/oily skin Hirsutism	**Absolute** None

SELECTED EXAMPLES OF PROGESTIN-ONLY METHODS

Progestin-Only Pill ("minipill")
- Micronor® 0.35 mg norethindrone
- taken daily at same time of day to ensure reliable effect; no pill free interval
- higher failure rate (1.1-13% with typical use, 0.51% with perfect use) than other hormonal methods
- ovulation inhibited only in 60% of women; most have regular cycles (but may cause oligo/amenorrhea)
- highly effective if also post-partum breastfeeding, or if >35 yr
- relies on the progestin effects on the cervical mucous and endometrial lining

Depo-Provera®
- injectable depot medroxyprogesterone acetate
- dose 150 mg IM q12-14wk (convenient dosing)
- initiate ideally within 5 d of beginning of normal menses, immediately postpartum in breastfeeding and non-breastfeeding women. Can consider quick start
- irregular spotting progresses to complete amenorrhea in 70% of women (after 1-2 yr of use)
- highly effective 99%; failure rate 0.3%
- suppresses ovulation very effectively
- side effect: decreased bone density (may be reversible)
- disadvantage: restoration of fertility may take up to 1-2 yr

Intrauterine Device

Table 11. IUS/IUD Contraceptive Methods

Mechanism of Action	Side Effects	Contraindications
Copper-Containing IUD (Nova-T®): mild foreign body reaction in endometrium toxic to sperm and alters sperm motility	**Both Copper and Progesterone IUD** Breakthrough bleeding Expulsion (5% in the 1st yr, greatest in 1st mo and in nulliparous women) Uterine wall perforation (1/1,000) on insertion If pregnancy occurs with an IUD, increased risk of ectopic Increased risk of PID (within first 10 d of insertion only)	**Absolute** **Both Copper and Progesterone IUD** Known or suspected pregnancy Undiagnosed genital tract bleeding Acute or chronic PID Lifestyle risk for STIs* Copper IUD Known allergy to copper Wilson's disease
Progesterone-Releasing IUS (Mirena®, Jaydess®): decidualization of endometrium and thickening of cervical mucus; minimal effect on ovulation		
Highly effective (95-99%); failure rate 0-1.2%	**Copper IUD:** increased blood loss and duration of menses, dysmenorrhea	**Relative** **Both Copper and Progesterone IUD** Valvular heart disease
Contraceptive effects last 5 yr Reversible, private, convenient May be used in women with contraindications to OCPs or wanting long-term contraception	**Progesterone IUD:** bloating, headache	Past history of PID or ectopic pregnancy Presence of prosthesis Abnormalities of uterine cavity, intracavitary fibroids Cervical stenosis Immunosuppressed individuals (e.g. HIV) **Copper IUD:** severe dysmenorrhea or menorrhagia

*Cervical swabs for gonorrhea and chlamydia should be done prior to insertion

Missed Progestin-Only Pills >3 h
Use back-up contraceptive method for at least 48 h; continue to take remainder of pills as prescribed

Missed Depo-Provera
- If last injection given 13-14 wk prior: give next injection immediately
- if >14 wk prior, do β-hCG
  - If β-hCG is positive, give EPC and no injection
  - If β-hCG is negative, give next injection right away and:
    - Intercourse occurred in last 5 d: give EPC, use back-up contraception for 7 d Repeat β-hCG in 3 wk
    - Intercourse occurred >5 d ago but within the last 14 d: use back-up contraception for 7 d Repeat β-hCG in 3 wk
    - Intercourse occurred >14 d ago: use back-up contraception for 7 d
  - No evidence of fetal abnormalities if conceived on DMPA
SOGC Committee Opinion on Missed Hormonal Contraceptives: New Recommendations.
JOGC 2008;30:1050-62. http://www.sogc.org/guidelines/documents/gui219EC00811.pdf

Steroidal Contraceptives and Bone Fractures in Women: Evidence from Observational Studies
Cochrane Database Syst Rev. 2015; 7
Purpose: Systematic review of observational studies assessing the association between hormonal contraceptive use and risk of fractures in women.
Results: Systematic review identified 14 observation studies (7 cohort and 7 case-control) that assessed hormonal contraceptives use and fracture risk. Analysis of six moderate to high quality studies, all of which analyzed OCs and fractures risk, suggest minimal association between OCs and fractures risk. There is some evi-dence that suggests higher fracture risk in certain subgroups, such as the long-term users. However, this evidence is minimal. Two-case control studies reported higher risk of fractures in those who use progestin only contraceptives. The first suggested higher fracture risk for DMPA ever-use (OR = 1.44). The second reports higher risk for any previous users (OR = 1.17)
Conclusion: Current evidence does not support an association between OCP use and fracture risk. However, there is some evidence suggesting DMPA may be associated with higher fracture risk in women.

Continuous or Extended Cycle vs. Cyclic Use of Combined Hormonal Contraceptives for Contraception
Cochrane DB Syst Rev 2014:7
Purpose: Systematic review of RCTs assessing the efficacy and side effects of cyclic administration vs. extended use (longer periods of active pills and/or shorter periods placebo) or continuous use (uninterrupted active pill administration) of combination oral contraceptives (COC).
Results: The initial review published in 2012 identified 12 RCTs that ultimately showed no difference between groups with regards to efficacy (pregnancy rates), safety, and compliance rates. Continuous or extended CHCs were shown to reduce menstrual symptoms (headaches, tiredness, bloating, and menstrual pain). In addition, 11 of 12 studies reported similar or improved bleeding patterns with continuous or extended cycles.
Conclusions: This recently published updated systematic review identified a further 4 RCTs, however, results did not change.

Committee Opinion No. 602: Depot Medroxyprogresterone Acetate and Bone Effects
Obstet Gynecol 2014(6): 1298-402.
- The effect of DMPA on BMD should neither prevent practitioners from prescribing DMPA nor limit its use to 2 consecutive yr.
- BMD loss due to DMPA appears to be substantially or fully reversible.
- Contraceptive implants and intrauterine devices that do not affect BMD should be considered as first-line for adolescents.
- Inform patients about benefits and the potential risks of DMPA, and encourage daily exercise, calcium and vitamin D intake.
- Routine BMD monitoring is not recommended for DMPA users.

Emergency Postcoital Contraception

Table 12. Emergency Contraceptive Methods

Method	Mechanism of Action	Side Effects	Contraindications
HORMONAL			
Yuzpe Method Used within 72 h of unprotected intercourse; limited evidence of benefit up to 5 d Ovral® 2 tablets then repeat in 12 h (ethinyl estradiol 100 μg/levonorgestrel 500 μg) Can substitute with any OCP as long as same dose of estrogen used 2% overall risk of pregnancy Efficacy decreased with time (e.g. less effective at 72 h than 24 h)	Unknown; theories include: Suppresses ovulation or causes deficient luteal phase Alters endometrium to prevent implantation Affects sperm/ova transport	Nausea (due to estrogen; treat with Gravol®) Irregular spotting	Pre-existing pregnancy (although not teratogenic) Caution in women with contraindications to OCP (although NO absolute contraindications)
"Plan B" Consists of levonorgestrel 750 μg q12h for 2 doses (can also take 2 doses together); taken within 72 h of intercourse. Can be taken up to 5 d Greater efficacy (75-95% if used within 24 h) and better side effect profile than Yuzpe method but efficacy decreases with time; 1st line if >24 h No estrogen thus very few contraindications/side effects (less nausea) Less effective in overweight individuals (>75 kg less effective, >80 kg not recommended)	Same as above	Same as above	Same as above
Ulipristal 30 mg PO within 5 d	Selective Progesterone Receptor Modulator (SPERM) with primarily antiprogestin activity: may delay ovulation by up to 5 d	Headache, hot flashes, constipation, vertigo, endometrial thickening	Same as above
NON-HORMONAL			
Postcoital IUD (Copper) Insert up to 7 d postcoitus Prevents implantation 1% failure rate Can use for short duration in higher risk individuals Mirena® IUS cannot be used as EPC	See Table 11	See Table 11	See Table 11

Any OCP can be used as EPC; 100 μg ethinyl estradiol PO q12h x 2 doses
- Levonorgestrel emergency contraception regimens are more effective and cause fewer side effects than the Yuzpe regimen
- Levonorgestrel emergency contraception single dose (1.5 mg) and the 2-dose levonorgestrel regimen (0.75 mg 12 h apart) have similar efficacy with no difference in side effects
SOGC Clinical Practice Guidelines: Emergency Contraception. *JOGC* 2012;34:870-878.
http://www.sogc.org/guidelines/documents/gui280CPG1209E_000.pdf

CMA Policy (1988)
"Induced abortion should be uniformly available to all women in Canada" and "there should be no delay in the provision of abortion services"

Terminations are generally done until the stage of viability (~23.5 wk), although this varies depending on the provider

Follow-up
- 3-4 wk post treatment to confirm efficacy (confirmed by spontaneous menses or pregnancy test)
- contraception counselling

Termination of Pregnancy

Definition
- active termination of a pregnancy before fetal viability (usually <500 g or <20 wk GA)

Indications
- inability to carry a pregnancy to term due to medical or social reasons (including patient preference)

Management
- medical
  - <9 wk: methotrexate + misoprostol
  - >12 wk: prostaglandins (intra- or extra-amniotically or IM) or misoprostol
- surgical
  - <12 wk: dilatation + vacuum aspiration ± curettage
  - >12 wk: dilatation and evacuation, early induction of labour
  - common complications: pain or discomfort
  - less common complications: hemorrhage, perforation of uterus, laceration of cervix, risk of infertility, infection/endometritis, Asherman's syndrome (adhesions within the endometrial cavity causing amenorrhea/infertility), retained products of conception
- counselling
  - supportive and counselling services
  - future contraception and family planning services
  - ensure follow-up

Pregnancy-Related Complications

Spontaneous Abortions

- see *Termination of Pregnancy* for therapeutic abortions

Table 13. Classification of Spontaneous Abortions

Type	History	Clinical	Management (± Rhogam®)
Threatened	Vaginal bleeding ± cramping	Cervix closed and soft	Watch and wait <5% go on to abort
Inevitable	Increasing bleeding and cramps ± rupture of membranes	Cervix closed until products start to expel, then external os opens	a) Watch and wait b) Misoprostol 400-800 μg PO/PV c) D&C ± oxytocin
Incomplete	Extremely heavy bleeding and cramps ± passage of tissue noticed	Cervix open	a) Watch and wait b) Misoprostol 400-800 μg PO/PV c) D&C ± oxytocin
Complete	Bleeding and complete passage of sac and placenta	Cervix closed, bleeding stopped	No D&C – expectant management
Missed	No bleeding (fetal death in utero)	Cervix closed	a) Watch and wait b) Misoprostol 400-800 μg PO/PV c) D&C ± oxytocin
Recurrent	≥3 consecutive spontaneous abortions		Evaluate mechanical, genetic, environmental, and other risk factors
Septic	Contents of uterus infected – infrequent		D&C IV broad spectrum antibiotics

Etiology of Recurrent Pregnancy Loss MAKE ME

Type	History
Mechanical	Uterine anomalies Congenital (septate uterus) Leiomyoma Endometrial polyps Intrauterine adhesions
Autoimmune	Immunologic Factors Antiphospholipid syndrome (blood tests: lupus anticoagulant, anti-cardiolipin Ab, anti-β2 glycoprotein-I)
Karyotype	Aneuploidy with increasing age or poor sperm quality Chromosomal rearrangements Check both parents Young mother, ≥3 miscarriages, FHx miscarriage/stillbirth/malformation
Endocrine	Poorly controlled disease Thyroid (associated with high antibody/hormone levels) DM (secondary to hyperglycemia, maternal vascular disease) PCOS
Maternal Infection	No infectious agent has been proven to cause recurrent pregnancy loss, though some cause sporadic loss (Listeria, toxoplasmosis, CMV, HSV)
Environment	Obesity, smoking, alcohol use, and caffeine consumption may contribute
Other	Prothrombotic conditions (i.e. thrombophilia)

Ectopic Pregnancy

Definition
- embryo implants outside of the endometrial cavity

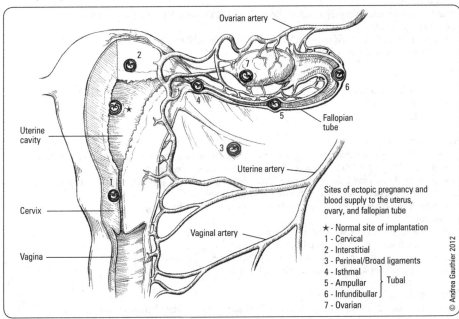

Figure 14. Sites of ectopic pregnancy implantation
Ampullary (70%) >> isthmal (12%) > fimbrial (11%) > ovarian (3%) > interstitial (2%) > abdominal (1%)

Epidemiology
- 1/100 pregnancies
- fourth leading cause of maternal mortality, leading cause of death in first trimester
- increase in incidence over the last 3 decades
- three commonest locations for ectopic pregnancy: ampullary (70%), isthmic (12%), fimbrial (11%)

DDx of Lower Abdominal Pain
- Urinary tract: UTI, kidney stones
- GI: diverticulitis, appendicitis
- Gyne: endometriosis, PID, fibroid (degenerating, infarcted, torsion), ovarian torsion, ovarian neoplasm, ovarian cyst, pregnancy-related

Clinical Features of Ectopic Pregnancy

4Ts and 1S
Temperature >38°C (20%)
Tenderness: abdominal (90%) ± rebound (45%)
Tenderness on bimanual examination, cervical motion tenderness
Tissue: palpable adnexal mass (50%) (half have contralateral mass due to lutein cyst)
Signs of pregnancy (e.g. Chadwick's sign, Hegar's sign)

More than half of patients with ectopic pregnancy have no risk factors

If Ectopic Pregnancy Ruptures
- Acute abdomen with increasing pain
- Abdominal distention
- Shock

Management of Abortions
- Always rule out an ectopic
- Always check Rh; if negative, give Rhogam®
- Always ensure patient is hemodynamically stable

Etiology
- 50% due to damage of fallopian tube cilia following PID
- intrinsic abnormality of the fertilized ovum
- conception late in cycle
- transmigration of fertilized ovum to contralateral tube

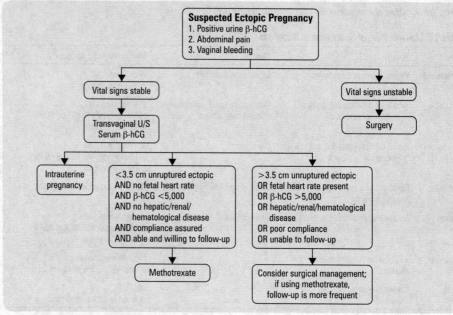

Figure 15. Algorithm for suspected ectopic pregnancy

Risk Factors
- previous ectopic pregnancy
- gynecologic
  - current IUD use – increased risk of ectopic if pregnancy occurs
  - history of PID (especially infection with *C. trachomatis*), salpingitis
  - infertility
- infertility treatment (IVF pregnancies following ovulation induction [7% ectopic rate])
- previous procedures
  - any surgery on fallopian tube (for previous ectopic, tubal ligation, etc.)
  - abdominal surgery for ruptured appendix, etc.
- smoking
- structural
  - uterine leiomyomas
  - adhesions
  - abnormal uterine anatomy (e.g. T-shaped uterus)

Investigations
- serial β-hCG levels; normal doubling time with intrauterine pregnancy is 1.6-2.4 d in early pregnancy
  - rise of <20% of β-hCG is 100% predictive of a non-viable pregnancy
  - prolonged doubling time, plateau, or decreasing levels before 8 wk implies nonviable gestation but does not provide information on location of implantation
  - 85% of ectopic pregnancies demonstrate abnormal β-hCG doubling
- ultrasound
  - U/S is only definitive if fetal cardiac activity is detected in the tube or uterus
  - specific finding on transvaginal U/S is a tubal ring
- suspect ectopic in case of empty uterus with β-hCG >5000 and no bleeding
- laparoscopy (sometimes used for definitive diagnosis)

Treatment
- goals of treatment: conservative (preserve tube if possible), maintain hemodynamic stability
- surgical = laparoscopy
  - linear salpingostomy an option if tube salvageable
  - salpingectomy if tube damaged or ectopic is ipsilateral recurrence
  - 15% risk of persistent trophoblast; must monitor β-hCG titres weekly until they reach non-detectable levels
  - consider Rhogam® if Rh negative
  - may require laparotomy if patient is unstable, extensive abdominal surgical history, etc.

- medical = methotrexate (for indications see Figure 4)
  - use 50 mg/m² body surface area; given in a single IM dose
  - this is 1/5 to 1/6 chemotherapy dose, therefore minimal side effects (reversible hepatic dysfunction, diarrhea, gastritis, dermatitis)
  - follow β-hCG levels weekly until β-hCG is non-detectable
    - plateau or rising levels suggest persisting trophoblastic tissue (requires further treatment)
  - 82-95% success rate, but up to 25% will require a second dose
  - tubal patency following methotrexate treatment approaches 80%

Prognosis
- 9% of maternal deaths during pregnancy
- 40-60% of patients will become pregnant again after surgery
- 10-20% will have subsequent ectopic pregnancy

Infertility

Epidemiology
- 10-15% of couples, must investigate both members of the couple

Female Factors

Etiology
- ovulatory dysfunction (15-20%)
  - hypothalamic (hypothalamic amenorrhea)
    - stress, poor nutrition, excessive exercise (even with presence of menstruation)
  - pituitary (prolactinoma, hypopituitarism)
    - PCOS
  - ovarian
    - premature ovarian failure
    - luteal phase defect (poor follicle production, premature corpus luteum failure, failed uterine lining response to progesterone), poorly understood
  - systemic diseases (thyroid, Cushing's syndrome, renal/hepatic failure)
  - congenital (Turner's syndrome, gonadal dysgenesis or gonadotropin deficiency)
- outflow tract abnormality (15-20%)
  - tubal factors (20-30%)
    - PID
    - adhesions (previous surgery, peritonitis, endometriosis)
    - ligation/occlusion (e.g. previous ectopic pregnancy)
  - uterine factors (<5%)
    - congenital anomalies, bicornuate uterus, septate uterus, prenatal DES exposure, intrauterine adhesions (e.g. Asherman's syndrome), fibroids/polyps (particularly intrauterine)
    - infection (endometritis, pelvic TB)
    - endometrial ablation
  - cervical factors (5%)
    - hostile or acidic cervical mucus, anti-sperm antibodies
    - structural defects (cone biopsies, laser or cryotherapy)
- endometriosis (15-30%)
- multiple factors (30%)
- unknown factors (10-15%)

Investigations
- ovulatory
  - day 3: FSH, LH, TSH, prolactin ± DHEA, free testosterone (if hirsute) add estradiol for proper FSH interpretation
  - day 21-23: serum progesterone to confirm ovulation
  - initiate basal body temperature monitoring (biphasic pattern)
  - postcoital test: evaluate mucus for clarity, pH, spinnbarkeit/fibrosity (rarely done)
- tubal factors
  - HSG (can be therapeutic – opens fallopian tube)
  - SHG (can be therapeutic; likely less – opens fallopian tube)
  - laparoscopy with dye insufflation (or tubal dye test)
- peritoneal/uterine factors
  - HSG/SHG, hysteroscopy
- other
  - karyotype

Interventions for Tubal Ectopic Pregnancy
Cochrane DB Syst Rev 2007;1:CD000324
Study: Cochrane Review of randomized controlled trials comparing treatments in women with tubal ectopic pregnancy.
Patients: Women with a diagnosis of tubal ectopic pregnancy.
Intervention: Surgery (salpingectomy/salpingostomy by open surgery or by laparoscopy), medical treatment, and expectant management.
Main Outcome: Primary treatment success, defined as an uneventful decline in serum β-hCG to undetectable levels by the initial treatment.
Results: Intramuscular MTX therapy and salpingostomy yielded similar treatment success rates (82-95% for MTX therapy vs. 80-92% for salpingostomy).

Infertility: inability to conceive or carry to term a pregnancy after one year of regular, unprotected intercourse
Primary infertility: infertility in the context of no prior pregnancies
Secondary infertility: infertility in the context of a prior conception
Generally, 75% of couples achieve pregnancy within 6 mo, 85% within 1 yr, 90% within 2 yr

Requirements for Conception
- Ovary
- Tube
- Cervix
- Endometrium
- Sperm

When Should Investigations Begin?
- <35 yr: after 1 yr of regular unprotected intercourse
- 35-40 yr: after >6 mo
- >40 yr: immediately
- Earlier if
  - History of PID
  - History of infertility in previous relationship
  - Prior pelvic surgery
  - Chemotherapy/radiation in either partner
  - Recurrent pregnancy loss
- Moderate-severe endometriosis

Controversial and Evolving Ethical Issues
- Infertility demands non-judgmental discussion
- Ethical issues surrounding therapeutic donor insemination in same sex couples, surrogacy, donor gametes, and other advanced reproductive technologies are still evolving and remain controversial
- If the doctor finds that certain treatment options lie outside of their moral boundaries, the infertile couple should be referred to another physician

Livebirth After Uterus Transplantation
Lancet 2015;385:607-16.
Purpose: Treatment for absolute uterine infertility. Eleven previous human uterus transplantations performed but all unsuccessful in producing livebirths.
Patient/Method: 35 yr old woman with congenital absence of uterus (Rokitansky syndrome) underwent transplantation of uterus donated from a living 61 yr old P2 woman. Implantation was performed using in vitro fertilization generated embryo derived from the recipient and her partner.
Results: Recipient and donor had uneventful postoperative recoveries. The recipient initiated menstruation 43 d after transplantation and her menstrual cycle remained regular, ranging from 26-36 d. Embryo transfer was performed 1 yr after transplantation, resulting in intrauterine pregnancy. The recipient was then treated with triple immunosuppressive therapy (tacrolimus, azathioprine, and corticosteroids), which was continued throughout her pregnancy. The patient experienced one episode of mild rejection during her pregnancy, which was treated with corticosteroids. Fetal growth paras and doppler studies were normal throughout her pregnancy. The patient was admitted at 31 + 5 wk for pre-eclampsia and a caesarean section was performed owing to abnormal fetal tracings. A male baby with normal birth weight (1775g) and APGAR scores was born.
Conclusions: Successful proof-of-concept uterus transplantation as treatment for uterine factor infertility using live uterus donation from a postmenopausal donor.

Treatment
- education: timing intercourse relative to ovulation (from 2 d prior to 2 d following presumed ovulation), every other day
- medical
  - ovulation induction
    - clomiphene citrate (Clomid®): estrogen antagonist causing a perceived decreased estrogen state, resulting in increased pituitary gonadotropins; which increases FSH and LH and induces ovulation (better results if anovulatory)
    - followed by β-hCG for stimulation of ovum release
  - may add
    - bromocriptine (dopamine agonist) if elevated prolactin
    - dexamethasone for hyperandrogenism (adult onset congenital adrenal hyperplasia)
    - metformin (for PCOS)
    - luteal phase progesterone supplementation for luteal phase defect (mechanism not completely understood)
    - anticoagulation and ASA (81 mg PO OD) for women with a history of recurrent spontaneous abortions (for antiphospholipid antibody syndrome)
    - thyroid replacement to keep TSH < 2.5
- surgical/procedural
  - tubuloplasty
  - lysis of adhesions
  - artificial insemination: intracervical insemination (ICI), intrauterine insemination (IUI), intrauterine tuboperitoneal insemination (IUTPI), intratubal insemination (ITI)
  - sperm washing
  - IVF (in vitro fertilization)
  - IFT (intrafallopian transfer)
  - GIFT* (gamete intrafallopian transfer): immediate transfer with sperm after oocyte retrieval
  - ZIFT* (zygote intrafallopian transfer): transfer after 24 h culture of oocyte and sperm
  - TET* (tubal embryo transfer): transfer after >24 h culture
  - ICSI (intracytoplasmic sperm injection)
  - IVM (in vitro maturation)
  - ± oocyte or sperm donors
  - ± pre-genetic screening for single gene defects in karyotype of zygote
  *not performed in Canada

Male Factors

- see Urology, U34

Normal Semen Analysis (WHO lower reference limits)
- Must be obtained after 2-7 d of abstinence
  - Volume 1.5 cc
  - Count 15 million/cc
  - Vitality 58% live
  - Motility 32% progressive, 40% total (progressive + non-progressive)
- Morphology 4.0% normal

Etiology
- varicocele (>40%)
- idiopathic (>20%)
- obstruction (~15%)
- cryptorchidism (~8%)
- immunologic (~3%)

Investigations
- semen analysis and culture
- postcoital (Huhner) test: rarely done

Polycystic Ovarian Syndrome

- also called chronic ovarian androgenism

Etiology

Polycystic Ovarian Syndrome – HAIR-AN
Hirsutism, **H**yper**A**ndrogenism, **I**nfertility, **I**nsulin **R**esistance, **A**canthosis **N**igricans

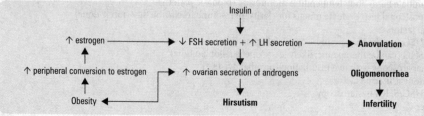

Figure 16. Pathophysiology of polycystic ovarian syndrome

Diagnosis
- Rotterdam diagnostic criteria: 2 of 3 required
  - oligomenorrhea/irregular menses for 6 mo
  - hyperandrogenism
    - clinical evidence - hirsutism or male pattern alopecia or
    - biochemical evidence - raised free testosterone
  - polycystic ovaries on U/S

Clinical Features
- average age 15-35 yr at presentation
- in adolescents, wait at least 1-2 yr to make diagnosis
- abnormal/irregular uterine bleeding, hirsutism, infertility, obesity, virilization
- acanthosis nigricans: browning of skin folds in intertriginous zones (indicative of insulin resistance)
- insulin resistance occurs in both lean and obese patients, family history of DM

Investigations
- goal: identify hyperandrogenism or chronic anovulation; and rule out specific pituitary or adrenal disease as the cause
- laboratory
  - prolactin, 17-hydroxyprogesterone, free testosterone, DHEA-S, TSH, free T4, androstenedione, SHBG
  - LH:FSH >2:1; LH is chronically high with FSH mid-range or low (low sensitivity and specificity)
  - increased DHEA-S, androstenedione and free testosterone (most sensitive), decreased SHBG
- transvaginal or transabdominal U/S: polycystic-appearing ovaries ("string of pearls" – 12 or more small follicles 2-9 mm, or increased ovarian volume)
- tests for insulin resistance or glucose tolerance
  - fasting glucose:insulin ratio <4.5 is consistent with insulin resistance (U.S. units)
  - 75 g OGTT yearly (particularly if obese)
- laparoscopy
  - not required for diagnosis
  - most common to see white, smooth, sclerotic ovaries with a thick capsule; multiple follicular cysts in various stages of atresia; hyperplastic theca and stroma
- rule out other causes of abnormal bleeding

Treatment
- cycle control
  - lifestyle modification (decrease BMI, increase exercise) to decrease peripheral estrone formation
  - OCP monthly or cyclic Provera® to prevent endometrial hyperplasia due to unopposed estrogen
  - oral hypoglycemic (e.g. metformin) if type 2 diabetic or if trying to become pregnant
  - tranexamic acid (Cyklokapron®) for menorrhagia only
- infertility
  - medical induction of ovulation: clomiphene citrate, human menopausal gonadotropins (HMG [Pergonal®]), LHRH, recombinant FSH, and metformin
    - metformin may be used alone or in conjuction with clomiphene citrate for ovulation induction
  - ovarian drilling (perforate the stroma), wedge resection of the ovary
  - bromocriptine (if hyperprolactinemia)
- hirsutism
  - any OCP can be used
    - Diane 35® (cyproterone acetate): antiandrogenic
    - Yasmin® (drospirenone and ethinyl estradiol): spironolactone analogue (inhibits steroid receptors)
  - mechanical removal of hair
  - finasteride (5-α reductase inhibitor)
  - flutamide (androgen reuptake inhibitor)
  - spironolactone: androgen receptor inhibitor

Gynecological Infections

Physiologic Discharge

- clear, white, flocculent, odourless discharge; pH 3.8-4.2
- smear contains epithelial cells, Lactobacilli
- increases with increased estrogen states: pregnancy, OCP, mid-cycle, PCOS, or premenarchal
- if increased in perimenopausal/postmenopausal woman, consider investigation for other effects of excess estrogen (e.g. endometrial cancer)

PCOS may be Confused with
- Late onset congenital adrenal hyperplasia (21-hydroxylase deficiency)
- Cushing's syndrome
- Ovarian and adrenal neoplasms
- Hyperprolactinemia
- Hypothyroidism

Clinical Signs of Endocrine Imbalance
- Menstrual disorder/amenorrhea (80%)
- Infertility (74%)
- Hirsutism (69%)
- Obesity (49%)
- Impaired glucose tolerance (35%)
- DM (10%)

Long-Term Health Consequences
- Hyperlipidemia
- Adult-onset DM
- Endometrial hyperplasia
- Infertility
- Obesity
- Sleep apnea

Use of Metformin in Polycystic Ovary Syndrome: A Meta-Analysis
Obstet Gynecol 2008;111(4):959-68.
Study: This meta-analysis of 17 RCTs assessed the efficacy of metformin or metformin in combination with clomiphene citrate in women with PCOS who were seeking pregnancy.
Main Outcomes: Ovulation, pregnancy, and live birth. Patients: 1,639 patients with PCOS were followed up for up to 12 mo.
Results: Compared to placebo, metformin increased the odds of ovulation (OR 2.94, 95% CI 1.43-6.02). However, when used alone, metformin did not significantly increase the odds of achieving pregnancy (OR 1.56, 95% CI 0.74-3.33). When compared to clomiphene alone, the combination of metformin and clomiphene increased the likelihood of ovulation (OR 4.39, 95% CI 1.94-9.96) and pregnancy (OR 2.67, 95% CI 1.45-4.94). The effect of combination therapy was most prominent in clomiphene-resistant and obese women with PCOS. Furthermore, the combination therapy had a higher likelihood of having a live birth compared to clomiphene alone, but this did not reach significance (OR 1.74, 95% CI 0.79-3.86).
Conclusions: Metformin increases the likelihood of ovulation. When used together with clomiphene, metformin increases the likelihood of both ovulation and pregnancy, especially in clomiphene-resistant and obese women.

Diagnostic Criteria for Polycystic Ovary Syndrome: Pitfalls and Controversies
JOGC 2008;8:671-679
At present, there is no clear-cut definition of biochemical hyperandrogenemia, particularly since there is dependence on poor atory standards for measuring androgens in women. Clinical signs of hyperandrogenism are ill-defined in women with PCOS, and diagnosis of both hirsutism and polycystic ovarian morphology remains subjective. There is also the inappropriate tendency to assign ovulatory status solely on basis of menstrual cycle history or poorly timed endocrine measurements. Therefore it is important as clinicians to recognize the multi-factorial and complex nature of PCOS and place this in the context of our present diagnostic limitations.

Vulvovaginitis

PREPUBERTAL VULVOVAGINITIS

- clinical features
  - irritation, pruritus
  - discharge
  - vulvar erythema
  - vaginal bleeding (specifically due to Group A Streptococci and *Shigella*)
- differential diagnosis
  - non-specific vulvovaginitis (25-75%)
  - infections (respiratory, enteric, systemic, sexually acquired)
  - foreign body (toilet paper most common)
  - Candida (if using diapers or chronic antibiotics)
  - pinworms
  - polyps, tumour (ovarian malignancy)
  - vulvar skin disease (lichen sclerosis, condyloma acuminata)
  - trauma (accidental straddle injury, sexual abuse)
  - psychosomatic vaginal complaints (specific to vaginal discharge)
  - endocrine abnormalities (specific to vaginal bleeding)
  - blood dyscrasia (specific to vaginal bleeding)
- etiology
  - infectious
    - poor hygiene, proximity of vagina to anus
    - recent infection (respiratory, enteric, systemic)
    - STI: investigate sexual abuse
  - non-specific
    - lack of protective hair and labial fat pads
    - lack of estrogenization
    - susceptible to chemicals, soaps (bubble baths), medications, and clothing
    - enuresis
- investigations
  - vaginal swab for culture (specifically state that it is a pre-pubertal specimen), pH, wet-mount, and KOH smear in adults only
- treatment
  - enhanced hygiene and local measures (handwashing, white cotton underwear, no nylon tights, no tight fitting clothes, no sleeper pajamas, sitz baths, avoid bubble baths, use mild detergent, eliminate fabric softener, avoid prolonged exposure to wet bathing suits, urination with legs spread apart)
  - A&D® dermatological ointment (vitamin A/D) to protect vulvar skin
  - infectious: treat with antibiotics for organism identified

Table 14. Other Common Causes of Vulvovaginitis in Prepubertal Girls

	Pinworms	Lichen Sclerosis	Foreign Body
Diagnosis	Cellophane tape test	Area of white patches and thinning of skin	
Treatment	Empirical treatment with mebendazole	Topical steroid creams	Irrigation of vagina with saline, may require local anesthesia or an exam under anesthesia

VAGINITISROPHIC / VAGINITIS

- clinical features
  - dyspareunia, postcoital spotting, mild pruritus
- investigations
  - atrophy is usually a visual diagnosis: thinning of tissues, erythema, petechiae, bleeding points, dryness on speculum exam
  - rule out malignancy, especially endometrial cancer
- treatment
  - local estrogen replacement (ideal): Premarin® cream, VagiFem® tablets, or Estring®
  - oral or transdermal hormone replacement therapy (if treatment for systemic symptoms is desired)
  - good hygiene

Vulvovaginitis
Vulvar and vaginal inflammation

Prepubertal and Adolescent Gynecological Infections: Legal Aspects of Confidentiality
- Clinicians who treat adolescents must be aware of federal, state, and provincial laws related to adolescent consent and confidentiality
- They must be aware of guidelines governing funding sources for particular services and be familiar with the consent and confidentiality policies of the facility in which they practice

There is no high quality evidence showing a link between vulvovaginal candidiasis and hygienic habits or wearing tight or synthetic clothing

Most common gynecological problem in prepubertal girls is non-specific vulvovaginitis, not yeast

INFECTIOUS VULVOVAGINITIS

Table 15. Infectious Vulvovaginitis

	Candidiasis	Bacterial Vaginosis (BV)	Trichomoniasis
Organisms	*Candida albicans* (90%) *Candida glabrata* (<5%) *Candida tropicalis* (<5%)	*Gardnerella vaginalis* *Mycoplasma hominis* Anaerobes: *Prevotella, Mobiluncus, Bacteroides*	*Trichomonas vaginalis* (flagellated protozoan)
Pathophysiology or Transmission	Predisposing factors include: Immunosuppressed host (DM, AIDS, etc.) Recent antibiotic use Increased estrogen levels (e.g. pregnancy, OCP)	Replacement of vaginal *Lactobacillus* with organisms above	Sexual transmission
Discharge	Whitish, "cottage cheese," minimal	Grey, thin, diffuse	Yellow-green, malodourous, diffuse, frothy
Other	20% asymptomatic	50-75% asymptomatic	25% asymptomatic
Signs/Symptoms	Intense pruritus Swollen, inflamed genitals Vulvar burning, dysuria, dyspareunia	Fishy odour, especially after coitus Absence of vulvar/vaginal irritation	Petechiae on vagina and cervix Occasionally irritated tender vulva Dysuria, frequency
pH	≤4.5	≥4.5	≥4.5
Saline Wetmount	KOH wetmount reveals hyphae and spores	>20% clue cells = squamous epithelial cells dotted with coccobacilli (*Gardnerella*) Paucity of WBC Paucity of *Lactobacilli* Positive whiff test: fishy odour with addition of KOH to slide (due to formation of amines)	Motile flagellated organisms Many WBC Inflammatory cells (PMNs)
Treatment	Clotrimazole, butoconazole, miconazole, terconazole suppositories, and/or creams for 1, 3, or 7 d treatments Treatment in pregnancy is usually topical Fluconazole 150 mg PO in single dose (can be used in pregnancy)	No treatment if non-pregnant and asymptomatic, unless scheduled for pelvic surgery or procedure **Oral** Metronidazole 500 mg PO bid x 7 d **Topical** Metronidazole gel 0.75% x 5 d OD (may be used in pregnancy) Clindamycin 2% 5 g intravaginally at bedtime for 7 d Probiotics (lactobacillus sp.): oral or topical alone or as adjuvant	Treat even if asymptomatic Metronidazole 2 g PO single dose or 500 mg bid x 7 d (alternative) Symptomatic pregnant women should be treated with 2 g metronidazole once
Other	Prophylaxis for recurrent infection includes boric acid, vaginal suppositories, luteal phase fluconazole Routine treatment of partner(s) not recommended (not sexually transmitted)	Associated with recurrent preterm labour, preterm birth, and postpartum endometritis Need to warn patients on metronidazole not to consume alcohol (disulfiram-like action) Routine treatment of partner(s) not recommended (not sexually transmitted)	Warnings accompanying metronidazole use Treat partner(s)

Sexually Transmitted Infections

- see Family Medicine, FM42

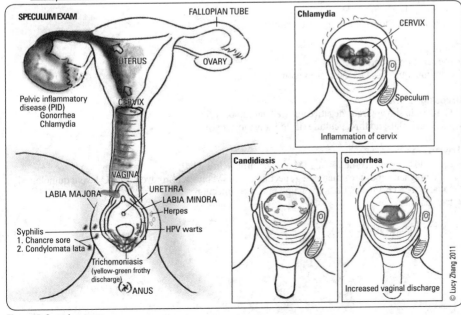

Figure 17. Speculum exam

CDC Notifiable Diseases
- Chancroid
- Chlamydia
- Gonorrhea
- Hepatitis A, B, C
- HIV
- Syphilis

Risk Factors for STIs
- History of previous STI
- Contact with infected person
- Sexually active individual <25 yr
- Multiple partners
- New partner in last 3 mo
- Lack of barrier protection use
- Street involvement (homelessness, drug use)

TRICHOMONIASIS
- see *Infectious Vulvovaginitis*, Table 15

CHLAMYDIA

Etiology
- Chlamydia trachomatis

Epidemiology
- most common bacterial STI in Canada
- often associated with *N. gonorrhoeae*

Clinical Features
- asymptomatic (80% of women)
- muco-purulent endocervical discharge
- urethral syndrome: dysuria, frequency, pyuria, no bacteria on culture
- pelvic pain
- postcoital bleeding or intermenstrual bleeding (particularly if on OCP and prior history of good cycle control)
- symptomatic sexual partner

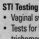

STI Testing
- Vaginal swab
- Tests for bacterial vaginosis, trichomoniasis, candida
- Cervical swab
- Tests for gonorrhea and chlamydia

Investigations
- cervical culture or nucleic acid amplification test
- obligate intracellular parasite: tissue culture is the definitive standard
- urine and self vaginal tests now available, which are equally or more effective than cervical culture

Treatment
- doxycycline 100 mg PO bid for 7 d or azithromycin 1 g PO in a single dose (may use in pregnancy)
- also treat gonorrhea because of high rate of co-infection
- treat partners
- reportable disease
- test of cure for chlamydia required in pregnancy (cure rates lower in pregnant patients) → retest 3-4 wk after initiation of therapy

Test of cure for *C. trachomatis* and *N. gonorrhoeae* is not routinely indicated Repeat testing if symptomatic, if compliance with treatment is uncertain, or if pregnant

Screening
- high risk groups
- during pregnancy
- when initiating OCP if sexually active (independent risk factor)

Complications
- acute salpingitis, PID
- Fitz-Hugh-Curtis syndrome (liver capsule inflammation)
- reactive arthritis (male predominance, HLA-B27 associated), conjunctivitis, urethritis
- infertility: tubal obstruction from low grade salpingitis
- ectopic pregnancy
- chronic pelvic pain
- perinatal infection: conjunctivitis, pneumonia

Etiology
- *Neisseria gonorrhoeae*
- symptoms and risk factors same as with chlamydia

Investigations
- Gram stain shows Gram-negative intracellular diplococci
- cervical, rectal, and throat culture (if clinically indicated)

Treatment
- single dose of ceftriaxone 250 mg IM plus azithromycin 1 g PO
  - if pregnant: above regimen or 2 g spectinomycin IM plus azithromycin 1 g PO (avoid quinolones)
  - also treat chlamydia, because of high rate of co-infection
- treat partners
  - reportable disease
  - screening as with chlamydia

HUMAN PAPILLOMAVIRUS

Etiology
- most common viral STI in Canada
- >200 subtypes, of which >30 are genital subtypes
- HPV types 6 and 11 are classically associated with anogenital warts/condylomata acuminata
- HPV types 16 and 18 are the most oncogenic (classically associated with cervical HSIL)
- types 16, 18, 31, 33, 35, 36, 45 (and others) associated with increased incidence of cervical and vulvar intraepithelial hyperplasia and carcinoma

Clinical Features
- latent infection
  - no visible lesions, asymptomatic
  - only detected by DNA hybridization tests
- subclinical infection
  - visible lesion found during colposcopy or on Pap test
- clinical infection
  - visible wart-like lesion without magnification
  - hyperkeratotic, verrucous or flat, macular lesions
  - vulvar edema

Investigations
- cytology
- koilocytosis: nuclear enlargement and atypia with perinuclear halo
- biopsy of lesions at colposcopy
- detection of HPV DNA subtype using nucleic acid probes (not routinely done but can be done in presence of abnormal Pap test to guide treatment)

Treatment
- patient administered
  - podofilox 0.5% solution or gel bid x 3 d in a row (4 d off) then repeat x 4 wk
  - imiquimod (Aldara®) 5% cream 3x/wk qhs x 16 wk
- provider administered
  - cryotherapy with liquid nitrogen: repeat q1-2wk
  - podophyllin resin in tincture of benzoin: weekly
  - trichloroacetic acid (TCA) or bichloroacetic acid weekly (80-90%); safe in pregnancy
  - surgical removal/laser
  - intralesional interferon

Prevention
- vaccination: Gardasil®, Cervarix® see Table 25, GY43
- condoms may not fully protect (areas not covered, must be used every time throughout entire sexual act)

HERPES SIMPLEX VIRUS OF VULVA

Etiology
- 90% are HSV-2, 10% are HSV-1

Clinical Features
- may be asymptomatic
- initial symptoms: present 2-21 d after contact
- prodromal symptoms: tingling, burning, pruritus
- multiple, painful, shallow ulcerations with small vesicles appear 7-10 d after initial infection (absent in many infected persons); lesions are infectious
- inguinal lymphadenopathy, malaise, and fever often with first infection
- dysuria and urinary retention if urethral mucosa affected
- recurrent infections: less severe, less frequent, and shorter in duration (usually only HSV-2)

Investigations
- viral culture preferred in patients with ulcer present, however decreased sensitivity as lesions heal
- cytologic smear (Tzanck smear) shows multinucleated giant cells, acidophilic intranuclear inclusion bodies
- HSV DNA PCR
- type specific serologic tests for antibodies to HSV-1 and HSV-2 (not available routinely in Canada)

Genital Warts During Pregnancy
- Condyloma tend to get larger in pregnancy and should be treated early (consider excision)
- C-section only if obstructing birth canal or risk of extensive bleeding
- Do not use imiquimod, podophyllin, or podofilox

Human Rights in Health Equity: Cervical Cancer and HPV Vaccines
Am J Law Med 2009;35:365-387
- While cervical cancer rates have drastically fallen in developed countries due to effective prevention and treatment, socially disadvantaged women within these countries remain disproportionately more likely to develop and die of cervical cancer.
- In most developing countries cervical cancer rates have risen or remained unchanged.
- Must recognize that cervical cancer disparities between race groups, urban and rural residence, and high and low socioeconomic status are attributed to disparate screening and vaccination coverage.
- Programs are implemented without sufficient attention to conditions that render screening less effective or inaccessible to disadvantaged social groups including: lack of information, undervaluing of preventive care, opportunistic delivery in limited health care settings, sexual health stigma, and related privacy concerns.

A 9-Valent HPV Vaccine Against Infection and Intraepithelial Neoplasia in Women
NEJM 2015;372:711-23.
Purpose: To determine the efficacy and immunogenicity of the qHPV (types 6, 11, 16, 18) vs. 9vHPV (five additional types 31, 33, 45, 52, 58) vaccines.
Method: International randomized, double-blinded phase 2B-3 study of 9vHPV vaccine in 14,215 women between ages of 16-26. Participants were randomized to the 9vHPV vaccine group or the qHPV vaccine group and each received a series of three IM injections (day 1, 2 and 6 months). Swabs of labial, vulvar, perineal, perianal, endocervical, and ectocervical tissue was obtained and used for HPV DNA testing/Pap smear.
Results: Rate of high-grade cervical, vulvar, or vaginal disease was 14.0 per 1,000 person-years in both vaccine groups. The rate of high-grade cervical, vulvar, or vaginal disease related to HPV-31, 33, 52, and 58 was 0.1 per 1,000 person-years in the 9vHPV group and 1.6 per 1,000 person-years in the qHPV group (95% CI = 80.9-99.8). Antibody responses to HPV-6, 11, 16, and 18 were not significantly different between the two vaccine groups although adverse events related to injection sites were more common in the 9vHPV group.
Conclusions: The 9vHPV vaccine was non-inferior to qHPV vaccine in preventing infection and disease related to HPV-6, 11, 16, and 18 and also covered additional oncogenic types HPV-31, 33, 45, 52, and 58 in a susceptible population.

HSV Infections During Pregnancy
- Antiviral suppression of women with first episode or history of HSV infections from 36 wk GA onward
- C-section should be performed on women who have active genital lesions at time of delivery
- Treatment: acyclovir 400 mg PO tid

Epidemiology of Genital Ulcers
HSV   70-80%
1° Syphilis 5%
Chancroid   <1%
(*Haemophilus ducreyi*)

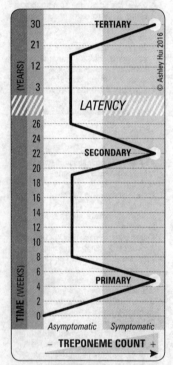

Figure 18. Natural history of syphilis infection

Treatment
- first episode
  - acyclovir 200 mg PO five times daily x 5-10 d, or famciclovir 250 mg PO tid x 7-10 5 d, or valacyclovir 1 g PO bid x 10 d
- recurrent episode
  - acyclovir 200 mg PO five times daily x 5 d, or famciclovir 125 mg PO bid x 5 d, or valacyclovir 500 mg PO bid OR 1 g PO OD x 3 d
- daily suppressive therapy
  - consider for > 6 recurrences per yr or one every 2 mo
  - acyclovir 400 mg PO bid, or famciclovir 250 mg bid, or valacyclovir 0.5-1 g PO OD
- severe disease: consider IV therapy: acyclovir 55 mg/kg IV over 60 min q8h
- education regarding transmission
- avoid contact from onset of prodrome until lesions have cleared
- use barrier contraception

SYPHILIS

Etiology
- *Treponema pallidum*

Classifications
- primary syphilis
  - 3-4 wk after exposure
  - painless chancre on vulva, vagina, or cervix
  - painless inguinal lymphadenopathy
  - serological tests usually negative, local infection only
- secondary syphilis (can resolve spontaneously)
  - 2-6 mo after initial infection
  - nonspecific symptoms: malaise, anorexia, headache, diffuse lymphadenopathy
  - generalized maculopapular rash: palms, soles, trunk, limbs
  - condylomata lata: anogenital, broad-based fleshy grey lesions
  - serological tests usually positive
- latent syphilis
  - no clinical manifestations; detected by serology only
- tertiary syphilis
  - may involve any organ system
  - neurological: tabes dorsalis, general paresis
  - cardiovascular: aortic aneurysm, dilated aortic root
  - vulvar gumma: nodules that enlarge, ulcerate and become necrotic (rare)
- congenital syphilis
  - may cause fetal anomalies, stillbirths, or neonatal death

Investigations
- aspiration of ulcer serum or node
- darkfield microscopy (most sensitive and specific diagnostic test for syphilis)
  - spirochetes
- non-treponemal screening tests (VDRL, RPR); nonreactive after treatment, can be positive with other conditions
- specific anti-treponemal antibody tests (FTA-ABS, MHA-TP, TP-PA)
  - confirmatory tests; remain reactive for life (even after adequate treatment)

Treatment
- treatment of primary, secondary, latent syphilis of <1 yr duration
  - benzathine penicillin G 2.4 million units IM single dose
  - treat partners, reportable disease
- treatment of latent syphilis of >1 yr duration
  - benzathine penicillin G 2.4 million units IM q1wk x 3 wk
- treatment of neurosyphilis
  - IV aqueous penicillin G 3-4 million units IM q4h x 10-14 d
- screening
  - high risk groups
  - in pregnancy (see Obstetrics, Table *Infections During Pregnancy*, OB29)

Complications
- if untreated, 1/3 will experience late complications

HIV
- see Infectious Diseases, ID27

Bartholin Gland Abscess

Etiology
- often anaerobic and polymicrobial
- *U. urealyticum, N. gonorrhoeae, C. trachomatis, E. coli, P. mirabilis, Streptococcus* spp., *S. aureus* (rare)
- blockage of duct

Clinical Features
- unilateral swelling and pain in inferior lateral opening of vagina
- sitting and walking may become difficult and/or painful

Treatment
- sitz baths, warm compresses
- antibiotics: cephalexin x 1 wk
- incision and drainage using local anesthesia with placement of Word catheter (10 French latex catheter) for 2-3 wk (or as long as stays insitu)
- marsupialization under general anesthetic – more definitive treatment
- rarely treated by removing gland

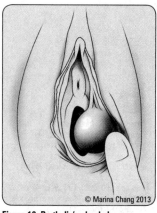

© Marina Chang 2013

Figure 19. Bartholin's gland abscess

Pelvic Inflammatory Disease

- up to 20% of all gynecology-related hospital admissions

Etiology
- causative organisms (in order of frequency)
  - *C. trachomatis*
  - *N. gonorrhoeae*
    - gonorrhea and chlamydia often co-exist
  - endogenous flora: anaerobic, aerobic, or both
    - *E. coli, Staphylococcus, Streptococcus, Enterococcus, Bacteroides, Peptostreptococcus, H. influenzae, G. vaginalis*
    - cause of recurrent PID
    - associated with instrumentation
  - *Actinomyces israelii* (Gram-positive, non acid-fast anaerobe)
    - 1-4% of PID cases associated with IUDs
  - others (TB, Gram-negatives, CMV, U. urealyticum, etc.)

Risk Factors
- age <30 yr
- risk factors as for chlamydia and gonorrhea
- vaginal douching
- IUD (within first 10 d after insertion)
- invasive gynecologic procedures (D&C, endometrial biopsy)

Clinical Presentation
- up to 2/3 asymptomatic: many subtle or mild symptoms
- common: fever >38.3° C, lower abdominal pain and tenderness, abnormal discharge: cervical or vaginal
- uncommon: N/V, dysuria, AUB
- chronic disease (often due to chlamydia)
  - constant pelvic pain
  - dyspareunia
  - palpable mass
  - very difficult to treat, may require surgery

Investigations
- blood work
  - β-hCG (must rule out ectopic pregnancy), CBC, blood cultures if suspect septicemia
- urine R&M
- speculum exam, bimanual exam
  - vaginal swab for Gram stain, C&S
  - cervical cultures for *N. gonorrhoeae, C. trachomatis*
  - endometrial biopsy will give definitive diagnosis (rarely done)
- ultrasound
  - may be normal
  - free fluid in cul-de-sac
  - pelvic or tubo-ovarian abscess
  - hydrosalpinx (dilated fallopian tube)
- laparoscopy (gold standard)
  - for definitive diagnosis: may miss subtle inflammation of tubes or endometritis

PID accounts for up to 20% of all gynecological hospital admissions

PID
Inflammation of the upper genital tract (above cervix) including endometrium, fallopian tubes, ovaries, pelvic peritoneum, ± contiguous structures

PID Diagnosis
Must have
- Lower abdominal pain
Plus one of
- Cervical motion tenderness
- Adnexal tenderness
Plus one or more of
- High risk partner
- Temperature >38°C
- Mucopurulent cervical discharge
- Positive culture for *N. gonorrhoeae, C. trachomatis, E. coli,* or other vaginal flora
- Cul-de-sac fluid, pelvic abscess or inflammatory mass on U/S or bimanual
- Leukocytosis
- Elevated ESR or CRP (not commonly used)

Treatment

- must treat with polymicrobial coverage
- inpatient if
  - moderate to severe illness
  - atypical infection
  - adnexal mass, tubo-ovarian mass, or pelvic abscess
  - unable to tolerate oral antibiotics or failed oral therapy
  - immunocompromised
  - pregnant
  - adolescent – first episode
  - surgical emergency cannot be excluded (e.g. ovarian torsion)
  - PID is secondary to instrumentation
  - recommended treatment
    - ◆ cefoxitin 2 g IV q6h (no longer available in U.S.A.) + doxycycline 100 mg IV/PO q12h or clindamycin 900 mg IV q8h + gentamicin 2 mg/kg IV/IM loading dose then gentamicin 1.5 mg/kg IV q8h maintenance dose
    - ◆ continue IV antibiotics for 24 h after symptoms have improved then doxycycline 100 mg PO bid to complete 14 d
    - ◆ percutaneous drainage of abscess under U/S guidance
    - ◆ when no response to treatment, laparoscopic drainage
    - ◆ if failure, treatment is surgical (salpingectomy, TAH/BSO)
- outpatient if
  - typical findings
  - mild to moderate illness
  - oral antibiotics tolerated
  - compliance ensured
  - follow-up within 48-72 h (to ensure symptoms not worsening)
  - recommended treatment
    - ◆ ceftriaxone 250 mg IM x 1 + doxycycline 100 mg PO bid x 14 d or cefoxitin 2 g IM x 1 + probenecid 1 g PO + doxycyline 100 mg PO bid ± metronidazole 500 mg PO bid x 14 d
    - ◆ ofloxacin 400 mg PO bid x 14 d or levofloxacin 500 mg PO OD x 14 d ± metronidazole 500 mg PO bid x 14 d
    - ◆ consider removing IUD after a minimum of 24 h of treatment
    - ◆ reportable disease
    - ◆ treat partners
    - ◆ consider re-testing for *C. trachomatis* and *N. gonorrhoeae* 4-6 wk after treatment if documented infection

Complications of Untreated PID

- chronic pelvic pain
- abscess, peritonitis
- adhesion formation
- ectopic pregnancy
- infertility
  - 1 episode of PID → 13% infertility
  - 2 episodes of PID → 36% infertility
- bacteremia
- septic arthritis, endocarditis

Toxic Shock Syndrome

- see Infectious Diseases, ID23

Risk Factors

- tampon use
- diaphragm, cervical cap, or sponge use (prolonged use, i.e. >24 h)
- wound infections
- post-partum infections
- early recognition and treatment of syndrome is imperative as incorrect diagnosis can be fatal

Clinical Presentation

- sudden high fever
- sore throat, headache, diarrhea
- erythroderma
- signs of multisystem organ failure
- refractory hypotension
- exfoliation of palmar and plantar surfaces of the hands and feet 1-2 wk after onset of illness

Alternative PID Treatments
For patients with contraindications to treatment with cephalosporins or quinolones, recent evidence suggests that a short course of azithromycin at a dose of either 250 mg PO daily for
1 wk or 1 g PO weekly for 2 wk combined with metronidazole is effective in achieving a clinical cure for acute PID
Source: Update to the Canadian Guidelines on Sexually Transmitted Infections. January 2010

Treat PID with **FOXY DOXY**
(cefoxitin + doxycycline)

PID Complications

I FACE PID
Infertility
Fitz-Hugh-Curtis syndrome
Abscesses
Chronic pelvic pain
Ectopic pregnancy
Peritonitis
Intestinal obstruction
Disseminated infection (sepsis, endocarditis, arthritis, meningitis)

Toxic Shock Syndrome
Multiple organ system failure due to *S. aureus* exotoxin (rare condition)

Treatment
- remove potential sources of infection (foreign objects and wound debris)
- debride necrotic tissues
- adequate hydration
- penicillinase-resistant antibiotics, e.g. cloxacillin
- steroid use controversial but if started within 72 h, may reduce severity of symptoms and duration of fever

Surgical Infections

Post-Operative Infections in Gynecological Surgery
- pelvic cellulitis
  - common post hysterectomy, affects vaginal vault
  - erythema, induration, tenderness, discharge involving vaginal cuff
  - treat if fever and leukocytosis with broad spectrum antibiotics, i.e. clindamycin and gentamicin
  - drain if excessive purulence or large mass
  - can result in intra-abdominal and pelvic abscess
- see General Surgery, Post-Operative Fever, GS7

Sexual Abuse

- see Family Medicine, FM26, Emergency Medicine, ER27

Sexuality and Sexual Dysfunction

SEXUAL RESPONSE
1. desire: energy that allows an individual to initiate or respond to sexual stimulation
2. arousal: physical and emotional stimulation leading to breast and genital vasodilation and clitoral engorgement
3. orgasm: physical and emotional stimulation is maximized, allowing the individual to relinquish their sense of control
4. resolution: most of the congestion and tension resolves within seconds, complete resolution may take up to 60 min

SEXUAL DYSFUNCTION

Etiology
- psychological or emotional: depression, abuse
- hormonal: menopause
- neurologic dysfunction: spinal cord injury
- vascular insufficiency: DM
- drug side effects: β-blockers
- trauma: episiotomy

Classification
- lack of desire (60-70% of women)
- lack of arousal
- anorgasmia (5-10%)
  - primary anorgasmia: never before achieved orgasm under any circumstances
  - secondary anorgasmia: was able to achieve orgasms before but now unable to
- dyspareunia (3-6%): painful intercourse, superficial or deep
  - vaginismus (15%)
  - vulvodynia
  - vaginal atrophy
  - vulvar vestibulitis: associated with history of frequent yeast infections
  - PID

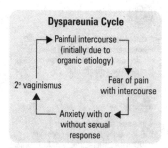

Figure 20. Dyspareunia Cycle

Treatment
- lack of desire: assess factors, rule out organic causes, relationship therapy, sensate focus exercises
- anorgasmia: self-exploration/pleasuring, relationship therapy if needed, bridging techniques (different sexual positions, clitoral stimulation during intercourse)
- dyspareunia
  - Kegel and reverse Kegel exercises
  - dilator treatment
  - comfort with self-exam
  - psychotherapy, other behavioural techniques
  - female on top position: allows for control of speed and duration
  - vestibulitis: remove local irritants, change in contraceptive methods, dietary changes (increased citrate, decreased oxalate), and vestibulectomy (rare)
  - vulvodynia: local moisturization, cold compresses, systemic nerve blocking therapy (amitriptyline, gabapentin) orally or topically, topical anesthetics, estrogen cream
  - pain clinic

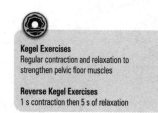

Kegel Exercises
Regular contraction and relaxation to strengthen pelvic floor muscles

Reverse Kegel Exercises
1 s contraction then 5 s of relaxation

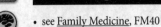

Menopause

- see <u>Family Medicine</u>, FM40

Definitions
- lack of menses for 1 yr
- types of menopause
  - physiological; average age 51 yr (follicular atresia)
  - premature ovarian failure; before age 40 (autoimmune disorder, infection, Turner's syndrome)
  - iatrogenic (surgical/radiation/chemotherapy)

Clinical Features
- associated with estrogen deficiency
  - vasomotor instability (tends to dissipate with time)
    - hot flushes/flashes, night sweats, sleep disturbances, formication, nausea, palpitations
  - urogenital atrophy involving vagina, urethra, bladder
    - dyspareunia, pruritus, vaginal dryness, bleeding, urinary frequency, urgency, incontinence
  - skeletal
    - osteoporosis, joint and muscle pain, back pain
  - skin and soft tissue
    - decreased breast size, skin thinning/loss of elasticity
  - psychological
  - mood disturbance, irritability, fatigue, decreased libido, memory loss

Investigations
- increased levels of FSH (>35 IU/L) on day 3 of cycle (if still cycling) and LH (FSH>LH)
- FSH level not always predictive due to monthly variation; use absence of menses for 1 yr to diagnose
- decreased levels of estradiol (later)

Treatment
- goal is for individual symptom management
  - vasomotor instability
    - HRT (first line), SSRIs, venlafaxine, gabapentin, propranolol, clonidine
    - acupuncture
  - vaginal atrophy
    - local estrogen: cream (Premarin®), vaginal suppository (VagiFem®), ring (Estring®)
    - lubricants (Replens®)
  - urogenital health
    - lifestyle changes (weight loss, bladder re-training), local estrogen replacement, surgery
  - osteoporosis
    - 1,000-1,500 mg calcium OD, 800-1,000 IU vitamin D, weight-bearing exercise, smoking cessation
    - bisphosphonates (e.g. alendronate)
    - selective estrogen receptor modifiers (SERMs): raloxifene (Evista®) – mimics estrogen effects on bone, avoids estrogen-like action on breast and uterine cancer; does not help hot flashes
    - HRT: second-line treatment (unless for vasomotor instability as well)
  - decreased libido
    - vaginal lubrication, counselling, androgen replacement (testosterone cream or the oral form Andriol®)
  - cardiovascular disease
    - management of cardiovascular risk factors
  - mood and memory
    - antidepressants (first line), HRT (augments effect)
  - alternative choices (not evidence-based, safety not established)
    - black cohosh, phytoestrogens, St. John's wort, gingko biloba, valerian, evening primrose oil, ginseng, Don Quai

Hormone Replacement Therapy

- see <u>Family Medicine</u>, FM40
- primary indication is treatment of menopausal symptoms (vasomotor instability)
- keep doses low (e.g. 0.3 mg Premarin®) and duration of treatment short (<5 yr)

HRT Components
- estrogen
- oral or transdermal (e.g. patch, gel)
- transdermal preferred for women with hypertriglyceridemia or impaired hepatic function, smokers, and women who suffer from headaches associated with oral HRT

Menopause
Occurrence of last spontaneous menstrual period, resulting from loss of ovarian function (loss of oocyte response to gonadotropins)

"Being in menopause"
Lack of menses for 1 yr

Perimenopause
Period of time surrounding menopause (2-8 yr preceding + 1 yr after last menses) characterized by fluctuating hormone levels, irregular menstrual cycles, and symptom onset

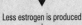

- 85% of women experience hot flashes
- 20-30% seek medical attention
- 10% are unable to work

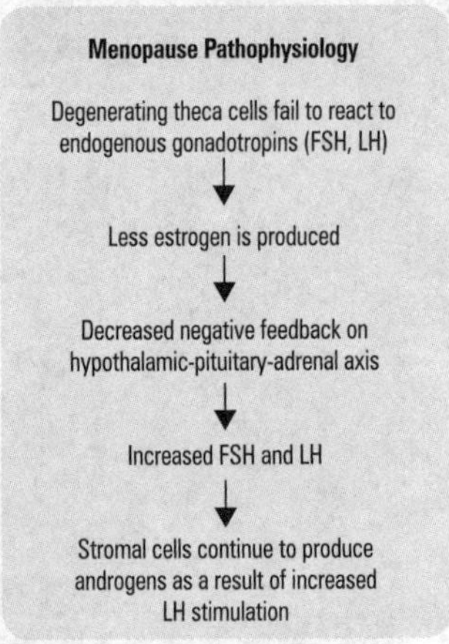

Menopause Pathophysiology

Degenerating theca cells fail to react to endogenous gonadotropins (FSH, LH)

↓

Less estrogen is produced

↓

Decreased negative feedback on hypothalamic-pituitary-adrenal axis

↓

Increased FSH and LH

↓

Stromal cells continue to produce androgens as a result of increased LH stimulation

Figure 21. Menopause pathophysiology

- Osteoporosis is the single most important health hazard associated with menopause
- Cardiovascular disease is the leading cause of death post-menopause

- Increased risk of breast cancer (RR 1.3) is associated with estrogen+progesterone HRT, but not with estrogen-only HRT
- All women taking HRT should have periodic surveillance and counselling regarding its benefits and risks

- low-dose (preferred dose: 0.3 mg Premarin®/25 μg Estradot® patch, can increase if necessary)
- progestin
- given in combination with estrogen for women with an intact uterus to prevent development of endometrial hyperplasia/cancer

Table 16. Examples of HRT Regimens

HRT Regimen	Estrogen Dose	Progestin Dose	Notes
Unopposed Estrogen	CEE 0.625 mg PO OD	None	If no intact uterus
Standard-dose	CEE 0.625 mg PO OD	MPA 2.5 mg PO OD, or micronized progesterone 100 mg PO OD	Withdrawal bleeding may occur in a spotty, unpredictable manner Usually abates after 6-8 mo due to endometrial atrophy Once patient has become amenorrheic on HRT, significant subsequent bleeding episodes require evaluation (endometrial biopsy)
Standard-dose Cyclic	CEE 0.625 mg PO OD	MPA 5-10 mg PO days 1-14 only, or micronized progesterone 200 mg PO OD days 1-14 only	Bleeding occurs monthly after day 14 of progestin (can continue for years) PMS-like symptoms (breast tenderness, fluid retention, headache, nausea) are more prominent with cyclic HRT
Pulsatile	CEE 0.625 mg PO OD	MPA low-dose	3 d on, 3 d off
Transdermal	Estroderm®-Estradiol 0.05 mg/d or 0.1 mg/d Estalis®-Estradiol 140 μg/d or 250 μg/d	Estroderm®-MPA 2.5 mg PO OD Estalis®-NEA 50 μg/d	Use patch twice weekly Can use oral progestins (Estroderm®) Combined patches available (Estalis®)
Topical	Estrace® 2-4 g/d x 1-2 wk, 1 g/d maintenance Premarin® 0.5-2 g/d for 21 d then off 7 d for vaginal atrophy, 0.5 g/d for 21 d then off 7 d or twice/wk for dyspareunia Estragyn® 2-4 g/d	Crinone® 4% or 8% (45 or 90 mg applicator)	If simultaneously taking oral estrogen tablet, may need to adjust dosing If intact uterus, also take progesterone

CEE = conjugated equine estrogen (e.g. Premarin®); MPA = medroxyprogesterone acetate (e.g. Provera®); NEA = norethindrone acetate
Consider lower dose regimens, PREMPRO® 0.45/1.5 (Premarin® 0.45 mg and Provera® 1.5 mg); Estrace® (topical 17β-estradiol) = 0.1 mg active ingredient/g; Premarin® (topical CEE) = 0.625 mg active ingredient/g; Estragyn® (topical estrone) = 1 mg active ingredient/g

Side Effects of HRT

- abnormal uterine bleeding
- mastodynia – breast tenderness
- edema, bloating, heartburn, nausea
- mood changes (progesterone)
- can be worse in progesterone phase of combined therapy

Contraindications to HRT

- absolute
  - acute liver disease
  - undiagnosed vaginal bleeding
  - known or suspected uterine cancer/breast cancer
  - acute vascular thrombosis or history of severe thrombophlebitis or thromboembolic disease
  - cardiovascular disease
- relative
  - pre-existing uncontrolled HTN
  - uterine fibroids and endometriosis
  - familial hyperlipidemias
  - migraine headaches
  - family history of estrogen-dependent cancer
  - chronic thrombophlebitis
  - DM (with vascular disease)
  - gallbladder disease, hypertriglyceridemia, impaired liver function (consider transdermal estrogen)
  - fibrocystic disease of the breasts

Absolute Contraindications to HRT

ABCD
Acute liver disease
Undiagnosed vaginal **B**leeding
Cancer (breast/uterine), **C**ardiovascular disease
DVT (thromboembolic disease)

Long-Term Hormone Therapy for Perimenopausal and Postmenopausal Women
Cochrane DB Syst Rev 2012;7:CD004143
Purpose: To determine the effect of long-term HRT on mortality, cardiovascular outcomes, cancer, gallbladder disease, fractures, cognition, and QOL in perimenopausal and postmenopausal women, during HRT use, and after cessation of HRT.
Results: 23 studies with 42,380 women included. 70% of the data from the WHI (1998) and HERS (1998). None of the studies focused on perimenopausal women. Combined continuous HRT: increased risk of coronary event after 1 yr (absolute risk 18/1,000, 95% CI 3-7), venous thromboembolism after 1 yr (AR 7/1,000, 95% CI 4-11), stroke after 3 yr (AR 18/1,000, 95% CI 14-23), breast cancer after 5.6 yr (AR 23/1,000, 95% CI 19-29), gallbladder disease after 5.6 yr (AR 27/1,000, 95% CI 21-34), and death from lung cancer after 5.6 yr use (AR 9/1,000, 95% CI 6-13). Estrogen only HRT: increased risk of venous thromboembolism after 1-2 yr use (AR 5/1,000, 95% CI 2-10; after 7 yr AR 21/1,000, 95% CI 16-28), stroke after 7 yr (AR 32/1,000, 95% CI 25-40), and gallbladder disease after 7 yr use (AR 45/1,000, 95% CI 36-57) and did not significantly affect the risk of breast cancer. Women >65 yr of age taking combined HRT had a statistically significant increase in the incidence of dementia after 4 yr use (AR 18/1,000, 95% CI 11-30). Women taking HRT had a decreased risk of fractures with combined HRT after 5.6 yr (AR 86/1,000, 95% CI 79-84) and 7.1 yr of estrogen only HRT (AR 102/1,000, 95% CI 91-112).
Conclusions: HRT is not indicated for primary or secondary prevention of cardiovascular disease or dementia. Although HRT is considered effective for the prevention of postmenopausal osteoporosis, it is generally recommended as an option only for women at significant risk, for whom non-estrogen therapies are unsuitable.

WOMEN'S HEALTH INITIATIVE (launched in 1991)

- two non-randomized studies investigating health risks and benefits of HRT in healthy postmenopausal women 50-79 yr old
  - continuous combined HRT (CEE 0.625 mg + MPA 2.5 mg OD) in 16,608 women with an intact uterus
  - estrogen-alone (CEE 0.625 mg) in 10,739 women with a previous hysterectomy
- both arms of the trial were stopped early because of evidence of increased risk of breast cancer, stroke, PE, and CHD in the combined HRT arm, and increased risk of stroke with no CHD benefits in the estrogen-alone arm
- the apparent increase in CHD was in disagreement with results of previous observational trial
- results of the WHI study have since been challenged and revision of how CHD was diagnosed led to loss of statistical significance of the results
- benefits and risks reported as number of cases per 10,000 women each year

Table 17. HRT Benefits vs. Risks

Benefits	Risks
Vasomotor Symptoms: less frequent and severe with use of either combined or estrogen-alone HRT	**Stroke**: 8 additional cases with combined HRT, and 12 additional cases for estrogen alone (WHI)
Osteoporosis: 5 fewer cases of hip fractures and 47 fewer cases of all fractures with combined HRT; 6 fewer cases of hip fractures with estrogen alone	**DVT/PE**: 18 additional cases with combined HRT, and 9 additional cases for estrogen-alone (WHI)
Colon Cancer: 6 fewer cases with combined HRT (WHI) One additional case with estrogen-alone	**CHD**: 7 additional MIs with combined HRT (WHI); secondary analysis suggests greater absolute risk for women aged >70 yr and for women who start HRT >10 yr post-menopause
	Breast Cancer: 8 additional cases with combined HRT (WHI) Risk only increased after >5 yr of combined HRT use; no increased risk for estrogen-alone
	Dementia and Mild Cognitive Impairment: 50% greater risk of developing dementia in women taking estrogen-alone after age 65; risk is greater for women taking combined HRT; risk of developing dementia was reduced for women taking HRT before age 65

Urogynecology

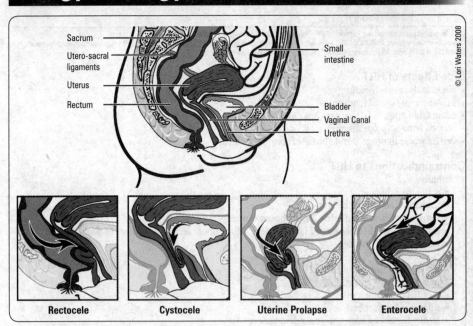

Figure 22. Pelvic anatomy

Rectocele Cystocele Uterine Prolapse Enterocele

Prolapse

Etiology
- relaxation, weakness, or defect in the cardinal and uterosacral ligaments which normally maintain the uterus in an anteflexed position and prevent it from descending through the urogenital diaphragm (i.e. levator ani muscles)
- related to
  - vaginal childbirth
  - aging
  - decreased estrogen (post-menopause)
  - following pelvic surgery
  - increased intra-abdominal pressure (obesity, chronic cough, constipation, ascites, heavy lifting)
  - congenital (rarely)
  - ethnicity (Caucasian women > Asian or African women)
  - collagen disorders

GENERAL CONSERVATIVE TREATMENT
(for pelvic relaxation/prolapse and urinary incontinence)
- Kegel exercises
- local vaginal estrogen therapy
- vaginal pessary (intravaginal suspension disc)

Table 18. Pelvic Prolapse

Type	Clinical Features	Treatment
Cystocele (protrusion of bladder into the anterior vaginal wall)	Frequency, urgency, nocturia Stress incontinence Incomplete bladder emptying ± associated increased incidence of UTIs – may lead to renal impairment	See above Anterior colporrhaphy ("anterior repair") Consider additional/alternative surgical procedure if documented urinary stress incontinence
Enterocele (prolapse of small bowel in upper posterior vaginal wall)		Similar to hernia repair Contents reduced, neck of peritoneal sac ligated, uterosacral ligaments, and levator ani muscles approximated
Rectocele (protrusion of rectum into posterior vaginal wall)	Straining/digitation to evacuate stool Constipation	See above Also laxatives and stool softeners Posterior colporrhaphy ("posterior repair"), plication of endopelvic fascia and perineal muscles approximated in midline to support rectum and perineum (can result in dyspareunia)
Uterine Prolapse (protrusion of cervix and uterus into vagina)	Groin/back pain (stretching of uterosacral ligaments) Feeling of heaviness/pressure in the pelvis Worse with standing, lifting Worse at the end of the day Relieved by lying down Ulceration/bleeding (particularly if hypoestrogenic) ± urinary incontinence	See above Vaginal hysterectomy ± surgical prevention of vault prolapse Consider additional surgical procedures if urinary incontinence, cystocele, rectocele, and/or enterocele are present
Vault Prolapse (protrusion of apex of vaginal vault into vagina, post-hysterectomy)		See above Sacralcolpopexy (vaginal vault suspension), sacrospinous fixation, or uterosacral ligament suspension

Urinary Incontinence

- see <u>Urology</u>, U5

STRESS INCONTINENCE

Definition
- involuntary loss of urine with increased intra-abdominal pressure (coughing, laughing, sneezing, walking, running)

Risk Factors for Stress Incontinence in Women
- pelvic prolapse
- pelvic surgery
- vaginal delivery
- hypoestrogenic state (post-menopause)
- age
- smoking
- neurological/pulmonary disease

Grading of Pelvic Organ Prolapse
- 0 = no descent during straining
- 1 = distal portion of prolapse >1 cm above level of hymen
- 2 = distal portion of prolapse ≤1 cm above or below level of hymen
- 3 = distal portion of prolapse >1 cm below level of hymen but without complete vaginal eversion
- 4 = complete eversion of total length of lower genital tract
- Procidentia: failure of genital supports and complete protrusion of uterus through the vagina

Pelvic Relaxation/Prolapse
Protrusion of pelvic organs into or out of the vagina

The only **true** hernia of the pelvis is an ENTEROCELE because peritoneum herniates with the small bowel

Treatment
- see *Prolapse, General Conservative Treatment*, GY37
- surgical
  - tension-free vaginal tape (TVT), tension-free obturator tape (TOT), prosthetic/fascial slings or retropubic bladder suspension (Burch or Marshall-Marchetti-Krantz procedures)

URGE INCONTINENCE

Definition
- urine loss associated with an abrupt, sudden urge to void
- "overactive bladder"
- diagnosed based on symptoms

Etiology
- idiopathic (90%)
- detrusor muscle overactivity ("detrusor instability")

Associated Symptoms
- frequency, urgency, nocturia, leakage

Treatment
- behaviour modification (reduce caffeine/liquid, smoking cessation, regular voiding schedule)
- Kegel exercises
- medications
  - anticholinergics: oxybutinin (Ditropan®), tolterodine (Detrol®), solifenacin (VESIcare®)
  - tricyclic antidepressants: imipramine

Gynecological Oncology

Uterus

ENDOMETRIAL CARCINOMA

Epidemiology
- most common gynecological malignancy in North America (40%); 4th most common cancer in women
- 2-3% of women develop endometrial carcinoma during lifetime
- mean age is 60 yr
- majority are diagnosed in early stage due to detection of symptoms
- 85-90% 5 yr survival for stage I disease
- 70-80% overall 5 yr survival for all stages

Risk Factors
- General: increasing age and FHx
- Type I: excess estrogen (estrogen unopposed by progesterone)
  - obesity
  - PCOS
  - unbalanced HRT (balanced HRT is protective)
  - nulliparity
  - late menopause (> 55 yr), early menarche
  - estrogen-producing ovarian tumours (e.g. granulosa cell tumours)
  - HNPCC (hereditary non-polyposis colorectal cancer)/Lynch II syndrome
  - tamoxifen
- Type II: not estrogen-related
  - possibly tamoxifen

Classification and Clinical Features
- Type I (well-differentiated endometrioid adenocarcinoma) ~80% of cases
  - postmenopausal bleeding in majority, abnormal uterine bleeding in majority of affected pre-menopausal women (menorrhagia, intermenstrual bleeding)
- Type II (serous, clear cell carcinoma, grade 3 endometrioid, undifferentiated, carcinosarcoma) ~15% of cases
  - may not present with bleeding in early stage, more likely to present with advanced stage disease with symptoms like ovarian cancer (i.e. bloating, bowel dysfunction, pelvic pressure)

Investigations
- endometrial sampling
  - office endometrial biopsy
  - D&C ± hysteroscopy
- ± pelvic ultrasound (in women where adequate endometrial sampling not feasible without invasive methods)
- not acceptable as alternative to pelvic exam or endometrial sampling to rule out cancer

Urge Incontinence
Urine loss associated with an abrupt, sudden urge to void

Rule Out Neurological Causes of Urge Incontinence
- MS
- Herniated disc
- DM

Incidence of Malignant Gynecological Lesions in North America
endometrium > ovary > cervix > vulva > vagina > fallopian tube

Risk Factors for Endometrial Cancer

COLD NUT
Cancer (ovarian, breast, colon)
Obesity
Late menopause
Diabetes mellitus
Nulliparity
Unopposed estrogen: PCOS, anovulation, HRT
Tamoxifen: chronic use

Postmenopausal bleeding = endometrial cancer until proven otherwise (95% present with vaginal bleeding)

An endometrial thickness of 5 mm or more is considered abnormal in a postmenopausal woman with vaginal bleeding

Table 19. FIGO Staging of Endometrial Cancer (2009)

Stage	Description	Stage	Description
I	Confined to corpus	IIIC	Metastasis to pelvic ± para-aortic LNs
IA	No or less than half myometrial invasion	IIIC1	Positive pelvic LN
IB	Invades through ≥½ of myometrium	IIIC2	Positive para-aortic LN ± positive pelvic LNs
II	**Tumour invades cervical stroma, but does not extend beyond uterus***	**IV**	**Invasion of bladder ± bowel mucosa ± distant metastases**
		IVA	
III	**Local and/or regional spread of tumour**	IVB	Invasion of bladder ± bowel mucosa
IIIA	Invasion of serosa, corpus uteri ± adnexae		Distant mets, including intra-abdominal mets ± inguinal LNs
IIIB	Vaginal ± parametrial involvement		

FIGO: International Federation of Gynecology and Obstetrics
*Note: endocervical glandular involvement is now considered as Stage I (previously Stage II)

Treatment
- surgical: hysterectomy/bilateral salpingo-oophorectomy (BSO) and pelvic washings ± pelvic and para-aortic node dissection ± omentectomy
  - goals: diagnosis, staging, treatment, defining optimal adjuvant treatment
  - laparoscopic approach associated with improved quality of life (optimal for most patients)
- adjuvant radiotherapy (for improved local control in patients at risk for local recurrence) and adjuvant chemotherapy (in patients at risk for distant recurrence or with metastatic disease): based on presence of poor prognostic factors in definitive pathology
- chemotherapy: often used for recurrent disease (especially if high grade or aggressive histology)
- hormonal therapy: progestins can be used for recurrent disease (especially if low grade)

UTERINE SARCOMA
- rare; 2-6% of all uterine malignancies
- arise from stromal components (endometrial stroma, mesenchymal or myometrial tissues)
- behave more aggressively and are associated with worse prognosis than endometrial carcinoma; 5-yr survival is 35%
- vaginal bleeding is most common presenting symptom

Prognostic Factors
Most important is FIGO stage
Other Prognostic Factors:
- Age
- Grade
- Histologic subtype
- Depth of myometrial invasion
- Presence of lymphovascular space involvement (LVSI)
- Hormone receptor status

Complications of Therapy
- Surgical site infection
- Lymphedema
- Radiation fibrosis
- Cystitis
- Proctitis

Uterine Sarcoma – Symptoms
BAD-P
Bleeding
Abdominal distention
Foul smelling vaginal **D**ischarge
Pelvic Pressure

A rapidly enlarging uterus, especially in a postmenopausal woman, should prompt consideration of leiomyosarcoma

Table 20. Summary of Uterine Sarcoma Subtypes and Features

Type	Epidemiology	Features	Diagnosis	Treatment
PURE TYPE				
1. Leiomyosarcoma	Accounts for 40% Average age of presentation is 55 yr but may present in premenopausal woman Often coexists with benign leiomyomata (fibroids) 50% arise within a fibroid ("sarcomatous degeneration")	Histologic distinction from leiomyoma 1. Increased mitotic count (>10 mitoses/10 high power fields) 2. Tumour necrosis 3. Cellular atypia Rapidly enlarging fibroids in a premenopausal woman Enlarging fibroids in a postmenopausal woman	Often post-operatively after uterus removed for presumed fibroids Stage using FIGO 2009 staging for leiomyosarcomas and ECC	Hysterectomy/BSO usually No routine pelvic lymphadenectomy Adjuvant chemotherapy may be used if tumour has spread beyond uterus Radiation therapy does not improve local control or survival Poor outcomes overall, even for early stage disease
2. Endometrial Stromal Sarcoma (ESS)	Accounts for 10-15% Usually presents in perimenopausal or postmenopausal women with abnormal uterine bleeding	Abnormal uterine bleeding Good prognosis	Diagnosed by histology of endometrial biopsy or D&C Stage using FIGO 2009 staging for leiomyosarcomas and ECC	Hysterectomy & BSO (remove ovaries as ovarian hormones may stimulate growth) No routine pelvic lymphadenectomy Adjuvant therapy based on stage and histologic features (hormones and/or radiation) Hormonal therapy (progestins) may be used for metastatic disease
3. Undifferentiated Sarcoma	Accounts for 5-10%	Severe nuclear pleomorphism, high mitotic activity, tumour cell necrosis, and lack smooth muscle or endometrial stromal differentiation Poor prognosis	Often found incidentally post-operatively for abnormal bleeding	Treatment primarily surgical Radiation and/or chemotherapy for advanced diseased or unresectable disease
MIXED TYPE				
4. Adenosarcoma	The rarest of the uterine sarcoma Mixed tumour of low malignant potential	Present with abnormal vaginal bleeding Polypoid mass in uterine cavity	Mixture of benign epithelium with malignant low-grade sarcoma Often found incidentally at time of hysterectomy for PMB Stage using FIGO 2009 staging for adenosarcoma	Treatment is surgical with hysterectomy and BSO
RECLASSIFIED				
5. Carcinosarcoma	Most common (43%) Recently reclassified as high grade endometrioid carcinoma with associated metaplasia of the mesenchyme, rather than arising separately from stroma	Both epithelial and stromal malignant elements present Tend to form bulky polypoid masses that often fill uterine cavity and extend into or through the endocervical canal – often have extrauterine disease at presentation	Diagnosed by histology of endometrial biopsy or D&C Stage using FIGO 2009 staging for endometrial cancer	Usually treated as "high grade endometrial carcinoma" since behaviour and treatment similar (i.e. surgical staging and resection of any gross metastatic disease, adjuvant chemotherapy and radiation)

Table 21. FIGO Staging of Uterine Sarcoma (2009)

Stage	Description	Stage	Description
I	**Tumour limited to uterus**	III	
IA	<5 cm	IIIA	Tumour invades abdominal tissues, one site
IB	>5 cm	IIIB	Metastasis to pelvic and/or para-aortic lymph nodes
		IIIC	Tumour invades bladder and/or rectum
II	**Tumour extends beyond uterus**	IV	
IIA	To the pelvis, adnexal involvement	IVA	Tumour invades bladder and/or rectum
IIB	To extra-uterine pelvic tissue	IVB	Distant metastasis

Ovary

BENIGN OVARIAN TUMOURS
- see Table 22
- many are asymptomatic
- usually enlarge slowly, if at all
- may rupture or undergo torsion, causing pain
  - pain associated with torsion of an adnexal mass usually originates in the iliac fossa and radiates to the flank
- peritoneal irritation may result from an infarcted tumour – rare

MALIGNANT OVARIAN TUMOURS
- see Table 22

Epidemiology
- lifetime risk 1.4%
- in women >50 yr, more than 50% of ovarian tumours are malignant
- causes more deaths in North America than all other gynecologic malignancies combined
- 4th leading cause of cancer death in women
- 65% epithelial; 35% non-epithelial
- 5-10% of epithelial ovarian cancers are related to hereditary predisposition

Risk Factors (for epithelial ovarian cancers)
- excess estrogen
  - nulliparity
  - early menarche/late menopause
- age
- family history of breast, colon, endometrial, ovarian cancer
- race: Caucasian

Protective Factors (for epithelial ovarian cancers)
- OCP: likely due to ovulation suppression (significant reduction in risk even after 1 yr of use)
- pregnancy/breastfeeding
- salpingectomy (prophylactic)
- BSO (prophylactic surgery performed for this reason in high risk women – i.e. BRCA mutation carriers)

Screening
- no effective method of mass screening
- routine CA-125 level measurements or U/S not recommended
  - high false positive rates
- controversial in high risk groups: transvaginal U/S and CA-125, starting age 30 (no consensus on interval)
  - familial ovarian cancer (>1 first degree relative affected, BRCA-1 mutation)
  - other cancers (e.g. endometrial, breast, colon)
  - BRCA-1 or BRCA-2 mutation: may recommend prophylactic bilateral oophorectomy after age 35 or when child-bearing is completed

Clinical Features
- most women with epithelial ovarian cancer present with advanced stage disease since often "asymptomatic" until disseminated disease (symptoms with early stage disease are vague and non-specific)
- when present, symptoms may include
  - abdominal symptoms (nausea, bloating, dyspepsia, anorexia, early satiety)
  - symptoms of mass effect
    - increased abdominal girth – from ascites or tumour itself
    - urinary frequency
    - constipation
  - postmenopausal bleeding; irregular menses if pre-menopausal (rare)

Ovaries are like GEMS
Germ-cell
Epithelial
Metastatic
Sex cord stromal

Most (70%) epithelial ovarian cancers present at stage III disease

Risk/Protective Factors for Epithelial Ovarian Cancer

NO CHILD
Nulliparity
OCP, breastfeeding, tubal ligation, hysterectomy (protective)
Caucasian
Family History
Increasing age (>40 yr)
Late menopause
Delayed child-bearing

Ovarian Tumour Markers
- Epithelial cell – CA-125
- Stromal
- Granulosa cell – inhibin
- Sertoli-Leydig – androgens
- Germ cell
- Dysgerminoma – LDH
- Yolk sac – AFP
- Choriocarcinoma – β-hCG
- Immature Teratoma – none
- Embryonal cell – AFP + β-hCG

Diagnosis of ovarian tumours requires surgical pathology

Any adnexal mass in postmenopausal women should be considered malignant until proven otherwise

Omental Cake: a term for ascites plus a fixed upper abdominal and pelvic mass; almost always signifies ovarian cancer

Low Malignant Potential (also called "Borderline") Tumours

- pregnancy, OCP, and breastfeeding are protective factors
- ~15% of all epithelial ovarian tumours
- tumour cells display malignant characteristics histologically, but no invasion is identified
- able to metastasize, but not commonly
- treated primarily with surgery (BSO/omental biopsy ± hysterectomy)
  - NO proven benefit of chemotherapy
- generally slow growing, excellent prognosis
  - 5 yr survival >99%
  - recurrences tend to occur late, may be associated with low grade serous carcinoma

Malignant Ovarian Tumour Prognosis
5 Year Survival
Stage I   75-95%
Stage II   60-75%
Stage III   23-41%
Stage IV   11%

Table 22. Ovarian Tumours

Type	Description	Presentation	Ultrasound/Cytology	Treatment
FUNCTIONAL TUMOURS (all benign)				
Follicular Cyst	Follicle fails to rupture during ovulation	Usually asymptomatic May rupture, bleed, tort, infarct causing pain ± signs of peritoneal irritation	4-8 cm mass, unilocular, lined with granulosa cells	Symptomatic or suspicious masses warrant surgical exploration Otherwise if <6 cm, wait 6 wk then re-examine as cyst usually regresses with next cycle OCP (ovarian suppression) – will prevent development of new cysts Treatment usually laparoscopic (cystectomy vs. oophorectomy, based on fertility choice)
Corpus Luteum Cyst	Corpus luteum fails to regress after 14 d, becoming cystic or hemorrhagic	More likely to cause pain than follicular cyst May delay onset of next period	Larger (10-15 cm) and firmer than follicular cysts	Same as for follicular cysts
Theca-Lutein Cyst	Due to atretic follicles stimulated by abnormal β-hCG levels	Associated with molar pregnancy, ovulation induction with clomiphene		Conservative Cyst will regress as β-hCG levels fall
Endometrioma	See *Endometriosis*, GY13			
Polycystic Ovaries	See *Polycystic Ovarian Syndrome*, GY24			
BENIGN GERM-CELL TUMOURS				
Benign Cystic Teratoma (dermoid)	Single most common ovarian germ cell neoplasm Elements of all 3 cell lines; contains dermal appendages (sweat and sebaceous glands, hair follicles, teeth)	May rupture, twist, infarct 20% bilateral 20% occur outside of reproductive yr	Smooth-walled, mobile, unilocular Ultrasound may show calcification which is pathognomonic	Treatment usually laparoscopic cystectomy; may recur
MALIGNANT GERM-CELL TUMOURS				
General Information	Rapidly growing, 2-3% of all ovarian cancers	Usually children and young women (<30 yr)		Surgical resection (often conservative unilateral salpingo-oophorectomy ± nodes) ± chemotherapy
Dysgerminoma	Produces LDH	10% bilateral		Usually very responsive to chemotherapy, therefore complete resection is not necessary for cure
Immature Teratoma	No tumour marker identified			
Gonadoblastoma				
EPITHELIAL OVARIAN TUMOURS (malignant or borderline)				
General Information	Derived from mesothelial cells lining peritoneal cavity Classified based on histologic type 80-85% of all ovarian neoplasms (includes malignant)		Varies depending on subtype	**Borderline** Cystectomy vs. unilateral salpingo-oophorectomy **Malignant** 1. Early stage (stage I): Hysterectomy/BSO/staging (omentectomy, peritoneal biopsies, washings, pelvic and para-aortic lymphadenectomy) 2. Advanced stage: Upfront cytoreductive (debulking) followed by adjuvant chemotherapy consisting of IV carboplatic/paclitaxel vs. intraperitoneal chemotherapy (stage III) neoadjuvant chemotherapy with IV carboplatin/paclitaxel, followed by delayed debulking with further adjuvant IV chemotherapy
Serous	Most common ovarian tumour 50% of all ovarian cancers 75% of epithelial tumours 70% benign	20-30% bilateral	Lining similar to fallopian tube epithelium Often multilocular Histologically contain Psamomma bodies (calcified concentric concretions)	

Table 22. Ovarian Tumours (continued)

Type	Description	Presentation	Ultrasound/Cytology	Treatment
EPITHELIAL OVARIAN TUMOURS (malignant or borderline)				
Mucinous	20% of epithelial tumours 85% benign	Rarely complicated by Pseudomyxoma peritoneii: implants seed abdominal cavity and produce large quantities of mucin	Resembles endocervical epithelium Often multilocular May reach enormous size	Poor response to chemotherapy If mucinous, remove appendix as well to rule out possible source of primary disease
SEX CORD STROMAL OVARIAN TUMOURS				
General Information				Surgical resection of tumour Chemotherapy may be used for unresectable metastatic disease
Fibroma/Thecoma (benign)	From mature fibroblasts in ovarian stroma	Non-functioning Occasionally associated with Meig's syndrome (benign ovarian tumour and ascites and pleural effusion)	Firm, smooth rounded tumour with interlacing fibrocytes	
Granulosa-Theca Cell Tumours (benign or malignant)	Can be associated with endometrial cancer Inhibin is tumour marker	Estrogen-producing → feminizing effects (precocious puberty, menorrhagia, postmenopausal bleeding)	Histologic hallmark of cancer is small groups of cells known as Call-Exner bodies	
Sertoli-Leydig Cell Tumour (benign or malignant)	Can measure elevated androgens as tumour markers	Androgen-producing → virilizing effects (hirsutism, deep voice, recession of front hairline)		
METASTATIC OVARIAN TUMOURS				
From GI Tract, Breast, Endometrium, Lymphoma	4-8% of ovarian malignancies Krukenberg tumour – metastatic ovarian tumour (usually GI tract, commonly stomach or colon, breast) with "signet-ring" cells			

Effects of Screening on Ovarian Cancer Mortality: The Prostate, Lung, Colorectal, and Ovarian Cancer Screening Randomized Controlled Trial
JAMA 2011;305:2295-2303
Objective: To evaluate the effect of screening for ovarian cancer with CA-125 and transvaginal ultrasound on mortality in the prostate, lung, ectal, and ovarian (PLCO) cancer screening trial.
Participants: 78,216 women aged 55-74 yr.
Study Groups: Intervention group – annual screening with CA-125 for 6 yr, transvaginal ultrasound for 4 yr; control group – no CA-125 or transvaginal ultrasound screening, received usual medical care.
Follow-up: Maximum 13 yr (median, 12.4 yr).
Outcome Measures: Mortality from ovarian cancer, including primary fallopian tube cancers. Secondary outcomes included ovarian cancer incidence and complications associated with screening, examinations, and diagnostic procedures.
Results: Of those diagnosed with ovarian cancer in the intervention and usual care group, the mortality was 3.1% and 2.6% respectively. 15% of women undergoing diagnostic evaluation following a false positive screening test suffered a complication of the procedure.
Conclusions: Simultaneous screening with CA-125 and transvaginal ultrasound compared with usual care did not reduce ovarian cancer mortality. Diagnostic evaluation following a false positive screening test was associated with complications.

Investigation of Suspicious Ovarian Mass

- women with suspected ovarian cancer based on history, physical, or investigations should be referred to a gynecologic oncologist
  - bimanual examination
    - ◆ solid, irregular, or fixed pelvic mass is suggestive of ovarian cancer
  - RMI (Risk of Malignancy Index) is best tool available to assess likelihood of ovarian malignancy and need for pre-operative gynecologic oncology referral (see sidebar, GY43)
- blood work: CA-125 for baseline, CBC, liver function tests, electrolytes, creatinine
- radiology
  - bone scan or PET scan not indicated
  - transvaginal ultrasound best to visualize ovaries
  - CT scan abdomen and pelvis to look for metastatic disease
- try to rule out other primary source if suspected, based on
  - occult blood per rectum: endoscopy ± barium enema
  - gastric symptoms, gastroscopy ± upper GI series
  - abnormal vaginal bleeding, endometrial biopsy to rule out concurrent endometrial cancer, colposcopy ± endocervical curettage to rule out cervical cancer if abnormal cervix
  - breast lesion identified or risk factors present: mammogram

Table 23. FIGO Staging for Primary Carcinoma of the Ovary (Surgical Staging) (2014)

Stage	Description
I	**Growth limited to the ovaries**
IA	1 ovary, no ascites, no tumour on external surface, capsule intact, negative washings
IB	2 ovaries, no ascites, no tumour on external surface, capsule intact
IC	1 or 2 ovaries with any of the following: surgical spill (IC1), capsule ruptured (IC2), tumour on ovarian surface (IC2), or malignant cells in ascites (IC3)
II	**Growth involving one or both ovaries with pelvic extension or primary peritoneal cancer**
IIA	Extension ± implants to uterus/tubes
IIB	Extension to other pelvic structures
III	**Tumour involving one or both ovaries with peritoneal implants outside the pelvis and/or positive retroperitoneal nodes**
IIIA	Positive retroperitoneal LNs and/or microscopic metastasis beyond pelvis
IIIA1	Positive retroperitoneal LNs
IIIA2	Microscopic, extrapelvic peritoneal involvement ± positive retroperitoneal LNs
IIIB	Macroscopic peritoneal metastasis beyond pelvis ≤2 cm, ± positive retroperitoneal LNs. Includes extension to capsule of liver/spleen
IIIC	Same as above but peritoneal metastasis >2 cm
IV	**Distant metastasis beyond peritoneal cavity**
IVA	Pleural effusion with positive cytology
IVB	Hepatic and/or splenic parenchymal metastasis or metastasis to extra-abdominal organs (inguinal LNs and LNs outside of abdominal cavity included)

FIGO = International Federation of Gynecology and Obstetrics

Cervix

BENIGN CERVICAL LESIONS
- Nabothian cyst/inclusion cyst
- no treatment required
- endocervical polyps
- treatment is polypectomy (office procedure)

MALIGNANT CERVICAL LESIONS

Epidemiology
- majority are SCC (95%); adenocarcinomas increasing (5%); rare subtypes include small cell, adenosquamous
- 8,000 deaths annually in North America
- annual Pap test reduces a woman's chance of dying from cervical cancer from 0.4% to 0.05%
- average age at presentation: 52 yr old

Etiology
- at birth, vagina is lined with squamous epithelium; columnar epithelium lines only the endocervix and the central area of the ectocervix (original squamocolumnar junction)
- during puberty, estrogen stimulates eversion of a single columnar layer (ectopy), thus exposing it to the acidic pH of the vagina, leading to metaplasia (change of exposed epithelium from columnar to squamous)
  - a new squamocolumnar junction forms as a result
- the transformation zone (TZ) is the area located between the original and the current squamocolumnar junction
- the majority of dysplasias and cancers arise in the TZ of the cervix
- must have active metaplasia in presence of inducing agent (HPV) to get dysplasia
- dysplasia → carcinoma *in situ* (CIS) → invasion
- slow process (~10 yr on average)
- growth is by local extension
- metastasis occurs late

Risk Factors
- HPV infection
  - see *Sexually Transmitted Infections*, GY27
  - high risk of neoplasia associated with types 16, 18
  - low risk of neoplasia associated with types 6, 11
  - >99% of cervical cancers contain one of the high risk HPV types
- high risk behaviours (risk factors for HPV infection)
  - multiple partners
  - other STIs (HSV, trichomonas)
  - early age at first intercourse
  - high risk male partner
- smoking
- poor screening uptake is the most important risk factor for cervical cancer in Canada
- at-risk groups include
  - immigrant Canadians
  - First Nations Canadians
  - geographically isolated Canadians
  - sex-trade workers
  - low socioeconomic status

Cervical Cancer Screening Guidelines (Pap Test)
- see <u>Family Medicine</u>, FM5

Clinical Features
- SCC: exophytic, fungating tumour
- adenocarcinoma: endophytic, with barrel-shaped cervix
- early
  - asymptomatic
  - discharge: initially watery, becoming brown or red
  - postcoital bleeding
- late
  - 80-90% present with bleeding: either postcoital, postmenopausal or irregular bleeding
  - pelvic or back pain (extension of tumour to pelvic walls)
  - bladder/bowel symptoms
- signs
  - friable, raised, reddened, or ulcerated area visible on cervix

Incorporation of Bevacizumab in the Primary Treatment of Ovarian Cancer
NEJM 2011;365:2473-2483
Purpose: To evaluate the effect of bevacizumab addition to standard front-line therapy for epithelial ovarian cancer.
Study: Double-blind, placebo-controlled phase 3 trial with patients with newly diagnosed stage III (incompletely resectable) or stage IV epithelial ovarian cancer who had undergone debulking surgery to receive one of three treatments. All three treatments included chemotherapy with intravenous paclitaxel plus carboplatin. Patients received chemotherapy with placebo, bevacizumab-initiation treatment (cycles 2-6 of 22 cycles) or bevacizumab-throughout (cycles 2-22).
Results: 1,873 participants. The median progression-free survival was 10.3 mo in the control group, 11.2 mo in the bevacizumab-initiation group, and 14.1 mo in the bevacizumab-throughout group. The rate of hypertension requiring medical therapy was higher in the bevacizumab-initiation group (16.5%) and bevacizumab-throughout group (22.9%) than in the control group (7.2%) as well as gastrointestinal wall disruption (2.8%, 2.6%, 1.2%, respectively).
Conclusions: The use of bevacizumab during and up to 10 mo after carboplatin and paclitaxel chemotherapy prolongs the median progression-free survival by about 4 mo in patients with advanced epithelial ovarian cancer.

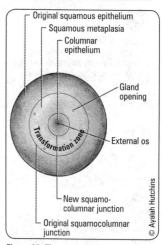

Figure 23. The cervix

Original squamous epithelium
Squamous metaplasia
Columnar epithelium
Gland opening
External os
New squamo-columnar junction
Original squamocolumnar junction
Transformation zone
© Ayalah Hutchins

A Risk of Malignancy Incorporating CA125, Ultrasound, and Menopausal Status for the Accurate Pre-Operative Diagnosis of Ovarian Cancer
BJOG 1990;97:922-929
RMI = U x M x CA-125
Ultrasound Findings (1 pt for each)
- Multilocular cyst
- Evidence of solid areas
- Evidence of metastases
- Presence of ascites
- Bilateral lesions
U = 1 (for U/S scores of 0 or 1)
U = 4 (for U/S scores of 2-5)
Menopausal Status
- Postmenopausal: M = 4
- Premenopausal: M = 1
Absolute Value of CA-125 Serum Level
- For RMI>200: Gynecologic oncology referral is recommended

Cervical cancer is most prevalent in developing countries and therefore is the only gynecologic cancer that uses clinical staging; this facilitates consistent international staging with countries that do not have technologies, such as CT and MRI

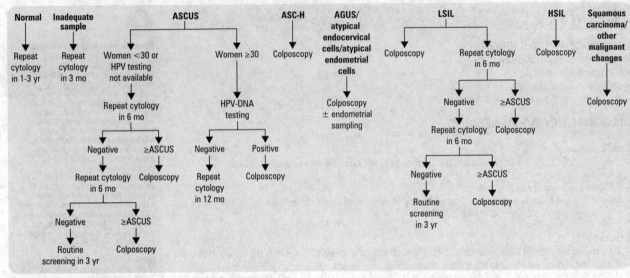

Figure 24. Decision making chart for Pap test (not applicable for adolescents)
Adapted from: Ontario Cervical Screening Practice Guidelines. May 2012. Cervical screening guidelines unique to each province

Diagnosis

- apply acetic acid and identify acetowhite lesions, punctation, mosaicism, and abnormal blood vessels to guide cervical biopsy
- endocervical curettage (ECC) if entire lesion is not visible or no lesion visible
- diagnostic excision (LEEP) if
  - lesion extends into endocervical canal
  - positive ECC
  - discrepancy between Pap test results and colposcopy
  - microinvasive carcinoma
- consider cold knife conization (in OR) if glandular abnormality suspected based on cytology or colposcopic findings due to concern for margin interpretation
- tests permitted for FIGO clinical staging include: physical exam (including examination under anesthesia), cervical biopsy (including cone biopsy), proctoscopy/cystoscopy, IVP, ultrasound liver/ kidneys, CXR, LFTs
- MRI and/or CT and/or PET scan often done to facilitate planning of radiation therapy, results do not influence clinical stage

The Bethesda Classification System is based on cytological results of a Pap test that permits the examination of cells but not tissue structure. Cervical intraepithelial neoplasia (CIN) or cervical carcinoma is a histological diagnosis, requiring a tissue sample via biopsy of suspicious lesions seen during colposcopy

With development of hypertension early in pregnancy (i.e. <20 wk), think gestational trophoblastic disease

Causes of Elevated CA-125
- Age influences reliability of test as a tumour marker
- 50% sensitivity in early stage ovarian cancer (poor) – therefore not good for screening

Malignant
- Gyne: ovary, uterus
- Non-Gyne: pancreas, stomach, colon, rectum

Non-Malignant
- Gyne: benign ovarian neoplasm, endometriosis, pregnancy, fibroids, PID
- Non-Gyne: cirrhosis, pancreatitis, renal failure

CA-125 is indicated for monitoring response to treatment

Cervical Cancer Prognosis 5-yr Survival
Stage 0   99%
Stage I   75%
Stage II   55%
Stage III 30%
Stage IV   7%
Overall   50-60%

Table 24. FIGO Staging Classification of Cervical Cancer (Clinical Staging) (2009)

Stage	Description
I	**Confined to cervix**
IA	Microinvasive (diagnosed only by microscopy)
IA1	Stromal invasion not >3 mm deep, not >7 mm wide
IA2	3-5 mm deep; not >7 mm wide
IB	Clinically visible lesion confined to cervix, or microscopic lesion >IA
IB1	Clinically visible lesion ≤4 mm in greatest dimension
IB2	Clinically visible lesion >4 mm in greatest dimension
II	**Beyond uterus but not to the pelvic wall or lower 1/3 of vagina**
IIA	No obvious parametrial involvement
IIA1	Clinically visible lesion ≤4 mm in greatest dimension
IIA2	Clinically visible lesion >4 mm in greatest dimension
IIB	Obvious parametrial involvement
III	**Extends to pelvic wall, and/or involves lower 1/3 of vagina and/or causes hydronephrosis or non-functioning kidney**
IIIA	Involves lower 1/3 vagina but no extension into pelvic side wall
IIIB	Extension into pelvic side wall and/or hydronephrosis or non-functioning kidney
IV	**Carcinoma has extended beyond true pelvis or has involved (biopsy proven) the mucosa of the bladder or rectum**
IVA	Spread of the growth to adjacent organs (bladder or rectum)
IVB	Distant metastases

Treatment: Prevention and Management

Prevention: HPV Vaccine

- two vaccines currently approved (Gardasil®, Cervarix®)

Table 25. Comparison of Two Vaccines against Human Papillomavirus (HPV)

	Gardasil®	Cervarix®
Viral Strains Covered	6, 11, 16, 18	16, 18
Route of Administration	IM	IM
Schedule of Dosing	0, 2, 6 mo	0, 1, 6 mo
Side Effects	Local: redness, pain, swelling General: headache, low grade fever, GI upset	Local: redness, pain, swelling General: headache, low grade fever, GI upset
Approved Age	Females age 9-45, males age 9-26	Females age 10-25
Contraindications	Pregnant women and women who are nursing (limited data)	

*Gardasil-9 also covers types 31, 33, 45, 52, and 58; also used to prevent genital wards

Efficacy of Human Papillomavirus (HPV)-16/18 AS04-Adjuvanted Vaccine Against Cervical Infection and Precancer Caused by Oncogenic HPV Types (PATRICIA): Final Analysis of a Double-Blind, Randomized Study in Young Women
Lancet 2009;374:301-314
Study: Phase III double-blind, controlled RCT.
Patients: 18,644 women aged 15-25.
Selected Outcomes: Development of HPV-16/18 associated CIN II+ was the primary outcome. Secondary to this were persistence of infections with HPV-16, HPV-18, or other oncogenic HPV types.
Selected Results: Efficacy against development of HPV-16/18 associated CIN II+ was 98.1% (p<0.0001). High levels of cross-protection were observed for persistent infection with HPV-31 and HPV-45 and HPV-31 or HPV-45 associated CIN II+.
Conclusions: The HPV-16/18 AS04-adjuvanted vaccine protected against HPV-16/18 associated CIN II+ lesions and lesions associated with HPV-31, HPV-33, and HPV-45.

- should be administered before onset of sexual activity (i.e. before exposure to virus) for optimal benefit of vaccination
- may be given at the same time as hepatitis B or other vaccines using a different injection site
- not for treatment of active infections
- most women will not be infected with all four types of the virus at the same time, therefore vaccine is still indicated for sexually active females or those with a history of previous HPV infection or HPV-related disease
- conception should be avoided until 30 d after last dose of vaccination

Table 26. Management of Patients Abnormal Cervical Histology and Cervical Cancer

	Management
CIN I	Preferred option for biopsy-proven CIN I is observation Repeat assessment and cytology in 12 mo Management according to cytology results If after HSIL or AGC: Cytology and histology should be reviewed If discrepancy remains, excisional biopsy may be considered
CIN II and CIN III	Women ≥25 yr: CIN II or III should be treated Excisional procedures preferred for CIN III Those with positive margins should have follow-up with colposcopy and directed biopsies and/or endocervical curettage Treatment for recurrent CIN II or III should be by excision Women <25 yr: Pathologist should be asked to clarify whether lesion is CIN II or CIN III CIN II: observe with colposcopy at 6-mo intervals for up to 24 mo before treatment considered CIN III: should be treated During pregnancy: CIN II or III suspected or diagnosed during pregnancy, repeat colposcopy and treatment delayed until 8-12 wk after delivery
Stage IA1 (no LVSI)	Trachelectomy (removal of only the cervix) if future fertility desired (and lesion ≤2 cm) Simple hysterectomy if future fertility is not desired
Stage IA2, IB1	Typically treated with radical hysterectomy and pelvic lymphadenectomy (sentinel nodes under study) Equal cure rates may be obtained with primary radiation therapy; advantage of surgery: may accurately stage and grade and more targeted adjuvant therapy Advantage is that ovaries can be spared if pre-menopausal For fertility preservation, may have radical trachelectomy (removal of cervix and parametria) and nodes instead of radical hysterectomy for early-stage disease Concurrent chemoradiation therapy if adverse high risk prognostic factors on radical surgical specimen, such as: positive pelvic lymph nodes, positive parametria, and/or positive margins
Stages IB2 (>4 cm), II, III, IV	Primary chemoradiation therapy PET/CT to grade: evaluate pelvic and para-aortic nodes For positive nodes on PET: primary chemoradiation with extended field RT Hysterectomy generally not suggested following primary treatment with curative intent

Abnormal Pap Tests in Pregnancy

- incidence: 1/2,200
- Pap test at all initial prenatal visits
- if abnormal Pap or suspicious lesion, refer to colposcopy
- if diagnostic conization required, should be deferred until second trimester (T2) to minimize risk of pregnancy loss
- if invasive cancer ruled out, management of dysplasia deferred until completion of pregnancy (may deliver vaginally)
- if invasive cancer present, management depends on prognostic factors, degree of fetal maturity, and patient wishes
  - general recommendations in T1: consider pregnancy termination, management with either radical surgery (hysterectomy vs. trachelectomy if desires future fertility), or concurrent chemoradiation therapy
  - recommendations in T2/T3: delay of therapy until viable fetus and C/S for delivery with concurrent radical surgery or subsequent concurrent chemoradiation therapy

Vulva

BENIGN VULVAR LESIONS

Non-Neoplastic Disorders of Vulvar Epithelium
- biopsy is necessary to make diagnosis and/or rule out malignancy
- hyperplastic dystrophy (squamous cell hyperplasia)
  - surface thickened and hyperkeratotic
  - pruritus most common symptom
  - typically postmenopausal women
  - treatment: 1% fluorinated corticosteroid ointment bid for 6 wk
- lichen sclerosis
  - subepithelial fat becomes diminished; labia become thin, atrophic, with membrane-like epithelium and labial fusion
  - pruritus, dyspareunia, burning
  - 'figure of 8' distribution
  - most common in postmenopausal women but can occur at any age
  - treatment: ultrapotent topical steroid 0.05% clobetasol x 2-4 wk then taper down, can consider long term suppression twice a week
- mixed dystrophy (lichen sclerosis with epithelial hyperplasia)
  - hyperkeratotic areas with areas of thin, shiny epithelium
  - treatment: fluorinated corticosteroid ointment

Tumours
- papillary hidradenoma, nevus, fibroma, hemangioma

MALIGNANT VULVAR LESIONS

Epidemiology
- 5% of genital tract malignancies
- 90% SCC; remainder melanomas, basal cell carcinoma, Paget's disease, Bartholin's gland carcinoma
  - Type I disease: HPV-related (50-70%)
    - more likely in younger women
    - 90% of VIN contain HPV DNA (usually types 16, 18)
  - Type II disease: not HPV-related, associated with current or previous vulvar dystrophy
    - usually postmenopausal women

Risk Factors
- HPV infection
- vulvar intraepithelial neoplasia (VIN): precancerous change which presents as multicentric white or pigmented plaques on vulva (may only be visible at colposcopy)
  - progression to cancer rarely occurs with appropriate management
  - treatment: local excision (i.e. superficial vulvectomy ± split thickness skin grafting to cover defects if required) vs. ablative therapy (i.e. laser, cauterization) vs. local immunotherapy (imiquimod)

Clinical Features
- many patients asymptomatic at diagnosis (many also deny or minimize symptoms)
- most lesions occur on the labia majora, followed by the labia minora (less commonly on the clitoris or perineum)
- localized pruritus or lesion most common
- less common: raised red, white or pigmented plaque, ulcer, bleeding, discharge, pain, dysuria
- patterns of spread
  - local
  - groin lymph nodes (usually inguinal → pelvic nodes)
  - hematogenous

Any suspicious lesion of the vulva should be biopsied

Investigations
- ± colposcopy
- ALWAYS biopsy any suspicious lesion

Prognosis
- depends on stage – particularly nodal involvement (single most important predictor followed by tumour size)
- lesions >4 cm associated with poorer prognosis
- overall 5 yr survival rate: 79%

Vagina

BENIGN VAGINAL LESIONS
- inclusion cysts
  - cysts form at site of abnormal healing of laceration (e.g. episiotomy)
  - no treatment required
- endometriosis
  - dark lesions that tend to bleed at time of menses
  - treatment: excision
- Gartner's duct cysts
  - remnants of Wolffian duct, seen along side of cervix
  - treatment: conservative unless symptomatic
- urethral diverticulum
  - can lead to recurrent urethral infection, dyspareunia
  - treatment: surgical correction if symptomatic

MALIGNANT VAGINAL LESIONS

Epidemiology
- primary carcinomas of the vagina represent 2-3% of malignant neoplasms of the female genital tract
- 80-90% are SCC
- more than 50% diagnosed between 70-90 yr old

Risk Factors
- associated with HPV infection (analogous to cervical cancer)
- increased incidence in patients with prior history of cervical and vulvar cancer

Investigations
- cytology
  - significant false negative rate for existing malignancy (i.e. if gross lesion present, biopsy!)
- colposcopy
- Schiller test (normal squamous epithelium takes up Lugol's iodine)
- biopsy, partial vaginectomy (wide local excision for diagnosis)
- rule out disease on cervix, vulva, or anus (most vaginal cancers are actually metastatic from one of these sites)
- staging

Clinical Features

Table 27. Clinical Features of Malignant Vaginal Lesions

Type	Clinical Features
Vaginal Intra-Epithelial Neoplasia (VAIN)	Grades: analogous to cervical dysplasia
Squamous Cell Carcinoma (SCC)	Most common site is upper 1/3 of posterior wall of vagina Asymptomatic Painless discharge and bleeding Vaginal discharge (often foul-smelling) Vaginal bleeding especially during/post-coitus Urinary and/or rectal symptom 2° to compression
Adenocarcinoma	Most are metastatic, usually from cervix, endometrium, ovary, or colon Most primaries are clear cell adenocarcinomas 2 types: non-DES and DES syndrome

Fallopian Tube

- least common site for carcinoma of female reproductive system (0.3%)
- usually serous epithelial carcinoma
- recently considered to be origin of serous ovarian cancer
- more common in fifth and sixth decade

Clinical Features
- classic triad present in minority of cases, but very specific
  - watery discharge (most specific) = "hydrops tubae profluens"
  - vaginal bleeding or discharge in 50% of patients
  - crampy lower abdominal/pelvic pain
  - most patients present with a pelvic mass (see *Ovarian Tumours*, GY40 for guidelines regarding diagnosis/investigation)

Treatment
- as for malignant epithelial ovarian tumours

Gestational Trophoblastic Disease/Neoplasia

- refers to a spectrum of proliferative abnormalities of the trophoblast

Epidemiology
- 1/1,000 pregnancies
- marked geographic variation – as high as 1/125 in Taiwan
- 80% benign, 15% locally invasive, 5% metastatic
- cure rate >95%

HYDATIDIFORM MOLE (Benign GTD)

Complete Mole
- most common type of hydatidiform mole
- diffuse trophoblastic hyperplasia, hydropic swelling of chorionic villi, no fetal tissues, or membranes present
- 46XX or 46XY, chromosomes completely of paternal origin (90%)
- 2 sperm fertilize empty egg or 1 sperm with reduplication
- 15-20% risk of progression to malignant sequelae
- risk factors
  - geographic (South East Asia most common)
  - others (maternal age >40 yr, β-carotene deficiency, vitamin A deficiency) – not proven
- clinical features
- often present during apparent pregnancy with abnormal symptoms/findings

With development of hypertension early in pregnancy (i.e. <20 wk), think gestational trophoblastic disease

  - vaginal bleeding (97%)
  - excessive uterine size for LMP (51%)
  - theca-lutein cysts >6 cm (50%)
  - preeclampsia (27%)
  - hyperemesis gravidarum (26%)
  - hyperthyroidism (7%)
  - β-hCG >100,000 IU/L
  - no fetal heart beat detected

Partial (or Incomplete) Mole
- focal trophoblastic hyperplasia and hydropic villi are associated with fetus or fetal parts
- often triploid (XXY, XYY, XXX) with chromosome complement from both parents
  - usually related to single ovum fertilized by two sperm
- low risk of progression to malignant sequelae (<4%)
- associated with fetus, which may be growth-restricted, and/or have multiple congenital malformations
- clinical features
  - typically present similar to threatened/spontaneous/missed abortion
  - pathological diagnosis often made after D&C

Investigations
- quantitative β-hCG levels (tumour marker) abnormally high for gestational age
- U/S findings
  - if complete: no fetus (classic "snow storm" due to swelling of villi)
  - if partial: molar degeneration of placenta ± fetal anomalies, multiple echogenic regions corresponding to hydropic villi, and focal intrauterine hemorrhage
- CXR (may show metastatic lesions)
- features of molar pregnancies at high risk of developing persistent GTN post-evacuation
  - local uterine invasion as high as 31%
  - β-hCG >100,000 IU/L
  - excessive uterine size
  - prominent theca-lutein cysts

Treatment
- suction D&C with sharp curettage and oxytocin
- Rhogam® if Rh negative
- consider hysterectomy (if patient no longer desires fertility)
- prophylactic chemotherapy of no proven benefit
- chemotherapy for GTN if develops after evacuation

Follow-Up
- contraception required to avoid pregnancy during entire follow-up period
- serial β-hCGs (as tumour marker) every week until negative x 3 (usually takes several wk), then monthly for 6-12 mo prior to trying to conceive again
- increase or plateau of β-hCG indicates GTN → patient needs chemotherapy

GTN (MALIGNANT GTD)

Invasive Mole or Persistent GTN

- diagnosis made by rising or plateau in β-hCG, development of metastases following treatment of documented molar pregnancy
- histology: molar tissue from D&C
- metastases are rare (4%)

Choriocarcinoma

- often present with symptoms from metastases
- highly anaplastic, highly vascular
- no chorionic villi, elements of syncytiotrophoblast and cytotrophoblast
- may follow molar pregnancy, abortion, ectopic, or normal pregnancy

Placental-Site Trophoblastic Tumour

- rare aggressive form of GTN
- abnormal growth of intermediate trophoblastic cells
- low β-hCG, production of human placental lactogen (hPL), relatively insensitive to chemotherapy

CLASSIFICATION of GTN

- non-metastatic
  - ~15% of patients after molar evacuation
  - may present with abnormal bleeding
  - all have rising or plateau of β-hCG
  - negative metastases on staging investigations
- metastatic
  - 4% patients after treatment of complete molar pregnancy
  - metastasis more common with choriocarcinoma which tends toward early vascular invasion and widespread dissemination
  - if signs or symptoms suggest hematogenous spread, do not biopsy (they bleed)
    - lungs (80%): cough, hemoptysis, CXR lesion(s)
    - vagina (30%): vaginal bleeding, "blue lesions" on speculum exam
    - pelvis (20%): rectal bleeding (if invades bowel), U/S lesion(s)
    - liver (10%): elevated LFTs, U/S or CT findings
    - brain (10%): headaches, dizziness, seizure (symptoms of space-occupying lesion), CT/MRI findings
  - highly vascular tumour → bleeding → anemia
  - all have rising or plateau of β-hCG
  - classification of metastatic GTN
    - divided into good prognosis and bad prognosis
    - features of bad prognosis
      - long duration (>4 mo from antecedent pregnancy)
      - high pre-treatment β-hCG titre: >100,000 IU/24 h urine or >40,000 IU/L of blood
      - brain or liver metastases
      - prior chemotherapy
      - metastatic disease following term pregnancy
    - good prognosis characterized by the absence of each of these features

Lungs are #1 site for malignant GTN metastases; when pelvic exam and chest x-ray are negative, metastases are uncommon

Investigations – For Staging

- blood work: CBC, electrolytes, creatinine, β-hCG, TSH, LFTs
- imaging: CXR, U/S pelvis, CT abdo/pelvis, CT brain
- if suspect brain metastasis but CT brain negative, consider lumbar puncture for CSF β-hCG
- ratio of plasma β-hCG:CSF β-hCG <60 indicates metastases

Table 28. FIGO Staging and Management of Malignant GTN

Stage	Findings	Management

I	Disease confined to uterine corpus	Single agent chemotherapy for low risk disease (WHO score ≤6)
		  1st line: pulsed – actinomycin D (Act-D) IV q2wk
		  Alternatives: MTX-based regimen
		  20% of patients need to switch to alternate single-agent regimen due to failure of β-hCG to return to normal
		Combination chemotherapy (EMA-CO: etoposide, MTX, ACT-D, cyclophosphamide, vincristine) if high risk (WHO score ≥7) or if resistant to single agent chemotherapy
		Can consider hysterectomy if fertility not desired or placental-site trophoblastic tumour

II	Metastatic disease to genital structures	As above
III	Metastatic disease to lungs with or without genital tract involvement	As above
IV	Distant metastatic sites including brain, liver, kidney, GI tract	Usually high risk (EMA-CO) with surgical resection of sites of disease Persistence/resistance to chemotherapy Consider radiation for brain mets

Table 29. WHO Prognostic Score for GTD (2011)

Prognostic Factor	Score			
	0	1	2	4
Maternal Age	>40	40		
Antecedent Pregnancy	Mole	Abortion	Term	
Interval (end of Antecedent Pregnancy to chemotherapy in months)	<4	4-6	7-13	>13
HCG IU/1	<103	103-104	104-105	>105
Number of Metastases	0	1-4	5-8	>8
Site of Metastases	Lung	Spleen, kidney	GI tract	Brain, liver
Largest Tumour Mass		3-5 cm	>5 cm	
Prior Chemotherapy			Single drug	Two drug

Follow-up (for GTN)
- contraception for all stages to avoid pregnancy during entire follow-up period
- stage I, II, III
  - weekly β-hCG until 3 consecutive normal results
  - then monthly x 12 mo
- stage IV
  - weekly β-hCG until 3 consecutive normal results
  - then monthly x 24 mo

GTN Diagnosis
- β-hCG plateau: <10% drop in β-hCG over four values in 3 wk (e.g. days 1, 7, 14, and 21) OR
- β-hCG rise >20% in any two values over two wk or longer (e.g. measure at days 1, 7, 14) OR
- β-hCG persistently elevated >6 mo OR
- metastases on workup

Common Medications

Table 30. Common Medications

Drug Name (Brand Name)	Action	Dosing Schedule	Indications	Side Effects (S/E), Contraindications (C/I), Drug Interactions (D/I)
acyclovir (Zovirax®)	Antiviral; inhibits DNA synthesis and viral replication	**First Episode:** 400 mg PO tid x 7-10 d **Recurrence:** 400 mg PO tid x 5 d	Genital herpes	**S/E:** headache, GI upset **D/I:** zidovudine, probenecid
bromocriptine (Parlodel®)	Dopaminomimetic Agonist at D2R Antagonist at D1R Acts directly on anterior pituitary cells to inhibit synthesis and release of prolactin	**Initial:** 1.25-2.5 mg PO qhs with food Then: increase by 2.5 mg every 2-7 d as needed until optimal therapeutic response **Usual Range:** 1.5-15 mg OD For IVF: **Initial:** 1.25 mg/d PO between days 4-6 of follicular phase **Then:** 2.5 mg/d until 3 d after onset menstruation	Galactorrhea + amenorrhea 2° to hyperprolactinemia Prolactin-dependent menstrual disorders and infertility Prolactin-secreting adenomas (microadenomas, prior to surgery of macroadenomas) IVF	**S/E:** N/V, headache, postural hypotension, somnolence **C/I:** uncontrolled HTN, pregnancy-induced HTN, CAD, breastfeeding **D/I:** domperidone, macrolides, octreotide
clomiphene citrate (Clomid®)	Increases output of pituitary gonadotropins which induces ovulation	50 mg OD x 5 d Try 100 mg or 160 mg OD if ineffective 3 courses = adequate trial	Patients with persistent ovulatory dysfunction (e.g. amenorrhea, PCOS) who desire pregnancy	**S/E:** Common – hot flashes, abdominal discomfort, exaggerated cyclic ovarian enlargement, accentuation of Mittelschmerz Rare – ovarian hyperstimulation syndrome, multiple pregnancy, visual blurring, birth defects **C/I:** pregnancy, liver disease, hormone-dependent tumours, ovarian cyst, undiagnosed vaginal bleeding
clotrimazole (Canesten®)	Antifungal; disrupt fungal cell membrane	**Tablet:** 100 mg/d intravaginally x 7 d or 200 mg/d x 3 d or 500 mg x 1 dose **Cream** (1 or 2%): 1 applicator intravaginally qhs x 3-7 d **Topical:** apply bid x 7 d	Vulvovaginal candidiasis	**S/E:** vulvar/vaginal burning
danazol (Cyclomen® – CAN) (Danocrine® – US)	Synthetic steroid that inhibits pituitary gonadotropin output and ovarian steroid synthesis Has mild androgenic properties	200-800 mg in 2-3 divided doses Used for 3-6 mo Biannual hepatic U/S required if >6 mo use	Endometriosis 1° menorrhagia/DUB	**S/E:** weight gain, acne, mild hirsutism, hepatic dysfunction **C/I:** pregnancy, undiagnosed vaginal bleeding, breastfeeding, severely impaired renal/hepatic/cardiac function, porphyria, genital neoplasia, thromboembolic disease **D/I:** warfarin, carbamazepine, cyclosporine, tacrolimus, anti-hypertensives

Table 30. Common Medications (continued)

Drug Name (Brand Name)	Action	Dosing Schedule	Indications	Side Effects (S/E), Contraindications (C/I), Drug Interactions (D/I)
doxycycline	Tetracycline derivative; inhibit protein synthesis	100 mg PO bid x ≥7 d	Chlamydia, gonococcal infection, syphilis	**S/E**: GI upset, hepatotoxicity **C/I**: pregnancy, severe hepatic dysfunction **D/I**: warfarin, digoxin
fluconazole (Diflucan®)	Antifungal; disrupt fungal cell membrane	150 mg PO x 1 dose	Vulvovaginal candidiasis unresponsive to clotrimazole	**S/E**: headache, rash, N/V, abdominal pain, diarrhea **D/I**: terfenadine, cisapride, astemizole, hydrochlorothiazide, phenytoin, warfarin, rifampin
leuprolide (Lupron®)	Synthetic GnRH analog. Induces reversible hypoestrogenic state	3.75 mg IM q1mo or 11.25 mg IM q3mo Usually ≤6 mo, check bone density if >6 mo Retreatment with Lupron® alone not recommended because of effects on bone density	Endometriosis Leiomyomata DUB Precocious puberty	**S/E**: hot flashes, sweats, headache, vaginitis, reduction in bone density, acne, GI upset **C/I**: pregnancy, undiagnosed vaginal bleeding, breastfeeding
menotropin (Pergonal®)	Human gonadotropin with FSH and LH effects; induce ovulation and stimulate ovarian follicle development	75-150 U of FSH and LH IM OD x 7-12 d, then 10,000 U hCG one day after last dose	Infertility	**S/E**: bloating, irritation at injection site, abdominal/pelvic pain, headache, N/V, multiple pregnancy **C/I**: primary ovarian failure, intracranial lesion (e.g. pituitary tumour), uncontrolled thyroid/adrenal dysfunction, ovarian cyst (not PCOS), pregnancy, undiagnosed uterine bleeding
metronidazole (Flagyl®)	Bactericidal; forms toxic metabolites which damage bacterial DNA	2 g PO x 1 dose or 500 mg PO bid x 7 d	Bacterial vaginosis, trichomonas vaginitis	**S/E**: headache, dizziness, N/V, diarrhea, disulfiram-like reaction (flushing, tachycardia, N/V) **C/I**: pregnancy (1st trimester) **D/I**: cisapride, warfarin, cimetidine, lithium, alcohol, amiodarone, milk thistle, carbamazepine
oxybutinin (Ditropan®)	Anticholinergic – relaxes bladder smooth muscle, inhibits involuntary detrusor contraction	5 or 10 mg/d PO May increase doses by 5 mg weekly to a max of 30 mg/d	Overactive bladder (urge incontinence)	**S/E**: dry mouth/eyes, constipation, palpitations, urinary retention, dizziness, headache **C/I**: glaucoma, GI ileus, severe colitis, obstructive uropathy, use with caution if impaired hepatic/renal function
tolterodine (Detrol®)	Anticholinergic	1-2 mg PO bid	Overactive bladder (urge incontinence)	**S/E**: anaphylaxis, psychosis, tachycardia, dry mouth/eyes, headache, constipation, urinary retention, chest pain, abdominal pain **C/I**: glaucoma, gastric/urinary retention, use with caution if impaired hepatic/renal function
tranexamic acid (Cyklokapron®)	Anti-fibrinolytic, reversibly inhibits plasminogen activation	1-1.5 g tid-qid for first 4 d of cycle Max 4 g/d Ophthalmic check if used for several wk	Menorrhagia	**S/E**: N/V, diarrhea, dizziness, rare cases of thrombosis, abdominal pain, MSK pain **C/I**: thromboembolic disease, acquired disturbances of colour vision, subarachnoid hemorrhage, age <15 yr
ulipristal acetate (Fibristal®)	Selective progesterone receptor modulator (SPRM)	5 mg PO OD for max 3 mo; first tablet taken anytime during first 7 days of menstruation	Leiomyoma (pre-operative)	**S/E**: headache, hot flushes, constipation, vertigo, endometrial thickening **C/I**: pregnancy, undiagnosed vaginal bleeding, any gyne cancer
urofollitropin (Metrodin®)	FSH	75 U/d SC x 7-12d	Ovulation induction in PCOS	**S/E**: ovarian enlargement or cysts, edema and pain at injection site, arterial thromboembolism, fever, abdominal pain, headache, multiple pregnancy **C/I**: primary ovarian failure, intracranial lesion (e.g. pituitary tumour), uncontrolled thyroid/adrenal dysfunction, ovarian cyst (not PCOS), pregnancy, abnormal uterine bleeding
combined oral contraceptive pill (OCP)	Ovulatory suppression by inhibiting LH and FSH. Decidualization of endometrium. Thickening of cervical mucus to prevent sperm penetration		Contraception Disorders of menstruation	See Tables 8-12
intrauterine device (IUD) copper IUD (Nova-T®) progesterone-releasing IUD (Mirena®, Jaydess®)	**Copper IUD**: mild foreign body reaction in endometrium which is toxic to sperm and alters sperm motility **Progesterone-releasing IUD**: decidualization of endometrium and thickening of cervical mucus, may suppress ovulation	Contraceptive effects last 3 yrs (Jaydess); up to 5 yr (Copper IUD, Mirena)	Same as above	See Table 8-12

References

Agency for Healthcare Research and Quality, Rockville, MD. Available from: http://www.ahrq.gov/clinic/utersumm.htm.

American Psychiatric Association. Diagnostic and statistical manual of mental disorders, 5th ed. Washington: American Psychiatric Publishing, 2013.

Anderson GL, Limacher M, Assaf AR, et al. (WHI Steering Committee). Effects of conjugated equine estrogen in postmenopausal women with hysterectomy – Women's Health Initiative randomized controlled trial. JAMA 2004;291:1701-1712.

ARHP Quick Reference Guide for Clinicians. Managing premenstrual symptoms. June 2008.

Bélisle S, Blake J, Basson R, et al. Canadian consensus conference on menopause, 2006 update. JOGC 2006;28(2 Suppl 1):S1-S94.

Bentley J, Bertrand M, Brydon L, et al. SOGC Joint Clinical Practice Guidelines. Colposcopic management of abnormal cervical cytology and histology, 2012. JOGC 2012;284;1188-1202.

Berek JS, Hacker NF. Gynecologic oncology, 5th ed. Lippincott Williams & Wilkins, 2010.

Brännström M, Johannesson L, et al. Livebirth after uterus transplantation. Lancet 2015;385:607-16.

Burger RA, Brady MF, Bookman MA, et al. Incoporation of bevacizumab in the primary treatment of ovarian cancer. NEJM 2011;365:2473-2483.

Buys SS, Partridge E, Black A, et al. Effect of screening on ovarian cancer mortality: the prostate, lung, colorectal and ovarian (PLCO) cancer screening randomized control trial. JAMA 2011;305:2295-2303.

Canadian Consensus Conference on Menopause, 2006 Update. JOGC 2006;171.

Centers for Disease Control and Prevention (CDC). Recommendations on the use of quadrivalent human papillomavirus vaccine in males – Advisory Committee on Immunization Practices (ACIP), 2011. MMWR 2011;60:1705-1708.

Creanga AA, Bradley HM, McCormick C, et al. Use of metformin in polycystic ovary syndrome: a meta-analysis. Obstet Gynecol 2008;111:959-968.

Cunningham FG, McDonald PC, Gant NF. Williams obstetrics, 14th ed. Appleton and Lange, 1993.

Davey E, Barratt A, Irwig L, et al. Effect of study design and quality of unsatisfactory rates, cytology classifications, and accuracy in liquid-based versus conventional cervical cytology: a systematic review. Lancet 2006;367:122-132.

Davis V, Dunn S. Emergency postcoital contraception. SOGC Clinical Practice Guidelines July 2000;82.

Dickey R. Managing contraceptive pill patients, 9th ed. EMIS Inc: Medical Publishers, 1998.

Donnez J, Tomaszewski J, Vasquez F, et al. Ulipristal acetate versus leuprolide acetate for uterine fibroids NEJM 2012;366(5):421-432.

Duffy JM, Arambage K, Correa FJ, et al. Laparoscopic surgery for endometriosis. Cochrane DB Syst Rev 2014;4:CD011031.

Erdman JN. Human rights in health equity: Cervical cancer and HPV vaccines. Am J Law & Medicine 2009;35:365-387.

Espeland MA, Rapp SR, Shumaker SA, et al. Conjugated equine estrogens and global cognitive function in postmenopausal women – Women's Health Initiative memory study. JAMA 2004;291:2959-2968.

Guilbert E, Boroditsky R, Black A, et al. Canadian consensus guideline on continuous and extended hormonal contraception. J Obstet Gyn Canada 2007;29:S1-S32.

Hacker NF, Moore JG. Essentials of obstetrics and gynecology, 2nd ed. WB Saunders, 1992.

Hulley S, Grady D, Bush T, et al. Randomized trial of estrogen plus progestin for secondary prevention of coronary heart disease in postmenopausal women. JAMA 1998;280:605-613.

Jacobs I, Oram D, Fairbanks J, et al. A risk of malignancy incorporating CA125, ultrasound and menopausal status for the accurate preoperative diagnosis of ovarian cancer. BJOG 1990;97:922-929.

Jick SS, Hernandez RK. Risk of non-fatal venous thromboembolism in women using oral contraceptives containing drospirenone compared with women using oral contraceptives containing levonorgestrel: case-control study using United States claims data. BMJ 2011;342:d2151.

Joura EA, Giuliano AR, et al. A 9-valent HPV vaccine against infetion and intraepithelial neoplasia in women. NEJM 2015;372:711-23.

Klipping C, Duijkers I, Trummer D, et al. Suppression of ovarian activity with a drospirenone-containing oral contraceptive in a 24/4 regimen. Contraception 2008;78:16-25.

Lidegaard O, Lokkegaard E, Jensen A, et al. Thrombotic stroke and myocardial infarction with hormonal contraception. NEJM 2012;366:2257-2266.

Lipscomb GH, McCord ML, Stovall TG, et al. Predictors of success of methotrexate treatment in women with tubal ectopic pregnancies. NEJM 2001;341:1974-1978.

Lopez LM, Chen M, Mullins S, et al. Steroidal contraceptives and bone fractures in women: evidence from observational studies. Cochrane DB Syst Rev 2012;8:CD009849.

Luciano AA, Solima RG. Ectopic pregnancy: from surgical emergency to medical management. Ann NY Acad Sci 2001;943:235-254.

Lujan ME, Chizen DR, Pierson RA. Diagnostic criteria for polycystic ovary syndrome: pitfalls and controversies. JOGC 2008;30(8):671-9.

Maclennan AH, Broadbent JL, Lester S, et al. Oral oestrogen and combined oestrogen/progetogen therapy versus placebo for hot flushes. Cochrane DB Syst Rev 2004;18.

Management of uterine fibroids. Summary, Evidence Report/Technology Assessment: Number 34. AHRQ Publication No. 01-E051, January 2001.

Manson JE, Martin KA. Postmenopausal hormone replacement therapy. NEJM 2001;345:34-40.

Mantha S, Karp R, Raghavan V, et al. Assessing the risk of venous thromboembolic events in women taking progestin-only contraception: a meta-analysis. BMJ 2012; 345:e4944.

Marchbanks PA, Aneger JF, Coulman CB, et al. Risk factors for ectopic pregnancy: a population based study. JAMA 1998;259:1823-1827.

Marjoribanks J, Farguhar C, Roberts H, et al. Long term hormone therapy for perimenopausal and postmenopausal women. Cochrane DB Syst Rev 2012;7:CD004143.

Martin JL, Williams KS, Abrams KR, et al. Systematic review and evaluation of methods of assessing urinary incontinence. Health Technol Assess 2006;10:1-132,iii-iv.

National guideline for the treatment of bacterial vaginosis. Clinical Effectiveness Group (Association of Genitourinary Medicine and the Medical Society for the Study of Venereal Diseases). Sex Transm Infect 1999;75:S1 6-8.

Ontario Cervical Screening Practice Guidelines. June 2005. Available from: http://www.cancercare.on.ca/index – cervical screening.htm.

Ouellet-Hellstram R, Graham DJ, Staffa JA, et al. Combined hormonal contraceptives (CHCs) and the risk of cardiovascular disease endpoints. CHC-CVD final report 111022v2.

Paley PJ. Screening for the major malignancies affecting women: current guidelines. Am J Obstet Gynecol 2001;184:1021-1030.

Public Health Agency of Canada, 2010. Canadian guidelines on sexually transmitted infections. (Updated January 2010). Available from: http://www.phac-aspc.gc.ca/std-mts/sti-its/cgsti-ldcits/index-eng.php.

Public Health Agency of Canada, 2011. Public health information update on the treatment of gonococcal infection. Available from: http://www.phac-aspc.gc.ca/std-mts/sti-its/alert/2011/alert-gono-eng.php.

PHAC National Advisory Committee on Immunization (NACI). Update on human papillomavirus (HPV) vaccines. Canada Communicable Disease Report 2012;38:ACS-1.

Rambout L, Hopkins L, Hutton B, et al. Prophylactic vaccination against human papillomavirus infection in women: a systematic review of randomized controlled trials. CMAJ 2007;177(5):469-479.

Ratner S, Ofri D. Menopause and hormone replacement therapy. West J Med 2001;175:32-34.

Reid R. Oral contraceptives and the risk of venous thromboembolism: an update. SOGC Clinical Practice Guideline. JOGC 2010;32:1192-1197.

Rimsza ME. Counselling the adolescent about contraception. Pediatr Rev 2003;24:162-170.

Rossouw JE, Prentice RL, Manson JE, et al. Postmenopausal hormone therapy and risks of cardiovascular disease by age and years since menopause. JAMA 2007;297:1465-1477.

Seeger JD, Loughlin J, Eng PM, et al. Risk of thromboembolism in women taking ethinylestradiol/drospirenone and other oral contraceptives. Obstet Gynecol 2007;110:587-593.

Sexuality and U. Society of Obstetricians and Gynaecologists of Canada. Available from: http://www.sexualityandu.ca.

Shapter AP. Gestational trophoblastic disease. Obs Gynecol Clin North Am 2001;28:805-817.

Shumaker SA, Legault C, Kuller L, et al. Conjugated equine estrogens and incidence of probable dementia and mild cognitive impairment in postmenopausal women – Women's Health Initiative memory study. JAMA 2004; 291:2947-2958.

SOGC Clinical Practice Guidelines: Abnormal Uterine Bleeding in Pre-Menopausal Women. JOGC May 2013;35(5 eSupple):S1-S28.

SOGC Clinical Practice Guidelines: Emergency Contraception. JOGC Sep 2012;34(9):870-878. Available from: http://www.sogc.org/guidelines/documents/gui280CPG1209E_000.pdf

SOGC Committee Opinion on Missed Hormonal Contraceptives: New recommendations. JOGC 2008;30:1050-1062. Available from: http://www.sogc.org/guidelines/documents/gui219ECO0811.pdf.

SOGC News Release. New recommendations from national ob/gyn society address Depo-Provera, bone loss. May 2006. Available from: http://www.sogc.org/media/pdf/advisories/dpma-may2006_e.pdf.

Tingulstad S, Hagen B, Skjeldestad FE, et al. The risk of malignancy index to evaluate potential ovarian cancers in local hospitals. Obstet Gynecol 1999;93:448-452.

Wooltorton E. The Evra (ethanyl estradiol/norelgestromin) contraceptive patch: estrogen exposure concerns. CMAJ 2006;174:164-165.

Wooltorton E. Medroxyprogesterone acetate (Depo-Provera) and bone mineral density loss. JAMA 2005;172:746.

Hematology

Ryan Chan, Tejas Desai, and **Brent Parker,** chapter editors
Claudia Frankfurter and **Inna Gong,** associate editors
Brittany Prevost and **Robert Vanner,** EBM editors
Dr. Michelle Sholzberg and **Dr. Martina Trinkaus,** staff editors

Acronyms

AFib	atrial fibrillation	HIT	heparin-induced thrombocytopenia	PNH	paroxysmal nocturnal hemoglobinuria
AFLP	acute fatty liver of pregnancy	HMWK	high molecular weight kinonogen	PT	prothrombin time
AIHA	autoimmune hemolytic anemia	HUS	hemolytic uremic syndrome	PTT	partial thromboplastin time
ALL	acute lymphoblastic leukemia	IMF	idiopathic myelofibrosis	PV	polycythemia vera
AML	acute myeloid leukemia	IPC	intermittent pneumatic compression	RAEB	refractory anemia with excess blasts
ANC	absolute neutrophil count	IPSS	international prognostic scoring system	RARS	refractory anemia with ringed sideroblasts
APC	activated protein C	ITP	immune thrombocytopenic purpura	RBC	red blood cell
APCR	activated protein C resistance	LMWH	low molecular weight heparin	RCMD	refractory cytopenia with multilineage dysplasia
APS	antiphospholipid antibody syndrome	MAHA/TMA	microangiopathic hemolytic anemia/thrombotic	RCMD-RS	refractory cytopenia with multilineage dysplasia and
BM	bone marrow		microangiopathy		ringed sideroblasts
CBC	complete blood count	MCH	mean corpuscular Hb	RDW	RBC distribution width
CLL	chronic lymphocytic leukemia	MCHC	mean corpuscular Hb concentration	SPEP	serum protein electrophoresis
CML	chronic myeloid leukemia	MCV	mean corpuscular volume	SCT	stem cell transplantation
DIC	disseminated intravascular coagulation	MDS	myelodysplastic syndromes	sTfR	soluble transferrin receptor
EPO	erythropoietin	MF	myelofibrosis	TIBC	total iron binding capacity
ESR	erythrocyte sedimentation rate	MGUS	monoclonal gammopathy of unknown significance	TPO	thrombopoietin
ET	essential thrombocythemia	MM	multiple myeloma	TTP	thrombotic thrombocytopenic purpura
FNA	fine needle aspiration	MPN	myeloproliferative neoplasm	UFH	unfractionated heparin
G6PD	glucose-6-phosphate dehydrogenase	MPV	mean platelet volume	UPEP	urine protein electrophoresis
G-CSF	granulocyte-colony stimulating factor	MUGA	multi-gated acquisition	VTE	venous thromboembolism
GSH	glutathione	NHL	non-Hodgkin lymphoma	vWD	von Willebrand disease
HA	hemolytic anemia	PCC	prothrombin complex concentrates	VWF	von Willebrand factor
Hb	hemoglobin	Ph	Philadelphia chromosome	WBC	white blood cell
Hct	hematocrit	PK	prekallikrein	WHO	World Health Organization

Basics of Hematology

Erythrocyte: carries oxygen from lungs to peripheral tissues

Reticulocyte: immature erythrocyte

Neutrophil: granulocyte integral in innate immunity; main cell in acute inflammation

Eosinophil: involved in response to parasites (especially helminths) and allergic response

Basophil: granulocyte mainly involved in allergy and parasitic infection

Lymphocyte: integral cell in adaptive immunity

Monocyte: involved in innate immunity; can differentiate into macrophage or dendritic cell

Platelet: mediator of primary hemostasis

Plasma: liquid component of blood containing water, proteins, coagulation factors, and immunoglobulins

Serum: equivalent to plasma minus clotting factors and fibrinogen

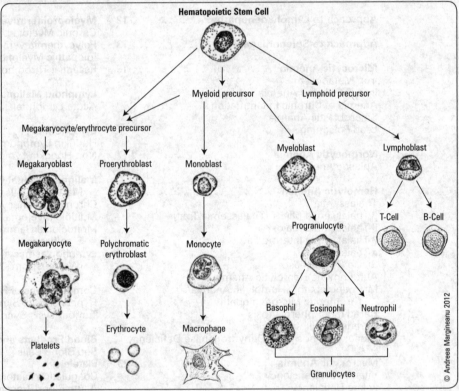

© Andreea Margineanu 2012

Figure 1. Hematopoiesis

- over 10^{11} blood cells are produced daily
- sites of hematopoiesis in adults: pelvis, sternum, vertebral bodies, cranium
- lifespan of mature cells in blood
  - erythrocytes (90-120 d), neutrophils (~1 d), platelets (7-10 d), lymphocytes (varies – memory cells persist for years)
- role of lymphoid organs
  - spleen: part of reticuloendothelial system, sequesters aged RBCs, removes opsonized cells, site of antibody production
  - thymus: site of T-cell maturation, involutes with age
  - lymph nodes: sites of B and T-cell activation (adaptive immune response)

Complete Blood Count

Table 1. Common Terms Found in the CBC

Test	Definition	Normal Values*
Red Blood Cell (RBC) Count	The number of RBCs per volume of blood	$4.2\text{-}6.9 \times 10^6/\text{mm}^3$
Hemoglobin (Hb)	Amount of oxygen-carrying protein in the blood	130-180 g/L (male) 120-160 g/L (female)
Hematocrit (Hct)	Percentage of a given volume of whole blood occupied by packed RBCs	45%-62% (male) 37%-48% (female)
Mean Corpuscular Volume (MCV)	Measurement of RBC size	$80\text{-}100\ \mu m^3$
Mean Corpuscular Hb (MCH)	Amount of oxygen-carrying Hb inside RBCs	27-32 pg/cell
Mean Corpuscular Hb Concentration (MCHC)	Average concentration of Hb inside RBCs	32%-36%
RBC Distribution Width (RDW)	Measurement of variance in RBC size	11.0%-15.0%
White Blood Cell (WBC) Count	The number of WBCs per volume of blood	$4.3\text{-}10.8 \times 10^9/\text{mm}^3$
WBC Differential	Neutrophils Lymphocytes Monocytes Eosinophils Basophils	$1.8\text{-}7.8 \times 10^3/\text{mm}^3$ $0.7\text{-}4.5 \times 10^3/\text{mm}^3$ $0.1\text{-}1.0 \times 10^3/\text{mm}^3$ $0.0\text{-}0.4 \times 10^3/\text{mm}^3$ $0.0\text{-}0.2 \times 10^3/\text{mm}^3$
Platelet Count	The number of platelets per volume of blood	$150\text{-}400 \times 10^9/\text{mm}^3$
Mean Platelet Volume (MPV)	Measurement of platelet size	
Reticulocytes	Immature RBCs that contain no nucleus but have residual RNA	Normally make up 1% of total RBC count

*Normal values may vary depending on site and age

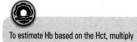

To estimate Hb based on the Hct, multiply by 3.3

Clinical Use of RDW
To distinguish the etiologies of microcytosis:
- Iron deficiency: increased RDW (anisocytosis) as cells are of varying sizes in iron deficiency
- Thalassemia minor: normal RDW (also expect a high RBC count) as cells are of similar size due to genetic defect in Hb

Approach to Interpreting a CBC

1. consider values in the context of individual's baseline
   up to 5% of population without disease may have values outside "normal" range
   an individual may display a clinically significant change from their baseline without violating "normal" reference range
2. is one cell line affected or are several?
   if all lines are low: pancytopenia (see *Pancytopenia*, H8)
   if RBCs and platelets are low: consider a MAHA/TMA (see *Microangiopathic Hemolytic Anemia/Thrombotic Microangiopathy*, H22)
   if single cell line affected: see *Common Presenting Problems*, H6

Blood Film Interpretation

RED BLOOD CELLS

Size
- microcytic (MCV <80 μm^3), normocytic (MCV = 80-100 μm^3), macrocytic (MCV >100 μm^3)
- anisocytosis: RBCs with increased variability in size (increased RDW)
  - iron deficiency anemia, hemolytic anemias, myelofibrosis, blood transfusion, MDS

Colour
- hypochromic: increase in size of central pallor (normal = less than 1/3 of RBC diameter)
  - iron deficiency anemia, anemia of chronic disease, sideroblastic anemia
- polychromasia: increased reticulocytes (pinkish-blue cells)
  - increased RBC production by bone marrow

Shape
- poikilocytosis: increased proportion of RBCs of abnormal shape
  - iron deficiency anemia, myelofibrosis, severe B_{12} deficiency, MDS, burns

Basics of Hematology

Table 2. Common Erythrocyte Shapes

Shape	Definition	Associated Conditions
Discocyte	Biconcave disc	Normal RBC
Spherocyte	Spherical RBC (due to loss of membrane)	Hereditary spherocytosis, immune hemolytic anemia, post-transfusion
Elliptocyte/Ovalcyte	Oval-shaped, elongated RBCs • Elliptocytes: the RBC long axis is ≥2x the length of the short axis • Ovalcytes: the RBC long axis is <2x the length of the short axis	Hereditary elliptocytosis, megaloblastic anemia, myelofibrosis, iron-deficiency, MDS (myelodysplastic syndrome)
Schistocyte (helmet cell, fragment)	Fragmented cells (due to traumatic disruption of membrane)	Microangiopathic hemolytic anemia (HUS, aHUS, TTP, DIC, preeclampsia, HELLP, malignant HTN), vasculitis, glomerulonephritis, prosthetic heart valve
Sickle Cell	Sickle-shaped RBC (due to polymerization of hemoglobin S)	Sickle cell disorders: HbSC, HbSS
Codocyte (target cell)	"Bull's eye" on dried film	Liver disease, hemoglobin SC, thalassemia, iron deficiency, asplenia
Dacrocyte (teardrop cell)	Single pointed end, looks like a teardrop	Myelofibrosis, thalassemia major, megaloblastic anemia, bone marrow infiltration
Acanthocyte (spur cell)	Distorted RBC with irregularly distributed thorn-like projections (due to abnormal membrane lipids)	Severe liver disease (spur cell anemia), starvation/anorexia, post-splenectomy
Echinocyte (burr cell)	RBC with numerous regularly spaced, small spiny projections	Uremia, HUS, burns, cardiopulmonary bypass, post-transfusion, storage artifact
Rouleaux Formation	Aggregates of RBC resembling stacks of coins (due to increased plasma concentration of high molecular weight proteins)	Pregnancy is most common cause (due to physiological increase in fibrinogen) Inflammatory conditions (due to polyclonal immunoglobulins) Plasma cell dyscrasias (due to monoclonal paraproteinemia, e.g. multiple myeloma, macroglobulinemia) Storage artifact

DIC = disseminated intravascular coagulation; HELLP = hemolysis, elevated liver enzymes, and low platelet count; HUS = hemolytic uremic syndrome; aHUS = atypical HUS; TTP = thrombotic thrombocytopenic purpura
Illustrations: Ayalah Hutchins and Merry Shiyu Wang 2012

Table 3. RBC Inclusions

Inclusions	Definition	Associated Conditions
Nucleus	Present in erythroblasts (immature RBCs)	Hyperplastic erythropoiesis (seen in hypoxia, hemolytic anemia), BM infiltration disorders, MPNs (MF)
Heinz Bodies	Denatured and precipitated hemoglobin	G6PD deficiency (post-exposure to oxidant), thalassemia, unstable hemoglobins
Howell-Jolly Bodies	Small nuclear remnant resembling a pyknotic nucleus	Post-splenectomy, hyposplenism (sickle cell disease), neonates, megaloblastic anemia
Basophilic Stippling	Deep blue granulations indicating ribosome aggregation	Thalassemia, heavy metal (Pb, Zn, Ag, Hg) poisoning, megaloblastic anemia, hereditary (pyrimidine 5'nucleotidase deficiency)
Sideroblasts	Erythrocytes with Fe containing granules in the cytoplasm	Hereditary, idiopathic, drugs, hypothyroidism (see *Sideroblastic Anemia*, H16), myelodysplastic syndrome, toxins (lead)

BM = bone marrow; MF = myelofibrosis; MPN = myeloproliferative neoplasm
Illustrations: Ayalah Hutchins and Merry Shiyu Wang 2012

WHITE BLOOD CELLS
- lymphocytes: comprise 30-40% of WBCs; great variation in "normal" lymphocyte morphology
- neutrophils
  - normally, only mature neutrophils (with 3-4 lobed nucleus) and band neutrophils (immediate precursor with horseshoe-shaped nucleus) are found in circulation
  - hypersegmented neutrophil: >5 lobes suggests megaloblastic process (B_{12} or folate deficiency)
  - left shift (increased granulocyte precursors)
    - seen in leukemoid reactions: acute infections, pregnancy, neonates, hypoxia, shock, myeloproliferative neoplasms (CML, MF)
- blasts
  - immature, undifferentiated precursors; associated with acute leukemia, MDS, G-CSF (growth factor that stimulates neutrophil production) use

Left Shift
Refers to an increase in granulocyte precursors in the peripheral smear (myelocytes, metamyelocytes, promyelocytes, blasts). If present, implies increased marrow production of granulocytes (e.g. inflammation, infection, G-CSF administration, CML)
The presence of predominantly blasts in the peripheral smear without cells between mature neutrophil and blast suggests clonal cell disorder (MDS, acute leukemias)
This is a MEDICAL EMERGENCY

Table 4. Abnormal White Blood Cells on Film

Appearance	Definition	Associated Conditions
Reed-Sternberg Cell	Giant, multinucleated B-lymphocyte, (classic 'owl-eye' morphology)	Primarily Hodgkin lymphoma, also seen in some non-Hodgkin lymphoma, CLL, and EBV infection
Smudge Cell	Lymphocytes damaged during blood film preparation indicating cell fragility	CLL and other lymphoproliferative disorders Pathognomonic in EBV infection
Auer Rod	Cytoplasmic inclusions that form long needles in the cytoplasm of myeloblasts	Pathognomonic for acute myeloid leukemia (AML)
Atypical Lymphocyte	Pale blue cytoplasm following RBC edges with pink granules	Viruses (particularly EBV) T-cell large granular lymphocyte leukemia (T-LGL)

EBV = Epstein-Barr virus , CLL = chronic lymphocytic leukemia
Illustrations: Ayalah Hutchins and Merry Shiyu Wang 2012

PLATELETS
- small, purple, anuclear cell fragments

Bone Marrow Aspiration and Biopsy

- sites: posterior iliac crest, sternum
- analyses: most often done together
  - aspiration: takes a fluid marrow sample for cellular morphology, flow cytometry, cytogenetics, molecular studies, microbiology (C&S, acid-fast bacilli, PCR)
    - note: differential diagnosis for a "dry tap": MF, hairy cell leukemia, bone marrow infiltration
  - biopsy: takes a sample of intact bone marrow to assess histology (architecture) and immunohistochemistry

Indications
- unexplained CBC abnormalities
- diagnosis and evaluation of infiltrating cancers: plasma cell disorders, leukemias, solid tumours
- diagnosis and staging of lymphoma or solid tumours
- evaluate iron metabolism and stores (gold standard, but rarely done)
- evaluate suspected deposition and storage disease (e.g. amyloidosis, Gaucher's disease)
- evaluate fever of unknown origin, suspected mycobacterial, fungal/parasitic infections, or granulomatous disease
- evaluate unexplained splenomegaly
- confirm normal bone marrow in potential allogenic hematopoietic cell donor

Important Considerations:
- consult a hematologist prior to conducting a bone marrow biopsy on a patient with an inherited (e.g. hemophilia, VWF disease) or acquired (e.g. DIC, anticoagulant therapy, coagulopathy of liver disease, severe thrombocytopenia) bleeding diathesis to determine if pro-hemostatic therapy is indicated pre-procedure
- do not perform a bone marrow biopsy if there is evidence of infection over the targeted skin site

Common Presenting Problems

Anemia

Definition
- a decrease in red blood cell (RBC) mass that can be detected by hemoglobin (Hb) concentration, hematocrit (Hct), and RBC count
  - adult males: Hb <130 g/L or Hct <0.41
  - adult females: Hb <120 g/L or Hct <0.36 (changes with pregnancy and trimester)

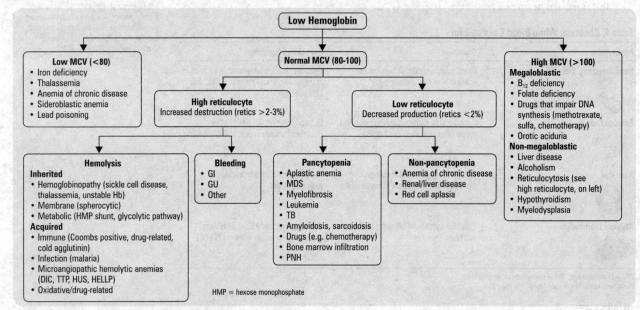

Figure 2. Approach to anemia – classification by size of RBC

Reticulocytes
- Reticulocytes are immature erythrocytes and are markers of erythrocyte production. (↑ colour, ↓ central pallor, ↑ size)
- The reticulocyte count should always be interpreted in the context of the Hb
- Should normally increase when there is a decrease in RBC
- With blood loss, reticulocytes should increase 2-3x initially and then 5-7x over the next week
- A normal reticulocyte count in anemia should be interpreted as a sign of decreased production, BM infiltration, or nutritional deficiency

Clinical Features
- history
  - symptoms of anemia: fatigue, headache, light-headedness, malaise, weakness, decreased exercise tolerance, dyspnea, palpitations, dizziness, tinnitus, syncope
  - acute vs. chronic, bleeding, systemic illness, diet (Fe, B12 sources), alcohol, family history
  - menstrual history: menorrhagia, menometrorrhagia
  - rule out pancytopenia (recurrent infection, mucosal bleeding, easy bruising)
- physical signs
  - HEENT: pallor in mucous membranes and conjunctiva at Hb <90 g/L (<9 g/dL), ocular bruits at Hb <55 g/L (<5.5 g/dL), angular chelosis, jaundice
  - cardiac: tachycardia, orthostatic hypotension, systolic flow murmur, wide pulse pressure, signs of CHF
  - dermatologic: ecchymosis, petechiae, pallor in palmar skin creases at Hb <75 g/L, jaundice (if due to hemolysis), nail changes (spooning), glossitis
  - splenomegaly, lymphadenopathy

Investigations
- rule out dilutional anemia (low Hb due to increased effective circulating volume)
- CBC with differential
- reticulocyte count and blood smear/film
- rule out nutritional deficit, gastrointestinal and genitourinary disease in iron deficiency anemia
- additional laboratory investigations as indicated (see *Microcytic Anemia*, H13, *Normocytic Anemia*, H17, *Hemolytic Anemia*, H18, and *Macrocytic Anemia*, H23)
- N.B. may have a mixed picture with multiple concomitant nutritional deficiencies

Erythrocytosis

Definition
- an increase in the number of RBCs: Hb >185 g/L or Hct >52% (males); Hb >165 or Hct >47% (females and African males)

Etiology
- relative/spurious erythrocytosis (decreased plasma volume): diuretics, severe dehydration, burns, "stress" (Gaisböck's syndrome)
- absolute erythrocytosis

Table 5. Etiology of Erythrocytosis

Primary	Secondary	Inappropriate Production of Erythropoietin
Polycythemia Vera (PV) (see *Polycythemia Vera*, H41)	**Physiologic (poor tissue oxygenation/ hypoxia)** Carbon monoxide poisoning Heavy smoking High altitude **Pulmonary Disease** COPD Sleep apnea Pulmonary hypertension **Cardiovascular Disease** R to L shunt (Eisenmenger syndrome) RBC defects (Hb with increased O_2 affinity, methemoglobinemia)	**Tumours** Hepatocellular carcinoma Renal cell carcinoma Cerebellar hemangioblastoma Pheochromocytoma Uterine leiomyoma Ovarian tumour **Other** Polycystic kidney disease Post-kidney transplant Hydronephrosis Androgens Exogenous erythropoietin

Clinical Features
- secondary to high red cell mass and hyperviscosity
  - headache, dyspnea, dizziness, tinnitus, visual disturbances, hypertensive symptoms, numbness/ tingling
  - symptoms of angina, congestive heart failure, aquagenic pruritus (only in MPNs)
- thrombosis (venous or arterial) or bleeding (seen with acquired vWD or acquired platelet dysfunction in MPNs)
- physical findings
  - splenomegaly ± hepatomegaly, facial plethora/ruddy complexion (70%) and/or palms, gout

Investigations
- serum erythropoietin (EPO): differentiates primary (low/normal) from other etiologies (elevated)
  - search for tumour as source of EPO as indicated (e.g. abdominal U/S, CT head)
  - JAK-2 mutation analysis: positive in >96% of cases of PV
    - only send if low/normal EPO level
- ferritin (iron deficiency can mask the diagnosis; if iron deficient with reticulocytosis, suggestive of PV)

Treatment
- if primary: see *Polycythemia Vera*, H41
- if secondary: treat underlying cause
  - O_2 for hypoxemia, CPAP for sleep apnea, surgery for EPO-secreting tumours
  - often cardiologists will be hesitant to treat high Hct in cyanotic patients

Thrombocytopenia

Definition
- platelet count <150 x10^9/L

Clinical Features
- history: mucocutaneous bleeding (easy bruising, gingival bleeding), epistaxis, peri-operative bleeding (including dental procedures), heavy menstrual bleeding, peripartum bleeding
- physical exam: bruising, petechiae, ecchymoses, non-palpable purpura, wet purpura
- see *Disorders of Primary Hemostasis*, H27 for complications

Investigations
- CBC and differential
- blood film
  - rule out pseudo-thrombocytopenia (platelet clumping or platelet satellitism)
  - decreased production: other cell line abnormalities, blasts, hypersegmented PMNs, leukoerythroblastic changes
  - increased destruction: large platelets (often seen in ITP), schistocytes (seen in MAHA/TMA)
- workup for nutritional deficiencies: B_{12}, RBC folate
- PT/INR, aPTT and fibrinogen if DIC suspected
- LFTs

Treatments
- life threatening bleeding: platelet transfusion (repeat CBC 1 h post-transfusion to confirm an appropriate rise in counts)
- if secondary: treat underlying cause
- ITP: see *Immune Thrombocytopenic Purpura*, H27

Rule-of-thumb: a deficit in all cell lines suggests decreased production, sequestration, or hemodilution, a deficit in platelets and RBCs suggests non-immune destruction, and an isolated thrombocytopenia suggests an immune-mediated process. In hospitalized patients, drugs and infection account for the majority of cases of thrombocytopenia

Must rule out factitious thrombocytopenia: platelet clumping (secondary to EDTA antibodies from collection tube). This can be seen on blood film and confirmed by repeating in a citrated sample (i.e. using a sodium citrate tube to collect blood, rather than EDTA)

References
APS: see Hematology, H34
Aplastic Anemia: see Hematology, H17
B₁₂/Folate Deficiency: see Hematology, H24/H25
DIC: see Hematology, H27
HIT: see Hematology, H29
HIV: see Infectious Diseases, ID27
ITP: see Hematology, H27
Myelodysplasia: see Hematology, H39
Preeclampsia: see Obstetrics, OB24
SLE: see Rheumatology, RH11

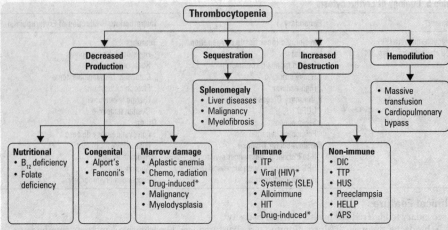

*In hospitalized patients most common causes of thrombocytopenia are drugs and infection

APS = antiphospholipid antibody syndrome; DIC = disseminated intravascular coagulation; HELLP = hemolysis, elevated liver enzymes, low platelet count; HIT = heparin induced thrombocytopenia; HUS = hemolytic uremic syndrome; ITP = idiopathic thrombocytopenic purpura; TTP = thrombotic thrombocytopenic purpura

Figure 3. Approach to thrombocytopenia   **Adapted from:** *Cecil Essentials of Medicine*

Thrombocytosis

Definition
- platelet count $>400 \times 10^9$/L
- primary thrombocytosis (uncommon): due to myeloproliferative neoplasms (e.g. CML, polycythemia vera, primary myelofibrosis, essential thrombocytosis; rarely associated with MDS)
- reactive/secondary thrombocytosis (common): acute phase reactant (e.g. surgery, inflammation, infection, trauma, bleeding, iron deficiency, neoplasms, ischemic injury)

Clinical Features
- history: trauma, surgery, splenectomy, infection, inflammation, bleeding, iron deficiency, prior diagnosis of chronic hematologic disorder, constitutional symptoms (malignancy)
- vasomotor symptoms: headache, visual disturbances, lightheadedness, atypical chest pain, acral dysesthesia, erythromelalgia, livedo reticularis, aquagenic pruritus
- clotting risk, bleeding risk (rare)
- physical exam: splenomegaly can be seen in myeloproliferative neoplasms (MPNs)

Investigations
- CBC, peripheral blood film, serum ferritin concentration
- non-specific markers of infection or inflammation (e.g. CRP, ESR, ferritin)
- if reactive process has been ruled out, bone marrow biopsy may be required to rule out MPN/MDS

Treatment
- primary: ASA ± cytoreductive agents (e.g. hydroxyurea, anagrelide, interferon-α)
- secondary: treat underlying cause

Pancytopenia

Definition
- a decrease in all hematopoietic cell lines

Clinical Features
- anemia: fatigue (see *Anemia*, H6)
- leukopenia: recurrent infections (see *Neutropenia*, H9)
- thrombocytopenia: mucosal bleeding (see *Thrombocytopenia*, H7)

Investigations
- CBC, peripheral blood film, serum ferritin concentration, B₁₂, folate
- non-specific markers of infection or inflammation (e.g. CRP, ESR, ferritin)
- work up as per Figure 4 and presenting symptoms/physical exam
- if reactive process has been ruled out, bone marrow biopsy may be required

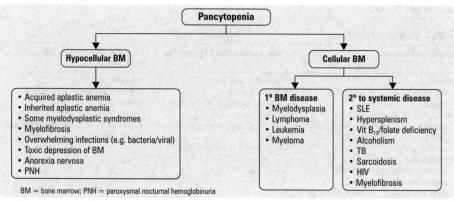

Figure 4. Approach to pancytopenia

Neutrophilia

Definition
• variable definition, but generally an absolute neutrophil count (ANC) >7.7 x 10^9/L (WHO definition)

Etiology
• primary neutrophilia
  ▪ chronic myeloid leukemia (CML)
  ▪ other myeloproliferative disorders: PV, ET, myelofibrosis
  ▪ hereditary neutrophilia (autosomal dominant)
  ▪ chronic idiopathic neutrophilia in otherwise healthy patients
  ▪ leukocyte adhesion deficiency
• secondary neutrophilia
  ▪ stress/exercise/epinephrine: movement of neutrophils from marginated pool into circulating pool
  ▪ obesity
  ▪ infection: leukocytosis with left shift ± toxic granulation, Döhle bodies (intra-cytoplasmic structures composed of agglutinated ribosomes)
  ▪ inflammation: e.g. rheumatoid arthritis (RA), IBD, chronic hepatitis, MI, PE, burns
  ▪ malignancy: hematologic (i.e. marrow invasion by tumour) and non-hematologic (especially large cell lung cancer)
  ▪ medications: glucocorticoids, β-agonists, lithium, G-CSF

Clinical Features
• look for signs and symptoms of fever, inflammation, malignancy to determine appropriate further investigations
  ▪ including lymphadenopathy and organomegaly
• examine oral cavity, teeth, peri-rectal area, genitals, and skin for signs of infection

Investigations
• CBC and differential: mature neutrophils or bands >20% of total WBC suggests infection/inflammation
• blood film: Döhle bodies, toxic granulation, cytoplasmic vacuoles in infection
• may require bone marrow biopsy if MPN suspected

Treatment
• directed at underlying cause

Neutropenia

Definition
• mild: ANC 1.0-1.5 x 10^9/L
• moderate: ANC 0.5-1.0 x 10^9/L (risk of infection starts to increase)
• severe: ANC <0.5 x 10^9/L
• profound: ANC <0.1 x 10^9/L for >7 d

Absolute Neutrophil Count (ANC) = WBC count x (%PMNs + %bands)

Beware of fever + ANC <0.5 x10^9/L = FEBRILE NEUTROPENIA

Prophylactic Hematopoietic Colony-Stimulating Factors on Mortality and Infection
Ann Intern Med 2007;147:400-411
Purpose: To review the effects of colony-stimulating factor (CSF) on mortality, infections, and febrile neutropenia in patients undergoing chemotherapy or stem-cell transplant (SCT).
Study Selection: 148 RCTs comparing the effects of CSFs to either placebo or no therapy were included. Prophylactic CSFs were given concurrently with or after initiation of chemotherapy.
Results: There were no differences in all-cause mortality or infection-related death between CSF and placebo groups. Compared to placebo or no therapy, CSFs reduced infection rate (median rate 38.9% vs. 43.1%; rate ratio 0.85), microbiologically documented infections (MR 23.5% vs. 28.6%; rate ratio 0.86), and febrile neutropenia (MR 25.3% vs. 44.2%; rate ratio 0.71).
Conclusions: Prophylactic CSFs decrease infection rates and episodes of febrile neutropenia in patients undergoing chemotherapy or SCT, but have no effect on mortality.

Etiology

Table 6. Etiology of Neutropenia

Decreased Production	Peripheral Destruction/Sequestration	Excessive Margination (Transient Neutropenia)
Infection Viral hepatitis, EBV, HIV, TB, typhoid, malaria **Hematological Diseases** Idiopathic, aplastic anemia, myelofibrosis, BM infiltration, cyclic, PNH, MDS, immune-mediated **Drug-Induced** Alkylating agents, antimetabolites, anticonvulsants, antipsychotics, anti-inflammatory agents, anti-thyroid drugs **Toxins/Chemicals** High dose radiation, benzene, DDT **Nutritional Deficiency** B_{12}, folate **Idiopathic** Constitutional neutropenia, benign cyclic neutropenia	Anti-neutrophil antibodies Spleen or lung trapping Autoimmune disorders: RA (Felty's syndrome), SLE Granulomatosis with polyangiitis (formerly Wegener's) Drugs: haptens (e.g. α-methyldopa)	Idiopathic (most common) Overwhelming bacterial infection Hemodialysis Cardiopulmonary bypass Racial variation (e.g. African or Ashkenazi Jewish descent)

Clinical Features
- fever, chills (only if infection present)
- infection by endogenous bacteria (e.g. *S. aureus*, gram negatives from GI and GU tract)
- painful ulceration on skin, anus, mouth, and throat following colonization by opportunistic organisms
- avoid digital rectal exam

Investigations
- dependent on degree of neutropenia, history, and symptoms
- ranges from observation with frequent CBCs to bone marrow aspiration and biopsy

Treatment
- regular dental care: chronic gingivitis and recurrent stomatitis major sources of morbidity
- treatment of febrile neutropenia (see Infectious Diseases, ID45)
- in severe immune-mediated neutropenia, G-CSF may increase neutrophil counts
  - if no response to G-CSF, consider immunosuppression (e.g. steroids, cyclosporine, methotrexate)

G-CSF = Neupogen® = Filgrastim

Lymphocytosis

Definition
- absolute lymphocyte count >4.0 x 10^9/L

Etiology
- infection (reactive lymphocytosis)
  - viral infections (majority); particularly mononucleosis
  - TB, pertussis, brucellosis, toxoplasmosis
- smoking
- physiologic response to stress (e.g. trauma, status epilepticus)
- hypersensitivity (e.g. drugs, serum sickness)
- autoimmune (e.g. rheumatoid arthritis)
- neoplasm (e.g. ALL if blasts present, CLL, B cell lymphocytosis of undetermined significance)

Investigations
- CBC, peripheral smear assessing lymphocyte morphology

Treatment
- treat underlying cause

Presence of atypical lymphocytes suggests viral infection

Presence of smudge cells suggests a lymphoproliferative disorder if persistently elevated above 5.0 x10^9/L for >3 mo; consider flow cytometry of peripheral blood

Lymphopenia

Definition
- absolute lymphocyte count $<1.0 \times 10^9$/L

Etiology
- idiopathic CD4+ lymphocytopenia
- radiation
- HIV/AIDS, hepatitis B, hepatitis C
- malignancy/chemotherapeutic agents
- malnutrition, alcoholism
- autoimmune disease (e.g. SLE)

Clinical Features
- opportunistic infections (see <u>Infectious Diseases</u>, ID34)

Treatment
- treat underlying cause
- treat opportunistic infections aggressively and consider antimicrobial prophylaxis
  (see <u>Infectious Diseases</u>, ID30)

Eosinophilia

Definition
- absolute eosinophil count $>0.5 \times 10^9$/L

Etiology
- primary: due to clonal bone marrow disorder
  - if no primary etiology identified, classified as hypereosinophilic syndrome
    - 6 mo of eosinophilia (count $>1.5 \times 10^9$/L) with no other detectable causes and end organ damage
    - can involve heart, bone marrow, CNS
- secondary
  - most common causes are parasitic (usually helminth) infections and allergic reactions
  - less common causes
    - collagen vascular diseases (e.g. RA, polyarteritis nodosa, see <u>Rheumatology</u>, RH19)
    - respiratory causes (asthma, eosinophilic pneumonia, Churg-Strauss)
    - cholesterol emboli
    - hematologic malignancy: see *Chronic Myeloid Leukemia*, H40 and *Hodgkin Lymphoma*, H45
    - adrenal insufficiency, see <u>Endocrinology</u>, E33
    - medications (penicillins)
    - atopic dermatitis

> **Basophilia and/or Eosinophilia**
> Can be an indicator of CML or other myeloproliferative neoplasm, associated with pruritus due to excessive histamine production

Treatment
- treat underlying cause
- ensure strongyloides serology is collected to rule out infection before initiating steroids for patients at risk

Agranulocytosis

Definition
- severe depletion of granulocytes (neutrophils, eosinophils, basophils) from the blood and granulocyte precursors from bone marrow

Etiology
- associated with medications in 70% of cases: e.g. chemotherapy, clozapine, thionamides (antithyroid drugs), sulfasalazine, and ticlopidine
  - immune-mediated destruction of circulating granulocytes by drug-induced antibodies or direct toxic effects upon marrow granulocytic precursors

Clinical Features
- abrupt onset of fever, chills, weakness, and oropharyngeal ulcers

Prognosis
- high fatality without vigorous treatment

Investigations/Treatment
- discontinue offending drug
- pan-culture and screen for infection if patient is febrile (blood cultures x2, urine culture, and chest x-ray as minimum, initiate broad-spectrum antibiotics)
- consider bone marrow aspirate and biopsy if cause unclear
- consider G-CSF

Leukemoid Reaction

- blood findings resembling those seen in certain types of leukemia which reflect the response of healthy BM to cytokines released due to infection or trauma
- leukocytosis >50 x 10^9/L, marked left shift (myelocytes, metamyelocytes, bands in peripheral blood smear)

Approach to Lymphadenopathy

History
- constitutional/B-symptoms: seen in TB, lymphoma, other malignancies
- growth pattern: acute vs. chronic
- exposures: cats (cat scratch – *Bartonella henselae*), ticks (Lyme disease – *Borrelia burgdorferi*), high risk behaviours (HIV)
- joint pain/swelling, rashes (connective tissue disorder)
- pruritus (seen in Hodgkin lymphoma)
- medications (can cause serum sickness → lymphadenopathy)

Clinical Features
- determine if lymphadenopathy is localized or generalized
- localized: typically reactive or neoplastic
  - cervical (bacterial/mycobacterial infections, ENT malignancies, metastatic cancer)
  - supraclavicular
    - right (mediastinal, bronchogenic, esophageal cancer)
    - left (gastric, gall bladder, pancreas, renal, testicular/ovarian cancer)
  - axillary (cat scratch fever, breast cancer, metastatic cancer)
  - epitrochlear (infections, sarcoidosis, lymphoma)
  - check for splenomegaly, constitutional symptoms

Investigations
- CBC and differential, blood film
- if generalized, consider tuberculin test, HIV RNA, VDRL, Monospot®/EBV serology, ANA, imaging
- if localized and no symptoms suggestive of malignancy, can observe 3-4 wk (if no resolution → biopsy)
- excisional biopsy is preferred as it preserves node architecture (essential for diagnosing lymphoma)
- in areas difficult to access (retroperitoneal, mediastinal/hilar) multiple core biopsies may be more practical/feasible
- FNA should NOT be used for diagnostic purposes in lymphoproliferative disease (use excisional biopsy instead)
  - FNA is helpful for recurrence of solid tumour malignancy
  - imaging such as U/S or CT can provide more info, but generally adds little to diagnosis

Constitutional/B-Symptoms
- Unexplained temperature >38°C
- Unexplained weight loss (>10% of body weight in 6 mo)
- Night sweats

Drugs that can cause Lymphadenopathy
- Allopurinol
- Atenolol
- Captopril
- Carbamazepine
- Cephalosporins
- Gold
- Hydralazine
- Penicillin
- Phenytoin
- Primidone
- Pyrimethamine
- Quinidine
- Sulfonamides
- Sulindac

Table 7. Inflammatory vs. Neoplastic Lymph Nodes

Feature	Inflammatory	Neoplastic
Consistency	Rubbery	Firm/hard
Mobility	Mobile	Matted/immobile
Tenderness	Tender	Non-tender
Size	<2 cm	>2 cm

*Note: these classifications are not absolute; lymphoma and CLL nodes can feel rubbery and are frequently mobile, non-tender

Table 8. Differential Diagnosis of Generalized Lymphadenopathy

Reactive	Inflammatory	Neoplastic
Bacterial (TB, Lyme, brucellosis, cat scratch disease, syphilis)	Collagen disease (RA, dermatomyositis, SLE, vasculitis, Sjögren's)	Lymphoproliferative disorder/lymphoma Metastatic cancer Histiocytosis X
Viral (EBV, CMV, HIV)	Drug hypersensitivity	
Parasitic (toxoplasmosis)	Sarcoidosis, amyloidosis	
Fungal (histoplasmosis)	Serum sickness	

Approach to Splenomegaly

Table 9. Differential Diagnosis of Splenomegaly

Increased Demand for Splenic Function			Congestive	Infiltrative
Hematological	**Infectious**	**Inflammatory**	**Cirrhosis**	**Non-Malignant**
Nutritional anemias	Viral e.g. EBV, HIV/	SLE	Portal HTN	Benign metaplasia
Hemoglobinopathies	AIDS, CMV	Sarcoidosis	Portal vein obstruction	Cysts
Hemolysis	Bacterial	Felty syndrome	(including right heart failure)	Amyloidosis, Sarcoidosis
Spherocytosis	e.g. Bacterial	Still's disease	Splenic vein thrombosis	Hamartomas
Sequestration crisis	endocarditis, TB			Vascular abnormalities
Elliptocytosis	Parasitic			Lysosomal storage diseases
	e.g. Malaria,			(Gaucher's, Niemann-Pick)
	Histoplasmosis,			Glycogen storage diseases
	Leishmaniasis			**Malignant**
	Fungal			Leukemia (CML, CLL)
				Lymphoproliferative disease
				Hodgkin lymphoma
				Myeloproliferative disorders
				Metastatic tumour

The underlined conditions cause *massive splenomegaly* (spleen crosses midline or reaches pelvis)

Causes of Splenomegaly

CHINA
Cirrhosis/Congestion (portal HTN)
Hematological
Infectious
Neoplasm (malignant, non-malignant)
Autoimmune

History
- constitutional symptoms, feeling of fullness in LUQ, early satiety
- signs or symptoms of infection (e.g. mononucleosis) or malignancy
- history of liver disease, hemolytic anemia, or high-risk exposures

Clinical Features
- jaundice, petechiae
- signs of chronic liver disease
- percussion (Castell's sign, Traube's space, Nixon's method) and palpation
- associated lymphadenopathy or hepatomegaly
- signs of CHF

Investigations
- CBC and differential, blood film
- as indicated: liver enzymes (AST, ALT, ALP, GGT) and/or LFTs (platelet, INR, albumin, bilirubin), reticulocyte count, Monospot®/EBV, haptoglobin, LDH, infectious, and autoimmune workup
- imaging
  - ultrasound of abdomen/liver to assess for cirrhosis and portal vein thrombosis (if positive, refer to hepatology for evaluation)
  - echo for cardiac function
  - CT to rule out lymphoma and assess splenic lesions

Microcytic Anemia

- MCV <80 fL
- see Figure 2, *Approach to Anemia*, H6

Table 10. Iron Indices and Blood Film in Microcytic Anemia

	Lab Tests					Blood Film
	Ferritin	Serum Iron	TIBC	% saturation	RDW	
Iron Deficiency Anemia	↓↓	↓	↑	↓	↑ (>15)	Hypochromic, microcytic
Anemia of Chronic Disease	N/↑	↓	↓	N	N	Normocytic/microcytic
Sideroblastic Anemia	N/↑	↑	N	N/↑	↑	Dual population Basophilic stippling
Thalassemia	N/↑	N/↑	N	N/↑	N/↑	Hypochromic, microcytic Basophilic stippling Poikilocytosis

Causes of Microcytic Anemia

TAILS
Thalassemia
Anemia of chronic disease
Iron deficiency
Lead poisoning
Sideroblastic anemia

Iron Metabolism

Iron Intake (Dietary)
- average North American adult diet = 10-20 mg iron (Fe) daily
- steady state absorption is 5-10% (0.5-2 mg/d); enhanced by citric acid, ascorbic acid (vitamin C) and reduced by polyphenols (e.g. in tea), phytate (e.g. in bran), dietary calcium, and soy protein
- males have positive Fe balance; up to 20% of menstruating females have negative Fe balance

Iron Absorption and Transport
- dietary iron is absorbed in the duodenum (e.g. absorption impaired in IBD and Celiac disease)
- in circulation the majority of non-heme iron is bound to transferrin which transfers iron from enterocytes and storage pool sites (macrophages of the reticuloendothelial system and hepatocytes) to RBC precursors in the bone marrow

Iron Levels
- hepcidin is a hormone produced by hepatocytes that regulates systemic iron levels
  - binds to iron exporter ferroportin (on duodenal enterocytes and reticuloendothelial cells) and induces its degradation, thereby inhibiting iron export into circulation (diminished absorption of iron and iron trapping in reticuloendothelial system cells)
  - hepcidin production is:
    - increased in states of iron overload (inhibiting additional iron absorption) and inflammation (mediating anemia of chronic inflammation through iron trapping)
    - decreased in states where erythropoiesis is increased (e.g. hemolysis) or oxygen tension is low

Iron Storage
- ferritin
  - ferric iron (Fe^{3+}) complexed to a protein called apoferritin (hepatocytes are main ferritin storage site)
  - small quantities are present in plasma in equilibrium with intracellular ferritin
  - also an acute phase reactant – can be spuriously elevated despite low Fe stores in response to a stressor
- hemosiderin
  - aggregates or crystals of ferritin with the apoferritin partially removed
  - macrophage-monocyte system is main source of hemosiderin storage

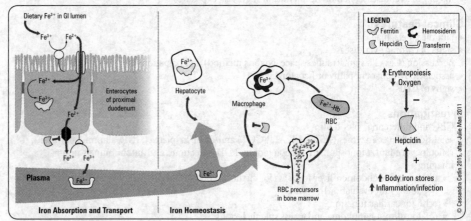

Figure 5. Iron metabolism

Iron Indices
- bone marrow aspirate: gold standard test for assessment of iron stores (rarely done)
- serum ferritin: most important blood test for iron stores
  - decreased in iron deficiency anemia
  - elevated in infection, inflammation, malignancy, liver disease, hyperthyroidism, and iron overload
- serum iron: measure of all non-heme iron present in blood
  - varies significantly daily
  - virtually all serum iron is bound to transferrin, only a trace is free or complexed in ferritin
- total iron binding capacity (TIBC): total amount of transferrin present in blood
  - normally, one third of TIBC is saturated with iron
  - high specificity for decreased iron, low sensitivity
- saturation
  - serum Fe divided by TIBC, expressed as a proportion or a percentage
- soluble transferrin receptor (sTfR)
  - reflects the availability of iron at the tissue level
  - the transferrin receptor is expressed on the surface of erythroblasts and is responsible for iron uptake – some is cleaved off and is present in circulation as sTfR
  - in iron deficient states more transferrin receptor is expressed on erythroblasts leading to an increase in sTfR
  - low in reduced erythropoiesis and iron overload
  - useful in determining iron deficiency in the setting of chronic inflammatory disorders (see *Iron Deficiency Anemia*)

Iron Deficiency Anemia

- see Pediatrics, P45
- most common cause of anemia in North America

Etiology
- increased demand
  - increased physiological need for iron in the body (e.g. pregnancy)
- decreased supply: dietary deficiencies (rarely the only etiology in the developed world)
  - cow's milk (infant diet), "tea and toast" diet (elderly), absorption imbalances, post-gastrectomy, malabsorption (IBD of duodenum, celiac disease, autoimmune atrophic gastritis, H.pylori infection)
- increased losses
  - hemorrhage
    - obvious causes: menorrhagia, abnormal uterine bleeding, frank GI bleed
    - occult: peptic ulcer disease, GI cancer
  - hemolysis
    - chronic intravascular hemolysis (e.g. PNH, cardiac valve RBC fragmentation)

Clinical Features
- iron deficiency may cause fatigue before clinical anemia develops
- signs/symptoms of anemia: see Anemia, H6
- brittle hair, nail changes (brittle, koilonychia)
- pica (appetite for non-food substances e.g. ice, paint, dirt)
- restless leg syndrome

Plummer-Vinson Syndrome
- Dysphagia (esophageal)
- Glossitis
- Iron deficiency anemia
- Stomatitis

Investigations
- iron indices, including soluble transferrin receptor
  - low ferritin (<18 µg/L) is diagnostic of iron deficiency
  - ferritin is an acute phase reactant and is elevated in the setting of inflammatory conditions and liver disease; serum ferritin <100 µg/L in these settings is suggestive of iron deficiency, necessitating further workup
- peripheral blood film
  - hypochromic microcytosis: RBCs have low Hb levels due to lack of iron
  - pencil forms, anisocytosis
  - target cells
- bone marrow (gold standard but rarely done)
  - iron stain (Prussian blue) shows decreased iron in macrophages and in erythroid precursors (sideroblasts)
  - intermediate and late erythroblasts show micronormoblastic maturation

Iron deficiency anemia is a common presentation of chronic lower GI bleeds (right-sided colorectal cancer, angiodysplasia, etc.)

In males and in post-menopausal women, a GI workup is always warranted (gastroscopy, colonoscopy)

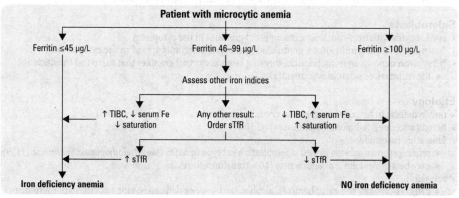

Figure 6. Approach to interpreting iron indices
Adapted from: Am Fam Physician 2007;75:671-678

Treatment
- treat underlying cause
- supplementation
  - oral (capsules, syrup)
    - ferrous sulphate 325 mg tid (65 mg elemental iron), ferrous gluconate 300 mg tid (35 mg elemental iron), or ferrous fumarate 300 mg tid (100 mg elemental iron)
    - supplement until anemia corrects, then continue for 3+ mo until serum ferritin returns to normal
    - oral iron should be taken with citrus juice (vitamin C) to enhance absorption
  - IV (iron sucrose or dextran) can be used if patient cannot tolerate or absorb oral iron
- monitoring response
  - reticulocyte count will begin to increase after one wk
  - Hb normalizes by 10 g/L per wk (if no blood loss)

Anemia of Chronic Inflammation

Etiology
- infection, malignancy, inflammatory and rheumatologic disease, chronic renal and liver disease, endocrine disorders (e.g. DM, hypothyroidism, hypogonadism, hypopituitarism)

Pathophysiology
- an anemia of underproduction due to impaired iron utilization (hepcidin is a key regulatory peptide)
    - hepatic hepcidin production is increased in inflammatory processes, trapping iron in enterocytes and macrophages (via ferroportin inhibition) (see Figure 5)
    - reduced plasma iron levels make iron relatively unavailable for new hemoglobin synthesis
    - marrow unresponsive to normal or slightly elevated EPO
- mild hemolytic component is often present i.e. RBC survival is modestly decreased

Investigations
- diagnosis of exclusion
- associated with elevation in acute phase reactants (ESR, CRP, fibrinogen, platelets)
- peripheral blood
    - mild: usually normocytic and normochromic
    - moderate: may be microcytic and normochromic
    - severe: may be microcytic and hypochromic
    - absolute reticulocyte count is frequently low, reflecting overall decrease in RBC production
- "classic" serum iron indices
    - serum iron and TIBC low, % saturation low
    - serum ferritin is normal or increased
- bone marrow
    - normal or increased iron stores
    - decreased or absent staining for iron in erythroid precursors

Treatment
- treat underlying disease
- only treat anemia in patients who can benefit from a higher hemoglobin
- IV iron if no benefit from PO iron (overcomes sequestration in enterocytes)
- erythropoietin indicated in chronic renal failure; not to be used if patient has concomitant curative solid tumour malignancy; ensure Hb target <110 g/L

Sideroblastic Anemia

- uncommon compared to iron deficiency anemia or anemia of chronic disease

Sideroblasts
- erythrocytes with iron-containing (basophilic) granules in the cytoplasm
- "normal": in healthy individuals, granules are small and randomly spread in the cytoplasm
- "ring": iron deposits in mitochondria, forming large, abnormal granules that surround the nucleus
    - the hallmark of sideroblastic anemia

Etiology
- due to defects in heme biosynthesis in erythroid precursors
- hereditary (rare): X-linked; median survival 10 yr
- idiopathic (acquired)
    - refractory anemia with ringed sideroblasts: a subtype of MDS (see *Myelodysplastic Syndromes*, H39)
    - may be a preleukemic phenomenon (10% transform to AML)
- reversible
    - drugs (isoniazid, chloramphenicol), alcohol, lead, copper deficiency, zinc toxicity, hypothyroidism

Clinical Features
- anemia symptoms (see *Anemia*, H6)
- hepatosplenomegaly, evidence of iron overload

Investigations
- serum iron indices
    - increased serum Fe^{2+}, normal TIBC, increased ferritin, increased sTfR
- blood film/bone marrow biopsy
    - ringed sideroblasts (diagnostic hallmark)
    - RBCs are hypochromic; can be micro-, normo-, or macrocytic
    - anisocytosis, poikilocytosis, basophilic stippling

Treatment

- depends on etiology
  - X-linked: high dose pyridoxine (vitamin B_6) in some cases
  - acquired: EPO and G-CSF
  - reversible: remove precipitating cause
- supportive transfusions for severe anemia

Lead Poisoning

Definition/Etiology

- blood lead levels greater than 80 µg/dL, possible symptomatology at 50 µg/dL
- identify source: consider occupational history, exposures history, utensil history

Clinical Features

- abdominal pain, constipation, irritability, difficulty concentrating

Treatment

- chelation therapy: dimercaprol and EDTA are first line agents

Normocytic Anemia

- MCV 80-100 fL
- see Figure 2, *Approach to Anemia*, H6

Aplastic Anemia

Definition

- destruction of hematopoietic cells of the bone marrow leading to pancytopenia and hypocellular bone marrow

Etiology

Table 11. Etiology of Aplastic Anemia

Congenital	Acquired	

Fanconi's anemia
Shwachman-Diamond syndrome
	Idiopathic
	  Often T-cell mediated
	Drugs
	  Dose-related (i.e. chemotherapeutics)
	  Idiosyncratic (chloramphenicol, anti-
	  malarials, phenylbutazone)
	Toxins
	  Benzene/organic solvents
	  DDT, insecticides
		Ionizing Radiation
		Post-Viral Infection
		  Parvovirus B19, EBV, HDV, HEV, HBV,
		  HHV6, HIV
		Autoimmune (rare)
		  SLE, Graft-versus-host disease
		Others
		  PNH, pregnancy, anorexia nervosa,
		  thymoma

Clinical Features

- can present acutely or insidiously
- symptoms of anemia (see *Anemia*, H6), thrombocytopenia (see *Thrombocytopenia*, H7), and/or infection
- ± splenomegaly and lymphadenopathy (depending on the cause)

Investigations

- exclude other causes of pancytopenia (see Figure 4), including PNH (overlap syndrome)
- CBC
  - anemia or neutropenia or thrombocytopenia (any combination) ± pancytopenia
  - decreased reticulocytes (<1% of the total RBC count)
- blood film
  - decreased number of normal RBCs
- bone marrow
  - aplasia or hypoplasia of marrow cells with fat replacement
  - decreased cellularity

Treatment

- remove offending agents
- supportive care (red cell and platelet transfusions, antibiotics)
  - judicious use so as to not increase the risk of immune sensitization to blood products
- immunosuppression (for idiopathic aplastic anemia)
  - anti-thymocyte globulin: 50-60% of patients respond
  - cyclosporine
- allogenic bone marrow transplant
- growth factors: e.g. Eltrombopag (TPO receptor agonist), G-CSF and EPO not effective

Consider lead poisoning in any child with microcytic anemia who lives in a house built before 1977

Features of Lead Poisoning

LEAD
Lead lines on gingivae and epiphyses of long bones on x-ray
Encephalopathy and **E**rythrocyte basophilic stippling
Abdominal colic and microcytic **A**nemia (sideroblastic)
Drops (wrist and foot drop)

Causes of Normocytic Anemia

ABCD
Acute blood loss
Bone marrow failure
Chronic disease
Destruction (hemolysis)

Hemolytic Anemia

Definition
- anemia due to a shortened survival of circulating RBCs, usually defined as <100 d
- uncommon cause for anemia (<5% of cases) with many etiologies (>200)

Classification
- hereditary
  - abnormal membrane (spherocytosis, elliptocytosis)
  - abnormal enzymes (pyruvate kinase deficiency, G6PD deficiency)
  - abnormal hemoglobin synthesis (thalassemias, hemoglobinopathies)
- acquired
  - immune
    - autoimmune: warm vs. cold autoimmune hemolytic anemias (AIHA), see Table 14 *Classification of AIHA*, H22
    - alloimmune: hemolytic disease of the fetus/newborn, post-transfusion
  - non-immune
    - MAHA/TMA, now known as TMA: thrombus in blood vessel causes RBCs to be sheared – associated with DIC, HUS, aHUS, TTP, preeclampsia/HELLP, vasculitides, malignant hypertension
    - other causes: PNH, hypersplenism, march hemoglobinuria (exertional hemolysis), infection (e.g. malaria), snake venoms, mechanical heart valves
- also classified as intravascular or extravascular
  - intravascular: MAHA/TMA (e.g. TTP, DIC), infections (malaria, *Clostridium*), and PNH
  - extravascular: RBCs are coated with antibodies (AIHA) or have an abnormal membrane structure/shape or inclusions

Clinical Features Specific to HA
- jaundice
- dark urine (hemoglobinuria, bilirubin)
- cholelithiasis (pigment stones)
- potential for an aplastic crisis (i.e. BM suppression in overwhelming infection)
- iron overload with extravascular hemolysis
- iron deficiency with intravascular hemolysis

Investigations

Table 12. Investigations for Hemolytic Anemia

Screening Tests	Tests Specific For Intravascular Hemolysis
Increased LDH	Schistocytes on blood film
Decreased haptoglobin	Free hemoglobin in serum
Increased unconjugated bilirubin	Methemalbuminemia (heme + albumin)
Increased urobilinogen	Hemoglobinuria (immediate)
Reticulocytosis	Hemosiderinuria (delayed) – most sensitive

Tests Specific for Extravascular Hemolysis
Direct Antiglobulin Test (direct Coombs)
Detects IgG or complement on the surface of RBC
Add anti-IgG or anti-complement Ab to patient's RBCs; positive if agglutination
Indications: hemolytic disease of newborn, AIHA, hemolytic transfusion reaction
Indirect Antiglobulin Test (indirect Coombs)
Detects antibodies in serum that can recognize antigens on RBCs
Mix patient's serum + donor RBCs + Coombs serum (anti-human Ig Ab); positive if agglutination
Indications: cross-matching donor RBCs, atypical blood group, blood group Ab in pregnant women, AIHA

Thalassemia

Definition
- defects in production of the α or β chains of hemoglobin
  - resulting imbalance in globin chains leads to ineffective erythropoiesis and hemolysis in the spleen or BM
- clinical manifestations and treatment depends on specific gene and number of alleles affected
- common features
  - increasing severity with increasing number of alleles involved
  - hypochromic microcytic anemia
  - basophilic stippling, abnormally shaped RBCs on blood film

On blood film schistocytes reflect an intravascular hemolysis while spherocytes usually reflect an extravascular hemolysis

Disruption of the heme breakdown pathway causes the **porphyria** disorders

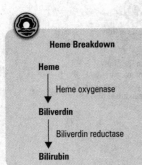

Heme Breakdown

Heme

↓ Heme oxygenase

Biliverdin

↓ Biliverdin reductase

Bilirubin

Laboratory Findings in HA
- ↑ retics
- ↓ haptoglobin
- ↑ unconjugated bilirubin
- ↑ urobilinogen
- ↑ LDH

Haptoglobin is a circulating protein that mops up free hemoglobin, allowing its clearance in the spleen; when there is abundant free hemoglobin, haptoglobin is consumed, and levels decrease

ThalasSEAmia
β-Thal → prevalent in Mediterranean
α-Thal → prevalent in South East Asia (SEA) and Africa (α = Asia, Africa)

Pathophysiology
- defect may be in any of the Hb genes
  - normally 4α genes in total; 2 on each copy of chromosome 16
  - normally 2β genes in total; 1 on each copy of chromosome 11
  - fetal hemoglobin, HbF ($\alpha_2\gamma_2$), switches to adult forms HbA ($\alpha_2\beta_2$) and HbA$_2$ ($\alpha_2\delta_2$) at 3-6 mo of life
  - HbA constitutes 97% of adult hemoglobin
  - HbA$_2$ constitutes 3% of adult hemoglobin

β-Thalassemia Minor (Thalassemia Trait)

Definition
- defect in single allele of β gene (heterozygous for one normal beta globin allele and one beta globin thalassemic allele)
- common in people of Mediterranean and Asian descent

Clinical Features
- usually asymptomatic; a palpable spleen is very rare

Investigations
- Hb (100-140 g/L), MCV(<70), Fe (normal), RBC count (normal)
- peripheral blood film – microcytosis basophilic stippling
- Hb electrophoresis
  - specific: HbA$_2$ increased to 3.5-5% (normal 1.5-3.5%)
  - non-specific: 50% have slight increase in HbF

Treatment
- no treatment required
- genetic counselling for patient and family

Microcytosis in β-Thal Minor
Microcytosis is much more profound and the anemia is much milder than that of iron deficiency

β-Thalassemia Major

Definition
- defect in both alleles of β gene (homozygous, autosomal recessive)

Pathophysiology
- ineffective chain synthesis leading to ineffective erythropoiesis, hemolysis of RBCs, and increase in HbF

Clinical Features
- initial presentation at age 6-12 mo when HbA (α_2/β_2) normally replaces HbF (α_2/γ_2)
  - severe anemia, jaundice
- iron overload progressing to hemochromatosis
  - secondary to repeated transfusions and ineffective erythropoiesis
  - leads to iron-induced organ damage (see Gastroenterology, G26)
- stunted growth and development (hypogonadal dwarf)
- gross hepatosplenomegaly (due to extramedullary hematopoiesis)
- radiologic changes (due to expanded marrow cavity) and extramedullary hematopoietic masses (erythroid tissue tumours)
  - skull x-ray has "hair-on-end" appearance
  - pathologic fractures common
- evidence of increased Hb catabolism (e.g. pigmented gallstones)
- death can result from
  - untreated anemia (should transfuse)
  - infection (should identify and treat early)
  - iron overload (common): late complication from repeated transfusions and ineffective erythropoiesis

Hemochromatosis Clinical Features

ABCDH
Arthralgia
Bronze skin
Cardiomyopathy, cirrhosis of liver
Diabetes (pancreatic damage)
Hypogonadism (anterior pituitary damage)

Investigations
- severe microcytic anemia (Hb <60 g/L)
- peripheral blood film: teardrop, target, hypochromic, microcytic
- Hb electrophoresis
  - HbA: 0-10% (normal >95%)
  - HbA$_2$ >2.5%
  - HbF: 90-100%

Treatment
- lifelong regular transfusions to suppress endogenous erythropoiesis
- iron chelation (e.g. deferoxamine, deferasirox, deferiprone) to prevent iron overload in organs and the formation of free radicals (which promote tissue damage and fibrosis)
- folic acid supplementation if not transfused
- allogenic bone marrow transplantation (potentially curative) or cord blood transplant
- splenectomy (now performed less frequently)

β-Thalassemia Intermedia

Definition
• clinical diagnosis in patients whose clinical manifestations are too mild to be classified as thalassemia major, but too severe to be classified as thalassemia minor

Clinical Features
• wide variety of clinical phenotypes
• in most cases of TI, both β-globin genes affected
• three main mechanisms account for the milder phenotype compared to thalassemia major: (1) subnormal (vs. absent) beta-chain synthesis, (2) increased number of gamma chains, (3) coinheritance of alpha thalassemia (in some cases)
• complications more commonly seen in TI than thalassemia major include extramedullary hematopoiesis, leg ulcers, gallstones, thrombosis, and pulmonary hypertension, and growth retardation

α-Thalassemia

Definition
• defect(s) in α genes
• similar geographic distribution as β-thalassemia, but higher frequency among Asians and Africans

Clinical Features
• 1 defective α gene (aa/a-): clinically silent; normal Hb, normal MCV
• 2 defective α genes (cis: aa/-- or trans: a-/a-): decreased MCV, normal Hb
  ▪ N.B. cis 2-gene deletion more common in Asia vs. trans 2-gene deletion more common in Africa – this leads to increased risk of fetal hydrops in offspring of Asian patients vs. African patients
• 3 defective α genes (a-/--): HbH (β4) disease; presents in adults, decreased MCV, decreased Hb, splenomegaly
• 4 defective α genes (--/--): Hb Barts (γ4) disease (hydrops fetalis); usually incompatible with life

Investigations
• peripheral blood film – screen for HbH inclusion bodies with supravital stain
• electrophoresis can be used to identify HgH disease, definitive diagnosis with DNA genotyping

Treatment
• depends on degree of anemia, referral for genetic/prenatal counselling
  ▪ 1 or 2 defective α genes: no treatment required
  ▪ HbH disease: similar to β-thalassemia intermedia
  ▪ HbBarts: no definitive treatment, majority of pregnancies terminated (fetal/maternal mortality risk), intrauterine transfusion, stem cell transplants

Sickle Cell Disease

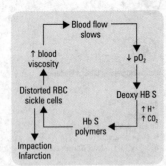

Figure 7. Pathophysiology of sickling

Definition
• autosomal recessive sickling disorders arise due to a mutant β-globin chain, most commonly caused by a Glu → Val substitution at position 6 (chromosome 11) resulting in HbS variant, rather than HbA (normal adult Hb)
  ▪ increased incidence of HbS allele with African or Mediterranean heritage (thought to be protective against malaria)
• sickle cell disease occurs when an individual has two HbS genes (homozygous, HbSS) or one HbS gene + another mutant β-globin gene (compound heterozygote) – most commonly HbS-β-thal and HbSC disease

Pathophysiology
• at low pO_2, deoxy HbS polymerizes leading to rigid crystal-like rods that distort membranes → 'sickles'
• the pO_2 level at which sickling occurs is related to the percentage of HbS present
• sickling aggravated by acidemia, increased CO_2, increased 2,3-DPG, fever, and osmolality
• fragile sickle cells then cause injury in two main ways
  1. fragile sickle cells hemolyze (nitric oxide depletion)
  2. occlusion of small vessels (hypoxia, ischemia-reperfusion injury)

Clinical Features
• HbAS (sickle cell trait): patient will be asymptomatic except during extreme hypoxia or infection increased risk of renal medullary carcinoma
• SCD-SS (HbSS)
  ▪ chronic hemolytic anemia
  ▪ jaundice in the first yr of life
  ▪ retarded growth and development ± skeletal changes
  ▪ splenomegaly in childhood; splenic atrophy in adulthood

- SCD-SS often presents with acute pain episode
  1. aplastic crises
     - toxins and infections (especially parvovirus B19) transiently suppress bone marrow
  2. splenic sequestration crises
     - usually in children; significant pooling of blood in spleen resulting in acute Hb drop and shock
     - uncommon in adults due to asplenia from repeated infarction
  3. vaso-occlusive crises (infarction)
     - may affect various organs causing ischemia-reperfusion injury (especially in back, chest, abdomen, and extremities), fever, and leukocytosis
     - can cause a stroke or a silent myocardial infarction
     - precipitated by infections, dehydration, rapid change in temperature, pregnancy, menses, and alcohol
  4. acute chest syndrome (see sidebar)
- SCD-SC (most common compound heterozygote)
  - 1:833 live births in African-Americans, common in West Africa
  - milder anemia than HbSS
  - similar complications as HbSS, although typically milder and less frequent (exception is proliferative sickle retinopathy, glomerulonephritis, and avascular necrosis)
  - spleen not always atrophic in adults

Investigations
- sickle cell prep (detects sickling of RBCs under the microscope in response to O_2 lowering agent): determines the presence of a HbS allele, but does not distinguish HbAS from HbSS
- Hb electrophoresis distinguishes HbAS, HbSS, HbSC, and other variants all newborns in developed countries typically screened for SCD

Table 13. Investigations for Sickle Cell Disease

	HbAS	HbSS
CBC	Normal	Increased reticulocytes, decreased Hb, decreased Hct
Peripheral Blood	Normal; possibly a few target cells	Sickled cells
Hb Electrophoresis	HbA fraction of 0.65 (65%) HbS fraction of 0.35 (35%)	No HbA, only HbS and HbF (proportions change with age); normal amount of HbA_2

Treatment
- genetic counselling
- HbAS: no treatment required
- HbSC: treatment as per HbSS, but is dictated by symptom severity
- HbSS
  1. folic acid to prevent folate deficiency
  2. hydroxyurea to enhance production of HbF
     - mechanism of action: stops repression of Hb-γ chains and/or initiates differentiation of stem cells in which this gene is active
     - presence of HbF in the SS cells decreases polymerization and precipitation of HbS
     - N.B. hydroxyurea is cytotoxic and may cause bone marrow suppression
  3. treatment of vaso-occlusive crisis
     - supportive care: oxygen, hydration (reduces viscosity), correct acidosis, analgesics/opiates
     - indication for exchange transfusion: Hb <50-60 g/L, SCD complications (acute chest syndrome, aplastic crisis, hepatic or splenic sequestration, stroke), prevention of complications, pre-operative
     - less routinely: antimicrobials for suspected infection
  4. prevention of crises
     - establish diagnosis
     - avoid conditions that promote sickling (hypoxia, acidosis, dehydration, fever)
     - vaccination in childhood (pneumococcus, meningococcus, *H. influenzae* b)
     - prophylactic penicillin (age 3 mo-5 yr)
     - good hygiene, nutrition, and social support
  5. screen for complications
     - regular blood work (CBC, reticulocytes, iron indices, BUN, LFTs, creatinine)
     - urinalysis annually (proteinuria, glomerulopathy)
     - transcranial doppler annually until 16 yr old (stroke prevention)
     - retinal examinations annually from 8 yr old (screen for retinopathy)
     - echocardiography once in late childhood/early adulthood (screen for pulmonary hypertension)

Acute Chest Syndrome
Affects 30% of patients with sickle cell disease and may be life threatening. Presentation includes dyspnea, chest pain, fever, tachypnea, leukocytosis, and pulmonary infiltrate on CXR. Caused by vaso-occlusion, infection, or pulmonary fat embolus from infarcted marrow

Organs Affected by Vaso-Occlusive Crisis

Organ	Problem
Brain	Ischemic or hemorrhagic stroke, vasculopathy
Eye	Hemorrhage, blindness
Liver	Infarcts, RUQ syndrome
Lung	Chest syndrome, long-term pulmonary hypertension
Gallbladder	Stones
Heart	Hyperdynamic flow murmurs
Spleen	Enlarged (child); atrophic (adult)
Kidney	Hematuria, loss of renal concentrating ability, proteinuria
Intestines	Acute abdomen
Placenta	Stillbirths
Penis	Priapism
Digits	Dactylitis
Femoral and Humeral Head	Avascular necrosis
Bone	Infarction, infection
Ankle	Leg ulcers

NIH Consensus Development Conference Statement: Hydroxyurea Treatment for Sickle Cell Disease
Ann Intern Med 2008;148:932-938
Efficacy: Strong evidence for adolescents and adults and there is emerging data supporting its use in children. In the single RCT, the Hb level was higher in hydroxyurea recipients than placebo recipients after 2 yr (difference, 6 g/L), as was HbF (absolute difference, 3.2%). The median number of painful crises was 44% lower than in the placebo arm. The 12 observational studies that enrolled adults reported a relative increase in HbF of 4-20% and a relative reduction in crisis rates by 68-84%. Hospital admissions declined by 18-32%.
Effectiveness: Data is limited. It seems to be highly effective but is currently underutilized.
Short-Term Harms (within 6 mo): Dose-related leukopenia, thrombocytopenia, anemia, and decreased reticulocyte count. Others include decreased sperm production and dry skin.
Long-Term Harms: Birth defects in offspring of people receiving the drug, growth delays in children receiving the drug, and cancer in both children and adults who receive the drug.

Autoimmune Hemolytic Anemia

Table 14. Classification of AIHA

	Warm (75-90% cases)	Cold
Antibody Allotype	IgG	IgM
Agglutination Temperature	37°C	4-37°C
Direct Coombs Test (direct anti-globulin test)	Positive for IgG ± complement	Positive for complement
Etiology	Idiopathic Secondary to lymphoproliferative disorder (e.g. CLL, Hodgkin lymphoma) Secondary to autoimmune disease (e.g. SLE) Drug-induced (e.g. penicillin, quinine, methyldopa)	Idiopathic Secondary to infection (e.g. mycoplasma pneumonia, EBV) Secondary to lymphoproliferative disorder (e.g. macroglobulinemia, CLL)
Blood Film	Spherocytes	Agglutination
Management	Treat underlying cause Corticosteroids Immunosuppression Splenectomy Folic acid Rituximab (2nd line to steroids)	Treat underlying cause Warm patient/avoid cold Rituximab regiments (1st line) Plasma exchange (2nd line for high IgM levels) Folic acid Low dose alkylating agents (chlorambucil, cyclophosphamide) or interferon may be useful but less effective

Microangiopathic Hemolytic Anemia/ Thrombotic Microangiopathy

Definition
- hemolytic anemia due to intravascular fragmentation of RBCs

Etiology
- see *Thrombotic Thrombocytopenic Purpura* and *Hemolytic Uremic Syndrome*, H30
- see Disseminated *Intravascular Coagulation*, H32
- eclampsia, HELLP syndrome, AFLP (see Obstetrics, OB25)
- malignant hypertension
- vasculitis
- malfunctioning heart valves
- metastatic carcinoma
- drugs (calcineurin inhibitors, quinine, simvastatin)
- infections (severe CMV or meningococcus)
- catastrophic antiphospholipid antibody syndrome

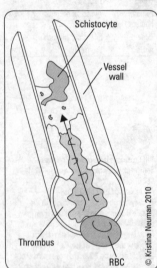

Schistocyte

Vessel wall

Thrombus

RBC

© Kristina Neuman 2010

Figure 8. Schistocyte

Investigations
- blood film: evidence of hemolysis, schistocytes
- hemolytic workup
- urine: hemosiderinuria, hemoglobinuria

Hereditary Spherocytosis

- most common type of hereditary hemolytic anemia
- abnormality in RBC membrane proteins (e.g. spectrin)
  - spleen makes defective RBCs more spherocytotic (and more fragile) by membrane removal; also acts as site of RBC destruction
- autosomal dominant with variable penetrance

Investigations
- blood film (shows spherocytes), osmotic fragility (increased), molecular analysis for spectrin gene

Treatment
- in severe cases, splenectomy and vaccination against pneumococcus, meningococcus, and *H. influenza* b (avoid in early childhood)

Hereditary Elliptocytosis

Definition/Etiology
- abnormality in spectrin interaction with other membrane proteins
- autosomal dominant
- 25-75% elliptocytes
- hemolysis is usually mild

Treatment
- immunizations; splenectomy for severe hemolysis

Glucose-6-Phosphate Dehydrogenase Deficiency

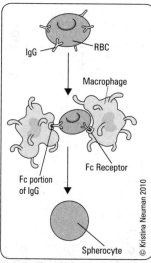

Figure 9. Spherocytosis secondary to AIHA

Definition
- deficiency in glucose-6-phosphate dehydrogenase (G6PD), corresponding to a lack of reduced glutathione (GSH) and leading to RBC sensitivity due to oxidative stress

Pathophysiology
- X-linked recessive, prevalent in individuals of African, Asian, and Mediterranean descent

Clinical Features
- frequently presents as episodic hemolysis precipitated by:
  - oxidative stress
  - drugs (e.g. sulfonamide, antimalarials, nitrofurantoin)
  - infection
  - food (fava beans)
- in neonates: can present as prolonged, pathologic neonatal jaundice

Investigations
- neonatal screening
- G6PD assay (may not be useful if result is normal)
  - should not be done in acute crisis when reticulocyte count is high (reticulocytes have high G6PD levels)
- blood film
  - Heinz bodies (granules in RBCs due to oxidized Hb); passage through spleen results in the generation of bite cells
  - may have features of intravascular hemolysis (e.g. RBC fragments)

Treatment
- folic acid
- stop offending drugs and avoid triggers
- transfusion in severe cases

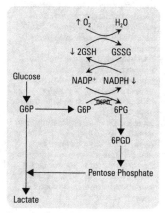

Figure 10. G6PD deficiency

Macrocytic Anemia

- MCV >100 fL
- see Figure 2, *Approach to Anemia*, H6

Table 15. Comparison Between Megaloblastic and Non-Megaloblastic Macrocytic Anemia

	Megaloblastic	Non-Megaloblastic
Morphology	Large, oval, nucleated RBC precursor Hypersegmented neutrophils	Large round RBC Normal neutrophils
Pathophysiology	Failure of DNA synthesis resulting in asynchronous maturation of RBC nucleus and cytoplasm	Reflects membrane abnormality with abnormal cholesterol metabolism

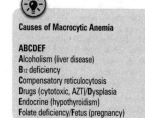

Causes of Macrocytic Anemia

ABCDEF
Alcoholism (liver disease)
B_{12} deficiency
Compensatory reticulocytosis
Drugs (cytotoxic, AZT)/Dysplasia
Endocrine (hypothyroidism)
Folate deficiency/Fetus (pregnancy)

Characteristics of Megaloblastic Macrocytic Anemia
- Pancytopenia
- Hypersegmented neutrophils
- Megaloblastic bone marrow

Vitamin B₁₂ Deficiency

B₁₂ (cobalamin) see Family Medicine – *Nutrition*, FM6
- binds to intrinsic factor (IF) secreted by gastric parietal cells
- absorbed in terminal ileum
- total body stores sufficient for 3-4 yr

Etiology

Table 16. Etiology of Vitamin B₁₂ Deficiency

Diet	Gastric	Intestinal Absorption	Genetic
Strict vegan More likely to present in pediatric population **Vegetarian in pregnancy** **Malnutrition**	**Mucosal atrophy** Gastritis, autoimmune **Pernicious anemia** (see below) **Post-gastrectomy**	**Malabsorption** Crohn's, celiac sprue, pancreatic insufficiency, *H. pylori* **Stagnant bowel** Blind loop, stricture **Fish tapeworm** **Resection of ileum** **Drugs** Neomycin, biguanides, PPI, N₂O anesthesia, metformin	**Transcobalamin II deficiency** **IF receptor defect**

Oral Vitamin B₁₂ vs. Intramuscular Vitamin B₁₂ for Vitamin B₁₂ Deficiency
Cochrane DB Syst Rev 2005;3:CD004655
Study: Systematic review. 2 RCTs met inclusion criteria; total 108 patients with follow-up from 90 d-4 mo.
Intervention: One study evaluated 1,000 μg of oral B₁₂ compared to 1,000 μg IM B₁₂ on the same dosing schedule. The other compared 2,000 μg daily oral B₁₂ to 1,000 μg IM B₁₂ on a less frequent dosing schedule. Neurological and hematological end points were evaluated.
Results: Meta-analysis was not attempted due to study heterogeneity. Both studies reported improvements in hematological and neurological end-points in both oral and IM groups. No significant difference was observed between groups in either study.
Conclusions: Limited data suggests high dose oral vitamin B₁₂ (1,000-2,000 μg) is equivalent to IM vitamin B₁₂ on the same or less frequent dosing schedule. This data is limited by small sample sizes and short follow-up periods. However, it suggests that a 3 to 4 month trial of oral supplementation is a reasonable first choice for patients with B₁₂ deficiency.

Pathophysiology of Pernicious Anemia
- auto-antibodies produced against gastric parietal cells leading to achlorhydria and lack of intrinsic factor secretion
- intrinsic factor is required to stabilize B₁₂ as it passes through the bowel
- decreased intrinsic factor leads to decreased ileal absorption of B₁₂
- may be associated with other autoimmune disorders (polyglandular endocrine insufficiency)
- most common in Northern European Caucasians, usually >30 yr old (median age of 60 yr old)

Clinical Features
- neurological (severity of anemia and neurological sequelae depends on deficiency)
  - peripheral neuropathy (variable reversibility)
    - usually symmetrical, affecting lower limbs more than upper limbs
  - cord (irreversible damage)
    - subacute combined degeneration
      - posterior columns: decreased vibration sense, proprioception, and 2-point discrimination, parasthesia
      - pyramidal tracts: spastic weakness, ataxia
  - cerebral (common, reversible with B₁₂ therapy)
    - confusion, delirium, dementia
  - cranial nerves (rare)
    - optic atrophy

Schilling Test

Part 1
- Tracer dose (1 μg) of radiolabeled B₁₂, given PO
- Flushing dose (1 mg) of unlabeled B₁₂ IM 1 h later to saturate tissue binders of B₁₂ thus allowing radioactive B₁₂ to be excreted in urine
- 24 h urine radiolabeled B₁₂ measured
- Normal >5% excretion (a normal excretion will only be seen if the low B₁₂ was due to dietary deficiency)

Part 2
- Same as part 1, but radiolabeled B₁₂ given with oral intrinsic factor
- Should be done only if first stage shows reduced excretion
- Normal test result (>5% excretion) = pernicious anemia
- Abnormal test result (<5% excretion) = intestinal causes (malabsorption)

Investigations
- CBC, reticulocyte count
  - anemia often severe ± neutropenia ± thrombocytopenia
  - MCV >110 fL
  - low reticulocyte count relative to the degree of anemia (<2%)
- serum B₁₂ and RBC folate
  - caution: low serum B₁₂ leads to low RBC folate because of failure of folate polyglutamate synthesis in the absence of B₁₂
  - alternatively, can measure elevated urine metabolites (methylmalonate, homocysteine)
- blood film
  - oval macrocytes, hypersegmented neutrophils
- bone marrow
  - hypercellularity
  - nuclear-cytoplasmic asynchrony in RBC precursors (less mature nuclei than expected from the development of the cytoplasm)
- bilirubin and LDH
  - elevated unconjugated bilirubin and LDH due to breakdown of cells in BM
- Schilling test (radiolabeled B₁₂ test, rarely done) to distinguish pernicious anemia from other causes
  - anti-intrinsic factor antibody, anti-parietal cell antibody

Treatment
- vitamin B₁₂ 1,000 μg IM or 1,000-1,200 μg PO if intestinal absorption intact, route and duration depends on cause
- less frequent, higher doses may be as effective (e.g. 1,000 μg IM q3mo)
- watch for hypokalemia and rebound thrombocytosis when treating severe megaloblastic anemia

Folate Deficiency

- uncommon in developed countries due to extensive dietary supplementation (enriched in flour)
- folate stores are depleted in 3-6 mo
- folate commonly found in green, leafy vegetables and fortified cereals

Etiology

Table 17. Etiology of Folate Deficiency

Diet/Deficiency	Malabsorption	Drugs	Increased Demand
Alcoholism	Celiac sprue	Anti-folates (methotrexate)	Pregnancy
Substance abuse	IBD	Anticonvulsants (phenytoin)	Hemolysis
Elderly/infants	Infiltrative bowel disease	Alcohol	Prematurity
Poor intake	Short bowel syndrome	Oral contraceptive	Exfoliative dermatitis/psoriasis
			Hemodialysis

Clinical Features

- anemia, mild jaundice, glossitis, diarrhea, confusion, pallor
- unlike B_{12} deficiency, folate deficiency has no neurologic manifestations
- consider social history, alcohol/drug abuse, very poor diet (e.g. elderly, depressed)

Investigations

- similar to B_{12} deficiency (CBC, reticulocytes, blood film, RBC folate, serum B_{12})
- if decreased RBC folate, rule out B_{12} deficiency as cause

Management

- folic acid 1-5 mg PO OD x 1-4 mo; then 1 mg PO OD maintenance if cause is not reversible

Never give folate alone to an individual with megaloblastic anemia because it will mask B_{12} deficiency and neurological degeneration will continue

Hemostasis

Stages of Hemostasis

1. Primary Hemostasis

- cellular defense – involves the platelet and VWF predominantly
- goal is rapid cessation of bleeding; main effect is on mucocutaneous bleeding
- vessel injury results in collagen/subendothelial matrix exposure and release of vasoconstrictors
- blood flow is impeded and platelets come into contact with damaged vessel wall (Figure 11a)
    - adhesion: platelets adhere to subendothelium via Von Willebrand factor (VWF)
    - activation: platelets are activated resulting in change of shape and release of ADP and thromboxane A_2
    - aggregation: these factors further recruit and aggregate more platelets resulting in formation of localized hemostatic plug

2. Secondary Hemostasis

- platelet plug is reinforced by production of fibrin clot (Figure 11b)
- extrinsic (initiation) pathway: initiation of coagulation in vivo
- intrinsic (amplification) pathway: amplification once coagulation has started via positive feedback
- both intrinsic and extrinsic pathways converge onto the common pathway which results in thrombin generation and fibrin formation

3. Fibrin Stabilization

- conversion from soluble to insoluble and stable clot

4. Fibrinolysis

- once healing initiated, clot dissolution via action of the fibrinolytic system

Normal hemostasis occurs as a result of the balance between procoagulant and anticoagulant factors

Phases of Hemostasis
- Primary hemostasis
- Secondary hemostasis
- Fibrin stabilization
- Fibrinolysis

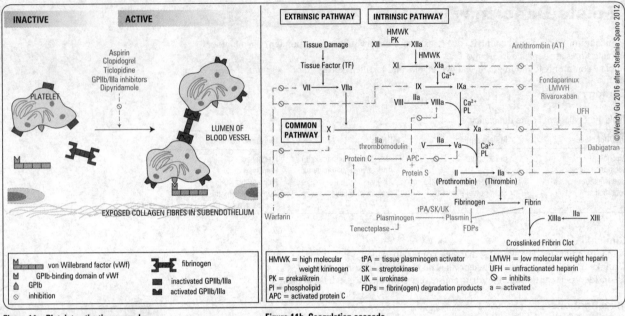

Figure 11a. Platelet activation cascade

Figure 11b. Coagulation cascade

Legend (Figure 11a):
- von Willebrand factor (vWf)
- GPIb-binding domain of vWf
- GPIb
- inhibition
- fibrinogen
- inactivated GPIIb/IIIa
- activated GPIIb/IIIa

Legend (Figure 11b):

HMWK = high molecular weight kininogen
PK = prekalikrein
Pl = phospholipid
APC = activated protein C
tPA = tissue plasminogen activator
SK = streptokinase
UK = urokinase
FDPs = fibrin(ogen) degradation products
LMWH = low molecular weight heparin
UFH = unfractionated heparin
⊘ = inhibits
a = activated

© Wendy Gu 2016 after Stefania Spano 2012

Tests of Secondary Hemostasis

PT/INR: **T**ennis is played outside (E**x**trinsic pathway)
PTT: **T**able **T**ennis is played inside (Intrinsic pathway)

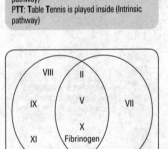

Figure 12. Clotting factors involved in PT and PTT

(Venn diagram, PTT circle: VIII, IX, XI, XII; PT circle: VII; common region: II, V, X, Fibrinogen)

Causes of an Prolonged PTT Without Bleeding include:
1. Early contact factor (Factor XII, HMWK, PK) deficiency
2. Lupus anticoagulant
3. Inappropriate blood draw
4. Heparin contamination
5. Erythrocytosis (laboratory artifact)

Consider PTT
- IV heparin, argatroban monitoring
- Hemophilia A/B, factor XI deficiency, severe VWF

Table 18. Commonly Used Tests of Hemostasis

Type of Hemostasis	Test	Reference Range	Purpose	Examples of Associated Diagnoses
Primary	Platelet count	150-400 x 10^9/L	To quantitate platelet number	Low in ITP, HUS/TTP, DIC
Secondary	aPTT	22-35 s	Measures intrinsic pathway (factors VIII, IX, XI, XII) and common pathway. Used to monitor heparin therapy	Prolonged in hemophilias A and B (if factor deficiency is below reagent threshold of detection) N.B. High if antiphospholipid antibodies (i.e. lupus anti-coagulant) are present
	PT	11-24 s	Measures extrinsic pathway (factor VII) and common pathway	Prolonged in vitamin K deficiency, vitamin K antagonist therapy (warfarin), factor VII deficiency
	INR	0.9-1.2	Used to monitor warfarin therapy and for assessment of hepatic function	
	Mixing studies		May differentiate inhibitors of clotting factor(s) from a deficiency in clotting factors. Mix patient's plasma with normal plasma in 1:1 ratio and repeat abnormal test	Normalization of clotting time if deficiency of single clotting factor (normalization may not occur if multiple clotting factors are deficient) Lack of normalization if inhibitor presence
Fibrinolysis	Euglobulin lysis time	N >90 min	Looks for accelerated fibrinolysis	May be accelerated in DIC or factor XIII deficiency. Decreased in hereditary deficiency of fibrinogen
Other	Fibrinogen D-dimer Specific factor assays (e.g. factor VIII) Lupus anticoagulant Thrombophilia tests (e.g. activated protein C resistance) Von Willebrand tests (VWF antigen, Ristocetin cofactor activity, factor VIII)			

Table 19. General Rules of Thumb: Signs and Symptoms of Disorders of Hemostasis

	Primary (Platelet, VWF)	Secondary (Coagulation)
Surface Cuts	Excessive, prolonged bleeding	Normal/slightly prolonged bleeding
Onset After Injury	Immediate	Delayed
Site of Bleeding	Superficial i.e. mucosal (nasal, gingival, GI tract, vaginal), skin	Deep i.e. joints, muscles Excessive post-traumatic
Lesions	Petechiae, ecchymoses	Hemarthroses, hematomas

Table 20. Lab Values in Disorders of Hemostasis

	PT	PTT	Platelet Count	Hemoglobin
Hemophilia A/B	N	↑	N	N*
VWD	N	±	N/↓	N*
DIC	↑	↑	↓	N/↓
Liver Failure	↑	N/↑	N/↓	N
ITP	N	N	↓	N
TTP	N	N	↓	↓

DIC = disseminated intravascular coagulation; ITP = idiopathic thrombocytopenic purpura; TTP = thrombotic thrombocytopenic purpura; VWD = von Willebrand disease;
* = anemia may develop from progressive iron deficiency and/or active bleeding

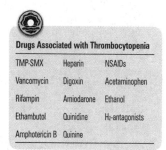

Consider PT/INR
- Warfarin
- Liver disease
- Risk factor for vitamin K deficiency (e.g. malabsorption, cholestasis, malnutrition)

Consider both PTT and PT/INR
- Suspected DIC
- Trauma patient, or requiring massive transfusion protocol
- Bleeding patient
- Patient receiving thrombolytic therapy

Disorders of Primary Hemostasis

Definition
- inability to form an adequate platelet plug due to
  - disorders of blood vessels
  - disorders of platelets: abnormal function/numbers
  - disorders of VWF

Classification

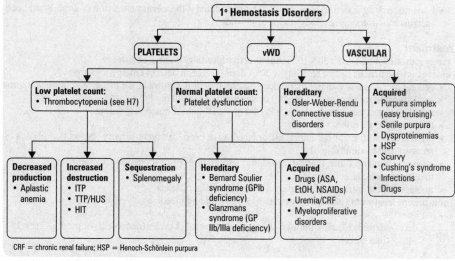

CRF = chronic renal failure; HSP = Henoch-Schönlein purpura

Figure 13. Approach to disorders of primary hemostasis

Drugs Associated with Thrombocytopenia

TMP-SMX	Heparin	NSAIDs
Vancomycin	Digoxin	Acetaminophen
Rifampin	Amiodarone	Ethanol
Ethambutol	Quinidine	H₂-antagonists
Amphotericin B	Quinine	

Immune Thrombocytopenia

Table 21. Features for Childhood vs. Adult Immune Thrombocytopenia

Features	Childhood ITP, see Pediatrics, P66	Adult ITP
Peak Age	2-6 yr	20-40 yr
Gender	None	F>M (3:1)
History of Recent Infection	Common	Rare
Onset of Bleed	Abrupt	Insidious
Duration	Usually wk	Months to yr
Spontaneous Remissions	80% or more	Uncommon

Terminology of ITP
- primary: isolated thrombocytopenia (platelet count <100x10⁹/L) with no other cause of thrombocytopenia
- secondary: thrombocytopenia associated with another condition (e.g. HIV, HCV, SLE, CLL)
- drug-induced: drug-dependent platelet antibodies causing platelet destruction

Mechanisms for HIV-associated Thrombocytopenia
- Direct effect of HIV on marrow
- Immune-mediated platelet destruction
- Some anti-retrovirals reduce platelet production

Classification of primary ITP
- acute: newly diagnosed (diagnosis to 3 mo)
- persistent: 3-12 mo from diagnosis
- chronic: >12 mo
- refractory: post-splenectomy

Pathophysiology
- primary or secondary ITP
- an acquired immune-mediated disorder (pathophysiology incompletely understood)
  - anti-platelet antibodies bind to platelet surface → increased splenic clearance
  - impaired platelet production
  - helper T-cell and cytotoxic T-cell activation also implicated in platelet destruction

Clinical Presentation
- variable presentation: asymptomatic, fatigue, minimal bruising, mucocutanous bleed, intracranial bleed
- assess for symptoms/signs suggesting a secondary cause

Investigations
- CBC and reticulocyte count: thrombocytopenia
- PT and aPTT: normal
- peripheral blood film: decreased platelets, giant platelets (rule out platelet clumping)
- HIV, HCV, *H. pylori* serology
- vitamin B_{12}, ANA, C3, C4, depending on clinical symptoms
- bone marrow aspirate and biopsy: increased number of megakaryocytes
  - recommended in patients >60 yr of age, pre-splenectomy or have failed traditional ITP therapy, those with systemic symptoms, an abnormal blood film
  - bone marrow aspirate and biopsy should be considered if there is any suspicion of diminished bone marrow function (e.g. myelodysplasia, infiltration)

Treatment
- rarely indicated if platelets >30 x 10^9/L unless active bleeding, trauma, or surgery
- **emergency treatment** (active bleeding [CNS, GI, or GU] or in need of emergency surgery)
  - general measures: stop drugs that reduce platelet function, control blood pressure, minimize trauma
  - corticosteroids: prednisone (1 mg/kg) or dexamethasone (40 mg PO x 4 d)
  - antifibrinolytic: tranexamic acid (1 g PO tid or 1 g IV q6h) if mucosal bleeding
  - IVIg 1 g/kg/d x 2 doses
  - platelet transfusion: for refractory, major bleeding or need for urgent surgery (expect that platelet recovery will be diminished)
  - emergency splenectomy: may be considered, vaccinations prior if possible (pneumococcus, meningococcus, *H. influenzae* b)
  - management of intracranial bleeding: IV steroids, IVIg, platelets
- **non-urgent treatment** (platelet count <20-30 x 10^9/L and no bleeding)
  - 1st line
    - corticosteroids (dexamethasone 40 mg qd x 4 days x 1-4 cycles (not weeks) or prednisone x 3 weeks then taper)
    - IVIg
    - anti-D: appropriate for Rh+ non-splenectomized patients, but can cause hemolysis (avoid if low Hb at baseline or if DAT is positive)
  - 2nd line
    - splenectomy (need vaccinations prior to splenectomy: pneumococcus, meningococcus, *H. influenzae* b)
    - rituximab
  - 3nd line
    - thrombopoietin (TPO) receptor agonists (romiplostim, eltrombopag) – may be considered for second line therapy if funding available
    - immunomodulating therapy (azathioprine, cyclophosphamide, danazol, vincristine)

Definitions of response to treatment
- complete response: platelet >100
- partial response: platelet 30-100
- no response: platelet <30

Prognosis
- ~20% will not attain a hemostatic platelet count after first and second line therapy
- fluctuating course
- overall relatively benign, life-expectancy similar to general population (however, risk of mortality from bleeding/infection increases with advancing age)
- major concern is spontaneous intracranial hemorrhage if platelet <5 x 10^9/L, more common in the elderly

Table 22. Heparin-Induced Thrombocytopenia (HIT)

Pathophysiology	Immune mediated Ab recognizes a complex of heparin and platelet factor 4 (PF4) leading to platelet activation via platelet Fc receptor and activation of coagulation system
Diagnosis	Suspected with intermediate or high probability HIT Score (Table 23) Confirm with ELISA testing and SRA testing
Onset of Decreased Platelets	5-15 d (if previously exposed to heparin within 100 d, HIT can develop in hours due to an anamnestic response)
Risk of Thrombosis	~30% to 50% (25% of events are arterial)
Clinical Features	Bleeding complications uncommon Venous thrombosis: DVT, PE, limb gangrene, cerebral sinus thrombosis Arterial thrombosis: MI, stroke, acute limb ischemia, organ infarct (mesentery, kidney) Heparin-induced skin necrosis (with LMWH) Acute platelet activation syndromes: acute inflammatory reactions (e.g. fever/chills, flushing, etc.) Transient global amnesia (rare)
Specific Tests	Re-test clinical scoring models can help rule-out HIT: 4-Ts (see Table 23) and the HIT Expert Probability (HEP) score 14C serotonin release assay (uses donor platelets with 14C serotonin and heparin with patient's plasma) ELISA for HIT-Ig (more sensitive, less specific than serotonin assay) Ultrasound of lower limb veins for DVT

Management	Clinical suspicion of HIT should prompt discontinuation of heparin and LWMH (specific tests take several days)
	Initiate anticoagulation with a non-heparin anticoagulant:
	    e.g. argatroban, danaparoid, fondaparinux, bivalirudin unless there is a strong contraindication (duration of treatment at least 2-3 mo if no thrombotic event, and at least 3-6 mo if thrombotic event has occurred)
	    Warfarin should only be restarted when platelet count >150 x 10⁹/L
	Allergy band and alert in patient records

Heparin-Induced Thrombocytopenia
- Heparin-induced thrombocytopenia (previously known as HIT type II): immune-mediated reaction following treatment with heparin leading to platelet and subsequent coagulation activation
- Heparin-associated thrombocytopenia (previously known at HIT type I): transient thrombocytopenia following administration of heparin

Heparin-Associated Thrombocytopenia (previously known as HIT type I)
- Direct heparin mediated platelet aggregation (non-immune)
- Platelets >100 X 10⁹/L
- Self-limited (no thrombotic risk)
- May continue with heparin therapy
- Onset 24-72 h

LMWH is also associated with HIT, but the risk is less than unfractionated heparin (2.6% in UFH vs. 0.2% in LMWH)

Table 23. The 4-T Pre-Test Clinical Scoring Model for HIT

Category	2 Points	1 Point	0 Points
1. Thrombocytopenia	Platelet count fall >50% AND platelet nadir ≥20 x 10⁹/L	Platelet count fall 30-50% OR platelet nadir 10-19 x10⁹/L	Platelet count fall <30% OR platelet nadir <10 x 10⁹/L
2. Timing of Platelet Count Fall	Clear onset between 5-10 d of heparin exposure OR platelet count fall at ≤1 d if prior heparin exposure within last 30 d	Consistent with fall in platelet count at 5-10 d but unclear (e.g. missing platelet counts) OR onset after day 10 OR fall ≤1 d with prior heparin exposure within 30-100 d	Platelet count fall after <4 d of heparin exposure, and no recent heparin
3. Thrombosis or Other Sequelae	Confirmed new thrombosis, skin necrosis, or acute systemic reaction after IV unfractionated heparin bolus	Progressive or recurrent thrombosis, non-necrotizing (erythematous) skin lesions, or suspected thrombosis that has not been proven	None
4. Other Causes for Thrombocytopenia	None apparent	Possible	Definite

6-8 points = high probability of HIT; 4-5 points = intermediate probability of HIT; 0-3 points = low probability of HIT
J Thromb Haemos 2006;4:759-765

Thrombotic Thrombocytopenic Purpura and Hemolytic Uremic Syndrome

Table 24. TTP and HUS

	TTP	HUS (see Pediatrics, P76)
Epidemiology	Predominantly adult	Predominantly children and elderly

Etiology	Deficiency of metalloproteinase that breaks down ultra-large VWF multimers: ADAMTS13
	    Congenital (genetic absence of ADAMTS-13)
	    Acquired (drugs, malignancy, transplant, HIV-associated, idiopathic)
		Shiga toxin (*E. coli* serotype O157:H7) in 90%
		Other bacteria, viruses, genetic causes, drugs

Clinical Features	1. Thrombocytopenia 2. MAHA/TMA 3. Neurological symptoms: headache, confusion, focal defects, seizures 4. Symptoms can be mild and non-specific	1. Severe thrombocytopenia 2. MAHA/TMA 3. Acute kidney injury 4. Bloody Diarrhea 5. GI prodrome
Investigations (both TTP, HUS)	CBC and blood film: decreased platelets and schistocytes PT, aPTT, fibrinogen: normal Markers of hemolysis: increased unconjugated bilirubin, increased LDH, decreased haptoglobin Negative Coombs test Creatinine, urea, to follow renal function ADAMSTS-13 gene, activity or inhibitor testing (TTP)	
Management	Medical emergency Plasma exchange ± steroids Platelet transfusion avoided unless life-threatening bleed (associated with microvascular thrombosis) Plasma infusion if plasmapheresis is not immediately available TTP mortality ~90% if untreated	Supportive therapy (fluids, RBC transfusion, nutrition, etc.) Some evidence for plasma exchange Possible role of Eculizumab (C5 antibody blocks complement activation) for neurologic symptoms

Note: atypical HUS is a complex disease with different etiology, treatment depends on genetic abnormalities

Von Willebrand Disease

Pathophysiology
- most common inherited bleeding disorder (prevalence of 1%)
- usually autosomal dominant (type 3 is autosomal recessive)
- women more commonly diagnosed (heavy menstrual bleeding, peripartum bleeding)
- qualitative defect or quantitative deficiency of VWF depending on type
  - VWF needed for platelet adhesion/aggregation and acts as chaperone for Factor VIII (extending its half-life in circulation), therefore abnormality of VWF can affect both primary and secondary hemostasis
  - VWF exists as a series of multimers ranging in size
    - largest multimers are most active in mediation of platelet adhesion/aggregation
    - both large and small multimers complex with Factor VIII
    - VWF levels vary according to blood group (non-group O patients have higher levels than group O patients)

Classification
- type 1: mild quantitative defect (decreased amount of VWF and proportional decrease in VWF activity) – 80% of cases
- type 2: qualitative defect (VWF activity disproportionally lower than quantity) – 20% of cases
- type 3: severe total quantitative defect (virtually no VWF produced), 1 per million

Clinical Features
- bleeding history is the single most important predictor of an underlying bleeding disorder
- validated, standardized bleeding assessment tools (e.g. ISTH-BAT) to facilitate exploration of the bleeding history
- mucocutaneous bleeding (easy bruising, epistaxis, heavy menstrual bleeding, peripartum bleeding, post-dental extraction bleeding, post-operative bleeding, gastrointestinal bleeding)
  - type 3 VWD patients can experience musculoskeletal bleeding due to significant deficiency in FVIII due to lack of FVIII chaperoning as VWF is absent

Investigations
- CBC, platelet, VWF:Antigen (determine how much VWF is present), VWF:Ristocetin cofactor activity (determine how well VWF bind to platelet), Factor VIII (determine how well VWF chaperon with FVIII), PTT
- tests to further categorize type/subtype of VWD: multimer analysis, ristocetin induced platelet agglutination, genetic studies

Pathophysiology of TTP
- Large VWF multimers secreted by endothelial cells are typically rapidly cleaved by ADAMTS-13 protease
- Congenital TTP is due to a genetic deficiency in ADAMTS-13
- Antibodies against ADAMTS-13 are present in acquired TTP (the more common form)

Differential Diagnosis of TTP
- DIC
- HUS
- aHUS
- HELLP
- Catastrophic antiphospholipid Ab syndrome
- Evans syndrome (AIHA + ITP)

Table 25. Investigations in VWD

Test	Expected Result	Test	Expected Result
PTT	N/↑	von Willebrand antigen	↓
Factor VIII	N/↓	Blood group	Affects antigen quantification (↓ in group O)
Plt Count	N/↓	vWF multimer analysis	Multimer variants
Ristocetin Activity	↓ (cofactor for vWF-Plt binding)		

Treatment
- desmopressin (DDAVP®) is effective treatment for 85-90% of patients with type 1 VWD and for some subtypes of type 2 VWD
  - causes release of VWF and Factor VIII from endothelial cells
  - variable efficacy depending on disease type; tachyphylaxis occurs after 4 consecutive doses
  - need to document responsiveness with "DDAVP challenge"
  - caution in children due to hyponatremia
- tranexamic acid (Cyklokapron®, antifibrinolytic) to stabilize clot formation
- VWF:FVIII concentrate (Humate P®, Wilate®) if DDAVP unresponsive/clinically ineffective or for severe bleeding episode
  - need to monitor VWF and factor VIII levels (very high factor VIII level can be prothrombotic)
- gynecologic focused care for heavy menstrual bleeding (NB estrogens have the added benefit of increasing VWF levels)

Consider VWD in all women with menorrhagia

VWD is the most common inheritable couagulation abnormality

Prognosis
- patients with mild type 1 VWD have auto-correction of VWF deficiency in pregnancy
- patients are best managed by a hematologist, ideally one who works in a Hemophilia Treatment Centre (HTC)

Disorders of Secondary Hemostasis

Definition
- inability to form an adequate fibrin clot
  - disorders of clotting factors or co-factors
  - disorders of proteins associated with fibrinolysis
- characterized by delayed bleeding, deep muscular bleeding, spontaneous hemarthroses

Table 26. Classification of Secondary Hemostasis Disorders

Hereditary	Acquired
Factor VIII: Hemophilia A, VWD	Liver disease
Factor IX: Hemophilia B (Christmas Disease)	DIC
Factor XI	Vitamin K deficiency
Other factor deficiencies are rare	Acquired inhibitors (FVIII most common)

Hemophilia A (Factor VIII Deficiency)

Pathophysiology
- X-linked recessive, 1/5,000 males
- mild (>5% of normal factor level), moderate (1-5%), severe (<1%)

Clinical Features
- see Table 19 – *Signs and Symptoms of Disorders of Hemostasis*, H26
- older patients may also have HIV or HCV from contaminated blood products

Investigations
- prolonged aPTT, normal INR (PT)
- decreased Factor VIII (<40% of normal)

Treatment
- desmopressin (DDAVP®) in mild hemophilia A
- Factor VIII concentrate for:
  prophylaxis
  on-demand (i.e. to treat a bleed)
- anti-fibrinolytic agents (e.g. tranexamic acid)

Hemophilia B (Factor IX Deficiency)

- X-linked recessive, 1/30,000 males; approximately half have severe disease (factor IX activity <1% of normal)
- clinical and laboratory features identical to hemophilia A (except decreased Factor IX)
- treatment: Factor IX concentrate (prophylaxis or on-demand), anti-fibrinolytic agents

Factor XI Deficiency

- autosomal recessive; more common in Ashkenazi Jewish population
- usually mild, often diagnosed in adulthood
- Factor XI level does not correlate with bleeding risk – risk of bleeding correlates with a previous history or family history of bleeding
- treatment: antifibrinolytic agents, frozen plasma, Factor XI concentrate

Liver Disease

- see Gastroenterology, G32

Pathophysiology
- deficient synthesis of all factors except VIII (also made in endothelium)
- aberrant or diminished synthesis of fibrinogen (factor I)
- diminished synthesis of natural anticoagulants and altered regulation of fibrinolysis

Investigations
- peripheral blood film: target cells
- primary hemostasis affected
  - thrombocytopenia 2° to hypersplenism, nutritional deficiency, direct bone marrow toxicity related to alcohol, diminished production from chronic viral infections (e.g. HCV), decreased production of thrombopoietin
- secondary hemostasis affected
  - elevated INR (PT), aPTT and TT, low fibrinogen in end-stage liver disease

Treatment
- supportive, treat liver disease, blood products if active bleeding (frozen plasma, platelets, cryoprecipitate)

Investigations in Liver Disease
Factor V, VII, VIII. Expect decreased V and VII because they have the shortest half-life. Factor VIII will be normal or increased because it is produced in the endothelium

Vitamin K Deficiency

Vitamin K Dependent Factors
Vitamin K antagonists (e.g. warfarin) affect function of these factors:
"1972 Canada vs. Soviets"
X, IX, VII, II proteins C and S

Etiology
- drugs
  - vitamin K antagonist (e.g. Warfarin) – diminished production of functional Factors II, VII, IX, X, proteins C and S
  - antibiotics eradicating gut flora, altering vitamin K uptake
- poor diet (especially in alcoholics) e.g. prolonged fasting or starvation
- biliary obstruction
- chronic liver disease (decreased stores)
- fat malabsorption (e.g. celiac disease, disorders of bile or pancreatic secretion, intestinal disease, CF)
- hemorrhagic disease of newborn, see Pediatrics, P46

Investigations
- INR (PT) is elevated out of proportion to elevation of the aPTT
- decreased Factors II, VII, IX, X (vitamin K-dependent)

PT should improve within 24 h of adequately dosed vitamin K repletion (onset is in 6-12 h); if not, search for other causes

Treatment
- hold anticoagulant if vitamin K antagonist on board
- vitamin K PO if no active bleeding
- if bleeding, give vitamin K 10 mg IV (reversal may take up to 12 hrs)
- if life-threatening bleeding and vitamin K antagonist used, give prothrombin complex concentrate (PCC) or FP if PCC contraindicated
  - PCCs are contraindicated if there is a previous history of HIT (heparin is within the PCC product)

American Society of Hematology Choosing Wisely Recommendation
Do not administer plasma or prothrombin complex concentrates for non-emergent reversal of vitamin K antagonists (e.g. outside of the setting of major bleeding, intracranial hemorrhage, or anticipated emergent surgery)

Disseminated Intravascular Coagulation

Definition
- excessive, dysregulated release of plasmin and thrombin leading to intravascular coagulation and depletion of platelets, coagulation factors and fibrinogen
- risk of life-threatening hemorrhage or thromboembolism

Etiology
- occurs as a complication of many other severe medical, surgical or obstetrical conditions
- widespread endothelial damage and extensive inflammatory cytokine release

DIC is a spectrum which may include thrombosis, bleeding, or both

Factor Levels in Acquired Coagulopathies

Factor	Liver Disease	Vitamin K Def	DIC
V	↓	N	↓
VII	↓	↓	↓
VIII	N/↑	N	↓

Table 27. Etiology of DIC

Activation of Procoagulant Activity	Endothelial Injury	Reticuloendothelial Injury	Vascular Stasis	Other

Antiphospholipid antibody syndrome (APS)
Intravascular hemolysis
  Incompatible blood, malaria
Tissue injury
  Obstetric complications, trauma, burns, crush injuries
Malignancy
  Solid tumours, hematologic malignancies (especially APML)
Snake venom, fat embolism, heat stroke
	Infections/sepsis
	Vasculitis
	Metastatic adenocarcinoma
	Aortic aneurysm
	Giant hemangioma
		Liver disease
		Splenectomy
			Hypotension
			Hypovolemia
			Pulmonary embolus
				Acute hypoxia/acidosis (check lactate)

Important Etiologies of DIC

OMITS
Obstetric complications
Malignancy
Infection
Trauma
Shock

Clinical Features
- presence of both hemorrhage and clotting

Table 28. Clinical Features of DIC

Signs of Microvascular Thrombosis	Signs of Hemorrhagic Diathesis
Neurological: multifocal infarcts, delirium, coma, seizures **Skin:** focal ischemia, superficial gangrene **Renal:** oliguria, azotemia, cortical necrosis **Pulmonary:** ARDS **GI:** acute ulceration **RBC:** microangiopathic hemolysis	Bleeding from any site in the body (2° to decreased platelets and clotting factors) **Neurologic:** intracranial bleeding **Skin:** petechiae, ecchymosis, oozing from puncture sites **Renal:** hematuria **Mucosal:** gingival oozing, epistaxis, massive bleeding

Levels of fibrinogen can still be normal in DIC as it is an acute phase reactant.
Serial fibrinogen levels should be measured to see if there is a trending decrease along with an increase in D-dimer

Investigations
- primary hemostasis: decreased platelets
- secondary hemostasis: prolonged INR (PT), aPTT, TT, decreased fibrinogen and other factors
- fibrinolysis: increased FDPs or D-dimers, short euglobulin lysis time (i.e. accelerated fibrinolysis)
- extent of fibrin deposition: urine output, RBC fragmentation

Treatment
- recognize early and treat underlying disorder - supportive measures: hemodynamic and/or ventilator support, aggressive hydration, RBC transfusion if severe bleed
- in hemorrhage: replacement of hemostatic elements with platelet transfusion, frozen plasma, cryoprecipitate
    - British Hematology Guidelines:
        - maintain platelets >50 x10⁹, hemoglobin >80 g/L, calcium between 2.2-2.7 mmol/L, and avoid hypothermia
        - 4-5 units of FP if INR >1.5 or aPTT >38
        - 10 units of cryoprecipitate if fibrinogen <1 g/L
        - 1 adult dose of buffy-coat platelets if <10 x10⁹ (<20 if febrile, <50 before invasive procedure)
- in thrombotic phase: UFH or LMWH in critically ill, non-bleeding patients

Differential Diagnosis of Elevated D-Dimer
- Arterial thromboembolic disease (MI, CVA, acute limb ischemia, AFib, intracardiac thrombus)
- Venous thromboembolic disease (DVT, PE)
- DIC
- Preeclampsia and eclampsia
- Abnormal fibrinolysis; use of thrombolytic agents
- Cardiovascular disease, CHF
- Severe infection/sepsis/inflammation
- Surgery/trauma (tissue ischemia, necrosis)
- Systemic inflammatory response syndrome
- Vasoocclusive episode of sickle cell disease
- Severe liver disease
- Malignancy
- Renal disease (nephrotic syndrome, acute/chronic renal failure)
- Normal pregnancy
- Venous malformation

Table 29. Screening Test Abnormalities in Coagulopathies

Increased INR Only	Increased PTT Only	Both Increased
Warfarin Vitamin K deficiency Factor VII deficiency Liver disease Factor VII inhibitors	Hemophilia A and B Heparin Antiphospholipid Ab Intrinsic factor inhibitors (e.g. FVIII) Factor XI and XII deficiency	Prothrombin deficiency Severe fibrinogen deficiency Factor V and X deficiency Severe liver disease Factor V and X, prothrombin, and fibrinogen inhibitors Excessive anticoagulation Severe vitamin K deficiency

Hypercoagulable Disorders

Hypercoagulability Workup – Venous Thrombosis
- work up for malignancy is suggested in the event of abnormal blood work, constitutional symptoms or physical exam suggestive of cancer
    - work up for hypercoagulable state is controversial and should only be done if it will alter treatment decisions
    - recommendations for a hypercoagulable work up include:
        - patients with recurrent or multiple thrombosis only if it will change management plans
        - warfarin-induced skin necrosis or neonatal purpura fulminans (protein C or S deficiency)
        - consider for patients with a family history of VTE who are considering OCP use
        - consider for patients who present with thrombosis at an unusual venous site only if it will change management plans
    - arterial thrombotic events have only been proven to be associated with APLA, HIT, JAK2 MPNs, and PNH

American Society of Hematology Choosing Wisely Recommendations
1. Do not test for thrombophilia in adult patients with venous thromboembolism occurring in the setting of major transient risk factors (surgery, trauma, or prolonged immobility)
2. Do not use inferior vena cava filters routinely in patients with acute venous thromboembolism

- work up
  - initial
    - CBC, blood smear, coagulation studies, liver/renal function, urinalysis, hemolysis markers (if anemic)
    - malignancy history, age appropriate cancer screening (see sidebar)
    - serology: antiphospholipid antibodies (APLA)
  - post-treatment (or ≥6 weeks, as protein levels depleted/consumed by clot)
    - antithrombin (not on heparin)
    - proteins C, S (not on warfarin)
- note: most of these tests do not change management, and a negative test does not rule out a hypercoagulable state
  - thus more focus on the reversible/treatable causes (APLA, cancer, etc.)

SELECTED CAUSES OF HYPERCOAGULABILITY LEADING TO VENOUS THROMBOEMBOLISM

Activated Protein C Resistance (Factor V Leiden)
- most common cause of hereditary thrombophilia
- 3-7% of European Caucasian population are heterozygotes
- point mutation in the Factor V gene (R506Q) results in resistance to inactivation of Factor Va by activated protein C

Prothrombin Gene Mutation (PT) G20210A
- 1-3% of European Caucasian population are heterozygotes
- G to A transposition at nucleotide position 20210 of the prothrombin gene promoter region results in increased levels of prothrombin, thus increased thrombin generation

Protein C and Protein S Deficiency
- protein C inactivates Factor Va and VIIIa using protein S as a cofactor
- protein C deficiency
  - homozygous or compound heterozygous: neonatal purpura fulminans
  - heterozygous
    - type I: decreased protein C levels
    - type II: decreased protein C activity
  - acquired: liver disease, sepsis, DIC, warfarin, certain chemotherapeutic agents
  - 1/3 of patients with warfarin necrosis have underlying protein C deficiency
- protein S deficiency
  - type I: decreased free and total protein S levels
  - type II: decreased protein S activity
  - type III: decreased free protein S levels
  - acquired: liver disease, DIC, pregnancy, nephrotic syndrome, inflammatory conditions, warfarin

Antithrombin Deficiency
- antithrombin slowly inactivates thrombin in the absence of heparin, rapidly inactivates thrombin in the presence of heparin
- autosomal dominant inheritance, urinary losses in nephrotic syndrome, or reduced synthesis in liver disease
- diagnosis must be made outside window of acute thrombosis and anticoagulation treatment (acute thrombosis, heparin, systemic disease all decrease antithrombin levels)
- deficiency may result in resistance to unfractionated heparin (LMWH may be considered, with monitoring of anti-Xa levels)
  - heparin resistance: suspect if >35,000 units of UFH required during 24 hour use

Elevated Factor VIII Levels
- an independent marker of increased incident and recurrent thrombotic risk, but levels can also be increased in numerous states as an acute phase reactant, therefore its clinical use is controversial

Congenital Dysfibrinogenemia
- may predispose to thromboembolic disease, bleeding or both

Disorders of Fibrinolysis
- includes congenital plasminogen deficiency, tissue plasminogen activator deficiency, although association with VTE risk is not clear

Antiphospholipid Antibody Syndrome (APS)
- definition: ≥1 clinical and ≥1 laboratory criteria
  - clinical: thrombosis, recurrent (>3) early pregnancy losses <10 weeks, one late fetal loss ≥10 weeks (morphologically normal), or premature birth before 34 wk due to (pre)eclampsia or placental insufficiency
  - laboratory (must be confirmed on two occasions, tested ≥12 wks apart): anticardiolipin antibodies, anti-β2 glycoprotein-I antibody, lupus anticoagulant

Common Causes of Hypercoagulability

CALM APES
Protein **C** deficiency
Antiphospholipid **A**b
Factor V **L**eiden
Malignancy
Antithrombin deficiency
Prothrombin G20210A
Increased Factor **V**III (Eight)
Protein **S** deficiency

Causes of Both Venous and Arterial Thrombosis include:
- Antiphospholipid antibodies
- Myeloproliferative neoplasms
- Heparin-induced thrombocytopenia
- Distal venous clot with patent foramen ovale
- Paroxysmal nocturnal hemoglobinuria

Protein C, protein S, and ATIII are decreased during acute thrombosis – therefore to test for deficiency, must be tested outside of this time period

Malignancy is a common cause of acquired hypercoagulability
Work up should include:
- Complete history and physical
- Routine blood work
- Urinalysis
- CXR
- Age appropriate screening: mammogram, Pap, PSA, colonoscopy
- Close follow-up
- No benefit with CT imaging

Although lupus anticoagulant prolongs PTT, this is a misnomer, as its main clinical feature is thrombosis

- mechanism: not well understood, antibodies interact with platelet membrane phospholipid causing increased activation; can also interfere with thrombin regulation, fibrinolysis, and inhibit the protein C pathway
- see Rheumatology, RH12

Venous Thromboembolism

Definition
- thrombus formation and subsequent inflammatory response in a superficial or deep vein
- superficial thrombophlebitis, deep vein thrombosis (DVT), and pulmonary embolism (PE)
- thrombi propagate in the direction of blood flow (commonly originating in calf veins)
- more common in lower extremity than upper extremity
- incidence ~1% if age >60 yr
- most important sequelae are pulmonary embolism (~50% chance with proximal DVT) and chronic venous insufficiency

Etiology (Virchow's Triad)
- endothelial damage
  - exposes endothelium to prompt hemostasis
  - leads to decreased inhibition of coagulation and local fibrinolysis
- venous stasis
  - immobilization (post-MI, CHF, stroke, post-operative) inhibits clearance and dilution of coagulation factors
- hypercoagulability
  - inherited (see *Hypercoagulable Disorders*, H33)
  - acquired
    - age (risk increases with age)
    - surgery (especially orthopedic, thoracic, GI, and GU)
    - trauma (especially fractures of spine, pelvis, femur or tibia, spinal cord injury)
    - neoplasms (especially lung, pancreas, colon, rectum, kidney, and prostate)
    - blood dyscrasias (myeloproliferative neoplasms, especially PV, ET), PNH, hyperviscosity (multiple myeloma, polycythemia, leukemia, sickle cell disease)
    - prolonged immobilization (CHF, stroke, MI, leg injury)
    - hormone related (pregnancy, OCP, HRT, SERMs)
    - APS
    - heart failure (risk of DVT greatest with right heart failure and peripheral edema)
- idiopathic (10-20% are later found to have cancer)

Clinical Features of DVT
- absence of physical findings does not rule out disease
- unilateral leg edema, erythema, warmth, and tenderness purple-blue
- palpable cord (thrombosed vein)
- phlegmasia alba dolens (white appearance) and phlegmasia cerula dolens (acute pain and edema) with massive thrombosis
- Homan's sign (pain with foot dorsiflexion) is unreliable

Differential Diagnosis of DVT
- muscle strain or tear, lymphangitis or lymph obstruction, venous valvular insufficiency, ruptured popliteal cysts, cellulitis, arterial occlusive disease

Investigations for DVT
- D-dimer test only useful to rule out DVT if negative with low clinical suspicion of disease and no other acute medical issues
- doppler ultrasound is most useful diagnostic test for DVT
  - sensitivity and specificity for proximal DVT ~95%
  - sensitivity for calf DVT ~70%
- other non-invasive tests include MRI and impedence plethysmography
- venography is the gold standard, but is expensive, invasive, and higher risk
- CTPA or V/Q scan if PE suspected

Post-Thrombotic Syndrome
- development of chronic venous stasis signs and symptoms secondary to a deep venous thrombosis
- symptoms: pain, venous dilatation, edema, pigmentation, skin changes, venous ulcers
- clinical severity can be estimated based on the Villalta score
- large impact on quality of life following a DVT
- treatment: extremity elevation, exercise, continuous compression stockings, intermittent pneumatic compression therapy, skin/ulcer care
- for clinical features and treatment of PE, see Respirology, R18

Risk of VTE in Hospitalized Patients Receiving Ineffective Antithrombotic Therapy

Risk Factor	RR (95% CI)	P-value
Age >75 yr	1.79 (1.18-2.71)	0.007
Cancer	1.58 (1.01-2.51)	
Previous VTE	1.67 (1.01-2.77)	0.08
Obesity	0.94 (0.59-1.51)	0.91
Hormone therapy	0.51 (0.08-3.38)	0.70
Heart failure	.08 (0.72-1.62)	0.82
NYHA III	0.89 (0.55-1.43)	0.72
NYHA IV	1.48 (0.84-2.6)	0.27
Acute infectious disease	1.50 (1.00-2.26)	0.06
Acute rheumatic disease	1.45 (0.84-2.50)	0.27

Source: *JAMA* 2004;164:963-968

Virchow's Triad
- Endothelial damage
- Stasis
- Hypercoagulability

Wells' Score for DVT
Criteria (Score)
- Paralysis, paresis, or recent orthopedic casting of lower extremity (1)
- Recently bedridden (>3 d) or major surgery within past 4 wk (1)
- Localized tenderness in deep vein system (1)
- Swelling of entire leg (1)
- Calf swelling >3 cm than other leg (measured 10 cm below the tibial tuberosity) (1)
- Pitting edema greater in the symptomatic leg (1)
- Collateral non-varicose superficial veins (1)
- Active cancer or cancer treated within 6 mo (1)
- Alternative diagnosis more likely than DVT (e.g. Baker's cyst, cellulitis, muscle damage, superficial venous thrombosis) (-2)

Total Score Interpretation
3-8: High probability, 1-2: Moderate probability, -2-0: Low probability

Low-Molecular-Weight Heparin vs. Coumarin for the Prevention of Recurrent Venous Thromboembolism in Patients with Cancer
NEJM 2003;349:146-153
Study: RCT comparing the efficacy of LMWH (dalteparin) with an oral anti-coagulant agent (coumarin) in preventing recurrent thrombosis in patients with cancer.
Methods: Patients with cancer who had acute, symptomatic proximal DVT, PE, or both were randomly assigned to either dalteparin or coumarin treatment for 6 mo.
Results: 27 of 336 patients in the dalteparin group had recurrent VTE versus 53 of 336 patients in the coumarin group (hazard ratio, 0.48; p=0.002). The probability of recurrent thromboembolism at 6 mo was 9% and 17% in dalteparin and coumarin groups respectively. There was no significant difference in bleeding rates. The mortality rate was 39% in the dalteparin group and 41% in the coumarin group.
Conclusions: In patients with cancer and acute VTE, dalteparin was more effective than coumarin in decreasing the risk of recurrent thromboembolism without increasing the risk of bleeding.

Duration of Treatment with Vitamin K Antagonists in Symptomatic Venous Thromboembolism
Cochrane DB Syst Rev 2009;CD001367
Study: Meta-analysis of 8 RCTs (2,994 patients) comparing different durations of treatment with vitamin K antagonists in patients with symptomatic VTE.
Results: In patients treated with vitamin K antagonists for a prolonged period, the reduction in risk of recurrent VTE remained consistent regardless of the period of time since the index event (OR 0.18; 95% CI 0.13-0.26). In addition, there was no observed excess of VTE recurrences following cessation of prolonged treatment (i.e. rebound phenomenon) (OR 1.24; 95% CI 0.91-1.69). However, patients who received prolonged treatment had a persistent increase in their risk of major bleeding complications (OR 2.61; 95% CI 1.48-4.61).
Conclusion: Prolonged treatment with vitamin K antagonists leads to a consistent reduction in the risk of recurrent VTE for as long as therapy is continued. Therapy should be discontinued when the risk of harm from major bleeding (which remains constant over time) is of greater concern than the absolute risk of recurrent VTE (which declines over time). No specific recommendation was made regarding optimal duration of treatment.

Common Medications that Interact with Warfarin
- Acetaminophen (interference with vitamin K metabolism)
- Allopurinol
- NSAIDs (GI injury)
- Fluconazole
- Metronidazole
- Sulfamethoxazole
- Tamoxifen

Initiation of Warfarin Therapy Requires Bridging with Heparin Therapy for 4-5 Days
- 10 mg loading dose (for example) of warfarin causes a precipitous decline in protein C levels in first 36 h resulting in a transient hypercoagulable state
- Warfarin decreases Factor VII levels in first 48 h, INR is prolonged (most sensitive to Factor VII levels), however full antithrombotic effect is not achieved until Factor IX, X, and II are sufficiently reduced (occurs after ~4 d)

Low Risk Surgical Patients
<40 yr, no risk factors for VTE, general anesthetic (GA) <30 min, minor elective, abdominal, or thoracic surgery

Moderate Risk Surgical Patients
>40 yr, >1 risk factor for VTE, GA >30 min

High Risk Surgical Patients
>40 yr, surgery for malignancy or lower extremity orthopedic surgery lasting >30 min, inhibitor deficiency, or other risk factor

High Risk Medical Patients
Heart failure, severe respiratory disease, ischemic stroke and lower limb paralysis, confined to bed and have
>1 additional risk factor (e.g. active cancer, previous VTE, sepsis, acute neurologic disease, IBD)

Approach to Treatment of Venous Thromboembolism

Purpose
- prevent further clot extension (3 mo duration is optimal)
- prevent acute pulmonary embolism (occurs in up to 50% of untreated patients)
- reduce the risk of recurrent thrombosis (duration depends on presence of other risk factors)
- treatment of massive ileofemoral thrombosis with acute lower limb ischemia and/or venous gangrene (phlegmasia cerulea dolens)
- limit development of late complications (e.g. postphlebitic syndrome, chronic venous insufficiency, and chronic thromboembolic pulmonary HTN)

Initial Treatment
- low molecular weight heparin (LMWH)
  - administered SC, at least as effective as UFH with a lower bleeding risk
  - advantages: predictable dose response and fixed dosing schedule; lab monitoring not required; <1% HIT; safe and effective outpatient therapy
  - disadvantages: only partially reversible by protamine, long-term use associated with osteoporosis Costly!
  - renally cleared – must adjust dose in patients with renal dysfunction
- unfractionated heparin (UFH)
  - in patient with average risk of bleed; use hospital-based nomograms that use bleeding risk and patient weight to determine appropriate dose
  - advantages: rapidly reversible by protamine
  - disadvantages: must monitor aPTT or heparin levels with adjustment of dose to reach therapeutic level (~2x normal value); monitor platelet counts for development of HIT
- alternatives to LMWH and UFH
  - direct thrombin inhibitors (hirudin, lepirudin, argatroban), direct factor Xa inhibitors (apixaban, rivaroxaban)
  - thrombolytic drugs (e.g. streptokinase, tPA) reserved for acute limb/life-threatening thrombosis, and low bleeding risk

Long-Term Treatment
- anticoagulation therapy
  - warfarin
  - standard treatment; should be initiated with heparin overlap: dual therapy for at least 48 hours with INR > 2, due to initial prothrombotic state secondary to warfarin's inhibition of natural anticoagulants protein C/S, half life of vitamin K factors and risk of warfarin-induced skin necrosis
  - INR: warfarin dosed to maintain INR at 2-3, monitor twice weekly for 1-2wk. Discontinue heparin after INR>2.0 for 2 consecutive days
  - direct oral anticoagulants (DOACs)
    - apixaban or rivaroxaban; with no laboratory monitoring required, patients with CrCl > 50 ml/min
    - dabigatran (factor IIa inhibitor): LMWH or IV heparin for at least 5-10 days before initiating dabigatran, patients with CrCl >30 ml/min
    - important drug interactions to consider for DOACs (no relevant food interactions however)
  - cancer patients: LMWH more effective than warfarin at preventing recurrence of venous thrombosis in cancer patients
- duration of anticoagulant treatment
  - provoked VTE with transient risk factor: 3 mo
  - provoked VTE with ongoing risk factor: consider indefinite therapy with annual reassessment
  - first unprovoked VTE: at least 3mo, subsequent reassessment
  - unprovoked proximal DVT or PE: consider indefinite therapy with annual reassessment
  - second unprovoked VTE: consider indefinite therapy
  - cancer-associated DVT: at least 3 mo, longer if continued evidence of cancer
- IVC filters
  - temporary filter indicated only if acute DVT (<4 wk) with significant contraindications to anticoagulant therapy (i.e. active bleeding) or if require interruption of anticoagulation (i.e. for urgent surgery)
  - must be retrieved once safe to do so as filter is pro-thrombotic in the long-term (consider anticoagulation if not retrieved)
- special considerations
  - pregnancy: treat with LMWH during pregnancy, then LMWH or warfarin for 6 wk post-partum (minimum total anticoagulation time of 3-6 mo, but must include 6 wks post-partum, as this is a high risk period); avoid warfarin in pregnancy due to teratogenicity
  - surgery: avoid elective surgery in the first three months after a venous thromboembolic event
    - pre-operatively: IV heparin may be used up to 4-6 h pre-operatively
    - perioperatively: warfarin or DOACs discontinued for at least 3-5 d pre-operatively (consider mechanism of drug clearance)
      - surgery safe when INR <1.5 off of warfarin, normal PTT on dabigatran, drug-specific Xa level at zero for apixaban/ rivaroxaban/LMWH, normal PTT on IV unfractionated heparin

- post-operatively: IV heparin, LMWH, DOAC can be used for anticoagulation (consult with surgeon prior to re-initiation)
- for patients at high risk for thromboembolism (VTE <12 wk, recurrent VTE, antiphospholipid antibody syndrome, atrial fibrillation with prior stroke, mechanical heart valve), IV heparin or LMWH (bridging) should be given before and after the procedure while the INR is below 2.0

Prophylaxis
- see sidebar
- consider for those with a moderate to high risk of thrombosis without contraindications
- non-pharmacological measures include: early ambulation, elastic compression stockings (TEDs), intermittent pneumatic compression (IPC)
- UFH 5,000 IU SC bid, UFH 5,000 IU SC tid or LMWH as per hospital protocol (e.g. enoxaparin 40 mg SC daily, dalteparin 5000 U SC qid), DOACs for orthopedic surgery thromboprophylaxis

Contraindications and Adverse Reactions of Anticoagulant Therapy
- absolute: active bleeding, severe bleeding diathesis, or platelets <20-30 x 10^9/L (<20,000/mm³), intracranial bleeding, neuro or ocular surgery within <10 d
- relative: mild-moderate neurologic diathesis or thrombocytopenia, brain metastases, recent major trauma, major abdominal surgery within past 2 d, GI/GU bleed within 14 d, endocarditis, severe HTN (sBP >200 or dBP >120), recent stroke

Table 30. Contraindications of Anticoagulant Therapy

Absolute Contraindications to Treatment	Relative Contraindications to Treatment
Active bleeding	Mild-moderate bleeding diathesis or thrombocytopenia
Severe bleeding diathesis or platelet count <20 x 10⁹/L (<20,000/mm³)	Brain metastases
	Recent major trauma
Intracranial bleeding	Recent stroke
Neurosurgery or ocular surgery within 10 d	Major abdominal surgery within past 2 d
	GI/GU bleeding within 1-4 d
	Endocarditis
	Severe hypertension (sBP >200 or dBP >120)

Treatment of Pulmonary Embolism
- see Respirology, R18

Hematologic Malignancies and Related Disorders

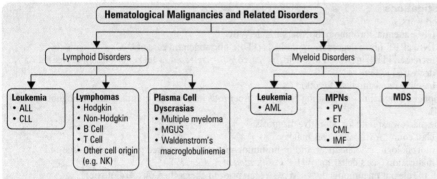

Figure 14. Overview of hematologic malignancies and related disorders

ALL = acute lymphocytic leukemia; AML = acute myeloid leukemia; CLL = chronic lymphocytic leukemia; CML = chronic myeloid leukemia; ET = essential thrombocythemia; IMF = idiopathic myelofibrosis; MDS = myelodysplastic syndromes; MGUS = monoclonal gammopathy of unknown significance; MPN = myeloproliferative neoplasms; PV = polycythemia vera

Myeloid Malignancies

Acute Myeloid Leukemia

Definition
- rapidly progressive malignancy characterized by failure of myeloid cells to differentiate beyond blast stage

Epidemiology
- incidence increases with age; median age of onset is 65 yr old; 80% of acute adult leukemias
- accounts for 10-15% of childhood leukemias

Typical Age of Presentation of Leukemias
- ALL: Children and older adults
- CML: 40-60 yr
- AML, CLL: >60 yr

Leukemia: malignant cells arise in bone marrow and may spread elsewhere (including blood, lymph nodes, and lymphoid tissue)
Lymphoma: malignant cells arise in lymph nodes and lymphoid tissues and may spread elsewhere (including blood and bone marrow) **BUT** the location where the malignant cells are found does not solely define the type of hematologic malignancy – classified based on the characteristics of the cell (histology, histochemistry, immunophenotyping, cytogenetics, molecular changes)

Acute Leukemia
Definition (WHO): presence of 20% blast cells or greater in bone marrow at presentation
Classification: divided into myeloid (AML) and lymphoid (ALL) depending on whether blasts are myeloblasts or lymphoblasts, respectively

2008 WHO Classification of AML and Related Neoplasms
- AML with recurrent genetic abnormalities
- AML with myelodysplasia-related changes
- Therapy-related myeloid neoplasms
- Myeloid sarcoma
- Myeloid proliferations related to Down syndrome
- Blastic plasmacytoid dendritic cell neoplasm
- AML, not otherwise specified (equivalent FAB classification)
  - Undifferentiated (M1)
  - Myeloblastic (M2)
  - Promyelocytic (M3)
  - Myelomonocytic (M4)
  - Monocytic (M5)
  - Erythroleukemic (M6)
  - Megakaryocytic (M7)
  - Acute basophilic leukemia
  - Acute panmyelosis with myelofibrosis

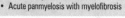

Auer rods are pathognomonic for AML

Risk Factors
- myelodysplastic syndromes (MDS), benzene, radiation, Down Syndrome, alkylating agents as treatment for previous malignancy

Pathophysiology
- etiology subdivided into
  - primary: *de novo*
  - secondary: hematologic malignancies (e.g. myeloproliferative disorders and MDS) or previous chemotherapeutic agents (e.g. alkylating agents)
- uncontrolled growth of blasts in marrow leads to
  - suppression of normal hematopoietic cells
  - appearance of blasts in peripheral blood – risk of leukostasis
  - accumulation of blasts in other sites (e.g. skin, gums)
  - metabolic consequences; tumour lysis syndrome

Clinical Features
- anemia, thrombocytopenia (associated with DIC in promyelocytic leukemia), neutropenia (even with normal WBC), leads to infections, fever
- accumulation of blast cells in marrow
  - skeletal pain, bony tenderness (especially sternum)
- organ infiltration
  - gingival hypertrophy (particularly myelomonocytic leukemia) – may present to dentist first
  - hepatosplenomegaly (in ALL)
  - lymphadenopathy (not marked in ALL)
  - gonads (in ALL)
  - skin: leukemia cutis or myeloid sarcoma
  - eyes: hemorrhages and/or whitish plaques, Roth spots, cotton wool spots, vision changes (uncommon)
- leukostasis/hyperleukocytosis syndrome (medical emergency)
  - large numbers of blasts interfere with circulation and lead to hypoxia and hemorrhage – can cause diffuse pulmonary infiltrates, CNS bleeding, respiratory distress, altered mental status, priapism
  - associated with AML more than ALL
- metabolic effects; aggravated by treatment (rare)
  - increased uric acid $\rightarrow$ nephropathy, gout
  - release of phosphate $\rightarrow$ decreased Ca^{2+}, decreased Mg^{2+}
  - release of procoagulants $\rightarrow$ DIC (higher risk in acute promyelocytic leukemia)
- decreased or normal K^+ before treatment, increased K^+ after treatment (from lysed cells)

Investigations
- blood work
  - CBC: anemia, thrombocytopenia, variable WBC
  - INR, aPTT, fibrin degradation products (FDP), fibrinogen (in case of DIC)
  - increased LDH, increased uric acid, increased PO_4^{3-} (released by leukemic blasts), decreased Ca^{2+}, decreased K^+
  - baseline renal and liver function tests
- peripheral blood film – circulating blasts with Auer rods (azurophilic granules) are pathognomonic for AML
- bone marrow aspirate for definitive diagnosis
  - blast count: AML >20% (normal is <5%)
  - morphologic, cytochemical, and/or immunotypic features are used to establish lineage and maturation (see sidebar for *WHO classification of AML*, H37)
- CXR to rule out pneumonia, ECG, MUGA scan prior to chemotherapy (cardiotoxic)

Treatment
- mainstay of treatment is chemotherapy (rapidly fatal without treatment)
- all AML subtypes are treated similarly, except acute promyelocytic leukemia (APL) with t(15:17) translocation
- all-trans-retinoic acid (ATRA) added to induce differentiation; arsenic trioxide + ATRA combination therapy for APL is non-inferior to traditional chemotherapy
- treatment strategy
  1. **Induction:** chemotherapy to induce complete remission of AML (see sidebar)
     - several possible regimens (e.g. cytarabine with anthracycline [daunorubicin])
     - patients with poor response to initial induction therapy – worse prognosis
     - must ensure reversal of DIC, platelet transfusions if <10
  2. **Consolidation:** to prevent recurrence
     - intensive consolidation chemotherapy
     - stem cell transplantation – autologous or allogeneic (younger patients with better performance status)
- consider acceleration with hematopoietic growth factors (e.g. G-CSF) if severe infection develops

Cure: survival that parallels age-matched population
Complete Remission: tumour load below threshold of detectable disease (normal peripheral blood film, normal bone marrow with <5% blasts, normal clinical state)

- supportive care
    - screening for infection via regular C&S of urine, stool, sputum, oropharynx, catheter sites, perianal area
    - fever: C&S of all orifices, CXR, start antibiotics
    - platelet and RBC transfusions (irradiated to prevent transfusion-related GVHD) ± EPO
    - prevention and treatment of metabolic abnormalities
        - allopurinol, rasburicase for prevention of hyperuricemia

Prognosis
- achievement of first remission
    - 70-80% if ≤60 yr old, 50% if >60 yr old
    - median survival 12-24 mo
    - prognosis is most related to 1) cytogenetics; classified as favourable, intermediate, or adverse and 2) molecular studies (i.e. NPM1+/FLT3- mutations)
    - prognosis depends on cytogenetics, age, performance status, prior cytotoxic agents or radiation therapy

Myelodysplastic Syndromes

Definition
- heterogeneous group of malignant stem cell disorders characterized by dysplastic and ineffective blood cell production resulting in peripheral cytopenias, and a variable risk of transformation to acute leukemias
- syndromes defined according to World Health Organization (WHO) classifications (see sidebar)

Pathophysiology
- disordered maturation: ineffective hematopoiesis despite presence of adequate numbers of progenitor cells in bone marrow (usually hypercellular); formed elements sometimes exhibit qualitative functional defects
- intramedullary apoptosis: programmed cell death within bone marrow
  both processes lead to reduced mature cells in periphery
- <30% develop AML

Risk Factors
- elderly, post-chemotherapy, exposures (benzene, tobacco, radiation), inherited genetic abnormalities
- occurs in 4/100,000 patients >60 yr old

Clinical Features
- insidious onset: associated with pancytopenia; most patients asymptomatic at diagnosis
- infections and bleeding out of proportion with peripheral blood counts

Investigations
- diagnosed by
    - anemia ± thrombocytopenia ± neutropenia
    - CBC and peripheral blood film
    - RBC: usually macrocytic with oval shaped red cells (macro-ovalocytes), decreased reticulocyte count
    - WBC: decreased granulocytes and abnormal morphology (e.g. bi-lobed or unsegmented nuclei = Pelger abnormality)
    - platelets: thrombocytopenia, abnormalities of size and cytoplasm (e.g. giant hypogranular platelets)
- bone marrow aspirate and biopsy with cytogenetic analysis required for definitive diagnosis
    - bone marrow: dysplastic and often normocellular/hypercellular
    - cytogenetics: high risk include partial or total loss of chromosomes 5, 7, and complex (>3 abnormalities)

Treatment
- **low risk** of transformation to acute leukemia (IPSS-R Very Low or Low)
    - erythropoietin stimulating agents weekly is first line in reducing transfusion requirements (EPO level must be <500)
    - lf 5q deletion based on cytogenics: lenalidomide PO
    - supportive care: RBC and platelet transfusion (consider iron chelation if frequent RBC transfusions)
- **high risk** of transformation to acute leukemia (IPSS-R Intermediate, High or Very High)
    - supportive care
    - stem cell transplantation if age <65 yr
    - epigenetic therapy: DNA methyltransferase inhibitors (e.g. 5-azacytidine), histone deacetylase inhibitors

Prognosis
- Revised International Prognostic Scoring System (IPSS-R) uses 5 factors to estimate mean survival:
    - cytology, % bone marrow blasts, hemoglobin, platelets, absolute neutrophil count
    - based on the calculated score, a patient's MDS prognostic risk is "Very Low", "Low", "Intermediate", "High", or "Very High" with a mean survival of 8.7, 5.3, 3.0, 1.6, and 0.8 yr, respectively

2008 WHO MDS Classification
- Refractory cytopenia with unilineage dysplasia
    - Refractory anemia
    - Refractory neutropenia
    - Refractory thrombocytopenia
- Refractory anemia with ringed sideroblasts (RARS)
- Refractory cytopenia with multilineage dysplasia (RCMD)
- Refractory cytopenia with multilineage dysplasia and ringed sideroblasts (RCMD-RS)
- Refractory anemia with excess blasts (RAEB)
- Myelodysplasic syndrome with isolated del (5q)
- Myelodysplasia unclassified (seen in cases of megakaryocyte dysplasia with fibrosis and others)
- Childhood myelodysplastic syndrome

MDS is a cause of macrocytic anemia

Use of Epoetin and Darbepoetin in Patients with Cancer
Blood 2008;111:25-41
Clinical practice guideline update by American Societies of Hematology and Clinical Oncology (2007).
Initial Recommendations
1. Initiate an erythropoiesis-stimulating agent (ESA) when hemoglobin (Hb) is 100 g/L (10 g/dL) in patients with palliative chemotherapy-associated anemia to decrease the need for transfusions.
2. Discontinue ESAs when patient not responding to treatment beyond 6-8 wk.
3. Monitor iron stores and supplement iron intake for ESA-treated patients when necessary.
4. Use ESAs cautiously with chemotherapy or in patients with an elevated risk for thromboembolic complications.
5. It is not recommended that ESA be used for therapy in patients with cancer who are not receiving chemotherapy, as it increases thromboembolic risks and lowers survival rate. Patients with low-risk myelodysplasia are an exception.

Myelodysplastic Syndromes
ineffective maturation
Myeloproliferative Neoplasms
overproduction of mature cells

Myeloproliferative Neoplasms

Definition
- clonal myeloid stem cell abnormalities leading to overproduction of one or more cell lines (leading to abnormalities in erythrocytes, platelets, and other cells of myeloid lineage)

Epidemiology
- mainly middle-aged and older patients (peak 60-80 yr)

Prognosis
- may develop marrow fibrosis with time
- all disorders may progress to AML

Table 31. Chronic Myeloproliferative Disorders

	CML	PV	IMF	ET
Hct	↓/N	↑↑	↓	N
WBC	↑↑	↑	↑/↓	N
Plt	↑/↓	↑	↑/↓	↑↑↑
Marrow Fibrosis	±	±	+++	±
Splenomegaly	+++	+	+++	+
Hepatomegaly	+	+	++	–
Genetic Association	bcr-abl mut. (95+%)	JAK2 mut. (96%)	JAK2 mut. (~50%) CALR mut (~30%)	JAK2 mut. (~50%) CALR mut (~30%)

CML = chronic myeloid leukemia; ET = essential thrombocythemia; IMF = idiopathic myelofibrosis; PV = polycythemia vera CALR = Calreticulin

Chronic Myeloid Leukemia

Definition
- myeloproliferative disorder characterized by increased proliferation of the granulocytic cell line without the loss of their capacity to differentiate

Basophilia is uncommon in other medical conditions

Epidemiology
- occurs in any age group (mostly middle age to elderly) with a median age of 65 yr

Pathophysiology
- Philadelphia chromosome (Ph)
  - translocation between chromosomes 9 and 22
  - the c-abl proto-oncogene is translocated from chromosome 9 to "breakpoint cluster region" (bcr) of chromosome 22 to produce bcr-abl fusion gene, an active tyrosine kinase

Clinical Features
- 3 clinical phases
  - **chronic phase:** 85% diagnosed here
    - few blasts (<10%) in peripheral film
    - ± slightly elevated eosinophils and basophils
    - no significant symptoms
  - **accelerated phase:** impaired neutrophil differentiation
    - circulating blasts (10-19%) with increasing peripheral basophils (pruritus)
    - CBC: thrombocytopenia <100 x 10⁹/L
    - cytogenetic evidence of clonal evolution
    - worsening constitutional symptoms and splenomegaly (extramedullary hematopoiesis)
  - **blast crisis:** more aggressive course, blasts fail to differentiate
    - blasts (>20%) in peripheral blood or bone marrow; reflective of acute leukemia (1/3 ALL, 2/3 AML)
- clinical presentation
  - 20-50% of patients are asymptomatic when diagnosed (incidental lab finding)
  - nonspecific symptoms
    - fatigue, weight loss, malaise, excessive sweating, fever
  - secondary to splenic involvement
    - early satiety, LUQ pain/fullness, shoulder tip pain (referred)
    - splenomegaly (most common physical finding)
  - anemia
  - bleeding: secondary to platelet dysfunction
  - pruritus, PUD: secondary to increased blood histamine
  - leukostasis, priapism, encephalopathy (rare): secondary to very elevated WBC (rare)

Investigations
- elevated WBC, decreased/normal RBC, increased/decreased platelets, increased basophils
  - WBC differential shows a bimodal distribution, with predominance of myelocytes and neutrophils

- peripheral blood film
  - leukoerythroblastic picture (immature red cells and granulocytes present, e.g. myelocytes and normoblasts)
  - presence of different mid-stage progenitor cells differentiates it from AML
- bone marrow
  - myeloid hyperplasia with left shift, increased megakaryocytes, mild fibrosis
- molecular and cytogenetic studies of bone marrow or peripheral blood for Philadelphia chromosome
- abdominal imaging for spleen size

Treatment
- **symptomatic**
  - allopurinol and antihistamines
- **chronic phase**
  - imatinib mesylate inhibits proliferation and induces apoptosis by inhibiting tyrosine kinase activity in cells positive for bcr-abl
    - if loss of response or intolerance (~40%), trial of 2nd generation TKIs: dasatinib or nilotinib
    - dasatinib and nilotinib may also be considered for first line management
  - interferon-α: may improve response to tyrosine kinase inhibitors; typically now only used for pregnant patients
  - hydroxyurea in palliative setting to reduce WBC
- **accelerated phase or blast phase**
  - refer for clinical trial or 2nd/3rd generation TKI and prepare for allogeneic stem cell transplant patients, in blast phase typically get standard AML induction
- stem cell transplantation may be curative: to be considered in young patients who do not meet therapeutic milestones
- treatment success is monitored based on therapeutic milestones
  - hematologic: improved WBC and platelet counts, reduced basophils
  - cytogenetic: undetectable Philadelphia-chromosome in the bone marrow
  - molecular: reduction/absence of *bcr-abl* transcripts in periphery and marrow

Prognosis
- survival dependent on response
  - those achieving complete cytogenetic response (CCR) on imatinib by 18 mo of therapy: 6 yr overall survival >90%
  - those who do NOT achieve CCR on imatinib: 6 yr overall survival of 66%
- acute phase (blast crisis – usually within 3-5 yr)
  - 2/3 develop a picture similar to AML
    - unresponsive to remission induction
  - 1/3 develop a picture similar to ALL
    - remission induction (return to chronic phase) achievable

Polycythemia Vera

Definition
- stem cell disorder characterized by elevated RBC mass (erythrocytosis) ± increased white cell and platelet production
- diagnosis (WHO 2008) requires either both major criteria plus one minor criteria OR the first major criterion plus 2 minor criteria
  - Major Criteria
    1. hemoglobin >185 g/L in men, >165 g/L in women or other evidence of increased red cell volume
    2. presence of JAK2 V617F or other functionally similar mutation such as JAK2 exon 12 mutation
  - Minor Criteria
    1. bone marrow biopsy showing hypercellularity for age with trilineage growth (panmyelosis) with prominent erythroid, granulocytic, and megakaryocytic proliferation
    2. serum erythropoietin level below the reference range for normal
    3. endogenous erythroid colony formation *in vitro*

Clinical Features
- symptoms are secondary to high red cell mass and hyperviscosity (see *Erythrocytosis*, H6)
- thrombotic complications: DVT, PE, Budd-Chiari (hepatic vein thrombosis), portal vein thrombosis, thrombophlebitis, increased incidence of stroke, MI
  - due to increased blood viscosity, increased platelet number and/or activity
  - bleeding complications: epistaxis, gingival bleeding, ecchymoses, and GI bleeding
  - if high platelet counts with associated acquired vWD
- erythromelalgia (burning pain in hands and feet and erythema of the skin)
  - associated with platelets >400 x 10^9/L
  - pathognomonic microvascular thrombotic complication in PV and ET
- pruritus, especially after warm bath or shower (40%)
  due to cutaneous mast cell degranulation and histamine release
- epigastric distress, PUD
  - due to increased histamine from tissue basophils, alterations in gastric mucosal blood flow due to increased blood viscosity

Chronic Myeloproliferative Neoplasias: Six Year Follow-Up of Patients Receiving Imatinib for the First-Line Treatment of CML
Leukemia 2009;23:1054-1061
Study: The Randomized Study of Interferon vs. STI571 (IRIS) trial enrolled patients with chronic phase chronic myeloid leukemia (CML-CP) to either imatinib (n=533) or interferon-α (IFN) plus cytarabine (n=553).
Results: Assessing the imatinib arm specifically at the sixth year point, there were no reports of disease progression to accelerated phase (AP) or blast crisis (BC), toxicity profile was unchanged, and cytogenetic response rate was 82%. Estimated event-free survival was 83% and rate of freedom from progression to AP and BC was 93%.
Conclusion: This 6-year update of IRIS demonstrates the efficacy and safety of imatinib as first-line therapy for CML patients.

Detection of the *bcr-abl* fusion gene is a diagnostic test for CML (present in over 90% of patients)

Erythromelalgia is a pathognomonic microvascular thrombotic complication in PV and ET

Cardiovascular Events and Intensity of Treatment in Polycythemia Vera
NEJM 2013;368:22-33
Study: Prospective, RCT, mean follow-up of 28.9 mo. Blinding not described.
Population: 365 patients with JAK2-positive polycythemia vera being treated with phlebotomy, hydroxyurea, or both.
Intervention: Patients were randomized to a target hematocrit <45% (low-hematocrit group) or 45-50% (high-hematocrit group).
Outcome: Composite of time until death from cardiovascular causes of major thrombotic events.
Results: The hazard ratio (HR) for the primary outcome was 3.91 (95% CI 1.45-10.53, p=0.007), while the HR for the primary outcome plus superficial venous thrombosis was 2.69 (95% CI 1.19-6.12, p=0.02) for the high-hematocrit vs. low-hematocrit group.
Conclusions: The hematocrit target of <45% was associated with a lower incidence of CV death, major thrombotic events, and superficial venous thrombosis in patients with polycythemia vera.

Efficacy and Safety of Low-dose Aspirin® in Polycythemia Vera
NEJM 2004;350:114-124
Study: Double-blind, placebo-controlled, RCT.
Participants: 518 patients with polycythemia vera (PV) with no clear indication for, or contraindication to, ASA therapy.
Intervention: Patients received either low-dose ASA 100 mg daily (n=253) or placebo (n=265) and were followed for up to 5 yr.
Primary Outcome: Cumulative rate of (I) nonfatal MI, nonfatal stroke, or death from cardiovascular causes and the cumulative rate of (II) the previous 3 plus PE and major venous thrombosis.
Results: Primary outcomes (I) and (II) were reduced with treatment compared to placebo (RR 0.41; p=0.09 and RR 0.4; p=0.03, respectively). There were no differences in overall or cardiovascular mortality and major bleeding episodes.
Conclusion: Low-dose ASA can safely prevent thrombotic complications in patients with PV.

- gout (hyperuricemia)
  - due to increased cell turnover
- characteristic physical findings
  - plethora (ruddy complexion) of face (70%), palms
  - splenomegaly (70%), hepatomegaly (40%)

Investigations
- see *Erythrocytosis*, H6
- must rule out secondary polycythemia if high Epo level

Treatment
- phlebotomy to keep hematocrit <45%
- hydroxyurea (prior thrombosis or symptoms, severe coronary artery disease, refractory to phlebotomy)
- low-dose Aspirin® (for antithrombotic prophylaxis, will also treat erythromelalgia)
- allopurinol: as needed
- antihistamines: as needed

Prognosis
- 10-20 yr survival with treatment
- complicated by thrombosis, hemorrhage, leukemic transformation (AML)

Idiopathic Myelofibrosis

Myelofibrosis can be either primary (idiopathic) or occur as a transformation of an antecedent PV or ET

Definition
- excessive bone marrow fibrosis leading to marrow failure
- characterized by anemia, extramedullary hematopoiesis, leukoerythroblastosis, teardrop red cells in peripheral blood and hepatosplenomegaly

Epidemiology
- rare, median age at presentation is 65 yr

Pathophysiology
- abnormal myeloid precursor postulated to produce dysplastic megakaryocytes that secrete fibroblast growth factors
  - stimulates fibroblasts and stroma to deposit collagen in marrow
- increasing fibrosis causes early release of hematopoietic precursors leading to:
  - leukoerythroblastic blood film (primitive RBCs and WBCs present in blood)
  - migration of precursors to other sites: extramedullary hematopoiesis (leading to hepatosplenomegaly)

A "leukoerythroblastic" blood film (RBC and granulocyte precursors) implies bone marrow infiltration with malignancy (e.g. leukemias, solid tumour metastases) or fibrosis (e.g. IMF)

Clinical Features
- anemia (severe fatigue is most common presenting complaint, pallor on exam in >60%)
- weight loss, fever, night sweats → secondary to hypermetabolic state
- splenomegaly (90%) → secondary to extramedullary hematopoiesis; may cause early satiety
- hepatomegaly (70%) → may get portal hypertension
- bone and joint pain → secondary to osteosclerosis, gout
- signs of extramedullary hematopoiesis (depends on organ involved)

IMF typically has a dry BM aspirate and teardrop RBCs (aspiration gives no blood cells)

Investigations
- CBC: anemia, variable platelets, variable WBC
- biochemistry: increased ALP (liver involvement, bone disease), increased LDH (2° to ineffective hematopoiesis), increased uric acid (increased cell turnover), increased B12 (2° to increased neutrophil mass)
- blood film: leukoerythroblastosis with teardrop RBCs, nucleated RBCs, variable polychromasia, large platelets, and megakaryocyte fragments
- JAK2 PCR and calreticulin PCR
- bone marrow aspirate: "dry tap" in as many as 50% of patients (no blood cells espirated)
- bone marrow biopsy (essential for diagnosis): fibrosis, atypical megakaryocytic hyperplasia, thickening and distortion of the bony trabeculae (osteosclerosis)

A Double-Blind, Placebo-Controlled Trial of Ruxolitinib for Myelofibrosis
NEJM 2012;366:799-807
Study: Double-blinded RCT of 309 patients with myelofibrosis randomized to ruxolitinib or placebo.
Outcome: Primary outcome was reduction in spleen volume of >35% at 24 wk. Secondary outcomes were durability of response, symptom burden, and overall survival.
Results: A greater proportion of patients on ruxolitinib had reduction in spleen volume >35% (41.9% vs. 0.7%) and this was sustained in 67% at 48 wk. Ruxolitinib also led to greater symptom improvement (45% vs. 5.3%) and less mortality (13 vs. 24). There was no difference in rate of discontinuation due to adverse events (11.0% vs. 10.6%) but anemia and thrombocytopenia were more common with ruxolitinib.
Conclusions: Ruxolitinib reduced spleen size, improved symptoms and improved survival, compared with placebo.

Treatment
- allogeneic stem cell transplant is potentially curative
- JAK2 inhibitors (Ruxolitinib)
- symptomatic treatment
  - transfusion for anemia
  - erythropoietin: 30-50% of patients respond
  - androgens for anemia (e.g. danazol has shown transient response with response rates of <30%)
  - hydroxyurea for splenomegaly, thrombocytosis, leukocytosis, systemic symptoms
    - interferon-α (as second line therapy)
    - splenectomy (as third line therapy; associated with high mortality and morbidity)
  - radiation therapy for symptomatic extramedullary hematopoiesis, symptomatic splenomegaly

Prognosis
- International Prognostic Scoring System (IPSS) for IMF uses 5 factors to determine mean survival
  - presence of constitutional symptoms; age >65; hemoglobin <100 g/L; leukocyte count >25,000/mm^3; circulating blast cells ≥1%
  - based on the calculated score, a patient's IMF is categorized as "low", "intermediate 1", "intermediate 2", or "high" with a mean survival of 135, 95, 48, and 27 mo respectively
- risk of transformation to AML (8-10%)

Essential Thrombocythemia

Definition
- overproduction of platelets in the absence of recognizable stimulus
- must rule out secondary thrombocythemia

Epidemiology
- increases with age; F:M = 2:1, but F=M at older age

Diagnosis (2008 WHO Criteria) requires meeting all four criteria:
1. sustained platelet count >450 x 10^9/L
2. bone marrow biopsy specimen showing proliferation mainly of the megakaryocytic lineage with increased number of enlarged, mature megakaryocytes; no significant increase or left shift of neutrophil granulopoiesis or erythropoiesis
3. not meeting WHO criteria for PV, primary myelofibrosis, *bcr-abl* CML, or myelodysplastic syndrome or other myeloid neoplasms
4. demonstration of JAK2 V617F or calreticulin (or in its absence another clonal marker), no evidence for reactive thrombocytosis

Clinical Features
- often asymptomatic
- vasomotor symptoms (40%)
  - headache (common), dizziness, syncope
  - erythromelalgia (burning pain of hands and feet, dusky colour, usually worse with heat, caused by platelet activation → microvascular thrombosis)
- thrombosis (arterial and venous)
- bleeding (often GI; associated with platelets >1,000 x 10^9/L)
- constitutional symptoms, splenomegaly
- pregnancy complications; increased risk of spontaneous abortion
- risk of transformation to AML (0.6-5%), myelofibrosis

Investigations
- CBC: increased platelets; may have abnormal platelet aggregation studies or VWD studies
- JAK2 PCR assay; if negative, CALR PCR assay
- bone marrow hypercellularity, megakaryocytic hyperplasia, giant megakaryocytes
- increased K$^+$, increased PO$_4^{3-}$ (2° to release of platelet cytoplasmic contents)
- diagnosis: exclude other myeloproliferative disorders and reactive thrombocytosis

Treatment
- low dose ASA if previous history of thrombotic event, ≥1 cardiovascular risk factors, older, or symptomatic
- cytoreductive therapy if thrombosis or thrombotic symptoms: hydroxyurea (HU) (1st line therapy), anagrelide, interferon-α, or ^{32}P (age >80 or lifespan <10 yr)

Lymphoid Malignancies

Acute Lymphoblastic Leukemia

Definition
- malignant disease of the bone marrow in which early lymphoid precursors proliferate and replace the normal hematopoietic cells of the marrow
- WHO subdivides ALL into two types depending on cell of origin
  1. B-cell: precursor B lymphoblastic leukemia
  2. T-cell: precursor T lymphoblastic leukemia
- the French-American-British (FAB) classification (L1, L2, L3) is no longer encouraged, as morphology is not prognostic

Etiology of Secondary Thrombocythemia
- Infection
- Inflammation (IBD, arthritis)
- Malignancy
- Hemorrhage
- Iron deficiency
- Hemolytic anemia
- Post splenectomy
- Post chemotherapy

Anagrelide vs. Hydroxyurea for **Essential Thrombocythemia: ANAHYDRET Study, A** Randomized Controlled Trial
Blood 2013;121:1720-8
Study: Prospective, non-inferiority, RCT. Majority of patients followed beyond 1 yr.
Population: 259 previously untreated, high-risk patients with essential thrombosis as per the WHO guidelines.
Intervention: Patients were randomized to receive either non-immediate release formulation of anagrelide or hydroxyurea.
Outcome: Examined platelet counts, hemoglobin levels, leukocyte counts, and occurrence of ET-related events.
Results: The hazard ratio (HR) of developing thrombocythemia was 1.19 (95% CI 0.61-2.30). The HR for a reduction of hemoglobin was 1.03 (95% CI 0.57-1.81), and 0.92 (95% CI 0.57-1.46) for leukocytosis. There was no statistical difference in occurrence of major or minor arterial or venous thrombosis, severe or minor bleeding events, or rate of discontinuation between the two arms.
Conclusions: In patients with ET, anagrelide is non-inferior to hydroxyurea in the prevention of thrombotic complications.

There is an asymptomatic "benign" form of essential thrombocythemia with a stable or slowly rising platelet count; treatment includes observation, ASA, sulfinpyrazone, or dipyridamole

75% of ALL occurs in children <6 yr old; second peak at age 40

Clinical Features
- see *Acute Myeloid Leukemia*, H37 for full list of symptoms
- distinguish ALL from AML based on Table 32
- clinical symptoms usually secondary to:
  - **bone marrow failure:** anemia, neutropenia (50% present with fever; also infections of oropharynx, lungs, perianal region), thrombocytopenia
  - **organ infiltration:** tender bones, lymphadenopathy, hepatosplenomegaly, meningeal signs (headache, N/V, visual symptoms; especially in ALL relapse)

Investigations
- CBC: increased leukocytes >10 x 10^9/L (occurs in 50% of patients); neutropenia, anemia, or thrombocytopenia
- may have increased uric acid, K^+, PO_4^{3-}, Ca^{2+}, LDH
- PT, aPTT, fibrinogen, D-dimers for DIC
- leukemic lymphoblasts lack specific morphological (no granules) or cytochemical features, therefore diagnosis depends on immunophenotyping
- cytogenetics: Philadelphia (Ph) chromosome in ~25% of adult ALL cases
- CXR: patients with ALL may have a mediastinal mass
- LP prior to systemic chemotherapy to assess for CNS involvement (ensure adequate platelet count and PT/PTT)

Treatment
- eliminate abnormal cloned cells
  1. **induction chemotherapy:** to induce complete remission (undetectable leukemic blasts, restore normal hematopoiesis)
  2. **consolidation and/or intensification of chemotherapy**
     - consolidation: continuing same chemotherapy to eliminate subclinical leukemic cells
     - intensification: high doses of different (non-cross-reactive) chemotherapy drugs to eliminate cells with resistance to primary treatment
  3. **maintenance chemotherapy:** low dose intermittent chemotherapy over prolonged period (2-3 yr) to prevent relapse
  4. **prophylaxis:** CNS radiation therapy or methotrexate (intrathecal or systemic)
- hematopoietic stem cell transplantation: potentially curative (due to pre-implant myeloablative chemoradiation and post-implant graft-versus-leukemia effect) but relapse rates and non-relapse mortality high

Prognosis
- depends on response to initial induction or if remission is achieved following relapse
- good prognostic factors: young, WBC <30 x 10^9/L, T-cell phenotype, absence of Ph chromosome, early attainment of complete remission
- achievement of first remission: 60-90%
- childhood ALL: 75% long-term remission (>5 yr)
  higher cure rates in children because of better chemotherapy tolerance, lower prevalence of *bcr-abl* fusion gene (associated with chemotherapeutic resistance)
- adult ALL: 30-40% 5-yr survival

Treatment of ALL vs. AML
- No proven benefit of maintenance chemotherapy in AML
- No routine CNS prophylaxis in AML

To Differentiate AML From ALL: Remember **Big** and Sm**ALL**

Table 32. Differentiating AML From ALL

AML	ALL
Big people (adults)	Small people (kids)
Big blasts	Small blasts
Big mortality rate	Small mortality rate (kids)
Lots of cytoplasm	Less cytoplasm
Lots of nucleoli (3-5)	Few nucleoli (1-3)
Lots of granules and Auer rods	No granules
Myeloperoxidase, Sudan black stain	PAS (periodic acid-Schiff)
Maturation defect beyond myeloblast or promyelocyte	Maturation defect beyond lymphoblast

Lymphomas

Definition
- collection of lymphoid malignancies in which malignant lymphocytes accumulate at lymph nodes and lymphoid tissues
  - leading to lymphadenopathy, extranodal disease, and constitutional symptoms

American Society of Hematology Choosing Wisely Recommendation
Limit surveillance CT scans in asymptomatic patients after curative-intent treatment for aggressive lymphoma

Table 33. Ann Arbor System for Staging Lymphomas

Stage	Description
I	Involvement of a single lymph node region OR extralymphatic organ/site (Stage IE)
II	Involvement of two or more lymph node regions or an extralymphatic site and one or more lymph node regions on same side of diaphragm
III	Involvement of lymph node regions on both sides of the diaphragm; may or may not be accompanied by single extra lymphatic site or splenic involvement
IV	Diffuse involvement of one or more extralymphatic organs including bone marrow

- subtypes
  A = absence of B-symptoms (see *Approach to Lymphadenopathy*, H12)
  B = presence of B-symptoms

- Ann Arbor staging can be used for both Hodgkin and non-Hodgkin lymphoma, but grade/histology is more important for non-Hodgkin lymphoma because the outcome differs significantly depending on type of lymphoma
- Prognostic scores are different for indolent versus aggressive lymphomas
- Highly aggressive lymphomas act like acute leukemias

Table 34. Chromosome Translocations

Translocation	Gene Activation	Associated Neoplasm
t(2;5)	ALK1 mutation	Anaplastic large cell lymphoma
t(8;14)	c-myc activation	Burkitt's lymphoma
t(14;18)	bcl-2 activation	Follicular lymphoma
t(11;14)	Overexpression of cyclin D1 protein	Mantle cell lymphoma
t(11;18)	MALT1 activation	Mucosa-associated lymphoid tissue (MALT)

Hodgkin Lymphoma

Definition
- malignant proliferation of lymphoid cells with Reed-Sternberg cells (thought to arise from germinal centre B-cells)

Hodgkin is distinguished from non-Hodgkin lymphoma by the presence of Reed-Sternberg cells

Epidemiology
- bimodal distribution with peaks at 20 yr and >50 yr
- association with Epstein-Barr virus in up to 50% of cases, causal role not determined

Clinical Features
- asymptomatic lymphadenopathy (70%)
  - non-tender, rubbery consistency
  - cervical/supraclavicular (60-80%), axillary (10-20%), inguinal (6-12%)
- splenomegaly (50%) ± hepatomegaly
- mediastinal mass
  - found on routine CXR, may be symptomatic (cough)
  - rarely may present with SVC syndrome, pleural effusion
- systemic symptoms
  - B symptoms (especially in widespread disease; fever in 30%), pruritus
- non-specific/paraneoplastic
  - alcohol-induced pain in nodes, nephrotic syndrome
- starts at a single site in lymphatic system (node), spreads first to adjacent nodes
  - disease progresses in contiguity with lymphatic system

Hodgkin lymphoma classically presents as a painless, non-tender, firm, rubbery enlargement of superficial lymph nodes, most often in the cervical region

Investigations
- CBC
  - anemia (chronic disease, rarely hemolytic), eosinophilia, lymphopenia, platelets normal or increased early, decreased in advanced disease
- biochemistry
  - HIV serology
  - liver enzymes and/or LFTs (liver involvement)
  - renal function tests (prior to initiating chemotherapy)
  - ALP, Ca^{2+} (bone involvement)
  - ESR, LDH (monitor disease progression)
- imaging
  - CXR, CT chest (lymph nodes, mediastinal mass), CT abdomen/pelvis (liver or spleen involvement), PET scans have replaced gallium scans

- cardiac function assessment (MUGA scan or echocardiography): for patients at high risk of pre-treatment cardiac disease (age >60, history of HTN, CHF, PUD, CAD, MI, CVA, malnourished), treatment can be cardiotoxic
  - PFTs: if history of lung disease (COPD, smoking, previous radiation to lung)
- excisional lymph node or core biopsy confirms diagnosis
- bone marrow biopsy to assess marrow infiltration (only necessary if B-symptoms, stage III or IV, bulky disease or cytopenia)

Treatment
- stage I-II: chemotherapy (ABVD) followed by involved field or involved site radiotherapy (XRT)
- stage III-IV: chemotherapy (ABVD) with XRT for bulky disease
- relapse, resistant to therapy: high dose chemotherapy, autologous stem cell transplant
  - PET scan results essential in clarifying disease response

Complications of Treatment
- cardiac disease: secondary to XRT, adriamycin is also cardiotoxic
- pulmonary disease: secondary to bleomycin (interstitial pneumonitis)
- infertility: recommend sperm banking
- secondary malignancy in irradiated field
  - <2% risk of MDS, AML (secondary to treatment, usually within 8 yr)
  - solid tumours of lung, breast; >8 yr after treatment
  - non-Hodgkin lymphoma
- hypothyroidism: post XRT

Prognosis
- Hasenclever adverse prognostic factors:
  1. serum albumin <40 g/L
  2. hemoglobin <105 g/L
  3. male
  4. stage IV disease
  5. age ≥45 yr
  6. leukocytosis (WBC >1.5 x 10^9/L)
  7. lymphocytopenia (lymphocytes <0.06 x 10^9/L or <8% of WBC count or both)
- prognostic score
  - each additional adverse prognostic factor decreases freedom from progression at 5 yr (FFP)

Non-Hodgkin Lymphoma

Definition
- malignant proliferation of lymphoid cells of progenitor or mature B- or T-cells

Classification
- multiple classification systems exist at present and may be used at different centres
- can originate from both B- (85%) and T- or NK- (15%) cells
  - B-cell NHL: e.g. diffuse large B-cell lymphoma, follicular lymphoma, Burkitt's lymphoma, mantle cell lymphoma
  - T-cell NHL: e.g. mycosis fungoides (skin), TCL-NOS, anaplastic large cell lymphoma
- WHO/REAL classification system: 3 categories of NHLs based on natural history
  - **indolent** (35-40% of NHL): e.g. follicular lymphoma, small lymphocytic lymphoma/CLL, mantle cell lymphoma
  - **aggressive** (~50% of NHL): e.g. diffuse large B-cell lymphoma
  - **highly aggressive** (~5% of NHL): e.g. Burkitt's lymphoma

Clinical Features
- painless superficial lymphadenopathy, usually >1 lymph node region
- usually presents as widespread disease (exception is aggressive lymphoma)
- constitutional symptoms not as common as in Hodgkin lymphoma
- cytopenia: anemia ± neutropenia ± thrombocytopenia can occur when bone marrow is involved
- abdominal signs
  - hepatosplenomegaly
  - retroperitoneal and mesenteric involvement (second most common site of involvement)
- oropharyngeal involvement in 5-10% with sore throat and obstructive apnea
- extranodal involvement: most commonly GI tract; also testes, bone, kidney
- CNS involvement in 1% (often with HIV)

Investigations
- CBC
  - normocytic normochromic anemia
  - autoimmune hemolytic anemia rare
  - advanced disease: thrombocytopenia, neutropenia, and leukoerythroblastic anemia
- peripheral blood film may show lymphoma cells

Treatment of HL depends on stage; treatment of NHL depends on histologic subtype

International Prognostic Factors Project 1998

Prognostic Factors	FFP
0	84%
1	77%
2	67%
3	60%
4	51%
5-7	42%

FFP = freedom from progression at 5 yr

NHL: Associated Conditions
- Immunodeficiency (e.g. HIV)
- Autoimmune diseases (e.g. SLE)
- Infections (e.g. EBV)

flow cytometry of peripheral blood lymphocytosis is valuable for low-grade NHL
biochemistry
- increase in uric acid
- abnormal LFTs in liver metastases
- increased LDH (rapidly progressing disease, poor prognostic factor)
staging: CT neck, chest, abdomen, pelvis and bone marrow biopsy
PET is useful for monitoring response to treatment and evaluation of residual tumour following therapy
in aggressive histological disease
diagnosed by
- lymph node biopsy: excisional biopsy preferred, FNA unreliable
- bone marrow biopsy: not optimal for diagnosis as BM involved in only 30% of high grade
  lymphomas

Treatment

localized disease (e.g. GI, brain, bone, head and neck)
- radiotherapy to primary site and adjacent nodal areas
- adjuvant chemotherapy
- surgery: splenic marginal zone lymphoma

indolent lymphoma: goal of treatment is symptom management
- watchful waiting
- radiation therapy for localized disease
- bendamustine plus rituximab, an anti-CD20 antibody, is superior to CHOP + rituximab (CHOP-R)
  for advanced stage disease (StIL trial)

aggressive lymphoma: goal of treatment is curative
- combination chemotherapy: CHOP is mainstay, plus rituximab if B-cell lymphoma
- radiation for localized/bulky disease
- CNS prophylaxis with high-dose methotrexate if certain sites involved (testicular)
- relapse, resistant to therapy: high dose chemotherapy, autologous SCT

highly aggressive lymphoma
- Burkitt lymphoma: short bursts of intensive chemotherapy "CODOX-M" chemotherapy regimen
  also often used ± IVAC with Rituximab
- CNS prophylaxis and tumour lysis syndrome prophylaxis

Common Chemotherapeutic Regimens
CHOP: cyclophosphamide,
hydroxydoxorubicin (Adriamycin®), vincristine
(Oncovin®), prednisone
VAD: vincristine, adriamycin, dexamethasone
ABVD: adriamycin, bleomycin, vinblastine,
dacarbazine
BEACOPP: bleomycin, etoposide, adriamycin,
cyclophosphamide, vincristine, procarbazine,
and prednisone

Complications

hypersplenism
infection
autoimmune hemolytic anemia and thrombocytopenia
vascular obstruction (from enlarged nodes)
bowel perforation
tumour lysis syndrome (particularly in very aggressive lymphoma) see *Tumour Lysis Syndrome*, H52

Prognosis

follicular lymphoma: Follicular Lymphoma International Prognostic Index is used (5 adverse prognostic
factors): age >60; >4 nodal areas; elevated LDH; Lugano stage III-IV; hemoglobin <120 g/L
- based on calculated risk, mean 5 yr survival ranges from 53-91%
- rarely curative, typically relapsing and remitting course with risk of transformation to aggressive
  lymphoma such as diffuse large B-cell lymphoma

diffuse large B-cell lymphoma: The International Prognostic Factor Index is used (5 adverse prognostic
factors): age >60; Ann Arbor stage (III-IV); performance status (ECOG/Zubrand 2-4); elevated LDH;
>1 extranodal site
- based on calculated risk, mean 5 yr survival ranges from 26-73%
- ~40% rate of cure

Table 35. Characteristics of Select Non-Hodgkin Lymphomas

	Follicular Lymphoma	Diffuse Large B-Cell Lymphoma (DLBCL)	Burkitt Lymphoma	Mantle Cell Lymphoma
Percentage of NHLs	22-30%	33%	<1% adult NHLs 30% childhood NHLs	6%
Genetic Mutation	Bcl-2 activation	Bcl-2, Bcl-6, MYC rearrangements	c-myc activation	Overexpression of cyclin D1 (Bcl-1 activation)
Classification	Indolent	Aggressive (high-grade)	Very aggressive	Indolent
Risk Factors	Middle-age – elderly	Previous CLL (Richter's transformation: 5% CLL patients progress to DLBCL)	1. Endemic: African origin, EBV-associated 2. Sporadic: no EBV 3. HIV-related: AIDS-defining illness	Male (M:F = 4:1)
Clinical Features	Widespread painless LAD* ± bone marrow involvement Frequent transformation to aggressive lymphoma Very responsive to chemoradiation treatment	Rapidly progressive LAD and extranodal infiltration 50% present at stage I/II, 50% widely disseminated	Endemic form: massive jaw LAD "Starry-sky" histology High risk of tumour lysis syndrome upon treatment	Often presents Stage IV with palpable LAD Involvement of GI tract (lymphomatosis polyposis), Waldeyer's Ring 5 yr survival 25%

*LAD = lymphadenopathy

Malignant Clonal Proliferations of Mature B-Cells

Table 36. Characteristics of B-Cell Malignant Proliferation

	CLL	Lymphoplasmacytic Lymphoma	Myeloma
Cell Type	Lymphocyte	Plasmacytoid	Plasma cell
Protein	IgM if present	IgM	IgG, A, light chain (rarely M, D, or E)
Lymph Nodes	Very common	Common	Rare
Hepatosplenomegaly	Common	Common	Rare
Bone Lesions	Rare	Rare	Common
Hypercalcemia	Rare	Rare	Common
Renal Failure	Rare	Rare	Common
Immunoglobulin Complications	Common	Rare	Rare

Rouleaux formation on peripheral blood smear, if not artifact, denotes hyperglobulinemia (but not necessarily monoclonality)

Chronic Lymphocytic Leukemia

Definition
- indolent disease characterized by clonal malignancy of mature B-cells

Epidemiology
- most common leukemia in Western world
- mainly older patients; median age 70 yr
- M>F

Pathophysiology
- accumulation of neoplastic lymphocytes in blood, bone marrow, lymph nodes, and spleen

Clinical Features
- 25% asymptomatic (incidental finding)
- 5-10% present with B-symptoms (≥1 of: unintentional weight loss ≥10% of body weight within previous 6 mo, temperature >38°C or night sweats for ≥2 wk without evidence of infection, extreme fatigue)
- lymphadenopathy (50-90%), splenomegaly (25-55%), hepatomegaly (15-25%)
- immune dysregulation: autoimmune hemolytic anemia (Coombs positive), ITP, hypogammaglobulinemia ± neutropenia
- bone marrow failure: late, secondary to marrow involvement by CLL cells

Investigations
- CBC: clonal population of B lymphocytes >5 x 10^9/L
- peripheral blood film
  - lymphocytes are small and mature
  - smudge cells
- flow cytometry (CD5, CD20dim, CD23)
- cytogenetics: FISH (dictates response therapy and prognosis)
- bone marrow aspirate
  - lymphocytes >30% of all nucleated cells
  - infiltration of marrow by lymphocytes in 4 patterns: nodular (10%), interstitial (30%), diffuse (35%, worse prognosis), or mixed (25%)

Smudge cells are artifacts of damaged lymphocytes from slide preparation

Natural History and Treatment
- natural history: indolent and incurable; most cases show slow progression
- small minority present with aggressive disease; usually associated with chromosomal abnormalities (e.g. p53 deletion)
- first line therapy is dictated by cytogenetic status and patient co-morbidities
  - observation if early, stable, asymptomatic
  - treatment options vary by region; ideal first line therapy should include a monoclonal CD20 agent (e.g. rituximab, obinutuzumab)
    - commonly fludarabine + cyclophosphamide+ rituximab (FCR) in fit patients with normal CrCl; bendamustine + rituximab (BR) in less fit
    - chlorambucil + anti-CD20 obinutuzumab in the elderly
  - corticosteroids, IVIg: especially for autoimmune phenomenaradiotherapy
- molecular therapies
  - Idelalisib – PI3K inhibitor
  - Ibrutinib – BTK (Bruton's tyrosine kinase) inhibitor

Prognosis
- 9 yr median survival, but varies greatly
- prognosis predicted by Rai staging and cytogenetic status
- low risk: lymphocytosis in blood and bone marrow only
- intermediate risk: lymphocytosis with enlarged nodes in any site or splenomegaly, hepatomegaly
- high risk: lymphocytosis with disease-related anemia (<110 g/L) or thrombocytopenia (<100 x 10^9/L)

Complications
- bone marrow failure
- immune complications: AIHA, ITP, immune deficiency (hypogammaglobulinemia, impaired T-cell function)
- polyclonal or monoclonal gammopathy (often IgM)
- hyperuricemia with treatment
- 5% undergo Richter's transformation: aggressive transformation to diffuse large B-cell lymphoma (see Table 35)

Multiple Myeloma

Definition
- neoplastic clonal proliferation of plasma cells producing a monoclonal immunoglobulin resulting in end organ dysfunction
- usually single clone of plasma cells, although biclonal myeloma also occurs; rarely non-secretory

Epidemiology
- incidence 3 per 100,000, most common plasma cell malignancy
- increased frequency with age; median age of diagnosis is 68 yr; M>F

Pathophysiology
- malignant plasma cells secrete monoclonal antibody
  - 95% produce M protein (monoclonal Ig = identical heavy chain + identical light chain, or light chains only)
    - IgG 50%, IgA 20%, IgD 2%, IgM 0.5%
    - 15-20% produce free light chains or light chains alone found in either:
      - serum as an increase in the quantity of either kappa or lambda light chain (with an abnormal kappa:lambda ratio)
      - urine has Bence-Jones protein
  - <5% are non-secretors

Clinical Features and Complications
- bone disease: pain (usually back), bony tenderness, pathologic fractures
  - lytic lesions are classical (skull, spine, proximal long bones, ribs)
  - increased bone resorption secondary to osteoclast activating factors such as PTHrP
- anemia: weakness, fatigue, pallor
  - secondary to bone marrow suppression
- weight loss
- infections
  - usually *S. pneumoniae* and Gram-negatives
  - secondary to suppression of normal plasma cell function
- hypercalcemia: N/V, confusion, constipation, polyuria, polydipsia
  - secondary to increased bone turnover
- renal disease/renal failure
  - most frequently causes cast nephropathy (see Nephrology, NP32)
- bleeding
  - secondary to thrombocytopenia, may see petechiae, purpura
  - can also be caused by acquired Von Willebrand disease
- extramedullary plasmacytoma
  - soft tissue mass composed of monoclonal plasma cells, purplish colour
- hyperviscosity: may manifest as headaches, stroke, angina, MI
  - secondary to increased viscosity caused by M protein
- amyloidosis
  - accumulation of insoluble fibrillar protein (Ig light chain) in tissues; can cause infiltration of any organ system: cardiac infiltration – diastolic dysfunction, cardiac arrhythmias, syncope, sudden death; GI involvement – malabsorption, beefy large or laterally scalloped tongue; neurologic involvement – orthostatic hypotension, carpal tunnel syndrome
  - may cause Factor X deficiency if fibrils bind Factor X → bleeding (raccoon eyes)
- neurologic disease: muscle weakness, pain, paresthesias
  - radiculopathy caused by vertebral fracture, extramedullary plasmacytoma
  - spinal cord compression (10-20% of patients) is a medical emergency

Multiple Myeloma

CRAB
Increased **C**alcium
Renal failure
Anemia
Bony lesions (lytic lesions or osteoporosis felt to be caused by myeloma)

Amyloid
The general term for a variety of proteinaceous materials that have a similar structural organization and are abnormally deposited in tissues

Found in a variety of clinical disorders and can cause systemic (e.g. MM [light chains]) or localized amyloidosis (e.g. Alzheimer disease [AB amyloid])

Routine urinalysis will not detect light chains as dipstick detects albumin. Need sulfosalicylic acid or 24 h urine protein for immunofixation or electrophoresis

Light Chain Disease
15% of MM produce only light chains. Renal failure is a major problem. Kappa > lambda light chain has better prognosis

Investigations
- CBC
  - normocytic anemia, thrombocytopenia, leukopenia
  - rouleaux formation on peripheral film
- biochemistry
  - increased Ca^{2+}, increased ESR, decreased anion gap, increased Cr, albumin, β2-microglobulin (as part of staging), proteinuria (24 h urine collection)
- monoclonal proteins
  - serum protein electrophoresis (SPEP): demonstrates monoclonal protein spike in serum in 80% (i.e. M protein)
  - urine protein electrophoresis (UPEP): demonstrates light chains in urine = Bence-Jones protein (15% secrete only light chains)
  - immunofixation: demonstrates M protein and identifies Ig type; also identifies light chains
  - serum free light chain quantification: kappa and lambda light chains, calculated ratio
- bone marrow aspirate and biopsy
  - often focal abnormality, greater than 10% plasma cells, abnormal morphology, clonal plasma cells; send for FISH or cytogenetics (prognostic implications)
- skeletal series (x-rays), MRI if symptoms of cord compression
  - presence of lytic lesions and areas at risk of pathologic fracture
  - bone scans are not useful since they detect osteoblast activity
- β2-microglobulin, LDH, and CRP are poor prognosticators

Diagnosis
- International Myeloma Working Group Criteria
  1. serum or urinary monoclonal protein
  2. presence of clonal plasma cells in bone marrow (>60% without "CRAB") or a plasmacytoma
  3. presence of end-organ damage related to plasma cell dyscrasia, such as:
     - increased serum Ca^{2+}
     - lytic bone lesions
     - anemia
     - renal failure

Treatment
- treatment is non-curative
- treatment goals
  - improvement in quality of life (improve anemia, reverse renal failure, bony pain)
  - prevention of progression and complications
  - increase overall survival
- autologous stem cell transplant if <65 yr old
  - usually preceded by 4-6 mo of cytoreductive therapy: steroid based with novel agents (i.e. immunomodulatory drugs or proteasome inhibitors)
- chemotherapy if >65 yr old or transplant-ineligible
  - melphalan, prednisone, cyclophosphamide and proteasome inhibitor (i.e. bortezomib)
- dexamethasone and bortezomib if ARF; bortezomib ± dexamethasone in light chain amyloidosis
- supportive management
  - bisphosphonates for those with osteopenia or lytic bone lesions (requires renal dosing)
  - local XRT for bone pain, spinal cord compression
  - kyphoplasty for vertebral fractures to improve pain relief and regain height
  - treat complications: hydration for hypercalcemia and renal failure, bisphosphonates for severe hypercalcemia, prophylactic antibiotics, erythropoietin for anemia, DVT prophylaxis
- all patients will relapse; choice of retreatment regimen depends on duration of remission, organ involvement, patient's comorbidities, and preferences

Prognosis
- ISS - International Staging System (β2-microglobulin and albumin) used to stage and estimate prognosis
- revised ISS for risk stratification: combination of original ISS, cytogenetic profile (i.e. p53 mutation associated with poor survival and resistance to chemotherapy) and LDH
- median survival based on stage, usually 3-7 yr

Monoclonal Gammopathy of Unknown Significance

Definition
- presence of M protein in serum in absence of any clinical or laboratory evidence of a plasma cell dyscrasia or lymphoproliferative disorders
  - incidence: 0.15% in general population, 5% of people >70 yr of age
  - asymptomatic

Serum Free Light Chain Ratio is an Independent Risk Factor for Progression in MGUS
Blood 2005;106:812-817
Purpose: To determine whether the presence of monoclonal free kappa or lambda immunoglobulin light chains in MGUS increases the risk of progression to malignancy.
Methods: Retrospective study with median follow-up of 15 yr. Baseline serum samples obtained from 1,383 MGUS patients seen at the Mayo clinic between 1960-1994. 1,148 baseline samples were obtained within 30 d of diagnosis.
Results: Malignant progression had occurred in 87 (7.6%) patients. In 379 (33%) patients, an abnormal serum free light chain (FLC) ratio was detected. There was a significantly higher risk of progression in patients with an abnormal FLC ratio relative to patients with a normal ratio (hazard ratio, 3.5; 95% CI 2.3-5.5; p<0.001). This finding was independent of the size and type of the serum monoclonal (M) protein. In high-risk MGUS patients (abnormal serum FLC ratio, non-IgG MGUS, high serum M protein level [≥1.5 gm/dL]), the risk of progression at 20 yr was 58% compared to 37% in high-intermediate-risk MGUS (two risk factors), 21% low-intermediate risk (with one risk factor) and 5% low-risk (no risk factors).
Conclusions: The presence of an abnormal FLC ratio is a clinically and statistically significant predictor of progression in MGUS. The low-risk subset of patients with MGUS accounts for 40% of all MGUS patients and have a small lifetime risk of progression, thus less follow-up can be justified.

Diagnosis
- presence of a serum monoclonal protein (M protein) at a concentration <30 g/L
- <10% plasma cells in bone marrow
- absence of hyperCalcemia, Renal insufficiency, Anemia, Bony disease related to the plasma cell proliferative process (absence of "CRAB")
- 0.3-1% of patients develop a hematologic malignancy each yr
  - patients with M protein peak ≥15 g/L or patients with IgA or IgM MGUS are at higher risk of malignant transformation
  - patients with abnormal serum free light chains ratio are at increased risk of malignant transformation
- monitor with annual history, physical, CBC, Cr, calcium, albumin, serum protein electrophoresis (considered pre-malignant)

Lymphoplasmacytic Lymphoma (Waldenstrom's Macroglobulinemia)

Definition
- proliferation of lymphoplasmacytoid cells
  - presence of monoclonal IgM paraprotein

Waldenstrom's macroglobulinemia accounts for 85% of all cases of hyperviscosity syndrome

Clinical Features
- chronic disorder of elderly patients; median age 64 yr
- symptoms: weakness, fatigue, bleeding (oronasal), weight loss, recurrent infections, dyspnea, CHF (triad of anemia, hyperviscosity, plasma volume expansion), neurological symptoms, peripheral neuropathy, cerebral dysfunction
- signs: pallor, splenomegaly, hepatomegaly, lymphadenopathy, retinal lesions
- key complication to avoid: hyperviscosity syndrome
  - because IgM (unlike IgG) confined largely to intravascular space

Investigations and Diagnosis
- bone marrow shows plasmacytoid lymphocytes
- bone lesions usually not present
- blood work rarely see hypercalcemia
- cold hemagglutinin disease possible: Raynaud's phenomenon, hemolytic anemia precipitated by cold weather
- normocytic anemia, rouleaux, high ESR if hyperviscosity not present

Treatment
- Bendamustine – R/R-CVP chemotherapy, alkylating agents (chlorambucil), nucleoside analogues (fludarabine), rituximab, or combination therapy
- corticosteroids
- plasmapheresis for hyperviscosity: acute reduction in serum IgM

Complications of Hematologic Malignancies

Hyperviscosity Syndrome

Definition
- refers to clinical sequelae of increased blood viscosity (when relative serum viscosity >5-6 units), resulting from increased circulating serum Igs or from increased cellular blood components in hyperproliferative disorders (e.g. multiple myeloma, leukemia, PV)
- Waldenstrom's macroglobulinemia accounts for 85% of cases

Clinical Features
- hypervolemia causing: CHF, headache, lethargy, dilutional anemia
- CNS symptoms due to decreased cerebral blood flow: headache, vertigo, ataxia, stroke
- retina shows venous engorgement and hemorrhages
- bleeding diathesis
  - due to impaired platelet function, absorption of soluble coagulation factors (e.g. nasal bleeding, oozing gums)
- ESR usually very low

Treatment
- plasmapheresis, chemotherapy

Tumour Lysis Syndrome

Definition
- group of metabolic complications that result from spontaneous or treatment-related breakdown of cancer cells
- more common in diseases with large tumour burden and high proliferative rate (high grade lymphoma, leukemia)

Clinical Features
- metabolic abnormalities
  - cells lyse, releasing K^+, uric acid, PO_4^{3-} (increased levels)
  - PO_4^{3-} binds Ca^{2+} (decreased Ca^{2+})
- complications
  - lethal cardiac arrhythmia (increased K^+)
  - acute kidney injury (formerly known as renal failure, see Nephrology, NP18)

Treatment
- prevention
  - aggressive IV hydration
  - alkalinization not recommended due to risk of calcium phosphate or xanthine precipitation in renal tubules
  - allopurinol or rasburicase
  - correction of pre-existing metabolic abnormalities
- dialysis

Blood Products and Transfusions

Blood Products
- RBCs, platelets and coagulation factors (frozen plasma [FP], cryoprecipitate, factor concentrates) are available for transfusion
- donated blood (1 U = 450-500 mL) is fractionated into these various components
  - centrifugation separates whole blood into RBCs and platelet-rich plasma
  - platelet-rich plasma is further fractionated into platelets and plasma
    - need to pool together multiple units to obtain therapeutic amounts
    - FP (previously known as FFP) is plasma frozen within 24 h of collection
    - cryoprecipitate is the high MW precipitate generated when FP is thawed at low temperatures

Specialized Products
- irradiated blood products
  - prevent proliferation of donor T-cells in potential or actual bone marrow transplant recipients
  - used for immunocompromised patients or for patients on purine analogue chemotherapy, first-degree relatives, HLA-matched products and intrauterine transfusions, Hodgkin lymphoma
- CMV-negative blood products
  - potential transplant recipients
  - neonates
  - AIDS patients
  - seronegative pregnant women

Red Blood Cells

Packed Red Blood Cells
- stored at 4°C
- transfuse within 42 d of collection, otherwise cell lysis may result in hyperkalemia
- infuse each unit over 2 h (max of 4 h)

Indications for Packed RBC Transfusion
- Hb <70 g/L; this may change as per patient's tolerance or symptoms
  - maintain Hb between 70 and 100 g/L during active bleeds
- consider maintaining a higher Hb for patients with:
  - CAD/unstable coronary syndromes
  - uncontrolled, unpredictable bleeding
  - impaired pulmonary function
  - increased O_2 consumption

Blood Groups

Group	Antigen (on RBC)	Antibody (in serum)
O	H	Anti-A, anti-B
A	A	Anti-B
B	B	Anti-A
AB	A and B	Nil

In Canada, blood products are leukodepleted via filtration immediately after donation; therefore it is considered:
- Low in lymphokines, resulting in a lower incidence of febrile nonhemolytic transfusion reactions
- CMV negative (because CMV is found in leukocytes)

1 unit of pRBC will increase Hb by approximately 10 g/L or increase Hct by 4%

American Society of Hematology Choosing Wisely Recommendation
Do not transfuse more than the minimum number of RBC units necessary to relieve symptoms of anemia or to return the patient to a safe hemoglobin range (70-80 g/L) in stable non-cardiac patients

Selection of Red Cells for Transfusion

- when anticipating an RBC transfusion, the following should be ordered:
  - group and screen: determines the blood group and Rh status of the recipient as well as the presence of autoantibodies vs. major/minor blood group antigens in the patient's serum
  - cross-match: involves mixing the recipient's blood with potential donor blood and looking for agglutination (takes 30-45 min)
- when blood is required, several options are available

  1st line: fully crossmatched blood, electronic crossmatch is becoming more widely used (not always available in emergency situations)

  2nd line: donor blood of the same group and Rh status as the recipient

  3rd line: O- blood for females of reproductive age; O+ blood for all others

Platelets

Table 37. Platelet Products

Product	Indication
Random donor (pooled)	Thrombocytopenia with bleeding
Single donor platelets	Potential BMT recipients
HLA matched platelets	Refractory to pooled or single donor platelets, presence of HLA antibodies

- stored at 20-24°C
- random donor platelets are transfused from a pool of 4 units; this should increase the platelet count by $\geq 15 \times 10^9$/L
- single donor platelets (transfused as single units) should increase the platelet count by $40\text{-}60 \times 10^9$/L
- if an increase in the platelet count is not seen post-transfusion: autoantibodies (i.e. ITP), alloantibodies, consumption (bleeding, sepsis), or hypersplenism may be present

Table 38. Indications for Platelet Transfusion

Plt (x 10^9/L)	Indications
<10	Non-immune thrombocytopenia
<20	Procedures not associated with significant blood loss
<50	Procedures associated with blood loss or major surgery (>500 mL EBL)
<100	Pre-neurosurgery or head trauma
Any	Platelet dysfunction (or antiplatelet agents) and marked bleeding

Relative Contraindications of Platelet Transfusion

- TTP, HIT, post-transfusion purpura, HELLP

Coagulation Factors

Table 39. Coagulation Factor Products

Product	Indication
Frozen plasma (FP)	Depletion of multiple coagulation factors (e.g. sepsis, DIC, dilution, TTP/HUS, liver disease), emergency reversal of life-threatening bleeding secondary to warfarin overdose
Cryoprecipitate (enriched fibrinogen, VWF, VIII, XIII)	Hemophilia A (Factor VIII deficiency) – use in emergencies Von Willebrand disease – use in emergencies Hypofibrinogenemia
Humate P or Wilate	Von Willebrand disease Hemophilia A
Factor VIII concentrate	Factor VIII deficiency (Hemophilia A)
Factor IX concentrate	Factor IX deficiency (Hemophilia B)
Recombinant factor VIIa	Factor VII deficiency with bleeding/surgery, Hemophilia A or B with inhibitors, Glanzmann thrombasthenia
Prothrombin complex concentrate; PCC (Octaplex, Beriplex®)	Reversal of warfarin therapy or vitamin K deficiency in bleeding patient or in patient requiring urgent (<6 h) surgical procedure, urgent non-specific "reversal" of direct Xa inhibitors
Activated prothrombin complex concentrate; aPCC (FEIBA)	Hemophilia A or B with inhibitors, urgent non-specific "reversal" of direct thrombin inhibitors

Transfusion Requirements in Critical Care (TRICC)
NEJM 1999;340:409-417
Study: Multicentre, RCT.
Participants: 838 critically ill patients with euvolemia after initial treatment and hemoglobin less than 9 g/dL within 72 h of ICU admission.
Intervention: Patients receiving a transfusion followed either (1) a restrictive strategy (RS; n=418) in which red cells were transfused if hemoglobin was less than 7.0 g/dL and then maintained at 7 to 9 g/dL or (2) a liberal strategy (LS; n=420) in which transfusions occurred when the hemoglobin was less than 10.0 g/dL and then maintained at 10 to 12 g/dL.
Primary Outcome: Mortality at 30 d and severity of organ dysfunction.
Results: Mortality rates at 30 d were similar between groups. However, mortality rates were significantly lower with the RS among less acutely ill patients (8.7% and RS group and 16.1% in LS group; p=0.03) and among those <55 yr of age (5.7% RS and 13% LS; p=0.02), but did not differ in a subgroup with clinically significant cardiac disease.
Conclusion: A RS of red cell transfusion is at least as effective as, and possibly superior to, a LS transfusion in critically ill patients.

Liberal or Restrictive Transfusion in High-Risk Patients After Hip Surgery (FOCUS)
NEJM 2011;365:2453-2462
Study: Multicentre RCT.
Participants: 2,016 patients aged greater than 50 yr with a history of or risk factors for cardiovascular disease and hemoglobin (Hb) level below 10 g/dL after hip-fracture surgery.
Intervention: Patients were randomly assigned to a liberal transfusion strategy (a Hb threshold of 10 g/dL) or a restrictive transfusion strategy (anemia symptoms or at physician discretion for a Hb level less than 8 g/dL).
Primary Outcome: Mortality or inability to walk across a room without human assistance on a 60 day follow-up.
Results: Primary outcome rates were 35.2% in the liberal transfusion strategy group and 34.7% in the restrictive transfusion strategy group. Rates of complications were similar in the two groups.
Conclusion: A liberal transfusion strategy did not reduce mortality rates or the inability to walk independently on 60 d follow-up compared to a restrictive transfusion strategy in elderly patients with high cardiovascular risk factors after hip surgery.

Acute Blood Transfusion Reactions

DDx of Post-Transfusion Fever
- Acute hemolytic transfusion reaction
- Febrile non-hemolytic transfusion reaction
- Bacterial contamination
- Allergy

DDx of Post-Transfusion Dyspnea
- Transfusion-associated circulatory overload (TACO)
- Transfusion-related acute lung injury (TRALI)
- Allergy (bronchospasm/anaphylaxis)

IMMUNE

Acute Hemolytic Transfusion Reactions
- ABO incompatibility resulting in intravascular hemolysis secondary to complement activation, occurs immediately after transfusion
- most commonly due to incorrect patient identification
- risk per unit of blood is <1 in 40,000
- presentation: fever, chills, hypotension, back or flank pain, dyspnea, hemoglobinuria
- acute renal failure (<24 h) and DIC
- treatment
  - stop transfusion
  - notify blood bank and check for clerical error
  - maintain BP with vigorous IV fluids ± inotropes
  - maintain urine output with diuretics, crystalloids, dopamine

Febrile Nonhemolytic Transfusion Reactions
- due to alloantibodies to WBC, platelets or other donor plasma antigens, and release of cytokines from blood product cells
- occurs within 0-6 h of transfusion
- risk per unit of blood is 1 in 100 (minor), 1 in 10,000 to 40,000 (severe)
- presents with fever ± rigors, facial flushing, headache, myalgia, hypotension
- treatment
  - rule out hemolytic reaction or infection
  - if temperature <38°C, continue with transfusion but decrease rate and give antipyretics
  - if temperature >38°C, stop transfusion, give antipyretics and anti-histamine

Allergic Nonhemolytic Transfusion Reactions
- alloantibodies (IgE) to proteins in donor plasma result in mast cell activation and release of histamine
- occurs mainly in those with history of multiple transfusions or multiparous women
- risk per unit of blood is 1 in 100
- presents mainly as urticaria and occasionally with fever
- can present as anaphylactoid reaction with bronchospasm, laryngeal edema, and hypotension, but this occurs mainly in IgA deficient patients that have anti-IgA antibodies
- treatment
  - mild: slow transfusion rate and give diphenhydramine
  - moderate to severe: stop transfusion, give IV diphenhydramine, steroids, epinephrine, IV fluids, and bronchodilators

Transfusion-Related Acute Lung Injury
- new-onset acute lung injury that occurs during transfusion or within 6 h of transfusion completion
  - insidious, acute onset of pulmonary insufficiency
  - profound hypoxemia (PaO_2/FiO_2 <300 mmHg)
  - bilateral pulmonary edema on CXR
  - pulmonary artery wedge pressure <18 mmHg
  - no clinical evidence of left atrial hypertension
- pathogenesis uncertain; perhaps due to binding of donor antibodies to WBC of recipient and release of mediators that increase capillary permeability in the lungs
- typically occurs 2-4 h post transfusion and resolves in 24-72 h
- risk per unit of blood is 1 in 10,000
  - is currently the leading cause of transfusion-related morbidity and mortality
- treatment: supportive therapy (oxygen)
- inform blood bank; patient and donor testing will be arranged

NONIMMUNE

Transfusion-Associated Circulatory Overload
- due to impaired cardiac function and/or excessive rapid transfusion
- presentation: dyspnea, orthopnea, hypotension, tachycardia, crackles at base of lung, and increased venous pressure
- incidence: 1 in 700 and is becoming more common
- treatment: transfuse at lower rate, give diuretics and oxygen

Bacterial Infection
- Gram positive: *S. aureus, S. epidermidis, Bacillus cereus*
- Gram negative: *Klebsiella, Serratia, Pseudomonas, Yersinia*
- overall risk is 1 in 100,000 for RBC and 1 in 10,000 for platelets
- never store blood >4 h after bag has left blood bank
- treatment: stop transfusion, blood cultures, IV antibiotics, fluids

Hyperkalemia
- due to K$^+$ release from stored RBC
- risk increases with storage time and if blood is irradiated and risk decreases if given fresh blood
- occurs in 5% of massively transfused patients
- treatment: see Nephrology, NP13

Citrate Toxicity
- occurs with massive transfusion in patients with liver disease – patients are unable to clear citrate from blood
- citrate binds to Ca^{2+} and causes signs and symptoms of hypocalcemia
- treatment: IV calcium gluconate (10 mL for every 2 units of blood)

Dilutional Coagulopathy
- occurs with massive transfusion (>10 units)
- pRBC contains no clotting factors, fibrinogen, cryoprecipitate, or platelets
- treatment: FP, cryoprecipitate, and platelets

Delayed Blood Transfusion Reactions

IMMUNE

Delayed Hemolytic
- due to alloantibodies to minor antigens such as Rh, Kell, Duffy, and Kidd
- level of antibody at time of transfusion is too low to cause hemolysis; later the level of antibody increases due to secondary stimulus and causes extravascular hemolysis
- occurs 5-7 d after transfusion
- presentation: anemia and mild jaundice
- treatment: no specific treatment required; important to note for future transfusion
- N.B. serologic transfusion reactions are the development of alloantibodies in the absence of frank hemolysis

Transfusion-Associated Graft Versus Host Disease
- transfused T-lymphocytes recognize and react against "host" (recipient)
- occurs 4-30 d following transfusion
- most patients already have severely impaired immune systems (e.g. Hodgkin lymphoma or leukemia)
- presentation: fever, diarrhea, liver function abnormalities, and pancytopenia
- can be prevented by giving irradiated blood products

NONIMMUNE

Iron Overload
- due to repeated transfusions over long period of time (e.g. β-thalassemia major)
- can cause secondary hemochromatosis
- treatment: iron chelators or phlebotomy if no longer requiring blood transfusion and not anemic

Viral Infection Risk
- HBV 1 in 1.1 to 1.7 million
- HCV 1 in 5 to 7 million
- HIV 1 in 8 to 12 million
- Human T-lymphotropic virus (HTLV) 1 in 1 to 1.3 million
- other infections include EBV, CMV, WNV (West Nile virus)

Common Medications

Antiplatelet Therapy

• see Figure 11a, *Platelet Activation Cascade*, H26

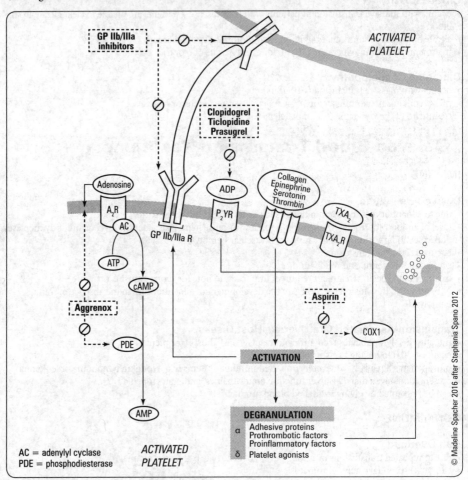

Figure 15. Mechanisms of action of antiplatelet therapy

Table 40. Antiplatelet Therapy

	Mechanism of Action	Dose/Route of Administration	Onset/Peak/ Duration	Specific Side Effects	Remarks
Aspirin® (ASA)	Irreversibly acetylates COX, inhibiting TXA2 synthesis, thus inhibiting platelet aggregation	Single loading 200-300 mg PO, followed by dose of 75-100 mg PO daily	Onset: 5-30 min Peak: 0.25-3 h Duration: 3-6 h	GI ulcer/bleeding Tinnitus Bronchospam Angioedema Reye's syndrome in pediatric patients	Indicated for stroke/MI prophylaxis Reduce incidence of recurrent MI Decrease mortality in post-MI patients Contraindicated in patients with GI ulcers
Aggrenox® (ASA + Dipyridamole)	Dipyridamole increases intracellular cAMP levels, which inhibits TXA2 synthesis, leading to decreased platelet aggregation	1 capsule PO bid	Peak: 75 min	H/A Dyspepsia N/V Abdominal pain Cardiac failure Hemorrhoids	More effective than ASA in secondary prevention of stroke Dipyridamole potentiates antiplatelet action of ASA
Clopidogrel (Plavix®)	Irreversibility inhibit ADP binding to platelets, thus decreased platelet aggregation	75-300 mg PO daily	Onset: 2 h Peak: 1 h	URI Chest pain H/A Flu-like syndrome Depression UTI GI hemorrhage Pancytopenia May cause TTP	Prevention of cardiovascular events in high-risk patients Clopidogrel is a prodrug requiring two-step activation to active metabolite CYP2C19 poor metabolizers have diminished response to clopidogrel Caution with hepatic/renal impairment
Prasugrel (Effient®)	Same as clopidogrel	5-10 mg PO daily	Onset: 30 min	Dizziness H/A Nervousness Blurry vision	Alternative to clopidogrel for prevention of cardiovascular events in high-risk patients Higher potency compared to clopidogrel No significant drug-drug interaction, although more data is required

Table 40. Antiplatelet Therapy (continued)

	Mechanism of Action	Dose/Route of Administration	Onset/Peak/ Duration	Specific Side Effects	Remarks
Ticagrelor (Brilinta®)	Reversibly inhibit ADP binding to platelets	90 mg PO daily	Onset: 1.5 h for prodrug, 2.5 h for active metabolite	Difficulty or labored breathing Shortness of breath Tightness in chest Dizziness	Alternative to clopidogrel for prevention of cardiovascular events in high-risk patients Higher potency compared to clopidogrel Ticagrelor is a prodrug that requires CYP3A4-mediated activation to active metabolite Drug-drug interactions with CYP3A4 inhibitors and inducers
Glycoprotein IIb/ IIIa Inhibitors (Reopro® [abciximab], Integrelin® [epti])	Blocking GP II/IIIa receptor inhibits fibrinogen and vWF binding, leading to decreased platelet aggregation	Variable IV	Variable	Hypotension Back pain N/V Chest pain Abdominal pain Thrombocytopenia	Used most commonly in cardiac catheterization Contraindicated in PUD Monitoring aPTT/activated clotting time

Anticoagulant Therapy

Table 41. Anticoagulant Therapy

	Mechanism of Action	Dose/Route of Administration	Onset/Peak/ Duration	Reversing Agent	Monitoring	Specific Side Effects	Remarks
Heparin	Accelerates inhibitory activity of antithrombin	As per hospital nomogram	Onset: 20-60 min Peak: 2-4 h	Protamine sulfate	aPTT (intrinsic pathway), UFH (anti-Xa) levels	Hemorrhage HIT Increased liver enzymes	Pregnancy: safe (does not cross placenta)
Warfarin	Vitamin K antagonist: inhibits production of II, VII, IX, X, proteins C and S	Individualized dosing by monitoring PT/INR PO	Onset: 36-48 h Peak: 1.5-3 d	IV vitamin K PCC FP	PT/INR maintain 2-3 (2.5-3.5 for mechanical valves)	Hemorrhage Cholesterol embolism syndrome Intraocular hemorrhage	Pregnancy: not used, can cross placenta (teratogenic)
LMWH (enoxaparin, dalteparin, tinzaparin)	Inhibits FXa	Variable SC/IV	Onset: 3-5 h Peak: 3-5 h Duration: 12 h	Partial reversibility with protamine sulfate	FXa in pediatrics, pregnancy and weight >150 kg	Hemorrhage Fever Increased liver enzymes <1% HIT	Increased bioavailability than heparin Can accumulate in patients low CrCl (<30 mL/min)
Fondaparinux	Indirect inhibitor of FXa (through antithrombin)	Variable SC daily	Onset: 2 h Peak: 2-3 h	Not reversible	None	Anemia Fever Nausea Rash	Heparin analogue Contraindicated in renal failure
Rivaroxaban	Direct FXa inhibitor	PO	Peak: 2-4 h	Not reversible	None	Syncope GI hemorrhage	Indicated in treatment of acute VTE (non-cancer patients), secondary VTE prevention, thromboprophylaxis in orthopedic patients and stroke prophylaxis in non-valvular AFib; ensure CrCl>30 mL/min
Apixaban	Direct FXa inhibitor	PO	Onset: 3-4h Peak: 3-4 h	Not reversible	None	Hemorrhage Nausea Anemia	Indicated for stroke prophylaxis in non-valvular AFib; Idiopathic VTE; ensure CrCl >30
Argatroban	Direct thrombin inhibitor	Variable IV	Onset: 5-10 min Duration: 20-40 min	Not reversible	aPTT	Dyspnea Hypotension Fever	Indicated for HIT and heparin resistance in the presence renal failure
Dabigatran	Direct thrombin inhibitor	150 mg PO bid	Peak: 1 h	Not reversible	None (prolonged aPTT can suggest residual drug on board)	GI upset Dyspepsia	Only indicated for AFib in Canada Contraindicated in renal failure, cancer patients, mechanical heart valves

Adverse Reactions of Heparin
- hemorrhage: depends on dose, age, and concomitant use of antiplatelet agents or thrombolytics
- heparin-induced thrombocytopenia: associated with venous or arterial thrombosis (see Table 22, H29)
- osteoporosis: with long-term use

Low Molecular Weight Heparin (enoxaparin, dalteparin, tinzaparin)
- increased bioavailability compared to normal heparin
- increased duration of action
- SC route of administration
- do not need to monitor aPTT
- adverse reactions less common than UFH
- patients with renal failure (CrCl <30 mL/min) can accumulate LMWH, therefore must adjust dose
- only partially reversible with protamine sulfate
- HIT is less common

Factor Xa Inhibitors Versus Vitamin K Antagonists for Preventing Cerebral or Systemic Embolism in Patients with Atrial Fibrillation
Cochrane DB Syst Rev. 2014;8:CD008980
Purpose: To review the evidence comparing factor Xa inhibitors with vitamin K antagonists for prevention of embolic events in patients with atrial fibrillation.
Study: Systematic review search 1950-2013, inclusive. Results included 10 RCTs, 42 084 patients, follow up for 12 wk to 1.9 yr.
Outcome: Stroke (hemorrhagic or ischemic) and non-CNS embolic event
Results: Factor Xa inhibitor treatment resulted in significantly fewer embolic events than dose adjusted warfarin treatment (OR 0.81; CI 0.72 to 0.91). There was no significant difference in rate of major bleeds between factor Xa inhibitors and warfarin treatment. Furthermore, factor Xa inhibitors resulted in significantly fewer intracranial bleeds and lower all-cause mortality.
Conclusions: Use of factor Xa inhibitor for anti-coagulation in patients with atrial fibrillation offered better protection against embolic events than warfarin. Factor Xa inhibitors also had equal or lower rates of adverse events.

Oral Direct Thrombin Inhibitors or Oral Factor Xa Inhibitors for the Treatment of Deep Vein Thrombosis
Cochrane DB Syst Rev 2015;6: CD010956
Purpose: To assess whether DTIs or factor Xa inhibitors are effective treatment for DVTs.
Study: Systematic review search 1950-2015, inclusive. Results included 11 RCTs, 27 945 patients, comparing DTIs or factor Xa inhibitors to standard treatment (heparin, wafarin, and similar)
Outcome: Recurrent DVT or PE.
Results: Separate meta-analyses of DTIs and factor Xa inhibitors showed that each was comparable to standard treatment in terms of DVT recurrence rates. Rates of fatal or non-fatal PE, and all-cause mortality were also not significantly different. Additionally, factor Xa inhibitors had lower rates of bleeding complications than standard treatment (OR 0.57; CI 0.43 to 0.76).
Conclusions: New oral treatment options, including direct thrombin inhibitors and factor Xa inhibitors represent reasonable and safe alternatives for acute.

Table 42. Recommended Therapeutic INR Ranges of Common Indications for Oral Anticoagulant Therapy

Indication	INR Range
Prophylaxis of venous thrombosis (high-risk surgery) Treatment of venous thrombosis Most cases of thrombosis with antiphospholipid antibody syndrome Treatment of pulmonary embolism Prevention of systemic embolism Tissue heart valves AMI (to prevent systemic embolism) Valvular heart disease Atrial fibrillation Bileaflet mechanical valve in aortic position	2.0-3.0
Mechanical prosthetic mitral valves (high risk)	2.5-3.5

AMI = acute myocardial infarction

Table 43. Recommended Management of a Supratherapeutic INR

INR	Bleeding Present	Recommended Action
>Therapeutic to 4.5	No	Lower warfarin dose OR Omit a dose and resume warfarin at a lower dose when INR is in therapeutic range OR No dose reduction needed if INR is minimally prolonged
>4.5 to 10.0	No	Omit the next 1 to 2 doses of warfarin, monitor INR more frequently and resume treatment at a lower dose when INR is in therapeutic range OR Omit a dose and administer 1 to 2.5 mg oral vit K in patients with increased risk of bleeding
>10.0	No	Hold warfarin and administer 5 to 10 mg oral vit K; monitor INR more frequently and administer more vit K as needed; resume warfarin at a lower dose when INR is in therapeutic range
Any	Serious or life threatening	Hold warfarin and administer 10 mg vit K by slow IV infusion; supplement with four-factor prothrombin complex concentrate; monitor and repeat as needed

Adapted from:. American College of Chest Physicians Evidence-Based Clinical Practice Guidelines. Chest 2012;(2 suppl):e152S

Chemotherapeutic and Biologic Agents Used in Oncology

Table 44. Selected Chemotherapeutic and Biologic Agents

Class	Example	Mechanism of Action or Target
Alkylating Agent	• chlorambucil, cyclophosphamide, melphalan (nitrogen mustards) • carboplatin, cisplatin • dacarbazine, procarbazine • busulfan • bendamustine	Damage DNA via alkylation of base pairs Leads to cross-linking of bases, abnormal base-pairing, DNA breakage
Antimetabolites	• methotrexate (folic acid antagonist) • 6-mercaptopurine, fludarabine (purine antagonist) • 5-fluorouracil (5-FU) (pyrimidine antagonist) • hydroxyurea • cytarabine	Inhibit DNA synthesis
Antibiotics	• adriamycin (anthracycline) • bleomycin • mitomycin C • daunorubicin	Interfere with DNA and RNA synthesis
Taxanes	• paclitaxel • docetaxel	Stabilize microtubules against breakdown once cell division complete
Vinca-alkaloids	• vinblastine • vincristine • vinorelbine	Inhibit microtubule assembly (mitotic spindles), blocking cell division
Topoisomerase Inhibitors	• irinotecan, topotecan (topo I) • etoposide (topo II)	Interfere with DNA unwinding necessary for normal replication and transcription
Steroids	• prednisone • dexamethasone	Immunosuppression
Purine Analogues	• fludarabine • cladribine	Interferes with DNA synthesis
Monoclonal Antibodies	• trastuzumab (Herceptin®) • bevacizumab (Avastin®) • rituximab (Rituxan®), ofatumumab (Arzerra®), obinutuzumab (Gayzva®) • cetuximab (Erbitux®)	HER2 antagonist VEGF antagonist CD20 antagonist EGFR antagonist
Small Molecule Inhibitors	• imatinib mesylate (Gleevec®) • dasatinib • nilotinib • erlotinib (Tarceva®) • gefitinib (Iressa®) • bortezomib (Velcade®) • sunitinib (Sutent®) • ibrutinib (Imbruvica®) • idealasib (Zyedlig®) • ruxolitinib (Jakavi®)	*Bcr-Abl* inhibitor *Bcr-Abl* inhibitor *Bcr-Abl* inhibitor EGFR antagonist EGFR antagonist 26S proteasome inhibitor VEGFR, PDGFR antagonist BTK inhibitor PI3K inhibitor JAK2 inhibitor

Landmark Hematology Trials

Trial	Reference	Results
Hematologic Malignancies and Related Disorders		
Hodgkin Lymphoma: ABVD vs. MOPP	*NEJM* 1992; 327:1478-84	In Hodgkin lymphoma, ABVD regimen has equal failure-free and overall survival to MOPP + ABVD, but less myelotoxicity; ABVD is standard chemotherapy for Hodgkin lymphoma
CHOP	*NEJM* 1993; 328:1002-6	In NHL, CHOP has lowest incidence of fatal toxic reactions and shows no significant difference from 3 other regimens in response or disease-free/overall survival; CHOP is the standard for advanced NHL
R-CHOP	*NEJM* 2002; 346:235-42	Addition of rituximab to CHOP increases complete response rate and prolongs event-free survival and overall survival in elderly with DLBCL
CML: Imatinib vs. IFN + Cytarabine	*NEJM* 2003; 348:994-1004	In patients with chronic-phase CML, imatinib was more effective than IFNα + cytarabine in inducing cytogenetic response and freedom from progression to accelerated phase/blast crisis
AZA-001	*Lancet Oncol* 2009; 10:223-32	Azacitidine increases overall survival in higher-risk myelodysplastic syndrome than conventional care
CLL8	*Lancet* 2010; 376:1164-74	Rituximab plus fludarabine and cyclophosphamide (FCR) improves progression-free and overall survival compared with fludarabine and cyclophosphamide alone (FC) in the treatment of CLL
VISTA	*JCO* 2010; 28:2259-66	Bortezomib plus melphalan and prednisone (MPV) is superior to melphalan and prednisone (MP) in overall survival of non-transplant-eligible multiple myeloma patients
MInT Group	*Lancet* 2011; 12:1013-1022	Rituximab added to CHOP-like chemotherapy improved long-term outcomes for young patients with good-prognosis DLBCL
StiL	*Lancet* 2013; 381(9873):1203-10	Bendamustine plus rituximab is superior to R-CHOP in terms of progression-free survival and fewer toxic effects in patients with previously untreated indolent lymphoma
Ibrutinib vs. Ofatumumab in previously treated CLL	*NEJM* 2014; 371:213-223	Ibrutinib, as compared with ofatumumab, significantly improved progression-free survival, overall survival, and response rate among patients with previously treated CLL or SLL
Thrombosis		
CLOT	*NEJM* 2003; 349:146-53	In patients with cancer and acute venous thromboembolism, LWMH was more effective than warfarin in reducing the risk of recurrent thromboembolism without increasing the risk of bleeding
PT1	*NEJM* 2005; 353:85-6	Hydroxyurea plus low-dose ASA is superior to anagrelide plus low-dose ASA for patients with essential thrombocythemia at high risk for vascular events
ESPIRIT	*Lancet* 2006; 367:1665-73	ASA plus dipyridamole is recommended over ASA alone as antithrombotic therapy after cerebral ischemia of arterial origin
Dabigatran vs. Warfarin in VTE	*NEJM* 2009; 361:2342-52	In the treatment of venous thromboembolism, dabigatran is as effective as warfarin and also has a similar safety profile; note: many problems in the trial, making it less pivotal in having drug approval
EINSTEIN-PE	*NEJM* 2012; 366: 1287-1297	Among patients with acute PE, rivaroxaban is noninferior to warfarin in preventing recurrent VTE, and is associated with similar bleeding rates
AMPLIFY	*NEJM* 2013; 369: 799-808	In patients with VTE who have completed 6-12 months of anticoagulation, long-term apixaban treatment reduces recurrent VTE or all-cause mortality without increasing rates of major bleeding.
RE-VERSE AD	*NEJM* 2015; 373:511-520	Idarucizumab for dabigatran reversal
Blood Products and Transfusion		
Platelet Transfusion Threshold	*NEJM* 1997; 337:1870-5	The risk of major bleeding in patients with AML undergoing induction chemotherapy was similar whether the platelet-transfusion threshold was set at 20 or 10; use of the lower threshold reduced platelet usage by 21.5%
TRICC BP	*NEJM* 1999; 340:409-17	A restrictive strategy of red-cell transfusion (when Hb <70) is at least as effective as and possibly superior to a liberal transfusion strategy (when Hb <100) in ICU patients; one possible exception is patients with an acute MI or unstable angina
Dose of Platelet Transfusion	*NEJM* 2010; 362:600-13	Low dose prophylactic platelet transfusion decreases total number of platelets transfused but increases number of transfusions but not incidence of bleeding in patients with hypoproliferative thrombocytopenia
Transfusion in High-Risk Patients after Hip Surgery	*NEJM* 2011; 365:2453-2462	A liberal transfusion strategy (Hb <100), as compared with a restrictive strategy (anemia symptoms or at physician discretion for Hb<80), did not reduce rates of death or inability to walk independently on 60-day follow-up or reduce in-hospital morbidity in elderly patients at high cardiovascular risk
Therapeutic Platelet Transfusion	*Lancet* 2012; 380:1309-16	Therapeutic platelet transfusions (when bleeding occurs) may be used if severe bleeding can be identified early in autologous stem-cell transplant patients; prophylactic transfusion (when platelets <10) should remain standard of care in AML patients
Transfusion Strategies for Acute Upper GI Bleeding	*NEJM* 2013; 368:11-21	As compared with a liberal transfusion strategy (Hb <90), a restrictive strategy (Hb<70) significantly improved outcomes in patients with acute upper gastrointestinal bleeding
Other		
MSH	*NEJM* 1995; 332:1317-22	Hydroxyurea is effective in reduction of complications and clinical manifestations of sickle cell disease
ITP: Dexamethasone	*NEJM* 2003; 349:831-6	A four-day course of high-dose dexamethasone is effective initial therapy for adults with immune thrombocytopenic purpura
CRASH-2	*Health Technol Assess* 2013; 17(10): 1-79	Early administration of TXA safely reduced the risk of death in bleeding trauma patients and is highly cost-effective. Treatment beyond 3 hours of injury is unlikely to be effective

References

American Society of Hematology Choosing Wisely Recommendations. http://www.choosingwisely.org/societies/american-society-of-hematology/

Armitage JO. Treatment of Non-Hodgkin's lymphoma. NEJM 1993;328:1023-1030.

Bataiile R, Harousseua J. Multiple myeloma. NEJM 1997;336:1657-1664.

Bates SM, Ginsberg JS. Treatment of deep-vein thrombosis. NEJM 2004;351:268-277.

Bazemore AW, Smucker DR. Lymphadenopathy and malignancy. Am Fam Phys 2002;66;2103-2110.

Bottomly SS. Causes of the hereditary and acquired sideroblastic anemias. Rose BD (editor). Waltham: UpToDate. 2006.

Brawley OW, Cornelius LJ, Edwards LR, et al. National Institutes of Health Consensus Development Conference Statement: hydroxyurea treatment for sickle cell disease. Ann Intern Med 2008;148:932-938.

Bruins Slot KM, Berge E. Factor Xa inhibitors versus vitamin K antagonists for preventing cerebral or systemic embolism in patients with atrial fibrillation. Cochrane DB Syst Rev. 2014;8:CD008980.

Callum JL. Idiopathic thrombocytopenia purpura. Available from: http://sunnybrook.ca/uploads/Idiopathic_Thrombocytopenia_Purpura.pdf

Callum JL, Pinkerton PH. Bloody easy, 3rd ed. Toronto: Sunnybrook and Women's College Health Sciences Centre, 2011. Blood transfusions, blood alternatives and transfusion reactions.

Canadian Blood Services Surveillance Report 2014. http://www.cps.ca/documents/position/transfusion-and-risk-of-infection-Canada

Canadian Pediatric Society. Transfusion and risk of infection in Canada: update 2012. Paediatr Child Health 17(10): e102-e111

Carson JL, Terrin ML, Noveck H, et al. Liberal or Restrictive Transfusion in High-Risk Patients after Hip Surgery. NEJM 2011;365:2453-2462.

Castellone DD. Saunders Manual of Clinical Laboratory Science. Philadelphia: WB Saunders, 1998. Evaluation of bleeding disorders.

Christiansen SC, Cannegieter SC, Koster T, et al. Thrombophilia, clinical factors, and recurrent thrombotic events. JAMA 2005;293:2353-2361.

Cines DB, Blanchette VS. Immune thrombocytopenic purpura. NEJM 2002;346:995-1008.

Coates TD, Baehner RL. Causes of neutrophilia. Rose BD (editor). Waltham: UpToDate. 2006.

Cohen K, Scadden DT. Non-Hodgkin's lymphoma: pathogenesis, clinical presentation, and treatment. Cancer Treat Res 2001;104:201-203.

Connolly SJ, Ezekowitz MD, Yusuf S, et al. Dabigatran versus warfarin in patients with atrial fibrillation. NEJM 2009;361:1139-1151.

Decousus H, Leizorovicz A, Parent F, et al. A clinical trial of vena caval filters in the prevention of pulmonary embolism in patients with proximal deep-vein thrombosis. NEJM 1998;338:409-415.

Driscoll MC. Sickle cell disease. Ped Rev 2007;28:259-286.

Druker BJ, Guilhot F, O'Brien SG, et al. Five-year follow-up of patients receiving imatinib for chronic myeloid leukemia. NEJM 2006;355:2408-2417.

EINSTEIN Investigators, Bauersachs R, Berkowitz SD, Brenner B, et al. Oral rivaroxaban for symptomatic venous thromboembolism. NEJM 2010; 362:2499-510.

Eriksson BI, Dahl OE, Rosencher N, et al. Dabigatran etexilate versus enoxaparin for prevention of venous thromboembolism after total hip replacement; a randomized, double-blind, non-inferiority trial. Lancet 2007;379:949-956.

Eriksson BI, Quinlan DJ, Eikelboom JW. Novel oral factor Xa and thrombin inhibitors in the management of thromboembolism. Ann Rev Med 2011;62:41-57.

Fleming RE, Ponka P. Iron overload in human disease. NEJM. 2012;366:348-59.

Geerts WH, Pineo GF, Heit JA, et al. Prevention of venous thromboembolism. Seventh ACCP conference on antithrombotic and thrombolytic therapy. Chest 2004;126L:3385-4005.

George JN. Treatment and prognosis of idiopathic thrombocytopenic purpura. Rose BD (editor). Waltham: UpToDate. 2005.

Goldman J. ABC of clinical haematology: chronic myeloid leukaemia. BMJ 1997;314:657.

Habermann TM, Steensma DP. Lymphadenopathy. Mayo Clinic Proc 2000;75:723-32.

Haddad H, Tyan P, Radwan A, et al. B-Thalassemia Intermedia: A Bird's-Eye View. Turk J Haematol 2014;31:5-16.

Hasenclever D, Diehl V. A prognostic score for advanced Hodgkin's disease. International prognostic factors project on advanced Hodgkin's disease. NEJM 1998;339:1506-1514.

Health Canada. Effects of lead on human health. Available from: http://www.hc-sc.gc.ca/ewh-semt/contaminants/lead-plomb/asked_questions-questions_posees-eng.php#exposure

Heaney ML, Golde DW. Myelodysplasia. NEJM 1999;340:1649-1660.

Jabbour E, Kantarjian HM, Saglio G, et al. Early response with dasatinib or imatinib in chronic myeloid leukemia: 3-year follow-up from a randomized phase 3 trial (DASISION). Blood 2014;123:494-500.

Kopko PM, Holland PV. Mechanisms of severe transfusion reactions. Transfus Clin Biol 2001;8:278-281.

Kovacs MJ, Rodger M, Anderson DR, et al. Comparison of 10-mg and 5-mg warfarin initiation monograms together with low-molecular-weight heparin for out patient treatment of acute venous thromboembolism. Ann Intern Med 2003;138:714-719.

Kyle RA, Rajkumar SV. Chemotherapy in multiple myeloma. Rose BD (editor). Waltham: UpToDate. 2006.

Kyle RA, Rajkumar SV. Clinical manifestations and diagnosis of Waldenstrom's macroglobulinemia. Rose BD (editor). Waltham: UpToDate. 2006.

Landaw SA. Approach to the adult patient with thrombocytopenia. Rose BD (editor). Waltham: UpToDate. 2006.

Leonardi-Bee J, Bath PM, Bousser MG, et al. Review: dipyridamole given with or without Aspirin® reduces recurrent stroke. ACP Journal Club 2005;143:10.

Liesner RJ, Machin SJ. ABC of clinical haematology: platelet disorders. BMJ 1997;314:809.

Liesner RJ, Goldstone AH. ABC of clinical haematology: the acute leukaemias. BMJ 1997;314:733.

Lo GK, Juhl D, Warkentin TE, et al. Evaluation of pretest clinical score (4-T's) for the diagnosis of heparin-induced thrombocytopenia in two clinical settings. J Thromb Haemost 2006;4:759-65.

Lowenberg B. Downing JR, Burnett A. Acute myeloid leukemia. NEJM 1999;341:1051-1062.

MabThera International Trial (MInT) Group. CHOP-like chemotherapy with or without rituximab in young patients with good-prognosis diffuse large-B-cell lymphoma: 6-year results of an open-label randomized study of the MInT Group. Lancet Oncol 2011;12:1013-1022.

Mackie IJ, Bull HA. Normal haemostasis and its regulation. Blood Rev 1989;3:237-250.

Markovic M, Majkic-Singh N, Subota V. Usefulness of soluble transferrin receptor and ferritin in iron deficiency and chronic disease. Scan J Clin Lab Invest 2005;65:571-576.

Mead GM. ABC of clinical haematology: malignant lymphomas and chronic lymphocytic leukaemia. BMJ 1997;314:1103.

Messinezy M, Pearson TC. ABC of clinical haematology: polycythaemia, primary (essential) thrombocythaemia and myelofibrosis. BMJ 1997;314:587.

Neunert C, Lim W, Crowther M, et al. The American Society of Hematology 2011 evidence-based practice guideline for immune thrombocytopenia. Blood 2011;117:4190-4207.

Pangalis GA, Vassilakopoulos TP, Boussiotis VA, et al. Clinical approach to lymphadenopathy. Semin Oncol 1993;20:570-582.

Pillot G, Chantler M, Magiera H, et al. (editors). The Washington Manual Hematology and Oncology Subspecialty Consult. Philadelphia: Lipincott Williams & Wilkins, 2004.

Pui C, Evans WE. Acute lymphoblastic leukemia. NEJM 1998;339:605-615.

Robertson L, Kesteven P, McCaslin JE. Oral direct thrombin inhibitors or oral factor Xa inhibitors for the treatment of deep vein thrombosis. Cochrane DB Syst Rev. 2015;6: CD010956.

Rozman C, Montserrat E. Chronic lymphocytic leukemia. NEJM 1995;333:1052-1057.

Sabatine MS (editor). Pocket medicine, 2nd ed. The Massachusetts General Hospital Handbook of Internal Medicine. Philadelphia: Lippincott Williams & Wilkins, 2004. Hematology-oncology.

Seiter K. Acute lymphoblastic leukemia. E-medicine 2015. Available from: http://emedicine.medscape.com/article/207631-overview

Sawyers C. Chronic myeloid leukemia. NEJM 1999;340:1330-1340.

Streiff MB, Smith B, Spivak JL. The diagnosis and management of polycythemia vera in the era since the Polycythemia Vera Study Group: a survey of American Society of Hematology members' practice patterns. Blood 2002;99:1144-1149.

Schulman S, Kearon C, Kakkar AK, et al. Dabigatran versus warfarin in the treatment of acute venous thromboembolism. NEJM 2009;361:2342-2352.

Tefferi A. Approach to the patient with thrombocytosis. Rose BD (editor). Waltham: UpToDate. 2006.

The Merck Manual. Section 11, Chapter 133: Platelet disorders.

Thomas RH. Hypercoagulability syndromes. Arch Intern Med 2001;161:2433-2439.

U.S. Consumer Product Safety Commission. Ban of lead-containing paint and certain consumer products bearing lead-containing paint. Available from: http://www.cpsc.gov/BUSINFO/regsumleadpaint.pdf.

Valentine KA, Hull RD. Clinical use of warfarin. Rose BD (editor). Waltham: UpToDate. 2006.

Valentine KA, Hull RD. Clinical use of heparin and low molecular weight heparin. Rose BD (editor). Waltham: UpToDate. 2006.

Vardiman JW, Thiele J, Arber DA, et al. The 2008 revision of the World Health Organization (WHO) classification of myeloid neoplasms and acute leukemia: rationale and important changes. Blood 2009;114:937-951.

Verstovsek S, Mesa RA, Gotlib J, et al. A Double-blind, placebo-controlled trial of ruxolitinib for Myelofibrosis. NEJM 2012;366:799-807.

Wells PS, Anderson DR, Rodger M, et al. Evaluation of D-dimer in the diagnosis of suspected deep-vein thrombosis. NEJM 2003;349:1227-1235.

Wilson SE, Watson HG, Crowther MA. Low-dose oral vitamin K therapy for the management of asymptomatic patients with elevated international normalized ratios: a brief review. CMAJ 2004;170:821-824.

ID | Infectious Diseases

Ilyse Darwish, David Kleinman and **Valerie Taylor**, chapter editors
Claudia Frankfurter and **Inna Gong**, associate editors
Brittany Prevost and **Robert Vanner**, EBM editors
Dr. Ari Bitnun, Dr. Andrea Boggild and **Dr. Susan Poutanen**, staff editors

Acronyms

AFB	acid-fast bacilli	GBS	group B *Streptococcus*	IE	infective endocarditis	RT-PCR	reverse transcription-PCR
AIDS	acquired immune deficiency syndrome	GC	gonococcus	IFN	interferon	SARS	severe acute respiratory syndrome
ANC	absolute neutrophil count	GNB	Gram negative bacilli	Ig	immunoglobulin	sBP	systolic blood pressure
AOM	acute otitis media	GP	Gram positive	INH	isoniazid	SIADH	syndrome of inappropriate
ARV	anti-retroviral	H. flu	*Haemophilus influenzae*	IVDU	intravenous drug use		antidiuretic hormone secretion
ART	anti-retroviral therapy	HAART	highly active anti-retroviral treatment	KOH	potassium hydroxide	Sn	sensitivity
BAL	bronchoalveolar lavage	HAV	hepatitis A virus	KSHV	Kaposi's sarcoma-associated herpes	Sp	specificity
BCG	Bacille Calmette-Guérin	HBc	HBV core antigen		virus	spp.	species
C&S	culture and sensitivity	HBeAg	HBV envelope antigen	LOC	level of consciousness	SRI	severe respiratory illness
CFU	colony forming units	HBsAg	HBV surface antigen	LP	lumbar puncture	STEC	Shiga toxin-producing *E. coli*
CMV	cytomegalovirus	HBV	hepatitis B virus	MERS	Middle Eastern respiratory syndrome	STI	sexually transmitted infection
CNS	central nervous system	HCC	hepatocellular carcinoma	MDR	multidrug resistance	TB	mycoplasma tuberculosis
CSF	cerebrospinal fluid	HCV	hepatitis C virus	MMR	measles/mumps/rubella	TIg	tetanus immune globulin
DEET	N,N-Diethyl-meta-toluamide	HDV	hepatitis D virus	MRSA	methicillin-resistant *S. aureus*	TMP/SMX	trimethoprim-sulfamethoxazole
DM	diabetes mellitus	HEV	hepatitis E virus	MSM	men who have sex with men	TNF	tumour necrosis factor
DVT	deep vein thrombosis	HHV	human herpes virus	O&P	ova and parasites	TORCH	toxoplasmosis, other, rubella,
EBV	Epstein-Barr virus	Hib	*Haemophilus influenzae* b	PCR	polymerase chain reaction		cytomegalovirus, HSV
EHEC	enterohemorrhagic *E. coli*	HIV	human immunodeficiency virus	PMN	polymorphonuclear leukocytes	TSS	toxic shock syndrome
EIEC	enteroinvasive *E. coli*	HPF	high power field	PNS	peripheral nervous system	URTI	upper respiratory tract infection
ETEC	enterotoxigenic *E. coli*	HRIg	human rabies immunoglobulin	PPD	purified protein derivative	UTI	urinary tract infection
FDP	fibrinogen degradation products	HSV	herpes simplex virus	RSV	respiratory syncytial virus	VRE	vancomycin-resistant *Enterococcus*
FUO	fever of unknown origin	HUS	hemolytic uremic syndrome	RTI	respiratory tract infection	VZV	varicella-zoster virus
GAS	group A *Streptococcus*						

Principles of Microbiology

Bacteriology

Bacteria Basics
- bacteria are prokaryotic cells that divide asexually by binary fission
- Gram stain divides most bacteria into two groups based on their cell wall
  - Gram positive (GP): thick, rigid layer of peptidoglycan
  - Gram negative (GN): thin peptidoglycan layer + thicker outer membrane composed of lipoproteins and lipopolysaccharides
    - clinical significance: GN thick outer membrane makes it resistant to penicillin's mechanism of action
- acid-fast bacilli (AFB): high mycolic acid content in cell wall, "acid fast" as washout phase with acid-alcohol is ineffective in acid-fast bacteria, e.g. *Mycobacteria, Nocardia*
- "atypical" bacteria: not seen on Gram stain and difficult to culture
  - obligate intracellular bacteria: e.g. *Chlamydia, Chlamydophilia*
  - bacteria lacking a cell wall: e.g. *Mycoplasma*
  - spirochetes: e.g. *Treponema pallidum*
- O_2 can be either vital or detrimental to growth
  - obligate aerobes: require O_2
  - obligate anaerobes: require environment without O_2
  - facultative anaerobes: can survive in environments with or without O_2

Mechanisms of Bacterial Disease
1. adherence to and colonization of skin or mucous membranes
   - fimbriae (pili): microfilaments extending through the cell wall attach to epithelial cells (e.g. *E. coli* in the urinary tract)
2. invasion or crossing epithelial barriers
3. evasion of host defense system through inhibition of
   - phagocytic uptake via polysaccharide capsule (e.g. *S. pneumoniae, N. meningitidis, H. influenzae*) or surface proteins (e.g. *Staphylococcus, Streptococcus*)
4. toxin production
   - exotoxins are secreted by living pathogenic bacteria and cause disease even if the bacteria is not present (e.g. *Clostridium*)
   - endotoxins are structural components of GN bacterial cell walls, and may be shed by live cells or released during cell lysis
5. intracellular growth
   - obligate intracellular: *Rickettsia, Chlamydia, Chlamydophilia*
   - facultative intracellular: *Salmonella, Neisseria, Brucella, Mycobacteria, Listeria, Legionella*
6. biofilm
   - an extracellular polysaccharide network forming mesh around the bacteria (e.g. *S. epidermidis*) which can coat prosthetic devices such as IV catheters

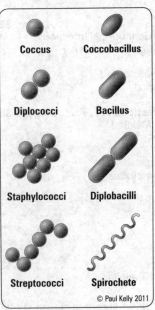

Coccus   **Coccobacillus**

Diplococci   **Bacillus**

Staphylococci   **Diplobacilli**

Streptococci   **Spirochete**

© Paul Kelly 2011

Figure 1. Bacteria morphology

Table 1. Common Bacteria

	Gram-Positive Bacteria		Gram-Negative Bacteria		Not Seen on Gram Stain	
	Cocci	Bacilli (rods)	Diplococci	Bacilli (rods)	Acid Fast	Others
Aerobes	*Staphylococcus* S. aureus S. saprophyticus S. epidermidis *Streptococcus* S. pneumoniae S. pyogenes (GAS) S. agalactiae (GBS) *Enterococcus* E. fecalis	*Bacillus* B. anthracis *Listeria* *Nocardia* (modified acid-fast positive)	*Neisseria* N. meningiditis N. gonorrhoeae *Moraxella* M. catarrhalis	*Enterobacteriaceae* E. coli, Salmonella, Shigella, Campylobacter, Yersinia *Klebsiella* *Legionella* *Pseudomonas* *Haemophilus* H. influenzae	*Mycobacteria* M. tuberculosis M. leprae M. avium complex M. bovis	Obligative intracellular *Rickettsiae* *Chlamydia* C. trachomatis *Chlamydophila* C. pneumoniae No cell wall *Mycoplasma* Spirochaete (spiral) *Treponema pallidum*
Anaerobes	*Peptostreptococcus*	*Clostridium* C. difficile, C. tetani, C. botulinum, C. perfringens		*Bacteroides* B. fragilis		

Table 2. Commensal Flora

Site	Organisms
Skin	Coagulase-negative staphylococci, *Corynebacterium, Propionibacterium acnes, Bacillus, S. aureus*
Oropharynx	Viridans group streptococci, *Haemophilus, Neisseria*, anaerobes (*Peptostreptococcus, Bacteroides, Veillonella, Fusobacterium, Actinomyces, Prevotella*)
Small Bowel	*E. coli*, anaerobes (low numbers)
Colon	*E. coli, Klebsiella, Enterobacter, Enterococcus*, anaerobes (*Bacteroides, Peptostreptococcus, Clostridium*)
Vagina	*Lactobacillus acidophilus*, viridans group streptococci, coagulase-negative staphylococci, facultative Gram-negative bacilli, anaerobes

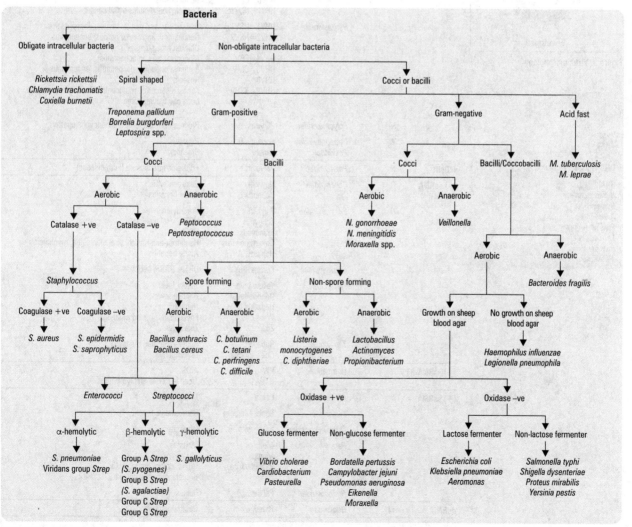

Figure 2. Laboratory identification of bacterial species

Virology

Viral Basics
- viruses are infectious particles consisting of RNA or DNA covered by a protein coat
  - infect cells and use host metabolic machinery to replicate
  - nucleic acid can be double stranded (ds) or single stranded (ss)
  - can be enveloped or naked
- virions are mature virus particles that can be released into the extracellular environment
- host susceptibility is governed by the host cell and virus surface proteins (viral tropism) and cellular immunity

Viral Disease Patterns
1. acute infections (e.g. adenovirus)
   - host cells are lysed in the process of virion release
   - some produce acute infections with late sequelae (e.g. measles virus subacute sclerosing panencephalitis)
2. chronic infections (>6 mo): (e.g. HBV, HIV)
   - host cell machinery is used to produce and chronically release virions
3. latent infections
   - viral genome remains latent in host cell nucleus
   - can reactivate (e.g. HSV, VZV)

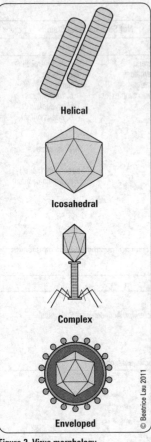

Helical

Icosahedral

Complex

Enveloped

© Beatrice Lau 2011

Figure 3. Virus morphology

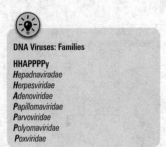

DNA Viruses: Families

HHAPPPPy
*He*padnaviradae
*He*rpesviridae
*A*denoviridae
*P*apillomaviridae
*P*arvoviridae
*P*olyomaviridae
*P*oxviridae

Table 3. Common Viruses

Nucleic Acid	Enveloped	Virus Family	Major Viruses	Medical Importance
dsDNA	N	*Adenoviridae*	Adenovirus	URTI Conjunctivitis Gastroenteritis
	N	*Papillomaviridae*	HPV1,4 HPV6,11 HPV16,18, etc.	Plantar warts Genital warts Cervical/anal dysplasia and cancer
	Y	*Herpesviridae*	HHV1=HSV1 HHV2=HSV2 HHV3=VZV HHV4=EBV HHV5=CMV HHV6* HHV8=KSHV	Oral, ocular, and genital herpes; encephalitis Genital, oral, and ocular herpes; encephalitis Chicken pox, shingles Mononucleosis, viral hepatitis Retinitis, pneumonitis, hepatitis, encephalitis Roseola Kaposi's sarcoma, multicentric Castleman's disease, body cavity lymphoma
	N	*Polyomaviridae*	JC virus	Progressive multifocal leukoencephalopathy
	Y	*Hepadnaviridae*	Hepatitis B	Hepatitis
	Y	*Poxviridae*	Variola	Smallpox
ssDNA	N	*Parvoviridae*	Parvovirus B19	Erythema infectiosum (Fifth disease)
(+) ssRNA	N	*Caliciviridae*	Norwalk Hepatitis E	Gastroenteritis Acute hepatitis
	N	*Picornaviridae*	Poliovirus Echovirus Rhinovirus Coxsackie virus Hepatitis A	Poliomyelitis URTIs, viral meningitis URTIs Hand-foot-and-mouth, viral meningitis, myocarditis Acute hepatitis
	Y	*Coronaviridae*	Coronavirus	URTIs, SARS, MERS
	Y	*Flaviviridae*	Yellow fever Dengue fever Hepatitis C West Nile Zika	Yellow fever Dengue fever Hepatitis Encephalitis, flaccid paralysis Zika fever
	Y	*Togaviridae*	Rubella Chikungunya	Rubella (German measles) Chikungunya
(+) ssRNA-RT	Y	*Retroviridae*	HIV HTLV-1	AIDS T-cell leukemia and lymphoma
(+) ssRNA	Y	*Arenaviridae*	Lassa	Lassa fever
	Y	*Filoviridae*	Ebola, Marburg	Hemorrhagic fever
	Y	*Orthomyxoviridae*	Influenza A, B, C	Influenza
	Y	*Paramyxoviridae*	Measles Mumps Parainfluenza RSV	Measles Mumps URTIs, croup, bronchiolitis Bronchiolitis, pneumonia
	Y	*Rhabdoviridae*	Rabies	Rabies
dsRNA	N	*Reoviridae*	Rotavirus	Gastroenteritis

Note: ___viridae = family, ___virus = genus, # = species (e.g. Retroviridae HIV-2)
*Roseolovirus, Herpes lymphotropic virus

Mycology

Fungal Basics
- fungi are eukaryotic organisms, they can have the following morphologies
    1. yeast (unicellular)
    2. moulds (also known as filamentous fungi) (multicellular with hyphae)
    3. dimorphic fungi (found as mould at room temperature but grow as yeast-like forms at body temperature)

Table 4. Membrane and Cell Wall Compositions

	Membrane Sterol	Cell Wall
Bacteria	–	Peptidoglycan
Human Cell	Cholesterol	–
Fungi	Ergosterol	Chitin (complex glycopolysaccharide)

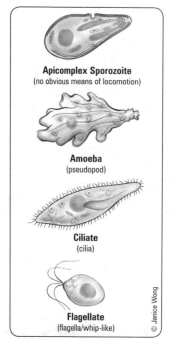

Figure 4. Common fungus morphology

Yeast

Mold: septate hyphae

Mold: non-septate hyphae

© Man-San Ma 2014 (after Janice Wong, 2012)

Mechanisms of Fungal Disease
- primary fungal infection by
    - overgrowth of normal flora (e.g. *Candida* species)
    - inhalation of fungal spores
    - traumatic inoculation into skin
- toxins produced by fungi (e.g. ingestion aflatoxins)
- allergic reactions to fungi (e.g. bronchopulmonary aspergillosis)

Parasitology

Parasite Basics
- **parasite:** an organism that lives in or on another organism (host) and damages the host in the process
- parasites with complex life cycles require more than one host to reproduce
    - reservoir host: maintains a parasite and may be the source for human infection
    - intermediate host: maintains the asexual stage of a parasite or allows development of the parasite to proceed through the larval stages
    - definitive host: allows the parasite to develop to the adult stage where reproduction occurs
- 2 major groups of parasites: protozoa and helminths
- see Tables 26 and 27 for examples of clinically important parasites

Table 5. Differences Between Protozoa and Helminths

Protozoa	Helminths
Unicellular	Multicellular
Motile trophozoite inactive cyst	Adult egg larva
Multiplication	No multiplication in human host
Eosinophilia unusual	Eosinophilia (proportional to extent of tissue invasion)*
Indefinite life span	Definite life span

*Adult Ascaris (roundworm) does not cause eosinophilia; migratory larval phases of Ascaris, however, cause high-grade eosinophilia

Apicomplex Sporozoite
(no obvious means of locomotion)

Amoeba
(pseudopod)

Ciliate
(cilia)

Flagellate
(flagella/whip-like)

© Janice Wong

Figure 5. Classification of protozoa based on movement

Characteristics of Parasitic Disease
- symptoms are usually proportional to parasite burden
- tissue damage is due to the parasite and host immune response
- chronic infections may occur with or without overt disease
- immunocompromised hosts are more susceptible to manifestations of infection, reactivation of latent infections, and more severe disease
- eosinophilia may suggest a parasitic infection

Parasite sampling may need to be repeated on a number of occasions before infection can be ruled out

Mechanisms of Parasitic Disease
1. mechanical obstruction (e.g. ascariasis, clonorchiasis)
2. competition with host for resources (e.g. anemia in hookworm disease, vitamin B_{12} deficiency in diphyllobothriasis)
3. cytotoxicity leading to abscesses and ulcers (e.g. amoebiasis, leishmaniasis)
4. inflammatory
    - acute hypersensitivity (e.g. pneumonitis in Loeffler's syndrome)
    - delayed hypersensitivity (e.g. egg granulomas in schistosomiasis)
    - cytokine-mediated (systemic illness of malaria, disseminated strongyloidiasis)
5. immune-mediated injury
    - autoimmune (e.g. myocarditis of Chagas disease, tissue destruction of mucocutaneous leishmaniasis)
    - immune complex (e.g. nephritis of malaria, schistosomiasis

Transmission of Infectious Diseases

Table 6. Mechanism of Transmission

Mechanism	Mode of Transmission	Examples	Preventative Measure
Contact	Direct physical contact, or indirect contact with a fomite	Skin-to-skin (MRSA) Sexual (*N. gonorrhoeae, C. trachomatis*, HSV, HIV) Blood-borne (HIV, HBV, HCV)	For patients in health care facilities: Contact precautions Barrier precautions Safe needlestick/sharp practices
Droplet/Contact	Respiratory droplets (>5 μm) can be projected short distances (≤2 m) and deposit on mucosal surfaces of the recipient (e.g. by coughing, sneezing, or talking); transmission can also occur by direct physical contact of respiratory fluids or indirect contact with a fomite contaminated with respiratory fluids	Influenza, mumps *N. meningitidis, Bordetella pertussis*	For patients in health care facilities: Contact/droplet precautions
Airborne	Airborne droplet nuclei (<5 μm) remain infectious over time and distance	*M. tuberculosis*, VZV, measles	For patients in health care facilities: Airborne precautions
Food/Waterborne	Ingestion of contaminated food or water	*V. cholerae, Salmonella*, HAV, HEV	Prophylactic vaccinations where available Ensure clean food/water supply For patients in health care facilities: Contact precautions used for admitted patients with fecal incontinence when stool is unable to be contained in diapers
Zoonotic	Disease transmission from animals to humans either directly or via an insect vector	Animals (rabies, Q fever) Arthropods (malaria, Lyme disease)	Prophylactic medications, vaccinations Protective clothing, insect repellent, mosquito nets, tick inspection
Vertical	Spread of disease from parent to offspring	Congenital syndromes (TORCH infections) Perinatal (HIV, HBV, GBS)	Prenatal screening Prophylactic treatment

Nosocomial Infections

- **nosocomial infections:** infections acquired >48 h after admission to a healthcare facility or within 30 d from discharge
- risk factors: prolonged hospital stay, antibiotic use, surgery, hemodialysis, intensive care, colonization with a resistant organism, immunodeficiency
- patients with nosocomial infections have higher mortality, longer hospital stays, and higher healthcare costs
- hand hygiene is an essential precaution

Table 7. Common Nosocomial Infectious Agents

Bacteria	Characteristics	Manifestation	Investigations	Management
Methicillin-Resistant *S. aureus* (MRSA)	Gram-positive cocci	Skin and soft tissue infection Bacteremia Pneumonia Endocarditis Osteomyelitis	Admission screening culture from nares and peri-anal region identifies colonization Culture of infection site CXR	Contact precautions For infection: vancomycin or daptomycin or linezolid To decolonize: 2% chlorhexidine wash OD (+ rifampin + (doxycycline or TMP/SMX) + mupirocin cream bid to nares) x 7 d
Vancomycin-Resistant *Enterococcus* (VRE)	Majority are *E. faecium* Resistant if minimum inhibitory concentration of vancomycin is ≥32 μg/mL	Rarely causes disease in healthy people UTI Bacteremia Endocarditis Meningitis	Rectal or perirectal swab OR stool culture for colonization Culture of infected site	Contact precautions* Ampicillin if susceptible Otherwise, linezolid, tigecycline, or daptomycin depending on site of infection No effective decolonization methods identified

Table 7. Common Nosocomial Infectious Agents (continued)

Bacteria	Characteristics	Manifestation	Investigations	Management
Clostridium difficile **(*C. difficile*)**	Releases exotoxins A and B Hypervirulent strain (NAP1/B1/027) has been responsible for increase in incidence and severity	Fever, nausea, abdominal pain Watery diarrhea ± occult blood Pseudomembranous colitis Severe: toxic megacolon Risk of bowel perforation Associated with antibiotic use Leukocytosis	Stool PCR for toxin A and B genes Stool immunoassay for toxins A and B (less sensitive than PCR) AXR (may see colonic dilatation) Sigmoidoscopy for pseudomembranes; avoid if known colonic dilatation	Contact precautions Stop culprit antibiotic therapy (primarily fluoroquinolones and cephalosporins) Supportive therapy (IV fluids) Mild-moderate disease: metronidazole PO x 10-14 d Severe disease: vancomycin PO x 10-14 d Toxic megacolon: metronidazole IV + vancomycin PO (as above) and general surgery consult
Extended Spectrum β-lactam Producers (ESBL producing *E. coli, K. pneumoniae*)	Resistant to most β-lactam antibiotics except carbapenams e.g. penicillins, aztreonam, and cephalosporins	UTI Pulmonary infection Bacteremia Liver abscess in susceptible patients Meningitis	Blood, sputum, urine, or aspirated body fluid culture Imaging at infection site (CXR, CT, U/S)	Carbapenems or non-β-lactam antibiotics can be used for empiric therapy

*the use of contact precautions for VRE varies depending on institutional policies

Respiratory Infections

Pneumonia

- see Pediatrics, P85

Definition
- infection of the lung parenchyma

Etiology and Risk Factors
- impaired lung defenses
  - poor cough/gag reflex (e.g. illness, drug-induced)
  - impaired mucociliary transport (e.g. smoking, cystic fibrosis)
  - immunosuppression (e.g. steroids, chemotherapy, AIDS/HIV, DM, transplant, cancer)
- increased risk of aspiration
  - impaired swallowing mechanism (e.g. impaired consciousness, neurologic illness causing dysphagia, mechanical obstruction)
- no organism identified in 75% of hospitalized cases, and >90% of ambulatory cases

When *Klebsiella* causes pneumonia; see red currant jelly sputum

3 As of *Klebsiella*
Aspiration pneumonia
Alcoholics and diabetics
Abscess in lungs

Table 8. Common Organisms in Pneumonia

Community-Acquired	Nosocomial	Aspiration	Immunocompromised Patients	Alcoholic
Typical Bacteria *Streptococcus pneumoniae* *Moraxella catarrhalis* *Haemophilus influenzae* *Staphylococcus aureus* GAS Atypical Bacteria *Mycoplasma pneumoniae* *Chlamydophila pneumoniae* *Legionella pneumophila* Viral Influenza virus Adenovirus	Enteric GNB (e.g. *E. coli*) *Pseudomonas aeruginosa* *S. aureus* (including MRSA)	Oral anerobes (e.g. *Bacteroides*) Enteric GNB (e.g. *E. coli*) *S. aureus* Gastric contents (chemical pneumonitis)	*Pneumocystis jiroveci* Fungi (e.g. *Cryptococcus*) *Nocardia* CMV HSV TB	*Klebsiella* Enteric GNB *S. aureus* Oral anaerobes (aspiration) TB

Aspiration pneumonias more commonly manifest as infiltrates in the right middle or lower lobes due to the larger calibre and more vertical orientation of the right bronchus

*See Pediatrics P86, Table for Common Causes and Treatment of Pneumonia at Different Ages

Clinical Features
- cough (± sputum), fever, pleuritic chest pain, dyspnea, tachypnea, tachycardia
- elderly often present atypically; altered LOC is sometimes the only sign
- evidence of consolidation (dullness to percussion, bronchial breath sounds, crackles)
- features of parapneumonic effusion (decreased air entry, dullness to percussion)
- complications: ARDS, lung abscess, parapneumonic effusion/empyema, pleuritis ± hemorrhage

Does This Patient Have Ventilator-Associated Pneumonia?
JAMA 2007;297:1583-1593
Study: Systematic review of articles describing the precision and accuracy of clinical, radiographic, and laboratory data to diagnose bacterial ventilator-associated pneumonia, which is the most common and fatal nosocomial complication of intensive care.
Results: The presence of a new infiltrate on radiography with 2 or more of purulent sputum, fever, or increased white blood cell count increases the likelihood of ventilator-associated pneumonia (LR 2.8, 95% CI 0.97-7.9). Fewer than 50% neutrophils on the cell count of lower pulmonary secretions make ventilator-associated pneumonia unlikely (LR 0.05-0.10).
Conclusions: Routine bedside evaluation with radiographic information provides suggestive, but not definitive, evidence of ventilator-associated pneumonia. Clinicians need to consider additional tests to provide further evidence for ventilator-associated pneumonia.

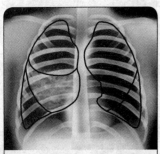

Lobar Pneumonia

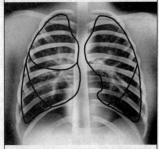

Bronchopneumonia

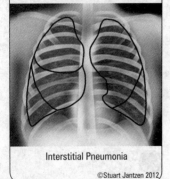

Interstitial Pneumonia

©Stuart Jantzen 2012

Figure 6. Lobar, broncho, and interstitial pneumonia

Investigations

- pulse oximetry to assess severity of respiratory distress
- CBC and differential, electrolytes, urea, Cr, ABG (if respiratory distress), troponin/CK, LFTs, urinalysis
- sputum Gram stain/C&S, blood C&S, ± serology/viral detection, ± pleural fluid C&S (if effusion >5 cm or respiratory distress)
- CXR±CT chest shows distribution (lobar consolidation or interstitial pattern), extent of infiltrate ± cavitation
- bronchoscopy ± washings for
  - (1) severely ill patients refractory to treatment and (2) immunocompromised patients

Treatment

- ABC, O₂, IV fluids, consider salbutamol (nebulized or MDI)
- determine prognosis and need for hospitalization and antibiotics

Criteria for Hospitalization

Table 9. CURB 65 Score – Pneumonia Clinical Prediction Tool

Component*	Measurement(s)	Points	Total Score	Mortality	Disposition
Confusion	Altered mental status	1	0-1	<5%	Can treat as outpatient
Urea/BUN	Urea >7 mmol/L or BUN >20 mg/dL	1	2-3	5-15%	Consider hospitalization
Respiratory Rate	>30 breaths/min	1	4-5	15-30%	Consider ICU
Blood Pressure	Systolic <90 or diastolic <60 mmHg	1			
Age	65 or older	1			

* A CRB-65 score may be applied in the community as its criteria depend on clinical assessment alone

Table 10. IDSA/ATS Community Acquired Pneumonia Treatment Guidelines 2007

Setting	Circumstances	Treatment
Outpatient	Previously well No antibiotic use in last 3 mo	Macrolide[1] OR Doxycycline
	Comorbidities[2] Antibiotic use in last 3 mo (use different class)	Respiratory fluoroquinolone[3] OR β-lactam[4] + Macrolide[1]
Inpatient	Ward	Respiratory fluoroquinolone[3]
	ICU	β-lactam[4] + (Macrolide[1] OR Respiratory fluoroquinolone[3])

1. **Macrolide:** azithromycin, clarithromycin, erythromycin
2. **Comorbidities:** chronic heart, lung, liver, or renal disease, DM, alcoholism, malignancy, asplenia, immunocompromised
3. **Respiratory fluoroquinolone:** moxifloxacin, gemifloxacin, levofloxacin
4. **β-lactam:** cefotaxime, ceftriaxone, ampicillin-sulbactam
IDSA: Infectious Diseases Society of America
ATS: American Thoracics Society

Table 11. IDSA/ATS Hospital/Ventilator/Healthcare-Associated Pneumonia Treatment Guidelines 2005

Setting	Treatment
No risk factors for multidrug resistance (MDR) Early onset (<5 d)	ceftriaxone OR levofloxacin, moxifloxacin, or ciprofloxacin OR ampicillin/sulbactam OR ertapenem

Late onset disease (≥5 d) or
With risk factors for MDR:
  Antibiotic use in last 3 mo
  High frequency of antibiotic resistance in the community or in the specific hospital unit
  Hospitalization >1 d in past 3 mo
  Residence in a nursing home or extended care facility
  Dialysis within 30 d
  Home wound care
  Family member with multidrug-resistant pathogen
  Immunosuppressive disease and/or therapy
	antipseudomonal cephalosporin (cefepime or ceftazidime)
	OR
	antipseudomonal carbepenem (imipenem or meropenem)
	OR
	β-lactam/β-lactamase inhibitor (piperacillin/tazobactam)
	PLUS
	antipseudomonal fluoroquinolone (ciprofloxacin or levofloxacin)
	OR
	aminoglycoside (amikacin, gentamicin, or tobramycin)
	PLUS for MRSA
	linezolid or vancomycin
	PLUS for *Legionella*
	ensure regime includes either a macrolide or a fluoroquinolone

Note: Always use directed therapy against specific organism if one is found on culture (e.g. blood, sputum, etc.)
Note: These guidelines may be less applicable in Canada given lower rates of antibiotic resistance among common nosocomial pathogens

Prevention

- Public Health Agency of Canada recommends the following
  - vaccine for influenza A and B annually for all ages ≥ 6 mo
  - pneumococcal polysaccharide vaccine (Pneumovax®) for all adults >65 yr and in younger patients 24 mo of age and older at high risk for invasive pneumococcal disease (e.g. functional or anatomic asplenia, congenital or acquired immunodeficiency)
  - pneumococcal conjugate vaccine (Prevnar-13®) for all children <5 yr, and for children and adolescents at high risk for invasive pneumococcal disease who are 5-17 yr and who have not previously received Prevnar-13® (CDC recommends giving Prevnar-13® to all adults at high risk for invasive pneumococcal disease)

Influenza

Definitions and Etiology

- influenza viruses A and B
- influenza A further divided into subtypes based on envelope glycoproteins
  - hemagglutinin (H) and neuraminidase (N)
- seasonal (epidemic) influenza
  - main circulating influenza viruses: influenza A (H1N1), influenza A (H3N2) and influenza B
  - associated with antigenic drift (gradual, minor changes due to random point mutations)
  - may create a new viral subtype resulting in a seasonal epidemic (disease prevalence is greater than expected)
  - outbreaks occur mainly during winter months (late December to early March)
- pandemic influenza
  - associated with antigenic shift: abrupt, major changes due to mixing of two different viral strains from different hosts
  - may create a new viral strain resulting in a pandemic outbreak (worldwide)
  - antigenic shift occurs only in type A
- transmission: droplet, possibly airborne

Table 12. Difference Between Influenza Strains

	Influenza A	Influenza B
Host(s)	Humans, birds, mammals	Humans only
Antigenic drift	Yes, new strains	Yes, new strains
Antigenic shift	Yes, new subtypes	No
Epidemics	Yes	Yes
Pandemics	Yes	No

Clinical Features

- incubation period 1-4 d and symptoms typically resolve in 7-10 days
- acute onset of systemic (fever, chills, myalgias, arthralgias, H/A, fatigue) and respiratory symptoms (cough, dyspnea, pharyngitis)
- complications: respiratory (viral pneumonia, secondary bacterial pneumonia, otitis media, sinusitis), muscular (rhabdomyolysis, myositis), neurologic (encephalitis, meningitis, transverse myelitis, Guillain-Barré syndrome)
- severe disease more likely in the elderly, children, pregnant women, patients with immunocompromise, asthma, COPD, CVD, diabetes and obesity

Investigations

- diagnosis is primarily clinical based on symptoms during the influenza season
- nasopharyngeal swabs for rapid antigen detection, DFA (Direct Fluorescent Antigen) detection, RT-PCR (gold standard)
- serology: rarely used for clinical management

Treatment and Prevention

- primarily supportive unless severe infection or high-risk of complications
- neuraminidase inhibitors: zanamivir (Relenza®) and oseltamivir (Tamiflu®) for treatment and prophylaxis against types A and B
  - decreases duration (by ~1 d) and severity of symptoms if given within 48 h of onset
  - treatment beyond 48 h time window may be warranted in immunosuppressed and critically ill patients
- vaccine for influenza A and B viruses is recommended annually for all ages ≥ 6 mo
  - vaccine is reformulated each year to reflect circulating influenza A and B strains

Does This Adult Patient Have Pneumonia? From The Rational Clinical Examination
JAMA 2009; http://www.jamaevidence.com/content/3485708
Study: Systematic review of articles assessing the sensitivity and specificity of clinical exam maneuvers for the diagnosis of adult community acquired pneumonia.
Results: The presence of fever or immunosuppression had a positive likelihood ratio (+LR) of 2, while a history of dementia had a +LR of 3; however, these traits are not confirmatory. The presence of an abnormality in any vital sign, including tachycardia, tachypnea, or fever had a +LR ranging from 2-4, which was not significantly affected by different cut-points. The absence of vital sign abnormality had a –LR ranging from 0.5-0.8. The combination of respiratory rate <30/min, heart rate <100/min, and temperature <37.8°C had a –LR of 0.18. Findings on chest exam raised the likelihood of diagnosis, but were uncommonly seen in studies. For example, presence of asymmetric respirations essentially confirmed the diagnosis, but was only present in 4% of patients. In patients with a clinical diagnosis, but normal radiograph, only ~10% will develop radiographic findings in 72 h.
Conclusions: Evidence suggests no single item on clinical history or physical exam is sufficient to rule in or out pneumonia without chest x-ray. Vital sign abnormalities were correlated with a diagnosis of pneumonia. Findings on chest exam significantly raised the likelihood of pneumonia, but were uncommonly seen in studies.

Beware! Do Not Confuse *H. influenzae* with Influenza Virus
H. influenzae: a bacterium (Types A, B, C, D, E, F, refer to capsule)
Influenza: a virus (Types A and B refer to strain)

Vaccines for Preventing Influenza in Healthy Adults
Cochrane DB Syst Rev 2014;CD001269
Study: Meta-analysis of 90 RCTs and quasi-RCTs evaluating influenza vaccines compared to placebo in healthy individuals aged 16-65 yr.
Results: The preventative effect of inactivated influenza vaccine on healthy adults is small: 40 people would need a vaccination to avoid one influenza-like illness and 71 people would need a vaccination to prevent one case of influenza. 15.6% of unvaccinated versus 9.9% of vaccinated people developed influenza-like symptoms: of these participants, only 2.4% and 1.1%, respectively, developed laboratory-confirmed influenza. Vaccination had a modest effect on working days lost, but no effects on hospitalization or complications. The effectiveness of live aerosol vaccinations on healthy adults is similar to that of inactivated influenza vaccines: 46 people would need a vaccination to avoid one influenza-like illness.
Conclusions: Influenza vaccines have a very modest effect in reducing influenza-like illness and working days lost in the general population.

Skin and Soft Tissue Infections

Cellulitis

Definition
- acute infection of the skin principally involving the dermis and subcutaneous tissue

Etiology
- common causative agents: *S. aureus*, β-hemolytic streptococci
- immunocompromised patients or water exposure: may also include GN rods and fungi
- risk factors
    - trauma with direct inoculation, recent surgery
    - peripheral vascular disease, lymphedema DM, cracked skin in feet/toes (tinea pedis)

Clinical Features
- pain, edema, erythema with indistinct borders ± regional lymphadenopathy, systemic symptoms (fevers, chills, malaise)
- can lead to ascending lymphangitis (visible red streaking in skin along lymphatics proximal to area of cellulitis)

Investigations
- CBC and differential, blood C&S if febrile
- skin swab ONLY if open wound with pus

Treatment
- antibiotics: cephalexin (broader coverage if risk factors for GN rods)
- if extensive erythema or systemic symptoms, consider cefazolin IV
- if MRSA is suspected, alternative therapy should be prescribed (see *A Simplified Look at Antibiotics*, ID47)
- limb rest and elevation may help reduce swelling

Necrotizing Fasciitis

Definition
- life- and limb-threatening infection of the deep fascia characterized by rapid spread

Etiology
- Two main forms
    - Type I: polymicrobial infection – aerobes and anaerobes (e.g. *S. aureus, Bacteroides, Enterobacteriaceae*)
    - Type II: monomicrobial infection with GAS, and less commonly *S. aureus*

Clinical Features
- pain out of proportion to clinical findings and beyond border of erythema
- edema, ± crepitus (subcutaneous gas from anaerobes), ± fever
- infection spreads rapidly
- patients may rapidly become very sick (tachycardia, hypotension, lightheadedness)
- late findings
    - skin turns dusky blue and black (secondary to thrombosis and necrosis)
    - induration, formation of hemorrhagic bullae

Investigations
- clinical/surgical diagnosis – do NOT wait for results of investigations before beginning treatment
- blood and tissue C&S
- serum CK (elevated CK usually means myonecrosis – a late sign)
- plain film x-ray (soft tissue gas may be visualized)
- surgical exploration for debridement of infected tissue

Treatment
- resuscitation with IV fluids
- emergency surgical debridement to confirm diagnosis and remove necrotic tissue (may require amputation)
- IV antibiotics
    - unknown organism: meropenem or piperacillin/tazobactam + clindamycin IV ± vancomycin if MRSA is considered
    - Type I (polymicrobial): piperacillin/tazobactam + clindamycin IV
    - Type II (monomicrobial): cefazolin (or cloxacillin) + clindamycin IV; with confirmed GAS infection, penicillin G + clindamycin IV
    - with Type II, evaluate for streptococcal toxic shock syndrome and the need for IVIg

Gastrointestinal Infections

Acute Diarrhea

- see Gastroenterology, G15 and Pediatrics, P33

Epidemiology
- one of the top five leading causes of death worldwide, according to the World Health Organization
- significant morbidity in developed countries (over 900,000 hospitalizations in the United States each year)

Definition
- passage of ≥3 loose or liquid stools/d OR >200 g stool/d for >2 d but ≤14 d

Approach to Acute Diarrhea
- rationale
  - the vast majority of acute diarrhea is caused by infection
  - in most cases, acute diarrheal illness is viral and/or self-limited, and lasts <3 d
  - investigations are costly and are necessary only in certain circumstances
- therefore, the evaluation of acute diarrhea involves
  - identifying characteristics of the illness or patient that warrant further investigation
  - assessing volume status to determine appropriate method of rehydration

Physical Exam
- volume status: appearance, level of alertness, pulse, BP, orthostatic vitals, JVP, mucous membranes, skin turgor, capillary refill
- abdominal exam: pain, guarding, peritoneal signs

Treatment
- rehydration is mainstay of treatment
  - oral rehydration therapy
  - IV rehydration if oral intake insufficient to replace fluid loss
- antidiarrheal agents reduce duration of diarrhea: loperamide, bismuth salicylate
  - delays excretion of causative pathogens
  - contraindications: diarrhea with fever, bloody stool or diarrhea caused by *C. difficile*
- antibiotic therapy is rarely indicated because
  - most acute diarrheal illness is viral and self-limited
  - antibiotics can eradicate normal gut flora, predisposing patient to *C. difficile* infection
  - antibiotics prolong the shedding of *Salmonella* and other causes of bacterial diarrhea
  - in EHEC infection, antibiotics may increase the risk of HUS

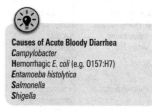

Causes of Acute Bloody Diarrhea
Campylobacter
Hemorrhagic *E. coli* (e.g. O157:H7)
Entamoeba histolytica
Salmonella
Shigella

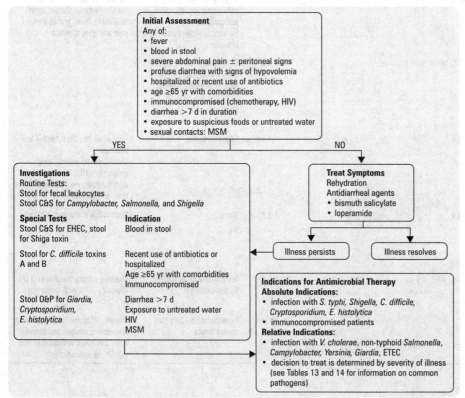

Figure 7. Approach to acute diarrhea

Table 13. Bacteria in Infectious Diarrhea

Pathogen	Source or Mode of Transmission	Incubation	Clinical Features				Duration	Antimicrobial Therapy	Notes
			Fever	Bloody Stool	Abdo Pain	N/V			
B. cereus – Type A (emetic)	Rice dishes	1-6 h	–	–	–	+	<12 h	None	Preformed exotoxin
B. cereus – Type B (diarrheal)	Meats, vegetables, dried beans, cereals	8-16 h	–	–	–	–	<24 h	None	Secondary endotoxin
Campylobacter jejuni	Uncooked meat, especially poultry	2-10 d	+	±	+	±	<1 wk	Macrolide or fluoroquinolone if diarrhea >1 wk, bloody diarrhea, or immunocompromised	Most common bacterial cause of diarrhea in Canada Associated with Guillain-Barré syndrome
Clostridium difficile	Can be normally present in colon in small numbers (primary risk factor for disease is exposure to antimicrobials)	Unclear	±	±	±	–	Variable	Stop culprit antibiotic therapy, if possible Supportive therapy (IV fluids) Mild-moderate disease: metronidazole PO x 10-14 d Severe disease: vancomycin PO x 10 - 14 d Toxic Megacolon: metronidazole IV + vancomycin PO (as above) and general surgery consult	Usually follows antibiotic treatment (especially clindamycin, fluoroquinolones, penicillins, cephalosporins) Can develop pseudomembranous colitis
Clostridium perfringens	Contaminated food, especially meat and poultry	8-12 h	±	–	+	–	<24 h	None	Clostridium spores are heat resistant Secondary enterotoxin
Enteroinvasive *E. coli* (EIEC)	Contaminated food/water	1-3 d	+	±	+	–	7-10 d	None	Relatively uncommon
Enterotoxigenic *E. coli* (ETEC)	Contaminated food/water	1-3 d	–	–	+	–	3 d	Fluoroquinolone or azithromycin for moderate to severe symptoms	Most common cause of traveller's diarrhea Heat-labile and heat-stable toxins
Enterohemorrhagic *E. coli* (EHEC/STEC) i.e. O157:H7	Contamination of hamburger, raw milk, drinking, and recreational water	3-8 d	–	+	±	±	5-10 d	None: antibiotics increase risk of HUS	Shiga toxin production Monitor renal function:10% develop HUS Antidiarrheals increase risk of HUS
Salmonella typhi *S. paratyphi* (i.e. Enteric Fever, Typhoid)	Fecal-oral Contaminated food/water, travel to endemic area	10-14 d	+	±	+	±	<5-7 d	Empiric treatment with ceftriaxone, ciprofloxacin, or azithromycin Fluoroquinolone resistance is increasing	*Salmonella typhi*: "Rose spot" rash (on anterior thorax, upper abdomen), fever, and abdominal pain precedes diarrhea
Non-typhoidal Salmonellosis *S. typhimurium*, *S. enteritidis*	Contaminated animal food products, especially eggs, poultry, meat, milk	12-72 h	+	±	+	+	3-7 d	Ciprofloxacin only in severe illness, extremes of age, joint prostheses, valvular heart disease, severe atherosclerosis, cancer, uremia	
Shigella dysenteriae	Fecal-oral Contaminated food/water	1-4 d	+	±	+	+	<1 wk	Fluoroquinolone	Very small inoculum needed for infection Complications include toxic megacolon, HUS Antidiarrheals may increase risk of toxic megacolon
Staphylococcus aureus	Unrefrigerated meat and dairy products (custard, pudding, potato salad, mayo)	2-4 h	–	–	+	+	1-2 d	None	Heat-stable preformed exotoxin
Vibrio cholerae	Contaminated food/water, especially shellfish	1-3 d	–	–	–	–	3-7 d	Tetracycline or quinolones (ciprofloxacin)	Massive watery diarrhea (1-3 L/d) Mortality <1% with treatment
Yersinia	Contaminated food Unpasteurized milk	5 d	+	±	+	±	Up to 3 wk	Fluoroquinolone only for severe illness	Majority of cases in children 1-4 yr Mesenteric adenitis and terminal ileitis can occur without diarrhea, mimicking appendicitis

Table 14. Parasites in Infectious Diarrhea

Pathogen	Source or Mode of Transmission	Incubation	Clinical Features				Duration	Antimicrobial Therapy	Notes
			Fever	Bloody Stool	Abdo Pain	N/V			
Cryptosporidium	Fecal-oral	7 d	±	−	−	+	1-20 d	Paromomycin + nitazoxanide	Immune reconstitution if immunosuppressed
Entamoeba histolytica	Worldwide endemic areas Fecal-oral	2-4 wk	±	+	−	+	Variable	Metronidazole + iodoquinol or paromomycin if symptomatic infection Only iodoquinol or paromomycin for asymptomatic cyst passage	If untreated, potential for liver abscess Sigmoidoscopy shows flat ulcers with yellow exudates
Giardia lamblia	Fecal-oral Contaminated food/water	1-4 wk	−	−	+	+	Variable	Metronidazole or nitazoxanide Treatment of asymptomatic carriers not recommended	Higher risk in: day care children, intake of untreated water ("beaver fever"), MSM, immunodeficiency (decreased IgA) May need duodenal biopsy

Table 15. Viruses in Infectious Diarrhea

Pathogen	Source or Mode of Transmission	Incubation	Clinical Features				Duration	Antimicrobial Therapy	Notes
			Fever	Bloody Stool	Abdo Pain	N/V			
Norovirus	Fecal-oral	24 h	−	−	+	+	24 h	None	Noroviruses includes Norwalk virus
Rotavirus	Fecal-oral	2-4 d	±	−	−	±	3-8 d	None	Can cause severe dehydration Virtually all children are infected by 3 yr of age Oral vaccine given at 2 and 4 mo of age

Traveller's Diarrhea

• see *Acute Diarrhea*, ID11

Epidemiology
• most common illness to affect travellers
• up to 50% of travellers to developing countries affected in first 2 wk and 10-20% after returning home

Etiology
• bacterial (80-90%): *E. coli* most common (ETEC), *Campylobacter, Shigella, Salmonella, Vibrio* (non-cholera); wide regional variation (e.g. *Campylobacter* more common in Southeast Asia)
• viral: norovirus, rotavirus, and astrovirus account for 5-8%
• protozoal (rarely): *Giardia, Entamoeba histolytica, Cryptosporidium,* and *Cyclospora* for ~10% in long-term travellers
• pathogen-negative traveller's diarrhea common despite exhaustive microbiological workup

Treatment
• rehydration is the mainstay of therapy
  ▪ rehydrate with sealed beverages
  ▪ in severe fluid loss use oral rehydration solutions (1 package in 1 L boiled or treated water)
• treat symptoms: antidiarrheal agents (e.g. bismuth salicylate, loperamide)
• empiric antibiotics in moderate or severe illness: ciprofloxacin or azithromycin or rifaximin
  ▪ note: there is increasing fluoroquinolone resistance in causative agents, especially in South and Southeast Asia

Prevention
• proper hygiene practices
  ▪ avoid consumption of: foods or beverages from establishments with unhygienic conditions (e.g. street vendors), raw fruits or vegetables without a peel, raw or undercooked meat and seafood
  ▪ avoid untreated water
• bismuth salicylate (Pepto-Bismol®): 60% effective (2 tablets qid according to CDC website)
• CDC Guidelines: antibiotic prophylaxis not recommended
  ▪ increased risk of infection with resistant organisms
  ▪ high risk groups (e.g. immunocompromised) likely to be infected with pathogen not covered by standard antimicrobial agents

Bismuth salicylate (Pepto-Bismol®) can cause patients to have black stools, which may be mistaken for melena

- Dukoral®: oral vaccine that offers protection against *V. cholerae* (efficacy ~80%) and ETEC (efficacy ~50-67%). Not recommended for routine use in travellers, but the PHAC recommends that it may be considered in short-term travellers >2 yr old who are high-risk (e.g. chronic illness) for whom there is an increased risk of serious consequences for traveller's diarrhea (e.g. chronic renal failure, CHF, type 1 DM, inflammatory bowel disease), immunosuppressed, history of repeat traveller's diarrhea, increased risk of acquiring traveller's diarrhea (gastric hypochlorhydria or young children >2 yr), or travellers to cholera endemic countries at increased risk of exposure
- Two vaccines against *Salmonella typhi* are available and their effectiveness is estimated to be between 50-70%

Chronic Diarrhea

- see Gastroenterology, G16

Peptic Ulcer Disease (*H. pylori*)

- see Gastroenterology, G11

Bone and Joint Infections

Septic Arthritis

Routes of Infection
- hematogenous
  - contiguous osteomyelitis common in children
- direct inoculation via skin/trauma
- iatrogenic (surgery, arthroscopy, arthrocentesis)

Etiology
- gonococcal
  - *N. gonorrhoeae*: previously accounted for 75% of septic arthritis in young sexually active adults
- non-gonococcal
  - *S. aureus*: affects all ages, rapidly destructive, accounts for most non-gonococcal cases of septic arthritis in adults (especially in those with rheumatoid arthritis)
  - *Streptococcus* species (Group A and B)
  - Gram-negatives: affect neonates, elderly, IV drug users, immunocompromised
  - *S. pneumoniae*: affects children
  - *Kingella kingae*: affects children aged <2 yr of age
  - *Haemophilus influenzae* type B (Hib) now rare due to Hib vaccine: consider in unvaccinated children
  - *Salmonella* spp.: characteristic of sickle cell disease
  - coagulase-negative *Staphylococcus* species: prosthetic joints
- if culture negative: partially-treated infection (prior to oral antibiotics), reactive arthritis, rheumatic fever, less common bacterial causes such as *Borrelia* spp. (Lyme disease) or *Tropheryma whipplei* (Whipple's disease), and non-infectious causes

Risk Factors
- gonococcal
  - age (<40 yr), multiple partners, unprotected intercourse, MSM
- non-gonoccocal
  - most affected children are previously healthy with no risk factors: occasionally preceding history of minor trauma
  - bacteremia (extra-articular infection with hematogenous seeding, endocarditis)
  - prosthetic joints/recent joint surgery
  - underlying joint disease (rheumatoid arthritis, osteoarthritis)
  - immunocompromise (DM, chronic kidney disease, alcoholism, cirrhosis)
  - loss of skin integrity (cutaneous ulcer, skin infection)
  - age >80 yr

Clinical Features of Gonococcal Arthritis
- two forms (although often overlap)
  - bacteremic form
  - systemic symptoms: fever, malaise, chills
  - gonococcal triad: migratory polyarthralgias, tenosynovitis, dermatitis (pustular skin lesions)
  - septic arthritis form
  - local symptoms in involved joint: swelling, warmth, pain, inability to bear weight, marked decrease in range of motion (see Rheumatology, RH5 for differential diagnosis)

Medical Emergency
Septic arthritis is a medical emergency! If untreated, rapid joint destruction will occur

Disseminated Gonococcal Infection Triad
- Migratory arthralgias
- Tenosynovitis next to inflamed joint
- Pustular skin lesions

Clinical Features of Non-Gonoccocal Arthritis
- acute onset of pain, swelling, warmth, decreased range of motion ± fever and chills
- most often in large weight-bearing joints (knee, hip, ankle) and wrists
- usually monoarticular (polyarticular risk factors: rheumatoid arthritis, endocarditis, GBS)

Investigations
- consider rheumatologic causes for monoarthritis (see <u>Rheumatology</u>, RH3)
- gonococcal: blood C&S, as well as endocervical, urethral, rectal, and oropharyngeal testing
- non-gonococcal: blood C&S
- arthrocentesis (synovial fluid analysis) is mandatory: CBC and differential, Gram stain, C&S, examine for crystals
    - infectious = opaque, increased WBCs (>15,000/mm³: likelihood of infection increases with increasing WBCs), PMNs >90%, culture positive
    - growth of *N. gonorrhoeae* from synovial fluid is successful in <50% of cases
- ± plain x-ray: assess for osteomyelitis, provides baseline to monitor treatment

Intra-articular steroids are contraindicated until septic arthritis has been excluded

Treatment
- medical
    - empiric IV antibiotics: specific choice depends on clinical scenario; for most adults, vancomycin + ceftriaxone is reasonable; for fully vaccinated children, cefazolin or cloxacillin IV unless MRSA is a consideration – delay may result in joint destruction
    - Gram stain and cultures guide subsequent treatment
    - gonococcal: ceftriaxone + azithromycin, for concurrent treatment of *C. trachomatis*
    - non-gonococcal: antibiotics against *Streptococcus* spp. (2-3 wk IV f/b PO), *S. aureus* (4 wk IV minimum), or GNB (4 wk)
- surgical drainage if (see <u>Orthopedics</u>, OR10)
    - persistent positive joint cultures on repeat arthrocentesis
    - hip joint involvement
    - prosthetic joint
- daily joint aspirations until culture sterile; no need to give intra-articular antibiotics
- physiotherapy

Prognosis
- gonococcal: responds well after 24-48 h of initiating antibiotics (usually complete recovery)
- non-gonococcal: in children, generally good outcome if treated promptly; in adults, up to 50% morbidity (decreased joint function/mobility)

Diabetic Foot Infections

Etiology
- neuropathy, peripheral vascular disease, and hyperglycemia contribute to foot ulcers that heal poorly, and are predisposed to infection
- organisms in mild infection: *S. aureus*, *Streptococcus* spp.
- organisms in moderate/severe infection: polymicrobial with aerobes (*S. aureus*, *Streptococcus*, *Enterococcus*, GNB) and anaerobes (*Peptostreptococcus*, *Bacteroides*, *Clostridium*)

Clinical Features
- not all ulcers are infected
- consider infection if: probe to bone (see below), ulcer present >30 d, recurrent ulcers, trauma, PVD, prior amputation, loss of protective sensation, renal disease, history of walking barefoot
- diagnosis of infected ulcer: ≥2 of the cardinal signs of inflammation (redness, warmth, swelling, pain) or the presence of pus
- ± crepitus, osteomyelitis, systemic toxicity
- visible bone or probe to bone → osteomyelitis
- infection severity
    - mild = superficial (no bone/joint involvement)
    - moderate = deep (beneath superficial fascia, involving bone/joint) or erythema >2 cm
    - severe = infection in a patient with systemic toxicity (fever, tachypnea, leukocytosis, tachycardia, hypotension)

Investigations
- curettage specimen from ulcer base, aspirate from an abscess or bone biopsy (results from superficial swabs do not represent organisms responsible for deeper infection)
- blood C&S if febrile
- assess for osteomyelitis by x-ray (although not sensitive in early stages) or MRI if high clinical suspicion
    - if initial x-ray normal, repeat 2-4 wk after initiating treatment to increase test sensitivity

Treatment
- evaluate for early surgical debridement ± revascularization or amputation
- eliminate/reduce pressure and provide regular local wound care
- mild: cephalexin or clindamycin

Does this Patient with Diabetes have Osteomyelitis of the Lower Extremity?
JAMA 2008;299:806-813
Study: Systematic literature review. 21 studies.
Population: 1,027 adult patients with DM being investigated for osteomyelitis.
Intervention: Various aspects of history, physical exam, laboratory tests, and diagnostic imaging studies versus bone biopsy.
Primary Outcome: Diagnostic utility.
Results: No studies examined any part of history taking. Temperature, ulcer characteristics (erythema, swelling, purulence), elevated WBC, skin swabs, and soft tissue cultures were not useful. Nuclear imaging has poor specificity for osteomyelitis (62%-88.5%), and MRIs have greater accuracy in detecting osteomyelitis.

Finding	(+) LR	(–) LR
Visualization of bone	9.2	0.70
Ulcer area >2 cm²	7.2	0.48
Probe-to-bone	6.4	0.39
Clinical judgment	5.5	0.54
ESR >70 mm/h	11	NS*
Plain radiographs	2.3	0.63
MRI	3.8	0.14

*NS = not significant

- moderate: clindamycin + ciprofloxacin or moxifloxacin PO, ceftriaxone or ertapenem IV ± MRSA coverage
- severe: piperacillin/tazobactam or meropenem IV ± vancomycin if MRSA known or suspected
- encourage glycemic control

Osteomyelitis

- see Orthopedics, OR9

Cardiac Infections

Infective Endocarditis

Definition
- infection of cardiac endothelium, most commonly the valves
- classifications: acute vs. subacute, native valve vs. prosthetic valve, right sided vs. left sided
- leaflet vegetations are made of platelet-fibrin thrombi, WBCs, and bacteria

Risk Factors and Etiology
- predisposing conditions
  - **high risk:** prosthetic cardiac valve, previous IE, congenital heart disease (unrepaired, repaired within 6 mo, repaired with defects), cardiac transplant with valve disease (surgically constructed systemic-to-pulmonary shunts or conduits)
  - moderate risk: other congenital cardiac defects, acquired valvular dysfunction, hypertrophic cardiomyopathy
  - low/no risk: secundum ASD or surgically repaired ASD < VSD, PDA, MV prolapse, ischemic heart disease, previous CABG
  - opportunity for bacteremia: IVDU, indwelling venous catheter, hemodialysis, poor dentition, DM, HIV
- frequency of valve involvement MV >> AV > TV > PV
  - but in 50% of IVDU-related IE the tricuspid valve is involved

Etiology of Culture-Negative Endocarditis
- HACEK (fastidious Gram-negative bacilli)
  Haemophilus parainfluenzae
  Aggregatibacter aphrophilus/
  Aggregatibacter actinomycetemcomitans
  Cardiobacterium hominis
  Eikenella corrodens
  Kingella kingae
- *Coxiella burnetii*
- *Bartonella* species
- *Tropheryma whipplei*
- Fungi
- Mycobacteria

Table 16. Microbial Etiology of Infective Endocarditis Based on Risk Factors

Native Valve	Intravenous Drug Users (IVDU)	Prosthetic Valve(recent surgery <2 mo)	Prosthetic Valve(remote surgery >2 mo)
Streptococcus[1] (36%)	*S. aureus* (68%)	*S. aureus* (36%)	*Streptococcus* (20%)
S. aureus (28%)	*Streptococcus* (13%)	*S. epidermidis* (17%)	*S. aureus* (20%)
Enterococcus (11%)	*Enterococcus*	Other	*S. epidermidis* (20%)
S. epidermidis	GNB	*Enterococcus*	*Enterococcus* (13%)
GNB	Candida	GNB	Other[2]
Other[2]	Other[3]	Other[2]	

Organisms in bold are the most common isolates
1. *Streptococcus* includes mainly viridans group streptococci
2. Other includes less common organisms such as:
   - *Streptococcus gallolyticus* (previously known as *S. bovis*; usually associated with underlying GI malignancy, cirrhosis)
   - Culture-negative organisms including nutritionally-deficient streptococci, HACEK, *Bartonella*, *Coxiella*, *Chlamydia*, *Legionella*, *Brucella*
   - *Candida*
3. IVDU endocarditis pathogens depend on substance used to dilute the drugs (i.e. tap water = *Pseudomonas*, saliva = oral flora, toilet water = GI flora)

Clinical Features
- systemic
  - fever (80-90%), chills, weakness, rigors, night sweats, weight loss, anorexia
- cardiac
  - dyspnea, chest pain, clubbing (subacute)
  - regurgitant murmur (new onset or increased intensity)
  - signs of CHF (secondary to acute MR, AR)
- embolic/vascular
  - petechiae over legs, splinter hemorrhages (linear, reddish-brown lesion within nail bed)
  - Janeway lesions (painless, 5 mm, erythematous, hemorrhagic pustular lesions on soles/palms)
  - focal neurological signs (CNS emboli), H/A (mycotic aneurysm)
  - splenomegaly (subacute)
  - microscopic hematuria, flank pain (renal emboli) ± active sediment
- immune complex
  - Osler's nodes (painful, raised, red/brown, 3-15 mm on digits)
  - glomerulonephritis
  - arthritis
  - Roth's spots (retinal hemorrhage with pale centre)

Clinical Features of Infective Endocarditis

FROM JANE
Fever
Roth's spots
Osler's nodes
Murmur
Janeway lesions
Anemia
Nail-bed hemorrhages (i.e. splinter hemorrhages)
Emboli

Diagnosis
- Modified Duke Criteria, see Table 17
  - definitive diagnosis if: 2 major, OR 1 major + 3 minor, OR 5 minor
  - possible diagnosis if: 1 major + 1 minor, OR 3 minor

Table 17. Modified Duke Criteria

Major Criteria (2)

1. Positive blood cultures for IE
- Typical microorganisms for IE from 2 separate blood cultures (*Streptococcus viridans*, HACEK group, *Streptococcus gallolyticus* (previously known as *S. bovis*), *Staphylococcus aureus*, community-acquired enterococci) OR
- Persistently positive blood culture, defined as recovery of a microorganism consistent with IE from blood drawn >12 h apart OR
- All of 3 or a majority of 4 or more separate blood cultures, with first and last drawn >1 h apart OR
- Single positive blood culture for *Coxiella burnetii* or antiphase I IgG antibody titer >1:800
2. Evidence of endocardial involvement
- Positive echocardiogram for IE (oscillating intracardiac mass on valve or supporting structures, or in the path of regurgitant jets, or on implanted material in the absence of an alternative anatomic explanation OR abscess OR new partial dehiscence of prosthetic valve) OR
- New valvular regurgitation (insufficient if increase or change in preexisting murmur)

Minor Criteria (5)

1. Predisposing condition (abnormal heart valve, IVDU)
2. Fever (38.0°C/100.4°F)
3. Vascular phenomena: major arterial emboli, septic pulmonary infarcts, mycotic aneurysms, ICH, conjunctival hemorrhages, Janeway lesions
4. Immunologic phenomena: glomerulonephritis, rheumatoid factor, Osler's nodes, Roth's spots
5. Positive blood culture but not meeting major criteria OR serologic evidence of active infection with organism consistent with IE

Investigations

- serial blood cultures: 3 sets (each containing one aerobic and one anaerobic sample) collected from different sites >1 h apart
  - persistent bacteremia is the hallmark of endovascular infection (such as IE)
- repeat blood cultures (at least 2 sets) after 48-72 h of appropriate antibiotics to confirm clearance
- blood work: CBC and differential (normochromic, normocytic anemia), ESR (increased), RF (+), BUN/Cr
- urinalysis (proteinuria, hematuria, red cell casts) and urine C&S
- ECG: prolonged PR interval may indicate perivalvular abscess
- echo findings: vegetations, regurgitation, abscess
  - TTE (poor sensitivity) inadequate in 20% (obesity, COPD, chest wall deformities)
  - TEE indicated if TTE is non-diagnostic in patients with at least possible endocarditis or if suspect prosthetic valve endocarditis or complicated endocarditis (e.g. paravalvular abscess/perforation) (~90% sensitivity)

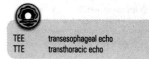

TEE   transesophageal echo
TTE   transthoracic echo

Treatment

- medical
  - usually non-urgent and can wait for confirmation of etiology before initiating treatment
  - empiric antibiotic therapy if patient is unstable; administer ONLY after blood cultures have been taken
    - first-line empiric treatment for native valve: vancomycin + gentamicin OR ceftriaxone
    - first line empiric treatment for prosthetic valve: vancomycin + gentamicin + cefepime + rifampin
  - targeted antibiotic therapy: antibiotic and duration (usually 4-6 wk) adjusted based on valve, organism, and sensitivities
  - monitor for complications of IE (e.g. CHF, conduction block, new emboli) and complications of antibiotics (e.g. interstitial nephritis)
  - prophylaxis only for high risk individuals listed above with dental procedures that may lead to bleeding OR invasive procedure of the respiratory tract that involves incision or biopsy of the respiratory mucosa, such as tonsillectomy and adenoidectomy OR procedures on infected skin, skin structure, or musculoskeletal tissue
    - dental/respiratory: amoxicillin single dose 30-60 min prior; clindamycin if penicillin-allergic
    - skin/soft tissue: cephalexin single dose 30-60 min prior; clindamycin if penicillin-allergic (modify based on etiology of skin/soft tissue infection)
- surgical
  - most common indication is refractory CHF
  - other indications include: valve ring abscess, fungal etiology, valve perforation, unstable prosthesis, ≥2 major emboli, antimicrobial failure (persistently positive blood cultures), mycotic aneurysm, Staphylococci on a prosthetic valve

Prognosis

- adverse prognostic factors: CHF, prosthetic valve infection, valvular/myocardial abscess, embolization, persistent bacteremia, altered mental status prognostic factors: CHF, prosthetic valve infection, valvular/myocardial abscess
- mortality: prosthetic valve IE (25-50%), non-IVDU *S. aureus* IE (30-45%), IVDU *S. aureus* or streptococcal IE (10-15%)

CNS Infections

Meningitis

- see Pediatrics, P59

Definition
- inflammation of the meninges

Etiology

Table 18. Common Organisms in Meningitis

	Bacterial		Viral	Fungal	Other
Age 0-4 wk	Age 1-23 mo	Age >2 yr			
GBS	GBS	S. pneumoniae	HSV-1, 2	Cryptococcus	Lyme disease
E. coli	E. coli	N. meningitidis	VZV	Coccidioides	Neurosyphilis
L. monocytogenes	S. pneumoniae	L. monocytogenes	Enteroviruses		TB
Klebsiella	N. meningitidis	(age >50 and	Parechoviruses		
	H. influenzae	comorbidities)	West Nile		

Brudzinski's Sign
Passive neck flexion causes involuntary flexion of hips and knees

Kernig's Sign
Resistance to knee extension when hip is flexed to 90º

Jolt Accentuation of H/A
Headache worsens when head turned horizontally at 2-3 rotations; more sensitive than Brudzinski's and Kernig's

Risk Factors
- lack of immunization against S. pneumoniae, H. influenzae type b in children
- most cases of bacterial meningitis are due to hematogenous spread from a mucosal surface (nasopharynx)
- direct extension from a parameningeal focus (otitis media, sinusitis) less common
- penetrating head trauma
- anatomical meningeal defects – CSF leaks
- previous neurosurgical procedures, shunts
- immunodeficiency (corticosteroids, HIV, asplenia, hypogammaglobulinemia, complement deficiency)
- contact with colonized or infected persons

CSF Gram Stain Findings
- S. pneumoniae – GP diplococci
- N. meningitidis – GN diplococci
- H. influenzae – Pleiomorphic GN coccobacilli
- L. monocytogenes – GP rods

Clinical Features
- neonates and children: fever, lethargy, irritability, vomiting, poor feeding
- older children and adults: fever, H/A, neck stiffness, confusion, lethargy, altered level of consciousness, seizures, focal neurological signs, N/V, photophobia, papilledema
- petechial rash in meningococcal meningitis, seen more frequently on trunk or lower extremities

Investigations
- blood work: CBC and differential, electrolytes (for SIADH), blood C&S
    - CSF: opening pressure, cell count + differential, glucose, protein, Gram stain, bacterial C&S
    - AFB, fungal C&S, cryptococcal antigen in immunocompromised patients, subacute illness, suggestive travel history or TB exposure
    - PCR for HSV, VZV, enteroviruses; in infants <6 mo, parechoviruses
    - WNV serology in blood and CSF during summer and early fall if viral cause suspected
- imaging/neurologic studies: CT, MRI, EEG if focal neurological signs present

Does this Adult Patient Have Acute Meningitis? From The Rational Clinical Examination
JAMA 2009; http://www.jamaevidence.com/content/3482857
Study: Systematic review of articles assessing the sensitivity and specificity of clinical exam maneuvers for the diagnosis of adult meningitis.
Results: In retrospective studies, sensitivity for headache was 68%, and 52% for nausea and vomiting. Sensitivity for physical exam findings is similarly low (fever: 87%, neck stiffness: 80%, altered mental status: 69%). Sensitivity for the combination of the classic triad of fever, neck stiffness, and altered mental status was 46%. In prospective studies, sensitivity of H/A was 92%, while sensitivity of N/V could not be pooled, and ranged from 32-70%. Brudzinski's and Kernig's signs had a sensitivity of 5% and Kernig's sign only 5-9%. Jolt accentuation had a sensitivity of 97%.
Conclusions: Data were heterogeneous, and lacked standardization of clinical exams. No single item on clinical history or physical exam was sufficient to rule out meningitis, including Kernig's and Brudzinski's signs, or the absence of the classic triad of fever, neck stiffness, and altered mental status meningitis. Jolt accentuation has high sensitivity, but further research is needed. LP may be performed safely without CT head in patients without altered LOC, no recent seizure, no history of CNS disease, not immunocompromised, and <60 yr.

Table 19. Typical CSF Profiles for Meningitis

CSF Analysis	Bacterial	Viral
Glucose (mmol/L)	Decreased	Normal
Protein (g/L)	Markedly Increased	Increased
WBC	500-10,000/μL	10-500/μL
Predominant WBC	Neutrophils	Lymphocytes

Treatment
- bacterial meningitis is a medical emergency: do not delay antibiotics for CT or LP
- empiric antibiotic therapy
    - age < wk: ampicillin + cefotaxime IV OR ampicillin ± an aminoglycoside IV
    - wk-3 mo: cefotaxime + vancomycin
    - age >3 mo: vancomycin
        - add ampicillin IV if risk factors for infection with L. monocytogenes present: age >50, alcoholism, immunocompromised
- steroids in acute bacterial meningitis: dexamethasone IV within 20 min prior to or with first dose of antibiotics
    - continue in those patients with proven pneumococcal meningitis
    - not recommended for patients with suspected bacterial meningitis in some resource-limited countries
    - not recommended for neonatal meningitis

Prevention
- see Pediatrics, P59
- immunization
  - children: immunization against *H. influenzae* type B (Pentacel®), *S. pneumoniae* (Synflorix®, Prevnar-13®), *N. meningitidis* (Menjugate®, Menactra®, Bexsero®)
  - adults: immunization against *N. meningitidis* in selected circumstances (outbreaks, travel, epidemics) and *S. pneumoniae* (Pneumovax®) for high-risk groups
- prophylaxis: close contacts of patients infected with *H. influenzae* type B should be treated with rifampin if they live with an inadequately immunized (<4 yr) or immunocompromised child (<18 yr); ciprofloxacin, rifampin, or ceftriaxone if close or household contact of a patient with *N. meningitidis*

Prognosis
- complications
  - H/A, seizures, cerebral edema, hydrocephalus, SIADH, residual neurological deficit (especially CN VIII), deafness, death
- mortality
  - *S. pneumoniae* 25%; *N. meningitidis* 5-10%; *H. influenzae* 5%
  - worse prognosis if: extremes of age, delays in diagnosis and treatment, stupor or coma, seizures, focal neurological signs, septic shock at presentation

Encephalitis

Definition
- inflammation of the brain parenchyma

Etiology
- identified in only 40-70% of cases
  - when cause is identified, the most common etiology is viral: HSV, VZV, EBV, CMV, enteroviruses, parechoviruses, West Nile and other arboviruses, influenza and other respiratory viruses, HIV, mumps, measles, rabies, polio
  - bacteria: *L. monocytogenes*, Mycobacteria, spirochetes (Lyme, syphillis), *Mycoplasma pneumoniae*
  - parasites: protozoa (e.g. *Toxoplasma*) and helminths (rare)
  - fungi: e.g. *Cryptococcus*
  - post-infectious (e.g. acute disseminated encephalomyelitis [ADEM])
  - auto-antibody mediated encephalitis
    - anti-N-methyl-D-aspartate (NMDA) receptor encephalitis most common
    - in adults, most autoantibody-mediated encephalitis cases are associated with malignancy

Pathophysiology
- acute inflammatory disease of the brain due to direct invasion or pathogen-initiated immune response
- viruses may reach the CNS via peripheral nerves (e.g. rabies, HSV)
- herpes simplex encephalitis
  - acute, necrotizing, asymmetrical hemorrhagic process with lymphocytic and plasma cell reaction which usually involves the medial temporal and inferior frontal lobes
  - associated with HSV-1, but can also be caused by HSV-2
- influenza and other respiratory viruses are associated with acute necrotizing encephalopathy (ANE); likely mediated by pathogen-initiated immune response

Clinical Features
- constitutional: fever, chills, malaise, N/V
- meningeal involvement (meningoencephalitis): H/A, nuchal rigidity
- parenchymal involvement: seizures, altered mental status, focal neurological signs
- herpes simplex encephalitis
  - acute onset (<1 wk) of focal neurological signs: hemiparesis, ataxia, aphasia, focal or generalized seizures
  - temporal lobe involvement: behavioural disturbance
  - usually rapidly progressive over several days and may result in coma or death
  - common sequelae: memory and behavioural disturbances

Investigations
- CSF: opening pressure, cell count and differential, glucose, protein, Gram stain, bacterial C&S, PCR for HSV, VZV, EBV, enteroviruses/parechoviruses, *M. pneumoniae*, and selectively for other less common etiologies
- serology: may aid diagnosis of certain causes of encephalitis (e.g. EBV, West Nile virus, rabies, *Bartonella henslae*)
- imaging/neurologic studies: CT, MRI, EEG to define anatomical sites affected
- invasive testing: brain tissue biopsy may be required for culture, histological examination, and immunocytochemistry (if diagnosis not clear via non-invasive means)
- findings in herpes simplex encephalitis (must rule out due to high mortality)
  - CT/MRI: medial temporal lobe necrosis
  - EEG: early focal slowing, periodic discharges

Public Health Agency of Canada Indications for Adult Immunization

Pneumococcal Polysaccharide Vaccine (i.e. Pneumovax®)
- >65 yr
- >2 yr, with chronic cardiovascular/ respiratory/hepatic/renal disorders, asplenia, sickle cell, or immunosuppression (8 wk after pneumococcal conjugate vaccine if <18 yr)

Meningococcal Quadrivalent Vaccine (Menactra® or Menomune®)
- Healthy young adults
- Asplenia
- Travellers to high-risk areas
- Military recruits or laboratory personnel
- Complement, factor D, or properdin deficiency or acquired terminal complement deficiency through receipt of eculizumab

Multicomponent meningococcal serogroup B vaccine (Bexsero®)
- Asplenia
- Military recruits or laboratory personnel
- Complement, factor D, or properdin deficiency, or acquired terminal complement deficiency through receipt of eculizumab

Meningitis and encephalitis patients can be distinguished based on their cerebral function. Cerebral function is abnormal in encephalitis patients (e.g. altered mental status, motor or sensory deficits, altered behaviour, speech or movement disorders), but may be normal in patients with meningitis. Note however, that there is considerable overlap between the two syndromes ("meningoencephalitis")

Treatment
- general supportive care
- monitor vital signs carefully
- IV acyclovir empirically until HSV encephalitis ruled out

Generalized Tetanus

- see Pediatrics, P4

Etiology and Pathophysiology
- caused by *Clostridium tetani*: motile, spore forming, anaerobic GP bacillus
- found in soil, splinters, rusty nails, GI tract (humans and animals)
- traumatic implantation of spores into tissues with low oxygenation (e.g. puncture wounds, burns, nonsterile surgeries or deliveries)
- upon inoculation, spores transform into *C. tetani* bacilli that produce tetanus toxin
  - toxin travels via retrograde axonal transport to the CNS where it irreversibly binds presynaptic neurons to prevent the release of inhibitory neurotransmitters (e.g. GABA)
  - net effect is the disinhibition of spinal motor reflexes which results in tetany and autonomic hyperactivity

Clinical Features
- generalized tetanus
  - initially present with painful spasms of masseters (trismus or "lockjaw")
  - sustained contraction of skeletal muscle with periodic painful muscle spasms (triggered by sensory stimuli, e.g. loud noises)
  - paralysis descends to involve large muscle groups (neck, abdomen)
  - apnea, respiratory failure, and death secondary to tonic contraction of pharyngeal and respiratory muscles
- autonomic hyperactivity
  - diaphoresis, tachycardia, HTN, fever as illness progresses

Investigations
- primarily a clinical diagnosis, often although not always with a history of a traumatic wound and lack of immunization
- culture wounds, CK may be elevated

Antimicrobial therapy (e.g. metronidazole) may fail to treat *C. tetani* unless adequate wound debridement is performed

Treatment
- stop toxin production
  - wound debridement to clear necrotic tissue and spores
  - antimicrobial therapy: IV metronidazole; IV penicillin G is an effective alternative
- neutralize unbound toxin with tetanus immune globulin (TIg)
- supportive therapy: intubation, spasmolytic medications (benzodiazepines), quiet environment, cooling blanket
- control autonomic dysfunction: α- and β-blockade (e.g. labetalol), magnesium sulfate

Prevention
- infection with *C. tetani* does not produce immunity – vaccinate patients on diagnosis
- tetanus toxoid vaccination (see Pediatrics, P4 and Emergency Medicine, ER17)

Rabies

Definition
- acute progressive encephalitis caused by RNA virus (genus *Lyssavirus* of the Rhabdoviridae family)

Etiology and Pathophysiology
- any mammal can transmit the rabies virus
  - most commonly transmitted by raccoon, skunk, bat, fox, cat, and dog; monkeys also a risk in the developing world
- transmission: breaching of skin by teeth or direct contact of infectious tissue (saliva, neural tissue) with skin or mucous membranes
  - almost all cases due to bites
- virus travels via retrograde axonal transport from PNS to CNS
- virus multiplies rapidly in brain, then spreads to other organs, including salivary glands
- development of clinical signs occurs simultaneously with excretion of rabies virus in saliva
  - infected animal can transmit rabies virus as soon as it shows signs of disease

Clinical Features
- five stages of disease
  1. incubation period
     - 1-3 mo on average (can range from days to years)

2. prodrome (<1 wk)
- influenza-like illness: low-grade fever, malaise, anorexia, N/V, H/A, sore throat
- pain, pruritus, and paresthesia may occur at wound site
- once prodromal symptoms develop, there is rapid, irreversible progression to death
  - progression from prodrome to coma and death may occur without an intervening acute neurologic syndrome
3. acute neurologic syndrome: 2 types (<1 wk)
  a. encephalitic (most common): hyperactivity, fluctuating LOC, hydrophobia, aerophobia, hypersalivation, fever, seizures
    - painful pharyngeal spasms on encountering gust of air or swallowing water cause aerophobia and hydrophobia, respectively
  b. paralytic: quadriplegia, loss of anal sphincter tone, fever
4. coma
- complete flaccid paralysis, respiratory and cardiovascular failure
5. death (within days to weeks of initial symptoms)

Investigations
- purpose of diagnosis by investigations is to limit patient contact with others and to identify others exposed to the infectious source
- ante-mortem: direct immunofluorescence or PCR on multiple specimens: saliva, skin biopsy, serum, CSF
- post-mortem: direct immunofluorescence in nerve tissue, presence of Negri bodies (inclusion bodies in neurons)

Treatment
- post-exposure prophylaxis depends on regional prevalence (contact Public Health) and circumstances surrounding injury
- 3 general principles
  - wound care: clean wound promptly and thoroughly with soap and running water
  - passive immunization: HRIG infiltrated into wound site, with any remaining volume administered IM in anatomical site distant from vaccine administration
  - active immunization: inactivated human diploid cell rabies virus vaccine (series of 4 shots post-exposure if not pre-immunized)
- treatment is supportive once victim manifests signs and symptoms of disease

Prevention
- pre-exposure vaccination
  - recommended for high risk persons: laboratory staff working with rabies, veterinarians, animal and wildlife control workers, long-term travellers to endemic areas
  - eliminates need for HRIG following an exposure, and reduces number of HDCV PEP shots from 4 to 2

Systemic Infections

Sepsis and Septic Shock

- see Respirology, R33

Definitions
- systemic inflammatory response syndrome (SIRS): 2 or more of
  1. temperature <36°C/96.8°F or >38°C/100.4°F
  2. heart rate >90 beats/min
  3. respiratory rate >20 breaths/min or $PaCO_2$ <32 mmHg
  4. WBC <4 x 10^9/L or >12 x 10^9/L or >10% bands
- sepsis: SIRS + proven or provable infection
- severe sepsis: sepsis + signs of end-organ dysfunction and hypoperfusion
- septic shock: severe sepsis + hypotension (<90 mmHg sBP), despite adequate fluid resuscitation

Pathophysiology
- causative agents are identified in only 50-70% of cases
- when organisms are identified, GP and GN organisms are the cause in 90% of cases
- primary bloodstream infection or secondary bacteremia → local immune response → immune cells release pro-inflammatory cytokines → immune response spreads beyond local environment → unregulated, exaggerated systemic immune response → vasodilation and hypotension → involvement of tissues remote from the site of injury/infection resulting in multiple major organ dysfunction → periodic immunoparalysis

Clinical Features
- history: fever, chills, dyspnea, cool extremities, fatigue, malaise, anxiety, confusion
- physical: abnormal vitals (fever, tachypnea, tachycardia, hypotension), local signs of infection

Investigations
- CBC and differential, electrolytes, BUN, creatinine, liver enzymes, ABG, lactate, INR, PTT, FDP, blood C&S x2, urinalysis, urine C&S and cultures of any wounds or lines
- CXR (other imaging depends on suspicion of focus of infection)

Treatment (see Respirology, R34)
- respiratory support: O₂ ± intubation
- cardiovascular support: IV fluids, ± norepinephrine + ICU
- IV antibiotics (empirical, depends on suspected source)
    - start with broad spectrum antibiotics (piperacillin/tazobactam or meropenem) ± additional agents depending on patient risk factors, suspected etiology of infection, and local microbial susceptibilities (± aminoglycoside for drug-resistant GNs or vancomycin for MRSA)
    - narrow once susceptibilities are known
- hydrocortisone IV in patients with septic shock unresponsive to fluid resuscitation and vasopressors

Leprosy (Hansen's Disease)

Etiology
- *Mycobacterium leprae*: obligate intracellular bacteria, slow-growing (doubling time 12.5 d), survives in macrophages
- bacteria transmitted from nasal secretions, potentially via skin lesions
- invades skin and peripheral nerves leading to chronic granulomatous disease

Clinical Features
- lesions involve cooler body tissues (e.g. skin, superficial nerves, nose, eyes, larynx)
- spectrum of disease determined by host immune response to infection
    i. paucibacillary "tuberculoid" leprosy (intact cell-mediated immune response)
    - ≤5 hypoesthetic lesions, usually hypopigmented, well-defined, dry
    - early nerve involvement, enlarged peripheral nerves, neuropathic pain
    - may be self-limited, stable, or progress over time to multibacillary "lepromatous" form
    ii. multibacillary "lepromatous" leprosy (weak cell-mediated immune response)
    - ≥6 lesions, symmetrical distribution
    - leonine facies (nodular facial lesions, loss of eyebrows, thickened ear lobes)
    - extensive cutaneous involvement, late and insidious nerve involvement causing sensory loss at the face and extremities
    iii. borderline leprosy
    - lesions and progression lies between tuberculoid and lepromatous forms

Investigations
- skin biopsy down to fat or slit skin smears for AFB staining, PCR
- histologic appearance: intracellular bacilli in spherical masses (lepra cells), granulomas involving cutaneous nerves

Treatment (WHO Treatment Regimens)
- paucibacillary: dapsone daily + rifampin monthly x 6 mo
- single skin lesion paucibacillary: single dose of rifampicin, ofloxacin, and minocycline
- multibacillary: dapsone + rifampin monthly + clofazimine monthly x 12 mo AND low dose clofazimine once daily x 12 mo
- treatment of leprosy can cause an immune reaction to killed or dying bacteria (e.g. erythema nodosum leprosum and reversal reaction): symptomatic management with NSAIDs if mild, prednisone with 6-12 wk taper if severe; thalidomide for erythema nodosum leprosum. Neuritis of reactions can lead to permanent nerve damage.

Prognosis
- curable with WHO-approved treatment regimens
- complications: muscle atrophy, contractures, trauma/superinfection of lesions, crippling/loss of limbs, erythema nodosum leprosum, social stigmatization due to clofazimine hyperpigmentation
- long post-treatment follow-up warranted to monitor for relapse and immune reactions

Lyme Disease

Etiology/Epidemiology
- spirochete bacteria: *Borrelia burgdorferi* (N. America), *B. garinii*, *B. afzelii* (Europe and Asia)
- transmitted by Ixodes tick
- reported in 49 of the 50 U.S. states, but most cases occur in the Northeast, the Midwest, and Northern California
- in Canada, reported in southern and southeastern Quebec, southern and eastern Ontario, southeastern Manitoba, New Brunswick and Nova Scotia, as well as southern British Columbia
- small rodents (mice) serve as primary reservoir, while larger animals (white-tailed deer) serve as hosts for ticks
- human contact usually May-August in fields with low brush near wooded areas
- infection usually requires >36 h tick attachment

BAKE a Key Lyme Pie
Bell's palsy
Arthritis
Kardiac block
Lyme
Erythema chronicum migrans

Clinical Features
- stage 1 (early localized stage: 7-14 d post-bite)
  - malaise, fatigue, H/A, myalgias
  - erythema migrans: expanding, non-pruritic bulls-eye (target) lesions (red with clear centre) on thigh/groin/axilla
- stage 2 (early disseminated stage): weeks post-infection
  - CNS: aseptic meningitis, CN palsies (CN VII palsy), peripheral neuritis
  - cardiac: transient heart block or myocarditis
- stage 3 (late persistent stage: months to years post-infection)
  - may not have preceding history of early stage infection
  - MSK: chronic monoarticular or oligoarticular arthritis
  - acrodermatitis chronicum atrophicans (due to *B. afzelii*)
  - neurologic: encephalopathy, meningitis, neuropathy

Investigations
- serology: ELISA, Western blot

Prevention
- use of protective clothing (tuck pants into socks), insect repellent, inspection for ticks and prompt removal of tick
- doxycycline prophylaxis within 72 h of removal of an engorged, Ixodes scapularis tick in hyperendemic area (local rate of infection of ticks ≥20%) for patients >8 yr who are not pregnant or lactating

Treatment
- stage 1: doxycycline/amoxicillin/cefuroxime
- stage 2-3: ceftriaxone

Toxic Shock Syndrome

Etiology
- superantigens produced by some strains of *S. aureus* or GAS cause widespread T-cell activation and pro-inflammatory cytokine release (IL-1, IL-6, TNF)
- course of disease is precipitous and leads to acute fever, shock, multiorgan failure
- Staphylococcal TSS involves the production of superantigen TSST-1 (toxic shock syndrome toxin 1)
- Streptococcal TSS involves the production of superantigens SPEA, SPEB, SPEC

Risk Factors
- Staphylococcal: tampon use, nasal packing, wound infections (e.g. postpartum vaginal or Cesarean or other surgical infections)
- Streptococcal: minor trauma, surgical procedures, preceding viral illness (e.g. chickenpox), use of NSAIDs

Clinical Features and Investigations
- acute onset
- Staphylococcal TSS
  - T >38.9°C
  - sBP <90 mmHg
  - diffuse erythroderma with subsequent desquamation, especially on palms and soles
  - involvement of 3 or more organ systems: GI (vomiting, diarrhea), muscular (myalgia, increased CK), mucous membranes (hyperemia), renal, hepatic, hematologic (thrombocytopenia), CNS (disorientation)
  - isolation of *S. aureus* is not required for diagnosis (*S. aureus* is rarely recovered from blood in TSS)

- Streptococcal TSS
  - sBP <90 mmHg
  - isolation of GAS from a normally sterile site (e.g. blood, pleural, tissue biopsy, or surgical wound)
  - ≥2 of coagulopathy, liver involvement, ARDS, soft tissue necrosis (necrotizing fasciitis, myositis, gangrene), renal impairment, erythematous macular rash that may desquamate

Treatment
- supportive: fluid resuscitation
- Staphylococcal: for methicillin-susceptible *S. aureus*: clindamycin + cloxacillin (IV); for MRSA: clindamycin + vancomycin x 10-14 d
- Streptococcal: IV penicillin and clindamycin and ± IVIg

Cat Scratch Disease

Etiology
- *Bartonella henselae*: intracellular bacteria
- cat-to-human transmission via cat scratch/bite

Clinical Features
- skin lesion appears 3-10 d post-inoculation
- may be followed by fever, tender regional lymphadenopathy
- in some patients, organism may disseminate causing fever of unknown origin, hepatosplenomegaly, retinitis, encephalopathy
- usually self-limited

Investigations
- serology, PCR, lymph node biopsy

Treatment
- supportive in most cases
- azithromycin x 10-14 d with lymphadenitis in patients with moderate-severe disease or immunodeficiency
- Combination therapy consisting of doxycycline or azithromycin plus rifampin often used for disseminated disease (neuroterinitis, hepatosplenic involvement)

Rocky Mountain Spotted Fever

Etiology
- *Rickettsia rickettsii*: obligate intracellular GN organism
- reservoir hosts: rodents, dogs
- vectors: *Dermacentor* ticks
- organisms cause inflammation of endothelial lining of small blood vessels, leading to small hemorrhages and thrombi
- can cause widespread vasculitis leading to H/A, and CNS changes; can progress to death if treatment is delayed

Clinical Features
- usually occurs in summer following tick bite
- influenza-like prodrome: acute onset fever, H/A, myalgia, N/V, anorexia
- macular rash appearing on day 2-4 of fever
  - begins on wrists and ankles, then spreads centrally to arms/legs/trunk/palms/soles
  - occasionally "spotless" (10% of patients)

Investigations
- skin biopsy and serology (indirect fluorescent antibody test)

Treatment
- doxycycline, usually 5-7 d (treat for 3 d after defervescence)

West Nile Virus

Epidemiology
- virus has been detected throughout the United States and much of southern Canada
- overall case-fatality rates in severe cases is ~10%

Transmission
- primarily from mosquitoes that have fed on infected birds (crows, blue jays)
- transplacental, blood products (rare), organ transplantation

Clinical Features
- most are asymptomatic
- most symptomatic cases are mild (West Nile fever): acute onset of H/A, back pain, myalgia, anorexia, maculopapular non-pruritic rash involving chest, back, arms
- severe complications: encephalitis, meningoencephalitis, and acute flaccid paralysis (especially in those >60 yr)

Investigations
- IgM antibody in serum or CSF (cross reactivity with yellow fever and Japanese encephalitis vaccines, and with dengue fever and St. Louis virus infection); may not reflect current illness as IgM antibody can last for >6 mo
- viral isolation by PCR from CSF, tissue, blood, and fluids (all have low sensitivity)
- CSF: elevated lymphocytes and protein if CNS involvement

Treatment and Prevention
- treatment: supportive
- prevention: mosquito repellant (DEET), drain stagnant water, community mosquito control programs

Syphilis

Etiology
- *Treponema pallidum*: thick motile spirochetes historically detectable by dark-field microscopy
- transmitted sexually, vertically, or parenterally (rare)

Argyll Robertson Pupil
Accommodates but does not react to light

Clinical Features
- see Dermatology, D31 and Gynecology, GY30
- multi-stage disease
  1. primary syphilis (3-90 d post-infection)
     - painless chancre at inoculation site (any mucosal surface)
     - regional lymphadenopathy
     - acute disease lasts 3-6 wk, 25% progress to secondary syphilis without treatment
  2. secondary syphilis = systemic infection (2-8 wk following chancre)
     - maculo-papular non-pruritic rash including palms and soles
     - generalized lymphadenopathy, low grade fever, malaise, H/A, aseptic meningitis, ocular/otic syphilis
     - condylomata lata: painless, wart-like lesion on palate, vulva, or scrotum (highly infectious)
  3. latent syphilis
     - asymptomatic infection that follows untreated primary/secondary syphilis
     - early latent (<1 yr post-infection) or late latent/unknown duration (>1 yr post-infection)
     - increased transmission risk with early latent; longer treatment duration required for late latent
  4. tertiary syphilis (1-30 yr post-infection)
     - gummatous syphilis: nodular granulomas of skin, bone, liver, testes, brain
     - aortic aneurysm and aortic insufficiency
     - neurosyphilis: dementia, personality changes, Argyll-Robertson pupils, tabes dorsalis
  5. congenital syphilis
     - causes spontaneous abortions, stillbirths, congenital malformations, developmental delay, deafness
     - most infected newborns are asymptomatic
     - clinical manifestation in early infancy include rhinitis (snuffles), lymphadenopathy, hepatosplenomegaly, pseudoparalysis (bone pain associated with osteitis)
     - late onset manifestations (>2 yr of age) include saddle nose, saber shins, Glutton joints, Hutchinson's teeth, mulberry molars, rhagades, CN VIII deafness, interstitial keratitis, juvenile paresis

Those with Untreated 1° or 2° Syphilis
1/3   cure
1/3   latent indefinitely
1/3   3° syphilis

Causes of False Positive VDRL and RPR Tests

Viruses (mononucleosis, hepatitis)
Drugs and substance abuse
Rheumatic fever
Lupus and leprosy

Patients with 2° or 3° syphilis treated with penicillin may experience a Jarisch-Herxheimer reaction. Lysis of organisms release pyrogens thought to cause fever, chills, myalgia, flu-like symptoms may last up to 24 h

Investigations
- screening tests: CMIA, CLIA, EIA (treponemal), RPR, or VDRL (non-treponemal)
- confirmatory tests: TPPA, FTA-ABS, MHA-TP, TPI, dark field microscopy with silver stain (rarely)
- LP for neurosyphilis if: seropositive and symptoms of neurosyphilis or treatment failure/other tertiary symptoms, or with HIV and late latent/unknown duration syphilis; consider in others
- for congenital syphilis, LP is essential; long bone x-rays may also be helpful

VDRL	Venereal Disease Research Laboratory
RPR	Rapid Plasma Reagin
EIA	Enzyme Immunoassay
CLIA	ChemiLuminescent ImmunoAssay
CMLA	ChemiLuminescent Microparticle ImmunoAssay
FTA-ABS	Fluorescent Treponema Antibody-Absorption
MHA-TP	Microhemagglutination Assay *T. pallidum*
TPPA	*T. pallidum* Particle Agglutination Assay

Treatment
- for 1°, 2°, early latent: benzathine penicillin G 2.4 million units IM x 1
- for 3°, late latent: benzathine penicillin G 2.4 million units IM weekly x 3
- if allergic to penicillin: doxycycline 100 mg PO bid x 14 d
- neurosyphilis: aqueous Penicillin G 18-24 million units/d IV x 14 d
- for congenital syphilis, penicillin G IV x 10 d
- see Family Medicine, FM43 for generalized STI workup

Tuberculosis

Etiology, Epidemiology, and Natural History
- 1/3 of the world's population is infected with TB
- contracted by aerosolized inhalation of *Mycobacterium tuberculosis*, a slow growing aerobe (doubling time = 18 h) that can evade innate host defenses, survive, and replicate in macrophages
- inhalation and deposition in the lung can lead to one of the following outcomes
  1. immediate clearance of the pathogen
  2. latent TB: asymptomatic infection contained by host immune defenses (represents 95% of infected people)
  3. primary TB: symptomatic, active disease (represents 5% of infected people)
  4. secondary TB: symptomatic reactivation of previously dormant TB (represents 5-10% of those with latent TB, most often within the first 2-3 yr of initial infection) at a pulmonary or extrapulmonary site

> **Tuberculous Polyserositis**
> pleural + pericardial + peritoneal effusions
> (usually from granuloma breakdown that spills TB into pleural cavity – very rare)

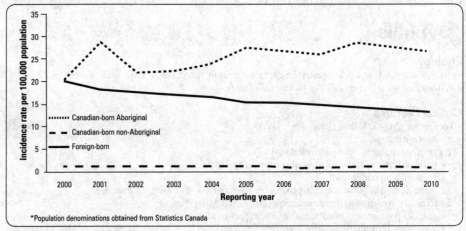

Figure 8. Tuberculosis statistics
Canadian Tuberculosis Standards, 7th ed.

Risk Factors
- social and environmental factors
  - travel or birth in a country with high TB prevalence (e.g. Asia, Latin America, Sub-Saharan Africa, Eastern Europe)
  - Aboriginal (particularly Inuit), crowded living conditions, low SES/homeless, IVDU
  - personal or occupational contact
- host factors
  - immunocompromised/immunosuppressed (especially HIV, including extremes of age)
  - silicosis
  - chronic renal failure requiring dialysis
  - malignancy and chemotherapy
  - substance abuse (e.g. drug use, alcoholism, smoking)

Clinical Features
- primary infection usually asymptomatic, although progressive primary disease may occur, especially in children and immunosuppressed patients
- secondary infection/reactivation usually produces constitutional symptoms (fatigue, anorexia, night sweats, weight loss) and site-dependent symptoms
  1. pulmonary TB
     - chronic productive cough ± hemoptysis
     - CXR consolidation or cavitation, lymphadenopathy
     - non-resolving pneumonia despite standard antimicrobial therapy
  2. miliary TB
     - widely disseminated spread especially to lungs, abdominal organs, marrow, CNS
     - CXR: multiple small 2-4 mm millet seed-like lesions throughout lung
  3. extrapulmonary TB
     - lymphadenitis, pleurisy, pericarditis, hepatitis, peritonitis, meningitis, osteomyelitis (vertebral = Pott's disease), adrenal (causing Addison's disease), renal, ovarian

Investigations
- screening for latent TB
  - PPD/Mantoux skin tests
    - both tests diagnose prior TB exposure; neither can diagnose or exclude active disease

- IFN-γ release assay (IGRA)
    - in patients previously infected with TB, T-cells produce increased amounts of IFN-γ when re-exposed to TB antigen
    - detects antigen not present in the BCG vaccine or in most types of non-tuberculous-mycobacteria (NTM), therefore fewer false positives
  - Canadian and American guidelines treat IGRAs as equivalent to the TB skin test and preferable in patients with a history of BCG vaccination or who may not return for a skin test reading
- diagnostic tests/investigations for active pulmonary TB
  - three sputum specimens (either spontaneous or induced) should be collected for acid-fast bacilli smear and culture; the three specimens can be collected on the same day, a minimum of 1 hour apart
  - BAL
  - CXR
    - nodular or alveolar infiltrates with cavitation (middle/lower lobe if primary, apical if secondary)
    - pleural effusion (usually unilateral and exudative) may occur independently of other radiograph abnormalities
    - hilar/mediastinal adenopathy (especially in children)
    - tuberculoma (semi-calcified well-defined solitary coin lesion 0.5-4 cm that may be mistaken for lung CA)
    - miliary TB (see clinical features)
    - evidence of past disease: calcified hilar and mediastinal nodes, calcified pulmonary focus, pleural thickening with calcification, apical scarring

Positive PPD Test
If induration at 48-72 h
>5 mm if immunocompromised, close contact with active TB
>10 mm all others; positive PPD → CXR; decision to treat depends on individual risk factors
False(–): poor technique, anergy, immunosuppression, infection <10 wk or remotely
False(+): BCG after 12 mo of age in a low-risk individual, NTM
Booster effect: initially false(–) result boost to a true(+) result by the testing procedure itself (usually if patient was infected long ago so had diminished delayed type hypersensitivity reaction or if history of BCG)

Prevention

- primary prevention
  - airborne isolation for active pulmonary disease
  - BCG vaccine
    - ~80% effective against pediatric miliary and meningeal TB
    - effectiveness in adults debated (anywhere from 0-80%)
    - recommended in high-incidence communities in Canada for infants in whom there is no evidence of HIV infection or immunodeficiency; widely used in other countries
- secondary prevention (defer in pregnancy unless mother is high risk)
  - likely INH-sensitive: isoniazid (INH) + pyridoxine (vit B6 to help prevent INH-associated neuropathy) x 9 mo
  - likely INH-resistant: rifampin x 4 mo

Treatment of Active Infection

- empiric therapy: INH + rifampin + pyrazinamide + ethambutol + pyridoxine
- pulmonary TB: INH + rifampin + pyrazinamide + ethambutol + pyridoxine x 2 mo (initiation phase), then INH + rifampin + pyridoxine x 4 mo in fully susceptible TB (continuation phase), total 6 mo
- extrapulmonary TB: same regimen as pulmonary TB but increase to 12 mo in bone/joint, CNS, and miliary/disseminated TB + corticosteroids for meningitis, pericarditis
- empiric treatment of suspected MDR (multidrug resistant) or XDR (extensively drug-resistant) TB requires referral to a specialist
  - MDR = resistance to INH and rifampin ± others
  - XDR = resistance to INH + rifampin + fluoroquinolone + ≥1 of injectable, second-line agents
    - very difficult to treat, global public health threat, 5 documented cases in Canada from 1997-2008
  - suspect MDR TB if previous treatment, exposure to known MDR index case, or immigration from a high-risk area
- note: TB is a reportable disease to Public Health (please see Public Health Agency of Canada website for more information: www.phac-aspc.gc.ca/tbpc-latb/pubs/tb-canada-7/index-eng.php)

HIV and AIDS

Epidemiology

HIV-1 is the predominant type in North America and most of the world

HIV-2 is found mainly in West Africa

Both lead to AIDS but HIV-2 is generally less virulent

Canadian Situation (Public Health Agency of Canada, 2013)
- estimated 71,300 Canadians living with HIV infection at the end of 2011, 25% unaware of HIV-positive status
- 2,090 new infections were reported in 2013: MSM account for 49.3% of cases, IVDU 12.8%

Global Situation (WHO and UNAIDS Core Epidemiology Slides, July 2014)
- estimated 35 million people living with HIV/AIDS in 2013
- estimated 2.1 million newly infected in 2013
- estimated 1.5 million AIDS-related deaths in 2013

p24 = capsid protein
gp41 = fusion and entry
gp120 = attachment to host T-cell

Homozygosity for A32 mutation in CCR5 gene confers relative resistance to HIV infection
Heterozygosity for A32 mutation in CCR5 gene associated with slower disease course

Definition and Pathophysiology

- HIV is a retrovirus that causes progressive immune system dysfunction which predisposes patients to various opportunistic infections and malignancies
- HIV virion includes an envelope (gp41 and gp120 glycoproteins), matrix (p17) and capsid (p24) enclosing 2 single-stranded copies of RNA + enzymes in its core
- virion glycoproteins bind CD4 and CXCR4/CCR5 on CD4+ T lymphocytes (T-helper cells) to fuse and enter the cells
- RNA converted to dsDNA by viral reverse transcriptase; dsDNA is integrated into host genome by viral integrase
- virus DNA transcribed and translated using host cell machinery, post-translational modifications include proteolytic activity of virally encoded protease enzymes
- newly produced virions bud out of host cell, incorporating host cell membrane; additional maturation steps are required before virion is considered infectious
- exact mechanisms of CD4 depletion incompletely characterized but likely include direct viral cytopathic effects, apoptosis, and increased cell turnover

Modes of Transmission

Table 20. Modes of Transmission by Site and Medium

HIV Invasion Site	Sub-Location	Transmission Medium	Transmission Probability per Exposure Event
Female genital tract	Vagina, ectocervix, endocervix	Semen	1 in 200 to 1 in 2,000
Male genital tract	Inner foreskin, penile urethra	Cervicovaginal and rectal secretions and desquamations	1 in 700 to 1 in 3,000
Intestinal tract	RectumUpper GI tract	Semen	1 in 20 to 1 in 300
		Semen	1 in 2,500
		Maternal blood/genital secretions (intrapartum)	1 in 5 to 1 in 10
		Breastmilk	1 in 5 to 1 in 10
Placenta	Chorionic villi	Maternal blood (intrauterine)	1 in 10 to 1 in 20
Blood stream		Contaminated blood products	95 in 100
		Sharp/needlestick injuries	1 in 150

Adapted with permission from Macmillan Publishers Ltd. *Nat Rev Immunology* 2008;8:447-457

NOTE: these estimates are for "all comers" i.e. they estimate transmission risk for anyone with HIV infection and do not take into account treatment status of the HIV+ person (in contrast to results of PARTNER study)

Natural History

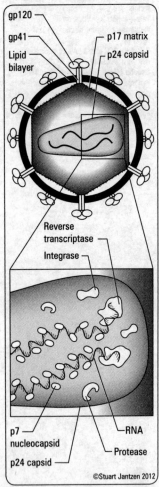

gp120
gp41
Lipid bilayer
p17 matrix
p24 capsid

Reverse transcriptase
Integrase

p7 nucleocapsid
RNA
Protease
p24 capsid

©Stuart Jantzen 2012

Figure 9. HIV viral particle

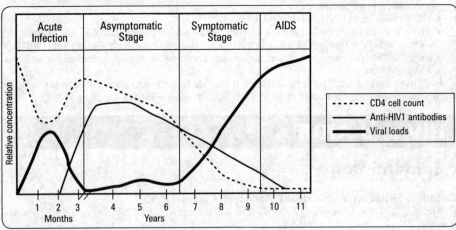

Figure 10. Relationships between CD4 T-cell count, viral load, and anti-HIV antibodies

Acute (Infection) Retroviral Syndrome
- 40-90% experience an acute "flu-like" illness (may include fever, pharyngitis, lymphadenopathy, rash, arthralgias, myalgias, H/A, GI symptoms, oral ulcers, weight loss) 2-6 wk post-exposure lasting 10-15 d
- hematologic disturbances (lymphopenia, thrombocytopenia)
- 10-20% present with aseptic meningitis; HIV RNA and/or p24 may be detected in CSF
- associated with a high level of plasma viremia and therefore high risk of transmission

Asymptomatic (Latent) Stage
- during latent phase, HIV infects and replicates in CD4+ T lymphocytes (lymph nodes)
- normal CD4 count in adults: 500-1,100 cells/mm^3
- CD4 count drops 60-100 cells/mm^3 per year
- by 10 yr post-infection, 50% have AIDS, 30% demonstrate milder symptoms, and <20% are asymptomatic if left untreated

AIDS Definition in Canada
- HIV-positive AND
- one or more of the clinical illnesses that characterize AIDS, including: opportunistic infections (e.g. PJP (previously PCP), esophageal candidiasis, CMV, MAC, TB, toxoplasmosis), malignancy (Kaposi's sarcoma, invasive cervical cancer), wasting syndrome OR
- CD4 <200 (or <15%); this is largely historical since ART can reverse CD4 count decline

Table 21. Symptomatic Stage (CD4 count thresholds for classic clinical manifestations)

CD4 Counts	Possible Manifestations
<500 cells/mm^3	Often asymptomatic Constitutional symptoms: fever, night sweats, fatigue, weight loss Mucocutaneous lesions: seborrheic dermatitis, HSV, VZV (shingles), oral hairy leukoplakia (EBV), candidiasis (oral, esophageal, vaginal), Kaposi's sarcoma (KS) Recurrent bacterial infections, especially pneumonia Pulmonary and extrapulmonary tuberculosis Lymphoma
<200 cells/mm^3	Pneumocystis jiroveci pneumonia (formerly PCP) KS Oral thrush Local and/or disseminated fungal infections: Cryptococcus neoformans, Coccidioides immitis, Histoplasma capsulatum
<100 cells/mm^3	Progressive multifocal leukoencephalopathy (PML) – JC virus CNS toxoplasmosis
<50 cells/mm^3	CMV infection: retinitis, colitis, cholangiopathy, CNS disease Mycobacterium avium complex (MAC) Bacillary angiomatosis (disseminated Bartonella) Primary central nervous system lymphoma (PCNSL)

Laboratory Diagnosis
- anti-HIV antibodies detectable after a median of 3 wk, virtually all by 3 mo (therefore 3 mo window period)
- initial screening test (3rd generation antibody test): enzyme linked immunosorbent assay (ELISA) detects serum antibody to HIV; sensitivity >99.5%
- increasingly, combination p24 antigen/HIV antibody tests (4th generation) used for screening; improved sensitivity in early or acute infection and sensitivity/specificity approach 100% for chronic infection
- confirmatory test: if positive screen, Western blot confirmation by detection of antibodies to at least two different HIV protein bands (p24, gp41, gp120/160); specificity >99.99%
- rapid (point of care) antibody tests: higher false positives, therefore need to confirm positive results with traditional serology
- p24 antigen: detection by ELISA may be positive during "window period"

Management of the HIV-Positive Patient

- verify positive HIV test
- complete baseline history and physical exam, then follow-up every 3-6 mo
- laboratory evaluation
  - routine CD4 count to measure status of the immune system
  - routine HIV-RNA levels (viral load)
    - also important indicator of effect of ART
  - baseline HIV resistance testing to guide ARV therapy
  - HLA-B*5701 genetic test to screen for abacavir hypersensitivity if considering abacavir in treatment regimen
  - CCR5 tropism testing if considering CCR5 antagonist in treatment regimen
  - baseline tuberculin skin test (PPD): induration greater than 5 mm is positive
  - baseline serologies (hepatitis A, B, and C, syphilis, toxoplasma, CMV, VZV)
  - routine biochemistry and hematology, CXR, urinalysis
  - annual fasting lipid profile and fasting glucose (due to ART side effects)

PARTNER Study: Risk of HIV Transmission Between Serodiscordant Couples with HIV+ Partner on ART
Preliminary results presented at Conference on Retroviruses and Opportunistic Infections 2014 (CROI 2014); final results due 2017
Participants: 740 serodiscordant heterosexual (60% of couples) and homosexual couples (40% of couples) that engage in sex without using condoms. The HIV- partner cannot be using pre- or post-exposure prophylaxis and the HIV+ partner must be on ART with an undetectable viral load.
Methods: Partners enrolled in the study are asked to independently complete a questionnaire on sexual behaviour with their partner every 3-6 mo. Additionally, if the HIV- partner seroconverts, a blood sample will be taken from each partner and the viruses genotyped for comparison. To remain in the study, the requirements for participation must be maintained.
Results: No HIV transmissions within couples from a partner with an undetectable viral load in an estimated 16,400 occasions of sex in MSM and 28,000 occasions of sex in the heterosexual couples. If the HIV+ partners had not been on treatment in this group, 50-100 (median: 86) transmissions would have been expected in the MSM group and 15 transmissions in heterosexual couples. In a couple whose sexual activity is considered as average for the group studied, there was a 95% chance that the greatest-possible risk of transmission from a partner was 0.45% per year as well as 1% per year from anal sex.

Seroconversion: Development of detectable anti-HIV antibodies

Window Period: Time between infection and development of anti-HIV antibodies; when serologic tests (ELISA, Western blot) are negative

All infants born to HIV infected mothers have positive ELISA tests because of circulating maternal anti-HIV antibodies, which disappear by 18 mo; early diagnosis is made by detection of HIV RNA in plasma

HLA-B*5701 Testing
Abacavir hypersensitivity reactions usually only occur in individuals carrying this HLA allele (~5-7% of Caucasians, lower prevalence in other ethnic groups). Routine screening for HLA-B*5701 at baseline and definitely prior to abacavir use

HIV Status
- CD4 count: progress and stage of disease
- Viral load: rate of progression

1° and 2° prophylaxis may be discontinued if CD4 count is above threshold for ≥6 mo while on ART

Anti-Retroviral pre-exposure prophylaxis (PrEP) for preventing HIV in high-risk individuals
Cochrane DB Syst Rev 2012 Jul 11;7:CD007189.
Purpose: To evaluate the efficacy of oral anti-retroviral prophylactic therapy in preventing HIV infection.
Study: Systematic review of 12 randomized controlled trials with 6 trials forming the core analysis.
Population: 9849 HIV-uninfected patients at high risk of contracting HIV including men who have sex with men, serodiscordant couples and others.
Outcome: New infection with HIV.
Results: Daily oral tenofovir disoproxil fumarate (TDF) plus emtricitabine (FTC) reduced the risk of HIV acquisition compared to placebo (RR 0.49; 95% CI 0.28-0.85). TDF alone also showed significant risk reduction in trials with fewer patients (RR 0.33; 95% CI 0.20-0.55). There was no significant increase in adverse events in any of the treatment groups. Sexual practices and adherence did not differ between treatment and placebo arms.
Conclusions: Pre-exposure prophylaxis with TDF with or without FTC effectively reduces the risk of HIV aquisition in high risk, HIV uninfected patients without causing significant adverse effects.

Reasons for Deterioration of a Patient with HIV/AIDS
• Opportunistic infections
• Neoplasms
• Medication-related toxicities
• Co-infections (e.g. HBV, HCV, STIs)
• Non-AIDS-related comorbidities (e.g. cardiovascular, renal, hepatic, neurocognitive, bone disease)

Treatment Failure
• Assess adherence
• Assess drug interactions
• Resistance testing
• Rule out opportunistic infections
• Rule out marrow suppression
• Construct new 3-drug regimen

• education
  ▪ regular follow-up on CD4 counts and viral loads (q3-6mo) as well as strict adherence to ART improves prognosis
  ▪ prevention of further transmission through safer sex and clean needles for injection drug use
  ▪ HIV superinfection (transmission of different HIV strains from another HIV+ person) does rarely occur so barrier protection during sex is still recommended
  ▪ discuss importance of disclosing HIV status to partners including risk of criminal prosecution of non-disclosure in jurisdictions where applicable
  ▪ connect to relevant community groups and resources
• health care maintenance
  ▪ assessment of psychosocial concerns and referral to psychiatry or social work if appropriate
  ▪ vaccines: influenza annually, 23-valent pneumococcal every 5 yr, HBV (if not immune), HAV (if seronegative)
  ▪ annual screening (PAP smear, STIs)
  ▪ management of comorbid conditions and provision of general primary care

Table 22. Prophylaxis Against Opportunistic Infections in HIV-infected Patients

Pathogen	Indication for Prophylaxis	Prophylactic Regimen
Pneumocystis jiroveci	CD4 count <200 cells/mm³ or history of oral candidiasis	TMP-SMX 1 SS or DS OD
Toxoplasma gondii	IgG antibody to *Toxoplasma* and CD4 count <100 cells/mm³	As per prophylaxis for pneumocystis
Mycobacterium tuberculosis	PPD reaction >5 mm or contact with case of active TB	INH + pyridoxine daily x 9 mo
Mycobacterium avium complex	CD4 count <50 cells/mm³	Azithromycin 1,200 mg q1wk

SS = single strength; DS = double strength
See 2002 USPHS/IDSA guidelines for preventing opportunistic infections among HIV-infected persons. Available from: http://aidsinfo.nih.gov/

Anti-Retroviral Treatment

Overall Treatment Principles
• recommended that all HIV+ patients initiate combination ART to restore and preserve immune function, reduce morbidity, prolong survival and prevent transmission
• patients starting ART should be committed to treatment and understand the importance of adherence; poor compliance can lead to viral resistance; may defer treatment on the basis of clinical and psychosocial factors on case by case basis
• consider results of baseline resistance testing and complete ART history before (re-) initiating ART
• goal: keep viral load below limit of detection i.e. <40 copies/mL (undetectable); viral load should decrease 10-fold within 4-8 wk, be undetectable by 6 mo, and restore immunological function
• strong evidence against intermittent ART or 'drug holidays'
• ART leads to 96% reduction in risk of transmitting HIV to sexual partners

ART Recommendations for Treatment of Naïve Patients
• 2 NRTIs + 1 INSTI/PI (boosted with ritonavir or cobicistat)

Treatment Failure
• defined clinically (HIV progression), immunologically (failure to increase CD4 count by 25-50 over first yr of treatment or CD4 decrease >100 over 1 yr), or virologically (failure to achieve viral load <40 copies/mL after 6 mo)
• ensure that viral load >40 is not just a transient viremia or 'blip'; confirm medication adherence, assess drug interactions, perform resistance testing

HIV and AIDS

Table 23. Anti-Retroviral Drugs

Class	Drugs	Mechanism	Adverse Effects
Nucleoside reverse transcriptase inhibitors (NRTIs)	zidovudine (AZT) lamivudine (3TC) stavudine (d4T) didanosine (ddl) abacavir (ABC) emtricitabine (FTC) tenofovir disoproxil fumarate (TDF) **Combination Tablets:** AZT/3TC (Combivir®) AZT/3TC/ABC (Trizivir®) ABC/3TC (Kivexa®) TDF/FTC (Truvada®)	Incorporated into the growing viral DNA chain, thereby competitively inhibiting reverse transcriptase and terminating viral DNA growth	Lactic acidosis Lipodystrophy Rash N/V/diarrhea Bone marrow suppression (AZT) Peripheral neuropathy (ddl, d4T) Drug-induced hypersensitivity (ABC) Pancreatitis (ddl/d4T) Myopathy (AZT)
Non-nucleoside reverse transcriptase inhibitors (NNRTIs)	efavirenz (EFZ) nevirapine (NVP) delavirdine (DLV) etravirine (ETR) rilpivirine (RPV)	Non-competitively inhibit function of reverse transcriptase, thereby preventing viral RNA replication	Rash, Stevens-Johnson syndrome CNS: dizziness, insomnia, somnolence, abnormal dreams (efavirenz) Hepatotoxicity (nevirapine – avoid in females with CD4 >250, men with CD4 >400) CYP3A4 interactions
Protease inhibitors (PIs)*	ritonavir (RTV) saquinavir (SQV) amprenavir (APV) nelfinavir (NFV) indinavir (IDV) atazanavir (ATV) fosamprenavir (FPV) lopinavir/ritonavir (Kaletra®) tipranavir (TPV) darunavir (DRV)	Prevent maturation of infectious virions by inhibiting the cleavage of polyproteins	Lipodystrophy, metabolic syndrome N/V/diarrhea Nephrolithiasis (indinavir) Rash (APV) Hyperbilirubinemia (atazanavir, indinavir) CYP3A4 interactions Hyperlipidemia
Fusion inhibitor	enfuvirtide (T-20)	Inhibit viral fusion with T-cells by inhibiting gp41, preventing cell infection	Injection site reactions, rash, infection, diarrhea, nausea, fatigue
CCR5 antagonist	maraviroc	Inhibit viral entry by blocking host CCR5 co-receptor	Fever, cough, dizziness
Integrase strand transfer inhibitors (INSTIs)	raltegravir elvitegravir dolutegravir	Inhibits integration of HIV DNA into the human genome thus preventing HIV replication	

*Standard of care is to pharmacologically boost most PIs with ritonavir to increase concentrations

Lactic Acidosis
- Occurs secondary to mitochondrial toxicity
- Symptoms include abdominal pain, fatigue, N/V, muscle weakness

Lipodystrophy
Body fat redistribution (mainly with old ARVs)
- Lipohypertrophy (e.g. dorsal fat pad, breast enlargement, increased abdominal girth) thought to be caused primarily by protease inhibitors
- Lipoatrophy (e.g. facial thinning, decreased adipose tissue in the extremities) is thought to be caused by thymidine analogue NRTIs such as d4T and AZT
- Metabolic abnormalities: lipids (increased LDL, increased TGs), glucose (insulin resistance, type 2 DM), increased risk of CVD

Single Tablet ART Regimens
- reduces pill burden and increases adherence
- generally better tolerated

Table 24. Single Tablet ART Regimens

Name	Contents	Common Side Effects
Atripla®	efavirenz/tenofovir/emtricitabine	psychiatric events, vivid dreams
Complera®	rilpivirine/emtricitabine/tenofovir	good side effect profile
Stribild®	elvitegravir/cobicistat/emtricitabine/tenofovir	good side effect profile
Triumeq®	Dolutegravir/abacavir/lamivudine	good side effect profile; use only in HLAB*5701 negative patients

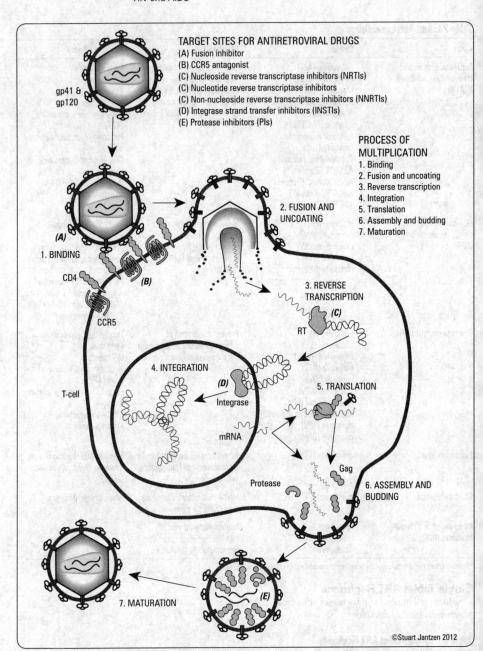

Figure 11. Mechanism of HIV replications

Prevention of HIV Infection

- education, including harm-reduction
  - safer sexual practices: condoms for vaginal and anal sex, barriers for oral sex
  - harm reduction for injection drug users: avoid sharing needles
- treatment of HIV+ women with ART during the 2nd and 3rd trimester of pregnancy and AZT during delivery followed by treatment of the infant for 4-6 wk (decreases maternal-fetal transmission from 25% to <3%)
- universal blood and body precautions for health care workers
  - post-exposure prophylaxis (PEP) after occupational (e.g. needle-stick injury) and non-occupational (e.g. consensual sex, sexual assault) exposure to HIV: 2- or 3-drug regimen initiated immediately (<72 h) after exposure and continuing for 4 wk
- recent data has demonstrated efficacy of pre-exposure prophylaxis (oral PrEP or topical microbicides) in preventing HIV
- ART associated with 96% reduction in risk of transmitting HIV to sexual partners
- screening of blood and organ donation

Types of Testing

1. Nominal/Name-Based HIV Testing
- person ordering the test knows the identity of the person being tested for HIV
- HIV test is ordered using the name of the person being tested
- person ordering the test is legally obligated to notify Public Health officials if test results are positive for HIV
- test result is recorded in the health care record of the person being tested

Early identification of HIV is essential for patients to receive the maximal benefit from ART

2. Non-Nominal/Non-Identifying HIV Testing
- similar to nominal/name-based testing on all points except:
- HIV test is ordered using a code or the initials of the person being tested

3. Anonymous Testing
- available at specialized clinics
- person ordering the HIV test does not know the identity of the person being tested
- HIV test is carried out using a unique non-identifying code that only the person being tested for HIV knows
- test results are not recorded on the health care record of the person being tested
- patient identification and notification of Public Health required to gain access to ART

HIV Pre- and Post-Test Counselling

- a diagnosis of HIV can be overwhelming and is often associated with stigma and discrimination
- consider pre- and post-test counselling, regardless of the results
- goals include: assessing risk, making informed decision to be tested, education to protect themselves and others from virus exposure, where to go for more information and support
- HIV+ patients should be connected with local support services

Fungal Infections

Skin and Subcutaneous Infections

Superficial Fungal Infections

- see <u>Dermatology</u>, D26

Dermatophytes

- see <u>Dermatology</u>, D26

Subcutaneous Fungal Infection

Pathophysiology
- fungi that naturally reside in soil and enter skin via traumatic break
- *Sporothrix schenckii*: most commonly affects gardeners injured by a rose thorn or splinter
  - causes subcutaneous nodule at point of entry
  - fungi may migrate up lymphatic vessels creating nodules along the way – "nodular lymphangitis"

Treatment
- oral azole (e.g. itraconazole)
- IV amphotericin B for severe or disseminated infection

Endemic Mycoses

Basics
- three major endemic mycoses in North America
  - histoplasmosis
  - blastomycosis
  - coccidioidomycosis

Histoplasmosis is commonly associated with exposure to chicken coops, bird roosts, and bat caves

- thermally dimorphic organisms: mould in cold temperature (e.g. soil) and yeast at higher temperature (e.g. tissue)
- infection occurs through inhalation of spores (soil, bird droppings, vegetation) or inoculation injury
- all can cause pneumonia and may disseminate hematogenously
- may reactivate or disseminate during immunocompromised states

Treatment
- common to all endemic mycoses
  - oral azole (e.g. itraconazole for mild-moderate local infection)
  - IV amphotericin B for systemic infection

Table 25. Endemic Mycoses

Disease	Endemic Region	Clinical Features	Investigations
Histoplasma capsulatum	Ohio and Mississippi River valleys in central USA, Ontario, Quebec; widespread	Asymptomatic (in most people) Primary pulmonary • Fever, cough, chest pain, H/A, myalgia, anorexia • CXR (acute): pulmonary infiltrates ± hilar lymphadenopathy • CXR (chronic): pulmonary infiltrates, cavitary disease Disseminated (rare) • Occurs primarily in immunocompromised patients • Spread to bone marrow (pancytopenia), GI tract (ulcers), lymph nodes (lymphadenitis), skin, liver, adrenals, CNS	Fungal culture, fungal stain Antigen detection (urine and serum) Serology
Blastomyces dermatitidis	States east of Mississippi River, Northern Ontario and along the Great Lakes	May be asymptomatic Primary: acute or chronic pneumonia • Fever, cough, chest pain, chills, night sweats, weight loss • CXR (acute): lobar or segmental pneumonia • CXR (chronic): lobar infiltrates, fibronodular interstitial disease Disseminated • Spread to skin (verrucous lesions that mimic skin cancer, ulcers, subcutaneous nodules), bones (osteomyelitis, osteolytic lesions), GU tract (prostatitis, epididymitis)	Sputum smear and culture Direct examination of clinical specimens for characteristic broad-based budding yeast (sputum, tissue, purulent material)
Coccidioides immitis	Deserts in southwest USA, northwest Mexico	Primary • "Valley fever": subacute fever, chills, cough, chest pain, sore throat, fatigue that lasts for weeks to months • Can develop hypersensitivity with arthralgias, erythema nodosum Disseminated • Rare spread to skin (ulcers), joints (synovitis), bones (lytic lesions), meninges (meningitis) • Common opportunistic infection in patients with HIV	Sputum culture Direct examination of clinical specimens for characteristic yeast (sputum, tissue, purulent material)

Opportunistic Fungi

Pneumocystis jiroveci (formerly *P. carinii*)
Pneumonia: PJP or PCP

Microbiology
- unicellular fungi
- previously classified as a protozoa

Transmission
- rarely person-to-person transmission
- most disease is due to reactivation of latent infection acquired by the respiratory route or reinfection by a different genotype
  - causes clinical disease in immunocompromised patients (steroid use, HIV)
  - 80% lifetime risk without prophylaxis (TMP/SMX) in HIV patients with CD4 count <200 cells/mm³

Clinical Features
- symptoms of pneumonia: fever, nonproductive cough, progressive dyspnea
- classic CXR

Investigations
- demonstration of organism in induced sputum, bronchoalveolar lavage, or endotracheal aspirate (if intubated)

CXR in *P. jiroveci*
- Bilateral, diffuse opacities
- CXR may be normal (20-30% cases)
- CT shows cysts (hence the name Pneumo"cystis") but almost never pleural effusions

Treatment and Prevention
- oxygen to keep SaO_2 >90%
- antimicrobial options
  - TMP/SMX (PO or IV)
  - dapsone and TMP
  - clindamycin and primaquine
  - pentamidine (IV)
  - atovaquone
- corticosteroids used as adjuvant therapy in those with severe hypoxia (pO_2 <70 mmHg or A-a gradient O_2 >35 mmHg)
- prophylactic TMP/SMX for those at high risk of infection (HIV patients when CD4 <200 cells/mm^3 or non-HIV immunocompromised patients under specific conditions)

Cryptococcus spp.

Microbiology
- encapsulated yeast found worldwide
- 2 human pathogenic species: *C. gattii, C. neoformans*

Transmission
- inhalation of airborne yeast from soil contaminated with pigeon droppings (*C. neoformans*) or certain tree species such as Eucalyptus or Douglas fir (*C. gattii*) → may cause local infection in lung → asymptomatic or pneumonia
- may also spread hematogenously to the CNS, skin, bones, and other organs
- *C. neoformans* tends to affect immunocompromised hosts
- *C. gattii* tends to affect immunocompetent hosts

C. gattii sees limited geographical distribution including Vancouver Island, Northern Australia, and Papua New Guinea

Clinical Features
- pulmonary
  - usually asymptomatic or self-limited pneumonitis
  - only 2% of HIV+ patients present with pulmonary symptoms including productive cough, chest tightness, and fever
- disseminated
  - frequently disseminates in HIV+ population
  - CNS: meningitis (leading cause of meningitis in patients with HIV)
  - skin: umbilicated papules that resemble large lesions of *Molluscum contagiosum*

Investigations
- serum cryptococcal antigen
- CSF for meningitis: India-ink stain, cryptococcal antigen test, culture to confirm

India-ink sensitivity for *Cryptococcus* is only 50% (higher in HIV patients); now replaced by cryptococcal antigen test in most laboratories

Treatment
- in patients with HIV who have cryptococcal meningitis or severe pulmonary disease:
  - amphotericin B (+ flucytosine) is used in the first 2 wk for induction therapy; limited duration due to side effects
  - switch to fluconazole for at least 8 wk as consolidation therapy, then continue at lower dose for prolonged maintenance

Candida albicans

Microbiology
- yeast forms with pseudohyphae germ tube formation at 37°C

Transmission
- normal flora of skin, mouth, vagina, and GI tract
- risk factors for overgrowth:
  - immunocompromised state (DM, corticosteroids)
  - ICU patients (broad-spectrum antibiotic use, central venous catheters, TPN)
  - obesity → maceration and moisture in intertriginous areas, pannus, under breasts

Clinical Features
- mucocutaneous
  - oral thrush, esophagitis (chest pain, odynophagia), vulvovaginitis (see Gynecology, GY26), balanitis, cutaneous (diaper rash, skin folds, folliculitis), chronic mucocutaneous
  - small satellite lesions beyond the margin of the rash
- invasive
  - candidemia, endophthalmitis, endocarditis, UTI (upper tract), hepatosplenic disease

Treatment
- thrush: nystatin suspension or pastilles for mild disease, fluconazole for severe disease
- vulvovaginal candidiasis: topical agents (imidazole or nystatin), oral fluconazole for recurrent disease
- cutaneous infection: topical imidazole
- opportunistic infections in HIV, other systemic infections: fluconazole or echinocandin
- chronic mucocutaneous: azoles

Aspergillus spp.

Microbiology
- branching septate hyphae
- common species causing disease include *A. fumigatus*, *A. flavus*

Transmission
- ubiquitous in the air and the environment
- *Aspergillus* produces a toxin called aflatoxin that contaminates nuts, grains, and rice

Clinical Features
- allergic bronchopulmonary aspergillosis (ABPA)
    - IgE-mediated asthma-type reaction with dyspnea, high fever, and transient pulmonary infiltrates
    - occurs more frequently in patients with asthma and allergies
- aspergilloma (fungus ball)
    - ball of hyphae in a preexisting lung cavity
    - symptoms range from asymptomatic to massive hemoptysis
    - CXR: round opacity surrounded by a thin lucent rim of air, often in upper lobes ("air crescent" sign)
- invasive aspergillosis
    - associated with prolonged and persistent neutropenia or transplantation
    - pneumonia – most common
    - may disseminate to other organs: brain, skin
    - severe symptoms with fever, cough, dyspnea, cavitation; fatal if not treated early and aggressively
    - CXR: local or diffuse infiltrates ± pulmonary infarction, pulmonary nodules with surrounding ground glass ("halo" sign)
- mycotoxicosis
    - aflatoxin produced by *A. flavus* (nuts, grains, rice)
    - results in liver hemorrhage, necrosis, and hepatocellular carcinoma formation

Treatment Options
- for invasive aspergillosis: voriconazole or amphotericin B
- surgical resection for aspergilloma
- corticosteroids ± itraconazole for ABPA

Parasitic Infections

Protozoa – Intestinal/Genitourinal Infections

Entamoeba histolytica (Amoebas)

Transmission
- reservoir: infected humans
- cysts by fecal-oral and food/waterborne transmission in areas of poor sanitation
- seen in immigrants, travellers, institutionalized individuals, Aboriginal Canadians, MSM

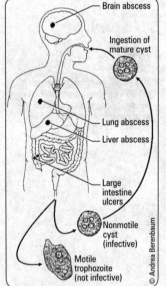

Figure 12. *Entamoeba* life cycle

Labels in figure: Brain abscess; Ingestion of mature cyst; Lung abscess; Liver abscess; Large intestine ulcers; Nonmotile cyst (infective); Motile trophozoite (not infective); © Andrea Berenbaum

Clinical Features
1. asymptomatic carriers
2. amoebic dysentery
    - abdominal pain, cramping, colitis, dysentery, low grade fever with bloody diarrhea secondary to local tissue destruction and ulceration of large intestine
3. amoebic abscesses (LINK to General Surgery "Liver Abscesses")
    - most common in liver (hematologic spread); presents with RUQ pain, weight loss, fever, hepatomegaly
    - can also occur in lungs and brain

Investigations
- serology, fecal/serum antigen testing, stool exam (for cysts and trophozoites), colon biopsy
- *E. histolytica* indistinguishable microscopically from the non-pathogen *E. dispar* (distinguish by specific stool antigen detection)

Treatment and Prevention
- metronidazole
- for invasive disease or cyst elimination: follow with iodoquinol or paromomycin
- aspiration of hepatic abscess if risk of cyst rupture, poor response to medical therapy, or diagnostic uncertainty
- asymptomatic cyst shedding: iodoquinol or paromomycin alone
- good personal hygiene, purification of water supply by boiling, filtration (not chlorination)

Giardia lamblia

Transmission
- reservoir: infected humans and other mammals
- food/waterborne (especially in the Rockies) and fecal-oral transmission of infectious cysts
- risk factors: travel, camping, institutions, day care centres, MSM

Clinical Features
- giardiasis ("beaver fever")
  - symptoms vary from asymptomatic to self-limited mild watery diarrhea to malabsorption syndrome (chronic giardiasis where the parasite coats the small intestine and thus prevents fat absorption)
  - nausea, malaise, abdominal cramps, bloating, flatulence, fatigue, weight loss, steatorrhea
  - no hematochezia (no invasion into intestinal wall), no mucous in stool

Investigations
- multiple stool samples (daily x 3 d) for microscopy, stool antigen used occasionally
- occasionally small bowel aspirate or biopsy

Treatment and Prevention
- metronidazole; nitazoxanide if symptomatic
- good personal hygiene and sanitation, water purification (iodine better than chlorination), outbreak investigation

Trichomonas vaginalis

Transmission
- sexual contact

Clinical Features
- often asymptomatic (10-50%), especially males (occasionally urethritis, prostatitis)
- trichomonas vaginitis (see <u>Gynecology</u>, GY26)
  - vaginal discharge (profuse, malodourous, yellow-green or grey, frothy), pruritus, dysuria, dyspareunia

Trichomonas causes 25% of vaginitis

Investigations
- wet mount (motile parasites), antigen detection, culture
- urine PCR to detect in males

Treatment
- metronidazole for patient and partner(s)

Cryptosporidium spp.

Transmission
- reservoir: infected humans and a wide variety of young animals
- fecal-oral transmission by ingestion of cysts; waterborne
- risk factors: summer and fall, young children (day care), MSM, contact with farm animals, immunodeficiency

Clinical Features
- range from self-limited watery diarrhea (immunocompetent) to chronic, severe, non-bloody diarrhea with N/V, abdominal pain, and anorexia resulting in weight loss and death (immunocompromised)

Investigations
- modified acid-fast stain of stool specimen, microscopic identification of oocysts in stool or tissue, stool antigen detection by direct fluorescent antibody

Treatment and Prevention
- supportive care
- in HIV, try HAART to restore immunity; if fails, try nitazoxanide
- good personal hygiene, water filtration

Blood and Tissue Infections

Plasmodium spp. (Malaria)

Malaria is the most common fatal infectious disease worldwide

Microbiology
- species include: *P. falciparum* (most common and most lethal), *P. vivax, P. ovale, P. malariae, P. knowlesi*
- complex life cycle: human host for asexual reproduction and mosquito for sexual reproduction
- sporozoites from mosquitoes infect human liver cells, where they multiply and are released as merozoites; merozoites infect RBCs and cause disease
- *P. ovale* and *P. vivax* can produce dormant hypnozoites in the liver that may cause relapsing malarial attacks by reactivating (entering the erythrocytic cycle) after many months

Transmission
- reservoir: infected human
- transmission by the night-biting female *Anopheles* mosquito, vertical transmission, and blood transfusion
- occurs in tropical/subtropical regions (sub-Saharan Africa, Oceania, South Asia, Central America, Southeast Asia, South America)

Clinical Features
- flu-like prodrome
- paroxysms of high spiking fever and shaking chills (due to synchronous systemic lysis of RBCs) (lasts several hours)
  - *P. vivax* and *P. ovale*: chills and fever x48 h but can be variable
  - *P. malariae*: chills and fever x72 h but can be variable
  - *P. falciparum*: less predictable fever interval, can be highly variable (>90% ill within 30 d)
- abdominal pain, diarrhea, myalgia, H/A, and cough
- hepatosplenomegaly and thrombocytopenia without leukocytosis

Complications
- *P. falciparum*: CNS involvement (cerebral malaria = seizures and coma), severe anemia, acute kidney injury, ARDS, primarily responsible for fatal disease
- *P. knowlesi*, and rarely *P. vivax*, can be fatal

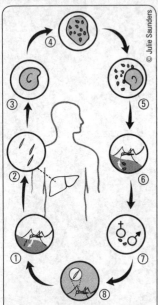

1. Sporozoites enter blood via mosquito bite, infect liver
2. Hepatic infiltration
3. Infect red blood cells
4. Trophozoite divides asexually many times to produce schizont (contains merozoites)
5. Red blood cell lyses and merozoites attack other red blood cells (chills and fever)
6. Male and female gametocytes (from merozoites) ingested by mosquito during bite
7. Male and female gametocytes (from merozoites) fuse in mosquito gut; produce ookinete
8. Ookinete matures into an oocyst which contains individual sporozoites; migrates to mosquito salivary glands

Figure 13. Life cycle of *Plasmodium* spp.

Investigations
- microscopy: blood smear q12-24h (x3) to rule out infection
  - thick smear (Giemsa stain) for presence of organisms
  - thin smear (Giemsa stain) for species identification and quantification of parasites
- rapid antigen detection tests

Treatment and Prevention
- *P. vivax, P. ovale*: chloroquine (and primaquine to eradicate liver forms)
- *P. vivax*, chloroquine resistant: atovaquone/proguanil + primaquine or quinine and doxycycline + primaquine
- *P. malariae, P. knowlesi*: chloroquine
- *P. falciparum*: most areas of the world show chloroquine resistance – check local resistance patterns
  - artemisinin combination therapy (e.g. artesunate + doxycycline or clindamycin or atovaquone/proguanil)
  - atovaquone/proguanil combination (Malarone®)
  - quinine + doxycycline or clindamycin
  - mefloquine and artemisinin resistance increasing in southeast Asia (check local resistance)
- prevention with antimalarial prophylaxis, covering exposed skin, bed nets, insect repellant

Drugs for Preventing Malaria in Travellers
Cochrane DB Syst Rev 2009;CD006491
Study: Cochrane Systematic Review. 8 RCTs.
Population: 4,240 non-immune adults and children traveling to regions with *P. falciparum* resistance to chloroquine.
Intervention: Atovaquone-proguanil, doxycycline, mefloquine, chloroquine-proguanil, or primaquine used for malaria prophylaxis.
Outcome: Efficacy, safety, and tolerability.
Results: Atovaquone-proguanil and doxycycline had similar adverse events. Atovaquone-proguanil had fewer overall (RR 0.72), GI (RR 0.54), and neuropsychiatric events (RR 0.49) than mefloquine. Doxycycline also had fewer neuropsychiatric events than mefloquine (RR 0.84).
Conclusion: Atovaquone-proguanil or doxycycline as prophylaxis against malaria is best tolerated in terms of adverse effects and mefloquine is associated with adverse neuropsychiatric outcomes.

Trypanosoma cruzi

Transmission
- found in Mexico, South America, and Central America
- transmission by Reduviid insect vector ("Kissing Bug"), which defecates on skin and trypomastigotes in the stool are rubbed into bite site by host
- also transmitted via placental transfer, organ donation, blood transfusion, and ingestion of contaminated food containing Reduviid insects (especially cane juice)

Clinical Features
- American trypanosomiasis (Chagas disease)
  - acute: usually asymptomatic, local swelling at site of inoculation ("Romana's sign"; usually around one eye) with variable fever, lymphadenopathy, cardiomegaly, and hepatosplenomegaly

- chronic indeterminate phase: asymptomatic but increasing levels of antibody in blood; most infected persons (60-70%) remain in this phase, and do not go on to manifest a determinate form of Chagas disease
- chronic determinate: leads to chronic dilated cardiomyopathy, esophagomegaly, and megacolon 10-25 yr after acute infection in 30-40% of infected individuals

Investigations
- wet prep and Giemsa stain of thick and thin blood smear, serology, PCR

Treatment and Prevention
- acute: nifurtimox or benznidazole
- indeterminate: increasing trend to treat as acute infection for children and adults under age 50 years
- chronic determinate: symptomatic therapy, surgery as necessary including heart transplant, esophagectomy, and colectomy; there may be a benefit to antiparasitic treatment
- insect control, bed nets

Toxoplasma gondii

Transmission
- acquired through exposure to cat feces (oocysts), ingestion of undercooked meat (tissue cysts), vertical transmission, organ transplantation, gardening without gloves (cat oocyst exposure), whole blood transfusions

Clinical Features
- congenital
  - result of acute primary infection of mother during pregnancy (see Obstetrics, OB29, *TORCH infection*)
  - stillbirth (rare), chorioretinitis, blindness, seizures, severe developmental delay, microcephaly
  - initially asymptomatic infant may develop reactivation of chorioretinitis as adolescent or adult blurred vision, scotoma, ocular pain, photophobia, epiphora, hearing loss, developmental delay
- acquired
  - usually asymptomatic or mononucleosis-like syndrome in immunocompetent patient
  - infection remains latent for life unless reactivation due to immunosuppression
- immunocompromised (most commonly AIDS with CD4 <200)
  - encephalitis with focal CNS lesions seen as single or multiple ring-enhancing masses on CT (H/A and focal neurological signs)
  - lymph node, liver, and spleen enlargement and pneumonitis
  - chorioretinitis

Investigations
- serology, CSF Wright-Giemsa stain, antigen or DNA detection (PCR); pathology provides definitive diagnosis
- immunocompromised patients: consider CT scan (ring-enhancing lesion in cortex or deep nuclei) and ophthalmologic examination
- negative serology in many AIDS patients (false negative due to decreased lymphocyte population)

Treatment and Prevention
- no treatment if: immunocompetent, not pregnant, no severe organ damage
- pregnancy: spiramycin to prevent transplacental transmission or pyrimethamine + sulfadiazine (add folinic acid), avoid undercooked meat and refrain from emptying cat litter boxes
- HIV: pyrimethamine + sulfadiazine (see *Prophylaxis*, ID30)
- eye disease, meningitis: corticosteroids
- proper hand hygiene, cook meat thoroughly to proper temperature

1/3 of Ontario's population is infected with *Toxoplasma gondii*

Classic Triad of Congenital Toxoplasmosis
- Chorioretinitis
- Hydrocephalus
- Intracranial calcifications

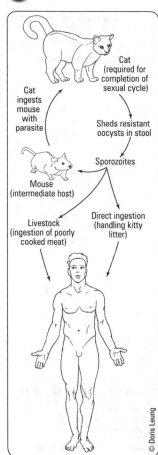
Figure 14. Life cycle of *Toxoplasma gondii*

Cat (required for completion of sexual cycle)

Cat ingests mouse with parasite

Sheds resistant oocysts in stool

Sporozoites

Mouse (intermediate host)

Direct ingestion (handling kitty litter)

Livestock (ingestion of poorly cooked meat)

© Doris Leung

Helminths

Roundworms – Nematodes

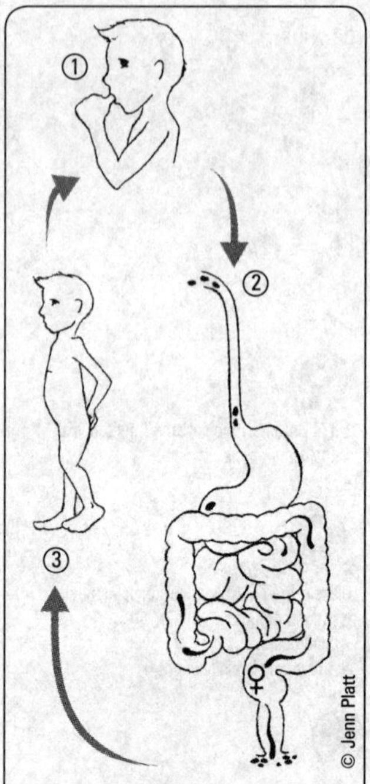

Table 26. Nematodes (Roundworms)

Nematode	Epidemiology	Transmission	Medical Importance	Treatment
Ascaris lumbricoides	Tropics	Human feces, ingestion of contaminated food or water containing eggs	Abdominal pain and intestinal obstruction from high worm burden Cough, dyspnea, pulmonary infiltrates from larval migration through lungs (Löffler's syndrome)	Mebendazole OR albendazole OR pyrantel pamoate
Trichuris trichiura (whipworm)	Tropics	Ingestion of eggs in soil	Diarrhea (± mucous, blood), abdominal pain, rectal prolapse, stunted growth	Mebendazole OR albendazole
Onchocerca volvulus	Africa, Latin America	Blackfly bite	River blindness (onchocerciasis), dermatitis	Ivermectin + doxycycline
Wuchereria bancrofti	Tropics	Mosquito bite	Damage to lymphatics resulting in lymphadenopathy, lymphedema, and elephantiasis Tropical pulmonary eosinophilia	Diethylcarbamazine + doxycycline
Loa Loa	Central Africa	Deer fly bite	Subcutaneous migration of worm, hyperresponsiveness in travellers	Diethylcarbamazine
Enterobius vermicularis (Pinworm)	Worldwide	Human host: fecal-oral self-inoculation and fomite person-to-person transfer Adult worms live in cecum and deposit eggs in perianal skin	Asymptomatic carriers or severe nocturnal perianal itching (pruritus ani) Occasional vaginitis, ectopic migration to appendix or other pelvic organs Abdominal pain, N/V with high worm burden	Sticky tape test: eggs adhere to tape applied to perianal skin (need 5-7 tests to rule out) Examination of perianal skin at night may reveal adult worms Usually no eosinophilia as no tissue invasion Mebendazole, albendazole; pyrantel in pregnancy Change underwear, bathe in morning, pajamas to bed, wash hands, trim fingernails Treat all family members simultaneously Reinfection common
Strongyloides stercoralis (Threadworm)	Subtropical, tropical, and temperate (including southern US)	Fecal contamination of soil: transmission via unbroken skin, walking barefoot Autoinfection: penetration of larvae through GI mucosa or perianal skin Adult worms live in mucosa of small intestine	One of few worms able to multiply in human host Mostly asymptomatic infection or can have pruritic dermatitis at site of larval penetration Transient pulmonary symptoms during pulmonary migration of larvae (eosinophilic pneumonitis = Löffler's syndrome) Abdominal pain, diarrhea, pruritis ani, larva currens (itchy rash) Hyperinfection: occasional fatal cases caused by massive auto-infection in immunocompromised host; immunoablative therapy, including high-dose corticosteroids, is the most common risk factor for disseminated infection	Ivermectin, 200 μg/kg/d PO x 2 doses (albendazole 400 mg PO bid x 7 d, less effective)

© Jenn Platt

1. Embryonated eggs ingested by humans
2. Larvae hatch in small intestine
3. Females migrate out anus at night

Figure 15. Life cycle of *Enterobius*

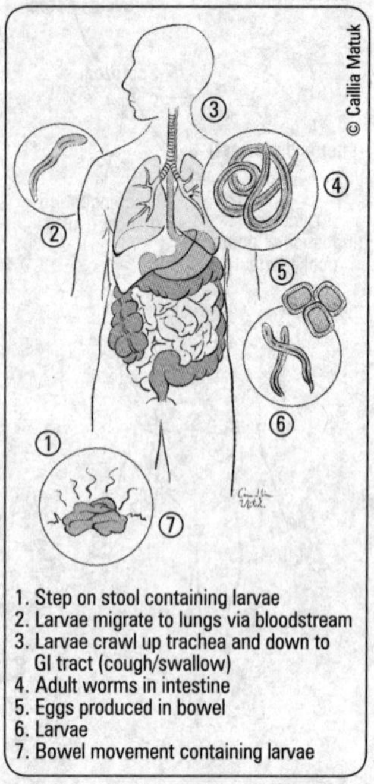

© Caillia Matuk

1. Step on stool containing larvae
2. Larvae migrate to lungs via bloodstream
3. Larvae crawl up trachea and down to GI tract (cough/swallow)
4. Adult worms in intestine
5. Eggs produced in bowel
6. Larvae
7. Bowel movement containing larvae

Figure 16. Life cycle of *Strongyloides*

Flatworms

Cestodes/Trematodes

Table 27. Cestodes/Trematodes (Flatworms)

	Epidemiology	Transmission	Medical Importance	Treatment
CESTODES				
Taenia solium	Developing countries	Undercooked pork (larvae), human feces (eggs)	Taeniasis: mild abdominal symptoms Cysticercosis: mass lesions in CNS, eyes, skin, seizures	Corticosteroids + albendazole for cysticercosis Antiepileptics if seizures Praziquantel for adult tapeworm in gut (taeniasis)
Taenia saginata	Developing countries	Undercooked beef (larvae)	Mild GI symptoms	Praziquantel
Diphyllobothrium latum	Europe, North America, Asia	Raw fish	B_{12} deficiency leading to macrocytic anemia and posterior column deficits	Praziquantel
Echinococcus granulosus	Rural areas Sheep-raising countries	Dog feces (eggs)	Liver/lung cysts (enlarge between 1-20 yr; may cause mass effect or rupture) Risk of anaphylaxis if cystic fluid released during surgical evacuation	Albendazole ± praziquantel alone Surgery + perioperative albendazole Percutaneous aspiration + perioperative albendazole
TREMATODES				
Clonorchis sinensis	Japan, Taiwan, China, SE Asia	Raw fish	Exists in bile ducts, causes inflammation and sometimes cholangiocarcinoma	Praziquantel
Schistosoma spp.	Africa, SE Asia, focal in Western Hemisphere	Fresh water exposure	Chronic sequelae secondary to long-term infection (e.g. chronic liver disease, SCC of the bladder)	Praziquantel

Trematodes/Flukes

Schistosoma spp.

Species
- *S. mansoni, S. hematobium, S. japonicum*

Transmission
- larvae (cercariae), released from snails, penetrate unbroken skin in infested fresh water
- adult worms live in terminal venules of bladder/bowel passing eggs into urine/stool
- eggs must reach fresh water to hatch; schistosomes cannot multiply in or pass between humans
  - more common in individuals from sub-Saharan Africa, South America, Asia, Caribbean, Eastern Mediterranean/North Africa

Clinical Features
- most asymptomatic; symptoms seen in travellers (nonimmune)
- swimmer's itch: pruritic skin rash at site of penetration (cercarial dermatitis)
- acute schistosomiasis (Katayama fever): hypersensitivity to migrating parasites (4-8 wk after infection)
  - fever, hives, H/A, weight loss, cough, abdominal pain, chronic diarrhea, high-grade eosinophilia

Complications of Chronic Infection
- *S. mansoni, S. japonicum*
  - worms in mesenteric vein, eggs in portal tracts of liver and bowel
  - heavy infections: intestinal polyps, portal and pulmonary HTN, splenomegaly (2° to portal HTN), hepatomegaly
- *S. hematobium*
  - worms in vesical plexus, eggs in distal ureter and bladder induce granulomas and fibrosis
  - hematuria and obstructive uropathy; associated with squamous cell bladder cancer
- neurologic complications: spinal cord neuroschistosomiasis (transverse myelitis), cerebral or cerebellar neuroschistosomiasis (increased ICP, focal CNS signs, seizures)
- pulmonary complications: granulomatous pulmonary endarteritis, pulmonary HTN, cor pulmonale; especially in patients with hepatosplenic involvement

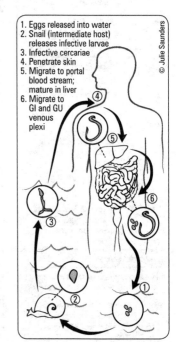

1. Eggs released into water
2. Snail (intermediate host) releases infective larvae
3. Infective cercariae
4. Penetrate skin
5. Migrate to portal blood stream; mature in liver
6. Migrate to GI and GU venous plexi

© Julie Saunders

Figure 17. Life cycle of *Schistosoma*

For up to date information on geographic and seasonal patterns of disease and travel advisories, check the website for the United States Centers for Disease Control and Prevention (wwwnc.cdc.gov/travel) or Foreign Affairs Canada (travel.gc.ca)

Investigations
- serology (high sensitivity and specificity), CBC (eosinophilia, anemia, thrombocytopenia)
- *S. mansoni, S. japonicum*: eggs in stool, liver U/S shows fibrosis, rectal biopsy
- *S. hematobium*: bladder biopsy, eggs in urine and occasionally stool, kidney and bladder U/S

Treatment and Prevention
- praziquantel
- add glucocorticoid if acute schistosomiasis or neurologic complications develop
- proper disposal of human fecal waste, molluscicide (pesticide against molluscs), avoidance of infested water
- do not swim in Lake Malawi

Ectoparasites

- scabies, lice
- see Dermatology, D27-28

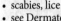

Travel Medicine

General Travel Precautions
- vector-borne: long sleeves, long pants, hats, repellents (containing permethrin) applied to clothes, belongings, and bed nets, and skin repellents (such as DEET) applied to exposed skin
- food/water: avoid eating raw meats/seafood, uncooked vegetables, and milk/dairy products; drink only bottled beverages, chlorinated water, boiled water
- recreation: caution when swimming in schistosomiasis-endemic regions (Lake Malawi), fresh water rafting/kayaking, beaches that may contain human/animal waste products, near storm drains, after heavy rainfalls
- prophylaxis: malaria (chloroquine, mefloquine, atovaquone + proguanil, doxycycline), traveller's diarrhea (bismuth salicylate)
- standard vaccines up to date (hepatitis B, MMR, tetanus/diphtheria, varicella, pertussis, polio, influenza)
- travel vaccines: hepatitis A/B, Japanese encephalitis, typhoid fever, yellow fever, rabies, ETEC, cholera
- sexually transmitted and blood-borne infections: safe sex practices, avoidance of percutaneous injury through razors, tattoos, piercings

Infectious Diseases to Consider
- vector borne: malaria, dengue fever, Chikungunya fever, yellow fever, spotted fever rickettsioses, West Nile virus, trypanosomiasis, Japanese encephalitis, tick-borne encephalitis, leishmaniasis
- sexually transmitted: HIV, HBV, acute HSV, syphilis, usual STIs
- zoonotic: rabies, hantavirus, tularemia, Q fever, anthrax, brucellosis
- airborne: TB
- food/water: HAV, HEV, brucellosis, typhoid, paratyphoid, amoebiasis, dysentery, traveller's diarrhea, cholera, *Campylobacter* spp.
- soil/water: schistosomiasis, strongyloidiasis, leptospirosis, cutaneous larva migrans, histoplasmosis, paracoccidioidomycosis

Fever in the Returned Traveller

Etiology
- commonly identified causes of fever in returning traveller
  - parasitic: malaria (20-30%)
  - viral: non-specific mononucleosis-like syndrome (4-25%), dengue (5%), viral hepatitis (3%)
  - bacterial: typhoid from *Salmonella* (2-7%), rickettsioses (3%)
  - diverse group of causative pathogens: traveller's diarrhea (10-20%), RTI (10-15%), UTI/STI (2-3%)
- febrile illness in travellers can be caused by routine infections that are common in non-travellers (e.g. URTI, UTI)
- less commonly, fever can be due to non-infectious causes (e.g. DVT, PE)

History
- pre-travel preparation
- travel itinerary: when, where, why, what, who, how?
  - dates of travel (determine incubation period)
  - season of travel: wet or dry
  - destination: country, region (urban or rural), environment (jungle, desert, etc.)
  - purpose of trip

Important Exposures

Insect Bites	
Mosquito	*Plasmodium* spp. (Malaria) Dengue Chikunguny Lymphatic filariasis (Elephantiasis) West Nile Encephalitis Yellow Fever Japanese Encephalitis
Tick	*Borrelia burgdorferi* (Lyme Disease) *Rickettsia rickettsii* (Rocky Mountain Spotted Fever)
Fly	*Trypanosoma brucei* spp. (African sleeping sickness) *Leishmania* spp. (Leishmaniasis) *Bartonella bacilliformis* (Bartonellosis)
Flea	*Yersinia* (Plague) *Tunga penetrans* (Tungiasis)

Mammal Bites	
Dog/Cat	Rabies, *Pasteurella*, anaerobes, *Streptococcus, S. aureus*
Human	*Streptococcus, S. aureus*, oral anaerobes, *Eikenella*

Oral Exposures	
Unpasteurized Milk	*Brucella* spp., non-tuberculous mycobacteria, *Salmonella, E. coli, Listeria*
Undercooked Meat/Fish	Enteric bacteria, helminths, protozoa
Water	Hepatitis A/E, Norwalk, cholera, *Salmonella, Shigella, Giardia*, poliovirus, *Cryptosporidium, Cyclospora*

Environmental Exposures	
Fresh Water	*Leptospira* spp., schistosomes, *Acanthamoeba, Naegleria fowleri*
Soil	Hookworms, *Toxocara* spp. (visceral larva migrans), *Leptospira interrogans* (leptospirosis)

Adapted with permission from *Lancet* 2003;361:1459-69

- persons visiting friends and family more likely to be exposed to local population and pathogens
  - style of travel: lodgings, camping, adventure travelling
  - local population: sick contacts
  - transportation: use of animals
- exposure history
  - street foods, untreated water: increased risk of traveller's diarrhea, enteric fever
  - uncooked meat/unpasteurized dairy: increased risk of parasitic infection
  - body fluids (sexual contacts, tattoos, piercings, IVDU, other injections)
  - increased risk of HBV, HCV, HIV, GC, *C. trachomatis*, syphilis
  - animal/insect bites: increased risk of malaria, dengue, rickettsioses, rabies
- fever pattern
- incubation period: use the earliest and latest possible dates of exposure to narrow the differential diagnosis and exclude serious infections
  - <21 d: consider malaria, typhoid fever, dengue fever, chikunguny, rickettsioses; exclude HBV, TB
  - >21 d: consider malaria, TB, typhoid fever; exclude dengue fever, chikungunya, traveller's diarrhea, rickettsioses
- body systems affected: GI, respiratory, CNS, skin

Fever in traveller from malaria endemic area is malaria until proven otherwise

Investigations
- all travellers with fever should undergo the following tests
  - blood work: CBC and differential, liver enzymes, electrolytes, creatinine, thick and thin blood smears x3 (for malaria), blood C&S
  - urine: urinalysis, urine C&S if dysuria or other localizing signs
- special tests based on symptoms, exposure history, and geography
  - stool: C&S, O&P
  - CXR
  - dengue serology for IgM

Table 28. Fever in the Returned Traveller

Illness	Geography/Timing	Pathogen	Incubation Period	Clinical Manifestations	Diagnosis	Treatment
Malaria	Africa India C. and S. America SE Asia Usually rural, night-biting mosquitoes	*Plasmodium falciparum* *Plasmodium vivax* *P. malariae* *P. ovale* *P. knowlesi*	7-30 d to mo or years	Fever and flu-like illness, (shaking chills, H/A, muscle aches, and fatigue) N/V and diarrhea Anemia and jaundice *Plasmodium falciparum*: (severe) kidney failure, seizures, mental confusion, prostration, coma, death, respiratory failure	Blood smear (thick and thin) x3 Rapid Diagnostic Test (with smear or PCR confirmation) Antigen detection PCR (mostly a research tool)	Artesunate (for severe disease) + malarone, doxycycline, or clindamycin Quinine sulfate + doxycycline or clindamycin Chloroquine + primaquine
Dengue	South East Asia Caribbean Usually urban, day-biting mosquitoes	Dengue viruses	3 d to 2 wk	Sudden onset of fever, H/A, retro-orbital pain, myalgias, and arthralgias Leukopenia Thrombocytopenia Hemorrhagic manifestations (rare in travellers)	Anti-dengue IgM positivity	Symptom relief: Acetaminophen (avoid using NSAIDs because of anticoagulant properties)
Typhoid (enteric fever)	Global but mostly Indian subcontinent	*Salmonella typhi* *Salmonella paratyphi*	3 to 60 d	Sustained fever 39°-40°C (103°-104°F) Abdominal pain, H/A, loss of appetite, cough, constipation	Stool, urine, or blood sample positive for *S. typhi* or *S. paratyphi*	Quinolone antibiotic (e.g. ciprofloxacin), ceftriaxone, or macrolide
Tick Typhus	Mediterranean South Africa India	*Rickettsia*	1 to 2 wk	Fever, H/A, fatigue, muscle aches, occasionally rash Eschar at site of tick bite Thrombocytopenia Elevated liver enzymes	Serology Presence of classic tick eschar	Doxycycline
TB	Global	*M. tuberculosis*	Variable	Fever, cough, hemoptysis	CXR Sputum culture and acid-fast stain	Ethambutol, isoniazid, pyrazinamide, rifampin, +/- pyridoxine (vit. B6)
Mononucleosis	Caribbean, C. and S. America	EBV or CMV	30 to 50 d	Malaise, fatigue, pharyngitis, lymphadenopathy, splenomegaly	Atypical lymphocytes on blood smear and positive heterophilic antibody (monospot) test	Acetaminophen or NSAIDs, fluids
Zika Virus Disease	Africa, SE Asia, S. America; spreading	Zika virus	Unknown, likely 3 to 12 d	Headache, malaise, muscle/joint pain, mild fever, rash, conjunctivitis	RT-PCR Serology	Rest, fluids, analgesics/antipyretics (avoid NSAIDs until Dengue ruled out)

Fever of Unknown Origin

Table 29. Classification of Fever of Unknown Origin (FUO) – Temp >38.3°C/101°F on several occasions

Classical FUO	Nosocomial FUO	Neutropenic FUO	HIV-associated FUO
Duration >3 wk	Hospitalized patient Infection not present/ incubating on admission	Neutrophil count <500/mL or is expected to fall to that level in 1-2	HIV infections Duration >4 wk for outpatients, >3 d for hospitalized patients
Diagnosis uncertain after 3 outpatient visits or 3 d in hospital or 1 wk of intensive ambulatory investigation	Diagnosis uncertain after 3 d of investigation, including at least 2 d incubation of cultures	Diagnosis uncertain after 3 d of investigation, including at least 2 d incubation of cultures	Diagnosis uncertain after 3 d of investigation, including at least 2 d incubation of cultures

Causes of Nosocomial FUO
B, C, D, E
Bacterial and fungal infections of respiratory tract and surgical sites
Catheters (intravascular and urinary)
Drugs
Emboli

Etiology of Classic FUO
- infectious causes (~30%)
    - TB: extra-pulmonary (most common), miliary, pulmonary (if pre-existing disease)
    - abscess: subphrenic, liver, splenic, pancreatic, perinephric, diverticular, pelvis, psoas
    - osteomyelitis
    - bacterial endocarditis (culture negative)
    - uncommon: viral (CMV, EBV), bacterial (brucellosis, bartonellosis), fungal (histoplasmosis, cryptococcosis), parasitic (toxoplasmosis, leishmaniasis, amoebiasis, malaria)
- neoplastic causes (~20%)
    - most commonly lymphomas (especially non-Hodgkin's) and leukemias, also multiple myeloma, myelodysplastic syndrome
    - solid tumours: RCC (most common), also breast, liver (hepatoma), colon, pancreas, or liver metastases
- collagen vascular diseases (~30%)
    - SLE, RA, rheumatic fever, vasculitis (temporal arteritis, PAN), JRA, Still's disease
- miscellaneous (~20%)
    - drugs, factitious fever
    - sarcoidosis, granulomatous hepatitis, IBD
    - hereditary periodic fever syndromes (such as familial Mediterranean fever)
    - venous thromboembolic disease: PE, DVT
    - endocrine: thyroiditis, thyroid storm, adrenal insufficiency, pheochromocytoma
- unknown in 30-50% despite detailed workup

Approach to Classic FUO

Drugs that may Cause Fever
- Anti-microbials (sulfonamides, penicillins, nitrofurantoin, antimalarials)
- Anti-hypertensives (hydralazine, methyldopa)
- Anti-epileptics (barbiturate, phenytoin)
- Anti-arrythmics (quinine, procainamide)
- Anti-inflammatories (NSAIDs)
- Anti-thrombotics (ASA)
- Anti-histamines
- Anti-thyroid

- careful history: travel, environmental/occupational exposures, infectious contacts, medication history, immunizations, TB history, sexual history, past medical history, comprehensive review of systems (including symptoms that resolved before interview)
- thorough physical exam: fever pattern, rashes (skin, mucous membranes), murmurs, arthritis, lymphadenopathy, organomegaly
- initial investigations as appropriate
    - blood work: CBC and differential, electrolytes, BUN, Cr, calcium profile, LFTs, ESR, CRP, muscle enzymes, RF, ANA, serum protein electrophoresis (SPEP), blood smear
    - cultures: blood (x2 sets), urine, sputum, stool C&S, O&P, other fluids as appropriate
    - serology: HIV, monospot, CMV IgM
    - imaging: CXR, abdominal imaging
- if there are diagnostic clues from any of the above steps, proceed with directed exam, biopsies or invasive testing as required, followed by directed treatment once a diagnosis is established
- if no diagnosis with the above, consider empiric therapy vs. watchful waiting
    - without intervention: patients that remain undiagnosed despite extensive workup have good prognosis
- immunocompromised hosts have increased susceptibility to infections from pathogens that are typically low virulence, commensal, or latent
- type of immunodeficiency predicts probable spectrum of agents

Infections in the Immunocompromised Host

Factors that Compromise the Immune System
- general: age (very young or elderly), malnutrition
- immune disease: HIV/AIDS, malignancies, asplenia (functional or anatomic), hypogammaglobulinemia, neutropenia
- DM
- iatrogenic: corticosteroids, chemotherapy, radiation treatment, anti-TNF therapy, other immunosuppressive drugs (e.g. in transplant patients)

Infections Associated with Asplenia
- *Haemophilus influenzae* type b
- *Streptococcus pneumoniae*
- *Neisseria meningitidis*
- *Salmonella*
- *Babesiosis*
- *Malaria*
- *Capnocytophaga canimorsus* (dog bite)

Table 30. Types of Immunodeficiency

Type	Conditions	Vulnerable To
Cell-Mediated Immunity	HIV, Hodgkin's, hairy cell leukemia, cytotoxic drugs, SCID, DiGeorge syndrome	Latent viruses Fungi Parasites
Humoral Immunity	CLL, lymphosarcoma, multiple myeloma, nephrotic syndrome, protein-losing enteropathy, burns, sickle cell anemia, asplenia, splenectomy, selective Ig deficiencies, Wiskott-Aldrich syndrome	Encapsulated organisms (*S. pneumoniae, H. influenzae, N. meningitidis, Salmonella typhi,* GBS)
Neutrophil Function	Myelodysplasia, paroxysmal nocturnal hemoglobinuria, radiation, cytotoxic drug therapy, C3 or C5 deficiencies, chronic granulomatous disease	Catalase-producing organisms (*Staphylococcus, Serratia, Nocardia, Aspergillus*)

Febrile Neutropenia

Definition
- fever (≥38.3°C/101°F or ≥38.0°C/100.4°F for ≥1 h) and one of
  - ANC <0.5 OR
  - ANC <1.0 but trending down to 0.5

ANC (absolute neutrophil count) = WBC x (%neutrophils + %bands)

Pathophysiology
- decreased neutrophil production
  - marrow: infection, aplastic/myelophthisic anemia, leukemia, lymphoma, myelodysplastic syndromes
  - iatrogenic: cancer chemotherapy, radiation, drugs
  - deficiencies: vitamin B_{12}, folate
- increased peripheral neutrophil destruction
  - autoimmune: Felty's syndrome, SLE, antineutrophil antibodies
  - splenic sequestration

Usual signs and symptoms of infection may be diminished because neutrophils are required for a robust inflammatory response; exam and x-ray findings may be more subtle

Epidemiology/Etiology
- most common life-threatening complication of cancer therapy
- 8 cases per 1,000 cancer patients per yr in the U.S.
- causative organism identified only 1/3 of the time
- GN (especially *Pseudomonas*) historically most common
- GP more common now
- fungal superinfection if neutropenia prolonged or if concurrent antibiotic use (especially *Candida, Aspergillus*)

WBC is lowest between 5-10 d after last chemotherapy cycle

Investigations
- examine for potential sites of infection: mucositis and line infections are most common
- do NOT perform DRE; examine perianal region
- blood C&S (x2 sets), urine C&S, culture all indwelling catheter ports, ± sputum C&S and NP swab for respiratory viruses
- CBC and differential, Cr, BUN, electrolytes, AST/ALT, total bilirubin

Prophylaxis against FN with G-CSF (granulocyte colony-stimulating factor) and GM-CSF (granulocyte-macrophage colony-stimulating factor) decreases hospitalization without affecting mortality (indicated if risk of FN 20% or if FN has occurred in a previous chemotherapy cycle)

Treatment
- most hospitals have their own specific protocol; one example is presented below

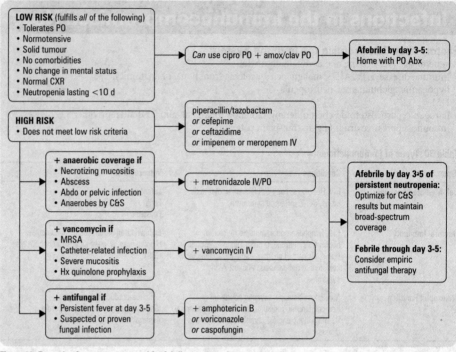

Figure 18. Example of treatment protocol for febrile neutropenia

Infections in Solid Organ Transplant Recipients

- infection is a leading cause of early morbidity/mortality in transplant recipients
- infection depends on degree of immunosuppression
- common infections <1 mo post-transplant
  - bacterial infection of wound/lines/lungs, herpetic stomatitis
- common infections >1 mo post-transplant
  - viral (especially CMV, EBV, VZV)
  - fungal (especially *Aspergillus, Cryptococcus, P. jiroveci*)
  - protozoan (especially *Toxoplasma*)
  - unusual bacterial/mycobacterial infections (especially TB, *Nocardia, Listeria*)

Prophylactic Vaccinations Given Before Transplant
- to all transplant patients: DTaP, pneumococcal, influenza, hepatitis A and B vaccines
- if low titre or poor documentation: MMR, polio, varicella vaccination (with booster 4-8 wk later)

Immune Reconstitution Syndrome

Definition
- a harmful inflammatory response directed against a previously acquired infection following a recovery of the immune system

Etiology
- paradoxical worsening of a successfully or partially treated opportunistic infection
- new onset response to a previously unidentified opportunistic infection
- the majority of cases are in HIV/AIDS or immunosuppressed patients starting anti-retroviral therapy or discontinuing immunosuppressive therapy; sudden recovery from an immunosuppressive state towards a pro-inflammatory state directed towards subclinical infection results in fever and inflammation
- can occur in response to multiple infections
  - *Mycobacteria* (*tuberculosis, avium* complex)
  - *Cryptococcus*
  - *Pneumocystis*
  - *Toxoplasma*
  - HBV and HCV
  - Herpes viruses (VZV reactivation, HSV, CMV)
  - JC virus (progressive multifocal leukoencephalopathy)
  - *Molluscum contagiosum*
- clinical features are dependent on the type and location of the pre-existing infection
- thought to be worse with quick increase in CD4 count and with lower pre-treatment CD4 count
- non-HIV conditions with documented IRS: solid organ transplant recipients, post-partum women, neutropenic patients, anti-TNF therapy

Epidemiology
- in HIV patients starting ART, IRS reported to affect ~10%

Investigations
- IRS is a diagnosis of exclusion
- rule out drug reaction, patient non-adherence, drug resistance

Treatment
- continue HAART therapy in HIV patients with mild-moderate symptoms, but consider discontinuation if symptoms are life-threatening or potentially irreversible
- treat underlying infection; initiate treatment for some infections prior to HAART initiation
- consider starting corticosteroids/NSAIDs to decrease inflammatory response

A Simplified Look at Antibiotics

- general overview, see Table 31 for more details

1. Penicillins

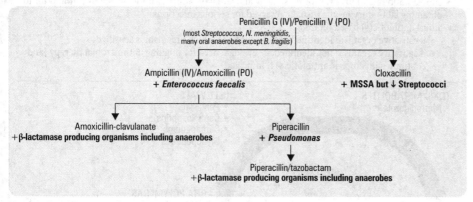

Figure 19. Penicillins

2. Cephalosporins (PO/IV)
- 1st generation: cephalexin/cefazolin (mostly GP, some GN)
- 2nd generation: cefuroxime/cefprozil (some GP and some GN, *anaerobes)
- 3rd generation: cefixime/cefotaxime, ceftriaxone (good Streptococcal coverage, mostly GN), and ceftazidime (no GP, mostly GN, *Pseudomonas*)
- 4th generation: --/cefepime (most GP, most GN, *Pseudomonas*)

3. Aminoglycosides (GN aerobic bacilli)
- gentamicin
- tobramycin
- amikacin

4. Macrolides (GP, *Haemophilus*, and atypical bacteria [*Legionella, Chlamydophila, Mycoplasma*])
- erythromycin
- clarithromycin
- azithromycin

5. Fluoroquinolones (GN – although resistance becoming a huge problem)
- ciprofloxacin (+ *Pseudomonas*)
- norfloxacin (for UTI only)
- respiratory fluoroquinolones (some GP, GN, "atypicals", *Legionella, Mycoplasma, Chlamydophila, Mycobacteria*)
  - levofloxacin, ofloxacin
  - moxifloxacin (+ anaerobes)

6. Carbapenems (broad coverage: GP, GN, and anaerobes)
- imipenem (+ *Pseudomonas*)
- meropenem (+ *Pseudomonas*)
- ertapenem

7. Others

- doxycycline/tetracycline (GP, syphilis, *Chlamydophila*, *Rickettsia*, *Mycoplasma*)
- tigecycline (for resistant GP infections, GN, anaerobes, *Chlamydophila*, *Rickettsia*, *Mycoplasma*)
- vancomycin (all GP and *C. difficile* – the oral form)
- linezolid (for resistant GP infections)
- daptomycin (for resistant GP infections)
- clindamycin (most GP, GN anaerobes)
- TMP/SMX (most *S. aureus* including: MRSA, GN aerobes, *Pneumocystis*)
- nitrofurantoin (GN bacilli, *S. saprophyticus*, *Enterococcus*)
- metronidazole (anaerobes including: *C. difficile*; *Trichomonas*, *Entamoeba*)
- treatment for *C. difficile*: metronidazole OR oral vancomycin; consider both in serious infection

Antimicrobials

Antibiotics

- empiric antibiotic therapy
  - choose antibiotic(s) to cover for most likely and lethal organisms for the type of infection prior to obtaining laboratory results (usually reserved for serious infections)
  - adjust antibiotic(s) based on C&S
    - if causative organism identified, use antibiotic to which organism is sensitive
    - if causative organism not identified, re-evaluate need for ongoing antimicrobial therapy (and continue with empiric antibiotic(s) if indicated)

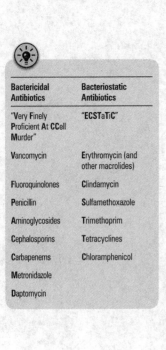

Reasons for Combination Therapy
- Polymicrobial infection
- Empiric therapy pending culture results
- Synergy for difficult to treat pathogens (e.g. *Enterococcus* spp. causing endocarditis)
- To prevent emergence of resistance

Bactericidal Antibiotics	Bacteriostatic Antibiotics
"Very Finely Proficient At CCell Murder"	"ECSTaTiC"
Vancomycin	Erythromycin (and other macrolides)
Fluoroquinolones	Clindamycin
Penicillin	Sulfamethoxazole
Aminoglycosides	Trimethoprim
Cephalosporins	Tetracyclines
Carbapenems	Chloramphenicol
Metronidazole	
Daptomycin	

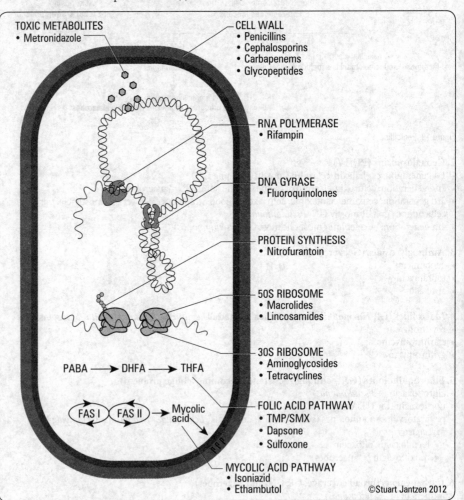

Figure 20. Mechanism of action of antibiotics

©Stuart Jantzen 2012

Table 31. Antibiotics

Class and Drugs	Coverage	Mechanism of Action	Adverse Effects	Indications	Contraindications
CELL WALL INHIBITORS					
Penicillins					
Benzyl penicillin - penicillin G IV/IM - penicillin V PO	GP <u>except</u> *Staphylococcus,* *Enterococcus,* *N. meningitidis,* Oral anaerobes Syphilis	Bactericidal: β-lactam inhibits cell wall synthesis by binding penicillin binding protein (PBP) preventing cross-linking of peptidoglycan	Immediate allergy (IgE): anaphylaxis, urticaria Late-onset allergy (IgG): urticaria, rash, serum sickness Interstitial nephritis Dose related toxicity: seizures Diarrhea	Mild to moderately severe infections caused by susceptible organisms including actinomycosis, streptococcal pharyngitis, streptococcal skin and soft tissue infections, pneumococcal pneumonia, syphilis	Hypersensitivity to penicillin cov
Aminopenicillin - ampicillin IV - amoxicillin PO (Amoxil®)	Same as penicillin AND *Enterococcus* *Listeria* selectively *H. influenzae,* *E. coli,* *K. pneumoniae*	See above	See above	Bacterial meningitis and endocarditis (IV ampicillin), acute otitis media (AOM), streptococcal pharyngitis, sinusitis, acute exacerbations of COPD, part of multidrug therapy for *H. pylori* treatment, Lyme disease, pneumococcal pneumonia; UTI (amoxicillin and ampicillin) for most enterococci and susceptible gram-negative pathogens	Hypersensitivity to penicillin or β-lactam antibiotics
Isoxazoylyl penicillin - cloxacillin - methicillin - nafcillin - oxacillin	Methicillin-sensitive *Staphylococcus aureus;* streptococci	See above	See above	Bacterial infections caused by staphylococci and streptococci including skin and soft-tissue infections	Hypersensitivity to cloxacillin or any penicillin
β-lactam/β-lactamase inhibitor combinations - amoxicillin-clavulanate (Clavulin®, Augmentin®) - piperacillin/tazobactam (Tazocin®)	Same as penicillin AND *Staphylococcus* *H. influenzae* *Enterococcus* Anaerobes (oral and gut)	β-lactamases prduced by certain bacteria inactivate β-lactams Lactamase inhibitors prevent this process, preserving antibacteral effect of β-lactams	See above	Various β-lactamase producing bacteria, Clavulin® sensitive bacteria including RTI, sinusitis, AOM, skin and soft tissue infections, UTI, and severe intra-abdominal and pelvic infections	Hypersensitivity to penicillin or cephalosporin History of Clavulin®-associated jaundice or hepatic dysfunction

Cephalosporins							
PO	**IV**	**GP**	**GN**	Bactericidal: β-lactam inhibits PBP, prevents cross-linking of peptidoglycan, less susceptible to penicillinases	10% penicillin allergy cross-reactivity Nephrotoxicity	Skin and soft tissue infections, prevention of surgical site infections (cefazolin); infections caused by susceptible organisms (especially *Staph* and *Strep* infections)	Hypersensitivity to cephalosporins or other β-lactam antibiotics
1° cephalexin (Keflex®)	cefazolin (Ancef®)	Good with the exception of *Enterococcus* and MRSA	*E. coli,* *Klebsiella,* *Proteus, H. influenzae* (not all isolates)				
2° cefuroxime (Ceftin®) cefprozil (Cefzil®)	cefuroxime (Zinacef®) cefoxitin^A	Weaker activity than 1°	More coverage than 1° (^Aincludes anaerobes)	See above	See above	Upper and lower respiratory tract infections; pneumococcal pneumonia; soft tissue infections	See above
3° cefixime (Suprax®)	ceftriaxone (Rocephin®) cefotaxime (Claforan®) ceftazidime^B (Fortaz®)	*S. aureus* + streptococcal coverage (cefotaxime and ceftriaxone) especially *S. pneumoniae*	Broad coverage (^Bincludes *Pseudomonas* for ceftazidime only)	See above	~1% penicillin allergy cross-reactivity	Community-acquired pneumonia (cefotaxime, ceftriaxone), gonorrhea (use ceftriaxone), community-acquired bacterial meningitis (ceftriaxone, cefotaxime); abdominal and pelvic infections (cefotaxime or ceftriaxone in combination with metronidazole); once-daily administration makes ceftriaxone convenient for outpatient IV therapy	Severe hypersensitivity (Type I) to other β-lactam antibiotics
4°	cefepime (Maxipine®)	Broad spectrum	Broad coverage including *Pseudomonas*	See above	See above	Empiric therapy for febrile neutropenia	See above

Table 31. Antibiotics (continued)

Class and Drugs	Coverage	Mechanism of Action	Adverse Effects	Indications	Contraindications
CELL WALL INHIBITORS					
Carbapenems					
imipenem (Primaxin®)	GP except MRSA GN including *Pseudomonas* + *Enterobacter*, ESBLs, anaerobes	β-lactam inhibits PBP and prevents cross-linking of peptidoglycan	Penicillin allergy cross-reactivity Seizures	Treatment of infections caused by GNB producing extended-spectrum β-lactamases, serious infections caused by susceptible organisms	Hypersensitivity to imipenem
meropenem (Merrem®)	See above; does not cover *Enterococcus*	See above	See above	See above	Hypersensitivity to β-lactams
ertapenem (Invanz®)	GP except *Enterococcus*, MRSA GN including *Enterobacter* (but not *Pseudomonas*), anaerobes	See above	See above	See above; once-daily administration makes it convenient for outpatient IV therapy	Hypersensitivity to β-lactams
Glycopeptides					
Vancomycin (Vancocin®)	GP including MRSA, not VRE *C. difficile* if PO	Glycopeptide sterically inhibits cell wall synthesis	Red Man Syndrome Nephrotoxicity Ototoxicity Thrombocytopenia	Severe or life-threatening GP infections, patients with β-lactam allergy May only be taken orally for severe *C. difficile* infection	Hypersensitivity to vancomycin
PROTEIN SYNTHESIS INHIBITORS (50S RIBOSOME)					
Macrolides					
erythromycin (Erybid®, Eryc®) *This agent is rarely used due to GI upset	GP except *Enterococcus* GN: *Legionella, B. pertussis* "Atypicals": *Chlamydophila*, *Mycoplasma*	Binds to 50S ribosomal subunit inhibiting protein synthesis	GI upset Acute cholestatic hepatitis Prolonged QT	Susceptible RTI, pertussis, diphtheria, Legionnaires' disease, skin and soft tissue infections	Hypersensitivity to erythromycin Concurrent therapy with astemizole, terfenadine
clarithromycin (Biaxin®)	See above, some mycobacteria	See above	See above	Susceptible RTI, skin infections, non-tuberculous mycobacterial infections, part of mulitdrug therapy for *H. pylori* treatment	Hypersensitivity to macrolides
azithromycin (Zithromax®)	See above, some mycobacteria	See above	See above	Susceptible RTI, acute exacerbations of COPD, community-acquired pneumonia, skin infections, *Campylobacter* infections if treatment indicated, chlamydia	Hypersensitivity to macrolides
Lincosamides					
clindamycin (Dalacin®)	GP except *Enterococcus*, most community-acquired MRSA Anaerobes	Inhibits peptide bond formation at 50S ribosome	Pseudomembranous colitis GI upset	Treatment of suspected or proven infections caused by GP, anaerobes including skin and skin structure infections, oropharyngeal infections, in combination with GN coverage for intra-abdominal and pelvic infections	Hypersensitivity to clindamycin Infants <30 d
chloramphenicol	GP GN Anaerobes	Inhibits peptidyl transferase action of tRNA at 50S ribosome	Aplastic anemia Grey Baby Syndrome	Serious infections by susceptible organisms when suitable alternatives are not available including meningococcal disease in patients with anaphylaxis to β-lactams	Hypersensitivity to chloramphenicol
linezolid (Zyvoxam®)	GP including VRE + MRSA	Binds 50S ribosome and prevents functional 70S initiation complex	HTN (acts as MAOI) Risks with prolonged use: myelosuppression optic neuropathy, peripheral neuropathy	Vancomycin-resistant *Enterococcus faecium* infections including intra-abdominal, skin and skin structure, and urinary tract infections, MRSA infections as outpatient therapy	Hypersensitivity to linezolid

Table 31. Antibiotics (continued)

Class and Drugs	Coverage	Mechanism of Action	Adverse Effects	Indications	Contraindications
PROTEIN SYNTHESIS INHIBITORS (30S RIBOSOME)					
Aminoglycosides					
gentamicin tobramycin amikacin (Amikin®)	GN (includes *Pseudomonas*)	Binds 30S subunit of ribosome inhibiting protein synthesis	Nephrotoxicity (reversible) Vestibular and ototoxicity (irreversible) Vestibular toxicity is the most important aminoglycoside toxicity	GN infections when alternatives do not exist, UTIs, used in low doses for synergy with β-lactams or with vancomycin for the treatment of serious enterococcal infections	Pre-existing hearing loss and renal dysfunction
Tetracyclines					
tetracycline (Apo-Tetra®, Nu-TetraT®) minocycline (MinocinT®) doxycycline (Doxycin®) tigecycline (Tygacil®)	GP Anaerobes "Atypicals": *Chlamydophila, Mycoplasma, Rickettsia, Borrelia burgdorferi Treponema* Malaria prophylaxis (doxycycline) Tigecycline has activity against MRSA, VRE, and ESBL-producing *E. coli/K. pneumoniae*	Binds 30S subunit of ribosome inhibiting protein synthesis	GI upset Hepatotoxicity Fanconi's syndrome Photosensitivity Teratogenic Yellow teeth and stunted bone growth in children	Rickettsial infections, *Chlamydophila*, acne (tetracycline, minocycline), PID (step-down), malaria prophylaxis (doxycycline)	Severe renal or hepatic dysfunction Pregnancy or lactation Children under 8 yr
TOPOISOMERASE INHIBITORS					
Fluoroquinolones (FQs)					
ciprofloxacin (Cipro®) norfloxacin (Apo-Norflox®) ofloxacin (Floxin®) Respiratory FQs: levofloxacin (Levaquin®) moxifloxacin (Avelox®)	Poor GP activity GN (includes *Pseudomonas*) Atypicals Levofloxacin and Moxifloxacin cover *S. pneumoniae* Moxifloxacin also covers many anaerobes	Inhibits DNA gyrase	H/A, dizziness Allergy Seizures Prolonged QT Dysglycemia (levofloxacin, moxifloxacin) Tendonitis Tendon rupture	Upper and lower RTI (not ciprofloxacin unless susceptible organism isolated), UTI, prostatitis (not moxifloxacin), bone and joint infections for susceptible organisms, skin and soft tissue infections (levofloxacin, moxifloxacin), infectious diarrhea, meningococcal prophylaxis, intra-abdominal infections (moxifloxacin, ciprofloxacin in combination with metronidazole or clindamycin), febrile neutropenia prophylaxis (ciprofloxacin, levofloxacin) or ciprofloxacin in combination with amoxicillin-clavulanate low management of "low-risk" febrile neutropenia	
OTHER					
Rifampin	GP cocci *N. meningitidis H. influenzae Mycobacteria*	Inhibits RNA polymerase	Hepatic dysfunction, P450 enzyme induction Orange tears/saliva/ urine	Part of multidrug treatment for active TB, alone for treatment of latent TB, part of multidrug treatment of other mycobacterial infections, endocarditis involving prosthetic valve or other prosthetic device infections in combination with other antibiotic agents, prophylaxis for those exposed to people with *N. meningitidis* or HiB meningitis	Jaundice Not to be used as monotherapy (except for prophylaxis)
Metronidazole (Flagyl®)	Anaerobes Protozoa	Forms toxic metabolites in bacterial cell which damage microbial DNA	Disulfiram-type reaction with EtOH Seizures Peripheral neuropathy	Protozoal infections (trichomoniasis, amoebiasis, giardiasis), bacterial vaginosis, anaerobic bacterial infections	
Daptomycin	GP, including MRSA and VRE	Hypothesized to bind to cell wall and form channels leading to intracellular K⁺ depletion	Skeletal muscle injury at high doses (elevated CPK) Peripheral neuropathy	Bacteremia, endocarditis, skin and soft tissue, and other infections due to resistant GP infections including MRSA and VRE	Known hypersensitivity

Table 31. Antibiotics (continued)

Class and Drugs	Coverage	Mechanism of Action	Adverse Effects	Indications	Contraindications
ANTI-METABOLITE					
Trimethoprim-Sulfamethoxazole (TMP/SMX) (Septra®, Bactrim®)	GP, especially *S. aureus* (including most MRSA) GN: enteric *Nocardia* Other: *Pneumocystis, Toxoplasmosis*	Inhibits folic acid pathway (TMP inhibits DHFR and SMX competes with PABA)	Hepatitis Stevens-Johnson syndrome Bone marrow suppression Hyperkalemia Drug toxicity (increases free levels of many drugs, including glyburide, warfarin)	Susceptible UTI, RTI, GI infections, skin and soft tissue infections caused by staphylococcal species, treatment and prophylaxis of *P. jiroveci* pneumonia	Hypersensitivity to TMP-SMX, sulfa drugs
nitrofurantoin (MacroBID®, (Macrodantin®)	*Enterococcus, S. saprophyticus* GN (coliforms)	Reactive metabolites inhibit ribosomal protein synthesis	Cholestasis, hepatitis Hemolysis if G6PD deficiency Interstitial lung disease with chronic use	Lower UTI; not pyelonephritis or bacteremia	Hypersensitivity to nitrofurantoin Anuria, oliguria, or significant renal impairment Pregnant patients during labour and delivery or when labour imminent Infants <1 mo of age
ANTI-MYCOBACTERIALS					
isoniazid (INH)	*Mycobacteria*	Inhibits mycolic acid synthesis	Hepatotoxicity Hepatitis Drug-induced SLE Peripheral neuropathy	Part of multidrug treatment for active TB, alone for treatment of latent TB	Drug-induced hepatitis or acute liver disease
rifampin (RIF)	*Mycobacteria*	Inhibits RNA polymerase	Hepatotoxicity P450 enzyme inducer Orange tears, saliva, urine	Part of multidrug treatment for active TB, alone for treatment of latent TB, part of multidrug treatment of other mycobacterial infections	Jaundice Not to be used monotherapy (except for prophylaxis)
ethambutol	*Mycobacteria*	Inhibits mycolic acid synthesis	Loss of central and colour vision	Part of multidrug treatment for active TB and other mycobacterial infections	Renal failure
pyrazinamide (PZA)	*Mycobacteria*	Unknown	Hepatotoxicity Gout Gastric irritation	Part of multidrug treatment for active TB	Severe hepatic damage or acute liver disease Patients with acute gout
SULFONES					
dapsone sulfoxone	*M. leprae, P. jiroveci, Toxoplasma*	Inhibit folic acid synthesis by competition with PABA	Rash Drug fever Agranulocytosis	Part of multidrug treatment for *M. leprae*, part of treatment for *P. jiroveci* pneumonia (with TMP), *P. jiroveci* pneumonia prophylaxis, toxoplasmosis prophylaxis with pyrimethamine	

Rifampin
- Good adjunct for treating prosthetic device infection (bacterial biofilm)
- Always used in combination with other antibiotics to reduce emergence of resistance

Table 32. Antibiotics for Selected Bacteria

Pseudomonas	S. aureus	Enterococcus	H. influenzae	Anaerobes
ciprofloxacin	cloxacillin (MSSA)	ampicillin	amoxicillin-clavulanate	metronidazole
gentamicin, tobramycin	1° cephalosporin (MSSA)	amoxicillin	2°/3° cephalosporin	clindamycin
piperacillin/tazobactam	clindamycin	vancomycin	macrolides (clarithromycin, azithromycin)	amoxicillin-clavulanate
ceftazidime	Cotrimoxazole (including MRSA)	nitrofurantoin (lower UTI)	levofloxacin	cefoxitin
cefepime	vancomycin (including MRSA)	linezolid for VRE	moxifloxacin	piperacillin/tazobactam
meropenem	linezolid (including MRSA)	daptomycin for VRE		moxifloxacin
imipenem	daptomycin (including MRSA)	tigecycline for VRE		ertapenem, imipenem, meropenem
	tigecycline (including MRSA)			

Antivirals

Table 33. Antivirals

Class and Drugs	Coverage	Mechanism of Action	Adverse Effects	Contraindications
ANTI-HERPESVIRUS				
acyclovir valacyclovir (Valtrex®) (prodrug of acyclovir)	HSV-1,2 VZV	Guanosine analog inhibits viral DNA polymerase	PO well-tolerated IV: nephrotoxicity, CNS	Hypersensitivity to acyclovir or valacyclovir
famciclovir (Famvir®) penciclovir	HSV-1,2 VZV	See above	H/A, nausea	Hypersensitivity to famciclovir or penciclovir
ganciclovir (Cytovene®) valganciclovir (prodrug of ganciclovir)	CMV HSV-1,2, VZV, HHV-6, EBV	See above	Heme: neutropenia, thrombocytopenia, anemia	Hypersensitivity to ganciclovir or valganciclovir Possible cross-hypersensitivity between acyclovir and valacyclovir
foscarnet	CMV Acyclovir-resistant HSV, VZV	Pyrophosphate analog inhibits viral DNA polymerase	Nephrotoxicity Anemia Electrolyte disturbance	Hypersensitivity to foscarnet
OTHER ANTIVIRALS				
(pegylated) interferon-α-2a or-2b	Chronic hepatitis B or C HPV	Inhibits viral protein synthesis	"Flu-like" syndrome Depression Bone marrow suppression	Hypersensitivity to any interferon Cannot use in combination with ribavirin if renal impairment
ribavirin (Virazole®)	Chronic hepatitis C RSV Lassa fever	Guanosine analog with multiple postulated mechanisms of action	Hemolytic anemia Rash, conjunctivitis Highly teratogenic	Pregnancy, women who may become pregnant or their partners Renal impairment
Cidofovir	Adenovirus CMV retinitis Acyclovir and foscarnet resistant HSV	Deoxycitidine analogue Inhibits DNA snythesis	Nephrotoxicity (proximal tubule dysfunction)	Renal failure; probenecid can reduce renal toxicity
lamivudine (Epivir®)	Chronic hepatitis B HIV	See *HIV and AIDS*, ID27	See *HIV and AIDS*, ID27	See *HIV and AIDS*, ID27
Tenofovir	Chronic hepatitis B HIV	See *HIV and AIDS*, ID27	See *HIV and AIDS*, ID27	See *HIV and AIDS*, ID27
Neuraminidase inhibitors: zanamivir (Relenza®) oseltamivir (Tamiflu®)	Influenza A and B: treatment and prophylaxis	Inhibits neuraminidase, an enzyme required for release of virus from infected cells and prevention of viral aggregation	GI: N/V, diarrhea Bronchospasm in zanamivir	Hypersensitivity to the neuraminidase inhibitors

Antifungals

Table 34. Antifungals

Class and Drugs	Coverage	Mechanism of Action	Adverse Effects	Contraindications
POLYENES				

amphotericin B	Endemic mycoses:
	  Histoplasmosis
	  Blastomycosis
	  Coccidioidomycosis
	Pulmonary:
	  Aspergillosis
	CNS:
	  Cryptococcus
		A polyene antimicrobial: inserts into fungal cytoplasmic membrane causing altered membrane permeability and cell death	Nephrotoxicity
			Hypo/hyperkalemia
			Infusion reactions: chills, fevers, H/A
			Peripheral phlebitis
				Renal impairment

nystatin (oral, topical)	Candidiasis: mucocutaneous, GI, oral (thrush), vaginal	See above Not absorbed from the GI tract	GI: N/V, diarrhea Highly toxic if given IV	
IMIDAZOLES				
clotrimazole (Canesten®)	Oral and vulvovaginal candidiasis Dermatomycoses	All azoles: inhibit ergosterol synthesis and thereby alter fungal cell membrane permeability	Pruritis, skin irritation	
miconazole (Monistat®, Micozole®)	Vulvovaginal candidiasis Dermatomycoses		Vaginal burning N/V	
ketoconazole (Nizoral®)	Dermatomycoses Seborrheic dermatitis		Pruritis, skin irritation GI nonspecific Results in decreased androgen and testosterone synthesis	Cross-sensitivity with other azoles possible Hepatic dysfunction Pregnant women or those that may become pregnant

Table 34. Antifungals (continued)

Class and Drugs	Coverage	Mechanism of Action	Adverse Effects	Contraindications
TRIAZOLES				
fluconazole (Diflucan®)	Candida infections (mucosal and invasive) Cryptococcal meningitis (step-down therapy)	All azoles: inhibit ergosterol synthesis and thereby alter fungal cell membrane permeability	Elevated liver enzymes GI nonspecific	Cross-sensitivity with other azoles unknown
itraconazole (Sporanox®)	Sporotrichosis Onychomycoses Endemic mycoses: Histoplasmosis Blastomycosis Coccidioidomycosis		Elevated liver enzymes Rash GI nonspecific HTN Hyperkalemia Peripheral edema	Cross-sensitivity with other azoles unknown Severe ventricular dysfunction
voriconazole (Vfend®)	Aspergillosis Candidiasis		Visual disturbance (30%) Hepatotoxicity Cutaneous photosensitivity Cutaneous squamous cell carcinoma with long-term use in immunosuppressed patients Prolonged QT Periostitis Neurologic toxicity	Cross-sensitivity with other azoles unknown May avoid or alter doses if co-administered with other CYP3A4 substrates, rifampin, carbamazepine, long-acting barbiturates, ritonavir, efavirenz, sirolimus, rifabutin, ergot alkaloids
posaconazole (Posanol®, Noxafil®)	Candidiasis Aspergillosis Mucormycosis		Elevated liver enzymes H/A Prolonged QT	Coadministration of cisapride, ergot alkaloids, pimozide, quinidine, or sirolimus
ALLYLAMINES				
terbinafine (Lamisil®)	Dermatomycoses Onychomycoses	Inhibits enzyme needed for ergosterol synthesis	Rash, local irritation GI nonspecific, transaminitis	Active liver disease
ECHINOCANDINS				
caspofungin micafungin anidulafungin	Refractory aspergillosis, candidemia (azole-resistant)	Inhibits 1-3 β-D-glucan synthesis (needed for fungal cell wall)	Hepatotoxicity Infusion and injection site reactions	

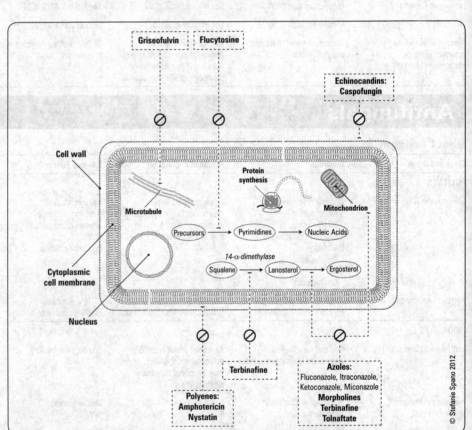

Figure 21. Mechanism of action of antifungals

Antiparasitics

Table 35. Antiparasitics

Class and Drugs	Coverage	Mechanism of Action	Adverse Effects	Contraindications
ANTIMALARIALS				
chloroquine	Malaria: treatment of erythrocytic phase of all five species of *Plasmodium* that infect humans Note: High resistance of *P. falciparum* and *P. vivax* in certain geographic areas	Inhibits parasite heme polymerase	CNS: blurred vision, retinopathy, dizziness Nonspecific GI (rare with prophylaxis)	Hypersensitivity to chloroquine or other 4-aminoquinoline Retinal or visual field changes due to 4-aminoquinoline
quinine	Malaria: treatment of all five species of *Plasmodium* that infect humans, including chloroquine-resistant *P. falciparum*		Cinchonism: ears (tinnitus, vertigo), eyes (visual disturbance), GI (N/V, diarrhea), CNS (H/A, fever) Hypoglycemia	Hypersensitivity to quinine, may have cross-sensitivity with quinidine Patients with G6PD deficiency, tinnitus, optic neuritis, hypoglycemia, history of blackwater fever or thrombocytopenic purpura due to quinine use
mefloquine (Lariam®)	Malaria: prophylaxis		CNS/Psych: irritability, nightmares, psychoses, suicide, depression, seizures, H/A	History of seizures, psychosis, severe anxiety or depression
primaquine	Malaria: treatment of liver hypnozoites of *P. vivax* and *P. ovale*; prophylaxis of all *Plasmodium* spp. *Pneumocystis jiroveci* (with clindamycin)	Interferes with mitochondrial function	Hemolytic anemia in G6PD deficient GI upset (take with food)	GI nonspecific G6PD deficiency Concurrent or recent use of quinacrine Pregnancy
atovaquone/proguanil (Malarone®)	Malaria: treatment and prophylaxis of *P. falciparum*	Inhibits mitochondrial electron transport and dihydrofolate reductase	N/V, anorexia, diarrhea, abdominal pain (take with food)	Hypersensitivity to atovaquone or proguanil Severe renal impairment
artemisinin derivatives (artemether, artesunate, etc.) Note: marketed primarily in endemic countries	Malaria: treatment of all *Plasmodium* spp. Severe malaria (IV artesunate) Typically used in combination with a longer-acting agent from above	Binds iron, leading to formation of free radicals that damage parasite proteins	Transient neurologic deficits (nystagmus, balance disturbance) Transient neutropenia (at high doses of oral artesunate) Transient neutropenia (at high doses of oral artesunate) Delayed hemolysis	Hypersensitivity to artemisinins
OTHER ANTI-PROTOZOAL				
iodoquinol (Diodoquin®)	Amoebiasis: *E. histolytica*, *Dientamoeba fragilis*, *Balantidium coli*, *Blastocystis hominis*	Contact amoebicide that acts in intestinal lumen by uncertain mechanism	GI: N/V, diarrhea, abdominal pain CNS: H/A, seizures, encephalitis	Hypersensitivity to any 8-hydroxy-quinoline or iodine Patients with hepatic damage or optic neuropathy Pregnancy
metronidazole	Amoebiasis, *T. vaginalis*, giardiasis, *D. fragilis*	See *Antibiotics*, ID47		
nitazoxanide	*Cryptosporidium*, giardiasis, cyclosporiasis	Interferes with parasite anaerobic metabolism	N/V, diarrhea, abdominal pain, H/A	Hypersensitivity to nitazoxanide
ANTI-HELMINTHICS				
praziquantel	*Schistosomiasis* and other flukes Tapeworms	Increases Ca^{2+} permeability of helminth cell membrane, causing paralysis and detachment	N/V, fever, dizziness	Ocular cysticercosis
albendazole	Intestinal roundworms *Neurocysticercosis* *Echinococcus* Hydatid disease	Inhibits glucose uptake into susceptible parasites	Elevated liver enzymes Alopecia GI nonspecific Agranulocytosis	Pregnancy Ocular cysticercosis or intraventricular cysticercosis
mebendazole (Vermox®)	Intestinal roundworms: pinworm, whipworm, hookworm, roundworm (e.g. *Ascaris*)	Inhibits microtubule formation and glucose uptake	Nonspecific GI	Pregnancy, infants
ivermectin	*Strongyloidiasis* *Onchocerciasis* Scabies	Interferes with polarization of nerve and muscles cells in susceptible parasites leading to paralysis	Nausea, bloating, diarrhea, myalgias, lightheadedness, H/A	Hypersensitivity to ivermectin Pregnancy
diethylcarbamazine	*Wuchereria bancrofti* *Loa loa*		Anorexia, N/V, H/A, drowsiness, encephalitis, retinal hemorrhage Mazzotti reaction if coinfected with onchocerciasis	Pregnancy Onchocerciasis

Quick Reference: Common Infections and Their Antibiotic Management

- see Family Medicine, FM49

References

Principles of Microbiology
Andreoli TE, Benjamin I, Griggs, et al. Cecil essentials of medicine, 8th ed. Philadelphia: WB Saunders, 2010.
Hawley LB. High yield microbiology and infectious diseases. Lippincott Williams & Wilkins, 2000.
Levinson W, Jawetz E. Medical microbiology and immunology: examination and board review, 7th ed. McGraw Hill, 2003.
Mandell GL, Bennett JE, Dolin R. Mandell, Douglas, and Bennett's principles and practice of infectious disease, 7th ed. Churchill Livingstone, 2009.
McGraw Hill. Harrison's Online. Available from: http://www.harrisonsonline.com.
Schaechter M, Engleberg N, Eisenstein B, et al. Mechanisms of microbial disease. Lippincott Williams & Wilkins, 1998.

Neurological Infections
Bloch KC, Glaser C. Diagnostic approaches for patients with suspected encephalitis. Curr Infect Dis Reports 2007;9:315-322.
Peterson LR, Marfin AA, Gubler DJ. West Nile virus. JAMA 2003;290:524-527.
Roberts L. Mosquitos and disease. Science 2002;298:82-83.
Rupprecht CE, Gibbons RV. Prophylaxis against rabies. NEJM 2004;351:2626-2635.
Rupprecht CE, Hanlon CA, Hemachudha T. Rabies re-examined. Lancet Infect Dis 2002;2:327-343.

Respiratory Infections
Dunbar LM, Wunderink RG, Habib MP, et al. High-dose, short-course levofloxacin for community-acquired pneumonia: a new treatment paradigm. Clin Infect Dis 2003;37:752-760.
H1N1 Flu. Centers for Disease Control and Prevention, 2009. Available from: http://www.cdc.gov/h1n1flu/.
H1N1 Flu Vaccine Information. Public Health Agency of Canada, 2009. Available from: http://www.phac-aspc.gc.ca/alert-alerte/h1n1/vacc/monovacc/index-eng.php.
Mandell LA, Wunderink RG, Anzueto A, et al. Infectious Diseases Society of America / American Thoracic Society Consensus guidelines on the management of community-acquired pneumonia in adults. Clin Infect Dis 2007;44(Suppl 2): S27-S72.

Cardiac Infections
Baddour LM, Wilson WR, Bayer AS, et al. Infective endocarditis: diagnosis, antimicrobial therapy, and management of complications. Circulation 2005;111:e394-e434.
Li JS, Sexton DJ, Mick N, et al. Proposed modifications to the Duke criteria for the diagnosis of infective endocarditis. Clin Infect Dis 2000;30:633-638.
Wilson W, Taubert KA, Gewitz M, et al. Prevention of infective endocarditis: guidelines from the American Heart Association. Circulation 2007;116:1736-1754.

Gastrointestinal Infections
Dupont HL. Bacterial diarrhea. NEJM 2009;361:1560-1569.
Gottlieb T, Heather CS. Diarrhea in adults (acute). Clinical Evidence 2011;02:901.
Jelinek T, Kollaritsch H. Vaccination with Dukoral against travelers' diarrhea (ETEC) and cholera. Expert Rev Vaccines 2008;7(5):561-567.
Pickering LK, Baker CJ, Long SS, et al. (editors). Red book: 2006 report of the committee on infectious diseases, 27th ed. Elk Grove Village: American Academy of Pediatrics, 2006.
Thielman NM, Guerrant RL. Acute infectious diarrhea. NEJM 2004;350:38-47.

Bone and Joint Infections
Butalia S, Palda VA, Sargeant RJ, et al. Does this patient with diabetes have osteomyelitis of the lower extremity? JAMA 2008;299:806-813.
Gilbert DN, Moellering RC, Eliopoulos GM, et al. The Sanford guide to antimicrobial therapy, 38th ed. 2008.
Hellman DB, Imboden JB. Musculoskeletal and immunologic disorders. 2010. McPhee SJ, Papadakis MA (editors). Current medical diagnosis and treatment. New York: McGraw-Hill, 2010.
Margaretten ME, Kohlwes J, Moore D, et al. Does this adult patient have septic arthritis? JAMA 2007;297:1478-1488.

Systemic Infections
Alejandria MM, Lansang MA, Dans LF, et al. Intravenous immunoglobulin for treating sepsis, severe sepsis and septic shock. Cochrane DB Syst Rev 2013;9:CD001090.
American College of Chest Physicians/Society of Critical Care Medicine Consensus Conference: definitions for sepsis and organ failure and guidelines for the use of innovative therapies in sepsis. Crit Care Med 1992;20:864-874.
Bernard GR, Vincent JL, LaTerre PF, et al. Efficacy and safety of recombinant human activated protein C for severe sepsis. NEJM 2001;344:699-709.
Fourrier F, Chopin C, Gouemand J, et al. Septic shock, multiple organ failure, and disseminated intravascular coagulation: compared patterns of antithrombin III, protein C and protein S deficiencies. Chest 1992;101:816-823.
Public Health Agency of Canada. Canadian tuberculosis standards, 6th ed. Ottawa: Public Health Agency of Canada, 2007.
Smieja MJ, Marchetti CA, Cook DJ, et al. Isoniazid for preventing tuberculosis in non-HIV infected persons. Cochrane DB Syst Rev 2000;2:CD001363.
Steere AC. Lyme disease. NEJM 2001;345:115-125.

HIV and AIDS
Guidelines for preventing opportunistic infections among HIV-infected persons – 2002. Recommendations of the U.S. Public Health Service and the Infectious Diseases Society of America. Available from: http://aidsinfo.nih.gov/ContentFiles/OIpreventionGL.pdf.
Guidelines for the use of anti-retroviral agents in HIV-1-infected adults and adolescents, 2006. Available from: http://aidsinfo.nih.gov/ContentFiles/AdultandAdolescentsGL.pdf.
Hammer SM, Saag MS, Schechter M, et al. Treatment for adult HIV infection: 2006 recommendations of the International AIDS Society: USA panel. JAMA 2006; 296:827-43.
Hladik F, McElrath MJ. Setting the stage: host invasion by HIV. Nat Rev Immunol 2008;8:447-457.
Moylett EH, Shearer WT. HIV: clinical manifestations. J Allergy Clin Immunol 2002;110:3-16.
Okwundu CI, Uthman OA, Okoromah CAN. Antiretroviral pre-exposure prophylaxis (PrEP) for preventing HIV in high-risk individuals. Cochrane Database of Syst Rev 2012; 7: CD007189.
Public Health Agency of Canada. HIV and AIDS in Canada. Summary: estimates of HIV prevalence and incidence in Canada, 2008. Ottawa: PHAC, 2009:1-3. Available from: http://www.phac-aspc.gc.ca/aids-sida/publication/index.html#surveillance.
WHO. AIDS epidemic update 2009. Available from: http://data.unaids.org/pub/EPISlides/2009/2009_epiupdate_en.pdf.
WHO. Case definitions of HIV for surveillance and revised clinical staging and immunological classification of HIV-related disease in adults and children, 2006. Available from: http://www.who.int/hiv/pub/vct/hivstaging/en/index.html.
Wilkinson D. Drugs for preventing tuberculosis in HIV infected persons. Cochrane DB Syst Rev 2000;4:CD000171.

Fungal Infections
Catherinot E, Lanternier F, Bougnoux ME, et al. Pneumocystis jiroveci pneumonia. Infect Dis Clin North Am 2010;24:107-138.
Bope ET, Kellerman R, Rakel RE. Conn's current therapy, 2nd ed. Philadelphia: Saunders, 2014.
Habif TP. Clinical dermatology, 5th ed. Philadelphia: Elsevier Inc. Mosby, 2009.
Hustan SM, Mody CH. Cryptococcus: an emerging respiratory mycosis. Clin Chest Med 2009;30:253-264.
Mandell GL, Bennett JE, Dolin R. Mandell, Douglas, and Bennett's principles and practice of infectious disease, 7th ed. Churchill Livingstone, 2009.
Pappas PG, Kauffman CA, Andes D, et al. Clinical practice guidelines for the management of candidiasis. Clin Infect Dis 2009;48:503-535.

Parasitic Infections
Center for Disease Control and Prevention. DPDX: identification and diagnosis of parasites of public health concern. Available from: http://www.dpd.cdc.gov/dpdx/Default.htm.
Croft MA, Jacquerioz FA. Drugs for preventing malaria in travelers. Cochrane DB Syst Rev 2009;4:CD006491.

Infections in the Immunocompromised Host

Freifeld AG, Bow EJ, Sepkowitz KA, et al. Clinical practice guideline for the use of antimicrobial agents in neutropenic patients with cancer: 2010 update by the Infectious Diseases Society of America. Clin Infect Dis 2011;52:e56-93.
Hughes WT, Armstrong D, Bodey GP, et al. Guidelines for the use of antimicrobial agents in neutropenic patients with cancer. Clin Infect Dis 2002;34:731-757.

Fever of Unknown Origin

Knockaert DC, Vanderschueren S, Blockmans D. Fever of unknown origin in adults: 40 years on. J Internal Med 2003;253:263-275.
Spira AM. Assessment of travellers who return home ill. Lancet 2003;361:1459-1469.

Nosocomial Infections

Pickering LK, Baker CJ, Long SS, et al. (editors). Red book: 2006 report of the committee on infectious diseases, 27th ed. Elk Grove Village: American Academy of Pediatrics, 2006. Staphylococcal infections.
Simor AE, Ofner-Agostini M, Gravel D, et al. Surveillance for methicillin-resistant staphylococcus aureus in Canadian hospitals – a report update from the Canadian Nosocomial Infection Surveillance Program. CCDR 2005;31(3):1-7.
Simor AE, Phillips E, McGeer A, et al. Randomized controlled trial of chlorhexidine gluconate for washing, intranasal mupirocin, and rifampin and doxycycline versus no treatment for the eradication of methicillin-resistant Staphylococcus aureus colonization. Clin Infect Dis 2007;44:178-185.

Travel Medicine

Boggild A, Ghesquiere W, McCarthy A. Fever in the returning international traveller initial assessment guidelines. Can Comm Dis Report 2011;37:1-15.
Freedman DO, Weld LH, Kozarsky PE, et al. Spectrum of disease and relation to place of exposure among ill returned travelers. NEJM 2006;354:119-1130.
Luzuriaga K, Sullivan J. Infectious mononucleosis. NEJM 2010;362:1993-2000.
Re VL, Gluckman SJ. Fever in the returned traveler. Am Fam Physician 2003;68:1343-50.
Ryan ET, Wilson ME, Kain KC. Illness after international travel. NEJM 2002;347:505-16.
Spira AM. Assessment of travellers who return home ill. Lancet 2003;361:1459-69.

Antimicrobials

e-CPS. Canadian Pharmacists Association, 2008. Available from: http://e-cps.pharmacists.ca.
MD Consult Drugs Online. Available from: http://home.mdconsult.com/das/drugs/.
Schlossberg D (editor). Current therapy of infectious disease, 2nd ed. St Louis: Mosby, 2001.

Antivirals

Mandell GL, Bennett JE, Dolin R. Mandell, Douglas, and Bennett's principles and practice of infectious disease, 7th ed. Churchill Livingstone, 2009.
Strategies for Management of Anti-retroviral Therapy (SMART) Study Group. CD4+ count-guided interruption of anti-retroviral treatment. NEJM 2006;355:2283-2296.

Notes

Medical Imaging

Armin Rahmani, Omid Shearkhani, and **Kota Talla**, chapter editors
Narayan Chattergoon and **Desmond She**, associate editors
Arnav Agarwal and **Quynh Huynh**, EBM editors
Dr. Nasir Jaffer and **Dr. Eugene Yu**, staff editors

Acronyms

¹⁸FDG	18-fluorodeoxyglucose	DTPA	diethylene triamine pentaacetic acid	LA	left atrium	POCUS	point-of-care ultrasound
AP	anteroposterior	DWI	diffusion-weighted image	LV	left ventricle	PTA	percutaneous transluminal angioplasty
ARDS	acute respiratory distress syndrome	ECD	ethyl cysteinate dimer	MAA	microaggregated albumin	PTC	percutaneous transhepatic cholangiography
AV	arteriovenous	ERCP	endoscopic retrograde cholangio-pancreatography	MAG3	mertiatide	RA	right atrium
AXR	abdominal x-ray			MCA	middle cerebral artery	RAIU	radioactive iodine uptake
BOOP	bronchiolitis obliterans organizing pneumonia	FLAIR	fluid-attenuated inversion recovery	MR	magnetic resonance	RV	right ventricle
		GI	gastrointestinal	MRA	magnetic resonance angiogram	SPECT	single photon emission computed tomography
CNS	central nervous system	GPA	granulomatosis with polyangiitis	MRCP	magnetic resonance cholangiopancreatography	SVC	superior vena cava
CSF	cerebrospinal fluid	HCC	hepatocellular carcinoma			TB	tuberculosis
CT	computed tomography	HIDA	hepatobiliary iminodiacetic acid	MRI	magnetic resonance imaging	TNK	tenecteplase
CTA	computed tomographic angiogram	HMPAO	hexamethylpropyleneamine oxime	MS	multiple sclerosis	tPA	tissue plasminogen activator
CVD	collagen vascular disease	HSG	hysterosalpingogram	MUGA	multiple gated acquisition	TRUS	transrectal ultrasound
CVP	central venous pressure	IBD	inflammatory bowel disease	PA	posteroanterior	TVUS	transvaginal ultrasound
CXR	chest x-ray	ICV	ileocecal valve	PBD	percutaneous biliary drainage	U/S	ultrasound
DEXA	dual-energy x-ray absorptiometry	IPF	interstitial pulmonary fibrosis	PET	positron emission tomography	VCUG	voiding cystourethrogram
DMSA	dimercaptosuccinic acid	IVP	intravenous pyelogram	PFT	pulmonary function test	V/Q	ventilation/perfusion
DSA	digital subtraction angiography	KUB	kidneys, ureters, bladder	PICC	peripherally-inserted central catheter		

Typical Effective Doses from Diagnostic Medical Exposures (in adults)*

Diagnostic Procedure Type	Equivalent Number of Chest X-Rays	Approximate Equivalent Period of Natural Background Radiation** (~3 mSv/yr)
X-Ray		
Skull	5	12 d
Cervical spine	10	3 wk
Thoracic spine	50	4 mo
Lumbar spine	75	6 mo
Chest (single PA film)	1	2 d
Shoulder	0.5	1 d
Mammography	20	7 wk
Abdomen	35	3 mo
Hip	35	3 mo
Pelvis	30	10 wk
Knee	0.25	<1 d
IVU	150	1 yr
Dual-energy x-ray absorptiometry (without/with CT)	0.5/2	<1 d/4 d
Upper GI series	300	2 yr
Small bowel series	250	20 mo
Barium enema	400	2.7 yr
CT		
Head	100	8 mo
Neck	150	1 yr
Spine	300	2 yr
Chest	350	2.3 yr
Chest (pulmonary embolism)	750	5 yr
Coronary angiography	800	5.3 yr
Abdomen	400	2.7 yr
Pelvis	300	2 yr
Radionuclide		
Brain (18FDG)	705	4.7 yr
Bone (99mTc)	315	2.1 yr
Thyroid (99mTc)	240	1.6 yr
Thyroid (123I)	95	8 mo
Cardiac rest-stress test		
(99mTc 1-d)	470	3 yr
(99mTc 2-d)	640	4 yr
Lung ventilation (133Xe)	25	2 mo
Lung perfusion (99mTc)	100	8 mo
Renal (99mTc)	90-165	7-13 mo
Liver-spleen (99mTc)	105	8.4 yr
Biliary tract (99mTc)	155	1 yr

*Source: *Radiology* 2008;248:254-263
**Calculated using average natural background exposure in Canada (Health Canada: http://www.hc-sc.gc.ca/hl-vs/iyh-vsv/environ/expos-eng.php)

Imaging Modalities

X-Ray Imaging
- x-rays, or Röentgen rays, are a form of electromagnetic energy of short wavelength
- as x-ray photons traverse matter, they can be absorbed (a process known as "attenuation") and/or scattered
- the density of a structure determines its ability to attenuate or "weaken" the x-ray beam
  - air < fat < water < bone < metal
- structures that have high attenuation (e.g. bone) appear white on the resulting images

Plain Films
- x-rays pass through the patient and interact with a detection device to produce a 2-dimensional projection image
- structures closer to the film appear sharper and less magnified
- contraindications: pregnancy (relative)
- advantages: inexpensive, non-invasive, readily available, reproducible, fast
- disadvantages: radiation exposure, generally poor at distinguishing soft tissues

Fluoroscopy
- continuous x-rays used for guiding angiographic and interventional procedures, in contrast examinations of the GI tract, and in the OR for certain surgical procedures (e.g. orthopedic, urological)
- on the fluoroscopic image, black and white are reversed so that bone and contrast agents appear dark and radiolucent structures appear light
- advantages: allows for real-time visualization of structures
- disadvantages: increased radiation dose; however, the use of pulsed fluoroscopy has reduced fluoroscopy time by 76% and radiation dose by 64% as compared with continuous fluoroscopy

Computed Tomography
- x-ray beam opposite a detector moves in a continuous 360° arc as patient is advanced through the imaging system
  - subsequent computer assisted reconstruction of anatomical structures from the axial plane
- attenuation is quantified in Hounsfield units:
  - subsequent computer assisted reconstruction of anatomical structures from the axial plane
  - adjusting the "window width" (range of Hounsfield units displayed) and "window level" (midpoint value of the window width) can maximally visualize certain anatomical structures (e.g. CT chest can be viewed using "lung", "soft tissue", and "bone" settings)
- contraindications: pregnancy (relative), contraindications to contrast agents (e.g. allergy, renal failure)
- advantages: delineates surrounding soft tissues, excellent at delineating bones and identifying lung/liver masses, may be used to guide biopsies, spiral/helical multidetector CT has fast data acquisition and allows 3D reconstruction, CTA is less invasive than conventional angiography
- disadvantages: high radiation exposure, soft tissue characterization is not as good in comparison with MRI, IV contrast injection, anxiety of patient when going through scanner, higher cost, and less available than plain film

Ultrasound

- high frequency sound waves are transmitted from a transducer and passed through tissues; reflections of the sound waves are picked up by the transducer and transformed into images
- reflection (or "echo") occurs when the sound waves pass through tissue interfaces of different acoustic densities
- structures are described based on their echogenicity; hyperechoic structures appear bright (U/S reflected) whereas hypoechoic structures appear dark (U/S waves not reflected back but pass through)
- higher U/S frequencies result in greater resolution but greater attenuation (i.e. deeper structures more difficult to visualize)
- artifacts: acoustic shadowing refers to the echo-free area located behind an interface that strongly reflects (e.g. tissue/air) or absorbs (e.g. tissue/bone) sound waves; enhancement refers to the increase in reflection amplitude (i.e. increased brightness) from objects that lie below a weakly attenuating structure (e.g. cyst)
- Duplex scan: grey-scale image that utilizes the Doppler effect to visualize the velocity of blood flow past the transducer
- Colour Doppler: assigns a colour based on the direction of blood flow
- advantages: relatively low cost, non-invasive, no radiation, real time imaging, may be used for guided biopsies, many different imaging planes (axial, sagittal), determines cystic versus solid
- disadvantages: highly operator-dependent, air in bowel may prevent imaging of midline structures in the abdomen, may be limited by patient habitus, poor for bone evaluation

Attenuation
Bone (= bright) > grey matter > white matter ("fatty" myelin) > CSF > air (= dark)

Magnetic Resonance Imaging

- non-invasive technique that does not use ionizing radiation
- able to produce images in virtually any plane
- patient is placed in a magnetic field; protons (H⁺) align themselves along the plane of magnetization due to intrinsic polarity. A pulsed radiofrequency beam is subsequently turned on which deflects all the protons off their aligned axes due to absorption of energy from the radiofrequency beam. When the radiofrequency beam is turned off, the protons return to their pre-excitation axis, giving off the energy they absorbed. This energy is measured with a detector and interpreted by a computer to generate MR images
- the MR image reflects the signal intensity picked up by the receiver. This signal intensity is dependent on:
  1. hydrogen density: tissues with low hydrogen density (e.g. cortical bone, lung) generate little to no MR signal compared to tissues with high hydrogen density (e.g. water)
  2. magnetic relaxation times (T1 and T2): reflect quantitative alterations in MR signal strength due to intrinsic properties of the tissue and its surrounding chemical and physical environment

Remember that water is "white" on **T2** as "World War II"

Methods to Reduce the Risk of Contrast Induced Nephropathy
- Optimal: 0.9% NaCl at 1 ml/kg/hr for 12 hr pre-procedure and 12 hr post-contrast administration
- For same day procedure: 0.9% NaCl or NaHCO3 at 3 ml/kg/hr for 1-3 hr pre-procedure and for 6 hr post-contrast administration

Table 1. Differences Between Diffusion, T1- and T2-Weighted MR Imaging

Imaging Techniques	Contrast Enhancements	Main Application	Advantages
Diffusion Weighted Imaging	Contrast dependent on the molecular motion of water. Decreased diffusion is hyperintense (bright), whereas increased diffusion is hypointense (dark)	Neuroradiology	Sensitive for detection of acute ischemic stroke and differentiating an acute stroke from other neurologic pathologies. Acute infarction appears hyperintense. Abscess collections also show restricted diffusion
T1-Weighted	Fluid is hypointense (dark) and fat is hyperintense (bright)	Body soft tissues	Often considered an anatomic scan since they provide a reference for functional imaging
T2-Weighted	Fluid is hyperintense (bright) and fat is hypointense (dark)	Body soft tissues	Often considered a pathologic scan since they will highlight edematous areas associated with certain pathologies

Positron Emission Tomography Scans

- non-invasive technique that involves exposure to ionizing radiation (~7 mSv)
- nuclear medicine imaging technique that produces images of functional processes in the body
- current generation models integrate PET and CT technologies into a single imaging device (PET-CT) that collects both anatomic and functional information during a single acquisition
- positron-producing radioisotope, such as 18FDG is chemically incorporated into a metabolically active molecule (e.g. glucose), injected into patient, which travels to target organ, accumulates in tissues of interest, and as radioactive substance begins to decay, gamma rays are produced which are detected by PET scanner
- contraindications: pregnancy
- advantages: shows metabolism and physiology of tissues (not only anatomic); in oncology allows diagnosis, staging, restaging; has predictive and prognostic value; can evaluate cardiac viability
- disadvantages: cost, ionizing radiation

Contraindications to IV Contrast

MADD Failure
Multiple myeloma
Adverse reaction previously
DM
Dehydration
Failure (renal, severe heart)

Contrast Enhancement

Table 2. Contrast Agents

Imaging Modality	Types	Advantages	Disadvantages	Contraindications
X-Ray/CT	1. Barium (oral or rectal)	Radioopaque substance which helps to delineate intraluminal anatomy, may demonstrate patency, lumen integrity, or large filling defects		Previous adverse reaction to contrast; barium enema is contraindicated in toxic megacolon, acute colitis, and suspected perforation
	2. Iodine (IV injection)	Delineates intraluminal anatomy, may demonstrate patency, lumen integrity, or large filling defects; under fluoroscopy, may also give information on function of an organ	Risk of nephrogenic systemic fibrosis in patients with end-stage renal disease	Previous adverse reaction to contrast, renal failure, DM, pregnancy, multiple myeloma, severe heart failure and dehydration eGFR <60 may require preventative measures and follow up
MRI	Gadolinium-Chelates (IV injection)	Shortens T1 relaxation time, thereby increasing signal intensity in T1-weighted sequences; gadolinium has some effect on T2-relaxation time; highlights highly vascular structures (e.g. tumours)	Risk of nephrogenic systemic fibrosis in patients with end-stage renal disease	Previous adverse reaction to contrast or if end-stage renal disease (relative contraindication)
U/S	Microbubbles (IV injection)	Since gas is highly echogenic, the microbubbles allow for echo-enhancement of a tissue		Contraindicated in individuals with right-to-left cardiac shunts or people with known hypersensitivity reactions

Chest Imaging

Chest X-Ray

Standard Views
- PA: anterior chest against film plate to minimize magnification of the heart size
- lateral: better visualization of retrocardiac space and thoracic spine (more sensitive at picking up pleural effusions)
  - helps localize lesions when combined with PA view
- AP: for bedridden patients (generally a lower quality film than PA because of enlarged cardiac silhouette)
- lateral decubitus: to assess for pleural effusion and pneumothorax in bedridden patients; however, POCUS can also be utilized for both these purposes
- lordotic: angled beam allowing better visualization of apices normally obscured by the clavicles and anterior ribs

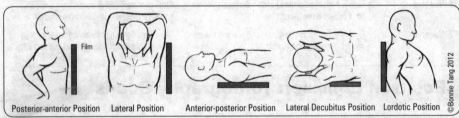

Posterior-anterior Position   Lateral Position   Anterior-posterior Position   Lateral Decubitus Position   Lordotic Position

©Bonnie Tang 2012

Figure 1. CXR views

Approach to CXR

Basics
- ID: patient name, MRN, sex, age
- date of exam
- markers: right and/or left
- technique: view (e.g. PA, AP, lateral), supine or erect
- indications for the study
- comparison: date of previous study for comparison (if available)
- quality of film: inspiration (6th anterior and 10th posterior ribs should be visible), penetration (thoracic spine should be visible) and rotation (clavicles vs. spinous process)

Analysis

- tubes and lines: check position and be alert for pneumothorax or pneumomediastinum
- soft tissues: neck, axillae, pectoral muscles, breasts/nipples, chest wall
  - nipple markers can help identify nipples (may mimic lung nodules)
  - amount of soft tissue, presence of masses and air (subcutaneous emphysema)
- abdomen (see *Abdominal Imaging*, MI10)
  - free air under the diaphragm, air-fluid levels, distention in small and large bowels
  - herniation of abdominal contents (i.e. diaphragmatic hernia)
- bones: C-spine, thoracic spine, shoulders, ribs, sternum, clavicles
  - lytic and blastic lesions and fractures
- mediastinum: trachea, heart, great vessels
  - cardiomegaly (cardiothoracic ratio >0.5), tracheal shift, tortuous aorta, widened mediastinum
- hila: pulmonary vessels, mainstem and segmental bronchi, lymph nodes
- lungs: lung parenchyma, pleura, diaphragm
  - comment on abnormal lung opacity, pleural effusions or thickening
  - right hemidiaphragm usually higher than left due to liver
  - right vs. left hemidiaphragm can be discerned on lateral CXR due to heart resting directly on left hemidiaphragm
- please refer to Toronto Notes' website for supplementary material on how to approach a CXR

Anatomy

Localizing Lesions for Parenchymal Lung Disease

- **silhouette sign**: loss of normal interfaces due to lung pathology (consolidation, atelectasis, mass), which can be used to localize disease in specific lung segments; note that pleural or mediastinal disease can also produce the silhouette sign)
- **spine sign**: on lateral films, vertebral bodies should appear progressively radiolucent as one moves down the thoracic vertebral column; if they appear more radioopaque, it is an indication of pathology (e.g. consolidation in overlying left lower lobe)
- **air bronchogram**: branching pattern of air filled bronchi on a background of fluid filled airspaces

Table 3. Localization Using the Silhouette Sign

Interface Lost	Location of Lung Pathology
SVC/right superior mediastinum	RUL
Right heart border	RML
Right hemidiaphragm	RLL
Aortic knob/left superior mediastinum	LUL
Left heart border	Lingula
Left hemidiaphragm	LLL

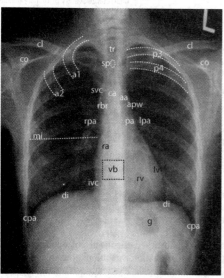

PA view

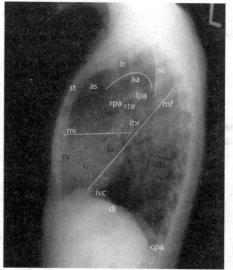

Lateral view

Legend

a1	anterior 1st rib
a2	anterior 2nd rib
aa	aortic arch
apw	aorto-pulmonary window
as	anterior airspace
ca	carina
cl	clavicle
co	coracoid process
cpa	costophrenic angle
di	diaphragm
g	gastric bubble
ivc	inferior vena cava
la	left atrium
lbr	left mainstem bronchus
lpa	left pulmonary artery
lv	left ventricle
mf	major fissure
mi	minor fissure
p3	posterior 3rd rib
p4	posterior 4th rib
pa	main pulmonary artery
ra	right atrium
rbr	right mainstem bronchus
rpa	right pulmonary artery
rv	right ventricle
sc	scapula
sp	spinous process
st	sternum
svc	superior vena cava
tr	trachea
vb	vertebral body

Figure 2. Location of fissures, mediastinal structures, and bony landmarks on CXR

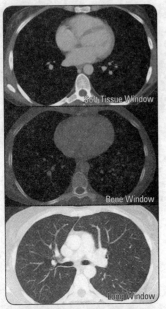

Figure 4. CT thorax windows

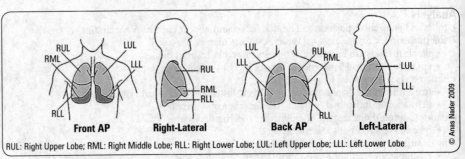

RUL: Right Upper Lobe; RML: Right Middle Lobe; RLL: Right Lower Lobe; LUL: Left Upper Lobe; LLL: Left Lower Lobe

Figure 3. Location of lobes of the lung

Computed Tomography Chest

Approach to CT Chest

- soft tissue window
  - thyroid, chest wall, pleura
  - heart: chambers, coronary artery calcifications, pericardium
  - vessels: aorta, pulmonary artery, smaller vasculature
  - lymph nodes: mediastinal, axillary
- bone window
  - vertebrae, sternum, manubrium, ribs: fractures, lytic lesions, sclerosis
- lung window
  - trachea: patency, secretions
  - bronchial trees: anatomic variants, mucus plugs, airway collapse
  - lung parenchyma: fissures, nodules, fibrosis/interstitial changes
  - pleural space: effusions
- please refer to Toronto Notes' website for supplementary material on how to approach a CT chest

Table 4. Types of CT Chest

	Advantage	Disadvantage	Contrast	Indication
Standard	Scans full lung very quickly (<1 min)	Poor at evaluating diffuse disease	±	CXR abnormality Pleural and mediastinal abnormality Lung cancer staging Follow up metastases Empyema vs. abscess
High Resolution	Thinner slices provide high definition of lung parenchyma	Only 5-10% lung is sampled	No	Hemoptysis Diffuse lung disease (e.g. sarcoidosis, hypersensitivity pneumonitis, pneumoconiosis) Pulmonary fibrosis Normal CXR but abnormal PFTs Characterize solitary pulmonary nodule
Low Dose	1/5th the radiation	Decreased detail	No	Screening Follow up infections, lung transplant, metastases
CTA	Iodinated contrast highlights vasculature	Contrast can cause severe allergic reaction and is nephrotoxic	Yes	PE Aortic aneurysms Aortic dissection

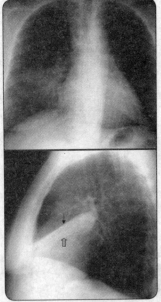

Figure 5. Atelectasis: RML collapse

DDx of Airspace Disease
- Pus (e.g. infections such as pneumonia, non-infectious inflammatory process)
- Fluid (e.g. pulmonary edema)
- Blood (e.g. pulmonary hemorrhage)
- Cells (e.g. bronchioalveolar carcinoma, lymphoma)
- Protein (e.g. alveolar proteinosis)

Lung Abnormalities

Atelectasis

- pathogenesis: collapse of alveoli due to restricted breathing, blockage of bronchi, external compression, or poor surfactant
- findings
  - increased opacity of involved segment/lobe, vascular crowding, silhouette sign, air bronchograms
  - volume loss: fissure deviation, hilar/mediastinal displacement, diaphragm elevation
  - compensatory hyperinflation of remaining normal lung
- differential diagnosis
  - obstructive (most common): air distal to obstruction is reabsorbed causing alveolar collapse
    - post-surgical, endobronchial lesion, foreign body, inflammation (granulomatous infections, pneumoconiosis, sarcoidosis, radiation injury), or mucous plug (cystic fibrosis)
  - compressive
  - tumour, bulla, effusion, enlarged heart, lymphadenopathy
  - traction (cicatrization): due to scarring, which distorts alveoli and contracts the lung
  - adhesive: due to lack of surfactant
    - hyaline membrane disease, prematurity

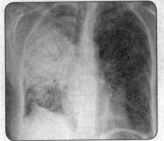

Figure 6. Air bronchograms in right lung

- passive (relaxation): a result of air or fluid in the pleural space
  - pleural effusion, pneumothorax
- management: in the absence of a known etiology, persisting atelectasis must be investigated (i.e. CT thorax) to rule out a bronchogenic carcinoma

Consolidation
- pathogenesis: fluid (water, blood), inflammatory exudates, protein, or tumour in alveoli
- findings
  - air bronchograms: lucent branching bronchi visible through opacification
  - airspace nodules: fluffy, patchy, poorly defined margins with later tendency to coalesce, may take on lobar or segmental distribution
  - silhouette sign
- differential diagnosis
  - fluid: pulmonary edema, blood (trauma, vasculitis, bleeding disorder, pulmonary infarct)
  - inflammatory exudates: bacterial infections, TB, allergic hypersensitivity alveolitis, BOOP, allergic bronchopulmonary aspergillosis, aspiration, sarcoidosis
  - protein: pulmonary alveolar proteinosis
  - tumour: bronchoalveolar carcinoma, lymphoma
- management: varies depending on the pattern of consolidation, which can suggest different etiologies; should also be done in the context of clinical picture

Interstitial Disease
- pathogenesis: pathological process involving the interlobular connective tissue (i.e. "scaffolding of the lung")
- findings
  - linear: fine lines caused by thickened connective tissue septae
    - Kerley A: long thin lines in upper lobes
    - Kerley B: short horizontal lines extending from lateral lung margin
    - Kerley C: diffuse linear pattern throughout lung
    - seen in pulmonary edema, lymphangitic carcinomatosis, and atypical interstitial pneumonias
  - nodular: 1-5 mm well-defined nodules distributed evenly throughout lung
    - seen in malignancy, pneumoconiosis and granulomatous disease (e.g. sarcoidosis, miliary TB)
  - reticular (honeycomb): parenchyma replaced by thin-walled cysts suggesting extensive destruction of pulmonary tissue and fibrosis
    - seen in IPF, asbestosis, and CVD
    - watch for pneumothorax as a complication
  - reticulonodular: combination of reticular and nodular patterns
  - may also see signs of airspace disease (atelectasis, consolidation)
- differential diagnosis
  - occupational/environmental exposure
    - inorganic: asbestosis, coal miner's pneumoconiosis, silicosis, berylliosis, talc pneumoconiosis
    - organic: hypersensitivity pneumonitis, bird fancier's lung, farmer's lung (mouldy hay), and other organic dust
  - autoimmune: CVD (e.g. rheumatoid arthritis, scleroderma, SLE, polymyositis, mixed connective tissue disease), IBD, celiac disease, vasculitis
  - drug-related: antibiotics (cephalosporins, nitrofurantoin), NSAIDs, phenytoin, carbamazepine, fluoxetine, amiodarone, chemotherapy (e.g. methotrexate), heroin, cocaine, methadone
  - infections: non-tuberculous mycobacteria, certain fungal infections
  - idiopathic: hypersensitivity pneumonitis, IPF, BOOP
  - for *Causes of Interstitial Lung Disease Classified by Distribution*, see <u>Respirology</u>, R13
  - management: high resolution CT thorax and biopsy

Pulmonary Nodule
- findings: round opacity ± silhouette sign
  - note: do not mistake nipple shadows for nodules; if in doubt, repeat CXR with nipple markers
- differential diagnosis
  - extrapulmonary density: nipple, skin lesion, electrode, pleural mass, bony lesion
  - solitary nodule
    - tumour: carcinoma, hamartoma, metastasis, bronchial adenoma
    - inflammation: histoplasmoma, tuberculoma, coccidioidomycosis
    - vascular: AV fistula, pulmonary varix (dilated pulmonary vein), infarct, embolism
  - multiple nodules: metastases, abscess, granulomatous lung disease (TB, fungal, sarcoid, rheumatoid nodules, silicosis, GPA)
- management: clinical information and CT appearance determine level of suspicion of malignancy
  - if high probability of malignancy, invasive testing (fine needle aspiration, transbronchial/transthoracic biopsy) is indicated
  - if low probability of malignancy, repeat CXR or CT in 1-3 mo and then every 6 mo for 2 yr; if no change, then >99% chance benign

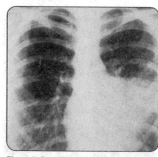

Figure 7. Consolidation: bacterial pneumonia

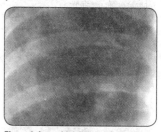

Figure 8. Interstitial disease: fine reticular pattern

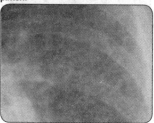

Figure 9. Interstitial disease: medium reticular pattern

DDx of Interstitial Lung Disease

FASSTEN (upper lung disease)
Farmer's lung (hypersensitivity pneumonitis)
Ankylosing spondylitis
Sarcoidosis
Silicosis
TB
Eosinophilic granuloma (Langerhans cell histiocytosis)
Neurofibromatosis

BAD RASH (lower lung disease)
BOOP
Asbestos
Drugs (nitrofurantoin, hydralazine, isoniazid, amiodarone, many chemotherapy drugs)
Rheumatological disease
Aspiration
Scleroderma
Hamman Rich (IPF) and idiopathic pulmonary fibrosis

DDx for Cavitating Lung Nodule

WEIRD HOLES
GPA (Wegener's)
Embolic (pulmonary, septic)
Infection (anaerobes, pneumocystis, TB)
Rheumatoid (necrobiotic nodules)
Developmental cysts (sequestration)
Histiocytosis
Oncological
Lymphangioleiomyomatosis
Environmental, occupational
Sarcoidosis

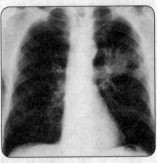

Figure 10. Pulmonary nodule: bronchogenic carcinoma

Table 5. Characteristics of Benign and Malignant Pulmonary Nodules

	Malignant	Benign
Margin	Ill-defined/spiculated ("corona radiata")	Well-defined
Contour	Lobulated	Smooth
Calcification	Eccentric or stippled	Diffuse, central, popcorn, concentric
Doubling Time	20-460 d	<20 d or >460 d
Other Features	Cavitation, collapse, adenopathy, pleural effusion, lytic bone lesions, smoking history	
Size	>3 cm	<3 cm
Cavitation	Yes, especially with wall thickness >15 mm, eccentric cavity and shaggy internal margins	No
Satellite Lesions	No	Yes

Pulmonary Vascular Abnormalities

Pulmonary Edema
- pathogenesis: fluid accumulation in the airspaces of the lungs
- findings
  - vascular redistribution/enlargement, cephalization, pleural effusion, cardiomegaly (may be present in cardiogenic edema and fluid overloaded states)
  - fluid initially collects in interstitium
    - ◆ loss of definition of pulmonary vasculature
    - ◆ peribronchial cuffing
    - ◆ Kerley B lines
    - ◆ reticulonodular pattern
    - ◆ thickening of interlobar fissures
  - as pulmonary edema progresses, fluid begins to collect in alveoli causing diffuse air space disease often in a "bat wing" or "butterfly" pattern in perihilar regions with tendency to spare the outermost lung fields
- differential diagnosis: cardiogenic (e.g. CHF), renal failure, volume overload, non-cardiogenic (e.g. ARDS)

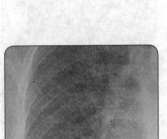

Figure 11. Peribronchial cuffing

Pulmonary Embolism
- pathogenesis: arterial blockage in the lungs due to emboli from pelvic or leg veins, rarely from PICC lines, ports, or air, fat, or amniotic fluid (difficult to diagnose on imaging except by combination of clinical history and CXR and CT findings of ARDS)
- findings
  - CXR: Westermark sign (localized pulmonary oligemia), Hampton's hump (triangular peripheral infarct), enlarged right ventricle and right atrium, atelectasis, pleural effusion, and rarely pulmonary edema
  - definitive imaging study: CT pulmonary angiography to look for filling defect in contrast-filled pulmonary arteries (emboli can be seen up to 4th order arterial branching)
  - V/Q scan: not a diagnostic study

Pleural Abnormalities

Pleural Effusion

Table 6. Sensitivity of Plain Film Views for Pleural Effusion

X-Ray Projection	Minimum Volume to Visualize
Lateral decubitus	25 mL: most sensitive
Upright lateral	50 mL: meniscus seen in the posterior costophrenic sulcus
PA	200 mL
Supine	Diffuse haziness

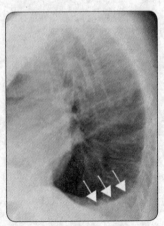

Figure 12. Pleural effusion in lateral view

- a horizontal fluid level is seen only in a hydropneumothorax (i.e. both fluid and air within pleural cavity)
- effusion may exert mass effect, shift trachea and mediastinum to opposite side, or cause atelectasis of adjacent lung
- U/S is superior to plain film for detection of small effusions and may also aid in thoracentesis, and POCUS is now standard of care in acute situations
- fluid level >1 cm on lateral decubitus film is indication to perform thoracentesis

Pneumothorax

- pathogenesis: gas/air accumulation within the pleural space resulting in separation of the lung from the chest wall
- findings
  - upright chest film allows visualization of visceral pleura as curvilinear line paralleling chest wall, separating partially collapsed lung from pleural air
  - more obvious on expiratory (increased contrast between lung and air) or lateral decubitus films (air collects superiorly)
  - more difficult to detect on supine film; look for the "deep (costophrenic) sulcus" sign, "double diaphragm" sign (dome and anterior portions of diaphragm outlined by lung and pleural air, respectively), hyperlucent hemithorax, sharpening of adjacent mediastinal structures
  - mediastinal shift may occur if tension pneumothorax
- differential diagnosis: spontaneous (tall and thin males, smokers), iatrogenic (lung biopsy, ventilation, CVP line insertion), trauma (associated with rib fractures), emphysema, malignancy, honeycomb lung
- management: needle decompression or chest tube insertion, repeat CXR to ensure resolution

Asbestos

- asbestos exposure may cause various pleural abnormalities including benign plaques (most common) that may calcify, diffuse pleural fibrosis, effusion, and malignant mesothelioma

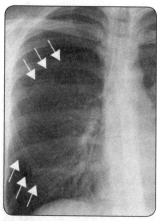

Figure 13. Pneumothorax

Mediastinal Abnormalities

Mediastinal Mass

- the mediastinum is divided into four compartments; this provides an approach to the differential diagnosis of a mediastinal mass
- anterior border formed by the sternum and posterior border by the heart and great vessels
  - 4 Ts: see sidebar
  - cardiophrenic angle mass differential: thymic cyst, epicardial fat pad, foramen of Morgagni hernia
- middle (extending behind anterior mediastinum to a line 1 cm posterior to the anterior border of the thoracic vertebral bodies)
  - esophageal carcinoma, esophageal duplication cyst, metastatic disease, lymphadenopathy (all causes), hiatus hernia, bronchogenic cyst
- posterior (posterior to the middle line described above)
  - neurogenic tumour (e.g. neurofibroma, schwannoma), multiple myeloma, pheochromocytoma, neurenteric cyst, thoracic duct cyst, lateral meningocele, Bochdalek hernia, extramedullary hematopoiesis
- superior boundaries (superiorly by thoracic inlet, inferiorly by plane of the sternal angle, anteriorly by manubrium, posteriorly by T1-T4, laterally by pleura)
- in addition, any compartment may give rise to lymphoma, lung cancer, aortic aneurysm or other vascular abnormalities, abscess, and hematoma

Enlarged Cardiac Silhouette

- heart borders
  - on PA view, right heart border is formed by right atrium; left heart border is formed by left atrium and left ventricle
  - on lateral view, anterior heart border is formed by right ventricle; posterior border is formed by left atrium (superior to left ventricle) and left ventricle
- cardiothoracic ratio = greatest transverse dimension of the central shadow relative to the greatest transverse dimension of the thoracic cavity
  - using a good quality erect PA chest film in adults, cardiothoracic ratio of >0.5 is abnormal
  - differential of ratio >0.5
    - cardiomegaly (myocardial dilatation or hypertrophy)
    - pericardial effusion
    - poor inspiratory effort/low lung volumes
    - pectus excavatum
- ratio <0.5 does not exclude enlargement (e.g. cardiomegaly + concomitant hyperinflation)
- pericardial effusion: globular heart with loss of indentations on left mediastinal border
- RA enlargement: increase in curvature of right heart border and enlargement of SVC
- LA enlargement: straightening of left heart border; increased opacity of lower right side of cardiovascular shadow (double heart border); elevation of left main bronchus (specifically, the upper lobe bronchus on the lateral film), distance between left main bronchus and "double" heart border >7 cm, splayed carina (late sign)
- RV enlargement: elevation of cardiac apex from diaphragm; anterior enlargement leading to loss of retrosternal air space on lateral; increased contact of right ventricle against sternum
- LV enlargement: displacement of cardiac apex inferiorly and posteriorly – "boot-shaped" heart

**Elevated Hemidiaphragm Suggests
PAL DIP**
Pregnancy
Atelectasis
Lung resection
Diaphragmatic paralysis
Intra-abdominal process
Pneumonectomy
Pleural effusion also may result in apparent elevation

**Depressed Hemidiaphragm Suggests
TALC**
Tumour
Asthma
Large pleural effusion
COPD

**DDx Anterior Mediastinal Mass
4 Ts**
Thyroid
Thymic neoplasm
Teratoma
Terrible lymphoma

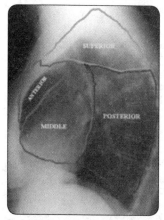

**Figure 14. Lateral CXR showing
4 mediastinal compartments**

Tubes, Lines, and Catheters

- ensure appropriate placement and assess potential complications of lines and tubes
- avoid mistaking a line/tube for pathology (e.g. oxygen rebreather mask for pneumothoraces)

Central Venous Catheter

- used for fluid and medication administration, vascular access for hemodialysis, and CVP monitoring
- tip must be located proximal to right atrium to prevent inducing arrhythmias or perforating wall of atrium
    - if monitoring CVP, catheter tip must be proximal to venous valves
- tip of well positioned central venous catheter projects over silhouette of SVC in a zone demarcated superiorly by the anterior first rib end and clavicle, and inferiorly by top of RA
- course should parallel course of SVC – if appears to bend as it approaches wall of SVC or appears perpendicular, catheter may damage and ultimately perforate wall of SVC
- complications: pneumothorax, bleeding (mediastinal, pleural), air embolism

Endotracheal Tube

- frontal chest film: tube projects over trachea and shallow oblique or lateral chest radiograph will help determine position in 3 dimensions
- progressive gaseous distention of stomach on repeat imaging is concerning for esophageal intubation
- tip should be located 4 cm above tracheal carina – avoids bronchus intubation and vocal cord irritation
- maximum inflation diameter <3 cm to avoid necrosis of tracheal mucosa and rupture – ensure diameter of balloon is less than tracheal diameter above and below balloon
- complications: aspiration (parenchymal opacities), pharyngeal perforation (subcutaneous emphysema, pneumomediastinum, mediastinitis)

Nasogastric Tube

- tip and sideport should be positioned distal to esophagogastric junction and proximal to gastric pylorus
- radiographic confirmation of tube is mandatory because clinical techniques for assessing tip position may be unreliable
- complications: aspiration (parenchymal opacities), intracranial perforation (trauma patients), pneumothorax

Swan-Ganz Catheter

- to monitor pulmonary capillary wedge pressure and to measure cardiac output for suspected LV dysfunction
- tip should be positioned within right or left main pulmonary arteries or in one of their large, lobar branches
- if tip is located more distally, increased risk of prolonged pulmonary artery occlusion resulting in pulmonary infarction or, rarely, pulmonary artery rupture
- complications: pneumothorax, bleeding (mediastinal, pleural), air embolism

Chest Tube

- in dorsal and caudal portion of pleural space to evacuate fluid
- in ventral and cephalad portions of pleural space to evacuate pneumothoraces
- tube may lie in fissure as long as functioning
- complications: lung perforation (mediastinal opacities)

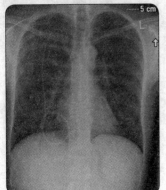

Figure 15. Well-positioned central venous catheter (CXR)

Abdominal Imaging

Abdominal X-Ray

- AXR 3 most common views: left lateral decubitus, supine, erect upright (see Figure 16)
- indications
    - acute abdomen: bowel perforation, toxic megacolon, bowel ischemia, small bowel obstruction, large bowel obstruction
    - chronic symptoms: constipation, calcifications (gallstones, renal stones, urinary bladder stones, etc.)
    - not useful in: GI bleeds, chronic anemia, vague GI symptoms

Anatomy

- abdomen divided into 2 cavities
    - peritoneal cavity: lined by peritoneum that wraps around most of the bowel, the spleen, and most of the liver; forms a recess lateral to both the ascending and descending colon (paracolic gutters)
    - retroperitoneal cavity: contains several organs situated posterior to the peritoneal cavity; the contour of these can often be seen on radiographs

3 Views of AXR
- Left lateral decubitus
- Supine
- Erect/Upright

Table 7. Differentiating Small and Large Bowel

Property	Small Bowel	Large Bowel
Mucosal Folds	Uninterrupted valvulae conniventes (or plicae circularis)	Interrupted haustra extend only partway across lumen
Location	Central	Peripheral (picture frame)
Maximum Diameter	3 cm	6 cm (9 cm at cecum)
Maximum Fold Thickness	3 mm	5 mm
Other	Rarely contains solid fecal material	Commonly contains solid fecal material

Approach to Abdominal X-Ray

- mnemonic: "Free ABDO"
- "Free": free air and fluid
  - free fluid
    - small amounts of fluid: increased distance between lateral fat stripes and adjacent colon may indicate free peritoneal fluid in the paracolic gutters
    - large amounts of fluid: diffuse increased opacification on supine film; bowel floats to centre of anterior abdominal wall
    - ascites and blood (hemoperitoneum) are the same density on the radiograph and therefore cannot be differentiated
    - free intraperitoneal air suggests rupture of a hollow viscus (anterior duodenum, transverse colon), penetrating trauma, or recent (<7 d) surgery
- "A": air in the bowel (can be normal, ileus, or obstruction)
  - volvulus – twisting of the bowel upon itself; from most to least common:
    - sigmoid: "coffee bean" sign (massively dilated sigmoid projects to right or mid-upper abdomen) with proximal dilation
    - cecal: massively dilated bowel loop projecting to left or mid-upper abdomen with small bowel dilation
    - gastric: rare
    - transverse colon: rare (usually young individuals)
    - small bowel: "corkscrew sign" (rarely diagnosed on plain films, seen best on CT)
  - toxic megacolon
    - manifestation of fulminant colitis
    - extreme dilatation of colon (>6.5 cm) with mucosal changes (e.g. foci of edema, ulceration, pseudopolyps), loss of normal haustral pattern
- "B": bowel wall thickening
  - increased soft tissue density in bowel wall, thumb-like indentations in bowel wall ("thumb-printing"), or a picket-fence appearance of the valvulae conniventes ("stacked coin" appearance)
  - may be seen in IBD, infection, ischemia, hypoproteinemic states, and submucosal hemorrhage
- "D": densities
  - bones: look for gross abnormalities of lower ribs, vertebral column, and bony pelvis
  - abnormal calcifications: approach by location
    - RUQ: renal stone, adrenal calcification, gallstone, porcelain gallbladder
    - RLQ: ureteral stone, appendicolith, gallstone ileus
    - LUQ: renal stone, adrenal calcification, tail of pancreas
    - LLQ: ureteral stone
    - central: aorta/aortic aneurysm, pancreas, lymph nodes
    - pelvis: phleboliths (i.e. calcified veins), uterine fibroids, bladder stones
- "O": organs
  - kidney, liver, gallbladder, spleen, pancreas, urinary bladder, psoas shadow
  - outlines can occasionally be identified because they are surrounded by more lucent fat, but all are best visualized with other imaging modalities (CT, MRI)

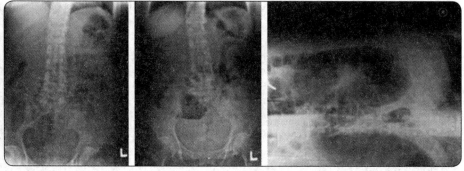

Figure 16. Normal AXRs: (left) supine anteroposterior AXR, (middle) upright anteroposterior AXR, and (right) left lateral decubitus AXR

Table 8. Abnormal Air on Abdominal X-Ray

Air	Appearance	Common Etiologies
Extraluminal Intraperitoneal (pneumoperitoneum)	Upright film: air under diaphragm Left lateral decubitus film: air between liver and abdominal wall Supine film: gas outlines of structures not normally seen: Inner and outer bowel wall (Rigler's sign) Falciform ligament Peritoneal cavity ("football" sign)	Perforated viscus Post-operative (up to 10 d to be resorbed)
Retroperitoneal	Gas outlining retroperitoneal structures allowing increased visualization: Psoas shadows Renal shadows	Perforation of retroperitoneal segments of bowel: duodenal ulcer, post-colonoscopy
Intramural (pneumatosis intestinalis)	Lucent air streaks in bowel wall, 2 types: 1. Linear 2. Rounded (cystoides type)	1. Linear: ischemia, necrotizing enterocolitis 2. Rounded/cystoides (generally benign): primary (idiopathic), secondary to COPD
Intraluminal	Dilated loops of bowel, air-fluid levels	Adynamic (paralytic) ileus, mechanical bowel obstruction
Loculated	Mottled, localized in abnormal position without normal bowel features	Abscess (evaluate with CT)
Biliary	Air centrally over liver	Sphincterotomy, gallstone ileus, erosive peptic ulcer, cholangitis, emphysematous cholecystitis
Portal Venous	Air peripherally over liver in branching pattern	Bowel ischemia/infarction

Table 9. Adynamic Ileus vs. Mechanical Obstruction

Feature	Adynamic Ileus	Mechanical Obstruction
Calibre of Bowel Loops	Normal or dilated	Usually dilated
Air-Fluid Levels (erect and left lateral decubitus films only)	Same level in the same single loop	Multiple air fluid levels giving "step ladder" appearance, dynamic (indicating peristalsis present), "string of pearls" (row of small gas accumulations in the dilated valvulae conniventes)
Distribution of Bowel Gas	Air throughout GI tract is generalized or localized In a localized ileus (e.g. pancreatitis, appendicitis), dilated "sentinel loop" remains in the same location on serial films, usually adjacent to the area of inflammation	Dilated bowel up to the point of obstruction (i.e. transition point) No air distal to obstructed segment "Hairpin" (180°) turns in bowel

Abdominal CT
- indications for plain CT: renal colic, hemorrhage
- indications for CT with contrast
  - IV contrast given immediately before or during CT to allow identification of arteries and veins
    - portal venous phase: indicated for majority of cases
    - biphasic (arterial and portal venous phases): liver, pancreas, bile duct tumours
    - caution: contrast allergy (may premedicate with steroids and antihistamine)
    - contraindication: impaired renal function, based on eGFR
  - oral contrast: barium or water soluble (water soluble if suspected perforation) given in most cases to demarcate GI tract
  - rectal contrast: given for investigation of colonic lesions

Approach to Abdominal Computed Tomography

- look through all images in gestalt fashion to identify any obvious abnormalities
- look at each organ/structure individually, from top to bottom evaluating size and shape of each area of increased or decreased density
- evaluate the following
  - soft tissue window
    - liver, gallbladder, spleen, and pancreas
    - adrenals, kidneys, ureters, and bladder
    - stomach, duodenum, small bowel mesentery, and colon/appendix
    - retroperitoneum: aorta, vena cava, and mesenteric vessels; look for adenopathy in vicinity of vessels
    - peritoneal cavity for fluid or masses
    - abdominal wall and adjacent soft tissue
  - lung window
    - visible lung (bases)
  - bone window
    - vertebrae, spinal cord, and bony pelvis

Colorectal Cancer: CT Colonography and Colonoscopy for Detection-Systematic Review and Meta-Analysis
Radiology 2011;259:393-405
Study: Systematic review and meta-analysis.
Population: 49 studies on 11,151 patients undergoing diagnostic study for detection of colorectal cancer (CRC).
Intervention: CT colonography (CTC) and optical colonoscopy (OC).
Main Outcome Measure: Sensitivity of CTC and OC for CRC.
Results: CTC has a sensitivity of 96.1% (95% CI 93.8%, 97.7%) and OC has a sensitivity of 94.7% (95% CI 90.4%, 97.2%) for the detection of CRC.
Conclusion: CTC is highly sensitive for the detection of CRC and may be a better modality for the initial investigation of suspected CRC, assuming reasonable specificity.

CT and Bowel Obstruction
- cause of bowel obstruction rarely found on plain films – CT is best choice for imaging
- the "3,6,9" rule is a very useful guide to determining when the bowel is dilated; the maximum diameter of the bowel is 3 cm for small bowel, 6 cm for large bowel, and 9 cm for cecum; this can also be useful to distinguish small and large bowel, and to assess for 'impending' cecal perforation (e.g. post-untreated Ogilvie's syndrome)
- closed-loop obstruction: an obstruction in two locations (usually small bowel) creating a loop of bowel segment obstructed both proximally and distally; complications (e.g. ischemia, perforation, necrosis) may occur quickly

CT Colonography (virtual colonoscopy)
- emerging imaging technique for evaluation of intraluminal colonic masses (i.e. polyps, tumours)
- two CT scans of the abdomen (prone and supine) after the instillation of carbon dioxide into a prepped colon
- computer reconstruction of 2D CT images into a 3D intraluminal view of the colon
- lesions seen on 3D images correlated with 2D axial images
- indications: surveillance in low-risk patients, incomplete colonoscopy, staging of obstructing colonic lesions

Contrast Studies

Table 10. Types of Contrast Studies

Study	Organ	Procedure Description	Assessment	Findings
Cine Esophagogram	Cervical esophagus	Contrast agent swallowed Recorded for later playback and analysis	Dysphagia, swallowing incoordination, recurrent aspiration, post-operative cleft palate repair	Aspiration, webs (partial occlusion), Zenker's diverticulum, cricopharyngeal bar, laryngeal tumour
Barium Swallow	Thoracic esophagus	Contrast agent swallowed under fluoroscopy, selective images captured	Dysphagia, rule out GERD, post esophageal surgery	Achalasia, hiatus hernia, esophagitis, cancer, esophageal tear
Upper GI Series	Thoracic esophagus, stomach, and duodenum	Double contrast study: 1. Barium to coat mucosa, then 2. Gas pills for distention Patient NPO after midnight	Dyspepsia, investigate possible upper GI bleed, weight loss/anemia, post gastric surgery	Ulcers, neoplasms, filling defects
Enterography & Enteroclysis (MRI or CT)	Entire small bowel	Enterography: patient drinks 1-2 L of sorbitol, psyllium, or barium solution to distend small bowel Enteroclysis: NJ tube used to pump barium, psyllium, or sorbitol contrast media directly into small bowel	IBD, malabsorption, weight loss/anemia, Meckel's diverticulum	Neoplasms, IBD, malabsorption, infection

Specific Visceral Organ Imaging

Liver
- U/S: assessment of cysts, abscesses, tumours, biliary tree
- CT ± IV: most popular procedure for imaging the liver parenchyma (primary liver tumours, metastases, cysts, abscesses, trauma, cirrhosis)
- MR: also excellent in evaluation of primary liver tumours, liver metastases, and other parenchymal conditions, and is particularly helpful in differentiating common benign hepatic hemangiomas from primary liver tumours and metastases
- elastography: measures shear wave velocity by U/S (Fibroscan) or MRI (MR elastography) to non-invasively quantify liver fibrosis
- findings
  - advanced cirrhosis: liver small and irregular (fibrous scarring, segmental atrophy, regenerating nodules)
  - portal HTN: increased portal vein diameter, collateral veins, splenomegaly (≥12 cm), portal vein thrombosis, recanalization of the umbilical vein
  - porto-systemic shunts: caput medusa, esophageal varices, spontaneous spleno-renal shunt
  - U/S: cirrhosis appears nodular and hyperechoic with irregular areas of atrophy of the right lobe and hypertrophy of the caudate or left lobes
  - CT: fatty infiltration appears hypodense
  - • in order to be visualized, some masses require contrast
- upon identifying a liver lesion on imaging (e.g. U/S), the follow-up imaging modality should be CT or MR. CT would be four-phase non-contrast, arterial, venous, and delayed to distinguish the common benign liver lesion hemangioma from other tumours

Normal liver appears denser than spleen on CT. If less dense, suspect fatty infiltration

Liver Mass DDx

5 Hs
HCC
Hydatid cyst
Hemangioma
Hepatic adenoma
Hyperplasia (focal nodular)

Revised Estimates of Diagnostic Test Sensitivity and Specificity in Suspected Biliary Tract Disease
Arch Intern Med 1998;154:2573-2581
Purpose: To assess the sensitivity and specificity of tests used to diagnose cholelithiasis and acute cholecystitis, including ultrasonography, oral cholecystography, radionucleotide scanning with Technetium, MRI, CT.
Study Characteristics: Meta-analysis of 30 studies evaluating the use of different imaging modalities in the diagnosis of biliary tract disease.
Participants: No limits.
Main Outcomes: Sensitivity and specificity of the different imaging modalities, using the gold standard of surgery, autopsy, or 3 mo clinical follow-up for cholelithiasis. For acute cholecystitis, pathologic findings, confirmation of an alternate disease, or clinical resolution during hospitalization for cholecystitis were used as the standard.
Results: For evaluating cholelithiasis, U/S had the best unadjusted sensitivity (0.97; 95% CI 0.95-0.99) and specificity (0.95, 95% CI 0.88-1.00) and adjusted (for verification bias) sensitivity (0.84; 95% CI 0.76-0.92) and specificity (0.99; 95% CI 0.97-1.00). For evaluating acute cholecystitis, radionucleotide scanning has the best sensitivity (0.97; 95% CI 0.96-0.98) and specificity (0.90; 95% CI 0.86-0.95).
Conclusions: U/S is the test of choice for diagnosing cholelithiasis and radionucleotide scanning is the superior test for diagnosing acute cholecystitis.

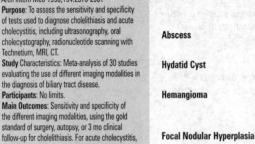

Table 11. Imaging of Liver Masses

Mass	U/S	CT
Metastases	Multiple masses of variable echotexture	Usually low attenuation on contrast enhanced scan
HCC	Single/multiple masses, or diffuse infiltration	Hypervascular enhances in arterial and washes out in venous phase with portal venous tumour thrombus
Abscess	Poorly defined, irregular margin, hypoechoic contents	Low-attenuation lesion with an irregular enhancing wall
Hydatid Cyst	Simple/multiloculated cyst	Low-attenuation simple or multiloculated cyst; calcification
Hemangioma	Homogeneous hyperechoic mass	Peripheral globular enhancement in arterial phase scans; central-filling and persistent enhancement on delayed scans
Focal Nodular Hyperplasia	Well-defined mass, central scar seen in 50%	Hypervascular mass in arterial phase and isoattenuation to liver in portal venous phase
Hepatic Adenoma	Most common in young women taking oral contraceptives. Well-defined mass with hyperechoic areas due to hemorrhage	Well-defined hypervascular lesion with enlarged central vessel becoming slightly isoattenuating in venous phase

Spleen
- U/S, CT, nuclear medicine scan (nuclear medicine only to distinguish ectopic splenic tissue from enhancing tumours)
- CT for splenic trauma (hemorrhage)

Pancreas
- tumours
  - U/S: mass is more echogenic than normal pancreatic tissue
  - CT: preferred modality for diagnosis/staging
- ductal dilation secondary to stone/tumour
  - MRCP: imaging of ductal system using MRI cholangiography; no therapeutic potential
  - ERCP: endoscope to inject dye into the biliary tree and x-ray imaging to assess pancreatic and biliary ducts; therapeutic potential (stent placement, stone retrieval); acute pancreatitis is a complication in 5% of diagnostic procedures and 10% of therapeutic procedures

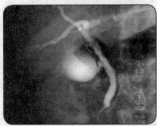

Figure 17. ERCP: biliary tree

Biliary Tree
- U/S: bile ducts usually visualized only if dilated, secondary to obstruction (e.g. choledocholithiasis, benign stricture, mass)
- CT: dilated intrahepatic ductules seen as branching, tubular structures following pathway of portal venous system
- MRCP, ERCP, PTC: further evaluation of obstruction and possible intervention

 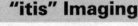 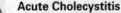

"itis" Imaging

Acute Cholecystitis
- pathogenesis: inflammation of gallbladder resulting from sustained gallstone impaction in cystic duct or, in the case of acalculous cholechystitis, due to gallbladder ischemia or cholestasis (see General Surgery, GS47)
- best imaging modality: U/S (best sensitivity and specificity); nuclear medicine (HIDA scan) can help diagnose cases of acalculous or chronic cholecystitis
- findings: thick wall, pericholecystic fluid, gallstones, dilated gallbladder, positive sonographic Murphy's sign
- management: cholecystectomy

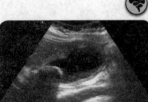

Figure 18. Ultrasound: inflamed gallbladder

Acute Appendicitis
- pathogenesis: luminal obstruction → bacterial overgrowth → inflammation/swelling → increased pressure → localized ischemia → gangrene/perforation → localized abscess or peritonitis (see General Surgery, GS27)
- best imaging modality: U/S or CT
- findings
  - U/S: thick-walled appendix, appendicolith, dilated fluid-filled appendix, non-compressible; may also demonstrate other causes of RLQ pain (e.g. ovarian abscess, IBD, ectopic pregnancy)
  - CT: enlargement of appendix (>6 mm in outer diameter), enhancement of appendiceal wall, adjacent inflammatory stranding, appendicolith; also facilitates percutaneous abscess drainage
- management: appendectomy

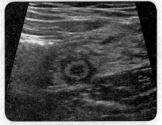

Figure 19. Ultrasound: inflamed appendix

Acute Diverticulitis
- pathogenesis: erosion of the intestinal wall (most commonly rectosigmoid) by increased intraluminal pressure or inspissated food particles → inflammation and focal necrosis → micro- or macroscopic perforation (see General Surgery, GS31)
- best imaging modality: CT is modality of choice, although U/S is sometimes used
- contrast: oral and rectal contrast given before CT to opacify bowel
- findings
  - cardinal signs: thickened wall, mesenteric infiltration, gas-filled diverticula, abscess
  - CT can be used for percutaneous abscess drainage before or in lieu of surgical intervention
  - sometimes difficult to distinguish from perforated cancer (therefore send abscess fluid for cytology and follow up with colonoscopy)
  - if chronic, may see fistula (most common to bladder) or sinus tract (linear or branching structures)
- management: ranges from antibiotic treatment to surgical intervention; can use imaging to follow progression

Acute Pancreatitis
- pathogenesis: activation of proteolytic enzymes within pancreatic cells leading to local and systemic inflammatory response (see Gastroenterology, G44); a clinical/biochemical diagnosis
- best imaging modality: imaging used to support diagnosis and evaluate for complications (diagnosis cannot be excluded by imaging alone)
  - U/S good for screening and follow-up
  - CT is useful in advanced stages and in assessing for complications (1st line imaging test)
- findings
  - U/S: hypoechoic enlarged pancreas (if ileus present, gas obscures pancreas)
  - CT: enlarged pancreas, edema, stranding changes in surrounding fat with indistinct fat planes, mesenteric and Gerota's fascia thickening, pseudocyst in lesser sac, abscess (gas or thick-walled fluid collection), pancreatic necrosis (low attenuation gas-containing non-enhancing pancreatic tissue), hemorrhage
- management: supportive therapy
  - CT-guided needle aspiration and/or drainage done for abscess when clinically indicated
  - pseudocyst may be followed by CT and drained if symptomatic

Chronic Pancreatitis
- pathogenesis: (see Gastroenterology, G45)
- best imaging modality: MRCP (can show calcification and duct obstruction)
- findings: U/S, CT scan, and MRI may show calcifications, ductal dilatation, enlargement of the pancreas and fluid collections (e.g. pseudocysts) adjacent to the gland

Angiography of Gastrointestinal Tract

- anatomy of the GI tract arterial blood supply branches
  - celiac artery: hepatic, splenic, gastroduodenal, left/right gastric
  - superior mesenteric artery: jejunal, ileal, ileo-colic, right colic, middle colic
  - inferior mesenteric artery: left colic, superior rectal
- imaging modalities
  - conventional angiogram: invasive (usual approach via femoral puncture), catheter used
    - flush aortography: catheter injection into abdominal aorta, followed by selective arteriography of individual vessels
  - CT angiogram: modality of choice, non-invasive using IV contrast (no catheterization required)

Genitourinary System and Adrenal

Urological Imaging

KUB (Kidney, Ureter, and Bladder X-ray)
- a frontal supine radiograph of the abdomen
- indication: useful in evaluation of radio-opaque renal stones (all stones but uric acid and indinavir), indwelling ureteric stents /catheters, and foreign bodies in abdomen
- findings: addition of IV contrast excreted by the kidney (intravenous urogram) allows greater visualization of the urinary tract, but has been largely replaced by CT urography

Abdominal CT

Renal Masses
- Bozniak classification for cystic renal masses
- class I-II: benign and can be disregarded
- class IIF: should be followed
- class III-IV: suspicious for malignancy, requiring additional workup

Computed Tomography and Ultrasonography to Detect Acute Appendicitis in Adults and Adolescents
Ann Intern Med 2004;141:537-546
Purpose: To review the diagnostic accuracy of CT and ultrasonography in the diagnosis of acute appendicitis.
Study Characteristics: Meta-analysis of 22 prospective studies evaluating the use of CT or ultrasonography, followed by surgical or clinical follow-up in patients with suspected appendicitis.
Participants: Age ≥14 with a clinical suspicion of appendicitis.
Main Outcomes: Sensitivity and specificity using surgery or clinical follow-up as the gold standard.
Results: CT (12 studies) had an overall sensitivity of 0.94 (95% CI 0.91-0.95) and a specificity of 0.95 (95% CI 0.93-0.96). Ultrasonography (14 studies) had an overall sensitivity of 0.86 (95% CI 0.83-0.88) and a specificity of 0.81 (95% CI 0.78-0.84).
Conclusions: CT is more accurate for diagnosing appendicitis in adults and adolescents, although verification bias and inappropriate blinding of reference standards were noted in the included studies.

Angiography requires active blood loss 1-1.5 mL/min under optimal conditions for a bleeding site to be visualized in cases of lower GI bleeding

Imaging Modality Based on Presentation
- Acute testicular pain = Doppler, U/S
- Amenorrhea = U/S, MRI (brain)
- Bloating = U/S, CT
- Flank pain = U/S, CT
- Hematuria = U/S, Cystoscopy, CT
- Infertility = HSG, MRI
- Lower abdominal mass = U/S, CT
- Lower abdominal pain = U/S, CT
- Renal colic = U/S, KUB, CT
- Testicular mass = U/S
- Urethral stricture = Urethrogram

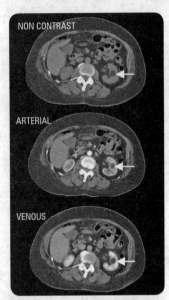

Figure 20. Triphasic CT of an angiomyolipoma: showing fat density with non-contrast scan, mildly enhancing with contrast

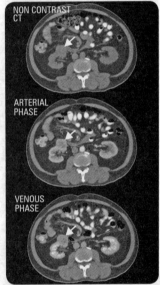

Figure 21. Triphasic CT of a renal cell carcinoma: showing arterial enhancing right renal lesion with venous washout (shunting)

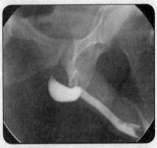

Figure 22. Retrograde urethrogram: demonstrating stricture in the membranous urethra

Table 12. Bozniak Classification for Cystic Renal Masses

Classes	Definition
Simple Renal Cysts	
Class I	Fluid-attenuating well-defined lesion, no septation, no calcification, no solid components, hair thin wall
Class II	Same as class I + fine calcification or moderately thickened calcification in septae or walls; also includes hyperdense cysts (<3 cm) that do not enhance with contrast
Complex Renal Cysts	
Class III	Thick irregular walls ± calcifications ± septated, enhancing walls or septa with contrast
Renal Cell Carcinoma	
Class IV	Same as class III + soft tissue enhancement with contrast (defined as >10 Hounsfield unit increase, characterizing vascularity) with de-enhancement in venous phase ± areas of necrosis

- **plain CT KUB indications**: general imaging of renal anatomy, renal colic symptoms, assessment of renal calculi (size and location), and hydronephrosis prior to urological treatment
- **CT urography indications**: investigation of cause of microscopic/gross hematuria, detailed assessment of urinary tracts (excretory phase), high sensitivity (95%) for uroepithelial malignancies of the upper urinary tracts, assessment of renal calculi
  phases: unenhanced, excretory
- **renal triphasic CT indications**: standard imaging for renal masses, allows accurate assessment of renal arteries and veins, better characterization of suspicious renal masses, especially in differentiating renal cell carcinoma from more benign masses, and pre-operative staging
    - **phases**: unenhanced, arterial and venous (nephrographic), excretory

Ultrasound

- indications: initial study for evaluation of kidney size and nature of renal masses (solid vs. cystic renal masses vs. complicated cysts); technique of choice for screening patients with suspected hydronephrosis (no IV contrast injection, no radiation to patient, and can be used in patients with renal failure); TRUS useful to evaluate prostate gland and guide biopsies; Doppler U/S to assess renal vasculature
- findings: solid renal masses are echogenic (bright on U/S), cystic renal masses have smooth well-defined walls with anechoic interior (dark on U/S), and complicated cysts have internal echoes within a thickened, irregular wall

Retrograde Pyelography

- indications: visualize the urinary collecting system via a cystoscope, ureteral catheterization, and retrograde injection of contrast medium, visualized by radiograph or fluoroscopy; ordered when the intrarenal collecting system and ureters cannot be opacified using intravenous techniques (patient with impaired renal function, high grade obstruction)
- findings: only yields information about the collecting systems (renal pelvis and associated structures), no information regarding the parenchyma of the kidney

Voiding Cystourethrogram

- bladder filled with contrast to the point where voiding is triggered
- fluoroscopy (continuous, real-time) to visualize bladder
- indications: children with recurrent UTIs, hydronephrosis, hydroureter, suspected lower urinary tract obstruction or vesicoureteral reflux
- findings: contractility and evidence of vesicoureteric reflux

Retrograde Urethrogram

- a small Foley catheter placed into penile urethral opening
- indications: used mainly to study strictures or trauma to the male urethra; first-line study if trauma with blood present at urethral meatus

MRI

- advantages: high spatial and tissue resolution, lack of exposure to ionizing radiation and nephrotoxic contrast agents
- indications: indicated over CT for depiction of renal masses in patients with previous nephron sparing surgery, patients requiring serial follow-up (less radiation dosage), patients with reduced renal function, patients with solitary kidneys, clinical staging of prostate cancer (endorectal coil MRI)

Renal Nuclear Scan

Table 13. Renal Scan Tests

Type of Test	Uses	Radionuclide
Renogram	assess renal function and collecting system: evaluation of renal failure, workup of urinary tract obstruction and renovascular HTN, investigation of renal transplant	IV 99mTc-pentetate (DTPA) or mertiatide (MAG3), and imaged at 1-3 s intervals with a gamma camera over the first 60 s to assess perfusion
Morphological	Assess renal anatomy: investigation of pyelonephritis and cortical scars	99mTc-DMSA 99mTc-glucoheptonate

Gynecological Imaging

Ultrasound
- transabdominal and transvaginal are the primary modalities, and are indicated for different scenarios
- transabdominal requires a full bladder to push out air containing loops of bowel
  - **indications**: good initial investigation for suspected pelvic pathology
- TVUS provides enhanced detail of deeper/smaller structures by allowing use of higher frequency sound waves at reduced distances
  - **indications**: improved assessment of ovaries, first trimester development, and ectopic pregnancies

Hysterosalpingogram
- performed by x-ray images of the pelvis after cannulation of the cervix and subsequent injection of opacifying agent
- **indications**: useful for assessing pathology of the uterine cavity and fallopian tubes, evaluating uterine abnormalities (e.g. bicornuate uterus), or evaluation of fertility (absence of flow from tubes to peritoneal cavity indicates obstruction)

CT/MRI
- **indications**: evaluating pelvic structures, especially those adjacent to the adnexa and uterus
- invaluable for staging gynecological malignancies and detecting recurrence

Sonohysterogram
- saline infusion sonohysterogram involves instilling fluid into the uterine cavity transcervically to provide enhanced endometrial visualization during TVUS examination
- **indications**: abnormal uterine bleeding, uterine cavity abnormalities that are suspected or noted on TVUS (e.g. leiomyomas, polyps, synechiae), congenital abnormalities of the uterine cavity, infertility, recurrent pregnancy loss
- **contraindications**: pregnancy, pelvic infection

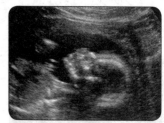
Figure 23. Transabdominal U/S: pregnancy, 18 wk fetus

Pregnancy should always be ruled out by β-hCG before CT of a female pelvis (or any organ system) is performed

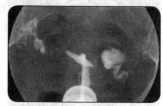
Figure 24. Hysterosalpingogram: left hydrosalpinx

Table 14. Typical and Atypical Findings on a Sonohysterogram

Finding	Typical	Atypical
Polyps	A well-defined, homogeneous, polypoid lesion isoechoic to the endometrium with preservation of the endometrial-myometrial interface	Atypical features include cystic components, multiple polyps, broad base, hypoechogenicity or heterogeneity
Leiomyoma	Well-defined, broad-based, hypoechoic, solid masses with shadowing. Overlying layer of endometrium is echogenic and distorts the endometrial-myometrial interface	Pedunculation or multilobulated surface
Hyperplasia and Cancer	Diffuse echogenic endometrial thickening without focal abnormality, although focal lesions can occur. Endometrial cancer is typically a diffuse process, but early cases can be focal and appear as a polypoid mass	
Adhesions	Mobile, thin, echogenic bands that cut across the endometrial cavity	Thick, broad-based bands that can completely obliterate the endometrial cavity, as in Asherman's syndrome

Adrenal Mass

- imaging modality: most often identified on CT scan as 'incidentaloma', can also use CT/MRI to distinguish benign from malignant masses

Table 15. Adrenal Mass Findings on CT and MRI

Factors	Adrenocortical Adenoma	Adrenocortical Carcinoma	Pheochromocytoma	Metastasis
Diameter (CT)	Usually ≤3 cm	Usually ≥4 cm	Usually >3 cm	Variable around <3 cm
Shape (CT)	Smooth margins and round/oval	Irregular with unclear margins	Round/oval with clear margins	Oval/irregular with unclear margins
Texture (CT)	Homogeneous	Heterogeneous with mixed densities	Heterogeneous with cystic areas	Heterogeneous with mixed densities
Vascularity (CT)	Not highly vascular	Usually vascular	Usually vascular	Usually vascular
Washout of Contrast Medium on CT	≥50% at 10 min	<50% at 10 min	<50% at 10 min	<50% at 10 min
Growth	Stable or very slow (<1 cm/yr)	Usually rapid (>2 cm/yr)	Slow (0.5-1 cm/yr)	Variable
Other Findings	Usually low density due to intracellular fat	Necrosis, calcifications, and hemorrhage	Hemorrhage	Occasionally hemorrhage
MRI on T2 Weighted Imaging	Isointense in relation to liver	Hyperintense in relation to liver	Markedly hyperintense in relation to liver	Hyperintense in relation to liver

Modality Based on Neuropathology Presentation
- Cognitive decline = CT
- Cord compression = MRI
- Decreased level of consciousness = CT
- Fish bone/other swallowed foreign body = CT
- Low back pain, radiculopathy = MRI
- Multiple sclerosis = MRI
- Neck infection = CT
- Orbital infection = CT
- Rule out bleed = CT
- Rule out aneurysm = CTA, MRA
- Seizure = CT
- Sinusitis = CT
- Stroke = CT, MRI
- Trauma = CT
- Weakness, systemically unwell = CT

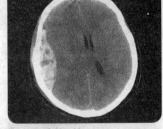

Figure 25. Epidural hematoma

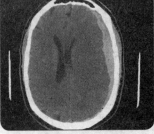

Figure 26. Subdural hematoma

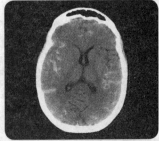

Figure 27. Subarachnoid hemorrhage

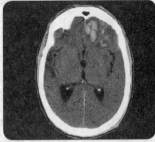

Figure 28. Intraparenchymal hemorrhage

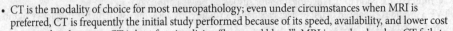

Neuroradiology

Modalities

- CT is the modality of choice for most neuropathology; even under circumstances when MRI is preferred, CT is frequently the initial study performed because of its speed, availability, and lower cost
  - acute head trauma: CT is best for visualizing "bone and blood"; MRI is used only when CT fails to detect an abnormality despite strong clinical suspicion
  - acute stroke: MRI ideal, CT most frequently used
  - suspected subarachnoid or intracranial hemorrhage
  - meningitis: rule out mass effect (e.g. cerebral herniation, shift) prior to lumbar puncture
  - tinnitus and vertigo: CT and MRI are used in combination to detect bony abnormalities and CN VIII tumours, respectively

Skull Films
- rarely performed, generally not indicated for non-penetrating head trauma
- **indications**: screening for destructive bony lesions (e.g. metastases), metabolic disease, skull anomalies, post-operative changes and confirmation of hardware placement, skeletal surveys, multiple myeloma

CT
- **indications**: excellent study for evaluation of bony and intracranial abnormalities
- often done first without and then with IV contrast to show vascular structures or anomalies
- vascular structures and areas of blood-brain barrier impairment are opaque (e.g. hyperattenuating or white/show enhancement) with contrast injection
  - when in doubt, look for circle of Willis or confluence of sinuses to determine presence of contrast enhancement
- posterior fossa can be obscured by extensive bony-related streak artifact
- rule out skull fracture, epidural hematoma (lenticular shape), subdural hematoma (crescentic shape), subarachnoid hemorrhage, space occupying lesion, hydrocephalus, and cerebral edema
- multiplanar imaging can be performed with newer generation of multidetector CT scanners

Myelography
- introduction of water-soluble, low-osmotic contrast media into subarachnoid space using lumbar puncture followed by x-ray or CT scan
- **indications**: excellent study for disc herniations, traumatic nerve root avulsions, patients with contraindication to MRI

MRI
- **indications**: shows brain and spinal soft tissue anatomy in fine detail, clearly distinguishes white from grey matter (especially T1-weighted series), multiplanar reconstruction helpful in pre-operative assessment

Cerebral Angiography/CT Angiography/MR Angiography
- **indications**: evaluation of vascular lesions such as atherosclerotic disease, aneurysms, vascular malformations, arterial dissection
- conventional DSA remains the gold standard for the assessment of neck and intracranial vessels; however, it is an invasive procedure requiring arterial (femoral) puncture; catheter manipulation has risk of vessel injury (e.g. dissection, occlusion, vasospasm, emboli)
- MRA methods (phase contrast, time of flight, gadolinium-enhanced) and CTA are much less invasive without actual risk to intracranial or neck vessels
- MRA and CTA are often used first as 'screening tests' for the assessment of subarachnoid hemorrhage, vasospasm, aneurysms

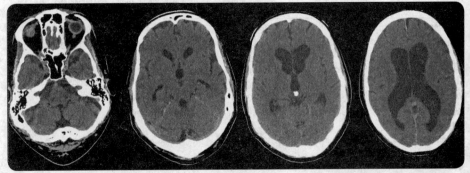

Figure 29. Hydrocephalus: ventricular dilatation (may see periventricular low attenuation due to transependymal CSF flow)

Table 16. Two Types of Hydrocephalus

Type	Cause
Communicating/Extra-Ventricular	Obstruction distal to the ventricles (e.g. at the level of the arachnoid granulations); imaging shows all ventricles dilated
Non-Communicating	Obstruction within the ventricular system (e.g. mass obstructing the aqueduct or foramen of Monro); imaging shows dilatation of ventricles proximal to the obstruction

Nuclear Medicine

- SPECT using ^{99m}Tc-exametazime (HMPAO) and ^{99m}Tc-bicisate (ECD) imaging assesses cerebral blood flow by diffusing rapidly across the blood brain barrier and becoming trapped within neurons proportional to cerebral blood flow
- 18FDG PET imaging assesses cerebral metabolic activity
- **indications**: differentiation of residual tumour vs. radiation necrosis; localizing of epileptic seizure foci; evaluation of atypical dementia

Approach to CT Head

- think anatomically, work from superficial to deep
- scan: confirm that the imaging is of the correct patient, whether contrast was used, if the patient is aligned properly, if there is artifact present
- skin/soft tissue: examine the soft tissue superficial to the skull, looking for thickening suggestive of hematoma or edema; also evaluate the ear, orbital contents (globe, fat, muscles), parotid, muscles of mastication (masseter, temporalis, pterygoids), visualized pharynx
- bone and airspace (use the bone window): check calvarium, visualize mandible, visualize C-spine (usually C1 and maybe part of C2) for fractures, absent bone, lytic/sclerotic lesions; inspect sinuses and mastoid air cells for opacity that may suggest fluid, pus, blood, tumour, or fracture; status of the orbital floor in cases of facial trauma (coronal series best)
- dura and subdural space: crescent-shaped hyperdensity in the subdural space suggests subdural hematoma; lentiform hyperdensity in the epidural space suggests epidural hematoma; check symmetry of dural thickness, where increased thickness may suggest the presence of blood
- parenchyma: asymmetry of the parenchyma suggests midline shift; poor contrast between grey and white matter suggests possible infarction, tumour, edema, infection, or contusion; hyperdensity in the parenchyma suggests enchancing lesions, intracerebral hemorrhage, or calcification; central grey matter nuclei (e.g. globus pallidus, putamen, internal capsule) should be visible, otherwise, suspect infarct, tumour, or infection
- ventricles/sulci/cisterns: examine position of ventricles for evidence of midline compression/shift; hyperdensities in the ventricles suggest ventricular/subdural hemorrhage; enlarged ventricles suggest hydrocephalus; obliteration of sulci may suggest presence of edema causing effacement, possible blood filling in the sulci, or tumour; cistern hyperdensities may suggest blood, pus, or tumour
- please refer to Toronto Notes' website for supplementary material on how to approach a head CT

Selected Pathology

- see <u>Neurosurgery</u>, NS4 for intracranial mass lesions
- see <u>Neurosurgery</u>, NS29 and <u>Plastic Surgery</u>, PL29 for head trauma
- see <u>Emergency Medicine</u>, ER7 for vertebral trauma
- see <u>Neurosurgery</u>, NS27 and <u>Orthopedics</u>, OR22 for degenerative spinal abnormalities

Cerebrovascular Disease (see <u>Neurology</u>, N26 and <u>Neurosurgery</u>, NS17)

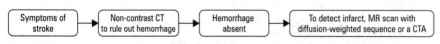

| Symptoms of stroke | → | Non-contrast CT to rule out hemorrhage | → | Hemorrhage absent | → | To detect infarct, MR scan with diffusion-weighted sequence or a CTA |

- pathogenesis of stroke: see <u>Neurology</u>, N48
- best imaging modality: infarcts best detected by MRI > CT
- findings of infarction
  - early changes
    - ◆ CT
      - usually normal within 6 h of infarction
      - edema (loss of grey-white matter differentiation – "insular ribbon" sign, effacement of sulci, mass effect)
      - within 24 h, development of low-density, wedge-shaped area of infarction extending to periphery (correlating to vascular territory distal to affected artery)
      - in case of ischemic stroke, may see hyperattenuating (bright) artery (hyperdense MCA sign) representing intravascular thrombus or embolus
      - in case of hemorrhagic stroke or transformation (common in basal ganglia and cortex), may see bright acute blood surrounded by edema

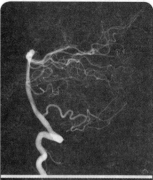

Figure 30. Vertebrobasilar circulation
(note the incidental basilar tip aneurysm)

Approach to the CT Head
Some = Scan
Sore = Skin/Soft Tissue
Brains = Bone/Airspace
Demonstrate = Dura/Subdural space
Pushed = Parenchyma
Ventricles = Ventricles/Sulci/Cisterns

Transient ischemic attacks are not associated with radiological findings

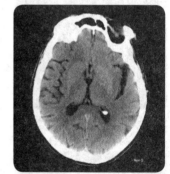

Figure 31. Insular Ribbon Sign (Left side)

Ddx for Ring Enhancing Cerebral Lesion

MAGIC DR
Metastasis
Abscess
Glioblastoma multiforme
Infarction (subacute/chronic)
Contusion/hematoma
Demyelinating disease (e.g. MS)
Radiation necrosis

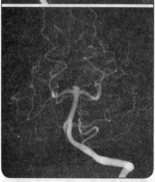

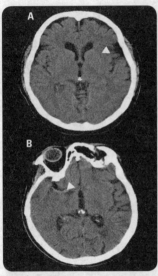

Figure 32. CT images of early infarct: (A) absence of left insular ribbon (B) hyperdense artery

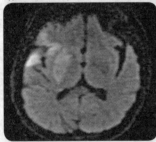

Figure 33. DWI of patient with right frontotemporal infarct

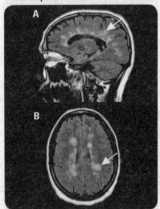

Figure 34. T2-weighted FLAIR: (A) sagittal (B) axial images of multiple sclerosis with periventricular "Dawson's Fingers"

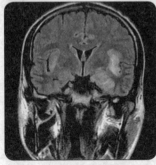

Figure 35. T2-weighted (FLAIR) coronal image of herpes simplex virus encephalitis affecting temporal lobes

- ♦ MRI
  - – edema with high signal on T2-weighted images and FLAIR image (loss of grey-white matter differentiation, effacement of sulci, mass effect)
  - – DWI shows acute high signal changes demonstrating restricted movement of water indicative of cytotoxic edema; usually indicates stroke damage before CT
  - – apparent diffusion coefficient image shows low signal intensity in acute ischemia (nadir 3-5 d, returns to baseline 1-4 wk)
  - ▪ subacute changes on CT and MRI
    - ♦ edema and mass effect more prominent
    - ♦ gyral enhancement with contrast indicative of blood-brain barrier breakdown
  - ▪ chronic changes on CT and MRI
    - ♦ encephalomalacia (parenchymal volume loss) with dilatation of adjacent ventricles
- • carotid artery disease
  - ▪ best imaging modality: Duplex Doppler U/S
  - ▪ other modalities: MRA or CTA if carotid angioplasty or endarterectomy is under consideration (conventional angiography reserved for inadequate MRA or CTA)

Multiple Sclerosis (see Neurology, N52)

- • best imaging modality: MRI has high sensitivity in diagnosing MS (>90%) but low specificity (71-74%)
- • findings
  - ▪ characteristic lesion on MRI is cerebral or spinal plaque
  - ▪ plaques typically found in periventricular region, corpus callosum (arranged at right angles to the corpus callosum), centrum semiovale, and to a lesser extent in deep white matter structures and basal ganglia
  - ▪ "Dawson's fingers" refers to perivenular regions of demyelination that are seen to radiate outwards into the deep periventricular region
  - ▪ plaques usually have ovoid appearance, hyperintense on T2 and hypointense on T1
  - ▪ conventional T2 may underestimate plaque size and overall plaque burden – advanced techniques (diffusion tensor imaging and MR spectroscopy) can be of use
  - ▪ perivascular and interstitial edema may be prominent
  - ▪ spinal cord lesions typical of MS
    - ♦ little or no cord swelling
    - ♦ unequivocal hyperintensity on T2-weighted sequences
    - ♦ size at least 3 mm but less than 2 vertebral segments in length
    - ♦ occupy only part of the cord in cross-section
    - ♦ focal (i.e. clearly delineated and circumscribed on T2-weighted sequences)

CNS Infections

- • leptomeningitis
  - ▪ pathogenesis: inflammation of the pia or arachnoid mater, most often secondary to hematogenous spread from infection or via organisms gaining access across areas not protected by the blood-brain barrier (choroid plexus or circumventricular organs)
    - ♦ pathogens include: *S. pneumoniae, H. influenzae, N. meningitidis, L. monocytogenes*
  - ▪ best imaging modality: MRI (T2-weighted/FLAIR) superior to CT
  - ▪ findings
    - ♦ meningeal enhancement (following the gyri/sulci, and/or basal cisterns), hydrocephalus (communicating), cerebral swelling, subdural effusion
    - ♦ a normal MRI does not rule out leptomeningitis
- • herpes simplex encephalitis (see Infectious Diseases, ID19)
  - ▪ pathogenesis: inflammation of the brain parenchyma secondary to infection with herpes simplex virus, asymmetrically affects the limbic regions of the brain (i.e. temporal lobes, orbitofrontal region, insula, and cingulate gyrus)
  - ▪ best imaging modality: MRI (T1- and T2-weighted)
  - ▪ findings
    - ♦ acute (within 4-5 d): asymmetric high intensity lesions on T2 MRI in temporal and inferior frontal lobes strongly suggestive
    - ♦ DDx: infarct, tumour, status epilepticus, limbic encephalitis
    - ♦ CT may show low density in temporal lobe and insula; rarely basal ganglia involvement
    - ♦ long-term may show parenchymal loss to affected areas
- • cerebritis/cerebral abscess
  - ▪ pathogenesis: an infection of the brain parenchyma (cerebritis) which can progress to a collection of pus (abscess), most frequently due to hematogenous spread of infectious organisms, commonly located in the distribution of the MCA
    - ♦ pathogens include: S. aureus (often in IV drug users, nosocomial), *Streptococcus*, Gram negative bacteria, Bacteroides
  - ▪ best imaging modality: MRI including DWI imaging series (abscess will be DWI positive); CT still used as a viable alternative
  - ▪ findings according to one of four stages of abscess formation
    - ♦ early cerebritis (1-3 d): inflammatory infiltrate with necrotic centre, low intensity on T1, high intensity on T2
    - ♦ late cerebritis (4-9 d): ring enhancement may be present
    - ♦ early capsule (10-13 d): ring enhancement
    - ♦ late capsule (14 d or greater): well demarcated ring-enhancing lesion, low intensity core, with mass effect; considerable edema around the lesion, seen as hyperintensity on T2

Musculoskeletal System

Modalities

- refer to MI2 for advantages and disadvantages of the following imaging modalities

Plain Film/X-Ray
- usually initial study used in evaluation of bone and joint disorders
- indications: fractures and dislocations, arthritis, assessment of malalignment, orthopedic hardware, and bone tumours (initial)
- minimum of two films orthogonal to each other (usually AP and lateral) to rule out a fracture
- image proximal and distal joints (particularly important with paired bones (e.g. radius/ulna)
- minimally effective in evaluating soft tissue injury

CT
- evaluation of fine bony detail
- indications: assessment of complex, comminuted, intra-articular or occult fractures including distal radius, scaphoid, skull, spine, acetabulum, calcaneus, and sacrum
- evaluation of soft tissue calcification/ossification

MRI
- indications: evaluation of internal derangement of joints (e.g. ligaments, joint capsule, menisci, labrum, cartilage), assessment of tendons and muscle injuries, characterization and staging of soft tissue and bony masses

Ultrasound
- indications: tendon injury (e.g. rotator cuff, Achilles tendon), detection of soft tissue masses and to determine whether cystic or solid, detection of foreign bodies, U/S guided biopsy and injections
- Doppler determines vascularity of structures

Nuclear Medicine (Bone Scintigraphy)
- determine the location and extent of bony lesions
- ^{99m}Tc-methylene diphosphonate localizes to areas of increased bone turnover or calcification – growth plate in children, tumours, infections, fractures, metabolic bone disease (e.g. Paget's), sites of reactive bone formation, and periostitis
- advantages: very sensitive, capable of imaging entire body with relatively low dose radiation
- disadvantages: low specificity, not widely available due to special requirements (e.g. gamma camera, radiopharmaceuticals)

Approach to Bone X-Rays

- identification: name, MRN, age of patient, type of study, region of investigation
- soft tissues: swelling, calcification/ossification
- joints: alignment, joint space, presence of effusion, osteophytes, erosions, bone density, overall pattern, and symmetry of affected joint
- bone: periosteum, cortex, medulla, trabeculae, density, articular surfaces, bone destruction, bone production, appearance of the edges or borders of any lesions

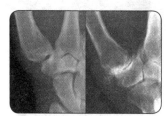

Figure 36. X-ray of first carpometacarpal joint: normal image (left) and osteoarthritis (right) with joint space narrowing and subchondral sclerosis

Trauma

Fracture/Dislocation
- description of fractures
- site of fracture (bone, region of bone, intra-articular vs. extra-articular)
- pattern of fracture line (simple vs. comminuted)
- displacement (distal fragment with reference to the proximal fragment)
- soft tissue involvement (calcification, gas, foreign bodies)
- type of fracture (stress vs. pathologic)
- for specific fracture descriptions and characteristics of fractures, see Orthopedics, OR4

Arthritis

Radiographic Hallmarks of Osteoarthritis
- joint space narrowing – typically non-uniform
- subchondral sclerosis
- subchondral cyst formation
- osteophytes

Radiographic Hallmarks of Rheumatoid Arthritis
- joint space narrowing – typically uniform
- soft tissue swelling
- erosions
- periarticular osteopenia

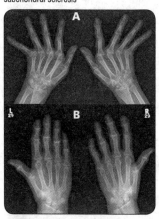

Figure 37. Rheumatoid arthritis (A) compared with osteoarthritis (B) changes on X-ray

Bone Tumour

Approach
- metastatic tumours to bone are much more common than primary bone tumours, particularly if age >40 yr
  - diagnosis usually requires a biopsy if primary not located
  - few benign tumours/lesions have potential for malignant transformation
  - MRI is good for tissue delineation and pre-operative assessment of surrounding soft tissues, neurovascular structures, and medullary/marrow involvement
  - plain film is less sensitive than other modalities but useful for assessing aggressiveness and constructing differential diagnosis

Considerations and Tumour Characteristics

- for specific bone tumours, see Orthopedics, OR45
- age – most common tumours by age group
  - <1 yr of age: metastatic neuroblastoma
  - 1-20 yr of age: Ewing's sarcoma in tubular bones
  - 10-30 yr of age: osteosarcoma and Ewing's tumour in flat bones
  - >40 yr of age: metastases, multiple myeloma, and chondrosarcoma
- multiplicity: metastases, myeloma, lymphoma, fibrous dysplasia, enchondromatosis
- location within bone

epiphysis: giant cell tumour, chondroblastoma, geode, eosinophilic granuloma, infection

metaphysis: simple bone cyst, aneurysmal bone cyst, enchondroma, chondromyxoid fibroma, nonossifying fibroma, osteosarcoma, chondrosarcoma

diaphysis: fibrous dysplasia, aneurysmal bone cyst, brown tumours, eosinophilic granuloma, Ewing's sarcoma

- expansile
  - aneurysmal bone cyst, giant cell tumour, enchondromas, brown tumours, metastases (especially renal and thyroid), plasmacytoma
- matrix mineralization
  - chondroid (popcorn calcification) or osseous
- margin/zone of transition: area between lesion and normal bone
- cortex: intact, disturbed
- periosteal reaction: onion-skinning, sunburst, Codman's triangle, periosteal neocortex
- soft tissue mass

Benign Lesions which may have Aggressive Features
- Osteomyelitis
- Osteoblastoma
- Aneurysmal bone cyst
- Langerhans cell histiocytosis
- Myositis ossificans

Periosteal Reaction
- "Onion skinning" = Ewing's sarcoma
- "Sunburst", "hair on end" = osteosarcoma
- "Codman's triangle" = osteosarcoma, Ewing's sarcoma, subperiosteal abscess

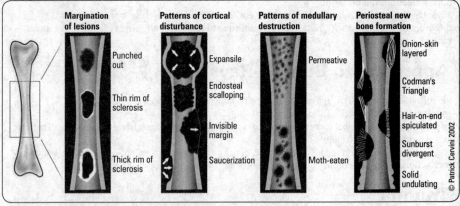

Figure 38. Radiographic appearance of bone remodelling and destruction processes

Table 17. Characteristics of Benign and Malignant Bone Lesions

Benign	Malignant
Thin sclerotic margin/sharp delineation of lesion	Poor delineation of lesion – wide zone of transition
Overlying cortex intact	Loss of overlying cortex/bony destruction
No or simple periosteal reaction	Periosteal reaction
No soft tissue mass	Soft tissue mass

Lytic = decreased density
Sclerotic = increased density

Metastatic Bone Tumours
- all malignancies have potential to metastasize to bone
- metastases are 20-30x more common than primary bone tumours
- metastasis can cause a lytic or a sclerotic reaction when seeding to bone
- when a primary malignancy is first detected, a bone scan is often part of the initial workup
- may present with pathological fractures or pain
- biopsy or determination of primary is the only way to confirm the diagnosis
- most common metastatic bone tumours: breast, prostate, lung, see Orthopedics, OR45

Table 18. Characteristic Bone Metastases of Common Cancers

Lytic	Sclerotic	Expansile	Peripheral
Breast	Prostate	Thyroid	Kidney
Lung	Breast	Renal	Lung
Thyroid	Lymphoma		Melanoma
Kidney	Lung		(KLM: flies to the periphery)
Multiple myeloma	Bowel		
	Medulloblastoma		
	Treated tumours		

Infection

Osteomyelitis
- MRI is the imaging modality of choice for demonstrating bone, bone marrow, and soft tissue abnormalities
- ^{99m}Tc, followed by ^{111}In labeled white cell scan or gallium radioisotope scan
- plain film changes visible 8-10 d after process has begun
  - soft tissue swelling
  - local periosteal reaction
  - pockets of air (from anaerobes) may be seen in the tissues, may also suggest necrotizing fasciitis
  - mottled and nonhomogeneous with a classic "moth-eaten" appearance
  - cortical destruction

Bone Abscess
- overlying cortex has periosteal new bone formation
- sharply outlined radiolucent area with variable thickness in zone of transition
- variable thickness periosteal sclerosis
- sequestrum: a piece of dead bone within a Brodie's abscess
- a sinus tract or cloaca may communicate between the abscess through the cortex to the surface of the bone
- best modality: MRI for bone, bone marrow, and soft tissue abnormalities; CT for sequestra and cortical erosions

Metabolic Bone Disease

Osteoporosis
- reduction in amount of normal bone mass; fewer and thinner trabeculae; diffuse process affecting all bones
- DEXA: gold standard for measuring bone mineral density
  - T-score: the number of standard deviations from the young adult mean, most clinically valuable
    - osteopenia: $-2.5 < \text{T-score} < -1$
    - osteoporosis: T-score ≤ -2.5
  - Z-score: the number of standard deviations from the age-matched mean
  - risk of fracture: related to bone mineral density, age, history of previous fractures, steroid therapy
  - diagnostic sensitivity of DEXA highest when bone mineral density measured at lumbar spine and proximal femur
- appearance on plain film
  - osteopenia: reduced bone density on plain films
    - may also be seen with osteomalacia, hyperparathyroidism, and disuse
  - compression of vertebral bodies
  - biconcave vertebral bodies ("codfish" vertebrae)
  - long bones have appearance of thinned cortex and increased medullary cavity
    - look for complications of osteoporosis (e.g. insufficiency fractures: hip, vertebrae, sacrum, pubic rami)
- see Endocrinology, E40

Osteoporosis
Reduced amount of bone

OsteoMalacia
Normal amount of bone, but reduced
Mineralization of normal osteoid

Osteomalacia/Rickets
- reduction in bone mineral density; normal amount of bone, but reduced mineralization of normal osteoid
- usually due to vitamin D deficiency, resulting in softening and bowing of long bones
- similar to osteoporosis, initial radiological appearance of osteopenia (coarse and poorly defined bone texture)
- "fuzzy", ill-defined trabeculae
- Looser's zones (pseudofracture)
  - characteristic radiologic feature
  - fissures or clefts at right angles to long bones and extending through cortex
  - DDx: chronic renal disease, fibrous dysplasia, hyperthyroidism, Paget's, osteodystrophy, X-linked hypophosphatemia

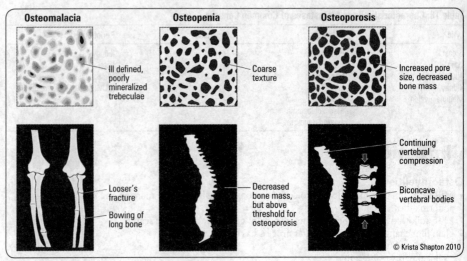

Figure 39. Osteomalacia, osteopenia, and osteoporosis

Hyperparathyroidism
- most common cause is renal failure (secondary hyperparathyroidism)
- chondrocalcinosis
- calcium crystal deposition in hyaline cartilage or fibrocartilage (including arteries and peri-articular soft tissue)
- resorption of bone typically in hands (subperiosteal and at tufts), sacroiliac joints (subchondral), skull ("salt and pepper" appearance), osteoclastoma (brown tumours)
- "rugger jersey spine": band-like osteosclerosis at superior/inferior margins of vertebral bodies

Paget's Disease
- abnormal remodelling involving single or multiple bones – especially skull, spine, pelvis
- 3 phases: 1st phase = lytic, 2nd phase = mixed (lytic/sclerotic), 3rd phase = sclerotic
- features
- coarsening of the trabeculae with bone expansion
- bone softening/bowing
- bone scan will reveal high activity, especially at bone ends
- thickened cortex
- see Endocrinology, E44

Nuclear Medicine

Brain

- ^{99m}Tc-exametazime (HMPAO) and ^{99m}Tc-bicisate (ECD) imaging used in SPECT to assess cerebral blood flow and cellular metabolism, taken up predominantly in grey matter; used for dementia, traumatic brain injury and to a lesser extent vasculitis, neuropsychiatric disorders and occasionally stroke; also the most commonly used tracers to confirm brain death (i.e. absent blood flow to the brain and absent uptake on delayed planar and SPECT images in brain and brainstem, assuming study is technically adequate); either tracer can be used for seizure imaging to assess for the most likely location of epileptogenic focus but usually must be made available for 24 hr and the patient followed by a nurse who is competent to administer the activity at the time of seizure
- PET imaging assesses metabolic activity most commonly with 18FDG; used for dementia imaging, grade and stage of brain tumours, occasionally for seizure disorder imaging, and vasculitis; PET imaging with amyloid tracers for diagnosis of Alzheimer's disease is becoming more common
- CSF imaging, intrathecal administration of ^{111}In DTPA to evaluate CSF leak or to differentiate normal pressure hydrocephalus from brain atrophy
- CSF shunt evaluation for obstruction (most commonly ventriculoperitoneal) with sterile or pyrogen free ^{99m}Tc (usually) or ^{111}In-DTPA; small quantity of activity is injected into the reservoir under sterile conditions and should flow freely into the peritoneal cavity by 45 min; maneuvers such as pumping the shunt, sitting the patient upright or ambulating are acceptable to encourage flow during this time
- adrenergic imaging of the heart with MIBG has been used to differentiate dementias with autonomic dysfunction (i.e. Lewy Body and Parkinson's disease) from other forms of dementia (i.e. autonomic impairment associated with decreased MIBG activity in the heart)

Thyroid

Radioactive Iodine Uptake (see Endocrinology, E21)
- index of thyroid function (trapping and organification of iodine)
- radioactive ^{131}I given PO to fasting patient (small quantity)
- measure percentage of administered iodine taken up by thyroid
- increased RAIU: toxic multinodular goitre, toxic adenoma, Graves' disease
- decreased RAIU: subacute thyroiditis, late Hashimoto's disease, exogenous thyroid hormone or iodine, falsely decreased in patient with recent radiographic contrast studies, high dietary iodine (e.g. seaweed, taking a "thyroid vitamin")
- **important** – iodine uptake helps in the differential of hyperthyroidism only, not hypothyroidism (exception is pediatrics)

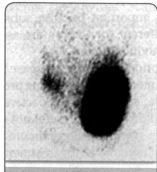

Thyroid Imaging (Scintiscan)
- ^{99m}Tc-pertechnetate IV or radioactive iodine (^{123}I); most Canadian sites use pertechnetate to reduce cost
- provides functional anatomic detail
- hot (hyperfunctioning) lesions: usually benign (e.g. adenoma, toxic multinodular goitre), cancer very unlikely (less than 1%)
- cold (hypofunctioning) lesions: cancer must be considered until biopsy negative even though only 6-10% are cancerous; decision to biopsy should be based on clinical and sonographic features
- isointense i.e. "warm" lesions: cancer must be considered as an isointense lesion may represent cold nodules superimposed on normal tissue; if cyst suspected, correlate with U/S

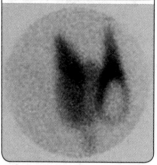

Radioiodine Ablation
- ^{131}I for Graves' disease, multinodular goitre, thyroid cancer (in the case of thyroid cancer, ablation performed at higher dose and after thyroidectomy)
- serum thyroglobulin used to detect recurrent thyroid cancer in a patient that has received ablation
- advice should be given for patient-specific precautions to remain away from family members and caregivers to reduce radiation exposure after thyroid ablation, do not initiate pregnancy for 6 mo, small risk of exophthalmos, thyroid storm, secondary malignancy

Pediatric Hypothyroidism
- pertechnetate thyroid scan can differentiate thyroid agenesis, hemiagenesis, lingular thyroid, organification defect, however should not wait for a diagnosis to start thyroid hormone replacement in a neonate; start immediately

Figure 40. Multinodular goitre (top). Cold nodule (bottom)

Respiratory

V/Q Scan
examine areas of lung in which ventilation and perfusion do not match
- ventilation scan
  - patient breathes radioactive gas (nebulized ^{99m}Tc-DTPA, ^{133}Xe, or most commonly Technegas) through a closed system, filling alveoli proportionally to ventilation
  - ventilation scan defects indicate: airway obstruction (i.e. air trapping), chronic lung disease, bronchospasm, tumour mass obstruction
- perfusion scan
  - radiotracer injected IV (^{99m}Tc-MAA) → trapped in pulmonary capillaries (0.1% of arterioles occluded) according to blood flow
  - relatively contraindicated in severe pulmonary HTN, right-to-left shunt, previous history of pneumonectomy, small child. In these cases fewer particles are usually given
- to rule out PE
  - indications: some institutions favour in pregnancy (lower radiation dose to breast than CT), or where CT contrast contraindicated (e.g. contrast allergy, renal failure)
  - areas of lung are well ventilated but not perfused (unmatched defect) are suspicious for acute infarction
  - defects are wedge-shaped, extend to periphery, usually bilateral and multiple
  - often reported as high probability (> 2 large i.e. segmental mismatched perfusion defects), intermediate, low, very low, or normal according to modified PIOPED II criteria although now are increasingly reported as PE present, indeterminate or normal
  - useful in finding clinically important emboli
  - decreased detection of incidentalomas commonly found on CT
- not valid for assessment of PE when patients have consolidation and the test can be limited by ventilatory problems (e.g. COPD), much like CT
- modified V/Q scan (perfusion only, lower dose contrast) may be used for pregnant patients if CXR is normal or If there are ventilatory problems

Ventilation Scan Defects Indicate
Airway obstruction, chronic lung disease, bronchospasm, tumour mass obstruction

Perfusion Scan Defects Indicate
Reduced blood flow due to PE, COPD, asthma, bronchogenic carcinoma, inflammatory lung diseases (pneumonia, sarcoidosis), mediastinitis, mucous plug, vasculitis

V/Q Scan
For PE investigation: normal scan makes PE unlikely
Probability of PE: high 80-100%, intermediate 20-80%, low <20%, very low <10%

Cardiac

Myocardial Perfusion Scanning

- to investigate coronary artery disease (CAD), assess treatment of CAD, pre op risk stratification, viability testing
- ^{99m}Tc-sestamibi, or ^{99m}Tc-tetrofosmin are used most commonly, thallium 201 was used previously but largely discontinued due to high radiation doses to patients and unfavourable imaging characteristics; today thallium still used for viability studies
- injected at peak exercise (85% max predicted heart rate by the Bruce protocol, chest pain, ECG changes) or after persantine challenge (vasodilator), or dobutamine infusion (chronotropic, again to 85% predicted heart rate); can be done as stress only protocol with optional rest or as stress and rest combined protocol (i.e. as 1 day or 2 day protocol)
- patients with left bundle usually given pharmacologic stress because EKG is difficult to interpret for ST changes and avoids a characteristic artifact
- pharmacologic stress contraindicated if BP is <90 systolic; persantine exacerbates asthma, so patients with asthma and wheeze who cannot exercise usually get dobutamine infusion; reverse persantine with aminophylline or caffeine
- persistent defect (at rest and stress) suggests infarction or myocardial scar; reversible defect (only during stress) suggests ischemia
- used to discriminate between reversible (ischemia) vs. irreversible (infarction) changes when other investigations are equivocal
- Courage trial indicates that patients with >10% ischemic myocardium benefit most from revascularization

- see <u>Cardiology and Cardiac Surgery</u>, C13

Radionuclide Ventriculography

- ^{99m}Tc tagged to red blood cells, tagged albumin is also acceptable
- first pass through RV → pulmonary circulation → LV; provides information about RV function, presence of shunts
- cardiac MUGA scan sums multiple cardiac cycles, usually at least 200 beats
- evaluation of LV function and regional wall motion, ejection fraction
- images are obtained by gating (synchronizing) the count acquisitions to the ECG signal
- can assess diastolic dysfunction
- provides information on ejection fraction (normal = 50-65%), ventricular volume, and wall motion
- indications: most commonly to monitor potential cardiac toxicity with chemotherapy or herceptin, as a gold standard of ejection fraction in defibrillator work up

Abdomen and Genitourinary System

HIDA Scan (Cholescintigraphy)

- IV injection of ^{99m}Tc-disofenin (DISIDA) or ^{99m}Tc-mebrofenin which is bound to protein, taken up, and excreted by hepatocytes into biliary system
- can be performed in non-fasting state but prefer NPO after midnight
- indicated in workup of cholecystitis when abdominal ultrasound result is equivocal:
    - acute cholecystitis: no visualization of gallbladder at 4 h or 1 hour after administration of morphine
    - chronic cholecystitis: no visualization of gallbladder at 1 h but seen at 4 h or after morphine administration
- gallbladder visualized when cystic duct is patent (rules out acute cholecystitis with >99% certainty), usually seen by 30 min to 1 h
- differential diagnosis of obstructed cystic duct: acute/chronic cholecystitis, decreased hepatobiliary function (commonly due to alcoholism), bile duct obstruction, parenteral nutrition, fasting less than 4 h or more than 24 h
- also used to assess bile leaks post-operatively or in trauma
- gallbladder ejection fraction (>38% is normal) can be measured after a fatty meal or CCK to assess for biliary dyskinesia

RBC Scan

- IV injection of radiotracer with sequential images of the abdomen (99mTc RBCs)
- GI bleed
    - if bleeding acutely at <0.5 mL/min, the focus of activity in the images generally indicates the site of the acute bleed, look for a change in shape and location on sequential image, requires active bleeding to localize
    - if bleeding acutely at >0.5 mL/min, use angiography (more specific)
- liver lesion evaluation
    - hemangioma has characteristic appearance: cold early (limited blood flow to lesion), fills in later (accumulation of tagged cells greater than surrounding liver parenchyma)

Other Important Nuclear Medicine Abdominal Tests

- Meckel's Scan: uses Tc 99m pertechnetate; give patient ranitidine premedication; Meckel's diverticulum contains gastric mucosa which will light up at the same time as the stomach and get brighter with time like stomach
- Indium 111 octreoscan: a somatostatin analog used for evaluation and staging of neuroendocrine tumours including carcinoid; gastrinoma and carcinoid tend to be more octeotide avid than insulinoma.
- Iodinated MIBG: a norepinephrine analog, used for pheochromocytoma, neuroblastoma and medullary thyroid cancer most commonly; limited cardiac applications as above
- solid and liquid gastric emptying: a standardized solid or liquid meal is labelled, usually with Tc 99m sulfur colloid and gastric emptying studied over time. There are normal ranges for solids and liquids

Urea Breath Test

- indication: diagnosis of gastric *Helicobacter pylori* infection
- patient administered 14C-labelled urea orally, urea metabolized by *H. pylori* to ammonia and $14CO_2$, 14C-labled CO_2 is measured via plastic filament detectors or liquid scintillation

Functional Renal Imaging

- evaluation of renal function and anatomy using ^{99m}Tc DTPA or Tc 99m MAG3
- frequently used to provide index of relative function between two kidneys
- frequently used in adults to assess for UPJ obstruction (by assessing the clearance half time with lasix), and assess renal transplants or as a nuclear GFR study in patients wanting to donate kidneys
- in children, imaging with Tc 99m DMSA is used to assess for pyelonephritis
- in children, the injection of tracer into the bladder via foley catheter is often used to assess for reflux

Bone

Bone Scan

- isotopes, usually ^{99m}Tc-diphosphonate
- radioactive tracer binds to hydroxyapatite of bone matrix
- increased binding when increased blood supply to bone and/or high bone turnover (active osteoblasts)
- indications: bone pain of unknown origin, staging or restaging of cancer with boney mets (or primary bone cancer), imaging of arthroplasty complications like loosening or infection, osteomyelitis imaging
- when used to assess for osteomyelitis, usually done in combination with gallium or white blood cell scan
- differential diagnosis of positive bone scan: bone metastases (breast, prostate, lung, thyroid), primary bone tumour, arthritis, fracture, infection, anemia, Paget's disease
- lytic lesions like multiple myeloma, renal cell cancer, eosinophilic granuloma: typically normal or cold (false negative); need a skeletal survey
- "superscan": increased bone uptake and poor renal uptake due to diffuse metastases (breast, prostate) or metabolic causes (i.e. renal osteodystrophy)

Interventional Radiology

Vascular Procedures

Angiography

- injection of contrast material through a catheter placed directly into an artery or vein to delineate vascular anatomy
- catheter can be placed into a large vessel (e.g. aorta, vena cava) for a "flush" or selectively placed into a branch vessel for more detailed examination of smaller vessels and specific organs
- indications: diagnosis of primary occlusive or stenotic vascular disease, aneurysms, coronary, carotid and cerebral vascular disease, PE, trauma, bleeding (GI, hemoptysis, hematuria), vascular malformations, as part of endovascular procedures (endovascular aneurysm repair, thrombolysis, stenting, and angioplasties)
- complications (<5% of patients): puncture site hematoma, infection, pseudoaneurysm, AV fistula, dissection, thrombosis, embolic occlusion of a distal vessel
- due to improved technology, non-invasive evaluation of vascular structures is being performed more frequently (colour Doppler U/S, CTA, and MRA)
- see *Neuroradiology*, MI18

Advanced ischemia patients should receive surgery rather than thrombolysis

Advanced ischemia patients should receive surgery rather than thrombolysis

Percutaneous Transluminal Angioplasty and Stents

- introduction and inflation of a balloon into a stenosed or occluded vessel to restore distal blood supply
- common alternative to surgical bypass grafting with 5-yr patency rates similar to surgery, depending on site
- renal, iliac, femoral, mesenteric, subclavian, coronary, and carotid artery stenoses are amenable to treatment
- vascular stents may help improve long-term results by keeping the vessel wall patent after angioplasty
- stents are also used for angioplasty failure or complications

Chemoembolization delivers chemotherapy directly into the tumour through its feeding blood supply and traps the drug in place by embolization

Thrombolytic Therapy for Pulmonary Embolism
Cochrane DB Syst Rev 2009;3:CD004437
Study: Systematic review of RCTs comparing thrombolytic therapy with placebo, heparin, or surgical intervention.
Patients: 679 patients with acute PE.
Intervention: Thrombolytics vs. heparin or placebo.
Outcome: Death rate, recurrence of PE, major and minor hemorrhagic events.
Results: Non-significant difference between thrombolytics and heparin or placebo in all measured outcomes. Rt-PA and heparin together reduced need for treatment for in-hospital events. Thrombolytics improved hemodynamic outcome, lung VQ scans, pulmonary angiography assessment, and echocardiograms greater than heparin. Need for further double-blinded RCTs.
Conclusion: We cannot conclude whether thrombolytic therapy is better than heparin for pulmonary embolism based on limited evidence found.

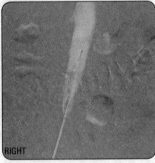

RIGHT

Figure 41. Retrievable IVC filter

Indications for Central Venous Access
FAT CAB
Fluids
Antibiotics
TPN
Chemotherapy
Administration of blood
Blood sampling

- stent grafts (metal mesh covered with durable fabric) may provide an alternative treatment option for aneurysms and AV fistulas
- complications: similar to angiography, but also includes vessel rupture

Thrombolytic Therapy
- may be systemic (IV) or catheter directed
- infusion of a fibrinolytic agent (urokinase, streptokinase, TNK, tPA – used most commonly) via a catheter inserted directly into a thrombus
- can restore blood flow in a vessel obstructed with a thrombus or embolus
- indications: treatment of ischemic limb (most common indication), early treatment of MI or stroke to reduce organ damage, treatment of venous thrombosis (DVT or PE)
- complications: bleeding, stroke, distal embolus, reperfusion injury with myoglobinuria and renal failure if advanced ischemia present

Embolization
- injection of occluding material into vessels
- permanent agents: amplatzer plugs, coils, glue, and onyx
- temporary: gel foam, autologous blood clots
- indications: management of hemorrhage (epistaxis, trauma, GI bleed, GU bleed), treatment of arteriovenous malformation, pre-operative treatment of vascular tumours (bone metastases, renal cell carcinoma), varicocele embolization for infertility, symptomatic uterine fibroids
- complications: post-embolization syndrome (pain, fever, leukocytosis), unintentional embolization of a non-target organ with resultant ischemia

Inferior Vena Cava Filter
- insertion of metallic "umbrellas" to mechanically trap emboli and prevent PE
- may be temporary (retrievable) or permanent
- inserted via femoral vein, jugular vein, or antecubital vein
- usually placed infrarenally to avoid renal vein thrombosis
- indications: contraindication to anticoagulation, failure of adequate anticoagulation (e.g. recurrent PE despite therapeutic anticoagulant levels), complication of anticoagulation

Central Venous Access
- variety of devices available
- PICC, external tunneled catheter (Hickman or dialysis catheters), subcutaneous port (Portacath®)
- indications: chemotherapy, TPN, long-term antibiotics, administration of fluids and blood products, blood sampling
- complications: venous thrombosis and central venous stenosis, infection including sepsis, pneumothorax

Nonvascular Interventions

Percutaneous Biopsy
- replaces open surgical procedure
- many sites are amenable to biopsy using U/S, fluoroscopy, CT or MR guidance
- complications: false negative (sampling error or tissue necrosis), pneumothorax in 30% of lung biopsies (chest tube required in ~5%), acute pancreatitis (pancreatic biopsies), bleeding from liver biopsies in patients with uncorrectable coagulopathies or ascites (can be minimized with transjugular approach)

Abscess Drainage
- placement of a drainage catheter into an infected fluid collection
- administer broad spectrum IV antibiotics prior to procedure
- routes: percutaneous (most common), transgluteal, transvaginal, transrectal
- complications: hemorrhage, injury to intervening structures (e.g. bowel), bacteremia, sepsis

Percutaneous Biliary Drainage/Cholecystostomy
- placement of drainage catheter ± metallic stent into obstructed biliary system (PBD) or gallbladder (cholecystostomy) for relief of jaundice or infection
- percutaneous gallbladder access can be used to crush or remove stones
- indications
  - cholecystostomy: acute cholecystitis
  - PBD: biliary obstruction secondary to stone or tumour, cholangitis
- complications
  - acute: sepsis, hemorrhage
  - long-term: tumour ingrowth and stent occlusion

Percutaneous Nephrostomy
- placement of catheter into renal collecting system
- indications: hydronephrosis, pyonephrosis, ureteric injury with or without urinary peritonitis (traumatic or iatrogenic)
- complications: bacteria and septic shock, hematuria due to pseudoaneurysm or AV fistulas, injury to adjacent organs

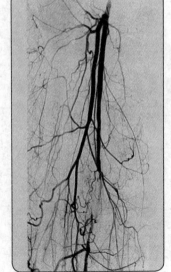

Figure 42. Femoral arteriogram: distal occlusion of superficial femoral artery

Gastrostomy/Gastrojejunostomy
- percutaneous placement of catheter directly into either stomach (gastrostomy) or through stomach into small bowel (transgastric jejunostomy)
- indications: inability to eat (most commonly CNS lesion e.g. stroke) or esophageal obstruction, decompression in gastric outlet obstruction
- complications: gastroesophageal reflux with aspiration, peritonitis, hemorrhage, bowel or solid organ injury

Radiofrequency Ablation
- U/S or CT guided probe is inserted into tumour, radiofrequency energy delivered through probe causes heat deposition and tissue destruction
- indications: hepatic tumours (HCC and metastases), renal tumours
- complications: destruction of neighbouring tissues and structures, bleeding

Breast Imaging

Modalities

Mammography

Description
- x-ray imaging of the breasts for screening in asymptomatic patients, or diagnosis of clinically-detected or screening-detected abnormalities (see General Surgery, GS56)
- routine evaluation involves two standard views: cranio-caudal and medial-lateral-oblique

Indications
- screening
  - begin screening from age 50 q2 yr
  - no strong data to support screening >70 yr, but may continue screening if in good general health
  - if <50, screening is only recommended for those with high risk of breast cancer
  - screening detects 2-8 cancers/1,000 women screened
- surveillance
  - follow-up of women with previous breast cancer
- diagnostic: includes mammography with special views and/or ultrasound
  - work-up of an abnormality that may be suggestive of breast cancer including a lump or thickening, localized nodularity, dimpling or contour deformity, a persistent focal area of pain, and spontaneous serous or sanguinous nipple discharge from a single duct
  - women with abnormal screening mammograms
  - suspected complications of breast implants

Table 19. Breast Imaging Reporting and Data System (BI-RADS®) Mammography Categories

Assessment Categories	Imaging Findings	Follow-Up Recommendations
BI-RADS 0	Incomplete	Additional imaging Comparison to prior films
BI-RADS 1	Negative	Routine screening
BI-RADS 2	Benign	Routine screening
BI-RADS 3	Probably benign Likelihood of malignancy is <2%	Unilateral mammogram at 6 mo
BI-RADS 4	Suspicious abnormality	Biopsy
BI-RADS 5	Highly suspicious of malignancy Likelihood of malignancy is 95%	Biopsy
BI-RADS 6	Malignancy confirmed by biopsy	Definitive therapy

Breast Ultrasound

Indications
- characterization of palpable abnormalities (ultrasound 1st line <30 yr and in lactating and pregnant women, >30 yr need mammogram 1st)
- further characterization of mammographic findings
- guidance for interventional procedures

Breast MRI

Description
- contrast enhanced MRI of the breasts
- sensitive for detecting invasive breast cancer (95-100%) but specificity variable (37-97%)
- for diagnosis, used only after mammography and U/S investigation
- use as a screening modality is limited to high risk patients, in conjunction with mammography

Indications
- "problem solving" of indeterminate findings following complete mammographic and ultrasound work up
- evaluation of patients with suspected silicone implant rupture and problems associated with breast implants
- evaluation of previously diagnosed breast cancer: positive margins, recurrence, response to chemotherapy
- High Risk Screening
  - known BRCA1 or BRCA2 mutation, or other gene predisposing to breast cancer or untested first-degree relative of a carrier of such a gene mutation
  - family history consistent with a hereditary breast cancer syndrome and/or estimated personal lifetime cancer risk >25%
  - high-risk marker on prior biopsy (atypical ductal hyperplasia, atypical lobular hyperplasia, lobular carcinoma in situ)
  - radiation therapy to chest (before age 30)

Breast Interventional Procedures

Description
- includes fine needle aspirate biopsy, core needle biopsy, stereotactic biopsy, MRI guided biopsy, abscess drainage, and cyst aspiration (see <u>General Surgery</u>, GS59)

Indications
- cystic mass: complex cyst, symptomatic, suspected abscess
- solid mass: confirm diagnosis of a lesion suspicious for malignancy (BI-RADS® Category 4 or 5)
- suspicious calcifications: confirm diagnosis of a lesion suspicious for malignancy (BI-RADS® Category 4 or 5) – stereotactic biopsy
- initial percutaneous biopsy procedure that was insufficient or discordant with imaging
- presurgical wire localization of a lesion

Breast Findings

Breast Masses
- definition: a space occupying lesion seen in two different projections; if seen in only a single projection it should be called an "asymmetry" until its three-dimensionality is confirmed

Table 20. Mammographic Features of Benign and Malignant Breast Masses

	Benign	Malignant
Shape	Oval, round, lobular	Irregular
Margin	Circumscribed, well-defined	Indistinct, microlobulated, spiculated
Density	Radiolucent (oil cyst, lipoma, fibrolipoma, galactocele, hamartoma)	Radiodense
Calcifications (± mass)	Popcorn (hyalinizing fibroadenoma), lucent centred (oil cyst/fat necrosis), layering (milk of calcium), vascular, round, scattered	Pleomorphic (vary in size and shape), amorphous (indistinct), fine linear, coarse heterogeneous, regional, segmental, clustered

Other Findings
- tubular density/dilated duct: branching tubular structures usually represent enlarged ducts (milk ducts); if they are clearly identified as such, these densities are of little concern
- intramammary lymph node: typical lymph nodes are circumscribed, reniform and often have a fatty notch and centre; usually less than 1 cm, and usually seen in the outer, often upper part of the breast; when these characteristics (particularly fatty centre or notch) are well seen, the lesion is almost always benign and insignificant
- focal asymmetry: area of breast density with similar shape on two views, but completely lacking borders and conspicuity of a true mass; must be carefully evaluated with focal compression to exclude findings of a true mass or architectural distortion
- if focal compression shows mass-like character, or if the area can be palpated, biopsy generally recommended

References

American College of Radiology (ACR) breast imaging reporting and data system atlas (BI-RADS atlas). Reston: American College of Radiology, 2003.
Brant WE, Helms CA. Fundamentals of diagnostic radiology. Philadelphia: Lippincott Williams and Wilkins, 1999.
Canadian Association of Radiologists (CAR) standard for breast imaging. Ottawa: Canadian Association of Radiologists, 1998.
Canadian Association of Radiologists (CAR) standard for performance of breast ultrasound examination. Ottawa: Canadian Association of Radiologists, 2003.
Canadian Association of Radiologists (CAR) standards for the performance of ultrasound-guided percutaneous breast interventional procedures. Ottawa: Canadian Association of Radiologists, 2003.
Chen MYM, Pope TL, Ott DJ. Basic radiology. New York: Lange Medical Books/McGraw Hill, 2004.
Daffner RH. Clinical radiology: the essentials. Baltimore: Williams & Wilkins, 1993.
Erkonen WE, Smith WL. Radiology 101. Philadelphia: Lippincott Williams & Wilkins, 2005.
Fleckenstein P, Tranun-Jensen J. Anatomy in diagnostic imaging, 2nd ed. Copenhagen: Blackwell Publishing, 2001.
Gay S, Woodcock Jr RJ. Radiology recall. Baltimore: Lippincott Williams & Wilkins, 2000.
Goldstein S. Saline infusion sonohysterogram. Rose BD (editor). Waltham: UpToDate. 2012.
Goodman LR. Felson's principles of chest roentgenology: a programmed text, 3rd ed. Philadelphia: Saunders Elsevier, 2007.
Joffe SA, Servaes S, Okon S, et al. Multi-detector row CT urography in the evaluation of hematuria. Radiographics 2003;23:1441-1455.
Juhl JH, Crummy AB, Kuhlman JE (editors). Paul and Juhl's essentials of radiologic imaging. Philadelphia: Lippincott-Raven, 1998.
Katz DS, Math KR, Groskin SA. Radiology secrets. Philadelphia: Hanley and Belfus, 1998.
Mettler FA Jr, Huda W, Yoshizumi TT, et al. Effective doses in radiology and diagnostic nuclear medicine: a catalog. Radiology 2008;248:254-263.
Novelline RA. Squire's fundamentals of radiology, 6th ed. Cambridge: Harvard University Press, 2004.
Ouellette H, Tetreault P. Clinical radiology made ridiculously simple. Miami: MedMaster, 2002.
Owen RJ, Hiremath S, Myers A, et al. Canadian Association of Radiologists consensus guidelines for the prevention of contrast-induced nephropathy: update 2012. Can Assoc Radiol J 2014;65:96-105.
Som PM, Curtin HD. Head and neck imaging, 3rd ed. St. Louis: Mosby, 1996.
Smith DL, Heldt JP, Richards GD, et al. Radiation exposure during continuous and pulsed fluoroscopy. J Endourol 2013;27(3):384-388.
Warner E, Messersmith H, Causer P, et al. Cancer Care Ontario's Program in Evidence-based Care. 2007. Magnetic resonance imaging screening of women at high risk for breast cancer: a clinical practice guideline. Available from: https://www.cancercare.on.ca/common/pages/UserFile.aspx?fileId=155763.
Warner E, Messersmith H, Causer P, et al. Magnetic resonance imaging screening of women at high risk for breast cancer: a clinical practice guideline. Program in Evidence-Based Care. Cancer Care Ontario, 2007.
Weissleder R, Rieumont MJ, Wittenberg J. Primer of diagnostic imaging, 2nd ed. Philadelphia: Mosby, 1997.
Young WF. Clinical practice. The incidentally discovered adrenal mass. NEJM 2007;356:601-610.

Notes

NP Nephrology

Elliot Lass, Jonathan Ripstein, and Roman Zyla, chapter editors
Claudia Frankfurter and Inna Gong, associate editors
Brittany Provost and Robert Vanner, EBM editors
Dr. Ramesh Prasad and Dr. Gemini Tanna, staff editors

Acronyms

ACEI	angiotensin converting enzyme inhibitor	CHF	congestive heart failure	GBM	glomerular basement membrane	R&M	routine and microscopy
ACR	albumin to creatinine ratio	CKD	chronic kidney disease	GFR	glomerular filtration rate	RAAS	renin-angiotensin-aldosterone system
ADH	antidiuretic hormone	Cr	creatinine	GN	glomerulonephritis	RBF	renal blood flow
AG	anion gap	CrCl	creatinine clearance	HCTZ	hydrochlorothiazide	RPF	renal plasma flow
AIN	acute interstitial nephritis	D5W	5% dextrose in water	HPF	high power field	RCC	renal cell carcinoma
AKI	acute kidney injury	DCT	distal convoluted tubule	HSP	Henoch-Schönlein purpura	RPGN	rapidly progressive glomerulonephritis
ANA	antinuclear antibody	DDAVP	1-desamino-8-d-arginine vasopressin	HTN	hypertension	RRT	renal replacement therapy
ARB	angiotensin receptor blocker	DI	diabetes insipidus	HUS	hemolytic uremic syndrome	RTA	renal tubular acidosis
ASA	acetylsalicylic acid	DIC	disseminated intravascular coagulation	IVP	intravenous pyelogram	SIADH	syndrome of inappropriate antidiuretic hormone
ASOT	anti-streptolysin-O titer	DKA	diabetic ketoacidosis	LOC	level of consciousness		
ATN	acute tubular necrosis	DM	diabetes mellitus	MDRD	modification of diet in renal disease	SLE	systemic lupus erythematosis
AVM	arteriovenous malformation	eGFR	estimated glomerular filtration rate	NS	normal saline	TBW	total body water
c-ANCA	cytoplasmic antineutrophil cytoplasmic antibody	ESR	erythrocyte sedimentation rate	p-ANCA	perinuclear anti-neutrophil cytoplasmic antibody	TIN	tubulointerstitial nephritis
		ESRD	end-stage renal disease			TTP	thrombotic thrombocytopenic purpura
C&S	culture and sensitivity	FF	filtration fraction	PCKD	polycystic kidney disease	UAG	urine anion gap
		FSGS	focal segmental glomerulosclerosis	PTH	parathyroid hormone	UTI	urinary tract infection

Basic Anatomy Review

Anatomy of the Kidney

- see Urology, U2

Renal Structure and Function

The Nephron
- basic structural and functional unit of the kidney, approximately 1 million per kidney
- 2 main components: glomerulus and attached renal tubule
- direction of blood flow: afferent arteriole → glomerular capillaries → efferent arteriole → vasa recta (the capillaries surrounding the tubules) → renal venules

Table 1. Major Kidney Functions

Function	Mechanism	Affected Elements
1. Waste Excretion	Glomerular filtration	Excretion of nitrogenous products of protein metabolism (urea, Cr)
	Tubular secretion	Excretion of organic acids (urate) and organic bases (Cr)
	Tubular catabolism	Breakdown and excretion of drugs (antibiotics, diuretics) and peptide hormones (most pituitary hormones, insulin, glucagon)
2. Electrolyte Balance and Osmoregulation	Tubular NaCl and water reabsorption	Controls volume status and osmolar balance
	Tubular K^+ secretion	Controls potassium concentration
	Tubular H^+ secretion	Acid-base balance
	HCO_3^- synthesis and reabsorption	Acid-base balance
	Tubular Ca^{2+}, Mg^{2+}, PO_4^{3-} transport	Alters Ca^{2+}, Mg^{2+}, PO_4^{3-} homeostasis
	Synthesize osmolytes	Increase osmolality of medullary cytoplasm to match medullary concentration gradient
3. Hormonal Synthesis	Erythropoietin production (cortex)	Red blood cell production
	Vitamin D activation: 25(OH)VitD converted to 1,25(OH)₂VitD (proximal tubule)	Calcium homeostasis
	Renin production (juxtaglomerular apparatus)	Alters vascular resistance and aldosterone secretion
4. Blood Pressure Regulation	Na^+ excretion	Alters ECF volume
	Renin production	Alters vascular resistance
5. Glucose Homeostasis	Gluconeogenesis (from lactate, pyruvate, and amino acids)	Glucose supply maintained in prolonged starvation
	Clearance and degradation of circulating insulin	Maintains glucose homeostasis

The Glomerulus
- site where blood constituents are filtered through to the kidney tubules for excretion or reabsorption
- filtration occurs across the glomerular filtration barrier (endothelium, GBM, podocytes) into Bowman's space
- particles are selectively filtered by size (<60 kDa) and charge (negative charge repelled)

- consists of following cell types
  1. Mesangial cells
     - structural cells that support the vascular tree; they are also contractile and produce vasoactive substances to help control blood flow
  2. Capillary endothelial cells
     - one of the cells of the glomerular filtration barrier; help form the plasma filtration apparatus due to their sinusoidal nature and glycocalyx; contribute to the production of the GBM
  3. Visceral epithelium (podocytes)
     - one of the cells of the glomerular filtration barrier; help form the plasma filtration apparatus due to their interdigitated foot process that form slit diaphragms; contribute to the production of the GBM
  4. Parietal epithelium
     - lines the interior of Bowman's capsule and contains a podocyte progenitor population
  5. Juxtaglomerular cells
     - smooth muscle cells in lining of afferent arteriole; produce, store and secrete renin

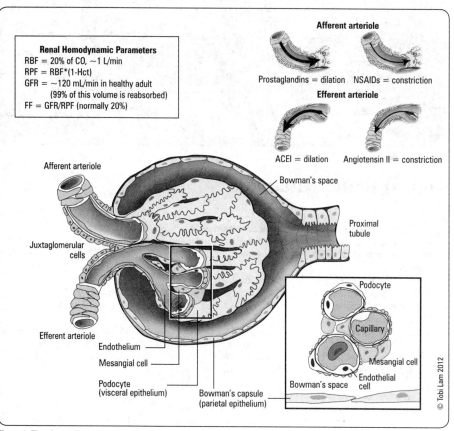

Renal Hemodynamic Parameters
RBF = 20% of CO, ~1 L/min
RPF = RBF*(1-Hct)
GFR = ~120 mL/min in healthy adult
      (99% of this volume is reabsorbed)
FF = GFR/RPF (normally 20%)

Afferent arteriole
Prostaglandins = dilation   NSAIDs = constriction

Efferent arteriole
ACEI = dilation   Angiotensin II = constriction

Afferent arteriole

Bowman's space

Proximal tubule

Juxtaglomerular cells

Podocyte

Capillary

Efferent arteriole

Endothelium

Mesangial cell

Mesangial cell

Endothelial cell

Bowman's space

Podocyte (visceral epithelium)

Bowman's capsule (parietal epithelium)

© Tobi Lam 2012

Figure 1. The glomerulus

The Renal Tubules

- reabsorption and secretion occur between the renal tubules and vasa recta forming urine for excretion
- each segment of the tubule selectively transports various solutes and water and is targeted by specific diuretics

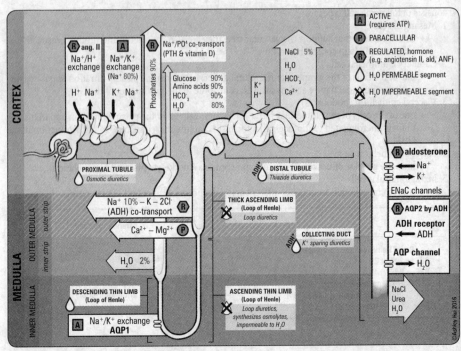

Figure 2. Tubular segments of the nephron

Renal Hemodynamics

- GFR
  - GFR is the sum of the filtration across all nephrons
  - the rate of fluid transfer between glomerular capillaries and Bowman's space
  - average 180 L/d, of which 99% is reabsorbed, giving a urine output of 1.0-1.5 L/d to match oral fluid intake
  - normal urine output is 0.5-2.0 ml/kg/h in adults
  - GFR is highest in early adulthood, and decreases thereafter starting around age 40
- renal autoregulation maintains constant GFR over mean arterial pressures of 70-180 mmHg
- 2 mechanisms of autoregulation
  - myogenic mechanism: release of vasoactive factors such as prostaglandins in response to changes in perfusion pressure (e.g. → perfusion pressure → afferent arteriolar constriction → ↓ GFR)
  - tubuloglomerular feedback: changes in Na+ delivery to macula densa lead to changes in afferent arteriolar tone (e.g. increased delivery causes afferent constriction)
- FF
  - percentage of RPF filtered across the glomeruli
  - expressed as a ratio: FF = GFR/RPF; normal = 0.2 or 20%
  - angiotensin II constricts renal efferent arterioles which increases FF, thereby maintaining GFR
- renin is released from juxtaglomerular apparatus in response to decreased RPF and maintain sodium balance

Glomerular Filtration Rate

GFR = $Kf (\Delta P - \Delta\Pi)$

Kf = ultrafiltration coefficient

ΔP = hydrostatic pressure difference between glomerular capillaries and Bowman's space

$\Delta\Pi$ = osmotic pressure difference between glomerular capillaries and Bowman's space

$\Delta P - \Delta\Pi$ = net outward pressure

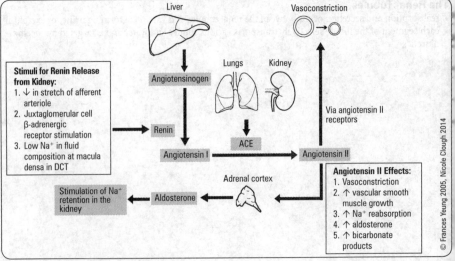

Figure 3. Renin-angiotensin-aldosterone system

Assessment of Renal Function

Measurement of Renal Function

- clinically, GFR is estimated using serum creatinine concentration, [Cr]
- inulin clearance is the gold standard for measuring GFR, but very rarely used clinically
- most renal functions decline in parallel with a decrease in GFR
- Cr is a metabolite of creatine (intermediate in muscle metabolism), therefore increased muscle mass increases Cr production
- Cr is freely filtered at the glomerulus with little tubular reabsorption
- tubular secretion of Cr varies based on level of renal function (10% to >50%)
- Cr filtered ≈ Cr excreted (at steady state)

Ways to Estimate GFR Using Serum Creatinine Concentration
1. Measure CrCl
    - calculation provides reasonable estimate of GFR
        - GFR/d = (urine [Cr] x 24 h urine volume)/(plasma [Cr])
        - must use same units for urine [Cr] and plasma [Cr]
2. Estimate CrCl using Cockcroft-Gault formula
    - serum Cr used along with age, gender, and weight (kg) to estimate GFR
    - overestimate GFR when renal function severely impaired
3. Estimate GFR using MDRD formula
    - most common way in which GFR is estimated (MDRD 7 equation)
    - complex formula incorporating age, gender, serum Cr, and African descent, but does not include weight
    - GFR is reported as mL/min/1.73 m² body surface area
    - underestimation of GFR at near normal values
4. Estimate GFR using CKD-EPI equation
    - the best current equation
    - calculated using serum Cr, age, sex, and race
    - overestimate GFR

Limitations of Using Serum Cr Measurements
1. must be in steady state
    - constant GFR and rate of production of Cr from muscles
    - sudden injury (e.g. AKI) may reduce GFR substantially, however, serum Cr will not immediately reflect sudden reduction in GFR until new Cr steady-state is reached
2. GFR must fall substantially before plasma [Cr] rises above normal laboratory range
    - with progressive renal failure, remaining nephrons compensate with hyperfiltration
    - GFR is relatively preserved despite significant structural damage
3. plasma [Cr] is influenced by the rate of Cr production
    - lower production with smaller muscle mass (e.g. female, elderly, low weight)
        - for example, consider plasma [Cr] of 100 μmol/L in both of these patients
            - 20 yr old man who weighs 100 kg, GFR = 144 mL/min
            - 80 yr old woman who weighs 50 kg, GFR = 30.6 mL/min
    - clinical correlation: GFR decreases with age but would not be reflected as a rise in serum Cr due to the age-associated decline in muscle mass
4. tubular secretion of Cr increases as GFR decreases
    - serum Cr and CrCl overestimate low GFR
    - certain drugs (cimetidine, trimethoprim) interfere with Cr secretion
5. errors in Cr measurement
    - very high bilirubin level causes [Cr] to be falsely low
    - acetoacetate (a ketone body) and certain drugs (cefoxitin) create falsely high [Cr]

Measurement of Urea Concentration
- urea is the major end-product of protein metabolism
- plasma urea concentration reflects renal function but should not be used alone as it is modified by a variety of other factors
- urea production reflects dietary intake of protein and catabolic rate; increased protein intake or catabolism (sepsis, trauma, GI bleed) causes urea level to rise
- ECF volume depletion causes a rise in urea independent of GFR or plasma [Cr]
- in addition to filtration, a significant amount of urea is reabsorbed along the tubule
- reabsorption is increased in hypernatremic states
- typical ratio of urea to [Cr] in serum is 1:12 in SI units (using mmol/L for urea and μmol/L for Cr)

$Cr_{filtered} = Cr_{excreted}$
$[Cr]_{plasma} \times GFR = [Cr]_{urine} \times$ urine flow rate (mL/min)
$GFR = \dfrac{[Cr]_{urine} \times \text{urine flow rate}}{[Cr]_{plasma}}$

At steady state $[Cr]_{serum} \propto 1/CrCl$

Cockcroft-Gault Formula
$CrCl\ (mL/min) = \dfrac{(\text{weight in kg}) (140\text{-age}) \times 1.23}{(\text{serum creatinine } (\mu mol/L)}$

Multiply above by 0.85 for females

MDRD Equation
$GFR\ (mL/min/1.73\ m^2) = 186 \times (S_{cr})^{-1.154} \times (Age)^{-0.203} \times (0.742\text{ if female}) \times (1.212\text{ if African American})$

Cystatin C
Cystatin C is a protease which is completely filtered by the glomerulus and is not affected by muscle mass; it is not currently used in clinical practice, but may be a more accurate way to measure renal function in the future, particularly in DM

Clinical Settings in which Urea Level is Affected Independent of Renal Function

Disproportionately High Urea
- Volume depletion (prerenal azotemia)
- GI hemorrhage
- High protein diet
- Sepsis
- Catabolic state with tissue breakdown
- Corticosteroid or cytotoxic agents

Disproportionately Low Urea
- Low protein diet
- Liver disease

Urinalysis

- use dipstick in freshly voided urine specimen to assess the following:

1. Specific Gravity
- ratio of the mass of equal volumes of urine/H2O
- range is 1.001 to 1.030
- values <1.010 reflect dilute urine, values >1.020 reflect concentrated urine
- value usually 1.010 in ESRD (isosthenuria: same specific gravity as plasma)

2. pH
- urine pH is normally between 4.5-7.0; if persistently alkaline, consider
  - RTA
  - UTI with urease-producing bacteria (e.g. *Proteus*)

3. Glucose
- freely filtered at glomerulus and reabsorbed in proximal tubule
- causes of glucosuria include
  1. hyperglycemia >9-11 mmol/L leads to filtration that exceeds tubular resorption capacity
  2. increased GFR (e.g. pregnancy)
  3. proximal tubule dysfunction (e.g. Fanconi's syndrome)

4. Protein
- dipstick only detects albumin; other proteins (e.g. Bence-Jones, Ig, Tamm-Horsfall) may be missed
- microalbuminuria (morning ACR of 2.0 - 20 mg/mmol) is not detected by standard dipstick, greater than these ranges would be macroalbuminuria (see *Diabetes*, NP31)
- sulfosalicylic acid detects all protein in urine by precipitation
- gold standard: 24 h timed urine collection for total protein

5. Leukocyte Esterase
- enzyme found in WBC and detected by dipstick
- presence of WBCs indicates infection (e.g. UTI) or inflammation (e.g. AIN)

6. Nitrites
- nitrates in urine are converted by some bacteria to nitrites
- high specificity but low sensitivity for UTI

7. Ketones
- positive in alcoholic/diabetic ketoacidosis, prolonged starvation, fasting

8. Hemoglobin
- positive in hemoglobinuria (hemolysis), myoglobinuria (rhabdomyolysis), and true hematuria (RBCs seen on microscopy)

Urine Microscopy

Table 2. Comparison of Urinary Sediment Findings

	Active Sediment = Suggestive of Parenchymal Kidney Disease	Bland Sediment = Less Likely Parenchymal Kidney Disease
Any one or more of the following seen on microscopy	Red cell casts	Only hyaline casts
	White cell casts	Small quantities of crystals
	Muddy-brown granular or epithelial cell casts	Small amount of bacteria
	>2 red cells per HPF	<2 red cells per HPF
	>4 white cells per HPF	<4 white cells per HPF

1. CELLS

Erythrocytes
- hematuria = greater than normal range of 2-3 RBCs per HPF
- dysmorphic RBCs and/or RBC casts suggest glomerular bleeding (e.g. proliferative GN)
- isomorphic RBCs, no casts suggest extraglomerular bleeding (e.g. bladder Ca)

Leukocytes
- pyuria = greater than upper limit of normal: 3 WBCs per HPF
- indicates inflammation or infection
- if persistent sterile pyuria present (i.e. negative culture), consider: chronic urethritis, prostatitis, interstitial nephritis, calculi, papillary necrosis, renal TB, viral infections

Eosinophils
- detected using Wright's or Hansel's stain (not affected by urine pH)
- consider AIN, atheroembolic disease

Oval Fat Bodies
- renal tubular cells filled with lipid droplets
- seen in heavy proteinuria (e.g. nephrotic syndrome)

2. CASTS
- cylindrical structures formed by intratubular precipitation of Tamm-Horsfall mucoprotein; cells may be trapped within the matrix of protein

Table 3. Interpretation of Casts

Casts	Interpretation
Hyaline casts	Physiologic (concentrated urine, fever, exercise)
RBC casts	Glomerular bleeding (GN, vasculitis)
WBC casts	Infection (pyelonephritis) Inflammation (interstitial nephritis)
Pigmented granular casts (heme granular casts, muddy brown)	ATN Acute GN
Fatty casts	Nephrotic Syndrome (>3.5 g/d)

3. CRYSTALS
- uric acid: consider acid urine, hyperuricosuria
- calcium phosphate: alkaline urine
- calcium oxalate: consider hyperoxaluria, ethylene glycol poisoning
- sulfur: sulfa-containing antibiotics

Urine Biochemistry

- commonly measure: Na^+, K^+, Cl^-, osmolality, and pH
- no "normal" values; electrolyte excretion depends on intake and current physiological state
- results must be interpreted in the context of a patient's current state, for example:
  1. ECF volume depletion: expect low urine $[Na^+]$ (kidneys should be retaining Na^+)
     - urine $[Na^+]$ >20 mmol/L suggests a renal problem or the action of a diuretic
     - urine $[Na^+]$ <20 mmol/L suggests a prerenal problem
  2. daily urinary potassium excretion rate should be decreased (<20 mmol/d) in hypokalemia
     - if higher than 20 mmol/d, suggests renal contribution to hypokalemia
- osmolality is useful to estimate the kidney's concentrating ability
- FE_{Na} refers to the fractional excretion of Na^+
  - FE_{Na} <1% suggests the pathology is prerenal
- urine pH is useful to grossly assess renal acidification
  - low pH (<5.5) in the presence of low serum pH is an appropriate renal response
  - a high pH in this setting might indicate a renal acidification defect (e.g. RTA)

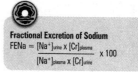

Fractional Excretion of Sodium
$$FE_{Na} = \frac{[Na^+]_{urine} \times [Cr]_{plasma}}{[Na^+]_{plasma} \times [Cr]_{urine}} \times 100$$

Electrolyte Disorders

Sodium Homeostasis

- hyponatremia and hypernatremia are disorders of water balance
  - hyponatremia usually suggests too much water in the ECF relative to Na^+ content
  - hypernatremia usually suggests too little water in the ECF relative to Na^+ content
- solutes (such as Na^+, K^+, glucose) that cannot freely traverse the plasma membrane contribute to effective osmolality and induce transcellular shifts of water
  - water moves out of cells in response to increased ECF osmolality
  - water moves into cells in response to decreased ECF osmolality
- ECF volume is determined by Na^+ content rather than concentration
  - Na^+ deficiency leads to ECF volume contraction
  - Na^+ excess leads to ECF volume expansion
- clinical signs and symptoms of hyponatremia and hypernatremia are secondary to cells (especially in the brain) shrinking (hypernatremia) or swelling (hyponatremia)

Table 4. Clinical Assessment of ECF Volume (Total Body Na⁺)

Fluid Compartment	Hypovolemic	Hypervolemic
Intravascular		
JVP	Decreased	Increased
Blood pressure	Orthostatic drop	Normal to increased
Auscultation of heart	Tachycardia	S3
Auscultation of lungs	Normal	Inspiratory crackles
Interstitial		
Skin turgor	Decreased	Normal/increased
Edema (dependent)	Absent	Present
Other		
Urine output	Decreased*	Variable
Body weight	Decreased	Increased
Hematocrit, serum protein	Increased	Decreased

*If there is a renal abnormality (e.g. osmotic diuresis), the urine output may be increased despite the presence of hypovolemia

Hyponatremia

If the urine osmolality is unknown, assume the urine is hypo-osmolar/dilute

- hyponatremia: serum [Na⁺] <135 mmol/L
- can be associated with hypo-osmolality (most common), iso-osmolality, or hyperosmolality
- consider if it is "appropriate" vs. "inappropriate" ADH secretion
- if appropriate ADH secretion, is it real vs. effective volume loss?

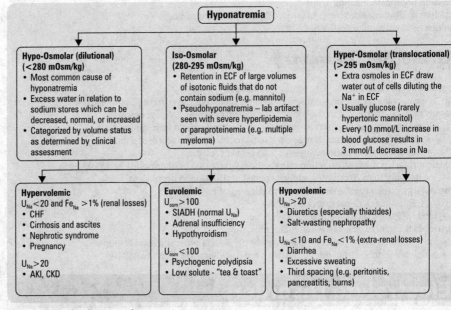

Figure 4. Approach to hyponatremia

Signs and Symptoms
- depend on degree of hyponatremia and more importantly, velocity of progression from onset
- hyponatremia = swollen cells
- acute hyponatremia (<24-48 h) more likely to be symptomatic
- chronic hyponatremia (>24-48 h) less likely to be symptomatic due to adaptation
  - adaptation: normalization of brain volume through loss of cellular electrolytes (within hours) and organic osmolytes (within days)
- adaptation is responsible for the risks associated with overly rapid correction
- neurologic symptoms predominate (secondary to cerebral edema): headache, nausea, malaise, lethargy, weakness, muscle cramps, anorexia, somnolence, disorientation, personality changes, depressed reflexes, decreased LOC

Complications
- seizures, coma, respiratory arrest, permanent brain damage, brainstem herniation, death
- risk of brain cell shrinkage with rapid correction of hyponatremia
  - can develop osmotic demyelination of pontine and extrapontine neurons; may be irreversible (e.g. central pontine myelinolysis: cranial nerve palsies, quadriplegia, decreased LOC)

Symptoms of Central Pontine Myelinolysis
- Cranial nerve palsies
- Quadriplegia
- Decreased LOC

Risk Factors for Osmotic Demyelination
- rise in serum [Na$^+$] with correction >8 mmol/L/24 hr if chronic hyponatremia
- associated hypokalemia and/or malnutrition (e.g. low muscle mass)
- if patient with hyponatremia and hypovolemia is given large volume of isotonic fluid (ADH is stimulated by hypovolemia; when hypovolemia is corrected, the ADH level falls suddenly causing sudden brisk water diuresis, and therefore rapid rise in serum Na$^+$ level)
- patient with psychogenic polydipsia, deprived of water

Investigations
- ECF volume status assessment (see Table 4)
- serum electrolytes, glucose, Cr
- serum osmolality, urine osmolality
- urine Na$^+$ (urine Na$^+$ <10-20 mmol/L suggests volume depletion as the cause of hyponatremia)
- assess for causes of SIADH (see Table 5)
- TSH, free T4, and cortisol levels
- consider CXR and possibly CT chest if suspect pulmonary cause of SIADH (e.g. paraneoplastic syndrome by small cell lung cancer)
- consider CT head if suspect CNS cause of SIADH

Treatment of Hyponatremia
- general measures for all patients
  1. treat underlying cause (e.g. restore ECF volume if volume depleted, remove offending drug, treat pain, nausea, etc.)
  2. restrict free water intake
  3. promote free water loss
  4. carefully monitor serum Na+, urine volume, and urine tonicity
  5. ensure frequently that correction is not occurring too rapidly
     - monitor urine output frequently: high output of dilute urine is the first sign of dangerously rapid correction of hyponatremia

A. Known Acute (known to have developed over <24-48 h)
- commonly occurs in hospital (dilute IV fluid, post-operative increased ADH)
- less risk from rapid correction since adaptation has not fully occurred
- if symptomatic
  - correct rapidly with 3% NaCl 1-2 cc/kg/h up to serum [Na$^+$] = 125-130 mmol/L
  - may need furosemide to address volume overload
- if asymptomatic, treatment depends on severity
  - if marked fall in plasma [Na$^+$], treat as symptomatic

B. Chronic or Unknown
  1. if severe symptoms (seizures or decreased LOC)
     - must partially correct acutely
     - aim for increase of Na$^+$ by 1-2 mmol/L/h for 4-6 h
     - limit total rise to 8 mmol/L in 24 h
     - IV 3% NaCl at 1-2 cc/kg/h
     - may need furosemide
  2. if asymptomatic
     - water restrict to <1 L/d fluid intake
     - consider IV 0.9% NS + furosemide (reduces urine osmolality, augments excretion of H$_2$O)
     - consider NaCl tablet or Oxocubes® as a source of Na$^+$
  3. refractory
     - furosemide and oral salt tablets
     - oral urea (osmotic aquaresis)
     - V2 receptor antagonists (e.g. tolvaptan)
  4. always pay attention to patient's ECF volume status – if already volume-expanded, unlikely to give NaCl (tablet or IV); if already volume-depleted, almost never appropriate to give furosemide

C. Options for Treatment of Overly-Rapid Correction
- give water (IV D5W)
- give ADH to stop water diuresis (DDAVP 1-2 µg IV)

Impact of IV Solution on Serum [Na+]
- formula to estimate the change in serum [Na$^+$] caused by retention of 1 L of any infusate [TBW = (for men) 0.6 x wt(kg); (for women) 0.5 x wt(kg)]

$$\text{change in serum } [Na^+] = \frac{\text{infusate } [Na^+] - \text{serum } [Na^+]}{TBW + 1\ L}$$

- formula assumes there are no losses of water or electrolytes

Beware of Rapid Correction of Hyponatremia
- Inadvertent rapid correction of hyponatremia can easily occur (e.g. patient with hyponatremia due to SIADH from nausea)
  - Anti-emetic given for relief of hyponatremia-induced nausea
  - ADH quickly turned off in the absence of nausea, the kidneys rapidly excrete the excess free water, and the serum [Na+] rises rapidly
- Patient at risk of osmotic demyelination
- High output dilute urine (>100 cc/h, <100 mOsm/L) in the setting of hyponatremia is usually the first sign of dangerously rapid correction of serum sodium

Correction of Na$^+$ in hyponatremia should not exceed 8 mmol/L/24 h unless definitely known to be <24-48 h duration; frequent monitoring of serum Na$^+$ and urine output is essential

Concentration of [Na$^+$] in Common Infusates
- [Na$^+$] in 0.45% NaCl = 77 mmol/L
- [Na$^+$] in 0.9% NaCl = 154 mmol/L
- [Na$^+$] in 3% NaCl = 513 mmol/L
- [Na$^+$] in 5% NaCl = 855 mmol/L
- [Na$^+$] in Ringer's lactate = 130 mmol/L
- [Na$^+$] in D5W = 0

SYNDROME OF INAPPROPRIATE ANTIDIURETIC HORMONE SECRETION
1. urine that is inappropriately concentrated for the serum osmolality
2. high urine sodium (>20-40 mmol/L)
3. high FE_{Na}

Table 5. Disorders Associated with SIADH

Cancer	Pulmonary	CNS	Drugs	Miscellaneous
Small cell cancer	Pneumonia	Mass lesion	Antidepressants	Post-operative state
Bronchogenic carcinoma	Lung abscess	Encephalitis	TCAs	Pain
Pancreatic	TB	Subarachnoid	SSRIs	Severe nausea
adenocarcinoma	Acute respiratory failure	hemorrhage	Antineoplastics	HIV
Hodgkin's lymphoma	Asthma	Stroke	Vincristine	
Thymoma	COPD	Head trauma	Cyclophosphamide	
Leukemia	Positive pressure	Acute psychosis	Anti-epileptics	
	ventilation	Acute intermittent	Carbamazepine	
		porphyria	Barbiturates	
			Chlorpropamide	
			ACEI	
			Other	
			DDAVP	
			Oxytocin	
			Nicotine	

Hypernatremia

- hypernatremia: serum [Na$^+$] >145 mmol/L
- too little water relative to total body Na$^+$; always a hyperosmolar state
- usually due to NET water loss, rarely due to hypertonic Na$^+$ gain
- less common than hyponatremia because patients are protected against hypernatremia by thirst and release of ADH

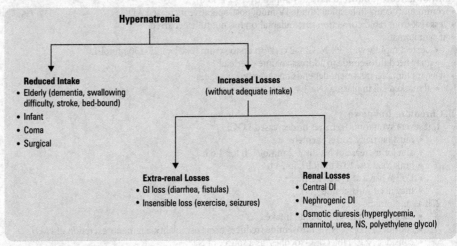

Figure 5. Approach to hypernatremia

Signs and Symptoms
- with acute hypernatremia no time for adaptation, therefore more likely to be symptomatic
- adaptive response: cells import and generate new osmotically active particles to normalize size
- due to brain cell shrinkage: altered mental status, weakness, neuromuscular irritability, focal neurologic deficits, seizures, coma, death
- ± polyuria, thirst, signs of hypovolemia

Complications
- increased risk of vascular rupture resulting in intracranial hemorrhage
- rapid correction may lead to cerebral edema due to ongoing brain hyperosmolality

Treatment of Hypernatremia
- general measures for all patients
  - give free water (oral or IV)
  - treat underlying cause
  - monitor serum Na$^+$ frequently to ensure correction is not occurring too rapidly
- if evidence of hemodynamic instability, must first correct volume depletion with NS bolus
- loss of water is often accompanied by loss of Na$^+$, but a proportionately larger water loss
- use formula to calculate free water H_2O deficit and replace
- encourage patient to drink pure water, as oral route is preferred for fluid administration

H₂O Deficit and TBW Equations
TBW = 0.6 x wt (kg) men
TBW = 0.5 x wt (kg) women

H$_2$O deficit = TBW x ([Na$^+$]plasma – 140) / 140

Correction of serum [Na$^+$] in hypernatremia should not exceed 12 mmol/L/24 h

1 L D5W approximately equals 1 L of free water
1 L 0.45% NS approximately equals 500 mL of free water

- if unable to replace PO or NG, correct H_2O deficit with hypotonic IV solution (IV D5W, 0.45% NS [half normal saline], or 3.3% dextrose with 0.3% NaCl ["2/3 and 1/3"])
- use formula (see *Hyponatremia*, NP8) to estimate expected change in serum Na^+ with 1 L infusate
- aim to lower $[Na^+]$ by no more than 12 mmol/L in 24 h (0.5 mmol/L/h)
- must also provide maintenance fluids and replace ongoing losses
- general rule: give 2 cc/kg/h of free water to correct serum $[Na^+]$ by about 0.5 mmol/L/h or 12 mmol/L/d

Diabetes Insipidus

- collecting tubule is impermeable to water due to absence of ADH or impaired response to ADH
- defect in central release of ADH (central DI) or renal response to ADH (nephrogenic DI)

Etiology
- central DI: neurosurgery, granulomatous diseases, trauma, vascular events, and malignancy
- nephrogenic DI: lithium (most common), hypokalemia, hypercalcemia, and congenital

Diagnosis
- urine osmolality inappropriately low in patient with hypernatremia (Uosm <300 mOsm/kg)
- serum vasopressin concentration may be absent or low (central), or elevated (nephrogenic)
- dehydration test: H_2O deprivation until loss of 3% of body weight or until urine osmolality rises above plasma osmolality; if urine osmolality remains <300 (fails to concentrate urine), most likely DI
- administer DDAVP (exogenous ADH) (10 μg intranasally or 2 μg SC or IV)
  - central DI: diagnosed if there is rise in urine osmolality, fall in urine volume
    - treat with DDAVP
  - nephrogenic DI: exogenous ADH fails to concentrate urine as kidneys do not respond
    - treat with water (IV D5W or PO water), thiazides may help as well (reduced ECF volume stimulates proximal tubular reabsorption of sodium and water, leading to less delivery of glomerular filtrate to ADH sensitive parts of renal tubule, and therefore lower urine volume results)

Potassium Homeostasis

- approximately 98% of total body K^+ stores are intracellular
- normal serum K^+ ranges from 3.5-5.0 mEq/L
- in response to K^+ load, rapid removal from ECF is necessary to prevent life-threatening hyperkalemia
- insulin, catecholamines, and acid-base status influence K+ movement into cells
  - aldosterone has a minor effect
- potassium excretion is regulated at the distal nephron
  - K^+ excretion = urine flow rate x urine $[K^+]$

Factors which Increase Renal K^+ Loss
- hyperkalemia
- increased distal tubular urine flow rate and Na^+ delivery (thiazides and loop diuretics)
- increased aldosterone activates epithelial sodium channels in cortical collecting duct, causing Na^+ reabsorption and K^+ excretion
- metabolic alkalosis (increases K^+ secretion)
- hypomagnesemia
- increased non-reabsorbable anions in tubule lumen: HCO_3^-, penicillin, salicylate (increased tubular flow rate increases K^+ secretion)

Hypokalemia

- serum $[K^+]$ <3.5 mEq/L

Signs and Symptoms
- usually asymptomatic, particularly when mild (3.0-3.5 mmol/L)
- N/V, fatigue, generalized weakness, myalgia, muscle cramps, and constipation
- if severe: arrhythmias, muscle necrosis, and rarely paralysis with eventual respiratory impairment
- arrhythmias occur at variable levels of K^+; more likely if digoxin use, hypomagnesemia, or CAD
- ECG changes are more predictive of clinical picture than serum $[K^+]$
  - U waves most important (low amplitude wave following a T wave)
  - flattened or inverted T waves
  - depressed ST segment
  - prolongation of Q-T interval
  - with severe hypokalemia: P-R prolongation, wide QRS, arrhythmias; increases risk of digitalis toxicity

Electrolyte Disorders

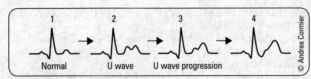

Figure 6. ECG changes in hypokalemia

- Hypokalemia often accompanied by metabolic alkalosis
- Potassium leaves cells, replaced by H^+
- Kidney tubular cells see high H^+, think acidosis and increase ammonium synthesis and excretion
- Increase in bicarbonate generation

Approach to Hypokalemia

1. emergency measures: obtain ECG; if potentially life threatening, begin treatment immediately
2. rule out transcellular shifts of K^+ as cause of hypokalemia
3. assess contribution of dietary K^+ intake
4. spot urine K:Cr (should be less than 1 in setting of hypokalemia)
   - if <1 consider GI loss
   - if >1 consider a renal loss
5. consider 24 h K^+ excretion
6. if renal K^+ loss, check BP and acid-base status
7. may also assess plasma renin and aldosterone levels, serum $[Mg^{2+}]$

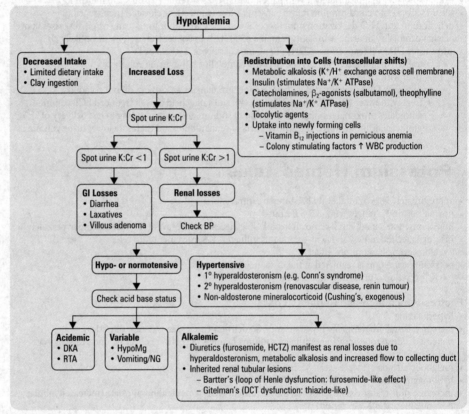

Figure 7. Approach to hypokalemia

Treatment

- treat underlying cause
- if true K^+ deficit, potassium repletion
  - oral sources – food, tablets (K-Dur™), KCl liquid solutions (preferable route if the patient tolerates PO medications)
  - IV – usually KCl in saline solutions, avoid dextrose solutions (may exacerbate hypokalemia via insulin release)
- max 40 mmol/L via peripheral vein, 60 mmol/L via central vein, max infusion 20 mmol/h
- K^+-sparing diuretics (triamterene, amiloride, spironolactone) can prevent renal K^+ loss
- restore Mg^{2+} if necessary
- if urine output and renal function are impaired, correct with extreme caution
- risk of hyperkalemia with potassium replacement especially high in elderly, diabetics, and patients with decreased renal function
- beware of excessive potassium repletion, especially if transcellular shift caused hypokalemia

Hyperkalemia

- serum $[K^+]$ >5.0 mEq/L

Signs and Symptoms
- usually asymptomatic but may develop nausea, palpitations, muscle weakness, muscle stiffness, paresthesias, areflexia, ascending paralysis, and hypoventilation
- impaired renal ammoniagenesis and metabolic acidosis
- ECG changes and cardiotoxicity (do not correlate well with serum $[K^+]$)
- peaked and narrow T waves
- decreased amplitude and eventual loss of P waves
- prolonged PR interval
- widening of QRS and eventual merging with T wave (sine-wave pattern)
- AV block
- ventricular fibrillation, asystole

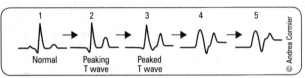

Figure 8. ECG changes in hyperkalemia

Table 6. Causes of Hyperkalemia

Factitious	Increased Intake	Transcellular Shift	Decreased Excretion
Sample hemolysis*	Diet	Intravascular hemolysis	Decreased GFR
Sample taken from vein	KCl tabs	Rhabdomyolysis	Renal failure
where IV KCl is running	IV KCl	Tumour lysis syndrome	Low effective circulating
Prolonged use of tourniquet	Salt substitute	Insulin deficiency	volume
Leukocytosis (extreme)		Acidemia	NSAIDs in renal insufficiency
Thrombocytosis (extreme)		Drugs	Normal GFR but
		β-blockers	hypoaldosteronism
		Digitalis overdose (blocks	
		Na^+/K^+ ATPase)	
		Succinylcholine	

*Most common

Table 7. Causes of Hyperkalemia with Normal GFR

Decreased Aldosterone Stimulus (low renin, low aldosterone)	Decreased Aldosterone Production (normal renin, low aldosterone)	Aldosterone Resistance (decreased tubular response)
Associated with diabetic nephropathy, NSAIDs, chronic interstitial nephritis, HIV	Adrenal insufficiency of any cause (e.g. Addison's disease, AIDS, metastatic cancer)	K^+-sparing diuretics
	ACEI	Spironolactone
	Angiotensin II receptor blockers	Amiloride
	Heparin	Triamterene
	Congenital adrenal hyperplasia with 21-hydroxylase deficiency	Renal tubulointerstitial disease

Approach to Hyperkalemia
1. emergency measures: obtain ECG, if life threatening begin treatment immediately
2. rule out factitious hyperkalemia; repeat blood test
3. hold exogenous K^+ (PO and IV) and any K^+ retaining medications
4. assess potential causes of transcellular shift
5. estimate GFR (calculate CrCl using Cockcroft-Gault)

In patients with DM and increased $[K^+]$ and hyperglycemia, often just giving insulin to restore euglycemia is sufficient to correct the hyperkalemia

Treatment
- acute therapy is warranted if ECG changes are present or if patient is symptomatic regardless of $[K^+]$
- tailor therapy to severity of increase in $[K^+]$ and ECG changes
  - $[K^+]$ <6.5 and normal ECG
    - treat underlying cause, stop K+ intake, increase the loss of K^+ via urine and/or GI tract
  - $[K^+]$ between 6.5 and 7.0, no ECG changes: add insulin to above regimen
  - $[K^+]$ >7.0 and/or ECG changes: first priority is to protect the heart, add calcium gluconate to above

1. Stabilize Myocardium
- calcium gluconate 1-2 amps (10 mL of 10% solution) IV
- antagonizes the membrane action of hyperkalemia, protects cardiac conduction system, no effect on serum $[K^+]$
- onset within minutes, lasts 30-60 min (may require repeat doses during treatment course of hyperkalemia)

Treatment of Hyperkalemia
C BIG K DROP
C – Calcium gluconate
BIG – β-agonist, Bicarbonate, Insulin, Glucose
K – Kayexalate®
DROP – Diuretics, Dialysis

Management of Patients with Acute Hyperkalemia
CMAJ 2010;182:1631-1635
Purpose: To review the evidence supporting different treatment options for acute hyperkalemia.
Study: Systematic review of updated research since 2005 Cochrane review, search 2003-2009 inclusive.
Results: Four new articles continued to support the acute usage of insulin and beta-agonists for shifting, and hemodialysis for elimination in severe and refractory hyperkalemia. One small randomized study comparing resins to laxatives was identified by the reviewers. It found no significant difference in serum potassium of the two groups in the 4 hours following administration. Study design was reportedly flawed; the resin group as a whole had lower initial serum concentration than the laxative control group.
Conclusion: Standard of care continues to include insulin, beta-agonists, and hemodialysis. There is no clear evidence supporting the use of resins, such as Kayexalate, for the acute management of hyperkalemia. Furthermore, prior studies have shown that resin usage can result in bowel obstruction and bowel necrosis.

2. Shift K+ into Cells
- regular insulin (Insulin R) 10-20 units IV, with 1-2 amp D50W (give D50W before insulin)
  - onset of action 15-30 min, lasts 1-2 h
  - monitor capillary blood glucose q1h because of risk of hypoglycemia
  - can repeat every 4-6 h
  - caution giving D50W before insulin if hyperkalemia is severe as it can cause a serious arrhythmia
- $NaHCO_3$ 1-3 ampules (given as 3 ampules of 7.5% or 8.4% $NaHCO_3$ in 1L D5W)
  - onset of action 15-30 min, transient effect, drives K^+ into cells in exchange for H^+
  - more effective if patient has metabolic acidosis
- β2-agonist (Ventolin®) in nebulized form (dose = 2 cc or 10 mg inhaled) or 0.5 mg IV
  - onset of action 30-90 min, stimulates Na^+/K^+ ATPase
  - caution if patient has heart disease as may result in tachycardia

3. Enhance K+ Removal from Body
- via urine (preferred approach)
  - furosemide (≥40 mg IV), may need IV NS to avoid hypovolemia
  - fludrocortisone (synthetic mineralocorticoid) if suspect aldosterone deficiency
- via gastrointestinal tract
  - cation-exchange resins: calcium resonium or sodium polystyrene sulfonate (Kayexalate®)
    - increasingly falling out of favour due to risk of colonic necrosis; works by binding Na^+ in exchange for K^+, and controversial how much K^+ is actually removed
    - lactulose or sorbitol PO to avoid constipation (must ensure that patient has a bowel movement after resin is administered - main benefit may be the diarrhea caused by lactulose)
  - Kayexalate® enemas with tap water
- dialysis (renal failure, life threatening hyperkalemia unresponsive to therapy)

Hyperphosphatemia

Definition
- serum phosphate >1.45 mmol/L
- critical role in the development of secondary hyperparathyroidism and renal osteodystrophy in patients with advanced CKD and on dialysis

Table 8. Etiology of Hyperphosphatemia

Increased Phosphate Load	Reduced Renal Clearance	Pseudohyperphosphatemia
GI intake (rectal enema, GI bleeding) IV phosphate load (K-Phos®, blood transfusion) Endogenous phosphate (tumour lysis syndrome, rhabdomyolysis, hemolysis, lactic and ketoacidosis)	Acute/chronic renal failure Hypoparathyroidism Acromegaly Tumour calcinosis (ability of kidney to specifically clear phosphate is defective)	Hyperglobulinemia Hyperlipidemia Hyperbilirubinemia

Clinical Features
- non-specific, include ectopic calcification, renal osteodystrophy

Treatment
- acute: hemodialysis if symptomatic ; aluminum hydroxide (use with extreme caution in renal failure)
- chronic: low PO_4^{3-} diet, phosphate binders (e.g. $CaCO_3$ or lanthanum carbonate or sevelamer with meals)

Hypophosphatemia

Definition
- serum phosphate <0.85 mmol/L

Table 9. Etiology of Hypophosphatemia

Inadequate Intake	Renal Losses	Excessive Skeletal Mineralization	Shift into ICF
Starvation Malabsorption (diarrhea, steatorrhea) Antacid use Alcoholism	Hyperparathyroidism Diuretics X-linked or AD hypophosphatemic rickets Fanconi syndrome Multiple myeloma Early post-kidney transplant	Osteoblastic metastases Post parathyroidectomy (referred to as 'hungry bone syndrome')	Recovery from metabolic acidosis Respiratory alkalosis Starvation refeeding (stimulated by insulin)

Symptoms usually present when phosphate <0.32 mmol/L (1.0 mg/dL)
Treat asymptomatic patients if phosphate <0.32 mmol/L

Severe burns can cause hypophosphatemia due to PO_4^{3-} losses through the skin

Clinical Features
- non-specific (CHF, coma, hypotension, weakness, defective clotting)

Treatment
- treat underlying cause
  - Oral PO_4^{3-}: 2-4 g/d divided bid-qid (start at 1 g/d to minimize diarrhea)
  - IV PO_4^{3-}: only for severely symptomatic patients or inability to tolerate oral therapy

Hypermagnesemia

Definition
- serum magnesium >0.85 mmol/L

Etiology
- AKI/CRF
- Mg^{2+}-containing antacids or enemas
- IV administration of large doses of $MgSO_4$ (e.g. for preeclampsia; see Obstetrics, OB24)

Clinical Features
- rarely symptomatic
- drowsiness, hyporeflexia, respiratory depression, heart block, cardiac arrest, hypotension

Treatment
- discontinue Mg^{2+}-containing products
- IV calcium (Mg^{2+}-antagonist) for acute reversal of magnesium toxicity
- dialysis if renal failure

Hypomagnesemia

Definition
- serum magnesium <0.70 mmol/L

Etiology

GI losses	Excess renal loss
Starvation/malabsorption	$2°$ hyperaldosteronism due to cirrhosis and CHF
Vomiting/diarrhea	Hyperglycemia
Alcoholism	Hypokalemia
Acute pancreatitis	Hypercalcemia
	Loop and thiazide-type diuretics
	Nephrotoxic medications
	Proton-pump inhibitors
	Early post-renal transplant

Clinical Features
- seizures, paresis, Chvostek and Trousseau signs, ECG changes (widened QRS, prolonged PR, T-wave abnormalities), and arrhythmias including Torsades de pointes

Treatment
- treat underlying cause
- **encourage increased dietary intake e.g. fruits**
- oral Mg^{2+} salts unless patients have seizures or other severe symptoms
- Mg^{2+} IM/IV; cellular uptake of Mg^{2+} is slow, therefore repletion requires sustained correction
- discontinue diuretics
  - in patients requiring diuretics, use a K^+-sparing diuretic to minimize magnesuria

You will be unable to correct hypokalemia or hypocalcemia without first supplementing magnesium if patient is hypomagnesemic

Acid-Base Disorders

- acid-base homeostasis influences protein function and can critically affect tissue and organ function with consequences to cardiovascular, respiratory, metabolic, and CNS function
- see Respirology, R6 for more information on respiratory acidosis/alkalosis
- normal concentration of HCO_3^- = 24 mEq/L (range: 22-30 mEq/L)
- normal pCO_2 = 40 mmHg (range: 36-44 mmHg)
- each acid base disorder has an appropriate compensation
  - inadequate compensation or overcompensation can indicate the presence of a second acid-base disorder (e.g. in metabolic acidosis, inadequate compensation means there is also respiratory acidosis; overcompensation means there is also respiratory alkalosis)

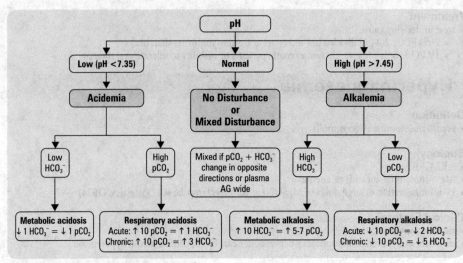

Figure 9. Approach to acid-base disorders

Approach

1. Identify the primary disturbance (see Figure 9)
- respiratory acidosis, metabolic acidosis, respiratory alkalosis, metabolic alkalosis

2. Evaluate compensation. If compensation is not appropriate, a second acid-base disorder is likely present
- compensation occurs in the same direction as the primary disturbance

3. Calculate Plasma AG
- $AG = [Na^+] - ([HCO_3^-] + [Cl-])$
- baseline = 12, normal range 10-14 mEq/L
- AG can be altered by plasma albumin level: for each 10 g/L fall in albumin, lower baseline AG by 3 mEq/L (e.g. if plasma [albumin]= 20 g/L, expect AG = 6 mEq/L)

4. If AG elevated, compare increase in AG with decrease in HCO₃⁻
- if increase in AG < decrease in HCO_3^-, there is a coexisting non-AG metabolic acidosis
- if increase in AG > decrease HCO_3^-, there is a coexisting metabolic alkalosis

5. Calculate Osmolar Gap
- osmolar gap = measured osmolality – calculated osmolality
   - calculated osmolality = $(2 \times [Na^+]) + [urea] + [glucose]$ (all units are in mmol/L)
   - normal osmolar gap <10
   - If OG >10, consider: methanol poisoning, ethylene glycol poisoning, or another cause of acidosis plus ethanol ingestion

Metabolic Acidosis

Etiology and Pathophysiology
1. Increased AG Metabolic Acidosis (4 types)
1. Lactic acidosis (2 types)
   - L-lactic acid
      - type A: due to tissue hypoperfusion (any cause of shock), ischemic bowel, profound hypoxemia
      - type B: non-hypoxic – multiple causes; the most common is failure to metabolize normally produced lactic acid in the liver due to severe liver disease; other causes include: excessive alcohol intake, thiamine deficiency, metformin accumulation (metformin interferes with electron transport chain), certain anti-retrovirals, large tumours, mitochondrial myopathies
   - D-lactic acid: rare syndrome characterized by episodes of encephalopathy and metabolic acidosis
      - occurs in the setting of carbohydrate malabsorption (e.g. short bowel syndrome), colonic bacteria metabolize carbohydrate load into D-lactic acid, diminished colonic motility and impaired D-lactate metabolism
2. Ketoacidosis
   - diabetic
   - starvation
   - alcoholic (decreased carbohydrate intake and vomiting)

Causes of Increased Osmolar Gap
- Methanol
- Ethylene glycol
- Ethanol
- Polyethelene glycol
- Mannitol
- Sorbitol

Useful Equations
- $AG = [Na^+] - [Cl-] - [HCO_3^-]$ (normal range = 10-14 mEq/L)
- Osmolar Gap = measured serum osmolality – calculated osmolality (normal <10 mEq/L)
   - "Two Salts and a Sticky BUN"
- Calculated Osmolality = $2[Na^+] + [Urea] + [Glucose] (+1.25[Ethanol])$

Causes of Increased AG Metabolic Acidosis
MUDPILES CAT
Methanol
Uremia
Diabetic ketoacidosis
Paraldehyde
Isopropyl alcohol/Iron/Ibuprofen/Indomethacin
Lactic acidosis
Ethylene glycol
Salicylates
Cyanide and **C**arbon monoxide
Alcoholic ketoacidosis
Toluene

3. Toxins
- methanol (toxic to brain and retina, can cause blindness and brain death): metabolized to formic acid
- ethylene glycol (toxic to brain and kidneys): metabolized to oxalic acid (envelope shaped crystals in urine) and multiple other acids
- salicylate (e.g. ASA) overdose: causes acidosis due to salicylic acid, and also accumulation of lactic acid (salicylate at toxic levels impairs electron transport chain) and ketoacid (salicylate activates fat breakdown)

4. Advanced renal failure (e.g. serum Cr increased at least 5x above baseline – a very low GFR causes anion retention, and renal disease leads to impaired bicarbonate production)

2. Normal AG Metabolic Acidosis (Hyperchloremic Acidosis)
- diarrhea (HCO_3^- loss from GI tract)
- RTA
  - type I RTA (distal): inability to secrete H^+ in collecting duct, leading to impaired excretion of ammonium into urine
  - type II RTA (proximal): impaired HCO_3^- reabsorption
  - type III RTA: combination of Types I and II and is extremely rare
  - type IV RTA: defective ammoniagenesis due to decreased aldosterone, hyporesponsiveness to aldosterone, or hyperkalemia
- to help distinguish renal causes from non-renal causes, use Urine AG = $(Na^+ + K^+) - Cl^-$
- calculation establishes the presence or absence of unmeasured positive ions (e.g. NH_4^+) in urine
  - if UAG <0, suggests adequate NH_4^+ excretion in urine (likely nonrenal cause: diarrhea)
  - if UAG >0, suggests problem is lack of NH_4^+ in urine (e.g. distal RTA)

Causes of Non-AG Metabolic Acidosis
HARDUP
Hyperalimentation
Acetazolamide
RTA*
Diarrhea*
Ureteroenteric fistula
Pancreaticoduodenal fistula
*Most common

Treatment of Metabolic Acidosis
1. treat underlying cause
   - fluid resuscitation and insulin for DKA
   - restore tissue perfusion for Type A lactic acidosis
   - ethanol/fomepizole ± dialysis for methanol or ethylene glycol poisoning
   - alkaline diuresis ± dialysis if ASA overdose
2. correct coexisting disorders of K^+ (see *Hyperkalemia*, NP13)
3. consider treatment with exogenous alkali (e.g. $NaHCO_3$) if
   - severe reduction in $[HCO_3^-]$ e.g. <8 mmol/L, especially with very low pH (<7)
   - no metabolizable anion (e.g. salicylate, formate, oxalate, or sulphate); note that lactate and ketoacid anions can be metabolized to HCO_3^-
- note: risks of sodium bicarbonate therapy
  - hypokalemia: causes K^+ to shift into cells (correct K^+ deficit first)
  - ECF volume overload: Na^+ load given with $NaHCO_3$, can exacerbate pulmonary edema
  - overshoot alkalosis: abrupt, poorly tolerated transition from overly aggressive alkali loading, partial conversion of accumulated organic anions to HCO_3^-, and persisting hyperventilation

3 Clinical Scenarios that Produce a Mixed Disorder with Near Normal pH
(e.g. increased AG metabolic acidosis + respiratory alkalosis)
- Cirrhosis
- ASA overdose
- Sepsis

Metabolic Alkalosis

Pathophysiology
- requires initiating event and maintenance factors
- precipitating factors
  - GI (vomiting, NG tube) or renal loss of H^+
  - exogenous alkali (oral or parenteral administration), milk alkali syndrome
  - diuretics (contraction alkalosis): decreased excretion of HCO_3^-, decreased ECF volume, therefore increased $[HCO_3^-]$
  - post-hypercapnia: renal compensation for respiratory acidosis is HCO_3^- retention, rapid correction of respiratory disorder results in transient excess of HCO_3^-
- maintenance factors
  - volume depletion: reduced GFR and increase proximal reabsorption of $NaHCO_3^-$ and increased aldosterone
  - hyperaldosteronism (1° or 2°): distal Na^+ reabsorption in exchange for K^+ and H^+ excretion leads to HCO_3^- generation; aldosterone also promotes hypokalemia
  - hypokalemia: transcellular K^+/H^+ exchange, stimulus for ammoniagenesis and HCO_3^- generation

Evaluate Compensation (identify co-existing respiratory acid-base disorders)
- hypoventilation (an upper limit to compensation exists – breathing cannot be stopped)

Treatment
- treat underlying cause
- correct underlying disease, replenish K^+ and Mg^{2+} deficits, and possibly K^+-sparing diuretic
- saline sensitive metabolic alkalosis (most common)
  - volume repletion ± carbonic anhydrase inhibitor (e.g. acetazolamide) to facilitate loss of HCO_3^- in urine
- saline resistant metabolic alkalosis
  - remove source of aldosterone or glucocorticoid ± spironolactone

Acute Kidney Injury

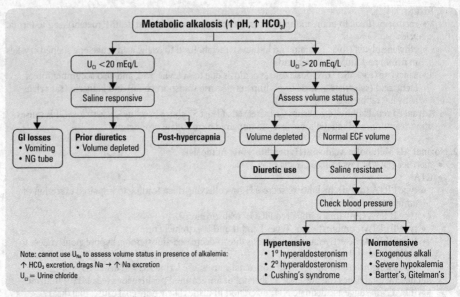

Figure 10. Approach to metabolic alkalosis

Note: cannot use U_{Na} to assess volume status in presence of alkalemia:
↑ HCO_3 excretion, drags Na → ↑ Na excretion
U_{Cl} = Urine chloride

The 2 most common causes of acute kidney injury in hospitalized patients are prerenal azotemia and ATN; remember that prerenal failure can lead to ATN

Acute Kidney Injury

Definition
- abrupt decline in renal function leading to increased nitrogenous waste products normally excreted by the kidney
- formerly known as acute renal failure

Clinical Presentation
- azotemia (increased BUN, Cr)
- abnormal urine volume: formally <0.5 ml/kg/h for >6 h but can manifest as anuria, oliguria, or polyuria

Approach to AKI

Clues to Prerenal Etiology
- Clinical: Decreased BP, increased HR, and orthostatic HR and BP changes
- Increased [urea] >> Increased [Cr]
- Urine [Na⁺] <10-20 mmol/L
- Urine osmolality >500 mOsm/kg
- Fractional excretion of Na⁺ <1%

Clues to Renal Etiology
- Appropriate clinical context
- Urinalysis positive for casts:
  Pigmented granular – ATN
  WBC – AIN
  RBC – GN
- Systemic features, anemia, thrombocytopenia, HTN, mild-moderate ECF volume overload

Clues to Postrenal Etiology
- Known solitary kidney
- Older man
- Recent retroperitoneal surgery
- Anuria
- Palpable bladder
- Ultrasound shows hydronephrosis

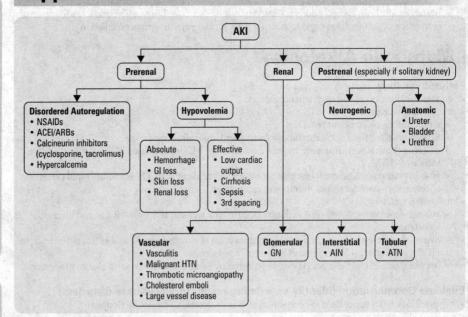

Figure 11. Approach to AKI

Differentiating Prerenal from ATN

	Prerenal	ATN
Urinalysis	Normal	RBC, pigmented granular casts
Urine [Na⁺]	<20	>20 mEq/L
Urine[Na⁺]/[Cr]	<20	>20
Urine osmolality	>500	<350 mOsm/kgH₂O
FeNa	<1%	>1%

Investigations
- blood work: CBC, electrolytes, Cr, urea (think prerenal if increase in urea is relatively greater than increase in Cr), Ca^{2+}, PO_4^{3-}
- urine dipstick: albumin, hemoglobin, WBC's, others: glucose, pH, urobilinogen, specific gravity
- urine volume, C&S, R&M: sediment, casts, crystals
- urinary indices: electrolytes, osmolality
- Foley catheterization (rule out bladder outlet obstruction)

- fluid challenge (e.g. fluid bolus to rule out most prerenal causes)
- imaging: abdomen U/S (assess kidney size, hydronephrosis, postrenal obstruction)
- indications for renal biopsy
  - diagnosis is not certain
  - prerenal azotemia or ATN is unlikely
  - oliguria persists >4 wk

Treatment
1. preliminary measures
   - prerenal
     - ◆ correct prerenal factors: optimize volume status and cardiac performance using fluids that will stay in the plasma subcompartment (NS, albumin, blood/plasma), hold ACEI/ARB (gently rehydrate when needed, e.g. CHF) and NSAIDs
   - renal
     - ◆ address reversible renal causes: discontinue nephrotoxic drugs, treat infection, and optimize electrolytes
     - ◆ correct ECF volume, supportive care, consider corticosteroid or immunosuppressive therapy
   - postrenal
     - ◆ consider obstruction: structural (stones, strictures) vs. functional (neuropathy)
     - ◆ for obstruction to cause AKI, must have functional solitary kidney or obstruction affecting both kidneys
     - ◆ treat with Foley catheter insertion, indwelling bladder catheter, nephrostomy, stenting
2. treat complications
   - fluid overload
     - ◆ NaCl restriction
     - ◆ high dose loop diuretics
   - hyperkalemia (see *Approach to Hyperkalemia*, NP13)
   - adjust dosages of medications cleared by kidney (e.g. amiodarone, digoxin, cyclosporin, tacrolimus, some antibiotics, and chemotherapeutic agents)
   - dialysis
3. definitive therapy depends on etiology

Prognosis
- high morbidity and mortality in patients with sustained AKI and multi-organ failure

Avoid NSAIDs in patients with diarrhea, heart failure or renal failure

Renal transplant is not a therapy for AKI

Drugs Implicated in Prerenal Azotemia
- Diuretics
- NSAIDs
- ACEI/ARBs

Parenchymal Kidney Diseases

Glomerular Diseases

HISTOLOGICAL TERMS OF GLOMERULAR CHANGES

Extent of Changes
- histological term describing the number of glomeruli affected in a given condition:
  - diffuse: majority of glomeruli abnormal
  - focal: some glomeruli affected
- histological term describing the extent to which individual glomeruli are affected in a given condition
  - global: entire glomerulus abnormal
  - segmental: only part of the glomerulus abnormal

Types of Changes
- proliferation: hyperplasia of one of the glomerular cell types (mesangial, endothelial, parietal epithelial), with or without inflammatory cell infiltration
  - crescent formation: parietal epithelial cell proliferation and mononuclear cell infiltration form crescent-shape in Bowman's space
- membranous changes: capillary wall thickening due to immune deposits or alterations in basement membrane

CLINICAL PRESENTATION OF GLOMERULAR DISEASE

Important Points to Remember
- glomerular diseases have diverse clinical presentations including hematuria, proteinuria, HTN, edema, and decreased GFR
  - each glomerulopathy presents as one of four major glomerular syndromes (these are NOT diagnoses)
    1. asymptomatic urinary abnormalities
       – proteinuria
       – hematuria
    2. nephritic syndrome
       – acute GN
       – rapidly progressive GN

3. nephrotic syndrome
4. ESRD
- glomerulopathies can be caused by a primary disease or can occur secondary to a systemic disease
- some glomerulopathies can present as more than one syndrome at different times

The Nephritic-Nephrotic Spectrum
- glomerular pathology can present with a clinical picture anywhere on a spectrum with pure nephritic and pure nephrotic syndromes at the extremes

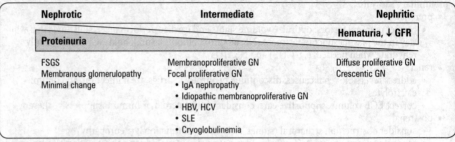

Nephrotic	Intermediate	Nephritic
		Hematuria, ↓ GFR
Proteinuria		
FSGS	Membranoproliferative GN	Diffuse proliferative GN
Membranous glomerulopathy	Focal proliferative GN	Crescentic GN
Minimal change	• IgA nephropathy	
	• Idiopathic membranoproliferative GN	
	• HBV, HCV	
	• SLE	
	• Cryoglobulinemia	

Figure 12. Spectrum of glomerular pathology

PROTEINURIA
- hallmark of nephrotic syndromes
- 24 h urine protein: gold standard to assess degree of proteinuria
- urine ACR: used to screen for diabetic nephropathy
- microalbuminuria
  - defined as ACR ≥2.0 mg/mmol
  - marker of vascular endothelial function
  - an important prognostic marker for kidney disease in DM and HTN (see *Diabetes*, NP31)
- microalbuminuria is the earliest sign of diabetic nephropathy
- composition of normal total urine protein
- upper limit of normal daily excretion of total protein is 150 mg/d
- upper limit of normal daily excretion of albumin is 30 mg/d
- the other normally excreted proteins are either filtered low molecular weight proteins (such as immunoglobulin light chains or β-2 microglobulin) or proteins secreted by the tubular epithelial cells (e.g. Tamm-Horsfall mucoprotein)

Sidebar

Pathologic Proteinuria

Tubulointerstitial
- Normally low molecular weight proteins (<60 kDa) pass through glomerular filtration barrier and are reabsorbed in proximal tubule
- Proximal tubule dysfunction causes impaired reabsorption and increased excretion of low molecular weight proteins
- Albumin (>60 kDa) is not affected; thus, edema is partly secondary to salt and water retention

Glomerular
- Normally, the filtration barrier is selectively permeable to size (<60 kDa) and charge (repels negative particles); thus, albumin is filtered to a very limited extent through a normal glomerulus
- Damage to any component of the glomerular filtration barrier results in loss of albumin and other high molecular weight proteins; thus, edema is secondary to hypoalbuminemia (low oncotic pressure), but also due to enhanced renal tubular reabsorption of filtered sodium and water (possibly due to filtered proteins stimulating the action of cortical collecting duct epithelial sodium channel)

Overflow
- Increased production of low molecular weight proteins which exceeds the reabsorptive capacity of the proximal tubule
- Plasma cell dyscrasias: produce light chain Ig (multiple myeloma, Waldenstrom's macroglobulinemia, monoclonal gammopathy of undetermined significance)

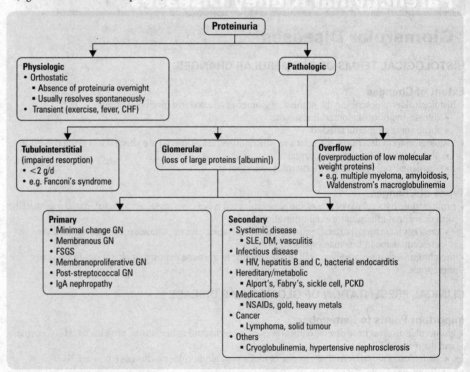

Figure 13. Classification of proteinuria

Table 10. Daily Excretion of Protein

Daily Excretion	Stage of Nephropathy	ACR
<150 mg total protein (and <30 mg albumin)	Normal	Less than 2.0 mg/mmol
30-300 mg albumin	Microalbuminuria	Greater than 2.0 mg/mmol
>3500 mg total protein/1.73m² BSA	Nephrotic range proteinuria	
Variable amount of proteinuria	Can be seen with glomerular disease	
Up to 2000 mg per d	Possible tubular disease because of failure to reabsorb filtered proteins	

Investigations
- urine R&M, C&S, urea, Cr
- further workup (if degree of proteinuria >0.5 g/d, casts, and/or hematuria)
  - CBC, glucose, electrolytes, 24 h urine protein, and Cr
  - urine and serum immunoelectrophoresis, abdominal/pelvic U/S
  - serology: ANA, RF, p-ANCA (MPO), c-ANCA (PR3), Hep B, Hep C, HIV, ASOT
- indications for nephrology referral
  - generally, if there is "heavy" proteinuria (ACR >30 mg/mmol), should refer to nephrologist
  - definitely if there is nephrotic syndrome: marked proteinuria >3.5 g/1.73m²/d with hypoalbuminemia (<35 g/L)

HEMATURIA
- hallmark of nephritic syndromes
- presence of blood or RBCs in urine
  - gross hematuria: pink, red, or tea-coloured urine
    - in gross hematuria, the urine should be centrifuged
      - if the sediment is red, true hematuria
      - if the supernatant is red, test for heme with a dipstick
        - if supernatant positive for heme: myoglobinuria or hemoglobinuria
        - if negative for heme: pseudohematuria; consider medications (e.g. rifampin), food dyes (e.g. beets), or metabolites (e.g. porphyria)
  - microscopic hematuria: blood in the urine that is invisible to the naked eye, >2-3 RBCs/HPF on microscopy

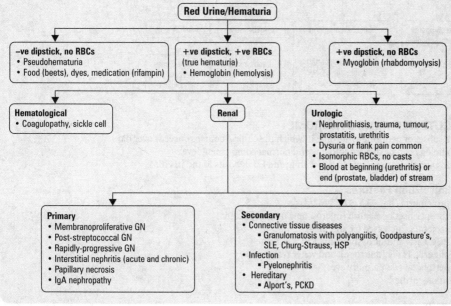

Figure 14. Approach to red urine

Investigations for Hematuria
- Hx and P/E: family history of nephrolithiasis, hearing loss (Alport Syndrome), cerebral aneurysm (PCKD), diet, recent URTI, irritative and obstructive urinary symptoms (UTI)
- urine R&M, C&S, urea, Cr
- renal U/S
- 24 h urine stone workup if there is a history of stone formation or if there is a stone noted on imaging: calcium, oxalate, citrate, magnesium, uric acid, cysteine
- further workup (if casts and/or proteinuria): CBC, electrolytes, 24 h urine protein and Cr, serology (ANA, RF, C3, C4, p-ANCA, c-ANCA, ASOT)
- consider urology consult and possible cystoscopy if not clearly a nephrologic source for hematuria or if >50 yr of age

Glomerular Syndromes

1. ASYMPTOMATIC URINARY ABNORMALITIES

Clinical/Lab Features
- often have rapid decline in GFR, anemia, elevated inflammatory markers, ECF volume replete or mildly overloaded
- proteinuria (usually <2 g/d) and/or microscopic or macroscopic hematuria
  - isolated proteinuria
    - can be postural
    - occasionally can signal beginning of more serious GN (e.g. FSGS, IgA nephropathy, amyloid, diabetic nephropathy)
  - hematuria with or without proteinuria
    - IgA nephropathy (Berger's disease): most common type of primary glomerular disease worldwide, usually presents after viral URTI
    - hereditary nephritis (Alport Syndrome – Type IV collagen mutation): X-linked nephritis often associated with sensorineural hearing loss; proteinuria <2 g/d
    - thin basement membrane disease: usually autosomal dominant, without proteinuria; benign
    - benign recurrent hematuria: hematuria associated with febrile illness, exercise, or immunization; a diagnosis of exclusion after other possibilities are ruled out

2. NEPHRITIC SYNDROME

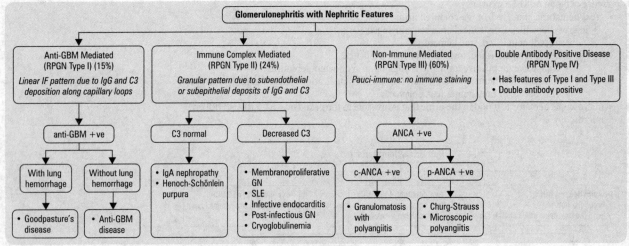

Figure 15. Approach to nephritic syndrome

ACUTE NEPHRITIC SYNDROME
- a subset of nephritic syndrome in which the clinical course proceeds over days
- etiology can be divided into low and normal complement levels
- frequently immune-mediated, with Ig and C3 deposits found in GBM

Clinical/Lab Features
- proteinuria (but <3.5 g/1.73 m2/d)
- abrupt onset hematuria (microscopic or macroscopic)
- azotemia (increased Cr and urea)
- RBC casts and/or dysmorphic RBCs in urine
- oliguria, HTN (due to salt and water retention)
- peripheral edema/puffy eyes
- smoky urine

Treatment
- depends on etiology
- pulse steroid therapy and other immunosuppression, BP control, monitoring for progression to end stage renal disease

RAPIDLY PROGRESSIVE GLOMERULONEPHRITIS/ CRESCENTIC GLOMERULONEPHRITIS
- a subset of nephritic syndrome in which the clinical course proceeds over weeks to months
- clinical diagnosis, not histopathological
- any cause of GN can present as RPGN (except minimal change disease)
- additional etiologies seen only as RPGN: anti-GBM Disease and granulomatosis with polyangiitis (previously called Wegener's granulomatosis)
- crescentic GN results from proliferation of parietal epithelial cells and is the most aggressive form of glomerular disease

Clinical/Lab Features
- fibrous crescents typically present on renal histopathology
- RBC casts and/or dysmorphic RBCs in urine
- classified by immunofluorescence staining
- Type I: Anti-GBM mediated (15% of cases)
- Type II: Immune Complex Mediated (24% of cases)
- Type III: Non-Immune Mediated (60% of cases)
- Type IV: Double Antibody Positive

Treatment and Prognosis
- treatment: underlying cause for postinfectious; corticosteroids + cyclophosphamide or other cytotoxic agent + plasmaphoresis in management of cases such as Anti-GBM Ab
- prognosis: 50% recovery with early treatment, depends on underlying cause

3. NEPHROTIC SYNDROME

Clinical/Lab Features
- heavy proteinuria (>3.5 g/1.73m2/d)
- hypoalbuminemia
- edema
- hyperlipidemia (elevated LDL cholesterol), lipiduria (fatty casts and oval fat bodies on microscopy)
- hypercoagulable state (due to antithrombin III, Protein C, and Protein S urinary losses)
- patient may report frothy urine
- glomerular pathology on renal biopsy
  - minimal change disease (or minimal lesion disease or nil disease) – e.g. glomeruli appear normal on light microscopy
  - membranous glomerulopathy
  - focal segmental glomerulosclerosis (FSGS)
  - membranoproliferative GN
  - nodular glomerulosclerosis
- each can be idiopathic or secondary to a systemic disease or drug (sirolimus can cause proteinuria without obvious glomerular pathology)

Table 11. Nephrotic Syndrome

	Minimal Change	Membranous Glomerulopathy	Focal Segmental Glomerulosclerosis	Membranoproliferative Glomerulonephritis	Nodular Glomerulosclerosis
Secondary Causes	Hodgkin's lymphoma	HBV, SLE, solid tumours (lung, breast, GI)	Reflux nephropathy, HIV, HBV, obesity, sickle cell disease	HCV, malaria, SLE, leukemia, lymphoma, shunt nephritis	DM, amyloidosis
Drug Causes	NSAIDs	Gold, penicillamine	Heroin		
Therapy	Steroids	Reduce BP, ACEI, steroids	Steroids, ACEI/ARB for proteinuria	Aspirin®, ACEI, dipyridamole (Persantine®) – controversial	Treat underlying cause

4. END STAGE RENAL DISEASE
- see *End Stage Renal Disease*, NP36

INVESTIGATIONS FOR GLOMERULAR DISEASE
- blood work
  - first presentation: electrolytes, Cr, urea, albumin, fasting lipids
  - determining etiology: CBC, ESR, serum immunoelectrophoresis, anti-GBM Disease, C3, C4, ANA, p-ANCA, c-ANCA, cryoglobulins, HBV and HCV serology, ASOT (anti-streptolysin titres), VDRL, HIV
- urinalysis: RBCs, WBCs, casts, protein
- 24 h urine for protein and CrCl
- radiology
  - CXR (infiltrates, CHF, pleural effusion)
  - renal U/S
- renal biopsy (percutaneous or open) if heavy proteinuria or renal insufficiency and cause is not obviously diabetic nephropathy
- urine immunoelectrophoresis
  - for Bence-Jones protein if proteinuria present

SECONDARY CAUSES OF GLOMERULAR DISEASE

Amyloidosis
- nodular deposits of amyloid in mesangium, usually related to amyloid light chain (AL)
- presents as nephrotic range proteinuria with progressive renal insufficiency
- can be primary or secondary
- secondary causes: multiple myeloma, TB, rheumatoid arthritis, malignancy

Systemic Lupus Erythematosus (see Rheumatology, RH11)
- lupus nephritis can present as any of the glomerular syndromes
- nephrotic syndrome with an active sediment is most common presentation
- GN caused by immune complex deposition in capillary loops and mesangium with resulting renal injury
- serum complement levels are usually low during periods of active renal disease
- children and males with SLE are more likely to develop nephritis

EULAR Recommendations for the Management of Systemic Lupus Erythematosus (SLE)
Ann Rheum Dis 2008;67:195-205
Lupus Nephritis Recommendations
Monitoring: Renal biopsy, urine sediment analysis, proteinuria, and kidney function may have independent predictive ability for clinical outcome in therapy of lupus nephritis but need to be interpreted in conjunction. Changes in immunological tests (anti-dsDNA, serum C3) have limited ability to predict response to treatment and may be used only as supplemental information.
Treatment: In patients with proliferative lupus nephritis, glucocorticoids in combination with immunosuppressive agents are effective against progression to end-stage renal disease. Long-term efficacy has been demonstrated only for cyclophosphamide-based regimens, which are associated with considerable adverse effects. In short- and medium-term trials, mycophenolate mofetil has demonstrated at least similar efficacy compared with pulse cyclophosphamide and a more favourable toxicity profile. Failure to respond by 6 mo should evoke discussions for intensification of therapy. Flares following remission are not uncommon and require diligent follow-up.
End-Stage Renal Disease: Dialysis and transplantation in SLE have long-term patient and graft-survival rates comparable with those observed in non-diabetic non-SLE patients, with transplantation being the method of choice.

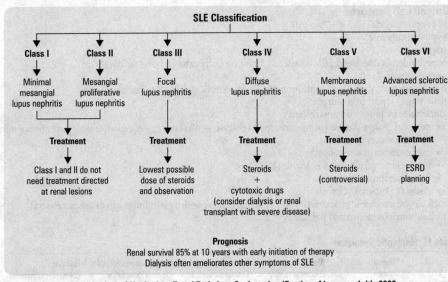

Figure 16. International Society of Nephrology/Renal Pathology Society classification of lupus nephritis 2003

Henoch-Schönlein Purpura
- seen more commonly in children
- purpura on buttocks and legs, abdominal pain, arthralgia, and fever
- IgA and C3 staining of mesangium
- usually benign, self-limiting course, 10% progress to CKD

Anti-GBM Disease
- Goodpasture Syndrome when lung and renal both involved
- antibodies against type IV collagen present in lungs and GBM
- present with RPGN type I and hemoptysis/dyspnea
- pulmonary hemorrhage more common in smokers and males
- treat with plasma exchange, cyclophosphamide, prednisone

ANCA-Associated Vasculitis
- c-ANCA most commonly associated with the clinical picture of granulomatosis with polyangiitis
- p-ANCA most commonly associated with the clinical picture of microscopic polyangiitis
- focal segmental necrotizing RPGN with no immune staining
- may be indolent or fulminant in progression
- vasculitis and granulomas rarely seen on renal biopsy
- treatment typically involves cyclophosphamide and prednisone

Cryoglobulinemia
- cryoglobulins: monoclonal IgM and polyclonal IgG which precipitate at reduced temperatures
- presents as purpura, fever, Raynaud's phenomenon, and arthralgias
- at least 50% of patients have hepatitis C
- renal disease seen in 40% of patients (isolated proteinuria/hematuria progressing to nephritic syndrome)
- most patients have decreased serum complement (C4 initially)
- treat hepatitis C, plasmapheresis
- overall prognosis: 75% renal recovery

Shunt Nephritis

- immune-complex mediated nephritis associated with chronically infected ventriculoatrial shunts inserted for treatment of hydrocephalus
- presents as acute nephritic syndrome with decreased serum complement
- nephrotic range proteinuria in 25% of patients
- treat by removing shunt and administering appropriate antibiotics

HIV-Associated Renal Disease

1. direct nephrotoxic effect of HIV infection, anti-retroviral drugs (e.g. tenofovir, indinavir), and other drugs used to treat HIV-associated infections
2. HIV-associated nephropathy
   - histology: focal and segmental glomerular collapse with mesangial sclerosis; "collapsing FSGS"
   - tubular cystic dilation and tubulo-reticular inclusions
   - clinical features: predominant in African American men, heavy proteinuria, progressive renal insufficiency
   - prognosis: kidney failure within 1 yr without treatment
   - therapy: short-term, high dose steroids, ACEI, HAART

Infective Endocarditis

- manifests as mild form of acute nephritic syndrome with decreased serum complement
- *S. aureus* is most common infecting agent
- treatment with appropriate antibiotics usually resolves GN

Hepatitis B

- can result in membranous nephropathy, polyarteritis nodosa, membranoproliferative GN

Hepatitis C

- can result in membranous nephropathy, cryoglobulinemia, and membranoproliferative GN

Syphilis

- can result in membranous GN

Tubulointerstitial Disease

TUBULOINTERSTITIAL NEPHRITIS

Definition

- cellular infiltrates affecting primarily the renal interstitium and tubular cells
- functional tubule defects are disproportionately greater than the decrease in GFR
- classified as acute or chronic

Signs and Symptoms

- manifestation of disease depends on site of tubule affected
  1. proximal tubule (e.g. multiple myeloma, heavy metals)
     - Fanconi syndrome: decreased reabsorption in proximal tubule causing glycosuria, aminoaciduria, phosphaturia, hyperuricosuria
     - proximal RTA (decreased bicarbonate absorption): Type II RTA
  2. distal tubule (e.g. amyloidosis, obstruction)
     - distal RTA (Type I RTA), usually hypokalemic
     - Na^+-wasting nephropathy
     - ± hyperkalemia leading to type IV RTA (where reduced renal bicarbonate production is caused by hyperkalemia)
  3. collecting duct (e.g. sickle cell anemia, analgesics, PCKD)
     - urinary concentrating defect leading to mild nephrogenic DI
     - polyuria

1. ACUTE TUBULOINTERSTITIAL NEPHRITIS

Definition

- rapid (days to weeks) decline in renal function
- 10-20% of all AKI

Etiology

- hypersensitivity
  1. antibiotics: β-lactams, sulfonamides, rifampin, quinolones, cephalosporins, fluoroquinolones
  2. other: NSAIDs, allopurinol, furosemide, thiazides, triamterene, PPIs, acyclovir, phenytoin, cimetidine

IgA nephropathy is the most common type of primary glomular disease worldwide

Features of Nephritic Syndrome

PHAROH
Proteinuria
Hematuria
Azotemia
RBC casts
Oliguria
HTN

Presentation of Nephrotic Syndrome
HELP
Hypoalbuminemia
Edema
Lipid abnormalities
Proteinuria

- infections
  - bacterial pyelonephritis, *Streptococcus*, brucellosis, *Legionella*, CMV, EBV, toxoplasmosis, leptospirosis, HIV, *Mycoplasma*
- immune
  - SLE, acute allograft rejection, Sjögren's syndrome, sarcoidosis, mixed essential cryoglobulinemia
- idiopathic

Pathophysiology
- acute inflammatory cell infiltrates into renal interstitium

Clinical Features
- AKI
- if hypersensitivity reaction: may see fever, skin rash, arthralgia, serum sickness-like syndrome (particularly rifampin)
- if pyelonephritis: flank pain and costovertebral angle (CVA) tenderness
- if drug reaction, AKI usually occurs 7- 10 days after exposure
- other signs and symptoms based on underlying etiology
- HTN and edema are uncommon

Findings
- urine
  - mild, non-nephrotic range proteinuria and microscopic hematuria
  - sterile pyuria, WBC casts
  - eosinophils if AIN
- blood work
  - increased Cr and urea
  - eosinophilia if drug reaction
  - normal AG metabolic acidosis (RTA)
  - hypophosphatemia, hyperkalemia, hyponatremia
- gallium scan often shows intense signal due to inflammatory infiltrate
- renal biopsy definitive

Treatment
- treat underlying cause (e.g. stop offending medications, antibiotics if pyelonephritis)
- corticosteroids (may be indicated in allergic or immune disease)

Prognosis
- recovery within 2 wk if underlying insult can be eliminated
- the longer the patient is in renal failure, the less likely they will have a full renal recovery

2. CHRONIC TUBULOINTERSTITIAL NEPHRITIS

Definition
- characterized by slowly progressive renal failure, moderate proteinuria, and signs of abnormal tubule function

Etiology
- persistence or progression of acute TIN
- urinary tract obstruction: most important cause of chronic TIN (tumours, stones, bladder outlet obstruction, vesicoureteral reflux)
- chronic pyelonephritis due to vesicoureteral reflux or UTI with obstruction
- nephrotoxins
  - exogenous
    - analgesics: NSAIDs (common), acetaminophen
    - cisplatin, lithium, cyclosporine, tacrolimus
    - heavy metals (lead, cadmium, copper, lithium, mercury, arsenic)
    - Chinese herbs (aristolochic acid)
  - endogenous
    - hypercalcemia, hypokalemia, oxalate, uric acid
- vascular disease: ischemic nephrosclerosis, atheroembolic disease
- malignancies: multiple myeloma, lymphoma
- granulomatous: TB, sarcoidosis, granulomatosis with polyangiitis
- immune: SLE, Sjögren's, cryoglobulinemia, Anti-GBM Disease, amyloidosis, renal graft rejection, vasculitis
- hereditary: cystic diseases of the kidney, sickle cell disease
- others: radiation, Balkan (endemic) nephropathy

Pathophysiology
- fibrosis of interstitium with atrophy of tubules, mononuclear cell inflammation

Signs and Symptoms
- dependent on underlying etiology

Findings
- normal AG metabolic acidosis
- hyperkalemia (out of proportion to degree of renal insufficiency)
- polyuria, nocturia
- partial or complete Fanconi's syndrome
- progressive renal failure with azotemia and uremia
- urine: mild proteinuria, few RBCs and WBCs, no RBC casts
- U/S: shrunken kidneys with irregular contours

Treatment
- stop offending agent or treat underlying disease
- supportive measures: correct metabolic disorders (Ca^{2+}, PO_4^{3-}) and anemia

3. ACUTE TUBULAR NECROSIS

Definition
- abrupt and sustained decline in GFR within minutes to days after ischemic/nephrotoxic insult
- GFR reduced (this serves the purpose of avoiding life-threatening urinary loss of fluid and electrolytes from non-functioning tubules)

Etiology

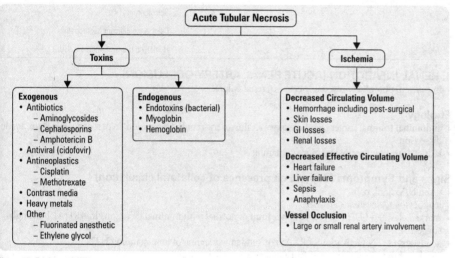

Figure 17. Etiology of ATN

Clinical Presentation
- typically presents as an abrupt rise in urea and Cr after a hypotensive episode, sepsis, rhabdomyolysis, or administration of nephrotoxic drug
- most common cause of non-prerenal AKI in hospitalized patients
- urine: high FE_{Na^+}, pigmented-granular casts

Risk Factors
- pre-existing chronic kidney disease, pre-existing cardiovascular disease, ECF volume depletion, multiple renal insults

Complications
- hyperkalemia: can occur rapidly and cause serious arrhythmias
- metabolic acidosis, decreased Ca^{2+}, increased PO_4^{3-}, hypoalbuminemia

Investigations
- blood work: CBC, electrolytes, Cr, urea, Ca^{2+}, PO_4^{3-}, blood gases
- urine: R&M, electrolytes, osmolality, microscopic urinalysis searching for pigmented granular casts
- ECG
- abdominal U/S
- rule out other causes of prerenal/postrenal azotemia and intrinsic AKI (GN, AIN, vasculitis)

Treatment
- largely supportive once underlying problem is corrected
- loop diuretics may help manage volume overload and reduce tubular metabolic requirements to allow for recovery (controversial)
- consider early dialysis in severe/rapidly progressing cases to prevent uremic syndrome

Meta-Analysis: Effectiveness of Drugs for Preventing Contrast-Induced Nephropathy
Ann Intern Med 2008;148:284-294
Purpose: To determine the effectiveness of N-acetylcysteine, theophylline, fenoldopam, dopamine, iloprost, statin, furosemide, or mannitol on preventing nephropathy.
Study Selection: RCTs that used these agents in patients receiving iodinated contrast.
Results: In the 41 RCTs included N-acetylcysteine (RR=0.62 [0.44-0.88]) and theophylline (RR=0.49 [0.23-1.06]) reduced the risk of nephropathy more than saline alone. Furosemide increased the risk (RR=3.27 [1.48-7.26]). Other agents did not affect risk of nephropathy.
Conclusion: N-acetylcysteine is more renoprotective than hydration alone.

Prevention
- correct fluid balance before surgical procedures
- for patients with chronic renal disease requiring radiographic contrast:
  - give N-acetylcysteine 600-1200 mg PO bid day before and day of procedure, give intravenous isotonic fluid (either NaCl or NaHCO₃)
  - isotonic NaHCO₃ at 3 mL/kg over 1 h before procedure and 1 mL/kg/h for 6 h post-procedure if not contraindicated
  - avoid giving diuretics, ACEI, cyclosporine on morning of procedure if possible
- use renal-adjusted doses of nephrotoxic drugs in patients with renal insufficiency

Vascular Diseases of the Kidney

LARGE VESSEL DISEASE

Table 12. Summary of Vascular Diseases

Large Vessel Disease	Medium Vessel Disease	Small Vessel Disease
Acute renal artery occlusion (infarct)	Kawasaki disease	Hypertensive nephrosclerosis
Renal artery stenosis (ischemia)	Polyarteritis nodosa	Atheroembolic renal disease
Renal vein thrombosis		Thrombotic microangiopathy
		Scleroderma
		Calcineurin inhibitor nephropathy
		Hemolytic Uremic Syndrome (HUS)

1. RENAL INFARCTION (ACUTE RENAL ARTERY OCCLUSION)
- important, potentially reversible cause of renal failure

Etiology
- abdominal trauma, surgery, embolism, vasculitis, extra-renal compression, hypercoagulable state, aortic dissection
- kidney transplant recipients more vulnerable

Signs and Symptoms (depend on presence of collateral circulation)
- fever, N/V, flank pain
- leukocytosis, elevated AST, ALP
- marked elevated LDH (LDH >4x upper limit of normal with minimal elevations in AST/ALT strongly suggestive)
- acute onset HTN (activation of RAAS) or sudden worsening of long-standing HTN
- renal dysfunction, e.g. elevated Cr (if bilateral, or solitary functioning kidney)

Investigations
- renal arteriography (more reliable but risk of atheroembolic renal disease)
- contrast-enhanced CT or MR angiography, duplex Doppler studies (operator dependent)

Treatment
- prompt localization of occlusion and restoration of blood flow
- anticoagulation, thrombolysis, percutaneous angioplasty or clot extraction, surgical thrombectomy
- medical therapy in the long-term to reduce risk (e.g. antihypertensives)

2. ISCHEMIC RENAL DISEASE (RENAL ARTERY STENOSIS)
- chronic renal impairment secondary to hemodynamically significant renal artery stenosis or microvascular disease
- significant cause of ESRD: 15% in patients >50 yr (higher prevalence if significant vascular disease)
- usually associated with large vessel disease elsewhere
- causes of renal artery stenosis
  - atherosclerotic plaques (90%): proximal 1/3 renal artery, usually males >55 yr, smokers
  - fibromuscular dysplasia (10%): distal 2/3 renal artery or segmental branches, usually young females (typical onset <30 yr)
- when there is decreased RBF, GFR is dependent on angiotensin II-induced efferent arteriolar constriction which raises the FF (GFR/RBF)
- most common cause of secondary HTN ("renovascular HTN"), 1-2% of all hypertensive patients
  - etiology
    - decreased renal perfusion of one or both kidneys leads to increased renin release and subsequent angiotensin production
    - increased angiotensin raises blood pressure in two ways
      1. causes generalized arteriolar constriction
      2. release of aldosterone increases Na+ and water retention
  - elevated blood pressure can in turn lead to further damage of kidneys and worsening HTN

Risk Factors
- >50 yr
- smoking
- other atherosclerotic disease (dyslipidemia, DM, diffuse atherosclerosis)

Signs and Symptoms
- severe/refractory HTN and/or hypertensive crises, with negative family history of HTN
- asymmetric renal size
- epigastric or flank bruits
- spontaneous hypokalemia (renin activation in under-perfused kidney)
- increasing Cr with ACEI/ARB
- flash pulmonary edema with normal LV function

Investigations
- must establish presence of renal artery stenosis and prove it is responsible for renal dysfunction
- duplex Doppler U/S (kidney size, blood flow): good screening test (operator dependent)
- digital subtraction angiography (risk of contrast nephropathy)
- CT or MR angiography (effective noninvasive tests to establish presence of stenosis, for MR avoid gadolinium contrast if eGFR <30 mL/min because of risk of systemic dermal fibrosis)
- ACEI renography (e.g. captopril renal scan)
- renal arteriography (gold standard)

Treatment
- surgical: percutaneous angioplasty ± stent, surgical revascularization, occasionally surgical bypass
- medical: BP lowering medications (ACEI is drug of choice if unilateral renal artery disease but contraindicated if bilateral renal artery disease)
- little or no benefit if therapy is late (e.g. kidney is already shrunken), however, therapy can be considered to save the opposite kidney if normal

3. RENAL VEIN THROMBOSIS

Etiology
- hypercoagulable states (e.g. nephrotic syndrome, especially membranous), ECF volume depletion, extrinsic compression of renal vein, significant trauma, malignancy (e.g. RCC), sickle cell disease
- clinical presentation determined by rapidity of occlusion and formation of collateral circulation

Signs and Symptoms
- acute: N/V, flank pain, hematuria, elevated plasma LDH, ± rise in Cr, sudden rise in proteinuria
- chronic: PE (typical first presenting symptom), increasing proteinuria and/or tubule dysfunction

Investigations
- renal venography (gold standard), CT or MR angiography, duplex Doppler U/S

Treatment
- thrombolytic therapy ± percutaneous thrombectomy for acute renal vein thrombosis
- anticoagulation with heparin then warfarin (1 yr or indefinitely, depending on risk factors)

MEDIUM VESSEL DISEASE

1. KAWASAKI DISEASE
- see Pediatrics, P92

2. POLYARTERITIS NODOSA
- see Rheumatology, RH19
- kidneys most commonly involved organ
- heterogenous impact on renal function
- pathologically can cause glomerular ischemia which manifests as mild proteinuria and hypertension

SMALL VESSEL DISEASE

1. HYPERTENSIVE NEPHROSCLEROSIS
- see Hypertension, NP34

2. ATHEROEMBOLIC RENAL DISEASE
- progressive renal insufficiency due to embolic obstruction of small- and medium-sized renal vessels by atheromatous emboli
- spontaneous or after renal artery manipulation (surgery, angiography, percutaneous angioplasty)
- anticoagulants and thrombolytics interfere with ulcerated plaque healing and can worsen disease

Stenting and Medical Therapy for Atherosclerotic Renal Artery Stenosis
NEJM 2014;370:13-22
Study: Multicentre, unblinded RCT, median follow-up of 43 mo.
Patients: 947 patients with atherosclerotic renal-artery stenosis who also have significant systolic HTN or CKD.
Intervention: Percutaneous revascularization (stenting) with medical therapy (statins, ARB, calcium channel blockers, HCTZ and BP control) versus medical therapy alone.
Outcomes: Occurrence of adverse CV or renal event (composite of death from CV or renal cause, MI, stroke, hospitalization for CHF, progressive renal insufficiency, or need for renal replacement therapy) and all-cause mortality.
Results: No significant difference in primary composite end point between participants who received stenting or those on medical therapy alone. No significant differences between the treatment groups in the rates of the individual components of the primary end point or in all-cause mortality.
Conclusion: Renal artery stenting did not confer a significant benefit with respect to the prevention of clinical events when added to comprehensive, multifactorial medical therapy in people with atherosclerotic renal artery stenosis and HTN or CKD.

Reduced Exposure to Calcineurin Inhibitors in Renal Transplantation (ELITE-Symphony Trial)
NEJM 2007;257:2562-2575
Study: Multicentre, RCT with 12 mo follow-up.
Patients: 1,645 patients scheduled to receive a single organ kidney transplant.
Intervention: Mycophenolate mofetil, corticosteroids, and either: 1) standard dose cyclosporine; 2) low dose cyclosporine with daclizumab induction; 3) low dose tacrolimus with daclizumab induction; 4) low dose sirolimus with daclizumab induction.
Primary Outcome: Estimated Cockcroft-Gault GFR 12 mo after transplantation.
Results: The tacrolimus arm showed significantly higher eGFR at 12 mo compared to all other arms (65.4 mL/min vs. 57.1, 59.4, 56.7 for arms 1, 2, 4 respectively, p≤0.001). The tacrolimus arm also showed decreased rates of acute rejection at 6 mo and 12 mo vs. all arms (p<0.001), improved allograft survival against standard dose cyclosporine and sirolimus, and decreased treatment failure against all other arms. There was no difference in overall patient survival between groups. Sirolimus had the highest incidence of lymphoceles, delayed wound healing, and serious adverse events; tacrolimus had significantly higher rates of new-onset DM; and cyclosporine regimes had the lowest incidence of diarrhea but highest opportunistic infection rates.
Conclusion: Immunosuppression regiments using low dose tacrolimus and daclizumab induction decrease nephrotoxicity while maintaining therapeutic immunosuppression in renal transplant patients.

- investigations
  - eosinophilia, eosinophiluria, and hypocomplementemia
  - renal biopsy: needle-shaped cholesterol clefts (due to tissue-processing artifacts) with surrounding tissue reaction in small-/medium-sized vessels
- treatment
  - no effective treatment; avoid angiographic and surgical procedures in patients with diffuse atherosclerosis, medical therapy for concomitant cardiovascular disease
- prognosis: poor overall, at least one third will develop ESRD

3. THROMBOTIC MICROANGIOPATHY
- see Hematology, H22
- etiologies include the spectrum of TTP-HUS, DIC, severe preeclampsia
- renal involvement more common in HUS than TTP
- renal involvement characterized by fibrin thrombi in glomerular capillary loops ± arterioles
- treatment
  - depends on cause
  - supportive therapy
  - TTP-HUS: plasma exchange, corticosteroids (splenectomy and rituximab if refractory)
- avoid platelet transfusions and ASA

4. CALCINEURIN INHIBITOR NEPHROPATHY
- cyclosporine and tacrolimus
- causes both acute reversible and chronic, largely irreversible nephrotoxicity
- major cause of kidney failure in other solid organ transplants (e.g. heart)
- acute: due to afferent and efferent glomerular capillary constriction leading to decreased GFR (tubular vacuolization)
  - prerenal azotemia
  - treatment: calcium channel blockers or prostaglandin analogs, reduce dose of cyclosporine or switch to another immunosuppressive drug
- chronic: result of obliterative arteriolopathy causing interstitial nephritis and CKD (striped fibrosis), less frequent now due to lower doses of calcineurin inhibitors

Analgesic Nephropathies

1. Vasomotor AKI
- clinically: develop prerenal azotemia within a few days of starting NSAID
- normally prostaglandins vasodilate afferent renal arteriole to maintain blood flow
- NSAIDs act by blocking cyclooxygenase enzyme, thereby preventing prostaglandin synthesis and causing renal ischemia
- more common in elderly, underlying renal disease, hypovolemia (diuretics, CHF, cirrhosis, nephrotic syndrome)
- treatment: discontinue NSAID, dialysis rarely needed

2. Acute Interstitial Nephritis
- fenoprofen (60%), ibuprofen, naproxen
- may be associated with minimal change glomerulopathy and nephrotic range proteinuria
- resolves eventually with discontinuation of NSAID, may require interval dialysis
- short-term high dose steroids (1 mg/kg/d of prednisone) may hasten recovery

3. Chronic Interstitial Nephritis
- due to excessive consumption of antipyretics (phenacetin or acetaminophen) in combination with NSAIDs
- seen in patients who also have emotional stress, psychiatric symptoms, and GI disturbance
- papillary necrosis
  - gross hematuria, flank pain, declining renal function
  - calyceal filling defect seen with IVP – "ring sign"
- increased risk of transitional cell carcinoma of renal pelvis
- good prognosis if discontinue analgesics

4. Acute Tubular Necrosis
- can be caused by acetaminophen
  - incidence of renal dysfunction is related to the severity of acetaminophen ingestion
- vascular endothelial damage can also occur
- both direct toxicity and ischemia contribute to the tubular damage
- renal function spontaneously returns to baseline within 1-4 wk
- dialysis may be required during the acute episode of ingestion

5. Other Effects of NSAIDs
- sodium retention (2° to reduced GFR)
- hyperkalemia, HTN (2° to hyporeninemic hypoaldosteronism)
- excess water retention (2° to loss of antagonistic effect of prostaglandins on ADH)

Systemic Disease with Renal Manifestation

Diabetes

- diabetic nephropathy: presence of microalbuminuria or overt nephropathy (e.g. macroalbuminuria) in patients with DM who lack indicators of other renal diseases
- most common cause of end-stage renal failure in North America
- 50% of patients with diabetes will develop nephropathy
- at diagnosis up to 30% of patients with type 2 DM have albuminuria (75% microalbuminuria, 25% overt nephropathy)
- microalbuminuria is a risk factor for progression to overt nephropathy and cardiovascular disease
- once macroalbuminuria is established, renal function declines, 50% of patients reach ESRD within 7-10 yr
- associated with HTN and diabetic retinopathy (especially type 1 DM) and/or neuropathy (especially type 2 DM)
- indication of possible non-diabetic cause of renal disease in patients with DM
    - rising Cr with little/no proteinuria
    - lack of retinopathy or neuropathy (microvascular complications)
    - persistent hematuria (microscopic or macroscopic)
    - signs or symptoms of systemic disease
    - inappropriate time course; rapidly rising Cr, renal disease in a patient with short duration of DM
    - family history of non-diabetic renal disease (e.g. PCKD, Alport's)

DM is one of the causes of ESRD that does not result in small kidneys at presentation of ESRD; the others are amyloidosis, HIV nephropathy, PCKD, and multiple myeloma

Abnormal Urine ACR Values from 2013 Canadian DM Association CPG
>2.0 mg/mmol in males and females

ACEI can cause hyperkalemia; therefore, be sure to watch serum K⁺, especially if patient has DM and renal insufficiency

DIABETIC RENAL COMPLICATIONS

1. Progressive Glomerulosclerosis
- classic diabetic glomerular lesion: Kimmelstiel-Wilson nodular glomerulosclerosis (15-20%)
- more common lesion is diffuse glomerulosclerosis with a uniform increase in mesangial matrix

Table 13. Stages of Diabetic Progressive Glomerulosclerosis

Stage 1	Stage 2	Stage 3	Stage 4
↑ GFR (120-150%) – compensatory hyperfiltration	Detectable microalbuminuria (0-300 mg/24 h)	Macroalbuminuria (>300 mg/24 h)	↑ proteinuria (>500 mg/24 h)
± slightly increased mesangial matrix	Albumin-Cr ratio (ACR) 2.0–20 mg/mmol (18-180 mg/d)	ACR >20 mg/mmol, (>180 mg/d)	↓ GFR
		Proteinuria (positive urine dipstick)	<20% glomerular filtration surface area present
	↑ mesangial matrix	Normal GFR	Sclerosed glomeruli
		↑↑↑ mesangial matrix	

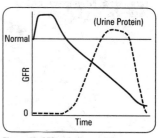

Figure 18. GFR and urine protein over time in DM

2. Accelerated Atherosclerosis
- common finding
- decreased GFR
- may increase angiotensin II production resulting in increased BP
- increased risk of ATN secondary to contrast media

3. Autonomic Neuropathy
- affects bladder leading to functional obstruction and urinary retention
- residual urine promotes infection
- obstructive nephropathy

4. Papillary Necrosis
- type 1 DM susceptible to ischemic necrosis of medullary papillae
- sloughed papillae may obstruct ureter
- can present as renal colic or with obstructive features ± hydronephrosis

2013 Canadian Diabetes Association Clinical Practice Guidelines on Chronic Kidney Disease in Diabetes
- screen for microalbuminuria with a random urine test for albumin to Cr ratio (ACR) and eGFR with a serum Cr (e.g. using MDRD equation)
    - type 1 DM: annually in post-pubertal individuals after 5 yr of diagnosis
    - type 2 DM: at diagnosis, then annually
    - if eGFR >60 mL/min or ACR <2.0 mg/mmol: there is no CKD, re-screen in 1 yr
    - if urine ACR >20.0 mg/mmol: diagnose CKD
    - if ACR <20.0 mg/mmol but >2.0 mg/mmol: order serum Cr for eGFR in 3 mo and 2 repeats of random urine ACRs over the next 3 mo; at 3 mo: if eGFR ≤60 ml/min or if >2/3 ACRs are >2.0 mg/mmol, diagnose CKD

Protein Restriction for Diabetic Renal Disease
Cochrane DB Syst Rev 2007;4:CD002181
Purpose: To review the effects of dietary protein restriction on the progression of diabetic nephropathy.
Study Selection: RCTs and before and after studies of the effects of restricted protein diet on renal function in subjects with DM. 12 studies were reviewed.
Results: The risk of end-stage renal disease or death was lower in patients on low-protein diet. In patients with type 1 DM no effect on GFR was noted in the low-protein diet group.

Renal Outcomes with Telmisartan, Ramipril, or Both in People at High Vascular Risk (ONTARGET Study)
Lancet 2008;372:547-553
Study: Prospective, multicentre, double-blind, RCT.
Participants: 25,620 patients with median follow-up of 56 mo.
Intervention: Patients received either ramipril (10 mg/d; n=8,576), telmisartan (80 mg/d; n=8,542), or a combination of both drugs (n=8,502).
Primary Outcome: Composite of dialysis, doubling of creatinine level, and death.
Results: The number of outcome events was similar for telmisartan (n=1,147) and ramipril (1,150; HR 1.00, 95% CI 0.92-1.09), but was increased with combination therapy (1,233; HR 1.09, 1.01-1.18, p=0.037). The need for dialysis or doubling of serum creatinine, was similar with telmisartan (189) and ramipril (174; HR 1.09, 0.89-1.34) and more frequent with combination therapy (212; HR 1.24, 1.01-1.51, p=0.038). Estimated GFR declined least with ramipril compared with telmisartan or combination therapy (p<0.001). The increase in urinary albumin excretion was less with telmisartan (p=0.004) and combination therapy (p=0.001) than with ramipril.
Conclusion: Renal outcomes were similar in both telmisartan and ramipril monotherapy. Combination therapy reduced proteinuria to a greater extent than monotherapy, but was associated with poorer renal outcomes.

- if CKD diagnosed, ordered urine R+M and dipstick, if negative then diagnose CKD in DM
- with CKD in DM: urine ACR and serum Cr (for eGFR) every 6 mo
- delay screening if transient cause of albuminuria or low eGFR
- evaluate for other causes of proteinuria, rule out non-diabetic renal disease
- avoid unnecessary potential nephrotoxins (NSAIDs, aminoglycosides, dye studies)

Priorities in the Management of Patients with DM
1. vascular protection for all patients with DM
   - ACEI, antiplatelet therapy (as indicated)
   - BP control, glycemic control, lifestyle modification, lipid control
2. optimization of BP in patients who are hypertensive
   - treat according to HTN guidelines
3. renal protection for DM patients with nephropathy (even in absence of HTN)
   - type 1 DM: ACEI
   - type 2 DM: CrCl >60 mL/min: ACEI or ARB – CrCl <60 mL/min: ARB
   - 2nd line agents: nondihydropyridine calcium channel blockers (diltiazem, verapamil)
   - combination of ACEI and ARB not recommended for proteinuria
- check serum Cr and K+ levels within 1 wk of initiating ACEI or ARB and at time of acute illness
- serum Cr can safely be allowed to rise up to 30% with initiation of ACEI or ARB, usually stabilizes after 2-4 wk, monitor for significant worsening of renal function or hyperkalemia
- if >30% rise in serum Cr or hyperkalemia, discontinue medication and consider 2nd line agent
- consider holding ACEI, ARB, and/or diuretic with acute illness and in women before becoming pregnant
- consider referral to nephrologist if ACR >60 mg/mmol, eGFR <30 mL/min, progressive kidney function loss, unable to achieve BP targets, or unable to stay on ACEI or ARB

Scleroderma

- see Rheumatology, RH13
- 50% of scleroderma patients have renal involvement (mild proteinuria, high Cr, HTN)
- renal involvement usually occurs early in the course of illness
- histology: media thickened, "onion skin" hypertrophy of small renal arteries, fibrinoid necrosis of afferent arterioles and glomeruli
- 10-15% of scleroderma patients have a "scleroderma renal crisis" (occurs in first few years of disease): malignant HTN, ARF, microangiopathy, volume overload, visual changes, HTN encephalopathy
- treatment: BP control with ACEI slows progression of renal disease

Multiple Myeloma

- see Hematology, H49
- malignant proliferation of plasma cells in the bone marrow with the production of immunoglobulins
- patients may present with severe bone disease and renal failure
- light chains are filtered at the glomerulus and appear as Bence-Jones proteins in the urine (monoclonal light chains)
- kidney damage can occur by several mechanisms
  - hypercalcemia
  - light chain cast nephropathy or "myeloma kidney"
  - hyperuricemia
  - infection
  - secondary amyloidosis
  - monoclonal Ig deposition disease
  - diffuse tubular obstruction
- light chain cast nephropathy
  - large tubular casts in urine sediment (light chains + Tamm-Horsfall protein)
  - proteinuria and renal insufficiency, can progress rapidly to kidney failure
- monoclonal Ig deposition disease
  - deposits of monoclonal Ig in kidney, liver, heart, and other organs
  - mostly light chains (85-90%)
  - causes nodular glomerulosclerosis (similar to diabetic nephropathy)
- lab features: increased BUN, increased Cr, urine protein immunoelectrophoresis positive for Bence-Jones protein (not detected on urine dipstick)
- poor candidates for kidney transplantation

Malignancy

- cancer can have many different renal manifestations
- kidney transplantation cannot be performed unless malignancy is cured
  - solid tumours: mild proteinuria or membranous GN
  - lymphoma: minimal change GN (Hodgkin's) or membranous GN (non-Hodgkin's)
  - renal cell carcinoma
  - tumour lysis syndrome: hyperuricemia, diffuse tubular obstruction, hyperkalemia, hyperphosphatemia, hypocalcemia, lactic acidosis
  - chemotherapy (especially cisplatin): ATN or chronic TIN
  - pelvic tumours/mets: postrenal failure secondary to obstruction
  - 2° amyloidosis
  - radiotherapy (radiation nephritis)

Chronic Kidney Disease

Definition

- progressive and irreversible loss of kidney function
- abnormal markers (Cr, urea)
  - GFR <60 mL/min for >3 mo; or
  - kidney pathology seen on biopsy; or
  - ultrasound: small shrunken kidneys <9 cm (normal 10-13 cm), increased cortical echogenicity

Clinical Features

- volume overload and HTN
- electrolyte and acid-base balance disorders (e.g. metabolic acidosis)
- uremia

Incidence of Etiologies of CKD

DM	42.9%
HTN	26.4%
Glomerulonephritis	9.9%
Other/Unknown	7.7%
Interstitial nephritis/ Pyelonephritis	4.0%
Cystic/Hereditary/Congenital	3.1%
Secondary GN/Vasculitis	2.4%

Table 14. Stages of CKD (KDIGO, 2013)

			Persistent Albuminuria Categories		
		GFR (mL/min/1.73m²)	A1 <30 mg/g <3 mg/mmol	A2 30-300 mg/g 3-30 mg/mmol	A3 >300 mg/g >30 mg/mmol
GFR Categories (mL/min/1.73m²)	G1	≥90	1 if CKD	1	2
	G2	60-89	1 if CKD	1	2
	G3a	45-59	1	2	3
	G3b	30-44	2	3	3
	G4	15-29	3	3	4+
	G5	<15 (kidney failure)	4+	4+	4+

The numbers in the boxes are a reflection of the risk of progression and are a guide to the frequency of monitoring/year
"D" is added to G5 for patients requiring dialysis
Classification is based on cause, GFR, and amount of albuminuria
Rate of progression and risk of complications are determined by the cause of CKD

Management of Complications of CKD
NEPHRON

N – Low-nitrogen diet
E – Electrolytes: monitor K⁺
P – pH: metabolic acidosis
H – HTN
R – RBCs: manage anemia with erythropoietin
O – Osteodystrophy: give calcium between meals (to increase Ca^{2+}) and calcium with meals (to bind and decrease PO_4^{3-})
N – Nephrotoxins: avoid nephrotoxic drugs (ASA, gentamicin) and adjust doses of renally excreted medications

Management of Chronic Kidney Disease

- diet
  - preventing HTN and volume overload
    - Na⁺ and water restriction
  - preventing electrolyte imbalances
    - K⁺ restriction (40 mmol/d)
    - PO_4^{3-} restriction (1 g/d)
    - avoid extra-dietary Mg^{2+} (e.g. antacids)
  - preventing uremia and potentially delaying decline in GFR
    - protein restriction with adequate caloric intake in order to limit endogenous protein catabolism
- medical
  - adjust dosages of renally excreted medications
  - HTN: ACEI (target 140/90 mmHg without DM and 130/80 mmHg with DM), loop diuretics when GFR <25 mL/min
  - dyslipidemia: statins (target LDL <2 mmol/L)
  - calcium and phosphate disorders
    - calcium supplements (e.g. TUMS®) treats hypocalcemia when given between meals and binds phosphate when given with meals
    - consider calcitriol (1,25-dihydroxy-vitamin D) if hypocalcemic
    - sevelamer (phosphate binder) if both hypercalcemic and hyperphosphatemic

Renin Angiotensin System Blockade and Cardiovascular Outcomes in Patients with Chronic Kidney Disease and Proteinuria: A Meta-Analysis
Am Heart J 2008;155:791-805
Purpose: To evaluate the role of RAS blockade in improving cardiovascular CV outcomes in patients with CKD.
Study Selection: RCT that analyzed CV outcomes in patients with CKD/proteinuria treated with RAS blockade (ACEI/ARB). RAS blockade-based therapy was compared with placebo and control therapy (β-blocker, calcium-channel blockers, and other antihypertensive-based therapy) in the study.
Results: Twenty-five trials (n=45,758) were included. Compared to placebo, RAS blockade reduced the risk of heart failure in patients with diabetic nephropathy. In patients with non-diabetic CKD, RAS blockade decreased CV outcome compared to control therapy.
Conclusions: RAS blockade reduced CV outcomes in diabetic nephropathy as well as non-diabetic CKD.

Effects of Lowering LDL Cholesterol with Simvastatin and Ezetimibe in Patients with Chronic Kidney Disease
Lancet 2011;377:2181-2192
Purpose: To assess the efficacy and safety of the combination of simvastatin and ezetimibe in patients with moderate to severe CKD.
Study: Randomized, double-blind trial with 9,270 patients with CKD with no known history of myocardial infarction or coronary vascularization. Patients were randomized to simvastatin 20 mg plus ezetimibe 10 mg daily versus matching placebo.
Primary Outcome: First major atherosclerotic event (non-fatal myocardial infarction or coronary death, non-hemorrhagic stroke, or any arterial revascularization procedure).
Results: The simvastatin plus ezetimibe group was associated with an average LDL cholesterol difference of 0.85 mmol/L during a median follow-up of 4.9 yr. There was a 17% proportional reduction in major atherosclerotic events in the simvastatin plus ezetimibe group compared to placebo.
Conclusions: Reducing LDL cholesterol with a treatment regimen of simvastatin plus ezetimibe safely reduced the incidence of major atherosclerotic events in patients with moderate to severe CKD.

- vitamin D analogues are being introduced in the near future
- cinacalcet for hyperparathyroidism (sensitizes parathyroid to Ca^{2+}, decreasing PTH)
- metabolic acidosis: sodium bicarbonate
- anemia: erythropoietin injections for Hb <90 g/L (9 g/dL) and target Hb between 90-105 g/L (9-10.5 g/dL)
- clotting abnormalities: DDAVP if patient has clinical bleeding or invasive procedures (acts to reverse platelet dysfunction)
- dialysis (hemodialysis, peritoneal dialysis)
  - indications include persistent and refractory hyperkalemia or metabolic acidosis, fluid overload, encephalopathy, persistent nausea and vomiting, evidence of malnutrition, pericarditis
- renal transplantation

Prevention of Progression
- as above
- control of HTN, DM (HbA1c <7%), cardiovascular risk factors (e.g. smoking cessation)
- avoid nephrotoxins such as NSAID's, COXIB's, IV contrast in patients with eGFR < 60 mL/min/1.73 m^2
- address reversible causes of AKI

Hypertension

- see Family Medicine, FM34
- HTN occurs in about 20% of population
- etiology classified as primary ("essential"; makes up 90% of cases) or secondary
- primary HTN can cause kidney disease (hypertensive nephrosclerosis), which may in turn exacerbate th HTN
- secondary HTN can be caused by renal parenchymal or renal vascular disease

Hypertensive Nephrosclerosis

Table 15. Chronic vs. Malignant Nephrosclerosis

	Chronic Nephrosclerosis	Malignant Nephrosclerosis
Histology	Slow vascular sclerosis with ischemic changes affecting intralobular and afferent arterioles	Fibrinoid necrosis of arterioles, disruption of vascular endothelium
Clinical Picture	Black race, underlying CKD, chronic hypertensive disease	Acute elevation in BP (dBP >120 mmHg) HTN encephalopathy
Urinalysis	Mild proteinuria, normal urine sediment	Proteinuria and hematuria (RBC casts)
Therapy	Blood pressure control, (target <140/90) with frequent follow-up	Lower dBP to 100-110 mmHg within 6-24 h More aggressive treatment can cause ischemic event Identify and treat underlying cause of HTN
Prognosis	Can progress to renal failure despite patient adherence	Lower survival if renal insufficiency develops

Renovascular Hypertension

- see *Vascular Diseases of the Kidney*, NP28

Renal Parenchymal Hypertension

- HTN secondary to GN, AIN, diabetic nephropathy, or any other chronic renal disease
- mechanism of HTN not fully understood but may include
  - excess RAAS activation due to inflammation and fibrosis in multiple small intra-renal vessels
  - production of unknown vasopressors, lack of production of unknown vasodilators, or lack of clearance of endogenous vasopressor
  - ineffective sodium excretion with fluid overload

Investigations
- as well as investigations for renovascular HTN, additional tests may include
  - 24 h urinary estimations of CrCl and protein excretion
  - imaging (U/S, CT)
  - serology for collagen-vascular disease
  - renal biopsy

Treatment
- most chronic renal disease is irreversible, but treatment of HTN can slow the progression of renal insufficiency
- control ECF volume: Na^+ restriction (2g/d intake), diuretic, dialysis with end-stage disease
- ACEI or ARB may provide added benefit (monitor K^+ and Cr) if there is significant proteinuria (>300 mg/

Cystic Diseases of the Kidney

- characterized by epithelium-lined cavities filled with fluid or semisolid debris within the kidneys
- includes: simple cysts (present in 50% of population >50), medullary cystic kidney, medullary sponge kidney, polycystic kidney disease (autosomal dominant and recessive), and acquired cystic kidney disease (in chronic hemodialysis patients)

Adult Polycystic Kidney Disease

- autosomal dominant; at least 2 genes: *PKD1* (chr 16p) and *PKD2* (chr 4q)
- *PKD1* (1:400), *PKD2* (1:1,000) accounts for about 10% of cases of renal failure
- patients generally heterozygous for mutant *PKD* gene but accumulate a series of second 'somatic hits' precipitating the condition
- *PKD* gene defect leads to abnormal proliferation and apoptosis of tubular epithelial cells leading to cyst growth
- most common extrarenal manifestations: multiple asymptomatic hepatic cysts (33%), mitral valve prolapse (25%), cerebral aneurysm (10%), diverticulosis
- polycystic liver disease rarely causes liver failure
- less common extrarenal manifestations: cysts in pancreas, spleen, thyroid, ovary, seminal vesicles, and aorta

Hypercalcemia complicates many cancers and can cause multiple kinds of renal disorders (renal vasoconstriction with reduced GFR, salt-wasting with volume depletion, risk of calcium kidney stones)

Signs and Symptoms
- often asymptomatic; discovered incidentally on imaging or by screening those with FHx
- acute abdominal flank pain/dull lumbar back pain
- hematuria (frequently initial sign is microscopic hematuria, otherwise gross hematuria)
- nocturia (urinary concentrating defect)
- rarely extra-renal presentation (e.g. ruptured berry aneurysm, diverticulitis)
- HTN (increased renin due to focal compression of intrarenal arteries by cysts) (60-75%)
- ± palpable kidneys

Extra-Renal Manifestations of PCKD
- Hepatic cysts
- Mitral valve prolapse
- Cerebral aneurysms
- Diverticulosis

Common Complications
- urinary tract and cyst infections, HTN, chronic renal failure, nephrolithiasis (5-15%), flank and chronic back pain

Clinical Course
- polycystic changes are always bilateral and can present at any age
- clinical manifestations rare before age 20-25
- kidneys are normal at birth but may enlarge to 10x normal size
- variable progression to renal functional impairment (ESRD in up to 50% by age 60)

Investigations
- radiographic diagnosis: best accomplished by renal U/S (enlarged kidneys, multiple cysts throughout renal parenchyma, increased cortical thickness, splaying of renal calyces)
- CT abdo with contrast (for equivocal cases, occasionally reveals more cystic involvement)
- gene linkage analysis for *PKD1* for asymptomatic carriers
- Cr, BUN, urine R&M (to assess for hematuria)

Treatment
- goal: to preserve renal function by prevention and treatment of complications
- educate patient and family about disease, its manifestations, and inheritance pattern
- genetic counselling: transmission rate 50% from affected parent
- prevention and early treatment of urinary tract and cyst infections (avoid instrumentation of GU tract)
- TMP/SMX, ciprofloxacin: able to penetrate cyst walls, achieve therapeutic levels
- adequate hydration to prevent stone formation
- avoid contact sports due to greater risk of injury to enlarged kidneys
- screen for cerebral aneurysms if family history of aneurysmal hemorrhages
- monitor blood pressure and treat HTN with ACEI
- dialysis or transplant for ESRD (disease does not recur in transplanted kidney)
- may require nephrectomy for symptomatic relief of pain or due to recurrent infections

Autosomal Recessive Polycystic Kidney Disease

- 1:20,000 incidence
- prenatal diagnosis by enlarged kidneys
- perinatal death from respiratory failure
- patients who survive perinatal period develop CHF, HTN, CKD
- treated with kidney and/or liver transplant

Medullary Sponge Kidney

- common, autosomal dominant, usually diagnosed in 4th-5th decades
- multiple cystic dilatations in the collecting ducts of the medulla
- renal stones, hematuria, and recurrent UTIs are common features
- an estimated 10% of patients who present with renal stones have medullary sponge kidney
- nephrocalcinosis on abdominal x-ray in 50% patients, often detect asymptomatic patients incidentally
- diagnosis: contrast filled medullary cysts on IVP leading to characteristic radial pattern ("bouquet of flowers"), "Swiss cheese" appearance on histological cross-section
- treat UTIs and stone formation as indicated
- does not result in renal failure

End Stage Renal Disease

- ESRD represents a decline in kidney function requiring renal replacement therapy which can occur over days to weeks (AKI), over months to years (CKD), or as a combination of the two

Presentation of End Stage Renal Disease

1. Volume Overload
- due to increase in total body Na^+ content
- signs: weight gain, HTN, pulmonary or peripheral edema

2. Electrolyte Abnormalities
- high
  - K^+ (decreased renal excretion, increased tissue breakdown)
  - PO_4^{3-} (decreased renal excretion, increased tissue breakdown)
  - Ca^{2+} (rare; happens during recovery phase after rhabdomyolysis-induced AKI or in settings where hypercalcemia contributes to renal failure, such as in multiple myeloma or sarcoidosis)
  - uric acid
- low
  - Na^+ (failure to excrete excessive water intake)
  - Ca^{2+} (decreased Vitamin D activation, hyperphosphatemia, hypoalbuminemia)
  - HCO_3^- (especially with sepsis or severe heart failure)

3. Uremic Syndrome
- manifestations result from retention of urea and other metabolites as well as hormone deficiencies

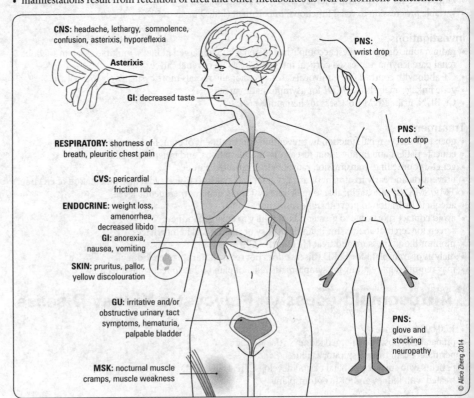

CNS: headache, lethargy, somnolence, confusion, asterixis, hyporeflexia

Asterixis

GI: decreased taste

PNS: wrist drop

RESPIRATORY: shortness of breath, pleuritic chest pain

CVS: pericardial friction rub

ENDOCRINE: weight loss, amenorrhea, decreased libido

GI: anorexia, nausea, vomiting

SKIN: pruritus, pallor, yellow discolouration

GU: irritative and/or obstructive urinary tract symptoms, hematuria, palpable bladder

MSK: nocturnal muscle cramps, muscle weakness

PNS: foot drop

PNS: glove and stocking neuropathy

© Alice Zheng 2014

Figure 19. Signs and symptoms of end stage renal disease

Complications
- CNS: decreased LOC, stupor, seizure
- CVS: cardiomyopathy, CHF, arrhythmia, pericarditis, atherosclerosis
- GI: peptic ulcer disease, gastroduodenitis, AVM
- hematologic: anemia, bleeding tendency (platelet dysfunction), infections
- endocrine
  - decreased testosterone, estrogen, progesterone
  - increased FSH, LH
- metabolic
  - renal osteodystrophy: secondary increased PTH due to decreased Ca^{2+}, high PO_4^{3-}, and low active vitamin D
    - osteitis fibrosa cystica
  - hypertriglyceridemia, accelerated atherogenesis
  - decreased insulin requirements, increased insulin resistance
- dermatologic: pruritus, ecchymosis, hematoma, calciphylaxis (vascular Ca^{2+} deposition)

Renal Replacement Therapy

Dialysis

Indications for Dialysis in Chronic Kidney Disease

Table 16. Indications for Dialysis

Absolute Indications	Relative Indications
Volume overload*	Anorexia
Hyperkalemia*	Decreased cognitive functioning
Severe metabolic acidosis*	Profound fatigue and weakness
Neurologic signs or symptoms of uremia (encephalopathy, neuropathy, seizures)	Severe anemia unresponsive to erythropoietin
Uremic pericarditis	Persistent severe pruritus
Refractory accelerated HTN	Restless leg syndrome
Clinically significant bleeding diathesis	Plasma Cr >1060 μmol/L or Urea >36 mmol/L
Persistent severe N/V	

*Unresponsive to medications

- **hemodialysis**: blood is filtered across a semipermeable membrane removing accumulated toxic waste products, solutes, excess fluid (ultrafiltration), and restoring buffering agents to the bloodstream
  - available as intermittent (e.g. 3x/wk), continuous (CVVHD) or sustained low efficiency (SLED)
  - can be delivered at home or in-centre, nocturnal
  - vascular access can be achieved through a central line, an artificial graft, or an AV fistula
- patients with CKD should be referred for surgery to attempt construction of a primary AV fistula when their eGFR is <20 mL/min, the serum Cr level quoted as >350 μmol/L, or within 1 yr of an anticipated need
- **peritoneal dialysis**: peritoneum acts as a semipermeable membrane similar to hemodialysis filter
  - advantages: independence, fewer stringent dietary restrictions, better rehabilitation rates
  - available as continuous ambulatory (CAPD; four exchanges per day) or cyclic (CCPD; machine carries out exchanges overnight)
- refer patients with chronic renal disease to a nephrologist early on to facilitate treatment and plan in advance for renal replacement therapy (RRT)

Table 17. Peritoneal Dialysis vs. Hemodialysis

	Peritoneal Dialysis	Hemodialysis
Rate	Slow	Fast
Location	Home	Hospital (usually)
Ultrafiltration	Osmotic pressure via dextrose dialysate	Hydrostatic pressure
Solute Removal	Concentration gradient and convection	Concentration gradient and convection
Membrane	Peritoneum	Semi-permeable artificial membrane
Method	Indwelling catheter in peritoneal cavity	Line from vessel to artificial kidney
Complications	Infection at catheter site Bacterial peritonitis Metabolic effects of glucose Difficult to achieve adequate clearance in patients with large body mass	Vascular access (clots, collapse) Bacteremia Bleeding due to heparin Hemodynamic stress of extracorporeal circuit Disequilibrium syndrome (headache, cerebral edema, hypotension, nausea, muscle cramps related to solute/water flux over short time)
Preferred When	Young, high functioning, residual renal function Success depends on presence of residual renal function	Bed-bound, comorbidities, no renal function Residual renal function not as important

How to Write Dialysis Orders (MUST BE INDIVIDUALIZED)
- Filter Type (e.g. F80)
- Length (e.g. 4 h 3x/wk or 2 h daily)
- Q Blood Flow (max 500 cc/min)
- Ultrafiltration (e.g. 2 L or to target dry weight)
- Na⁺ 140 (can be adjusted by starting at 155 and "ramping" down to minimize cramping)
- K⁺ (based on serum K⁺)

Serum K⁺	Dialysate
4-6	1.5
3.5-4	2.5
<3.5	3.5

- Ca²⁺ 1.25
- HCO₃⁻ 40
- Heparin (none, tight [500 U/h] or full [1000 U/h])
- IV fluid to support BP (e.g. NS)

When to Initiate Dialysis
CrCl <20 mL/min
- Educate patient regarding dialysis; if not a candidate for peritoneal dialysis, make arrangements for AV fistula
CrCl <15 mL/min
- Weigh risk and benefits for initiating dialysis
CrCl <10 mL/min
- Dialysis should be initiated

NOTE
- Cockcroft-Gault equation (or MDRD equation) should be used to measure kidney function
- Monitor for uremic complications
- Significant benefits in quality of life can occur if dialysis started before CrCl <15 mL/min
- It is unclear whether patients who start dialysis early have increased survival
- A preemptive transplant can be considered if patient is stable, in order to avoid dialysis

Source: National Kidney Foundation Kidney Disease Outcomes Quality Initiative

Commonly Used Immunosuppressive Drugs

Calcineurin inhibitors
- Cyclosporine
- Tacrolimus

Antiproliferative medications
- Mycophenolate mofetil
- Azathioprine

Other agents
- Sirolimus
- Prednisone

Anti-lymphocyte antibodies
- Thymoglobulin
- Basiliximab

Indications for Dialysis (refractory to medical therapy)

AE IOU
Acidosis
Electrolyte imbalance (K⁺)
Intoxication
Overload (fluid)
Uremia (encephalopathy, pericarditis, urea >35-50 mM)

Survival Benefit with Kidney Transplants from HLA-Incompatible Live Donors.
NEJM 2016;374:940-950
Purpose: To assess whether there is a survival advantage to receiving a kidney from HLA-incompatible donors compared to remaining on the waiting list for a possible matched deceased donor kidney.
Study: Retrospective, multi-centre analysis
Population: 1025 individuals who received HLA-incompatible live donor kidneys compared to two different controls: individuals waiting and possibly receiving a deceased donor kidney (N=5125), or individuals ultimately not receiving a kidney transplant (N=5125).
Outcome: Survival, tracked for up to 8 years.
Results: Individuals who received HLA incompatible kidneys had increased survival compared to either control group for time points at 1 year, 5 years, and 8 years post-transplant (p<0.001). After 8 years non-matched kidney recipients had 76.5% survival compared to 43.9% for individuals who ultimately did not receive a kidney transplant. Survival advantage was significant regardless of how the recipient anti-HLA antibodies were detected.
Conclusions: Individuals who received HLA-incompatible kidneys had significantly improved long-term survival compared to individuals who waited for compatible deceased donor kidneys.

Renal Transplantation

- provides maximum replacement of GFR
- preferred modality of RRT in CKD, not AKI
  - best way to reverse uremic signs and symptoms
  - renal transplantation has been shown to have improved long-term patient survival over dialysis
- native kidneys usually left in situ
- 2 types: deceased donor, living donor (related or unrelated)
- living donor transplants have been shown to have better outcomes than deceased donor transplants
- kidney transplanted into iliac fossa, transplant renal artery anastomosed to external iliac artery of recipient
- 1 yr renal allograft survival rates ≥90%

Complications

- acute rejection: graft site tenderness, rise in Cr, oliguria, ± fever, although symptoms are uncommon
- leading causes of late allograft loss: interstitial fibrosis/tubular atrophy (IFTA) and death with functioning graft
- #1 cause of mortality in transplanted patients is cardiovascular disease
- immunosuppressant drug therapy: side effects include infections, malignancy (skin, Kaposi's sarcoma, post-transplant lymphoproliferative disorder)
- de novo GN (usually membranous)
- new-onset DM (often due to prednisone use)
- cyclosporine or tacrolimus nephropathy (see *Small Vessel Disease*, NP29)
- chronic allograft nephropathy
- early allograft damage caused by episodes of acute rejection and acute peritransplant injuries
- immunologic and nonimmunologic factors (HTN, hyperlipidemia, age of donor, quality of graft, new onset DM)
- transplant glomerulopathy from antibody injury causes nephrotic proteinuria
- CMV (cytomegalovirus) infection and other opportunistic infections usually occur between 1 and 6 mo post-transplant
- BK virus (polyoma virus) nephropathy can result from over-immunosuppression and lead to graft loss

Common Medications

Table 18. Common Medications in Nephrology

Classification	Examples	Site of Action	Mechanism of Action (Secondary Effect)	Indication	Dosing	Adverse Effects
Loop Diuretics	furosemide (Lasix®) bumetanide (Bumex®/Buinex®) ethacrynate (Edecrin®) torsemide (Demadex®)	Thick ascending limb of Loop of Henle	↓ Na$^+$/K$^+$/2Cl$^-$ transport ± renal and peripheral vasodilatory effects (K$^+$ loss; ↑ H$^+$ secretion; ↑ Ca^{2+} excretion)	Management of edema secondary to CHF, nephrotic syndrome, cirrhotic ascites; ↑ free water clearance (e.g. in SIADH-induced hyponatremia), ↓ BP (less effective due to short action)	furosemide: edema: 20-80 mg IV/IM/PO q6-8h (max 600 mg/d) until desired response HTN: 20-80 mg/d PO OD/bid dosing	Allergy in sulfa-sensitive individuals Electrolyte abnormalities; hypokalemia, hyponatremia, hypocalcemia, hypercalciuria (with stone formation) Volume depletion with metabolic alkalosis Precipitates gouty attacks
Thiazide Diuretics	hydrochlorothiazide (HCTZ) chlorothiazide (Diuril®) indapamide (Lozol®, Lozide®) metolazone (Zaroxolyn®) chlorthalidone (Hygroton®)	Distal convoluted tubule	Inhibit Na$^+$/Cl$^-$ transporter (K$^+$ loss; ↑ H$^+$ secretion; ↑ Ca^{2+} excretion)	1st line for essential HTN Treatment of edema Idiopathic hypercalciuria and stones Diabetes insipidus (nephrogenic)	HCTZ: edema: 25-100 mg PO OD HTN: 12.5-25 mg PO OD (max 50 mg/d) nephrolithiasis/hypercalciuria: 25-100 mg OD	Hypokalemia Increased serum urate levels Precipitates gouty attacks, hypercalcemia Elevated lipids Glucose intolerance
Potassium-Sparing Diuretics	spironolactone (Aldactone®) triamterene (Dyrenium®) amiloride (Midamor®)	Cortical collecting duct (↓ Na$^+$ reabsorption)	Aldosterone antagonist (spironolactone) Block Na$^+$ channels (triamterene and amiloride)	Reduces K$^+$ loss caused by other diuretics Edema/hypervolemia Severe CHF, ascites (spironolactone), cystic fibrosis (amiloride ↓ viscosity of secretions)	spironolactone: 25-200 mg/d OD/bid dosing HTN: 50-200 mg/d OD/bid dosing Hyperaldosteronism: 100-400 mg/d OD/bid dosing amiloride: edema/HTN: 5-10 mg PO OD	Hyperkalemia (caution with ACEI) Triamterene can be nephrotoxic (rare) Nephrolithiasis Gynecomastia (estrogenic effect of spironolactone)
Combination Agents	Dyazide® (triamterene + HCTZ) Aldactazide® (spironolactone + HCTZ) Moduretic® (amiloride + HCTZ) Vaseretic® (enalapril + HCTZ) Zestoretic® (lisinopril + HCTZ)		Combination of ACEI and thiazide have a synergistic effect	Combine K$^+$-sparing drug with thiazide to reduce hypokalemia		
Osmotic Diuretics	mannitol (Osmitrol®) glycerol urea	Renal tubules (proximal and collecting duct)	Non-reabsorbable solutes increase osmotic pressure of glomerular filtrate – inhibits reabsorption of water and ↑ urinary excretion of toxic materials	To ↓ intracranial or intraoccular pressure Mobilization of excess fluid in renal failure or edematous states	mannitol: ↓ ICP: 0.25-2 g/kg IV over 30-60 min	Transient volume expansion Electrolyte abnormalities (↓/↑ Na$^+$, ↓/↑ K$^+$)

Table 18. Common Medications in Nephrology (continued)

Classification	Examples	Site of Action	Mechanism of Action (Secondary Effect)	Indication	Dosing	Adverse Effects
ACEI	ramipril (Altace®) enalapril (Vasotec®) lisinopril (Prinivil®) trandolapril (Mavik®) captopril (Capoten®)	Lungs Tissues diffusely	Inhibits angiotension converting enzyme, preventing formation of angiotensin II Prevents angiotensin II vasoconstricting vascular smooth muscle → ↓ BP Prevents angiotensin II mediated aldosterone release from adrenal cortex and action on proximal renal tubules → ↑ Na+ and H2O excretion → ↓ BP Reduces fibrosis and atherogenesis	HTN Cardioprotective effects (see Cardiology and Cardiac Surgery, C49) Renoprotective effects	ramipril: HTN: 2.5-20 mg PO OD/bid dosing renoprotective use; 10 mg PO OD trandolapril: HTN; 1-4 mg PO OD	Cough Asthma Hyperkalemia Angioedema Agranulocytosis (captopril) AKI Teratogenic
ARB	losartan (Cozaar®) candesartan (Atacand®) irbesartan (Avapro®) valsartan (Diovan®) telmisartan (Micardis®) eprosartan (Teveten®) olmesartan (Olmetec®)	Vascular smooth muscle, adrenal cortex, proximal tubules	Competitive inhibitor at the angiotensin II receptor: prevents angiotensin II vasoconstricting action on vascular smooth muscle → ↓ BP Prevents angiotensin II mediated aldosterone release from adrenal cortex and action on proximal renal tubules → ↑ Na+ and H2O excretion	HTN Cardioprotective effects (see Cardiology and Cardiac Surgery, C49) Renoprotective effects	HTN: losartan 25-100 mg PO OD candesartan 8-32 mg PO OD irbesartan 150-300 mg PO OD valsartan 80-320 mg PO OD telmisartan 20-80 mg PO OD eprosartan 400-800 mg PO OD olmesartan 20-40 mg PO OD	Hyperkalemia Caution – reduce dose in hepatic impairment AKI Teratogenic
Renin Antagonists	aliskiren (Rasilez®)	Direct renin antagonist	Inhibits renin production and activity Cardioprotective and renoprotective abilities being evaluated	HTN	aliskiren 150-300 mg PO OD	Hyperkalemia

Landmark Nephrology Trials

Trial	Reference	Results
4D	NEJM 2005; 353:238-48	Patients with type 2 DM receiving maintenance hemodialysis were randomized to 20 mg of atorvastatin per day or matching placebo; no difference in composite index of death from cardiac causes, nonfatal myocardial infarction, and stroke
AASK	JAMA 2001; 285:2719-28	Ramipril, compared with amlodipine, slows progression of hypertensive renal disease and proteinuria and may benefit patients without proteinuria as well
ACCOMPLISH	NEJM 2008; 359:2417-20	Combination treatment with an ACEI and a CCB (benazepril-amlodipine) was more successful than a combination of ACEI and a thiazide diuretic (benzapril-HCTZ) in reducing cardiovascular events in patients with HTN who were at risk for such events
ACEI and Diabetic	NEJM 1993; 329:1456-62	Captopril protects against deterioration in renal function in insulin-dependent diabetic nephropathy and is significantly more effective than blood pressure control alone
ALERT	Lancet 2003; 361:2024-31	The use of fluvastatin in renal transplant recipients did not significantly decrease the risk of the occurrence of a major adverse cardiac event (defined as cardiac death, non-fatal MI, or coronary intervention procedure) compared with placebo; however, there was a significant reduction in cardiac deaths or non-fatal MI
ALTITUDE	Early Termination (Unpublished Results; protocol – NDT 2009; 24:1663-71)	Combining Aliskiren with ACEI or ARB in high-risk patients with type 2 DM leads to increased incidence of nonfatal stroke, hyperkalemia, and hypotension
ASTRAL	NEJM 2009; 361:1953-62	Renal artery revascularization compared to medical therapy does not improve renal function, BP, renal or cardiovascular events, or mortality, and carries significant operative risks
AURORA	NEJM 2009; 360:1395-407	Patients receiving maintenance hemodialysis randomized to rosuvastatin 10 mg daily or placebo; rosuvastatin lowered the LDL cholesterol level but had no significant effect on the composite primary end point of death from cardiovascular causes, nonfatal myocardial infarction, or nonfatal stroke
BENEDICT	NEJM 2004; 351:1941-51	Treatment with ACEI trandolapril alone or trandolapril combined with verapamil decreased the incidence of microalbuminuria in patients with type 2 DM and HTN with normoalbuminuria
CHOIR	NEJM 2006; 355:2085-98	Patients with CKD were randomly assigned to receive a dose of epoetin alfa targeted to achieve a hemoglobin level of 135 g/L or 113 g/L; the higher target group had an increased risk of death, myocardial infarction, hospitalization for congestive heart failure (without renal replacement therapy), or stroke
CORAL	NEJM 2014; 370:13-22	Renal-artery stenting did not confer a significant benefit with respect to the prevention of renal or cardiac events when added to comprehensive, multifactorial medical therapy in people with atherosclerotic renal-artery stenosis and hypertension or chronic kidney disease
CREATE	NEJM 2006; 355:2071-84	Patients with CKD (15-35 mL/min) and mild to moderate anemia (110-125 g/L) were randomized to normal (130-150 g/L) or sub-normal (105-115 g/L) hemoglobin levels; early and complete correction of hemoglobin did not reduce the risk of cardiovascular events
DETAIL	NEJM 2004; 351:1952-61	The ARB telmisartan and the ACEI enalapril are equally effective in slowing renal function deterioration in type 2 DM with mild to moderate HTN and early nephropathy
ELITE-SYMPHONY	NEJM 2007; 357:2562-75	Daclizumab induction, MMF, steroids, and low-dose tacrolimus effectively maintain stable renal function following renal transplantation, without the negative effects on renal function commonly reported for standard CNI regimens
FHN	NEJM 2010;363:2287-300	Patients were randomized to dialysis 6x/wk (frequent) or 3x/wk (conventional); frequent hemodialysis was associated with improvement in composite outcomes of death, or change in left ventricular mass and death, or change in a physical-health composite score; frequent hemodialysis caused more frequent interventions related to vascular access
HEMO	NEJM 2002; 347:2010-19	Use of high dose dialysis or high flux membranes versus standard dose or low flux in thrice-weekly dialysis does not improve survival or outcomes; possible benefit in cardiac-related outcomes with high flux membranes

Landmark Nephrology Trials (continued)

Trial	Reference	Results
IDEAL	*NEJM* 2010; 363:609-19	Patients with progressive CKD and GFR between 10 and 15 mL/min randomized to initiate dialysis at GFR of 10-14 mL/min (early) or 5-7 mL/min (late); early initiation of dialysis in patients with stage G5 CKD was not associated with an improvement in survival or clinical outcomes
IDNT	*NEJM* 2001; 345:851-60	Treatment with irbesartan reduced the risk of developing end-stage renal disease and worsening renal function in patients with type 2 DM and diabetic nephropathy
IRMA	*NEJM* 2001; 345:870-8	Irbesartan is renoprotective independently of its blood pressure lowering effect in patients with type 2 DM and microalbuminuria
MDRD	*Ann Intern Med* 1995; 123:754-62	Patients with proteinuria of more than 1 g/d should have a target BP <125/75 mmHg; patients with proteinuria of 0.25 to 1.0 g/d should have a target BP <130/80 mmHg
ONTARGET	*Lancet* 2008; 372:547-53	Telmisartan and ramipril monotherapy reduced proteinuria and rise in Cr in patients with high vascular risk; combination of the two agents led to increased acute renal failure episodes, syncope, and hypotension
REIN	*Lancet* 1999; 354:359-64	In non-diabetic nephropathy, ACEI were renoprotective in patients with non-nephrotic range proteinuria
REIN2	*Lancet* 2005; 365:939-46	In non-diabetic nephropathy already on ACEI, no further benefit from intensified BP control (sBP/dBP<130/80 mmHg) by adding a CCB versus conventional BP control (dBP<90 mmHg) on ACEI alone
RENAAL	*NEJM* 2001; 345:861-9	Losartan conferred significant renal benefits in patients with type 2 DM and nephropathy and was generally well-tolerated
RENAL	*NEJM* 2009; 361:1627-38	High intensity continuous renal-replacement therapy in AKI does not improve survival or outcomes compared to low intensity treatment, and is associated with higher rates of hypophosphatemia
Rituximab in Children with Steroid-Dependent Nephrotic Syndrome	*JASN* 2015; 26 DOI: ASN.2014080799	Rituximab is non-inferior to steroids in maintaining remission in juvenile steroid dependent nephrotic syndrome
ROAD	*JASN* 2007; 18:1889-98	Uptitration of either ACEI benazepril or ARB losartan to optimal anti-proteinuria doses conferred benefit on renal outcome in patients without DM who had proteinuria and renal insufficiency
ROADMAP	*NEJM* 2011; 364:907-17	The use of the ARB olmesartan was more effective than placebo in delaying the onset of microalbuminuria in patients with type 2 DM, normoalbuminuria, and good blood pressure control; however, a higher rate of fatal cardiovascular events was found amongst patients with preexisting coronary heart disease in the olmesartan group
SHARP	*Lancet* 2011; 377:2181-92	Randomized placebo-controlled trial in patients with CKD and no history of MI or coronary revascularization took simvastatin 20 mg plus ezetimibe 10 mg daily versus matching placebo; simvastatin 20 mg plus ezetimibe 10 mg daily resulted in reduction of LDL cholesterol with associated reduction of major atherosclerotic events in patients with CKD
SPRINT	*NEJM* 2015; 373:2103-2116	A lower blood pressure target of 120/80 reduced the risk of composite cardiovascular events in a hypertensive patient population
TREAT	*NEJM* 2009; 361:2019-32	Patients with type 2 DM, CKD, and anemia were randomized to darbepoetin targeting a hemoglobin of 13 g/dL or placebo; darbepoetin did not reduce the risk of death, a cardiovascular event, or a renal event, and was associated with an increased risk of stroke
Tolvaptan in ADPKD	*NEJM* 2012; 367: 2407-18	Tolvaptan (vs. placebo) slowed the increase in total kidney volume and decline in kidney function over a 3-year period in patients with ADPKD but was associated with a higher discontinuation rate, due to adverse events

References

Adler SG, Salant DJ. An outline of essential topics in glomerular pathophysiology, diagnosis and treatment for nephrology trainees. Am J Kidney Dis 2003;42:395-418.
Androgue HJ, Madias NM. Management of life threatening acid-base disorders part I. NEJM 1999;338:26-33.
Androgue HJ, Madias NM. Management of life threatening acid-base disorders part II. NEJM 1999;338:107-111.
Androgue HJ, Madias NE. Hyponatremia. NEJM 2000;342:1581-1589.
Baigent C, Landray MJ, Reith C, et al. The effects of lowering LDL cholesterol with simvastatin plus ezetimibe in patients with chronic kidney disease (Study of Heart and Renal Protection): a randomized placebo-controlled trial. Lancet 2011;377:2181-2192.
Barnett AH, Bain SC, Bouter P, et al. Angiotensin-receptor blockade versus converting-enzyme inhibition in type 2 diabetes and nephropathy. NEJM 2004;351:1952-1961.
Brenner BM, Cooper ME, de Zeeuw D, et al. Effects of losartan on renal cardiovascular outcomes in patients with type 2 diabetes and nephropathy. NEJM 2001;345:861-869.
Canadian Diabetes Association Clinical Practice Guidelines Expert Committee. Can J Diabetes 2013;37(suppl 1):S1-S212.
Churchill DN, Blacke PG, Jindal KK, et al. Clinical practice guidelines for initiation of dialysis. Canadian Society of Nephrology. J Am Soc Nephrol 1999;10(Suppl 13):S238-291.
Cooper CJ, Murphy DP, Cutlip DE, et al. Stenting and medical therapy for atherosclerotic renal-artery stenosis. NEJM 2014;370:13-22.
Donadio JV, Grande JP. Medical progress: IgA nephropathy. NEJM 2002;347:738-748.
Elliott MJ, Ronksley PE, Clase CM, et al. Management of patients with acute hyperkalemia. CMAJ 2010;182:1631-1635
Gabow PA. Autosomal dominant polycystic kidney disease. NEJM 1993;329:332-342.
Greenberg AR. Primer on kidney diseases, 3rd ed. San Diego: Academic Press, 2001.
Hakim R, Lazarus M. Initiation of dialysis. J Am Soc Nephrol 1995;6:1319-1328.
Halperin ML, Goldstein MB, Kersey R, et al. Fluid, electrolyte, and acid-base physiology: a problem-based approach, 3rd ed. New York: Harcourt Brace, 1998.
Halperin ML, Kamel K. Potassium. Lancet 1998;352:135-140.
Hudson BG, Tryggvason K, Sundaramoorthy M, et al. Mechanisms of disease: Alport's syndrome, goodpasture's syndrome, and type IV collagen. NEJM 2003;348:2543-2556.
Johnson CA, Levey AS, Coresh J, et al. Clinical practice guidelines for chronic kidney disease in adults: Part II. Glomerular filtration rate, proteinuria, and other markers. Am Fam Phys 2004;70:1091-1097.
Johnson RJ, Feehally J (editors). Comprehensive clinical nephrology. New Nork: Mosby, 1999.
K/DOQI clinical practice guidelines for chronic kidney disease: evaluation, classification, and stratification: 2000 executive update. Available from: http://www. kidney.org/professionals/dogi/kdogi/toc.htm.
Keane WF, Garabed E. Proteinuria, albuminuria, risk assessment, detection, elimination (PARADE): a position paper of the National Kidney Foundation. Amer J Kid Dis 1999;33:1004-1010.
Lewis EJ, Hunsicker LG, Bain RP, et al. The effects of angiotensin-converting enzyme inhibition on diabetic nephropathy. NEJM 1993;329:1456-1462.
McFarlane P, Tobe S, Houlden R, et al. Nephropathy: Canadian Diabetes Association clinical practice guidelines expert committee. 2003. Available from:
Moist LM, Troyanov S, White CT, et al. Canadian Society of Nephrology Commentary on the 2012 KDIGO Clinical Practice Guideline for Anemia in CKD. Am J Kidney Dis 2013;62(5):860-73.
Myers A. Medicine, 4th ed. Baltimore: Lipincott Williams & Wilkins, 2001.
ONTARGET Investigators. Telmisartan, ramipril, or both in patients at high risk for vascular events. NEJM 2008;358:1547-1559.
Schiffl H, Lang SM, Fischer R. Daily hemodialysis and the outcome of acute renal failure. NEJM 2002;346:305-310.
Schreiber M. Seminars for year 3 University of Toronto Medicine clinical clerks on medicine: hyponatremia and hypernatremia. October 29, 2002.
Smith K. Renal disease: a conceptual approach. New York: Churchill Livingstone, 1987.
Thadhani R, Pascual M, Bonventre JV. Acute renal failure. NEJM 1996;334:1448-1460.
Wolfe RA, Ashby VB, Milford EL, et al. Comparison of mortality in all patients on dialysis, patients on dialysis awaiting transplantation, and recipients of a first cadaveric transplant. NEJM 1999;341(23):1725-30.

N

Neurology

Jane Liao, Anthony Wan, and Kirill Zaslavsky, chapter editors
Claudia Frankfurter and Inna Gong, associate editors
Brittany Prevost and Robert Vanner, EBM editors
Dr. Mark Boulos, Dr. Alfonso Fasano, Dr. Elizabeth Slow, and Dr. Peter Tai, staff editors

Acronyms

ACA	anterior cerebral artery	EOM	extraocular movement	LGB	lateral geniculate body	PPRF	paramedian pontine reticular formation
ACh	acetylcholine	EtOH	ethanol	LMN	lower motor neuron	PSP	progressives supranuclear palsy
AD	Alzheimer's disease	FEF	frontal eye field	LOC	level of consciousness	RAPD	relative afferent pupillary defect
ADL	activities of daily living	FTD	frontotemporal dementia	LP	lumbar puncture	REM	rapid eye movement
AED	antiepileptic drugs	GBS	Guillain-Barré syndrome	MCA	middle cerebral artery	RLS	restless legs syndrome
AION	acute ischemic optic neuropathy	GCA	giant cell arteritis	MG	myasthenia gravis	ROM	range of motion
ALS	amyotrophic lateral sclerosis	GCS	Glasgow coma scale	MLF	medial longitudinal fasciculus	SAH	subarachnoid hemorrhage
AVM	arteriovenous malformation	GPe	Globus pallidus pars externa	MMSE	mini mental status examination	SDH	subdural hematoma
AVPU	alert, verbal, pain, unresponsive	GPi	Globus pallidus pars interna	MoCA	Montreal cognitive assessment	SNc	substantia nigra pars compacta
CJD	Creutzfeldt-Jakob disease	HD	Huntington's disease	MS	multiple sclerosis	SNr	substantia nigra pars reticulata
CN	cranial nerve	IADL	instrumental activities of daily living	NCS	nerve conduction studies	STN	subthalamic nucleus
CNS	central nervous system	ICH	intracranial hemorrhage	NMJ	neuromuscular junction	TBI	traumatic brain injury
CRVO	central retinal vein occlusion	ICP	intracranial pressure	NPH	normal pressure hydrocephalus	TIA	transient ischemic attack
CSF	cerebral spinal fluid	IIH	idiopathic intracranial hypertension	PComm	posterior communicating artery	UMN	upper motor neuron
CVD	cerebrovascular disease	INO	internuclear ophthalmoplegia	PD	Parkinson's disease	VEGF	vascular endothelial growth factor
DBS	deep brain stimulation	IVIG	intravenous immunoglobulin	PICA	posterior inferior cerebral artery	VZV	varicella zoster virus
DLB	dementia with Lewy bodies	JC	John Cunningham virus	PLMS	periodic limb movement in sleep		
DM	diabetes mellitus	LEMS	Lambert-Eaton myasthenic syndrome	PPA	primary progressive aphasia		

Approach to the Neurological Complaint

Lesion Localization

- **cortical**
  - contralateral paresis (with differential effect on face and arm vs leg)
  - UMN injury (hyperreflexia, Babinski sign, spasticity, no atrophy)
  - cortical sensory loss (hemisensory loss, position sense, two-point discrimination, graphesthesia, stereognosis)
  - dominant hemisphere (aphasia, alexia, agraphia, acalculia, left-right disorientation)
  - non-dominant hemisphere (hemineglect, dysprosody, amusia, constructional apraxia)
  - homonymous hemianopia/quadrantanopia
  - gaze deviation (eyes look toward side of infarct)
  - seizure
  - agnosia (visual, auditory)
  - apraxia
  - alien hand syndrome
- **subcortical**
  - internal capsule: contralateral paresis with equal face, arm, leg involvement without sensory/cortical deficits; contralateral dysmetria/clumsiness and leg paresis
  - basal ganglia: pill-rolling tremor, bradykinesia, festinating gait, hemiballismus, chorea, dystonic posture
  - thalamus: dense sensory loss, contralateral severe pain
- **brainstem** (bulbar)
  - crossed hemiplegia or sensory loss (i.e. ipsilateral face, contralateral body)
  - ipsilateral cerebellar (dysmetria, rapid alternating movements, tandem gait)
  - nystagmus toward lesion, diplopia, INO (impaired adduction on contralateral gaze)
  - dysphagia, dysarthria
  - hearing loss, vertigo
- **cerebellum**
  - ipsilateral ataxia (unsteadiness, incoordination)
  - dysmetria, intention tremor
  - dysdiadochokinesia
  - wide-based gait, truncal titubation (staggering, reeling, lurching)
  - scanning speech (explosive speech with noticeable pauses and accentuated syllables)
  - nystagmus, distorted smooth pursuit, oscillopsia
- **spinal cord**
  - bilateral motor and/or sensory deficits below the lesion without facial involvement
  - ataxia, sensory level (sharp line below which there is decreased sensation); suspended "cape-like" sensory level
  - LMN signs (flaccid paresis, hypotonia, hyporeflexia, atrophy, fasciculations) at level of lesion; UMN signs below lesion (marked spasticity and Babinski)
  - bowel, bladder, sexual dysfunction
  - saddle anesthesia
  - ataxia
- **nerve root**
  - multiple peripheral nerve involvement
  - myotomal/dermatomal deficits
  - back/neck pain radiating to leg/arm

- **peripheral nerve**
  - distal "stocking-glove distribution" sensory loss
  - LMN signs (hypotonia, hyporeflexia, fasciculations, atrophy)
  - neuromuscular junction
  - fluctuating/fatiguable ocular (diplopia) and proximal muscle weakness
  - bulbar involvement (dysphonia, dysarthria)
- **muscle**
  - symmetric proximal weakness (climbing stairs, getting up from chair) without sensory deficits
  - muscle tenderness
  - muscle atrophy

The Neurological Exam

General Exam and Mental Status

- **vitals**: pulse (especially rhythm), BP, RR, temperature
- **H&N**: meningismus, head injury/bruises (signs of basal skull fracture: Battle's sign, raccoon eyes, hemotympanum, CSF rhinorrhea/otorrhea), tongue biting
- **CVS**: carotid bruits, heart murmurs
- **mental status**: orientation (person, place, time), LOC (GCS) (see <u>Emergency Medicine</u>, ER4)
  - GCS/15 – Motor/6, Verbal/5 (T= intubated), Eyes/4
- **cognition**
  - Folstein MMSE – /30 (note: dementia is a clinical diagnosis and is not diagnosed by cognitive testing)
  - MoCA – /30 (≥26 is considered normal)
  - frontal lobe testing (for perseveration – i.e. go/no-go test)
  - clock drawing

Cranial Nerve Exam

Table 1. Cranial Nerve Examination and Associated Deficits

Cranial Nerve	Recommended Physical Exams	Signs/Symptoms of Deficit
Olfactory (CN I)	Odor sensation: test each nostril separately	Anosmia (can be associated with loss of taste)
Optic (CN II)	Visual acuity: test each eye individually; best corrected vision Test visual fields Assess pupils: direct and consensual pupillary reaction (afferent), swinging flashlight test (for RAPD) Fundoscopy: optic disc edema and pallor, venous pulsations, hemorrhages Colour vision testing (Ishihara plates)	Blindness Absence of light reflexes, RAPD
Oculomotor (CN III)	Assess extraocular movements and nystagmus Test efferent limb of pupillary light response Assess size and shape of pupils; accommodation and saccadic eye movements Test for ptosis (levator palpebrae superioris)	Eyes deviated down and out; can demonstrate mydriasis
Trochlear (CN IV)	Test movement of superior oblique	Vertical diplopia; may tilt head towards unaffected side; affected eye cannot turn inward and downward
Trigeminal (CN V)	Test sensation above supraorbital ridge (V1), buccal area (V2), mandible (V3) Test corneal reflex (afferent limb) Assess motor function: temporalis, masseter, pterygoids, jaw jerk reflex	Loss of facial sensations and corneal reflex on stimulation ipsilaterally, weakness and wasting of muscles of mastication, deviation of open jaw to ipsilateral side; trigeminal neuralgia
Abducens (CN VI)	Test movement of lateral rectus	Horizontal diplopia, esotropia (convergent strabismus) and abductor paralysis of ipsilateral eye
Facial (CN VII)	Sensorimotor nerve function: to muscles of facial expression Test efferent limb of corneal reflex Visceral sensory nerve function: to anterior 2/3 of the tongue Visceral motor nerve function: to salivary and lacrimal glands	Paralysis of ipsilateral upper and lower facial muscles Loss of lacrimation Decreased salivation, dry mouth Loss of taste to anterior 2/3 of the tongue ipsilaterally LMN lesion = ipsilateral facial weakness UMN lesion = contralateral facial weakness, sparing the brow bilaterally

See Online Atlas for Cranial Nerves Exam, Motor Exam, and Sensory Exam Techniques

Battle's sign = mastoid ecchymosis
Raccoon eyes = periorbital ecchymosis

If patient has not brought their glasses, have them look through a pinhole for best corrected vision

When testing CN I, avoid noxious smells like ammonia, as this tests CN V

Screening Neurologic Exam
- mental status: orientation (person, place, time), obeys commands, GCS
- head and neck: examine for lacerations, contusions, deformities, signs of basal skull fracture, flex neck for meningismus if c-spine injury has been ruled out
- cranial nerve exam: visual fields ± fundoscopy, pupil size and reactivity, extraocular movements, facial strength, hearing to finger rub
- motor: power in deltoids, triceps, wrist extensors, hand interossei, iliopsoas, hamstrings, ankle dorsiflexors, pronator drift
- coordination: finger tapping, finger-to-nose, heel-knee-shin
- gait: tandem gait, heel walking
- reflexes: plantar, biceps, triceps, patellar, ankle, Babinski
- sensation: all 4 limbs, including double simultaneous stimulation, vibration sense at great toes

Table 1. Cranial Nerve Examination and Associated Deficits (continued)

Cranial Nerve	Recommended Physical Exams	Signs/Symptoms of Deficit
Vestibulocochlear (CN VIII)	Vestibular function - nystagmus, caloric reflexes Cochlear function - whisper test, Rinne, Weber	Vertigo, disequilibrium, and nystagmus Sensorineural hearing loss
Glossopharyngeal (CN IX)	Assess vocal cord function and gag reflex Assess taste to posterior third of the tongue (bitter and sour taste)	Loss of taste in posterior third of ipsilateral tongue Loss of gag reflex and dysphasia Unilateral lesion is rare
Vagus (CN X)	Assess vocal cord function and gag reflex Observe uvula deviation and palatal elevation Assess swallowing	Loss of gag reflex, dysphagia, hoarse voice Paralysis of soft palate (failed elevation) Deviation of uvula to contralateral side of lesion; anesthesia of pharynx and larynx ipsilaterally
Accessory (CN XI)	Assess strength of trapezius (shoulder shrug) and sternocleidomastoid muscles (head turn)	Ipsilateral shoulder weakness and turning head to opposite side
Hypoglossal (CN XII)	Inspect tongue for signs of lateral deviation, atrophy, fasciculations, asymmetry of movement and strength	Wasting of ipsilateral tongue muscles and deviation to ipsilateral side on protrusion

Motor Exam

- **bulk**: atrophy, asymmetry
- **tone**: hypotonia (flaccid), hypertonia (spasticity, rigidity, paratonia), cogwheeling
- **power**: pronator drift, asymmetric forearm rolling test (satellite sign)
- **reflexes**: deep tendon reflexes, abdominal reflexes, primitive reflexes, Babinski sign, Hoffmann reflex, clonus
- **abnormal movements**: tremors, chorea, dystonia, dyskinesia, hemiballism, myoclonus, athetosis, tics, fasciculations
- **abnormal posturing**: decorticate (upper extremity flexion, lower extremity extension), decerebrate (extremity extension)

Table 2. Localization of Motor Deficits

	LMN	UMN	Extrapyramidal
Muscle Tone	Flaccid	Spastic	Rigid
Involuntary Movements	Fasciculations	None	None
Reflexes	Decreased	Increased	Normal
Plantar Reflex	Down-going (flexor)	Up-going (extensor, i.e. Babinski sign)	Down-going (flexor)
Pattern of Muscle Weakness	Proximal, distal, or focal	**Pyramidal pattern**: look for hemiparetic gait (flexed arm, extended legs) Upper extremities: extensors weaker than flexors Lower extremities: flexors weaker than extensors	None

Table 3. Overview of Neuromuscular Diseases

	Motor Neuron Disease (i.e. ALS)	Peripheral Neuropathy	Neuromuscular Junction	Myopathy
SIGNS AND SYMPTOMS				
Weakness	Segmental and asymmetrical, distal → proximal	Distal (except GBS) but may be asymmetrical	Proximal and fatigable (e.g. MG), or weak then recovers (e.g. LEMS)	Proximal
Fasciculations	Yes	Yes	No	No
Reflexes	Increased	Decreased/absent	Normal	Normal (until late)
Sensory	No	Yes	No	No
Autonomic*	No	Yes	No	No
TESTS				
EMG	Denervation and reinnervation	Signs of demyelination ± axonal loss	Decremental response, Jitter on single fibre EMG	Small, short motor potentials
NCS	Normal	Abnormal	Normal	Normal
Muscle Enzyme	Normal	Normal	Normal	Increased

*e.g. orthostatic hypotension, anhidrosis, visual blurring, urinary hesitancy or incontinence, constipation, erectile dysfunction

CN Innervation of EOM
LR: CN VI, SO: CN IV, Other: CN III

Contraction of the left sternocleidomastoid turns the head right

Calorics: Brainstem Test
Describe nystagmus by direction of fast component

COWS
Cold
Opposite
Warm
Same

Upper Motor Neuron Tests
Babinski Reflex: 'Up-going' big toe ± fanning of toes indicates an UMN lesion
Hoffmann's Reflex: Flexion of IP joint of the thumb when tapping/flicking/flexing the nail of the index or ring finger may indicate an UMN lesion if asymmetrical
Pronator Drift: Unable to maintain full arm extension and supination; side of forearm pronation reflects contralateral pyramidal tract lesion; closing eyes accentuates effect

Pyramidal Pattern of Muscle Weakness (i.e. UMN)
Weaker arm extensors: shoulder abduction, elbow extension, wrist extension, finger extension, finger abduction
Weaker leg flexors: hip flexion, knee flexion, ankle dorsiflexion

Primitive Reflexes
Grasp, palmomental, root, glabellar tap, snout

Table 4. Approach to Strength Testing of Radiculopathies vs. Peripheral Neuropathies

How to use this table: For each nerve root, learn two (or more) peripheral nerves (and their associated muscles/movements). In radiculopathies, all associated peripheral nerves (and their movements) will be impaired, whereas in peripheral neuropathies, only one of the nerves (and its movement) will be impaired, sparing the other nerve. Particularly useful peripheral nerve "pairs" are bolded for emphasis.

Root	Peripheral Nerve	Movement	Muscle
C5	Axillary	Shoulder abduction	Deltoid
C6	Musculocutaneous (C5/6)	Elbow flexion	Biceps
	Radial (C6)	Elbow flexion	Brachioradialis
		Wrist extension	Extensor carpi radialis longus
C7	Radial	Elbow extension	Triceps
	Posterior interosseus	Finger extension	Extensor digitorum communis
C8, T1	**Median**	Thumb flexion	Flexor pollicis brevis (look for thenar wasting)
		Thumb abduction	Abductor pollicis brevis (look for thenar wasting)
		Opposition	Opponens pollicis (look for thenar wasting)
	Ulnar	Finger abduction	First dorsal interosseus (look for wasting in first dorsal webbed space)
L2, 3, 4	**Femoral**	Hip flexion	Iliopsoas
	Obturator	Hip adduction	Adductor muscles
L3, 4	Femoral (L3/4)	Knee extension	Quadriceps
	Deep peroneal (L4/5)	Dorsiflexion	Tibialis anterior
L5	Sciatic (L5, S1)	Hip extension	Gluteus maximus
	Tibial	Ankle inversion	Tibialis posterior
	Superficial peroneal	Ankle eversion	Peroneal muscles
	Deep peroneal	Big toe extension	Extensor hallucis longus
S1	Sciatic	Knee flexion	Hamstring muscles
	Tibial	Plantar flexion	Gastrocnemius and soleus

Sensory Exam

- **primary sensation**
  - spinothalamic tract: crude touch, pain, temperature
  - dorsal column-medial lemniscus pathway: fine touch, vibration, proprioception
- **cortical sensation**
  - graphesthesia, stereognosis, extinction, 2-point discrimination

Coordination Exam and Gait

- **coordination exam**
  - finger-to-nose, heel-to-shin, rapid alternating movements
- **stance and gait**
  - gait: antalgic, hemiplegic, ataxic, apraxic, festinating, foot drop, broad-based
  - tandem gait (heel-to-toe walking)
- **Romberg test**
  - pull test for postural instability

MRC Muscle Strength Scale
5 Full power
4 Submaximal power against resistance (ranging 4+, 4, 4-)
3 Full ROM against gravity without resistance
2 Full ROM with gravity removed
1 Muscle flicker
0 No muscle contraction

Deep Tendon Reflexes
Root	Muscle Tendon
C5/6	Biceps
C6	Brachioradialis
C7	Triceps
C8	Finger flexors
L2/3	Hip adductors
L3/4	Knee extensors
S1/2	Plantar flexion

Deep Tendon Reflex Scoring
0   Absent
1+ Depressed – elicited with reinforcement only
2+ Normal
3+ Increased
4+ Clonus (≥4 beats)

Interpreting a Slow or Uncoordinated Rapid Alternating Movement (RAM)
- Slow RAMs without fatiguing is suggestive of weakness (especially if it is asymmetric)
- Slow RAMs with fatiguing (i.e. decreasing amplitude over time) is suggestive of Parkinsonism
- Uncoordinated RAM is suggestive of cerebellar disorder (i.e. ataxia and irregularly irregular rhythm) or ideomotor apraxia

Common Cerebellar Findings
Frontal executive dysfunction/disinhibition, scanning speech, nystagmus, hypo- or hyper-metric saccades, hypotonia, pendular reflexes, intention tremor, ataxic finger-nose/heel-shin/tandem, wide based stance and gait, positive rebound
Midline cerebellar diseases: truncal ataxia
Lateral cerebellar hemisphere diseases: limb ataxia

Romberg Test
Stable with eyes open and closed = normal
Stable with eyes open, falls with eyes closed = positive Romberg, suggesting loss of joint position sense

Basic Anatomy Review

See Functional Neuroanatomy software

Basic Anatomy Review

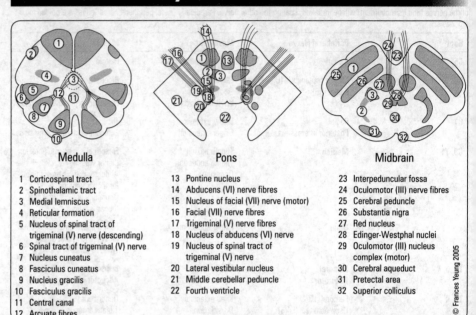

Medulla

1 Corticospinal tract
2 Spinothalamic tract
3 Medial lemniscus
4 Reticular formation
5 Nucleus of spinal tract of trigeminal (V) nerve (descending)
6 Spinal tract of trigeminal (V) nerve
7 Nucleus cuneatus
8 Fasciculus cuneatus
9 Nucleus gracilis
10 Fasciculus gracilis
11 Central canal
12 Arcuate fibres

Pons

13 Pontine nucleus
14 Abducens (VI) nerve fibres
15 Nucleus of facial (VII) nerve (motor)
16 Facial (VII) nerve fibres
17 Trigeminal (V) nerve fibres
18 Nucleus of abducens (VI) nerve
19 Nucleus of spinal tract of trigeminal (V) nerve
20 Lateral vestibular nucleus
21 Middle cerebellar peduncle
22 Fourth ventricle

Midbrain

23 Interpeduncular fossa
24 Oculomotor (III) nerve fibres
25 Cerebral peduncle
26 Substantia nigra
27 Red nucleus
28 Edinger-Westphal nuclei
29 Oculomotor (III) nucleus complex (motor)
30 Cerebral aqueduct
31 Pretectal area
32 Superior colliculus

© Frances Yeung 2005

Figure 1. Brainstem (axial view)

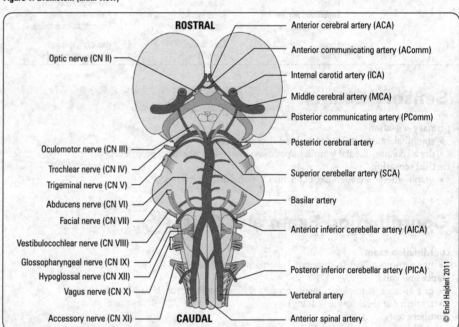

ROSTRAL

Optic nerve (CN II)

Oculomotor nerve (CN III)

Trochlear nerve (CN IV)

Trigeminal nerve (CN V)

Abducens nerve (CN VI)

Facial nerve (CN VII)

Vestibulocochlear nerve (CN VIII)

Glossopharyngeal nerve (CN IX)

Hypoglossal nerve (CN XII)

Vagus nerve (CN X)

Accessory nerve (CN XI)

CAUDAL

Anterior cerebral artery (ACA)

Anterior communicating artery (AComm)

Internal carotid artery (ICA)

Middle cerebral artery (MCA)

Posterior communicating artery (PComm)

Posterior cerebral artery

Superior cerebellar artery (SCA)

Basilar artery

Anterior inferior cerebellar artery (AICA)

Posteror inferior cerebellar artery (PICA)

Vertebral artery

Anterior spinal artery

© Enid Hajderi 2011

Figure 2. Brainstem (posterior view)

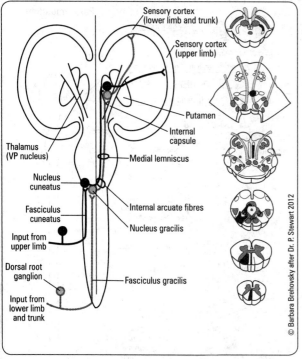

Figure 3. Discriminative touch pathway (dorsal column) from body

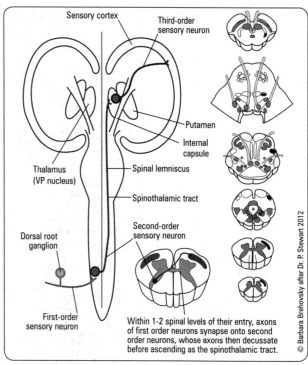

Figure 4. Spinothalamic tract from body

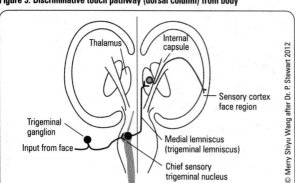

Figure 5. Discriminative touch pathway (dorsal column) from face

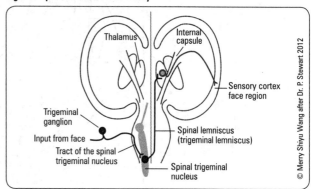

Figure 6. Spinothalamic tract pathway from face

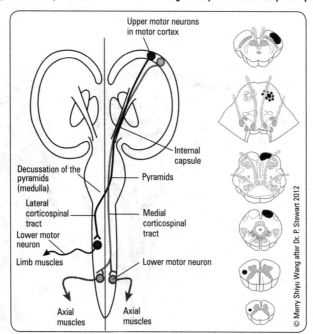

Figure 7. Corticospinal motor pathway

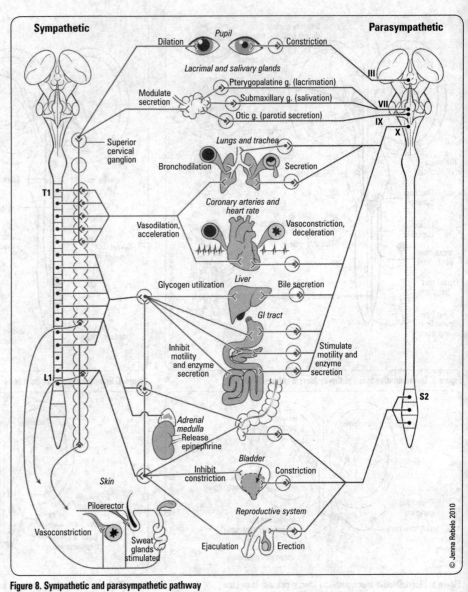

Figure 8. Sympathetic and parasympathetic pathway

Myotomes
C5 – Shoulder abduction/elbow flexion
C6 – Wrist extensors
C7 – Elbow extension
C8 – Finger flexion
T1 – Finger abduction
T2-9 – Intercostal (abdominal reflexes)
T9-10 – Upper abdominals
T11-12 – Lower abdominals
L2 – Hip flexion
L3 – Hip adduction
L4 – Knee extension and ankle dorsiflexion
L5 – Ankle dorsiflexion and big toe extension
S1 – Plantarflexion

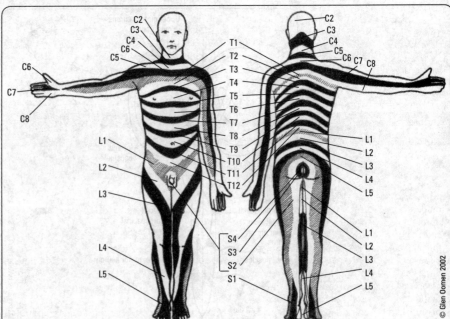

Figure 9. Dermatome map

Lumbar Puncture

Indications
- diagnostic: CNS infection (meningitis, encephalitis), inflammatory disorder (MS, Guillain-Barré, vasculitis), subarachnoid hemorrhage (if CT negative), CNS neoplasm (neoplastic meningitis)
- therapeutic: to administer anesthesia, chemotherapy, contrast media; to decrease ICP (pseudotumour cerebri, NPH)

Contraindications
- mass lesion causing increased ICP, could lead to cerebral herniation; CT first if suspect mass lesion
- infection over LP site/suspected epidural abscess
- low platelets (<50,000) or treatment with anticoagulation (high INR or aPTT)
- uncooperative patient

The needle for a LP is inserted into one of L3-4, L4-5, or L5-S1 interspaces

Complications
- tonsillar herniation (rare)
- SDH (rare)
- transient 6th nerve palsy (rare)
- post-LP headache (5-40%): worse when upright, better supine; generally onset within 24 h
  - prevention: smaller gauge (i.e. 22) needle, reinsert stylet prior to needle removal, blunt-ended needle
  - symptomatic treatment: caffeine and sodium benzoate injection
  - corrective treatment: blood patch (autologous)
- spinal epidural hematoma
- infection

Do not delay antibiotics while waiting for a LP if infection is suspected

LP Tubes
- **tube #1: cell count and differential:** RBCs, WBCs, and differential
  - xanthochromia (yellow bilirubin pigmentation implies recent bleed into CSF, diagnostic of SAH)
- **tube #2: chemistry:** glucose (compare to serum glucose) and protein
- **tube #3: microbiology:** Gram stain and C&S
  - specific tests depending on clinical situation/suspicion
    - viral: PCR for herpes simplex virus (HSV) and other viruses
    - bacterial: polysaccharide antigens of *H. influenzae, N. meningitidis, S. pneumoniae*
    - fungal: cryptococcal antigen, culture
    - TB: acid-fast stain, TB culture, TB PCR
- **tube #4:** cytology: for evidence of malignant cells
- **tube #5:** cell count: compare RBC count to that of tube #1
  - **note:** tube 4 or 5 can be sent for repeat cell count

RBCs in tube #1>>#5 → traumatic tap
RBCs in tube #1=#5 → SAH

Table 5. Lumbar Puncture Interpretation (Normal vs. Various Infectious Causes)

Condition	Colour	Protein	Glucose	Cells
NORMAL	Clear	<0.45 g/L	60% of serum glucose or >3.0 mmol/L	0-5 x 10^6/L
Viral Infection	Clear or opalescent	Normal or slightly increased <0.45-1 g/L	Normal	<1,000 x 10^6/L Lymphocytes mostly, some PMNs
Bacterial Infection	Opalescent yellow, may clot	>1 g/L	Decreased (<25% serum glucose or <2.0 mmol/L)	>1,000 x 10^6/L PMNs
Granulomatous Infection (tuberculosis, fungal)	Clear or opalescent	Increased but usually <5 g/L	Decreased (usually <2.0-4.0 mmol/L)	<1,000 x 10^6/L Lymphocytes

Approach to Common Presentations

Weakness

Approach
- **mode of onset:** abrupt (vascular, toxic, metabolic), subacute (neoplastic, infective, inflammatory), insidious (hereditary, degenerative, endocrine, neoplastic)
- **course:** worse at onset (vascular), progressive (neoplastic, degenerative, infective), episodic (vascular, inflammatory), activity dependent (NMJ, muscular)
- **pattern:** objective vs. subjective, generalized vs. localized, asymmetric vs. symmetric, proximal vs. distal, UMN vs. LMN, peripheral vs. myotomal
- **associated symptoms:** sensory symptoms, cortical symptoms, spinal symptoms (i.e. bowel/bladder dysfunction), signs/symptoms specific to various etiologies
- **history:** family history, developmental history, medications, risk factors, recent/preceding exposures
- **investigations for LMN:** NCS/EMG
- **investigations for UMN:** imaging (brain and/or spinal cord)

Differential Diagnosis
- objective muscle weakness; also, differentiate between true muscle weakness vs. fatigue
  - generalized
    - ◆ myopathy (proximal > distal weakness)
      - – endocrine: hypothyroidism, hyperthyroidism, Cushing's syndrome
      - – rheumatologic: polymyositis, vasculitis
      - – infectious: HIV, CMV, influenza
      - – other: collagen vascular disorders, steroids, statins, alcohol, electrolyte disorders
    - ◆ NMJ (MG, botulism, LEMS, organophosphate poisoning)
    - ◆ cachexia
  - localized
    - ◆ UMN (vasculitis, abscess, brain tumour, vitamin B12 deficiency, MS, stroke)
    - ◆ radicular pain (i.e. nerve root)
    - ◆ anterior horn cell (spinal muscular atrophy, ALS, polio, paraneoplastic, lead toxicity)
    - ◆ peripheral neuropathy (peroneal muscle atrophy, GBS, leprosy, amyloid, myeloma, DM, lead toxicity)
- no objective muscle weakness
  - chronic illness (cardiac, pulmonary, anemia, infection, malignancy)
  - depression, deconditioning
- if loss of passive motion, consider intra-articular, peri-articular, or extra-articular causes

Numbness/Altered Sensation

Approach
- positive sensory symptoms: paresthesia/dysesthesia = tingling, pins and needles, prickling, burning, stabbing
- negative sensory symptoms: hypoesthesia/anesthesia = numbness, diminution, or absence of feeling
- determine distribution of sensory loss:
  - nerve root vs. peripheral nerve
  - symmetric stocking-glove pattern (indicative of distal symmetric polyneuropathy)
  - dissociated sensory loss: dorsal column (fine touch, proprioception, vibration) vs. spinothalamic tract (pain and temperature)
- investigations: NCS, vitamin B12 levels, imaging based on associated findings

Differential Diagnosis
- cerebral: stroke, demyelination, tumour
  - associated symptoms: hemiplegia, aphasia, apraxia
- brainstem: stroke, demyelination, tumour
  - associated symptoms: diplopia, vertigo, dysarthria, dysphagia
- spinal cord/radiculopathy: cord infarction, tumour, MS, syringomyelia, vitamin B12 deficiency, disc lesion
  - associated symptoms: back/neck pain, weakness (paraparesis or Brown-Séquard pattern)
- neuropathy: focal compressive neuropathy (based on location and distribution), DM, uremia, vasculitis, vitamin B12 deficiency, HIV, Lyme disease, alcohol, paraneoplastic, amyloid

Gait Disturbance

Approach
1. Characterization of the gait disturbance
   - posture, stride length, width between feet, height of step, stability of pelvis, symmetry, arm swing, elaborate/inconsistent movements, standing from sitting
2. Identification of accompanying neurologic signs
   - full neurological exam required (diagnosis often can be made by P/E alone)
3. Identify red flags
   - sudden onset, cerebellar ataxia, paresis (hemi-, para- or quadri-), bowel/bladder incontinence
4. Workup
   - based on etiology – requires blood work, neuroimaging, and urgent neurologist referral

---

Central Motor Systems

3 components to the control of gait:
- Pyramidal: main outflow from cortex to spinal cord
- Extrapyramidal: basal ganglia inhibits excess movements
- Cerebellum: affects coordination of gait

Table 6. Types of Gait Disturbance

Location	Description	Disorder
Visual Loss	Broad based gait with tentative steps	Cataract surgery without lens replacement
Proprioceptive Loss	Sensory ataxia: wide-based with high stepping posture and positive Romberg	Demyelinating neuropathies, paraneoplastic syndrome, tabes dorsalis, MS, compressive myelopathy, B12 deficiency
Peripheral Vestibular Lesion 1. Acute 2. Bilateral	1. Vestibular ataxia 2. Disequilibrium	1. Tumour, trauma, infectious, Ménière's disease 2. Ototoxic drugs
Peripheral Nerve Disorder 1. Foot drop 2. Lumbosacral radiculopathy	Steppage gait	Acquired/hereditary peripheral neuropathy, compressive peroneal neuropathy, L4-5 radiculopathy
Myopathies	Waddling gait: broad based, short stepped gait with pronounced lumbar lordosis, rotation of pelvis	Progressive muscular dystrophy
Pyramidal/Corticospinal Tract Lesion 1. Unilateral 2. Bilateral	Spastic gait: spastic foot drop, circumduction, scissoring of legs or toe walking with bilateral circumduction	Unilateral: stroke (ischemic/hemorrhagic) Bilateral: cervical spondylosis, cerebral palsy, spinal cord tumour, combined spinal cord degeneration, MS, motor neuron disease
Basal Ganglia	1. Parkinsonian gait: small paces, stooped posture, reduced armswing 2. Choreic/hemiballistic/dystonic gait	Infarct, Huntington's, Sydenham's chorea, Wilson's disease, SLE, neuroleptic medications, polycythemia vera, genetic dystonia
Cerebellar Disorder	Cerebellar ataxic gait: wide-based without high stepping; veers to side of lesion Alcoholic gait	Primary and secondary neoplasm, toxins (alcohol), vitamin E deficiency, hypothyroid, hypoxia, hypoglycemia, paraneoplastic syndrome

Cranial Nerve Deficits

CN I: Olfactory Nerve

Clinical Features
- absence of sense of smell associated with a loss of taste

Differential Diagnosis
- **nasal**: physical obstruction
  - heavy smoking, chronic rhinitis, sinusitis, neoplasms, septal deformity, choanal atresia, vestibular stenosis, foreign body
- **olfactory neuroepithelial**: destruction of receptors or their axon filaments
  - influenza, herpes simplex, interferon treatment of hepatitis C virus, atrophic rhinitis (leprosy)
- **central**: lesion of olfactory pathway
  - Kallmann syndrome, albinism, head injury, cranial surgery, SAH, chronic meningeal inflammation, meningioma, aneurysm, PD, stroke, MS
- **endocrine/metabolic**
  - DM, adrenal hypo/hyperfunction, pseudohypoparathyroidism, hypothyroidism, renal/liver failure, vitamin deficiency

CN II: Optic Nerve

- see *Neuro-Ophthalmology*, N14

CN III: Oculomotor Nerve

Clinical Features
- ptosis, resting eye position is "down and out" (depressed and abducted), pupil dilated (mydriasis)
- vertical and horizontal diplopia; paralysis of adduction, elevation, and depression

Differential Diagnosis
- **PComm aneurysm**: early mydriasis, then CN III palsy
- **cavernous sinus** (internal carotid aneurysm, meningioma, sinus thrombosis): associated with deficits in other CNs near the cavernous sinus
- **midbrain lesion**: complete unilateral CN III palsy with bilateral weakness of the superior rectus and ptosis with contralateral pyramidal signs ± mydriasis
- **orbital lesion**: associated with optic neuropathy, chemosis, proptosis
- **other**: inflammatory, infection, neoplasia, uncal herniation, trauma

If anosmia is not associated with loss of taste, consider malingering

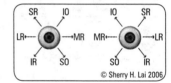

Figure 10. Diagnostic positions of gaze to isolate primary action of each muscle

Kallmann syndrome is a congenital disorder of anosmia and hypogonadotropic hypogonadism

Pupillary constrictor fibres run along outside of nerve, whereas vasculature is contained within nerve
For CN III palsy with a reactive pupil, always think ischemic cause ("pupil sparing")
For CN III palsy with mydriasis, think compressive lesion

Lesions involving the cavernous sinus can lead to cranial nerve palsies of III, IV, VI, V1, and V2 as well as orbital pain and proptosis

DDx of CN III Palsy

iCAM
ischemic
Cavernous sinus
Aneurysm (PComm, internal carotid)
Midbrain lesion

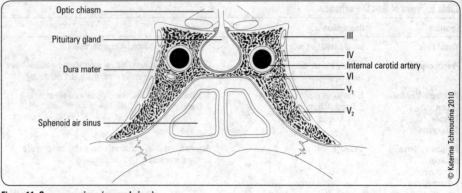

Figure 11. Cavernous sinus (coronal view)

CN IV is the only cranial nerve that decussates at midline and exits posteriorly
A CN IV lesion may cause a contralateral deficit if lesion affects the nucleus

CN IV is at risk of trauma during neurosurgical procedures involving the midbrain because of its long intracranial course

Distinguishing CN III, IV, and VI Lesions

	III	IV	VI
Diplopia	Oblique	Vertical	Horizontal
Exacerbating	Near target	Looking down	Far target
Head Tilt	Up and rotated away	Down and flexed away	Rotated towards

Jaw deviation is towards the side of a LMN CN V lesion

CN VI has the longest intracranial course and is vulnerable to increased ICP, creating a false localizing sign

Forehead is spared in a UMN CN VII lesion due to bilateral innervation of CN VII nuclei from cerebral hemispheres for the frontalis

When screening for dysphagia and assessing aspiration risk, the presence of a gag reflex is insufficient; the correct screening test is to observe the patient drinking water from a cup while observing for any coughing, choking, or "wetness" of voice

CN IV: Trochlear Nerve

Clinical Features
- vertical and torsional diplopia; defect of intorsion and depression
- patient may complain of difficulty going down stairs or reading

Differential Diagnosis
- common: ischemic (DM, HTN), idiopathic, trauma (TBI or surgical), congenital
- other: cavernous sinus lesion, superior orbital fissure (tumour, granuloma)

CN V: Trigeminal Nerve

Clinical Features
- ipsilateral facial numbness, weakness of muscles of mastication (V3 only) with pterygoid deviation towards the side of the lesion

Differential Diagnosis
- **brainstem**: ischemia, tumour, syringobulbia, demyelination
- **peripheral**: tumour, aneurysm, chronic meningitis, metastatic infiltration of nerve
- **trigeminal ganglion**: acoustic neuroma, meningioma, fracture of middle fossa
- **cavernous sinus**: carotid aneurysm, meningioma, sinus thrombosis
- **trauma**
- note: other CN V lesions that cause facial pain = trigeminal neuralgia, herpes zoster

CN VI: Abducens Nerve

Clinical Features
- resting inward deviation (esotropia)
- horizontal diplopia; defect of lateral gaze

Differential Diagnosis
- **pons** (infarction, hemorrhage, demyelination, tumour): associated with facial weakness and contralateral pyramidal signs
- **tentorial orifice** (compression, meningioma, trauma): false localizing sign of increased ICP
- **cavernous sinus**: carotid aneurysm, meningioma, sinus thrombosis
- **ischemia of CN VI**: DM, temporal arteritis, HTN, atherosclerosis
- **congenital**: Duane's syndrome

CN VII: Facial Nerve

Clinical Features
- **LMN lesion**: ipsilateral facial weakness (facial droop, flattening of forehead, inability to close eyes, flattening of nasolabial fold)
- **UMN lesion**: contralateral facial weakness with forehead sparing (due to bilateral frontalis innervation)
- impaired lacrimation, decreased salivation, numbness behind auricle, hyperacusis, taste dysfunction of anterior 2/3 of tongue

Differential Diagnosis
- **idiopathic** = Bell's palsy, 80-90% of cases (see Otolaryngology, OT22)
  - most often related to HSV, but other viruses may be implicated (CMV, herpes zoster, EBV)
- **other**: temporal bone fracture, EBV, Ramsay Hunt (VZV), otitis media/mastoiditis, sarcoidosis, DM mononeuropathy, parotid gland disease, Lyme meningitis, HIV

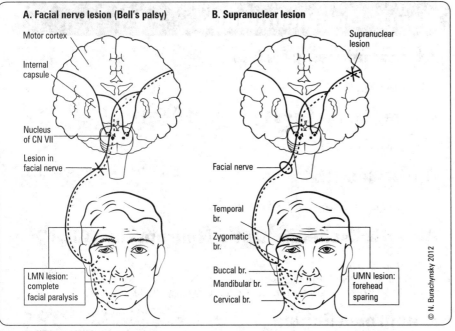

A. Facial nerve lesion (Bell's palsy)

Motor cortex

Internal capsule

Nucleus of CN VII

Lesion in facial nerve

LMN lesion: complete facial paralysis

B. Supranuclear lesion

Supranuclear lesion

Facial nerve

Temporal br.

Zygomatic br.

Buccal br.

Mandibular br.

Cervical br.

UMN lesion: forehead sparing

© N. Burachynsky 2012

Figure 12. UMN vs. LMN facial nerve palsy

Facial Nerve Branch Memory Aid
To Zanzibar By Motor Car
Temporal
Zygomatic
Buccal
Mandibular
Cervical

Differential Diagnosis of Lower Cranial Nerve Deficits (CN IX, X, XI, XII)
Intracranial/Skull Base: meningioma, neurofibroma, metastases, osteomyelitis, meningitis
Brainstem: stroke, demyelination, syringobulbia, poliomyelitis, astrocytoma
Neck: trauma, surgery, tumours

Normal swallowing is initiated when the tongue moves a bolus back into the palatal archway. Tongue movements are innervated exclusively by CN XII. The bolus stimulates the soft palate to elevate and the bolus is deflected into the oropharynx. Next the pharyngeal constrictors contract, the larynx elevates, and the vocal cords close. Swallowing depends on afferent information via CN V, IX, and X and motor action via CN V, VII, IX, X, and XII.
Connections in the nucleus of the tractus solitarius in the medulla (in proximity to the respiratory centre) act as the swallowing centre. Swallowing and breathing are coordinated to prevent aspiration

CN VIII: Vestibulocochlear Nerve

- see Otolaryngology, OT14

CN IX: Glossopharyngeal Nerve

Clinical Features
- unilateral lesion is rare
- taste dysfunction in posterior 1/3 of tongue
- absent gag reflex and dysphagia

Disorders
- glossopharyngeal neuralgia: sharp paroxysmal pain of posterior pharynx radiating to ear, triggered by swallowing
  - treated with carbamazepine or surgical ablation of CN IX

CN X: Vagus Nerve

Clinical Features
- oropharyngeal dysphagia (transfer dysphagia) due to palatal and pharyngeal weakness
  - neuromuscular causes of dysphagia
    - CNS: stroke, cerebral palsy, tumour, trauma, PD, AD, MS
    - CN: DM, laryngeal nerve palsy, polio, ALS
    - myopathic/NMJ: dermatomyositis, polymyositis, MG, sarcoidosis
  - other causes of dysphagia: see Gastroenterology, G8
- dysarthria: inability to produce understandable speech due to impaired phonation and/or resonance

Uvula deviation is away from the side of a LMN CN X lesion due to impaired ipsilateral palatal elevation

CN XI: Accessory Nerve

Clinical Features
- LMN lesion: paralysis of ipsilateral trapezius and sternocleidomastoid (ipsilateral shoulder drop, weakness on turning head to contralateral side)
- UMN lesion: paralysis of ipsilateral sternocleidomastoid and contralateral trapezius

CN XI is vulnerable to damage during neck surgery

CN XII: Hypoglossal Nerve

Clinical Features
- LMN lesion: tongue deviation towards lesion; ipsilateral tongue atrophy and fasciculations (if chronic)
- UMN lesion: tongue deviation away from lesion; absence of atrophy and fasciculations

Neuro-Ophthalmology

Abnormalities of Vision

- see Ophthalmology

Acute Visual Loss

- see Ophthalmology, OP3

Optic Neuritis

NAION can be caused by use of sildenafil (Viagra®) in rare cases

- see *Optic Disc Edema below, Multiple Sclerosis*, N52

Anterior Ischemic Optic Neuropathy (AION)

If you suspect the diagnosis of giant cell arteritis do not wait for biopsy results, begin treatment immediately

- see *Optic Disc Edema*
- **non-arteritic (NAION):** due to atherosclerosis
- **arteritic (AAION):** due to giant cell arteritis (see Rheumatology, RH20)

Amaurosis Fugax

- see Ophthalmology, OP35 and *Stroke*, N48

Central Retinal Vein Occlusion

- see Ophthalmology, OP22

Optic Disc Edema

Table 7. Common Causes of Optic Disc Edema

	Optic Neuritis	Papilledema	AION	CRVO
Age	<50 yr	Any	>50 yr but usually >70 yr	>50 yr
Vision	Rapidly progressive monocular central vision loss (↓ acuity and colour vision) with recovery	Late visual loss	Painless unilateral acute field defect over hours to days with ↓ colour vision	Painless unilateral variable vision loss
Symptoms	Pain (especially with eye movement)	H/A, N/V, local neurological deficits	If GCA: H/A, scalp tenderness, jaw claudication, weight loss, fatigue	Cardiovascular risk factors
Pupil	RAPD	No RAPD	RAPD	± RAPD
Fundus	Disc swelling if anterior Normal disc if retrobulbar	Bilateral disc swelling, retinal hemorrhage, no venous pulsations	Pale segmental disc edema, retinal dot, flame hemorrhages	Swollen disc, venous engorgement, retinal hemorrhage
Etiologies	MS, viral	Increased ICP	Giant cell arteritis Non-arteritic: atherosclerosis	Associated with vasculopathy, thrombus
Investigations	MRI with gadolinium	Emergent CT; LP if CT is normal to measure opening pressure	CBC, ESR, CRP, temporal artery biopsy	Fluorescein angiogram and coherence tomography
Treatment	IV methylprednisolone	Treat cause	Consider ASA if non-arteritic; steroids if arteritic	Optimize risk factors, reduce IOP, ± laser, ± VEGF inhibitors

Optic Disc Atrophy

- **etiologies**: glaucoma, AION, compressive tumour, optic neuritis, Leber's hereditary optic neuropathy, congenital
- **presentation**: disc pallor, low visual acuity, peripheral vision defect, decreased colour vision
- **treatment**: none (irreversible), aim to prevent

Abnormalities of Visual Field

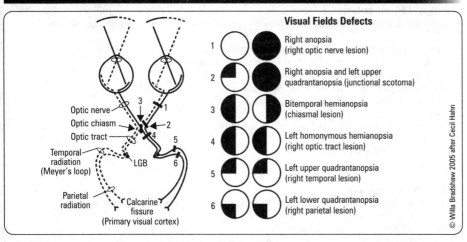

Visual Fields Defects

1. Right anopsia (right optic nerve lesion)
2. Right anopsia and left upper quadrantanopsia (junctional scotoma)
3. Bitemporal hemianopsia (chiasmal lesion)
4. Left homonymous hemianopsia (right optic tract lesion)
5. Left upper quadrantanopsia (right temporal lesion)
6. Left lower quadrantanopsia (right parietal lesion)

© Willa Bradshaw 2005 after Cecil Hahn

Figure 13. Characteristic visual field defects with lesions along the visual pathway

Bitemporal Hemianopsia DDx by Age
- Children: craniopharyngioma
- Middle aged (20s to 50s): pituitary mass
- Elderly (>60 yr): meningioma

In homonymous hemianopsia, more congruent deficits are caused by more posterior lesions; macular sparing may occur with occipital lesions

A lesion in a cerebral hemisphere causes eyes to "look away" from the hemiplegia, and to look towards the lesion
A lesion in the brainstem causes the eyes to "look toward" the side of the hemiplegia, and to look away from the lesion

Check all hemiplegic patients for homonymous hemianopsia (ipsilateral to side of hemiplegia)

Abnormalities of Eye Movements

Disorders of Gaze

Pathophysiology
- horizontal gaze: FEF → contralateral PPRF (midbrain/pons) → eyes saccade away from FEF
- vertical gaze: cortex → rostral interstitial nucleus in the MLF (midbrain)

Clinical Features
- unilateral lesion in one FEF → eyes deviate toward the side of the lesion
  - can be overcome with doll's eye maneuver
- unilateral lesion in the PPRF → eyes deviate away from the lesion
  - cannot be overcome with doll's eye maneuver if CN VI nucleus lesion as well
- seizure involving a FEF: eyes deviate away from the focus

Etiology
- common: infarcts (frontal or brainstem), MS, tumours

Internuclear Ophthalmoplegia

Pathophysiology
- results from a lesion in MLF which disrupts coordination between CN VI nucleus in pons and the contralateral CN III nucleus in midbrain → disrupts conjugate horizontal gaze

Clinical Features
- horizontal diplopia on lateral gaze, oscillopsia
- gaze away from the side of the lesion: ipsilateral adduction defect and contralateral abduction nystagmus
- cannot be overcome by caloric testing
- accommodation reflex intact
- may be bilateral (especially in MS)

Etiology
- common: MS, brainstem infarct

Investigations
- MRI

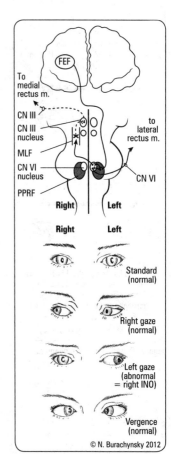

Figure 14. Internuclear ophthalmoplegia

Diplopia

Etiology – Monocular
- mostly due to relatively benign optical problems (refractive error, cataract) or functional

Etiology – Binocular (due to ocular misalignment)
- muscle: Graves' ophthalmopathy, EOM restriction/entrapment
- neuromuscular junction: MG (see *Myasthenia Gravis*, N38)
- cranial nerve palsy (see *Cranial Nerve Deficits*, N11)
- INO (see *Internuclear Ophthalmoplegia*, N15)
- other
  - orbital trauma (orbital floor fracture), tumour, infection, inflammation
  - Miller-Fisher variant of GBS
  - Wernicke's encephalopathy
  - leptomeningeal disease

Approach to Diplopia
- monocular (diplopia when one eye open) vs. binocular (diplopia when both eyes open)
- horizontal vs. vertical vs. oblique diplopia
- direction of gaze that exacerbates diplopia
- corrective head movements

Workup
- may observe isolated 4th or 6th nerve palsy for a few weeks, but workup if persistent or other symptoms develop
- indications for neuroimaging
  - bilateral or multiple nerve involvement
  - severe sudden onset headache (rule out aneurysm)

Diplopia worse at the end of the day suggests myasthenia gravis (e.g. fatigable)

If diplopia is only on extremes of gaze, cover each eye in isolation during extremes of gaze
The covered eye that makes the lateral image disappear is the pathological one

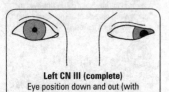

Left CN III (complete)
Eye position down and out (with ptosis and pupillary dilation)

Left Sympathetic Pathway
Horner's syndrome: ptosis, miosis, and anhydrosis

CN IV
Difficulty looking down and in (i.e. looking down at a golf ball – think CN Fore!)

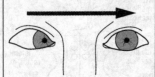

Left CN VI
Difficulty looking laterally

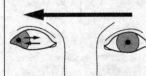

Left Medial Longitudinal Fasciculus
Internuclear ophthalmoplegia (INO): Difficulty adducting ipsilateral eye and horizontal nystagamus in abducted contralateral eye

© Minyan Wang 2012

Figure 15. Abnormal eye movement

Nystagmus

- definition: rapid, involuntary, small amplitude movements of the eyes that are rhythmic in nature
- direction of nystagmus is labelled by the **rapid** component of the eye movement
- can be categorized by movement type (pendular, jerking, rotatory, coarse) or as physiological vs. pathological

Table 8. Nystagmus Features

	Peripheral (Vestibular)	Central (Brainstem)
Direction	Unidirectional, fast phase away from the lesion	May be bilateral/unidirectional
Nystagmus	Usually horizontal	Usually vertical
Gaze Fixation	Relieves nystagmus	Does not relieve nystagmus
Vertigo	Severe	Mild
Auditory Symptoms	Common	Extremely rare
Other Neurological Signs	Absent	Often present
DDx	Benign paroxysmal positional vertigo, vestibular neuritis, Ménière's disease, toxicity, trauma, Ramsay Hunt syndrome	MS, vascular (brainstem/cerebellar), neoplastic/paraneoplastic

Abnormalities of Pupils

- see Ophthalmology, OP28

Nutritional Deficiencies and Toxic Injuries

- sufficient nutritional intake is required for optimal nervous system functioning; deficiencies in the following key nutrients, among others, may impair central and peripheral nervous system function (potential neurological symptoms are provided)

Table 9. Nutritional Deficiency Features and Management

Vitamin Deficiency	Neurological Clinical Manifestation	Investigation	Treatment*
Vitamin B12	Paresthesias and sensory ataxia are the most common initial symptoms Myelopathy (Subacute Combined Degeneration), peripheral neuropathy Neuropsychiatric: memory impairment, change in personality, delirium, and psychosis Optic neuropathy	Serum cobalamin Serum methylmalonic acid Serum homocysteine	IM Vitamin B12 1,000 μg for 5 d, then once per month or oral B12 1,000 μg/d
Folate	Myelopathy, peripheral neuropathy May be clinically indistinguishable from Vitamin B12 deficiency	Serum folate Homocysteine	Oral folate 1 mg tid initially; 1 mg daily thereafter
Copper	Myelopathy, pyramidal signs (e.g. brisk muscle stretch reflexes at the knees and extensor plantar responses) Severe sensory loss	Serum copper and ceruloplasmin; urinary copper	Discontinue zinc; oral copper 8 mg/d for 1 wk; 6 mg/d for 1 wk; 4 mg/d for 1 wk; 2 mg/d thereafter
Vitamin E	Ophthalmoplegia, retinopathy, spinocerebellar syndrome with peripheral neuropathy (with signs of cerebellar ataxia)	Serum vitamin E; ratio serum vitamin E to sum of cholesterol and triglycerides	Vitamin E 2,200 mg/kg/d oral or IM
Thiamine	Three manifestations include: beriberi (dry and wet), infantile beriberi, Wernicke-Korsakoff syndrome Alcoholism is a cause of reduced thiamine intake and deficiency	Clinical diagnosis; brain MRI	Thiamine 100 mg IV followed by 50-100 mg IV or IM until nutritional status stable
Pyridoxine (Vitamin B6)	Painful sensorimotor peripheral neuropathy	Serum pyridoxal phosphate	Pyridoxine 50-100 mg daily
Niacin (Vitamin B3)	Pellagra: Encephalopathy, dementia, coma, and peripheral neuropathy	Urinary excretion niacin metabolites	Nicotinic acid 25-50 mg daily oral or IM

*IM = intramuscular; IV = intravenous

- it is also important to consider occupational neurotoxic syndromes secondary to exposure to pesticides, solvents, and metals. Encephalopathy, extrapyramidal features, neurodegenerative diseases, and peripheral neuropathy are commonly encountered. Onset and progression of neurological diseases should be temporally related to neurotoxin exposure. Main toxins associated with neurotoxicity are listed below

Table 10. Selected Occupational Neurotoxic Syndromes

Toxin	Associated Occupations	Characteristic Neurological Findings
Organic Solvents	Printer, spray painters, industrial cleaners, paint or glue manufacturers, graphic industry, electronic industry, plastic industry	Nausea, H/A, concentration difficulty Long-term exposure may lead to "chronic solvent-induced encephalopathy", characterized by mild-to-severe cognitive impairment
Pesticides (e.g. insecticides, fungicides, rodenticides, fumigants, herbicides)	Agricultural work, pesticide manufacturing and formulating employees, highway and railway workers, green house, forestry and nursery workers	Parkinson's disease risk increased by ~70% following pesticide exposure
Heavy Metals (e.g. lead, mercury, manganese, aluminum, arsenic)	Battery and metal production (e.g. solder, pipes), chemical and electronic application industries, steel manufacturing, welders, alloy workers, transportation, packaging, construction	**Lead**: delayed/reversed development, permanent learning disabilities, peripheral neuropathy, seizures, coma, death from encephalopathy (rare) **Mercury**: psychiatric disturbances, ataxia, visual loss, hearing loss, tiredness, memory disturbances **Manganese**: psychiatric symptoms, hallucinations ("manganese madness"), extrapyramidal features, dystonia, parkinsonism (manganism) **Aluminum**: implicated in Alzheimer's pathogenesis **Arsenic**: sleeplessness/sleepiness, irritability, H/A, spasms in muscle extremities and muscle fatigue
Gases (e.g. carbon dioxide, nitrous oxide, formaldehyde)	Anesthesia, disinfection, manufacture of illuminating gas and water-gas	Cognitive/behavioural and emotional symptoms, parkinsonian syndromes

Neurologic Complications due to Toxic Injuries Related to Bariatric Surgery
- deficiencies of both fat- and water-soluble vitamins may occur following malabsorptive bariatric surgery
- patients who have undergone malabsorptive surgery should be monitored for late metabolic complications and neurological manifestations

Seizure Disorders and Epilepsy

Seizure

Stroke is the most common cause of late-onset (>50 yr) seizures, accounting for 50-80% of cases

Definitions
- **seizure**: transient neurological dysfunction caused by excessive activity of cortical neurons, resulting in paroxysmal alteration of behaviour and/or EEG changes
  - can be symptom of acute insult to the brain such as: alcohol and illicit drug use/withdrawal, brain injury/abnormality (tumour, trauma, vascular), CNS infection, fever (children), metabolic (hypoglycemia, electrolyte abnormalities, liver/renal failure), medications, OR be a manifestation of epilepsy
- **epilepsy**: chronic condition characterized by two or more unprovoked seizures, or underlying predisposition to seizures in a patient who has already had at least one seizure
  - etiologies: genetic, structural (e.g. prior stroke, tumour, meningo/encephalitis, perinatal insult, vascular malformation, malformation of cortical development, neurodegenerative), or unknown

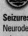

Seizures and Dementia
Neurodegenerative diseases can underlie seizures; conversely, seizures can be a cause of dementia

Classification

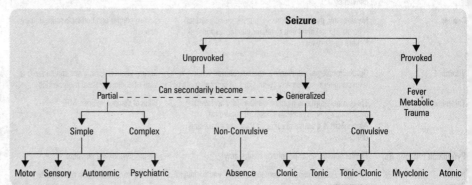

Figure 16. Classification of seizures
NOTE: seizures can also be classified using age of onset (childhood/adolescence, adulthood/late [i.e. >age 30]), setting (sleep, upon awakening), EEG (focal, generalized)

Clinical Features
- **partial (focal) seizures**
  - simple or complex can secondarily generalize, or simple → complex → generalized seizures
  - **simple (focal without loss of awareness)**
    - motor: postural, phonatory, forceful turning of eyes and/or head, focal muscle rigidity/jerking ± Jacksonian march (spreading to adjacent muscle groups)
    - sensory: unusual sensations affecting vision, hearing, smell, taste, or touch
    - autonomic: epigastric discomfort, pallor, sweating, flushing, piloerection, pupillary dilatation
    - psychiatric: symptoms rarely occur without impairment of consciousness and are more commonly complex partial

Temporal lobe epilepsy is suggested by an aura of fear, olfactory or gustatory hallucinations, and visceral or déjà vu sensations
Frontoparietal cortex seizures are suggested by contralateral focal sensory or motor phenomena

  - **complex (focal with loss of awareness)**
    - patient may appear to be awake but with impairment of awareness
    - classic complex seizure is characterized by automatisms such as chewing, swallowing, lip-smacking, scratching, fumbling, running, disrobing, and other stereotypic movements
    - other forms: dysphasic, dysmnesic (déjà vu), cognitive (disorientation of time sense), affective (fear, anger), illusions, structured hallucinations (music, scenes, taste, smells), epigastric fullness
- **generalized seizures**
  - **absence (petit mal)**: usually seen in children, unresponsive for 5-10 s with arrest of activity, staring, blinking or eye-rolling, no post-ictal confusion; 3 Hz spike and slow wave activity on EEG
  - **clonic**: repetitive rhythmic jerking movements
  - **tonic**: muscle rigidity in flexion or extension
  - **tonic-clonic (grand mal)**
    - may have prodrome of unease or irritability hours to days before the episode
    - tonic ictal phase: muscle rigidity
    - clonic ictal phase: repetitive violent jerking of face and limbs, tongue biting, cyanosis, frothing, incontinence
    - post-ictal phase: flaccid limbs, extensor plantar reflexes, headache, confusion, aching muscles, sore tongue, amnesia, elevated serum CK lasting hours; may have focal paralysis (Todd's paralysis).
  - **myoclonic**: sporadic contractions localized to muscle groups of one or more extremities
  - **atonic**: loss of muscle tone leading to drop attack

Table 11. Classic Factors Differentiating Seizure, Syncope and Pseudoseizure

Characteristic	Seizure	Syncope	Pseudoseizure* (Psychogenic non-epileptic seizure)
Timing	Day or night	Day	Day; other people present
Onset	Sudden, in any position	Gradual; Upright position (not recumbent)	Provoked by emotional disturbance or suggestion
Prodrome	Possible specific aura	Lightheadedness, pallor, diaphoresis	Variable
Duration	Brief or prolonged	Brief	Often prolonged
Incontinence	Common	Possible but rare	Rare
Post-Ictal	Occurs in tonic-clonic or complex partial	No	Variable, often none
Motor Activity	Synchronous, stereotypic, automatisms (common in absence and complex partial), lateral tongue biting, eyes rolled back	Occasional brief jerks	Opisthotonos, rigidity, eye closure, irregular extremity movements, shaking head, pelvic thrust, crying, geotropic eye movements, tongue biting at the tip
Injury	Common	Rare unless from fall	Rare
EEG	Usually abnormal; ± interictal discharges	Normal	Normal

*Pseudoseizures do not rule out seizures (not uncommon to have both)

- alcoholic withdrawal seizures may occur up to 2 days from the last exposure to alcohol (see Emergency Medicine, ER54)

Investigations
- CBC, electrolytes, fasting blood glucose, Ca^{2+}, Mg^{2+}, ESR, Cr, liver enzymes, CK, prolactin
- also consider toxicology screen, EtOH level, AED level (if applicable)
- CT/MRI (if new seizure without identified cause or known seizure history with new neurologic signs/symptoms)
- LP (if fever or meningismus)
- EEG

Treatment
- avoid precipitating factors
- indications for antiepileptic drugs (AED): 2 or more unprovoked seizures, known organic brain disease, EEG with epileptiform activity, first episode of status epilepticus, abnormal neurologic examination or findings on neuroimaging
- psychosocial issues: stigma of seizures, education of patient and family, status of driver's license, pregnancy issues
- safety issues: driving, operating heavy machinery, bathing, swimming alone
- refer for evaluation for possible surgical treatment if focal and refractory

Status Epilepticus

- **definition**: unremitting seizure or successive seizures without return to a baseline state of greater than 5 min
- **complications**: anoxia, cerebral ischemia and cerebral edema, MI, arrhythmias, cardiac arrest, rhabdomyolysis and renal failure, aspiration pneumonia/pneumonitis, death (20%)
- **initial measures**: ABCs, vitals, monitors, capillary glucose (STAT), ECG, nasal O_2, IV NS, IV glucose, IV thiamine, ABGs (if respiratory distress/cyanotic)
- **blood work**: electrolytes, Ca^{2+}, Mg^{2+}, PO_4^{3-}, glucose, CBC, toxicology screen, EtOH level, AED levels
- **focused history**: onset, past history of seizures, drug and alcohol ingestion, past medical history, associated symptoms, witnesses/collateral history
- **physical exam** (once seizures controlled): LOC, vitals, HEENT (nuchal rigidity, head trauma, tongue biting, papilledema), complete neurological exam, signs of neurocutaneous disorders, decreased breath sounds, cardiac murmurs or arrhythmias, urinary incontinence, MSK exam (rule out injuries)
- **post-treatment stabilization**: CT head, EEG, Foley catheter to monitor urine output, urine toxicology screen, monitor for rhabdomyolysis, and IV fluids to maintain normal cerebral perfusion pressure

Antiepileptic Drugs
- **focal and most generalized seizures**
  - valproate (Depakene®), lamotrigine (Lamictal®), levetiracetam (Keppra®), topiramate (Topamax®), phenobarbital (Phenobarb®), primidone, zonisamide, rufinamide (Banzel®), felbamate, benzodiazepines
- **primarily focal seizures (± 2° generalization)**
  - carbamazepine (Tegretol®), phenytoin (Dilantin®), gabapentin (Neurontin®), lacosamide (Vimpat®), oxcarbazepine (Trileptal®), eslicarbazepine acetate (Aptiom®), pregabalin (Lyrica®), tiagabine (Gabitril®), vigabatrin (Sabril®)
- **absence seizure**: ethosuximide (Zarontin®)

DDx of Convulsions
Syncope, pseudoseizure, hyperventilation, panic disorder, TIA, hypoglycemia, movement disorder, alcoholic blackouts, migraines (confusional, vertebrobasilar), narcolepsy (cataplexy)

Note that frontal seizures (rare) can look like a pseudoseizure due to odd motor activity that may occur

By law, the Ministry of Transportation in most provinces must be contacted for all patients who have had a seizure; patients will have their license suspended until seizure free for 6 mo; commercial drivers face a longer wait

EEG findings suggestive of epilepsy: abnormal spikes, polyspike discharges, spike-wave complexes

20-59% of first EEG are positive in epilepsy; 59-92% of epilepsy is picked up with repeated EEGs; normal interictal EEGs do not rule out epilepsy

Medical Emergency: Status epilepticus can cause irreversible brain damage without treatment

The most common causes of status epilepticus are failure to take AEDs and first presentation of epilepsy
Status epilepticus as a result of EtOH withdrawal is rare, despite it being a very common cause of seizures

Rule out non-convulsive status epilepticus in any patient who is still unconscious >20 min post-ictal; order a stat EEG if unsure

Complex partial status epilepticus can resemble schizophrenia or psychotic depression

Teratogenicity of anticonvulsants includes neural tube defects, cleft palate, urogenital malformations, and heart defects. Advise patient planning pregnancy to take 5 mg/d of folic acid. Optimize AEDs with lowest possible dose associated with good seizure control, preferably monotherapy if possible. Risk of fetal malformations with AEDs is 2x general population; highest risk associated with valproic acid and/or 2+ concurrent AEDs. Consider pre-conception AED levels if patient is well-controlled, monthly serum levels during pregnancy, and titrate AED to maintain pre-conception serum levels. Refer to high risk OB for intrapartum fetal screening

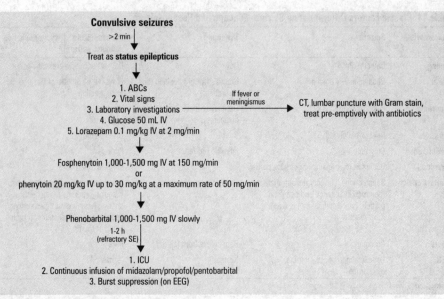

Figure 17. Status epilepticus treatment algorithm

Behavioural Neurology

- see Psychiatry, PS19

Acute Confusional State/Delirium

Table 12. Selected Intracranial Causes of Acute Confusion

	Etiology	Key Clinical Features	Investigations
Vascular	Subarachnoid hemorrhage	Thunderclap H/A, increased ICP, meningismus	CT, LP Angiography if CT and LP negative
	Stroke/TIA	Focal neurological signs	CT
Infectious	Meningitis	Fever, H/A, nausea, photophobia, meningismus	CT, LP
	Encephalitis	Fever, H/A, ± seizure Focal neurological signs	CT, LP MRI
	Abscess	Increased ICP Focal neurological signs	CT with contrast (often ring enhancing lesion)
Traumatic	Diffuse axonal shear, epidural hematoma, SDH	Trauma Hx Increased ICP Focal neurological signs	CT MRI
Autoimmune	Acute CNS vasculitis	Skin rash, active joints	ANA, ANCA, RF MRI Angiography
	Paraneoplastic encephalitis (anti-NMDA-R)	Onset: Psychiatric features, memory loss, seizures Delayed: Movement disorder, and changes in BP, HR, and temperature	CSF (test for presence of antibodies)
Neoplastic	Mass effect/edema, hemorrhage, seizure	Increased ICP Focal neurological signs Papilledema	CT MRI
Seizure	Status epilepticus	*See Seizure Disorders and Epilepsy, N18*	EEG
Primary Psychiatric	Psychotic disorder, mood disorder, anxiety disorder	No organic signs or symptoms	No specific tests
Other	Drugs (e.g. cocaine)	Chest pain, cough with black sputum, new-onset seizure, HTN, increased ICP, dyspnea	Vital signs Serum chemistry and electrolyte analysis
	Medications (with anticholinergic side effects)	Flushing, dry skin and mucous membranes, mydriasis with loss of accommodation	Serum chemistry and electrolyte analysis
	Neuroleptic Malignant Syndrome	Antipsychotic medication use Muscle rigidity Hyperthermia Autonomic instability	Serum chemistry and electrolyte analysis

Mild Neurocognitive Disorder (Mild Cognitive Impairment)

Definition
- cognitive impairment not meeting criteria of Major Neurocognitive Disorder
- measurable deficit in at least one cognitive domain reported by patient or others without impairment in ADLs
- amnestic (precursor to AD) vs. non-amnestic

Epidemiology
- mild NCD: 2-10% at age 65 yr and 5-25% by age 85 yr

Risk Factors
- vascular: hypertension, diabetes mellitus, obesity, cardiac disease, apolipoprotein E epsilon 4 genotype

Clinical Features
- cognitive impairment
  - particularly in amnestic subtype
  - important to ascertain that memory complaints represent change from baseline
  - patients with mild NCD are often troubled by memory symptoms in comparison to patients with dementia
- neuropsychiatric symptoms
  - depression (50%), irritability, anxiety, aggression, and apathy

Investigations
- establish a baseline for follow-up
- clinical interview with patient and his/her caregivers is the cornerstone of mild NCD evaluation
- neuropsychological testing
  - MMSE or MoCA; should not be used in isolation
  - if abnormal, follow-up in one year to monitor cognitive and functional decline
- neuroimaging
  - role uncertain
  - most advocate for a non-contrast brain CT to evaluate for structural abnormalities (CVD, SDH, NPH, or mass lesion)
- other testing
  - exclude treatable conditions and underlying psychiatric conditions

Treatment
- watch and wait
- no evidence for cholinesterase inhibitors, anti-inflammatory agents, vascular risk factor modification, exercise, cognitive interventions

Prognosis
- 10% progress to major NCD per yr
- typically progress to major NCD over a period of 2-3 yr

Delirium is a medical emergency carrying significant risk of morbidity and mortality; it is characterized by acute onset, disorientation, fluctuating level of consciousness, poor attention, and marked psychomotor changes

Visual hallucinations more commonly indicate organic disease

Major Neurocognitive Disorder (formerly Dementia)

- see Psychiatry, PS20 and Geriatric Medicine, GM4

Definition
- an acquired, generalized, and (usually) progressive impairment of cognitive function associated with impairment in ADLs/iADLs (i.e. shopping, food preparation, finances, medication management)
- diagnosis of major NCD requires presence of significant cognitive decline from a previous level of performance in one or more cognitive domains (complex attention, executive function, learning and memory, language, perceptual-motor, or social cognition) based on:
  - A) concern of the individual or a knowledgeable informant AND
  - B) a substantial impairment in cognitive performance either documented by standardized neuropsychological testing, or quantified clinical assessment
- see Psychiatry, PS19 for DSM-5 diagnostic criteria
- in comparison, mild NCD does not affect ADLs
  - mild NCD represents an intermediate stage between major NCD and normal aging

Epidemiology
- major NCD: 1-2% at age 65 yr and reaching as high as 30% by age 85 yr
- note
  - major NCD due to Alzheimer's disease is uncommon before age 60 yr
  - major NCD due to frontotemporal lobar degeneration has an earlier onset and represents a progressively smaller fraction of all NCDs with age

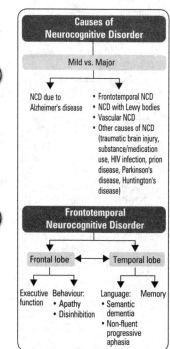

Figure 18. Major NCD classification

Sensitivity and Specificity

Tool	Sensitivity	Specificity
MMSE	87%	82%
Clinical Judgment	85%	82%
DSM IV	76%	80%

Vitamin B₁₂ Deficiency Symptoms
- Macrocytic anemia, pallor, SOB, fatigue, chest pain, palpitations
- Confusion or change in mental status (if advanced)
- Decreased vibration sense
- Distal numbness and paresthesia
- Weakness with UMN findings
- Diarrhea, anorexia

Major NCD Considerations for Management

ABCDs
Affective disorders, **A**DLs
Behavioural problems
Caretaker, **C**ognitive medications and stimulation
Directives, **D**riving
Sensory enhancement (glasses/hearing aids)

Most common causes of rapidly progressive neurodegenerative dementia (less than 4 yr survival): CJD, frontal temporal lobar dementia, tauopathies, diffuse Lewy body disease, and AD
Arch Neurol 2009;66:201-207
Head turning sign: when patient looking at his/ her caregiver for answers after being asked a question in clinical interviews
60% sensitivity, 98% specificity for diagnosis of cognitive Impairment

Early Signs of Major NCD	Normal Aging
Forgetting the names of close relations	Forgetting the names of acquaintances
Increased frequency of forgetting	Briefly forgetting part of an experience
Repeating phrases/ stories in the same conversation	Not putting away things properly
Unpredictable mood changes	Mood changes in response to appropriate causes
Decreased interest in activities and difficulty making choices	Changes in usual interests

Etiology
- see Table 13 for selected causes of major NCD
- reversible causes: alcohol (intoxication or withdrawal, Wernicke's encephalopathy), medication (benzodiazepines, anticholinergics), heavy metal toxicity, hepatic or renal failure, B12 deficiency, glucose, cortisol, thyroid dysfunction, NPH, depression (pseudodementia), intracranial tumour, SDH, hypercalcemia (secondary to elevated PTH)
- must rule out delirium

History
- "geriatric giants"
  - confusion/incontinence/falls
  - memory and safety (wandering, leaving doors unlocked, leaving stove on, losing objects, driving)
  - behavioural (mood, anxiety, psychosis, suicidal ideation, personality changes, aggression)
  - polypharmacy and compliance (sedative hypnotics, antipsychotics, antidepressants, anticholinergics)
- ADLs and IADLs
- cardiovascular, endocrine, neoplastic, renal ROS, head trauma history
- alcohol, smoking
- collateral history

Physical Exam
- blood pressure
- hearing and vision
- neurological exam with attention to signs of parkinsonism, UMN findings
- general physical exam with focus on CVD, patient-specific risk factors and history
- MMSE or MoCA, clock drawing, frontal lobe testing (go/no-go, word lists, similarities, proverb)

Investigations
- rule out reversible causes
  - CBC (note MCV for evidence of alcohol use and B12 deficiency), glucose, TSH, B12, RBC folate
  - electrolytes, LFTs, renal function, lipids, serum calcium
  - CT head, MRI as indicated, SPECT (optional)
  - as clinically indicated: VDRL, HIV, ANA, anti-dsDNA, ANCA, ceruloplasmin, copper, cortisol, toxicology, heavy metals
- issues to consider
  - failure to cope, fitness to drive, caregiver capacity and wellbeing, power of attorney, legal will, advanced medical directives, patient and caregiver safety

Table 13. Selected Causes of Major NCD (Dementia)

Etiology	Key Clinical Features	Investigations
PRIMARY DEGENERATIVE		
Alzheimer's disease	Memory impairment Aphasia, apraxia, agnosia	CT or MRI, SPECT
Dementia with Lewy bodies	Visual hallucinations Parkinsonism Fluctuating cognition	CT or MRI, SPECT
Frontotemporal dementia (e.g. Pick's disease)	Behavioural presentation: Disinhibition, perseveration, decreased social awareness, mental rigidity, memory relatively spared Language presentation: Progressive non-fluent aphasia, semantic dementia	CT or MRI, SPECT
Huntington's disease	Chorea	Genetic testing
VASCULAR		
Vascular cognitive impairment (previously Multi-infarct dementia)	Bradyphrenia without features of parkinsonism (slow thinking, slow rate of learning, slow gait) Dysexecutive syndrome May be abrupt onset Stepwise deterioration is classic but progressive deterioration is most common	CT or MRI, SPECT
CNS vasculitis	Systemic signs and symptoms of vasculitis	ANA; ANCA; RF CT or MRI Angiography

Table 13. Selected Causes of Major NCD (Dementia) (continued)

Etiology	Key Clinical Features	Investigations
INFECTIOUS		
Chronic meningitis	Fever, H/A, nausea Meningismus Localizing neurological deficits	CT, LP
Chronic encephalitis	Fever, headache	CT or MRI
Chronic abscess	Increased ICP Localizing neurological deficits	CT with contrast
HIV	See Infectious Diseases, ID27	HIV serology
Creutzfeldt-Jakob disease	Rapidly progressive, myoclonus	EEG, CT or MRI, LP
Syphilis	Ataxia, myoclonus, tabes dorsalis	LP, CT, or MRI VDRL
TRAUMATIC		
Diffuse axonal shear, epidural hematoma, subdural hematoma, SDH	Trauma Hx Increased ICP, papilledema Localizing neurological signs	CT
RHEUMATOLOGIC		
SLE	See Rheumatology, RH11	MRI ANA, anti-dsDNA
NEOPLASTIC		
Mass effect/edema, hemorrhage, seizure Paraneoplastic encephalitis	Increased ICP Localizing neurological signs Systemic symptoms of cancer	CT with contrast MRI Anti-Hu antibodies
OTHER		
Normal pressure hydrocephalus	Gait disturbances Urinary incontinence See Neurosurgery, NS8	CT or MRI

Cholinesterase Inhibitors for Dementia with Lewy Bodies (DLB), Parkinson's Disease Dementia (PDD) and Cognitive Impairment in Parkinson's Disease (CIND-PD)
Cochrane DB Syst Rev 2012;3:CD006504
Study: Meta-analysis of RCTs assessing efficacy of treatment with cholinesterase inhibitors in DLB, PDD, and CIND-PD.
Results: The six trials (n=1,236) included demonstrated therapeutic benefit of cholinesterase inhibitors for global assessment, cognitive function, behavioural disturbance, and activities of daily living. Cholinesterase inhibitors were associated with increased adverse events (OR 1.64) and drop out (OR 1.94). Adverse events were more common with rivastigmine but not with donepezil. Fewer deaths occurred in the treatment group (OR 0.28).
Conclusion: Current evidence supports use of cholinesterase inhibitors for patients with PDD but its role in DLB and CIND-PD is still unclear.

Major or Mild NCD due to Alzheimer's Disease

- see Psychiatry, PS20

Definition
- beyond criterion for NCD, the core features of Alzheimer's disease include an insidious onset and gradual progression of cognitive and behavioural symptoms
- typical presentation: amnestic
  - mild phase: impairment in memory and learning sometimes accompanied with deficits in executive function
  - moderate-severe phase: visuoconstructional/perceptual-motor ability and language may also be impaired
  - social cognition tends to be preserved until late in the course of the disease
- atypical nonamnestic presentation (one of the following):
  1. aphasia: language disturbance
  2. apraxia: impaired ability to carry out motor activities despite intact motor function
  3. agnosia: failure to recognize or identify objects despite intact sensory function

4 As and one D of AD
Anterograde amnesia
Aphasia
Apraxia
Agnosia
Disturbance in executive function
(Anterograde amnesia plus at least one of the other features is required for AD diagnosis)

Pathophysiology
- genetic factors
  - minority (<7%) of AD cases are familial (autosomal dominant)
  - 3 major genes for autosomal dominant AD have been identified:
    - amyloid precursor protein (chromosome 21), presenilin 1 (chromosome 14), presenilin 2 (chromosome 1)
  - the E4 polymorphism of apolipoprotein E (APOE) is a susceptibility genotype (E2 is protective)
  - note: APOE cannot serve as a diagnostic marker because it is only a risk factor and neither necessary nor sufficient for disease occurrence
- pathology (although not necessarily specific for AD)
  - gross pathology
    - diffuse cortical atrophy, especially frontal, parietal, and temporal lobes (hippocampi)

Down syndrome predisposes to early onset of Alzheimer's (i.e. age of ~40) due to three copies of the amyloid gene (APP)

- microscopic pathology
    - senile plaques (extracellular deposits of amyloid in the grey matter of the brain)
    - loss of synapses
    - neurofibrillary tangles (intracytoplasmic paired helical filaments with amyloid and hyperphosphorylated Tau protein)
    - loss of cholinergic neurons in nucleus basalis of Meynert that project diffusely throughout the cortex
- biochemical pathology
    - 50-90% reduction in action of choline acetyltransferase

Epidemiology
- 1/12 of population 65-75 yr of age
- up to 1/3 population >85 yr of age
- accounts for 60-90% of all dementias (depending on setting and diagnostic criteria)

Risk Factors
- age is the largest risk factor
- genetic susceptibility polymorphism: apolipoprotein E4 increases risk and decreases age of onset
- other factors include: traumatic brain injury, family history, Down syndrome, low education, and vascular risk factors (e.g. smoking, HTN, hypercholesterolemia, DM)

Clinical Features
- cognitive impairment
    - memory impairment for newly acquired information (early)
    - deficits in language, abstract reasoning, and executive function
- behavioural and psychiatric manifestations (80% of those with major NCD)
    - mild NCD: major depressive disorder and/or apathy
    - major NCD: psychosis, irritability, agitation, combativeness, and wandering
- motor manifestations (late)
    - gait disturbance, dysphagia, incontinence, myoclonus, and seizures

Investigations
- perform investigations to rule out other potentially reversible causes of dementia
- EEG: usually normal, may observe generalized slowing (nonspecific)
- MRI: preferential atrophy of the hippocampi and precuneus of the parietal lobe; dilatation of lateral ventricles; widening of cortical sulci
- SPECT: hypoperfusion in temporal and parietal lobes
- PET imaging using Pittsburgh compound B (PIB) as a tracer enables imaging of beta-amyloid plaque in neuronal tissue

Treatment
- acetylcholinesterase inhibitors have been shown to slow decline in cognitive function
    - donepezil, rivastigmine, galantamine
    - relative contraindications: bradycardia, heart block, arrhythmia, CHF, CAD, asthma, COPD, ulcers, or risk factors for ulcers and/or GI bleeding
    - galantamine is contraindicated in patients with hepatic/renal impairment
- memantine is an NMDA-receptor antagonist that has some benefits in later stage AD (i.e. when MMSE <17)
- symptomatic management
    1. pharmacologic
        - low dose neuroleptics for agitation (neuroleptics may worsen cognitive decline)
        - trazodone for sleep disturbance
        - antidepressants (SSRIs)
    2. non-pharmacologic
        - redirection
        - explore inciting factors for behaviour and modify behaviour of patient or caregiver
        - family support and day care facilities

Prognosis
- mean duration of survival after diagnosis is approximately 10 yr, reflecting the advanced age of the majority of individuals rather than the course of the disease
- in those who survive the full course, death commonly results from aspiration

Cognitive Effects of Atypical Antipsychotic Medications in Patients with Alzheimer's Disease: Outcomes from CATIE-AD
Am J Psychiatry 2011;168:831-839
Study: 421 outpatients with Alzheimer's disease and psychosis or agitated/aggressive behaviour were randomized to receive olanzapine, quetiapine, risperidone, or placebo in a multicentre double-blinded RCT. MMSE and Alzheimer's Disease Assessment Scale (ADAS) scores were measured at 36 wk.
Results: Patients receiving atypical antipsychotics exhibited a faster rate of cognitive decline as measured by MMSE scores (– 0.067/wk vs. -0.007/wk). They also had a significantly faster decline compared to placebo on a composite measure of ADAS, MMSE, and various other cognitive tests (-0.011/wk vs. -0.001/wk).
Conclusions: Long-term use of atypical antipsychotics for behavioural symptoms and psychosis in dementia patients is associated with greater rates of cognitive decline.

Major or Mild NCD with Lewy Bodies
(formerly Dementia with Lewy Bodies)

Definition
- A NCD characterized by progressive cognitive impairment (with early changes in complex attention and executive function) and recurrent complex visual hallucinations
- core diagnostic features
  - fluctuating cognition with pronounced variations in attention and alertness
  - recurrent visual hallucinations that are well formed and detailed
  - spontaneous features of parkinsonism, with onset subsequent to development of cognitive decline (rest tremor may be absent in DLB, but otherwise same classic features of Parkinson's disease)
- suggestive/supportive features
  - rapid eye movement (REM) sleep behaviour disorder
  - severe sensitivity to neuroleptic medications (rigidity, neuroleptic malignant syndrome, extrapyramidal symptoms)
  - repeated falls, syncope, or transient episodes of unexplained loss of consciousness
  - auditory or other nonvisual hallucinations, systematic delusions, and depression

Etiology and Pathogenesis
- Lewy bodies (eosinophilic cytoplasmic inclusions) found in both cortical and subcortical structures
- mixed DLB and AD pathology is common

Diagnostically Suggestive Markers
- low striatal dopamine transporter uptake on SPECT or PET
- relative preservation of medial temporal structures on CT/MRI

Epidemiology
- 0.1-5% of the general elderly population
- Lewy bodies are present in 20-35% of all dementia cases (more common in males)

Treatment
- acetylcholinesterase inhibitors (e.g. donepezil)

Prognosis
- average duration of survival 5-7 yr

Major or Mild Frontotemporal NCD
(formerly Frontotemporal Dementia)

Definition
- refers to a group of disorders caused by progressive cell degeneration in the brain's frontal or temporal lobes
  - deficits in executive function (e.g. poor mental flexibility, abstract reasoning, response inhibition, planning/organization, increased distractibility) with relative sparing of learning, memory and perceptual-motor function
- there are several variants of FTD each with specific core symptoms
- "probable" is distinguished from "possible" frontotemporal NCD by:
  - evidence of causative frontotemporal NCD genetic mutation, from either family history or genetic testing
  - evidence of disproportionate frontal and/or anterior temporal atrophy on MRI or CT
  - evidence of frontal and/or anterior temporal hypoperfusion or hypometabolism on PET or SPECT

Behavioural Variant FTD
- most common variant
- insidious onset: must show progressive deterioration of behaviour and/or cognition by observation or history
- typically early symptom presentation (i.e. within the first 3 yr)
- three out of the following symptoms must be present and persistent/recurrent:
  - behavioural disinhibition (socially inappropriate behaviour, impulsive, careless)
  - apathy or inertia
  - loss of sympathy or empathy (diminished response to others' needs/feelings, social interest)
  - preservative, stereotyped, or compulsive/ritualistic behaviour
  - hyperorality and dietary changes (binge eating, increased consumption of alcohol/cigarettes or inedible objects)

Language Variants (Primary Progressive Aphasia)
- prominent decline in language ability, in the form of speech production, word finding, object naming, grammar, or word comprehension
- three subtypes
  - nonfluent/agrammatic variant PPA (NFAV-PPA) or progressive nonfluent aphasia (PNFA): non-fluent, laboured articulation/speech, anomia, preserved single word comprehension, word-finding deficit, impaired repetition
  - semantic variant PPA (SV-PPA) or semantic dementia (SD): fluent, normal rate, anomia, impaired single word comprehension, intact repetition, use words of generalization ("thing") or supraordinate categories ("animal" for "dog")
  - logopenic progressive aphasia (LPA): naming difficulty and impaired repetition

FTD Movement Disorders
- corticobasal degeneration (CBD) (see Parkinsonism)
- progressive supranuclear palsy (PSP) (see Parkinsonism)

Etiology and Pathogenesis
- unknown, however there is likely a genetic/familial component (40% have family history of early onset NCD)
- genetic variants: MAPT gene (Tau), PGRN gene (progranulin), VCP gene, TARDBP gene (TDP-43), CHMP2D gene
- unlike AD, FTD does not show amyloid plaques or neurofibrillary tangles, instead it is characterized by severe atrophy and specific neuronal inclusion bodies
- gross changes: atrophy in the frontal and anterior temporal lobes; cortical thinning; possible ventricular enlargement
- histological changes: gliosis, swollen neurons, microvacuolation, inclusion bodies in neurons/glia (Tau or TDP-43)

Epidemiology
- fourth most common cause of dementia (5% of all dementia cases)
- common cause of early-onset NCD in individuals younger than 65 yr

Prognosis
- median survival being 6-11 yr after symptoms onset and 3-4 yr after diagnosis
- survival is shorter and decline is faster than in typical Alzheimer's disease

Major or Mild Vascular NCD

Definition
- diagnosis of major or mild NCD with determination of CVD as the dominant if not exclusive pathology that accounts for the cognitive deficits
- vascular etiology suggested by one of the following:
  - onset of cognitive deficits is temporally related to one or more cerebrovascular events
  - evidence for decline is prominent in complex attention (including processing speed) and frontal-executive function
- neuroimaging evidence of cerebrovascular disease comprises one or more of the following:
  - one or more large vessel infarct or hemorrhage
  - a strategically placed single infarct or hemorrhage (e.g. angular gyrus, thalamus, basal forebrain)
  - two or more lacunar infarcts outside the brainstem
  - extensive and confluent white matter lesions
- for mild vascular NCD: history of a single stroke or extensive white matter disease is sufficient
- for major vascular NCD: history of two or more strokes, a strategically placed stroke, or a combination of white matter disease and one or more lacunae is generally necessary
- associated features supporting diagnosis: personality and mood changes, abulia, depression, emotional lability, and psychomotor slowing

Etiology and Pathogenesis
- major risk factors are the same as those for CVD (i.e. HTN, DM, smoking, obesity, high cholesterol levels, high homocysteine levels, other risk factors for atherosclerosis, atrial fibrillation, and conditions increasing risk of cerebral emboli)
- major or mild vascular NCD with gradual onset and slow progression is generally due to small vessel disease leading to lesions in white matter, basal ganglia, and/or thalamus
- cognitive deficits can be attributed to disruption of cortical-subcortical circuits

Epidemiology
- second most common cause of NCD
- prevalence estimates for vascular dementia/NCD range from 0.2-13% (by age 70), 16% (ages 80+) to 44.6% (ages 90+)
- higher prevalence in African Americans compared to Caucasians and East Asians
- prevalence higher in males than in females

Creutzfeldt-Jakob Disease

- rare degenerative fatal brain disorder caused by prion proteins causing spongiform changes, astrocytosis, and neuronal loss
- most common forms are sporadic (85%), hereditary (5-10%), and acquired (<1%)
- investigations: CSF analysis, MRI brain (cortical and/or subcortical FLAIR changes), EEG (periodic complexes)
- definitive diagnosis is by brain biopsy
- no treatments currently exist

Prion proteins have a normal form and an infectious form, which results from conversion of the protein from alpha-helix (normal) to beta-pleated sheet (abnormal); these abnormally folded proteins aggregate leading to neuronal loss

Aphasia

Definition
- an acquired disturbance of language characterized by errors in language production, writing, comprehension, or reading

Neuroanatomy of Aphasia
- Broca's area (posterior inferior frontal lobe) involved in language production (expressive)
- Wernicke's area (posterior superior temporal lobe) involved in comprehension of language (receptive)
- angular gyrus is responsible for relaying written visual stimuli to Wernicke's area for reading comprehension
- arcuate fasciculus association bundle connects Wernicke's and Broca's areas

>99% of right-handed people have left hemisphere language representation

70% of left-handed people have left hemisphere language representation, 15% have right hemisphere representation, and 15% have bilateral representation

Assessment of Language
- assessment of context
  - handedness (writing, drawing, toothbrush, scissors), education level, native language, learning difficulties
- assessment of aphasia
  - spontaneous speech (fluency, paraphasias, repetition, naming, comprehension – auditory and reading, writing, neologisms)

Types of Paraphasias
Semantic ("chair" for "table")
Phonemic ("clable" for "table")

Aphasia localizes the lesion to the dominant cerebral hemisphere

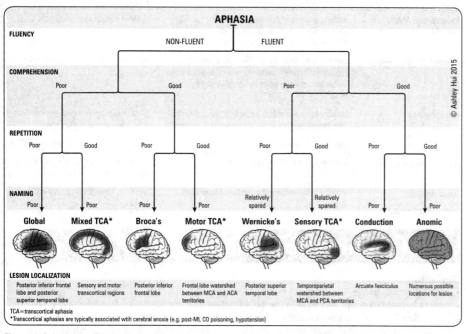

Figure 19. Aphasia classification

Apraxia

Definition
- inability to perform skilled voluntary motor sequences that cannot be accounted for by weakness, ataxia, sensory loss, impaired comprehension, or inattention

Clinicopathological Correlations

Table 14. Apraxia

	Description	Tests	Hemispheres
Ideomotor	Inability to perform skilled learned motor sequences	Blowing out a match; combing one's hair	Left
Ideational	Inability to sequence actions	Preparing and mailing an envelope	Right and left
Constructional*	Inability to draw or construct	Copying a figure	Right and left
Dressing*	Inability to dress	Dressing	Right

*Refers specifically to the inability to carry out the learned movements involved in construction, drawing, or dressing; not merely the inability to construct, draw, or dress. Many skills aside from praxis are needed to carry out these tasks

Agnosia

Definition
- disorder in the recognition of the significance of sensory stimuli in the presence of intact sensation and naming

Clinicopathological Correlations

Table 15. Agnosias

	Description	Lesion
Apperceptive Visual Agnosia	Inability to name or demonstrate the use of an object presented visually 2° to distorted visual perception Recognition by touch remains intact	Bilateral temporo-occipital cortex
Associative Visual Agnosia	Inability to name an object presented visually 2° to disconnect between visual cortex and language areas Visual perception is intact as demonstrated by visual matching	Bilateral inferior temporo-occipital junction
Prosopagnosia	Inability to recognize familiar faces in the presence of intact visual perception and intact auditory recognition	Bilateral temporo-occipital areas or right inferior temporo-occipital region
Colour Agnosia	Inability to perceive colour	Bilateral inferior temporo-occipital lesions
Impaired Stereognosis	Inability to identify objects by touch	Anterior parietal lobe in the hemisphere opposite the affected hand
Finger Agnosia	Inability to recognize, name, and point to individual fingers	Dominant hemisphere parietal-occipital lesions

> **Parietal Lobe Lesions**
> - Lesions of the dominant parietal lobe are characterized by Gerstmann's syndrome: acalculia, agraphia, finger agnosia, and left-right disorientation
> - Lesions of the non-dominant parietal lobe are characterized by neglect, anosognosia, and asomatognosia
> - Cortical sensory loss (graphesthesia, astereognosis, impaired 2 point discrimination and extinction) can be seen with left or right parietal lesions

> - Extent of retrograde amnesia correlates with severity of injury
> - Regained from most distant to recent memories

Mild Traumatic Brain Injury

Definition
- mild TBI = concussion
- trauma induced transient alteration in mental status that may involve loss of consciousness
- hallmarks of concussion: confusion and amnesia, which may occur within minutes
- loss of consciousness (if present) must be less than 30 min, initial GCS must be between 13-15, and post-traumatic amnesia must be less than 24 h

Epidemiology
- 75% of TBIs are estimated to be mild; remainder are moderate or severe (see <u>Neurosurgery</u>, NS30 and <u>Emergency Medicine</u>, ER8)
- highest rates in children 0-4 yr, adolescents 15-19 yr, and elderly >65 yr

Clinical Features
- impairments following mild TBI
  - somatic: headache, sleep disturbance, nausea, vomiting, blurred vision
  - cognitive dysfunction: attentional impairment, reduced processing speed, drowsiness, amnesia
  - emotion and behaviour: impulsivity, irritability, depression
- severe concussion: may precipitate seizure, bradycardia, hypotension, sluggish pupils
- associated conditions: brain contusion, diffuse axonal injury, C-spine injury

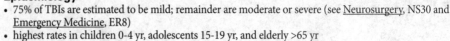

Investigations
- neurological exam to identify focal neurologic deficits
- neurocognitive assessment
  - simple orientation questions are inadequate to detect cognitive changes
  - initial assessment of severity is determined by
    - Glasgow Coma Scale: mild: 13-15, moderate: 9-12, severe: 3-8
  - sideline evaluation: Standardized Assessment of Concussion, Westmead Post-Traumatic Amnesia Scale, Sport Concussion Assessment Tool
- neuroimaging
  - x-ray of skull: not indicated for routine evaluation of MTBI
  - CT head as indicated by Canadian CT Head Rules (see Emergency Medicine, ER8)
  - MRI not indicated in initial evaluation – indicated in presence of continued or worsening symptoms despite normal CT

Treatment
- observation for first 24 h after mild TBI in all patients because of risk of intracranial complications
- emergency department for assessment if any loss of consciousness or persistent symptoms
- hospitalization with normal CT if GCS <15, seizures, or bleeding diathesis; or abnormal CT scan
- early rehabilitation to maximize outcomes
  - OT, PT, SLP, vestibular therapy, driving, therapeutic recreation
- pharmacological management of headaches, pain, depression
- CBT, relaxation therapy
- follow Return to Play guidelines (www.thinkfirst.ca)

Prognosis
- most recover from mild TBI with minimal treatment, but some experience long-term consequences
- athletes with a previous concussion are at increased risk of subsequent concussion and cumulative brain injury
- repeat TBI can lead to life threatening cerebral edema (controversially known as second impact syndrome) or permanent impairment
- sequelae include
  - post-concussion syndrome: dizziness, headache, neuropsychiatric symptoms, cognitive impairment (usually resolves within weeks to months)
  - post-traumatic headaches: begin within 7 d of injury
  - post-traumatic epilepsy: approximately 2% risk of epilepsy post-mild TBI, prophylactic anticonvulsants not effective
  - post-traumatic vertigo

Neuro-Oncology

Paraneoplastic Syndromes

- see Endocrinology, E48

Tumours of the Nervous System

- see Neurosurgery, NS37

Movement Disorders

Function of the Basal Ganglia

- the cerebral cortex initiates movement via excitatory (glutamatergic) projections to the striatum, which then activate two pathways: direct and indirect
- direct: cortex → striatum → GPi/SNr → thalamus → motor cortex
  - activation of this pathway removes the inhibitory effect of the GPi on the thalamus, letting the thalamus activate the cortex and ultimately allowing movement
- indirect: cortex → striatum → GPe → STN → GPi/SNr → thalamus → motor cortex
  - activation of this pathway causes inhibition of the thalamus and ultimately prevents movement

Movement Disorders

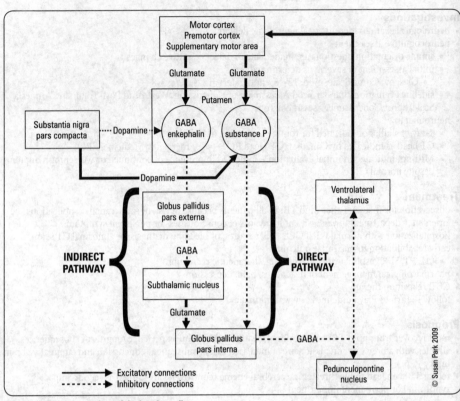

Figure 20. Neural connections of the basal ganglia

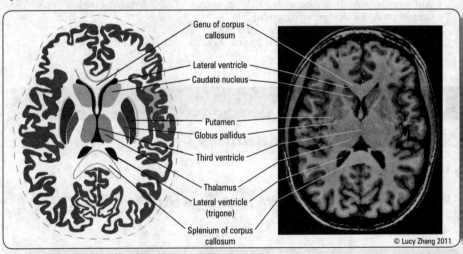

Figure 21. Horizontal section of basal ganglia

Overview of Movement Disorders

Table 16. Movement Disorder Definitions

Akathisia	Subjective generalized restlessness relieved by voluntary stereotypic movements (e.g. squirming)
Asterixis	Transient loss of muscle tone (negative myoclonus)
Athetosis	Slow writhing movements, especially distally
Bradykinesia	Slow and/or small amplitude of movements
Chorea	Brief, flowing, irregular movements; can appear purposeful in milder forms
Dysdiadochokinesia	Inability to smoothly perform rapidly alternating movements
Dyskinesia	Any involuntary movement, but the term is often used to describe the stereotypical movements that come with long-term neuroleptic use (tardive dyskinesia)
Dystonia	Co-contraction of agonist and antagonist muscles causing sustained twisting movements which can be tonic (dystonic postures) or phasic (dystonic movements)
Freezing	Episodes of halted motor action, especially during repetitive actions (eg. walking)
Hemiballismus	Unilateral violent flinging movement
Myoclonus	Brief muscle group contraction that is either focal, segmental, or generalized
Myokymia	Spontaneous, fine, fascicular contraction of muscle
Tachykinesia	Acceleration of movements
Tics	Stereotyped and brief repetitive actions due to inner urge; can be suppressed; can be phonic (vocal) or motor
Tremor	Rhythmic and involuntary alternating muscle contractions

Movement Disorders

Differential Diagnoses

1. Tremor

Table 17. Approach to Tremors

	Resting	Action-Postural	Action-Intention
Body Part	UE>jaw>LE>head	UE>head>LE>tongue	UE>voice>LE
Characteristics	3-7 Hz pill rolling	6-12 Hz fine tremor	<5 Hz coarse tremor
Worse with Associated Sx	Rest while concentrating "TRAP"	Sustained posture (outstretched arms) ± Autosomal dominant FHx	Finger to nose Cerebellar findings
DDx	PD, Parkinsonism, Wilson's disease, mercury poisoning	Physiologic, essential, hyperthyroidism, hyperglycemia, heavy metal poisoning, CO poisoning, drug toxicity, sedative/alcohol withdrawal	Cerebellar disorders, Wilson's disease, MS, anticonvulsants, alcohol, sedatives
Treatment	Carbidopa-levodopa (Sinemet®), surgery, DBS	Propranolol, primidone, topiramate, and other anticonvulsants	Treat underlying cause

2. Chorea: Huntington's disease (HD), HD-like syndromes, neuroacanthocytosis, SLE, APLA syndrome, Wilson's disease, CVD, tardive dyskinesia, senile chorea, Sydenham's chorea, pregnancy chorea (chorea gravidarum)

3. Dystonia
- **primary dystonia**: familial, sporadic (torticollis, blepharospasm, writer's cramp)
- **dystonia-plus syndromes**: dopa-responsive dystonia, myoclonus-dystonia
- **secondary dystonia**: thalamotomy, stroke, CNS tumour, demyelination, PNS injury, drugs/toxins (L-dopa, neuroleptics, anticonvulsants, Mn, CO, cyanide, methanol)
- **heredodegenerative dystonias**: Parkinsonian disorders, Wilson's disease, Huntington's disease

4. Myoclonus
- **physiologic myoclonus**: hiccups, nocturnal myoclonus
- **essential myoclonus**: myoclonus-dystonia with minimal or no occurrence of dystonia
- **epileptic myoclonus**
- **symptomatic myoclonus**
- **degenerative disorders**: Wilson's disease, Huntington's disease, Corticobasal degeneration
- **infectious disorders**: CJD, viral encephalitis, AIDS-dementia complex
- **metabolic disorders**: drug intoxication/withdrawal, hypoglycemia, hyponatremia, HHS, hepatic encephalopathy, uremia, hypoxia
- **focal brain damage**: head injury, stroke, mass

In some cases, dystonias may only occur during voluntary movement and sometimes only during specific activities such as writing, chewing, or speaking (task-specific dystonia)

Hemiballismus is most often due to a vascular lesion of the contralateral subthalamic nucleus

Myoclonus is often stimulus-sensitive as it can be induced by sudden noise, movement, light, visual threat, or pinprick

In a young patient (<45) must do TSH (thyroid disease), ceruloplasmin (Wilson's disease), and CT/MRI (cerebellar disease) as indicated by type of tremor

The majority of essential tremor does not need treatment

Alcohol
- Dampens essential tremor
- Potentiates intention tremor during abstinence (delirium tremens)
- Does not improve resting tremor of PD

Most common cause of chorea is drug therapy for PD (L-dopa induced dyskinesias)

Palatal myoclonus can result from lesion to the Dentato-Rubro-Olivary tract, and is associated with an audible clicking and tremor of other facial muscles

Parkinson's Disease

Key Parkinsonian Features

TRAP
Tremor (resting)
Rigidity
Akinesia/bradykinesia
Postural instability

Etiology
- **sporadic**: combination of oxidative stress to dopaminergic neurons, environmental toxins (e.g. pesticides), accelerated aging, genetics
- **familial** (10%): autosomal dominant α-synuclein or LRRK2 mutations, autosomal recessive parkin, PINK1 or DJ-1mutation (juvenile onset)
- **MPTP** (neurotoxin)

Epidemiology
- prevalence of 0.3% in industrialized countries, but rises with increased age
- second most common neurodegenerative disorder, after Alzheimer's
- mean age of onset is 60 yr

2015 MDS Clinical Diagnostic Criteria for PD
"Clinically Established PD" requires:
- Cardinal Parkinsonism Manifestations: Bradykinesia with either rest tremor or rigidity
- 2 or more supportive criteria (clear and dramatic beneficial response to dopaminergic therapy, levodopa-induced dyskinesia, rest tremor of a limb, olfactory loss/cardiac sympathetic denervation on MIBG scintigraphy)
- No absolute exclusion criteria and no red flags (see full diagnostic criteria - Postuma et al (2015). Mov Disord.)

Associated Factors
- **risk**: family history, male, head injury, rural living, exposure to certain neurotoxins
- **protective**: coffee drinking, smoking, NSAID use, estrogen replacement in post-menopausal women

Pathophysiology
- loss of dopaminergic neurons in pars compacta of substantia nigra, thus reduced dopamine in striatum leading to disinhibition of the indirect pathway and decreased activation of the direct pathway causing increased inhibition of cortical motor areas
- α-synucleinopathy: α-synuclein accumulates in Lewy bodies and causes neurotoxicity in substantia nigra

Clinical Features
- positive motor
  - resting tremor: asymmetric 4-5 Hz "pill-rolling" tremor, especially in hands
  - rigidity: lead-pipe rigidity with cogwheeling due to superimposed tremor
- negative motor
  - bradykinesia: slow, small amplitude movements, fatiguing of rapid alternating movements, difficulty initiating movement
- related findings: masked facies, hypophonia, aprosody (monotonous speech), dysarthria, micrographia, shuffling gait with decreased arm swing
- freezing of gait: occurs with walking triggered by initiating stride or barriers/destinations, lasting seconds
- postural instability: late finding presenting as falls
- cognition: bradyphrenia (slow to think/respond), dementia (late finding)
- behavioural: decreased spontaneous speech, depression, sleep disturbances, anxiety
- autonomic: constipation, urinary retention, sexual dysfunction, orthostatic hypotension, clinostatic hypertension

Consider an Alternative Diagnosis if Atypical Parkinsonism
- Poor response to levodopa
- Abrupt onset of symptoms
- Rapid progression
- Early falls
- Early autonomic dysfunction
- Symmetric symptoms at onset
- Early age of onset (<50 yr)
- Early cognitive impairment
- FHx of psychiatric/dementing disorders
- Recent diagnosis of psychiatric disease
- History of encephalitis
- Unusual toxin exposure
- Extensive travel history

Treatment
- **pharmacologic**
  - mainstay of treatment: levodopa/carbidopa (Sinemet®) or levodopa/benserazide (Prolopa®). Levodopa is a dopamine precursor; carbidopa and benserazide decreases peripheral metabolism of levodopa, decreasing side effects and increasing half-life of levodopa
    - levodopa-related fluctuation: delayed onset of response (affected by mealtime), end-of-dose deterioration ("wearing-off"), random oscillations of on-off symptoms
    - major complication of levodopa is dyskinesia
  - treatment of early PD: dopamine agonists, amantadine, MAOI
  - adjuncts: dopamine agonists, MAOI, anticholinergics (especially if prominent tremors), COMT inhibitors
- **surgical:** thalamotomy, pallidotomy, DBS (thalamic, pallidal, subthalamic)
- **psychiatric**

Other Parkinsonian Disorders

Dopamine Agonist Therapy in Early Parkinson's Disease
Cochrane DB Syst Rev 2009;2:CD006564
Study: Meta-analysis of trials of dopamine agonists in early Parkinson's disease.
Results: Twenty-nine trials were included (n=5,247). Dopamine agonists were found to have decreased motor side effects (dyskinesia [OR 0.51], dystonia [OR 0.64], motor fluctuations [OR 0.75]) compared to levodopa, but provided poorer symptom control compared to levodopa. Also, other side effects were increased (constipation [OR 1.59], hallucinations [OR 1.69], dizziness [OR 1.45]).
Conclusion: Dopamine agonists have fewer motor side effects than levodopa, but provide worse symptom control and increased rate of other side effects.

- **NCD with Lewy bodies** (see *Behavioural Neurology*, N25)
- **progressive supranuclear palsy**: tauopathy with limited vertical gaze (downgaze more specific), early falls, axial rigidity and akinesia, dysarthia, and dysphagia
- **corticobasal syndrome**: tauopathy with varied presentations but classically presents with unilateral parkinsonism, dystonia/myoclonus, apraxia ± "alien limbs" phenomenon; may also present as progressive non-fluent aphasia
- **multiple system atrophy**: synucleinopathy presenting as either cerebellar predominant (MSA-C, previously olivopontocerebellar atrophy) or parkinsonism predominant (MSA-P, previously nigrostriatal degeneration); both are associated with early autonomic dysfunction (previously Shy-Drager syndrome)
- **vascular parkinsonism**: multi-infarct presentation with gait instability and lower body parkinsonism; less likely associated with tremor

Huntington's Disease

Etiology and Pathogenesis
- genetics: autosomal dominant CAG repeats (with anticipation) in Huntington's gene on Chromosome 4, which leads to accumulation of defective protein in neurons
- pathology: global cerebral atrophy, especially affecting the striatum, leading to increased activity of the direct pathway, and decreased activity of the indirect pathway

Epidemiology
- North American prevalence 4-8/100,000
- mean age of onset 35-44 yr; but varies with degree of anticipation from 5-70 yr

Clinical Features
- typical progression: insidious onset with clumsiness, fidgetiness, and irritability, progressing over 15 yr to major NCD, psychosis, and chorea
  - major NCD: progressive memory impairment and loss of intellectual capacity
  - chorea: begins as movement of eyebrows and forehead, shrugging of shoulders, and parakinesia (pseudo-purposeful movement to mask involuntary limb jerking)
  - progresses to dance-like or ballism, and in late stage is replaced by dystonia and rigidity
  - mood changes: irritability, depression, anhedonia, impulsivity, bouts of violence
- Juvenile-onset HD (Westphal variant) characterized by Parkinsonism and dystonia

Investigations
- MRI: enlarged ventricles, atrophy of cerebral cortex and caudate nucleus
- genetic testing
  - expansion of the cytosine-adenine-guanine (CAG) trinucleotide repeats in the HTT gene
  - CAG repeats on chromosome 4p16.3 that encodes the protein huntingtin

Treatment
- no disease altering treatment
- psychiatric symptoms: antidepressants and antipsychotics
- chorea: neuroleptics and benzodiazepines
- dystonia: botulinum toxin

Dystonia

Epidemiology
- third most common movement disorder after Parkinson's disease and essential tremor

Clinical Features
- symptoms exacerbated by fatigue, stress, emotions; relieved by sleep or specific tactile/proprioceptive stimuli ('geste antagoniste', e.g. place hand on face for cervical dystonia)
- more likely to be progressive and generalize if younger onset or leg dystonia

Treatment
- local medical: botulinum toxin
- systemic medical: anticholinergics (benztropine), muscle relaxants (baclofen), benzodiazepines, dopamine depletors (tetrabenazine); dopamine for dopa-responsive dystonia
- surgical: surgical denervation of affected muscle, stereotactic thalamotomy (unilateral dystonia), posteroventral pallidotomy, or DBS

Tic Disorders

Definition
- a tic is a sudden, rapid, recurrent, nonrhythmic, stereotyped motor movement or vocalization
- common criteria
  - tics may wax and wane in frequency but have persisted for an extended period of time
  - onset before age 18 yr
  - disturbance is not attributable to the physiological effects of a substance or another medical condition

Clinical Classification
- **Tourette's disorder**: multiple motor and one or more vocal tics that have persisted for more than 1 yr since onset
- **persistent (chronic) motor or vocal tic disorder**: single or multiple motor or vocal tics (but not both motor and vocal) that have persisted for more than 1 yr since onset
- **provisional tic disorder**: single or multiple motor and/or vocal tics present for <1 yr since first tic onset
- **other specified or unspecified tic disorder**: symptoms characteristic of a tic disorder but do not meet full criteria
- **secondary tic disorders**: encephalitis, CJD, Sydenham's chorea, head trauma, drugs, mental retardation syndromes

Motor vs. Vocal Tics
- simple tics: short duration (milliseconds)
- complex tics: longer (seconds), more purposeful and often include a combination of simple tics
- motor tics
  - simple: blinking, head jerking, shoulder shrugging, extension of the extremities
  - dystonic: bruxism (grinding teeth), abdominal tension, sustained mouth opening
  - complex: copropraxia (obscene gestures), echopraxia (imitate gestures), throwing, touching
- vocal tics
  - simple: blowing, coughing, grunting, throat clearing
  - complex: coprolalia (shout obscenities), echolalia (repeat others' phrases), palilalia (repeat own phrases)

Treatment
- dopamine blockers, dopamine depletors (tetrabenazine), clonidine, clonazepam, DBS

Tourette's Syndrome (Gilles de la Tourette's Syndrome)

Definition According to DSM V
1. presence of both multiple motor and one or more vocal tics at some point during the illness, although not necessarily concurrently
2. tics may wax and wane in frequency but have persisted for more than 1 yr since first tic onset (with no tic-free periods greater than 3 mo)
3. onset is before age 18 yr
4. not due to effect of a substance or another medical condition

Epidemiology
- estimated prevalence among adolescents 3-8 per 1,000 school-age children; M:F = 2:1 to 4:1

Signs and Symptoms
- tics: wide variety that wax and wane in type and severity; can be voluntarily suppressed for some time but are preceded by unpleasant sensation that is relieved once tic is carried out
  - can be worsened by anxiety, excitement, and exhaustion; better during calm focused activities
- psychiatric: compulsive behaviour (associated with OCD and ADHD), hyperactive behaviour, 'rages', sleep-wake disturbances, learning disabilities

Treatment
- same as tics (dopamine blockers, dopamine depletors, clonidine, clonazepam, DBS)

Prognosis
- typically begins between ages 4-6
- peak severity occurs between ages 10-12, with a decline in severity during adolescence (50% are tic-free by 18 yr of age)
- tic symptoms, however, can manifest similarly in all age groups and across the lifespan

Cerebellar Disorders

Clinico-Anatomic Correlations
- **vermis**: trunk/gait ataxia
- **cerebellar lobe** (i.e. lateral): rebound phenomenon, scanning dysarthria, dysdiadochokinesia, dysmetria, nystagmus

Symptoms and Signs of Cerebellar Dysfunction
- nystagmus: observe during extraocular movement testing (most common is gaze-evoked nystagmus)
- dysarthria (ataxic): abnormal modulation of speech velocity and volume – elicit scanning/telegraphic/slurred speech on spontaneous speech
- ataxia: broad-based, uncoordinated, lurching gait
- dysmetria: irregular placement of voluntary limb or ocular movement
- dysdiadochokinesia: impairment of rapid alternating movements (e.g. pronation – supination task)
- postural instability: truncal ataxia on sitting, titubation (rhythmic rocking of trunk and head), difficulty with tandem and broad-based gait
- intention tremor: typically orthogonal to intended movement, and increases as target is approached
- hypotonia: decreased resistance to passive muscular extension (occurs shortly after injury to lateral cerebellum)
- pendular patellar reflex: knee reflex causes pendular motion of leg (occurs after injury to cerebellar hemispheres); pendular reflexes at triceps
- rebound phenomenon: overcorrection after displacement of a limb
- hypometric and hypermetric saccades

Wernicke-Korsakoff Syndrome

- see Psychiatry, PS24
- note that alcohol can also cause a cerebellar ataxia separate from thiamine deficiency; this ataxia can be due to cerebellar atrophy or alcohol polyneuropathy

Cerebellar Ataxias

Congenital Ataxias

- early onset non-progressive ataxias associated with various syndromes as well as developmental abnormalities (e.g. Arnold-Chiari malformation, Dandy-Walker cysts)

Hereditary Ataxias

- **autosomal recessive**: includes Friedrich's ataxia, ataxia telangiectasia, vitamin E deficiency
  - Friedrich's ataxia: prevalence 2/100,000; typical onset between 8 and 15 yr
    - signs: gait and limb ataxia, weakness, areflexia, extensor plantar reflex, impaired proprioception and vibration, dysarthria
    - death in 10-20 yr from cardiomyopathy or kyphoscoliotic pulmonary restriction
- **autosomal dominant**: most commonly spinocerebellar ataxias (SCAs) (Over 30 types, most common SCAs due to CAG repeats)
  - signs: ataxia and dysarthria; , chorea, polyneuropathy, pyramidal and/or extrapyramidal features, „ dementia

Acquired Ataxias

- **neurodegeneration** (e.g. multiple system atrophy)
- **systemic**: alcohol, celiac sprue, hypothyroidism, Wilson's, thiamine deficiency
- **toxins**: carbon monoxide, heavy metals, lithium, anticonvulsants, solvents
- **vascular**: infarct, bleed, basilar migraine
- **autoimmune**: MS, Miller-Fischer (GBS)

Vertigo

- see Otolaryngology, OT12

Motor Neuron Disease

Amyotrophic Lateral Sclerosis (Lou Gehrig's Disease)

Definition

- progressive neurodegenerative disease that causes UMN and LMN symptoms and is ultimately fatal

Etiology

- idiopathic (most), genetic (5-10% familial, especially SOD1 mutation, other: C9orf72, TARDBP)

Pathology

- disorder of anterior horn cells of spinal cord, cranial nerve nuclei, and corticospinal tract

Epidemiology

- 5/100,000; incidence increases with age

Clinical Features

- limb motor symptoms: segmental and asymmetrical UMN and LMN symptoms
- bulbar findings: dysarthria (flaccid or spastic), dysphagia, tongue atrophy and fasciculations, facial weakness and atrophy
- pseudobulbar affect, frontotemporal dementia (up to 10%)
- sparing of sensation, ocular muscles, and sphincters

Investigations

- EMG: chronic denervation and reinnervation, fasciculations
- NCS: to rule out peripheral neuropathy (i.e. multifocal motor neuropathy with conduction block)
- CT/MRI: to rule out cord disease/compression

The only interventions that have been shown to extend survival in ALS are riluzole and use of BiPAP

Red Flags Inconsistent with ALS
Sensory sx, predominant pain, bowel or bladder incontinence, cognitive impairment, ocular muscle weakness

Denervation on EMG
Fibrillations, positive sharp waves, complex repetitive discharges; reinnervation – increased amplitude and duration of motor units

Treatment
- riluzole (modestly slows disease progression)
- symptomatic relief
  - spasticity/cramping: baclofen, tizanidine (Zanaflex®), regular exercise, and physical therapy
  - sialorrhea: TCA (i.e. amitriptyline), sublingual atropine drops, parotid/submandibular Botox® (rare)
  - pseudobulbar affect: dextromethorphan/quinidine, TCA, SSRI
- non-pharmacologic: high caloric diet, ventilatory support (especially BiPAP), early nutritional support (i.e. PEG tube), rehabilitation (PT, OT, SLP), psychosocial support

Prognosis
- median survival 3 yr; death due to respiratory failure

Other Motor Neuron Diseases

- degenerative
  - **progressive muscular atrophy (progressive bulbar palsy):** only LMN symptoms with asymmetric weakness, later onset than ALS, 5-10% of patients in ALS centres
  - **primary lateral sclerosis (progressive pseudobulbar palsy):** UMN symptoms, later onset, not fatal with variable disability; 5-10% of patients in ALS centres
  - **spinal muscular atrophy:** pediatric disease with symmetric LMN symptoms
- infectious
  - **post-polio syndrome, West Nile infection:** residual asymmetric muscle weakness, atrophy

Peripheral Neuropathies

Diagnostic Approach to Peripheral Neuropathies
1. differentiate: motor vs. sensory vs. autonomic vs. mixed
2. pattern of deficit: symmetry; focal vs. diffuse; upper vs. lower limb; cranial nerve involvement
3. temporal pattern: acute vs. chronic; relapsing/remitting vs. constant vs. progressive
4. history: PMH, detailed FHx, exposures (e.g. insects, toxins, sexual, travel), systemic symptoms
5. detailed peripheral neuro exam: LMN findings, differentiate between root and peripheral nerves, cranial nerves, respiratory status

Diabetic Neuropathies
- Peripheral neuropathy: pain or loss of sensation in a glove and stocking distribution (hands and feet affected before arms and legs)
- Autonomic: anhidrosis, orthostatic hypotension, impotence, gastroparesis, bowel and bladder dysfunction
- Mononeuropathy multiplex: nerve infarct or compression
- Cranial neuropathy: CN III (pupil sparing) > IV > VI
- Lumbosacral plexopathy

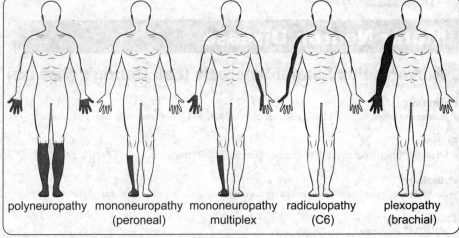

polyneuropathy   mononeuropathy   mononeuropathy   radiculopathy   plexopathy
                 (peroneal)   multiplex   (C6)   (brachial)

Figure 22. Pattern of distribution for peripheral neuropathies

Tinel's Sign
Tap lightly over the median nerve at the wrist, the patient's symptoms of carpal tunnel will be elicited in a positive test

Phalen's Test
Hold both wrists in forced flexion (with the dorsal surfaces of the hands pressed against each other) for 30-60 s; test is positive if symptoms of carpal tunnel are elicited

DDx of Demyelinating Neuropathy
GBS, CIDP, paraproteinemia, diphtheria, amiodarone, Charcot-Marie-Tooth, storage diseases, pressure palsy predisposition, paraneoplastic

Classification
- **monoradiculopathy**: dermatomal deficit due to single nerve root lesion
  - due to disc herniation or root compression causing radicular pain
  - little tactile anesthesia, as dermatomes overlap
- **polyradiculopathy**: multiple dermatome deficits due to multiple nerve root lesions
  - one type is cauda equina syndrome (lumbosacral roots)
- **plexopathy**: deficit matching distribution of a nerve plexus
  - brachial plexopathy
    - upper (C5-C7): LMN sx of shoulder and upper arm muscles (Erb's palsy)
    - lower (C8-T1): LMN sx and sensory sx of forearm and hand (Klumpke's palsy)
    - DDx: trauma, idiopathic neuritis, tumour infiltration, radiation, thoracic outlet syndrome (i.e. cervical rib)
  - lumbosacral plexopathy (rare, especially unilateral)
    - DDx: idiopathic neuritis, infarction (i.e. DM), compression

- **mononeuropathy**: single nerve deficit
  - **carpal tunnel syndrome** (most common): compression of median nerve at wrist
    - symptoms: wrist pain, paresthesia first 3 and ½ digits, ± radiation to elbow, worse at night
    - signs: Tinel's sign, Phalen's test, thenar muscle wasting, sensory deficit
    - EMG and NCS: slowing at wrist (both motor and sensory)
    - etiology: entrapment, pregnancy, DM, gammopathy, rheumatoid arthritis, thyroid disease
  - **Bell's palsy** (most common cranial neuropathy): see <u>Otolaryngology</u>, OT22
  - other less common mononeuropathies due to entrapment/compression: ulnar (compression at elbow), median (at pronator teres), radial (at spiral groove of humerus), obturator (from childbirth), peroneal (due to crossing legs or surgical positioning), posterior tibial (tarsal canal)
- **mononeuropathy multiplex**: deficit affecting multiple discrete nerves (asymmetric)
  - must rule out vasculitis or collagen vascular disease; consider MMN (multifocal motor neuropathy) or MADSAM (multifocal acquired demyelinating sensory and motor neuropathy)
- **polyneuropathy**: symmetrical distal stocking-glove pattern
  - symmetrical distal sensorimotor deficit affecting longest fibres first (stocking-glove distribution), hypotonia; progression of dysesthesia early and weakness later
  - etiology: DM (most common), renal disease, substances, toxins, genetics, SLE, HIV, leprosy, alcohol, B12 deficiency, uremia
  - **chronic inflammatory demyelinating polyneuropathy (CIDP)**
    - chronic relapsing sensorimotor polyneuropathy with increase protein in CSF and demyelination (shown on EMG/NCS)
    - course is fluctuating, in contrast with the acute onset of GBS
    - treatment: first-line is prednisone; alternatives are plasmapheresis, IVIG, and azathioprine

Table 18. Differential Diagnosis of Symmetric Polyneuropathy

	Etiology	Mechanism	Course	Modalities	Investigations
Vascular	PAN	Ischemic	Chronic	S/M	See <u>Rheumatology</u>, RH19
	SLE	Ischemic	Chronic	S/M	See <u>Rheumatology</u>, RH11
	RA	Ischemic	Chronic	S/M	See <u>Rheumatology</u>, RH8
Infectious	HIV	Axonal/demyelination	Chronic	S/A	HIV serology
	Leprosy	Infiltrative	Acute	S/A	Leprosy serology Nerve biopsy
	Lyme	Axonal/demyelination	Chronic	M	Lyme serology
Immune	GBS	Demyelination	Acute	M	LP (↑ protein; no ↑ cells)
	CIDP	Demyelination	Chronic	S/M	LP (↑ protein)
Hereditary	HMSN	Axonal/demyelination	Chronic	S/M	Genetic testing
Neoplastic	Paraneoplastic	Axonal/demyelination	Chronic	S/M	Paraneoplastic antibodies
	Myeloma	Axonal/demyelination	Chronic	S/M	SPEP Skeletal bone survey
	Lymphoma	Axonal	Chronic	M	SPEP Bone marrow biopsy
	Monoclonal gammopathy	Demyelination	Chronic	S/M	SPEP Bone marrow biopsy
Toxin	EtOH	Axonal	Sub-acute	S/M	GGT, MCV
	Heavy metals (i.e. lead)	Axonal	Sub-acute	S/M	Urine heavy metals
	Medications	Axonal	Sub-acute	S/M	Drug levels
Metabolic	DM	Ischemic/axonal	Chronic	S/A	Fasting glucose, HbA1c, 2 h OGTT
	Hypothyroidism	Axonal	Chronic	S/M	TSH, T3, T4
	Renal failure	Axonal	Chronic	S/A	Electrolytes, Cr, BUN
Nutritional	B12 deficiency	Axonal	Sub-acute	S/M	Vitamin B12
Other	Porphyria	Axonal	Sub-acute	M	Urine porphyrins
	Amyloid	Axonal	Sub-acute	S	Nerve biopsy

A = autonomic; CIDP = chronic inflammatory demyelinating polyneuropathy; GGT = gamma-glutamyl transferase; HMSN = hereditary motor sensory neuropathy; M = motor; OGTT = oral glucose tolerance test; PAN = polyarteritis nodosa; RA = rheumatoid arthritis; S = sensory; SLE = systemic lupus erythematosus; SPEP = serum protein electrophoresis

Axonal neuropathies have decreased amplitude on NCS; demyelinating neuropathies have decreased velocity on NCS

Ototoxic drugs (e.g. aminoglycosides) should not be given to diabetics
Sensory neuropathy of the feet prevent them from adequately compensating for loss of vestibular function

IVIG and plasmapheresis lead to more rapid improvement, less intensive care and less ventilation, but do not change mortality or relapse rate

Evaluation of Distal Symmetric Polyneuropathy: Role of Laboratory and Genetic Testing
Neurology 2009;72:185-192
Screening Lab Tests: Blood glucose, serum B12 with metabolites, serum protein immunofixation electrophoresis.
Genetic Testing: Indicated for cryptogenic polyneuropathy exhibiting classic hereditary neuropathy phenotype. Screen for CMT1A duplication/deletion and Cx32 mutations.

GBS is a neurological emergency due to risk of imminent respiratory failure

The most common antecedent infection in GBS is *Campylobacter jejuni*

Miller-Fischer Variant of GBS – Triad
- Ophthalmoplegia
- Ataxia
- Areflexia

Guillain-Barré Syndrome
- **definition**: acute rapidly evolving demyelinating inflammatory polyradiculoneuropathy that often starts in the distal lower limbs and ascends
- **etiology**
  - autoimmune attack and damage to peripheral nerve myelin
  - sometimes preceded by viral/bacterial infections
- **signs and symptoms**
  - sensory: distal and symmetric paresthesias, loss of proprioception and vibration sense, neuropathic pain
  - motor: weakness starting distally in legs, areflexia
  - autonomic: blood pressure dysregulation, arrhythmias, bladder dysfunction
- **investigations**
  - CSF: albuminocytologic dissociation (high protein, normal WBC)
  - EMG/NCS: conduction block, differential or focal (motor > sensory) slowing, decreased F-wave, sural sparing
- **subtypes**
  1. acute inflammatory demyelinating polyneuropathy (AIDP)
  2. acute motor-sensory axonal neuropathy (AMSAN)
  3. acute motor axonal neuropathy (AMAN)
- **treatment**
  - IVIG or plasmapheresis, ± pain management, monitor vitals and vital capacity
- **prognosis**
  - peak of symptoms at 2-3 wk, resolution at 4-6 wk
  - 5% mortality (higher if require ICU); up to 15% have permanent deficits

Neuromuscular Junction Diseases

Clinical Approach to Disorders of the Neuromuscular Junction

Neuromuscular Junction Disease
Diseases of the neuromuscular junction typically feature prominent fatigability
Fatigability can be tested by holding the arms out or by holding the gaze in the upward position (especially in MG)
Muscle weakness due to fatigability will improve with rest or ice

Table 19. Common Disorders of the Neuromuscular Junction

	Myasthenia Gravis	Lambert-Eaton	Botulism
Ocular/Bulbar Paresis	+	–	++ (early)
Limb Weakness	+	+	+
Fatigability	+	+	+
Post-Exercise Enhancement	–	+	+
Reflexes	N	↓	↓
Anticholinergic Sx	–	+	++
Sensory Sx	–	–	–
Associated Conditions	Thymoma	Small cell carcinoma	GI S&S
Repetitive EMG Stimulation	Decremental response	Incremental response	↑ (rapid stimulation) ↓ (slow stimulation)

Myasthenia Gravis

Etiology and Pathophysiology
- progressive autoimmune disorder due to anti-AChR or anti-MuSK antibodies, resulting in early saturation at the NMJ and inadequate muscle activation with increasing nerve stimulation
- 15% of patients with MG have associated thymic neoplasia, 85% have thymic hyperplasia

Epidemiology
- bimodal age of onset – 20s (mostly women) and 60s (mostly men)

Clinical Features
- fatigable, symmetric or asymmetric weakness without reflex changes, sensory changes, or coordination abnormalities
- ocular (diplopia/ptosis), bulbar (dysarthria/dysphagia), and/or proximal limb weakness
- symptoms may be exacerbated by infection, pregnancy, menses, and various drugs
- respiratory muscle weakness may lead to respiratory failure

Investigations
- edrophonium (Tensilon®) test
- assess for improvement over 2 min following edrophonium injection
- EMG
  - repetitive stimulation → decremental response
  - single fibre electromyography shows increased jitter (80-100% sensitivity)

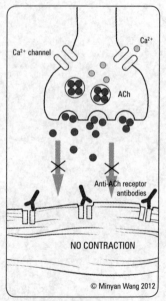

Figure 23. Myasthenia gravis

Ca²⁺ channel

Ca²⁺

ACh

Anti-ACh receptor antibodies

NO CONTRACTION

© Minyan Wang 2012

- spirometry – forced vital capacity may be used to monitor adequacy of respiratory effort over time
- anti-acetylcholine receptor antibody assay (70-80% sensitivity)
- anti-MuSK antibody may be used if seronegative for anti-AChR antibody
- CT/MRI to screen for thymoma/thymic hyperplasia

Treatment
- thymectomy - 85% of patients show improvement or remission
- symptomatic relief
- acetylcholinesterase inhibitors (e.g. pyridostigmine)
- does not affect primary pathologic process so rarely results in control of disease when used alone
- immunosuppression
- steroids are mainstay of treatment (70-80% remission rate)
- azathioprine, cyclophosphamide, and mycophenolate as adjuncts or as steroid sparing therapy
- short-term immunomodulation (for crises) – IVIG and plasmapheresis

Prognosis
- 30% eventual spontaneous remission
- with treatment, life expectancy is equal to that of a person without MG, but quality of life may vary

Tensilon® is a drug that inhibits acetylcholinesterase. It improves muscle function immediately in myasthenia gravis, but not in a cholinergic crisis
This test is infrequently used; when performed, a crash cart should be nearby as respiratory difficulty and/or bradycardia may occur

Lambert-Eaton Myasthenic Syndrome

Etiology and Pathophysiology
- autoimmune disorder due to antibodies against presynaptic voltage-gated calcium channels, causing decreased ACh release at the NMJ
- 50-66% are associated with small cell carcinoma of the lung

Clinical Features
- weakness of skeletal muscles without sensory or coordination abnormalities, proximal and lower muscles more affected
- reflexes are diminished or absent, but increase after active muscle contraction
- bulbar and ocular muscles affected in 25% (vs. 90% in MG)
- prominent anticholinergic autonomic symptoms (dry mouth > impotence > constipation > blurred vision)

Investigations
- edrophonium test → no response
- EMG
  - rapid (>10 Hz) repetitive stimulation → incremental response
  - post-exercise facilitation → an incremental response with exercise
- screen for malignancy, especially small cell lung cancer

Treatment
- tumour removal
- acetylcholine modulation
  - increased acetylcholine release (3,4-diaminopyridine)
  - decreased acetylcholine degradation (pyridostigmine)
- immunomodulation - steroids, plasmapheresis, IVIG

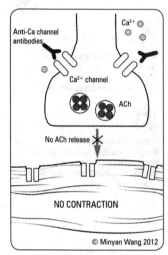

Figure 24. Lambert-Eaton myasthenic syndrome (LEMS)

Botulism

Etiology and Pathophysiology
- caused by a toxin produced by spores of Clostridium botulinum bacteria, which can enter through wounds or by ingestion
- infantile botulism is the most common form, and is usually from ingestion of honey or corn syrup

Clinical Features
- occur 6-48 h after ingestion
- CN paralysis: ptosis, extraocular muscle weakness, dilated poorly reactive pupils, dysarthria, jaw weakness, dysphagia
- autonomic dysfunction: nausea, orthostatic hypotension, constipation (paralytic ileus), bladder distension
- anticholinergic symptoms: dry mouth, constipation, urinary retention
- spreads to trunk and limbs: symmetric weakness with paralysis and absent/decreased deep tendon reflexes
- pattern of paresis often starts with GI symptoms, then extraocular muscle weakness, then dysphagia, then limbs and respiratory involvement; all associated with dry mouth.
- rarely respiratory distress, potentially advancing to respiratory failure

Investigations
- blood test for toxin, stool culture
- CT/MRI to rule out stroke, lesion (normal in botulism)

Treatment
- botulinum anti-toxin – good prognosis with prompt treatment
- supportive therapy as required

Myopathies

Clinical Approach to Muscle Diseases

Myopathies are characterized by prominent symmetric proximal weakness and absent sensory changes

Good Questions to Assess Proximal Weakness
- Legs: climbing stairs, stand from sit
- Arms: reach above head, wash hair

Common Medications that Cause Myopathy: steroids, statins, anti-retrovirals, thyroxine, fibrates, cyclosporine, ipecac
Common Drugs that Cause Myopathy: ethanol, cocaine, heroin

Table 20. Myopathies

	Etiology	Key Clinical Features	Key Investigations
Inflammatory	Polymyositis (see Rheumatology, RH15)	Myalgias Pharyngeal involvement	↑ CK Biopsy: endomysial infiltrates; necrosis
	Dermatomyositis (see Rheumatology, RH15)	Myalgias Characteristic rashes Can be paraneoplastic	↑ CK Biopsy: perifascicular atrophy
	Sarcoidosis	See Respirology, R14	ACE level Biopsy: granulomas
	Inclusion body myositis	Weak quadriceps and deep finger flexors	↑ CK Biopsy: inclusion bodies
Endocrine	Thyroid (↑ or ↓) Cushing's syndrome Parathyroid (↑ or ↓)	See Endocrinology, E32	TSH, serum cortisol, calcium panel
Toxic	Medication	Medication or toxin history	Toxicology screen
	Critical illness myopathy	ICU patient Hx steroids and nondepolarizing paralyzing agents Failure to wean from ventilation	Biopsy: selective loss of thick myosin filaments
Infectious	Parasitic, bacterial, or viral	Myalgias Inflammatory myopathy	↑ myoglobin
Hereditary Dystrophy	Duchenne (see Pediatrics, P43)	Early onset (Duchenne and Becker)	Dystrophin analysis: absent
	Becker (see Pediatrics, P39)	Progressive proximal muscle weakness Calf pseudohypertrophy	Dystrophin analysis: abnormal
	Myotonic dystrophy	Distal myopathy Myotonia Genetic anticipation	Genetic testing
Hereditary Metabolic	McArdle's	Exercise-related myalgias, cramping, and myoglobuminuria	↑ lactate ↑ serum/urinary myoglobin post-exercise
Hereditary Periodic Paralysis	"Channelopathy"	Episodic weakness Normal between attacks	Normal, ↑ or ↓ K^+
Hereditary Mitochondrial	MERRF	Myoclonus, generalized seizures, dementia, myopathy	Biopsy: ragged red fibres Increased lactate
	MELAS	Pediatric onset, stroke-like symptoms, episodic vomiting, dementia	
	Kearns Sayre	Progressive ophthalmoplegia, retinal pigment degeneration, cardiac conduction abnormalities	

MELAS = mitochondrial encephalomyopathy, lactic acidosis, and stroke-like episodes; MERRF = mitochondrial encephalomyopathy with ragged red fibres

Myotonic Dystrophy

Etiology and Pathophysiology
- unstable trinucleotide (CTG) repeat in DMK gene (protein kinase) at 19q13.3, number of repeats correlates with severity of symptoms, autosomal dominant

Epidemiology
- most common adult muscular dystrophy, prevalence 3-5/100,000

Clinical Features
- appearance: ptosis, bifacial weakness, frontal baldness (including women), triangular face giving a drooping/dull appearance
- physical exam
  - distribution of weakness: distal weaker than proximal (in contrast to other myopathies), steppage gait
  - myotonia: delayed relaxation of muscles after exertion (elicit by tapping on thenar muscles with hammer)
  - cardiac: 90% have conduction defects (1° heart block; atrial arrhythmias)
  - respiratory: hypoventilation 2° to muscle weakness
  - ocular: subcapsular cataracts, retinal degeneration, decreased intraocular pressure
  - other: DM, infertility, testicular atrophy
  - EMG: subclinical myotonia – long runs with declining frequency and amplitude

Treatment and Prognosis
- no cure, progressive, death usually around 50 yr
- management of myotonia: phenytoin

Pain Syndromes

Approach to Pain Syndromes

Definitions
- **nociceptive pain**: pain arising from normal activation of peripheral nociceptors
- **neuropathic pain**: pain arising from direct injury to neural tissue, bypassing nociceptive pathways
- **spontaneous pain**: unprovoked burning, shooting, or lancinating pain
- **paresthesia**: spontaneous abnormal non-painful sensation (e.g. tingling)
- **dysesthesia**: evoked pain with inappropriate quality or excessive quantity
- **allodynia**: a dysesthetic response to a non-noxious stimulus
- **hyperalgesia**: an exaggerated pain response to a noxious stimulus

Non-Pharmacological Management
- physical (PT, acupuncture, chiropractic manipulation, massage)
- psychoeducational (CBT, family therapy, education, psychotherapy)

Medical Pain Control
- combination multi-modal therapy is important
- primary analgesics: acetaminophen, NSAIDs (often used for soft tissue injuries, strains, sprains, headaches, and arthritis), opiates
- adjuvants: antidepressants (TCAs, SSRIs), anticonvulsants (gabapentin, carbamazepine, pregabalin), baclofen, sympatholytics (phenoxybenzamine), α2-adrenergic agonists (clonidine)

Surgical Pain Control
- peripheral ablation: nerve blocks, facet joint denervation
- direct delivery: implantable morphine pump
- central ablation: stereotactic thalamotomy, spinal tractotomy, or dorsal root entry lesion
- DBS or dorsal column stimulation

Neuropathic Pain

Definition
- pain resulting from a disturbance of the central or peripheral nervous system

Epidemiology
- affects up to 6% of people (2 million Canadians)

- Pinprick sensation mediated by Aδ fibres
- Pain due to tissue damage is mediated by C fibres

WHO Pain Ladder
- **Mild Pain**: Non-opioid (acetaminophen and/or NSAID) ± adjuvant
- **Moderate Pain**: Opioid for mild to moderate pain (codeine/oxycodone) + non-opioid ± adjuvant
- **Severe Pain**: Opioid for moderate to severe pain (morphine/hydromorphone) + non-opioid ± adjuvant

Axonal regeneration is directed by intact nerve sheaths; if the nerve sheath is damaged, axons grow without direction, become tangled and form a neuroma, which can result in ectopic electrical impulses and neuropathic pain

Symptoms and Signs
- hyperalgesia/allodynia
- subjectively described as burning, heat/cold, pricking, electric shock, perception of swelling, numbness
- can be spontaneous or stimulus evoked
- distribution may not fall along classical neuro-anatomical lines
- associated issues: sleep difficulty, anxiety/stress/mood alteration

Causes of Neuropathic Pain
- **sympathetic**: complex regional pain syndrome
- **non-sympathetic**: damage to peripheral nerves
  - **systemic disease**: DM, thyroid disease, renal disease, rheumatoid arthritis, multiple sclerosis
  - **nutritional/toxicity**: alcoholism, pernicious anemia, chemotherapy
  - **infectious**: post-herpetic, HIV
  - **trauma/compression**: nerve entrapment, trigeminal neuralgia, post-surgical, nerve injury, cervical/lumbar radiculopathy, plexopathy
- **central**: abnormal CNS activity
  - phantom limb, post spinal cord injury, post stroke, MS

Treatment
- identify/treat underlying cause
- **pharmacotherapy**
  - Stepwise approach (Canadian Pain Society, 2014)
    - 1st line: Gabapentinoids, TCA, SNRI
    - 2nd line: Tramadol, opioid analgesics
    - 3rd line: Cannabinoids
    - 4th line: Fourth-line agents: topical lidocaine (second line for postherpetic neuralgia), methadone, lamotrigine, lacosamide, tapentadol, botulinum toxin
- **common non-pharmacologic therapies**
  - neuropsychiatry: CBT, psychotherapy
  - rehabilitation: physiotherapy
- **surgical therapies**: dorsal column neurostimulator, DBS (thalamus)

Trigeminal Neuralgia

Clinical Features
- recurrent episodes of sudden onset, excruciating unilateral paroxysmal shooting "electric" pain in trigeminal root territory (V3>V2>>V1)
- may have normal sensory exam
- pain lasts seconds/minutes over days/weeks; may remit for wk/mo
- triggers: touching face, eating, talking, cold wind, shaving, applying make-up

Etiology
- **classic TN**: idiopathic
- **secondary TN**: compression by tortuous blood vessel (superior cerebellar artery), cerebellopontine angle tumour (5%), MS (5%)

Epidemiology
- F>M; usually middle-aged and elderly

Diagnosis
- clinical diagnosis
- investigate for secondary causes, which are more likely if bilateral TN or associated sensory loss
  - MRI to rule out structural lesion, MS, or vascular lesion

Treatment
- first line: carbamazepine or oxcarbazepine
- second line: baclofen or lamotrigine
- narcotics not generally recommended
- if medical treatment fails: trigeminal ganglion percutaneous technique, gamma knife, invasive percutaneous denervation (radiofrequency/glycerol), percutaneous balloon microcompression, microvascular decompression

Postherpetic Neuralgia

Herpes Zoster of Trigeminal Nerve
Typically involves V1 (ophthalmic division)
Hutchinson's Sign
Tip of nose involvement predicts corneal involvement

Clinical Features
- pain persisting in the region of a cutaneous outbreak of herpes zoster
- constant deep ache or burning, intermittent spontaneous lancinating/jabbing pain, allodynia
- distribution: thoracic, trigeminal, cervical > lumbar > sacral
- associated impaired sleep, decreased appetite, decreased libido

Etiology and Pathogenesis
- destruction of the sensory ganglion neurons (e.g. dorsal root, trigeminal, or geniculate ganglia) secondary to reactivation of herpes zoster infection

Epidemiology
- incidence in those with zoster increases with age (2% in <60 yr, 19% in >70 yr)
- risk factors: older age, greater acute pain, greater rash severity

Prevention
- varicella zoster vaccine (Varivax®) in childhood reduces incidence of varicella zoster
- herpes zoster vaccine (Zostavax®) reduces incidences of shingles, PHN, and other herpetic sequel (currently recommended in Canada for those >60 yr old)

Treatment
- medical: TCA (i.e. amitriptyline), anti-convulsants (i.e. pregabalin, gabapentin), analgesia (i.e. opiates, lidocaine patch), intrathecal methylprednisolone, topical capsaicin
  - early treatment of acute herpes zoster with antivirals (acyclovir; longer-acting famciclovir and valacyclovir more effective)
  - treatment of herpes zoster with corticosteroids DOES NOT decrease PHN
- surgical: spinal tractotomy, dorsal root entry zone lesion, DBS of thalamus

Painful Diabetic Neuropathy

- see Endocrinology, E13

Approach
- determine if pain is neuropathic or vascular
- more likely neuropathic if pain present at rest and improves with walking, pain is sharp/tingling, more in feet than calves

Treatment
- Level A: pregabalin
- Level B: venlafaxine, duloxetine, amitriptyline, gabapentin, valproate, rarely opioids, capsaicin

Complex Regional Pain Syndromes

Clinical Features
- presence of an initiating noxious event (MI, stroke)
- continuing pain, allodynia, or hyperalgesia with pain disproportionate to inciting event
- evidence during the course of symptoms of edema, changes in skin blood flow or abnormal vasomotor activity
- absence of conditions that would otherwise account for degree of pain and dysfunction
- other features can include edema, osteoporosis, hyperhidrosis, hair loss, fascial thickening

Classification
- CRPS type I (reflex sympathetic dystrophy): minor injuries of limb or lesions in remote body areas precede onset of symptoms
- CRPS type II (causalgia): injury of peripheral nerves precedes the onset of symptoms

Investigations
- trial of differential neural blockade may be helpful in diagnosis
- autonomic testing (evidence of sympathetic dysfunction)
- bone scan, plain radiography, MRI

Prevention
- early mobilization after injury/infarction

Treatment
- goal of treatment: to facilitate function
- conservative treatment: education, support groups, PT/OT, smoking cessation
- medical: topical capsaicin, TCA, NSAID, tender point injections with corticosteroid/lidocaine, gabapentin/pregabalin/lamotrigine, calcitonin or bisphosphonates, oral corticosteroids
- surgical: paravertebral sympathetic ganglion blockade
- refer to pain management clinic

Headache

- see <u>Emergency Medicine</u>, ER23 and <u>Family Medicine</u>, FM32

If CT is negative but clinically there is suspicion of SAH or meningitis, perform an LP

Clinical Approach
- history
    - pain characteristics: onset, frequency, duration, intensity, location, radiation, other specific features (e.g. worse in AM, worse with bending/cough/Valsalva)
    - associated symptoms: visual changes, change in mental status, nausea/vomiting, fever, meningismus, photophobia, phonophobia, TMJ popping/clicking, jaw claudication, neurological symptoms
    - precipitating/alleviating factors (triggering factors, analgesics), medications (especially nitrates, CCBs, NSAIDs, anticoagulants), PMH, FHx
    - red flags (possible indications for CT scan/further investigation): new-onset headache (especially if age <5 or >50), quality worse/different than previous headaches, sudden and severe ('thunderclap'), immunocompromised, fever, focal neurological deficits, trauma
- physical exam
    - vitals (including BP and temp), Kernig's/Brudzinski's, MSK examination of head and neck
    - HEENT: fundi (papilledema, retinal hemorrhages), red eye, temporal artery tenderness, sinus palpation, TMJ
    - full neurological exam (including LOC, orientation, pupils (symmetry), and focal neurological deficits)
    - **red flags**: papilledema, altered LOC, fever, meningismus, focal neurological deficits, signs of head trauma

Headache DDx

ER VISIT
Eye (acute angle closure glaucoma, sinusitis)
Recurrent/Chronic (migraine, tension, cluster, TMJ disease, cervical OA)
Vascular (SAH, ICH, temporal arteritis)
Infectious (meningitis, encephalitis)
Systemic (anemia, anoxia, CO, pre-eclampsia)
ICP (mass/abscess, HTN encephalopathy, pseudotumour cerebri)
Trauma (concussion, SDH, EDH)

Classification
- primary
    - tension, migraine, cluster, other autonomic cephalgias
- secondary
    - cervical OA, TMJ syndrome, SAH, ICH, stroke, venous sinus thrombosis, meningitis/encephalitis, trauma, increased ICP (space-occupying lesion, malignant HTN or pseudotumour cerebri), temporal arteritis, sinusitis, acute-angle closure glaucoma, pre-eclampsia, post LP, drugs/toxins (e.g. nitroglycerin use and analgesia withdrawal); all can be associated with serious morbidity or mortality

Acute and Preventive Pharmacologic Treatment of Cluster Headache
Neurology 2010;75:463-473
Study: Meta-analysis of prospective, double-blind, RCTs of pharmacologic agents for prevention or treatment of CH.
Results: 27 trials were included. Sumatriptan 6 mg SC, zolmitriptan nasal spray 5-10 mg, and 100% oxygen 6-12 L/min received Level A recommendation for acute treatment. For prevention, Level B recommendations were given for intranasal civamide 100 µg daily and suboccipital steroid injections.
Conclusion: Sumatriptan, zolmitriptan, and mid flow oxygen are effective acute treatments for CH.

Antiepileptics in Migraine Prophylaxis: An Updated Cochrane Review
Cephalalgia 2015; 35:51-62
Purpose: To review the evidence for anticonvulsants in migraine prophylactics.
Study: Systematic meta-analysis of 37 published and 3 unpublished prospective, controlled trials of regular use of anticonvulsants to prevent migraines and or improve quality of life related to migraines.
Results: Sodium valproate and topiramate were associated with a reduction of 4 and 1 days of headache per month, respectively, and patients taking either drug were more than two times as likely to experience greater than 50% reduction in headache frequency, versus placebo. Neither drug was associated with undue rates of adverse events, though higher doses of topiramate were associated with increased adverse events. There is insufficient evidence of efficacy other antiepileptic drugs, including gabapentin, for migraine prophylaxis.
Conclusions: Daily sodium valproate 400 mg and topiramate 50 mg are well tolerated and effective in prophylactic treatment of migraine headache in adults.

Table 21. Headaches – Selected Primary Types

	Tension-Type	Migraine	Cluster
Prevalence	70%	~10-20%	<1%
Age of Onset	15-40	10-30	20-40
Sex Bias	F>M	F>M	M>F
Family History	None	+++	+
Location	Bilateral frontal Nuchal-occipital	Unilateral > bilateral Fronto-temporal	Retro-orbital
Duration	Minutes – days	Hours – days	10 min-2 h
Onset/Course	Gradual; worse in PM	Gradual; worse in PM	Daily attacks for weeks to months; more common early AM or late PM
Quality	Band-like; constant	Throbbing	Constant, aching, stabbing
Severity	Mild-moderate	Moderate-severe	Severe (wakes from sleep)
Triggers/Provoking	Depression Anxiety Noise Hunger Sleep deprivation	Noise/light Caffeine/alcohol Hunger Stress Sleep deprivation	Light EtOH
Palliating	Rest	Rest	Walking around
Associated Sx	No vomiting No photophobia	Nausea/vomiting Photo/phonophobia Aura	Red watery eye Nasal congestion or rhinorrhea Unilateral Horner's
Management	Non-pharmacological Psychological counselling Physical modalities (e.g. heat, massage) Pharmacological Simple analgesics Tricyclic antidepressants	Acute Rx ASA NSAIDs Triptans Ergotamine Prophylaxis TCA Anticonvulsants Propranolol	Acute Rx O₂ Sumatriptan (nasal or injection) Prophylaxis Verapamil Lithium Methysergide Prednisolone

Table 22. Prophylactic Management of Migraine Headaches

Class	Drug	Evidence	Contraindications	Side Effects
Beta-blockers	Propranolol Timolol Metoprolol	A A B	Asthma, DM (mask hypoglycemia) CHF	Fatigue Depression Light-headedness
TCA	Amitriptyline Nortriptyline	A C	Heart disease, glaucoma *Avoid in elderly	Sedation Dry mouth Weight gain Light-headedness
CCBs	Flunarizine	A	Depression, obesity	Weight gain, depression, PD (rare)
	Verapamil	B	Heart disease	Weight gain (4.5-9 kg), constipation
AED	Valproate	A	Liver, renal, pancreatic disease	Weight gain, tremor, alopecia, teratogenic: neural tube defect
	Topiramate + folic acid supplement	A	Renal disease	Paresthesia, weight loss, cognitive: memory loss, difficulty concentrating, renal stone (rare)

Table 23. Headaches – Selected Serious but Rare Secondary Types

	Meningeal Irritation	Increased ICP	Temporal Arteritis
Age of Onset	Any age	Any age	>60 yr
Location	Generalized	Any location	Temporal
Onset/Course	Meningitis: hours-days		
SAH: thunderclap onset	Gradual; worse in AM	Variable	
Severity	Severe	Severe	Variable; can be severe
Provoking	Head movement	Lying down Valsalva Head low Exertion	Jaw claudication
Associated Sx	Neck stiffness Photophobia Focal deficits (e.g. CN palsies)	N/V Focal neuro symptoms Decreased level of consciousness	Polymyalgia rheumatica Visual loss
Physical Signs	Kernig's sign Brudzinski's sign Meningismus	Focal neuro symptoms Papilledema	Temporal artery changes: Firm, nodular, incompressible Tender
Management	CT/MRI with gadolinium LP, antibiotics for bacterial meningitis	CT/MRI and treatment to reduce pressure See Neurosurgery, NS4	Prednisone See Rheumatology, RH20
Etiology	Meningitis, SAH	Tumour, IIH, malignant HTN	Vasculitis (GCA)

IIH = idiopathic intracranial HTN

Migraine Headaches

Definition (Common Migraine)
- ≥5 attacks fulfilling each of the following criteria
    - 4-72 h duration
    - 2 of the following: unilateral, pulsating, moderate-severe (interferes with daily activity), aggravated by routine physical activity
    - 1 of the following: nausea/vomiting, photophobia/phonophobia/osmophobia

Epidemiology
- 18% females, 6% males; frequency decreases with age (especially at menopause)

Etiology and Pathophysiology
- theories of migraine etiology
    - depolarizing wave of "cortical spreading depression" across the cerebral cortex that may cause an aura (e.g. visual symptoms due to wave through occipital cortex) and also activate trigeminal nerve afferent fibres
    - possible association with vasoconstriction/dilation
- significant genetic contribution
- **triggers**: stress, sleep excess/deprivation, drugs (estrogen, nitroglycerin), hormonal changes, caffeine withdrawal, chocolate, tyramines (e.g. red wine), nitrites (e.g. processed meats)

The oral contraceptive pill is contraindicated with complicated migraine due to risk of stroke

Migraine auras can mimic other causes of transient neurological deficits (e.g. TIAs and seizures)

"Menstrual Migraine" Subtype
Migraine headache that is associated with the onset of menstruation – usually 2 d before to 3 d after the onset of menstrual bleeding

If patient presents to ED with severe migraine and N/V – consider treating with IV antiemetics (chlorpromazine, prochlorperazine)

Pharmacological Treatments for Acute Migraine
Pain 2002;97:247-257
Study: Meta-analysis of 54 double-blind, placebo-controlled RCTs of pharmacologic treatment of acute migraine of moderate to severe intensity (21,022 patients in total).
Data Extraction: Number of patients, dosing regimens, details of study design, and timing or type of rescue medication. Outcomes include headache relief at 1 and 2 h, freedom from pain at 2 h, sustained relief for 24 h, and adverse effects within 24 h.
Main Results: Data were available for 9 oral medications, 2 intranasal medications, and subcutaneous sumatriptan. For H/A relief at 2 h, all interventions were effective except Cafergot®, with NNTs ranging from 2.0 for sumatriptan 6 mg SC to 5.4 for naratriptan 2.5 mg. The lowest NNT for oral medication was 2.6 for eletriptan 80 mg. For patients pain free at 2 h, the lowest NNT was 2.1 for sumatriptan 6 mg SC, with the lowest NNT for oral medication being 3.1 for rizatriptan 10 mg. For sustained relief over 24 h NNT ranged from 2.8 for eletriptan 80 mg to 8.3 for rizatriptan 5 mg. Side effects could not be analyzed systematically. There were no drug-to-drug comparisons.
Conclusion: Overall, most treatments were effective. Subcutaneous sumatriptan and oral triptans were most effective.

Signs and Symptoms
- stages of uncomplicated migraine
  1. prodrome (hours to days before headache onset)
  2. aura
  3. headache
  4. postdrome
- aura
  - fully reversible symptom of focal cerebral dysfunction lasting <60 min
  - examples: visual disturbance (fortification spectra – zigzags; scintillating scotomata – spots), unilateral paresthesia and numbness or weakness, aphasia
- prodrome/postdrome: appetite change, autonomic symptoms, altered mood, psychomotor agitation/retardation
- classification of migraines
  - common migraine: no aura
  - classic migraine: with aura (headache follows reversible aura within 60 min)
  - complicated migraine: with severe/persistent sensorimotor deficits
    - examples: basilar-type migraine (occipital headache with diplopia, vertigo, ataxia, and altered level of consciousness), hemiplegic/hemisensory migraine, ophthalmoplegic migraine
  - acephalgic migraine (i.e. migraine equivalent): aura without headache

Treatment
- avoid triggers
- mild to moderate migraine
  - 1st line: NSAIDs (ibuprofen, naproxen)
- moderate to severe migraine
  - triptans (most effective), ergots (dihydroergotamine, DHE)
- migraine prophylaxis: anticonvulsants (divalproex, topiramate, gabapentin), TCA (amitriptyline, nortriptyline), propranolol, calcium channel blocker (verapamil)

Sleep Disorders

Overview of Sleep

Definition
- newborn: 18 h sleep (50% REM), adolescents: 10 h, adults: 7-9 h but most get insufficient amounts
- many elderly have reduced sleep as a consequence of underlying sleep disorders

Sleep Architecture
- **polysomnogram (PSG) measures:** EEG, eye movements (electro-oculogram – EOG), EMG, respiratory effort, oxygenation, ECG

Elements of Sleep History
- Initiation of sleep
- Events prior to bed
- Lights
- Latency (estimated)
- Restless legs
- Hallucinations
- Maintaining sleep
- Number of wakeups/night
- Sleep walking/talking
- Snoring/gasping
- Dreams/nightmares
- Consequences of sleep
- Restorative
- Morning headache
- Falling asleep in inappropriate setting

Table 24. Sleep Stage Characteristics

	EEG	EOG	Muscle Tone	Other Characteristics
Waking State	Alpha waves: high frequency (8-12 Hz), low voltage	Rapid, blinking	High	
Stage N1 (~5%)	Less than 50% Alpha waves (see above), mixed with slow wave activity	Slow, roving eye movements	High, but gradually dropping	Marker for very light quality sleep or sleep disruption
Stage N2 (~50%)	K complexes (high voltage negative and positive discharges) with sleep spindles (11-16 Hz)	Still	High	
Stage N3 (previously 3 and 4)/Slow Wave/Delta Sleep (~20%)	Delta waves: low frequency (<2 Hz), high voltage (>75 μV)	Still	Low	Homeostatic sleep Reduced BP, HR, cardiac output, RR Growth hormone release
Rapid Eye Movement (REM) Sleep (~25%)	Sawtooth waves, mixed frequency, low voltage	Rapid eye movements	Very low	Irregular respiration Arrhythmias, heart rate variation Classical dreaming state

Disturbances of Alertness and Sleep

Coma
- see Neurosurgery, NS33

Insomnia
- **definition/criteria**
  - difficulty initiating or maintaining sleep, or waking up earlier than desired (leading to sleep that is chronically non-restorative/poor quality) despite adequate opportunity and circumstances for sleep
- **types**
  - sleep state misperception, psychophysiologic insomnia (learned sleep-preventing associations – i.e. clock watching), fatal familial insomnia (rare prion protein mutation causing autonomic dysfunction), idiopathic (lifelong difficulty)
  - **secondary causes**
    - ◆ psychiatric disorders (80% of psychiatric patients): anxiety and depression (see Psychiatry, PS27)
    - ◆ neurologic disorders: neurodegenerative disease, epilepsy, neuromuscular disorders, many others
    - ◆ sleep disorders: restless legs syndrome (sleep initiation difficulties), sleep apnea (sleep maintenance difficulties)
    - ◆ medical conditions: pregnancy, cardiorespiratory (COPD/HF), GERD, pain (arthritis, fibromyalgia, cancer)
    - ◆ drugs/toxins: caffeine, alcohol, stimulants, antidepressants, glucocorticoids, sedative withdrawal
- **treatment**
  - sleep log, sleep hygiene, stimulus control, sleep restriction, relaxation response, CBT

> **Drug Effects on Wakefulness and Sleep**
> - Antihistamines associated with increased sleepiness
> - Stimulants increase arousal
> - Caffeine (an adenosine antagonist) increases wakefulness
> - Benzodiazepines reduce slow wave sleep
> - Antidepressants (TCA/MAOI/SSRI) reduce REM, prolong REM latency
> - Alcohol may hasten sleep onset but associated with increased arousals

Sleep Apnea
- **definition**
  - disorder of breathing in sleep associated with sleep disruption and consequent excessive somnolence (or drowsiness)
- **epidemiology**
  - >2-4% of the population
  - correlated with obesity
  - significant morbidity: HTN, stroke, heart failure, sleepiness, mortality (accidents)
- **types**
  - obstructive sleep apnea
  - central sleep apnea: no effort to breath over 10 s
  - mixed apnea: starts as central, but eventually becomes obstructive
- **etiology of central apnea**: heart failure, opiates, brainstem pathology, myotonic dystrophy
- **etiology of obstructive apnea**: collapse of airway due to low muscle tone in deep and REM sleep
- **diagnosis**: apnea hypopnea index (AHI) or respiratory disturbance index (RDI) should be <5 in the normal state
- **treatment**: conservative measures, dental devices, CPAP (common), surgery (rare), ensure driving safety

> Avoid sleep medications (especially in elderly patients) due to increased risk of falls, pseudodepression, and memory loss

Restless Leg Syndrome (RLS) and Periodic Limb Movement in Sleep (PLMS)
- **definition**
  - urge to move accompanied by uncomfortable sensations that begin or worsen with rest, are partially or totally relieved with movement, and are worse in evening/night; these features cannot be accounted for by another medical/behavioural condition
  - RLS refers to sensation
  - PLMS refers to the manifestation
- **epidemiology**: 10% North Americans, 90% of RLS have PLMS, 50% of patients with PLMS have RLS
- **etiology**: central (spasticity), peripheral nervous system (radiculopathy, neuropathy), pregnancy, iron deficiency, alcohol use
- **treatment**
  - underlying contributors (iron and B12 supplementation), dopaminergic agonists (first line), clonazepam (causes tachyphylaxis), opioids (only exceptional circumstances)
  - NOT recommended: levodopa/carbidopa (Sinemet®), causes augmentation

Narcolepsy
- **definition/clinical features**: excessive daytime sleepiness (all narcolepsy), cataplexy = loss of muscle tone with emotional stimuli (pathognomonic), sleep paralysis (unable to move upon wakening), hypnagogic hallucinations (vivid dreams or hallucinations at sleep onset)
- **epidemiology**: prevalence 1:2,000, onset in adolescence/early adulthood; life-long disorder
- **etiology**: presumed autoimmune attack on orexin/hypocretin system, post head injury, MS, hypothalamic tumours; rarely familial
- **diagnosis**: based on clinical history + multiple sleep latency test findings of short sleep latency <8 min and REM within 15 min of sleep onset on 2/4 naps
- **treatment**
  - sleep hygiene and scheduled brief naps, restricted driving
  - alerting agents: modafinil (non-amphetamine stimulant), stimulant (i.e. methylphenidate)
  - anticataplectic: TCAs, SSRIs, sodium oxybate

Parasomnias
- **definition/clinical features**: unusual behaviours in sleep with clinical features appropriate to stage of sleep
- **etiology**: in elderly, REM sleep behaviour disorder may be associated with PD; in children, slow wave sleep arousals (sleep walking) may be associated with sleep disordered breathing
- **diagnosis**: clinical history in children, polysomnography in adults to exclude nocturnal seizures
- **treatment**: behavioural management (safety, adequate sleep); clonazepam for REM sleep behaviour, tonsillectomy if appropriate in children

Circadian Rhythm
- **definition/clinical features**: abnormalities based on time of day rather than sleep (i.e. jet lag, shift work)
- **diagnosis**: clinical history

CNS Infections

- see Infectious Diseases, ID18

Spinal Cord Syndromes

- see Neurosurgery, NS27

Stroke

Terminology

Hypertension Encephalopathy
Acute severe HTN (typically dBP >130 or sBP >200) can cause hypertensive encephalopathy – abnormal fundoscopic exam (papilledema, hemorrhages, exudates, cotton-wool spots), focal neurologic symptoms, N/V, visual disturbances, and change in LOC

- **stroke**: sudden onset of neurological deficits of a vascular basis with infarction of CNS tissue
  - infarction is permanent tissue injury (confirmed by neuroimaging)
- **TIA**: sudden onset of neurological deficits of a vascular basis without infarction (i.e. no imaging evidence of stroke)
  - may present with amaurosis fugax (transient monocular painless vision loss)

Pathophysiology

Consider transfer of acute stroke patient to a designated stroke centre for neuroprotective or thrombolytic therapy if the patient is seen in first few hours

- two major types: ischemic (~80%) and hemorrhagic (~20%)

1. Ischemic
- arterial thrombosis: thrombus formation in artery (local/in situ)
  - large vessel: stenosis or occlusion of the internal carotid artery, vertebral, or intracranial arteries
    - mechanism: insufficient blood flow beyond lesion (hemodynamic stroke)
    - underlying processes: atherosclerosis (most common cause), dissection, and vasculitis
  - small vessel/lacunar
    - mechanism: chronic HTN and DM cause vessel wall thickening and decreased luminal diameter
    - affects mainly small penetrating arteries (primarily basal ganglia, internal capsule, and thalamus)

Early seizure activity occurs in 5-25% of patients after ICH

- cardioembolic: blockage of cerebral arterial blood flow due to particles originating from a cardiac source
  - atrial fibrillation (most common), rheumatic valve disease, prosthetic heart valves, recent MI, fibrous and infectious endocarditis
- systemic hypoperfusion (global cerebral ischemia)
  - inadequate blood flow to brain, usually secondary to cardiac pump failure (e.g. cardiac arrest, arrhythmia, or MI)
  - primarily affects watershed areas (between the major cerebral arterial territories)

Cerebral venous sinus thrombosis should be considered in the differential diagnosis of stroke and headache. It is an uncommon cause of either, but is associated with high morbidity and mortality. Patients often present with headache alone, but can also have seizures, focal neurological deficits, or cranial nerve palsies. This is diagnosed with MRV or CTV. Treatment is typically anticoagulation with heparin initially, then transition to warfarin

2. Hemorrhagic
- intracerebral hemorrhage
  - mechanisms
    - hypertensive (most common): rupture of small microaneurysms (Charcot-Bouchard aneurysms) causing intraparenchymal hemorrhage; most common sites: putamen, thalamus, cerebellum, and pons
    - other: trauma, amyloid angiopathy (associated with lobar hemorrhage), vascular malformations, vasculitis, drug use (cocaine or amphetamines)
  - subarachnoid hemorrhage see Neurosurgery, NS17

20-40% of patients with ischemic stroke may develop hemorrhagic transformation within 1 wk after the initial infarction

Blood work should only delay treatment if: patient is on anticoagulants, low platelet count suspected, abnormal electrolytes suspected, or any bleeding abnormality suspected

Stroke Syndromes According to Vascular Territory

- **ACA**: contralateral leg paresis, sensory loss, cognitive deficits (e.g. apathy, confusion, and poor judgment)
- **MCA**: proximal occlusion involves:
  1. contralateral weakness and sensory loss of face and arm
  2. cortical sensory loss
  3. may have contralateral homonymous hemianopia or quadrantanopia
  4. if dominant (usually left) hemisphere: aphasia
  5. if non-dominant (usually right) hemisphere: neglect
  6. eye deviation towards the side of the lesion and away from the weak side
- **PCA**
  1. contralateral hemianopia or quadrantanopia
  2. midbrain findings: CN III and IV palsy/pupillary changes, hemiparesis
  3. thalamic findings: sensory loss, amnesia, decreased level of consciousness
  4. if bilateral: cortical blindness or prosopagnosia
  5. hemiballismus
- **basilar artery**
  - proximal (usually thrombosis): impaired EOM, vertical nystagmus, reactive miosis, hemi- or quadriplegia, dysarthria, locked-in syndrome, coma
  - distal (usually embolic, i.e. top of the basilar sydrome): somnolence, memory and behaviour abnormalities, oculomotor deficit
- **PICA (lateral medullary or Wallenberg syndrome):** ipsilateral ataxia, ipsilateral Horner's, ipsilateral facial sensory loss, contralateral limb impairment of pain and temperature sensation, nystagmus, vertigo, nausea/vomiting, dysphagia, dysarthria, hiccups
- **medial medullary infarct** (anterior spinal artery, which can be associated with anterior cord infarct): contralateral hemiparesis (facial sparing), contralateral impaired proprioception and vibration sensation, ipsilateral tongue weakness
- **lacunar infarcts** (deep hemispheric white matter; involving deep penetrating arteries of MCA, circle of Willis, basilar, and vertebral arteries)
  - pure motor hemiparesis (posterior limb of internal capsule): contralateral arm, leg, and face
  - pure sensory loss (ventral thalamic): hemisensory loss
  - ataxic hemiparesis (ventral pons or internal capsule): ipsilateral ataxia and leg paresis
  - dysarthria-clumsy hand syndrome (ventral pons or genu of internal capsule): dysarthria, facial weakness, dysphagia, mild hand weakness and clumsiness

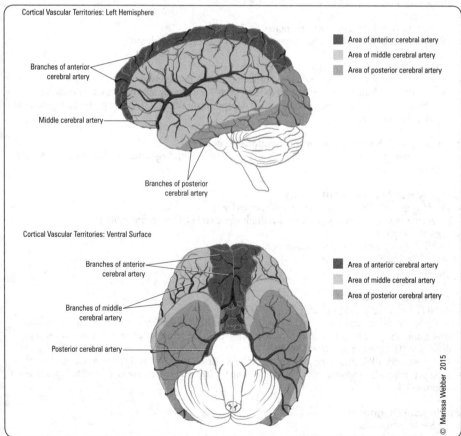

Figure 25. Vascular territories

Stroke mimics: drug intoxication, infections, migraines, metabolic, seizures, tumours.

Suspect an alternate diagnosis if: fever, decreased LOC, fluctuating symptoms, gradual onset, no focal neurological symptoms, and/or positive symptoms

Infarcted area of brain tissue can often appear normal on CT during the first several hours after the onset of stroke

Oral Direct Thrombin Inhibitors or Oral Factor Xa Inhibitors for the Treatment of Deep Vein Thrombosis
Cochrane DB Syst Rev 2015;6: CD010956
Purpose: To assess whether DTIs or factor Xa inhibitors are effective treatment for DVTs.
Study: Systematic review search 1950-2015, inclusive. Results included 11 RCTs, 27 945 patients, comparing DTIs or factor Xa inhibitors to standard treatment (heparin, wafarin, and similar).
Outcome: Recurrent DVT or PE.
Results: Separate meta-analyses of DTIs and factor Xa inhibitors showed that each was comparable to standard treatment in terms of DVT recurrence rates. Rates of fatal or non-fatal PE, and all-cause mortality were also not significantly different. Additionally, factor Xa inhibitors had lower rates of bleeding complications than standard treatment (OR 0.57; CI 0.43 to 0.76).
Conclusions: New oral treatment options, including direct thrombin inhibitors and factor Xa inhibitors represent reasonable and safe alternatives for acute.

The National Institute of Health Stroke Scale (NIHSS) is a standardized clinical examination that determines the severity of an acute stroke; it can also be used to monitor response to treatment over time
The scale uses 11 items that evaluate:
- Level of consciousness
- Visual system
- Motor system
- Sensory system
- Language abilities
Scoring (x/42):
0=no stroke
1-4=mild stroke
5-15=moderate stroke
15-20=moderate to severe stroke
21-42=severe stroke
rtPA is typically considered if score ≥6, but some stroke neurologists will administer rtPA with lower NIH stroke scale scores

Aspect Score: 10-point quantitative score to assess ischemic changes on CT scan
• 10/10 is normal and <4/10 signifies high risk of bleed with rtPA
• Subtract 1 point for each of following structures if abnormal within the ischemic hemisphere: caudate, lentiform, insula, internal capsule, MCA 1, 2, 3, 4, 5, 6 regions

If rtPA given at stroke onset, delay acute antiplatelet/anticoagulation treatment by 24 h

Absolute Contraindications to rtPA
Hx: improving sx, minor sx, seizure at stroke onset, recent major surgery (within 14 d) or trauma, recent GI or urinary hemorrhage (within 21 d), recent LP or arterial puncture at noncompressible site, PMHx ICH, sx of SAH/pericarditis/MI, pregnancy
P/E: sBP ≥185, dBP ≥110, aggressive treatment to decrease BP, uncontrolled serum glucose, thrombocytopenia
Ix: hemorrhage or mass on CT, high INR or aPTT

Factor Xa Inhibitors Versus Vitamin K Antagonists for Preventing Cerebral or Systemic Embolism in Patients with Atrial Fibrillation
Cochrane DB Syst Rev. 2014;8:CD008980
Purpose: To review the evidence comparing factor Xa inhibitors with vitamin K antagonists for prevention of embolic events in patients with atrial fibrillation.
Study: Systematic review search 1950-2013, inclusive. Results included 10 RCTs, 42 084 patients, follow up for 12 weeks to 1.9 years.
Outcome: Stroke (hemorrhagic or ischemic) and non-CNS embolic event
Results: Factor Xa inhibitor treatment resulted in significantly fewer embolic events than dose adjusted warfarin treatment (OR 0.81; CI 0.72 to 0.91). There was no significant difference in rate of major bleeds between factor Xa inhibitors and warfarin treatment. Furthermore, factor Xa inhibitors resulted in significantly fewer intracranial bleeds and lower all-cause mortality.
Conclusions: Use of factor Xa inhibitor for anti-coagulation in patients with atrial fibrillation offered better protection against embolic events than warfarin. Factor Xa inhibitors also had equal or lower rates of adverse events.

High-Dose Atorvastatin after Stroke or Transient Ischemic Attack (SPARCL Trial)
NEJM 2006;355:549-559
Method: Multicentre double-blind RCT.
Population: 4,731 patients with stroke or TIA within 1-6 mo before study entry, LDL 100-190 mg/dL, no coronary heart disease.
Intervention: 80 mg atorvastatin PO OD or placebo.
Outcome: First non-fatal or fatal stroke over 5 yr. Results: Patients receiving atorvastatin had a lower rate of stroke (ARI 2.2%, hazard ratio 0.84; p=0.03). There was a five yr absolute reduction in risk of 3.5% (p=0.002). There was no significant change in mortality rate, but a small significant increase in the risk of hemorrhagic stroke.
Conclusions: High-dose atorvastatin decreases overall incidence of strokes and cardiovascular events in patients with a history of recent stroke or TIA.

Evaluating for Occult Atrial Fibrillation – CRYSTAL AF Trial
NEJM 2014: 370:2478-2486.
Patients with a cryptogenic ischemic stroke or TIA and no evidence of atrial fibrillation on ECG and Holter monitoring may benefit from ambulatory cardiac monitoring with subcutaneous implantable loop recorder or external loop recorder for several weeks.

Assessment and Treatment of Ischemic Stroke

General Assessment
• ABCs, full vital sign monitoring, capillary glucose (Accu-Chek®), urgent CODE STROKE if <4.5 h from symptom onset (for possible thrombolysis)
• level of consciousness (knows age, month, obeys commands), dysarthria, dysnomia (cannot name objects)
• gaze preference, visual fields, facial palsy
• arm drift, leg weakness, ataxia
• sensation to pinprick, extinction/neglect
• history
  ▪ onset: time when last known to be awake and symptom free
  ▪ mimics to rule out: seizure/post-ictal, hypoglycemia, migraine, conversion disorder
• investigations
  ▪ non-contrast CT head (STAT): to rule out hemorrhage and assess extent of infarct
  ▪ ECG: to rule out atrial fibrillation (cardioembolic cause)
  ▪ carotid dopplers, echocardiogram
  ▪ CBC, electrolytes, creatinine, PTT/INR, blood glucose, lipid profile
• imaging (i.e. CT ± MR or CT angiography) signs of stroke
  ▪ loss of cortical white-grey differentiation
  ▪ sulcal effacement (i.e. mass effect decreases visualization of sulci)
  ▪ hypodensity of parenchyma
  ▪ insular ribbon sign
  ▪ hyperdense MCA sign

ACUTE STROKE MANAGEMENT

1. Thrombolysis
• rtPA (recombinant tissue plasminogen activator)
• given **within 4.5 h** of acute ischemic stroke onset provided there are clinical indications and no contraindications to use
• indications and contraindications (see sidebar)

2. Anti-Platelet Therapy
• give at presentation of TIA or stroke if rtPA not received
• antiplatelet agents
  ▪ ASA: recommended dose 81 mg chewed
  ▪ if patient intolerant to ASA, use other antiplatelet agent (i.e. clopidogrel)

3. Acute Anti-Coagulant Therapy
• for patients with TIA or stroke and atrial fibrillation, if rtPA not received:
  ▪ recommend IV heparin (or ensuring INR between 2-3 if already anticoagulated on warfarin)
  ▪ may delay initiation of oral anticoagulation depending on size of infarct and presence of petechial/frank hemorrhage

4. Intra-arterial Thrombectomy by Interventional Radiology
• early thrombectomy improves outcomes in ischemic stroke with large artery occlusions of the proximal anterior circulation

Other Acute Management Issues
• avoid hyperglycemia which can increase the infarct size
• lower temperature if febrile (febrile stroke: think septic emboli from endocarditis)
• prevent complications
  ▪ NPO if dysphagia (to be reassessed by SLP)
  ▪ DVT prophylaxis if bed-bound
  ▪ initiate rehabilitation early

Blood Pressure Control
• do **NOT** lower the blood pressure unless the HTN is severe
• antihypertensive therapy is withheld for 48-72 hr (permissive hypertension) after thromboembolic stroke unless sBP >220 mmHg or dBP >120 mmHg, or in the setting of acute MI, renal failure, aortic dissection (IV labetalol first-line if needed)
• acutely elevated BP is necessary to maintain brain perfusion to the ischemic penumbra
• most patients with an acute cerebral infarct are initially hypertensive and their BP will fall spontaneously within 1-2 d

Etiological Diagnosis
• further investigations
  ▪ additional neuroimaging (MRI)
  ▪ vascular imaging: CTA/MRA/carotid dopplers
  ▪ cardiac tests: echocardiogram, Holter monitoring
  ▪ correct etiological diagnosis is critical for appropriate secondary prevention strategies

Primary and Secondary Prevention of Ischemic Stroke

Anti-Platelet Therapy
- primary prevention
  - no firm evidence for a protective role for antiplatelet agents for low-risk patients without a prior stroke/TIA
- secondary prevention
  - initial choice: ASA
  - if cerebrovascular symptoms while on ASA or if unable to tolerate ASA: Aggrenox® (ESPRIT trial), clopidogrel (CAPRIE trial)

Carotid Stenosis
- primary prevention (asymptomatic)
  - carotid endarterectomy is controversial: if stenosis >60%, risk of stroke is 2% per yr; carotid endarterectomy reduces the risk of stroke by 1% per yr (but 5% risk of complications)
- secondary prevention (previous stroke/TIA in carotid territory)
  - carotid endarterectomy clearly benefits those with symptomatic severe stenosis (70-99%), and is less beneficial for those with symptomatic moderate stenosis (50-69%) (NASCET trial), see Vascular Surgery, VS7
- according to the CREST trial, endarterectomy and carotid stenting have similar benefits in a composite endpoint of reduction of stroke, MI, and death; however, in the periprocedural period, stenting results in a higher rate of stroke, while endarterectomy results in a higher rate of MI

Atrial Fibrillation
- primary and secondary prevention with anticoagulation
  - classical risk stratification used CHADS2 score (0-6), but Stroke 2014 guidelines recommend that virtually all patients with atrial fibrillation without contraindication be anticoagulated
    - 0 (low risk, 1.9% annual stroke risk): antiplatelet
    - 1 (intermediate risk, 2.8% annual stroke risk): anticoagulant or antiplatelet – patient specific decision
    - >2 (high risk, 4-18.2% annual stroke risk): anticoagulant
  - anticoagulation therapy
    - warfarin (titrate to INR 2-3)
    - dabigatran (110 or 150 mg PO bid), apixaban (2.5 or 5 mg PO bid) or rivaroxaban (15 or 20 mg PO daily) may be alternatives to warfarin, but should be used cautiously; Praxbind reversal agent for dagibatran if necessary

Hypertension
- primary prevention
  - targets: BP <140/90 (or <130/80 for diabetics or renal disease); high risk but without diabetes, target sBP < 120 (SPRINT trial)
  - ACEI: ramipril 10 mg PO OD is effective in patients at high risk for cardiovascular disease (HOPE trial)
- secondary prevention
  - ACEI and thiazide diuretics are recommended in patients with previous stroke/TIA (PROGRESS trial)

Hypercholesterolemia
- primary prevention
  - statins in patients with CAD or at high risk for cardiovascular events, even with normal cholesterol (CARE trial)
- secondary prevention
  - statins – high dose atorvastatin (SPARCL trial) but lower doses may be more appropriate if patient cannot tolerate high dose

Diabetes
- ideal management: HbA1c <7%, fasting blood glucose between 4 and 7

Smoking
- primary prevention: smoking increases risk of stroke in a dose-dependent manner
- secondary prevention: after smoking cessation, the risk of stroke decreases to baseline within 2-5 yr

Physical Activity
- beneficial effect of regular physical activity has a dose-related response in terms of intensity and duration of activity

Stroke Rehabilitation
- individualized based on severity and nature of impairment; may require inpatient program and continuation through home care or outpatient services
- multidisciplinary approach includes dysphagia assessment and dietary modifications, communication rehabilitation, cognitive and psychological assessments including screen for depression, therapeutic exercise programs, assessment of ambulation and evaluation of need for assistive devices, splints or braces, vocational rehabilitation

CHADS²
Stroke risk stratification for patients with atrial fibrillation
CHF (1 point)
HTN sBP >160 mmHg/treated HTN (1 point)
Age >75 yr (1 point)
DM (1 point)
Prior Stroke or TIA (2 points)

Carotid endarterectomy needs to be done within 2 wk of the ischemic event for the most benefit

ABCD² Score
To predict/identify individuals at high risk of stroke following TIA
Age: 1 point for age >60 yr
Blood pressure (at presentation):
1 point for HTN
(>140/90 mmHg at initial evaluation)
Clinical features: 2 points for unilateral weakness, 1 point for speech disturbance without weakness
Duration of symptoms: 1 point for 10-59 min, 2 points for >60 min
DM: 1 point
Stroke risk: 0-3: low risk, 4-5: moderate risk, 6-7: high risk

Long-Term Results of Stenting vs. Endarterectomy for Carotid-Artery Stenosis
NEJM 2016; 374:1021-1031
Study: Patients were randomly assigned to stenting or endarterectomy and assessed every 6 months for up to 10 years.
Population: 2502 patients at 117 centres with carotid-artery stenosis.
Outcome: Primary composite outcome was stroke, myocardial infarction, or death during periprocedural period or subsequent ipsilateral stroke.
Results: There was no significant difference in outcomes of either primary composite endpoint (HR 1.10; 95% CI 0.83-1.44) or post-procedural stroke (HR 0.99; 95%CI 0.64-1.52) in patients treated with stenting or endarterectomy. Asymptomatic and symptomatic patients showed no significant between-group differences in either endpoint.
Conclusions: The rate of periprocedural stroke, myocardial infarction, death, and subsequent ipsilateral stroke did not differ between carotid-artery stenosis patients treated with stenting or endarterectomy at 10 years of follow-up.

Endovascular Treatment vs. Medical Care Alone for Ischaemic Stroke: Systematic Review and Meta-Analysis
BMJ 2016;353:i1754
Purpose: To evaluate the evidence for endovascular intervention in the treatment of ischaemic stroke.
Study: Systematic review and meta-analysis of 10 randomized-controlled trials of 2925 patients testing the efficacy and safety of adjunctive endovascular intervention in patients suffering acute, ischaemic stroke in the anterior circulation versus medical therapy, including thrombolysis, alone.
Results: The 7 RCTs published or presented in 2015 were without significant heterogeneity and formed the basis for the analysis. The majority of patients (86%) received stent retrievers and experienced higher than expected rates of recanalization (>58%). Risk ratio for good functional outcomes was 1.56 (95%CI 1.38-1.75) and 0.86 for mortality (95% CI 0.69-1.06). There was no difference in symptomatic intracranial hemorrhage following therapy.
Conclusions: Endovascular therapy is safe and improves functional outcomes when added to medical care with thrombolysis when administered within 6-8 hours of large vessel, anterior circulation ischaemic stroke. A trend towards improved mortality exists with complete follow-up results of several key trials pending.

ACE Inhibitor in Stroke Prevention – HOPE Trial
NEJM 2000;342:145-153
Study: Randomized, blinded, placebo-controlled trial. Mean follow-up 5 yr.
Patients: 9,297 patients ≥55 yr (mean age 66 yr, 73% men) who had evidence of vascular disease or DM plus one other cardiovascular risk factor and who were not known to have a low ejection fraction or heart failure.
Intervention: Ramipril 10 mg daily orally vs. matching placebo.
Main Outcomes: Stroke, MI, or death from cardiovascular causes.
Results:

Outcome	RRR (95%CI)	NNT (CI)
Stroke	32% (16-44)	67 (43-145)
MI, stroke, or CV mortality	22% (14-30)	26 (19-43)
All-cause mortality	16% (5-25)	56 (32-195)

Treatment with ramipril reduced the risk of stroke (3.4% vs. 4.9%; RR 0.68; p<0.001).
Conclusions: In adults at high risk for cardiovascular events, ramipril reduced the risk of stroke, as well as other vascular events and overall mortality. In addition, ACEI reduce risk of stroke beyond their hypertensive effect.

Cerebral Hemorrhage

- **definition**: intracranial bleeding into brain tissue
- **etiology**: head trauma, hemorrhagic stroke

Investigations
- general investigations: see *Assessment and Treatment of Ischemic Stroke*, N50
- further investigations
  - LP (if suspect subarachnoid hemorrhage despite negative CT)
  - may require cerebral angiogram if suspect aneurysm or AVM
  - if typical location for hypertensive hemorrhage, repeat CT head in 4-6 wk after hemorrhage has resolved to rule out an underlying lesion

Treatment
- medical
  - anti-hypertensives: no conclusive BP target ranges for managing ICH exist; 2010 AHA/ASA guidelines suggest that reducing sBP to as low as 140 mmHg with IV anti-hypertensives is safe and appropriate management (target sBP 140-160 systolic)
  - ICP lowering medical management (if necessary): see <u>Neurosurgery</u>, NS4
- surgical: see <u>Neurosurgery</u>, NS20

Neurocutaneous Syndromes

- see <u>Pediatrics</u>, P84

Multiple Sclerosis

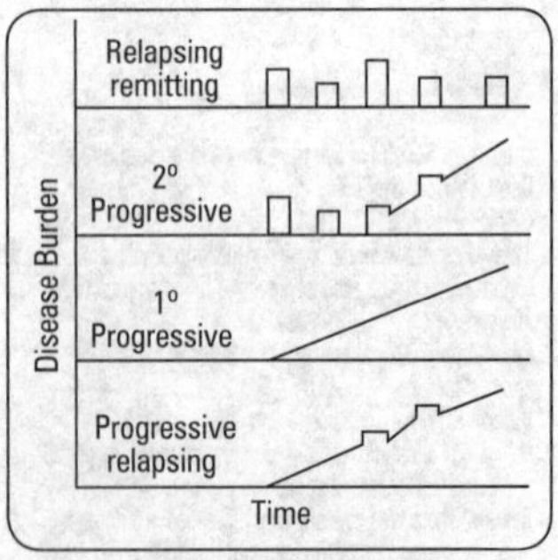

Definition
- a chronic inflammatory disease of the CNS characterized by relapsing remitting, or progressive neurologic symptoms due to inflammation, demyelination, and axonal degeneration

Clinical Patterns of MS
- relapsing remitting (RRMS) 85%, primary progressive (PPMS) 10%, progressive relapsing (PRMS) 5%, secondary progressive (SPMS)
- benign MS (BMS): retrospective diagnosis made after 15 years of mild disease, with no evidence of worsening (in functional ability and MRI)
- most RRMS goes on to become SPMS

MS Variants
- **Devic's = neuromyelitis optica (NMO):** severe optic neuritis and extensive transverse myelitis extending >3 vertebral segments (NMO antibody positive)
- **clinically isolated syndrome (CIS):** single MS-like episode, which may progress to MS
- **tumefactive MS:** solitary lesion >2 cm mimicking neoplasms on MRI
- **fulminant MS (Marburg):** rapidly progressive and fatal MS associated with severe axonal damage, inflammation, and necrosis
- **pediatric MS:** onset of MS before the age of 18
  - epidemiology: rare (1.35-2.5 per 100,000 children)
  - presentation: more likely to present with isolated optic neuritis, isolated brainstem syndrome or symptoms of encephalopathy compared to adults
  - course: 98% have RRMS
  - diagnosis and treatment similar to adult MS
  - differential diagnosis: in the setting of nonspecific CSF abnormalities and MRI evidence of white matter lesion, rule out ADEM, optic neuritis, transverse myelitis, neuromyelitis optica, CNS malignancies, leukodystrophies, and mitochondrial disease
- **acute disseminated encephalomyelitis (ADEM):** monophasic demyelinating disorder with multifocal neurologic symptoms seen mainly in children often following infection or vaccination

Etiology
- **genetic**
  - polygenetic: the HLA-DRB1 gene has been demonstrated to be a genetically susceptible area
  - 30% concordance for monozygotic twins, 2-4% risk in offspring of affected mother or father
- **environmental**
  - MS is more common in regions with less sun exposure and lower stores of vitamin D (Europe, Canada, US, New Zealand, SE Australia)
  - MS has also been linked to certain viruses (EBV is associated with MS)

Figure 26. Clinical patterns of MS

Most symptoms in MS are due to cord, brainstem, and optic nerve lesions

Chronic Cerebrospinal Venous Insufficiency (CCSVI)
A theory proposed in 2008 describing abnormal venous blood flow in patients with MS; while some RCTs are still underway, recent studies have largely discredited this highly controversial theory. That is, studies indicate no connection between CCSVI and MS

The Expanded Disability Status Scale (EDSS) is used as a measure of disability progression and is scored from 0 to 10 based on the neurologic exam and ambulation

Epidemiology
- onset 17-35 yr; F:M = 3:1
- PPMS occurs in an older population with F=M

Diagnosis for RRMS
- demonstration of both dissemination in time and space based on the revised McDonald criteria (2010)
  - dissemination in time: 2 or more attacks, simultaneous presence of asymptomatic gadolinium enhancing and non-enhancing MRI lesions at any time, or a new T2 and/or gadolinium-enhancing lesion(s) on follow-up MRI
  - dissemination in space: ≥1 T2 lesions on MRI in at least 2 of the 4 CNS regions (periventricular, juxtacortical, infratentorial, or spinal cord) or developing a second attack that implicates a different CNS region

Clinical Features
- symptoms include numbness, visual disturbance (optic neuritis), weakness, spasticity, diplopia (e.g. INO), impaired gait, vertigo, bladder dysfunction
- **Lhermitte's sign:** flexion of neck causes electric shock sensation down back into limbs indicating cervical cord lesion
- **Uhthoff's phenomenon:** worsening of symptoms (classically optic neuritis) in heat
- SPMS: classically weakness of legs in pyramidal distribution paired with cerebellar findings of arms (i.e. intention tremor)
- symptoms not commonly found in MS: visual field defects, aphasia, apraxia, progressive hemiparesis
- relapse: acute/subacute onset of clinical dysfunction that peaks from days to weeks, followed by remission with variable symptom resolution (symptoms must last at least 24 h)
- in RRMS, average 0.4 to 0.6 relapses/yr, but higher disease activity in 1st yr of disease

Investigations
- **MRI:** demyelinating plaques appear as hyperintense lesions on T2 weighted MRI, with active lesions showing enhancement with gadolinium
  - typical locations: periventricular, corpus callosum, cerebellar peduncles, brainstem, juxtacortical region, and dorsolateral spinal cord
  - Dawson's fingers: periventricular lesions extending into corpus callosum
  - cranial MRI is more sensitive than spinal MRI
- **CSF:** oligoclonal bands in 90%, increased IgG concentration
- **evoked potentials (visual/auditory/somatosensory):** delayed but well-preserved wave forms

Treatment
- **acute treatment:** methylprednisolone 1,000 mg IV daily x 3-7 d (no taper required); if poor response to corticosteroids may consider plasma exchange
- **disease modifying therapy (DMT)**
  - goals: decrease relapse rate, decrease progression of disability, slow accumulation of MRI lesions
  - first line: teriflunomide, interferon-β (injection: Betaseron®, Avonex®, Rebif®), glatiramer acetate (injection: Copaxone®), BG-12 (Tecfidera®)
  - second line: natalizumab (Tysabri®) (monthly IV infusion), fingolimod (Gilenya®)
    - ◆ increased risk of progressive multifocal leukoencephalopathy (PML)
  - CIS: early treatment with interferons may delay potential second attack
  - RRMS: DMT reduces rate of relapse by about 30%
  - PPMS/SPMS: no proven efficacy of DMTs
- **symptomatic treatment**
  - spasticity: baclofen, tizanidine, dantrolene, benzodiazepine, botulinum toxin
  - bladder dysfunction: oxybutynin
  - pain: TCA, carbamazepine, gabapentin
  - fatigue: amantadine, modafinil, methylphenidate
  - depression: antidepressant, lithium
  - constipation: high fibre intake, stool softener, laxatives
  - sexual dysfunction: sildenafil (Viagra®), tadalafil (Cialis®), vardenafil (Levitra®, Staxyn®)
- **education and counselling:** MS Society, support groups, psychosocial issues

Prognosis
- good prognostic indicators: female, young, RRMS, presenting with optic neuritis, low burden of disease on initial MRI, low rate of relapse early in disease
- PPMS: poor prognosis, higher rates of disability, poor response to therapy

Fingolimod for Relapsing-Remitting Multiple Sclerosis
Cochrane DB Syst Rev 2016; 4:CD009371
Purpose: Systematic literature review of the evidence for fingolimod in treatment of relapsing-remitting multiple sclerosis.
Study: Meta-analysis of six randomized controlled trials (n=5152 patients) of the benefits and harms of fingolimod and other disease modifying drugs in treatment of relapsing-remitting multiple sclerosis.
Results: Compared to placebo and interferon beta-1a, fingolimod increases the probability of being relapse free at 24 months (RR 1.44 vs. placebo, RR 1.18 vs. interferon beta-1a) but has little to no effect on disability progression (RR 1.07 vs. placebo, RR 1.02 vs. interferon beta-1a). Fingolimod use was associated with a higher incidence of adverse events and discontinuation within 6 months.
Conclusions: Fingolimod significantly reduces disease activity in relapse-remitting multiple sclerosis compared to placebo but does not prevent disability. Its use is associated with adverse events and requires close patient monitoring, particularly within the first 6 months. Further study is needed to assess the benefits of fingolimod versus other disease modify drugs.

Recombinant Interferon Beta or Glatiramer Acetate for Delaying Conversion of the First Demyelinating Event to Multiple Sclerosis
Cochrane DB Syst Rev 2008; 2:CD005278
Study: Meta-analysis of RCTs of clinically isolated syndrome (CIS) patients treated with immunomodulatory drugs.
Primary Outcomes: Proportion of patients converting to clinically definite MS and adverse effects.
Results: Three trials (n=1,160) tested the efficacy of interferon (IFN-α) and no trial tested glatiramer acetate (GA). A pooled odds ratio (OR) of 0.53 (95% CI 0.40-0.71, p<0.0001) for patients on IFN vs. placebo at 1 yr. Two year follow-up odds ratio was 0.52 (95% CI 0.38-0.70, p<0.0001). There was no significant increase in adverse events for those on IFN-α.
Conclusions: IFN-α treatment can delay progression to clinically definite MS in patients with CIS over 2 yr.

Risk of Natalizumab-Associated Progressive Multifocal Leukoencephalopathy
NEJM 2012; 366:1870-1880
Purpose: To assess the risk of progressive multifocal leukoencephalopathy (PML) in multiple sclerosis patients treated with natalizumab.
Study: A retrospective analysis funded of clinical studies, a Swedish patient registry and post-marketing sources, funded by Biogen Idec and Elan Pharmaceuticals.
Population: 99, 571 patients with relapsing-remitting multiple sclerosis treated with natalizumab.
Results: 212 of 99, 571 natalizumab-treated patients developed PML (2.1 cases per 1000 patients). Of the 54 PML patients with pre-diagnosis samples, all were positive for anti-JC antibodies. The highest risk of PML was in patients positive for anti-JC antibodies, treated with immunosuppressants prior to natalizumab, and had received 25-48 months of natalizumab (11.1 cases per 1000 patients). Patients negative for anti-JC antibodies were at lowest risk of PML (0.09 cases per 1000 patients).
Conclusions: In multiple sclerosis patients treated with natalizumab, those with positive anti-JC antibodies, lengthy treatment with natalizumab, and prior use of immunosuppressants, together or independently, were at highest risk of developing PML.

Common Medications

Table 25. Common Medications – Major Issues

Indications	Mechanism of Action/ Class	Generic Name	Trade Name	Dosing	Contraindications	Side Effects
Parkinson's Disease	Dopamine precursor	levodopa + carbidopa	Sinemet®	Carbidopa 25 mg/ levodopa 100 mg PO tid Maximum 200 mg carbidopa and 2,000 mg levodopa per day	Narrow-angle glaucoma, use of MAO inhibitor in last 14 d, history of melanoma or undiagnosed skin lesions	Nausea, hypotension, hallucinations, dyskinesias in last 14 d, history of melanoma or undiagnosed skin lesions
	Dopamine agonist	bromocriptine	Parlodel®	1.25 mg PO bid, increase by 2.5 mg/d q2-4wk, up to 10-30 mg PO tid	Concomitant use of potent inhibitors of CYP3A4, uncontrolled HTN, ischemic heart disease, peripheral vascular disease; caution with renal or hepatic disease	Hypotension, N/V, dizziness, constipation, diarrhea, abdominal cramps, H/A, nasal congestion, drowsiness, hallucinations
	MAO B inhibitor	selegiline	Eldepryl®	5 mg PO bid	Concomitant use of meperidine or tricyclic antidepressants	H/A, insomnia, dizziness, nausea, dry mouth, hallucinations, confusion, orthostatic hypotension increased akinesia, risk of hypertensive crisis with tyramine-containing foods
Myasthenia Gravis	Acetylcholinesterase inhibitor	pyridostigmine	Mestinon®	600 mg/d PO divided in 5-6 doses Range 60-1,500 mg/d	GI or GU obstruction	Nausea, vomiting, diarrhea, abdominal cramps, increased peristalsis, increased salivation, increased bronchial secretions, miosis, diaphoresis, muscle cramps, fasciculations, muscle weakness
Acute Migraine	Triptan (selective 5-hydroxytryptamine receptor agonist)	sumatriptan	Imitrex®	25-100 mg PO prn, maximum 200 mg/d	Hemiplegic/basilar migraine, ischemic heart disease, CVD, uncontrolled HTN, use of ergotamine/5-HT1 agonist in past 24 h, use of MAO inhibitor in last 14 d, severe hepatic disease	Vertigo, chest pain, flushing, sensation of heat, hypertensive crisis, peripheral vascular disease, coronary artery vasospasm, cardiac arrest, nausea, vomiting, H/A, hyposalivation, fatigue
	Ergot (5-HT1D receptor agonist)	dihydroergotamine	Migranal®	Nasal spray 0.5 mg/ spray, maximum 4 sprays/d	Hemiplegic/basilar migraine, high-dose ASA therapy, uncontrolled HTN, ischemic heart disease, peripheral vascular disease, severe hepatic or renal dysfunction, use of triptans in last 24 h, use of MAO inhibitors in last 14 d	Coronary artery vasospasm, transient myocardial ischemia, myocardial infarction, ventricular tachycardia, ventricular fibrillation; may cause significant rebound H/A
Migraine Prophylaxis	Anticonvulsant	topiramate	Topamax®	25 mg OD PO (in evening); may increase weekly by 25 mg/d to a max 50 mg bid		Sedation, mood disturbance, cognitive dysfunction, anorexia, nausea, diarrhea, paresthesias, metabolic acidosis, glaucoma, SJS/TEN
	β-blocker	propranolol	Inderal®	80 mg/d divided every 6-8 h; increase by 20-40 mg/dose every 3-4 wk to max 160-240 mg/d in divided doses q6-8h	Uncompensated CHF, severe bradycardia or heart block, severe COPD or asthma	Fatigue, cognitive dysfunction, disturbed sleep, rashes, dyspepsia, dry eyes, heart failure, bronchospasm, risk of acute tachycardia and HTN if withdrawal
Epilepsy	Anticonvulsant for partial ± 2° generalization, generalized tonic-clonic	carbamazepine	Tegretol®	Start at 100-200 mg PO OD-tid, increase by 200 mg/d up to 800-1,200 mg/d	History of bone marrow depression, hepatic disease, hypersensitivity to the drug, use of MAO inhibitor in last 14 d	Drowsiness, H/A, unsteadiness, dizziness, N/V, skin rash, agranulocytosis/aplastic anemia (rare)
	Anticonvulsant for partial, tonic-clonic, status epilepticus	phenytoin	Dilantin®	100 mg PO tid, maintenance dose up to 200 mg PO tid SE: 10-15 mg/kg IV loading dose then maintenance doses of 100 mg PO or IV q6-8h	Hypersensitivity, pregnancy, breastfeeding; caution with P-450 interactions	Hypotension, SJS/TEN, SLE-type symptoms, gingival hypertrophy, peripheral neuropathy, H/A, blood dyscrasias, nystagmus, N/V, constipation, sedation, teratogenic
	Anticonvulsant for partial or generalized, absence seizures	valproic acid	Depakene® Apo-Valproic®	10-15 mg/kg/d PO in divided doses, increase incrementally until therapeutic dose to max of 60 mg/kg/d	Hypersensitivity, hepatic disease, urea cycle disorders	Hepatic failure, H/A, somnolence, alopecia, N/V, diarrhea, tremor, diplopia, thrombocytopenia, hypothermia, pancreatitis, encephalopathy
	Anticonvulsant for absence seizures	ethosuximide	Zarontin®	500 mg/d PO, increase by 250 mg every 4-7 d to max 1.5 g/d in divided doses	Hypersensitivity (succinimides)	CNS depression, blood dyscrasias, SLE, SJS, GI symptoms

Table 25. Common Medications – Major Issues (continued)

Indications	Mechanism of Action/ Class	Generic Name	Trade Name	Dosing	Contraindications	Side Effects
Stroke Prevention in AF	Anticoagulant (direct thrombin inhibitor)	dabigatran	Pradaxa®	110 mg PO bid or 150 mg PO bid	CrCl <30 mL/min, significant hemostatic impairment or CNS lesions within 6 mo with high risk of bleeding	Dyspepsia, gastritis, bleeding
	Anticoagulant (Factor Xa inhibitor)	rivaroxaban	Xarelto®	15 mg PO daily or 20 mg PO daily	Concomitant anticoagulant, hepatic disease, pregnancy, strong CYP3A4 and P-gp inhibitors e.g. itraconazole, ritonavir	Bleeding
	Anticoagulant (Factor Xa inhibitor)	apixaban	Eliquis®	2.5 mg PO bid or 5 mg PO bid	Active bleeding, gastrointestinal bleeding, recent cerebral infarction, active peptic ulcer disease with recent bleeding, hepatic disease with coagulopathy	Bleeding (conjunctival, gastrointestinal, gingival, contusion, hematoma, epistaxis, hematuria)
Mild to Moderate AD or DLB	Cholinesterase Inhibitor	donepezil	Aricept®	5 mg PO OD, may increase to 10 mg PO OD after 4-6 wk	Hypersensitivity to donepezil or to piperidine derivatives	Diarrhea, N/V, insomnia, muscle cramps, fatigue, anorexia, HTN, syncope, AV block
Multiple Sclerosis	MS Disease Modifying Therapy	interferon-β-1b interferon-β-1a SC interferon-β-1a IM	Betaseron® Rebif® Avonex®	0.25 mg (8 MU) SC every other day 44 μg SC 3 times/wk 30 μg IM once weekly	Pregnancy, hypersensitivity to natural or recombinant interferon-β	Injection site reactions, injection site necrosis, flu-like symptoms (fever, chills, myalgia; tend to decrease over time)
	MS Disease Modifying Therapy	glatiramer acetate	Copaxone®	20 mg SC OD	Hypersensitivity to glatiramer or mannitol	Injection site reactions, nausea, transient chest pain, vasodilation
	MS Disease Modifying Therapy	natalizumab	Tysabri®	300 mg IV given over 1 h, every 4 wk	Hypersensitivity to natalizumab, progressive multifocal leukoencephalopathy (PML)	Rash, nausea, arthralgia, H/A, infections, rare risk of PML and melanoma
	MS Disease Modifying Therapy	fingolimod	Gilenya®	0.5 mg PO OD	Not available	Diarrhea, transaminitis, H/A, bradyarrhythmia, lymphopenia
Spasticity (i.e. MS)	Muscle Relaxant – Antispastic	baclofen	Lioresal®	5 mg PO tid, increase by 15 mg/d q3d to max dose 80 mg/d in three divided doses	Hypersensitivity to baclofen	Transient drowsiness, daytime sedation, dizziness, weakness, fatigue, convulsions, constipation, nausea

Landmark Neurology Trials

Trial	Reference	Results
NASCET	*NEJM* 1991;7:445-53	Patients with symptomatic carotid stenosis of 70-99% benefited more from carotid endarterectomy than best medical therapy
Interferon-β Multiple Sclerosis Study Group Trial	*Neurology* 1993;43:655-61	Interferon-β-1b reduces relapse rate and severity of relapses in RRMS
NINDS rtPA	*NEJM* 1995;333:1581-7	rtPA reduces mortality and long-term disability when administered within 3 h of acute stroke
SPARCL	*NEJM* 2006;355:549-59	The observed benefit of statins in cardiovascular disease is also extended to patients with a recent stroke or TIA
ECASS 3	*NEJM* 2008;359:1317-29	rtPA improved clinical outcomes when administered within 3 to 4.5 h of acute ischemic stroke
PROFESS	*NEJM* 2008;359:1238-51	ASA + dipyridamole and clopidogrel showed similar benefits in secondary stroke prevention
RELY	*NEJM* 2009;361:1139	Dabigatran superior to warfarin for stroke prevention in patients with atrial fibrillation
ROCKET-AF	*NEJM* 2011;365:883-891	Rivaroxaban noninferior to warfarin stroke prevention in patients with atrial fibrillation
ERS	*NEJM* 2011;365:981-992	Apixaban superior to warfarin for stroke prevention in patients with atrial fibrillation
CREST	*NEJM* 2010;363:11-23	Carotid stenting and endarterectomy had similar benefits in reduction of stroke, MI, and death in carotid stenosis, but in the periprocedural period, stenting had a higher rate of stroke, while endarterectomy had a higher rate of MI
INTERACT2	*NEJM* 2013;368:2355-65	Intensive lowering of blood pressure (sBP<140) in spontaneous intracerebral hemorrhage did not improve mortality or severe disability but improved functional outcomes (odds ratio for greater disability, 0.87; 95% CI, 0.77 to 1.00; P=0.04)
MR CLEAN	*NEJM* 2015;372:11-20	Intra-arterial treatment (intra-arterial thrombolysis, mechanical treatment, or both) for emergency revascularization administered within 6 h after stroke onset was effective and safe for acute ischemic stroke caused by proximal intracranial occlusion of the anterior circulation

References

Coma
Bhidayasiri R, Waters MF, Giza CC. Neurological differential diagnosis: a prioritized approach. Massachusetts: Blackwell Publishing, 2005. 71-72.
Kasper DL, Braunwald E, Fauci AS, et al. (editors). Harrison's principles of internal medicine, 16th ed. Toronto: McGraw-Hill Companies, 2005. 1629-1630.

Common Presenting Complaints
Bhidayasiri R, Waters MF, Giza CC. Neurological differential diagnosis: a prioritized approach. Massachusetts: Blackwell Publishing, 2005. 12-13, 305-314.

Drug Information
Compendium of Pharmaceuticals and Specialties 2010. Ottawa: Canadian Pharmacists Association, 2010.
Lexi-Comp Online™. Hudson: Lexi-Comp, 2011.

Epilepsy
Ambati BK, Smith WT, Azer-Bentsianov MT. Residents' manual of medicine. Hamilton: BC Decker, 2001. 203-205.
Ferri FF. Practical guide to the care of the medical patient. St. Louis: Mosby, 2001. 617-619.
Lowenstein DH, Alldredge BK. Status epilepticus. NEJM 1998;338:970-976.

General
Aminoff MJ, Greenberg DA, Simon RP. Lange: clinical neurology, 6th ed. Toronto: McGraw-Hill, 2009.
Ettinger AB, Weisbrot DM. Neurologic Differential Diagnosis: a Case-Based Approach. Cambridge: Cambridge University Press, 2014.
Mumenthaler M, Mattle H. Fundamentals of neurology. Thieme: Stuttgart and New York, 2006.
Scherokman B, Selwa L, Alguire PC. Approach to common neurological symptoms in internal medicine: AAN core curricula. 2011.
Yamada KA, Awadalla S. The Washington manual of medical therapeutics, 31st ed. New York: Lippincott Williams & Wilkins. 531-534.

Headache
Mulleners WM, McCrory DC, and Linde M. Antiepileptics in migraine prophylaxis: An updated Cochrane review. Cephalagia 2015; 135: 51-62.
Detsky ME, McDonald DR, Baerlocher MO, et al. Does this patient with headache have a migraine or need neuroimaging? JAMA 2006;296:1274-1283.
Francis GJ, Becker WJ, Pringsheim TM. Acute and preventive pharmacologic treatment of cluster headache. Neurology 2010;75:463-473.
Headache Classification Subcommittee of the International Headache Society. The international classification of headache disorders, 2nd ed. Cephalalgia 2004;24(S1):9-160.
Oldman AD, Smith LA, McQuay HJ, et al. Pharmacological treatments for acute migraine: quantitative systematic review. Pain 2002;97:247-257.

Movement Disorders
Bayard M, Avonda T, Wadzinski J. Restless legs syndrome. Am Fam Physician 2008; 78:235-40.
Centers for Disease Control and Prevention (CDC). Diagnosis and management of foodborne illnesses: a primer for physicians and other health care professionals. MMWR Recomm Rep 2004;53(RR-4):1-33.
England JD, Gronseth G, Franklin G, et al. Practice Parameter: evaluation of distal symmetric polyneuropathy: role of laboratory and genetic testing (an evidence-based review). Neurology 2009;72:185-192.
Hughes AJ, Daniel SE, Kilford L, et al. Accuracy of clinical diagnosis of idiopathic Parkinson's disease: a clinico-pathological study of 100 cases. J Neurol Neurosurg Psychiatry 1992;55:181-184.
Stowe RL, Ives NJ, Clarke CE, et al. Dopamine agonist therapy in early Parkinson's disease. Cochrane DB Syst Rev 2008:CD006564.
Walkup JT, Ferrao Y, Leckman JF, et al. Tic disorders: some key issues for DSM-V. Depression and Anxiety 2010:600-610.
Postuma RB, Berg D, Stern M, et al. MDS clinical diagnostic criteria for Parkinson's disease. Mov Disord. 2015 Oct;30(12):1591-601.

Multiple Sclerosis
Ambati BK, Smith WT, Azer-Bentsianov MT. Residents' manual of medicine. Hamilton: BC Decker, 2001. 211-213.
Bloomgren G, Richman S, Hotermans C, et al. Risk of Natalizumab-Associated Progressive Multifocal Leukoencephalopathy. NEJM 2012; 366:1870-1880.
Carpenter CCJ, Griggs RC, Loscalzo J (editors). Cecil essentials of medicine, 5th ed. Philadelphia: WB Saunders, 2001. 973-976.
Clerico M, Faggiano F, Palace J, et al. Recombinant interferon beta or glatiramer acetate for delaying conversion of the first demyelinating event to multiple sclerosis. Cochrane DB Syst Rev 2009:CD005278.
Ferri FF. Practical guide to the care of the medical patient. St. Louis: Mosby, 2001. 654-656.
La Mantia L, Tramacere I, Firwana B, et al. Fingolimod for relapsing-remitting multiple sclerosis. Cochrane Database of Systematic Reviews 2016; CD009371.
Noseworthy JH, Lucchinetti C, Rodriguez M, et al. Multiple sclerosis. NEJM 2000;343:938-952.
Olek MJ (editor). Multiple sclerosis: etiology, diagnosis, and new treatment strategies. New Jersey: Humana Press, 2005. 36-40, 57, 131, 222-223.
Polman CH, Reingold SC, Edan G, et al. Diagnostic criteria for multiple sclerosis: 2005 revisions to the "McDonald Criteria". Ann Neurol 2005;58:840-846.
Samuels MA, Feske SK (editors). Office practice of neurology, 2nd ed. Philadelphia: Elsevier Science, 2003. 410-411.
The TRANSFORMS Study Group. Oral fingolimod or intramuscular interferon for relapsing MS. NEJM 2010;362:402-415.
Vosoughi R, Freedman MS. Therapy of MS. Clin Neurol Neurosurg 2010;112:365-385.

Neurocognitive Disorders (Dementia)
Feldman HH, Jacova C, Robillard A, et al. Diagnosis and treatment of dementia: diagnosis. CMAJ 2008;178:825-836.
Josephs KA, Ahlskog JE, Parisi JE, et al. Rapidly progressive neurodegenerative dementias. Arch Neurol 2009;66:201-207.
McKeith IG, Dickson DW, Lowe J, et al. Consortium on DLB. Diagnosis and management of dementia with Lewy bodies: third report of the DLB consortium. Neurology 2005;65:1863-1872.
Neary D, Snowden JS, Gustafson L, et al. Frontotemporal lobar degeneration: a consensus on clinical diagnostic criteria. Neurology 1998;51:1546-1554.
Patterson C, Feightner JW, Garcia A, et al. Diagnosis and treatment of dementia: risk assessment and primary prevention of Alzheimer disease. CMAJ 2008;178:548-556.
Rascovsky K, Hodges JR, Knopman D, et al. Sensitivity of revised diagnostic criteria for the behavioural variant of frontotemporal dementia. Brain 2011;134:2456-2477.
Rolinski M, Fox C, Maidment I, et al. Cholinesterase inhibitors for dementia with Lewy bodies, Parkinson's disease dementia and cognitive impairment In Parkinson's disease. Cochrane DB Syst Rev 2012:CD006504.
Vigen CL, Mack WJ, Keefe RS, et al. Cognitive effects of atypical antipsychotic medications in patients with Alzheimer's disease: outcomes from CATIE-AD. Am J Psychiatry 2011;168:831-839.
Zerr I, Pocchiari M, Collins S, et al. Analysis of EEG and CSF 14-3-3 proteins as aids to the diagnosis of Creutzfeldt-Jakob disease. Neurology 2000;55:811-815.
Zerr I, Kallenberg K, Summers DM, et al. Updated clinical diagnostic criteria for sporadic Creutzfeldt-Jakob disease. Brain 2009;132:2659-2668.

Pain
Chen N, Li Q, Zhang Y, et al. Vaccination for preventing postherpetic neuralgia. Cochrane DB Syst Rev 2011:CD007795.
Coen PG, Scott F, Leedham-Green M, et al. European Journal of Pain 2006;10:695-700.
Marcus D. Chronic pain - a primary guide to practical management. New Jersey: Humana Press, 2005. 111-128.
Salinas RA, Alvarez G, Daly F, et al. Corticosteroids for Bell's palsy (idiopathic facial paralysis). Cochrane DB Syst Rev 2010:CD001942.
Vargas-Schaffer G. Is the WHO analgesic ladder still valid? Twenty-four yr of experience. Can Fam Phys 2010;56:514-517.

Spinal Cord Syndrome
Wagner R, Jagoda A. Neurologic emergencies: spinal cord syndromes. Emerg Med Clinic N Am 1997;15:699-711.

Stroke
Adams HP Jr., Bendixen BH, Kappelle LJ, et al. Classification of subtype of acute ischemic stroke. Definitions for use in a multicenter clinical trial. Stroke 1993;24:35-41.
Bhatt DL, Fox KA, Hacke W, et al. Clopidogrel and Aspirin® versus Aspirin® alone for the prevention of atherothrombotic events. NEJM 2006;354:1706-1717.
Brott TG, Howard G, Roubin GS, et al. Long-Term Results of Stenting versus Endarterectomy for Carotid-Artery Stenosis. NEJM 2016; 374:1021-1031.
Bruins Slot KM, Berge E. Factor Xa inhibitors versus vitamin K antagonists for preventing cerebral or systemic embolism in patients with atrial fibrillation. Cochrane DB Syst Rev. 2014;8:CD008980.
CAPRIE Steering Committee. A randomized, blinded, trial of clopidogrel versus Aspirin® in patients at risk of ischaemic events (CAPRIE). Lancet 1996;348:1329-1339.
Connolly SJ, Ezekowitz MD, Yusuf S, et al. Dabigatran versus warfarin in patients with atrial fibrillation. NEJM 2009;361:1139-1151.

Diener HC, Bogousslavsky J, Brass LM, et al. Aspirin® and clopidogrel compared with clopidogrel alone after recent ischaemic stroke or transient ischaemic attack in high-risk patients (MATCH): randomized, double-blind, placebo-controlled trial Lancet 2004;364:331-337.
Frontera W, Silver J. Essentials of physical medicine and rehabilitation. Philadelphia: Hanley and Belfus, 2002. 778-782.
Gage BF, Waterman AD, Shannon W, et al. Validation of clinical classification schemes for predicting stroke: results from the National Registry of Atrial Fibrillation. JAMA 2001;285:2864-2870.
Johnston SC, Rothwell PM, Nguyen-Huynh MN, et al. Validation and refinement of scores to predict very early stroke risk after transient ischaemic attack. Lancet 2007;369:283-292.
Lindsay K, Bone I. Neurology and neurosurgery illustrated. Philadelphia: Churchill Livingstone, 2003. 244.
Mullins ME, Lev MH, Scheillingerhout D, et al. Intracranial hemorrhage complicating acute stroke: how common is hemorrhagic stroke on initial head CT scan and how often is initial clinical diagnosis of acute stroke eventually confirmed? Am J Neuroradiol 2005;26:2207-2212.
Stroke Unit Trialists' Collaboration. Organized inpatient (stroke unit) care for stroke. Cochrane DB Syst Rev 2009:CD000197.
Passero S, Rocchi R, Rossi S, et al. Seizures after spontaneous supratentorial intracerebral hemorrhage. Epilepsia 2002;43:1175-1180.
Pexman JH, Barber PA, Hill MD, et al. Use of the Alberta Stroke Program Early CT Score (ASPECTS) for assessing CT scans in patients with acute stroke. Am J Neuroradiol 2001;22:1534-1542.
Program early CT score (ASPECTS) for assessing CT scans in patients with acute strokes. AMJ Neuroradiol 2001;22:1534-1542.
Robertson L, Kesteven P, McCaslin JE. Oral direct thrombin inhibitors or oral factor Xa inhibitors for the treatment of deep vein thrombosis. Cochrane DB Syst Rev. 2015;6: CD010956.
Rodrigues FB, Neves JB, Caldeira D, et al. Endovascular treatment versus medical care alone for ischaemic stroke: systematic review and meta-analysis. BMJ 2016; 353:i1754.
The ESPRIT Study Group. Aspirin® plus dipyridamole versus Aspirin® alone after cerebral ischaemia of arterial origin (ESPRIT): randomized controlled trial. Lancet 2006;367:1665-1673.
The Heart Outcomes Prevention Evaluation Study Investigators. Effects of an ACEI, ramipril, on cardiovascular events in high-risk patients. NEJM 2000;342:145-153.
The National Institute of Neurological Disorders and Stroke rt-PA Stroke Study Group. Tissue plasminogen activator for acute ischemic stroke. NEJM 1995;333:1581-1588.
The National Institute of Neurological Disorders and Stroke rt-PA Stroke Study Group. Effects of tissue plasminogen activator for acute ischemic stroke at one year. NEJM 1999;340:1781-1787.

Traumatic Brain Injury
Anderson-Barnes VC, Weeks SR, Tsao JW. Mild traumatic brain injury update. Continuum 2010;16(6):17-23.

Notes

Alan Chalil, Laureen Hachem, and **Ryan Muir**, chapter editors
Dhruvin Hirpara and **Sneha Raju**, associate editors
Valerie Lemieux and **Simran Mundi**, EBM editors
Dr. Todd Mainprize and **Dr. Eric Massicotte**, staff editors

Acronyms

AVF	arteriovenous fistula	EEG	electroencephalography	LOC	loss of consciousness	SAH	subarachnoid hemorrhage
AVM	arteriovenous malformation	EMG	electromyography	LP	lumbar puncture	SDH	subdural hemorrhage
BBB	blood brain barrier	EVD	external ventricular drain	MAP	mean arterial pressure	SIADH	syndrome of inappropriate antidiuretic hormone
CBF	cerebral blood flow	GCS	Glasgow coma scale	MLS	midline shift		
CSF	cerebral spinal fluid	GPi	globus pallidus pars interna	NC	neurogenic claudication	SPECT	single photon emission computed tomography
CPA	cerebellar pontine angle	H/A	headache	NPH	normal pressure hydrocephalus		
CPP	cerebral perfusion pressure	IC	internal capsule	OPLL	ossification of posterior longitudinal ligament	SRS	stereotactic radiosurgery
CVR	cerebral vascular resistance	ICF	intracellular fluid	PAG	periaqueductal grey matter	STN	subthalamic nucleus
DBS	deep brain stimulation	ICH	intracerebral hemorrhage	PET	positron emission tomography	UMN	upper motor neuron
DI	diabetes insipidus	ICP	intracranial pressure	PLL	posterior longitudinal ligament	VPL	ventral posterolateral
ECF	extracellular fluid	IVH	intraventricular hemorrhage	PNET	primitive neuroectodermal tumour	VPM	ventral posteromedial
ECT	electroconvulsive therapy	LMN	lower motor neuron	PVG	periventricular grey matter	WBRT	whole brain radiation therapy

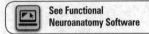 See Functional Neuroanatomy Software

Basic Anatomy Review

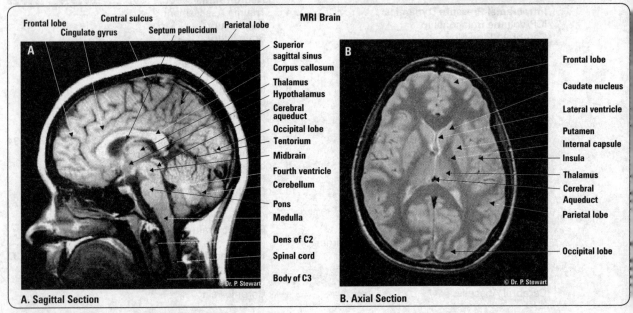

Figure 1. Magnetic resonance imaging (MRI) neuroanatomy
Stewart P, et al. Functional Neuroanatomy (Version 2.1). Health Education Assets Library 2005

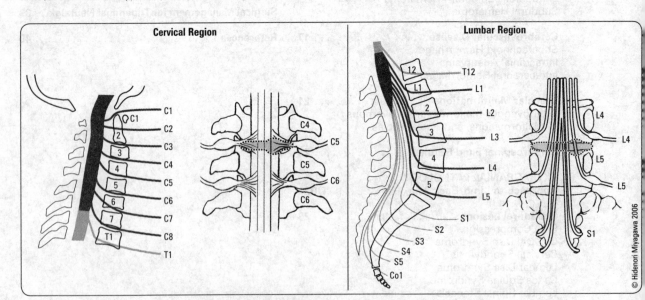

Figure 2. Relationship of nerve roots to vertebral level in the cervical and lumbar spine
Note: AP views depict left-sided C4-5 and L4-5 disc herniation, and correlating nerve root impingement

© Hidenori Miyagawa 2006

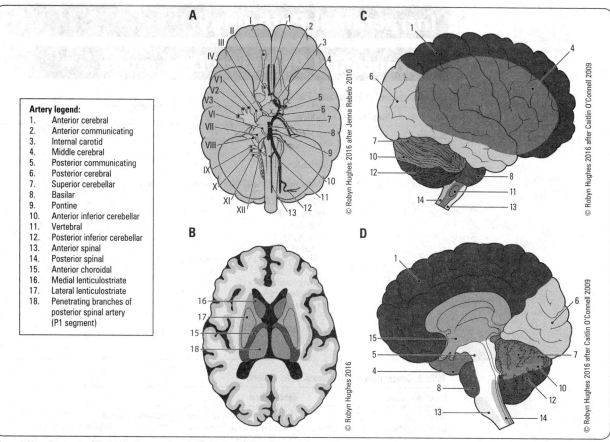

Figure 3. Vascular supply of the brain. Please see legend for artery names. 3A. Circle of Willis, most common variant. 3B. Vascular territories of the brain and brainstem, saggital view, seen laterally. 3C. Vascular territories of the brain and brainstem, saggital view, seen medially

Differential Diagnoses of Common Neurosurgical Presentations

Intracranial Mass Lesions

Tumour
Metastasis
Astrocytoma
Meningioma
Vestibular schwannoma (acoustic neuroma)
Pituitary adenoma
Primary CNS lymphoma

Pus/Inflammation
Cerebral abscess, extradural abscess, subdural empyema
Encephalitis (see Infectious Diseases, ID19)
Tumefactive MS

Blood
Extradural (epidural) hematoma
Subdural hematoma
Ischemic stroke
Hemorrhage: SAH, ICH, IVH

Cyst
Arachnoid cyst
Dermoid cyst
Epidermoid cyst
Colloid cyst (3rd ventricle)

Disorders of the Spine

Extradural
Degenerative: disc herniation, canal stenosis, spondylolisthesis/spondylolysis
Infection/inflammation: osteomyelitis, discitis
Ligamentous: ossification of posterior longitudinal ligament (OPLL)
Trauma: mechanical compression/instability, hematoma
Tumours (55% of all spinal tumours): lymphoma, metastases (lymphoma, lung, breast, prostate), neurofibroma

Intradural Extramedullary
Vascular: dural arteriovenous fistula, subdural hematoma (especially if on anticoagulants)
Tumours (40% of all spinal tumours): meningioma, schwannoma, neurofibroma

Intradural Intramedullary
Tumours (5% of all spinal tumours): astrocytomas, ependymomas, hemangioblastomas and dermoids
Syringomyelia: trauma, congenital, idiopathic
Infectious/inflammatory: TB, sarcoid, transverse myelitis
Vascular: AVM, ischemia

Peripheral Nerve Lesions

Neuropathies
Traumatic
Entrapments
Iatrogenic
Inflammatory
Tumours

Artery legend:
1. Anterior cerebral
2. Anterior communicating
3. Internal carotid
4. Middle cerebral
5. Posterior communicating
6. Posterior cerebral
7. Superior cerebellar
8. Basilar
9. Pontine
10. Anterior inferior cerebellar
11. Vertebral
12. Posterior inferior cerebellar
13. Anterior spinal
14. Posterior spinal
15. Anterior choroidal
16. Medial lenticulostriate
17. Lateral lenticulostriate
18. Penetrating branches of posterior spinal artery (P1 segment)

Intracranial Pathology

Intracranial Pressure Dynamics

Table 1. Approach to Intracranial Pathology

Issue	Time Frame	Features
Vascular	Sudden	No H/A = occlusive H/A = hemorrhagic
Metabolic	Hours to days	Affects entire CNS
Infectious	Days to weeks	Often a source of infection or immunodeficiency on history
Tumour	Months	Increased ICP: Initially → H/A Constant Progressive Severe Worse in morning and/or wakes from sleep As ICP increases: Blurry vision Projectile vomiting Severely raised ICP: Cushing's reflex 1. Bradycardia 2. HTN 3. Respiratory irregularity

Table 2. Consequences of Common Brain Lesions

Location of Lesion	Consequence
Frontal Lobe Usually large lesions produce symptoms	Disinhibition, abulia, apathy, executive dysfunction, deficits in orientation and judgment, ± primitive reflex re-emergence, ± contralateral upper motor neuron signs (upgoing Babinski reflex and pronator drift)
Frontal Eye Fields	Gaze deviation toward side of a destructive lesion Gaze deviation away from irritative lesion (i.e. seizure)
Broca's Area Posterior inferior frontal gyrus of dominant hemisphere	Non-fluent, dysarthric, aphasia Repetition impaired Comprehension spared
Occipital Lobe	Contralateral homonamous hemianopsia
Parietal Lobe Either side Dominant side (Left) Non-dominant side (Right)	 Cortical sensory loss, lower homonamous quadrantanopia Aphasias, Gerstmann's syndrome Hemispatial neglect, apraxias, agnosias
Temporal Lobe	Hippocampus: anterograde amnesia Upper homonymous hemianopia Wernicke's aphasia
Wernicke's Area Posterior superior temporal gyrus of dominant hemisphere	Fluent aphasia Repetition impaired Comprehension impaired
Basal Ganglia	Resting tremor Chorea Athetosis
Subthalamic Nucleus	Contralateral hemiballismus
Brainstem	Absent reflexes: oculocephalic, oculovestibular, corneal, gag, and cough Dorsal midbrain: Parinaud's syndrome (supranuclear upward gaze palsy) Pontine base: locked-in syndrome Below red nucleus: decerebrate posture Above red nucleus: decorticate posture Reticular activating system (midbrain): reduced level of arousal Cerebellar pontine angle: tinnitus, disequilibrium, ataxia and other CN V, VII, VIII deficits
Cerebellar Hemisphere	Intention tremor Ipsilateral limb ataxia Fall towards side of lesion
Cerebellar Vermis	Truncal ataxia Dysarthria

ICP/Volume Relationship

- Monro-Kellie Doctrine: the brain is encased in a rigid skull with constant intracranial volume consisting of CSF, blood and brain
- the increase in one constituent will: 1) necessitate the redistribution of CSF, blood and/or brain and 2) increase ICP
- compensatory mechanisms initially maintain a normal ICP
  - **immediate**: egression of CSF through foramen magnum to spinal canal, displacement of venous blood from sinuses into jugular veins
- once compensation is exhausted, ICP rises exponentially (Figure 4):
  - **late**: displacement of arterial blood (decreased CPP) eventually leading to ischemia, increasing brain edema or expanding mass displaces parenchyma into compartments under less pressure (Table 3)
  - **end**: cessation of cerebral perfusion when ICP>MAP, cerebral herniation down into foramen magnum

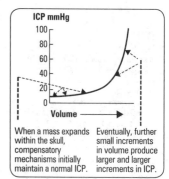

When a mass expands within the skull, compensatory mechanisms initially maintain a normal ICP. Eventually, further small increments in volume produce larger and larger increments in ICP.

Figure 4. ICP volume curve
Adapted from: Lindsay KW, et al. Neurology and neurosurgery illustrated. © 2004. With permission from Elsevier

Cerebral Blood Flow

- brain receives about 15% of cardiac output (~750 mL/min)
- CBF is the vital parameter for brain function and depends on cerebral perfusion pressure (CPP) and cerebral vascular resistance (CVR)
- CPP is dependent on the difference between mean arterial pressure (MAP) and Intracranial Pressure (ICP) (Normal CPP > 50 mmHg)
- cerebral autoregulation: mechanism that maintains constant CBF despite changes in CPP, unless:
  - high ICP such that CPP <40 mmHg
  - MAP >150 mmHg or MAP <50 mmHg
  - increased CO_2 = increased CBF via vasodilation
  - O_2 <50 mmHg = increased CBF via vasodilation
  - brain injury: e.g. SAH, severe trauma

CBF = CPP / CVR
CPP = MAP – ICP

MAP Targets in Trauma
TBI: MAP >80 mmHg
SCI: MAP between 85-90 mmHg in first 7d post injury

ICP Measurement

- normal ICP 10-15 mmHg for adult, 3-7 mmHg for child, 1.5-6 mmHg for infant; varies with patient position
  - moderate elevation >20 mmHg
  - severe elevation >40 mmHg

Acute Monitoring
- **indications include**: severe TBI (GCS<8T) + abnormal CT; normal CT under some conditions
- **methods**: many methods, but "gold standard" is intraventricular catheter, aka external ventricular drain (EVD), is the most accurate and allows therapeutic drainage of CSF

Chronic Monitoring
- fibreoptic monitor (intraventricular, intraparenchymal, subdural), subarachnoid bolt (Richmond screw), and epidural monitor

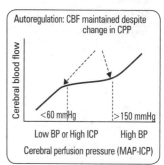

Autoregulation: CBF maintained despite change in CPP

Cerebral blood flow

<60 mmHg   >150 mmHg
Low BP or High ICP   High BP
Cerebral perfusion pressure (MAP-ICP)

Figure 5. Cerebral autoregulation curve
Adapted from: Lindsay KW, et al. Neurology and neurosurgery illustrated. © 2004. With permission from Elsevier

Elevated ICP

Etiology
- **increased intracranial brain volume**
  - intracranial mass (tumour, cyst)
  - cerebral edema
    - vasogenic: BBB compromised (encephalitis, meningitis, hypertensive encephalopathy, tumour, late ischemia, status epilepticus)
    - cytotoxic: BBB intact (cell death in: early ischemia, brain injury, encephalitis, status epilepticus)
    - interstitial: transudaton of CSF into peri-ventricular white matter in hydrocephalus
    - osmotic: osmotic gradient increases intracellular free H_2O (acute hyponatremia, hepatic encephalopathy)
  - other space occupying lesions: depressed skull fracture, foreign body, pus/empyema
- **increased intracranial blood volume**
  - space occupying blood: epidural and subdural hematomas, intraparenchymal and subarachnoid hemorrhages
  - venous obstruction (venous sinus thrombosis, superior vena cava syndrome, cor pulmonale, venous sinus compression)
  - impaired autoregulation (hypotension, HTN, brain injury, status epilepticus)
  - vasodilatation (increased pCO_2/decreased pO_2/decreased extracellular pH)
  - cranial dependency
- **increased intracranial CSF volume**
- increased production (rare): choroid plexus papilloma
- hydrocephalus: obstructive vs non-obstructive (see Table 6)
- idiopathic intracranial HTN (pseudotumour cerebri) – see *Idiopathic Intracranial Hypertension, NS7*

Lumbar puncture can be used for ICP monitoring, though it is not the most accurate. LP can precipitate tonsillar and uncal herniation with elevated ICP and is absolutely contraindicated with known/suspected intracranial mass

Consider Monitoring ICP in the Following Situations
- Patients with an abnormal head CT (SAH, hematoma, contusion, basal cistern compression, swelling, and herniation) and GCS score ≤ 8 after CPR
Or
- Patients with a normal head CT and GCS score of ≤8 AND the presence of two or more of the following:
- >40 yr
- Unilateral or bilateral motor posturing
- sBP <90 mmHg
- Post-operative monitoring
- Investigation of NPH

Cautioned medication use in elevated ICP
- Nitroprusside – can raise ICP in patients with intracranial mass lesions due to direct vasodilation (arterial>venous)
- Nitroglycerine – can raise ICP via vasodilation but less so than Nitroprusside because venous>arterial
- Succinylcholine – induced fasciculations may increase ICP

Blood Brain Barrier
Glucose and amino acids cross slowly
Non-polar/lipids cross fast

Infarction/neoplasm → destroy tight junctions → vasogenic edema

Cushing's Triad of Acute Raised ICP
(full triad seen in 1/3 of cases)
- Hypertension
- Bradycardia (late finding)
- Irregular respiratory pattern

Papilledema
- Optic disc swelling with blurred margins (most commonly bilateral)
- Larger blind spot

Clinical Features

Table 3. Clinical Features of Elevated ICP

Clinical Features	Acutely Elevated ICP	Chronic Progressive ICP Elevation
Headache	Both aggravated by stooping, coughing, straining Morning headaches: vasodilatation due to increased CO_2 with recumbency	
Nausea and Vomiting	Present in both, though greater predilection in acutely elevated ICP	
Level of Consciousness	Lethargy if ICP = dBP or midbrain compression	Normal or modestly reduced LOC, confusion
GCS	Significant decline in GCS Best index to monitor progress and predict outcome of acute intracranial process (see *Neurotrauma*, NS29)	Can be unchanged or modestly decreased
Optic Disc Changes	Subtle changes suggesting papilledema (subtle elevations in disc margin, mild disc hyperemia) ± retinal hemorrhages (may take 24-48 h to develop)	Obvious papilledema
Visual Changes	Often not affected initially, however visual obscurations, flickering or blurring can occur	Optic atrophy/blindness due to chronic papilledema Enlarged blind spot, if advanced → episodic constrictions of visual fields ("grey-outs") Differentiate from papillitis (usually unilateral with decreased visual acuity)
Extra-Occular Movements	CN VI palsy: due to long intracranial course, more sensitive to ICP changes and thus earlier sign of acutely increased ICP Often falsely localizing (causative lesion remote to nerve) **Upward gaze palsy and sunset eyes** (especially in children with obstructive hydrocephalus)	Often full EOM
Herniation Syndromes	Often occur (see Table 4)	Present if acute on chronic presentation
Neurologic Deficits	Focal deficits present	Focal deficits can be present

Investigations
- patients with suspected elevated ICP require an urgent CT/MRI to identify etiology, assess for midline shift/herniation
- ICP monitoring where appropriate

Herniation Syndromes

Table 4. Herniation Syndromes

Herniation Syndrome	Definition	Etiology	Clinical Features
1. Subfalcine	Cingulate gyrus herniates under falx	Lateral supratentorial lesion	Usually asymptomatic Warns of impending transtentorial herniation Risk of ACA compression
2. Central Tentorial (Axial)	Displacement of diencephalon through tentorial notch	Supratentorial midline lesion Diffuse cerebral swelling Late uncal herniation	Small pupils, moderately dilated, fixed (rostral to caudal deterioration), sequential failure of diencephalon, medulla Decreased LOC (midbrain compression), EOM/upward gaze impairment ("sunset eyes"): compression of pretectum and superior colliculi (Parinaud's syndrome) Risk of PCA compression Brainstem (Duret) hemorrhage: secondary to shearing of basilar artery perforating vessels Diabetes insipidus (traction on pituitary stalk and hypothalamus), end-stage sign
3. Lateral Tentoria (Uncal)	Uncus of temporal lobe herniates down through tentorial notch	Lateral supratentorial lesion (often rapidly expanding traumatic hematoma)	Ipsilateral non-reactive dilated pupil (earliest, most reliable sign) + ipsilateral EOM paralysis, ptosis (CN III compression) Decreased LOC (midbrain compression) Risk of PCA compression Contralateral hemiplegia ± extensor (upgoing) plantar response ± ipsilateral hemiplegia ("Kernohan's notch" – a false localizing sign resulting from pressure from the edge of the tentorium on the contralateral cerebral peduncle)
4. Upward	Cerebellar vermis herniates through tentorial incisura	Posterior fossa mass, brainstem or cerebellar infarction, exacerbated by ventriculostomy or VP shunt	Cerebellar infarct (superior cerebellar artery [SCA] compression) Hydrocephalus(cerebral/sylvian aqueduct compression)
5. Tonsillar	Cerebellar tonsils herniate through foramen magnum	Infratentorial lesion Following central tentorial herniation Following LP in presence of intracranial mass lesion	Neck stiffness and head tilt (tonsillar impaction) Decreased LOC (midbrain compression) Flaccid paralysis Respiratory irregularities, respiratory arrest (compression of medullary respiratory centres) Blood pressure instability (compression of medullary cardiovascular centres)

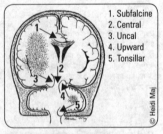

1. Subfalcine
2. Central
3. Uncal
4. Upward
5. Tonsillar

© Heidi Maj

Figure 6. Herniation types

Treatment of Elevated ICP

- **treatment principle**: treat primary etiology (i.e. remove mass lesions, ensure adequate ventilation for example in ARDS)
- if elevated ICP persists following treatment of primary cause, consider therapy when ICP >20 mmHg
- **targets**: ICP <20 mmHg, CPP >65 mmHg, MAP >90 mmHg

Treatment of Elevated ICP

ICP HEAD
Intubate
Calm (sedate)/Coma
Place drain/Paralysis
Hyperventilate
Elevate head
Adequate BP
Diuretic (mannitol)

Table 5. Management of Elevated ICP

Consideration	Intervention	Rationale
Conservative Measures		
Position	Elevate head of bed at 30° Maintain neck in neutral position	Increases 1. Jugular venous patency 2. intracranial venous outflow with minimal effect on MAP
Prevent Hypotension	PRN: fluid, vasopressors, dopamine, norepinephrine	Maintains CBF
Normocarbia	Ventilate to pCO₂ 35-40 mmHg	Prevents vasodilatation
Adequate O₂	Target pO₂ >60 mmHg	Prevents hypoxic brain injury
Osmolar Diuresis	Mannitol 20% IV solution 1-1.5 g/kg, then 0.25 g/kg q6h to serum osmolarity of 315-320 Acts in 15-30 min, maintain sBP >90 mmHg	Increase serum tonicity → osmotically drives fluid out of brain
Corticosteroids	Dexamethasone	Decrease vasogenic edema over subsequent days around brain tumour, abscess, blood No proven value in head injury or stroke
Aggressive Measures		
Sedation	Light = barbituates/codeine Heavy = fentanyl/MgSO4	Reduces sympathetic tone Reduces HTN induced by muscle contraction
Paralysis	Vecuronium	Reduces sympathetic tone Reduces HTN induced by muscle contraction
Barbiturate-Induced Coma	Phentobarbital 10 mg/kg over 30 min, then 1 mg/kg q1h continuous infusion	Reduce CBF and metabolism Decreases mortality, but no affect on neurologic outcome No role for the use of hypothermia in head injury
Hyperventilate	Target pCO₂ 30-35 mmHg	Decreases CBF and thus ICP but use for brief periods only
Drain CSF	Insert EVD (if acute) or shunt Drain 3-5 mL CSF	Reduces intracranial volume
Decompression	Decompressive craniectomy	Allows brain to swell while reducing risk of herniation

Idiopathic Intracranial Hypertension (Pseudotumour Cerebri)

Definition
- raised ICP with papilledema, but without: mass, hydrocephalus, infection, or hypertensive encephalopathy (diagnosis of exclusion)

Etiology
- unknown (majority), but associated with:
  - dural sinus thrombosis
  - **habitus/diet:** obesity, hypervitaminosis A
  - **endocrine:** reproductive age, menstrual irregularities, Addison's/Cushing's disease
  - **hematologic:** iron deficiency anemia, polycythemia vera
  - **drugs:** steroid withdrawal, tetracycline, amiodarone, lithium, nalidixic acid, oral contraceptive
- risk factors overlap with those of venous sinus thrombosis; similar to those for gallstones ("fat, female, fertile, forties")

Epidemiology
- incidence: general population ~1-2/100,000 per year; obese women of childbearing age 19-21/100,000

Clinical Features
- **symptoms**: H/A in >90%, nausea, pulsatile intracranial noise, impaired vision, diploplia can occur with CN VI palsy
- **signs**: CN VI palsy can occur (otherwise no neurologic deficits), visual acuity and field deficits, papilledema, optic atrophy
- **morbidity**: risk of blindness, which is not reliably correlated to duration, symptoms or clinical course
- **clinical course**: usually self-limited, recurrence in 10%, chronic in some

Investigations
- **MRI-brain** (with and without contrast): slit like ventricles, but otherwise normal
  - rule out: venous sinus thrombosis, mass, infection, hydrocephalus
- **LP findings**: 1. Opening pressure >20 mm H_2O 2. Normal CSF analysis
- **ophthalmologic**: fields, acuity, papilledema

Treatment
- **lifestyle change**: encourage weight loss, fluid/salt restriction
- **pharmacotherapy**: acetazolamide (decreases CSF production), thiazide diuretic, or furosemide; discontinue offending medications
- **surgery**: if above fail, serial LPs, shunts, optic nerve sheath decompression (if progressive impairment of visual acuity)
- **long term**: 2 yr follow-up, repeat imaging to rule out occult tumour, ophthalmology follow-up

Hydrocephalus

- for hydrocephalus in children, see *Pediatric Neurosurgery*, NS35

CSF production = CSF reabsorption = ~ 500 mL/d in normal adults
Normal CSF volume ~150 mL (50% spinal, 50% intracranial → 25 mL intraventricular, 50 mL subarachnoid)

Definition
- accumulation of excess CSF in the brain, functionally divided into obstructive and communicating
- flow of CSF: produced by choroid plexus, lateral ventricles → foramen of Monroe → 3rd ventricle → cerebral/sylvian aqueduct → 4th ventricle → foramina of Luschka (lateral) and Magendie (medial) → subarachnoid space where CSF is re-absorbed by arachnoid villi/granulations into dural venous sinuses

Etiology
- **impaired CSF dynamics**
  a. obstruction of CSF flow
  b. decreased CSF absorption
  c. increased CSF production (rarely in choroid plexus papilloma – 0.4-1% of intracranial tumours)
- congenital and acquired causes

Epidemiology
- estimated prevalence 1-1.5%; incidence of congenital hydrocephalus ~1-2/1,000 live births

Classification

Table 6. Classification of Hydrocephalus

Disorder	Definition	Etiology	Findings on CT/MRI
Obstructive (Non-Communicating) Hydrocephalus	CSF Circulation blocked within ventricular system proximal to the arachnoid granulations	**Acquired** **Aqueductal Stenosis**: adhesions after infection, hemorrhage; gliosis, tumour (e.g. medulloblastoma) **Intraventricular lesions**: tumours, e.g. 3rd ventricle colloid cyst, hematoma Mass causing tentorial herniation causing aqueduct/4th ventricle compression **Others**: neurosarcoidosis, abscess/granulomas, arachnoid cysts **Congenital** Primary aqueductal stenosis, Dandy-Walker malformation, Arnold-Chiari malformation, myelomeningocele, encephalocele (see *Pediatric Neurosurgery*, NS35-36)	Ventricular enlargement proximal to block (enlarged temporal horns, ballooning frontal and/or occipital horns, enlarged 3rd ± 4th ventricles) Periventricular hypodensity/lucency (transependymal migration of CSF forced into extracellular space) Sulcal effacement, reduced visibility of sylvian and interhemispheric fissures
Non-Obstructive (Communicating) Hydrocephalus	Most commonly CSF absorption blocked at extraventricular site = arachnoid granulations, rarely CSF absorption is overwhelmed by increased production	Post-infectious (#1 cause) → meningitis, abscess, cysticercosis Post-hemorrhagic (#2 cause) → SAH, IVH, traumatic Leptomeningeal carcinomatosis – metastatic meningitis Choroid plexus papilloma Idiopathic → normal pressure hydrocephalus	All ventricles dilated
Normal Pressure Hydrocephalus (NPH)	Persistent ventricular dilatation in the context of normal CSF pressure	Idiopathic (50%) Others: subarachnoid hemorrhage, meningitis, trauma, radiation-induced	Enlarged ventricles without increased prominence of cerebral sulci
Hydrocephalus *Ex Vacuo*	Ventricular enlargement resulting from atrophy of surrounding brain tissue	Normal aging Degenerative dementias see <u>Neurology</u>, N21 (Alzheimer's, Frontal Temporal, Creutzfeldt-Jacob Disease)	Enlarged ventricles and sulci Cerebral atrophy

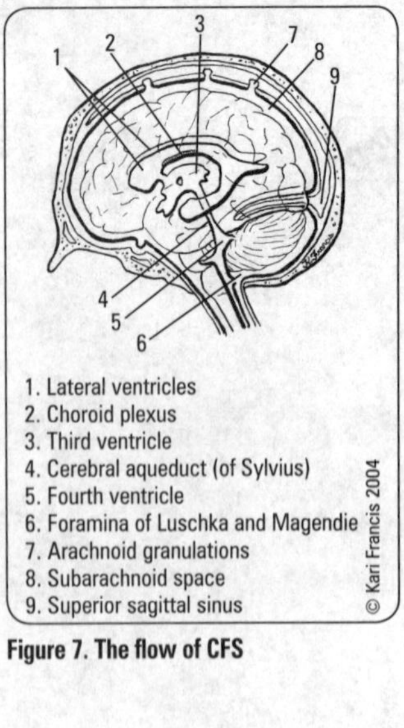

1. Lateral ventricles
2. Choroid plexus
3. Third ventricle
4. Cerebral aqueduct (of Sylvius)
5. Fourth ventricle
6. Foramina of Luschka and Magendie
7. Arachnoid granulations
8. Subarachnoid space
9. Superior sagittal sinus

© Kari Francis 2004

Figure 7. The flow of CFS

Clinical Features

- acute hydrocephalus: signs and symptoms of acutely elevated ICP (see Table 3)
- chronic/gradual onset hydrocephalus: (weeks to months) (i.e. NPH) presents with a classic triad
  - **Ataxia** (magnetic gait) + apraxia (pressure of ventricle on lower extremity motor fibres → gait disturbance)
  - **Incontinence** (pressure on cortical bowel/bladder centre)
  - **Dementia** (pressure on frontal lobes)

Investigations

- **imaging**
  - **CT/MRI** findings (see Table 6)
  - **ultrasound** (through anterior fontanelle in infants): ventriculomegaly, size and location of lesions (e.g. IVH)
  - mantleradionuclide cisternography can test CSF flow and absorption rate (unreliable)
- **ICP monitoring** (e.g. LP, EVD) may be used to investigate NPH and test response to shunting (lumbar tap test)

Treatment

- external ventricular drain (EVD)
- intermittent LPs for transient **communicating** hydrocephalus (SAH, IVH in premature infants)
- **surgical**: surgical removal of obstruction (if possible) or excision of choroid plexus papilloma
- eliminating obstruction (i.e. excision of mass, posterior fossa decompression for Chiari Malformation)
- endoscopic
  - endoscopic third ventriculostomy (ETV) ± choroid plexus cauterization (for obstructive hydrocephalus)
  - endoscopic placement of aqueductal stent
- shunt
  - ventriculoperitoneal (VP): most common shunt
  - ventriculopleural (VPl)
  - ventriculoatrial (VA)
  - lumboperitoneal: for communicating hydrocephalus and pseudotumour cerebri

Shunt Complications

Table 7. Shunt Complications

Complication	Etiology	Clinical Features	Investigations
Obstruction (most common) Proximal Catheter Valve Distal Catheter	Obstruction by choroid plexus Buildup of proteinaceous accretions, blood, cells (inflammatory or tumour) Infection Disconnection or damage	Acute hydrocephalus signs and symptoms of Increased ICP	"Shunt series" (plain x-rays of entire shunt that only rule-out disconnection, break, tip migration) CT Radionuclide "shuntogram"
Infection (3-6%)	S. epidermidis S. aureus P. acnes Gram-negative bacilli	Fever, N/V, anorexia, irritability Meningitis Peritonitis Signs and symptoms of shunt obstruction Shunt nephritis (VA shunt)	CBC Blood culture Tap shunt for CandS (LP usually NOT recommended)
Overshunting (10% over 6.5 yr)	Slit ventricle syndrome, collapse of ventricles leading to occlusion of shunt ports by ependymal lining Chronic or recurring headaches often relieved when lying down CT/MRI Slit-like ventricles on imaging Subdural hematoma Collapsing brain tears bridging veins (especially common in NPH patients)	Asymptomatic Headaches, vomiting, somnolence	CT
	Secondary craniosynostosis (children): apposition and overlapping of the cranial sutures in an infant following decompression of hydrocephalus	Abnormal head shape	Clinical CT
Seizures (5.5% risk in 1st yr, 1.1% after 3rd yr)	Ventricular shunts only		EEG
Inguinal Hernia (17% incidence with VP shunt inserted in infancy) ± skin breakdown over hardware	Increased intraperitoneal pressure/fluid results in hernia becoming apparent	Inguinal swelling, discomfort	U/S

Classic Triad of NPH Progression

AID
Ataxia/Apraxia of gait
Incontinence
Dementia

Important Features to Note on CT and MRI (± contrast enhancement)
- Lesions (± edema, necrosis, hemorrhage)
- Midline shifts and herniations
- Effacement of ventricles and sulci (often ipsilateral), basal cisterns
- Single or multiple (multiple implies metastasis)

Complications of Specific Hydrocephalus Treatments
1. VP Shunt – intra-abdominal cysts, adhesions, ascites
2. VA Shunt – greater infection risk, septicemia, emboli
3. VPl Shunt – pleural effusion, hydrothorax, respiratory distress
4. LP Shunt – radiculopathy, CSF leaks, adhesions, arachnoiditis
5. ETV – 56% success rate, hypothalamic injury, traumatic basilar aneurysm

DDx for Ring Enhancing Lesion on CT with Contrast

MAGICAL DR
Metastases*
Abscess*
Glioblastoma (high grade astrocytoma)*
Infarct
Contusion
AIDS (toxoplasmosis)
Lymphoma
Demyelination
Resolving hematoma, Radiation Necrosis
(*3 most common diagnoses)

Ring Enhancing Lesions in Patients with HIV
DDx: Toxoplasmosis or CSN Lymphoma
Tx: Pyrimethamine and Sulfadiazine; later brain biopsy if no resolution with antimicrobial
Primary CNS lymphoma reported in 6-20% of HIV infected patients

Primary Sources of Metastatic Brain Tumours
Lung　　　44%
Breast　　10%
Kidney (RCC)　7%
GI　　　　6%
Melanoma　3%

Brain Metastasis
~1/3 of all adult brain tumours
Well circumscribed, often at grey-white matter junction

Primary Brain Tumours
Rarely undergo metastasis
Adults = mostly supratentorial
Children = mostly infratentorial

New onset communicating hydrocephalus in a patient with cancer should raise the suspicion of leptomeningeal carcinomatosis

Tumours

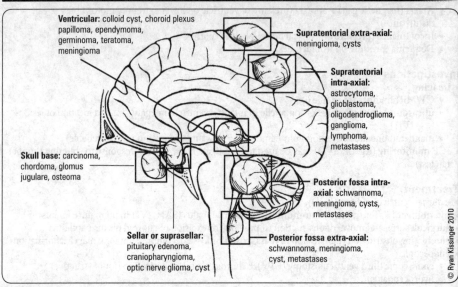

Figure 8. Tumours

Classification
- primary vs. metastatic, intra-axial (parenchymal) vs. extra-axial, supratentorial vs. infratentorial, adult vs. pediatric
- benign: non-invasive, but can be devastating due to expansion of mass in fixed volume of skull (mass effect)
- malignant: implies rapid growth, invasiveness, but rarely extracranial metastasis
- classification of nervous system tumours (* = most common)
  - **neuroepithelial**
    - astrocytic tumours: astrocytoma*, glioblastoma
    - oligodendroglial tumours: oligodendroglioma
    - oligoastrocytic tumours: oligoastrocytoma
    - neuronal and mixed neuronal-glial tumours: ganglion cell tumours, cerebral neurocytomas/neuroblastomas
    - embryonal tumours: medulloblastoma, primitive neuroectodermal tumours (PNET)
    - other: pineal, ependymal, and choroid plexus tumours
  - **meningeal**: meningiomas*, mesenchymal, hemangioblastomas
  - **cranial and paraspinal nerves**: schwannoma, neurofibroma
  - **lymphomas and hematopoietic**: primary CNS lymphoma, plasmacytoma
  - **germ cell**: germinomas, teratomas, choriocarcinomas
  - **sellar region**: craniopharyngiomas, spindle cell oncocytoma, pituitary adenomas*
  - **cysts**: epidermoid/dermoid cysts, colloid cysts
  - **local extension**: chordomas, glomus jugulare tumours
  - **metastatic tumours***: lung (small cell),* breast*
- familial syndromes associated with CNS tumours
  - **von Hippel-Lindau**: hemangioblastoma of cerebellum, brainstem and spinal cord, retina; renal cysts, pheochromocytomas
  - **tuberous sclerosis**: giant cell astrocytoma; cortical tuber; suependymal nodules and calcifications on CT
  - **neurofibromatosis type 1**: optic glioma, neurofibroma astrocytoma,
  - **neurofibromatosis type 2**: vestibular schwannoma, meningioma, ependymoma, astrocytoma
  - **Li-Fraumeni**: astrocytoma, PNET; many other tumours too (sarcomas, breast cancer, leukemia)
  - **Turcot syndrome**: glioblastoma multiforme, medulloblastoma, pineoblastoma
  - **multiple endocrine neoplasia type 1** (MEN-1): pituitary adenoma

Investigations
- CT, MRI, stereotactic biopsy (tissue diagnosis), metastatic workup, tumour markers (i.e. germ cell tumours)

Treatment
- conservative: serial Hx, Px, imaging for slow growing/benign lesions
- medical: corticosteroids to reduce cytotoxic cerebral edema, pharmacologic (i.e. pituitary adenoma)
- surgical: total or partial excision (decompressive, palliative), shunt if hydrocephalus
- radiotherapy: conventional fractionated radiotherapy (XRT), stereotactic radiosurgery (e.g. Gamma Knife®)
- chemotherapy: e.g. alkylating agents (i.e. Vincristine, cyclophosphamide, etc.)

Table 8. Tumour Location: Etiology and Clinical Presentation

	Supratentorial	Infratentorial (Posterior Fossa)
Etiology		
Age <15 yr Incidence: 2-5/100,000/yr 60% infratentorial	Astrocytoma (all grades) (50%) Craniopharyngioma (2-5%) Others: pineal region tumours, choroid plexus tumours, ganglioglioma, DNET	Medulloblastoma (15-20%) Cerebellar astrocytoma (15%) Ependymoma (9%) Brainstem astrocytoma
Age >15 yr 80% supratentorial	High grade astrocytoma (12-15%, e.g. GBM) Metastasis (15-30%, includes infratentorial) Meningioma (15-20%) Low grade astrocytoma (8%) Pituitary adenoma (5-8%) Oligodendroglioma (5%) Other: colloid cyst, CNS lymphoma, dermoid/epidermoid cysts	Metastasis Acoustic neuroma (schwannoma) (5-10%) Hemangioblastoma (2%) Meningioma
Clinical Presentation		
Shared Features (from elevated ICP)	**Headache**: usually worse in AM and made worse with straining, coughing **Nausea/Vomiting** **Papilledema** **Diploopia** - CN VI palsy	
Specific Features	**Seizure**: commonly the first symptom Progressive neurological deficits (70%) Frontal lobe: hemiparesis, dysphasia, personality changes, cognitive changes Temporal lobe: auditory/olfactory hallucinations, memory deficits, contralateral superior quadrantanopsia **Mental Status Change**: depression, apathy, confusion, lethargy "Tumour TIA" – stroke like symptoms caused by a) occlusion of vessel by tumour cells, b) hemorrhage, c) 2° to "steal phenomenon" - blood is shunted from ischemic regions to non-ischemic regions Endocrine disturbance - with pituitary tumours (see Endocrinology, E19)	Brainstem involvement: cranial nerve deficits and long tract signs **Nausea/Vomiting**: compression on vagal nucleus/area postrema **Diplopia**: direct compression CN VI **Vertigo** **Nystagmus** **Truncal Ataxia + Titubation**: cerebellar vermis lesions **Limb Ataxia, dysmetria, intention tremor**: cerebellar hemisphere lesions **Obstructive hydrocephalus** more common than supratentorial lesions

Metastatic Tumours

- most common brain tumour seen clinically
- 15-30% of cancer patients present with cerebral metastatic tumours
  - most common sources: lungs, breast
  - other sources: kidney, thyroid, stomach, prostate, testis, melanoma
- hematogenous spread most common

Location
- 80% are hemispheric, often at grey-white matter junction or temporal-parietal-occipital lobe junction (likely emboli spreading to terminal MCA branches)

Investigations
- identify primary tumour
  - metastatic workup (CXR, CT chest/abdo, abdominal U/S, bone scan, mammogram)
- CT with contrast → round, well-circumscribed, often ring enhancing, ++ edema, often multiple
- MRI more sensitive, especially for posterior fossa
- consider biopsy in unusual cases or if no primary tumour identified

Treatment
- medical
  - phenytoin (or levetiracetam) for seizure prophylaxis if patient presents with seizure
  - dexamethasone to reduce edema given with ranitidine
  - chemotherapy (e.g. small cell lung cancer), but difficult delivery across BBB
- radiation
  - stereotactic radiosurgery: for discrete, deep-seated/inoperable tumours
  - multiple lesions: use WBRT; consider stereotactic radiosurgery if <3 lesions
  - post-operative WBRT is commonly used
- surgical
  - single/solitary lesions: use surgery and radiation

Prognosis
- median survival without treatment once symptomatic is ~1 mo, with optimal treatment 6-9 mo but varies depending on primary tumour type

Guideline on the Management of Newly Diagnosed Brain Metastasis(es) (American Society for Radiation Oncology)
Pract Radiat Oncol 2012;2:210-225
Prognostic Factors
Three prognostic groups based on 1,200 patients:
Class I – Karnofsky performance status (KPS) ≥70 yr, <65 yr with controlled primary (3 mo stability on imaging or newly diagnosed), no extracranial metastases (median survival 7.1 mo).
Class II – everything else (median survival 4.2 mo).
Class III – KPS <70 (median survival 2.3 mo).
Summary of Evidence for Single and Multiple Brain Metastasis(es)
1) For patients with good performance status (e.g. KPS ≥70), limited extracranial disease and resectable metastasis, complete resection improves the probability of extended survival. WBRT in addition to resection improves local and overall brain control but does not affect overall survival or duration of functional independence.
2) For patients with a good prognosis (>3 mo expected survival), single brain metastases <4 cm in size, good performance status, and controlled extracranial disease, the addition of radiosurgery to WBRT improves survival when compared with WBRT alone.
3) In patients with a good prognosis and up to 4 brain metastases <4 cm in size, radiosurgery added to WBRT improves lesion site and overall brain control compared with WBRT alone, but does not influence survival. Therefore, WBRT alone may be considered in these patients.
4) The use of radiosurgery boost to WBRT may improve KPS and decrease the need for steroids at 6 mo in patients with up to 3 brain metastases.
5) For selected patients with poor life expectancy (<3 mo), the use of WBRT may or may not significantly improve symptoms from brain metastases. Comfort measures, or short course (20 Gy in 5 daily fractions) WBRT are reasonable options.
6) There is no evidence of a survival benefit with the combined use of radiosensitizers with WBRT.
7) Although chemotherapy trials have reported improved response rates with combined chemotherapy and WBRT, the addition of chemotherapy leads to increased toxicity and does not improve survival. The routine use of chemotherapy in the management of brain metastases is not generally recommended.

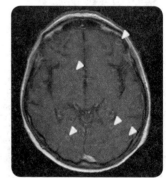

Figure 9. Multiple brain metastases
(see arrows)

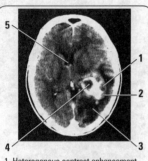

1. Heterogenous contrast enhancement
2. Ill-defined borders (infiltrative)
3. Peritumoural edema
4. Central necrosis
5. Compression of ventricles, midline shift

Figure 10. High grade astrocytoma on CT

Comparison of a Strategy Favouring Early Surgical Resection vs. a Strategy Favouring Watchful Waiting in Low-Grade Gliomas
JAMA (2012) 308(18): 1881-8
Purpose: To examine "watchful waiting" vs. early surgical resection of low grade gliomas.
Study: A population-based parallel cohort study was undertaken between two hospitals that each favoured different management approaches for low grade gliomas (biopsy and watchful waiting vs. early surgical resection).
Results: 66 patients were included from the watchful waiting hospital and 87 patients from the early resection centre. Median follow-up was 7.0 and 7.1 years at each centre. The two groups were equivalent in terms of baseline parameters. Overall, survival was significantly better with early surgical resection (watchful waiting: median survival of 5.9 years 95% CI, 4.5-7.3 vs. early resection: median survival was not reached due to prolonged length of life, p<0.01).
Conclusions: Early surgical resection of low grade-gliomas is associated with better overall survival as compared to watchful waiting.

Bevacizumab Plus Radiotherapy-Temozolamide for Newly Diagnosed Glioblastoma
NEJM 2014;370:709-722
Purpose: To evaluate the effect of combined bevacizumab and radiotherapy-temozolamide in the treatment of newly diagnosed glioblastoma.
Study: Patients with supratentorial glioblastoma randomly assigned to receive intravenous bevacizumab or placebo plus radiotherapy and oral temozolamide for 30 wk total in cycles, followed by bevacizumab or placebo monotherapy. Outcomes were progression-free survival and overall survival.
Results: 458 patients in bevacizumab group, 463 patients in placebo. The median progression-free survival was longer in the bevacizumab group compared with placebo (10.6 mo vs. 6.2 mo, HR 0.64, 95% CI 0.55-0.74), although overall survival did not differ significantly between groups (HR 0.88, 95% CI 0.76-1.02). Baseline health-related QOL and performance status were maintained longer in the bevacizumab group although there was a higher frequency of adverse events.
Conclusions: The addition of bevacizumab to radiotherapy-temozolamide improves progression-free survival but not overall survival in patients with glioblastoma.

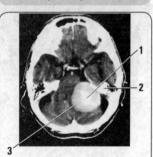

1. Homogenous contrast enhancement
2. Dural attachment
3. Distinct margins

Figure 11. Meningioma on CT

Astrocytoma

- most common primary intra-axial brain tumour, common in 4th-6th decades

Table 9. World Health Organization Astrocytoma Grading System

	Typical CT/MRI Findings	Survival
I – Pilocytic astrocytoma	± mass effect, ± enhancement	>10 yr, cure if gross total resection
II – Low grade/diffuse	Mass effect, no enhancement	5 yr
III – Anaplastic	Complex enhancement	1.5-2 yr
IV – Glioblastoma multiforme (GBM)	Necrosis (ring enhancement)	12 mo, 10% at 2 yr

Clinical Features
- sites: cerebral hemispheres >> cerebellum, brainstem, spinal cord
- symptoms: recent onset of new/worsening H/A, N/V, seizure, ± focal deficits or symptoms of increased ICP

Investigations
- CT/MRI with contrast: variable appearance depending on grade
  - hypodense on CT, hypointense on T1 MRI, hyperintense on T2 MRI
  - low grade: most do not enhance and have calcification on CT
  - high grade: most enhance with CT contrast dye/gadolinium

Treatment
- **low grade diffuse astrocytoma**
  - close follow-up, radiation, chemotherapy, and surgery all valid options
  - dedifferentiation to more malignant grade; typically occurs faster when diagnosed after age 45
  - surgery: not curative, trend towards better outcomes
  - radiotherapy alone or post-operative prolongs survival (retrospective evidence)
  - chemotherapy: usually reserved for tumour progression
- **high grade astrocytomas** (anaplastic astrocytoma and GBM)
  - goal is to prolong "quality" survival
  - **surgery**
    - gross total resection: maximal safe resection + fractionated radiation with 2 cm margin + concomitant and adjuvant temozolomide
      - except: nearing end-of-life; or extensive brainstem, bilateral, or dominant lobe GBM involvement
    - stereotactic biopsy if resection not possible, followed by fractioned radiation with 2 cm margin
  - **expectant** (based on functional impairment – Karnofsky score <70; patient's/family's wishes)
  - **chemotherapy:** ~20% response rate, temozolomide (agent of choice); better response to temozolomide predicted by MGMT gene hypermethylation
- **multiple gliomas:** WBRT ± chemotherapy

Meningioma

- most common *primary* intracranial tumour (14-19%), arise from arachnoid membrane
- often calcified, cause hyperostosis of adjacent bone
- classically see Psammoma bodies on histology
- location: 70% occur along the parasagittal convexity, falx cerebri, and sphenoid bone; other locations: tuberculum sellae, foramen magnum, olfactory groove, and CP angle

Clinical Features
- middle aged, slight female predominance (M:F = 1:1.8), high progesterone receptors (increase in size with pregnancy)
- many are asymptomatic; when symptoms occur focal neurologic deficits specific to location, ± seizures, symptoms of increased ICP

Investigations
- **CT with contrast:** homogeneous, densely enhancing, along dural border ("dural tail"), well circumscribed, usually solitary (10% multiple, likely with loss of NF2 gene/22q12 deletion)
- **MRI with contrast:** characterization of mass and provides a better assessment of the patency of dural venous sinuses
- **angiography**
  - most are supplied by external carotid feeders (meningeal vessels)
  - can assess venous sinus involvement, "tumour blush" commonly seen (prolonged contrast image)

Treatment
- **conservative management:** asymptomatic and/or non-progressive on CT/MRI
- **surgery:** curative if complete resection and indicated when symptomatic and/or documented growth on serial CT/MRI

- **endovascular**: embolization for highly vascularized, likely bloody, tumours to facilitate surgery
- **radiation**: SRS may be an option for lesions <3 cm partially occluding the superior sagittal sinus; SRS or XRT for non-resectable, recurrent atypical/malignant meningiomas

Prognosis
- >90% 5 yr survival, recurrence rate variable (often ~10-20%)
- depends on extent of resection (Simpson's classification)

WHO Classification of Meningioma (by histology)
Grade 1: low risk of recurrence
Grade 2: intermediate risk of recurrence
Grade 3: high risk of recurrence

Vestibular Schwannoma (Acoustic Neuroma)

- slow-growing (average of 1-10 mm/yr), benign posterior fossa tumour (8-10% of tumours)
- arises from vestibular nerve of CN VIII in internal auditory canal, expanding into bony canal and cerebello-pontine angle (CPA)
- if bilateral, diagnostic of neurofibromatosis type II
- epidemiology: 1.5/100,000; all age groups affected, peaks at 4th-6th decades

Progressive unilateral or asymmetrical sensorineural hearing loss = acoustic neuroma until proven otherwise

Clinical Features
- **early clinical triad**: (tumour <2 cm) unilateral progressive hearing loss 98%, tinnitus, and disequilibrium (compression of CN VIII)
- **later clinical features**
  - tumour usually >2 cm: otalgia, facial numbness + weakness, changes to taste (due to CN V and VII compression)
  - tumour usually >4 cm: ataxia, H/A, N/V, diploplia, cerebellar signs (due to brainstem compression; ± obstructive hydrocephalus)

Investigations
- MRI with gadolinium or T2 FIESTA sequence (>98% sensitive/specific); CT with contrast 2nd choice
- audiogram, brainstem auditory evoked potentials, caloric tests

Treatment
- expectant: serial imaging (CT/MRI q6mo) and audiometry
- radiation: stereotactic radiosurgery or fractionated radiotherapy
- surgery: if lesion >3 cm, brainstem compression, edema, hydrocephalus
- curable if complete resection (almost always possible)
- operative complications: CSF leak, meningitis, required shunt; CN V, VII, VIII dysfunction (proportional to tumour size; only significant CNVIII disability if bilateral)

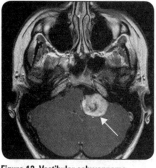

Figure 12. Vestibular schwannoma
(tumour in cerebello-pontine angle)

Pituitary Adenoma

- primarily from anterior pituitary, 3rd-4th decades, M=F, associated with MEN-1 syndrome
- incidence in autopsy studies approximately 20%
- **classification**
  - microadenoma <1 cm; macroadenoma ≥1 cm
  - endocrine active (functional/secretory) vs. inactive (non-functional)
    - most common functional: prolactinomas, adrenocorticotropic, growth-hormone producing
  - differential diagnosis: parasellar tumours (e.g. craniopharyngioma, tuberculum sellae meningioma), carotid aneurysm

Clinical Features
- **mass effects**
- H/A
- bitemporal hemianopsia (compression of optic chiasm); hydrocephalus (3rd ventricle compression)
- invasive adenomas: CN III, IV, V1, V2, VI palsy (cavernous sinus compression); proptosis and chemosis (cavernous sinus occlusion)
- **endocrine effects** (see Endocrinology, E19)
  - **hyperprolactinemia** (prolactinoma): infertility, amenorrhea, galactorrhea, decreased libido
  - **ACTH production**: Cushing's disease, hyperpigmentation
  - **GH production**: acromegaly/gigantism
  - **panhypopituitarism**: due to compression of pituitary (hypothyroidism, hypoadrenalism, hypogonadism)
  - **diabetes insipidus** (DI) – rare, except in apoplexy
- **pituitary apoplexy** (sudden expansion of mass due to hemorrhage or necrosis)
  - abrupt onset H/A, visual disturbances, ophthalmoplegia, reduced mental status, panhypopituitarism and DI
  - CSF rhinorrhea and seizures (rare)
  - signs and symptoms of subarachnoid hemorrhage (rare)

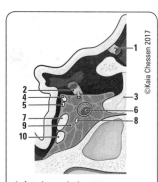

1. Anterior cerebral artery
2. Internal carotid artery (cerebral part)
3. Pituitary gland
4. Oculomotor nerve
5. Trochlear nerve
6. Internal carotic artery (cavernous part)
7. Ophthalmic nerve
8. Abducent nerve
9. Cavernous sinus
10. Maxillary nerve

Figure 13. Cavernous Sinus

Go Look For The Adenoma Please – GH, LH, FSH, TSH, ACTH, Prolactin
A compressive adenoma in the pituitary will impair hormone production in this order (i.e. GH-secreting cells are most sensitive to compression)

Investigations
- formal visual fields, CN testing
- endocrine tests (prolactin level, TSH, 8 AM cortisol, fasting glucose, FSH/LH, IGF-1), electrolytes, urine electrolytes, and osmolarity
- imaging (MRI with and without contrast)

Treatment
- **medical**
  - for apoplexy: rapid corticosteroid administration ± surgical decompression
  - for prolactinoma: dopamine agonists (e.g. bromocriptine)
  - for Cushing's: serotonin antagonist (cyproheptadine), inhibition of cortisol production (ketoconazole)
  - for acromegaly: somatostatin analogue (octreotide) ± bromocriptine
  - endocrine replacement therapy
- **surgical**
  - trans-sphenoidal, trans-ethmoidal, and less commonly trans-cranial approaches (i.e. for significant suprasellar extension)
- **post-operative concerns**: DI, adrenal insufficiency (AI), CSF leak
  - **DI and AI**: AM cortisol, serum sodium and osmolality, urine output and specific gravity (treatment - AI: glucocorticoids; DI: desmopressin/DDAVP)
  - **CSF rhinorrhea**: test for beta transferrin

Pus

Sources of Pus/Infection
- four routes of microbial access to CNS
  1. hematogenous spread (most common): arterial and retrograde venous
     - adults: chest is #1 source (lung abscess, bronchiectasis, empyema)
     - children: congenital cyanotic heart disease with R to L shunt
     - immunosuppression (AIDS – toxoplasmosis)
  2. direct implantation (dural disruption)
     - trauma
     - iatrogenic (e.g. following LP, post-operative)
     - congenital defect (e.g. dermal sinus)
  3. contiguous spread (adjacent infection): from air sinus, naso/oropharynx, surgical site (e.g. otitis media, mastoiditis, sinusitis, osteomyelitis, dental abscess)
  4. spread from PNS (e.g. viruses: rabies, herpes zoster)
- common examples
  - epidural abscess: in cranial and spinal epidural space, associated with osteomyelitis
    - treatment: immediate drainage and antibiotics, surgical emergency if cord compression
  - subdural empyema: bacterial/fungal infection, due to contiguous spread from bone or air sinus, progresses rapidly
    - treatment: surgical drainage and antibiotics, 20% mortality
  - meningitis, encephalitis (see Infectious Diseases, ID19)
  - cerebral abscess

Cerebral Abscess

Definition
- pus in brain substance, surrounded by tissue reaction (capsule formation)

Etiology
- modes of spread: 10-60% of patients have no cause identified
- pathogens
  - *Streptococcus* (most common), often anaerobic or microaerophilic
  - *Staphylococcus* (penetrating injury)
  - Gram-negatives, anaerobes (*Bacteroides, Fusobacterium*)
  - in neonates: *Proteus* and *Citrobacter* (exclusively)
  - immunocompromised: fungi and protozoa (*Toxoplasma, Nocardia, Candida albicans, Listeria monocytogenes, Mycobacterium*, and *Aspergillus*)

Risk Factors
- lung abnormalities (infection, AV fistulas; especially Osler-Weber-Rendu syndrome [i.e. hereditary hemorrhagic telengiectasia])
- congenital coronary heart disease: R-to-L shunt bypasses pulmonary filtration of micro-organisms
- bacterial endocarditis
- penetrating head trauma
- immunosuppression (e.g. AIDS)
- dental abscess

Clinical Features
- focal neurological signs and symptoms
  - H/A, decreased LOC; hemiparesis and seizures in 50%
- mass effect, increased ICP and sequelae (cranial enlargement in children)
- hemiparesis and seizures in 50%
- ± signs and symptoms of systemic infection (low-grade fever, leukocytosis)

Complications
- with abscess rupture: ventriculitis, meningitis, venous sinus thrombosis
- CSF obstruction
- transtentorial herniation

Investigations
- CT scan often first test in emergency department
- MRI
  - imaging of choice
  - apparent diffusion coefficient (ADC) used to differentiate abscess (black) from tumour (white)
- WBC/ESR may be normal, blood cultures rarely helpful and LP contraindicated if large mass
- CSF: non-specific (high ICP, high WBC, high protein, normal carbohydrate), rarely helpful, usually negative culture

Treatment
- aspiration ± excision and send for Gram stain, acid fast bacillus (AFB), CandS, fungal culture
- excision preferable if location suitable
- antibiotics
  - empirically: vancomycin + ceftriaxone + metronidazole or chloramphenicol or rifampin (6-8 wk therapy)
  - revise antibiotics when CandS known
- anti-convulsants (1-2 yr)
- follow-up CT is critical (do weekly initially, more frequent if condition deteriorates)

Prognosis
- mortality with appropriate therapy ~10%, permanent deficits in ~50%

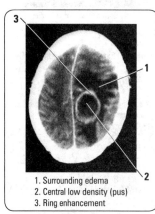

1. Surrounding edema
2. Central low density (pus)
3. Ring enhancement

Figure 14. Cerebral abscess on CT

Blood

Table 10. Comparison of Epidemiology and Etiology of Intracranial Bleeds

Types of Hematoma/ Hemorrhage	Etiology	Epidemiology	Clinical Features	CT Features	Treatment	Prognosis
Epidural Hematoma	Skull fracture causing middle meningeal bleed	M>F (4:1), associated with trauma	Lucid interval before LOC	Hyperdense lenticular mass with sharp margins, usually limited by suture lines	Craniotomy	Good with prompt management (Note: respiratory arrest can occur from uncal herniation)
Acute SDH	Ruptured subarachnoid bridging vessels	Age >50, associated with trauma	No lucid interval, hemiparesis, pupillary changes	Hyperdense crescentic mass, crossing suture lines	Craniotomy if bleed >1 cm thick	Poor
Chronic SDH	Ruptured subarachnoid bridging vessels	Age >50, EtOH abusers, anti-coagulated	Often asymptomatic, minor H/A, confusion, signs of increased ICP	Hypodense crescentic mass, crossing suture lines	Burr hole to drain; craniotomy if recurs	Good
SAH	Trauma, spontaneous (aneurysms, idiopathic, AVM)	Age 55-60 20% cases under age 45	Sudden onset thunderclap H/A, signs of increased ICP	Hyperdense blood in cisterns/fissures (sensitivity decreases over time)	Conservative: NPO, IV NS, ECG, Foley, BP 120-150, vasospasm prophylaxis (nimodipine); open vs. endovascular surgery to repair if rebleed	Poor: 50% mortality 30% of survivors have moderate to severe disability
ICH	HTN, vascular abnormality, tumours, infections, coagulopathy	Age >55, male, drug use (cocaine, EtOH, amphetamine)	TIA-like symptoms, signs of increased ICP	Hyperdense intraparenchymal collection	Medical: decrease BP, control ICP Surgical: craniotomy	Poor: 44% mortality due to cerebral herniation

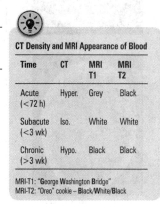

CT Density and MRI Appearance of Blood

Time	CT	MRI T1	MRI T2
Acute (<72 h)	Hyper.	Grey	Black
Subacute (<3 wk)	Iso.	White	White
Chronic (>3 wk)	Hypo.	Black	Black

MRI-T1: "George Washington Bridge"
MRI-T2: "Oreo" cookie – Black/White/Black

Blood

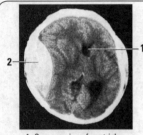

1. Compression of ventricles (midline shift)
2. Blood

Figure 15. Extradural hematoma on CT

Poor Prognostic Indicators for Epidural Hematoma
- Older age
- Low GCS on admission
- Pupillary abnormalities (especially non-reactive)
- Longer delay in obtaining surgery (if needed)
- Post-operative elevated ICP

Compression of ventricles and midline shift

Blood

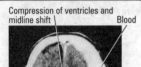

Acute

Old blood

Chronic

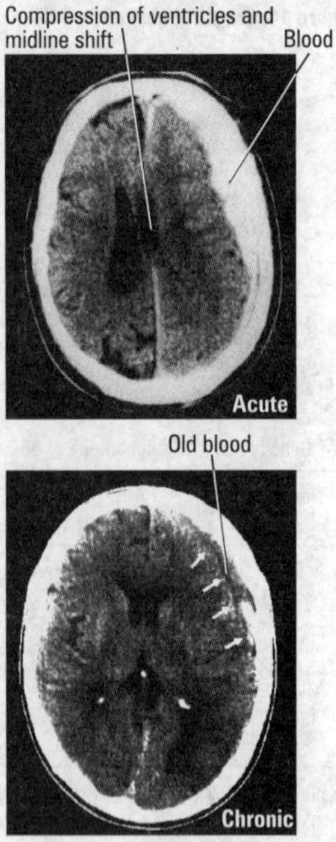

Figure 16. Subdural hematoma on CT

Use of Drains vs. No Drains After Burr-Hole Evacuation of Chronic Subdural Hematoma: A Randomized Control Trial
Lancet 2009;374:1067-1073
Purpose: To examine the effect of drains on recurrence rates of chronic subdural hematoma (SDH) and clinical outcomes.
Study: RCT with 269 patients ≥18 yr of age with chronic SDH. Half of the patients were randomly assigned to receive a subdural drain and the other half no drain after evacuation.
Results: Recurrence occurred in 9.3% of people with a drain and 24% without (p=0.003; 95% CI 0.14-0.70). Although rates of complications were the same between the study groups, mortality at 6 mo was 8.6% in the group receiving a drain and 18.1% in the group not receiving a drain (p=0.042; 95% CI 0.1-0.99).
Conclusions: Use of drains after burr-hole drainage of chronic SDH is safe and associated with a reduced recurrence and mortality at 6 mo.

Extradural ("Epidural") Hematoma

Etiology
- temporal-parietal skull fracture: 85% are due to ruptured middle meningeal artery; remainder of cases are due to bleeding from middle meningeal vein, dural sinus, or bone/diploic veins

Epidemiology
- young adult, M>F = 4:1; rare before age 2 or after age 60
- 1-4% of traumatic head injuries

Clinical Features
- classic sequence (seen in <30%): post-traumatic reduced LOC, a lucid interval of several hours, then obtundation, hemiparesis, ipsilateral pupillary dilatation, and coma
- signs and symptoms depend on severity but can include H/A, N/V, amnesia, altered LOC, aphasia, seizures, HTN, and respiratory distress
- deterioration can take hours to days

Investigations
- CT without contrast: "lenticular-shaped" usually limited by suture lines but not limited by dural attachments

Treatment
- admission, close neurological observation with serial CT indicated if all of the following are present
  - small volume clot, minimal midline shift (MLS <5 mm), GCS >8, no focal deficit
- otherwise, craniotomy to evacuate clot, follow up CT
- mannitol pre-operative if elevated ICP or signs of brain herniation

Prognosis
- good with prompt management, as the brain is often not damaged
- worse prognosis if bilateral Babinski or decerebration pre-operative
- death is usually due to respiratory arrest from uncal herniation (injury to the midbrain)

Subdural Hematoma

Table 11. Comparison of Epidemiology and Etiology of Acute and Chronic SDH

	Acute SDH	Chronic SDH
Time Course	1-2 d after bleeding onset	≥15 d after bleeding onset
Etiology	Rupture of vessels that bridge the subarachnoid space (e.g. cortical artery, large vein, venous sinus) or cerebral laceration	Many start out as acute SDH Blood within the subdural space evokes an inflammatory response: Fibroblast invasion of clot and formation of neomembranes within days → growth of neocapillaries → fibrinolysis and liquefaction of blood clot (forming a hygroma) Course is determined by the balance of rebleeding from neomembranes and resorption of fluid
Risk Factors	Trauma, acceleration-deceleration injury, anticoagulants, alcohol, cerebral atrophy, infant head trauma	Older, alcoholics, patients with CSF shunts, anticoagulants, coagulopathies
Clinical Features	No lucid period, signs and symptoms can include: altered LOC, pupillary Irregularity, hemiparesis	Often due to minor injuries or no history of injury May present with minor H/A, confusion, language difficulties, TIA-like symptoms, symptoms of raised ICP ± seizures, progressive dementia, gait problem Obtundation disproportionate to focal deficit; "the great imitator" of dementia, tumours
Investigations	CT: Hyperdense concave "crescentic" mass, crossing suture lines	CT: hypodense (liquefied clot), crescentic mass
Treatment	Craniotomy if clinically symptomatic, if hematoma > 1 cm thick, or if MLS>5 mm (optimal if surgery <4 h from onset Otherwise observe with serial imaging	Seizure prophylaxis only if post-traumatic seizure Reverse coagulopathies Burr hole drainage of liquefied clot indicated if symptomatic or thickness >1 cm; craniotomy if recurs more than twice
Prognosis	Poor overall since the brain parenchyma is often injured (mortality range is 50-90%, due largely to underlying brain injury) Prognostic factors: initial GCS and neurologica status, post operative ICP	Good overall as brain usually undamaged, but may require repeat drainage

Cerebrovascular Disease

Ischemic Cerebral Infarction (80%)
- embolic, thrombosis of intracerebral arteries, vasculitis, hypercoagulability, etc. (see <u>Neurology</u>, N48)

Intracranial Hemorrhage (20%)
- SAH, spontaneous ICH, IVH

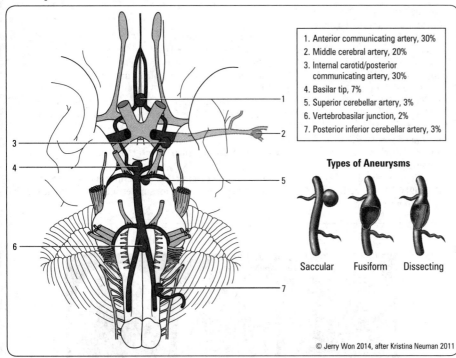

1. Anterior communicating artery, 30%
2. Middle cerebral artery, 20%
3. Internal carotid/posterior communicating artery, 30%
4. Basilar tip, 7%
5. Superior cerebellar artery, 3%
6. Vertebrobasilar junction, 2%
7. Posterior inferior cerebellar artery, 3%

Types of Aneurysms

Saccular   Fusiform   Dissecting

© Jerry Won 2014, after Kristina Neuman 2011

Figure 17. Aneurysms of the Circle of Willis

Hemicraniectomy in Older Patients with Extensive Middle-Cerebral-Artery Stroke
NEJM 2014;370:1091-1100
Purpose: To determine if early decompressive hemicraniectomy reduces mortality among patients >60 yr.
Study: 112 patients >60 yr (median age 70 yr) with malignant MCA infarction randomly assigned to conservative ICU treatment versus hemicraniectomy. Endpoint was survival without severe disability (modified Rankin scale score 0-4).
Results: The proportion of patients who survived without severe disability was 38% in the hemicraniectomy group and 18% in the control group (OR 2.91, 95% CI 1.06-7.49). Modified Rankin scale scores in hemicraniectomy versus control group in terms of percentages of patients: 0-2 (0%, 0%), 3 or moderate disability (7%, 3%), 4 or moderate severe disability (32%, 15%), 5 or severe disability (28%, 13%) and 6 or death (33%, 70%). Infections were more frequent in the hemicraniectomy group and herniation more frequent in the control group.
Conclusions: Hemicraniectomy increased survival without severe disability among patients >60 yr with a malignant MCA infarction.

Subarachnoid Hemorrhage

Definition
- bleeding into subarachnoid space (intracranial vessel between arachnoid and pia)

Etiology
- trauma (most common)
- spontaneous
  - ruptured aneurysms (75-80%)
  - idiopathic (14-22%)
  - AVMs (4-5%)
- coagulopathies (iatrogenic or primary), vasculitides, tumours, cerebral artery dissections (<5%)

Epidemiology
- ~10-28/100,000 population/yr
- peak age 55-60, 20% of cases occur under age 45

Risk Factors
- HTN
- pregnancy/parturition in patients with pre-existing AVMs, eclampsia
- oral contraceptive pill
- substance abuse (cigarette smoking, cocaine, alcohol)
- conditions associated with high incidence of aneurysms (see *Intracranial Aneurysms*, NS19)

Clinical Features of Spontaneous SAH
- sudden onset (seconds) of severe "thunderclap" H/A usually following exertion and described as the "worst headache of my life" (up to 97% sensitive, 12-25% specific)
- N/V, photophobia
- meningismus (neck pain/stiffness, positive Kernig's and Brudzinski's sign)
- decreased LOC (due to either raised ICP, ischemia, seizure)
- focal deficits: cranial nerve palsies (CN III, IV), hemiparesis
- ocular hemorrhage in 20-40% (due to sudden raised ICP compressing central retinal vein)

Hunt and Hess Grade
(clinical grading scale for SAH)

Grade	Description
1	No Sx or mild H/A and/or mild meningismus
2	Grade 1 + CN palsy
3	Confusion/lethargy, mild hemiparesis, or aphasia
4	GCS <15 but >8, moderate-severe hemiparesis, mild rigidity
5	Coma (GCS <9), decerebrate, moribund appearance

Mortality of Grade 1-2 20%, increased with grade

Nontraumatic Subarachnoid Hemorrhage in the Setting of Negative Cranial Computed Tomography Results: External Validation of a Clinical and Imaging Prediction Rule
Ann Emerg Med 2012;59:460-8.e1-7.doi:10.1016
Background: Two rules for SAH diagnosis exist. A clinical prediction rule states that patients with acute severe H/A but without the clinical variables age ≥40 yr, neck pain, loss of consciousness, or onset of H/A with exertion are at low risk for SAH. An imaging prediction rule bases diagnosis on non-contrast cranial CT for patients within 6 h of H/A onset.
Methods: Matched case-control study of 55 patients at 21 emergency departments between 2000 and 2011, and diagnoses were verified by lumbar puncture.
Results: The clinical prediction rule for diagnosis of SAH was 97.1% sensitive, 22.7% specific, and had a negative likelihood ratio of 0.13. Using the imaging prediction rule resulted in a false negative rate of 20%.
Conclusions: Performing the clinical and imaging rules together has the potential for maximizing sensitivity of prediction and reducing rates of lumbar puncture, but using imaging alone can result in missed cases.

Calcium Antagonists for Aneurysmal Subarachnoid Hemorrhage
Cochrane DB Syst Rev 2007;3:CD000277
Introduction: This study looked to review the evidence in regards to whether calcium antagonists improve the outcome in patients with aneurysmal subarachnoid hemorrhage.
Methods/Population: The review included 3,361 patients presenting with aneurysmal subarachnoid hemorrhage from 16 RCTs comparing treatment with calcium antagonists vs. control from 1980 to March 2006.
Results: The results were based mainly on one large trial of oral nimodipine, which showed a RR of 0.67 (95% CI 0.55-0.81) and the evidence for other calcium agonists was not statistically significant.
Conclusion: The authors endorse the use of oral nimodipine in patients with aneurysmal subarachnoid hemorrhage.

- reactive HTN
- sentinel bleeds
  - represents undiagnosed SAH
  - SAH-like symptoms lasting <1 d ("thunderclap H/A")
  - may have blood on CT or LP
  - ~30-60% of patients with full blown SAH give history suggestive of sentinel bleed within past 3 wk
- differential diagnosis: sentinel bleed, dissection/thrombosis of aneurysm, venous sinus thrombosis, benign cerebral vasculitis, benign exertional H/A

Investigations
- non-contrast CT – for diagnosis of SAH
  - 98% sensitive within 12 h, 93% within 24 h; 100% specificity
  - may be negative if small bleed or presentation delayed several days
  - acute hydrocephalus, IVH, ICH, infarct or large aneurysm may be visible
- lumbar puncture (highly sensitive) – for diagnosis of SAH if CT negative but high suspicion:
  - elevated opening pressure (>18 cm H₂O)
  - bloody initially, xanthochromic supernatant with centrifugation ("yellow") by ~12 h, lasts 2 wk
  - RBC count usually >100,000/mm³ without significant drop from first to last tube (in contrast to traumatic tap)
  - elevated protein due to blood breakdown products
- four vessel cerebral angiography ("gold standard" for aneurysms)
  - demonstrates source of SAH in 80-85% of cases
  - angiogram negative SAH: repeat angiogram in 7-14 d, if negative → "perimesencephalic SAH"
- MRA and CTA: sensitivity up to 95% for aneurysms, CTA>MRA for smaller aneurysms and delineating adjacent bony anatomy

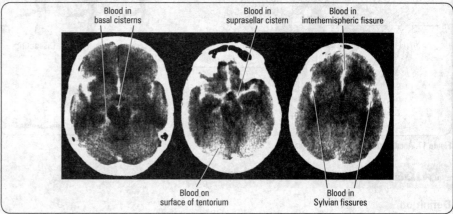

Figure 18. Diagnosis of SAH

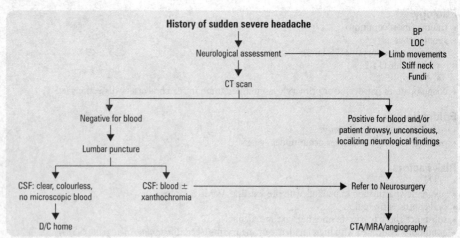

Figure 19. Approach to SAH

Treatment
- admit to ICU or NICU
  - oxygen/ventilation prn
  - NPO, bed rest, elevate head of bed 30°, minimal external stimulation, neurological vitals q1h
  - aim to maintain sBP = 120-150 (balance of vasospasm prophylaxis, risk of rebleed, risk of hypotension since CBF autoregulation impaired by SAH)
  - cardiac rhythm monitor, Foley prn, strict monitoring of ins and outs

- medications
  - IV NS with 20 mmol KCl/L at 125-150 cc/h
  - nimodipine 60 mg PO/NG q4h x 21 d for delayed cerebral ischemia neuroprotection; may discontinue earlier if patient is clinically well
  - •seizure prophylaxis: levetiracetam (Keppra®) 500 mg PO/IV q12h x 1 wk
  - mild sedation prn

Complications

- vasospasm: vasoconstriction and permanent pathological vascular changes in response to vessel irritation by blood – can lead to delayed cerebral ischemia and death
  - onset: 4-14 d post-SAH, peak at 6-8 d; most commonly due to SAH, rarely due to ICH/IVH
  - clinical features (new onset ischemic deficit): confusion, decreased LOC, focal deficit (speech or motor e.g. pronator drift)
  - risk factors: large amount of blood on CT (high Fisher grade), smoking, increased age, HTN
  - "symptomatic" vasospasm in 20-30% of SAH patients
  - "radiographic" vasospasm in 30-70% of arteriograms performed 7 d following SAH
  - diagnosed clinically, and/or with transcranial Doppler (increased velocity of blood flow)
  - risk of cerebral infarct and death
  - treatment
    - hyperdynamic ("triple H") therapy using fluids and pressors, usually after ruptured aneurysm has been clipped/coiled
    - direct vasodilation via angioplasty or intra-arterial verapamil for refractory cases
- hydrocephalus (15-20%): due to blood obstructing arachnoid granules
  - can be acute or chronic, requires extraventricular drain (EVD) or shunt, respectively
- neurogenic pulmonary edema
- hyponatremia: due to cerebral salt wasting (increased renal sodium loss and ECFV loss), not SIADH
- diabetes insipidus
- cardiac: arrhythmia (>50% have ECG changes), MI, CHF

Risk of Recurrent Subarachnoid Hemorrhage, Death, or Dependence and Standardized Mortality Ratios after Clipping or Coiling of an Intracranial Aneurysm in the International Subarachnoid Aneurysm Trial (ISAT): Long-Term Follow-Up
Lancet Neurol 2009;8:427-433
Objective: To assess the long-term risk of death, disability, and rebleeding in patients randomly assigned to clipping or endovascular coiling after rupture of an intracranial aneurysm in the follow-up of the ISAT trial.
Methods: Randomized controlled trial comparing endovascular coiling treatment with craniotomy and clipping for ruptured intracranial aneurysms in 2,143 patients who were considered eligible for either modality of therapy. Annual follow-up was done for a mean length of 9 yr to assess long-term survival and dependency.
Results: 10 patients in the coiled group and 3 patients in the clipped group had rebled from the original aneurysm. In patients with ruptured intracranial aneurysms suitable for both treatments, the survival rate at 5 yr after endovascular coiling was higher at 89% vs. 86% for neurosurgical clipping (relative risk 0.77, p=0.03). The likelihood of independence at 5 yr following treatment is the same for both groups (83% for coiling vs. 82% for clipping).
Conclusions: The risk of death at 5 yr was significantly lower in the coiled group than it was in the clipped group. There was a small increased risk of recurrent bleeding from a coiled aneurysm compared with a clipped aneurysm.

Prognosis

- 10-15% mortality before reaching hospital, overall 50% mortality (majority within first 2-3 wk)
- 30% of survivors have moderate to severe disability
- a major cause of mortality is rebleeding, for untreated aneurysms:
  - risk of rebleed: 4% on first day, 15-20% within 2 wk, 50% by 6 mo
  - if no rebleed by 6 mo, risk decreases to same incidence as unruptured aneurysm (2%)
  - only prevention is early clipping or coiling of "cold" aneurysm
  - rebleed risk for "perimesencephalic SAH" is approximately same as for general population

Intracranial Aneurysms

Epidemiology

- prevalence 1-4% (20% have multiple)
- F>M; age 35-65 yr

Risk Factors

- autosomal dominant polycystic kidney disease (15%)
- fibromuscular dysplasia (7-21%)
- AVMs
- connective tissue diseases (Ehlers-Danlos, Marfan)
- family history
- bacterial endocarditis
- Osler-Weber-Rendu syndrome (hereditary hemorrhagic telangiectasia)
- atherosclerosis and HTN
- trauma

Types

- saccular (berry)
  - most common type
  - located at branch points of major cerebral arteries (Circle of Willis)
  - 85-95% in carotid (anterior) system, 5-15% in vertebrobasilar (posterior) circulation
- fusiform
  - atherosclerotic
  - more common in vertebrobasilar system, rarely rupture
- infectious
  - secondary to any infection of vessel wall, 20% multiple
  - 60% *Streptococcus* and *Staphylococcus*
  - 3-15% of patients with bacterial endocarditis

Development of the PHASES Score for Prediction of Risk of Rupture of Intracranial Aneurysms: A Pooled Analysis of Six Prospective Cohort Studies
Lancet Neurol 2014;13:59-66
Purpose: The construction of an algorithm for estimating 5 yr aneurysm rupture risk.
Study: Systematic review and analysis of patient data. 8,382 patients, 6 prospective cohort studies. Outcome was SAH.
Results: Predictors of aneurysm rupture were age, HTN, history of subarachnoid hemorrhage, aneurysm size, aneurysm location, and geographical region. In North America and European populations, the 5 yr risk of rupture ranged from 0.25% in individuals <70 yr without vascular risk factors and with ICA aneurysm <7 mm to >15% in patients ≥70 yr with HTN, a history of SAH, and >20 mm posterior circulation aneurysm. Finnish and Japanese people had a 3.6- and 2.8-fold higher risk of rupture, respectively, compared with North American and European populations.
Conclusions: The PHASES score may help to predict risk of rupture for incidental intracranial aneurysms.

Long-Term, Serial Screening for Intracranial Aneurysms in Individuals with a Family History of Aneurysmal Subarachnoid Hemorrhage: A Cohort Study
Lancet Neurol 2014;13:385-392
Purpose: To examine the yield of long-term serial screening for intracranial aneurysms for individuals with a positive family history of aneurysmal subarachnoid hemorrhage (aSAH) (two or more first degree relatives who have had aSAH or unruptured intracranial aneurysms).
Study: Screening results from April 1 1993 to April 1 2013 were reviewed in a cohort study. MRA or CTA was done from age 16-18 to 65-70 yr. After a negative screen, individuals were advised to contact the clinic in 5 yr for follow up.
Results: Aneurysms were identified in 11% of individuals at first screening (n=458), 8% at second screening (n=261), 5% at third screening (n=128), and 5% at fourth screening (n=63). Smoking (OR 2.7, 95% CI 1.2-5.9), history of previous aneurysms (3.9, 1.2-12.7), and familial history of aneurysms (3.5, 1.6-8.1) were significant risk factors for aneurysm at first screening. History of previous aneurysms was the only significant risk factor for aneurysms at follow-up screening (HR 4.5, 95% CI 1.1-18.7).
Conclusions: The benefit of long-term screening in individuals with a family history of aSAH is substantial up to and after 10 yr of follow-up and two initial negative screens.

Table 12. Five Year Cumulative Rupture Risk in Unruptured Aneurysms Based on Size and Location

	Cavernous Carotid	AC/MC/IC	Vertebrobasilar/PC/PComm
<7 mm	0%	0%	2.5%
7-12 mm	0%	2.6%	14.5%
13-24 mm	3%	14.5%	18.4%
≥24 mm	6.4%	40%	50%

AC = anterior cerebral/anterior communicating artery; IC = internal carotid artery; MC = middle cerebral artery; PC = posterior cerebral artery; PComm = posterior communicating artery. Lancet 2003;362:103-110

Clinical Presentation
- rupture (90%), most often SAH, but 30% ICH, 20% IVH, 3% subdural bleed
- sentinel hemorrhage ("thunderclap H/A") → requires urgent clipping/coiling to prevent catastrophic bleed
- mass effect (giant aneurysms)
    - internal carotid or anterior communicating aneurysm may compress:
        - the pituitary stalk or hypothalamus causing hypopituitarism
        - the optic nerve or chiasm producing a visual field defect
    - basilar artery aneurysm may compress midbrain, pons (limb weakness), or CN III
    - posterior communicating artery aneurysm may produce CN III palsy
    - intracavernous aneurysms (CN III, IV, V1, V2, VI)
- distal embolization (e.g. amaurosis fugax)
- seizures
- H/A (without hemorrhage)
- incidental CT or angiography finding (asymptomatic)

Investigations
- CT angiogram (CTA), magnetic resonance angiography (MRA), cerebral angiogram

Treatment
- **ruptured aneurysms**
    - overall trend towards better outcome with early surgery or coiling (48-96 h after SAH)
    - treatment options: surgical placement of clip across aneurysm neck, trapping (clipping of proximal and distal vessels), thrombosing using Guglielmi detachable coils (coiling) or flow diversion stents, wrapping (last resort)
    - choice of surgery vs. coiling not yet well defined: consider location, size, shape, and tortuosity of the aneurysm, patient comorbidities, age, and neurological condition; in general:
        - coiling: posterior > anterior circulation, deep/eloquent location, basilar artery bifurcation/apex, older age, presence of comorbidities, presence of vasospasm
        - clipping: superficial > deep, broad aneurysmal base, branching arteries at the aneurysm base, tortuosity/atherosclerosis of afferent vessels, dissection, hematoma, acute brainstem compression
- **unruptured aneurysms**
    - average 1% annual risk of rupture: risk dependent on size and location of aneurysm
    - no clear evidence on when to operate: need to weigh life expectancy
    - risk of morbidity/mortality of SAH (20%-50%) vs. surgical risk (2%-5%)
    - generally treat unruptured aneurysms >10 mm
    - consider treating when aneurysm 7-9 mm in middle-aged, younger patients or patients with a family history of aneurysms
    - follow smaller aneurysms with serial angiography

Intracerebral Hemorrhage

Definition
- hemorrhage within brain parenchyma, accounts for ~10% of strokes
- can dissect into ventricular system (IVH) or through cortical surface (SAH)

Location of ICH
Basal Ganglia/Internal Capsule (50%)
Thalamus (15%)
Cerebral White Matter (15%)
Cerebellum/Brainstem – usually pons (15%)
Other (5%)

Etiology
- HTN (usually causes bleeds at putamen, thalamus, pons, and cerebellum)
- hemorrhagic transformation (reperfusion post stroke, surgery, strenuous exercise, etc.)
- vascular anomalies
    - aneurysm, AVMs, and other vascular malformations (see *Vascular Malformations*, NS21)
    - venous sinus thrombosis
    - arteriopathies (cerebral amyloid angiopathy, lipohyalinosis, vasculitis)
- tumours (1%): often malignant (e.g. GBM, lymphoma, metastases)
- drugs (amphetamines, cocaine, alcohol, anticoagulants, etc.)
- coagulopathy (iatrogenic, leukemia, TTP, aplastic anemia)
- CNS infections (fungal, granulomas, herpes simplex encephalitis)
- post trauma (immediate or delayed, frontal and temporal lobes most commonly injured via coup-contrecoup mechanism)
- eclampsia
- post-operative (post-carotid endarterectomy cerebral reperfusion, craniotomy)
- idiopathic

Epidemiology
- 12-15 cases/100,000 population/yr

Risk Factors
- increasing age (mainly >55 yr)
- male gender
- HTN
- Black/Asian > Caucasian
- previous CVA of any type (23x risk)
- both acute and chronic heavy alcohol use; cocaine, amphetamines
- liver disease
- anticoagulants

Clinical Features
- TIA-like symptoms often precede ICH, can localize to site of impending hemorrhage
- gradual onset of symptoms over minutes-hours, usually during activity
- H/A, N/V, and decreased LOC are common
- specific symptoms/deficits depend on location of ICH

Investigations
- hyperdense blood on non-contrast CT
- CTA routine, if spot sign demonstrated there is high likelihood of clot growth

Treatment
- **medical**
  - decrease MAP to pre-morbid level or by ~20% (target BP 140/90)
  - check PTT/INR, and correct coagulopathy
  - control raised ICP (see *Intracranial Pressure Dynamics*, NS4)
  - levetiracetam/phenytoin for seizure prophylaxis
  - follow electrolytes (SIADH common)
  - angiogram to rule out vascular lesion unless >45 yr, known HTN, and putamen/thalamic/posterior fossa ICH (yield ~0%)
- **surgical**
  - craniotomy with evacuation of clot, treatment of source of ICH (i.e. AVM, tumour, cavernoma), ventriculostomy to treat hydrocephalus
  - indications
    - ◆ symptoms of raised ICP or mass effect
    - ◆ rapid deterioration (especially if signs of brainstem compression)
    - ◆ favourable location (e.g. cerebellar, non-dominant hemisphere)
    - ◆ young patient (<50 yr)
    - ◆ if tumour, AVM, aneurysm, or cavernoma suspected (resection or clip to decrease risk of rebleed)
  - contraindications
    - ◆ small bleed: minimal symptoms, GCS >10
    - ◆ poor prognosis: massive hemorrhage (especially dominant lobe), low GCS/coma, lost brainstem function
    - ◆ medical reasons (e.g. very elderly, severe coagulopathy, difficult location [e.g. basal ganglia, thalamus])

Prognosis
- 30-d mortality rate 44%, mostly due to cerebral herniation
- rebleed rate 2-6%, higher if HTN poorly controlled

Vascular Malformations

Types
- arteriovenous malformations (AVMs)
- cavernous malformations (= cavernomas, cavernous hemangiomas/angiomas)
- venous angioma
- capillary telangiectasias
- arteriovenous fistula (AVF) (carotid-cavernous fistula, dural AVF, vein of Galen aneurysm)
- "angiographically occult vascular malformations" (any type, 10% of malformations)

ICH Risk Factors

CALL HARM
CVA past history
Age (>55 yr)
Liver disease
Liquid blood (anticoagulated)
HTN
Alcohol, cocaine, amphetamines
Race (Black/Asian > Caucasian)
Male

Decompressive Hemicraniectomy in Patients with Supratentorial Intracerebral Hemorrhage
Stroke 2012 Dec;43(12):3207-11
Purpose: Assess the feasibility and safety of decompressive craniectomy (DC) without clot evacuation in intracerebral hemorrhage (ICH).
Methods: Retrospective analysis (2012-2010) of patients with supratentorial ICH treated with DC without hematoma evacuation and matched controls treated with best medical management. Outcomes were dichotomized into good (modified Rankin Scale 0-4) and poor (modified Rankin Scale 5-6).
Results: Of the 12 patients were treated by DC (mean age 48, mean hematoma volume 61.3mL, mean GCS 8, 4 patients had signs of herniation), 9 had good, 3 had poor outcomes, and 3 patients died (25% vs. 53% in control group).
Conclusions: DC is feasible and may reduce mortality in patients with ICH. Larger prospective study is needed to assess safety and efficacy.

Decompressive Hemicraniectomy Without Clot Evacuation in Dominant-Sided Intracerebral Hemorrhage with ICP Crisis
Neurosurg Focus 2013 May;34(5):E4
Purpose: Assess utility of decompressive hemicraniectomy (DC) in intracerebral hemorrhage (ICH) without clot evacuation in patients with supratentorial, dominant-sided lesions.
Methods: Prospective study of patients (n=5) presenting with spontaneous supratentorial dominant-sided ICH treated by DC without clot evacuation for recalcitrant elevated ICP compared to all patients presenting with ICH and matched controls treated with best medical management.
Results: Patient median age was 43 yrs; ICH etiology was hypertension in 4 of 5 patients and systemic lupus erythematosys vasculitis in 1 patient. On admission the median GCS was 7, median ICH volume was 53 cm³, and median midline shift was 7.6 mm. There was decrease in midline shift (median -2.7 mm) and increase in GCS score (median +1) one day following surgery. At discharge, median GCS was 10 and all patients were alive. At six mo post-ICH, 1 patient died, 2 were functionally dependent, and 2 were functionally independent. Outcomes for DC patients were good compared to all patients with supratentorial ICH and compared to matched controls managed medically.
Conclusions: DC without clot evacuation appears feasible in patients with large ICH and requires further investigation.

Spetzler-Martin AVM Grading Scale

Item	Score
Size	
0-3 cm	1
3.1-6.0 cm	2
>6 cm	3
Location	
Noneloquent	0
Eloquent	1
Deep Venous Drainage	
Not present	0
Present	1

AVM grades calculated by adding the 3 individual Spetzler-Martin Scale scores from the above table. e.g. a 2 cm tumour in noneloquent location without deep venous drainage = Grade I

Arteriovenous Malformations, Cavernous Malformations, and Dural Fistulas

Untreated Clinical Course of Cerebral Cavernous Malformations: A Prospective, Population-Based Cohort Study
Lancet Neurol 2012;11:217-224
Purpose: To determine whether or not the risk of hemorrhage and focal neurological deficits from cerebral cavernous malformations (CCMs) is influenced by factors such as sex and CCM location.
Methods: Population-based study to identify CCM diagnoses in residents of Scotland from 1999-2003. Primary outcome was a composite of intracranial hemorrhage and focal neurological deficit related to CCM.
Results: 139 patients with at least one CCM. The 5 yr risk of a first hemorrhage was lower than the risk of recurrent hemorrhage (2.4% vs. 29.5%; p<0.0001) during 1,177 person-years of follow-up. For the primary outcome, the 5 yr risk of a first event was lower than the risk of recurrence (9.3% vs. 42.4%; p<0.0001). The annual risk of recurrence of the primary outcome declined from 19.8% in yr 1 to 5.0% in yr 5 and was higher for women than men.
Conclusions: The risk of recurrent hemorrhage or focal neurological deficit from a CCM is greater than the risk of a first event, is greater for women, and declines over 5 yr.

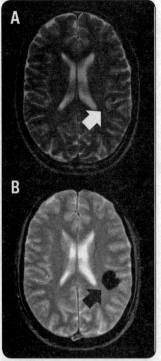

Figure 20. MRI of cavernous malformation
A. T2 weighted imaging MRI
B. Gradient echo sequencing MRI

Table 13. Comparison of Pathoetiology, Clinical Presentation, and Treatment of Arteriovenous Malformations, Cavernous Malformations, and Dural Fistula's

	Arteriovenous Malformation	Cavernous Malformations	Dural Fistulas
Definition	Tangle of abnormal vessels/arteriovenous shunts, with no intervening capillary beds or brain parenchyma; usually congenital	Benign vascular hamartoma consisting of irregular sinusoidal vascular channels located within the brain without intervening neural tissue or associated large arteries/veins. Several genes now described: CCM1, CCM2, CCM3	Fistula's connecting dural arteries to dural veins or the dural sinus. Frequently described to occur at the transverse and cavernous sinuses, but can be found at every cranial dural sinus. Hypothesized to be related to venous sinus thrombosis formation, and subsequent microvascular shunt formation within the dura between arteries and veins
Epidemiology	Prevalence ~0.14%, M:F = 2:1, average age at diagnosis = 33 yr. 15-20% of patients with hereditary hemorrhagic telengiectasia (Osler-Weber-Rendu syndrome) will have cerebral AVMs	Prevalence of 0.1-0.2%, both sporadic and hereditary forms described	Unknown true incidence. Constitute 10-15% of all intracranial vascular abnormalities
Clinical Features	Hemorrhage (40-60%): small AVMs are more likely to bleed due to direct high pressure AV connections. Seizures (50%): more common with larger AVMs. Mass effect. Focal neurological signs secondary to ischemia (high flow → "steal phenomena"). Localized headache, increased ICP. Bruit (especially with dural AVMs). May be asymptomatic ("silent")	Seizures (60%), progressive neurological deficit (50%), hemorrhage (20%), H/A. Often an incidental finding. Hemorrhage risk less than AVM, usually minor bleeds	Asymptomatic, pulsatile tinnitus if involving sigmoid or transverse sinuses, bruits, headache. Carotid cavernous involvement classically produces proptosis, chemosis, and bruits. Symptoms of SAH, SDH, or ICH
Investigations	MRI (flow void), MRA. Angiography (7% will also have one or more associated aneurysms)	T2WI MRI (non-enhancing) gradient echo sequencing (best for diagnosis)	Non-enhanced CT to r/o hemorrhage. MRI; however, this does not demonstrate the arterial supply to the fistula. Angiography remains the gold standard
Treatment	Decreases risk of future hemorrhage and seizure. Surgical excision is treatment of choice. SRS (stereotactic radiosurgery) is preferred for small (<3 cm) or very deep lesions. Endovascular embolization (glue, balloon) can be curative (5%) or used as adjuvant to surgery or SRS in larger lesions. Conservative (e.g. palliative embolization, seizure control if necessary)	Surgical excision. Only appropriate for symptomatic lesions that are surgically accessible (supratentorial lesions are less likely to bleed than infratentorial lesions)	Approach is dependent on size, location and symptoms, and includes: Conservative treatment, Neuroradiological endovascular interventions, Radiation therapy, Surgery, Combination of the above
Prognosis	10% mortality, 30-50% morbidity (serious neurological deficit) per bleed. Risk of major bleed in untreated AVMs: 2-4% per year		8.1% annual risk of hemorrhage. 6.9% annual risk for non-hemorrhagic neurological deficit. 10.4% mortality rate

Cerebrospinal Fluid Fistulas

Etiology
- cranial or spinal
- traumatic: after head trauma, iatrogenic (post-transsphenoidal surgery, post skull base surgery)
- nontraumatic: high pressure (hydrocephalus, tumour), normal pressure (bone erosion secondary to infection, congenital defect)

Clinical Features
- otorrhea or rhinorrhea (clear fluid)
- low pressure headaches (worse when sitting up)
- confirmatory testing for CSF: beta transferrin test, quantitative glucose analysis of fluid, "ring sign", "reservoir sign"

Investigations
- CT (detect pneumocephalus, fractures, skull base defects), water contrast CT cisternography

Treatment
- lower ICP (avoid straining, acetazolamide to reduce CSF production, modest fluid restriction)
- persistent leak: may require continuous lumbar drainage via percutaneous catheter
- surgical indications: traumatic leak lasting > 2wks, spontaneous leaks, delayed onset of leak after trauma or surgery, leaks complicated by meningitis

EXTRACRANIAL PATHOLOGY

Approach to Limb/Back Pain

- see Orthopedics, OR23

Extradural Lesions

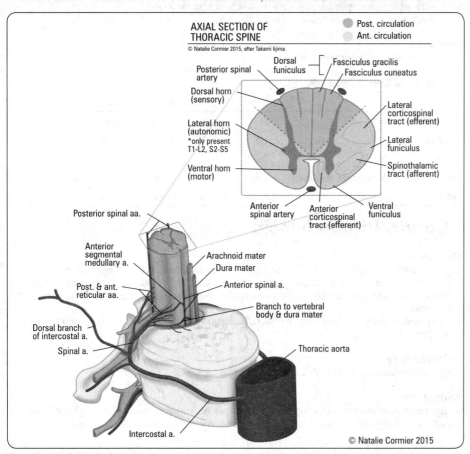

Figure 21. Vascular supply of spinal cord

Suspect CSF fistula in patients with otorrhea or rhinorrhea after head trauma or recurrent meningitis

Ring Sign: If CSF is stringed with blood. Allow CSF to drain onto the surrounding sheets; positive if clear in centre with surrounding blood coloured ring (double ring sign)
Reservoir sign: Gush of CSF leaks out in certain head positions; aka teapot sign (not specific or sensitive)

Stereotactic Radiosurgery for Cavernous Malformations
J Neurosurg 2000;93:987-991
Introduction: The use of radiosurgery for treatment of cerebral cavernous malformations (CM) is controversial. The safety and efficacy of CM radiosurgery is described.
Methods: Retrospective review of 17 patients with CM who underwent radiosurgery over a 10 yr period. All patients had at least 2 documented hemorrhages prior to therapy.
Results: Annual hemorrhage rate 51 mo preceding surgery was 40.1% compared to 8.8% in first 2 yr after radiosurgery and 2.9% thereafter. However, 41% of patients developed a permanent radiation-related morbidity.
Conclusions: Impossible to conclude that radiosurgery protects patients with CMs against future hemorrhage.

RED FLAGS for Back Pain
BACK PAIN
Bowel/**B**ladder (retention or incontinence)
Anesthesia (saddle)
Constitutional symptoms
Khronic disease
Parasthesia
Age >50 yr or <20 yr
IV drug use
Neuromotor deficits
Cauda Equina
- Urinary retention or incontinence, fecal incontinence or loss of anal sphincter tone, saddle anesthesia, uni/bilateral, leg weakness/pain
Malignancy
- Age >50 yr, previous Hx of cancer, pain unrelieved by bed rest, constitutional symptoms
Infection
- Increased ESR, IV drug use, immunosuppressed, fever
Compression Fracture
- Age >50 yr, trauma, prolonged steroid use

Sensory Fibres
Fasciculus gracilis/cuneatus: proprioception, fine touch, vibration
Spinothalamic tract: pain and temperature
Motor Fibres
Corticospinal tract: skilled movements

Disc herniations impinge the nerve root at the level below the interspace (i.e. C5-6 disc affects the C6 nerve root)

Root Compression

Differential Diagnosis
- herniated disc
- neoplasm (neurofibroma, schwannoma)
- synovial cyst, abscess
- hypertrophic bone/spur

Cervical Disc Syndrome

Etiology
- nucleus pulposus herniates through annulus fibrosus and impinges upon nerve root, most commonly at C6-C7 (C7 root)

Clinical Features
- pain in arm follows nerve root distribution, worse with neck extension, ipsilateral rotation, and lateral flexion (all compress the ipsilateral neural foramen)
- LMN signs and symptoms
- central cervical disc protrusion causes myelopathy as well as nerve root deficits

Investigations
- if red flags: C-spine x-ray, CT, MRI (imaging of choice)
- only consider EMG, nerve conduction studies if diagnosis uncertain and presenting more as peripheral nerve issue

Treatment
- **conservative**
  - no bedrest unless severe radicular symptoms
  - activity modification, patient education (reduce sitting, lifting)
  - physiotherapy, exercise programs focus on strengthening core muscles
  - analgesics, NSAIDs are more efficacious
  - avoid cervical manipulation, like traction
- **surgical indications**
  - anterior cervical discectomy is usual approach
  - intractable pain despite adequate conservative treatment for >3 mo
  - progressive neurological deficit

Prognosis
- 95% improve spontaneously in 4-8 wk

Table 14. Lateral Cervical Disc Syndromes

	C4-5	C5-6	C6-7	C7-T1
Root Involved	C5	C6	C7	C8
Incidence	2%	19%	69%	10%
Sensory	Shoulder	Thumb	Middle finger	Ring finger, 5th finger
Motor	Deltoid, biceps, supraspinatus	Biceps	Triceps	Digital flexors, intrinsics
Reflex	No change	Biceps, brachioradialis	Triceps	Finger jerk (Hoffmann's sign)

Cervical Spondylosis

Cervical spondylotic myelopathy is the most common cause of spinal cord impairment

Definition
- progressive degenerative process of cervical spine leading to canal stenosis – congenital spinal stenosis, degeneration of intervertebral discs, hypertrophy of lamina, dura, or ligaments, subluxation, altered mobility, telescoping of the spine due to loss of height of vertebral bodies, alteration of normal lordotic curvature
- resultant syndromes: mechanical neck pain, radiculopathy (root compression), myelopathy (spinal cord compression)

Epidemiology
- typically begins at age 40-50, M>F, most commonly at the C5-C6 > C6-C7 levels

Pathogenesis
- any of: disc degeneration/herniation, osteophyte formation, ossification, and hypertrophy of ligaments
- pathophysiology includes static compression, dynamic compression, and vascular compromise

Clinical Features
- insidious onset of mechanical neck pain exacerbated by excess vertebral motion (particularly rotation and lateral bending with a vertical compressive force – Spurling's test)
- the earliest symptoms are gait disturbance and lower extremity weakness or stiffness
- occipital H/A is common
- radiculopathy may involve 1 or more roots, and symptoms include neck, shoulder and arm pain, paresthesias and numbness
- cervical spondylotic myelopathy (CSM) may present with
  - weakness (upper > lower extremity), lower extremity weakness (corticospinal tracts) is most worrisome complaint
  - decreased dexterity, loss of fine motor control
  - sensory changes
  - UMN findings such as hyperreflexia, clonus, and Babinski reflex
  - funicular pain, characterized by burning and stinging ± Lhermitte's sign (lightning-like sensation down the back with neck flexion)

Investigations
- x-ray of cervical spine ± flexion/extension (alignment, fractures)
- MRI most useful for determination of compression of the neural element
- CT is only used for better determination of bony anatomy (i.e. OPLL)
- EMG/nerve conduction studies reserved for peripheral nerve investigation

Treatment
- nonsurgical: prolonged immobilization with cervical bracing (limit movement to minimize cumulative trauma to spinal cord), bed rest, anti-inflammatory medications
- surgical: anterior approach (anterior cervical discectomy or corpectomy), posterior approach (decompressive cervical laminectomy)
- surgical indications: myelopathy with motor impairment, progressive neurologic impairment, intractable pain
- complete remission almost never occurs. Surgical decompression may stop progression of disease

Lumbar Disc Syndrome

Etiology
- posteriolaterally herniated disc compressed nerve root exiting BELOW the level of the disc or the traversing nerve root
- far lateral disc herniation compressed nerve root AT the level of the disc or the exiting nerve root
- central herniation causes cauda equina or lumbar stenosis (neurogenic claudication)

Clinical Features
- initialy back pain, then leg pain > back pain
- limited back movement (especially forward flexion) due to pain
- motor weakness, dermatomal sensory changes, decreased reflexes
- exacerbation with valsalva; relief with flexing the knee or thigh
- nerve root tension signs
  - straight leg raise (SLR, Lasegue's test) or crossed SLR (pain should occur at less than 60°) suggests L5, S1 root involvement
  - femoral stretch test suggests L2, L3, or L4 root involvement

Investigations
- MRI is modality of choice
- x-ray spine (only to rule out other lesions), CT (bony anatomy)
- myelogram and post-myelogram CT (only if MRI is contraindicated)

Treatment
- conservative (same as cervical disc disease)
- surgical indications: same as cervical disc + cauda equina syndrome

Prognosis
- 95% improve spontaneously within 4-8 wk
- do not follow patients with serial MRIs; clinical status is more important at guiding management

Table 15. Lateral Lumbar Disc Syndromes

	L3-4	L4-5	L5-S1
Root Involved	L4	L5	S1
Incidence	<10%	45%	45%
Pain	Femoral pattern	Sciatic pattern	Sciatic pattern
Sensory	Medial leg	Dorsal foot to hallux Lateral leg	Lateral foot
Motor	Tibialis anterior (dorsiflexion)	Extensor hallucis longus (hallux extension)	Gastrocnemius, soleus (plantar flexion)
Reflex	Knee jerk	Medial hamstrings	Ankle jerk

Efficacy and Safety of Surgical Decompression in Patients with Cervical Spondylotic Myelopathy: Results of the AOSpine North America Prospective Multi-centre Study
J Bone Joint Surg Am. 2013 Sep 18;95(18):1651-8
Purpose: Evaluate impact of surgical decompression on functional, QOL, and disability outcomes 1-yr post-surgery in patients with cervical spondylotic myelopathy.
Methods: 278 patients with mild to severe symptomatic cervical spondylotic myelopathy and MRI evidence of spinal cord compression were followed for 1 yr following surgical decompression. Outcomes (mJOA score, Nurick grade, Neck Disability Index, Short Form-36v2) were compared to preoperative values. Treatment-related complication data was collected.
Results: There was significant improvement (P<0.05) from baseline in mJOA score, Nurick grade, NDI score, and all SF-36v2 health dimensions other than general health. 18.7% of patients experienced complications with no significant differences among the severity groups.
Conclusion: Surgical decompression of cervical spondylotic myelopathy is associated with improved function, disability, and QOL outcomes at 1 yr.

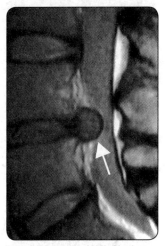

Figure 22. T2 weighted MRI of lumbar disc herniation

Lumbar Disc Herniation: What are Reliable Criterions Indicative for Surgery?
Orthopedics 2009;32:589-597
1) The only clear indication for early surgery in LDH is cauda equina syndrome.
2) Pain may also be an indication for surgery. If conservative treatment is intended, it should be considered for at least 2 mo but not beyond 1 yr if the patient shows minimal improvement, since the beneficial effects of surgery will diminish after this period.
3) The type of herniation on MRI is not relevant to the decision of whether or not to operate on patients with LDH.
4) Although paresis is often a red flag symptom for patients with LDH, neither the magnitude nor the duration of paresis should be used as an indication for early surgery.

Magnetic Resonance Imaging in Follow-Up Assessment of Sciatica
NEJM 2013;368:999-1007
Background: Follow-up MRI is a controversial method for monitoring sciatica in patients with known lumbar-disc herniation.
Methods: Participants (n=283) were recruited from a simultaneous, parallel, randomized study comparing surgery and conservative care for sciatica (the Sciatica Trial). MRI and clinical assessment were undertaken pre-treatment and 1 yr post-treatment randomization to visualize disc herniation and evaluate outcome.
Results: At 1 yr, disc herniation was visible in 35% with a favourable outcome (complete, or nearly complete symptom resolution) and in 33% with an unfavourable outcome (p=0.70). A favourable outcome was reported in 85% of patients with disc herniation and 83% without disc herniation (p=0.70).
Conclusions: Anatomical abnormalities visible on repeated MRI 1 yr after treatment for sciatica due to lumbar-disc herniation could not distinguish patients with resolution of their symptoms from patients still experiencing symptoms.

Causes of Cauda Equina Syndrome
- Lumbar disc herniation
- Spinal stenosis
- Spinal tumour
- Epidural abscess
- Hematoma
- Trauma

Table 16. Differentiating Conus Medullaris Syndrome from Cauda Equina Syndrome

	Conus Medullaris Syndrome	Cauda Equina Syndrome
Onset	Sudden, bilateral	Gradual, unilateral
Spontaneous Pain	Rare, if present usually bilateral, symmetric in perineum or thighs	Severe, radicular type: in perineum, thighs, legs, back, or bladder
Sensory Deficit	Saddle; bilateral and symmetric; sensory dissociation	Saddle; no sensory dissociation; may be unilateral and asymmetric
Motor Deficit	Symmetric; paresis less marked;	
fasciculations may be present	Asymmetric; paresis more marked; atrophy may be present; fasciculations rare	
Reflexes	Only ankle jerk absent (preserved knee jerk)	Knee and ankle jerk may be absent
Autonomic Symptoms (bladder dysfunction, impotence, etc.)	Urinary retention and atonic anal sphincter prominent early; impotence frequent	Sphincter dysfunction presents late; impotence less frequent

Cauda Equina Syndrome

Etiology
- compression or irritation of lumbosacral nerve roots below conus medullaris (below L2 level)
- decreased space in the vertebral canal below L2
- common causes: herniated disc ± spinal stenosis, vertebral fracture, and tumour

Clinical Features
- usually acute (develops in less than 24 h); rarely subacute or chronic
- motor (LMN signs)
  - weakness/paraparesis in multiple root distribution
  - reduced deep tendon reflexes (knee or ankle)
- autonomic
  - urinary retention (or overflow incontinence) and/or fecal incontinence due to loss of anal sphincter tone
- sensory
  - low back pain radiating to legs (sciatica) aggravated by Valsalva maneuver and by sitting; relieved by lying down
  - bilateral sensory loss or pain: depends on the level affected
  - saddle area (S2-S5) anesthesia
  - sexual dysfunction (late finding)

Investigations
- urgent MRI to confirm compression of S2-S3-S4 nerve root by a large disc herniation
- post-void residual very helpful to determine if true retention is present; volumes controversial but anything over 250 cc in a healthy individual is cause for concerns

Treatment
- surgical decompression (<48 h) to preserve bowel, bladder, and sexual function, and/or to prevent progression to paraplegia

Prognosis
- markedly improves with surgical decompression
- recovery correlates with function at initial presentation: if patient is ambulatory, likely to continue to be ambulatory; if unable to walk, unlikely to walk after surgery

Lumbar Spinal Stenosis

Etiology
- congenital narrowing of spinal canal combined with degenerative changes (herniated disc, hypertrophied facet joints, and ligamentum flavum)

Clinical Features
- gradually progressive back and leg pain with standing and walking that is relieved by sitting or lying down (neurogenic claudication – 60% sensitive)
- neurologic exam may be normal, including straight leg raise test

Investigations
- MRI is the optimal investigation to confirm and localize the level of stenosis (unlike nerve root compression which can be localized with clinical exam)

Treatment
- conservative: NSAIDs, analgesia
- surgical: laminectomy with root decompression (the role of fusion may need to be considered if the amount of bone removed with the laminectomy results in destabilization)

Neurogenic Claudication

Etiology
- ischemia of lumbosacral nerve roots secondary to vascular compromise and increased demand from exertion, often associated with lumbar stenosis

Clinical Features
- dermatomal pain/paresthesia/weakness of buttock, hip, thigh, or leg initiated by standing or walking
- slow relief with postural changes (sitting >30 min), NOT simply exertion cessation
- induced by variable degrees of exercise or standing
- may be elicited with lumbar extension, but may not have any other neurological findings, no signs of vascular compromise (e.g. ulcers, poor capillary refill, etc.)

Investigations
- bicycle test may help distinguish neurogenic claudication (NC) from vascular claudication (the waist-flexed individuals on the bicycle with NC can last longer)

Treatment
- same as for lumbar spinal stenosis

> **Key Features of Neurogenic vs. Vascular Claudication**
> **Neurogenic Claudication**: dermatomal distribution with positional relief occurring over minutes
> **Vascular Claudication**: sclerotomal distribution with relief occurring with rest over seconds

Intradural Intramedullary Lesions

Syringomyelia (Syrinx)

Definition
- cystic cavitation of the spinal cord
- presentation is highly variable, usually progresses over months to years
- initially pain, weakness; later atrophy and loss of pain and temperature sensation

Etiology
- 70% are associated with Chiari I malformation, 10% with basilar invagination
- post-traumatic
- tumour
- tethered cord

Clinical Features
- nonspecific features for any intramedullary spinal cord pathology
  - initially pain, weakness, atrophy, loss of pain and temperature in upper extremities (central syrinx) with progressive myelopathy over years
  - sensory loss with preserved touch and proprioception in a band-like distribution at the level of cervical syrinx
  - dysesthetic pain often occurs in the distribution of the sensory loss
  - LMN arm/hand weakness or wasting
  - painless neuropathic arthropathies (Charcot's joints), especially in the shoulder and neck due to loss of pain and temperature sensation

Investigations
- MRI is best method, myelogram with delayed CT

Treatment
- treat underlying cause (e.g. posterior fossa decompression for Chiari I, surgical removal of tumour if causing a syrinx)
- rarely does the syrinx need to be shunted, only when progressive and size allows for insertion of tube

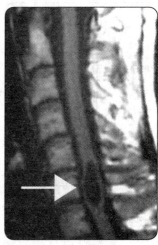

Figure 23. T1 weighted MRI of syringomyelia

Spinal Cord Syndromes

Complete Spinal Cord Lesion
- bilateral loss of motor/sensory and autonomic function at ≥4 segments below lesion/injury, with UMN signs
- about 3% of patients with complete injuries will develop some recovery within 24 h, beyond 24 h, no distal function will recover

Incomplete Spinal Cord Lesion
- any residual function at ≥4 segments below lesion
- signs include sensory/motor function in lower limbs and "sacral sparing" (perianal sensation, voluntary rectal sphincter contraction)

> **American Spinal Injury Association Impairment Scale**
>
> | Grade | Description |
> | --- | --- |
> | A | complete, no motor/sensory below neurological level including S4/5 |
> | B | incomplete, sensory but not motor function preserved below neurological level including S4/5 |
> | C | incomplete, motor function preserved below neurological level, and more than half of the key muscles below neurological level have a muscle grade <3 |
> | D | incomplete, motor function preserved below neurological level, and more than half of the key muscles below neurological level have a muscle grade ≥3 |
> | E | normal motor and sensory function |

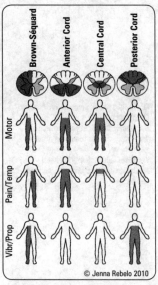

Figure 24. Spinal cord lesion syndromes

Table 17. Comparison Between Incomplete Spinal Cord Lesion Syndromes

Syndrome	Etiology	Motor	Sensory
Brown-Séquard	Hemisection of cord	Ipsilateral LMN weakness at the lesion Ipsilateral UMN weakness below the lesion	Ipsilateral loss of vibration and proprioception Contralateral loss of pain and temperature Preserved light touch
Anterior Cord	Anterior spinal artery compression or occlusion	Bilateral LMN weakness at the lesion Bilateral UMN weakness below the lesion Urinary retention	Preserved vibration and proprioception Bilateral loss of pain and temperature Preserved light touch
Central Cord (most common)	Syringomyelia, tumours, spinal hyperextention injury	Bilateral motor weakness: Upper limb weakness (LMN lesion) > Lower limb weakness (UMN lesion) Urinary retention	Variable bilateral suspended sensory loss Loss of pain and temperature > loss of vibration and proprioception
Posterior Cord	Posterior spinal artery infarction, trauma	Preserved	Bilateral loss of vibration, proprioception, light touch at and below the lesion Preserved pain and temperature

Peripheral Nerves

- see Neurology, N36

Classification

Table 18. Seddon's Classification of Peripheral Nerve Injury

Nerve Injury	Description	Recovery
Neurapraxia (class I)	Axon structurally intact but fails to function	Within hours to months (average 6-8 wk)
Axonotmesis (class II)	Axon and myelin sheath disrupted but endoneurium and supporting structures intact → Wallerian degeneration of axon segment distal to injury	Spontaneous axonal recovery at 1 mm/d, max at 1-2 yr
Neurotmesis (class III)	Nerve completely transected	Need surgical repair for possibility of recovery

Etiology
- ischemia
- nerve entrapment – nerve compressed by nearby anatomic structures, often secondary to localized, repetitive mechanical trauma with additional vascular injury to nerve

Investigations
- clinical exam: power, sensation, reflexes, localization via Tinel's sign (paresthesias elicited by tapping along the course of a nerve)
- electrophysiological studies: EMG, nerve conduction study (assess nerve integrity and monitoring recovery after 2-3 wk post-injury)
- labs: blood work, CSF
- imaging: C-spine, chest/bone x-rays, myelogram, CT, magnetic resonance neurography, angiogram if vascular damage is suspected

Treatment
- early neurosurgical consultation if injury is suspected

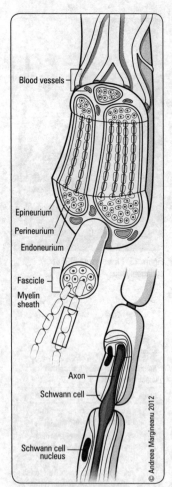

Figure 25. Peripheral nerve structure

Table 19. Treatment by Injury Type

Injury	Treatment
Entrapment	Conservative: prevent repeated stress/injury, physiotherapy, NSAIDs, local anesthesia/steroid injection Surgical: nerve decompression ± transposition for progressive deficits, muscle weakness/atrophy, failure of medical management
Stretch/contusion	Follow-up clinically for recovery; exploration if no recovery in 3 mo
Axonotmesis	If no evidence of recovery, resect damaged segment Prompt physical therapy and rehabilitation to increase muscle function, maintain joint ROM, maximize return of useful function Recovery usually incomplete
Neurotmesis	Surgical repair of nerve sheath unless known to be intact (suture nerve sheaths directly if ends approximate or nerve graft [usually sural nerve]) Clean laceration: early exploration and repair Contamination or associated injuries: tag initially with nonabsorbable suture, reapproach within 10 d

Complications

- neuropathic pain: with neuroma formation
- complex regional pain syndrome: with sympathetic nervous system involvement

SPECIALTY TOPICS

Neurotrauma

Trauma Management (see <u>Emergency Medicine</u>, ER8)

Indications for Intubation in Trauma

1. depressed LOC (patient cannot protect airway): usually GCS ≤8
2. need for hyperventilation
3. severe maxillofacial trauma: patency of airway is doubtful
4. need for pharmacologic paralysis for evaluation or management
   - if basal skull fracture suspected, avoid nasotracheal intubation as may inadvertently enter brain
   - note: intubation prevents patient's ability to verbalize for determining GCS

Trauma Assessment

Initial Management

ABCs of Trauma Management

- see <u>Emergency Medicine</u>, ER8

Neurological Assessment

Mini-History

- period of LOC, post-traumatic amnesia, loss of sensation/function, type of injury/accident

Neurological Exam

- GCS
- head and neck (lacerations, bruises, basal skull fracture signs, facial fractures, foreign bodies)
- spine (palpable deformity, midline pain/tenderness)
- eyes (pupillary size and reactivity)
- brainstem (breathing pattern, CN palsies)
- cranial nerve exam
- motor exam, sensory exam (only if GCS is 15), reflexes
- sphincter tone
- record and repeat neurological exam at regular intervals

Investigations

- spinal injury precautions (cervical collar) are continued until C-spine is cleared
- C,T,L-spine x-rays
   - AP, lateral, odontoid views for C-spine (must see from C1 to T1; swimmer's view if necessary) or CT
   - rarely done: oblique views looking for pars interarticularis fracture ("Scottie dog" sign)
- CT head and upper C-spine (whole C-spine if patient unconscious) look for fractures, loss of mastoid or sinus air spaces, blood in cisterns, pneumocephalus
- cross and type, ABG, CBC, drug screen (especially alcohol)
- chest and pelvic x-ray as indicated

Treatment

Treatment for Minor Head Injury

- observation over 24-48 h
- wake every hour
- judicious use of sedatives or pain killers during monitoring period

Treatment for Severe Head Injury (GCS ≤8)

- clear airway and ensure breathing (if GCS ≤8, intubate)
- secure C-spine
- maintain adequate BP
- monitor for clinical deterioration
- monitor and manage increased ICP if present (see *Herniation Syndromes*, NS6)

Glasgow Coma Scale

Eye Response	Verbal Response	Motor Response
4 spontaneous	5 oriented	6 obeys commands
3 opens eyes to voice	4 confused	5 localizes to pain
2 opens eyes to pain	3 inappropriate words	4 withdraws from pain
1 no eye opening	2 incomprehensible sounds	3 flexion to pain (decorticate posturing)
	1 no response	2 extension to pain (decerebrate posturing)
	T intubated	1 no response

Best response for each component recorded individually (e.g. E3V3M5)
≥13 is mild injury; 9-12 is moderate injury; ≤8 is severe injury

- Never do lumbar puncture in head injury unless increased ICP has been ruled out
- All patients with head injury have C-spine injury until proven otherwise
- Suspect hematoma in alcoholic-related injuries
- Low BP after head injury means injury elsewhere
- Must clear spine both radiologically AND clinically

Assessment of Spine CT/X-Ray (Parasagittal View)
ABCDS
Alignment (columns: anterior vertebral line, posterior vertebral line, spinolaminar line, posterior spinous line)
Bone (vertebral bodies, facets, spinous processes)
Cartilage
Disc (disc space and interspinous space)
Soft tissues

Comparative Effectiveness of Using Computed Tomography Alone to Exclude Cervical Spine Injuries in Obtunded or Intubated Patients: Meta-Analysis of 14,327 Patients with Blunt Trauma
J Neurosurg 2011;115:541-549
Purpose: To determine the effectiveness of helical CT alone (vs. CT and adjuvant imaging such as MR) to diagnose acute unstable cervical spine injury following blunt trauma.
Results: 17 studies with 14,327 patients total. Sensitivity and specificity for modern CT were both >99.9% (95% CI 0.99 -1.00 for both). The negative predictive value of a normal CT scan was 100% (95% CI 0.96-1.00) and accuracy was not affected by the global severity of injury, CT slice thickness, or study quality.
Conclusions: CT alone is sufficient to detect unstable cervical spine injuries in trauma patients and adjuvant imaging is unnecessary with a negative CT scan result. Consequently, if a CT scan is negative for acute injury, the cervical collar may be removed from obtunded or intubated trauma patients.

The Canadian CT Head Rule for Patients with Minor Head Injury
Lancet 2001;357:1391-1396
CT Head is only required for patients with minor head injuries with any one of the following:
High Risk (for neurological intervention)
- GCS score <15 at 2 h after injury.
- Suspected open or depressed skull fracture.
- Any sign of basal skull fracture (hemotympanum, "raccoon" eyes, cerebrospinal fluid otorrhea/ rhinorrhoea, Battle's sign).
- Vomiting ≥2 episodes.
- Age ≥65 yr.
Medium Risk (for brain injury on CT)
- Amnesia after impact >30 min.
- Dangerous mechanism (pedestrian struck by motor vehicle, occupant ejected from motor vehicle, fall from height >3 feet or five stairs).
Minor Head Injury is defined as witnessed loss of consciousness, definite amnesia, or witnessed disorientation in a patient with a GCS score of 13-15.

A Trial of Intracranial-Pressure Monitoring in Traumatic Brain Injury
NEJM 2012;367:2471-2481
Background: ICP monitoring is frequently used to monitor severe traumatic brain injury, but controversy exists over whether it is beneficial.
Methods: Study sample (n=324 patients, ≥13 yr) consisted of those who had severe traumatic brain injury and were being treated in ICU in Bolivia or Ecuador. Patients were randomly assigned to one management group:
1. ICP-monitoring based management.
2. Management based on imaging and clinical examination.
Primary outcome was a composite of survival time, impaired consciousness, functional status (at 3, 6 mo), and neuropsychological status (at 6 mo).
Results: No significant difference between management groups based on primary outcome, 6-mo mortality, median length of ICU stay, or occurrence of serious adverse events. However, duration of brain-specific treatments (e.g. use of hyperosmolar fluids or hyperventilation) higher in the imaging-clinical examination group (4.8 d vs. 3.4 d, p=0.002).
Conclusion: Maintaining monitored ICP at 20 mmHg or less is not superior to care based on imaging and clinical examination.

Admission required if
- skull fracture (indirect signs of basal skull fracture, see *Head Injury*)
- confusion, impaired consciousness, concussion with >5 min amnesia
- focal neurological signs, extreme H/A, vomiting, seizures
- unstable spine
- use of alcohol
- poor social support

Head Injury

Epidemiology
- M:F = 2-3:1

Pathogenesis
- acceleration/deceleration: contusions, subdural hematoma, axon and vessel shearing/mesencephalic hematoma
- impact: skull fracture, concussion, epidural hematoma
- penetrating: worse with high velocity and/or high missile mass
  - low velocity: highest damage to structures on entry/exit path
  - high velocity: highest damage away from missile tract

Scalp Injury
- rich blood supply
- considerable blood loss (vessels contract poorly when ruptured)
- minimal risk of infection due to rich vascularity

Skull Fractures
- depressed fractures: double density on skull x-ray (outer table of depressed segment below inner table of skull), CT with bone window is gold standard
- simple fractures (closed injury): no need for antibiotics, no surgery
- compound fractures (open injury): increased risk of infection, surgical debridement within 24 h is necessary
  - internal fractures into sinus may lead to meningitis, pneumocephalus
  - risk of operative bleed may limit treatment to antibiotics
- basal skull fractures: not readily seen on x-ray, rely on clinical signs
  - retroauricular ecchymoses (Battle's sign)
  - periorbital ecchymoses (raccoon eyes)
  - hemotympanum
  - CSF rhinorrhea, otorrhea (suspect CSF if halo or target sign present); suspect with Lefort II/III midface fracture

Cranial Nerve Injury
- most traumatic causes of cranial nerve injury do not warrant surgical intervention
- surgical intervention
  - CN II: local eye/orbit injury
  - CN III, IV, VI: if herniation secondary to mass
  - CN VIII: repair of ossicles
- CN injuries that improve
  - CN I: recovery may occur in a few months; most do not improve
  - CN III, IV, VI: majority recover
  - CN VII: recovery with delayed lesions
  - CN VIII: vestibular symptoms improve over weeks, deafness usually permanent (except when resulting from hemotympanum)

Arterial Injury
- e.g. carotid-cavernous (C-C) fistula, carotid/vertebral artery dissection

Intracranial Bleeding
- see *Blood*, NS15 and *Cerebrovascular Disease*, NS17

Brain Injury

Primary Impact Injury
- mechanism of injury determines pathology: penetrating injuries, direct impact
  - low velocity: local damage
  - high velocity: distant damage possible (due to wave of compression), concussion
- **concussion**: a trauma-induced alteration in mental status
  - American Academy of Neurology (AAN) Classification
  - no parenchymal abnormalities on CT

- **coup** (damage at site of blow) and **contrecoup** (damage at opposite site of blow)
  - acute decompression causes cavitation followed by a wave of acute compression
- **contusion** (hemorrhagic)
  - high density areas on CT ± mass effect
  - commonly occurs with brain impact on bony prominences (inferior frontal lobe, pole of temporal lobe)
- **diffuse axonal injury/shearing**
  - wide variety of damage results
  - may tear blood vessels (hemorrhagic foci)
  - often the cause of decreased LOC if no space-occupying lesion on CT

Secondary Pathologic Processes
- same subsequent biochemical pathways for each traumatic etiology
- delayed and progressive injury to the brain due to
  - high glutamate release → NMDA receptor activation → cytotoxic cascade
  - cerebral edema
  - intracranial hemorrhages
  - ischemia/infarction
  - raised ICP, intracranial HTN
  - hydrocephalus

Extracranial Conditions
- hypoxemia
  - due to trauma to the chest, upper airway, brainstem
  - extremely damaging to vulnerable brain cells
  - leads to ischemia, raised ICP
- hypercarbia
  - leads to raised ICP (secondary to vasodilation)
  - systemic hypotension
  - caused by blood loss (e.g. ruptured spleen)
  - loss of cerebral autoregulation leads to decreased CPP, ischemia
- hyperpyrexia
  - leads to increased brain metabolic demands → ischemia
- fluid and electrolyte imbalance
  - iatrogenic (most common)
  - SIADH caused by head injury
  - diabetes insipidus (DI)
  - may lead to cerebral edema and raised ICP
- coagulopathy

Intracranial Conditions
- raised ICP due to traumatic cerebral edema OR traumatic intracranial hemorrhage

Brain Injury Outcomes
- mildly traumatic (GCS 13-15): post-concussive symptoms: H/A, fatigue, dizziness nausea, blurred vision, diplopia, memory impairment, tinnitus, irritability, low concentration; 50% at 6 wk, 14% at 1 yr
- moderately traumatic (GCS 9-12): proportional to age (>40) and CT findings; 60% good recovery, 26% moderately disabled, 7% severely disabled, 7% vegetative/dead
- severe (GCS ≤8): difficult to predict, correlates with post-resuscitation GCS (especially motor) and age

Late Complications of Head/Brain Injury

- seizures: 5% of head injury patients develop seizures
  - incidence related to severity and location of injury (increased with local brain damage or intracranial hemorrhage)
  - post-traumatic seizure may be immediate, early, or late
  - presence of early (within first wk) post-traumatic seizure raises incidence of late seizures
- meningitis: associated with CSF leak from nose or ear
- hydrocephalus: acute hydrocephalus or delayed normal pressure hydrocephalus (NPH)

Spinal Cord Injury

- see Orthopedics, OR22 and Emergency Medicine, ER9

NEUROGENIC AND SPINAL SHOCK
1. neurogenic shock: hypotension that follows SCI (sBP usually ≤80 mmHg) caused by
   - interruption of sympathetics (unopposed parasympathetics) below the level of injury
   - loss of muscle tone due to skeletal muscle paralysis below level of injury → venous pooling (relative hypovolemia)
   - blood loss from associated wounds (true hypovolemia)

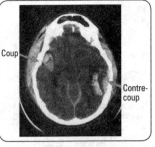

Figure 26. CT showing coup-contrecoup injury

AAN Classification
Grade 1: altered mental status <15 min
Grade 2: altered mental status >15 min
Grade 3: any loss of consciousness

SIADH → hyponatremia
DI → hypernatremia

Concussion Grades

AAN Grade	Management Options
1	Examine 15 min for amnesia and other symptoms Return to normal activity if symptoms clear within 15 min
2	Remove from activity for 1 d, then re-examine CT or MRI if H/A or other symptoms worsen or last >1 wk Return to normal activity after 1 wk without symptoms
3	Emergent neurological exam + imaging; if initial exam is normal, may go home with close follow-up Admit if any signs of pathology or persistent abnormal mental status CT or MRI if H/A or other symptoms If brief loss of consciousness (<1 min), return to normal activity after 1 wk without symptoms If prolonged loss of consciousness (>1 min), return to normal activity only after 2 wk without symptoms

Resolution of spinal shock is indicated by the return of reflexes (most commonly the bulbocavernous reflex)

Pharmacological Therapy for Acute Spinal Cord Injury: Congress of Neurological Surgeons (CNS) and American Association of Neurological Surgeons (AANS) Guidelines
Neurosurgery 2013;72(Suppl 2):93-105
Level I Recommendations
• No Class I or Class II medical evidence supports the use of methylprednisone in the treatment of acute SCI. Several Class II and Class III studies have been published stating inconsistent effects of methylprednisone likely related to random chance or selection bias.
• Administration of GM-1 ganglioside (Sygen) for the treatment of acute SCI is not recommended.

Early vs. Delayed Decompression for Traumatic Cervical Spinal Cord Injury: Results of the Surgical Timing in Acute Spinal Cord Injury Study (STASCIS)
PLoS ONE 2012;7:e32037. doi:10.1371/journal.pone.0032037
Introduction: This study sought to determine the relative effectiveness of early (<24 h after injury) versus late (≥24 h after injury) decompressive surgery following a traumatic cervical spinal cord injury (SCI).
Methods/Population: A prospective cohort study completed in 2002-2009 involving 6 North American institutions. Participants were 16-80 yr with a cervical SCI. Outcomes evaluated were changes in American Spinal Injury Association Impairment Scale (AIS) grade at 6 mo follow-up, complications, and mortality.
Results: Of 313 participants enrolled, 182 underwent early surgery and 131 underwent late surgery. 222 participants were available for follow-up at 6 mo. The odds of at least 2 grade AIS improvement were greater for those who had early surgery compared to those with late surgery (OR = 2.83, 95% CI 1.10, 7.28). Mortality was observed for each group during the first 30 d post injury. No statistically significant differences were observed for complications (p=0.21).
Conclusion: Early decompression surgery following a SCI is safe and associated with higher AIS improvement at 6 mo following injury.

A New Classification of Thoracolumbar Injuries: The Importance of Injury Morphology, the Integrity of the Posterior Ligamentous Complex, and Neurological Status
Spine 2005;30:2325-2333
Introduction: To devise a practical and comprehensive classification system to assist in clinical decision of operative or non-operative thoracolumbar injuries.
Methods/Population: Spine trauma specialists contributed factors that were deemed important for clinical decisions regarding thoracolumbar trauma.
Results: A new classification system called the Thoracolumbar Injury Classification and Severity Score (TLICS) was devised based on three parameters: 1) morphology of the injury determined radiographically, 2) integrity of posterior ligamentous complex, and 3) neurological status.
Conclusion: An easy to apply and clinically relevant decision making tool regarding thoracolumbar trauma.

2. spinal shock: transient loss of all neurologic function below the level of the spinal cord injury, causing flaccid paralysis and areflexia for variable periods

Whiplash-Associated Disorders
• definition: traumatic injury to the soft tissue structures in the region of the cervical spine due to hyperflexion, hyperextension, or rotational injury to the neck

Initial Management of SCI
• major causes of death in SCI are aspiration and shock
• the following patients should be treated as having a SCI until proven otherwise:
• all victims of significant trauma
• minor trauma patients with decreased LOC or complaints of neck or back pain, weakness, abdominal breathing, numbness/tingling, or priapism

Stabilization and Initial Evaluation in the Hospital
1. ABCs, immobilization (backboard/head strap), oxygenation, Foley catheter to urometer, temperature regulation
2. hypotension: maintain sBP >90 mmHg with pressors (dopamine), hydration, and atropine
   ◆ DVT prophylaxis
3. monitor CBC/electrolytes
4. focused history (see *Trauma Assessment*, NS29)
5. spine palpation: point tenderness or deformity
6. motor level assessment (including rectal exam for voluntary anal sphincter contraction)
7. sensory level assessment: pinprick, light touch, and proprioception
8. evaluation of reflexes
9. signs of autonomic dysfunction: altered level of perspiration, bowel or bladder incontinence, priapism
10. radiographic evaluation
    ◆ 3 views C-spine x-rays (AP, lateral, and odontoid) to adequately visualize C1 to C7-T1 junction
    ◆ flexion-extension views to disclose occult instability
    ◆ CT scan (bony injuries) typically most trauma centres use CT as the modality of choice for looking at fractures, very sensitive with the high resolution scanners
    ◆ MRI mandatory if neurological deficits (soft tissue injuries)

Medical Management Specific to SCI
• option: methylprednisolone (given within 8 h of injury) this is controversial and you need to confer with Neurosurgery service
• ± decompression in acute, non-penetrating SCI

Fractures of the Spine

FRACTURES AND FRACTURE-DISLOCATIONS OF THE THORACIC AND LUMBAR SPINE
• assess ligamentous instability using flexion/extension x-ray views of ± MRI
• thoracolumbar spine unstable if 4/6 segments disrupted (3 columns divided into left and right)
  ▪ anterior column: anterior half of vertebral body, disc, and anterior longitudinal ligament
  ▪ middle column: posterior half of vertebral body, disc, and posterior longitudinal ligament
  ▪ posterior column: posterior arch, facet joints, pedicle, lamina and supraspinous, interspinous, and ligamentum ligaments

Types of Injury

Table 20. Denis Classification of Spinal Trauma

Fracture Type	Description
Compression Fracture (58%)	Produced by flexion Posterior ligament complex (supraspinous and interspinous ligaments, ligamentum flavum, and intervertebral joint capsules) remain intact Fractures are stable but lead to kyphotic deformity

Burst Fracture (17%)	Stable: anterior and middle columns parted with bone retropulsed nearby
	    Hallmark is pedicle widening on AP x-ray
	    Spinal cord (seen on x-ray and CT); posterior column is uninjured
	Unstable: same as the stable but with posterior column disruption (usually ligamentous)

Flexion Distraction Injury (6%)	Hyperflexion and distraction of posterior elements Middle and posterior columns fail in distraction Classic: Chance = horizontal fracture through posterior arch, pedicles, posterior vertebral body Can be purely ligamentous, i.e. through PLL and disc
Fracture-Dislocation (6%)	Anterior and cranial dislocation of superior vertebral body → 3 column failure Three types: (1) flexion-rotation, (2) flexion-distraction, (3) shear/hyperextension (rare)

Management of Thoracolumbar Injury
- severity and management based on TLICS classification

FRACTURES OF THE CERVICAL SPINE

Types of Injury

Table 21. Fracture Patterns of the Cervical Spine

Fracture Type	Description
C1 Vertebral Fracture (Jefferson fracture)	Vertical compression forces the occipital condyles of the skull down on the C1 vertebra (atlas), pushing the lateral masses of the atlas outward and disrupting the ring of the atlas Also can cause an occipital condylar fracture

Odontoid Fracture	Causes C1 and odontoid of C2 to move independently of C2 body
	This occurs because
	   Normally C1 vertebra and odontoid of C2 are a single functional unit
	   Alar and transverse ligaments on posterior aspect of odontoid usually remain intact after injury
	Patients often report a feeling of instability and present holding their head with their hands
	Type II fracture the most common

C2 Vertebral Fracture (hangman fracture)	Bilateral fracture through the pars interarticularis of C2 with subluxation of C2 on C3 (spondylolisthesis of axis) Usually neurologically intact
Clay-Shoveler Fracture	Avulsion of spinous process, usually C6 or C7

Imaging
- AP spine x-ray (open-mouth and lateral view), CT

Treatment
- immobilization in cervical collar or halo vest until healing occurs (usually 2-3 mo)
- Type II and III odontoid fractures
- consider surgical fixation for comminution, displacement, or inability to maintain alignment with external immobilization
- confirm stability after recovery with flexion-extension x-rays

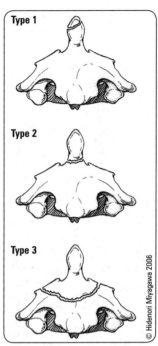

Figure 27. Odontoid fracture classification

Neurologically Determined Death

Definition
- irreversible and diffuse brain injury resulting in absence of clinical brain function
- cardiovascular activity may persist for up to 2 wk

Criteria of Diagnosis
- prerequisites: no CNS depressant drugs/neuromuscular blocking agents, no drug intoxication/poisoning, temperature >32°C, no electrolyte/acid-base/endocrine disturbance
- absent brainstem reflexes: pupillary light reflex, corneal reflexes, oculocephalic response, caloric responses (e.g. no deviation of eyes to irrigation of each ear with 50 cc of ice water – allow 1 min after injection, 5 min between sides), pharyngeal and tracheal reflexes, cough with tracheal suctioning, absent respiratory drive at PaCO$_2$ >60 mmHg or >20 mmHg above baseline (apnea test)
- 2 evaluations separated by time, usually performed by two specialists (e.g. anesthetist, neurologist, neurosurgeon)
- confirmatory testing: flat EEG, absent perfusion assessed with cerebral angiogram

Coma

Definition
- an unrousable state in which patients show no meaningful response to environmental stimuli

Pathophysiology
- lesions affecting the cerebral cortex bilaterally, the reticular activating system (RAS) or their connecting fibres
- focal supratentorial lesions do not alter consciousness except by herniation (compression on the brainstem or on the contralateral hemisphere) or by precipitating seizures

Classification
- structural lesions (tumour, pus, blood, infarction, CSF): 1/3 of comas
  - supratentorial mass lesion: leads to herniation
  - infratentorial lesion: compression of or direct damage to the RAS or its projections

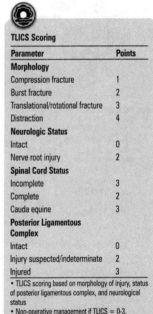

TLICS Scoring

Parameter	Points
Morphology	
Compression fracture	1
Burst fracture	2
Translational/rotational fracture	3
Distraction	4
Neurologic Status	
Intact	0
Nerve root injury	2
Spinal Cord Status	
Incomplete	3
Complete	2
Cauda equine	3
Posterior Ligamentous Complex	
Intact	0
Injury suspected/indeterminate	2
Injured	3

- TLICS scoring based on morphology of injury, status of posterior ligamentous complex, and neurological status
- Non-operative management if TLICS = 0-3, operative management if TLICS = 5+, either operative or non-operative if TLICS = 4

- metabolic disorders/diffuse hemispheric damage: 2/3 of comas
  - deficiency of essential substrates (e.g. oxygen, glucose, vitamin B12)
  - exogenous toxins (e.g. drugs, heavy metals, solvents)
  - endogenous toxins/systemic metabolic diseases (e.g. uremia, hepatic encephalopathy, electrolyte imbalances, thyroid storm)
  - infections (meningitis, encephalitis)
  - trauma (concussion, diffuse shear axonal damage)

Investigations and Management

- ABCs
- labs: electrolytes, extended electrolytes, TSH, LFTs, Cr, BUN, toxin screen, glucose
- CT/MRI, LP, EEG

Persistent Vegetative State

Definition

- a condition of complete unawareness of the self and the environment accompanied by sleep-wake cycles with either complete or partial preservation of hypothalamic and brainstem autonomic function
- "awake but not aware"
- follows comatose state

Etiology/Prognosis

- most commonly caused by cardiac arrest or head injury
- due to irreversible loss of cerebral cortical function but intact brainstem function
- average life expectancy is 2-5 yr

Pediatric Neurosurgery

Spinal Dysraphism

Table 22. Summary of Spinal Dysraphic Anomolies

	SPINA BIFIDA OCCULTA	MENINGOCELE (SPINA BIFIDA APERTA)	MYELOMENINGOCELE (SPINA BIFIDA APERTA)
Definition	Congenital absence of a spinous process and a variable amount of lamina No visible exposure of meninges or neural tissue	Herniation of meningeal tissue and CSF through a defect in the spine, without associated herniation of neural tissue	Herniation of meningeal and CNS tissue through a defect in the spine
Epidemiology	15-20% of the general population; most common at L5 or S1	0.1-0.2% of live births	0.1-0.2% of live births
Etiology		Failure of fusion of posterior neural arch	Primary failure of neural tube closure
Clinical Features	No obvious clinical signs Presence of lumbosacral cutaneous abnormalities (dimple, sinus, port-wine stain, or hair tuft) should increase suspicion of an underlying anomaly (lipoma, dermoid, diastematomyelia)	Most common in lumbosacral area Usually no disability, low incidence of associated anomalies, and hydrocephalus	Sensory and motor changes distal to anatomic level producing varying degrees of weakness Urinary and fecal incontinence Hydrocephalus (65-85% of patients) Most have Type II Chiari malformation (see *Chiari Malformations*, NS36)
Investigations	Plain film: absence of the spinous process and minor amounts of the neural arch U/S, MRI to exclude spinal anomalies	Plain films, CT, MRI, U/S, echo, GU investigations	Plain films, CT, MRI, U/S, echo, GU investigations
Treatment	Requires no treatment	Surgical excision and tissue repair	Surgical closure to preserve neurologic status and prevent CNS infections Closure *in utero* shown to decrease hydrocephalus and improve post natal motor scores
Prognosis	Generally good prognosis	Good prognosis with surgical treatment	Operative mortality close to 0%, 95% 2-yr survival 80% have IQ >80 (but most are 80-95), 40-85% ambulatory, 3-10% have normal urinary continence Early mortality: usually due to Chiari malformation complications (respiratory arrest, aspiration), late mortality: due to shunt malfunction

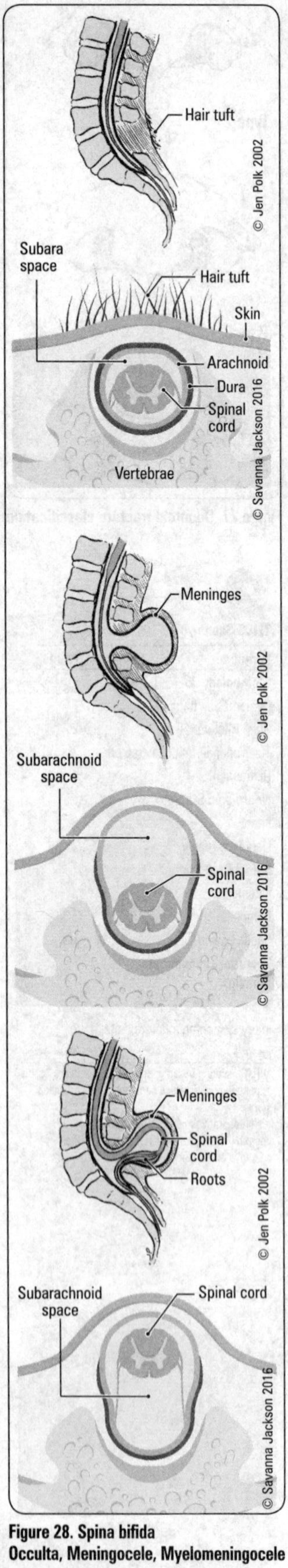
Hair tuft
© Jen Polk 2002
Subara space
Hair tuft
Skin
Arachnoid
Dura
Spinal cord
Vertebrae
© Savanna Jackson 2016
Meninges
© Jen Polk 2002
Subarachnoid space
Spinal cord
© Savanna Jackson 2016
Meninges
Spinal cord
Roots
© Jen Polk 2002
Subarachnoid space
Spinal cord
© Savanna Jackson 2016

Figure 28. Spina bifida Occulta, Meningocele, Myelomeningocele

Intraventricular Hemorrhage

- see Pediatrics, P68

Hydrocephalus in Pediatrics

Etiology
- congenital
  - aqueductal anomalies, primary aqueductal stenosis in infancy
  - secondary gliosis due to intrauterine viral infections (mumps, varicella, TORCH)
  - Dandy-Walker malformation (2-4%)
  - Chiari malformation, especially Type II
  - myelomeningocele
- acquired
  - post meningitis
  - post hemorrhage (SAH, IVH)
  - masses (vascular malformation, neoplastic)

Clinical Features
- symptoms and signs of hydrocephalus are age related in pediatrics
- increased head circumference (HC), bulging anterior fontanelle, widened cranial sutures
- irritability, lethargy, poor feeding, and vomiting
- "cracked pot" sound on cranial percussion
- scalp vein dilation (increased collateral venous drainage)
- sunset sign – forced downward deviation of eyes
- episodic bradycardia and apnea

Investigations
- skull x-ray, U/S, CT, MRI, ICP monitoring

Treatment
- similar to adults (see *Hydrocephalus Treatment*, NS9)

Dandy-Walker Malformation

Definition
- atresia of foramina of Magendie and Luschka, resulting in:
  - complete or incomplete agenesis of the cerebellar vermis with widely separated, hypoplastic cerebellar hemispheres
  - posterior fossa cyst, enlarged posterior fossa
  - dilatation of 4th ventricle (also 3rd and lateral ventricles)
- associated anomalies
  - hydrocephalus (90%)
  - agenesis of corpus callosum (17%)
  - occipital encephalocele (7%)

Epidemiology
- 2-4% of pediatric hydrocephalus

Clinical Features
- 20% are asymptomatic, seizures occur in 15%
- symptoms and signs of hydrocephalus combined with a prominent occiput in infancy
- ataxia, spasticity, poor fine motor control common in childhood

Investigations
- ultrasound, CT, MRI

Treatment
- asymptomatic patients require no treatment
- associated hydrocephalus requires surgical treatment
- e.g. ventriculoperitoneal (VP) shunt, cystoperitoneal (CP) shunt, lumboperitoneal (LP) shunt, ventriculoatrial (VA) shunt, lumbar drain

Prognosis
- 75-100% survival, 50% have normal IQ

Chiari Malformations

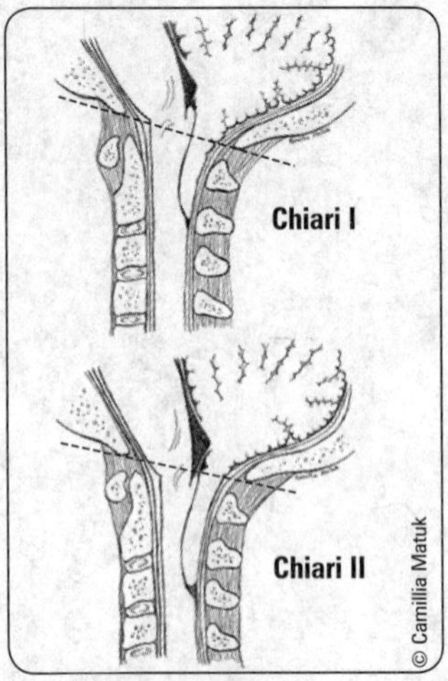

Definition
- malformations at the medullary-spinal junction

Etiology
- unclear, likely maldevelopment/dysgenesis during fetal life

Categories

Chiari I

Chiari II

© Camillia Matuk

Figure 29. Chiari malformations

Table 23. Categories of Chiari Malformations

	Type I	Type II
Definition	Cerebellar tonsils lie below the level of the foramen magnum	Part of cerebellar vermis, medulla, and 4th ventricle extend through the foramen magnum often to midcervical region
Epidemiology	Average age at presentation 15 yr	Present in infancy
Clinical Features	Many are aysmptomatic Pain (69%), weakness (56%), numbness (52%), loss of temperature sensation (40%) Central cord syndrome (65%) Foramen magnum compression syndrome (22%), Cerebellar syndrome (11%), Syringomyelia (50%), Hydrocephalus (10%)	Findings due to brainstem and lower cranial nerve dysfunction Neurogenic dysphagia (69%), apnea (58%), stridor (56%), aspiration (40%), arm weakness (27%), downbeat nystagmus Respiratory arrest is the most common cause of mortality Usually associated with myelomingocele and hydrocephalus
Investigations	MRI	MRI
Treatment	Symptomatic patients (early surgery recommended; <2 yr post symptom onset) → suboccipital craniectomy, duraplasty	Preserved When symptomatic, check the shunt first. Then consider surgical decompression (which does not reverse intrinsic brainstem abnormalities) → cervical laminectomy, duraplasty

Craniosynostosis

Definition
- premature closure of the cranial suture(s)

Classification
- sagittal (most common): long narrow head with ridging sagittal suture (scaphocephaly)
- coronal: expansion in superior and lateral direction (brachiocephaly)
- metopic (trigonocephaly)
- lambdoid: least common

Epidemiology
- 0.6/1,000 live births, most cases are sporadic; familial incidence is 2% of sagittal and 8% of coronal synostosis

Clinical Features
- skull deformity, raised ICP ± hydrocephalus
- ophthalmologic problems due to increased ICP or bony abnormalities of the orbit
- must differentiate between positional plagiocephaly (secondary to back sleeping)

Investigations
- plain radiographs, CT scan

Treatment
- parental counselling about nature of deformity, associated neurological symptoms
- surgery for cosmetic purposes, except in cases of elevated ICP (≥2 sutures involved)

Pediatric Brain Tumours

- see *Tumours*, NS10

Epidemiology
- 20% of all pediatric cancers (second only to leukemia)
- 60% of pediatric brain tumours are infratentorial
- pediatric brain tumours arise from various cellular lineages
  - glia: low-grade astrocytoma (supra- or infratentorial), anaplastic astrocytoma, glioblastoma multiforme (largely supratentorial) (see *Astrocytoma*, NS12)
  - primitive nerve cells: supratentorial PNET
    - 90% of neonatal brain tumours, infratentorial (medulloblastoma), pineal gland (pineoblastoma)
  - non-neuronal cells: germ cell tumour, craniopharyngioma, dermoid, meningioma, neurinoma (schwanoma), pituitary adenoma, others

Most Common Pediatric Brain Tumours
Astrocytoma, low grade
Supratentorial
Infratentorial
Medulloblastoma
Ependymoma
Gliobastoma

Clinical Features
- vomiting, seizure, macrocrania, hydrocephalus
- developmental delay, poor feeding, failure to thrive
- often initially escapes diagnosis due to expansile cranium and neural plasticity in children

Table 24. Overview of Childhood Primary Brain Tumours

Pilocytic (low grade) Astrocytoma	Usually in posterior fossa Well circumscribed Benign, good prognosis
Medulloblastoma	A primitive neuroectodermal tumour (PNET) In cerebellum → compresses 4th ventricle → hydrocephalus Highly malignant
Ependymoma	In 4th ventricle → hydrocephalus Poor prognosis
Hemangioblastoma	Often cerebellar Associated with von Hippel-Lindau syndrome with retinal angiomas Can produce EPO → secondary polycythemia
Craniopharyngioma	Causes bitemporal hemianopsia (thus often confused with pituitary adenoma) Most common supratentorial childhood tumour Benign

Functional Neurosurgery

Movement Disorders

- see Neurology, *Tremor*, N31, *Parkinson's Disease*, N32, *Dystonia*, N33, and *Multiple Sclerosis*, N52

Table 25. Surgical Targets for Movement Disorders

Disorder	Indications	Procedures	Outcomes	Morbidity
Parkinson's Disease	Intractable contralateral bradykinesia/tremor Failure of medical management (advanced disease) Drug-induced dyskinesias (see dystonia, below)	Simultaneous, bilateral surgery/stimulation is most common Preferred target: anterodorsal subthalamic nucleus (STN) Other targets: stereotactic ablation (pallidotomy)/stimulation of posteroventral globus pallidus pars interna (GPi) Caudal zona incerta Parkinsonian tremor: stereotactic ablation (thalamotomy)/stimulation of ventral intermediate (Vim) nucleus of thalamus	39-48% improvement in Unified Parkinson's Disease Rating Scale (UPDRS) scores Reduced dosage of medications (STN) More effective than medical management in advanced PD Early intervention may reduce severity, course, and progression of disease Of little benefit for patients with atypical presentations	Intracerebral hemorrhage, infection, seizure (1%-4%) Paresthesias Involuntary movements Cognitive functioning: decreased lexical fluency, impaired executive function (STN > GPi) Psychiatric: depression, mania, anxiety, apathy (STN > GPi)
Dystonia	Contralateral primary (generalized) dystonias; cervical and tardive dystonias (GPi) Contralateral secondary dyskinesia (i.e. drug-induced: L-dopa, neuroleptics; STN)	Preferred target (primary dystonia): stereotactic ablation (pallidotomy/stimulation of posteroventral GPi Secondary dystonia: stimulation of anterodorsal STN Stimulation of ventral posterior lateral (VPL) thalamic nucleus	Primary dystonia: 51% reduction in Burke-Fahn-Marsden Dystonia Scale (BFMDS) score Secondary dystonia: 62-89% improvement in dystonias Delayed effects: weeks to months	Intracerebral hemorrhage, infection, seizure (1%-4%) Minor effects on cognitive functioning (especially decreased lexical fluency; STN > GPi)
Tremor	Contralateral appendicular ET (first disorder to be treated by DBS; DBS is viable alternative to Rx) Intention tremor (IT) resulting from demyelination of cerebellar outflow tracts (e.g. in multiple sclerosis) Brainstem tremor (Holmes tremor)	Preferred target: stereotactic ablation (thalamotomy)/stimulation of Vim nucleus of thalamus Other targets: stimulation of caudal zona incerta Parkinsonian tremor: stimulation of anterodorsal STN	Durable reductions in essential tremor rating scale (ETRS) scores Reduced dosage of medications Conflicting data on vocal/facial tremor	Intracerebral hemorrhage, infection, seizure (1%-4%) Paresthesias/pain Dysarthria Ataxia Minor effects on cognitive functioning (especially decreased lexical fluency) Tolerance may develop over time

Neuropsychiatric Disorders

- see <u>Neurology</u>, N34 and <u>Psychiatry</u> for Tourette's Syndrome, Obsessive Compulsive Disorder and Depression

Table 26. Surgical Targets for Neuropsychiatric Disorders

Disorder	Indications	Procedures	Outcomes	Morbidity
Obsessive Compulsive Disorder (OCD)	Severe symptoms refractory to medical management	Anterior capsulotomy/ stimulation of the anterior limb of the internal capsule (IC)	Currently under investigation Reportedly 25-75% response rate	Intracerebral hemorrhages (1-2%) Mild effects on cognitive functioning Anxiety ± panic disorder (case report)
Tourette's Syndrome	Severe symptoms refractory to medical management	Stimulation of midline intralaminar nuclei of the thalamus Stimulation of motor and limbic portions of GPi Stimulation of the anterior limb of the IC	Currently under investigation Reportedly >70% reduction in vocal or motor tics + urge	Intracerebral hemorrhages (1-2%) Mild sexual dysfunction
Major Depressive Disorder (MDD)	Severe depression refractory to medical management and ECT	Stimulation of the subgenual cingulate cortex	Currently under investigation Reportedly 60% response rate; 35% remission rate	Intracerebral hemorrhages (1-2%) Pain, H/A Worsening mood, irritability

Chronic Pain

Table 27. Surgical Targets for Chronic Pain

Disorder	Indications	Procedures	Outcomes	Morbidity
Neuropathic Pain	Severe, intractable, organic neuropathic pain (e.g. post-stroke pain, phantom limb pain, trigeminal neuralgia, chronic low-back pain, complex regional pain syndrome)	Preferred target: stimulation of the contralateral VPL VPM thalamic nuclei ± periventricular/ periaqueductal grey matter (PVG/PAG) Other targets: stimulation of the contralateral IC Stimulation of the contralateral motor cortex	47% improvement in perception of pain intensity Less favourable results in central pain syndromes and poorly localized pain	Intracerebral hemorrhages (1-2%) Paresthesia Anxiety ± panic disorder
Nociceptive Pain	Severe, intractable, organic nociceptive pain	Bilateral (most common) stimulation of the PVG/PAG	Reportedly 63% improvement in perception of pain intensity	Intracerebral hemorrhages (1-2%) Paresthesia Anxiety ± panic disorder

Surgical Management of Epilepsy

- see <u>Neurology</u>, N19 for the medical treatment of epilepsy

Indications
- medically refractory seizures, usually defined as seizures resistant to two first line anti-seizure medications used in succession
- identification of a distinct epileptogenic region through clinical history, EEG, MRI, and neuropsychological testing; other localizing investigations include magnetoencephalography, SPECT, and PET
- if a distinct epileptogenic region cannot be identified, the patient may be a candidate for a palliative procedure such as corpus callosotomy

Procedure
- adults: resection of the hippocampus and parahippocampal gyrus for mesial temporal lobe epilepsy arising from mesial temporal sclerosis
- children: resection of an epileptogenic space-occupying lesion
- hemispherectomy and corpus callosotomy are less common

Outcomes
- 41-79% of adult patients are seizure free for 5 yr after temporal lobe resection
- 58-78% of children are seizure free after surgery
- surgery is associated with improvements in preexisting psychiatric conditions such as depression and anxiety, as well as improvement in quality of life measures

Morbidity
- 0.4-4% of surgical patients will have partial hemianopsia, aphasia, motor deficit, sensory deficit, or cranial nerve palsy following anteromedial temporal lobectomies
- most patients will have some decline in verbal memory following dominant temporal lobectomy and in visuospatial memory in non-dominant temporal resection
- the degree of memory decline stabilizes after 1-2 yr

Predictors
- positive predictive factors for seizure freedom following anteromedial temporal lobectomy
  - hippocampal sclerosis (unilateral)
  - focal localization of interictal epileptiform discharges
  - absence of pre-operative generalized seizures
  - tumoural cause
  - complete resection of the lesion

A Randomized, Controlled Trial of Surgery for Temporal Lobe Epilepsy
NEJM 2001;345:311-318
Introduction: This RCT evaluates the efficacy and safety of neurosurgery for temporal lobe epilepsy. **Methods**: 80 patients with poorly controlled temporal lobe epilepsy were randomized for surgery (n=40) or for continued treatment with antiepileptic drugs (n=40). The primary outcome was freedom from seizures that impair awareness of self and surroundings during the period of 1 yr. Secondary outcomes included frequency and severity of seizures, quality of life, disability and death. **Results**: The surgical group had higher cumulative proportion of patients without seizures impairing awareness compared to the medical group (p<0.01). The surgical group also had lower seizure frequency (p<0.001) and better quality of life (p<0.001). 4 patients in the surgical group had adverse effects (thalamic infarct, n=1; wound infection, n=1; verbal memory decline impairment occupation, n=2). One patient in the medical group died; no patients died in the surgical group. **Conclusions**: In patients with poorly controlled temporal-lobe epilepsy, surgery is superior to prolonged medical therapy.

Surgical Management for Trigeminal Neuralgia

- reserved for cases refractory to medical management; see <u>Neurology</u>, N42 for medical management

Surgical Options
- trigeminal nerve branch procedures
  - local blocks (phenol, alcohol)
  - neurectomy of the trigeminal branch
  - nerve branches
    - V1 block at the supraorbital, supratrochlear nerves
    - V2 block at the foramen rotundum or infraorbital nerves
    - V3 block at the foramen ovale
- percutaneous trigeminal rhizotomy
  - glycerol injection
  - mechanotrauma via catheter balloon
- radiofrequency thermocoagulation
- Gamma Knife® radiosurgery
- microvascular decompression
  - posterior fossa craniotomy with microsurgical exploration of the root entry zone, displacement of the vessel impinging on the nerve with placement of non-absorbable Teflon® felt

References

Adzick N, Thom E, Spong C, et al. A randomized trial of prenatal versus postnatal repair of myelomeningocele. NEJM 2011;364:993-1004.

Ahn NU, Ahn UM, Nallamshetty L, et al. Cauda equina syndrome in ankylosing spondylitis (the CES-AS syndrome): meta-analysis of outcomes after medical and surgical treatments. J Spinal Disord 2001;14:427-433.

Al-Shahi Salman R, Hall JM, Horne MA, et al. Untreated clinical course of cerebral cavernous malformations: a prospective, population-based cohort study. Lancet Neurol 2012;11:217-224.

Asgeir SJ, Kristin SM, Roar K, et al. Comparison of a strategy favouring early surgical resection vs a strategy of watchful waiting in low-grade gliomas. JAMA 2012;308:1881-1888.

Barker FG 2nd, Ogilvy CS. Efficacy of prophylactic nimodipine for delayed ischemic deficit after subarachnoid hemorrhage: a metaanalysis. J Neurosurg 1996;84:405-414.

Barnett H, Taylor W, Eliasziw M, et al. Benefit of carotid endarterectomy in patients with symptomatic moderate or severe stenosis. NEJM 1998;339:1415-1425.

Bor AS, Rinkel GJ, van Norden J, et al. Long-term, serial screening for intracranial aneurysms in individuals with a family history of aneurysmal subarachnoid haemorrhage: a cohort study. Lancet Neurol 2014;13:385-392.

Bracken MB, Shepard MJ, Holford TR, et al. Methylprednisolone or tirilazad mesylate administration after acute spinal cord injury: 1-year follow up. Results of the third National Acute Spinal Cord Injury randomized controlled trial. J Neurosurg 1998;89:699-706.

Cakir B, Schmidt R, Reichel H, et al. Lumbar disk herniation: what are reliable criterions indicative for surgery? Orthopedics 2009;32:589-597.

Chesnut RM, Temkin N, Carney N, et al. A trial of intracranial-pressure monitoring in traumatic brain injury. NEJM 2012;367:2471-2481.

Chinot OL, Wick W, Mason W, et al. Bevacizumab plus radiotherapy-temozolamide for newly diagnosed glioblastoma. NEJM 2014;370:709-722.

Crossman AR, Neary D. Neuroanatomy: an illustrated colour text. Toronto: Churchill Livingston, 1998.

Dorhout Mees SM, Rinkel GJ, Feigin VL, et al. Calcium antagonists for aneurysmal subarachnoid haemorrhage. Cochrane DB Syst Rev 2007;3:CD000277.

Edlow J, Caplan L. Avoiding pitfalls in the diagnosis of subarachnoid hemorrhage. NEJM 2000;342:29-36.

el Barzouhi A, Vleggeert-Lankamp CL, Lycklama à Nijeholt GJ, et al. Magnetic resonance imaging in follow-up assessment of sciatica. NEJM 2013;368:999-1007.

Executive Committee for the Asymptomatic Carotid Atherosclerosis Study (ACAS). Endarterectomy for asymptomatic carotid artery stenosis. JAMA 1995;273:1421-1428.

Fehlings MG, Tator CH. An evidence-based review of surgical decompression for acute spinal cord injury: rationale, indications, and timing based on experimental and clinical studies. J Neurosurg 1999;91(1 Suppl):1-11.

Fehlings MG, Vaccaro A, Wilson JR, et al. Early versus delayed decompression for traumatic cervical spinal cord injury: results of the surgical timing in acute spinal cord injury dtudy (STASCIS). PLoS ONE 2012;7:e32037. doi:10.1371/journal.pone.0032037.

Fitzgerald MJT. Neuroanatomy: basic and clinical, 3rd ed. Philadelphia: WB Saunders, 1997.

Goetz CG, Pappert EJ. Textbook of clinical neurology, 1st ed. Toronto: WB Saunders, 1999.

Greenberg MS. Handbook of neurosurgery, 7th ed. New York: Thieme Medical Publishers, 2010. Greving JP, Wermer MJ, Brown RD Jr, et al. Development of the PHASES score for prediction of risk of rupture of intracranial aneurysms: a pooled analysis of six prospective cohort studies. Lancet Neurol 2014;13:59-66.

Hurlbert RJ, Hadley MN, Walters BC, et al. Pharmacological therapy for acute spinal cord injury. Neurosurgery 2013;72(Suppl 2):93-105.

International Study of Unruptured Intracranial Aneurysms Investigators. Unruptured intracranial aneurysms – risk of rupture and risks of surgical intervention. NEJM 1998;339:1725-1733.

Juttler E, Unterberg A, Woitzik J, et al. Hemicraniectomy in older patients with extensive middle-cerebral-artery stroke. NEJM 2014;370:1091-1100.

Kitchen N, McKhann II GM, Manji H. Clinical neurology and neurosurgery. Thieme Medical Publishers, 2003.

Kun LE. Brain tumours: challenges and directions. Pediat Clin N Am 1997;44:907-917.

Lindsay KW, Bone I. Neurology and neurosurgery illustrated. New York: Churchill Livingstone, 2004.

Mark DG, Hung YY, Offerman SR, et al. Nontraumatic subarachnoid hemorrhage in the setting of negative cranial computed tomography results: external validation of a clinical and imaging prediction rule. Ann Emerg Med 2012;pii:S0196-0644:1508-1509.

Molyneux AJ, Kerr RS, Birks J, et al. Risk of recurrent subarachnoid haemorrhage, death, or dependence and standardised mortality ratios after clipping or coiling of an intracranial aneurysm in the International Subarachnoid Aneurysm Trial (ISAT): long-term follow-up. Lancet Neurol 2009;8:427-433.

MRC Asymptomatic Carotid Surgery Trial (ACST) Collaborative Group. Prevention of disabling and fatal strokes by successful carotid endarterectomy in patients without recent neurological symptoms: randomized controlled trial. Lancet 2004;363:1491-1502.

Nieuwenhuys R, Voogd J, van Huijzen C. The human central nervous system, 3rd ed. New York: Springer-Verlag, 1988.

Ogilvy CS, Stieg PE, Awad I, et al. Recommendations for the management of intracranial arteriovenous malformations. Circulation 2001;103:2644-2657.

Panczkowski DM, Tomycz ND, Okonkwo DO. Comparative effectiveness of using computed tomography alone to exclude cervical spine injuries in obtunded or intubated patients: meta-analysis of 14,327 patients with blunt trauma. J Neurosurg 2011;115:541-549.

Portenoy RK, Lipton RB, Foley KM. Back pain in the cancer patient: an algorithm for evaluation and management. Neurology 1987;37:134-138.

Porter PJ, Willinsky RA, Harper W, et al. Cerebral cavernous malformations: natural history and prognosis after clinical deterioration with or without hemorrhage. J Neurosurg 1997;87:190-197.

Ross J, Al-Shahi Salman R. Interventions for treating brain arteriovenous malformations in adults. Cochrane DB Syst Rev 2010;7:CD003436.

Saal JS, Saal JA, Yurth EF. Nonoperative management of herniated cervical intervertebral disc with radiculopathy. Spine 1996;21:1877-1883.

Santarius T, Kirkpatrick PJ, Ganesan D, et al. Use of drains versus no drains after burr-hole evacuation of chronic subdural haematoma: a randomised control trial. Lancet 2009;374:1067-1073.

Sayer FT, Kronvall E, Nilsson OG. Methylprednisolone treatment in acute spinal cord injury: the myth challenged through a structured analysis of published literature. Spine 2006;6:335-343.

Shapiro S. Medical realities of cauda equina syndrome secondary to lumbar disc herniation. Spine 2000;25:348-351.

Shemie S, Doig C, Dickens B, et al. Severe brain injury to neurological determination of death: Canadian forum recommendations. CMAJ 2006;174:S1-30.

Spencer S, Huh L. Outcomes of epilepsy surgery in adults and children. Lancet Neurol 2008;7:525-37.

Spetzler RF, Martin NA. A proposed grading system for arteriovenous malformations. J Neurosurg 1986;65:476-83.

Stiell IG, Wells GA, Vandemheen K, et al. The Canadian CT head rule for patients with minor head injury. Lancet 2001;357:1391-1396.

The North American Symptomatic Carotid Endarterectomy Trial (NASCET). Beneficial effects of carotid endarterectomy in symptomatic patients with high-grade carotid stenosis. NEJM 1991;325:445-453.

Tsao MN, Rades D, Wirth A, et al. Radiotherapeutic and surgical management for newly diagnosed brain metastasis(es): an American radiation oncology evidence-based guideline. Pract Radiat Oncol 2012;2:210-225.

Vaccaro AR, Lehman RA, Hurlbert RJ, et al. A new classification of thoracolumbar injuries: The importance of injury morphology, the integrity of the posterior ligamentous complex, and neurological status. Spine 2005; 30: 2325-2333.

Walton JGR, Hutchinson M, McArdle MJF, et al. Aids to the examination of the peripheral nervous system. London: Bailliere Tindall, 1986.

Wiebe S, Blume WT, Girvin JP, et al. Effectiveness and efficiency of surgery for temporal lobe epilepsy study group. A randomized, controlled trial of surgery for temporal-lobe epilepsy. NEJM 2001;345:311-318.

OB Obstetrics

Karyn Medcalf, Erica Pascoal, and **Adam Rosen**, chapter editors
Dhruvin Hirpara and **Sneha Raju**, associate editors
Valerie Lemieux and **Simran Mundi**, EBM editors
Dr. Richard Pittini and **Dr. Amanda Selk**, staff editors

Acronyms

AC	abdominal circumference	EFW	estimated fetal weight	IUFD	intrauterine fetal death	PG	plasma glucose
ACOG	American Congress of Obstetricians and Gynecologists	FDP	fibrin degradation products	IUGR	intrauterine growth restriction	PPD	postpartum depression
		FHR	fetal heart rate	IVH	intraventricular hemorrhage	PPH	postpartum hemorrhage
AFI	amniotic fluid index	FISH	fluorescence *in situ* hybridization	L/S	lecithin-sphingomyelin ratio	PPROM	preterm premature rupture of membranes
AFLP	acute fatty liver of pregnancy	FL	femur length	LLDP	left lateral decubitus position		
AFV	amniotic fluid volume	FM	fetal movement	LMP	last menstrual period	PROM	premature rupture of membranes
AP	anteroposterior	FPG	fasting plasma glucose	MSAFP	maternal serum α-fetoprotein	PTL	preterm labour
APS	antiphospholipid antibody syndrome	FTS	first trimester screen	MSS	maternal serum screen	RDS	respiratory distress syndrome
BPP	biophysical profile	GA	gestational age	MTX	methotrexate	ROM	rupture of membranes
C/S	Cesarean section	GBS	Group B *Streptococcus*	NIPT	non-invasive prenatal testing	SFH	symphysis fundal height
CPD	cephalopelvic disproportion	GDM	gestational diabetes mellitus	NST	non-stress test	SOGC	Society of Obstetricians and Gynaecologists of Canada
CTG	cardiotocography	GTN	gestational trophoblastic neoplasia	NTDs	neural tube defects		
CVS	chorionic villus sampling	HC	head circumference	NTUS	nuchal translucency ultrasound	SVD	spontaneous vaginal delivery
D&C	dilatation and curettage	HELLP	hemolysis, elevated liver enzymes, low platelets	OA	occiput anterior	TENS	transcutaneous electrical nerve stimulation
DIC	disseminated intravascular coagulation			OGTT	oral glucose tolerance test		
DVT	deep vein thrombosis	IGF	infant growth factors	oNTD	open neural tube defect	TPN	total parenteral nutrition
ECV	external cephalic version	IMM	intramyometrial	OP	occiput posterior	UTI	urinary tract infection
EDC	estimated date of confinement	IOL	induction of labour	OT	occiput transverse	VBAC	vaginal birth after Cesarean
EFM	electronic fetal monitoring	IPS	integrated prenatal screen	PAPP-A	pregnancy-associated plasma protein a		

Basic Anatomy Review

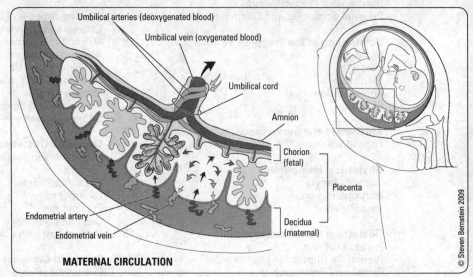

Figure 1. Placental blood flow

Placenta
- site of fetal nutritive, respiratory, and excretory function
- discoid mass composed of fetal (chorion frondosum) and maternal (decidua basalis) tissues divided by fissures into cotyledons (lobules) on the uterine side
- produces hormones such as progesterone, placental lactogen, estrogen, relaxin, β-hCG, and IGFs
- poor implantation can lead to spontaneous abortion
- abnormal location, implantation, or detachment can lead to antepartum hemorrhage (see *Obstetrical Hemorrhage*, OB13)

Pregnancy

Diagnosis of Pregnancy

History
- symptoms: amenorrhea, nausea and/or vomiting, breast tenderness, urinary frequency, and fatigue
- obstetrical and gynecological history
- obtain the year, location, mode of delivery, duration of labour, sex, gestational age, birth weight, and complications of every pregnancy; organize into GTPAL format
  - **Gravidity (G)**
    - G: total number of pregnancies of any gestation (multiple gestation=one pregnancy)
  - includes current pregnancy, abortions, ectopic pregnancies, and hydatidiform moles

- **Parity (TPAL)**
  - **T**: number of term infants delivered (>37 wk)
  - **P**: number of premature infants delivered (20-36+6 wk)
  - **A**: number of abortions (loss of intrauterine pregnancy prior to viability of fetus <20 wk and/or <500 g fetal weight)
    - induced (therapeutic) and spontaneous (miscarriage)
  - **L**: number of living children

Physical Signs
- Goodell's sign: softening of the cervix (4-6 wk)
- Chadwick's sign: bluish discolouration of the cervix and vagina due to pelvic vasculature engorgement (6 wk)
- Hegar's sign: softening of the cervical isthmus (6-8 wk)
- uterine enlargement
- breast engorgement, areolae darkening, and prominent vascular patterns

Investigations
- β-hCG: peptide hormone composed of α and β subunits produced by placental trophoblastic cells – maintains the corpus luteum during pregnancy
  - positive in serum 9 d post-conception, positive in urine 28 d after first day of LMP
  - plasma levels usually double every 1.4-2.0d, peak at 8-10 wk, then fall to a plateau until delivery
    - levels less than expected suggest: ectopic pregnancy, abortion, inaccurate dates, and some normal pregnancies
    - levels greater than expected suggest: multiple gestation, molar pregnancy, Trisomy 21, or inaccurate dates
- U/S
  - transvaginal
    - 5 wk amenorrhea: gestational sac visible
    - 6 wk: fetal pole visible
    - 7-8 wk: fetal heart activity visible
  - transabdominal
    - 6-8 wk: intrauterine pregnancy visible

β-hCG Rule of 10s
10 IU at time of missed menses
100,000 IU at 10 wk (peak)
10,000 IU at term

Trimesters
- T1 (first trimester): 0-14 wk
- T2 (second trimester): 14-28 wk
- T3 (third trimester): 28-42 wk
- Normal pregnancy term: 37-42 wk

Maternal Physiologic Adaptations to Pregnancy

Table 1. Physiologic Changes During Pregnancy

Skin	Increased pigmentation of perineum and areola, chloasma (pigmentation changes under eyes and on bridge of nose), linea nigra (midline abdominal pigmentation),spider angiomas, palmar erythema due to increased estrogen, striae gravidarum due to connective tissue changes
Cardiovascular	Hyper-dynamic circulation Increased CO, HR, and blood volume Decreased blood pressure: decreased PVR and decreased venous return from enlarging uterus compressing IVC and pelvic veins Increased venous pressure leads to risk of varicose veins, hemorrhoids, leg edema
Hematologic	Hemodilution causes physiologic anemia and apparent decrease in hemoglobin and hematocrit Increased leukocyte count but impaired function leads to improvement in autoimmune diseases Gestational thrombocytopenia: mild (platelets >70,000/μL) and asymptomatic, normalizes within 2-12 wk following delivery Hypercoagulable state: increased risk of DVT and PE but also decreased bleeding at delivery
Respiratory	Increased incidence of nasal congestion Increased O_2 consumption to meet increased metabolic requirements Elevated diaphragm (i.e. patient appears more "barrel-chested") Increased minute ventilation leads to decreased CO_2 resulting in mild respiratory alkalosis that helps CO_2 diffuse across the placenta from fetal to maternal circulation Decreased TLC, FRC, and RV No change in VC and FEV_1
Gastrointestinal	GERD due to increased intra-abdominal pressure and progesterone (causing decreased sphincter tone and delayed gastric emptying) Increased gallstones due to progesterone causing increased gallbladder stasis Constipation and hemorrhoids due to progesterone causing decreased GI motility
Genitourinary	Increased urinary frequency due to increased total urinary output Increased incidence of UTI and pyelonephritis due to urinary stasis (see *Urinary Tract Infection*, OB28) Glycosuria that can be physiologic especially in the 3rd trimester; must test for GDM Ureters and renal pelvis dilation (R>L) due to progesterone-induced smooth muscle relaxation and uterine enlargement Increased CO and thus increased GFR leads to decreased creatinine (normal in pregnancy 35-44 mmol/L), uric acid, and BUN
Neurologic	Increased incidence of carpal tunnel syndrome and Bell's palsy
Endocrine	Thyroid: moderate enlargement (not clinically detectable) and increased basal metabolic rate Increased total thyroxine and thyroxine binding globulin (TBG) Free thyroxine index and TSH levels are normal Adrenal: maternal cortisol rises throughout pregnancy (total and free) Calcium: decreased total maternal Ca^{2+} due to decreased albumin Free ionized Ca^{2+} (i.e. active) proportion remains the same due to parathyroid hormone (PTH), results in increased bone resorption and gut absorption, increased bone turnover (but no loss of bone density due to estrogen inhibition)

Antepartum Care

- provided by obstetrician, family doctor, midwife, or multidisciplinary team (based on patient preference and risk factors)

Family doctors and midwives to consider OB consultation if:
- Insulin-dependent GDM
- VBAC
- HTN
- Multiple gestation
- Malpresentation
- Active antepartum hemorrhage
- PTL/PPROM
- Failure to progress/descend
- Induction/augmentation if high risk
- Tears: 3rd or 4th degree
- Retained placenta

Note: Guidelines vary by institution and by provincial midwifery colleges

Advise all women capable of becoming pregnant to supplement their diet with 0.4 mg/d of folic acid (CTFPHC Grade II-2-A Evidence)

Prenatal and genetic screening are voluntary and require proper counselling and informed consent before proceeding
HIV is done automatically in some provinces as opt-out testing, need to inform patient

Preconception Counselling

- 3-8 wk GA is a critical period of organogenesis, so early preparation is vital
- **past medical history**: optimize illnesses and medications prior to pregnancy (see *Medical Complications of Pregnancy*, OB25, and *Medications*, OB10)
- **supplementation**
  - folic acid: encourage diet rich in folic acid and supplement 8-12 wk preconception until end of T1 to prevent NTDs
    - 0.4-1 mg daily in all women; 5 mg if previous NTD, antiepileptic medications, DM, or BMI >35 kg/m^2
- iron supplementation, prenatal vitamins
- **risk modification**
  - lifestyle: balanced nutrition and physical fitness
  - medications: discuss teratogenicity of medications so they may be adjusted or stopped if necessary
  - infection screening: rubella, HBsAg, VDRL, Pap smear, gonorrhea/chlamydia, HIV, TB testing based on travel and health care worker, history of varicella or vaccination, parvovirus immunity if exposed to small children, cytomegalovirus immunity if health care worker, toxoplasmosis serology if cats or gardening last pertussis vaccine
  - genetic testing as appropriate for high risk groups (see *Prenatal Screening*, Table 2); consider genetics referral in known carriers, recurrent pregnancy loss/stillbirth, family members with developmental delay, birth anomalies, genetic diseases
  - social: smoking, alcohol, drug use, domestic violence (see <u>Family Medicine</u>, FM11, FM12, FM26)

Initial Prenatal Visit

- usually within 8-12 wk of the first day of LMP or earlier if <20 or >35 yr old, bleeding, very nauseous, or other risk factors present

In history of previous pregnancies, **ALWAYS** ask:
GTPAL
Year
Sex
Weight
Gestational age (GA)
Mode of delivery
Length of labour
Complications

History
- gestational age by dates from the first day of the LMP
  - Naegle's rule: 1st day of LMP + 7 d – 3 mo
  - e.g. LMP = 1 Apr 2014, EDC = 8 Jan 2015 (modify if cycle >28 d by adding number of d >28)
- if LMP unreliable, get a dating ultrasound which could coincide with nuchal translucency at ~12 wk
- dates should change if T1 U/S is greater than 5 days in difference from LMP due date
- history of present pregnancy (e.g. bleeding, N/V) and all previous pregnancies
- past medical, surgical, and gynecological history
- prescription and non-prescription medications
- family history: genetic diseases, birth defects, multiple gestation, consanguinity
- social history: smoking, alcohol, drug use, domestic violence (see <u>Family Medicine</u>, FM11, FM12, FM26)

Ask every woman about abuse – not just those whose situations raise suspicion of abuse AND ask as early as possible in pregnancy

Physical Exam
- complete physical exam to obtain baseline patient information – BP and weight important for interpreting subsequent changes

Investigations
- blood work
  - CBC, blood group and Rh status, antibody screen, infection screening as per preconception counselling
- urine R&M, midstream urine C&S
  - screen for bacteriuria and proteinuria
- pelvic exam
  - pap smear (only if required according to patient history and provincial screening guidelines), cervical or urine PCR for *N. gonorrhoeae* (GC) and *C. trachomatis*

Nausea and Vomiting

Epidemiology
- affects 50-90% of pregnant women
- often limited to T1 but may persist

Toronto Notes 2017 Antepartum Care Obstetrics OB5

Management
- rule out other causes of N/V
- weigh frequently, assess level of hydration, test urine for ketones
- **non-pharmacological**
  - avoid mixing fluids and solids, frequent small meals (bland, dry, salty better tolerated)
  - electrolyte oral solutions (Pedialyte®, Gatorade®)
  - stop prenatal vitamins (folic acid must continue until >12 wk)
  - increase sleep/rest
  - ginger (maximum 1,000 mg/d)
  - acupuncture, acupressure
- **pharmacological**
  - first line: Diclectin® (10 mg doxylamine succinate with vitamin B6) 4 tablets PO daily to maximum of 8 tablets
  - if no improvement, try dimenhydrinate (50-100 mg q4-6h PO), followed by hydroxyzine, pyridoxine, phenothiazine, or metoclopramide
  - vitamin B6 lollipops
  - if patient dehydrated, assess fluid replacement needs and resuscitate accordingly
- **severe/refractory**
  - consider homecare with IV fluids and parenteral anti-emetics, hospitalization

Hyperemesis Gravidarum

Definition
- intractable N/V, usually presents in T1 then diminishes; occasionally persists throughout pregnancy
- affects ~1% of pregnancies

Etiology
- multifactorial with hormonal, immunologic, and psychologic components
- rapidly rising β-hCG ± estrogen levels may be implicated

Investigations
- rule out systemic causes: GI inflammation, pyelonephritis, thyrotoxicosis
- rule out other obstetrical causes: multiple gestation, GTN, HELLP syndrome
- CBC, electrolytes, BUN, creatinine, LFTs, urinalysis
- ultrasound

Management
- thiamine supplementation may be indicated
- non-pharmacological (see *Nausea and Vomiting*)
- pharmacological options
  - Diclectin® (for dosage, see *Nausea and Vomiting*)
  - Dimenhydrinate can be safely used as an adjunct to Diclectin® (1 suppository bid or 25 mg PO qid)
  - other adjuncts: hydroxyzine, pyridoxine, phenothiazine, metoclopramide
  - also consider: ondansetron or methylprednisolone
  - if severe: admit to hospital, NPO initially then small frequent meals, correct hypovolemia, electrolyte disturbance, and ketosis, TPN (if very severe) to reverse catabolic state

Complications
- maternal
- dehydration, electrolyte and acid-base disturbances
- Mallory-Weiss tear
- Wernicke's encephalopathy, if protracted course
- death
- fetal: usually none, IUGR is 15x more common in women losing >5% of pre-pregnancy weight

Subsequent Prenatal Visits

Timing
- for uncomplicated pregnancies, SOGC recommends q4-6wk until 30 wk, q2-3wk from 30 wk, and q1-2 from 36 wk until delivery

Assess at Every Visit
- estimated GA
- history: fetal movements, uterine bleeding, leaking, cramping, questions, concerns
- physical exam: BP, weight gain, SFH, Leopold's maneuvers (T3) for lie, position, and presentation of fetus
- investigations: urinalysis for glucosuria, proteinuria; fetal heart rate starting at 10-12 wk using Doppler U/S

Symphysis Fundal Height

SFH < Dates
- Date miscalculation
- IUGR
- Fetal demise
- Oligohydramnios
- Early engagement

SFH > Dates
- Date miscalculation
- Multiple gestation
- Polyhydramnios
- LGA (familial, DM)
- Fibroids

Leopold's Maneuvers

- performed after 30-32 wk gestation
- first maneuver: to determine which fetal part is lying furthest away from the pelvic inlet
- second maneuver: to determine the location of the fetal back
- third maneuver: to determine which fetal part is lying above the pelvic inlet
- fourth maneuver: to locate the fetal brow

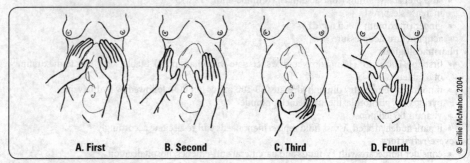

A. First   **B. Second**   **C. Third**   **D. Fourth**

© Emilie McMahon 2004

Figure 2. Leopold's maneuvers (T3)
Reprinted with permission from Essentials of Clinical Examination Handbook, 6th ed. Lincoln, McSheffrey, Tran, Wong

Prenatal Screening and Diagnostic Tests

Screening Tests

- testing should only occur following counselling and with the informed consent from the patient

Table 2. High-Risk Population Screening Tests

Disease (Inheritance)	Population(s) at Risk	Screening Test(s)
Thalassemia (AR)	**Mediterranean, South East Asian, Western Pacific**, African, Middle Eastern, Caribbean, South American	CBC (MCV and MCH), Hb electrophoresis, or HPLC
Sickle Cell (AR)	**African, Caribbean**, Mediterranean, Middle Eastern, Indian, South American	CBC (MCV and MCH), Hb electrophoresis, or HPLC
Cystic Fibrosis (CF) (AR)	Family history of CF in patient or partner or medical condition linked to CF like male infertility	CFTR gene DNA analysis
Tay Sachs Disease (AR)	Ashkenazi Jewish*, French Canadians, Cajun	Enzyme assay HEXA, or DNA analysis HEXA gene
Fragile X Syndrome (X-linked)	Family history – confirmed or suspected	DNA analysis: FMR-1 gene

AR = autosomal recessive; HEXA = hexosaminidase A; HPLC = high performance liquid chromatography
*If both partners are Ashkenazi Jewish, test for Canavan disease and Familial Dysautonomia (FD); if family history of a specific condition, look for carrier status: e.g. Gaucher, CF, Bloom syndrome, Niemann-Pick disease, etc. In all cases, if both partners positive, refer for genetic counselling

Table 3. Gestation-Dependent Screening Investigations

Gestational Age (wk)	Investigations	Details
8-12	Dating U/S, possible Pap smear, chlamydia/gonorrhea cultures, urine C&S, HIV, VDRL, HepBSAg, Rubella IgG, Parvovirus IgM or IgG if high risk (small child at home or daycare worker/primary teacher), Varicella IgG if no history of disease/immunization, CBC, blood group and screen	
>10	NIPT	Measures cell free fetal DNA in maternal circulation
10-12	CVS	
11-14	FTS IPS Part 1	Measures 1. Nuchal translucency on U/S 2. β-hCG 3. PAPP-A
11-14	Nuchal translucency U/S	
15-16 to term	Amniocentesis	
15-20	IPS Part 2 (or MSAFP only for patients who did FTS earlier)	Measures 1. MSAFP 2. β-hCG 3. Unconjugated estrogen (estriol or μE3) 4. Inhibin A

Routine T2 U/S at 18-22 wk Helps Determine
- Number of fetuses
- GA (if no prior U/S)
- Location of placenta
- Fetal anomalies

Table 3. Gestation-Dependent Screening Investigations (continued)

Gestational Age (wk)	Investigations	Details
15-20	MSS (or MSAFP only for patients who did FTS earlier)	Measures 1. MSAFP 2. β-hCG 3. Unconjugated estrogen (estriol or μE3) 4. Inhibin A
18-20 to term	Fetal movements (quickening)	
18-20	U/S for dates, fetal growth, and anatomy assessment	
24-28	Gestational Diabetes Screen 50 g OGCT	See *Diabetes Mellitus*, OB26
28	Repeat CBC RhIG for all Rh negative women	
35-37	GBS screen	See *Group B Streptococcus*, OB27
6 wk postpartum	Discuss contraception, menses, breastfeeding, depression, mental health, support Physical exam: breast exam, pelvic exam including Pap smear (only if due as per provincial screening)	

Maternal serum screen is also referred to as Triple Screen; if Inhibin A is also tested, it is referred to as Quadruple Screen

DDx of Increased MSAFP
- Incorrect GA
- >1 fetus (e.g. twins)
- Fetal demise
- oNTD
- Abdominal wall defects (e.g. omphalocele)

DDx of Decreased MSAFP
- Incorrect GA
- Gestational trophoblastic neoplasia
- Missed abortion
- Chromosomal anomalies
- Maternal DM

Ultrasound Screening
- 8-12 wk GA: Dating Ultrasound (most accurate form of pregnancy dating)
  - measurement of crown-rump length (margin of error ± 5 d)
  - change EDC to U/S date if >5 d discrepancy from EDC based on LMP
- 11-14 wk GA: NTUS
  - measures the amount of fluid behind the neck of the fetus
  - early screen for Trisomy 21 (may also detect cardiac and other aneuploidies like Turner's syndrome)
  - NT measurement is necessary for the FTS and IPS Part 1
- 18-20 wk GA: Growth and Anatomy U/S (margin of error ± 10 d)
- earlier or subsequent ultrasounds performed when medically indicated

Symphysis Fundal Height (SFH)
12 wk   Uterine fundus at pubic symphysis
20 wk   Fundus at umbilicus, SFH should be within 2 cm of GA between 20-36 wk

Non-Invasive Prenatal Testing (NIPT)
- analyses maternal blood for circulating cell free fetal DNA (ccffDNA) at 10 wk GA onwards. Requires dating ultrasound for accuracy

Advantage
- in high risk women (>age 35) highly sensitive for Trisomy 21 (>99.5%), specificity (>99.8%)-can also look for trisomy 18, 13 and some X and Y disorders as well as common microdeletions
- not harmful to the pregnancy, results available in 7-10 day

Disadvantages
- does not screen for oNTD
- high cost to patient (only covered in some provinces in certain cases)
- unclear how accurate yet in low risk women (<35)
- need to confirm with invasive testing
- Does not test for all aneuploidy

Table 4. Comparison of FTS, MSS, and IPS

FTS	MSS	IPS
11-14 wk	15-20 wk	11-13 wk U/S-Nuchal Translucency 11-14 wk: FTS blood 15-20 wk : MSS blood including inhibin
Risk estimate for 1. Down syndrome (Trisomy 21): increased NT, increased β-hCG, decreased PAPP-A 2. Trisomy 18 : increased NT, decreased PAPP-A, decreased β-hCG	Risk estimate for 1. oNTD: increased MSAFP (sensitivity 80-90%) 2. Trisomy 21: decreased MSAFP, increased β-hCG, decreased μE3 (sensitivity 65%) 3. Trisomy 18: decreased MSAFP, decreased β-hCG, decreased μE3, decreased inhibin (sensitivity 80%)	Risk estimate for oNTD, Trisomy 21, Trisomy 18 Sensitivity ~85-90% 2% false positive rate Patients with positive screen should be offered U/S and/or amniocentesis or NIPT (covered in some provinces, self-pay in others)
Note: does not measure risk of open neural tube defect (oNTD) and should be combined with MSAFP at 15-20 wk Useful where patient wants results within the first trimester More accurate estimate of Down syndrome risk than MSS, sensitivity ~85% (when combined with age) 5% false positive rate Patients with positive screen should be offered CVS, amniocentesis, or NIPT (covered in some provinces, self-pay in others)	Only offered alone if patient missed the time window for IPS or FTS 8% baseline false positive rate for Trisomy 21, lower for oNTD and Trisomy 18 Patients with positive screen should be offered U/S, amniocentesis, or NIPT (covered in some provinces, self-pay in others)	

Note: In twins, FTS, MSS, and IPS are not applicable; screen with NT, NIPT for chromosomal abnormalities and MSAFP for oNTDs

Diagnostic Tests

Indications
- age >35 yr (increased risk of chromosomal anomalies)
- risk factors in current pregnancy
  - abnormal U/S
  - abnormal prenatal screen (IPS, FTS, or MSS)
- past history/family history of
  - chromosomal anomaly or genetic disease
  - either parent a known carrier of a genetic disorder or balanced translocation
  - consanguinity
  - >3 spontaneous abortions

AMNIOCENTESIS
- U/S-guided transabdominal extraction of amniotic fluid

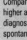

Compared to CVS, amniocentesis has a higher accuracy of prenatal cytogenetic diagnosis (99.8% vs. 97.5%) and lower risk of spontaneous abortion (0.5% vs. 1-2%)

Indications
- identification of genetic anomalies (15-16 wk gestation) as per indications above
- confirmation of positive NIPT testing
- positive FTS/IPS
- assessment of fetal lung maturity (T3) via the L/S ratio (lecithin:sphingomyelin)
  - if >2:1, RDS is less likely to occur

Advantages
- also screens for oNTD (acetylcholinesterase and amniotic AFP) – 96% accurate
- in women >35 yr, the risk of chromosomal anomaly (1/180) is greater than the risk of miscarriage from the procedure
- more accurate genetic testing than CVS

Disadvantages
- 1/400-1/500 risk of procedure related pregnancy loss
- results take 14-28 d; FISH can be done on chromosomes X, Y, 21, 13, 18 to give preliminary results in 48 h

Risk Factors for Neural Tube Defects

GRIMM
Genetics: family history of NTD (risk of having second child with NTD is increased to 2-5%), consanguinity, chromosomal (characteristic of Trisomy 13, 18, and 21)
Race: European Caucasians > African Americans, 3-fold higher in Hispanics
Insufficient vitamins: zinc and folate
Maternal chronic disease (e.g. DM)
Maternal use of antiepileptic drugs

General population risk for NTD is 0.1%

CHORIONIC VILLUS SAMPLING
- biopsy of fetal-derived chorion using a transabdominal needle or transcervical catheter at 10-12 wk

Advantages
- enables pregnancy to be terminated earlier than with amniocentesis
- rapid karyotyping and biochemical assay within 48 h, including FISH analysis
- high sensitivity and specificity

Disadvantages
- 1-2% risk of procedure related pregnancy loss
- does not screen for oNTD
- 1-2% incidence of genetic mosaicism "false negative" results

ISOIMMUNIZATION SCREENING

Definition
- isoimmunization: antibodies (Ab) produced against a specific RBC antigen (Ag) as a result of antigenic stimulation with RBC of another individual

Etiology
- maternal-fetal circulation normally separated by placental barrier, but sensitization can occur and can affect the current pregnancy, or more commonly, future pregnancies
- Anti-Rh Ab produced by a sensitized Rh-negative mother can lead to fetal hemolytic anemia
- Risk of isoimmunization of an Rh-negative mother with an Rh-positive ABO-compatible infant is 16%
- sensitization routes
- incompatible blood transfusions
- previous fetal-maternal transplacental hemorrhage (e.g. ectopic pregnancy, abruption)
- invasive procedures in pregnancy (e.g. prenatal diagnosis, cerclage, D&C)
- any type of abortion
- labour and delivery

Rh Antibody Titre
A positive titre (≥1:16) indicates an increased risk of fetal hemolytic anemia

Investigations
- screening with indirect Coombs test at first visit for blood group, Rh status, and antibodies
- Kleihauer-Betke test used to determine extent of fetomaternal hemorrhage by estimating volume of fetal blood volume that entered maternal circulation
- detailed U/S for hydrops fetalis
- MCA dopplers are done to assess degree of fetal anemia or if not available bilirubin is measured by serial amniocentesis to assess the severity of hemolysis
- cordocentesis for fetal Hb should be used cautiously (not first line)

Prophylaxis
- exogenous Rh IgG (Rhogam® or WinRho®) binds to Rh antigens of fetal cells and prevents them from contacting maternal immune system
- Rhogam® (300 µg) given to all Rh negative and antibody screen negative women in the following scenarios
  - routinely at 28 wk GA (provides protection for ~12 wk)
  - within 72 h of the birth of an Rh positive fetus
  - with any invasive procedure in pregnancy (CVS, amniocentesis)
  - in ectopic pregnancy
  - with miscarriage or therapeutic abortion
  - with an antepartum hemorrhage
- a Betke-Kleihauer test or Flow cytometry can be used to determine whether more than 300 µg of RhIg is required (>30 ml fetal blood)
- if Rh negative and Ab screen positive, follow mother with serial monthly Ab titres throughout pregnancy +ultrasounds± serial amniocentesis as needed (Rhogam® has no benefit)

Standard dose of 300 µg of Rhogam® sufficient for 30 mL of fetal blood. Give additional 10 µg of Rhogam® for every mL of fetal blood over 30 mL

Treatment
- falling biliary pigment warrants no intervention (usually indicative of either unaffected or mildly affected fetus)
- intrauterine transfusion of O-negative pRBCs may be required for severely affected fetus or early delivery of the fetus for exchange transfusion

Complications
- anti-Rh IgG can cross the placenta and cause fetal RBC hemolysis resulting in fetal anemia, CHF, edema, ascites
- severe cases can lead to fetal hydrops (edema in at least two fetal compartments due to fetal heart failure secondary to anemia) or erythroblastosis fetalis (moderate to severe immune-mediated hemolytic anemia)

Counselling of the Pregnant Woman

Nutrition

- Canada's Food Guide to Healthy Eating suggests
  - 3-4 servings of milk products daily (greater if multiple gestation)
  - a daily caloric increase of ~100 cal/d in the 1st trimester, ~300 cal/d in the second and third trimesters and ~450 cal/d during lactation
  - daily multivitamin should be continued in the 2nd trimester for women who do not consume an adequate diet; otherwise routine vitamin supplementation is not necessary (avoid excess vitamin A)
- nutrients important during pregnancy
  - folate: 0.4 mg/d for first 12 wk (5 mg/d if high risk)
    - supports increase in blood volume, growth of maternal and fetal tissue, decreases incidence of NTD
    - foods rich in folic acid include: spinach, lentils, chick peas, asparagus, broccoli, peas, brussels sprouts, corn, and oranges
  - calcium: 1200-1500 mg/d
    - maintains integrity of maternal bones, skeletal development of fetus, breast milk production
  - vitamin D: 1,000 IU
    - promotes calcium absorption
  - iron: 0.8 mg/d in T1, 4-5 mg/d in T2, and >6 mg/d in T3
    - supports maternal increase in blood cell mass, supports fetal and placental tissue
    - required amounts exceed normal body stores and typical intake, and therefore need supplemental iron
    - iron is the only known nutrient for which requirements during pregnancy cannot be met by diet alone (see *Iron Deficiency Anemia*, OB25)
  - essential fatty acids – supports fetal neural and visual development
    - contained in vegetable oils, margarines, peanuts, fatty fish

Caffeine
- diuretic and stimulant that readily crosses placenta
- less than 300 mg/d is not thought to contribute to miscarriage or preterm birth (ACOG)
  - relationship between caffeine and IUGR is unknown (ACOG)
  - SOGC states 1-2 cups/d are safe during pregnancy

Sources of Caffeine
- 5 oz cup coffee: 40-180 mg
- 5 oz brewed tea: 20-90 mg
- 12 oz cola: 46 mg
- Red Bull®: 67 mg
- Dark chocolate bar: 10 mg
- 8 oz hot chocolate: 5 mg

Herbal Teas and Preparations
- not enough scientific information about safety of various herbs and herbal products to recommend their use during pregnancy
- some herbal teas can have toxic or pharmacological effects on the mother or fetus
- chamomiles have been reported to exhibit adverse effects on the uterus
- raspberry leaf tea often used at term to promote labour

Herbal Teas Considered Safe in Moderation (2-3 cups/d)
- Citrus peel
- Ginger
- Lemon balm
- Linden flower – not with prior cardiac condition
- Orange peel
- Rose hip

Foodborne Illnesses
- microbiological contamination of food may occur through cross-contamination and/or improper food handling
  - listeriosis (Listeria monocytogenes) and toxoplasmosis (Toxoplasma gondii) are of concern during pregnancy
  - avoid consumption of raw meats, fish, shellfish, poultry, hotdogs, raw eggs, and unpasteurized dairy products
  - avoid unpasteurized soft cheeses, deli meats, smoked salmon, and pates as they may be sources of Listeria
- chemical contamination of food
  - current guideline for mercury of 0.5 ppm in fish is not considered harmful for the general population, including pregnant women
  - Health Canada advises pregnant women to limit consumption of top predator fish such as shark, swordfish, king mackeral, tilefish

Lifestyle

- exercise under physician guidance; "talk test" = should be able to speak while exercising; avoid supine position after 20 weeks GA
- absolute contraindications
  - ruptured membranes, preterm labour, hypertensive disorders of pregnancy, incompetent cervix, IUGR, multiple gestations (>3), placenta previa after 28th wk, persistent 2nd or 3rd trimester bleeding, uncontrolled type I DM, uncontrolled thyroid disease, or other serious cardiovascular, respiratory, or systemic disorder
- relative contraindications
  - previous preterm birth, mild/moderate cardiovascular or respiratory disorder, anemia (Hb ≤10 g/dL), malnutrition or eating disorder, twin pregnancy after 28th wk, other significant medical conditions
- weight gain: optimal gain depends on pre-pregnancy BMI (varies from 6.8-18.2 kg)
- work: strenuous work, extended hours and shift work during pregnancy may be associated with greater risk of low birth weight, prematurity, and spontaneous abortion
- air travel is acceptable in second trimester; airline cut off for travel is 36-38 wk gestation depending on the airline, to avoid giving birth on the plane
- sexual intercourse: may continue, except in patients at risk for: abortion, preterm labour, or placenta previa; breast stimulation may induce uterine activity and is discouraged in high-risk patients near term
- smoking: assist/encourage to reduce or quit smoking
  - increased risk of decreased birth weight, placenta previa/abruption, spontaneous abortion, preterm labour, stillbirth
- alcohol: no amount of alcohol is safe in pregnancy; encourage abstinence from alcohol during pregnancy; alcohol increases incidence of abortion, stillbirth, and congenital anomalies
  - fetal alcohol syndrome (see Pediatrics, P24)
- cocaine: microcephaly, growth retardation, prematurity, abruptio placentae

Expected Weight Gain

BMI (kg/m²)	Weight (kg)
<19	12.7-18.2
19-25	11.3-15.9
>25	6.8-11.3

General Rule: 1-3.5 kg/wk during T1, then 0.45 kg/wk until delivery

Medications

- most drugs cross the placenta to some extent
- very few drugs are teratogenic, but very few drugs have proven safety in pregnancy
- use any drug with caution and only if necessary
- analgesics: acetaminophen preferable to ASA or ibuprofen

Drug Resources During Pregnancy and Breastfeeding
- Motherisk at the Hospital for Sick Children in Toronto: www.motherisk.org
- Hale T. Medications and mothers' milk, 11th ed. Pharmasoft Publishing, 2004

Table 5. Documented Adverse Effects, Contraindicated

Contraindicated Medication	Adverse Effect
ACEI	Fetal renal defects, IUGR, oligohydramnios
Tetracycline	Stains infant's teeth, may affect long bone development
Retinoids (e.g. Accutane®)	CNS, craniofacial, cardiac, and thymic anomalies
Misoprostol	Mobius syndrome (congenital facial paralysis with or without limb defects, spontaneous abortion, preterm labour)

Table 6. Documented Adverse Effects, Weigh Benefits vs. Risks, and Consider Medication Change

Medication	Adverse Effect
Phenytoin	Fetal hydantoin syndrome in 5-10% (IUGR, mental retardation, facial dysmorphogenesis, congenital anomalies)
Valproate	oNTD in 1%
Carbamazepine	oNTD in 1-2%
Lithium	Ebstein's cardiac anomaly, goitre, hyponatremia
Warfarin	Increased incidence of spontaneous abortion, stillbirth, prematurity, IUGR, fetal warfarin syndrome (nasal hypoplasia, epiphyseal stippling, optic atrophy, mental retardation, intracranial hemorrhage)
Erythromycin	Maternal liver damage (acute fatty liver)
Sulpha drugs	Anti-folate properties, therefore theoretical risk in T1; risk of kernicterus in T3
Chloramphenicol	Grey baby syndrome (fetal circulatory collapse 2° to toxic accumulation)

Immunizations

Intrapartum
- administration is dependent on the risk of infection vs. risk of immunization complications
- safe: tetanus toxoid, diphtheria, influenza, hepatitis B, pertussis
- avoid live vaccines (risk of placental and fetal infection): polio, measles/mumps/rubella, varicella
- contraindicated: oral typhoid
- the public health agency of Canada recommends:
  - all pregnant women receive the influenza vaccine
  - all pregnant women at 26 weeks of pregnancy or later, who have not received a dose of pertussis-containing vaccine in adulthood, should receive Tdap vaccination in pregnancy

Postpartum
- rubella vaccine for all non-immune mothers
- hepatitis B vaccine should be given to infant within 12 h of birth if maternal status unknown or positive – follow-up doses at 1 and 6 mo
- any vaccine required/recommended is generally safe postpartum

Radiation

- ionizing radiation exposure is considered teratogenic at high doses
  - if indicated for maternal health, should be done
- imaging not involving direct abdominal/pelvic high dosage is not associated with adverse effects
  - higher dosage to fetus: plain x-ray of lumbar spine/abdomen/pelvis, barium enema, CT abdomen, pelvis, lumbar spine
- most investigations involve minimal radiation exposure
- radioactive isotopes of iodine are contraindicated
- no known adverse effects from U/S or MRI (long-term effects of gadolinium unknown, avoid if possible)

Table 7. Approximate Fetal Doses from Common Diagnostic Procedures

Examination	Estimated Fetal Dose (rad)	Number of Exams Safe in Pregnancy
Plain Film		
Abdomen	0-14	35
Pelvis	0-11	45
Lumbar spine	0-17	29
Thoracic spine	0.009	555
Chest (2 views)	<0.001	5000
CT		
Abdomen	0-8	6
Pelvis	2-5	2
Lumbar spine	0-24	20
Chest	0.006	833

Adapted from: Cohen-Kerem, et al. 2005 and Valentin 2000

Radiation in Pregnancy
- Necessary amount to cause miscarriage: >5 rads
- Necessary amount to cause malformations: >20-30 rads

Antenatal Fetal Surveillance

Fetal Movements

- patients will generally first notice fetal movement ("quickening") at 18-20 wk in primigravidas; can occur 1-2 wk earlier in multigravidas; can occur 1-2 wk later if placenta is implanted on the anterior wall of uterus
- if the patient is concerned about decreased fetal movement, she is counselled to choose a time when the fetus is normally active to count movements (usually recommended after 26 wk)
- all high risk women should be told to do FM counts
  - if there is a subjective decrease in fetal movement, try drinking juice, eating, changing position, or moving to a quiet room and count for 2 h; ≥6 movements in 2 h expected
  - if there are <6 movement counts in 2 h, patient should present to labour and delivery triage

NON-STRESS TEST

Definition
- FHR tracing ≥20 min using an external Doppler to assess FHR and its relationship to fetal movement (see *Fetal Monitoring in Labour*, OB33)

Indication
- any suggestion of uteroplacental insufficiency or suspected compromise in fetal well-being

Table 8. Classification of Antepartum Non-Stress Test

Parameter	Normal NST (Previously "Reactive")	Atypical NST (Previously "Non-Reactive")	Abnormal NST (Previously "Non-Reactive")
Baseline	110-160 bpm	100-110 bpm or >160 bpm for <30 min Rising baseline	Bradycardia <100 bpm Tachycardia >160 for >30 min Erratic baseline
Variability	6-25 bpm (moderate) ≤5 (absent or minimal) for <40 min	5 (absent or minimal) for 40-80 min	≤5 for 80 min Sinusoidal 25 bpm for >10 min
Decelerations	None or occasional variable <30 s	Variable decelerations 30-60 s duration	Variable decelerations >60 s Late deceleration(s)
Accelerations in Term Fetus	2 accelerations with acme of ≥15 bpm, lasting 15 s over <40 min of testing	2 accelerations with acme of ≥15 bpm, lasting 15 s in 40-80 min	<2 accelerations with acme of ≥15 bpm, lasting 15 s in >80 min
Accelerations in Preterm Fetus (<32 wk)	>2 accelerations with acme of >10 bpm, lasting 10 s in <40 min	<2 accelerations with acme of >10 bpm, lasting 10 s in 40-80 min	<2 accelerations with acme of >10 bpm, lasting 10 s in >80 min
Action	FURTHER ASSESSMENT OPTIONAL, based on total clinical picture	FURTHER ASSESSMENT REQUIRED	URGENT ACTION REQUIRED An overall assessment of the situation and further investigation with U/S or BPP is required; some situations will require delivery

Adapted from: *SOGC*, Fetal Health Surveillance: Antepartum and Intrapartum Consensus Guideline, September 2007

Operating Characteristics
- false positive rate depends on duration; false negative rate = 0.2-0.3%

Interpretation
- normal: at least 2 accelerations of FHR >15 bpm from the baseline lasting >15 s, in 20 min
- abnormal: <2 accelerations of FHR in 40 min
- if no observed accelerations or fetal movement in the first 20 min, stimulate fetus (fundal pressure, acoustic/vibratory stimulation) and continue monitoring for 30 min
- if NST abnormal, then perform BPP

BIOPHYSICAL PROFILE

Definition
- U/S assessment of the fetus ± NST

Indications
- abnormal or atypical NST
- post-term pregnancy
- decreased fetal movement
- IUGR
- any other suggestion of fetal distress or uteroplacental insufficiency

Operating Characteristics
- false positive rate ≤30%, false negative rate = 0.1%

Table 9. Scoring of the BPP

Parameter	Reassuring (2 points)
Tone (Limb Extension then Flexion)	At least one episode of limb extension followed by flexion
Movement	Three discrete movements
Breathing	At least one episode of breathing lasting at least 30 s
AFV*	Fluid pocket of 2 cm in 2 axes

*AFV is a marker of chronic hypoxia, all other parameters indicate acute hypoxia

Reassuring BPP (8/8)

LAMB
Limb extension + flexion
AFV 2 cm x 2 cm
Movement (3 discrete)
Breathing (one episode x 30 s)

Interpretation
- 8: perinatal mortality rate 1:1,000; repeat BPP as clinically indicated
- 6: perinatal mortality 31:1,000; repeat BPP in 24 h
- 0-4: perinatal mortality rate 200:1,000; deliver fetus if benefits of delivery outweigh risks

Obstetrical Hemorrhage

Definition
- vaginal bleeding from 20 wk to term

Differential Diagnosis
- bloody show (shedding of cervical mucous plug) – most common etiology in T3
- placenta previa
- abruptio placentae – most common pathological etiology in T3
- vasa previa
- cervical lesion (cervicitis, polyp, ectropion, cervical cancer)
- uterine rupture
- other: bleeding from bowel or bladder, abnormal coagulation

Table 10. Comparison of Placenta Previa and Abruptio Placentae

	Placenta Previa	Abruptio Placentae
Definition	Abnormal location of the placenta near, partially, or completely over the internal cervical os	Premature separation of a normally implanted placenta after 20 wk GA
Etiology	Idiopathic	Idiopathic
Epidemiology	0.5-0.8% of all pregnancies	1-2% of all pregnancies
Risk Factors	History of placenta previa (4-8% recurrence risk) Multiparity Increased maternal age Multiple gestation Uterine tumour (e.g. fibroids) or other uterine anomalies Uterine scar due to previous abortion, C/S, D&C, myomectomy	Previous abruption (recurrence rate 5-16%) Maternal HTN (chronic or gestational HTN in 50% of abruptions) or vascular disease Cigarette smoking (>1 pack/d), excessive alcohol consumption, cocaine Multiparity and/or maternal age >35 yr PPROM Rapid decompression of a distended uterus (polyhydramnios, multiple gestation) Uterine anomaly, fibroids Trauma (e.g. motor vehicle collision, maternal battery)
Bleeding	PAINLESS	Usually PAINFUL

Placenta Previa

Definition
- placenta implanted in the lower segment of the uterus, presenting ahead of the leading pole of the fetus
- placental position is described in relation to the internal os as "mm away" or "mm of overlap"

Clinical Features
- PAINLESS bright red vaginal bleeding (recurrent), may be minimized and cease spontaneously, but can become catastrophic
- mean onset of bleeding is 30 wk GA, but onset depends on degree of previa
- **physical exam**
  - uterus soft and non-tender
  - presenting fetal part high or displaced
  - FHR usually normal
  - shock/anemia correspond to degree of apparent blood loss

Greater than 20 of overlap over the internal os in the third trimester of pregnancy is highly predictive of the need for a C/S. Any degree of overlap after 35 wk is an indication for a C/S

- **complications**
    - fetal
        - perinatal mortality low but still higher than with a normal pregnancy
        - prematurity (bleeding often dictates early C/S)
        - intrauterine hypoxia (acute or IUGR)
        - fetal malpresentation
        - PPROM
        - risk of fetal blood loss from placenta, especially if incised during C/S
    - maternal
        - <1% maternal mortality
        - hemorrhage and hypovolemic shock, anemia, acute renal failure, pituitary necrosis (Sheehan syndrome)
        - placenta accreta – especially if previous uterine surgery, anterior placenta previa
        - hysterectomy

Investigations

- transvaginal U/S is more accurate than transabdominal U/S at diagnosing placenta previa at any gestational age
- if the placenta lies between 20 mm of overlap and 20 mm away from the internal os after 20 wk transvaginal ultrasounds should be repeated in the third trimester as continued change in the placental location is likely

Do NOT perform a vaginal exam until placenta previa has been ruled out by U/S

Management

- goal: keep pregnancy intrauterine until the risk of delivery < risk of continuing pregnancy
- stabilize and monitor
    - maternal stabilization: large bore IV with hydration, O_2 for hypotensive patients
    - maternal monitoring: vitals, urine output, blood loss, blood work (hematocrit, CBC, INR/PTT, platelets, fibrinogen, FDP, type and cross match)
    - electronic fetal monitoring
    - U/S assessment: when fetal and maternal condition permit, determine fetal viability, gestational age, and placental status/position
- Rhogam® if mother is Rh negative
- determine extent of fetomaternal transfusion so that appropriate dose of Rhogam® can be given
- GA <37 wk and minimal bleeding: expectant management
    - admit to hospital
    - limited physical activity, no douches, enemas, or sexual intercourse
    - consider corticosteroids for fetal lung maturity
    - delivery when fetus is mature or hemorrhage dictates
- GA ≥37 wk, profuse bleeding, or L/S ratio is >2:1 – deliver by C/S

Abruptio Placentae

Definition

- premature partial or total placental detachment caused by bleeding at the decidual-placental interface
- occurring >20 wks gestation

Clinical Features

- classification
    - total (fetal death inevitable) vs. partial
    - external/revealed/apparent: blood dissects downward toward cervix
    - internal/concealed/occult (20%): blood dissects upward toward fetus
    - most are mixed
- presentation
    - usually PAINFUL (80%) vaginal bleeding (bleeding not always present if abruption is concealed), uterine tenderness, uterine contractions/hypertonus
    - pain: sudden onset, constant, localized to lower back and uterus
    - shock/anemia out of proportion to apparent blood loss
    - ± fetal distress, fetal demise (15% present with demise), bloody amniotic fluid (fetal presentation typically normal)
    - ± coagulopathy

Abruptio placentae is the most common cause of DIC in pregnancy

Complications

- fetal complications: perinatal mortality 25-60%, prematurity, intrauterine hypoxia
- maternal complications: <1% maternal mortality, DIC (in 20% of abruptions), acute renal failure, anemia, hemorrhagic shock, pituitary necrosis (Sheehan syndrome), amniotic fluid embolus

Investigations

- clinical diagnosis, U/S not sensitive for diagnosing abruption (sensitivity = 15%)

Management
- maternal stabilization: large bore IV with hydration, O_2 for hypotensive patients
- maternal monitoring: vitals, urine output, blood loss, blood work (hematocrit, CBC, PTT/PT, platelets, fibrinogen, FDP, type and cross match)
- EFM
- blood products on hand (red cells, platelets, cryoprecipitate) because of DIC risk
- Rhogam® if Rh negative
  - Kleihauer-Betke test may confirm abruption
- mild abruption
  - GA <37 wk: use serial Hct to assess concealed bleeding, deliver when fetus is mature or when hemorrhage dictates
  - GA ≥37 wk: stabilize and deliver
- moderate to severe abruption
  - hydrate and restore blood loss and correct coagulation defect if present
  - vaginal delivery if no contraindication and no evidence of fetal or maternal distress OR fetal demise
  - C/S if live fetus and fetal or maternal distress develops with fluid/blood replacement, labour fails to progress or if vaginal delivery otherwise contraindicated

Kleihauer-Betke Test
Quantifies fetal cells in the maternal circulation

Vasa Previa

Definition
- unprotected fetal vessels pass over the cervical os; associated with velamentous insertion of cord into membranes of placenta or succenturiate (accessory) lobe

Epidemiology
- 1 in 5,000 deliveries – higher in twin pregnancies

Clinical Features
- PAINLESS vaginal bleeding and fetal distress (tachy- to bradyarrhythmia)
- 50% perinatal mortality, increasing to 75% if membranes rupture (most infants die of exsanguination)

Investigations
- Apt test (NaOH mixed with the blood) can be done immediately to determine if the source of bleeding is fetal (supernatant turns pink) or maternal (supernatant turns yellow)
- Wright stain on blood smear and look for nucleated red blood cells (in cord, not maternal blood)

Management
- emergency C/S (since bleeding is from fetus, a small amount of blood loss can have catastrophic consequences)

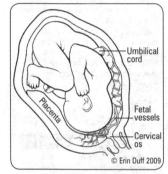

Figure 3. Vasa previa

Obstetrical Complications

Preterm Labour

Definition
- labour between 20 and 37 wk gestation

Etiology
- idiopathic (most common)
- maternal: infection (recurrent pyelonephritis, untreated bacteriuria, chorioamnionitis), HTN, DM, chronic illness, mechanical factors, previous obstetric, gynecological, and abdominal surgeries, socio-environmental (poor nutrition, smoking, drugs, alcohol, stress)
- maternal-fetal: PPROM (common), polyhydramnios, placenta previa, placental abruption, or placental insufficiency
- fetal: multiple gestation, congenital abnormalities of fetus, fetal hydrops, stress
- uterine: incompetent cervix, excessive enlargement (hydramnios, multiple gestation), malformations (intracavitary leiomyomas, septate uterus, mullerian duct abnormalities)

Epidemiology
- preterm labour complicates about 10% of pregnancies

Risk Factors
- prior history of spontaneous PTL is the most important risk factor
- prior history cervical excisions (LEEPs/cone biopsy) or mechanical dilatation (D&C)
- cervical length: measured by transvaginal U/S (cervical length >30 mm has high negative predictive value for PTL before 34 wk)
- identification of bacterial vaginosis and ureaplasma urealyticum infections; routine screening not supported by current data but it is reasonable to screen high risk women
- family history of preterm birth

Preterm labour is the most common cause of neonatal mortality in the US

Positive fetal fibronectin in cervicovaginal fluid (>50 ng/mL) at 24 wk gestation predicted spontaneous PTL at <34 wk with sensitivity of 23%, specificity of 97%, PPV of 25%, NPV of 96%

Tocolytics for Preterm Premature Rupture of Membranes
Cochrane DB Syst Rev 2014;2:CD007062
Purpose: To assess the potential benefits and harms of tocolysis in women with PPROM.
Selection Criteria: Pregnant women with singleton pregnancies and PPROM (23-36 wk and 6 d GA).
Results: 8 studies with 408 women total. Prophylactic tocolysis with PPROM was associated with increased overall latency, without additional benefits for maternal/neonatal outcomes. For women with PPROM before 34 wk, there was a significantly increased risk of chorioamnionitis in women who received tocolysis. Neonatal outcomes were not significantly different.
Conclusion: Although there are limitations to the studies, there is currently insufficient evidence to support tocolytic therapy for women with PPROM, as there was an increase in maternal chorioamnionitis without significant benefits to the infant.

Cerclage for Short Cervix on Ultrasonography in Women With Singleton Gestations and Previous Preterm Birth
Obstet Gynecol 2011;117:663-671
Purpose: To determine if cerclage prevents preterm birth (<35 wk gestation) and perinatal mortality and morbidity among women with previous spontaneous preterm birth, asymptomatic singleton gestation, and short cervical length (<25 mm before 24 wk gestation) on transvaginal ultrasonography.
Methods: Meta-analysis of randomized trials identified using searches on MEDLINE, PUBMED, EMBASE, and the Cochrane Library.
Results: 5 trials included. Preterm birth was significantly lower among women receiving cerclage vs. those not (RR = 0.70, 95% CI 0.55-0.89). Cerclage also significantly reduced preterm birth before 24, 28, 32, and 37 wk gestation. Perinatal mortality and morbidity were significantly lower in the cerclage group (RR = 0.64, 95% CI 0.45-0.91).
Conclusions: Cerclage significantly prevents preterm birth and perinatal mortality and morbidity in this specific group of women.

Antenatal Betamethasone for Women at Risk for Late Preterm Delivery
N Engl J Med 2016 Apr; 374(14): 1311-20.
Purpose: This was a randomized trial comparing betamethasone (n = 1429) to placebo (n=1402) in the treatment of women with a singleton preg-nancy between 34 to 36 + 5/7 weeks that were at high risk of delivery. Composite endpoints assessing the need for respiratory support within 72 hours of birth were used to measure treatment effectiveness. Specifically these endpoints included: supplemental oxygen, extracorporeal mem-brane oxygenation (ECMO), mechanical ventilation, and CPAP or high-flow nasal cannula.
Results: The primary outcome occurred less frequently in those who received betamethasone (11.6% vs 14.4%, RR 0.8, p = 0.02). Treatment with betamethasone also significantly reduced additional respiratory complications, bronchopulmonary dysplasia, transient tachypnea of the newborn, and surfactant use.
Conclusion: Treating women (GA 34 to 36 + 5/7 weeks) who are at risk of delivery with betamethasone reduces the risk of neonatal complications.

Predicting PTL
- fetal fibronectin: a glycoprotein in amniotic fluid and placental tissue
  - positive if >50 ng/mL; NPV > PPV
  - in symptomatic women (i.e. preterm contractions), fetal fibronectin is most effectively combined with U/S detecting cervical length
  - if cervical length is not short and fetal fibronectin is negative, preterm labour is highly unlikely

Clinical Features
- regular contractions (2 in 10 min, >6/h)
- cervix >1 cm dilated, >80% effaced, or length <2.5 cm

Management
A. Initial
- transfer to appropriate facility if stable
- hydration (NS at 150 mL/h)
- bed rest in LLDP
- sedation (morphine)
- avoid repeated pelvic exams (increased infection risk)
- U/S examination of fetus (GA, BPP, position, placenta location, estimated fetal weight)
- prophylactic antibiotics; (for GBS) important to consider if PPROM (e,g, erythromycin controversial but may help to delay delivery)

B. Suppression of Labour – Tocolysis
- does not inhibit preterm labour completely, but may delay delivery (used for <48 h) to allow for betamethasone valerate (Celestone®) and/or transfer to appropriate centre for care of the premature infant
- requirements (all must be satisfied)
  - preterm labour
  - live, immature fetus, intact membranes, cervical dilatation of <4 cm
  - absence of maternal or fetal contraindications
- contraindications
  - maternal: bleeding (placenta previa or abruption), maternal disease (HTN, DM, heart disease), preeclampsia or eclampsia, chorioamnionitis
  - fetal: erythroblastosis fetalis, severe congenital anomalies, fetal distress/demise, IUGR, multiple gestation (relative)
- agents
  - calcium channel blockers: nifedipine
    - 20 mg PO loading dose followed by 20 mg PO 90 min later
    - 20 mg can be continued q3-8h for 72 h or to a max of 180 mg
    - 10 mg PO q20min x 4 doses
    - contraindications: nifedipine allergy, hypotension, hepatic dysfunction, concurrent beta-mimetics or $MgSO_4$ use, transdermal nitrates, or other antihypertensive medications
  - prostaglandin synthesis inhibitors: indomethacin
    - 1st line for early preterm labour (<30 wk GA) or polyhydramnios
    - 50-100 mg PR loading dose followed by 50 mg q6h x 8 doses for 48 hours
  - magnesium sulphate
    - was previously used for tocolysis; currently, only indicated for prevention of eclampsia or for neuroprotection if preterm delivery is inevitable between 24 and 31+6 wks GA for neuroprotection
    - 4 g IV loading dose followed by 1g q1h maintenance until birth

C. Enhancement of Fetal Pulmonary Maturity
- betamethasone valerate (Celestone®) 12 mg IM q24h x 2 doses or dexamethasone 6 mg IM q12h x 4 doses
  - 28-36+6 wk GA: reduces incidence of RDS
  - 24-28 wk GA: reduces severity of RDS, overall mortality and rate of IVH
  - specific maternal contraindications: active TB

D. Cervical Cerclage
- definition: placement of cervical sutures at the level of the internal os, usually at the end of the first trimester or in the second trimester and removed in the third trimester
- indications: cervical incompetence (i.e. cervical dilation and effacement in the absence of increased uterine contractility)
  - emerging evidence indicates that progesterone suppositories are superior to cerclage in preventing preterm labour not due to cervical incompetence; (neither is effective in multiple gestations)
- diagnosis of cervical incompetence
  - obstetrical Hx: silent cervical dilation, 2nd trimester losses, procedures on cervix
  - ability of cervix to hold an inflated Foley catheter during a hysterosonogram
- proven benefit in the prevention of PTL in women with primary structural abnormality of the cervix (e.g. conization of the cervix, connective tissue disorders)

Prognosis
- prematurity is the leading cause of perinatal morbidity and mortality
- 30 wk or 1,500 g (3.3 lb) = 90% survival
- 33 wk or 2,000 g (4.4 lb) = 99% survival
- morbidity due to asphyxia, hypoxia, sepsis, RDS, intraventricular cerebral hemorrhage, thermal instability, retinopathy of prematurity, bronchopulmonary dysplasia, necrotizing enterocolitis

Prevention of Preterm Labour
- currently there are no agents approved by Health Canada to arrest preterm labour
- preventative measures: good prenatal care, identify pregnancies at risk, treat silent vaginal infection or UTI, patient education
- transvaginal ultrasound of cervical length is recommended only for high-risk pregnancies and only before 30 weeks GA

Premature Rupture of Membranes

Definitions
- PROM: prelabour rupture of membranes at any GA
- prolonged ROM: >24 h elapsed between rupture of membranes and onset of labour
- preterm ROM: ROM occurring before 37 wk gestation
- PPROM: preterm (before 37 wk) AND prelabour rupture of membranes

Risk Factors
- maternal: multiparity, cervical incompetence, infection (cervicitis, vaginitis, STI, UTI), family history of PROM, low socioeconomic class/poor nutrition
- fetal: congenital anomaly, multiple gestation
- other risk factors associated with PTL

Clinical Features
- history of fluid gush or continued leakage

Investigations
- sterile speculum exam (avoid introduction of infection)
  - pooling of fluid in the posterior fornix
  - may observe fluid leaking out of cervix on cough/Valsalva ("cascade")
- nitrazine (basic amniotic fluid turns nitrazine paper blue)
  - low specificity as can be positive with blood, urine, or semen
- ferning (high salt in amniotic fluid evaporates, looks like ferns under microscope)
- U/S to rule out fetal anomalies, assess GA, presentation and BPP

Management
- admit for expectant management and monitor vitals q4h, daily BPP and WBC count
- avoid introducing infection by minimizing examinations
  - consider administration of betamethasone valerate (Celestone*) to accelerate maturity if <34 wk and up to 36+6 weeks if no evidence of infection
  - consider tocolysis for 48 h to permit administration of steroids if PPROM induces labour
- screen women for UTIs, STIs, GBS carriage and treat with appropriate antibiotics if positive
- if not in labour or labour not indicated, consider antibiotics: penicillins or macrolide antibiotics are the antibiotics of choice
- deliver urgently if evidence of fetal distress and/or chorioamnionitis

Table 11. PROM Management

Degree of Prematurity	Management
<24 wk	Consider termination (poor outcome due to pulmonary hypoplasia)
24-25 wk	Individual consideration with counselling of parents regarding risks to preterm infants
26-34 wk	Expectant management as prematurity complications are significant
34-36 wk	"Grey zone" where risk of death from RDS and neonatal sepsis is the same
≥37 wk	Induction of labour since the risk of death from sepsis is greater than RDS

Prognosis
- varies with gestational age
- 90% of women with PROM at 28-34 wk GA go into spontaneous labour within 1 wk
- 50% of women with PROM at <26 wk GA go into spontaneous labour within 1 wk
- complications: cord prolapse, intrauterine infection (chorioamnionitis), premature delivery, limb contracture

Membrane Status determined by
- Pooling of fluid on speculum exam
- Increased pH of vaginal fluid (nitrazine test)
- Ferning of fluid under light microscope
- Decreased AFV on U/S

Antibiotic Therapy in Preterm Premature Rupture of the Membranes
J Obstet Gynaecol Can. 2009; 31(9) 863-7.
Study: A review of recent systematic reviews, randomized control trials/controlled trials, and observational studies assessing the use of antibiotics in PPROM.
Recommendations:
1. Following PPROM at ≤32 weeks' gestation, antibiotics should be administered to women who are not in labour in order to prolong pregnancy and to decrease maternal and neonatal morbidity. (I-A)
2. The use of antibiotics should be gestational-age dependent. The evidence for benefit is greater at earlier gestational ages (< 32 weeks). (I-A)
3. For women with PPROM at >32 weeks' gestation, administration of antibiotics to prolong pregnancy is recommended if fetal lung maturity can not be proven and/or delivery is not planned. (I-A)
4. Antibiotic regimens may consist of an initial parenteral phase followed by an oral phase, or may consist of only an oral phase. (I-A)
5. Antibiotics of choice are penicillins or macrolide antibiotics (erythromycin) in parenteral and/or oral forms. (I-A) In patients allergic to penicillin, macrolide antibiotics should be used alone. (III-B)
6. The following two regimens may be used (the two regimens were used in the largest PPROM randomized controlled trials that showed a decrease in both ma-ternal and neonatal morbidity): (1) ampicillin 2 g IV every 6 hours and erythromycin 250 mg IV every 6 hours for 48 hours followed by amoxicillin 250 mg orally every 8 hours and erythromycin 333 mg orally every 8 hours for 5 days (I-A); (2) erythromycin 250 mg orally every 6 hours for 10 days (I-A)
7. Amoxicillin/clavulanic acid should not be used because of an increased risk of necrotizing enterocolitis in neonates exposed to this antibiotic. Amoxicillin with-out clavulanic acid is safe. (I-A)
8. Women presenting with PPROM should be screened for urinary tract infections, sexually transmitted infections, and group B *Streptococcus* carriage, and treated with appropriate antibiotics if positive. (II-2B)

*Evidence was approved by the Maternal Fetal Medicine Committee and Infectious Disease Committee of the Society of Obstetricians and Gynecologists of Canada

Prolonged Pregnancy

Definition
- pregnancy >42 wk GA

Epidemiology
- 41 wk GA: up to 27%
- >42 wk GA: 5.5%

Etiology
- most cases idiopathic
- anencephalic fetus with no pituitary gland
- placental sulfatase deficiency (X-linked recessive condition in 1/2,000-1/6,000 infants) – rare

Clinical Features
- postmaturity syndrome (10-20% of post-term pregnancies): fetal weight loss, reduced subcutaneous fat, scaling, dry skin from placental insufficiency, long thin body, open-eyed, alert and worried look, long nails, palms and soles wrinkled)
- with increasing GA, higher rates of: intrauterine infection, asphyxia, meconium aspiration syndrome, placental insufficiency, placental aging and infarction, macrosomia, dystocia, fetal distress, operative deliveries, pneumonia, seizures, and requirement of NICU admission, and stillbirth

Management
- GA 39 wk with advanced maternal age (>40yo): consideration should be given to IOL due to increased risk of stillbirth
- GA 40-41 wk: expectant management
  - no evidence to support IOL or C/S unless other risk factors for morbidity are present (see prognosis)
- GA >41 wk: offer IOL if vaginal delivery is not contraindicated
  - IOL shown to decrease C/S, fetal heart rate changes, meconium staining, macrosomia, and death when compared with expectant management
- GA >41 wk and expectant management elected: serial fetal surveillance
  - fetal movement count by the mother
  - BPP q3-4d
- if AFI is decreased, labour should be induced

Prognosis
- if >42 wk, perinatal mortality 2-3x higher (due to progressive uteroplacental insufficiency)
- morbidity increased with HTN in pregnancy, DM, abruption, IUGR, and multiple gestation

Intrauterine Fetal Death

Definition
- fetal death in utero after 20 wk GA

Epidemiology
- occurring in 1% of pregnancies

Etiology
- 50% idiopathic
- 50% secondary to HTN, DM, erythroblastosis fetalis, congenital anomalies, umbilical cord or placental complications, intrauterine infection, APS

Clinical Features
- decreased perception of fetal movement by mother
- SFH and maternal weight not increasing
- absent fetal heart tones on Doppler (not diagnostic)
- high MSAFP
- on U/S: no fetal heart rate. Depending on timing of death may see skull collapse, brain tissue retraction, empty fetal bladder, non-filled aorta, poor visualization of midline flax

Management
- diagnosis: absent cardiac activity and fetal movement on U/S required for diagnosis
- determine secondary cause
  - maternal: HbA1c, fasting glucose, TSH, Kleihauer-Betke, VDRL, ANA, CBC, anticardiolipins, antibody screens, INR/PTT, serum/urine toxicology screens, cervical and vaginal cultures, TORCH screen
  - fetal: karyotype, cord blood, skin biopsy, genetics evaluation, autopsy, amniotic fluid culture for CMV, parvovirus B19, herpes
  - placenta: pathology, bacterial cultures

DIC: Generalized Coagulation and Fibrinolysis Leading to Depletion of Coagulation Factors

Obstetrical Causes
- Abruption
- Gestational HTN
- Fetal demise
- PPH

DIC-specific Blood Work
- Platelets
- aPTT and PT
- FDP
- Fibrinogen

Treatment
- Treat underlying cause
- Supportive
- Fluids
- Blood products
- FFP, platelets, cryoprecipitate
- Consider anti-coagulation as VTE prophylaxis

Treatment
- <12 wk: dilation and curettage
- 13-20 wk: dilation and evacuation or sometimes IOL
- >20 wk: induction of labour
- monitor for maternal coagulopathy (10% risk of DIC)
- parental psychological care/bereavement support as per hospital protocol
- comprehensive discussion within 3 mo about final investigation and post-mortem results, help make plans for future pregnancies

Intrauterine Growth Restriction

Definition
- infant weight <10th percentile for GA or <2,500 g at term

Etiology/Risk Factors
- 50% unknown
- maternal causes
  - malnutrition, smoking, drug abuse, alcoholism, cyanotic heart disease, type 1 DM, SLE, pulmonary insufficiency, previous IUGR (25% risk, most important risk factor), chronic HTN
- maternal-fetal
  - any disease causing placental insufficiency
  - includes gestational HTN, chronic renal insufficiency, gross placental morphological abnormalities (infarction, hemangiomas, placenta previa, abnormal cord insertion), prolonged gestation
- fetal causes
  - TORCH infections, multiple gestation, congenital anomalies / chromosomal abnormalities (10%)

TORCH
Toxoplasmosis
Others: e.g. syphilis
Rubella
CMV
HSV
- See Table 12, OB20

Clinical Features
- symmetric/type I (25-30%): occurs early in pregnancy
  - reduced growth of both head and abdomen
  - head:abdomen ratio may be normal (>1 up to 32 wk; =1 at 32-34 wk; <1 after 34 wk GA)
  - usually associated with congenital anomalies or TORCH infections
- asymmetric/type II (70%): occurs late in pregnancy
  - fetal abdomen is disproportionately smaller than fetal head
  - brain is spared, therefore head:abdomen ratio increased
  - usually associated with placental insufficiency
  - more favourable prognosis than type I
- complications
  - prone to meconium aspiration, asphyxia, polycythemia, hypoglycemia, hypocalcemia, hyperphosphatemia hyponatremia, and mental retardation
  - greater risk of perinatal morbidity and mortality

Differential Diagnosis of Incorrect Uterine Size for Dates
- Inaccurate dates
- Early descent of presenting part (engagement)
- Maternal: DM
- Maternal-fetal: polyhydramnios, oligohydramnios
- Fetal: abnormal karyotype, IUGR, macrosomia, fetal anomaly, abnormal lie, multiple gestation

Investigations
- SFH measurements at every antepartum visit
- if mother at high risk or SFH lags >2 cm behind GA
  - U/S for biparietal diameter, head and abdominal circumference ratio, femur length, fetal weight, and AFV (decrease associated with IUGR), decrease in the rate of growth
  - ± BPP
  - Doppler analysis of umbilical cord blood flow

Management
- prevention via risk modification prior to pregnancy is ideal
- modify controllable factors: smoking, alcohol, nutrition, and treat maternal illness
- bed rest in LLDP
- serial BPP (monitor fetal growth) and determine cause of IUGR, if possible
- delivery when extrauterine existence is less dangerous than continued intrauterine existence (abnormal function tests, absent growth, severe oligohydramnios) especially if GA >34 wk
- liberal use of C/S since IUGR fetus withstands labour poorly

Macrosomia

Definition
- infant weight >90th percentile for a particular GA or >4,000 g

Etiology/Risk Factors
- maternal obesity, GDM, past history of macrosomic infant, prolonged gestation, multiparity

Clinical Features
- increased risk of perinatal mortality
- CPD and birth injuries (shoulder dystocia, fetal bone fracture) more common
- complications of DM in labour (see Table 15, OB27)

Investigations
- serial SFH
- further investigations if mother at high risk or SFH >2 cm ahead of GA
- U/S predictors
  - polyhydramnios
  - third trimester AC >1.5 cm/wk
  - HC/AC ratio <10th percentile
  - FL/AC ratio <20th percentile

Management
- prophylactic C/S is a reasonable option where EFW >5,000 g in non-diabetic woman and EFW >4,500 g in diabetic woman
  - no evidence that prophylactic C/S improves outcomes
- risks and benefits of early induction (risk of C/S vs. risk of dystocia) must be weighed in diabetic mothers, as current research is unclear

Polyhydramnios/Oligohydramnios

Table 12. Polyhydramnios and Oligohydramnios

	Polyhydramnios	Oligohydramnios
Definition	AFI >25 cm U/S: single deepest pocket >8 cm	AFI <5 cm U/S: single deepest pocket ≤2 cm

Etiology	Idiopathic most common
	Maternal
	  Type 1 DM: abnormalities of transchorionic flow
	Maternal-fetal
	  Chorioangiomas
	  Multiple gestation
	  Fetal hydrops (increased erythroblastosis)
	Fetal
	  Chromosomal anomaly (up to 2/3 of fetuses have severe polyhydramnios)
	  Respiratory: cystic adenomatoid malformed lung
	  CNS: anencephaly, hydrocephalus, meningocele
	  GI: tracheoesophageal fistula, duodenal atresia, facial clefts (interfere with swallowing)
		Idiopathic most common
		Maternal
		  Uteroplacental insufficiency (preeclampsia, nephropathy)
		  Medications (ACEI)
		Fetal
		  Congenital urinary tract anomalies (renal agenesis, obstruction, posterior urethral valves)
		  Demise/chronic hypoxemia (blood shunt away from kidneys to perfuse brain)
		  IUGR
		  Ruptured membranes: prolonged amniotic fluid leak
		  Amniotic fluid normally decreases after 35 wk

Epidemiology	Occur in 0.2-1.6% of all pregnancies	Occur in ~4.5% of all pregnancies Severe form in <0.7% Common in pregnancies >41 wk (~12%)

Clinical Features and Complications	Uterus large for dates, difficulty palpating fetal parts and hearing FHR
	Maternal complications
	  Pressure symptoms from overdistended uterus (dyspnea, edema, hydronephrosis)
	Obstetrical complications
	  Cord prolapse, placental abruption, malpresentation, preterm labour, uterine dysfunction, and PPH
		Uterus small for dates
		Fetal complications
		  15-25% have fetal anomalies
		  Amniotic fluid bands (T1) can lead to Potter's facies, limb deformities, abdominal wall defects
		Obstetrical complications
		  Cord compression
		  Increased risk of adverse fetal outcomes
		  Pulmonary hypoplasia (late-onset)
		  Marker for infants who may not tolerate labour well

Management	Determine underlying cause
	  Screen for maternal disease/infection
	  Complete fetal U/S evaluation
	Depends on severity
	  Mild to moderate cases require no treatment
	  If severe, hospitalize and consider therapeutic amniocentesis
		Always warrants admission and investigation
		  Rule out ROM
		  Fetal monitoring (NST, BPP)
		  U/S Doppler studies (umbilical cord and uterine artery)
		Maternal hydration with oral or IV fluids to help increase amniotic fluid
		Injection of fluid via amniocentesis will improve condition for ~1 wk – may be most helpful for visualizing any associated fetal anomalies
		Consider delivery if term
		Amnio-infusion may be considered during labour via intrauterine catheter

Prognosis	2-5 fold increase in risk of perinatal mortality	Poorer with early onset High mortality related to congenital malformations and pulmonary hypoplasia when diagnosed during T2

Multi-Fetal Gestation and Malpresentation

Epidemiology
- incidence of twins is 1/80 and triplets 1/6,400 in North America
- 2/3 of twins are dizygotic (fraternal)
  - risk factors for dizygotic twins: IVF, increased maternal age, newly discontinued OCP, ethnicity (e.g. certain African regions)
- monozygous twinning occurs at a constant rate worldwide (1/250)
- determine zygosity by number of placentas, thickness of membranes, sex, blood type

Clinical Features

Table 13. Complications Associated with Multiple Gestation

Maternal	Uteroplacental	Fetal
Hyperemesis gravidarum	Increased PROM/PTL	Prematurity*
GDM	Polyhydramnios	IUGR
Gestational HTN	Placenta previa	Malpresentation
Anemia	Placental abruption	Congenital anomalies
Increased physiological stress on all	PPH (uterine atony)	Twin-twin transfusion
systems	Umbilical cord prolapse	Increased perinatal morbidity and mortality
Increased compressive symptoms	Cord anomalies	Twin interlocking (twin A breech, twin B
C/S	(velamentous insertion, 2 vessel cord)	vertex)
		Single fetal demise

*Most common cause of perinatal mortality in multiple gestation

The Ps of Multiple Gestation Complications

Increased rates of
Puking
Pallor (anemia)
Preeclampsia/PIH
Pressure (compressive symptoms)
PTL/PROM/PPROM
Polyhydramnios
Placenta previa/abruptio
PPH/APH
Prolonged labour
Cord Prolapse
Prematurity
MalPresentation
Perinatal morbidity and mortality
Parental distress
Postpartum depression

Management
- U/S determination of chorionicity must be done within first trimester (ideally 8-12 wk GA)
- increased antenatal surveillance
  - serial U/S q 2-3wk from 24 wk GA to assess growth (uncomplicated diamniotic dichorionitic)
  - increased frequency of ultrasounds in monochorionic diamniotic and monochorionic monoamniotic twins
  - Doppler flow studies weekly if discordant fetal growth (>30%)
  - BPP as needed
- may attempt vaginal delivery if twin A presents as vertex, otherwise C/S (40-50% of all twin deliveries, 15% of cases have twin A delivered vaginally and twin B delivered by C/S)
- mode of delivery depends on fetal weights, GA, presentation

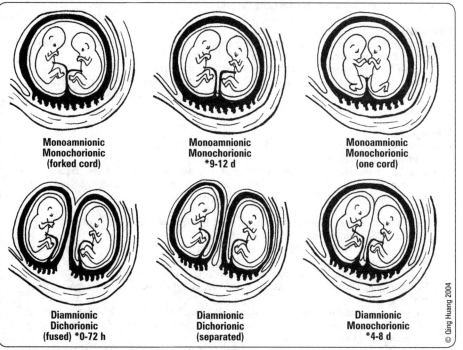

Monoamnionic	Monoamnionic	Monoamnionic
Monochorionic	Monochorionic	Monochorionic
(forked cord)	*9-12 d	(one cord)

Diamnionic	Diamnionic	Diamnionic
Dichorionic	Dichorionic	Monochorionic
(fused) *0-72 h	(separated)	*4-8 d

© Qing Huang 2004

Figure 4. Classification of twin pregnancies　　　*Indicates time of cleavage

Twin-Twin Transfusion Syndrome

Definition
- formation of placental intertwin vascular anastomoses cause arterial blood from donor twin to pass into veins of the recipient twin

Epidemiology
- 10% of monochorionic twins
- concern if >30% discordance in estimated fetal weight

Clinical Features
- donor twin: IUGR, hypovolemia, hypotension, anemia, oligohydramnios
- recipient twin: hypervolemia, HTN, CHF, polycythemia, edema, polyhydramnios, kernicterus in neonatal period

Investigations
- detected by U/S screening, Doppler flow analysis

Management
- therapeutic serial amniocentesis to decompress polyhydramnios of recipient twin and decrease pressure in cavity and on placenta
- intrauterine blood transfusion to donor twin if necessary
- laparoscopic occlusion of placental vessels
- fetoscopic laser ablation of placental vascular anastomoses when indicated and if available

Breech Presentation

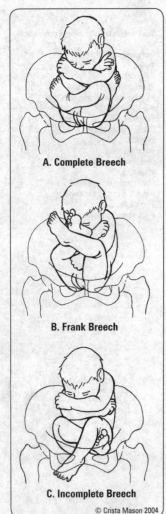

A. Complete Breech

B. Frank Breech

C. Incomplete Breech

© Crista Mason 2004

Figure 5. Types of breech presentation

Criteria for Vaginal Breech Delivery
- Frank or complete breech, GA >36 wk
- EFW 2,500-3,800 g based on clinical and U/S assessment (5.5–8.5 lb)
- Fetal head flexed
- Continuous fetal monitoring
- 2 experienced obstetricians, assistant, and anesthetist present
- Ability to perform emergency C/S within 30 min if required

Definition
- fetal buttocks or lower extremity is the presenting part as determined on U/S
- complete (10%): hips and knees both flexed
- frank (60%): hips flexed, knees extended, buttocks present at cervix
- most common type of breech presentation
- most common breech presentation to be delivered vaginally
- incomplete (30%): both or one hip flexed and both or one knee present below the buttocks, feet or knees present first (footling breech, kneeling breech)

Epidemiology
- occurs in 3-4% of pregnancies at term (25% <28 wk)

Risk Factors
- maternal: pelvis (contracted), uterus (shape abnormalities, intrauterine tumours, fibroids, previous breech), pelvic tumours causing compression, grand multiparity
- maternal-fetal: placenta (previa), amniotic fluid (poly-/oligohydramnios)
- fetal: prematurity, multiple gestation, congenital malformations (found in 6% of breeches; 2-3% if in vertex presentations), abnormalities in fetal tone and movement, aneuploidy, hydrocephalus, anencephalus

Management
- ECV: repositioning of singleton fetus within uterus under U/S guidance
  - overall success rate of 65%
  - criteria: >36 wk GA, singleton, unengaged presenting part, reactive NST, not in labour
  - contraindications: previous T3 bleed, prior classical C/S, previous myomectomy, oligohydramnios, PROM, placenta previa, abnormal U/S, suspected IUGR, HTN, uteroplacental insufficiency, nuchal cord
  - risks: abruption, cord compression, cord accident, ROM, labour, fetal bradycardia requiring C/S (<1% risk), alloummunization, fetal death 1:5,000
  - method: tocometry, followed by U/S guided transabdominal manipulation of fetus with constant fetal heart monitoring
  - if patient Rh negative, give Rhogam® prior to procedure
  - better prognosis if multiparous, good fluid volume, small baby, skilled obstetrician, posterior placenta
    - pre- or early labour ultrasound to assess type of breech presentation, fetal growth, estimated weight, placenta position, attitude of fetal head (flexed is preferable); if ultrasound unavailable, recommend C/S
- ECV and elective C/S should be presented as options with the risks and benefits outlined; obtain informed consent

- method for vaginal breech delivery
  - encourage effective maternal pushing efforts
  - at delivery of after-coming head, assistant must apply suprapubic pressure to flex and engage fetal head
  - delivery can be spontaneous or assisted; avoid fetal traction
  - apply fetal manipulation only after spontaneous delivery to level of umbilicus
- C/S recommended if: the breech has not descended to the perineum in the second stage of labour after 2 h, in the absence of active pushing, or if vaginal delivery is not imminent after 1 h of active pushing
- contraindications to vaginal breech delivery:
  - cord presentation
  - clinically inadequate maternal pelvis
  - fetal factors incompatible with vaginal delivery (e.g. hydrocephalus), macrosomia, fetal growth restriction

Prognosis
- regardless of route of delivery, breech infants have lower birth weights and higher rates of perinatal mortality, congenital anomalies, abruption, and cord prolapse

Hypertensive Disorders of Pregnancy

Hypertension in Pregnancy

- hypertensive disorders of pregnancy are classified as either pre-existing or gestational HTN

PRE-EXISTING HYPERTENSION

Definition
- BP >140/90 prior to 20 wk GA, persisting >7 wk postpartum
- essential HTN is associated with an increased risk of gestational HTN, abruptio placentae, IUGR, and IUFD

GESTATIONAL HTN

Definition
- sBP >140 or dBP >90 developing after 20th wk GA in the absence of proteinuria in a woman known to be normotensive before pregnancy

Risk Factors
- maternal factors
  - primigravida (80-90% of gestational HTN), first conception with a new partner, PMHx or FHx of gestational HTN
  - DM, chronic HTN, or renal insufficiency
  - obesity
  - antiphospholipid syndrome
  - extremes of maternal age (<18 or >35 yr)
  - previous stillbirth or IUFD
- fetal factors
  - IUGR or oligohydramnios
  - GTN
  - multiple gestation
  - fetal hydrops "mirror syndrome"

Clinical Evaluation of HTN in Pregnancy
- in general, clinical evaluation should include the mother and fetus
- **evaluation of mother**
  - body weight
  - central nervous system
    - presence and severity of headache
    - visual disturbances – blurring, scotomata
    - tremulousness, irritability, somnolence
    - hyperreflexia
  - hematologic
    - bleeding, petechiae
  - hepatic
    - RUQ or epigastric pain
    - severe N/V
  - renal
    - urine output and colour
  - lonon-dependent edema (i.e. hands and face)

Vaginal Delivery of Breech Presentation
SOGC Clinical Practice Guidelines 2009;226;557-566
Objective: To discuss risks and benefits of trial of labour versus planned C/S, with selection criteria, management, and delivery techniques for trial of vaginal breech birth.
Evidence: Randomized trials, prospective cohort studies and select cohort studies from Medline search for long-term outcomes and epidemiology of vaginal breech delivery.
Summary: Higher risk of perinatal mortality and short-term neonatal morbidity can be associated with vaginal breech birth as compared to elective C/S. However, careful case selection (including term singleton breech fetuses and clinically adequate maternal pelvis) and labour management may achieve a similar safety level as elective C/S (~2 per 1,000 births perinatal mortality, ~2% short-term neonatal morbidity). Specific protocols for vaginal breech delivery should be followed: continuous fetal heart monitoring, assessment for adequate progress in labour, no induction of labour recommended, emergency C/S available, if required, and health care providers with requisite skills and experience. Informed consent for the preferred delivery method should be obtained.

Ominous Symptoms of HTN in Pregnancy
RUQ pain, headache, and visual disturbances

Hypertension in Pregnancy

Adverse Maternal Conditions
- sBP >160 mmHg
- dBP >100 mmHg
- HELLP
- Cerebral hemorrhage
- Renal dysfunction: oliguria <500 mL/d
- Left ventricular failure, pulmonary edema
- Placental abruption, DIC
- Symptoms
- Abdominal pain, N/V
- Headaches, visual problems
- SOB, chest pain
- Eclampsia: convulsions

Adverse Fetal Conditions
- IUGR
- Oligohydramnios
- Absent/reversed umbilical artery end diastolic flow
- Can result in:
  - Fetal disability and/or death

I-A Evidence-Recommendation Highlights of SOGC Clinical Practice Guidelines
Diagnosis, Evaluation, and Management of the Hypertensive Disorders of Pregnancy
J Obstet Gynaecol Can 2014;36(5):416-438
- For BP measurement, Korotkoff phase V should be used to designate the dBP.
- Calcium supplementation (of at least 1g/d, orally) is recommended for women with low dietary intake of calcium (<600 mg/d). (I-A)
- For preeclampsia prevention among increased risk women, low-dose Aspirin® (75-100 mg/d) is recommended until delivery.
- Umbilical artery Doppler velocimetry should be part of the antenatal fetal surveillance in preeclampsia.
- Initial antihypertensive therapy for severe HTN (sBP >160 or dBP ≥110) should be with labetalol, nifedipine, or hydralazine.
- Initial antihypertensive therapy for non-severe HTN (BP 140-159/90-109 mmHg) should be with methyldopa, β-blockers, or calcium channel blockers.
- Antenatal corticosteroids for fetal lung maturation should be considered for all women with preeclampsia before 34 wk gestation.
- In a planned vaginal delivery with an unfavourable cervix, cervical ripening should be used.
- Oxytocin 5 units IV or 10 units IM should be used as part of the management during the third stage of labour, particularly in the presence of thrombocytopenia or coagulopathy.
- MgSO₄ is the recommended first-line treatment for eclampsia.
- MgSO₄ is the recommended eclampsia prophylaxis in severe preeclampsia.

- **evaluation of fetus**
  - fetal movement
  - fetal heart rate tracing – NST
  - ultrasound for growth
  - BPP
  - Doppler flow studies

Laboratory Evaluation of Gestational Hypertension
- CBC
- PTT, INR, fibrinogen – especially if surgery or regional anaesthetics are planned
- ALT, AST
- creatinine, uric acid
- 24 h urine collection for protein or albumin:creatinine ratio

Complications
- maternal
- liver and renal dysfunction
- seizure "eclampsia"
- abruptio placentae
- left ventricular failure/pulmonary edema
- DIC (release of placental thromboplastin consumptive coagulopathy)
- HELLP syndrome
- hemorrhagic stroke (50% of deaths)
- fetal (2° to placental insufficiency)
- IUGR, prematurity, abruptio placentae, IUFD

Management
- for non-severe HTN (149-159/90 to 105) target a BP of 130-155/80-105 in women without comorbidities or <140/90 in women with comorbidities
- for both pre-existing and gestational HTN, labetalol 100-400 mg PO bid-tid, nifedipine XL preparation 20-60 mg PO od, or α-methyldopa 250-500 mg PO bid-qid
- for severe HTN (BP>160/110), give one of:
  - labetalol 20 mg IV then 20-80 mg IV q30min (max 300 mg)(then switch to oral)
  - nifedipine 5-10 mg capsule q30min
    - hydralazine 5 mg IV, repeat 5-10 mg IV q30min or 0.5 to 10 mg/hr IV, to a maximum of 20 mg IV (or 30 mg IM)
- no ACEI, ARBs, diuretics, prazosin, or atenolol
- pre-existing HTN and gestational HTN without any deterioration can be followed until 37 wk then decide to induce shortly thereafter

PREECLAMPSIA

Definition
- pre-existing or gestational HTN with new onset proteinuria or adverse conditions

Risk Factors
- nulliparity
- preeclampsia in a previous pregnancy
- age >40 yr or <18 yr
- FHx of preeclampsia
- chronic HTN
- chronic renal disease
- antiphospholipid antibody syndrome or inherited thrombophilia
- vascular or connective tissue disease
- DM (pre-gestational and gestational)
- obesity
- hydrops fetalis "mirror syndrome"
- unexplained fetal growth restriction
- abruptio placentae
- there is a potential for further deterioration to severe preeclampsia as defined above

Preeclampsia Investigations
- CBC
- AST, ALT
- INR and aPTT (if regional anesthesia planned)
- Cr
- Urine (24 h protein collection or albumin/creatinine ratio)
- Uric acid

Management
- depends on GA, possible threat of seizures
- if stable and no adverse factors, may admit and follow, ± decide to deliver as approaching 34-36 wk (must weigh risks of fetal prematurity vs. risks of developing severe preeclampsia/eclampsia)
- for severe preeclampsia, stabilize and deliver
- if severe preeclampsia during labour, increase maternal monitoring: hourly input and output, urine dip q12h, hourly neurological vitals, and increase fetal monitoring (continuous FHR monitoring)
- antihypertensive therapy
  - labetalol 20 mg IV then 20-80 mg IV q30min (max 300 mg)(then switch to oral)
  - nifedipine 5-10 mg capsule q30min
    - hydralazine 5 mg IV, repeat 5-10 mg IV q30min or 0.5 to 10 mg/hr IV, to a maximum of 20 mg IV (or 30 mg IM)

- seizure prevention
  - $MgSO_4$
  - postpartum management
  - risk of seizure highest in first 24 h postpartum – continue $MgSO_4$ for 12-24 h after delivery
  - vitals q1h
  - consider HELLP syndrome
  - most return to a normotensive BP within 2 wk

ECLAMPSIA

Definition
- the occurrence of one or more generalized convulsions and/or coma in the setting of preeclampsia and in the absence of other neurologic conditions

Epidemiology
- an eclamptic seizure occurs in approximately 0.5% of mildly preeclamptic women and 2-3% of severely preeclamptic women

Risk Factors
- same as risk factors for preeclampsia

Clinical Manifestations
- eclampsia is a clinical diagnosis
- typically tonic-clonic and lasting 60-75 s
- symptoms that may occur before the seizure include persistent frontal or occipital headache, blurred vision, photophobia, right upper quadrant or epigastric pain, and altered mental status
- in up to one third of cases, there is no proteinuria or blood pressure <140/90 mmHg prior to the seizure
- in general, women with typical eclamptic seizures who do not have focal neurologic deficits or prolonged coma do not require diagnostic evaluation including imaging

Management
- ABCs
- roll patient into LLDP
- supplemental O_2 via face mask to treat hypoxemia due to hypoventilation during convulsive episode
- aggressive antihypertensive therapy for sustained diastolic pressures ≥105 mmHg or systolic blood pressures ≥160 mmHg with hydralazine or labetalol
- prevention of recurrent convulsions: to prevent further seizures and the possible complications of repeated seizure activity (e.g. rhabdomyolysis, metabolic acidosis, aspiration pneumonitis, etc.)
- $MgSO_4$ is now the drug of choice, with previously used agents including diazepam and phenytoin
- the definitive treatment of eclampsia is DELIVERY, irrespective of gestational age, to reduce the risk of maternal morbidity and mortality from complications of the disease
- mode of delivery is dependent on clinical situation and fetal-maternal condition

HELLP Syndrome
Hemolysis
Elevated Liver enzymes
Low Platelets

Note
Eclampsia prior to 20 wk of gestation is rare and should raise the possibility of an underlying molar pregnancy or antiphospholipid syndrome

Differential Diagnosis of Cause for Seizure in a Pregnant Woman
- Stroke
- Hypertensive disease (hypertensive encephalopathy, pheochromocytoma)
- Space-occupying lesion of the CNS
- Metabolic disorders (hypoglycemia, SIADH)
- Infection (meningitis, encephalitis)
- Thrombotic thrombocytopenic purpura or thrombophilia
- Idiopathic epilepsy
- Use of illicit drugs
- Cerebral vasculitis

Medical Complications of Pregnancy

Iron and Folate Deficiency Anemia

Table 14. Iron Deficiency and Folate Deficiency Anemia

	Iron Deficiency Anemia	Folate Deficiency Anemia
Etiology	See Hematology, H15	See Hematology, H25
Epidemiology	Responsible for 80% of causes of non-physiologic anemia during pregnancy	Incidence varies from 0.5-25% depending on region, population, diet
Clinical Features	See Hematology, H15	See Hematology, H25
Investigations	See Hematology, H15	See Hematology, H25
Management	Prevention (non-anemic): 30 mg elemental iron/d (met by most prenatal vitamins) Treatment (anemic): 30-120 mg elemental iron/d 325 mg ferrous fumarate = 106 mg elemental Fe^{2+}; 325 mg ferrous sulfate = 65 mg elemental Fe^{2+}; 325 mg ferrous gluconate = 36 mg elemental Fe^{2+} Polysaccharide-Iron Complex = 150 mg elemental Fe/capsule	Prevention: 0.4-1 mg folic acid PO daily for 1-3 mo preconceptually and throughout T1, or 5 mg folic acid per day with past history of oNTD, DM, or antiepileptic medication use
Complications	Maternal: angina, CHF, infection, slower recuperation, preterm labour Fetal: decreased oxygen carrying capacity leading to fetal distress, IUGR, and low birth weight	Maternal: decreased blood volume, N/V, anorexia Fetal: neural tube defects in T1, low birth weight, prematurity
Notes	Mother needs 1 g of elemental iron per fetus; this amount exceeds normal stores + dietary intake Iron requirements increase during pregnancy due to fetal/placental growth (500 mg), increased maternal RBC mass (500 mg), and losses (200 mg) – more needed for multiple gestations	Minimum daily requirement is 0.4 mg Most often associated with iron deficiency anemia Folic acid is necessary for closure of neural tube during early fetal development (by day 28 of gestation)

Diabetes Mellitus

Epidemiology
- 2-4% of pregnancies are complicated by DM

Classification of Diabetes Mellitus
- type 1 and type 2 DM (see Endocrinology, E7)
- GDM: onset of DM during pregnancy (usually around 24-28 wk GA)

Etiology
- type 1 and type 2 DM
- GDM: anti-insulin factors produced by placenta and high maternal cortisol levels create increased peripheral insulin resistance → leading to GDM and/or exacerbating pre-existing DM

MANAGEMENT

A. TYPE 1 and TYPE 2 DM

Preconception
- pre-plan and refer to high-risk clinic
- optimize glycemic control
- counsel patient on potential risks and complications
- evaluate for diabetic retinopathy, neuropathy, CAD

Pregnancy
- if already on oral medication, generally switch to insulin therapy
  - continuing glyburide or metformin controversial
  - teratogenicity unknown for other oral anti-hyperglycemics
- tight glycemic control
  - insulin dosage may need to be adjusted in T2 due to increased demand and increased insulin resistance
- monitor as for normal pregnancy plus initial 24 h urine protein and creatinine clearance, retinal exam, HbA1c
  - HbA1c: >140% of pre-pregnancy value associated with increased risk of spontaneous abortion and congenital malformations
- increased fetal surveillance (BPP, NST), consider fetal ECHO to look for cardiac abnormalities

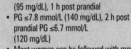

Monitoring Glucose Levels
- Frequent measurements of blood glucose during pregnancy are advised for women with type 1 or 2 DM to help prevent or treat both hypoglycemia and hyperglycemia, and also improves neonatal outcome
- Aim for FPG ≤5.3 mmol/L (95 mg/dL), 1 h post prandial
- PG ≤7.8 mmol/L (140 mg/dL), 2 h post prandial PG ≤6.7 mmol/L (120 mg/dL)
- Most women can be followed with monthly HbA1c determinations

Labour
- timing of delivery depends on fetal and maternal health and risk factors (i.e. must consider size of baby, lung maturity, maternal blood glucose, and blood pressure control)
- can wait for spontaneous labour if blood glucose well-controlled and BPP normal
- induce by 38-39 wk
- type of delivery
  - increased risk of cephalopelvic disproportion (CPD) and shoulder dystocia with babies >4,000 g (8.8 lbs)
  - consider elective C/S for predicted birthweight >4,500 g (9.9 lbs) (controversial)
- monitoring
  - during labour monitor blood glucose q1h with patient on insulin and dextrose drip
  - aim for blood glucose between 3.5-6.5 mmol/L to reduce the risk of neonatal hypoglycemia

Postpartum
- insulin requirements dramatically drop with expulsion of placenta (source of insulin antagonists)
- no insulin is required for 48-72 h postpartum in most type 1 DM
- monitor glucose q6h, restart insulin at two-thirds of pre-pregnancy dosage when glucose >8 mmol/L

B. GESTATIONAL DM

Post-prandial blood glucose values seem to be the most effective at determining the likelihood of macrosomia or other adverse pregnancy outcomes

Risk Factors for GDM
- Age >25 yr
- Obesity
- Ethnicity (Aboriginal, Hispanic, Asian, African)
- FHx of DM
- Previous history of GDM
- Previous child with birthweight >4.0 kg
- Polycystic ovarian syndrome
- Current use of glucocorticoids
- Essential HTN or pregnancy-related HTN

Screening and Diagnosis
- all pregnant women between 24-28 wk GA (or at any stage if high risk)
- 2 screening options
  - 1-step screening with fasting 75 g OGTT; GDM if ≥1 of:
    - FPG ≥ 5.1 mmol/L
    - 1h PG ≥ 10.0 mmol/L
    - 2h PG ≥ 8.5 mmol/L
  - 2-step screening (recommended by the Canadian Diabetes Association)
    - Step 1: Perform a random nonfasting 50 g OGCT
      - 1h PG < 7.8 mmol/L is normal
      - 1h PG ≥ 11.1 mmol/L is GDM
      - if 1h PG 7.8-11.0 mmol/L, proceed to Step 2
    - Step 2: Perform a fasting 75 g OGTT, GDM if ≥1 of:
      - FPG ≥ 5.3 mmol/L
      - 1h PG ≥ 10.6 mmol/L
      - 2h PG ≥ 9.0 mmol/L

Management
- first line is management through diet modification and increased physical activity
- initiate insulin therapy if glycemic targets not achieved within 2 wk of lifestyle modification alone
- glycemic targets: FPG <5.3 mmol/L, 1h PG <7.8 mmol/L, 2h PG <6.7 mmol/L
- oral agents can be used in pregnancy but is off-label and should be discussed with patient
- stop insulin and diabetic diet postpartum
- follow up with 75 g OGTT by 3 months postpartum, counsel about lifestyle modifications, and perform glucose challenge test q2 yr

Prognosis
- most maternal and fetal complications are related to hyperglycemia and its effects

Long-Term Maternal Complications
- type 1 and type 2 DM: risk of progressive retinopathy and nephropathy
- GDM: 50% risk of developing type 2 DM in next 20 yr

Table 15. Complications of DM in Pregnancy

Maternal	Fetal
Obstetric HTN/preeclampsia (especially if pre-existing nephropathy/proteinuria): insulin resistance is implicated in etiology of HTN Polyhydramnios: maternal hyperglycemia leads to fetal hyperglycemia, which leads to fetal polyuria (a major source of amniotic fluid)	**Growth Abnormalities** Macrosomia: maternal hyperglycemia leads to fetal hyperinsulinism resulting in accelerated anabolism IUGR: due to placental vascular insufficiency
Diabetic Emergencies Hypoglycemia Ketoacidosis Diabetic coma	**Delayed Organ Maturity** Fetal lung immaturity: hyperglycemia interferes with surfactant synthesis (respiratory distress syndrome)
End-Organ Involvement or Deterioration (occur in type 1 DM and type 2 DM, not in GDM) Retinopathy Nephropathy	**Congenital Anomalies (occur in type 1 DM and type 2 DM, not in GDM)** 2-7x increased risk of cardiac (VSD), NTD, GU (cystic kidneys), GI (anal atresia), and MSK (sacral agenesis) anomalies due to hyperglycemia Note: Pregnancies complicated by GDM do not manifest an increased risk of congenital anomalies because GDM develops after the critical period of organogenesis (in T1)
Other Pyelonephritis/UTI: glucosuria provides a culture medium for E. coli and other bacteria Increased incidence of spontaneous abortion (in type 1 DM and type 2 DM, not in GDM): related to pre-conception glycemic control	**Labour and Delivery** Preterm labour/prematurity: most commonly in patients with HTN/preeclampsia Preterm labour is associated with poor glycemic control but the exact mechanism is unknown Increased incidence of stillbirth Birth trauma: due to macrosomia, can lead to difficult vaginal delivery and shoulder dystocia
	Neonatal Hypoglycemia: due to pancreatic hyperplasia and excess insulin secretion in the neonate Hyperbilirubinemia and jaundice: due to prematurity and polycythemia Hypocalcemia: exact pathophysiology not understood, may be related to functional hypoparathyroidism Polycythemia: hyperglycemia stimulates fetal erythropoietin production

Group B *Streptococcus*

Epidemiology
- 15-40% vaginal carrier rate

Risk Factors (for neonatal disease)
- GBS bacteriuria during current pregnancy even if treated
- previous infant with invasive GBS infection
- preterm labour <37 wk
- ruptured membranes >18 h before delivery
- intrapartum maternal temperature ≥38°C
- positive GBS screen between 35-37 weeks GA in current pregnancy

Clinical Features
- not harmful to mother
- risk of vertical transmission (neonatal sepsis, meningitis or pneumonia, and death)

Indications for Intrapartum Antibiotic GBS Prophylaxis
Centres for Disease Control and Prevention. Prevention of Perinatal Group B Streptococcal Disease. MMWR 2010;59(RR-10):14
- Previous infant with invasive GBS disease.
- GBS bacteriuria during any trimester of the current pregnancy.
- Positive GBS vaginal-rectal screening culture in late gestation during current pregnancy.
- Unknown GBS status at the onset of labour (culture not done, incomplete, or results unknown) and any of the following:
- Delivery at <37 wk gestation.
- Amniotic membrane rupture ≥18 h.
- Intrapartum temperature ≥38.0°C (≥ 100.4°F).
- Intrapartum nucleic-acid amplification test positive for GBS.

Investigations
- offer screening to all women at 35-37 wk with vaginal and anorectal swabs for GBS culture

Treatment
- treatment of maternal GBS at delivery decreases neonatal morbidity and mortality
- indications for antibiotic prophylaxis: positive GBS screen, GBS in urine, or previous infant with GBS disease or GBS status unknown and one of the other risk factors
- antibiotics for GBS prophylaxis
  - penicillin G 5 million units IV then 2.5 million units IV q4h until delivery
  - penicillin allergic but not at risk for anaphylaxis: cefazolin 2 g IV then 1 g q8h
  - penicillin allergic and at risk for anaphylaxis: vancomycin 1 g IV q12h until delivery
- if fever, broad spectrum antibiotic coverage is advised

Urinary Tract Infection

Treat asymptomatic bacteriuria in pregnancy because of increased risk of progression to cystitis, pyelonephritis, and probable increased risk of preterm labour

Epidemiology
- most common medical complication of pregnancy
- asymptomatic bacteriuria in 2-7% of pregnant women, more frequently in multiparous women
- note: asymptomatic bacteriuria should be treated in pregnancy due to increased risk of pyelonephritis and preterm labour

Etiology
- increased urinary stasis from mechanical and hormonal (progesterone) factors
- organisms include GBS as well as those that occur in non-pregnant women

Clinical Features
- may be asymptomatic
- dysuria, urgency, and frequency in cystitis
- fever, flank pain, and costovertebral angle tenderness in pyelonephritis

Investigations
- urinalysis, urine C&S
- cystoscopy and renal function tests in recurrent infections

Management
- uncomplicated UTI
- first line: amoxicillin (250-500 mg PO q8h x 7 d)
- alternatives: nitrofurantoin (100 mg PO bid x 7 d)
- follow with monthly urine cultures
- pyelonephritis
- hospitalization and IV antibiotics

Prognosis
- complications if untreated: acute cystitis, pyelonephritis, and possible preterm labour
- recurrence is common

Infections During Pregnancy

Table 16. Infections During Pregnancy

Infection	Agent	Source of Transmission	Greatest Transmission Risk to Fetus	Effects on Fetus	Effects on Mother	Diagnosis	Management
Chicken Pox	Varicella zoster virus (herpes family)	To mom: direct, respiratory To baby: transplacental	13-30 wk GA, and 5 d pre- to 2 d post-delivery	Congenital varicella syndrome (limb aplasia, chorioretinitis, cataracts, cutaneous scars, cortical atrophy, IUGR, hydrops), preterm labour	Fever, malaise, vesicular pruritic lesions	Clinical, ± vesicle fluid culture, ± serology	VZIG for mother if exposed, decreases congenital varicella syndrome Note: do not administer vaccine during pregnancy (live attenuated vaccine)
*CMV	DNA virus (herpes family)	To mom: blood/organ transfusion, sexual contact To baby: transplacental, during delivery, breast milk	T1-T3	5-10% develop CNS involvement (mental retardation, cerebral calcification, hydrocephalus, microcephaly, deafness, chorioretinitis)	Asymptomatic or flu-like	Serologic screen; isolate virus from urine or secretion culture	No specific treatment; maintain good hygiene and avoid high risk situations
Erythema Infectiosum (Fifth Disease)	Parvovirus B19	To mom: respiratory, infected blood products To baby: transplacental	10-20 wk GA	Spontaneous abortion (SA), stillbirth, hydrops *in utero*	Flu-like, rash, arthritis; often asymptomatic	Serology, viral PCR, maternal AFP; if IgM present, follow fetus with U/S for hydrops	If hydrops occurs, consider fetal transfusion
Hepatitis B	DNA virus	To mom: blood, saliva, semen, vaginal secretions To baby: transplacental, breast milk	T3 10% vertical transmission if asymptomatic and HBsAg +ve; 85-90% if HBsAg and HBeAg +ve	Prematurity, low birth weight, neonatal death	Fever, N/V, fatigue, jaundice, elevated liver enzymes	Serologic screening for all pregnancies	Rx neonate with HBIG and vaccine (at birth, 1, 6 mo); 90% effective
*Herpes Simplex Virus	DNA virus	To mom: intimate mucocutaneous contact To baby: transplacental, during delivery	Delivery (if genital lesions present); less commonly *in utero*	Disseminated herpes (20%); CNS sequelae (35%); self-limited infection	Painful vesicular lesions	Clinical diagnosis	Acyclovir for symptomatic women, suppressive therapy at 36 wk controversial Suggested C/S if active genital lesions, even if remote from vulva
HIV	RNA retrovirus	To mom: blood, semen, vaginal secretions To baby: in utero, during delivery, breast milk	1/3 in utero, 1/3 at delivery, 1/3 breastfeeding	IUGR, preterm labour, PROM	See <u>Infectious Diseases</u>, ID27	Serology, viral PCR All pregnant women are offered screening	Triple anti-retroviral therapy decreases transmission to <1% Elective C/S: no previous antiviral Rx or monotherapy only, viral load unknown or >500 RNA copies/mL, unknown prenatal care, patient request
*Rubella	ssRNA togavirus	To mom: respiratory droplets (highly contagious) To baby: transplacental	T1	SA or congenital rubella syndrome (hearing loss, cataracts, CV lesions, MR, IUGR, hepatitis, CNS defects, osseous changes)	Rash (50%), fever, posterior auricular or occipital lymphadenopathy, arthralgia	Serologic testing; all pregnant women screened (immune if titre >1:16); infection if IgM present or >4x increase in IgG	No specific treatment; offer vaccine following pregnancy Do not administer during pregnancy (live attenuated)
Syphilis	Spirochete (*Treponema pallidum*)	To mom: sexual contact To baby: transplacental	T1-T3	Risk of preterm labour, multisystem involvement, fetal death	See <u>Infectious Diseases</u>, ID25	VDRL screening for all pregnancies; if positive, requires confirmatory testing	Pen G 2.4 million U IM x 1 dose if early syphilis, 3 doses if late syphilis, monitor VDRL monthly If Pen G allergic: Clindamycin 900 mg IV q8h
*Toxoplasmosis	Protozoa (*Toxoplasma gondii*)	To mom: raw meat, unpasteurized goat's milk, cat feces/urine To baby: transplacental	T3 (but most severe if infected in T1); only concern if primary infection during pregnancy	Congenital toxoplasmosis (chorioretinitis, hydrocephaly, intracranial calcification, MR, microcephaly) NB: 75% initially asymptomatic at birth	Majority subclinical; may have flu-like symptoms	IgM and IgG serology; PCR of amniotic fluid	Self-limiting in mother; spiramycin decreases fetal morbidity but not rate of transmission

* Indicates TORCH infection

Venous Thromboembolism

Epidemiology
- incidence of 12.1/10, 000 (DVT), and 5.4/10,000 (PE)
- increased risk VTE throughout pregnancy with highest risk of DVT in third trimester and post-partum period and highest risk of PE post-partum (first 6 weeks)

Risk Factors

- previous VTE, age >35, obesity, infection, bedrest/immobility, shock/dehydration, thrombophilias (see Hematology, H35)

Table 17. Risk Factors for VTE Specific to Pregnancy

Hypercoagulability	Stasis	Endothelial
II, V, VII, VIII, IX, X, XII, fibrinogen Increased platelet aggregation Decreased protein S, tPA, factors XI, XIII	**Increased Factors** Increased resistance to activated protein C Antithrombin can be normal or reduced Increased venous distensibility Decreased venous tone 50% decrease in venous flow in lower extremity by T3 Uterus is mechanical impediment to venous return	Vascular damage at delivery (C/S or SVD) Uterine instrumentation Peripartum pelvic surgery

Clinical Features
- most DVTs occur in the iliofemoral or calf veins with a predilection for the left leg
- signs of a pulmonary embolism are non-specific (as in non-pregnant women)
- unexplained spontaneous fetal loss

Investigations
- duplex venous Doppler sonography for DVT
- CXR and V/Q scan or spiral CT for PE

Management
- before initiating treatment, obtain a baseline CBC including platelets, and aPTT
- warfarin is contraindicated during pregnancy due to its potential teratogenic effects
- unfractionated heparin
  - bolus of 5,000 IU followed by an infusion of ~30,000 IU/24h
  - measure aPTT 6 h after the bolus
  - maintain aPTT at a therapeutic level (1.5-2x normal)
  - repeat q24h once therapeutic
  - heparin-induced thrombocytopenia (HIT) uncommon (3%) but serious complication
  - LMWH can also be used in pregnancy
- compression stockings
- poor evidence to support a recommendation for or against avoidance of prolonged sitting
- VTE prophylaxis
  - women on long-term anticoagulation: full therapeutic anticoagulation throughout pregnancy and for 6-12 wk postpartum
  - women with a non-active PMHx of VTE: unfractionated heparin regimens suggested
  - insufficient evidence in pregnancy to recommend routine use of LMWH for all patients
  - current prophylaxis regimens for acquired thrombophilias (e.g. APS syndrome) include low dose Aspirin® in conjunction with prophylactic heparin

Virchow's Triad for VTE
- Hypercoagulable state
- Stasis
- Endothelial damage

Normal Labour and Delivery

Definition of Labour

- true labour: regular, painful contractions of increasing intensity associated with progressive dilatation and effacement of cervix and descent of presenting part, or progression of station
  - preterm (>20 to <36+6 wk GA)
  - term (37-41+6 wk GA)
  - postterm (>42 wk GA)
- false labour (Braxton-Hicks contractions): irregular contractions, with unchanged intensity and long intervals, occur throughout pregnancy and not associated with any cervical dilatation, effacement, or descent
  - often relieved by rest or sedation

The Cervix

- dilatation: latent phase (0-4 cm, variable time); active phase (4-10 cm)
- effacement: thinning of the cervix by percentage or length of cervix (cm)
- consistency: firm vs. soft
- position: posterior, mid or anterior
- application: contact between the cervix and presenting part (i.e. well or poorly applied)
- see *Bishop Score* (Table 22, OB36)

The Fetus

- **fetal lie**: orientation of the long axis of the fetus with respect to the long axis of the uterus (longitudinal, transverse, oblique)
- **fetal presentation**: fetal body part closest to the birth canal
    - breech (complete, frank, incomplete) (see Figure 5, OB22)
    - cephalic (vertex/occiput, face, asynclitic, brow)
    - transverse (shoulder)
    - compound (fetal extremity prolapses along with presenting part)
        - all except vertex are considered malpresentations (see *Obstetrical Complications*, OB15)
- **fetal position**: position of presenting part of the fetus relative to the maternal pelvis
    - OA: most common presentation ("normal") – left OA most common
    - OP: most rotate spontaneously to OA; may cause prolonged second stage of labour
    - OT: leads to arrest of dilatation
        - normally, fetal head enters maternal pelvis and engages in OT position
        - subsequently rotates to OA position (or OP in a small percentage of cases)
- **attitude**: flexion/extension of fetal head relative to shoulders
    - brow presentation: head partially extended (requires C/S)
    - face presentation: head fully extended
        - mentum posterior always requires C/S, mentum anterior can deliver vaginally
- **station**: position of presenting bony part relative to ischial spines – determined by vaginal exam
    - at ischial spines = station 0 = engaged
    - -5 to -1 cm above ischial spines or
    - +1 to +5 cm below ischial spines
    - alternatively stations can be placed on a scale from -3 to +3

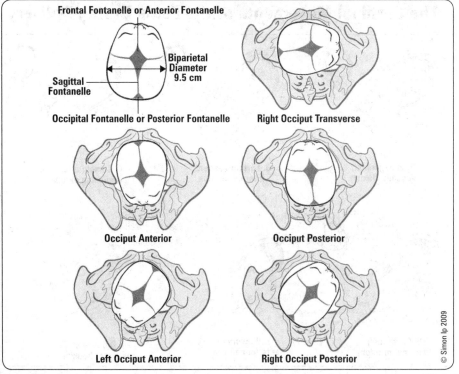

Figure 6. Fetal positions

Course of Normal Labour*

Stage	Nulliparous	Multiparous
First	6-18 h	2-10 h
Second	30 min-3 h	5-30 min
Third	5-30 min	5-30 min

* - without epidural

Signs of Placental Separation
- Gush of blood
- Lengthening of cord
- Uterus becomes globular
- Fundus rises

Continuous Support for Women During Childbirth
Cochrane DB Syst Rev 2011;16:CD003766
Study: Systematic review of 21 RCTs from 11 countries, 15,061 women in labour.
Intervention: Continuous support during labour vs. usual care.
Outcome: Effects on mothers and their babies.
Results: Continuous intrapartum support increased likelihood of shorter labour, spontaneous vaginal birth, decrease in analgesia use, and a decrease in dissatisfaction with childbirth experience. Greatest benefit when provider is not a health care professional. Continuous support was also associated with decreased likelihood to have a Cesarean or instrumental vaginal birth, regional analgesia, or a baby with a low 5 min APGAR score.

Four Stages of Labour

First Stage of Labour (0 – 10 cm cervical dilation)
- latent phase
  - uterine contractions typically infrequent and irregular
  - slow cervical dilatation (usually to 4 cm) and effacement
- active phase
  - rapid cervical dilatation to full dilatation (nulliparous ≥1.0 cm/h, multiparous ≥1.2 cm/h)
  - phase of maximum slope on cervical dilatation curve
  - painful, regular contractions q2-3min, lasting 45-60 s
  - contractions strongest at fundus

Second Stage of Labour (10 cm dilation – delivery of the baby)
- from full dilatation to delivery of the baby, duration varies based on parity, contraction quality, and type of analgesia
- mother feels a desire to bear down and push with each contraction
- women may choose a comfortable position that enhances pushing efforts and delivery
  - upright (semi-sitting, squatting) and LLDP are supported in the literature
- progress measured by descent

Third Stage of Labour (delivery of the baby – delivery of the placenta)
- from baby's birth to separation and expulsion of the placenta
- can last up to 30 min before intervention indicated
- demonstrated by gush of fresh blood, umbilical cord lengthening, uterine fundus changing shape (firm and globular) and rising upward
- active management: start oxytocin IV drip, or give 10 U IM or 5 mg IV push after delivery of anterior shoulder in anticipation of placental delivery, otherwise give after delivery of placenta
- routine oxytocin administration in third stage of labour can reduce the risk of PPH by >40%

Fourth Stage of Labour
- first postpartum hour
- monitor vital signs and bleeding, repair lacerations
- ensure uterus is contracted (palpate uterus and monitor uterine bleeding)
- inspect placenta for completeness and umbilical cord for presence of 2 arteries and 1 vein
- 3rd and 4th stages of labour most dangerous to the mother (i.e. hemorrhage)

The Cardinal Movements of the Fetus During Delivery

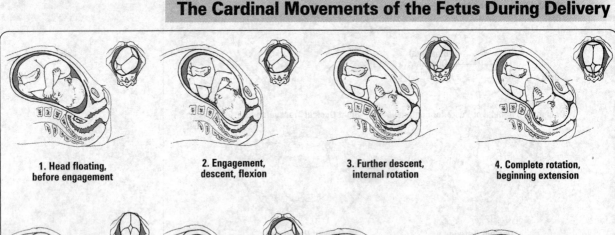

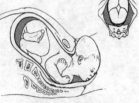

1. Head floating, before engagement

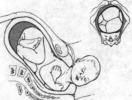

2. Engagement, descent, flexion

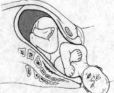

3. Further descent, internal rotation

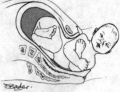

4. Complete rotation, beginning extension

5. Complete extension

6. Restitution (external rotation)

7. Delivery of anterior shoulder

8. Delivery of posterior shoulder

© Danielle Bader

Figure 7. Cardinal movements of fetus during delivery
Adapted from illustration in Williams Obstetrics, 19th ed

Analgesic and Anesthetic Techniques in Labour and Birth

- pain or anxiety leads to high endogenous catecholamines, which produce a direct inhibitory effect on uterine contractility

Non-Pharmacologic Pain Relief Techniques
- reduction of painful stimuli
  - maternal movement, position change, counter-pressure, abdominal compression
- activation of peripheral sensory receptors
  - superficial heat and cold
  - immersion in water during labour
  - touch and massage, acupuncture, and acupressure
  - TENS
  - intradermal injection of sterile water
  - aromatherapy
- enhancement of descending inhibitory pathways
  - attention focusing and distraction
  - hypnosis
  - music and audio analgesia
  - biofeedback

Pharmacologic Methods (see <u>Anesthesia and Perioperative Medicine</u>, A26)
- nitrous oxide (e.g. self-administered Entonox®)
- narcotics (usually combined with anti-emetic)
- pudendal nerve block
- perineal infiltration with local anesthetic
- regional anesthesia (epidural block, combined spinal-epidural, spinal)

Fetal Monitoring in Labour

- see online **Fetal Heart Rate Tutorial**

Vaginal Exam
- membrane status
- cervical effacement (thinning), dilatation, consistency, position, application
- fetal presenting part, position, station
- bony pelvis size and shape
- monitor progress of labour at regular intervals and document in a partogram

Intrapartum Fetal Monitoring
- intermittent fetal auscultation with Doppler device q15-30min for 1 min in first stage active phase following a contraction, q5min during second stage when pushing has begun
- continuous electronic FHR monitoring reserved for abnormal auscultation, prolonged labour, and labour which is induced or augmented, meconium present, multiple gestation/fetal complication
  - use of continuous electronic monitoring shown to lead to higher intervention rates and no improvement in outcome for the neonate when used routinely in all patients (ie no risk factors)
  - techniques for continuous monitoring include external (Doppler) vs. internal (fetal scalp electrode) monitoring
- fetal scalp sampling should be used in conjunction with electronic FHR monitoring and contraction monitoring (CTG) to resolve the interpretation of abnormal or atypical patterns

Electronic FHR Monitoring
- FHR measured by Doppler; contractions measured by tocometer
- described in terms of baseline FHR, variability (short-term, long-term), and periodicity (accelerations, decelerations)

- **Baseline FHR**
- normal range is 110-160 bpm
- parameter of fetal well-being vs. distress

- **Variability**
- physiologic variability is a normal characteristic of FHR
- variability is measured over a 15 min period and is described as: absent, minimal (<6 bpm), moderate (6-25 bpm), marked (>25 bpm)
- normal variability indicates fetal acid-base status is acceptable
- can only be assessed by electronic fetal monitoring (CTG)
- variability decreases intermittently even in healthy fetus
- see Table 19, OB34

Approach to the Management of Abnormal FHR

POISON – ER
Position (left lateral decubitus position)
O₂ (100% by mask)
IV fluids (corrects maternal hypotension)
Fetal **S**calp stimulation
Fetal **S**calp electrode
Fetal **S**calp pH
Stop **O**xytocin
Notify MD
Vaginal **E**xam to rule out cord prolapse
Rule out fever, dehydration, drug effects, prematurity
• If above fails, consider C/S

Continuous CTG as a Form of EFM for Fetal Assessment During Labour
Cochrane DB Syst Rev 2013;5:CD006066
Purpose: To examine the effectiveness of continuous electronic fetal monitoring or cardiotocography during labour.
Selection Criteria: Randomized and quasi-randomized controlled trials comparing continuous CTG (with and without fetal blood sampling) to a) no fetal monitoring, b) intermittent auscultation, or c) intermittent CTG.
Results: 13 trials, 37,000 women. Continuous CTG compared with intermittent auscultation showed no difference in overall perinatal death rate or cerebral palsy rates. Nonetheless, neonatal seizures were halved (RR 0.50, 95% CI 0.31-0.80) and there was a significant increase in Cesarean sections with CTG (RR 1.63, 95% CI 1.29-2.07) and instrumental vaginal birth (RR 1.15, 95% CI 1.01-1.33).
Conclusion: Continuous CTG may reduce the incidence of neonatal seizures, but has no effect on cerebral palsy rates, infant mortality, or other measures of neonatal well-being. Continuous CTG was also associated with an increase in Cesarean sections and instrumental deliveries.

- **Periodicity**
- accelerations: increase of ≥15 bpm for ≥15 s, in response to fetal movement or uterine contraction (or ≥10 bpm for ≥10 s if <32 wk GA)
- decelerations: 3 types, described in terms of shape, onset, depth, duration recovery, occurrence, and impact on baseline FHR and variability

Table 18. Factors Affecting Fetal Heart Rate

	Fetal Tachycardia (FHR >160 bpm)	Fetal Bradycardia (FHR <110 bpm)	Decreased Variability
Maternal Factors	Fever, hyperthyroidism, anemia, dehydration	Hypothermia, hypotension, hypoglycemia, position, umbilical cord occlusion	Infection Dehydration
Fetal Factors	Arrhythmia, anemia, infection, prolonged activity, chronic hpoxemia, congenital anomalies	Rapid descent, dysrhythmia, heart block, hyopoxia, vagal stimulation (head compression), hypothermia, acidosis	CNS anomalies Dysrhythmia Inactivity/sleep cycle, preterm fetus
Drugs	Sympathomimetics	β-blockers Anesthetics	Narcotics, sedatives Magnesium sulphate, β-blockers
Uteroplacental	Early hypoxia (abruption, HTN) Chorioamnionitis	Late hypoxia (abruption, HTN) Acute cord prolapse Hypercontractility	Hypoxia

Table 19. Comparison of Decelerations

Early Decelerations

- Uniform shape with onset early in contraction, returns to baseline by end of contraction, mirrors contraction (nadir occurs at peak of contraction)
- Gradual deceleration and return to baseline
- Often repetitive; no effect on baseline FHR or variability
- Benign, due to vagal response to head compression

Rule of 60s Suggesting Severe Variable Decelerations
Deceleration to <60 bpm
>60 bpm below baseline
>60 s in duration with slow return to baseline

Variable Decelerations

- Variable in shape, onset, and duration
- Most common type of periodicity seen during labour
- Often with abrupt drop in FHR >15 bpm below baseline (>15 s, <2 min); usually no effect on baseline FHR or variability
- Due to cord compression or, in second stage, forceful pushing with contractions

Complicated Variable Decelerations

- FHR drop <70 bpm for >60 s
- Loss of variability or decrease in baseline after deceleration
- Biphasic deceleration
- Slow return to baseline
- Baseline tachycardia or bradycardia
- May be associated with fetal academia

Late Decelerations

- Uniform shape with onset, nadir, and recovery occurring after peak of contraction, slow return to baseline
- May cause decreased variability and change in baseline FHR
- Due to fetal hypoxia and acidemia, maternal hypotension, or uterine hypertonus
- Usually a sign of uteroplacental insufficiency (an ominous sign)

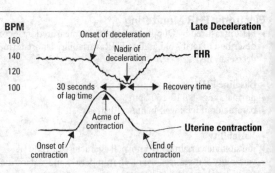

Table 20. Classification of Intrapartum EFM Tracings

	Normal Tracing (Category 1)	Atypical Tracing* (Category 2)	Abnormal Tracing* (Category 3)
Baseline	110-160 bpm	Bradycardia 100-110 bpm Tachycardia >160 for 30-80 min Rising baseline	Bradycardia <100 bpm Tachycardia >160 bpm for >80 min Erratic baseline
Variability	6-25 bpm ≤5 bpm for <40 min	≤5 bpm for 40-80 min	<5 bpm for >80 min ≥25 bpm for >10 min
Decelerations	None Early decelerations Occasional uncomplicated variable decelerations	Repetitive (≥3) uncomplicated variable decelerations Occasional late decelerations Any prolonged deceleration (2-3 min)	Repetitive (≥3) complicated variable decelerations Repetitive late decelerations Any prolonged deceleration (≥3 min)
Accelerations	Accelerations spontaneous or during scalp stimulation	Absent with scalp stimulation	Nearly absent
Action	EFM may be interrupted for ≤30 min if mother/fetus stable	Further assessment required	Action required: review clinical situation, obtain scalp pH, prepare for possible delivery

Adapted from *SOGC* Guidelines, September 2008
*Previous classification was "reassuring" vs. "non-reassuring", but distinction is now made between tracings that have some concerning changes but do not require immediate action (atypical) versus those with major concerns requiring immediate intervention (abnormal)

Fetal Scalp Blood Sampling

- cervix must be adequately dilated
- indicated when atypical or abnormal fetal heart rate is suggested by clinical parameters including heavy meconium or moderately to severely abnormal FHR patterns, including unexplained low variability, repetitive late decelerations, complex variable decelerations, fetal cardiac arrhythmias
- done by measuring pH or more recently fetal lactate
  - pH ≥7.25: normal, repeat if abnormal FHR persists
  - pH 7.21-7.24: repeat assessment in 30 min or consider delivery if rapid fall since last sample
  - pH ≤7.20: indicates fetal acidosis, delivery is indicated
- contraindications
  - known or suspected fetal blood dyscrasia (hemophilia, von Willebrand disease)
  - active maternal infection (HIV, genital herpes)

Fetal Oxygenation

- uterine contractions during labour decrease uteroplacental blood flow, which results in reduced oxygen delivery to the fetus
- most fetuses tolerate this reduction in flow and have no adverse effects
- distribution of oxygen to the fetus depends on maternal, uteroplacental, and fetal factors
- fetal response to hypoxia/asphyxia:
  - decreased movement, tone, and breathing activities
  - anaerobic metabolism (decreased pH)
  - transient fetal bradycardia followed by fetal tachycardia
  - redistribution of fetal blood flow
    - increased flow to brain, heart, and adrenals
    - decreased flow to kidneys, lungs, gut, liver, and peripheral tissues
    - increase in blood pressure

Table 21. Factors Affecting Fetal Oxygenation

Factor	Mechanism	Example
Maternal	Decreased maternal oxygen carrying capacity	Significant anemia (iron deficiency, hemoglobinopathies), carboxyhemoglobin (smokers)
	Decreased uterine blood flow	Hypotension (blood loss, sepsis), regional anesthesia, maternal positioning
	Chronic maternal conditions	Vasculopathies (SLE, type 1 DM, chronic HTN), antiphospholipid syndrome, cyanotic heart disease, COPD
Uteroplacental	Uterine hypertonus	Placental abruption, hyperstimulation secondary to oxytocin, prostaglandins, or normal labour
	Uteroplacental dysfunction	Placental abruption, placental infarction (dysfunction marked by IUGR, oligohydramnios, abnormal Doppler studies), chorioamnionitis, placental edema (DM, hydrops), placental senescence (post-dates)
Fetal	Cord compression	Oligohydramnios, cord prolapse, or entanglement
	Decreased fetal oxygen carrying capacity	Significant anemia (isoimmunization, feto-maternal bleed), carboxyhemoglobin (exposure to smokers)

Induction of Labour

Definition
- artificial initiation of labour in a pregnant woman prior to spontaneous initiation to deliver the fetus and placenta

Prerequisites for Labour Induction
- capability for C/S if necessary
- maternal
  - inducible/ ripe cervix: short, thin, soft, anterior cervix with open os
  - if cervix is not ripe, use prostaglandin vaginal insert (Cervidil®), prostaglandin gel (Prepidil®), misoprostol (Cytotec®) or Foley catheter
- fetal
  - normal fetal heart tracing
  - cephalic presentation
  - adequate fetal monitoring available
- likelihood of success determined by Bishop score (Table 22)
  - cervix considered unfavourable if <6
  - cervix favourable if ≥6
  - score of 9-13 associated with high likelihood of vaginal delivery

Table 22. Bishop Score

Cervical Characteristic	0	1	2	3
Position	Posterior	Mid	Anterior	–
Consistency	Firm	Medium	Soft	–
Effacement (%)	0-30	40-50	60-70	≥80
Dilatation (cm)	0	1-2	3-4	≥5
Station of Fetal Head	-3	-2	-1, 0	+1, +2, +3

Indications
- post-dates pregnancy (generally >41 wk) = most common reason for induction
- maternal factors
  - DM = second most common reason for induction
  - gestational HTN
  - other maternal medical problems, e.g. renal or lung disease, chronic hypertension, cholestasis or pregnancy
  - maternal age over 40
- maternal-fetal factors
  - isoimmunization, PROM, chorioamnionitis, post-term pregnancy
- fetal factors
  - suspected fetal jeopardy as evidenced by biochemical or biophysical indications
  - fetal demise, IUGR, oligo/polyhydraminos, anomalies requiring surgical intervention, twins
  - previous still birth, low PAPP-A

Risks
- failure to achieve labour and/or vaginal birth
- uterine hyperstimulation with fetal compromise or uterine rupture
- maternal side effects to medications
- uterine atony and PPH

Contraindications
- maternal
  - prior classical or inverted T-incision C/S or uterine surgery (e.g. myomectomy)
  - unstable maternal condition
  - active maternal genital herpes
  - invasive cervical carcinoma
  - pelvic structure deformities
- maternal-fetal
  - placenta previa or vasa previa
  - cord presentation
- fetal
  - fetal distress, malpresentation /abnormal lie, preterm fetus without lung maturity

Induction is indicated when the risk of continuing pregnancy exceeds the risks associated with induced labour and delivery

Induction vs. Augmentation
Induction is the artificial initiation of labour
Augmentation promotes contractions when spontaneous contractions are inadequate

Consider the Following Before Induction
- Indication for induction
- Contraindications
- GA
- Cervical favourability
- Fetal presentation
- Potential for CPD
- Fetal well-being/FHR
- Membrane status

Induction Methods

CERVICAL RIPENING

Definition
- use of medications or other means to soften, efface, and dilate the cervix, increases likelihood of successful induction
- ripening of an unfavourable cervix (Bishop score <6) is warranted prior to induction of labour

Methods
- intravaginal prostaglandin PGE2 gel (Prostin® gel): long and closed cervix
- recommended dosing interval of prostaglandin gel is every 6 to 12 h up to 3 doses
- intravaginal PGE2 (Cervidil®): long and closed cervix, may use if ROM
- continuous release, can be removed if needed
- controlled release PGE2
- intravaginal PGE1 Misoprostol (Cytotec®): long and closed cervix
- inexpensive, stored at room temperature
- more commonly used in 2nd trimester termination of pregnancy
- Foley catheter placement to mechanically dilate the cervix

INDUCTION OF LABOUR

Amniotomy
- artificial rupture of membranes (amniotomy) to stimulate prostaglandin synthesis and secretion; may try this as initial measure if cervix is open and soft, the membranes can be felt, and if the head is present at the cervix
- few studies address the value of amniotomy alone for induction of labour
- amniotomy plus intravenous oxytocin: more women delivered vaginally at 24 h than amniotomy alone (relative risk = 0.03) and had fewer instrumental vaginal deliveries (relative risk = 5.5)

Oxytocin
- oxytocin (Pitocin®): 10 U in 1L NS, run at 0.5-2 mU/min IV increasing by 1-2 mU/min q20-60min to a max of 36-48 mU/min
- reduces rate of unsuccessful vaginal deliveries within 24 h when used alone (8.3% vs. 54%, RR 0.16)
- ideal dosing regime of oxytocin is not known
- current recommendations: use the minimum dose to achieve active labour and increase q30min as needed
- reassessment should occur once a dose of 20 mU/min is reached
- potential complications
- hyperstimulation/tetanic contraction (may cause fetal distress or rupture of uterus)
- uterine muscle fatigue, uterine atony (may result in PPH)
- vasopressin-like action causing anti-diuresis

Augmentation of Labour

- augmentation of labour is used to promote adequate contractions when spontaneous contractions are inadequate and cervical dilatation or descent of fetus fails to occur
- oxytocin (0.5-2 mU/min IV increasing by 1-2 mU/min q20-60min to a max of 36-48 mU/min)

Abnormalities and Complications of Labour and Delivery

Meconium in Amniotic Fluid

Epidemiology
- present early in labour in 10% of pregnancies
- in general, meconium may be present in up to 25% of all labours; usually NOT associated with poor outcome, but extra care is required at time of delivery to avoid aspiration. Concern if fluid changes from clear to meconium stained. Always abnormal if seen in preterm patient

Etiology
- likely cord compression ± uterine hypertonia
- may indicate undiagnosed breech
- increasing meconium during labour may be a sign of fetal distress

Features
- may be watery or thicker (particulate)
- light yellow/green or dark green-black in colour

Evidence for Cervical Ripening Methods (SOGC Guidelines)
- Meta-analysis of five trials has concluded that the use of oxytocin to ripen the cervix is not effective
- Since the best dose and route of misoprostol for labour induction with a live fetus are not known and there are concerns regarding hyperstimulation, the use of misoprostol for induction of labour should be within clinical trials only (Level Ib evidence) or in cases of intrauterine fetal death to initiate labour

Intravaginal PGE2 (Cervidil®) Compared to Intravaginal Prostaglandin Gel
4 RCTs have compared the two with varying results, depending on the dosing regime of gel used.
Theoretical advantages of Cervidil®:
- Slow, continuous release
- Only one dose required
- Ability to use oxytocin 30 min after removal vs 6 hours for gel
- Ability to remove insert if required (i.e. excessive uterine activity)

Oxytocin t1/2 = 3-5 min

Provided there are no contraindications, oxytocin is utilized to improve uterine contraction strength and/or frequency

Treatment
- call respiratory therapy, neonatology, or pediatrics to delivery room
- oropharynx suctioning upon head expulsion or immediately after delivery if baby not breathing spontaneously (do NOT stimulate infant before)
- consider amnioinfusion of ~800 mL of IV NS over 50-80 min during active stage of labour and a maintenance dose of ~3 mL/min until delivery
- closely monitor FHR for signs of fetal distress

Abnormal Progression of Labour (Dystocia)

Definition
- expected patterns of descent of the presenting part and cervical dilatation fail to occur in the appropriate time frame; can occur in all stages of labour
- during active phase: >4 h of <0.5 cm/h
- during 2nd stage: >1 h with no descent during active pushing

The 4 Ps of Dystocia
Power
Passenger
Passage
Psyche

Etiology
- **Power** (leading cause): contractions (hypotonic, incoordinate), inadequate maternal expulsive efforts
- **Passenger**: fetal position, attitude, size, anomalies (hydrocephalus)
- **Passage**: pelvic structure (CPD), maternal soft tissue factors (tumours, full bladder or rectum, vaginal septum)
- **Psyche**: hormones released in response to stress may contribute to dystocia; psychological and physiological stress should be evaluated as part of the management once dystocia has been diagnosed

Management
- confirm diagnosis of labour (rule out false labour)
- search for factors of CPD
- diagnosed if adequate contractions measured by intrauterine pressure catheter (IUPC) with no descent/dilatation for >2 h
- management: if CPD ruled out, IV oxytocin augmentation ± amniotomy

Risks of Dystocia
- inadequate progression of labour is associated with an increased incidence of:
    - maternal stress
    - maternal infection
    - postpartum hemorrhage
    - need for neonatal resuscitation
    - fetal compromise (from uterine hyperstimulation)
    - uterine rupture
    - hypotension

Shoulder Dystocia

Definition
- fetal anterior shoulder impacted above symphysis pubis after fetal head has been delivered
- life threatening emergency

Etiology/Epidemiology
- incidence 0.15-1.4% of deliveries
- occurs when breadth of shoulders is greater than biparietal diameter of the head

Risk Factors
- maternal: obesity, DM, multiparity, previous shoulder dystocia
- fetal: prolonged gestation, macrosomia (especially if associated with GDM)
- labour
    - prolonged 2nd stage
    - instrumental midpelvic delivery

Presentation
- "turtle sign": head delivered but retracts against inferior portion of pubic symphysis
- complications
    - fetal
        - hypoxic ischemic encephalopathy (chest compression by vagina or cord compression by pelvis can lead to hypoxia)
        - brachial plexus injury (Erb's palsy: C5-C7; Klumpke's palsy: C8-T1), 90% resolve within 6 mo
        - fracture (clavicle, humerus, cervical spine)
        - death
    - maternal
        - perineal injury
        - PPH (uterine atony, lacerations)
        - uterine rupture

Treatment
- goal: to displace anterior shoulder from behind symphysis pubis; follow a stepwise approach of maneuvers until goal achieved
- other options
  - cleidotomy (deliberate fracture of neonatal clavicle)
  - Zavanelli maneuver: replacement of fetus into uterine cavity and emergent C/S
  - symphysiotomy

Prognosis
- 1% risk of long-term disability for infant

Umbilical Cord Prolapse

Definition
- descent of the cord to a level adjacent to or below the presenting part, causing cord compression between presenting part and pelvis

Etiology/Epidemiology
- increased incidence with prematurity/PROM, fetal malpresentation (~50% of cases), low-lying placenta, polyhydramnios, multiple gestation, CPD
- incidence: 1/200 – 1/400 deliveries

Presentation
- visible or palpable cord
- FHR changes (variable decelerations, bradycardia, or both)

Treatment
- emergency C/S
- O$_2$ to mother, monitor fetal heart
- alleviate pressure of the presenting part on the cord by elevating fetal head with a pelvic exam (maintain this position until C/S)
- keep cord warm and moist by replacing it into the vagina ± applying warm saline soaks
- roll mom onto all fours
- position mother in Trendelenburg or knee-to-chest position
- if fetal demise or too premature (<22 wk), allow labour and delivery

Uterine Rupture

Etiology/Epidemiology
- associated with previous uterine scar (in 40% of cases), hyperstimulation with oxytocin, grand multiparity, and previous intrauterine manipulation
- generally occurs during labour, but can occur earlier with a classical incision
- 0.5-0.8% incidence, up to 12% with classical incision

Presentation
- prolonged fetal bradycardia – most common presentation
- acute onset of constant lower abdominal pain, may not have pain if receiving epidural analgesia
- hyper or hypotonic uterine contractions
- vaginal bleeding
- intra-abdominal hemorrhage
- sudden loss of fetal descent

Risk Factors
- uterine scarring (i.e. previous uterine surgeries including Cesarean (especially classical incision), perforation with D&C, myomectomy)
- excessive uterine stimulation (i.e. protracted labour, oxytocin, prostaglandins)
- uterine trauma (i.e. operative equipment, ECV)
- multiparity
- uterine abnormalities
- placenta accreta

Treatment
- rule out placental abruption
- immediate delivery for fetal survival
- maternal stabilization (may require hysterectomy), treat hypovolemia

Complications
- maternal mortality 1-10%
- maternal hemorrhage, shock, DIC
- amniotic fluid embolus
- hysterectomy if uncontrollable hemorrhage
- fetal distress, associated with 50% fetal mortality

- 1/3 of protraction disorders develop into 2° arrest of dilatation due to CPD
- 2/3 of protraction disorders progress through labour to vaginal delivery

Umbilical Cord Accident Causes
- Nuchal cord
- Type A (looped)
- Type B (hitched)
- Body loop
- Single artery
- True knot
- Torsion
- Velamentous
- Short cord <35 cm
- Long cord >80 cm

Maternal Mortality Causes
- Thromboembolism
- Cardiac event
- Suicide
- Sepsis
- Ectopic pregnancy
- HTN
- Amniotic fluid embolism
- Hemorrhage

* In Canada (2013), lifetime risk of maternal death is 1 in 5,200

Amniotic Fluid Embolus

Definition
- amniotic fluid debris in maternal circulation triggering an anaphylactoid immunologic response

Etiology/Epidemiology
- rare intrapartum or immediate postpartum complication
- 60-80% maternal mortality rate, accounts for 10% of all maternal deaths
- leading cause of maternal death in induced abortions and miscarriages
- 1/8,000-1/80,000 births

Risk Factors
- placental abruption
- rapid labour
- multiparity
- uterine rupture
- uterine manipulation

Differential Diagnosis
- pulmonary embolus, drug-induced anaphylaxis, septic shock, eclampsia, HELLP syndrome, abruption, chronic coagulopathy

Presentation
- sudden onset of respiratory distress, cardiovascular collapse (hypotension, hypoxia), and coagulopathy
- seizure in 10%
- ARDS and left ventricular dysfunction seen in survivors

Management
- supportive measures (high flow O_2, ventilation support, fluid resuscitation, inotropic support, ± intubation), coagulopathy correction
- ICU admission

Chorioamnionitis

Definition
- infection of the chorion, amnion, and amniotic fluid typically due to ascending infection by organisms of normal vaginal flora

Etiology/Epidemiology
- incidence 1-5% of term pregnancies and up to 25% in preterm deliveries
- ascending from vagina
- predominant microorganisms include: GBS, *Bacteroides* and *Prevotella* species, *E. coli*, and anaerobic *Streptococcus*

Risk Factors
- prolonged ROM, long labour, multiple vaginal exams during labour, internal monitoring
- bacterial vaginosis and other vaginal infections

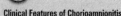

Clinical Features of Chorioamnionitis
- Temperature
- Tachycardia (maternal or fetal)
- Tenderness (uterine)
- Foul discharge

Clinical Features
- maternal fever, maternal or fetal tachycardia, uterine tenderness, foul, and purulent cervical discharge

Investigations
- CBC: leukocytosis
- amniotic fluid: leukocytes or bacteria

Treatment
- IV antibiotics
  - ampicillin (2 g IV q6h) and gentamicin (1.5 mg/kg q8h)
  - anaerobic coverage (i.e. clindamycin if C/S)
- expedient delivery regardless of gestational age

Complications
- bacteremia of mother or fetus, wound infection if C/S, pelvic abscess, infant meningitis

Operative Obstetrics

Operative Vaginal Delivery

Definition
- forceps or vacuum extraction

Indications
- fetal
  - atypical or abnormal fetal heart rate tracing, evidence of fetal compromise
  - consider if second stage is prolonged as this may be due to poor contractions or failure of fetal head to rotate
- maternal
  - need to avoid voluntary expulsive effort (e.g. cardiac/cerebrovascular disease)
  - exhaustion, lack of cooperation, and excessive analgesia may impair pushing effort

Contraindications
- non-vertex cephalic presentation (i.e. Brow or face)
- unengaged head
- cervix incompletely dilated

Forceps

Outlet Forceps Position
- head visible between labia in between contractions
- sagittal suture in or close to AP diameter
- rotation cannot exceed 45°

Low Forceps Position
- presenting part at station +2 or greater
- subdivided based on whether rotation less than or greater than 45 degrees

Mid Forceps Position
- presenting part below spines but above station +2

Types of Forceps
- Simpson or Tucker-McLane forceps for OA presentations
- Kielland (rotational) forceps when rotation of head is required
- Piper forceps for breech

Vacuum Extraction

- traction instrument used as alternative to forceps delivery; aids maternal pushing
- contraindications: <34 wk GA (<2500 g), fetal head deflexed, fetus requires rotation, fetal condition (e.g. bleeding disorder)

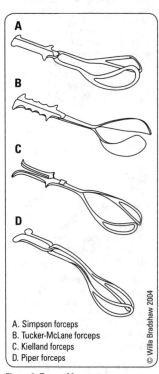

A. Simpson forceps
B. Tucker-McLane forceps
C. Kielland forceps
D. Piper forceps

© Willa Bradshaw 2004

Figure 8. Types of forceps

Table 23. Advantages and Disadvantages of Forceps versus Vacuum Extraction

	Forceps	Vacuum Extraction
Advantages	Higher overall success rate for vaginal delivery Decreased incidence of fetal morbidity	Easier to apply Less anesthesia required Less maternal soft-tissue injury compared to forceps
Disadvantages	Greater incidence of maternal injury	Contraindicated if fetus at risk for coagulation defect Suitable only for vertex presentations Maternal pushing required Contraindicated in preterm delivery
Complications	Maternal: anesthesia risk, lacerations, injury to bladder, uterus, or bone, pelvic nerve damage, PPH, infections Fetal: fractures, facial nerve palsy, trauma to face/scalp, intracerebral hemorrhage, cephalohematoma, cord compression	Increased incidence of cephalohematoma and retinal hemorrhages, and jaundice compared to forceps Subgaleal hemorrhage, Subaponeurotic hemorrhage, Soft tissue trauma

Risk Factors for Primary and Subsequent Anal Sphincter Lacerations
Am J Obstet Gynecol 2007;196:344
Objective: Assess effects of pregnancy, delivery method, and parity on risk of primary and secondary anal sphincter laceration in women with 1st vaginal delivery (VD), VBAC, or 2nd VD.
Methods: Retrospective cohort study of all deliveries at one hospital from 1995-2002. Conclusion: 20,674 live singleton deliveries were included. Women with first VD and VBAC both had OR 5.1 for laceration compared to 2nd VD. Forceps and midline episiotomy significantly increased risk of laceration for all 3 groups. Second stage of labour >2 h only increased risk for 1st VD. Factors that had no significant increase in risk: infant birth weight >3,500 g and vacuum delivery. Women with prior anal sphincter laceration are at 3x increased risk for subsequent sphincter laceration, compared with women with prior vaginal delivery without sphincter laceration.

Lacerations

- first degree: involves skin and vaginal mucosa but not underlying fascia and muscle
- second degree: involves fascia and muscles of the perineal body but not the anal sphincter
- third degree: involves the anal sphincter (partial IIIa or complete IIIb)
- fourth degree: extends through the anal sphincter into the rectal mucosa

Episiotomy

Definition
- incision in the perineal body at the time of delivery
- essentially a controlled second degree laceration
- midline: incision through central tendinous portion of perineal body and insertions of superficial transverse perineal and bulbocavernosus muscle
  - heals better, but increases risk of 3rd/4th degree tears
- mediolateral: incision through bulbocavernosus, superficial transverse perineal muscle, and levator ani
  - reduced risk of extensive tear but more painful
  - easier to repair

Indications
- to relieve obstruction of the unyielding perineum
- to expedite delivery (e.g. abnormal FHR pattern)
- instrumental delivery
- controversial between practitioners as to whether it is preferable to make a cut or let the perineum tear as needed
- current evidence suggests letting perineum tear and then repair as needed (restricted use)

Complications
- infection, hematoma, extension into anal musculature or rectal mucosa, fistula formation, incontinence

Cesarean Delivery

Epidemiology
- incidence 20-25%

Indications
- maternal: obstruction, active herpetic lesion on vulva, invasive cervical cancer, previous uterine surgery (past C/S is most common), underlying maternal illness (eclampsia, HELLP syndrome, heart disease)
- maternal-fetal: failure to progress, placental abruption or previa, vasa previa
- fetal: abnormal fetal heart tracing, malpresentation, cord prolapse, certain congenital anomalies

Types of Cesarean Incisions
- skin
  - transverse (i.e. Pfannensteil)
    - decreased exposure and slower entry
    - improved strength and cosmesis
  - vertical midline
    - rapid peritoneal entry and increased exposure
    - increased dehiscence
- uterine
  - low transverse (most common): in noncontractile lower segment
    - decreased chance for rupture in subsequent pregnancies
  - low vertical
    - used for very preterm infants, poorly developed maternal lower uterine segment
  - classical (rare): in thick, contractile segment
    - used for transverse lie, fetal anomaly, >2 fetuses, lower segment adhesions, obstructing fibroid, morbidly obese patients

Risks/Complications
- complications related to general anesthesia* (e.g. aspiration)
- hemorrhage (average blood loss ~1,000 cc)
- infection (UTI, wound, endometritis)
  - single dose prophylactic antibiotic should be used (e.g. cefazolin 1-2 g)
- injury to surrounding structures (bowel, bladder, ureter, uterus)
- thromboembolism (DVT, PE)
- increased recovery time/hospital stay
- maternal mortality (<0.1%)

Vaginal Birth After Cesarean

TRIAL OF LABOUR AFTER CESAREAN

- should be recommended if no contraindications after previous low transverse incision
- success rate varies with indication for previous C/S (generally 60-80%)
- risk of uterine rupture (<1% with low transverse incision)

Contraindications

- previous classical, inverted T, or unknown uterine incision, or complete transection of uterus (6% risk of rupture)
- history of uterine surgery (e.g. myomectomy) or previous uterine rupture
- multiple gestation
- non-vertex presentation or placenta previa
- inadequate facilities or personnel for emergency C/S

VBAC
- Rate of successful VBAC ranges from 60-82%
- No significant difference in maternal deaths or hysterectomies between VBAC or C/S
- Uterine rupture more common in VBAC group
- Evidence regarding fetal outcome is lacking

Safety of vaginal birth after Cesarean section: A systematic review. *Obstet Gynecol* 2004;103:420-9

Puerperal Complications

- puerperium: 6 wk period of adjustment after pregnancy when pregnancy-induced anatomic and physiologic changes are reversed

Postpartum Hemorrhage

Definition

- loss of >500 mL of blood at the time of vaginal delivery, or >1,000 mL with C/S
- early (immediate) – within first 24 h postpartum
- late (delayed) – after 24 h but within first 6 wk

Epidemiology

- incidence 5-15%

Etiology (4 Ts)

1. **Tone** (uterine atony)
   - most common cause of PPH
   - avoid by giving oxytocin with delivery of the anterior shoulder or placenta
   - occurs within first 24 h
   - due to
     - overdistended uterus (polyhydramnios, multiple gestations, macrosomia)
     - uterine muscle exhaustion (prolonged or rapid labour, grand multiparity, oxytocin use, general anaesthetic)
     - uterine distortion (fibroids, placenta previa, placental abruption)
     - intra-amniotic infection (fever, prolonged ROM)
2. **Tissue**
   - retained placental products (membranes, cotyledon or succenturiate lobe)
   - retained blood clots in an atonic uterus
   - gestational trophoblastic neoplasia
   - abnormal placentation
3. **Trauma**
   - laceration (vagina, cervix, uterus), episiotomy, hematoma (vaginal, vulvar, retroperitoneal), uterine rupture, uterine inversion
4. **Thrombin**
   - coagulopathy (pre-existing or acquired)
     - most identified prior to delivery (low platelets increases risk)
     - includes hemophilia, DIC, Aspirin* use, ITP, TTP, vWD (most common)
     - therapeutic anti-coagulation

Uterine atony is the most common cause of PPH

DDx of Early PPH – 4 Ts
Tone (atony)
Tissue (retained placenta, clots)
Trauma (laceration, inversion)
Thrombin (coagulopathy)

DDx of Late PPH
Retained products
± endometritis
Sub-involution of uterus

Investigations

- assess degree of blood loss and shock by clinical exam
- explore uterus and lower genital tract for evidence of tone, tissue, or trauma
- may be helpful to observe red-topped tube of blood – no clot in 7-10 min indicates coagulation problem

Management

- ABCs , call for help
- 2 large bore IVs, run crystalloids wide open
- CBC, coagulation profile, cross and type pRBCs
- treat underlying cause
- Foley catheter to empty bladder and monitor urine output

Medical Therapy
- oxytocin 5U IV bolus (20-40 U/250 mL in crystalloid) with delivery of anterior shoulder or infusion of 20 U in 1000ml crystalloid @ 50ml/hr or can give 10 U IM if CV collapse or IV access not possible
- methylergonavine maleate (ergotamine) 0.25 mg IM/IMM q5min up to 1.25 mg; can be given as IV bolus of 0.125 mg (may exacerbate HTN)
- carboprost (Hemabate®), a synthetic PGF-1α analog 250 μg IM/IMM q15min to max 2 mg (major prostaglandin side effects and contraindicated in cardiovascular, pulmonary, renal, and hepatic dysfunction)
- misoprostol 600-800 μg po/sl (faster) or pr/pv (side effect: pyrexia if >600 μg)
- tranexamic acid (Cyklokapron®) 1 g IV, an antifibrinolytic

Local Control
- bimanual massage: elevate the uterus and massage through patient's abdomen
- uterine packing (mesh with antibiotic treatment)
- Bakri Balloon for tamponade: may slow hemorrhage enough to allow time for correction of coagulopathy or for preparation of an OR

Surgical Therapy (Intractable PPH)
- D&C (beware of vigorous scraping which can lead to Asherman's syndrome)
- embolization of uterine artery or internal iliac artery by interventional radiologist
- laparotomy with bilateral ligation of uterine artery (may be effective), internal iliac artery (not proven), ovarian artery, or hypogastric artery, compression sutures (B-Lynch or Cho sutures)
- hysterectomy last option with angiographic embolization if post-hysterectomy bleeding

Retained Placenta

Definition
- placenta undelivered after 30 min postpartum

Etiology
- placenta separated but not delivered
- abnormal placental implantation (placenta accreta, placenta increta, placenta percreta)

Risk Factors
- placenta previa, prior C/S, post-pregnancy curettage, prior manual placental removal, uterine infection

Clinical Features
- risk of postpartum hemorrhage and infection

Investigations
- explore uterus
- assess degree of blood loss

Management
- 2 large bore IVs, type and screen
- Brant maneuver (firm traction on umbilical cord with one hand applying suprapubic pressure cephalad to avoid uterine inversion by holding uterus in place)
- oxytocin 10 IU in 20 mL NS into umbilical vein
- manual removal if above fails
- D&C if required
- Ancef 2 g IV if manual removal or D&C

Uterine Inversion

Definition
- inversion of the uterus through cervix ± vaginal introitus

Etiology/Epidemiology
- often iatrogenic (excess cord traction with fundal placenta)
- excessive use of uterine tocolytics
- more common in grand multiparous (lax uterine ligaments)
- 1/1,500-1/2,000 deliveries

Clinical Features
- can cause profound vasovagal response with bradycardia, vasodilation, and hypovolemic shock
- shock may be disproportionate to maternal blood loss

Management
- urgent management essential, call anesthesia
- ABCs: initiate IV crystalloids

- can use tocolytic drug (see *Management of Preterm Labour*, OB16) or nitroglycerin IV to relax uterus and aid replacement
- replace uterus without removing placenta
- remove placenta manually and withdraw slowly
- IV oxytocin infusion (only after uterus replaced)
- re-explore uterus
- may require general anesthetic ± laparotomy

Postpartum Pyrexia

Definition
- fever >38°C on any 2 of the first 10 d postpartum, except the first day

Etiology
- endometritis
- wound infection (check C/S and episiotomy sites)
- mastitis/engorgement
- UTI
- atelectasis
- pneumonia
- DVT, pelvic thombophlebitis

Investigations
- detailed history and physical exam, relevant cultures
- for endometritis: blood and genital cultures

Treatment
- depends on etiology
  - infection: empiric antibiotics, adjust when sensitivities available
    - endometritis: clindamycin + gentamycin IV
    - mastitis: cloxacillin or cephalexin
    - wound infection: cephalexin, frequent sitz baths for episiotomy site infection
  - DVT: anticoagulants
- prophylaxis against post-C/S endometritis: administer 2g of Cephazolin IV 30 minutes prior to skin incision

ENDOMETRITIS
- definition: infection of uterine myometrium and parametrium
- clinical features: fever, chills, abdominal pain, uterine tenderness, foul-smelling discharge, or lochia
- treatment: depends on infection severity; oral antibiotics if well, IV with hospitalization in moderate to severe cases

VENOUS THROMBOEMBOLISM
- see *Venous Thromboembolism*, OB30

Etiology of Postpartum Pyrexia

B-5W
Breast: engorgement, mastitis
Wind: atelectasis, pneumonia
Water: UTI
Wound: episiotomy, C/S site infection
Walking: DVT, thrombophlebitis
Womb: endometritis

Risk Factors for Endometritis
C/S, intrapartum chorioamnionitis, prolonged labour, prolonged ROM, multiple vaginal examinations

Mastitis

- definition: inflammation of mammary glands
- must rule out inflammatory carcinoma, as indicated
- differentiate from mammary duct ectasia: mammary duct(s) beneath nipple clogged and dilated ± ductal inflammation ± nipple discharge (thick, grey to green), often postmenopausal women

Table 24. Lactational vs. Non-Lactational Mastitis

	Lactational	Non-Lactational
Epidemiology	More common than non-lactational Often 2-3 wk postpartum	Periductal mastitis most common Mean age 32 yr
Etiology	S. aureus	May be sterile May be infected with S. aureus or other anaerobes Smoking is risk factor May be associated with mammary duct ectasia
Symptoms	Unilateral localized pain Tenderness Erythema	Subareolar pain May have subareolar mass Discharge (variable colour) Nipple inversion
Treatment	Heat or ice packs Continued nursing/pumping Antibiotics (cloxacillin/cephalexin) (Erythromycin if pen-allergic)	Broad-spectrum antibiotics and I&D Total duct excision (definitive)
Abscess	Fluctuant mass Purulent nipple discharge Fever, leukocytosis Discontinue nursing, IV antibiotics (nafcillin/oxacillin), I&D usually required	If mass does not resolve, FNA to exclude cancer and U/S to assess presence of abscess Treatment includes antibiotics, aspiration, or I&D (tends to recur) May develop mammary duct fistula A minority of non-lactational abscesses may occur peripherally in breast with no associated periductal mastitis (usually S. aureus)

Postpartum Mood Alterations

POSTPARTUM BLUES
- 40-80% of new mothers, onset day 3-10; extension of the "normal" hormonal changes and adjustment to a new baby
- self-limited, should resolve by 2 wk
- manifested by mood lability, depressed affect, increased sensitivity to criticism, tearfulness, fatigue, irritability, poor concentration/despondency, anxiety, insomnia

POSTPARTUM DEPRESSION
- definition: major depression occurring in a woman within 6 mo of childbirth (see Psychiatry, PS12)
- epidemiology: 10-15%, risk of recurrence 50%
- risk factors
  - personal or family history of depression (including PPD)
  - prenatal depression or anxiety
  - stressful life situation
  - poor support system
  - unwanted pregnancy
  - colicky or sick infant
- clinical features: suspect if the "blues" last beyond 2 wk, or if the symptoms in the first 2 wk are severe (e.g. extreme disinterest in the baby, suicidal or homicidal/infanticidal ideation)
- assessment: Edinburgh Postnatal Depression Scale or other
- treatment: antidepressants, psychotherapy, supportive care, ECT if refractory
- prognosis: interferes with bonding and attachment between mother and baby so it can have long-term effects

POSTPARTUM PSYCHOSIS
- definition: onset of psychotic symptoms over 24-72 h within first month postpartum, can present in the context of depression
- epidemiology: rare (0.2%)

Postpartum Care

Postpartum Office Visit at 6 Weeks

Care of Mother (The 10 Bs)
- Be careful: do not use douches or tampons for 4-6 wk post-delivery
- Be fit: encourage gradual increases in walking, Kegel exercises
- Birth control: assess for use of contraceptives; breastfeeding is NOT an effective method of birth control (see Gynecology, GY16, for more detail about different contraceptive options postpartum)
- Bladder: assess for urinary incontinence, maintain high fluid intake
- Blood pressure: especially if gestational HTN
- Blood tests: glucose, CBC (for anemia as sign of hematomas, retained placenta)
- Blues: (see Postpartum Mood Alterations)
- Bowel: fluids and high-fibre foods, bulk laxatives; for hemorrhoids/perineal tenderness: pain meds, doughnut cushion, Sitz baths, ice compresses
- Breast and pelvic exam: watch for Staphylococcal or Streptococcal mastitis/abscess, ± Pap smear at 6 wk

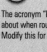

The acronym "**BUBBLES**" for what to ask about when rounding on postpartum care. Modify this for C/S or vaginal delivery.

Baby care and breastfeeding (latch, amount)
Uterus – firm or boggy?
Bladder function – Voiding well? Dysuria?
Bowel function – Passing gas or stool? Constipated?
Lochia or discharge – Any blood?
Episiotomy/laceration/incision – Pain controlled?
Symptoms of VTE – Dyspnea? Calf pain?

Physiological Changes Postpartum
- uterus weight rapidly diminishes through catabolism, cervix loses its elasticity and regains firmness
  - should involute ~1 cm below umbilicus per day in first 4-5 d, reaches non-pregnant state in 4-6 wk postpartum
- ovulation resumes in ~45 d for non-lactating women and within 3-6 mo for lactating women and sometimes later
- lochia: normal vaginal discharge postpartum, uterine decidual tissue sloughing
  - decreases and changes in colour from red (lochia rubra; presence of erythrocytes, 3-4 d) → pale (lochia serosa) → white / yellow (lochia alba; residual leukorrhea) over 3-6 wk
  - foul-smelling lochia suggests endometritis

Breastfeeding Problems
- inadequate milk: consider domperidone
- breast engorgement: cool compress, manual expression/pumping
- nipple pain: clean milk off nipple after feeds, moisture cream, topical steroid if needed
- mastitis: treat promptly (see Postpartum Pyrexia, OB45)
- inverted nipples: makes feeding difficult
- maternal medications: may require pediatric consultation (see Breastfeeding and Drugs)

Bladder Dysfunction
- pelvic floor prolapse can occur after vaginal delivery
- stress or urge urinary incontinence common
- increased risk with instrumental delivery or prolonged second stage
- conservative management: pelvic floor retraining with Kegel exercises/pelvic physiotherapy, vaginal cone, or pessaries, lifestyle modifications (e.g. limit fluid, caffeine intake)
- surgical management: minimally invasive procedures (tension-free vaginal tape, transobturator tape, midurethral sling)

Puerperal Pain
- "after pains" common in first 3 d due to uterine contractions; encourage simple analgesia
- ice packs can be used on perineum if painful
- encourage regular analgesia and stool softener

Breastfeeding and Drugs

Table 25. Drug Safety During Breastfeeding

Safe During Breastfeeding	Contraindicated When Breastfeeding
Analgesics (e.g. acetaminophen, NSAIDs)	Chloramphenicol (bone marrow suppression)
Anticoagulants (e.g. heparin)	Cyclophosphamide (immune system suppression)
Antidepressants (e.g. sertraline, fluoxetine, TCAs)	Sulphonamides (in G6PD deficiency, can lead to hemolysis)
Antiepileptics (e.g. phenytoin, carbamazepine, valproic acid)	Nitrofurantoin (in G6PD deficiency, can lead to hemolysis)
Antihistamines	Tetracycline
Antimicrobials (e.g. penicillins, aminoglycosides, cephalosporins)	Lithium
β-adrenergics (e.g. propranolol, labetalol)	Phenindione
Insulin	Bromocriptine
Steroids	Anti-neoplastics and immunosuppresants
OCP (low dose) – although may decrease breast milk production	Psychotropic drugs (relative contraindication)

Breastfeeding: Contraindicated Drugs

BREAST
Bromocriptine/Benzodiazepines
Radioactive isotopes/Rizatriptan
Ergotamine/Ethosuximide
Amiodarone/Amphetamines
Stimulant laxatives/Sex hormones
Tetracycline/Tretinoin

Common Medications

Table 26. Common Medications

Drug Name (Brand Name)	Dosing Schedule	Indications/Comments
betamethasone valerate (Celestone®)	12 mg IM q24h x 2 doses	Enhancement of fetal pulmonary maturity for PTL
carboprost (Hemabate®)	0.25 mg IM/IMM q15min; max 2 mg	Treatment of uterine atony
cefazolin	2 g IV then 1 g q8h	GBS prophylaxis (penicillin allergic and not at risk for anaphylaxis)
clindamycin	900 mg IV q8h	Used in endometritis
dexamethasone	6 mg IM q12h x 4 doses	Enhancement of fetal pulmonary maturity for PTL
dinoprostone (Cervidil®: PGE2 impregnated thread)	10 mg PV (remove after 12 h) max 3 doses	Induction of labour Advantage: can remove if uterine hyperstimulation
doxylamine succinate (Diclectin®)	2 tabs qhs + 1 tab qAM + 1 tab qPM max 8 tabs/d	Each tablet contains 10 mg doxylamine succinate with vitamin B6 Used for hyperemesis gravidarum
erythromycin	500 mg IV q6h	GBS prophylaxis (penicillin allergic and at risk for anaphylaxis)
folic acid	0.4-1 mg PO OD x 1-3 mo preconception and T1 5 mg PO OD with past Hx of NTD/risks for NTD	Prevention of oNTD
methotrexate	50 mg/m² IM or 50 mg PO x 1 dose	For ectopic pregnancy or medical abortion
methylergonavine maleate (Ergotamine®)	0.25 mg IM/IMM q5min up to 1.25 mg or IV bolus 0.125 mg	Treatment of uterine atony
misoprostol (Cytotec®)	600-1000 µg PR x 1 dose 400 µg PO/SL x 1 dose or 800 µg PV x 1 dose, 3-7 d after methotrexate	For treatment of PPH For medical abortion/retained products of conception Also used for NSAID-induced ulcers (warn patients of contraindications)
oxytocin (Pitocin®)	0.5-2.0 mU/min IV, or 10 U/L NS increase by 1-2 mU/min q20-60min max 36-48 mU/min 10 U IM at delivery of anterior shoulder and of placenta 20 U/L NS or RL IV continuous infusion	Augmentation of labour (also induction of labour) Prevention of uterine atony Treatment of uterine atony
Penicillin G	5 million U IV then 2.5 million U IV q4h until delivery	GBS prophylaxis
PGE2 gel (Prostin® gel)	0.5 mg PV q6-12h; max 3 doses	Induction of labour

Rh IgG (Rhogam®)	300 µg IM x 1 dose	Given to Rh negative women
		  Routinely at 28 wk GA
		  Within 72 h of birth of Rh+ fetus
		  Positive Kleihauer-Betke test
		  With any invasive procedure in pregnancy
		  Ectopic pregnancy
		  Antepartum hemorrhage
		  Miscarriage or therapeutic abortion (dose: 50 µg IM only)

Misoprostol (Cytotec®) is also indicated to protect against NSAID-induced gastric ulcers in non-pregnant individuals. The use of misoprostol for cytoprotection is contraindicated in pregnancy; warn female patients of this contraindication

References

American College of Obstetricians and Gynecologists. Available from: www.acog.org.
The Society of Obstetricians and Gynaecologists of Canada. Available from: www.sogc.org.
Alfirevic Z, Devane D, Gyte GM. Continuous cardiotocography (CTG) as a form of electronic fetal monitoring (EFM) for fetal assessment during labour. Cochrane DB Syst Rev 2013;5:CD006066.
Antenatal Corticosteroid Therapy for Fetal Maturation. SOGC clinical practice guidelines policy statement. December 1995:53.
Arsenault M, Lane CA. Guidelines for the management of nausea and vomiting in pregnancy. SOGC Clinical Practice Guidelines Committee Opinion 2002;120:1-7.
Banti S et al. From the third month of pregnancy to 1 year postpartum. Prevalence, incidence, recurrence, and new onset of depression. Results from the perinatal depression-research&screening unit study. Compr Psychiatry. 2011 Jul;52(4):343-51. Epub 2010 Sep 23.
Baskett T. Essential management of obstetric emergencies, 3rd ed. Bristol: Clinical Press, 1999.
Bastian LA, Piscitelli JT. Is this patient pregnant? Can you reliably rule in or rule out early pregnancy by clinical examination? JAMA 1997;278:586-591.
Berghella V, Odibo AO, Tolosa JE. Cerclage for prevention of preterm birth in women with a short cervix found on transvaginal examination: a randomized trial. Am J Obstet Gynecol 2004;191:1311-1317.
Berghella V, Rafael TJ, Szychowski JM, et al. Cerclage for short cervix on ultrasonography in women with singleton gestations and previous preterm birth: a meta-analysis. Obstet Gynecol 2011;117:663-671.
Blenning CE, Paladine H. An approach to the postpartum office visit. Am Fam Physician 2005;72(12):2491-2496.
Boucher M. Mode of delivery for pregnant women infected by the human immunodeficiency virus. Clinical Practice Guidelines Policy Statement 2001:101.
Boucher M, Gruslin A. The reproductive care of women living with hepatitis C infection. Clinical Practice Guidelines Policy Statement 2000:96.
Bricker L, Luckas M. Amniotomy alone for induction of labour. Cochrane DB Syst Rev 2000;(4):CD002862.
Carroli G, Mignini L. Episiotomy for vaginal birth. Cochrane DB Syst Rev 2009;1:CD000081.
Chamberlain G, Zander L. Induction. BMJ 1999;318:995-998.
Chamberlain G, Steer P. Labour in special circumstances. BMJ 1999;318:1124-1127.
Chamberlain G, Steer P. Obstetric emergencies. BMJ 1999;318:1342-1345.
Chamberlain G, Steer P. Operative delivery. BMJ 1999;318:1260-1264.
Chamberlain G, Steer P. Unusual presentations and positions and multiple pregnancy. BMJ 1999;318:1192-1194.
Chodirker BN, Cadrin C, Davies GAL, et al. Canadian guidelines for prenatal diagnosis. Techniques of prenatal diagnosis. SOGC Clinical Practice Guidelines 2001:105.
Chyu JK, Strassner HT. Prostaglandin E2 for cervical ripening: a randomized comparison of cervidil vs. prepidil. Am J Obstet Gynecol 1997;177:606-611.
Cohen-Kerem R, Nulman I, Abramow-Newerly M, et al. Diagnostic radiation in pregnancy: perception versus true risks. JOGC 2005;28:43-48.
Crane J. Induction of labour at term. SOGC Clinical Practice Guidelines 2001;107:1-12.
Farrell S, Chan MC, Schulz JA. Midurethral minimally invasive sling procedures for stress urinary incontinence. SOGC Clinical Practice Guidelines 2008;213:728-733.
Findley I, Chamberlain G. Relief of pain. BMJ 1999;318:927-930.
Ford HB, Schust DJ. Recurrent pregnancy loss: etiology, diagnosis, and therapy. Rev Obstet Gynecol 2009;2:76-83.
Gagnon A, Wilson R. Obstetrical complications associated with abnormal maternal serum markers analytes. SOGC Clinical Practice Guidelines 2008;216:918-932.
Gavin NI et al. Perinatal depression: a systematic review of prevalence and incidence.Obstet Gynecol. 2005 Nov;106(5 Pt 1):1071-83.
Goldenberg RL, Culhane JF, Iams JD, et al. Epidemiology and causes of preterm birth. Lancet 2008;371;75-84.
Guise JM, Berlin M, McDonagh M, et al. Safety of vaginal birth after cesarean: a systematic review. Obstet Gynec 2004;103:420-429.
Hajenius PJ, Mol F, Mol BW, et al. Interventions for tubal ectopic pregnancy. Cochrane DB Syst Rev 2007;1:CD000324.
Hamilton P. Care of the newborn in the delivery room. BMJ 1999;318:1403-1406.
Hennessey MH, Rayburn WF, Stewart JD, et al. Preeclampsia and induction of labour: a randomized comparision of prostaglandin E2 as an intracervical gel, with oxytocin immediately, or as a sustained-release vaginal insert. Am J Obstet Gynecol 1998;179:1204-1209.
Hod M, Bar J, Peled Y, et al. Antepartum management protocol. Timing and mode of delivery in gestational diabetes. Obstet Gynecol 2009;113:206-217.
Hodnett ED, Gates S, Hofmeyr GJ, et al. Continuous support for women during childbirth. Cochrane DB Syst Rev 2011;2:CD003766.
Howarth GR, Botha DJ. Amniotomy plus intravenous oxytocin for induction of labour. Cochrane DB Syst Rev 2001;3:CD003250.
Kelly AJ, Tan B. Intravenous oxytocin alone for cervical ripening and induction of labour. Cochrane DB Syst Rev 2001;3:CD003246.
Kent N. Prevention and treatment of venous thromboembolism (VTE) in obstetrics. SOGC Clinical Practice Guidelines 2000;95:2-8.
Koren G. Motherisk update: Caffeine during pregnancy? Canadian Family Phys 2000;46:801-803.
Kotaska A, Menticoglou S, Gagnon R, et. al. Vaginal delivery of breech presentation. SOGC Clinical Practice Guidelines 2009;226;557-566.
Langlois S, Ford J, Chitayat D. Carrier screening for thalassemia and hemoglobinopathies in Canada. J Obstet Gynaecol Can 2008;217;950-959.
Langlois S, Wilson R. Carrier screening for genetic disorders in individuals of Ashkenazi Jewish descent. SOGC Clinical Practice Guidelines 2006;177;324-332.
Ling F, Duff P. Obstetrics and Gynecology, Principles for practice. USA: McGraw-Hill Companies, 2002.
Liston R, Sawchuck D, Young D. Fetal health surveillance: antepartum and intrapartum consensus guideline. SOGC Clinical Practice Guidelines 2007;197:S1-60.
Lowder JL, Burrows LJ, Krohn MA, et al. Risk factors for primary and subsequent anal sphincter lacerations: a comparison of cohorts by parity and prior mode of delivery. Am J Obstet Gynecol 2007;196:344.e1-5.
Luckas M, Bricker L. Intravenous prostaglandin for induction of labour. Cochrane DB Syst Rev 2000;4:CD002864.
Mackeen AD, Seibel-Seamon J, Muhammad J, et al. Tocolytics for preterm premature rupture of membranes. Cochrane DB Syst Rev 2014;2:CD007062.
Magee LA, Helewa M, Moutquin J-M, et al. Diagnosis, evaluation, and management of the hypertensive disorders of pregnancy. J Obstet Gynaecol Can 2008;30:S1-48.
Menezes EV, Yakoob MY, Soomro T, et al. Reducing stillbirths: prevention and management of medical disorders and infections during pregnancy. BMC Pregnancy Childbirth 2009;9(Suppl 1):S4.
Menticoglou S, Gagnon R, Kotaska A. Vaginal delivery of breech presentation. SOGC Clinical Practice Guidelines 2009;226;557-566.
Ministry of Health and Long Term Care and Canadian Medical Association. Antenatal record 1. Ontario.
Ministry of Health and Long Term Care and Canadian Medical Association. Antenatal record 2. Ontario.
Money D, Dobson S. The prevention of early-onset group B streptococcal disease. SOGC Clinical Practice Guidelines 2004;149:826-832.
Morgan S, Koren G. Is caffeine consumption safe during pregnancy? Can Fam Physician 2013;59(4):361-362.
Mottola MF, Wolfe LA, MacKinnon K, et al. Exercise in pregnancy and the postpartum period. SOGC Clinical Practice Guidelines 2003;129:1-7.
Mount Sinai Hospital. First trimester combined screening program. 2001.
Nicolaides KH, Syngelaki A, Ashoor G, et al. Noninvasive prenatal testing for fetal trisomies in a routinely screened first-trimester population. Am J Obstet Gynecol 2012;207(5):374.
North York General Hospital Genetics Program. Integrated prenatal screening. 1999.
Ottinyer WS, Menara MK, Brost BC. A randomized control trial of prostaglandin E2 intracervical gel and a slow release vaginal pessary for preinduction cervical ripening. Am J Obstet Gynecol 1998;179:349-353.
Ross S, Robert M. Conservative management of urinary incontinence. SOGC Practice Guidelines 2006;186:1113-1118.
Schrag SJ, Zell ER, Lynfield R, et al. A population-based comparison of strategies to prevent early-onset group B streptococcal disease in neonates. NEJM 2002;347:233-239.
Schuurmans N, Gagne G, Ezzat A, et al. Healthy beginnings: guidelines for care during pregnancy and childbirth. Clinical Practice Guidelines Policy Statement 1998:71:1-65.
Steer P, Flint C. Physiology and management of normal labour. BMJ 1999;318:793-796.
Steer P, Flint C. Preterm labour and premature rupture of membranes. BMJ 1999;318:1059-1062.
Stewart D. A broader context for maternal mortality. CMAJ 2006;74;302-303.
Stewart JD, Rayburn WF, Farmer KC, et al. Effectiveness of prostaglandin E2 intracervical gel (prepidil) with immediate oxytocin vs. vaginal insert (cervidil) for induction of labour. Am J Obstet Gynecol 1998;179:1175-1180.
Summers A, Langlois S, Wyatt P, et al. Prenatal screening for fetal aneuploidy. SOGC Clinical Practice Guidelines 2007;187:146-161.
Thompson D, Berger H, Feig D, et al. Diabetes and Pregnancy. Can J Diabetes 2013;37:S168-S183.
Van den Hof M, Crane J. Ultrasound cervical assessment in predicting preterm birth. SOGC Clinical Practice Guidelines 2001;102:1-4.
Verani JR, McGee L, Schrag SJ. Prevention of perinatal group B streptococcal disease. MMWR 2010;59(No.RR-10):1-32.
Zander L, Chamberlain G. Place of birth. BMJ 1999;318:721-723.
Zhang J, Bowes WA Jr, Fortney JA. Efficacy of external cephalic version: a review. Obstet Gynecol 1993;82(2):306-312.

OP Ophthalmology

Aaron Chan, Eli Kisilevsky, and **Alex Tam**, chapter editors
Dhruvin Hirpara and **Sneha Raju**, associate editors
Valerie Lemieux and **Simran Mundi**, EBM editors
Dr. Iqbal K. Ahmed, Dr. Wai-Ching Lam, and **Dr. Marisa Sit,** staff editors

Acronyms 2

Basic Anatomy Review 2

Differential Diagnoses of Common Presentations . . .3
Loss of Vision
Red Eye
Ocular Pain
Floaters
Flashes of Light (Photopsia)
Photophobia (Severe Light Sensitivity)
Diplopia (Double Vision)
Ocular Problems in the Contact Lens Wearer
Acute Painless Vision Loss

Ocular Emergencies 5

The Ocular Examination 5

Optics 7

The Orbit 9
Globe Displacement
Preseptal Cellulitis
Orbital Cellulitis

Lacrimal Apparatus 10
Dry Eye Syndrome (Keratoconjunctivitis Sicca)
Epiphora (Excessive Tearing)
Dacryocystitis
Dacryoadenitis

Lids and Lashes 11
Lid Swelling   Hordeolum (Stye)
Ptosis   Chalazion
Trichiasis   Blepharitis
Entropion   Xanthelasma
Ectropion

Conjunctiva 13
Pinguecula
Pterygium
Subconjunctival Hemorrhage
Conjunctivitis

Sclera 15
Episcleritis
Scleritis

Cornea 16
Foreign Body
Corneal Abrasion
Recurrent Erosions
Corneal Ulcer
Herpes Simplex Keratitis
Herpes Zoster Ophthalmicus
Keratoconus
Arcus Senilis
Kayser-Fleischer Ring

The Uveal Tract 19
Uveitis

Lens 20
Cataracts
Dislocated Lens (Ectopia Lentis)

Vitreous 21
Posterior Vitreous Detachment
Vitreous Hemorrhage
Endophthalmitis and Vitritis

Retina 22
Central/Branch Retinal Artery Occlusion
Central/Branch Retinal Vein Occlusion
Retinal Detachment
Retinitis Pigmentosa
Age-Related Macular Degeneration

Glaucoma 25
Primary Open-Angle Glaucoma
Normal Tension Glaucoma
Secondary Open Angle Glaucoma
Primary Angle-Closure Glaucoma
Secondary Angle-Closure Glaucoma

Pupils 28
Pupillary Light Reflex
Pupil Abnormalities
Dilated Pupil (Mydriasis)
Constricted Pupil (Miosis)
Relative Afferent Pupillary Defect

Malignancies 31
Lid Carcinoma
Malignant Melanoma
Metastases

Ocular Manifestations of Systemic Disease 32
HIV/AIDS
Other Systemic Infections
Diabetes Mellitus
Hypertension
Multiple Sclerosis
TIA/Amaurosis Fugax
Graves' Disease
Connective Tissue Disorders
Giant Cell Arteritis/Temporal Arteritis
Sarcoidosis

Pediatric Ophthalmology 36
Strabismus
Amblyopia
Leukocoria
Retinoblastoma
Retinopathy of Prematurity
Nasolacrimal System Defects
Ophthalmia Neonatorum
Congenital Glaucoma

Ocular Trauma 39
Blunt Trauma
Penetrating Trauma
Hyphema
Blow-Out Fracture
Chemical Burns

Ocular Drug Toxicity 41

Common Medications 42

References 44

Acronyms

AION	anterior ischemic optic neuropathy	EOM	extraocular movement	OHT	ocular hypertension	RD	retinal detachment
AMD	age-related macular degeneration	FML	fluorometholone	PACG	primary angle-closure glaucoma	ROP	retinopathy of prematurity
BCVA	best corrected visual acuity	GAT	Goldmann applanation tonometry	PDR	proliferative diabetic retinopathy	RPE	retinal pigment epithelium
BRAO	branch retinal artery occlusion	GCA	giant cell arteritis	PDT	photodynamic therapy	SLE	systemic lupus erythematosus
BRVO	branch retinal vein occlusion	HRT	Heidelberg retinal tomography	PERRLA	pupils equal, round, and reactive to light	SPK	superficial punctate keratitis
C:D	cup to disc ratio	INO	internuclear ophthalmoplegia		and accommodation	TIA	transient ischemic attack
CMV	cytomegalovirus	IOL	intraocular lens	POAG	primary open-angle glaucoma	VEGF	vascular endothelial growth factor
CRAO	central retinal artery occlusion	IOP	intraocular pressure	PRK	photorefractive keratectomy	YAG	yttrium aluminium garnet
D	diopter	LASIK	laser-assisted in situ keratomileusis	PVD	posterior vitreous detachment		
DM	diabetes mellitus	MS	multiple sclerosis	RA	rheumatoid arthritis		
DR	diabetic retinopathy	OCT	optical coherence tomography	RAPD	relative afferent pupillary defect		

Basic Anatomy Review

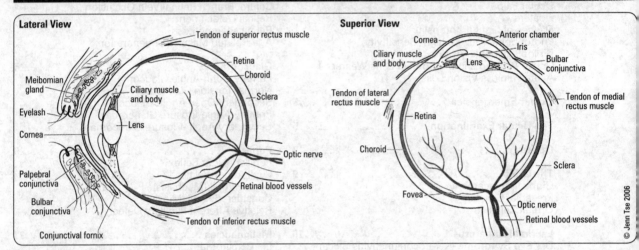

Figure 1. Anatomy of the eye

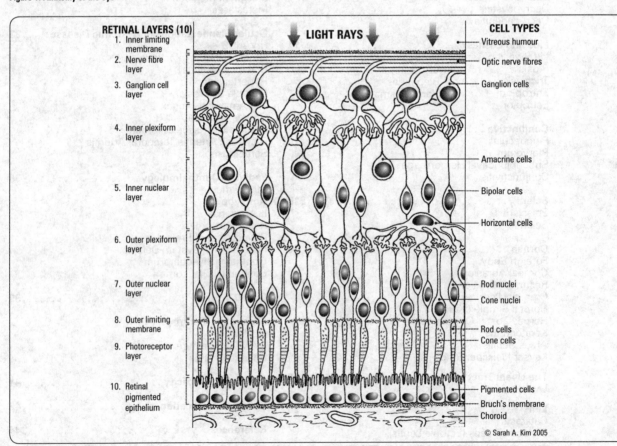

Figure 2. Layers of the retina

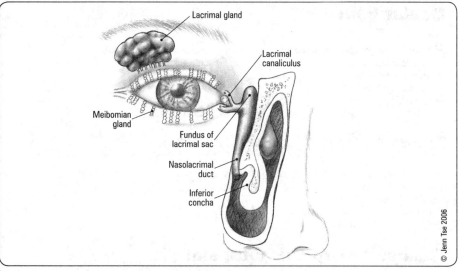

Figure 3. Tear drainage from the eye (lacrimal apparatus)

Differential Diagnoses of Common Presentations

Loss of Vision

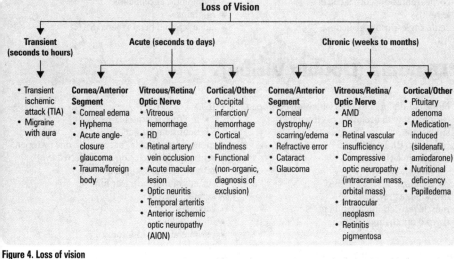

Figure 4. Loss of vision

Top 3 Differential Diagnosis of Acute Loss of Vision
- Vitreous hemorrhage
- Retinal artery/vein occlusion
- Retinal detachment

Top 3 Differential Diagnosis of Chronic Loss of Vision
Reversible
- Cataract
- Refractive error
- Corneal dystrophy
Irreversible
- AMD
- Glaucoma
- DR
Note: Anti-VEGF treatment for exudative AMD and diabetic macular edema may reverse some vision loss

Red Eye

- lids/orbit/lacrimal system
  - hordeolum/chalazion
  - blepharitis
  - entropion/ectropion
  - foreign body/laceration
  - dacryocystitis/dacryoadenitis
- conjunctiva/sclera
  - subconjunctival hemorrhage
  - conjunctivitis
  - dry eyes
  - pterygium
  - episcleritis/scleritis
  - preseptal/orbital cellulitis
- cornea
  - foreign body (including contact lens)
  - keratitis
  - abrasion, laceration
  - ulcer
- anterior chamber
  - anterior uveitis (iritis, iridocyclitis)
  - acute glaucoma
  - hyphema (blood in anterior chamber)
  - hypopyon (pus in anterior chamber)
- other
  - trauma
  - post-operative
  - endophthalmitis
  - pharmacologic (e.g. prostaglandin analogs)

Ocular Pain

- differentiate from eye fatigue (asthenopia)
- ocular surface disease
- herpes zoster prodrome
- trauma/foreign body
- blepharitis
- keratitis
- corneal abrasion, corneal ulcer
- acute glaucoma
- acute uveitis
- scleritis
- episcleritis
- optic neuritis

Floaters

- PVD (often secondary to age-related vitreous syneresis)
- vitreous hemorrhage
- retinal tear/detachment
- intermediate uveitis (pars planitis)
- posterior uveitis (chorioretinitis)

Flashes of Light (Photopsia)

- PVD (often secondary to age-related vitreous syneresis)
- retinal tear/detachment
- migraine with aura

Photophobia (Severe Light Sensitivity)

- corneal abrasion, corneal ulcer
- keratitis
- acute angle-closure glaucoma
- iritis
- meningitis, encephalitis
- migraine
- subarachnoid hemorrhage (SAH)

Diplopia (Double Vision)

- binocular diplopia (occurs with both eyes open, eliminated with occlusion of either eye)
- strabismus
- CN palsy (III, IV, VI)
  - ischemia (DM)
  - tumour
  - trauma
- myasthenia gravis
- muscle restriction/entrapment
- thyroid ophthalmopathy
- INO
  - multiple sclerosis
  - brainstem infarct
- monocular diplopia (occurs with one eye open, remains with occlusion of unaffected eye)
- refractive error/astigmatism
- strands of mucus in tear film
- keratoconus
- cataracts
- dislocated lens
- peripheral laser iridotomy

Ocular Problems in the Contact Lens Wearer

- solution hypersensitivity
- tight lens syndrome
- corneal abrasion
- giant papillary conjunctivitis/contact lens allergy
- SPK from dry eyes
- limbal stem cell deficiency
- corneal neovascularization
- sterile corneal infiltrates (immunologic)
- infected ulcers (*Pseudomonas*, *Acanthamoeba*)

Acute Painless Vision Loss

- vitreous hemorrhage
- retinal artery/vein occlusion
- RD
- AION
- optic neuritis
- amaurosis fugax/TIA/stroke

Table 1. Common Differential Diagnoses of Red Eye

	Conjunctivitis	Acute Iritis	Acute Glaucoma	Keratitis (Corneal Abrasion/Ulcer)
Discharge	Bacterial: purulent Viral: serous/mucoid Allergic: mucous	No	No	Profuse tearing
Pain	±	++ (dull/achy)	+++ (nausea)	++ (sharp)
Photophobia	No	+++	+	++
Blurred Vision	No	++	+++	Varies
Pupil	Normal	Smaller	Fixed in mid-dilation	Same or smaller
Injection	Conjunctiva with			
limbal Pallor	Ciliary flush	Diffuse	Diffuse	
Cornea	Normal	Keratic precipitates	Cloudy	Infiltrate, edema,
epithelial Defects				
IOP	Normal	Varies	Increased markedly	Normal or increased
Anterior Chamber	Normal	+++ Cells and flare	Shallow	Cells and flare or normal
Other	Large, tender pre-auricular node(s) if viral	Posterior synechiae	Coloured halos Nausea and vomiting	

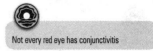

Not every red eye has conjunctivitis

Ocular Emergencies

These require urgent consultation to an ophthalmologist for management

Sight Threatening
- lid/globe lacerations
- chemical burn
- corneal ulcer
- gonococcal conjunctivitis
- acute iritis
- acute glaucoma
- CRAO
- intraocular foreign body
- RD (especially when macula threatened)
- endophthalmitis
- GCA

Life Threatening
- proptosis (rule out cavernous sinus fistula or thrombosis)
- CN III palsy with dilated pupil (intracranial aneurysm or externally compressive neoplastic lesion)
- papilledema (elevated increased intracranial pressure work up)
- orbital cellulitis
- leukocoria: white reflex (absent red reflex, must rule out retinoblastoma)

The Ocular Examination

Visual Acuity – Distance
- Snellen Acuity (Figure 5) = $\dfrac{\text{testing distance (usually 20 ft or 6 m)}}{\text{smallest line patient can read on the chart}}$
    - e.g. 20/40 = what the patient can see at 20 feet (numerator), what a "normal" person can see at 40 feet (denominator)
- distance visual acuity should be tested with distance glasses on in order to obtain best corrected visual acuity
- testing hierarchy for low vision: Snellen acuity (20/x) → counting fingers at a given distance (CF) → hand motion (HM) → light perception with projection (LP with projection) → light perception (LP) → no light perception (NLP)
- legal blindness is BCVA that is ≤20/200 in best eye
- minimum visual requirements to operate a non-commercial automobile in Ontario are: 20/50 BCVA with both eyes open and examined together, 120° continuous horizontal visual field, and 15° continuous visual field above and below fixation

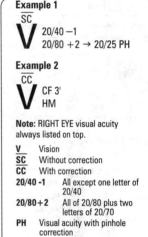

Example 1

$\overline{SC}$

V   20/40 −1
    20/80 +2 → 20/25 PH

Example 2

$\overline{CC}$

V   CF 3'
    HM

Note: RIGHT EYE visual acuity always listed on top.

V	Vision
SC	Without correction
CC	With correction
20/40 -1	All except one letter of 20/40
20/80+2	All of 20/80 plus two letters of 20/70
PH	Visual acuity with pinhole correction
CF	Counting fingers
HM	Hand motion

Figure 5. Ophthalmology nomenclature for VA

OD = oculus dexter = right eye
OS = oculus sinister = left eye
OU = oculus uterque = both eyes

Snellen visual acuity of 20/20 equates to "normal" vision

Normal Infant and Child Visual Acuity
- 6-12 mo: 20/120
- 1-2 yr: 20/80
- 2-4 yr: 20/20

For patients with dark irides, test pupils using an ophthalmoscope focused on the red reflex; this will provide a better view than using a penlight

Ocular Changes for Near Fixation
• Eye convergence
• Pupil constriction
• Lens accommodation

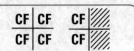

RIGHT EYE fields drawn on right side;
LEFT EYE fields drawn on left side
(as if seen through patient's eyes).

CF Able to count fingers in specified quadrant with peripheral vision

/// Gross visual field deficit in specified quadrant using peripheral vision

Figure 6. Ophthalmology nomenclature for visual fields by confrontation

4 Ps of Inspection
Pupil: shape, size, symmetry
Position: esotropia, exotropia, central
Ptosis
Primary nystagmus

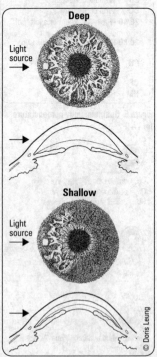

Figure 7. Estimation of anterior chamber depth

Visual Acuity – Near
• use pocket vision chart (Rosenbaum Pocket Vision Screener)
• record Jaeger (J) or Point number and testing distance (usually 30 cm) e.g. J2 @ 30 cm
• conversion to distance VA possible (e.g. immobile patient, no distance chart available)

Visual Acuity for Infants, Children, Non-English Speakers, and Dysphasics
• newborns
  ▪ VA cannot be tested conventionally
• 3 mo-3 yr (can only assess visual function, not acuity)
  ▪ test each eye for fixation symmetry using an interesting object
  ▪ normal function noted as "CSM" = central, steady, and maintained
• 3 yr until alphabet known
  ▪ pictures or letter cards/charts such as HOTV or Sheridan-Gardner test (children point to optotypes on a provided matching card)
  ▪ tumbling "E" chart

Colour Vision
• test with Ishihara pseudoisochromatic plates
• record number of correctly identified plates presented to each eye, specify incorrect plates
• important for testing optic nerve function (e.g. optic neuritis, chloroquine use, thyroid ophthalmopathy)
• note: red-green colour blindness is sex-linked and occurs in 7-10% of males

VISUAL FIELDS
• test "visual fields by confrontation" (4 quadrants, each eye tested separately) for estimation of visual field loss
• accurate, quantifiable assessment with automated visual field testing (Humphrey or Goldmann) or Tangent Screen
• use Amsler grid (each eye tested separately) to check for central or paracentral scotomas (blindspots) in patients with AMD

PUPILS
• use reduced room illumination with patient focusing on distant fixed object to prevent near reflex
• examine pupils for shape, size, symmetry, and reactivity to light (both direct and consensual response)
• test for RAPD with swinging flashlight test, check by reverse RAPD if one pupil non-reactive
• test pupillary constriction portion of near reflex by bringing object close to patient's nose
• "normal" pupil testing often noted as PERRLA (pupils equal, round, and reactive to light and accommodation)

ANTERIOR CHAMBER DEPTH
• shine light tangentially from temporal side
• if >2/3 of nasal side of iris in shadow → shallow anterior chamber

The van Herick Method (Slit Lamp technique)
• shine thin-angled slit beam onto the peripheral cornea of each eye, view at a 60° angle from the beam
• estimate depth between the posterior surface of the cornea and the iris as a proportion of corneal thickness
• ratios ≤1/4 implies risk of occludable angle; however, if >1/4 this does not rule out.
• gonioscopy, as performed by an ophthalmologist, is gold-standard for assessing anterior chamber depth

EXTRAOCULAR MUSCLES

Alignment
• Hirschberg corneal reflex test
• examine in primary position of gaze (i.e. straight ahead) with patient focusing on distant object
• shine light into patient's eyes from ~30 cm away
• corneal light reflex should be at the same position on each cornea
• strabismus testing as indicated (cover test, cover-uncover test, prism testing) (see *Strabismus*, OP6)

Movement
• examine movement of eyeball through six cardinal positions of gaze
• ask patient if diplopia or pain is present in any position of gaze
• observe for horizontal, vertical, or rotatory nystagmus (rhythmic, oscillating movements of the eye)
• resolving horizontal nystagmus at end-gaze is usually normal

Diplopia
• See Neurology – *Neuro-ophthalmology Diplopia*

SLIT-LAMP EXAMINATION

Ocular Adnexa
- lids, lashes, lacrimal system

Anterior Segment
- conjunctiva / sclera
- cornea
  - fluorescein dye: stains de-epithelialized cornea; dye appears fluorescent green with cobalt blue filtered light
  - Rose Bengal dye: stains devitalized corneal epithelium
- anterior chamber / angle (Van Herick)
- iris / pupil
- lens (assess for cataract)
- anterior vitreous

Posterior Segment (requires 78D or 90D lens)
- vitreous
- optic disc (colour, C:D ratio, sharpness of disc margin)
- macula (~1.5-2 disc diameters temporal to disc), fovea (foveal light reflex)
- retinal vessels
- retinal background

TONOMETRY
- measurement of IOP
- normal range is 9-21 mmHg (average 15 mmHg)
- IOP has diurnal variation, so always record the time of day at which the measurement was taken
- commonly measured by
  - Goldmann Applanation Tonometry (GAT): clinical gold standard, performed using the slit-lamp with special tip (prism)
  - Tono-Pen®: benefit is portability and use of disposable probe tips; use when cornea is scarred/asymmetric (GAT inaccurate)
  - air puff (non-contact and least reliable)
- use topical anesthetic for GAT and Tono-Pen®; apply fluorescein dye when using GAT

DIRECT OPHTHALMOSCOPY
- best performed with pupils dilated (for list of mydriatics and cycloplegics see Table 11, OP42)
  1. assess red reflex
     - light reflected off the retina produces a "red reflex" when viewed from ~1 foot away
     - anything that interferes with the passage of light will diminish the red reflex (e.g. large vitreous hemorrhage, cataract, retinoblastoma)
  2. examine the posterior segment of the eye
     - vitreous
     - optic disc (colour, C:D ratio, sharpness of disc margin)
     - macula (~1.5-2 disc diameters temporal to disc), fovea (foveal light reflex)
     - retinal vessels
     - retinal background
- contraindications to pupillary dilatation
  - shallow anterior chamber – can precipitate acute angle-closure glaucoma
  - iris-supported anterior chamber lens implant
  - potential neurologic abnormality requiring pupil evaluation
  - use caution with cardiovascular disease – mydriatics may cause tachycardia

Optics

REFRACTION
- two techniques used
  - flash/streak retinoscopy: refractive error determined objectively by the examiner using lenses and retinoscope
  - manifest: subjective trial using loose lenses or a phoropter (device the patient looks through that is equipped with lenses)
  - cycloplegic: manifest refraction with accommodation temporarily paralyzed with mydriatics
- a typical lens prescription would contain
  - sphere power in dioptre (measurement of refractive power of lens, equal to reciprocal of focal length in metres)
  - cylinder power in dioptre to correct astigmatism
  - axis of cylinder in degrees
  - "add" (bifocal/progressive reading lens) for presbyopes
  - e.g. -1.50 + 1.00 x 120 degrees, add +2.00

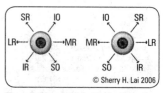

Figure 8. Diagnostic positions of gaze for isolated primary actions of extraocular muscles

Extraocular Muscle Innervations

LR6 SO4 AE3
Lateral Rectus via CN **VI**
Superior Oblique via CN **IV**
All Else via CN **III** (superior, medial, and inferior rectus, inferior oblique)

Aqueous Flare
- Resembles dust particles in a beam of light
- Results from protein leaking from blood vessels
- Distinguish from aqueous cells (individual cells in anterior chamber)

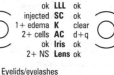

Note: RIGHT EYE drawn on the left, LEFT EYE drawn on the right (as if looking at patient's face)

ok	**LLL**	ok
injected	**SC**	ok
1+ edema	**K**	clear
2+ cells	**AC**	d+q
ok	**Iris**	ok
2+ NS	**Lens**	ok

— Eyelids/eyelashes
— Conjunctiva/sclera/episclera
— Cornea/Iris/anterior surface of lens

LLL	Lids, lashes, lacrimal
SC	Sclera, conjunctiva
K	Cornea
AC	Anterior chamber
d+q	Deep (not shallow) and quiet (no cells in AC)
NS	Nuclear sclerosis (cataract)

Ⓝ D/M/V
(normal disc, macula, vessels)

C:D 0.3   C:D 0.4

C:D	Cup : Disc ratio
x	Fovea

Any abnormality or pathology is drawn on the sketch in the appropriate location, and is labelled (e.g. trichiasis, conjunctivitis/episcleritis/scleritis, corneal abrasion/ulcer, foreign body, etc.)

© Tobi Lam 2012

Figure 9. Slit-lamp examination note

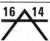

Note: RIGHT EYE IOP always listed on top. Always include time.

Note method used to measure IOP (GAT, Tono-Pen®, airpuff).

Figure 10. Tonometry

Central Corneal Thickness (CCT)
Average CCT = 550 μm
By GAT, IOP is over-estimated with thick corneas and under-estimated with thin corneas

Myopia

LMN
Long globe
Myopic
Negative correction/Nearsighted

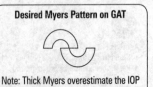

Desired Myers Pattern on GAT

Note: Thick Myers overestimate the IOP and are a result of excess fluorescein

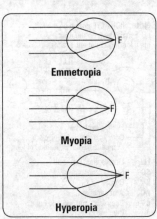

Figure 11. Emmetropia and refractive errors

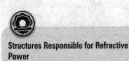

Structures Responsible for Refractive Power
• Cornea (2/3)
• Lens (1/3)

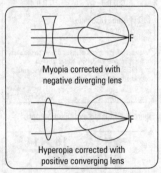

Figure 12. Correction of refractive errors

REFRACTIVE EYE SURGERY
• permanently alters corneal refractive properties by ablating tissue to change curvature of the cornea
• used for correction of myopia, hyperopia, and astigmatism
• common types include PRK and LASIK
• potential risks/side-effects: infection, under/overcorrection, decreased night vision (nyctalopia), corneal haze, dry eyes, regression, complete sever of corneal flap (LASIK only)

Table 2. Optics

	Pathophysiology	Clinical Features	Treatment	Complications
Emmetropia	Image of distant objects focus exactly on the retina	No refractive error		
Myopia	Globe too long relative to refractive mechanisms, or refractive mechanisms too strong. Light rays from distant object focus in front of retina → blurring of (distance) vision	"Nearsightedness" Usually presents in 1st or 2nd decade, stabilizes in 2nd and 3rd decade; rarely begins after age 25 except in patients with DM or cataracts. Blurring of distance vision; near vision usually unaffected. Prevalence: 30-40% in U.S. population	Correct with negative diopter/concave/"negative" lenses to diverge light rays. Refractive eye surgery	Retinal tear/detachment, macular hole, open angle glaucoma. Other complications that are not prevented with refractive correction
Hyperopia	Globe too short relative to refractive mechanisms, or refractive mechanisms too weak. Light rays from distant object focus behind retina → blurring of near ± distant vision. May be developmental or due to any etiology that shortens globe	"Farsightedness" Youth: usually do not require glasses (still have sufficient accommodative ability to focus image on retina), but may develop accommodative esotropia (see Strabismus, OP36). 30s-40s: blurring of near vision due to decreased accommodation, may need reading glasses. >50s: blurring of distance vision due to severely decreased accommodation	When symptomatic, correct with positive diopter/convex/"plus" lenses to converge light rays. Refractive eye surgery	Angle-closure glaucoma, particularly later in life as lens enlarges
Astigmatism	Light rays not refracted uniformly in all meridians due to non-spherical surface of cornea or non-spherical lens (e.g. football-shaped). **Two types** Regular – curvature uniformly different in meridians at right angles to each other. Irregular – distorted cornea caused by injury, keratoconus (cone-shaped cornea), corneal scar, or severe dry eye	Affects ~30% of population, with prevalence increasing with age. Mild astigmatism unnoticeable. Higher amounts of astigmatism may cause blurry vision, squinting, asthenopia, or headaches	Correct with cylindrical lens (if regular), try contact lens (if irregular). Refractive eye surgery	
Presbyopia	Normal aging process (>40 yr). Hardening/reduced deformability of lens results in decreased accommodative ability. Accommodative power is 14D at age 10, diminishes to 3.5D by age 40 yr. Near images cannot be focused onto the retina (focus is behind the retina as in hyperopia)	If initially emmetropic, person begins to hold reading material farther away, but distance vision remains unaffected. If initially myopic, person removes distance glasses to read. If initially hyperopic, symptoms of presbyopia occur earlier	Correct with positive diopter/convex/"plus" lenses for reading	
Anisometropia	Difference in refractive errors between eyes			Second most common cause of amblyopia in children

The Orbit

Globe Displacement

Table 3. Exophthalmos (Proptosis) and Enophthalmos

	Exophthalmos (Proptosis)	Enophthalmos
Definition	Anterior displacement (protrusion) of the globe Exophthalmos generally refers to an endocrine etiology or protrusion of >18 mm (as measured by a Hertel exophthalmometer) Proptosis generally refers to other etiologies (e.g. cellulitis) or protrusion of <18 mm	Posterior displacement (retraction) of the globe
Investigations	CT/MRI head/orbits, ultrasound orbits, thyroid function tests	CT/MRI orbits
Etiology	Note: rule out pseudoexophthalmos (e.g. lid retraction) Graves' disease (unilateral or bilateral, most common cause in adults) Orbital cellulitis (unilateral, most common cause in children) 1° or 2° orbital tumours Orbital/retrobulbar hemorrhage Cavernous sinus thrombosis or fistula	"Blow-out" fracture (see Ocular Trauma, OP39) Orbital fat atrophy Congenital abnormality Metastatic disease

Preseptal Cellulitis

- infection of soft tissue anterior to orbital septum

Etiology
- usually follows periorbital trauma or dermal infection

Clinical Features

Table 4. Clinical Features of Preseptal and Orbital Cellulitis

Finding	Preseptal Cellulitis	Orbital Cellulitis
Fever	May be present	Present
Lid edema	Moderate to severe	Severe
Conjunctival injection	Absent	Present
Chemosis	Absent or mild	Marked
Proptosis	Absent	Present
Pain on eye movement	Absent	Present
Ocular mobility	Normal	Decreased
Vision	Normal	Diminished ± diplopia
RAPD	Absent	May be seen if severe
Leukocytosis	Moderate	Marked
ESR	Normal or elevated	Elevated
Additional findings	Skin infection	Sinusitis, dental abscess

Role of Oral Corticosteroids in Orbital Cellulitis
Am J Ophthalmol 2013;156:178-183
Purpose: To evaluate the role of oral corticosteroids as an anti-inflammatory adjunct for the treatment of orbital cellulitis.
Study: RCT. Patients with acute onset (within 14 d) of orbital cellulitis with or without abscess. 21 patients total (7 patients in group 1: standard intravenous antibiotics; 14 patients in group 2: adjuvant steroids).
Results: Patients in group 2 showed earlier resolution of periorbital edema, conjunctival chemosis, pain, proptosis, and EOM deficits, including decreased duration of intravenous antibiotics and hospital stay (p<0.05 for all).
Conclusion: The use of oral steroids as an adjunct to intravenous antibiotics for orbital cellulitis may decrease inflammatory symptoms with a low risk of worsening infection.

Treatment
- systemic antibiotics (suspect *H. influenzae* in children; *S. aureus* or *Streptococcus* in adults)
  - e.g. amoxicillin-clavulanic acid
- if severe or child <1 yr, treat as orbital cellulitis

Orbital Cellulitis

- **OCULAR** and **MEDICAL EMERGENCY**
- inflammation of orbital contents posterior to orbital septum
- common in children, elderly, and immunocompromised

Etiology
- usually secondary to sinus/facial/tooth infections or trauma, can also arise from preseptal cellulitis

Clinical Features (see Table 4)

Orbital cellulitis is life-threatening if untreated (mortality of 17-20% without antibiotic use); prompt diagnosis and treatment is essential

Treatment
- admit, blood cultures x2, orbital CT, IV antibiotics (ceftriaxone + vancomycin) for 1 wk
- surgical drainage of abscess with close follow-up, especially in children

Complications
- optic nerve inflammation, cavernous sinus thrombosis, meningitis, and brain abscess with possible loss of vision, death

Lacrimal Apparatus

- tear film made up of three layers
  - outer oily layer (reduces evaporation): secreted by the Meibomian glands
  - middle watery layer (forms the bulk of the tear film): constant secretion from conjunctival glands and reflex secretion by lacrimal gland with ocular irritation or emotion
  - inner mucinous layer (aids with tear adherence to cornea): secreted by conjunctival goblet cells
- tears drain from the eyes through the upper and lower lacrimal puncta → superior and inferior canaliculi → lacrimal sac → nasolacrimal duct → nasal cavity behind inferior concha (Figure 3)

Dry Eye Syndrome (Keratoconjunctivitis Sicca)

Etiology
- aqueous-deficient (lacrimal pathology)
  - Sjögren syndrome (autoimmune etiology e.g. RA, SLE)
  - non-Sjögren syndrome (idiopathic age-related disease; lacrimal gland scarring e.g. trachoma; decreased secretion e.g. contact lenses, CN VII palsy, anticholinergics, antihistamines, diuretics, β-blockers)
- evaporative (normal lacrimal function, excessive evaporation of aqueous layer)
  - Meibomian gland dysfunction (posterior blepharitis)
  - vitamin A deficiency (xerophthalmia with goblet cell dysgenesis)
  - eyelid abnormalities e.g. ectropion, CN VII palsy (decreased blinking)
  - preserved topical ocular medications
  - contact lenses, allergic conjunctivitis
- mixed etiologies is common

Clinical Features
- dry eyes, red eyes, foreign body sensation, blurred vision, tearing
- slit-lamp exam: decreased tear meniscus, decreased tear break-up time (normally should be 10 s), punctate staining of cornea with fluorescein

Investigations
- surface damage observed with fluorescein/Rose Bengal staining
- decreased distance in Schirmer's test

Complications
- erosions and scarring of cornea

Long-term use of artificial tears with preservatives should be avoided when treating dry eyes

Treatment
- medical: preservative-free artificial tears up to q1h and ointment at bedtime (preservative toxicity becomes significant if used >q1h PRN), mild corticosteroid
  - for severe cases, cyclosporine ophthalmic emulsion 0.05% (Restasis®) can be used
- procedural: punctal occlusion (punctal plug insertion), lid taping, tarsorrhaphy (sew lids together) if severe
- treat underlying cause

Epiphora (Excessive Tearing)

Excessive tearing can be caused by dry eyes – if the tear quality is insufficient, "reflex tearing" may occur

Etiology
- emotion, pain
- environmental stressor (cold, wind, pollen, sleep deprivation)
- lid/lash malposition: ectropion, entropion, trichiasis
- inflammatory: conjunctivitis, dacryoadenitis, uveitis, keratitis, corneal foreign body
- dry eyes (reflex tearing)
- lacrimal drainage obstruction (congenital failure of canalization, aging, rhinitis, dacryocystitis)
- paradoxical gustatory lacrimation reflex (crocodile tears)

Investigations
- using fluorescein dye, examine for punctal reflux by pressing on canaliculi
- Jones dye test: fluorescein placed in conjunctival cul-de-sac, and cotton applicator placed in nose to detect flow (i.e. rule out lacrimal drainage obstruction)

Treatment
- lid repair for ectropion or entropion
- eyelash removal for trichiasis
- punctal irrigation (dilation and irrigation)
- nasolacrimal duct probing (infants)
- tube placement: temporary (Crawford) or permanent (Jones)
- surgical: dacryocystorhinostomy – forming a new connection between the lacrimal sac and the nasal cavity

Dacryocystitis

- acute or chronic infection of the lacrimal sac
- most commonly due to obstruction of the nasolacrimal duct
- commonly associated with S. aureus, S. pneumoniae, Pseudomonas species

Clinical Features
- pain, swelling, redness over lacrimal sac at medial canthus
- epiphora, crusting, ± fever
- digital pressure on the lacrimal sac may extrude pus through the punctum
- in the chronic form, epiphora may be the only symptom

Treatment
- warm compresses, nasal decongestants, systemic and topical antibiotics
- if chronic, obtain cultures by aspiration
- once infection resolves, consider dacryocystorhinostomy

Dacryoadenitis

- inflammation of the lacrimal gland (outer third of upper eyelid)
- acute causes: S. aureus, mumps, EBV, herpes zoster, *N. gonorrhoeae*
- chronic causes (often bilateral): lymphoma, leukemia, sarcoidosis, tuberculosis, thyroid ophthalmopathy

Clinical Features
- pain, swelling, tearing, discharge, redness of the outer region of the upper eyelid
- chronic form is more common and may present as painless enlargement of the lacrimal gland

Treatment
- supportive: warm compresses, oral NSAIDs
- systemic antibiotics if bacterial cause
- if chronic, treat underlying disorder

Lids and Lashes

Lid Swelling

Etiology
- commonly due to allergy, with shriveling of skin between episodes
- dependent edema on awakening (e.g. CHF, renal or hepatic failure)
- orbital venous congestion due to mass or cavernous sinus fistula
- dermatochalasis (loose skin due to aging or heredity)
- lid cellulitis, thyroid disease (e.g. myxedema), trauma, chemosis

Ptosis

- drooping of upper eyelid

Etiology
- aponeurotic: disinsertion or dehiscence of levator aponeurosis (most common)
  - associated with advancing age, trauma, surgery, pregnancy, chronic lid swelling
- mechanical
  - incomplete opening of eyelid due to mass or scarring
- neuromuscular
  - myasthenia gravis (neuromuscular palsy), myotonic dystrophy
  - CN III palsy
  - Horner's syndrome (see *Constricted Pupil, Horner's Syndrome*, OP30)
- congenital
- pseudoptosis (e.g. dermatochalasis, enophthalmos, contralateral exophthalmos)
- drugs (e.g. high dose opioids, heroin abuse, pregabalin)

Treatment
- surgery (e.g. blepharoplasty, levator resection, Müller's muscle resection, frontalis sling)

Trichiasis

- eyelashes turned inwards
- may result from entropion, involutional age change, chronic inflammatory lid diseases (e.g. blepharitis), trauma, burns
- patient complains of red eye, foreign body sensation, significant discomfort, tearing
- may result in corneal ulceration and scarring

Treatment
- topical lubrication, repeat eyelash epilation, electrolysis, cryotherapy

Entropion

- lid margin turns in towards globe causing tearing, foreign body sensation, and red eye
- most commonly affects lower lid
- may cause corneal abrasions with secondary corneal scarring

Etiology
- involutional (aging)
- cicatricial (herpes zoster, surgery, trauma, burns)
- orbicularis oculi muscle spasm
- congenital

Treatment
- lubricants, evert lid with tape, surgery

Testing for Entropion
Forced lid closure: Ask patient to tighten lid then open. In entropion, lid rolls inwards

Ectropion

- lid margin turns outward from globe causing tearing and possibly exposure keratitis

Etiology
- involutional (aging)
- paralytic (CN VII palsy)
- cicatricial (burns, trauma, surgery)
- mechanical (lid edema, tumour, herniated fat)
- congenital

Treatment
- topical lubrication, eyelid taping overnight, surgery

Testing for Ectropion
Snapback test: Pull eyelid inferiorly. In ectropion, lid remains away from globe

Hordeolum (Stye)

- acute inflammation of eyelid gland: either Meibomian glands (internal lid), glands of Zeis (modified sweat gland) or Moll (modified sebaceous gland in external lid)
- infectious agent is usually S. aureus
- painful, red swelling of lid

Treatment
- warm compresses, lid care, gentle massage
- topical antibiotics are typically ineffective
- usually resolves within 2 weeks, but may require incision and drainage.

Hordeolum vs. Chalazion
Hordeolums are due to an infectious etiology, whereas chalazions are granulomatous inflammation

Chalazion

- chronic granulomatous inflammation of Meibomian gland often preceded by an internal hordeolum
- acute inflammatory signs are usually absent
- differential diagnosis: basal cell carcinoma, sebaceous cell adenoma, Meibomian gland carcinoma

Treatment
- warm compresses
- if no improvement after 1 mo, consider incision and curettage
- chronic recurrent lesion must be biopsied to rule out malignancy

Blepharitis

- inflammation of lid margins

Etiology
- two main types
- staphylococcal (*S. aureus*): ulcerative, dry scales
- seborrheic: no ulcers, greasy scales

Clinical Features
- itching, tearing, foreign body sensation
- thickened, red lid margins, crusting, discharge with pressure on lids ("toothpaste sign")

Complications
- recurrent hordeola
- conjunctivitis
- keratitis (from poor tear film)
- corneal ulceration and neovascularization

Treatment
- warm compresses and lid scrubs with diluted "baby shampoo"
- topical or systemic antibiotics as needed
- if severe, ophthalmologist may prescribe a short course of topical corticosteroids, omega-3 fatty acids

Xanthelasma

- eyelid xanthoma (lipid deposits in dermis of lids)
- appear as pale, slightly elevated yellowish plaques or streaks
- most commonly on the medial upper lids, often bilateral
- associated with hyperlipidemia (~50% of patients)
- common in the elderly, more concerning in the young

Treatment
- excision for cosmesis only, commonly recurs

Conjunctiva

- thin, vascular mucous membrane
- bulbar conjunctiva: lines sclera to limbus (junction between cornea and sclera)
- palpebral (tarsal) conjunctiva: lines inner surface of eyelid

Pinguecula

- yellow-white subepithelial deposit of hyaline and elastic tissue adjacent to the nasal or temporal limbus, sparing the cornea
- associated with sun and wind exposure, aging
- benign, sometimes enlarges slowly
- may be irritating due to abnormal tear film formation over the deposits
- surgery for cosmesis only
- irritative symptoms may be treated with lubricating drops

Pterygium

- fibrovascular, triangular, wing-like encroachment of epithelial tissue onto the cornea,
- may induce astigmatism, decrease vision
- excision for chronic inflammation, threat to visual axis, cosmesis
- irritative symptoms may be treated with lubricating drops
- one-third recur after excision, lower recurrence with conjunctival autograft (~5%)

Subconjunctival Hemorrhage

- blood beneath the conjunctiva, otherwise asymptomatic
- idiopathic or associated with trauma, Valsalva maneuver, bleeding disorders, HTN, anticoagulation
- give reassurance if no other ocular findings, resolves spontaneously in 2-3 wk
- 360 degree involvment should be highly suspicious for globe rupture
- if recurrent, consider medical/hematologic workup

Conjunctivitis

Types of Discharge
- Allergic: mucoid
- Viral: watery
- Bacterial: purulent
- Chlamydial: mucopurulent

- Follicles are usually seen in viral and chlamydial conjunctivitis
- Papillae are usually seen in allergic and bacterial conjunctivitis

Antibiotics vs. Placebo for Acute Bacterial Conjunctivitis
Cochrane DB Syst Rev 2012;9:CD001211
Purpose: To assess the benefits and harms of antibiotic therapy in the management of acute bacterial conjunctivitis.
Criteria: RCTs with any form of antibiotic treatment compared with placebo including topical, systemic or combined (e.g. antibiotics and steroids) antibiotic treatments.
Results: 11 RCTs, 3,673 participants. Topical antibiotics improve early (2-5 d) clinical and microbiological remission rates (RR 1.36, 95% CI 1.15-1.61; RR 1.55; 95% CI 1.37-1.76) and benefit clinical remission and microbiological cure rates at a late time point (6-10 d) (RR 1.21, 95% CI 1.10-1.33; RR 1.37, 95% CI 1.24-1.52). By 6-10 d 41% of cases had resolved in the placebo group. No serious outcomes were reported in any group.
Conclusion: The use of antibiotic eye drops is associated with modestly improved rates of clinical and microbiological remission in comparison to placebo. Antibiotic eye drops should therefore be considered in order to speed the resolution of symptoms and infection although acute bacterial conjunctivitis is frequently self-limiting.

Etiology
- infectious
- bacterial, viral, chlamydial, gonococcal, fungal, parasitic
- non-infectious
- allergic: atopic, seasonal, giant papillary conjunctivitis (contact lens wearers)
- toxic: irritants, dust, smoke, irradiation
- secondary to another disorder: dacryocystitis, dacryoadenitis, cellulitis, systemic inflammatory disease

Clinical Features
- red eye (conjunctival injection often with limbal pallor), chemosis, corneal subepithelial infiltrates
- itching, foreign body sensation, tearing, discharge, crusting of lashes in the morning, lid edema
- ± preauricular and/or submandibular nodes
- follicles: pale lymphoid elevations of the conjunctiva, overlain by vessels
- papillae: fibrovascular elevations of the conjunctiva with central network of finely branching vessels (cobblestone appearance)

ALLERGIC CONJUNCTIVITIS

Atopic
- associated with rhinitis, asthma, dermatitis, hay fever
- small papillae, chemosis, thickened and erythematous lids, corneal neovascularization
- seasonal (pollen, grasses, plant allergens)
- treatment: cool compresses, antihistamine, mast cell stabilizer (e.g. ketotifen, olopatadine), topical corticosteroids

Giant Papillary Conjunctivitis
- immune reaction to mucus debris on lenses in contact lens wearers
- large papillae form on superior palpebral conjunctiva
- treatment: clean, change or discontinue use of contact lens, topical corticosteroids

Vernal Conjunctivitis
- large papillae (cobblestones) form on superior palpebral conjunctiva with corneal ulcers and keratitis
- seasonal (warm weather)
- occurs in children, lasts for 5-10 yr then resolves
- treatment: consider topical steroid, topical cyclosporine (by ophthalmologist)

VIRAL CONJUNCTIVITIS (Pink Eye)
- presents with itchiness, pain and swelling
- serous discharge, lid edema, follicles, pseudomembranes
- subepithelial corneal infiltrates
- preauricular node often palpable and tender
- initially unilateral, often progresses to the other eye
- mainly due to adenovirus – highly contagious for up to 12 d

Treatment
- cool compresses, topical lubrication
- usually self-limiting (7-12 d)
- proper hygiene is important to prevent transmission

BACTERIAL CONJUNCTIVITIS
- purulent discharge, lid swelling, papillae, conjunctival injection, chemosis
- common agents include *S. aureus*, *S. pneumoniae*, *H. influenzae* and *M. catarrhalis*
- in neonates or if sexually active must consider *N. gonorrhoeae* (invades cornea to cause keratitis)
- *C. trachomatis* is the most common cause in neonates

Treatment
- topical broad-spectrum antibiotic
- systemic antibiotics if indicated, especially in neonates and children
- usually a self-limited course of 10-14 d if no treatment, 1-3 d with treatment

GONOCOCCAL AND CHLAMYDIAL CONJUNCTIVITIS
- caused by *N. gonorrhoeae* and *C. trachomatis*, respectively
- affects sexually active individuals, neonates (*ophthalmia neonatorum*) in first 5 days of life when caused by gonorrhea (shorter incubation period) and days 3-14 of life when caused by chlamydia (longer incubation period)
- newborn prophylaxis with 0.5% erythromycin ointment no longer recommended
- causes trachoma and inclusion conjunctivitis (different serotypes)

- Enlarged lymph nodes suggest infectious etiology, especially viral or chlamydial conjunctivitis
- Temporal conjunctival lymphatics drain to preauricular nodes, and nasal to submandibular nodes

Trachoma
- leading infectious cause of blindness in the world
- severe keratoconjunctivitis leads to corneal abrasion, ulceration, and scarring
- initially, follicles on superior palpebral conjunctiva
- treatment: oral azithromycin and topical tetracycline

Inclusion Conjunctivitis
- chronic conjunctivitis with follicles and subepithelial infiltrates
- most common cause of conjunctivitis in newborns
- newborn prophylaxis with 0.5% erythromycin ointment no longer recommended
- treatment: oral azithromycin, tetracycline, doxycycline

Sclera

- white fibrous outer protective coat of the eye, composed of irregularly distributed collagen bundles
- continuous with the cornea anteriorly and the dura of the optic nerve posteriorly
- episclera is a thin layer of vascularized tissue between the sclera and conjunctiva

Episcleritis

- immunologically mediated inflammation of episclera
- 1/3 bilateral; simple (80%) or nodular (20%)
- more frequent in women than men (3:1)

Etiology
- mostly idiopathic
- associated with collagen vascular diseases, infections (herpes zoster, herpes simplex, syphilis), inflammatory bowel disease, rosacea, atopy

Clinical Features
- may have discomfort and pain associated with red eye (often interpalpebral),
- sectoral or diffuse injection of radially-directed vessels, chemosis, small mobile nodules
- blanches with topical phenylephrine (constricts superficial conjunctival vessels)

Treatment
- generally self-limited, recurrent in 2/3 of cases
- topical steroid for 3-5 d if painful (prescribed and monitored by ophthalmologist)
- oral NSAID

Scleritis

- usually bilateral: diffuse, nodular, or necrotizing
- anterior scleritis: pain radiating to face, may cause scleral thinning, in some cases necrotizing
- posterior scleritis: rapidly progressive blindness, may cause exudative RD
- more common in women and elderly

Etiology
- may be a manifestation of systemic disease
- collagen vascular disease, e.g. SLE, RA, ankylosing spondylitis
- granulomatous, e.g. tuberculosis, sarcoidosis, syphilis
- metabolic, e.g. gout, thyrotoxicosis
- infectious, e.g. *S. aureus, S. pneumoniae, P. aeruginosa*, herpes zoster
- chemical or physical agents, e.g. thermal, alkali, or acid burns
- idiopathic

Clinical Features
- severe pain, photophobia, red eye, decreased vision
- pain is best indicator of disease progression
- inflammation of scleral, episcleral, and conjunctival vessels
- may have anterior chamber cells and flare, corneal infiltrate, scleral thinning, scleral edema
- sclera may have a blue hue (best seen in natural light), due to rearranged scleral fibres
- failure to blanch with topical phenylephrine

Treatment
- **vision threatening** – needs to be referred to ophthalmology
- systemic NSAID or topical or systemic steroid
- treat underlying etiology

Preventing Ophthalmia Neonatorum
Paediatr Child Health 2015;20(2):93-96
The use of silver nitrate as prophylaxis for neonatal ophthalmia was instituted in the late 1800s to prevent the devastating effects of neonatal ocular infection with Neisseria gonorrhoeae. At that time – during the preantibiotic era – many countries made such prophylaxis mandatory by law. Today, neonatal gonococcal ophthalmia is rare in Canada, but ocular prophylaxis for this condition remains mandatory in some provinces/territories. Silver nitrate drops are no longer available and erythromycin, the only ophthalmic antibiotic eye ointment currently available for use in newborns, is of questionable efficacy. Ocular prophylaxis is not effective in preventing chlamydial conjunctivitis. Applying medication to the eyes of newborns may result in mild eye irritation and has been perceived by some parents as interfering with mother-infant bonding. Physicians caring for newborns should advocate for rescinding mandatory ocular prophylaxis laws. More effective means of preventing *ophthalmia neonatorum* include screening all pregnant women for gonorrhea and chlamydia infection, and treatment and follow-up of those found to be infected. Mothers who were not screened should be tested at delivery. Infants of mothers with untreated gonococcal infection at delivery should receive ceftriaxone. Infants exposed to chlamydia at delivery should be followed closely for signs of infection.

To differentiate between episcleritis and scleritis, place a drop of phenylephrine 2.5% (Mydfrin®; AK-Dilate®) in the affected eye. Re-examine the vascular pattern 10-15 min later; in episcleritis the episcleral vessels should blanch with phenylephrine

Scleromalacia Perforans
- Asymptomatic anterior necrotizing scleritis without inflammation
- Strongly associated with RA
- May result in scleral thinning
- Traumatic perforation can easily occur – examine eye very gently

Learn the Layers of the Cornea
ABCDE
Anterior epithelium
Bowman's Membrane
Corneal Stroma
Dua's Layer, Descemet's Membrane
Endothelium

A new corneal layer was discovered by H. Dua in 2013 and is characterized as a pre-Descemet's membrane

Foreign body behind lid may cause multiple vertical corneal epithelial abrasions due to blinking

Topical analgesics should only be used to facilitate examination. They should NEVER be used as treatment for any ocular problem

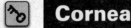

Cornea

- function
  - transmission of light
  - refraction of light (2/3 of total refractive power of eye)
  - barrier against infection, foreign bodies
- transparency due to avascularity, uniform collagen structure and deturgescence (relative dehydration)
- 6 layers (anterior to posterior): epithelium, Bowman's membrane, stroma, Dua's layer, Descemet's membrane, endothelium (dehydrates the cornea; dysfunction leads to corneal edema)
- extensive sensory fibre network (V1 distribution); therefore abrasions are very painful

Foreign Body

- foreign material in or on cornea
- may have associated rust ring if metallic
- patients may note pain, tearing, photophobia, foreign body sensation, red eye
- signs include foreign body, conjunctival injection, epithelial defect that stains with fluorescein, corneal edema, anterior chamber cells/flare

Complications
- abrasion, infection, ulcer, scarring, rust ring, secondary iritis

Treatment
- remove under magnification using local anesthetic and sterile needle or refer to ophthalmology for removal under magnification (depending on depth and location)
- treat as per corneal abrasion

Corneal Abrasion

- epithelial defect usually due to trauma (e.g. fingernails, paper, twigs), contact lens (Figure 14)

Clinical Features (Table 5)
- pain, redness, tearing, photophobia, foreign body sensation
- de-epithelialized area stains with fluorescein dye
- pain relieved with topical anesthetic (DO NOT use for treatment- risk of corneal melt)

Complications
- infection, ulceration, recurrent erosion, secondary iritis

Corneal abrasions from organic matter (e.g. twig, finger nail, etc.) have higher recurrence, even years later

Treatment
- topical antibiotic (drops or ointment), abrasion from organic material should be covered against pseudomonas
- consider topical NSAID (caution due to risk of corneal melt with prolonged use), cycloplegic (relieves pain and photophobia by paralyzing ciliary muscle), patch
- most abrasions clear spontaneously within 24-48 h

Recurrent Erosions

- recurrent episodes of pain, photophobia, foreign body sensation with a spontaneous corneal epithelial defect
- usually occurs upon awakening
- associated with improper adherence of epithelial cells to the underlying basement membrane

Corneal Abrasion: To Patch or Not to Patch
Patching for corneal abrasion.
Cochrane DB Syst Rev 2006;2:CD004764
Patching is not indicated for simple corneal abrasions, measuring <10 mm There is no improvement in healing rates on days 1-3, no changes in reported pain and no difference in the use of antibiotics between the patch and non-patch groups

Etiology
- previous traumatic corneal abrasion
- corneal dystrophy
- idiopathic

Treatment
- as for corneal abrasion until re-epithelialization occurs
- topical hypertonic saline ointment at bedtime for 3 mo, topical lubrication
- bandage contact lens, anterior stromal puncture or phototherapeutic keratectomy for chronic recurrences

Corneal Ulcer

Etiology
- local necrosis of corneal tissue due to infection
- infection is usually bacterial, rarely viral, fungal, or protozoan (*Acanthamoeba*)
- secondary to corneal exposure, abrasion, foreign body, contact lens use (50% of ulcers)
- also associated with conjunctivitis, blepharitis, keratitis, vitamin A deficiency

Clinical Features
- pain, photophobia, tearing, foreign body sensation, decreased VA (if central ulcer)
- corneal opacity that necroses and forms an excavated ulcer with infiltrative base
- overlying corneal epithelial defect that stains with fluorescein
- may develop corneal edema, conjunctival injection, anterior chamber cells/flare, hypopyon, corneal hypoesthesia (in viral keratitis)
- bacterial ulcers may have purulent discharge, viral ulcers may have watery discharge

Complications
- decreased vision, corneal perforation, iritis, endophthalmitis

Investigations
- Seidel test: fluorescein drop on the cornea under cobalt blue filter is used to detect leaking penetrating lesions; any aqueous leakage will dilute the green stain at site of wound

Treatment
- urgent referral to ophthalmology
- culture prior to treatment
- topical antibiotics every hour
- must treat vigorously to avoid complications

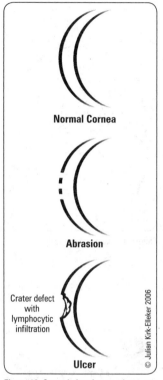

Normal Cornea

Abrasion

Crater defect with lymphocytic infiltration

Ulcer

© Julian Kirk-Elleker 2006

Figure 13. Corneal abrasion vs. ulcer

Table 5. Corneal Abrasion vs. Corneal Ulcer

	Abrasion	Ulcer
Time Course	Acute (instantaneous)	Subacute (days)
History of Trauma	Commonly	Rare
Cornea	Clear	White, necrotic area
Iris Detail	Clear	Obscured
Corneal Thickness	Normal	May have crater defect/thinning
Extent of Lesion	Limited to epithelium	Extension into stroma

Abrasion vs. Ulcer on Slit-Lamp
An abrasion appears clear while an ulcer is more opaque

Herpes Simplex Keratitis

- usually HSV type 1 (90% of population are carriers)
- may be triggered by stress, fever, sun exposure, immunosuppression

Clinical Features
- pain, tearing, foreign body sensation, red eye, may have decreased vision, eyelid edema
- corneal hypoesthesia
- dendritic (thin and branching) lesion with terminal end bulbs in epithelium that stains with fluorescein

Complications
- corneal scarring (can lead to loss of vision)
- chronic interstitial keratitis due to penetration of virus into stroma
- secondary iritis, secondary glaucoma

Treatment
- topical antiviral such as trifluridine, orsystemic antiviral such as acyclovir
- dendritic debridement
- NO STEROIDS initially – may exacerbate condition
- ophthalmologist must exercise caution if adding topical steroids for chronic keratitis or iritis

Steroid treatment for ocular disorders should only be prescribed and supervised by an ophthalmologist, as they can impair corneal healing, exacerbate herpetic keratitis, and elevate IOP

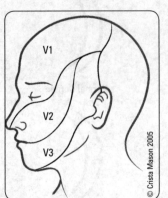

Figure 14. Trigeminal distribution

To detect keratoconus, look for bulging of the lower eyelid when the patient looks downward (Munson's sign)

Herpes Zoster Ophthalmicus

- dermatitis in the dermatomal distrubtion of (CN V1) that is typically unilateral and respects the midline
- Hutchinson's sign: if tip of nose is involved (nasociliary branch of V1) then globe will be involved in ~75% of cases
- if no nasal involvement, eye is involved in 1/3 of patients

Clinical Features
- pain, tearing, photophobia, red eye
- corneal edema, pseudodendrite, SPK
- corneal hypoesthesia

Complications
- corneal keratitis, ulceration, perforation and scarring
- secondary iritis, secondary glaucoma, cataract
- muscle palsies (rare) due to CNS involvement
- occasionally severe post-herpetic neuralgia

Treatment
- oral antiviral (acyclovir, valcyclovir, or famciclovir) immediately
- topical steroids, cycloplegia as indicated for keratitis, iritis
- erythromycin ointment if conjunctival involvement

Keratoconus

- bilateral paracentral thinning (ectasia) and bulging of the cornea resulting in a conical shape
- usually sporadic but can be associated with Down's syndrome, atopy, contact lens use and vigorous eye rubbing
- associated with breaks in Descemet's and Bowman's membrane
- results in decreased vision from irregular astigmatism, scarring and stromal edema

Treatment
- attempt correction with spectacles and/or rigid gas permeable contact lens
- corneal collagen cross-linking treatment to halt disease progression
- intrastromal corneal ring segments can help flatten the corneal cone
- penetrating keratoplasty (corneal transplant) as last resort

Arcus Senilis

- hazy white ring in peripheral cornea, <2 mm wide, clearly separated from limbus
- common, bilateral, benign corneal degeneration due to lipid deposition, part of the aging process
- may be associated with hypercholesterolemia if age <40 yr, check lipid profile
- no associated visual symptoms, complications or treatment necessary

Kayser-Fleischer Ring

- brown-yellow-green pigmented ring in peripheral cornea, starting inferiorly
- due to deposition of copper pigment in Descemet's membrane
- associated with Wilson's disease
- no associated symptoms or complications of ring
- treat underlying disease

The Uveal Tract

- uveal tract (from anterior to posterior) = iris, ciliary body, choroid
- vascularized, pigmented middle layer of the eye, between the sclera and the retina

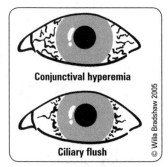

Conjunctival hyperemia

Ciliary flush

© Willa Bradshaw 2005

Figure 15. Conjunctival hyperemia vs. ciliary flush

Uveitis

- uveal inflammation which may involve one, two, or all three parts of the tract
- idiopathic or associated with autoimmune, infectious, granulomatous, malignant causes
- should be managed by an optometrist or ophthalmologist
- anatomically classified as anterior uveitis, intermediate uveitis, posterior uveitis, or panuveitis based on primary site of inflammation

Table 6. Anatomic Classification of Uveitis

	Anterior Uveitis (Iritis)	Intermediate Uveitis	Posterior Uveitis
Location	Inflammation of iris, usually accompanied by cyclitis (inflammation of ciliary body), both = iridocyclitis. Usually unilateral	The vitreous is the major site of the inflammation	Inflammation of the choroid and/or retina

Etiology	Usually idiopathic
	Connective tissue diseases :
	    HLA-B27: reactive arthritis, ankylosing spondylitis, psoriatic arthritis, inflammatory bowel disease
	    Non-HLA-B27: juvenile idiopathic arthritis
	Infectious: syphilis, Lyme disease, toxoplasmosis, TB, HSV, herpes zoster
	Other: sarcoidosis, trauma, large abrasion, post ocular surgery
		Mostly idiopathic, secondary causes include sarcoidosis, Lyme disease, and multiple sclerosis	Bacterial: syphilis, tuberculosis
			Viral: herpes simplex virus, CMV in AIDS
			Fungal: histoplasmosis, candidiasis
			Parasitic: toxoplasmosis (most common cause), toxocara
			Immunosuppression may predispose to any of the above infections
			Autoimmune: Behçet's disease (triad of oral ulcers, genital ulcers, and posterior uveitis)
			Malignancies (masquerade syndrome): metastatic lesions, malignant melanoma

Clinical Features	Photophobia (due to reactive spasm of inflamed iris muscle), ocular pain, tenderness of the globe, brow ache (ciliary muscle spasm), decreased VA, lacrimation Ciliary flush (perilimbal conjunctival injection), miosis (spasm of sphincter muscle) Anterior chamber "cells" (WBC in anterior chamber due to anterior segment inflammation) and "flare" (protein precipitates in anterior chamber secondary to inflammation), hypopyon (collection of neutrophilic exudates inferiorly in the anterior chamber) Occasionally keratic precipitates (clumps of cells on corneal endothelium) Iritis typically reduces IOP because ciliary body inflammation causes decreased aqueous production; however, severe iritis, or iritis from herpes simplex and zoster may cause an inflammatory glaucoma (trabeculitis)	Insidious onset of blurred vision, accompanied by vitreous floaters Initial symptoms are usually unilateral but inflammatory changes are usually bilateral and asymmetric Associated with anterior uveitis, most severe cases of secondary intermediate uveitis Vitreous cells, condensations, and snowballs (vitreous aggregates of inflammatory cells) Posterior segment 'snowbank' = grey-white fibrovascular plaque at the pars plana	Painless as choroid has no sensory innervation Often no conjunctival or scleral injection present Decreased VA Floaters (debris and inflammatory cells) Vitreous cells and opacities Hypopyon formation

Complications	Inflammatory glaucoma
	Posterior synechiae
	    Adhesions of posterior iris to anterior lens capsule
	    Indicated by an irregularly shaped pupil
	    If occurs 360°, can lead to angle closure glaucoma
	    Peripheral anterior synechiae (rare): adhesions of iris to cornea → secondary angle closure glaucoma
	Cataracts
	Band keratopathy (with chronic iritis)
	Superficial corneal calcification keratopathy
	Macular edema with chronic iritis
		Cystoid macular edema (30% of cases), cataract, and glaucoma	Macular edema
			Vitritis
			Neovascularization
			Visual field loss/scotoma

Treatment	Mydriatics: dilate pupil to prevent formation of posterior synechiae and to decrease pain from ciliary spasm Steroids: topical, sub-tenon, or systemic Systemic analgesia If recurrent episodes, extensive medical workup may be indicated to rule out secondary causes	Systemic or sub-tenon/intravitreal steroids and immunosuppressive agents Vitrectomy, cryotherapy, or laser photocoagulation to the "snowbank"	Steroids: sub-tenon, intravitreal, or systemic if indicated (e.g. threat of vision loss)

Lens

- consists of an outer capsule surrounding a soft cortex and a firm inner nucleus

Cataracts

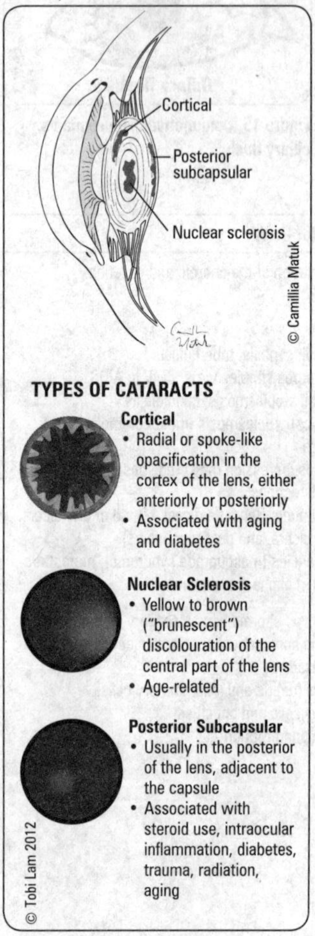

- any opacity of the lens, regardless of etiology
- most common cause of reversible blindness worldwide
- types: nuclear sclerosis, cortical, posterior subcapsular

Etiology
- acquired
  - age-related (over 90% of all cataracts)
  - cataract associated with systemic disease (may have juvenile onset)
    - DM
    - metabolic disorders (e.g. Wilson's disease, galactosemia, homocystinuria)
    - hypocalcemia
  - traumatic (may be rosette shaped)
  - intraocular inflammation (e.g. uveitis)
  - toxic (steroids, phenothiazines)
  - radiation
- congenital
  - high myopia
  - present with altered red reflex or leukocoria
  - treat promptly to prevent amblyopia

Clinical Features
- gradual, painless, progressive decrease in VA
- glare, dimness, halos around lights at night, monocular diplopia
- "second sight" phenomenon: patient is more myopic than previously noted, due to increased refractive power of the lens (in nuclear sclerosis only)
  - patient may read without previously needed reading glasses
- diagnosis by slit-lamp exam
- may impair view of retina during fundoscopy

Treatment
- medical: no role for medical management
- surgical: definitive treatment
  - indications for surgery
    - to improve visual function in patients whose vision loss leads to functional impairment
    - to aid management of other ocular disease (e.g. cataract that prevents adequate retinal exam or laser treatment of DR)
    - congenital or traumatic cataracts
  - phacoemulsification (phaco = lens)
  - most commonly used surgical technique
  - post-operative complications
    - RD, endophthalmitis, dislocated IOL, macular edema, glaucoma, posterior capsular opacification

Dislocated Lens (Ectopia Lentis)

Etiology
- associated with Marfan's Syndrome, Ehlers-Danlos type VI, homocystinuria, syphilis, lens coloboma (congenital cleft due to failure of ocular adnexa to complete growth)
- traumatic

Clinical Features
- decreased VA
- may get monocular diplopia
- iridodenesis (quivering of iris with movement)
- direct ophthalmoscopy may elicit abnormal red reflex

Complications
- cataract, glaucoma, uveitis

Treatment
- surgical correction ± lens replacement

Figure 16. Types of cataracts

© Camillia Matuk

TYPES OF CATARACTS

Cortical
- Radial or spoke-like opacification in the cortex of the lens, either anteriorly or posteriorly
- Associated with aging and diabetes

Nuclear Sclerosis
- Yellow to brown ("brunescent") discolouration of the central part of the lens
- Age-related

Posterior Subcapsular
- Usually in the posterior of the lens, adjacent to the capsule
- Associated with steroid use, intraocular inflammation, diabetes, trauma, radiation, aging

© Tobi Lam 2012

Femtosecond Laser-Assisted Cataract Surgery Compared with Conventional Cataract Surgery
Clin Experiment Ophthalmol 2013 Jul;41(5):455-62.
Purpose: Compare the safety and efficacy of femtosecond laser-assisted to conventional phacoemulsification cataract surgery.
Methods: Non-randomized prospective trial of 400 patients undergoing cataract surgery comparing phacoemulsification time and intraoperative complication rates with intention to treat analysis.
Results: Effective phacoemulsification time was reduced by 70% in the fentosecond laser treated group (P<0.0001) seen in all grades of cataract severity and there was no significant difference in intraoperative complication rates between groups.
Conclusion: Fentosecond laser-assisted cataract surgery may allow greater efficiency and short-term safety when compared to conventional surgery. Long term safety is not yet known.

Vitreous

- clear gel (99% water plus collagen fibrils, glycosaminoglycans, and hyaluronic acid) that fills the posterior segment of eye
- normally adherent to optic disc, pars plana, and along major retinal blood vessels

Posterior Vitreous Detachment

Etiology
- central vitreous commonly shrinks and liquefies with age (syneresis)
- during syneresis, molecules that hold water condense causing vitreous floaters
- liquid vitreous moves between posterior vitreous gel and retina
- vitreous is peeled away and separates from the internal limiting membrane of the neurosensory retina posterior to the vitreous base

Clinical Features
- floaters, flashes of light

Complications
- traction at areas of abnormal vitreoretinal adhesions may cause retinal tears/detachment
- retinal tears/detachment may cause vitreous hemorrhage if bridging retinal blood vessel is torn
- complications more common in high myopes and following ocular trauma (blunt or perforating)

Treatment
- acute onset of PVD requires a dilated fundus exam to rule out retinal tears/detachment
- no specific treatment available for floaters/flashes of light

Weiss Ring: formed by glial tissue around the optic disc that remains attached to the detached posterior vitreous

Floaters: "bugs", "cobwebs", or "spots" of vitreous condensation that move with eye position

Although most floaters are benign, new or markedly increased floaters or flashes of light require a dilated fundus exam to rule out retinal tears/detachment

Vitreous Hemorrhage

- bleeding into the vitreous cavity

Etiology
- PDR
- retinal tear/detachment
- PVD
- retinal vein occlusion
- trauma

Clinical Features
- sudden loss of VA
- may be preceded by "shower" of many floaters and/or flashes of light
- ophthalmoscopy: no red reflex if large hemorrhage, retina not visible due to blood in vitreous

Treatment
- ultrasound (B-scan) to rule out RD
- expectant: in non-urgent cases (e.g. no RD), blood usually resorbs in 3-6 mo
- surgical: vitrectomy ± RD repair ± retinal endolaser to possible bleeding sites/vessels

Any time a vitreous or retinal hemorrhage is seen in a child, must rule out child abuse

Endophthalmitis and Vitritis

- intraocular infection: acute, subacute, or chronic

Etiology
- most commonly a post-operative complication; risk following cataract surgery is <0.1%
- also due to penetrating injury to eye (risk is 3-7%), endogenous spread, and intravitreal injections
- etiology usually bacterial, may be fungal

Clinical Features
- painful, red eye, photophobia, discharge
- severely reduced VA, lid edema, proptosis, corneal edema, anterior chamber cells/flare, hypopyon, reduced red reflex
- may have signs of a ruptured globe (severe subconjunctival hemorrhage, hyphema, decreased IOP, etc.)

Treatment (see *Ocular Trauma*, OP39)
- **OCULAR EMERGENCY**: presenting vision best indicates prognosis
- LP or worse: admission, immediate vitrectomy, and intravitreal antibiotics to prevent loss of vision
- HM or better: vitreous tap for culture and intravitreal antibiotics
- topical fortified antibiotics

Remember to inquire about tetanus status in post-traumatic endophthalmitis

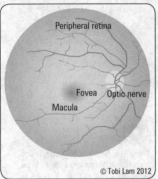

Peripheral retina

Fovea   Optic nerve

Macula

© Tobi Lam 2012

Figure 17. Retina

Retina

- composed of two parts (Figure 2)
  - neurosensory retina: comprises 9 of the 10 retinal layers, including the photoreceptors and the ganglion cell layer
  - retinal pigmented epithelium (RPE) layer: external to neurosensory retina
- macula: rich in cones (for colour vision); most sensitive area of retina
- fovea: centre of macula; responsible for detail, fine vision, lacks retinal vessels
- optic disc: collection of retinal nerve fibre layers forming optic nerve (CN2)
- ora serrata: irregularly-shaped, anterior margin of the retina (cannot be visualized with direct ophthalmoscope)

Central/Branch Retinal Artery Occlusion

Etiology
- emboli from carotid arteries or heart (e.g. arrhythmia, endocarditis, valvular disease)
- thrombus
- temporal arteritis

Clinical Features
- sudden, painless (except in GCA), severe monocular loss of vision
- RAPD
- patient may have experienced transient episodes in the past (amaurosis fugax)
- fundoscopy
  - "cherry-red spot"
  - retinal pallor
  - cotton wool spots (retinal infarcts)
  - cholesterol emboli (Hollenhorst plaques) – usually located at arteriole bifurcations

Hallmark of CRAO
"Cherry-red spot" located at centre of macula (visualization of unaffected highly vascular choroid through the thin fovea)

Treatment
- **OCULAR EMERGENCY**: attempt to restore blood flow within 2 h (irreversible retinal damage if >90 min of complete CRAO)
- massage the globe (compress eye with heel of hand for 10 s, release for 10 s, repeat for 5 min) to dislodge embolus
- decrease IOP
  - topical β-blockers
  - IV acetazolamide
  - IV mannitol (draws fluid from eye)
  - drain aqueous fluid – anterior chamber paracentesis (carries risk of infection, lens puncture)
- Nd:YAG laser embolectomy
- intra-arterial or intra-venous thrombolysis

Treatment for a central retinal artery occlusion (CRAO) must be initiated within 2 h of symptom onset for any hope of restoring vision

Central/Branch Retinal Vein Occlusion

- second most frequent "vascular" retinal disorder after DR
- usually a manifestation of a systemic disease (e.g. HTN, DM)
- thrombus occurs within the lumen of the blood vessel

The "blood and thunder" appearance on fundoscopy is very specific for CRVO

Predisposing Factors
- arteriosclerotic vascular disease
- HTN
- DM
- glaucoma
- hyperviscosity (e.g. polycythemia rubra vera, sickle-cell disease, lymphoma, leukemia)
- drugs (e.g. oral contraceptive pill, diuretics)

There is an 8-10% risk of developing CRVO or BRVO in other eye

Clinical Features
- painless, monocular, gradual or sudden vision loss
- ± RAPD
- fundoscopy
  - "blood and thunder" appearance
  - diffuse retinal hemorrhages, cotton wool spots, venous engorgement, swollen optic disc, macular edema
- two fairly distinct groups
  - venous stasis/non-ischemic retinopathy
  - no RAPD, VA ~20/80
  - mild hemorrhage, few cotton wool spots
  - resolves spontaneously over weeks to months
  - may regain normal vision if macula intact

GENEVA Phase 3 Trials in BRVO and CRVO
Ophthalmology 2010;117:1134-1146
Randomized sham-controlled trial of dexamethasone intravitreal implant in patients with macular edema due to retinal vein occlusion.
Dexamethasone intravitreal implant reduces the risk of vision loss and improves the speed and incidence of visual improvement in eyes with macular edema 2° to BRVO and CRVO.

- hemorrhagic/ischemic retinopathy
  - usually older patient with deficient arterial supply
  - RAPD, VA ~20/200, reduced peripheral vision
  - more hemorrhages, cotton wool spots, congestion
  - poor visual prognosis

Complications
- neovascularization of retina and iris (secondary rubeosis), leading to secondary glaucoma
- vitreous hemorrhage
- macular edema

Treatment
- treatment available for complications of CRVO/BRVO including retinal laser photocoagulation and anti-VEGF and/or corticosteroid injection

Retinal Detachment

- cleavage in the plane between the neurosensory retina and the RPE
- three types
  - rhegmatogenous (most common)
    - caused by a tear or hole in the neurosensory retina, allowing fluid from the vitreous to pass into the subretinal space
    - tears may be caused by PVD, degenerative retinal changes, trauma, or iatrogenically
    - incidence increases with advancing age, in high myopes, and after ocular surgery/trauma
  - tractional
    - caused by vitreal, epiretinal, or subretinal membrane pulling the neurosensory retina away from the underlying RPE
    - found in conditions such as DR, CRVO, sickle cell disease, ROP, and ocular trauma
  - exudative
    - caused by damage to the RPE resulting in fluid accumulation in the subretinal space
    - main causes are intraocular tumours, posterior uveitis, central serous retinopathy

Clinical Features
- sudden onset
- flashes of light
  - due to mechanical stimulation of the retinal photoreceptors
- floaters
- hazy spots in the line of vision which move with eye position, due to drops of blood from torn vessels bleeding into the vitreous
- curtain of blackness/peripheral field loss
  - darkness in one field of vision when the retina detaches in that area
- loss of central vision (if macula "off")
- decreased IOP (usually 4-5 mmHg lower than the other, normal eye)
- ophthalmoscopy: detached retina is grey-white with surface blood vessels, loss of red reflex
- ± RAPD

Treatment
- prophylactic: symptomatic tear (flashes or floaters) can be sealed off with laser/cryotherapy
- therapeutic
  - rhegmatogenous
    - scleral buckle procedure
    - pneumatic retinopexy
    - vitrectomy plus injection of gas (injection of silicone oil in cases of recurrent detachment)
  - tractional
    - vitrectomy ± membrane removal/scleral buckling/injection of intraocular gas or silicone oil as necessary
  - exudative
    - treat underlying cause

Complications
- loss of vision, vitreous hemorrhage, recurrent RD
- a RD is an emergency, especially if the macula is still attached (macula "on")
- prognosis for visual recovery varies inversely with the amount of time the retina is detached and whether the macula is attached or not

Retinitis Pigmentosa

- hereditary degenerative disease of the retina manifested by rod > cone photoreceptor degeneration and retinal atrophy
- many forms of inheritance, most commonly autosomal recessive (60%)

Efficacy and Safety of Widely Used Treatments for Macular Oedema Secondary to Retinal Vein Occlusion: A Systematic Review
BMC Ophthalmol 2014;14:7
Purpose: To assess the efficacy of widely used treatments for macular oedema (MO) secondary to retinal vein occlusion (RVO). MO secondary to RVO can cause vision loss due to blockage of the central retinal vein (CRVO) or a branch retinal vein (BRVO).
Outcomes: Mean change in best corrected visual acuity (BCVA) from baseline and/or number of patients gaining at least 10 letters from baseline to 6 mo or equivalent time point.
Results: 14 unique RCTs identified. Ranibizumab 0.5 mg produced greater improvements in BCVA at 6 mo compared to sham in BRVO (mean difference 11 letters; 95% CI 7.83-14.17) and CRVO (mean difference 14 letters; 95% CI 10.51-17.69). Improvements in BCVA were also observed with dexamethasone intravitreal implant (IVT) 0.7 mg compared with sham in patients with BRVO or CRVO (mean difference 2.5 letters; 95% CI 0.7-4.3). The difference was significant with BRVO alone, but not CRVO alone. At 36 mo in a large prospective RCT, a greater proportion of patients with BRVO gained >15 letters with laser therapy versus no treatment (OR 3.16; 95% CI 1.25-8.00), whereas no difference was observed in a 9 mo end point smaller study. Three studies showed no benefit for laser therapy in CRVO.
Conclusions: Both ranibizumab and dexamethasone IVT show significant improvements over previously accepted standard of care (laser therapy) for the treatment of BRVO and CRVO.

Superotemporal retina is the most common site for horseshoe tears

Retinitis Pigmentosa Inherited Forms
- Autosomal recessive: most common
- Autosomal dominant: best prognosis
- X-linked: worst prognosis

Triad of Retinitis Pigmentosa
APO
Arteriolar narrowing
Perivascular bony-spicule pigmentation
Optic disc pallor

Clinical Features
- night blindness, decreased peripheral vision ("tunnel vision"), decreased central vision (macular changes), glare (from posterior subcapsular cataracts, common)

Investigations
- fundoscopy: areas of "bone-spicule" pigment clumping in mid-periphery of retina, narrowed retinal arterioles, pale optic disc
- electrophysiological tests: electroretinography (ERG) and electrooculography (EOG) assist in diagnosis

Treatment
- no treatments available to reverse the condition; cataract extraction improves visual function; vitamin A and vitamin E supplementation can reduce progression of disease in some patients

Age-Related Macular Degeneration

- leading cause of irreversible blindness in the Western world, associated with increasing age, usually bilateral but asymmetric

Classification
- **Non-Exudative/"Dry" (Non-Neovascular) AMD**
  - most common type of AMD (90% of cases)
  - slowly progressive loss of visual function
  - drusen: yellow-white deposits between the RPE and Bruch's membrane (area separating inner choroidal vessels from RPE)
  - RPE atrophy: coalescence of depigmented RPE, clumps of focal hyperpigmentation, or hypopigmentation
  - may progress to neovascular AMD

- **Exudative/"Wet" (Neovascular) AMD**
  - 10% of AMD, but 80% of AMD that results in severe vision loss
  - choroidal neovascularization: drusen predisposes to breaks in Bruch's membrane causing subsequent growth and proliferation of new, fine choroidal vessels
  - may lead to serous detachment of overlying RPE and retina, hemorrhage and lipid precipitates into subretinal space
  - can also lead to an elevated subretinal mass due to fibrous metaplasia of hemorrhagic RD leads to disciform scarring and severe central vision loss

Risk Factors
- female
- increasing age
- family history
- smoking
- Caucasian race
- blue irides

Clinical Features
- variable degree of progressive central vision loss
- metamorphopsia (distorted vision characterized by straight parallel lines appearing convergent or wavy) due to macular edema

Investigations
- Amsler grid: held at normal reading distance with glasses on, assesses macular function
- fluorescein angiography: assess type and location of choroidal neovascularization – pathologic new vessels leak dye
- OCT retinal imaging

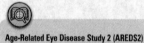

Age-Related Eye Disease Study 2 (AREDS2)
Lutein + zeaxanthin and omega-3 fatty acids for AMD: the Age-Related Eye Disease Study 2 (AREDS2) randomized clinical trial. *JAMA* 2013 May 15;309(19):2005-2015
Addition of lutein+zeaxanthin, DHA+EPA, or both to the AREDS formulation in primary analyses didn't reduce risk of progression to advance AMD. However, because of the potential increased incidence of lung cancer in former smokers, lutein+zeaxanthin could be an appropriate carotenoid substitute in the AREDS formulation.

Treatment
- non-neovascular "dry" AMD
  - monitor, Amsler grid allows patients to check for metamorphopsia
  - low vision aids (e.g. magnifiers, closed-circuit television)
  - anti-oxidants, green leafy vegetables
  - sunglasses/visors
  - see Age-related Eye Disease Study 2 (AREDS2) in sidebar
- neovascular "wet" AMD
  - see *Common Medications*, OP42
  - intravitreal injection of anti-VEGF
    - pegaptanib (Macugen®), ranibizumab (Lucentis®), bevacizumab (Avastin®), aflibercept (Eylea®) (see *VEGF Inhibitors*, OP43)
  - laser photocoagulation for neovascularization
  - no definitive treatment for disciform scarring
  - photodynamic therapy with verteporfin (Visudyne®)
    - IV injection of verteporfin followed by low intensity laser to area of choroidal neovascularization

Glaucoma

Definition
- progressive, pressure-sensitive, optic neuropathy involving characteristic structural changes to optic nerve head with associated visual field changes
- commonly associated with high IOP, but not required for diagnosis

Background
- aqueous is produced by the ciliary body and drains into the episcleral veins via the trabecular meshwork and the Canal of Schlemm
- an isolated increase in IOP is termed ocular hypertension (OHT) - should be followed for increased risk of developing glaucoma
- pressures >21 mmHg are at increased risk of developing glaucoma
- loss of peripheral vision most commonly precedes central vision loss
- Structural changes commonly precedes functional changes

Investigations
- VA testing
- slit-lamp exam to assess anterior chamber depth with gonioscopic lens to assess angle patency
- ophthalmoscopy to assess the disc features
- tonometry to measure IOP
- visual field testing
- pachymetry to measure corneal thickness
- follow-up includes optic disc examination, IOP measurement, and visual field testing to monitor course of disease

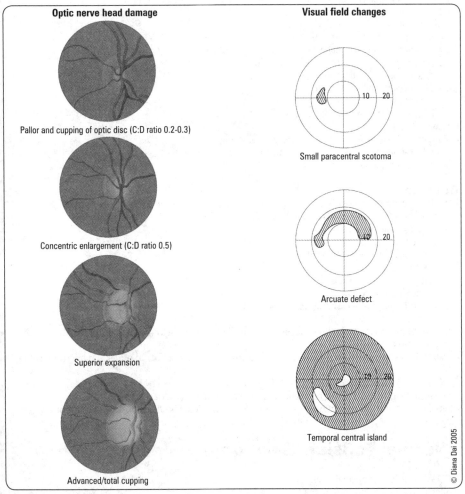

Figure 18. Glaucomatous damage

Optic nerve head damage:
- Pallor and cupping of optic disc (C:D ratio 0.2-0.3)
- Concentric enlargement (C:D ratio 0.5)
- Superior expansion
- Advanced/total cupping

Visual field changes:
- Small paracentral scotoma
- Arcuate defect
- Temporal central island

© Diana Dai 2005

Ten Year Follow-Up of Age-Related Macular Degeneration in the Age-Related Eye Disease Study: AREDS Report No. 36
JAMA Ophthalmol 2014 Mar;132(3):272-7
Study: Randomized clinical trial.
Objective: To describe 10 yr progression rates to intermediate or advanced AMD.
Patients: Age-related eye disease study (AREDS) participants were observed for an additional 5 yr after RCT completion. Participants aged 55-80 yr with no AMD or AMD of varying severity (n = 4,757) were followed up in the AREDS trial for a median duration of 6.5 yr. When the trial ended, 3,549 of the 4,203 surviving participants were followed for 5 additional yr.
Intervention: Treatment with antioxidant vitamins and minerals.
Main Outcome: Development of varying stages of AMD and changes in visual acuity.
Results: The risk of progression to advanced AMD increased with increasing age (p=0.01) and severity of drusen. Women (p=0.005) and current smokers (p<0.001) were at increased risk of neovascular AMD. In the oldest participants with the most severe AMD status at baseline, the risks of developing neovascular AMD and central geographic atrophy by 10 yr were 48.1% and 26.0%, respectively. Similarly, rates of progression to large drusen increased with increasing severity of drusen at baseline, with 70.9% of participants with bilateral medium drusen progressing to large drusen and 13.8% to advanced AMD in 10 yr. Median visual acuity at 10 yr in eyes that had large drusen at baseline but never developed advanced AMD was 20/25; eyes that developed advanced AMD had a median visual acuity of 20/200.
Conclusion: The natural history of AMD demonstrates relentless loss of vision in persons who developed advanced AMD.

Average IOP = 15 ± 3 mmHg
Normal C:D ≤0.4
Suspect glaucoma if C:D ratio >0.6, C:D ratio differs between eyes by >0.2, or cup approaches disc margin

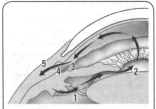
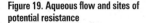

1. Ciliary body processes
2. Pupillary block
3. Pretrabecular
4. Trabecular and Canal of Schlemm
5. Post-trabecular

© Janice Wong

Figure 19. Aqueous flow and sites of potential resistance

Primary Open-Angle Glaucoma

- most common form, >95% of all glaucoma cases
- due to obstruction of aqueous drainage within the trabecular meshwork and its drainage into the Canal of Schlemm
- insidious and asymptomatic, screening is critical for early detection

Risk Factors for POAG
A FIAT
Age
Family history
IOP
African descent
Thin cornea

Major Risk Factors
- ocular hypertension (IOP>21 mmHg)
- age: prevalence at 40 yr is 1-2% and at 80 yr is 10%
- ethnicity: African descent
- familial (2-3x increased risk); polygenic
- thin central cornea (OHTS trial)

Minor Risk Factors
- myopia
- HTN
- DM
- hyperthyroidism (Graves' disease)
- chronic topical ophthalmic steroid use in steroid responders – yearly eye exams recommended if >4 wk of steroid use
- previous ocular trauma
- anemia/hemodynamic crisis (ask about blood transfusions in past)

Open- and Closed-Angle Glaucoma

POAG	PACG
• Common (95%)	• Rare (5%)
• Chronic course	• Acute onset
• Painless eye without redness	• Painful red eye
• Moderately ↑ IOP	• Extremely ↑ IOP
• Normal cornea and pupil	• Hazy cornea
• No N/V	• Mid-dilated pupil unreactive to light
• No halos around light	• ± N/V, abdominal pain
	• Halos around light

Clinical Features
- asymptomatic initially
- insidious, painless, gradual rise in IOP due to restriction of aqueous outflow
- bilateral, but usually asymmetric
- earliest signs are optic disc changes
  - increased C:D ratio (vertical C:D >0.6)
  - significant C:D asymmetry between eyes (>0.2 difference)
  - thinning, notching of the neuroretinal rim
  - flame shaped disc hemorrhage
  - 360° of peripapillary atrophy
  - nerve fibre layer defect
  - large vessels become nasally displaced
- visual field loss
- slow, progressive, irreversible loss of peripheral vision
- paracentral defects, arcuate scotoma, and nasal step are characteristics (Figure 19)
- late loss of central vision if untreated

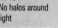

Elevated IOP is the only modifiable risk factor that has been proven to prevent progression of glaucoma. Treatment of patients with ocular hypertension but no signs of glaucoma also benefit from a reduction in risk of development of glaucoma

Treatment
- medical treatment: decrease IOP by increasing the drainage and/or decreasing the production of aqueous (see *Glaucoma Medications*, Table 12, OP42)
  - increase aqueous outflow
    - topical cholinergics
    - topical prostaglandin analogues
    - topical α-adrenergics
  - decrease aqueous production
    - topical β-blockers
    - topical and oral carbonic anhydrase inhibitor
    - topical α-adrenergics
- laser trabeculoplasty, cyclophotocoagulation in order to achieve selective destruction of ciliary body (for refractory cases)
- trabeculectomy: creation of a new outflow tract from anterior chamber to under conjunctiva forming a bleb
- minimally invasive glaucoma surgery (MIGS): implantation of IOP lowering drainage devices (e.g. iStent) through an ab interno microincisional approach during cataract surgery
- serial optic nerve head examinations, IOP measurements, and visual field testing to monitor disease course

The Ocular Hypertension Treatment Study
Arch Ophthalmol-Chic 2002;120:701-713
Study: Randomized clinical trial.
Patients: 1,636 patients with no evidence of glaucomatous damage, aged 40-80 yr, and with IOP between 24-32 mmHg in one eye and between 21-32 mmHg in the other eye.
Intervention: Randomized to observation or treatment with commercially available topical ocular hypotensive medication.
Main Outcome: Development of visual field abnormality or optic disc deterioration attributed to POAG.
Results: Mean reduction in IOP in the medication group was 22.5% ± 9.9% vs. 4.0% ± 11.6% in the observation group. At 5 yr the probability of developing POAG was 4.4% in the medication group and 9.5% in the observation group (p<0.0001).
Conclusions: Topical ocular hypotensive medication was effective in delaying or preventing the onset of POAG in individuals with elevated IOP.

Normal Tension Glaucoma

- POAG with IOP in normal range
- often found in women >60 but may occur earlier
- associated with migraines, peripheral vasospasm, systemic nocturnal hypotension, sleep apnea
- damage to optic nerve may be due to vascular insufficiency

Treatment
- treat reversible causes

Secondary Open Angle Glaucoma

- increased IOP secondary to ocular/systemic disorders that obstruct the trabecular meshwork
- steroid-induced glaucoma
- traumatic glaucoma
- pigmentary dispersion syndrome
- pseudoexfoliation syndrome

Primary Angle-Closure Glaucoma

- 5% of all glaucoma cases
- peripheral iris bows forward obstructing aqueous access to the trabecular meshwork
- sudden forward shift of the lens-iris diaphragm causes pupillary block, and results in imparied drainage leading to a sudden rise in IOP

Risk Factors
- hyperopia: small eye, big lens – large lens crowds the angle
- age >70 yr
- female
- family history
- more common in people of Asian and Inuit descent
- mature cataracts
- shallow anterior chamber
- pupil dilation (topical and systemic anticholinergics, stress, darkness)

Clinical Features
- red, painful eye = **RED FLAG**
- unilateral, but other eye increased risk
- decreased visual acuity, vision acutely blurred from corneal edema
- halos around lights
- nausea and vomiting, abdominal pain
- fixed, mid-dilated pupil
- marked increase in IOP; may be noticeable even to palpation (>40 mmHg)
- shallow anterior chamber ± cells in anterior chamber

Complications
- irreversible loss of vision within hours to days if untreated
- permanent peripheral anterior synechiae, resulting in permanent angle closure

Treatment
- **OCULAR EMERGENCY**: refer to ophthalmologist for acute angle closure glaucoma
  - aqueous suppressants and hyperosmotic agents
- medical treatment (see *Glaucoma Medications*, Table 12, OP42)
  - miotic drops (pilocarpine) to reverse pupillary block
  - multiple topical IOP-lowering agents
  - hypserosmotic agents such as oral glycerine, or IV mannitol
- laser iridotomy is definitive

Secondary Angle-Closure Glaucoma

Uveitis
- inflamed iris adheres to lens (posterior synechiae)

Neovascular Glaucoma
- abnormal blood vessels develop on surface of iris (rubeosis iridis), in the angle, and within the trabecular meshwork
- due to retinal ischemia associated with PDR or CRVO
- treatment with laser therapy to retina reduces neovascular stimulus to iris and angle vessels

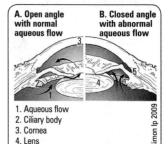

Figure 20. Normal open angle vs. angle-closure glaucoma

A. Open angle with normal aqueous flow

B. Closed angle with abnormal aqueous flow

1. Aqueous flow
2. Ciliary body
3. Cornea
4. Lens
5. Blocked trabecular meshwork

© Simon Ip 2009

Rule of Fours
1/4 of general population using topical steroid for 4 wk, 4 x/d will develop an increase in IOP

Angle Closure Glaucoma
BACH
Tx with miotics and β-blockers **A**drenergics
Cholinergics
Hyperosmotic agents

Collaborative Normal Tension Glaucoma Study
Curr Opin Ophthalmol 2003;14:86-90
Treatment aimed at lowering IOP by 30% in patients with normal tension glaucoma tends to reduce the rate of visual field loss. Due to variability in disease progression and a significant group that shows no visual field loss at 5 yr despite no treatment, further studies are needed to delineate which subgroups may benefit most from treatment.

Medical Interventions for Primary Open-Angle Glaucoma and Ocular Hypertension
Cochrane DB Syst Rev 2007;4:CD003167
Study: Cochrane systematic review of 26 trials and meta-analysis of 10 trials investigating the effectiveness of topical pharmacological therapies for POAG or OHT.
Patients: 4,979 participants randomized in 26 trials. Patients had OHT with IOP >21 mmHg or open angle glaucoma.
Intervention: Topical eye medications, including β-blockers, dorzolamide, brimonidine, pilocarpine, and epinephrine vs. each other and placebo.
Main Outcome: Reduction of progression or prevention of onset of visual field defects.
Results: Meta-analysis on all trials that tested drugs against placebo or untreated controls demonstrated that lowering IOP reduces incidence of glaucomatous visual field defects, with an odds ratio of 0.62 (95% CI 0.47-0.81). However, this result is of limited practical use since different therapies were pooled. No single drug demonstrated significant visual field protection. However, as a class, β-blockers showed borderline significance in reducing onset of glaucoma in patients with OHT when compared to placebo, with an OR of 0.67 (95% CI 0.45-1.00).
Conclusion: Lowering IOP can reduce progression of visual field defects in patients with OHT.

5 Targets of Retinal Signals
• Pre-tectal nucleus (pupillary reflex/eye movements)
• Lateral geniculate body of thalamus
• Superior colliculus (eye movements)
• Suprachiasmatic nucleus (optokinetic)
• Accessory optic system (circadian rhythm)

Pupils

- pupil size is determined by the balance between the sphincter muscle and the dilator muscle
- sphincter muscle is innervated by the parasympathetic nervous system carried by CN III
- dilator muscle is innervated by the sympathetic nervous system (SNS)
  - first order neuron = hypothalamus → brainstem → spinal cord
  - second order/preganglionic neuron = spinal cord → sympathetic trunk via internal carotid artery → superior cervical ganglion in neck
  - third order/postganglionic fibres originate in the superior cervical ganglion, neurotransmitter is norepinephrine
    - as a diagnostic test, 4-10% cocaine prevents the re-uptake of norepinephrine, and will cause dilation of normal pupil, but not one with loss of sympathetic innervation (Horner's Syndrome)
- see Neurology, Figure 8, N8

Pupillary Light Reflex

- light shone directly into eye travels along optic nerve (CN II, afferent limb) → optic tracts → bilateral midbrain
- impulses enter bilaterally in midbrain via pretectal area and Edinger-Westphal nuclei
- nerve impulses then travel down CN III (efferent limb) bilaterally to reach the ciliary ganglia, and finally to the iris sphincter muscle, which results in the direct and consensual light reflexes

α1 – Pupillary dilator muscle contraction (Mydriasis)
β2 – Ciliary muscle relaxation (Non-accommodation); increased aqueous humour production
M3 – Pupillary sphincter contraction (Miosis); increased ciliary muscle contraction (Accommodation)

Pupil Abnormalities

Denervation Hypersensitivity
- when post-ganglionic fibres are damaged, the understimulated end-organ attempts to compensate by developing an excess of neuroreceptors and becomes hypersensitive
- postganglionic parasympathetic lesions (i.e. Adie's pupil)
  - pupil will constrict with 0.125% pilocarpine (cholinergic agonist), normal pupil will not
- postganglionic sympathetic lesions (this test is used to differentiate between pre- and post-ganglionic lesions in Horner's syndrome)
  - pupil will dilate with 0.125% epinephrine, normal pupil will not

Local Disorders of Iris
- posterior synechiae (adhesions between iris and lens) due to iritis can present as an abnormally shaped pupil
- ischemic damage (e.g. post-acute angle-closure glaucoma) usually occurs at 3 and 9 o'clock positions resulting in a vertically oval pupil that reacts poorly to light
- trauma (e.g. post-intraocular surgery)

Anisocoria
- unequal pupil size
- idiopathic/physiologic anisocoria
- 20% of population
- round, regular, <1 mm difference
- pupils reactive to light and accommodation
- responds normally to mydiatrics/miotics
- post eye surgery
- see Table 7 for other causes of anisocoria

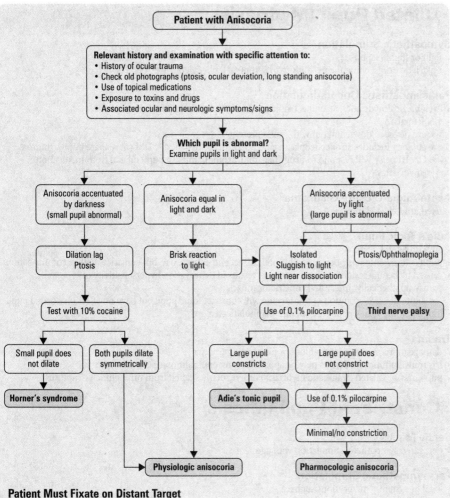

Patient Must Fixate on Distant Target

Figure 21. Approach to anisocoria
Reproduced with permission from: Kedar S, Biousse V, Newman NJ. Approach to the patient with anisocoria. In: UpToDate, Rose, BD (editor), UpToDate, Waltham, MA, 2011. Copyright 2011 UpToDate, Inc. For more information visit www.uptodate.com.

Table 7. Summary of Conditions Causing Anisocoria

	Features	Site of Lesion	Light and Accommodation	Anisocoria	Mydriatics/Miotics	Effect of Pilocarpine
ABNORMAL MIOTIC PUPIL (impaired pupillary dilation)						
Argyll-Robertson Pupil	Irregular, usually bilateral	Midbrain	Poor in light; better to accommodation		Dilates/Constricts	
Horner's Syndrome	Round, unilateral, ptosis, anhydrosis, pseudoenophthalmos	Sympathetic system	Both brisk	Greater in dark	Dilates/Constricts	
ABNORMAL MYDRIATIC PUPIL (impaired pupillary constriction)						
Adie's Tonic Pupil	Irregular, larger in bright light	Ciliary ganglion	Poor in light, better to accommodation	Greater in light	Dilates/Constricts	Constricts (hypersensitivity to dilute pilocarpine)
CN III Palsy	Round	Superficial CN III	± fixed (acutely) at 7-9 mm	Greater in light	Dilates/Constricts	Constricts
Mydriatic Pupil	Round, uni- or bilateral	Iris sphincter	Fixed at 7-8 mm	Greater in light	No effect	Will not constrict

CN III palsy with pupillary involvement may be associated with a posterior communicating artery aneurysm

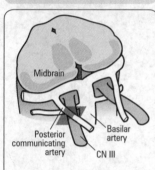

Midbrain

Posterior communicating artery

Basilar artery

CN III

Normal

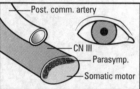

Post. comm. artery

CN III

Parasymp.

Somatic motor

Externally Compressive CN III Lesion

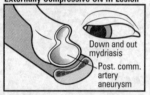

Down and out mydriasis

Post. comm. artery aneurysm

Central Vascular CN III Lesion

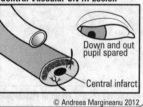

Down and out pupil spared

Central infarct

© Andreea Margineanu 2012

Figure 22. CN III lesions with and without mydriasis

Horner's MAP
Miosis
Anhydrosis
Ptosis

Dilated Pupil (Mydriasis)

Sympathetic Stimulation
- fight or flight response
- mydriatic drugs: epinephrine, dipivefrin (Propine®), phenylephrine

Parasympathetic Understimulation
- cycloplegics/mydriatics: atropine, tropicamide, cyclopentolate (parasympatholytic)
- CN III palsy
  - eye deviated down and out with ptosis present
  - etiology includes stroke, neoplasm, aneurysm, acute rise in ICP, DM (may spare pupil), trauma
  - CN III palsy will respond to drugs (e.g. pilocarpine), unlike a pupil dilated from medication (mydriatics)

Acute Angle-Closure Glaucoma
- fixed, mid-dilated pupil

Adie's Tonic Pupil
- 80% unilateral, F>M
- pupil is tonic or reacts poorly to light (both direct and consensual) but constricts with accommodation
- caused by benign lesion in ciliary ganglion; results in denervation hypersensitivity of parasympathetically innervated constrictor muscle
  - dilute (0.125%) solution of pilocarpine will constrict tonic pupil but have no effect on normal pupil
- long-standing Adie's pupils are smaller than unaffected eye

Trauma
- damage to iris sphincter from blunt or penetrating trauma
- iris transillumination defects may be apparent using ophthalmoscope or slit-lamp
- pupil may be dilated (traumatic mydriasis) or irregularly shaped from tiny sphincter ruptures

Constricted Pupil (Miosis)

Senile Miosis
- decreased sympathetic stimulation with age

Parasympathetic Stimulation
- local or systemic medications such as:
  - cholinergic agents: pilocarpine, carbachol
  - cholinesterase inhibitor: phospholine iodide
  - opiates, barbiturates

Horner's Syndrome
- lesion in sympathetic pathway
- difference in pupil size greater in dim light, due to decreased innervation of adrenergics to iris dilator muscle
- associated with ptosis, anhydrosis of ipsilateral face/neck
- application of cocaine 4-10% (blocks reuptake of norepinephrine) to eye does not result in pupil dilation (vs. physiologic anisocoria), therefore confirms diagnosis
- hydroxyamphetamine 1% (stimulates norepinephrine release) will dilate pupil if central or preganglionic lesion, not postganglionic lesion
- postganglionic lesions result in denervation hypersensitivity, which will cause pupil to dilate with 0.125% epinephrine, whereas normal pupil will not
- causes: carotid or subclavian aneurysm, brainstem infarct, demyelinating disease, cervical or mediastinal tumour, Pancoast tumour, goitre, cervical lymphadenopathy, surgical sympathectomy, Lyme disease, cervical ribs, tabes dorsalis, cervical vertebral fractures

Iritis
- miotic pupil initially
- later, may be irregularly shaped pupil due to posterior synechiae
- later stages non-reactive to light

Argyll-Robertson Pupil
- both pupils irregular and <3 mm in diameter, ± ptosis
- does not respond to light stimulation
- responds to accommodation (light-near dissociation)
- suggestive of neurosyphilis or other conditions (DM, encephalitis, MS, chronic alcoholism, CNS degenerative diseases)

Other Causes
- optic neuritis, retinal lesions

Relative Afferent Pupillary Defect

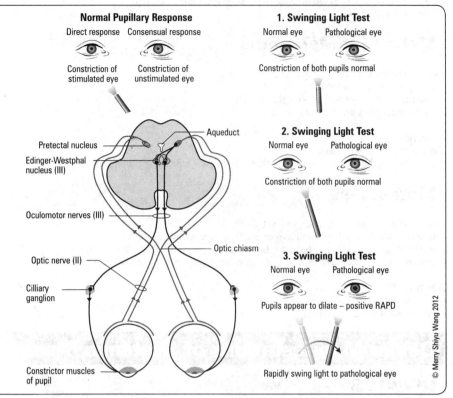

Figure 23. Relative afferent pupillary defect

- also known as Marcus Gunn pupil
- impairment of direct pupillary response to light, caused by a lesion in visual afferent (sensory) pathway anterior to optic chiasm
- differential diagnosis: large RD, BRAO, CRAO, CRVO, advanced glaucoma, optic nerve compression, optic neuritis (most common)
- does not occur with media opacity (e.g. corneal edema, cataracts)
- pupil reacts poorly to light and better to accommodation
- test: swinging flashlight
  - if light is shone in the affected eye, direct and consensual response to light is decreased
  - if light is shone in the unaffected eye, direct and consensual response to light is normal
  - if the light is moved quickly from the unaffected eye to the affected eye, "paradoxical" dilation of both pupils occurs
  - observe red reflex, especially in patients with dark irides
- if the defect is bilateral there is no RAPD, as dilation is measured relative to the other eye

Cataracts never produce an RAPD

It is possible to have RAPD and normal vision at the same time, e.g. in damaged superior colliculus caused by thalamic hemorrhage

Differentiate RAPD from physiologic pupillary athetosis ("hippus"), which is rapid, rhythmic fluctuations of the pupil, with equal amplitude in both eyes

Malignancies

- uncommon site for 1° malignancies
- see *Retinoblastoma*, OP38

Lid Carcinoma

Etiology

- basal cell carcinoma (rodent ulcer) (90%)
  - spread via local invasion, rarely metastasizes
  - ulcerated centre, indurated base with pearly rolled edges, telangiectasia
- squamous cell carcinoma (<5%)
  - spread via local invasion, may also spread to nodes and metastasize
  - ulceration, keratosis of lesion
- sebaceous cell carcinoma (1-5%)
  - often masquerades as chronic blepharitis or recurrent chalazion
  - highly invasive, metastasize
- Kaposi's sarcoma, malignant melanoma, Merkel cell tumour, metastatic tumour

Treatment
- incisional or excisional biopsies
- may require cryotherapy, radiotherapy, chemotherapy, immunotherapy
- surgical reconstruction

Malignant Melanoma

To Find Small Ocular Melanoma

TFSOM
T – Thickness > 2mm
F – Subretinal Fluid
S – Symptoms – Vision changes
O – Orange pigment
M – Margin within 3 mm of optic disc

- most common 1° intraocular malignancy in adults
- more prevalent in Caucasians
- arise from uveal tract, 90% choroidal melanoma
- hepatic metastases predominate

Treatment
- imaging to investigate spread
- depending on the size of the tumour, either radiotherapy, enucleation, limited surgery

Metastases

- most common intraocular malignancy in adults
- most commonly from breast and lung in adults, neuroblastoma in children
- usually infiltrate the choroid, but may also affect the optic nerve or extraocular muscles
- may present with decreased or distorted vision, irregularly shaped pupil, iritis, hyphema

Treatment
- local radiation, chemotherapy
- enucleation if blind, painful eye

Ocular Manifestations of Systemic Disease

HIV/AIDS

- up to 75% of patients with AIDS have ocular manifestations

External Ocular Signs
- Kaposi's sarcoma
  - secondary to human herpes virus 8 (HHV-8), affects conjunctiva of lid or globe
  - differential diagnosis: subconjunctival hemorrhage (non-clearing), hemangioma
- multiple molluscum contagiosum
- herpes simplex/zoster keratitis

Retina
- HIV retinopathy (most common)
  - cotton wool spots in >50% of HIV patients
  - intraretinal hemorrhage
- CMV retinitis
  - ocular opportunistic infection developed when severely immunocompromised (CD4 count ≤50)
  - a necrotizing retinitis, with retinal hemorrhage and vasculitis, "brushfire" or "pizza pie" appearance
  - presents with scotomas (macular involvement and RD), blurred vision, and floaters
  - untreated infection will progress to other eye in 4-6 wk
  - treatment: virostatic agents (e.g. gancyclovir or foscarnet) via IV or intravitreal injection
- necrotizing retinitis
  - from herpes simplex virus, herpes zoster, toxoplasmosis
  - disseminated choroiditis
  - *Pneumocystis carinii, Mycobacterium avium intracellulare, Candida*

Other Systemic Infections

- herpes zoster
  - see *Herpes Zoster*, OP18
- candidal endophthalmitis
  - fluffy, white-yellow, superficial retinal infiltrate that may eventually result in vitritis
  - may present with inflammation of the anterior chamber
  - treatment: systemic amphotericin B, oral fluconazole

- toxoplasmosis
  - focal, grey-yellow-white, chorioretinal lesions with surrounding vasculitis and vitreous infiltration (vitreous cells)
  - can be congenital (transplacental) or acquired (caused by *Toxoplasma gondii* protozoa transmitted through raw meat and cat feces)
  - congenital form more often causes visual impairment (more likely to involve the macula)
  - treatment: pyrimethamine, sulfonamide, folinic acid, or clindamycin. Consider adding steroids if severe inflammation (vitritis, macular or optic nerve involvement)

Diabetes Mellitus

- most common cause of blindness in young people in North America
- loss of vision due to
  - progressive microangiopathy leading to macular edema
  - progressive DR → neovascularization → traction → RD and vitreous hemorrhage
  - rubeosis iridis (neovascularization of the iris) leading to neovascular glaucoma (poor prognosis)
  - macular ischemia

Macular edema is the most common cause of visual loss in patients with background DR

DIABETIC RETINOPATHY

Background
- altered vascular permeability (loss of pericytes, breakdown of blood-retinal barrier, thickening of basement membrane)
- predisposition to retinal vessel obstruction (CRAO, CRVO, and BRVO)

Classification
- **non-proliferative**: increased vascular permeability and retinal ischemia
  - microaneurysms
  - dot and blot hemorrhages
  - hard exudates (lipid deposits), non-specific for DR
  - macular edema
- **advanced non-proliferative (or pre-proliferative)**
  - non-proliferative findings plus:
    - venous beading (in ≥2 of 4 retinal quadrants)
    - intraretinal microvascular anomalies (IRMA) in 1 of 4 retinal quadrants
      - IRMA: dilated, leaky vessels within the retina
    - cotton wool spots (nerve fibre layer infarcts)
- **proliferative**
  - 5% of patients with DM will reach this stage
  - neovascularization of iris, disc, retina to vitreous
    - neovascularization of iris (rubeosis iridis) can lead to neovascular glaucoma
    - vitreous hemorrhage, bleeding from fragile new vessels, fibrous tissue can contract causing tractional RD
  - high risk of severe vision loss secondary to vitreous hemorrhage, RD

Expanded 2 Year Follow-Up of Ranizumab Plus Prompt or Deferred Laser or Triamcinuclone Plus Prompt Laser for Diabetic Macular Edema
Ophthalmology 2011;118:609-614
Ranibizumab (Lucentis®) with prompt or deferred laser is more effective than intravitreal corticosteroid injections + laser or laser alone with sustained efficacy up to 24 mo.

Screening Guidelines for Diabetic Retinopathy
- type 1 DM
  - screen for retinopathy beginning annually 5 yr after disease onset
  - annual screening indicated for all patients over 12 yr and/or entering puberty
- type 2 DM
  - initial examination at time of diagnosis, then annually
- pregnancy
  - ocular exam in 1st trimester, close follow-up throughout as pregnancy can exacerbate DR
  - gestational diabetics are not at risk for DR

Clinically significant macular edema is defined as thickening of the retina at or within 500 μm of the centre of the macula

Presence of DR in
Type 1 DM
- 25% after 5 yr
- 60% after 10 yr
- >80% after 15 yr
Type 2 DM
- 20% at time of diagnosis
- 60% after 20 yr

Treatment
- Diabetic Control and Complications Trial (DCCT)
  - tight control of blood sugar decreases frequency and severity of microvascular complications
- blood pressure control
- focal laser for clinically significant macular edema
- intravitreal injection of corticosteroid or anti-VEGF for foveal involved diabetic macular edema
- panretinal laser photocoagulation for PDR: reduces neovascularization, hence reducing the angiogenic stimulus from ischemic retina by decreasing retinal metabolic demand → reduces risk of blindness
- vitrectomy for non-clearing vitreous hemorrhage and tractional RD in PDR
- vitrectomy before vitreous hemorrhage does not improve the visual prognosis

Lens Changes
- earlier onset of senile nuclear sclerotic and cortical cataracts
- may get hyperglycemic cataract, due to sorbitol accumulation (rare)
- changes in blood glucose levels (poor control) can suddenly cause refractive changes by 3-4 diopters

Effects of Medical Therapies on Retinopathy Progression in Type 2 DM
NEJM 2010;363:233-244
Purpose: To determine whether or not intensive glycemic control, combination therapy for dyslipidemia, and intensive blood-pressure control may limit the progression of DR in persons with type 2 DM.
Methods: RCT with 10,251 participants with type 2 DM at high risk of cardiovascular disease. Intensive or standard treatment for glycemia (glycated hemoglobin level <6.0% or 7.0-7.9%), dyslipidemia (160 mg daily fenofibrate plus simvastatin or placebo plus simvastatin), or systolic blood-pressure control (target <120 or <140 mm Hg).
Results: Rates of progression of DR at 4 yr were 7.3% with intensive glycemia treatment vs. 10.4% with standard therapy (OR 0.67; 95% CI 0.51-0.87); 6.5% with fenofibrate for intensive dyslipidemia therapy vs. 10.2% with placebo (OR 0.60; 95% CI 0.42-0.87) and 10.4% with intensive blood-pressure therapy vs. 8.8% with standard therapy (OR 1.23; 95% CI 0.84-1.79).
Conclusions: Intensive glycemic control and intensive combination treatment of dyslipidemia, but not intensive blood-pressure control, reduced the rate of DR.

Extraocular Muscle Palsy
- usually CN III infarct
- pupil usually spared in diabetic CN III palsy, but ptosis is observed
- may involve CN IV and VI
- usually recover within few months

Optic Neuropathy
- visual acuity loss due to infarction of optic disc/nerve

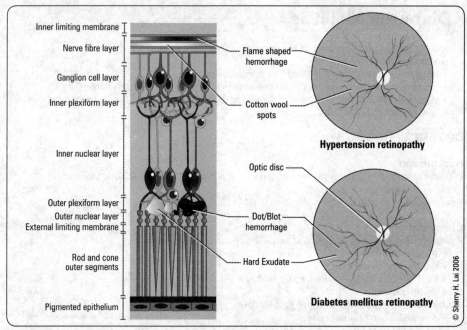

Figure 24. DM vs. HTN retinopathy

Hypertension

- retinopathy is the most common ocular manifestation
- chronic HTN retinopathy: arteriovenous (AV) nicking, blot retinal hemorrhages, microaneurysms, cotton wool spots
- acute HTN retinopathy: retinal arteriolar spasm, superficial retinal hemorrhage, cotton wool spots, optic disc edema

Table 8. Keith-Wagener-Barker Classification

Group 1	Mild arterial narrowing
Group 2	Obvious arterial narrowing with focal irregularities
Group 3	Group 2 characteristics plus: Cotton wool spots Hemorrhage and/or exudate
Group 4	Group 3 plus papilledema

Multiple Sclerosis

- see Neurology, N52

Corticosteroids for Treating Optic Neuritis
Cochrane DB Syst Rev 2012;4:CD001430
Purpose: To assess the effects of corticosteroids on visual recovery in patients with acute optic neuritis.
Results/Conclusions: 6 RCTs, 750 participants. Follow-up at 6 mo or one yr. There is no conclusive evidence of benefit with respect to recovery to normal visual acuity, visual field or contrast sensitivity with either intravenous or oral corticosteroids at the doses evaluated in included trials.

Clinical Features
- blurred vision and decreased colour vision: secondary to optic neuritis
- central scotoma: due to damage to papillomacular bundle of retinal nerve fibres
- diplopia: secondary to INO
- RAPD, ptosis, nystagmus, uveitis, optic atrophy, optic neuritis
- white matter demyelinating lesions of optic nerve on MRI

Treatment
- IV steroids with taper to oral form for optic neuritis
  - DO NOT treat with oral steroids in isolation as this increases likelihood of eventual development of MS

TIA/Amaurosis Fugax

- sudden, transient blindness from intermittent vascular compromise
- ipsilateral carotid most frequent embolic source
- typically monocular, lasting <5-10 min
- Hollenhorst plaques (glistening microemboli seen at branch points of retinal arterioles)

Graves' Disease

- ophthalmopathy occurs despite control of thyroid gland status
- ocular manifestations occur secondary to sympathetic overdrive and/or specific inflammatory infiltrate of the orbital tissue

The most common cause of unilateral or bilateral proptosis in adults is Graves' disease

Clinical
- initial inflammatory phase is followed by a quiescent cicatricial phase

Progression of Signs and Symptoms of Graves' Ophthalmopathy

NO SPECS
No signs/symptoms
Only signs (lid retraction, lid lag)
Soft tissue swelling (periorbital edema)
Proptosis (exophthalmos)
Extraocular muscle weakness (causing diplopia)
Corneal exposure
Sight loss

Treatment
- treat hyperthyroidism
- monitor for corneal exposure and maintain corneal hydration
- manage diplopia, proptosis and compressive optic neuropathy with one or a combination of:
    - steroids (during acute phase)
    - orbital bony decompression
    - external beam radiation of the orbit
- consider strabismus and/or eyelid surgical procedures once acute phase subsides

Connective Tissue Disorders

- RA, juvenile idiopathic arthritis, SLE, Sjögren syndrome, ankylosing spondylitis, polyarteritis nodosa
- most common ocular manifestation: dry eyes (keratoconjunctivitis sicca)

Giant Cell Arteritis/Temporal Arteritis

- see Rheumatology, RH20

Clinical Features
- more common in women >60 yr
- abrupt monocular loss of vision, pain over the temporal artery, jaw claudication, scalp tenderness, constitutional symptoms, and past medical history of polymyalgia rheumatica
- ischemic optic atrophy
- 50% lose vision in other eye if untreated

ESR in Temporal Arteritis
Males > age/2
Females > (age + 10)/2

Diagnosis
- temporal artery biopsy + increased ESR (ESR can be normal, but likely 80-100 in first hour), increased CRP
- if biopsy of one side is negative, biopsy the other side

Does this Patient have Temporal Arteritis?
JAMA 2002;287:92-101
Rule in: jaw claudication and diplopia on history, temporal artery beading, prominence of the artery and tenderness over the artery on exam.
Rule out: no temporal artery abnormalities on exam, normal ESR.

Treatment
- high dose corticosteroid to relieve pain and prevent further ischemic episodes
- if diagnosis of GCA is suspected clinically: start treatment + perform temporal artery biopsy to confirm diagnosis within 2 wk of initial presentation (**DO NOT WAIT TO TREAT**)

Sarcoidosis

- granulomatous uveitis with large "mutton fat" keratitic precipitates and posterior synechiae
- neurosarcoidosis: optic neuropathy, oculomotor abnormalities, visual field loss

Treatment
- steroids and mydriatics

Pediatric Ophthalmology

Strabismus

- ocular misalignment in one or both eyes, can be found in up to 3% of children
- classification
  - manifest (constant) vs. latent (hidden) alignment.
  - comitant (deviation equal in all positions of gaze) vs. incomitant (deviation worse in certain positions)
  - described in direction of deviation relative to the fixating eye
- distinguish from pseudostrabismus (prominent epicanthal folds, hypertelorism)
- complications: amblyopia, cosmesis

Strabismus in children under 4 mo of age sometimes resolves, particularly if the deviation is intermittent, variable, or measures <40 prism diopters

All children with strabismus and/or possible reduced vision require prompt referral to an ophthalmologist

HETEROTROPIA

- manifest deviation
- deviation not corrected by the fusion mechanism (i.e. deviation is apparent when the patient is using both eyes)

Types

- exo- (lateral deviation), eso- (medial deviation)
- hyper- (upward deviation), hypo- (downward deviation)
- esotropia = "crossed-eyes"; exotropia = "wall-eyed"

Tests

- Hirschberg test (corneal light reflex): positive if the light reflex on both corneas is asymmetrical
  - light reflex lateral to central cornea indicates esodeviation; light reflex medial to central cornea indicates exodeviation
  - false positives occur if visual axis and anatomic pupillary axis of the eye are not aligned (angle κ)
- cover test
- the deviation can be quantified using prisms

HETEROPHORIA

- latent deviation
- deviation corrected in the binocular state by the fusion mechanism (i.e. deviation not seen when patient is focusing with both eyes)
- Hirschberg test will be normal (light reflexes symmetrical)
- very common – majority are asymptomatic
- may be exacerbated or become manifest with asthenopia (eye strain, fatigue)

Tests

- cover-uncover test
- alternate cover test
  - alternating the cover between both eyes reveals the total deviation, both latent and manifest
  - maintain cover over one eye for 2-3 s before rapidly shifting to other eye

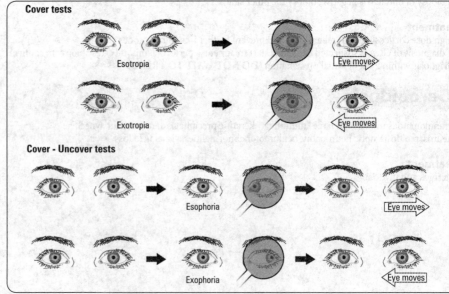

Figure 25. Cover and cover-uncover tests for detection of tropias and phorias

© Lori Waters 2005

Table 9. Paralytic vs. Non-Paralytic Strabismus

Clinical Characteristics	Paralytic Strabismus	Nonparalytic Strabismus
Definition	Incomitant strabismus	Concomitant strabismus
Onset	Often sudden but may be gradual or congenital	Usually gradual or shortly after birth; rarely sudden
Age of Onset	Any age; most often acquired	Usually during infancy

Etiology	Reduction or restriction in range of eye movements due to:
	  Neural (CN III, IV, VI): ischemia (e.g. DM), MS, aneurysm, brain tumour, trauma
	  Muscular: myasthenia gravis (neuromuscular junction pathology), Graves' disease
	  Structural: restriction or entrapment of extraocular muscles due to orbital inflammation, tumour, fracture of the orbital wall
		Develops early in childhood
		No restriction in range of eye movements
		Monocular, alternating, or intermittent

Diplopia	Common	Uncommon; image from the misaligned eye is suppressed
Visual Acuity in Other Eye	Usually unaffected in the other eye, unless CN II is involved	Deviated eye may become amblyopic if not treated when the child is young Amblyopia treatment rarely successful after age 8-10 yr Amblyopia usually does not develop if child has alternating strabismus or intermittency, which allows neural pathways for both eyes to develop
Possibility of Amblyopia	Uncommon	Common
Neurologic Findings or Systemic Disease	May be present	Usually absent

Accommodative Esotropia

- normal response to approaching object is the triad of the near reflex: convergence, accommodation and miosis
- hyperopes must constantly accommodate – excessive accommodation can lead to esotropia in young children via over-activation of the near reflex
- average age of onset is 2.5 yr
- usually reversible with correction of refractive error

Non-Accommodative Esotropia

- accounts for 50% of childhood strabismus
- most are idiopathic
- may be due to monocular visual impairment (e.g. cataract, corneal scarring, anisometropia, retinoblastoma) or divergence insufficiency (ocular misalignment that is greater at distance fixation than at near fixation)

Amblyopia

Definition

- a neurodevelopmental visual disorder with unilateral (or less commonly, bilateral) reduction of best corrected visual acuity that cannot be attributed only and directly to the effect of a structural abnormality of the eye.
- it is caused by abnormal visual experience early in life and cannot be remedied immediately by spectacle glasses alone
- in approximately half of the cases, amblyopia is secondary to strabismus (mainly esotropia). Other causes may include uncorrected refractive errors, anisometropia (asymmetric refractive errors), and concomitant structural ocular problems

Detection

- "Holler Test": young child upset if good eye is covered
- quantitative visual acuity by age 3-4 yr using picture charts and/or matching game (Sheridan-Gardiner), testing each eye separately
- amblyopia treatment less successful after age 8-10 yr, but a trial should be given no matter what age
- prognosis: 90% will have good vision restored and maintained if treated <4 yr old

Etiology and Management
- strabismus
  - correct with glasses for accommodative esotropia
  - occlusion therapy (see below)
  - surgery: recession (weakening) – moving muscle insertion further back on the globe; or resection (strengthening) – shortening the muscle
  - botulinum toxin for single muscle weakening
  - after ocular alignment is restored (glasses, surgery, botulinum toxin), patching is frequently necessary to maintain vision until ~8 yr of age
- anisometropia
  - amblyopia usually in the more hyperopic eye
  - the more emmetropic (normal refraction) eye receives a clear image while the less emmetropic eye receives a blurred image; input from the blurred eye is cortically suppressed and visual pathway fails to develop normally
  - treat with glasses to correct refractive error
  - patching is required if visual acuity difference persists after 4-8 wk of using glasses
- deprivation amblyopia
  - occlusion due to ptosis, cataract, retinoblastoma, corneal opacity
  - occlusion amblyopia: prolonged patching of good eye may cause it to become amblyopic

Occlusion Therapy
- patching the good eye to force the brain to use the non-dominant eye and redevelop its vision
- atropine cycloplegic drops to impair accommodation and blur vision of the better seeing eye

Risks
- permanent loss of vision in the affected eye
- possibility of injury to "remaining" good eye
- safety glasses or polycarbonate lenses recommended if visual acuity in worse eye is <20/50
- loss of stereopsis

Leukocoria

- white reflex (red reflex is absent)

Differential Diagnosis
- cataract
- retinoblastoma
- retinal coloboma
- ROP
- persistent hyperplastic primary vitreous or persistent fetal vasculature
- Coat's disease (exudative retinal telangiectasis)
- toxocariasis
- RD

Retinoblastoma

- most common primary intraocular malignancy in children
- incidence: 1/15,000; sporadic or genetic transmission; screening of siblings/offspring essential
- unilateral (2/3) or bilateral (1/3)
- malignant – direct or hematogenous spread
- diagnosis
  - often presents with leukocoria or strabismus
  - U/S or CT scan may demonstrate calcified mass (present in most cases)

Treatment
- radiotherapy, chemotherapy combined with laser, cryopexy, and/or enucleation

Retinopathy of Prematurity

- vasoproliferative retinopathy that is a major cause of blindness in the developed world

Risk Factors
- non-black race (black infants have lower risk of developing ROP)
- low gestational age, birth weight <1500 g
- high oxygen exposure after birth (iatrogenic)

Classification (ROP Staging)
- stage 1: faint demarcation line at the junction between the vascularized and avascular retina
- stage 2: elevated ridge

Retinal Zones
- Zone I: circle with radius twice the distance from the disc to the macula (most difficult to treat)
- Zone II: annulus from zone I to nasal extent of retina (nasal ora serrata)
- Zone III: remaining retina

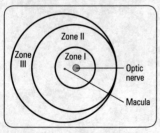

Figure 26. Zones of the retina in ROP

- stage 3: extra-retinal fibrovascular tissue extending into vitreous
- stage 4: partial RD (4A: macula "on", 4B: macula "off")
- stage 5: total RD
- plus (+) disease: dilatation and tortuosity of retinal vessels
- threshold disease: stage 3+ in zones 1 or 2 with 5 continuous or 8 cumulative clock hours of ROP involvement

Treatment
- threshold disease is treated with cryotherapy or laser (laser is now the standard treatment, with better refractive outcome), off label anti-VEGF intravitreal injections
- ROP beyond threshold level is either watched carefully (usually stage 4A) or treated with vitrectomy/ scleral buckle

Prognosis
- higher incidence of myopia among ROP infants, even if treated successfully
- stage 4B and 5 have poor prognosis for visual outcome despite treatment

Nasolacrimal System Defects

- congenital obstruction of the nasolacrimal duct (failure of canalization), usually occurs at 1-2 mo of age
- epiphora, crusting, discharge, recurrent conjunctivitis
- can have reflux of mucopurulent material from lacrimal punctum when pressure is applied over lacrimal sac

Treatment
- massage over lacrimal sac at medial corner of eyelid
- vast majority spontaneously resolve in 9-12 mo, otherwise consider referral for duct probing

Ophthalmia Neonatorum

- newborn conjunctivitis in first mo of life
- causes
  - toxic: silver nitrate, erythromycin
  - infectious: bacterial (e.g. *N. gonorrhoeae* – most common, *C. trachomatis*), herpes simplex virus
- diagnose using stains and cultures

Treatment
- systemic antibiotics with possible hospitalization if infectious etiology
- topical prophylaxis, most commonly with erythromycin (or silver nitrate), is required by law at birth

Congenital Glaucoma

- due to inadequate development of the filtering mechanism of the anterior chamber angle

Clinical Features
- cloudy cornea, increased IOP
- photophobia, epiphora
- buphthalmos (large cornea, "ox eye", secondary to increased IOP), blepharospasm

Treatment
- filtration surgery is required soon after birth to prevent blindness

Ocular Trauma

Blunt Trauma

- caused by blunt object such as fist, squash ball
- history: injury, ocular history, drug allergy, tetanus status
- exam: VA first, pupil size and reaction, EOM (diplopia), external and slit-lamp exam, ophthalmoscopy
- if VA normal or slightly reduced, globe less likely to be perforated
- if VA reduced may be perforated globe, corneal abrasion, lens dislocation, retinal tear
- bone fractures
  - blow out fracture: restricted EOM, diplopia, enophthalmos (sunken eye)
  - ethmoid fracture: subcutaneous emphysema of lid
- lids: swelling, laceration, emphysema
- conjunctiva: subconjunctival hemorrhage
- cornea: abrasion – detect with fluorescein staining and cobalt blue filter using slit-lamp or ophthalmoscope

Efficacy of Intravitreal Bevacizumab for Stage 3+ Retinopathy of Prematurity (ROP)
NEJM 2011;364:603-615
Study: Randomized controlled clinical trial.
Patients: 150 infants born at gestational age ≤30 wk and birth weight ≤1500 g.
Intervention: Randomized to conventional laser therapy or intravitreal bevacizumab monotherapy.
Main Outcome: Recurrence of ROP in one or both eyes requiring retreatment before 54 wk postmenstrual age.
Results: ROP recurrence was lower in the bevacizumab group (6 of 140 eyes [4%]) vs. the laser-therapy group (32 of 146 eyes [22%]) (p=0.002). A significant treatment effect was found for zone I ROP (p=0.003).
Conclusions: Intravitreal bevacizumab monotherapy is beneficial for infants with zone I state 3+ ROP and allows continued development of peripheral retinal vessels following treatment.

Gonococcal infection is the most serious threat to sight as it can rapidly penetrate corneal epithelium, causing corneal ulceration

Epiphora in children – rule out congenital glaucoma

Always test VA first – medicolegal protection

Refer if You Observe Any of These Signs
- Decreased VA
- Shallow anterior chamber
- Hyphema
- Abnormal pupil
- Ocular misalignment
- Retinal damage

- anterior chamber: assess depth, hyphema, hypopyon
- iris: prolapse, iritis
- lens: cataract, dislocation
- retinal tear/detachment

Penetrating Trauma

Management of Suspected Globe Rupture
CAN'T forget
CT orbits
Ancef (cefazolin) ± Aminoglycoside IV
NPO
Tetanus status

- include ruptured globe ± prolapsed iris, intraocular foreign body
- rule out intraocular foreign body, especially if history of "metal striking metal", orbit CT
- **OCULAR EMERGENCY**: initial management - REFER IMMEDIATELY
  - ABCs
  - don't press on eye globe!
  - don't check IOP if possibility of globe rupture
  - check vision, diplopia
  - apply rigid eye shield to minimize further trauma
  - keep head elevated 30-45° to keep IOP down
  - keep NPO
  - tetanus status
  - give IV antibiotics
    - selecting appropriate agents depends on the mechanism of injury; Gram-positive bacteria are more commonly involved than Gram-negative; retained intraocular foreign objects increase the risk of infections with Bacillus species, whereas exposure to vegetable matter increase the risk of a fungal etiology

Post-Traumatic Infectious Endophthalmitis
Surv Ophthalmol 2011;56:214-251
- Delayed primary repair (>24 h after open globe injury) increases risk for post-traumatic endophthalmitis in the absence of an intraocular foreign body (IOFB).
- If IOFB present, early vitrectomy and IOFB removal must be performed within 24 h of injury.
- Extreme pain with hypopyon and vitritis indicate endophthalmitis until proven otherwise, and samples must be obtained.
- Treat with empirical intravitreal and intravenous antibiotic guided by nature of trauma, and adjust based on culture.

Hyphema

- blood in anterior chamber often due to damage to root of the iris
- may occur with blunt trauma

Treatment
- refer to ophthalmology
- shield and bedrest x 5 d or as determined by ophthalmologist
- sleep with head upright
- may need surgical drainage if hyphema persists or if re-bleed

Shaken Baby Syndrome
Syndrome of findings characterized by absence of external signs of abuse with respiratory arrest, seizures, or coma. Ocular exam findings are important diagnostically for Shaken Baby Syndrome. These findings include extensive retinal and vitreous hemorrhages that occur during the shaking process and are extremely rare in accidental trauma. A detailed fundoscopic exam or an ophthalmology referral should be conducted for all infants in whom abuse is suspected

Complications
- risk of re-bleed highest on days 2-5, resulting in secondary glaucoma, corneal staining, and iris necrosis
- never prescribe Aspirin®, as it increases the risk of a re-bleed

Blow-Out Fracture

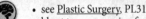

- see Plastic Surgery, PL31
- blunt trauma causing fracture of orbital floor and herniation of orbital contents into maxillary sinus
- orbital rim remains intact
- inferior rectus and/or inferior oblique muscles may be incarcerated at fracture site
- infraorbital nerve courses along the floor of the orbit and may be damaged

Classic Signs of Blow-Out
- Enophthalmos
- Decreased upgaze (IR trapped)
- Cheek anesthetized (infraorbital nerve trapped)

Clinical Features
- pain and nausea at time of injury
- diplopia, restriction of EOM
- infraorbital and upper lip paresthesia (CN V2)
- enophthalmos (sunken eye), periorbital ecchymoses

Investigations
- plain films: Waters' view and lateral
- CT: anteroposterior and coronal view of orbits

Treatment
- refrain from coughing, blowing nose
- systemic antibiotics may be indicated
- surgery if fracture >50% orbital floor, diplopia not improving, or enophthalmos >2 mm
- may delay surgery if the diplopia improves

Chemical Burns

- alkali burns have a worse prognosis than acid burns because acids coagulate tissue and inhibit further corneal penetration
- poor prognosis if cornea opaque, likely irreversible stromal damage
- even with a clear cornea initially, alkali burns can progress for weeks (thus, very guarded prognosis)

Treatment
- immediately irrigate at site of accident with water or buffered solution
  - IV drip for at least 20-30 min with eyelids retracted in emergency department
  - swab upper and lower fornices to remove possible particulate matter
- do not attempt to neutralize because the heat produced by the reaction will damage the cornea
- cycloplegic drops to decrease iris spasm (pain) and prevent secondary glaucoma (due to posterior synechiae formation)
- topical antibiotics and patching
- topical steroids (by ophthalmologist) to decrease inflammation, use for <2 wk (in the case of a persistent epithelial defect)

Fluorescein lights up alkali so you can detect it and assess whether it has been removed

Ocular Drug Toxicity

Table 10. Drugs with Ocular Toxicity

Amiodarone	Corneal microdeposits and superficial keratopathy (vortex keratopathy) Rare: ischemic optic neuropathy
Atropine, benztropine	Pupillary dilation (risk of angle closure glaucoma)
Bisphosphonates (Fosamax®, Actonel®)	Inflammatory eye disease (iritis, scleritis, episcleritis)
Chloroquine, hydroxychloroquine	Bull's eye maculopathy Vortex keratopathy
Chlorpromazine	Anterior subcapsular cataract
Contraceptive pills	Decreased tolerance to contact lenses Migraine Optic neuritis Central vein occlusion, benign increase intracranial pressure
Digitalis	Yellow vision Blurred vision
Ethambutol	Optic neuropathy
Haloperidol (Haldol®)	Oculogyric crises Blurred vision
Indomethacin	Superficial keratopathy
Interferon	Retinal hemorrhages and cotton wool spots
Isoniazid	Optic neuropathy
Nalidixic acid	Papilledema
Steroids	Posterior subcapsular cataracts Glaucoma Papilledema (systemic steroids) Increased severity of HSV infections (geographic ulcers) Predisposition to fungal infections
Sulphonamides, NSAIDs	Stevens-Johnson syndrome
Tamsulosin (Flomax®)	Intraoperative Floppy Iris Syndrome, which can complicate cataract surgery
Tetracycline	Papilledema (associated with pseudotumour cerebri)
Thioridazine	Pigmentary degeneration of retina
Vigabatrin	Retinal deposition with macular sparing, peripheral visual field loss
Vitamin A toxicity	Papilledema
Vitamin D toxicity	Band keratopathy

Common Medications

TOPICAL OCULAR DIAGNOSTIC DRUGS

Fluorescein Dye
- water soluble orange-yellow dye
- green under cobalt blue light (ophthalmoscope or slit-lamp)
- absorbed in areas of epithelial loss (ulcer or abrasion)
- also stains mucus and contact lenses

Rose Bengal Stain
- stains devitalized epithelial cells and mucus

Anesthetics
- e.g. proparacaine HCl 0.5%, tetracaine 0.5%
- indications: removal of foreign body and sutures, tonometry, examination of painful cornea
- toxic to corneal epithelium (inhibit mitosis and migration) and can lead to corneal ulceration and scarring with prolonged use, therefore **NEVER** prescribe

Mydriatics
- dilate pupils
- two classes
  - cholinergic blocking (e.g. tropicamide – Mydriacyl®)
    - dilation plus cycloplegia (loss of accommodation) by paralysis of iris sphincter and the ciliary body
    - indications: refraction, ophthalmoscopy, therapy for iritis
  - adrenergic stimulating (e.g. phenylephrine HCl 2.5%)
    - stimulate pupillary dilator muscles, no effect on accommodation
    - usually used with tropicamide for additive effects
    - side effects: HTN, tachycardia, arrhythmias

Green	Cholinergics
Red	Anti-Cholinergics
White	Anaesthetics, Antibiotics, Artificial tears, Steroids
Yellow	Beta-Blockers
Blue	Beta-Blocker combinations
Purple	Alpha-Agonists
Teal	Prostaglandins
Orange	Carbonic Anhydrase Inhibitors
Tan	Fluoroquinolones
Grey	NSAIDs
Pink	Anti-inflammatories, Steroids

Table 11. Mydriatic Cycloplegic Drugs and Duration of Action

Drugs	Duration of Action
Tropicamide (Mydriacyl®) 0.5%, 1%	4-5 h
Cyclopentolate HCL 0.5%, 1%	3-6 h
Homatropine HBr 1%, 2%	3-7 d
Atropine sulfate 0.5%, 1%	1-2 wk
Scopolamine HBr 0.25%, 5%	1-2 wk

GLAUCOMA MEDICATIONS

Table 12. Glaucoma Medications

Drug Category	Dose	Effect	Comment/Side Effects
α-Agonist **Non-selective** • epinephrine HCl 1% (Epifrin®) • dipivalyl epinephrine 0.1% (Propine®) **α2-selective** • brimonidine 0.2% (Alphagan®) • apraclonidine 0.5% (Iopidine®)	1 gtt OS/OD bid/tid	1. Non-selective: ↓ aqueous production + ↑ TM outflow 2. Selective: ↓ aqueous production + ↑ uveoscleral outflow	1. Non-selective: mydriasis, macular edema, tachycardia 2. Selective: contact allergy, hypotension in children
β-Blocker **Non-selective** • timolol (Timoptic®) • levobunolol (Betagan®) **β1-selective** betaxolol (Betoptic®)	1 gtt OS/OD qd/bid	↓ aqueous production	**Bronchospasm (caution in asthma/COPD)** ↑ CHF Bradycardia, hypotension. depression, heart block, impotence
Carbonic Anhydrase Inhibitor • dorzolamide (Trusopt®) • brinzolamide (Azopt®) • oral: acetazolamide (Diamox®), methazolamide (Neptazane®)	1 gtt OS/OD tid Diamox®: 500 mg PO bid	↓ aqueous production	**Must ask about sulfa allergy** Generally local side effects with topical preparations Oral: diuresis, fatigue, paresthesias, GI upset, etc.
Parasympathomimetic (cholinergic stimulating) • pilocarpine (Pilopine®) • carbachol (Isopto Carbachol®)	1-2 gtts OS/OD tid/qid	↑ TM outflow	Miosis ↓ night vision ↑ GI motility, brow ache, headache ↓ heart rate
Prostaglandin Analogues • latanoprost (Xalatan®) • travaprost (Travatan®) • bimatoprost (Lumigan®)	1 gtt OS/OD qhs	↑ uveoscleral outflow (uveoscleral responsible for 20% of drainage)	Iris colour change Periorbital skin pigmentation Lash growth Conjunctival hyperemia

Cosopt® = timolol + dorzolamide; Xalacom® = timolol + lantanoprost; Combigan® = timolol + brimonidine; DuoTrav® = tinolol + travaprost; gtt = drop, gtts = drops

WET AGE-RELATED MACULAR DEGENERATION MEDICATIONS

VEGF Inhibitors
- block VEGF which prevents ocular angiogenesis and further development of choroidal neovascularization
- administered via intravitreal injections
- pegaptanib (Macugen®) is a selective anti-VEGF targeting VEGF isoform 165 (no longer widely used)
- ranibizumab (Lucentis®) is a non-selective anti-VEGF agent
- aflibercept (Eylea®) is an VEGF "trap" agent that binds VEGF-A and placental growth factor
- bevacizumab (Avastin®) is another non-selective anti-VEGF agent but is only FDA approved for metastatic breast cancer, colorectal cancer, and non-small cell lung cancer; therefore, its widespread ophthalmologic use is off-label

TOPICAL OCULAR THERAPEUTIC DRUGS

NSAIDs
- used for less serious chronic inflammatory conditions
- e.g. ketorolac (Acular®), diclofenac (Voltaren®), nepafenac (Nevanac®) drops

Anti-Histamines
- used to relieve red and itchy eye, often in combination with decongestants
- sodium cromoglycate – stabilizes membranes

Decongestants
- weak adrenergic stimulating drugs (vasoconstrictor)
- e.g. naphazoline, phenylephrine (Isopto Frin®)
- rebound vasodilation with overuse; rarely can precipitate angle closure glaucoma

Antibiotics
- indications: bacterial conjunctivitis, keratitis, or blepharitis
- commonly as topical drops or ointments, may give systemically
- e.g. sulfonamide (sodium sulfacetamide, sulfisoxazole), gentamicin (Garamycin®), erythromycin, tetracycline, bacitracin, polymyxin B, fluoroquinolones (ciprofloxacin [Ciloxan®], ofloxacin [Ocuflox®], moxifloxacin [Vigamox®], gatifloxacin [Zymar®])

Corticosteroids
- e.g. fluorometholone (FML®), betamethasone, dexamethasone (Maxidex®), prednisolone (Predsol® 0.5%, Pred Forte® 1%), rimexolone (Vexol®), loteprednol etabonate 0.5% (Lotamax®), difluprednate (Durezol®)
- primary care physicians should avoid prescribing topical corticosteroids due to risk of glaucoma, cataracts, and reactivation of HSV keratitis
- complications
  - potentiates HSV keratitis and fungal keratitis as well as masks symptoms
  - increased IOP, more rapidly in steroid responders (within weeks)
  - posterior subcapsular cataract (within months)

References

ACCORD Study Group; ACCORD Eye Study Group, Chew EY, Ambrosius WT, Davis MD, et al. Effects of medical therapies on retinopathy progression in type 2 diabetes NEJM 2010;363:233-244

Age-Related Eye Disease Study Research Group. A randomized, placebo-controlled, clinical trial of high-dose supplementation with vitamins C and E, beta carotene, and zinc for age-related macular degeneration and vision loss: AREDS report no. 8. Arch Ophthalmol 2001;119:1417-1436.

Anderson DR, Normal Tension Glaucoma Study. Collaborative normal tension glaucoma study. Curr Opin Ophthalmol 2003;14:6-90.

Atlas of ophthalmology. Available from: www.atlasophthalmology.com/atlas/frontpage.jsf.

Bhagat N, Nagori S, Zarbin M. Post-traumatic Infectious Endophthalmitis. Surv Ophthalmol 2011;56:214-51.

Bradford C. Basic ophthalmology for medical students and primary care residents, 7th ed. San Francisco: American Academy of Ophthalmology, 1999.

CATT Research Group, Martin DF, Maguire MG, Ying GS, et al. Ranibizumab and bevacizumab for neovascular age-related macular degeneration. NEJM 2011;364:1897-1908.

Elman MJ, Bressler NM, Qin H, et al. Expanded 2-year follow-up of ranibizumab plus prompt or deferred laser or triamcinolone plus prompt laser for diabetic macular edema. Ophthal 2011;118:609-614.

Friedman N, Pineda R, Kaiser P. The Massachusetts eye and ear infirmary illustrated manual of ophthalmology. Toronto: WB Saunders, 1998.

Gal RL, Vedula SS, Beck R. Corticosteroids for treating optic neuritis. Cochrane DB Syst Rev 2012;4:CD001430.

Glanville J, Patterson J, McCool R, et al. Efficacy and safety of widely used treatments for macular oedema secondary to retinal vein occlusion: a systematic review. BMC Ophthalmol 2014;14:7.

Haller JA, Bandello F, Belfort R Jr, et al. Randomized, sham-controlled trial of dexamethasone intravitreal implant in patients with macula edema due to retinal vein occlusion. Ophthal 2010;117:1134-1146.

Heijl A, Leske MC, Bengtsson B, et al. Reduction of intraocular pressure and glaucoma progression: results from the early manifest glaucoma trial. Arch Opthalmol 2002;120:1268-1279.

Kanski JJ. Clinical Ophthalmology: A systematic approach, 6th ed. Oxford: Butterworth-Heinemann, 2007.

Lichter PR, Musch DC, Gillespie BW, et al. Interim clinical outcomes in the collaborative initial glaucoma treatment study comparing initial treatment randomized to medications or surgery. Ophthal 2001;108:1943-1953.

Maguire AM, High KA, Auricchio A, et al. Age-dependent effects of RPE65 gene therapy for Leber's congenital amaurosis: a phase 1 dose-escalation trial. Lancet 2009;374:1597-1605.

Mintz-Hittner HA, Kennedy KA, Chuang AZ, BEAT-ROP Cooperative Group. Efficacy of intravitreal bevacizumab for stage 3+ retinopathy of prematurity. NEJM 2011;364:603-615.

Pushker N, Tejwani LK, Bajaj MS, et al. Role of oral corticosteroids in orbital cellulitis. Am J Ophthalmol 2013;156:178-183.

Rayapudi S, Schwartz SG, Wang X, et al. Vitamin A and fish oils for retinitis pigmentosa Cochrane DB Syst Rev 2013;12:CD008428

Sheikh A, Hurwitz B, van Schayck CP, et al. Antibiotics versus placebo for acute bacterial conjunctivitis. Cochrane DB Syst Rev 2012;9:CD001211.Smetana GW, Shmerling RH. Does this patient have temporal arteritis? JAMA 2002;287:92-101.

Stein R, Stein H. Management of ocular emergencies, 4th ed. Montreal: Mediconcept, 2006.

Tasman W, Jaegar EA. Duane's ophthalmology, 2011 ed. Philadelphia: Lippincott Wiliams & Wilkins, 2010.

Turner A, Rabiu M. Patching for corneal abrasion. Cochrane DB Syst Rev 2006;2:CD004764.

University of Michigan Kellogg Eye Centre. Available from: www.kellogg.umich.edu/theeyeshaveit/index.html.

Vass C, Hirn C, Sycha T, et al. Medical interventions for primary open-angle glaucoma and ocular hypertension. Cochrane DB Syst Rev 2007;4:CD003167.

Vedula SS, Krzystolik MG. Antiangiogenic therapy with anti-vascular endothelial growth factor modalities for neovascular age-related macular degeneration. Cochrane DB Syst Rev 2008;2:CD005139.

Wilhelmus KR. Antiviral treatment and other therapeutic interventions for herpes simplex virus epithelial keratitis. Cochrane DB Syst Rev 2010;12:CD002898.

Wilson FM. Practical ophthalmology: a manual for beginning residents, 4th ed. American Academy of Ophthalmology, 2005.

Wong AM. New concepts concerning the neural mechanisms of amblyopia and their clinical implications. Can J Opthalmol 2012;47:399-409.

OR | Orthopedics

Aaron Gazendam and **Graeme Hoit**, chapter editors
Dhruvin Hirpara and **Sneha Raju**, associate editors
Valerie Lemieux and **Simran Mundi**, EBM editors
Dr. Jeremy A. Hall and **Dr. Herbert P. von Schroeder**, staff editors

Acronyms

ABI	ankle brachial index	DRUJ	distal radioulnar joint	MT	metatarsal	RSD	reflex sympathetic dystrophy
AC	acromioclavicular	DVT	deep vein thrombosis	MTP	metatarsophalangeal	SCFE	slipped capital femoral epiphysis
ACL	anterior cruciate ligament	EtOH	ethanol/alcohol	MVC	motor vehicle collision	SLAP	superior lateral, anterior posterior
AIN	anterior interosseous nerve	FAI	femoroacetabular impingement	NVS	neurovascular status	SN	sensitivity
AP	anterior posterior	FOOSH	fall on outstretched hand	NWB	non-weight bearing	THA	total hip arthroplasty
ARDS	acute respiratory distress syndrome	GA	general anesthetic	OA	osteoarthritis	TKA	total knee arthroplasty
AVN	avascular necrosis	HO	heterotopic ossification	ORIF	open reduction internal fixation	TSA	total shoulder arthroplasty
CA	coracoacromial	I&D	incision and drainage	PCL	posterior cruciate ligament	WB	weight bearing
CC	coracoclavicular	IM	intramedullary	PIN	posterior interosseous nerve	#	fracture
CRPS	complex regional pain syndrome	LCL	lateral collateral ligament	RA	rheumatoid arthritis		
DDH	developmental dysplasia of the hip	MCL	medial collateral ligament	ROM	range of motion		

Basic Anatomy Review

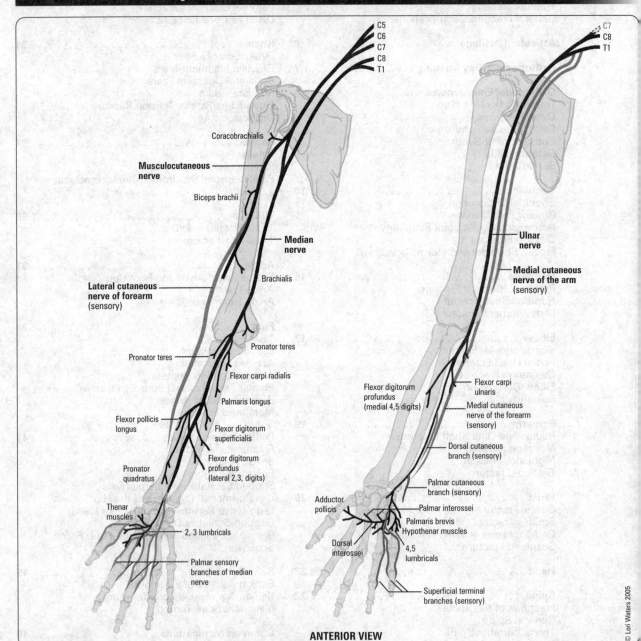

ANTERIOR VIEW

© Lori Waters 2005

Figure 1. Median, musculocutaneous, and ulnar nerves: innervation of upper limb muscles

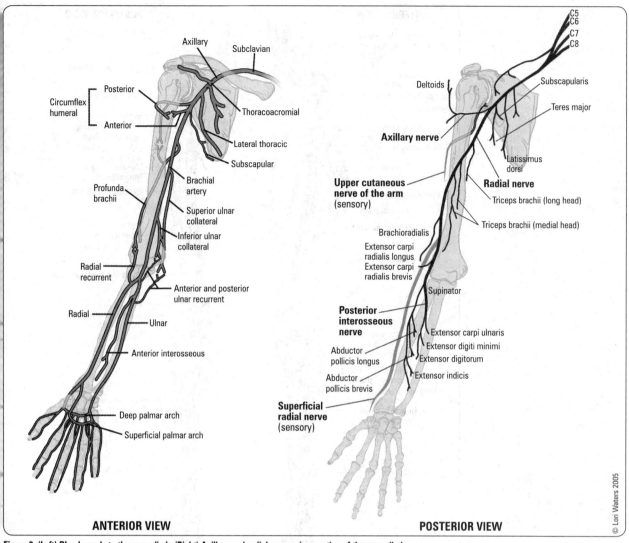

Figure 2. (Left) Blood supply to the upper limb, (Right) Axillary and radial nerves: innervation of the upper limb

Table 1. Sensory and Motor Innervation of the Nerves in the Upper and Lower Extremities

Nerve	Motor	Sensory	Nerve Roots
Axillary	Deltoid/Teres Minor	Lateral Upper Arm (Sergeant's Patch)	C5, C6
Musculocutaneous	Biceps/Brachialis	Lateral Forearm	C5, C6
Radial	Triceps Wrist/Thumb/Finger Extensors	Lateral Dorsum of the Hand Medial Upper Forearm	C5, C6, C7, C8
Median	Wrist Flexors and Abductors Flexion of the 1st-3rd Digits	Volar Thumb to Radial half of 4th Digit	C6, C7
Ulnar	Wrist Flexors and Adductors Flexion of the 4th-5th Digits	Medial Forearm Medial Dorsum and Volar of Hand (Ulnar half of 4th and 5th Digit)	C8, T1
Tibial	Ankle Plantar Flexion Knee Flexion Great Toe Flexion	Sole of Foot	L5, S1
Superficial Peroneal	Ankle Eversion	Dorsum of Foot	L5, S1
Deep Peroneal	Ankle Dorsiflexion and Inversion Great Toe Extension	1st Web Space	L5, S1
Sural		Lateral Foot	S1, S2
Saphenous		Anteromedial Ankle	L3, L4

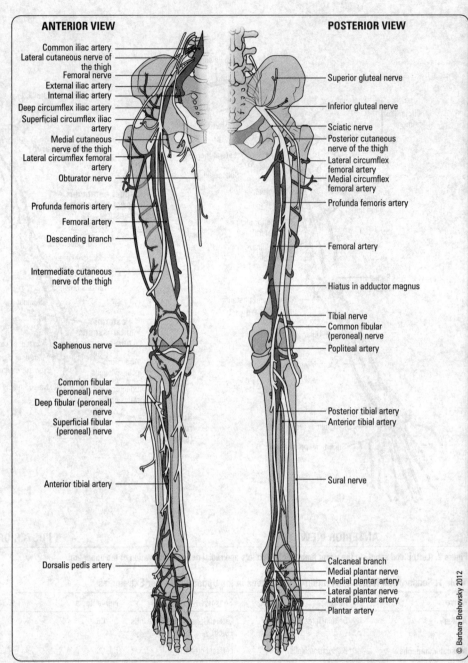

ANTERIOR VIEW

Common iliac artery
Lateral cutaneous nerve of the thigh
Femoral nerve
External iliac artery
Internal iliac artery
Deep circumflex iliac artery
Superficial circumflex iliac artery
Medial cutaneous nerve of the thigh
Lateral circumflex femoral artery
Obturator nerve
Profunda femoris artery
Femoral artery
Descending branch
Intermediate cutaneous nerve of the thigh
Saphenous nerve
Common fibular (peroneal) nerve
Deep fibular (peroneal) nerve
Superficial fibular (peroneal) nerve
Anterior tibial artery
Dorsalis pedis artery

POSTERIOR VIEW

Superior gluteal nerve
Inferior gluteal nerve
Sciatic nerve
Posterior cutaneous nerve of the thigh
Lateral circumflex femoral artery
Medial circumflex femoral artery
Profunda femoris artery
Femoral artery
Hiatus in adductor magnus
Tibial nerve
Common fibular (peroneal) nerve
Popliteal artery
Posterior tibial artery
Anterior tibial artery
Sural nerve
Calcaneal branch
Medial plantar nerve
Medial plantar artery
Lateral plantar nerve
Lateral plantar artery
Plantar artery

© Barbara Brehovsky 2012

Figure 3. Nerves and arteries of lower limbs

Fractures – General Principles

Fracture Description

1. Name of Injured Bone

2. Integrity of Skin/Soft Tissue
- closed: skin/soft tissue over and near fracture is intact
- open: skin/soft tissue over and near fracture is lacerated or abraded, fracture exposed to outside (or contaminated - such as the bowel) environment, or contaminated (i.e. bowel)
- signs: continuous bleeding from puncture site or fat droplets in blood are suggestive of an open fracture

3. Location (Figure 5)
- epiphyseal: end of bone, forming part of the adjacent joint
- metaphyseal: the flared portion of the bone at the ends of the shaft
- diaphyseal: the shaft of a long bone (proximal, middle, distal)
- physis: growth plate

4. Orientation/Fracture Pattern

- transverse: fracture line perpendicular (<30° of angulation) to long axis of bone; result of direct high energy force
- oblique: angular fracture line (30°- 60° of angulation); result of angular or rotational force
- butterfly: fracture site fragment which looks like a butterfly
- segmental: a separate segment of bone bordered by fracture lines; result of high energy force
- spiral: complex, multi-planar fracture line; result of rotational force, low energy
- comminuted/multi-fragmentary: >2 fracture fragments
- intra-articular: fracture line crosses articular cartilage and enters joint
- avulsion: tendon or ligament tears/pulls off bone fragment; often in children, high energy
- compression/impacted: impaction of bone; typical sites are vertebrae or proximal tibia
- torus: a buckle fracture of one cortex, often in children (see Figure 50, OR41)
- greenstick: an incomplete fracture of one cortex, often in children (see Figure 50, OR41)
- pathologic: fracture through bone weakened by disease/tumour

5. Alignment of Fracture Fragments

- nondisplaced: fracture fragments are in anatomic alignment
- displaced: fracture fragments are not in anatomic alignment
- distracted: fracture fragments are separated by a gap (opposite of impacted)
- impacted: fracture fragments are compressed, resulting in shortened bone
- angulated: direction of fracture apex (e.g. varus/valgus)
- translated/shifted: percentage of overlapping bone at fracture site
- rotated: fracture fragment rotated about long axis of bone

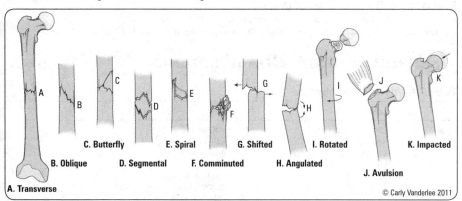

C. Butterfly   **E. Spiral**   **G. Shifted**   **I. Rotated**   **K. Impacted**

B. Oblique   **D. Segmental**   **F. Comminuted**   **H. Angulated**

J. Avulsion

A. Transverse   © Carly Vanderlee 2011

Figure 4. Fracture types

Approach to Fractures

1. **Clinical Assessment**
   - ABCs, primary survey and secondary survey (ATLS protocol)
     - rule out other fractures/injuries
     - rule out open fracture
   - AMPLE history (minimum): Allergies, Medications, Past medical history, Last meal, Events surrounding injury
     - mechanism of injury
     - previous significant injury or surgery to affected area
     - consider pathologic fracture with history of only minor trauma
   - physical exam: look (deformity, soft tissue integrity); feel (maximal tenderness, NVS-document best possible neurovascular exam, avoid ROM/moving injured area to prevent exacerbation)
2. **Analgesia**
3. **Imaging** (see *Orthopedic X-Ray Imaging*, OR7)
4. **Splint Extremity**
5. **Management: Closed vs. Open Reduction**
   1. obtain the reduction (for appropriate IV sedation see Table 27, OR48)
      - closed reduction
        - apply traction in the long axis of the limb
        - reverse the mechanism that produced the fracture
        - reduce with IV sedation and muscle relaxation (fluoroscopy can be used if available)
      - indications for open reduction
        - "NO CAST"
        - other indications include
          - failed closed reduction
          - not able to cast or apply traction due to site (e.g. hip fracture)
          - pathologic fractures
          - potential for improved function with ORIF
      - ALWAYS re-check and document NVS after reduction and obtain post-reduction x-ray

Displacement
Refers to position of the distal fragment relative to the proximal fragment

Varus/Valgus Angulation
Varus = Apex away from midline
Valgus = Apex toward midline

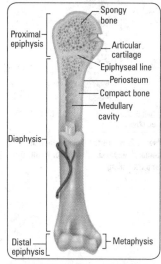

Spongy bone
Articular cartilage
Epiphyseal line
Periosteum
Compact bone
Medullary cavity
Proximal epiphysis
Diaphysis
Distal epiphysis
Metaphysis

Figure 5. Schematic diagram of the long bone

Quick Motor Nerve Exam
"Thumbs Up": PIN (Radial Nerve)
"OK Sign": AIN (Median Nerve)
"Spread Fingers": Ulnar Nerve

X-Ray Rule of 2s
2 sides = bilateral
2 views = AP + lateral
2 joints = joint above + below
2 times = before + after reduction

Reasons for Splinting
- Pain control
- Reduces further damage to vessels, nerves, and skin and may improve vascular status
- Decreases risk of inadvertently converting closed to open fracture
- Facilitates patient transport

Indications for Open Reduction

NO CAST
Non-union
Open fracture
Neurovascular **C**ompromise
Displaced intra-**A**rticular fracture
Salter-Harris 3,4,5
Poly**T**rauma

Buck's Traction
A system of weights, pulleys, and ropes that are attached to the end of a patient's bed exerting a longitudinal force on the distal end of a fracture, improving its length, alignment, and rotation

2. maintain the reduction
  - external stabilization: splints, casts, traction, external fixator
  - internal stabilization: percutaneous pinning, extramedullary fixation (screws, plates, wires), IM fixation (rods)
  - follow-up: evaluate bone healing
3. rehabilitate to regain function and avoid joint stiffness

Fracture Healing

Normal Healing

Weeks 0-3	Hematoma, macrophages surround fracture site
Weeks 3-6	Osteoclasts remove sharp edges, callus forms within hematoma
Weeks 6-12	Bone forms within the callus, bridging fragments
Months 6-12	Cortical gap is bridged by bone
Years 1-2	Normal architecture is achieved through remodelling

Figure 6. Stages of bone healing

Evaluation of Healing: Tests of Union
- clinical: no longer tender to palpation or stressing on physical exam
- x-ray: trabeculae cross fracture site, visible callus bridging site on at least 3 of 4 cortices

General Fracture Complications

Table 2. General Fracture Complications

	Early	Late
Local	Compartment syndrome Neurological injury Vascular injury Infection Implant failure Fracture blisters	Mal-/non-union AVN Osteomyelitis HO Post-traumatic OA Joint stiffness/adhesive capsulitis CRPS type I/RSD
Systemic	Sepsis DVT PE ARDS secondary to fat embolism Hemorrhagic shock	

Articular Cartilage

Properties
- 2-4 mm layer covering ends of articulating bones, provides nearly frictionless surface
- avascular (nutrition from synovial fluid), aneural, alymphatic

ARTICULAR CARTILAGE DEFECTS

Etiology
- overt trauma, repetitive minor trauma (such as repetitive ankle sprains or patellar maltracking); common sports injury
- degenerative conditions such as early stage OA or osteochondritis dissecans

Clinical Features
- similar to symptoms of OA (joint line pain with possible effusion, etc.)
- often have predisposing factors, such as ligament injury, malalignment of the joint (varus/valgus), obesity, bone deficiency (AVN, osteochondritis dissecans, ganglion bone cysts), inflammatory arthropathy, and familial osteoarthropathy
- may have symptoms of locking or catching related to the torn/displaced cartilage

Investigations
- x-ray (to rule out bony defects and check alignment)
- MRI
- diagnostic arthroscopy (treatment is often guided by what is seen during arthroscopy)

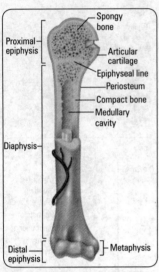

Figure 7. Heterotopic ossification of femoral diaphysis after femur fracture and IM nailing

Heterotopic Ossification
The formation of bone in abnormal locations (e.g. in muscle), secondary to pathology

Wolff's Law
Bone remodels itself to over time in response to mechanical load to better withstand loading stressors placed upon it

Avascular Necrosis
Ischemia of bone due to disrupted blood supply; most commonly affecting the femoral neck, talus neck or proximal scaphoid.

Fracture Blister
Formation of vesicles or bullae that occur on edematous skin overlying a fractured bone

Table 3. Outerbridge Classification of Chondral Defects

Grade	Chondral Damage
I	Softening and swelling of cartilage
II	Fragmentation and fissuring <1/2" in diameter
III	Fragmentation and fissuring >1/2" in diameter
IV	Erosion of cartilage down to bone

Treatment
- individualized
  - patient factors (age, skeletal maturity, activity level, etc.)
  - defect factors (Outerbridge Classification, subchondral bone involvement, etc.)
- non-operative
  - rest, NSAIDs, bracing
- operative
  - microfracture, osteochondral grafting (autograft or allograft), autologous chondrocyte implantation

Orthopedic X-Ray Imaging

General Principles
- x-ray 1 joint above and 1 below
- obtain at least 2 orthogonal views ± specialized views

CRPS/RSD
An exaggerated response to an insult in the extremities; characterized by symptoms of hyperalgesia and allodynia, with signs of autonomic dysfunction (temperature asymmetry, mottling, hair or nail changes)

Table 4. Orthopedic X-Ray Imaging

Site	Injury	X-Ray Views
Shoulder	Anterior dislocation Posterior dislocation AC Frozen shoulder	AP Axillary ± stress view with 10 lb in hand Trans-scapular Zanca view (10-15 cephalic tilt)
Arm	Humerus #	AP Lateral Trans-scapular Axillary
Elbow/Forearm	Supracondylar # Radial head # Monteggia # Night stick # Galeazzi #	AP Lateral
Wrist	Colles' # Smith # Scaphoid #	AP Lateral Scaphoid (wrist extension and ulnar deviation x 2 wk)
Pelvis	Pelvic #	AP pelvis Inlet and outlet views Judet views (obturator and iliac oblique for acetabular #)
Hip	Femoral head/neck # Intertrochanteric # Arthritis SCFE FAI	AP Lateral Frog-leg lateral Dunn
Knee	Knee dislocation Femur/tibia # Patella # Patella dislocation Patella femoral syndrome Tibia shaft #	AP standing, lateral Skyline – tangential view with knees flexed at 45° to see patellofemoral joint
Ankle	Ankle #	AP Lateral Mortise view: ankle at 15° of internal rotation
Foot	Talar # Calcanial #	AP Lateral Harris Axial
Spine	Compression # Burst # Cervical spine #	AP spine AP odontoid Lateral Oblique Swimmer's view: lateral view with arm abducted 180° to evaluate C7-T1 junction if lateral view is inadequate Lateral flexion/extension view: evaluate subluxation of cervical vertebrae

Orthopedic Emergencies

Trauma Patient Workup

Etiology
- high energy trauma e.g. MVC, fall from height
- may be associated with spinal injuries or life-threatening visceral injuries

Clinical Features
- local swelling, tenderness, deformity of the limbs, and instability of the pelvis or spine
- decreased level of consciousness, hypotension/hypovolemia
- consider involvement of EtOH or other substances

Investigations
- trauma survey (see Emergency Medicine, ER7, ER15)
- x-rays: lateral cervical spine, AP chest, AP pelvis, AP and lateral of all bones suspected to be injured
- CT is also utilized to inspect for musculoskeletal injuries in the trauma setting
- other views of pelvis: AP, inlet, and outlet; Judet views for acetabular fracture (for *Classification of Pelvic Fractures* see Table 18, OR27)

Treatment
- ABCDEs and initiate resuscitation for life threatening injuries
- assess genitourinary injury (rectal exam/vaginal exam mandatory)
- external or internal fixation of all fractures
- DVT prophylaxis

Complications
- hemorrhage – life threatening (may produce signs and symptoms of hypovolemic shock)
- fat embolism syndrome (SOB, hypoxemia, petechial rash, thrombocytopenia, and neurological symptoms)
- venous thrombosis – DVT and PE
- bladder/urethral/bowel injury
- neurological damage
- persistent pain/stiffness/limp/weakness in affected extremities
- post-traumatic OA of joints with intra-articular fractures
- sepsis if missed open fracture

Open Fractures

- fractured bone and hematoma in communication with the external or contaminated environment

Emergency Measures
- ABCs, primary survey and resuscitation as needed
- removal of obvious foreign material
- irrigate with normal saline if grossly contaminated
- cover wound with sterile dressings
- immediate IV antibiotics
- tetanus toxoid or immunoglobulin as needed
- reduce and splint fracture
- NPO and prepare for OR (blood work, consent, ECG, CXR)
  - operative irrigation and debridement within 6-8 h to decrease risk of infection
  - traumatic wound often left open to drain but vacuum-assisted closure dressing may be used
  - re-examine with repeat irrigation and debridement in 48 h

Table 5. Gustilo Classification of Open Fractures

Gustilo Grade	Length of Open Wound	Description	Prophylactic Antibiotic Regimen
I	<1 cm	Minimal contamination and soft tissue injury Simple or minimally comminuted fracture	First generation cephalosporin (cefazolin) for 3 d If allergy use floroquinolone If MRSA positive use vancomycin
II	1-10 cm	Moderate contamination Moderate soft tissue injury	As per Grade I
III*	>10 cm	IIIA: Extensive soft tissue injury with adequate ability of soft tissue to cover wound IIIB: Extensive soft tissue injury with periosteal stripping and bone exposure; inadequate soft tissue to cover wound IIIC: Vascular injury/compromise	First generation cephalosporin (cefazolin) for 3 d plus Gram-negative coverage (gentamicin) for at least 3 d For soil contamination, penicillin is added for clostridial coverage

*Any high energy, comminuted fracture, shot gun, farmyard/soil/water contamination, exposure to oral flora, or fracture >8 h old is immediately classified as Grade III

Orthopedic Emergencies

VON CHOP
Vascular compromise
Open fracture
Neurological compromise/cauda equina syndrome
Compartment syndrome
Hip dislocation
Osteomyelitis/septic arthritis
Unstable **P**elvic fracture

Controversies in Initial Management of Open Fractures
Scand J Surg 2014;103(2):132-137
Study: Literature review examining the initial management of open fractures. 40 studies included.
Findings:
- A first generation cephalosporin (or clindamycin) should be administered upon arrival. In general, 24 h of antibiotics after each debridement is sufficient to reduce infection rates.
- Although cultures are taken from delayed (>24 h) or infected injuries, it may not be necessary to routinely take post-debridement cultures in open fractures.
- Open fractures should be debrided as soon as possible although the "6-hr rule" is not generally valid.
- Wounds should be closed within 7 d once soft tissue has stabilized and all non-viable tissue removed.
- Negative pressure wound therapy (NPWT) has been shown to decrease infection rates in open fractures.

33% of patients with open fractures have multiple injuries

Antibiotics for Preventing Infection in Open Limb Fractures
Cochrane DB Syst Rev 2004;1:CD003764
Purpose: To review the evidence regarding the effectiveness of antibiotics in the initial treatment of open fractures of the limbs.
Methods: Randomized or quasi randomized controlled trials comparing antibiotic treatment with placebo or no treatment in preventing acute wound infection were identified and reviewed. Data were extracted and pooled for analysis.
Results: Eight studies (n=1,106) were reviewed. The use of antibiotics had a protective effect against early infection compared with no antibiotics or placebo (RRR=0.43, 95% CI 0.29, 0.65; ARR=0.07, 95% CI 0.03=0.10).
Conclusions: Antibiotics reduce the incidence of early infections in open fractures of the limbs.

Cauda Equina Syndrome

- see <u>Neurosurgery</u>, NS26

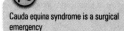
Cauda equina syndrome is a surgical emergency

Compartment Syndrome

- increased interstitial pressure in an anatomical compartment (forearm, calf) where muscle and tissue are bounded by fascia and bone (fibro-osseous compartment) with little room for expansion
- interstitial pressure exceeds capillary perfusion pressure leading to muscle necrosis (in 4-6 h) and eventually nerve necrosis

Etiology

- intracompartmental: fracture (particularly tibial shaft or paediatric supracondylar and forearm fractures)
  - Reperfusion injury, crush injury or ischemia
- extracompartmental: constrictive dressing (circumferential cast), poor position during surgery, circumferential burn

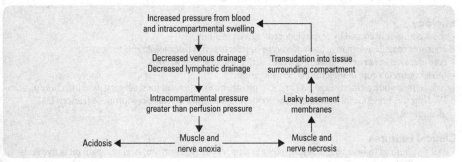

Figure 8. Pathogenesis of compartment syndrome

Clinical Features

- pain out of proportion to injury (typically first symptom)
- pain with active contraction of compartment
- pain with passive stretch (most sensitive)
- swollen, tense compartment
- suspicious history

- **5 Ps**: late sign – do not wait for these to develop to make the diagnosis!

Most important sign is increased pain with passive stretch. Most important symptom is pain out of proportion to injury

5 Ps of Compartment Syndrome
Pain: out of proportion for injury and not relieved by analgesics
- Increased pain with passive stretch of compartment muscles
Pallor: late finding
Paresthesia
Paralysis: late finding
Pulselessness: late finding

Investigations

- usually not necessary as compartment syndrome is a clinical diagnosis
- in children or unconscious patients where clinical exam is unreliable, compartment pressure monitoring with catheter AFTER clinical diagnosis is made (normal = 0 mmHg; elevated ≥30 mmHg or [measured pressure – dBP] ≤30 mmHg)

Treatment

- non-operative
  - remove constrictive dressings (casts, splints), elevate limb at the level of the heart
- operative
  - urgent fasciotomy
  - 48-72 h post-operative: wound closure ± necrotic tissue debridement

Complications

- Volkmann's ischemic contracture: ischemic necrosis of muscle, followed by secondary fibrosis and finally calcification; especially following supracondylar fracture of humerus
- rhabdomyolysis, renal failure secondary to myoglobinuria

Osteomyelitis

- bone infection with progressive inflammatory destruction

Etiology

- most commonly caused by *Staphylococcus aureus*
- mechanism of spread: hematogenous (most common) vs. direct-inoculation vs. contiguous focus
- risk factors: recent trauma/surgery, immunocompromised patients, DM, IV drug use, poor vascular supply, peripheral neuropathy

Plain Film Findings of Osteomyelitis
- Soft tissue swelling
- Lytic bone destruction*
- Periosteal reaction (formation of new bone, especially in response to #)*
*Generally not seen on plain films until 10-12 d after onset of infection

Rapid progression of signs and symptoms (over hours) necessitates need for serial examinations

Acute osteomyelitis is a medical emergency which requires an early diagnosis and appropriate antimicrobial and surgical treatment

Most commonly affected joints in descending order
knee → hip → elbow → ankle → sternoclavicular joint

Plain Film Findings in a Septic Joint
• Early (0-3 d): usually normal; may show soft-tissue swelling or joint space widening from localized edema
• Late (4-6 d): joint space narrowing and destruction of cartilage

Serial C-reactive protein (CRP) can be used to monitor response to therapy

Does This Adult Patient Have Septic Arthritis?
JAMA 2007;297(13):1478-1488
Purpose: To review the accuracy and precision of the clinical evaluation for the diagnosis of nongonococcal bacterial arthritis.
Methods: Review of 14 studies including 6242 patients of which 653 had positive synovial culture (gold standard diagnostic tool for septic arthritis).
Results/Conclusions: Age, diabetes mellitus, rheumatoid arthritis, joint surgery, hip or knee prosthesis, skin infection, and human immunodeficiency virus type 1 infection significantly increase the probability of septic arthritis. Joint pain, history of joint swelling, and fever are useful clinical findings in identifying patients with a monoarticular arthritis who may have septic arthritis. Laboratory findings from an arthrocentesis are also required and helpful prior to Gram stain and culture. The presence of increased WBC increases the likelihood ratio (for counts <25 000/μL: LR, 0.32; 95% CI, 0.23-0.43; for counts ≥25 000/μL: LR, 2.9; 95% CI, 2.5-3.4; for counts ≥100 000/μL: LR, 28.0; 95% CI, 12.0-66.0). A polymorphonuclear cell count of ≥90% increases the LR of septic arthritis by 3.4 while an PMN cell count of < 90% reduces the LR by 0.34.

Posterior Shoulder Dislocation
Up to 60-80% are missed on initial presentation due to poor physical exam and radiographs

Clinical Features

• symptoms: pain and fever
• on exam: erythema, tenderness, edema common ± abscess/draining sinus tract; impaired function/WB

Diagnosis

• see <u>Medical Imaging</u>, MI23
• workup includes: WBC and diff, ESR, CRP, blood culture, aspirate culture/bone biopsy

Table 6. Treatment of Osteomyelitis

Acute Osteomyelitis	Chronic Osteomyelitis
IV antibiotics 4-6 wk; started empirically and adjusted after obtaining blood and aspirate cultures ± surgery (I&D) for abscess or significant involvement ± hardware removal (if present)	Surgical debridement Antibiotics: both local (e.g. antibiotic beads) and systemic (IV)

Septic Joint

• joint infection with progressive destruction if left untreated

Etiology

• most commonly caused by Staphylococcus aureus in adults
• consider coagulase-negative *Staphylococcus* in patients with prior joint replacement
• consider *Neisseria gonorrhoeae* in sexually active adults and newborns
• most common route of infection is hematogenous
• risk factors: young/elderly (age >80 yr), RA, prosthetic joint, recent joint surgery, skin infection/ulcer, IV drug use, previous intra-articular corticosteroid injection, immune compromise (cancer, DM, alcoholism)

Clinical Features

• inability/refusal to bear weight, localized joint pain, erythema, warmth, swelling, pain on active and passive ROM, ± fever

Investigations

• x-ray (to rule out fracture, tumour, metabolic bone disease), ESR, CRP, WBC, blood cultures
• joint aspirate: cloudy yellow fluid, WBC >50,000 with >90% neutrophils, protein level >4.4 mg/dL, joint glucose level < 60% blood glucose level, no crystals, positive Gram stain results
• listen for heart murmur (to reduce suspicion of infective endocarditis, use Duke Criteria)

Treatment

• IV antibiotics, empiric therapy (based on age and risk factors), adjust following joint aspirate C&S results
• non-operative
  ▪ therapeutic joint aspiration, serially if necessary (if early diagnosis and joint superficial)
• operative
  ▪ arthroscopic/open irrigation and irrigation and drainage ± decompression

Shoulder

Shoulder Dislocation

• complete separation of the glenohumeral joint; may be anterior or posterior

Investigations

• anterior dislocation x-rays (AP, trans-scapular, axillary views)
• posterior dislocation x-rays (AP, trans-scapular, axillary) or CT scan

Table 7. Anterior and Posterior Shoulder Dislocation

	Anterior Shoulder Dislocation (>90%)	Posterior Shoulder Dislocation (5%)
MECHANISM		
	Abducted arm is externally rotated/hyperextended, or blow to posterior shoulder Involuntary, usually traumatic; voluntary, atraumatic	Adducted, internally rotated, flexed arm FOOSH 3 Es (epileptic seizure, EtOH, electrocution) Blow to anterior shoulder
CLINICAL FEATURES		
Symptoms	Pain, arm slightly abducted and externally rotated with inability to internally rotate	Pain, arm is held in adduction and internal rotation; external rotation is blocked
Shoulder Exam	"Squared off" shoulder Positive apprehension test: patient looks apprehensive with gentle shoulder abduction and external rotation to 90o since humeral head is pushed anteriorly and recreates feeling of anterior dislocation (see Figure 13) Positive relocation test: a posteriorly directed force applied during the apprehension test relieves apprehension since anterior subluxation is prevented Positive sulcus sign: presence of subacromial indentation with distal traction on humerus indicates inferior shoulder instability (see Figure 13)	Anterior shoulder flattening, prominent coracoid, palpable mass posterior to shoulder Positive posterior apprehension ("jerk") test: with patient supine, flex elbow 90° and adduct, internally rotate the arm while applying a posterior force to the shoulder; patient will "jerk" back with the sensation of subluxation (see Figure 13) Note: the posterior apprehension test is used to test for recurrent posterior instability, NOT for acute injury
Neurovascular Exam Including	Axillary nerve: sensory patch over deltoid and deltoid contraction Musculocutaneous nerve: sensory patch on lateral forearm and biceps contraction	Full neurovascular exam as per anterior shoulder dislocation
RADIOGRAPHIC FINDINGS		
Axillary View	Humeral head is anterior	Humeral head is posterior
Trans-scapular 'Y' View	Humeral head is anterior to the centre of the "Mercedes-Benz"sign	Humeral head is posterior to centre of "Mercedes-Benz" sign
AP View	Sub-coracoid lie of the humeral head is most common	Partial vacancy of glenoid fossa (vacant glenoid sign) and >6 mm space between anterior glenoid rim and humeral head (positive rim sign), humeral head may resemble a lightbulb due to internal rotation (lightbulb sign)
Hill-Sachs and Bony Bankart Lesions	± Hill-Sachs lesion: compression fracture of posterior humeral head due to forceful impaction of an anteriorly dislocated humeral head against the glenoid rim (see Figure 12) ± bony Bankart lesion: avulsion of the anterior glenoid labrum (with attached bone fragments) from the glenoid rim (see Figure 12)	± reverse Hill-Sachs lesion (75% of cases): divot in anterior humeral head ± reverse bony Bankart lesion: avulsion of the posterior glenoid labrum from the bony glenoid rim
TREATMENT		
	Closed reduction with IV sedation and muscle relaxation Traction-countertraction: assistant stabilizes torso with a folded sheet wrapped across the chest while the surgeon applies gentle steady traction Stimson: while patient lies prone with arm hanging over table edge, hang a 5 lb weight on wrist for 15-20 min Hippocratic method: place heel into patient's axilla and apply traction to arm Cunningham's method: low risk, low pain; if not successful try above methods Obtain post-reduction x-rays Check post-reduction NVS Sling x 3 wk (avoid abduction and external rotation), followed by shoulder rehabilitation (dynamic stabilizer strengthening)	Closed reduction with sedation and muscle relaxation Inferior traction on a flexed elbow with pressure on the back of the humeral head Obtain post-reduction x-rays Check post-reduction NVS Sling in abduction and external rotation x 3 wk, followed by shoulder rehabilitation (dynamic stabilizer strengthening)

Prognosis
- recurrence rate depends on age of first dislocation
- <20 yr = 65-95%; 20-40 yr = 60-70%; >40 yr = 2-4%

Specific Complications
- rotator cuff or capsular or labral tear (Bankart/SLAP lesion), shoulder stiffness
- injury to axillary nerve/artery, brachial plexus
- recurrent/unreduced dislocation (most common complication)

There are 4 Joints in the Shoulder
glenohumeral, AC, sternoclavicular (SC), scapulothoracjc
Shoulder passive ROM: abduction – 180°, adduction – 45°, flexion – 180°, extension – 45°, int. rotation – level of T4, ext. rotation – 40-45°

Factors Causing Shoulder Instability
- Shallow glenoid
- Loose capsule
- Ligamentous laxity
Frequency of Dislocations
- Anterior shoulder > Posterior shoulder
- Posterior hip > Anterior hip
The glenohumeral joint is the most commonly dislocated joint in the body since stability is sacrificed for motion

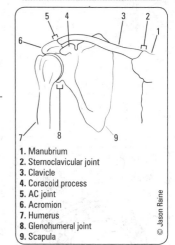

1. Manubrium
2. Sternoclavicular joint
3. Clavicle
4. Coracoid process
5. AC joint
6. Acromion
7. Humerus
8. Glenohumeral joint
9. Scapula

Figure 9. Shoulder joints

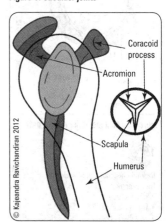

Figure 10. Mercedes-Benz

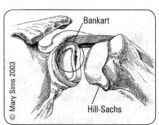

Figure 11. Posterior view of anterior dislocation causing Hill-Sachs and Bankart lesions

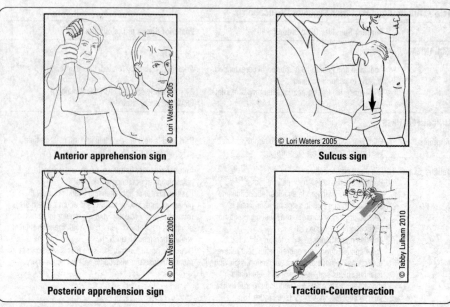

Figure 12. Shoulder maneuvers

Rotator Cuff Disease

- rotator cuff consists of 4 muscles that act to stabilize humeral head within the glenoid fossa

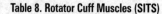

Table 8. Rotator Cuff Muscles (SITS)

Muscle	Muscle Attachments		Nerve Supply	Muscle Function
	Proximal	Distal		
Supraspinatus	Scapula	Greater tuberosity of humerus	Suprascapular nerve	Abduction
Infraspinatus	Scapula	Greater tuberosity of humerus	Suprascapular nerve	External rotation
Teres Minor	Scapula	Greater tuberosity of humerus	Axillary nerve	External rotation
Subscapularis	Scapula	Lesser tuberosity of humerus	Subscapular nerve	Internal rotation and adduction

SPECTRUM OF DISEASE: IMPINGEMENT, TENDONITIS, MICRO OR MACRO TEARS

Etiology
- anything that leads to a narrow subacromial space
- most commonly, a relative imbalance of rotator cuff and larger shoulder muscles allowing for superior translation and subsequent wear of the rotator cuff muscle tendons
  - glenohumeral muscle weakness leading to abnormal motion of humeral head
  - scapular muscle weakness leading to abnormal motion of acromion
  - acromial abnormalities such as congenital narrow space or osteophyte formation or Type III acromion morphology
    1. outlet/subacromial impingement: "painful arc syndrome", compression of rotator cuff tendons (primarily supraspinatus) and subacromial bursa between the head of the humerus and the undersurface of acromion, AC joint, and CA ligament
    2. bursitis and tendonitis
    3. rotator cuff thinning and tear if left untreated

Clinical Features
- insidious onset, but may present as an acute exacerbation of chronic disease, night pain and difficulty sleeping on affected side
- pain worse with active motion (especially overhead); passive movement generally permitted
- weakness and loss of ROM especially between 90°-130° (e.g. trouble with overhead activities)
- tenderness to palpation over greater tuberosity
- rule out bicep tendinosis: Speed test; SLAP lesion: O'Brien's test

Investigations
- x-ray: AP view may show high riding humerus relative to glenoid indicating large tear, evidence of chronic tendonitis
- MRI: coronal/sagittal oblique and axial orientations are useful for assessing full/partial tears and tendinopathy ± arthrogram: geyser sign (injected dye leaks out of joint through rotator cuff tear)
- arthrogram: can assess full thickness tears, difficult to assess partial tears

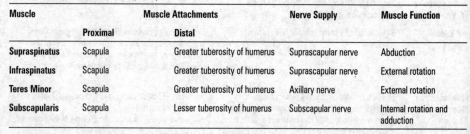

Figure 13. Muscles of the rotator cuff

Treatment

- non-operative
  - for mild ("wear") or moderate ("tear") cases
  - physiotherapy, NSAIDs ± steroid injection
- operative
  - indication: severe ("repair")
  - impingement that is refractory to 2-3 mo physiotherapy and 1-2 corticosteroid injections
  - arthroscopic or open surgical repair (i.e. acromioplasty, rotator cuff repair)

Table 9. Rotator Cuff Special Tests

Test	Examination	Positive Test
Jobe's Test	Supraspinatus: place the shoulder in 90° of abduction and 30° of forward flexion and internally rotate the arm so that the thumb is pointing toward the floor	Weakness with active resistance suggests a supraspinatus tear
Lift-off Test	Subscapularis: internally rotate arm so dorsal surface of hand rests on lower back; patient instructed to actively lift hand away from back against examiner resistance (use Belly Press Test if too painful)	Inability to actively lift hand away from back suggests a subscapularis tear
Posterior-Cuff Test	Infraspinatus and teres minor: arm positioned at patient's side in 90° of flexion; patient instructed to externally rotate arm against the resistance of the examiner	Weakness with active resistance suggests posterior cuff tear
Neer's Test	Rotator cuff impingement: passive shoulder flexion	Pain elicited between 130-170° suggests impingement
Hawkins-Kennedy Test	Rotator cuff impingement: shoulder flexion to 90° and passive internal rotation	Pain with internal rotation suggests impingement
Painful Arc Test	Rotator cuff tendinopathy: patient instructed to actively abduct the shoulder	Pain with abduction >90° suggests tendinopathy
Speed's Test	Apply resistance to the forearm when the arm is in forward flexion with the elbows fully extended.	Pain in the bicipital groove
O'Brien's Test	SLAP lesion: forward flexion of the arm to 90 degrees while keeping the arm extended. Arm is adducted 10-15 degrees. Internally rotate the arm so thumb is facing down and apply a downward force. Repeat the test with arm externally rotated	Pain or clicking in the glenohumoral joint in internal rotation but not external rotation

Ruling in Rotator Cuff Tears – 98% probability of rotator cuff tear if all 3 of the following are present:
- Supraspinatus weakness
- External rotation weakness
- Positive impingement sign(s)

Diagnosis of rotator cuff tears. *Lancet* 2001; 357:769-770

Does this Patient with Shoulder Pain have Rotator Cuff Disease? The Rational Clinical Examination Systematic Review
JAMA 2013;310:837-847
Study: 5 studies of sufficient quality including 30-203 shoulders and a prevalence of RCD ranging from 33-81%.
Results/Conclusions: Among pain provocation tests, a positive painful arc test had the greatest specificity and sensitivity (SP 81%, SN 71%) Among strength tests, a positive external rotation lag test and internal rotation lag test were the most accurate for full-thickness tears (SP 47%, SN 94%; SP 97%, SN 83% respectively). The internal rotation lag test was therefore also the most accurate for identifying patients without a full-thickness tear. A positive drop arm test is helpful to identify patients with RCD (SN 24%, SP 93%).

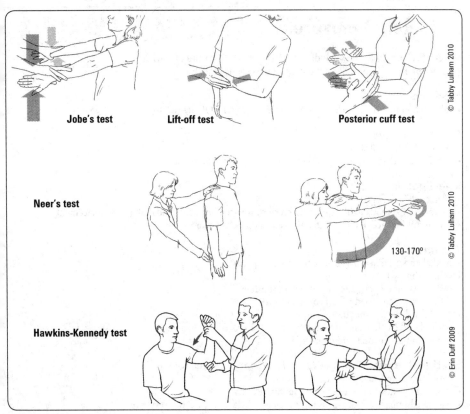

Figure 14. Rotator cuff tests

Acromioclavicular Joint Pathology

- subluxation or dislocation of AC joint
- 2 main ligaments attach clavicle to scapula: AC and CC ligaments

Mechanism
- fall onto shoulder with adducted arm or direct trauma to point of shoulder

Clinical Features
- pain with adduction of shoulder and/or palpation over AC joint
- palpate step deformity between distal clavicle and acromion (with dislocation)
- limited ROM

Investigations
- x-rays: bilateral AP, Zanca view (10-15° cephalic tilt), axillary

Treatment
- **non-operative**
  - sling 1-3 wk, ice, analgesia, early ROM and rehabilitation
- **operative**
  - indication: Rockwood Class IV-VI (III if labourer or high level athlete)
  - number of different approaches involving AC/CC ligament reconstruction or screw/hook plate insertion

Pneumothorax or pulmonary contusion are potential complications of severe AC joint dislocation

Table 10. Rockwood Classification of Acromioclavicular Joint Separation

Grade	Features	Treatment
I	Joint sprain, absence of complete tear of either ligament	Non-operative
II	Complete tear of AC ligament, incomplete tear of CC ligament, without marked elevation of lateral clavicular head	Non-operative
III	Complete tear of AC and CC ligaments, >5 mm elevation at AC joint, superior aspect of acromion is below the inferior aspect of the clavicle	Most non-operative, operative if labourer or high level athlete Will heal with step deformity, although most fully functional in 4-6 mo
IV-VI	Based on the anatomical structure the displaced clavicle is in proximity with	Operative in most cases

Clavicle Fracture

- incidence: proximal (5%), middle (80%), or distal (15%) third of clavicle
- common in children (unites rapidly without complications)

Mechanism
- fall on shoulder (87%), direct trauma to clavicle (7%), FOOSH (6%)

Clinical Features
- pain and tenting of skin
- arm is clasped to chest to splint shoulder and prevent movement

Investigations
- evaluate NVS of entire upper limb
- x-ray: AP, 45° cephalic tilt (superior/inferior displacement), 45° caudal tilt (AP displacement)
- CT: useful for medial physeal fractures and sternoclavicular injury

Associated Injuries with Clavicle Fractures
- Up to 9% of clavicle fractures are associated with other fractures (most commonly rib fractures)
- Majority of brachial plexus injuries are associated with proximal third fractures

Treatment
- medial and middle third clavicle fractures
- simple sling x 1-2 wk
- early ROM and strengthening once pain subsides
- if fracture is shortened >2 cm consider ORIF
- distal third clavicle fractures
- undisplaced (with ligaments intact): sling x 1-2 wk
- displaced (CC ligament injury): ORIF

Specific Complications (see *General Fracture Complications*, OR6)
- cosmetic bump usually only complication
- shoulder stiffness, weakness with repetitive activity
- pneumothorax, brachial plexus injuries, and subclavian vessel (all very rare)

Frozen Shoulder (Adhesive Capsulitis)

- disorder characterized by progressive pain and stiffness of the shoulder usually resolving spontaneously after 18 mo

Mechanism
- primary adhesive capsulitis
  - idiopathic, usually associated with DM
  - usually resolves spontaneously in 9-18 mo
- secondary adhesive capsulitis
  - due to prolonged immobilization
  - shoulder-hand syndrome: CRPS/RSD characterized by arm and shoulder pain, decreased motion, and diffuse swelling
  - following MI, stroke, shoulder trauma
  - poorer outcomes

Clinical Features
- gradual onset (weeks to months) of diffuse shoulder pain with:
  - decreased active AND passive ROM
  - pain worse at night and often prevents sleeping on affected side
  - increased stiffness as pain subsides: continues for 6-12 mo after pain has disappeared

Investigations
- x-ray: AP (neutral, internal/external rotation), scapular Y, axillary
  - may be normal, or may show demineralization from disease

Treatment
- freezing phase
  - active and passive ROM (physiotherapy)
    - NSAIDs and steroid injections if limited by pain
- thawing phase
  - manipulation under anesthesia and early physiotherapy
    - arthroscopy for debridement/decompression

Conditions Associated with an Increased Incidence of Adhesive Capsulitis
- Prolonged immobilization (most significant)
- Female gender
- Age >49 yr
- DM (5x)
- Cervical disc disease
- Hyperthyroidism
- Stroke
- MI
- Trauma and surgery
- Autoimmune disease

Stages of Adhesive Capsulitis
1. Freezing phase: gradual onset, diffuse pain (lasts 6-9 mo)
2. Frozen phase: decreased ROM impacting functioning (lasts 4-9 mo)
3. Thawing phase: gradual return of motion (lasts 5-26 mo)

Humerus

Proximal Humeral Fracture

Mechanism
- young: high energy trauma (MVC)
- elderly: FOOSH from standing height in osteoporotic individuals

Clinical Features
- proximal humeral tenderness, deformity with severe fracture, swelling, painful ROM, bruising extends down arm and chest

Investigations
- test axillary nerve function (deltoid contraction and skin over deltoid)
- x-rays: AP, trans-scapular, axillary are essential
- CT scan: to evaluate for articular involvement and fracture displacement

Classification
- Neer classification is based on 4 fracture locations or 'parts'
- displaced: displacement >1 cm and/or angulation >45°
- the Neer system regards the number of displaced fractures, not the fracture line, in determining classification
- ± dislocated/subluxed: humeral head dislocated/subluxed from glenoid

Treatment
- treat osteoporosis if needed
- non-operative
  - nondisplaced: broad arm sling immobilization, begin ROM within 14 d to prevent stiffness
  - minimally displaced (85% of patients) - closed reduction with sling immobilization x 2 wk, gentle ROM
- operative
  - ORIF (anatomic neck fractures, displaced, associated dislocated glenohumeral joint)
  - hemiarthroplasty or reverse TSA may be necessary, especially in elderly

Specific Complications (see *General Fracture Complications*, OR6)
- AVN, nerve palsy (45%; typically axillary nerve), malunion, post-traumatic arthritis

Neer Classification
Based on 4 parts of humerus
- Greater Tuberosity
- Lesser Tuberosity
- Humeral Head
- Shaft

One-part fracture: any of the 4 parts with none displaced
Two-part fracture: any of the 4 parts with 1 displaced
Three-part fracture: displaced fracture of surgical neck + displaced greater tuberosity or lesser tuberosity
Four-part fracture: displaced fracture of surgical neck + both tuberosities

Anatomic neck fractures disrupt blood supply to the humeral head and AVN of the humeral head may ensue

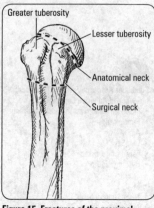

Figure 15. Fractures of the proximal humerus

Acceptable Humeral Shaft Deformities for Non-Operative Treatment
- <20° anterior angulation
- <30° varus angulation
- <3 cm of shortening

Risk of radial nerve and brachial artery injury

The anterior humeral line refers to an imaginary line drawn along the anterior surface of the humeral cortex that passes through the middle third of the capitellum when extended inferiorly. In subtle supracondylar fractures the anterior humeral line is disrupted, typically passing through the anterior third of the capitellum

Humeral Shaft Fracture

Mechanism
- high energy: direct blows/MVC (especially young); low energy: FOOSH, twisting injuries, metastases (in elderly)

Clinical Features
- pain, swelling, weakness ± shortening, motion/crepitus at fracture site
- must test radial nerve function before and after treatment: look for drop wrist, sensory impairment dorsum of hand

Investigations
- x-ray: AP and lateral radiographs of the humerus including the shoulder and elbow joints

Treatment
- in general, humeral shaft fractures are treated non-operatively
- non-operative
  - ± reduction; can accept deformity due to compensatory ROM of shoulder
  - hanging cast (weight of arm in cast provides traction across fracture site) with collar and cuff sling immobilization until swelling subsides, then Sarmiento functional brace, followed by ROM
- operative
  - indications: see "NO CAST" (OR5), pathological fracture, "floating elbow" (simultaneous unstable humeral and forearm fractures)
  - ORIF: plating (most common), IM rod insertion, external fixation

Specific Complications (see *General Fracture Complications*, OR6)
- radial nerve palsy: expect spontaneous recovery in 3-4 mo, otherwise send for EMG
- non-union: most frequently seen in middle 1/3
- decreased ROM
- compartment syndrome

Distal Humeral Fracture

Mechanism
- young: high energy trauma (MVC)
- elderly: FOOSH

Clinical Features
- elbow pain and swelling
- assess brachial artery

Investigations
- x-ray: AP and lateral of humerus and elbow
- CT scan: helpful when suspect shear fracture of capitulum or trochlea

Classification
- supracondylar, distal single column, distal bicolumnar and coronal shear fractures

Treatment
- goal is to restore ROM 30-130° flexion (unsatisfactory outcomes in 25%)
- non-operative
  - cast immobilization (in supination for lateral condyle fracture; pronation for medial condyle fractures)
- operative
  - indications: displaced, supracondylar, bicolumnar
  - closed reduction and percunatneous pinning; ORIF; total elbow arthroplasty (bicolumnar in elderly)

Elbow

Supracondylar Fracture

- subclass of distal humerus fracture: extra-articular, fracture proximal to capitulum and trochlea, usually transverse
- most common in pediatric population (peak age ~7 yr old), rarely seen in adults
- AIN (median nerve) injury commonly associated with extension type

Mechanism
- >96% are extension injuries via FOOSH (e.g. fall off monkey bars); <4% are flexion injuries

Clinical Features
- pain, swelling, point tenderness
- neurovascular injury: assess median and radial nerves, radial artery (check radial pulse)

Investigations
- x-ray: AP, lateral of elbow
  - disruption of anterior humeral line suggests supracondylar fracture
  - fat pad sign: a sign of effusion and can be indicative of occult fracture

Treatment
- reduction indications: evidence of arterial obstruction, unacceptable angulation, displaced (>50%)
- non-operative
  - nondisplaced: long arm plaster slab in 90° flexion x 3 wk
- operative
  - indications: displaced, vascular injury, open fracture
  - requires percutaneous pinning followed by limb cast with elbow flexed <90o
  - in adults, ORIF is necessary

Specific Complications (see *General Fracture Complications*, OR6)
- stiffness is most common
- brachial artery injury (kinking can occur if displaced fracture), median or ulnar nerve injury, compartment syndrome (leads to Volkmann's ischemic contracture), malalignment cubitus varus (distal fragment tilted into varus)

Radial Head Fracture

- a common fracture of the upper limb in young adults

Mechanism
- FOOSH with elbow extended and forearm pronated

Clinical Features
- marked local tenderness on palpation over radial head (lateral elbow)
- decreased ROM at elbow, ± mechanical block to forearm pronation and supination
- pain on pronation/supination

Investigations
- x-ray: enlarged anterior fat pad ("sail sign") or the presence of a posterior fat pad indicates effusion which could occur with occult radial head fractures

Table 11. Classification and Treatment of Radial Head Fractures

Mason Class	Radiographic Description	Treatment
1	Nondisplaced fracture	Elbow slab or sling x 3-5 d with early ROM
2	Displaced fracture	ORIF if: angulation >30°, involves ≥1/3 of the radial head, or if ≥3 mm of joint incongruity exists
3	Comminuted fracture	Radial head excision ± prosthesis (if ORIF not feasible)
4	Comminuted fracture with posterior elbow dislocation	Radial head excision ± prosthesis

Specific Complications (see *General Fracture Complications*, OR6)
- myositis ossificans – calcification of muscle
- recurrent instability (if MCL injured and radial head excised)

Three Joints at the Elbow
- Humeroradial joint
- Humeroulnar joint
- Radioulnar joint

Normal carrying angle of elbow is ~10° of valgus

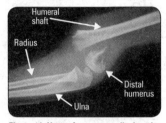

Figure 16. X-ray of transverse displaced supracondylar fracture of humerus with elbow dislocation

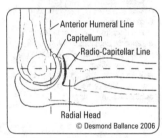

Figure 17. Lateral view of elbow

Terrible Triad
- Radial head fracture
- Coronoid fracture
- Elbow dislocation

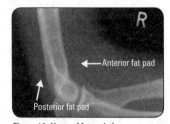

Figure 18. X-ray of fat pad sign

To avoid stiffness do not immobilize elbow joint >2-3 wk

Olecranon Fracture

Mechanism
- direct trauma to posterior aspect of elbow (fall onto the point of the elbow) or FOOSH

Clinical Features
- localized pain, palpable defect
- ± loss of active extension due to avulsion of triceps tendon

Investigations
- x-ray: AP and lateral (require true lateral to determine fracture pattern)

Treatment
- non-operative
  - non-displaced (<2 mm, stable): cast x 3 wk (elbow in 90° flexion) then gentle ROM
- operative
  - displaced: ORIF (plate and screws or tension band wiring) and early ROM if stable

Elbow Dislocation

- third most common joint dislocation after shoulder and patella
- anterior capsule and collateral ligaments disrupted

Mechanism
- elbow hyperextension via FOOSH or valgus/supination stress during elbow flexion
- usually the radius and ulna are dislocated together, or the radius head dislocates and the ulna remains ("Monteggia")
- 80% are posterior/posterolateral, anterior are rare and usually devastating

Clinical Features
- elbow pain, swelling, deformity
- flexion contracture
- ± absent radial or ulnar pulses

Investigations
- x-ray: AP and lateral views

Treatment
- assess NVS before reduction: brachial artery, median and ulnar nerves (can become entrapped during manipulation)
- non-operative
  - closed reduction under conscious sedation (post-reduction x-rays required)
  - Parvin's method: patient lies prone with arm hanging down; apply gentle traction downwards on wrist, as olecranon slips distally, gently lift up the arm at elbow to reduce joint
  - long-arm splint with forearm in neutral rotation and elbow in 90° flexion
  - early ROM (<2 wk)
- operative
  - indications: complex dislocation or persistent instability after closed reduction
  - ORIF

Specific Complications (see *General Fracture Complications*, OR6)
- stiffness (loss of extension), intra-articular loose body, neurovascular injury (ulnar nerve, median nerve, brachial artery), radial head fracture
- recurrent instability uncommon

Epicondylitis

- lateral epicondylitis = "tennis elbow", inflammation of the common extensor tendon as it inserts into the lateral epicondyle
- medial epicondylitis = "golfer's elbow", inflammation of the common flexor tendon as it inserts into the medial epicondyle

Mechanism
- repeated or sustained contraction of the forearm muscles/chronic overuse

Clinical Features
- point tenderness over humeral epicondyle and/or distal to it
- pain upon resisted wrist extension (lateral epicondylitis) or wrist flexion (medial epicondylitis)
- generally a self-limited condition, but may take 6-18 mo to resolve

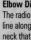

Elbow Dislocation
The radio-capitellar line refers to an imaginary line along the longitudinal axis of the radial neck that passes through the centre of the capitellum regardless of the degree of elbow flexion. If the radio-capitellar line does not pass through the centre of the capitellum a dislocation should be suspected

Tennis Elbow = laTeral epicondylitis; pain associated with exTension of wrist

Treatment
- non-operative (very good outcomes)
  - rest, ice, NSAIDs
  - use brace/strap
  - physiotherapy, stretching, and strengthening
  - corticosteroid injection
- operative
  - indication: failed 6-12 mo conservative therapy
  - percutaneous or open release of common tendon from epicondyle

Elbow Joint Injection
Inject at the centre of the triangle formed by the lateral epicondyle, radial head, and olecranon

Forearm

Radius and Ulna Shaft Fractures

Mechanism
- high energy direct or indirect (MVA, fall from height, sports) trauma
- fractures usually accompanied by displacement due to high force

Clinical Features
- deformity, pain, swelling
- loss of function in hand and forearm

Investigations
- x-ray: AP and lateral of forearm ± oblique of elbow and wrist
- CT if fracture is close to joint

Treatment
- goal is anatomic reduction since imperfect alignment significantly limits forearm pronation and supination
- ORIF with plates and screws; closed reduction with immobilization usually yields poor results for displaced forearm fractures (except in children)

Specific Complications (see *General Fracture Complications*, OR6)
- soft tissue contracture resulting in limited forearm rotation – surgical release of tissue may be warranted

Monteggia Fracture

- fracture of the proximal ulna with radial head dislocation and proximal radioulnar joint injury
- more common and better prognosis in the pediatric age group when compared to adults

Mechanism
- direct blow on the posterior aspect of the forearm
- hyperpronation
- fall on the hyperextended elbow

Clinical Features
- pain, swelling, decreased rotation of forearm ± palpable lump at the radial head
- ulna angled apex anterior and radial head dislocated anteriorly (rarely the reverse deformity occurs)

Investigations
- x-ray: AP, lateral elbow, wrist and forearm

Treatment
- adults: ORIF of ulna with indirect radius reduction in 90% of patients (ORIF of radius if unsuccessful)
- splint and early post-operative ROM if elbow completely stable, otherwise immobilization in plaster with elbow flexed for 6 wk
- pediatrics: attempt closed reduction and immobilization in plaster with elbow flexed for Bado Type I-III, surgery for Type IV

Specific Complications (see *General Fracture Complications*, OR6)
- PIN: most common nerve injury; observe for 3 mo as most resolve spontaneously
- radial head instability/redislocation
- radioulnar synostosis

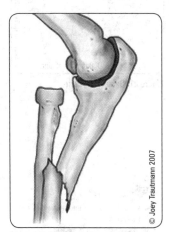
Figure 19. Monteggia fracture

In all isolated ulna fractures, assess proximal radius to rule out a Monteggia fracture

Bado Type Classification of Monteggia Fractures
Based on the direction of displacement of the dislocated radial head, generally the same direction as the apex of the ulnar fracture
Type I: anterior dislocation of radial head and proximal/middle third ulnar fracture (60%)
Type II: posterior dislocation of radial head and proximal/middle third ulnar fracture (15%)
Type III: lateral dislocation of radial head and metaphyseal ulnar fracture (20%)
Type IV – combined: proximal fracture of the ulna and radius, dislocation of the radial head in any direction (<5%)

Nightstick Fracture

- isolated fracture of ulna without dislocation of radial head

Mechanism
- direct blow to forearm (e.g. holding arm up to protect face)

Treatment
- non-operative
  - non-displaced
  - below elbow cast (x 10 d) followed by forearm brace (~8 wk)
- operative
  - displaced
  - ORIF if >50% shaft displacement or >10° angulation

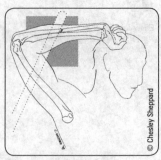
Figure 20. Nightstick fracture
© Chesley Sheppard

For all isolated radius fractures assess DRUJ to rule out a Galeazzi fracture

Galeazzi Fracture

- fracture of the distal radial shaft with disruption of the DRUJ
- most commonly in the distal 1/3 of radius near junction of metaphysis/diaphysis

Mechanism
- hand FOOSH with axial loading of pronated forearm or direct wrist trauma

Clinical Features
- pain, swelling, deformity and point tenderness at fracture site

Investigations
- x-ray: AP, lateral elbow, wrist and forearm
- shortening of distal radius >5 mm relative to the distal ulna
- widening of the DRUJ space on AP
- dislocation of radius with respect to ulna on true lateral

Treatment
- all cases are operative
  - ORIF of radius; afterwards assess DRUJ stability by balloting distal ulna relative to distal radius
  - if DRUJ is stable and reducible, splint for 10-14 d with early ROM encouraged
  - if DRUJ is unstable, ORIF or percutaneous pinning with long arm cast in supination x 6 wk

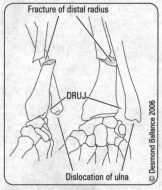
Fracture of distal radius

DRUJ

Dislocation of ulna

Figure 21. Galeazzi fracture
© Desmond Ballance 2006

Wrist

Colles' Fracture

- extra-articular transverse distal radius fracture (~2 cm proximal to the radiocarpal joint) with dorsal displacement ± ulnar styloid fracture
- most common fracture in those >40 yr, especially in women and those with osteoporotic bone

Mechanism
- FOOSH

Clinical Features
- "dinner fork" deformity
- swelling, ecchymoses, tenderness

Investigations
- x-ray: AP and lateral wrist

Treatment
- goal is to restore radial height (13 mm), radial inclination (22°), volar tilt (11°) as well as DRUJ stability and useful forearm rotation
- non-operative
  - closed reduction (think opposite of the deformity)
    - hematoma block (sterile prep and drape, local anesthetic injection directly into fracture site) or conscious sedation
    - closed reduction: 1) traction with extension (exaggerate injury), 2) traction with ulnar deviation, pronation, flexion (of distal fragment – not at wrist)
    - dorsal slab/below elbow cast for 5-6 wk
    - x-ray at 1 wk, 3 wk and at cessation of immobilization to ensure reduction is maintained
  - obtain post-reduction films immediately; repeat reduction if necessary

Indications for surgical management of Colles' Fracture
- Displaced intra-articular fracture
- Comminuted
- Severe osteoporosis
- Dorsal angulation >5° or volar tilt >20°
- >5 mm radial shortening

ORIF Colles' Fracture if Post-Reduction Demonstrates
- Radial shortening >3 mm or,
- Dorsal tilt >10° or,
- Intra-articular displacement/step-off >2 mm

- operative
  - indication: failed closed reduction, or loss of reduction
  - percutaneous pinning, external fixation or ORIF

Smith's Fracture

- volar displacement of the distal radius (i.e. reverse Colles' fracture)

Mechanism
- fall onto the back of the flexed hand

Investigations
- x-ray: AP and lateral wrist

Treatment
- usually unstable and needs ORIF
- if patient is poor operative candidate, may attempt non-operative treatment
  - closed reduction with hematoma block (reduction opposite of Colles')
  - long-arm cast in supination x 6 wk

Complications of Wrist Fractures

- most common complications are poor grip strength, stiffness, and radial shortening
- distal radius fractures in individuals <40 yr of age are usually highly comminuted and are likely to require ORIF
- 80% have normal function in 6-12 mo

Table 12. Early and Late Complications of Wrist Fractures

Early	Late
Difficult reduction ± loss of reduction	Malunion, radial shortening
Compartment syndrome	Painful wrist secondary to ulnar prominence
Extensor pollicis longus tendon rupture	Frozen shoulder ("shoulder-hand syndrome")
Acute carpal tunnel syndrome	Post-traumatic arthritis
Finger swelling with venous block	Carpal tunnel syndrome
Complications of a tight cast/splint	CRPS/RSD

Scaphoid Fracture

Epidemiology
- common in young men; not common in children or in patients beyond middle age
- most common carpal bone injured
- may be associated with other carpal or wrist injuries (e.g. Colles' fracture)

Mechanism
- FOOSH: impaction of scaphoid on distal radius, most commonly resulting in a transverse fracture through the waist (65%), distal (10%), or proximal (25%) scaphoid

Clinical Features
- pain with resisted pronation
- tenderness in the anatomical "snuff box", over scaphoid tubercle, and pain with long axis compression into scaphoid
- usually nondisplaced

Investigations
- x-ray: AP, lateral, scaphoid views with wrist extension and ulnar deviation
- ± CT or MRI
- bone scan rarely used
- note: a fracture may not be radiologically evident up to 2 wk after acute injury, so if a patient complains of wrist pain and has anatomical snuff box tenderness but a negative x-ray, treat as if positive for a scaphoid fracture and repeat x-ray 2 wk later to rule out a fracture; if x-ray still negative order CT or MRI

Treatment
- early treatment critical for improving outcomes
- non-operative
  - non-displaced (<1 mm displacement/<15° angulation): long-arm thumb spica cast x 4 wk then short arm cast until radiographic evidence of healing is seen (2-3 mo)
- operative
  - displaced: ORIF with headless/countersink compression screw is the mainstay treatment

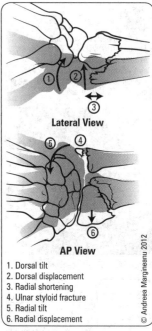

1. Dorsal tilt
2. Dorsal displacement
3. Radial shortening
4. Ulnar styloid fracture
5. Radial tilt
6. Radial displacement

Figure 22. Colles' fracture and associated bony deformity

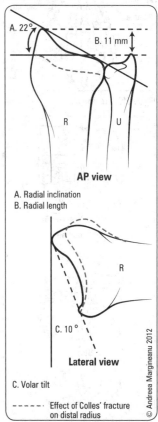

A. Radial inclination
B. Radial length

C. Volar tilt

- - - - - Effect of Colles' fracture on distal radius

Figure 23. Normal wrist angles + wrist angles in Colles' fracture
Note the relative shortening of the radius relative to the ulna on AP view in Colles' fracture

Scaphoid Fracture Special Tests
Tender snuff box: 100% sensitivity, but 29% specific as positive with many other injuries of radial aspect of wrist with FOOSH

Hand

The proximal pole of the scaphoid receives as much as 100% of its arterial blood supply from the radial artery that enters at the distal pole. A fracture through the proximal third disrupts this blood supply and results in a high incidence of AVN/non-union

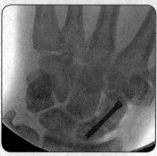

Figure 24. ORIF left scaphoid

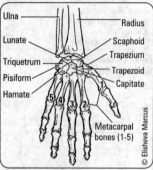

Figure 25. Carpal bones

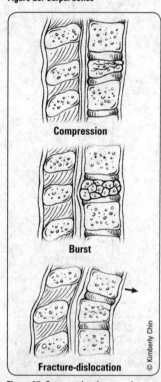

Figure 27. Compression, burst, and dislocation fractures

Specific Complications (see *General Fracture Complications*, OR6)
• most common: non-union/mal-union (use bone graft from iliac crest or distal radius with fixation to heal)
• AVN of the proximal fragment
• delayed union (recommend surgical fixation)
• scaphoid nonunion advanced collapse (SNAC) – chronic nonunion leading to advanced collapse and arthritis of wrist

Prognosis
• proximal fifth fracture: AVN rate 100%; proximal third fracture: AVN rate 33%
• waist fractures have healing rates of 80-90%
• distal third fractures have healing rates close to 100%

Hand

• see Plastic Surgery, PL22

Spine

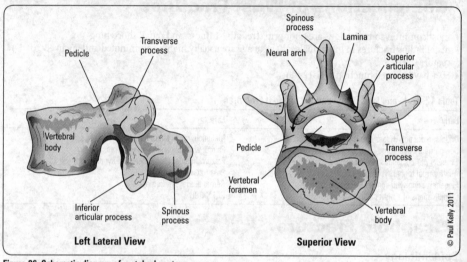

Figure 26. Schematic diagram of vertebral anatomy
Adapted from: Moore KL, Agur AMR. Essential Clinical Anatomy, 3rd ed. Philadephia: Lippincott Williams and Wilkins, 2007. p274

Fractures of the Spine

• see Neurosurgery, NS32

Cervical Spine

General Principles
• C1 (atlas): no vertebral body, no spinous process
• C2 (axis): odontoid = dens
• 7 cervical vertebrae; 8 cervical nerve roots
• nerve root exits above vertebra (i.e. C4 nerve root exits above C4 vertebra), C8 nerve root exits below C7 vertebra
• radiculopathy = impingement of nerve root
• myelopathy = impingement of spinal cord

Special Testing
• compression test: pressure on head worsens radicular pain
• distraction test: traction on head relieves radicular symptoms
• Valsalva test: Valsalva maneuver increases intrathecal pressure and causes radicular pain

Table 13. Cervical Radiculopathy/Neuropathy

Root	C5	C6	C7	C8
Motor	Deltoid Biceps Wrist extension	Biceps Brachioradialis	Triceps Wrist flexion Finger extension	Interossei Digital flexors
Sensory	Axillary nerve (patch over lateral deltoid)	Thumb	Index and middle finger	Ring and little finger
Reflex	Biceps	Biceps Brachioradialis	Triceps	Finger jerk

X-Rays for C-Spine
- AP spine: alignment
- AP odontoid: atlantoaxial articulation
- lateral
  - vertebral alignment: posterior vertebral bodies should be aligned (translation >3.5 mm is abnormal)
  - angulation: between adjacent vertebral bodies (>11° is abnormal)
  - disc or facet joint widening
  - anterior soft tissue space (at C3 should be ≤3 mm; at C4 should be ≤8-10 mm)
- oblique: evaluate pedicles and intervertebral foramen
- ± swimmer's view: lateral view with arm abducted 180° to evaluate C7-T1 junction if lateral view is inadequate
- ± lateral flexion/extension view: evaluate subluxation of cervical vertebrae

Differential Diagnosis of C-Spine Pain
- neck muscle strain, cervical spondylosis, cervical stenosis, RA (spondylitis), traumatic injury, whiplash, myofascial pain syndrome

C-SPINE INJURY
- see <u>Neurosurgery</u>, NS31

Thoracolumbar Spine

General Principles
- spinal cord terminates at conus medullaris (L1/2)
- individual nerve roots exit below pedicle of vertebra (i.e. L4 nerve root exits below L4 pedicle)

Special Tests
- straight leg raise: passive lifting of leg (30-70°) reproduces radicular symptoms of pain radiating down posterior/lateral leg to knee ± into foot
- Lasegue maneuver: dorsiflexion of foot during straight leg raise makes symptoms worse or, if leg is less elevated, dorsiflexion will bring on symptoms
- femoral stretch test: with patient prone, flexing the knee of the affected side and passively extending the hip results in radicular symptoms of unilateral pain in anterior thigh

Table 14. Lumbar Radiculopathy/Neuropathy

Root	L4	L5	S1
Motor	Quadriceps (knee extension + hip adduction) Tibialis anterior (ankle inversion + dorsiflexion)	Extensor hallucis longus Gluteus medius (hip abduction)	Peroneus longus + brevis (ankle eversion) Gastrocnemius + soleus (plantar flexion)
Sensory	Medial malleolus	1st dorsal webspace and lateral leg	Lateral foot
Screening Test	Squat and Rise	Heel Walking	Walking on Toes
Reflex	Knee (patellar)	Medial hamstring*	Ankle (Achilles)
Test	Femoral stretch	Straight leg raise	Straight leg raise

*Unreliable

Differential Diagnosis of Back Pain
1. mechanical or nerve compression (>90%)
   - degenerative (disc, facet, ligament)
   - peripheral nerve compression (disc herniation)
   - spinal stenosis (congenital, osteophyte, central disc)
   - cauda equina syndrome
2. others (<10%)
   - neoplastic (primary, metastatic, multiple myeloma)
   - infectious (osteomyelitis, TB)
   - metabolic (osteoporosis)
   - traumatic fracture (compression, distraction, translation, rotation)
   - spondyloarthropathies (ankylosing spondylitis)
   - referred (aorta, renal, ureter, pancreas)

DEGENERATIVE DISC DISEASE
- loss of vertebral disc height with age resulting in
  - bulging and tears of annulus fibrosus
  - change in alignment of facet joints
  - osteophyte formation

Mechanism
- compression over time with age

Clinical Features
- axial back pain without radicular symptoms
- pain worse with axial loading and flexion
- negative straight leg raise

Investigations
- x-ray, MRI, provocative discography

Treatment
- non-operative
  - staying active with modified activity
  - back strengthening
  - NSAIDs
  - do not treat with opioids; no proven efficacy of spinal traction or manipulation
- operative – rarely indicated
  - decompression ± fusion
  - no difference in outcome between non-operative and surgical management at 2 yr

SPINAL STENOSIS
- narrowing of spinal canal <10 mm
- congenital (idiopathic, osteopetrosis, achondroplasia) or acquired (degenerative, iatrogenic – post spinal surgery, ankylosing spondylosis, Paget's disease, trauma)

Clinical Features
- ± bilateral back and leg pain
- neurogenic claudication
- ± motor weakness
- normal back flexion; difficulty with back extension (Kemp sign)
- positive Straight leg raise, pain not worse with Valsalva

Investigations
- CT/MRI reveals narrowing of spinal canal, but gold standard = CT myelogram

Treatment
- non-operative
  - vigorous physiotherapy (flexion exercises, stretch/strength exercises), NSAIDs, lumbar epidural steroids
- operative
  - indication: non-operative failure >6 mo
  - decompressive surgery

Table 15. Differentiating Claudication

	Neurogenic	Vascular
Aggravation	With standing or exercise Walking distance variable	Walking set distance
Alleviation	Change in position (usually flexion, sitting, lying down)	Stop walking
Time	Relief in ~10 min	Relief in ~2 min
Character	Neurogenic ± neurological deficit	Muscular cramping

MECHANICAL BACK PAIN
- back pain NOT due to prolapsed disc or any other clearly defined pathology

Clinical Features
- dull backache aggravated by activity and prolonged standing
- morning stiffness
- no neurological signs

Cauda equina syndrome and ruptured aortic aneurysms are causes of low back pain that are considered surgical emergencies

Treatment
- symptomatic (analgesics, physiotherapy)
- prognosis: symptoms may resolve in 4-6 wk, others become chronic

LUMBAR DISC HERNIATION

- tear in annulus fibrosus allows protrusion of nucleus pulposus causing either a central, posterolateral, or lateral disc herniation, most commonly at L5-S1 > L4-5 > L3-4
- 3:1 male to female
- only 5% become symptomatic
- usually a history of flexion-type injury

Clinical Features

- back dominant pain (central herniation) or leg dominant pain (lateral herniation)
- tenderness between spinous processes at affected level
- muscle spasm ± loss of normal lumbar lordosis
- neurological disturbance is segmental and varies with level of central herniation
  - motor weakness (L4, L5, S1)
  - diminished reflexes (L4, S1)
  - diminished sensation (L4, L5, S1)
- positive straight leg raise
- positive contralateral SLR
- positive Lasegue and Bowstring sign
- cauda equina syndrome (present in 1-10%): surgical emergency

Investigations

- x-ray, MRI, consider a post-void residual volume to check for urinary retention; post-void >100 mL should heighten suspicion for cauda equine syndrome

Treatment

- non-operative
  - symptomatic
    - extension protocol
    - NSAIDS
- operative
  - indication: progressive neurological deficit, failure of symptoms to resolve within 3 mo or cauda equina syndrome due to central disc herniation
  - surgical discectomy
- prognosis
- 90% of patients improve in 3 mo with non-operative treatment

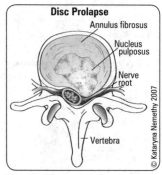

Disc Prolapse

Figure 29. Disc herniation causing nerve root compression

Neurogenic claudication is position dependent; vascular claudication is exercise dependent

MRI abnormalities (e.g. spinal stenosis, disc herniation) are quite common in both asymptomatic and symptomatic individuals and are not necessarily an indication for intervention without clinical correlation

Table 16. Types of Low Back Pain

| | **Mechanical Back Pain** | | **Direct Nerve Root Compression** | |
	Disc Origin	**Facet Origin**	**Spinal Stenosis**	**Root Compression**
Pain Dominance	Back	Back	Leg	Leg
Aggravation	Flexion	Extension, standing, walking	Exercise, extension, walking, standing	Flexion
Onset	Gradual	More sudden	Congenital or acquired	Acute leg ± back pain
Duration	Long (weeks, months)	Shorter (days, weeks)	Acute or chronic history (weeks to months)	Short episodes Attacks (minutes)
Treatment	Relief of strain, exercise	Relief of strain, exercise	Relief of strain, exercise + surgical decompression if progressive or severe deficit	Relief of strain, exercise + surgical decompression if progressive or severe deficit

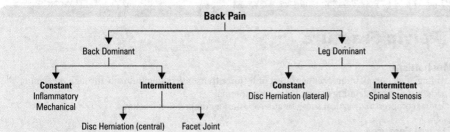

Figure 28. Approach to back pain

SPONDYLOLYSIS

Definition

- defect in the pars interarticularis with no movement of the vertebral bodies

Mechanism

- trauma: gymnasts, weightlifters, backpackers, loggers, labourers

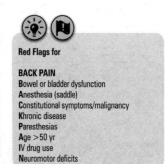

Red Flags for

BACK PAIN
Bowel or bladder dysfunction
Anesthesia (saddle)
Constitutional symptoms/malignancy
Khronic disease
Paresthesias
Age >50 yr
IV drug use
Neuromotor deficits

Sciatica
- Most common symptom of radiculopathy (L4-S3)
- Leg dominant, constant, burning pain
- Pain radiates down leg ± foot
- Most common cause = disc herniation

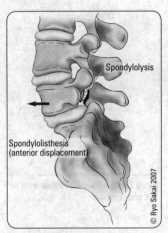

Figure 30. Spondylolysis, spondylolisthesis

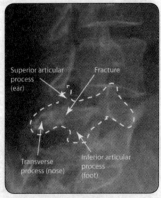

Figure 31. "Scottie dog" fracture

Clinical Features
- activity-related back pain, pain with unilateral extension (Michelis' test)

Investigations
- oblique x-ray: "collar" break in the "Scottie dog's" neck
- bone scan
- CT scan

Treatment
- non-operative
    - activity restriction, brace, stretching exercise

ADULT ISTHMIC SPONDYLOLISTHESIS

Definition
- defect in pars interarticularis causing a forward translation or slippage of one vertebra on another usually at L5-S1, less commonly at L4-5

Mechanism
- congenital (children), degenerative (adults), traumatic, pathological, teratogenic

Clinical Features
- lower back pain radiating to buttocks relieved with sitting
- neurogenic claudication
- L5 radiculopathy
- Meyerding Classification (percentage of slip)

Investigations
- x-ray (AP, lateral, obliques flexion-extension views), MRI

Treatment
- non-operative
    - activity restriction, bracing, NSAIDS
- operative
    - see Table 17

Table 17. Classification and Treatment of Spondylolisthesis

Class	Percentage of Slip	Treatment
1	0-25%	Symptomatic operative fusion only for intractable pain
2	25-50	Same as above
3	50-75	Decompression for spondylolisthesis and spinal fusion
4	75-100	Same as above
5	>100	Same as above

Specific Complications
- may present as cauda equina syndrome due to roots being stretched over the edge of L5 or sacrum

Pelvis

Pelvic Fracture

Mechanism
- young: high energy trauma, either direct or by force transmitted longitudinally through the femur
- elderly: fall from standing height, low energy trauma
- lateral compression, vertical shear, or anteroposterior compression fractures

Clinical Features
- pain, inability to bear weight
- local swelling, tenderness
- deformity of lower extremity
- pelvic instability

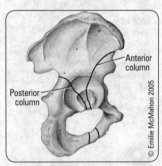

Figure 32. Pelvic columns

Investigations
- x-ray: AP pelvis, inlet and outlet views, Judet views (obturator and iliac oblique for acetabular fracture)
  - 6 cardinal radiographic lines of the acetabulum: ilioischial line, iliopectineal line, tear drop, roof, posterior rim, anterior rim
- CT scan useful for evaluating posterior pelvic injury and acetabular fracture
- assess genitourinary injury (rectal exam, vaginal exam, hematuria, blood at urethral meatus)
  - if involved, the fracture is considered an open fracture

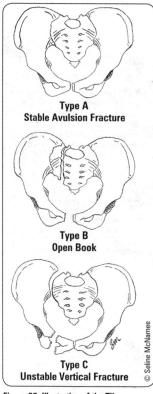

Classification

Table 18. Tile Classification of Pelvic Fractures

Type	Stability	Description
A	Rotationally stable Vertically stable	A1: fracture not involving pelvic ring (ex: avulsion or iliac wing fracture) A2: minimally displaced fracture of pelvic ring (e.g. ramus fracture) A3: transverse sacral fracture
B	Rotationally unstable Vertically stable	B1: open book (external rotation) B2: lateral compression – ipsilateral B2-1: with anterior ring rotation/displacement through ipsilateral rami B2-2: with anterior ring rotation/displacement through non-ipsilateral rami (bucket-handle) B3: bilateral
C	Rotationally unstable Vertically unstable	C1: unilateral C1-1: iliac fracture, C1-2: sacroiliac fracture-dislocation C1-3: sacral fracture C2: bilateral with 1 side type B and 1 side type C C3: bilateral both sides type C

Treatment
- ABCDEs
- non-operative treatment: protected weight bearing
  - indication: stable fracture
- emergency management
  - IV fluids/blood
  - pelvic binder/sheeting
  - external fixation vs. emergent angiography/embolization
  - ± laparotomy (if FAST/DPL positive)
- operative treatment: ORIF
  - indications
    - unstable pelvic ring injury
    - disruption of anterior and posterior SI ligament
    - symphysis diastasis >2.5 cm
    - vertical instability of the posterior pelvis
    - open fracture

Specific Complications (see *General Fracture Complications*, OR6)
- **hemorrhage (<u>life-threatening</u>)**
- injury to rectum or urogenital structures
- obstetrical difficulties, sexual and voiding dysfunction
- persistent SI joint pain
- post-traumatic arthritis of the hip with acetabular fractures
- high risk of DVT/PE

Type A
Stable Avulsion Fracture

Type B
Open Book

Type C
Unstable Vertical Fracture

© Seline McNamee

Figure 33. Illustration of the Tile classification of pelvic fractures

Hip

Hip Dislocation

- full trauma survey (see <u>Emergency Medicine</u>, *Patient Assessment/Management*, ER2)
- examine for neurovascular injury PRIOR to open or closed reduction
- reduce hip dislocations within 6 h to decrease risk of AVN of the femoral head
- hip precautions (no extreme hip flexion, adduction, internal or external rotation) for 6 wk post-reduction
- see *Hip Dislocation Post-Total Hip Arthroplasty*, OR29

ANTERIOR HIP DISLOCATION
- mechanism: posteriorly directed blow to knee with hip widely abducted
- clinical features: shortened, abducted, externally rotated limb
- treatment
  - closed reduction under conscious sedation/GA
  - post-reduction CT to assess joint congruity

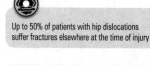

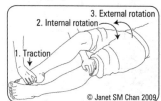

3. External rotation
2. Internal rotation
1. Traction

© Janet SM Chan 2009

Figure 34. Rochester method

POSTERIOR HIP DISLOCATION
- most frequent type of hip dislocation
- mechanism: severe force to knee with hip flexed and adducted
  - e.g. knee into dashboard in MVC
- clinical features: shortened, adducted, internally rotated limb
- treatment
  - closed reduction under conscious sedation/GA only if no associated femoral neck fracture or ipsilateral displacement
  - ORIF if unstable, intra-articular fragments or posterior wall fracture
  - post-reduction CT to assess joint congruity and fractures
  - if reduction is unstable, put in traction x 4-6 wk

COMPLICATIONS FOR ALL HIP DISLOCATIONS
- post-traumatic OA
- AVN of femoral head
- fracture of femoral head, neck, or shaft
- sciatic nerve palsy in 25% (10% permanent)
- HO
- thromboembolism – DVT/PE

Hip Fracture

General Features
- acute onset of hip pain
- unable to weight-bear
- shortened and externally rotated leg
- painful ROM

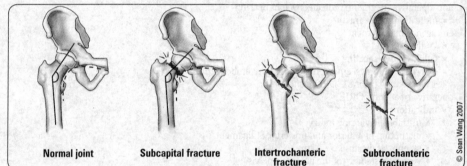

© Sean Wang 2007

Normal joint   Subcapital fracture   Intertrochanteric fracture   Subtrochanteric fracture

Figure 35. Subcapital, intertrochanteric, subtrochanteric fractures

Table 19. Overview of Hip Fractures

Fracture Type	Definition	Mechanism	Special Clinical Features	Investigations	Treatment	Complications
Femoral Neck (Subcapital)	Intracapsular (See Garden Classification, Table 20)	Young: MVC, fall from height Elderly: fall from standing, rotational force	Same as general	X-Ray: AP hip, AP pelvis, cross table lateral hip	See Table 20	DVT, non-union, AVN, dislocation
Intertrochanteric Stable: intact posteromedial cortex Unstable: non-intact posteromedial cortex	Extracapsular fracture including the greater and lesser trochanters and transitional bone between the neck and shaft	Same as femoral neck fracture Direct or indirect force transmitted to the intertrochanteric area	Ecchymosis at back of upper thigh	X-Ray: AP pelvis, AP/lateral hip	Closed reduction under fluoroscopy then dynamic hip screw or IM nail	DVT, varus displacement of proximal fragment, malrotation, non-union, failure of fixation device
Subtrochanteric	Fracture begins at or below the lesser trochanter and involves the proximal femoral shaft	Young: high energy trauma Elderly: osteopenic bone + fall, pathological fracture	Ecchymosis at back of upper thigh	X-Ray: AP pelvis, AP/lateral hip and femur	Closed/open under fluoroscopy then plate fixation or IM nail	Malalignment, non-union, wound infection

Table 20. Garden Classification of Femoral Neck Fractures

Type	Displacement	Extent	Alignment	Trabeculae	Treatment
I	None	"Incomplete"	Valgus or neutral	Malaligned	Internal fixation to prevent displacement (valgus impacted fracture)
II	None	Complete	Neutral	Aligned	Internal fixation to prevent displacement
III	Some	Complete	Varus	Malaligned	Young: ORIF Elderly: hemi-/total hip arthroplasty
IV	Complete	Complete	Varus	Aligned	Young: ORIF Elderly: hemi-/total hip arthroplasty

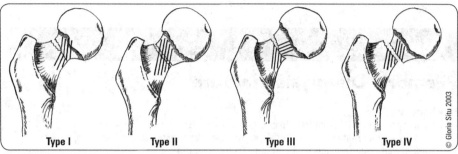

Figure 36. Garden classification of femoral neck fractures

Arthritis of the Hip

Etiology
- OA, inflammatory arthritis, post-traumatic arthritis, late effects of congenital hip disorders, or septic arthritis

Clinical Features
- pain (groin, medial thigh) and stiffness aggravated by activity, better with rest in OA
- RA: morning stiffness >1 h, multiple joint swelling, hand nodules
- decreased ROM (internal rotation is lost first)
- crepitus
- effusion
- ± fixed flexion contracture leading to apparent limb shortening (Thomas test)
- ± Trendelenburg sign

Investigations
- x-ray: weight bearing views of affected joint
  - OA: joint space narrowing, subchondral sclerosis, subchondral cysts, osteophytes
- RA: osteopenia, erosion, joint space narrowing, subchondral cysts,
- blood work: ANA, RF

Treatment
- non-operative
  - weight reduction, activity modification, physiotherapy, analgesics, walking aids
- operative
  - indication: advanced disease
  - realign = osteotomy; replace = arthroplasty; fuse = arthrodesis
- complications with arthroplasty: component loosening, dislocation, HO, thromboembolism, infection, neurovascular injury, limb length discrepancy
- arthroplasty is standard of care in most patients with hip arthritis

Hip Dislocation Post-Total Hip Arthroplasty

- occurs in 1-4% of primary THA and 10-16% of revision THAs
- risk factors: neurological impairment, post-traumatic arthritis, revision surgery, substance abuse

Mechanism
- THA that is unstable when hip is flexed, adducted and internally rotated, or extended and externally rotated (avoid flexing hip >90° or crossing legs for ~6 wk after surgery)

Investigations
- x-ray: AP pelvis, AP and lateral hip

Treatment
- non-operative
  - closed reduction: external abduction splint to prevent hip adduction (most often)
- operative
- indication: 2 or more dislocations with evidence of polyethylene wear, malalignment, hardware failure
  - revision THA
  - conversion to hemiarthroplasty with a larger femoral head
  - resection arthroplasty is a last resort

Complications
- sciatic nerve palsy in 25% (10% permanent)
- HO
- infection

DVT Prophylaxis in Elective THA
(continue 10-35 d post-operative)
Fondaparinux, low molecular weight heparin, or Coumadin

Femur

Femoral Diaphysis Fracture

Mechanism
- high energy trauma (MVC, fall from height, gunshot wound)
  - pathologic as a result malignancy, osteoporosis, bisphosphonate use
- in children, can result from low energy trauma (spiral fracture)

Clinical Features
- shortened, externally rotated leg (if fracture displaced)
- inability to weight-bear
- often open injury, always a Gustilo III (see Table 5, OR8)
- Winquist and Hansen classification

Investigations
- x-ray: AP pelvis, AP/lateral hip, femur, knee

It is important to rule out ipsilateral femoral neck fracture as they occur in 2-6% of femoral diaphysis fractures and are reportedly missed in 19-31% of cases

Treatment
- non-operative (uncommon)
  - indication: non-displaced femoral shaft fractures in co-morbid patients
  - long leg cast
- operative
  - ORIF with anterograde IM nail (most common) or retrograde IM nail, external fixator for unstable patients, open fractures, or highly vascular areas, or plate and screws for open growth plates within 24 h
  - early mobilization and strengthening

Complications
- blood loss
- fat embolism leading to ARDS
- extensive soft tissue damage
- ipsilateral hip dislocation/fracture (2-6%)
- nerve injury

Distal Femoral Fracture

- fractures from articular surface to 5cm above metaphyseal flare

Mechanism
- direct high energy force or axial loading
- three types: extra articular, partial articular, complete articular

Clinical Features
- extreme pain
- knee effusion (hemarthrosis)
- neurovascular deficits can occur with displaced fracture

Investigations
- x-ray: AP, lateral
- CT, angiography if diminished pulses

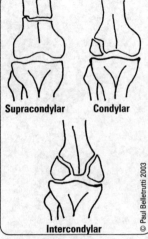

Supracondylar   Condylar

Intercondylar

© Paul Belletrutti 2003

Figure 37. Distal femoral fractures

Treatment

- non-operative (uncommon)
  - indication: non-displaced extra-articular fracture
    - ◆ hinged knee brace
- operative
  - indication: displaced fracture, intra-articular fracture, non-union
    - ◆ ORIF or retrograde IM nail if supracondylar and non-comminuted
    - ◆ early mobilization and strengthening

Specific Complications (see *General Fracture Complications*, OR6)

- femoral artery tear
- popliteal artery injury
- nerve injury
- extensive soft tissue injury
- angulation deformities

Knee

Evaluation of Knee

Common Complaints

- locking, Instability and swelling
  - torn meniscus/loose body in joint
- pseudo-locking: limited ROM without mechanical block
  - effusion, muscle spasm after injury, arthritis
- painful clicking (audible)
  - torn meniscus
- giving way: instability
  - cruciate ligament or meniscal tear, patellar dislocation

Special Tests of the Knee

- anterior and posterior drawer tests
  - demonstrate ACL and PCL, respectively
    - ◆ knee flexed at 90°, foot immobilized, hamstrings released
    - ◆ if able to sublux tibia anteriorly (anterior drawer test), then ACL may be torn
    - ◆ if able to sublux tibia posteriorly (posterior drawer test), then PCL may be torn
    - ◆ anterior drawer test for ACL: 3.8 positive likelihood ratio, 0.30 negative likelihood ratio
- Lachmann test
  - demonstrates torn ACL
  - hold knee in 10-20° flexion, stabilizing the femur
  - try to sublux tibia anteriorly on femur
  - similar to anterior drawer test, more reliable due to less muscular stabilization
  - for ACL: 25.0 positive likelihood ratio, 0.1 negative likelihood ratio
- Thessaly test
  - demonstrates meniscal tear
  - patient stands flat footed on one leg while the examiner provides his or her hands for balance. The patient then flexes the knee to 20° and rotates the femur on the tibia medially and laterally three times while maintaining the 20° flexion
  - positive for a meniscal tear if the patient experiences medial or lateral joint line discomfort
  - for medial meniscus: 29.67 positive likelihood ratio, 0.11 negative likelihood ratio
  - for lateral meniscus: 23.0 positive likelihood ratio, 0.083 negative likelihood ratio
- posterior sag sign
  - demonstrates torn PCL
  - may give a false positive anterior draw sign
  - flex knees and hips to 90°, hold ankles and knees
  - view from the lateral aspect
  - if one tibia sags posteriorly compared to the other, its PCL is torn
- pivot shift sign
  - demonstrates torn ACL
  - start with the knee in extension
  - internally rotate foot, slowly flex knee while palpating and applying a valgus force
  - if incompetent ACL, tibia will sublux anteriorly on femur at start of maneuver. During flexion, the tibiwill reduce and externally rotate about the femur (the "pivot")
  - reverse pivot shift (start in flexion, externally rotate, apply valgus and extend knee) suggests torn PCL
  - composite assessment for ACL: 25.0 positive likelihood ratio, 0.04 negative likelihood ratio
  - composite assessment for PCL: 21.0 positive likelihood ratio, 0.05 negative likelihood ratio

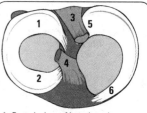

1. Posterior horn of lateral meniscus
2. Anterior horn of lateral meniscus
3. PCL
4. ACL
5. Posterior horn of medial meniscus
6. Anterior horn of medial meniscus

© Jenn Platt 2004

Figure 38. Diagram of the right tibial plateau

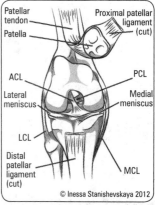

Patellar tendon
Proximal patellar ligament (cut)
Patella
ACL
PCL
Lateral meniscus
Medial meniscus
LCL
Distal patellar ligament (cut)
MCL

© Inessa Stanishevskaya 2012

Figure 39. Knee ligament and anatomy

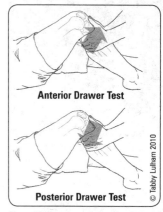

Anterior Drawer Test

Posterior Drawer Test

© Tabby Lulham 2010

Figure 40. Anterior and posterior drawer test

6 Degrees of Freedom of the Knee
- Flexion and extension
- External and internal rotation
- Varus and valgus angulation
- Anterior and posterior glide
- Medial and lateral shift
- Compression and distraction

On physical exam of the knee, do not forget to evaluate the hip

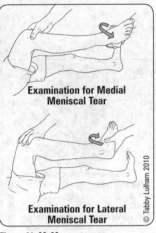

Examination for Medial Meniscal Tear

Examination for Lateral Meniscal Tear

© Tabby Lulham 2010

Figure 41. McMurray test

- **collateral ligament stress test**
    - palpate ligament for "opening" of joint space while testing
    - with knee in full extension, apply valgus force to test MCL, apply varus force to test LCL
    - repeat tests with knee in 20° flexion to relax joint capsule
    - opening in 20° flexion due to MCL damage only
    - opening in 20° of flexion and full extension is due to MCL, cruciate, and joint capsule damage
- **tests for meniscal tear**
    - joint line tenderness
        - ◆ joint line pain when palpated
        - ◆ palpate one side at a time and watch patient's eyes
        - ◆ for meniscal tear: 0.9 positive likelihood ratio, 1.1 negative likelihood ratio
    - crouch compression test
        - ◆ joint line pain when squatting (anterior pain suggests patellofemoral pathology)
    - McMurray's test useful collaborative information
        - ◆ with knee in flexion, palpate joint line for painful "pop/click"
        - ◆ internally rotate foot, varus stress, and extend knee to test lateral meniscus
        - ◆ externally rotate foot, valgus stress, and extend knee to test medial meniscus
        - ◆ for meniscal tear: 1.3 positive likelihood ratio, 0.8 negative likelihood ratio
    - composite assessment for meniscal tears: 2.7 positive likelihood ratio, 0.4 negative likelihood ratio

X-Rays
- AP standing, lateral
- skyline: tangential view with knees flexed at 45° to see patellofemoral joint
- 3-foot standing view: useful in evaluating leg length and varus/valgus alignment
- Ottawa Knee Rules (see Emergency Medicine, ER16)

Cruciate Ligament Tears

- ACL tear much more common than PCL tear

Table 21. Comparison of ACL and PCL Injuries

	Anterior Cruciate Ligament	Posterior Cruciate Ligament
Anatomy	From medial wall of lateral femoral condyle to the anteromedial and posterolateral intercondyloid eminence of the tibial plateau	Lateral wall of medial femoral condyle to posterior intercondyloid eminence of the tibial plateau
Mechanism	Sudden deceleration Hyperextension and internal rotation of tibia on femur (i.e. "plant and turn")	Sudden posterior displacement of tibia when knee is flexed or hyperextended (e.g. dashboard MVC injury)
History	Audible "pop" Immediate swelling Knee "giving way" Inability to continue activity	Audible "pop" Immediate swelling Pain with push off Cannot descend stairs
Physical	Effusion (hemarthrosis) Posterolateral joint line tenderness Positive anterior drawer Positive Lachmann Pivot shift Test for MCL, meniscal injuries	Effusion (hemarthrosis) Anteromedial joint line tenderness Positive posterior drawer Reverse pivot shift Other ligamentous, bony injuries
Treatment	Stable knee with minimal functional impairment: immobilization 2-4 wk with early ROM and strengthening High demand lifestyle: ligament reconstruction	Unstable knee or young person/high-demand lifestyle: ligament reconstruction

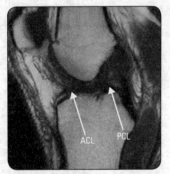

Figure 42. T1 MRI of torn ACL and PCL

ACL   PCL

Collateral Ligament Tears

Mechanism
- valgus force to knee = MCL tear
- varus force to knee = LCL tear

Clinical Features
- swelling/effusion
- tenderness above and below joint line medially (MCL) or laterally (LCL)
- joint laxity with varus or valgus force to knee
    - laxity with endpoint suggests a partial tear
    - laxity with no endpoint suggests a complete tear
- test for other injuries (e.g. O'Donoghue's unhappy triad), common peroneal nerve injury

O'Donoghue's Unhappy Triad
- ACL rupture
- MCL rupture
- Meniscal damage (medial and/or lateral)

Investigations
- x-ray: AP and lateral; MRI

Treatment
- non-operative
  - partial tear: immobilization x 2-4 wk with early ROM and strengthening
  - complete tear: immobilization at 30° flexion
- operative
  - indication: multiple ligamentous injuries
  - surgical repair of ligaments

Partial ligamentous tears are much more painful than complete ligamentous tears

Meniscal Tears

- medial tear much more common than lateral tear

Mechanism
- twisting force on knee when it is partially flexed (e.g. stepping down and turning)
- requires moderate trauma in young person but only mild trauma in elderly due to degeneration

Meniscal repair is done if tear is peripheral with good vascular supply, is a longitudinal tear and 1-4cm in length
Partial meniscectomy is done with tears not amenable to repair (complex, degenerative, radial)

Clinical Features
- immediate pain, difficulty weight-bearing, instability, and clicking
- increased pain with squatting and/or twisting
- effusion (hemarthrosis) with insidious onset (24-48 h after injury)
- joint line tenderness medially or laterally
- locking of knee (if portion of meniscus mechanically obstructing extension)

Investigations
- MRI, arthroscopy

Tissue Sources for ACL Reconstruction
- Hamstring
- Middle 1/3 patellar tendon (bone-patellar-bone)
- Allograft (e.g. cadaver)

Treatment
- non-operative
  - indication: not locked
  - ROM and strengthening (NSAIDs)
- operative
  - indication: locked or failed non-operative treatment
  - arthroscopic repair/partial meniscectomy

ACL tear more common than PCL tear
MCL tear more common than LCL tear

Quadriceps/Patellar Tendon Rupture

Mechanism
- sudden forceful contraction of quadriceps during an attempt to stop
- more common in obese patients and those with pre-existing degenerative changes in tendon
- DM, SLE, RA, steroid use, renal failure on dialysis

Clinical Features
- inability to extend knee or weight-bear
- possible audible "pop"
- patella in lower or higher position with palpable gap above or below patella respectively
- may have an effusion

Patella alta = high riding patella
Patella baja (infera) = low riding patella

Investigations
- ask patient to straight leg raise (unable with complete rupture)
- knee x-ray to rule out patellar fracture, MRI to distinguish between complete and partial tears
- lateral view: patella alta with patella tendon rupture, patella baja (infera) with quadriceps tendon rupture

Treatment
- non-operative
  - indication: incomplete tears with preserved extension of knee
  - immobilization in brace
- operative
  - indication: complete ruptures with loss of extensor mechanism
- early surgical repair: better outcomes compared with delayed repair (>6 wk post injury)
- delayed repair complicated by quadriceps contracture, patella migration, and adhesions

Dislocated Knee

Mechanism
- high energy trauma
- by definition, caused by tears of multiple ligaments

Clinical Features
- classified by relation of tibia with respect to femur
    - anterior, posterior, lateral, medial, rotary
- knee instability
- effusion
- pain
- ischemic limb
- Schenck classification

Schenck Classification
Type 1: single ligament injury (ACL or PCL)
Type 2: Injury to ACL and PCL
Type 3: Injury to ACL, PCL
         and either MCL or LCL
Type 4: Injury to ACL, PCL, MCL, LCL
Type 5: Multiligamentous injury
         with periarticular fracture

Investigations
- x-ray: AP, lateral, skyline
- associated radiographic findings include tibial plateau fracture dislocations, proximal fibular fractures, and avulsion of fibular head
- ABI (abnormal if <0.9)
- arteriogram or CT angiogram if abnormal vascular exam (such as abnormal pedal pulses)

Treatment
- urgent closed reduction
- complicated by interposed soft tissue
- assessment of peroneal nerve, tibial artery, and ligamentous injuries
- emergent operative repair if vascular injury, open fracture or dislocation, non-reducible dislocation, compartment syndrome
- knee immobilization x 6-8 wk

Specific Complications
- high incidence of associated injuries
- popliteal artery tear
- peroneal nerve injury
- capsular tear
- chronic: instability, stiffness, post-traumatic arthritis

Patella

Patellar Fracture

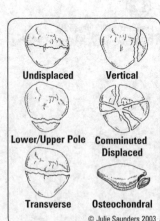

Undisplaced   Vertical

Lower/Upper Pole   Comminuted
                    Displaced

Transverse   Osteochondral
© Julie Saunders 2003

Figure 43. Types of patellar fractures

Complications
- Symptomatic wiring
- Loss of reduction
- Osteonecrosis (proximal fragment)
- Hardware failure
- Knee stiffness
- Nonunion
- Infection

Mechanism
- direct blow to the patella: fall, MVC (dashboard)
- indirect trauma by sudden flexion of knee against contracted quadriceps

Clinical Features
- marked tenderness
- inability to extend knee or straight leg raise
- proximal displacement of patella
- patellar deformity
- ± effusion/hemarthrosis

Investigations
- x-rays: AP, lateral, skyline
- do not confuse with bipartite patella: congenitally unfused ossification centres with smooth margins on x-ray at superolateral corner

Treatment
- non-operative
    - indication: non-displaced (step-off <2-3 mm and fracture gap <1-4 mm)
        ◆ straight leg immobilization 1-4 wk with hinged knee brace, weight bearing as tolerated
        ◆ progress in flexion after 2-3 wk
        ◆ physiotherapy: quadriceps strengthening when pain has subsided
- operative
    - indication: displaced (>2 mm), comminuted, disrupted extensor mechanism
    - ORIF, if comminuted may require partial/complete patellectomy
- goal: restore extensor mechanism with maximal articular congruency

Patellar Dislocation

Mechanism
- usually a non-contact twisting injury
- lateral displacement of patella after contraction of quadriceps at the start of knee flexion in an almost straight knee joint
- direct blow, e.g. knee/helmet to knee collision

Risk Factors

- young, female
- obesity
- high-riding patella (patella alta)
- genu valgus

- Q-angle (quadriceps angle) ≥20°
- shallow intercondylar groove
- weak vastus medialis
- tight lateral retinaculum
- ligamentous laxity (Ehlers-Danlos)

Clinical Features
- knee catches or gives way with walking
- severe pain, tenderness anteromedially from rupture of capsule
- weak knee extension or inability to extend leg unless patella reduced
- positive patellar apprehension test
  - passive lateral translation results in guarding and patient apprehension
- often recurrent, self-reducing
- concomitant MCL injury
- increased Q-angle
- J-sign

Investigations
- x-rays: AP, lateral, skyline view of patella
- check for fracture of medial patella (most common) and lateral femoral condyle

Treatment
- non-operative first
  - NSAIDs, activity modification, and physical therapy
  - short-term immobilization for comfort then 6 wk controlled motion
  - progressive weight bearing and isometric quadriceps strengthening
- operative
  - indication: if recurrent or if loose bodies present
  - surgical tightening of medial capsule and release of lateral retinaculum, possible tibial tuberosity transfer, or proximal tibial osteotomy

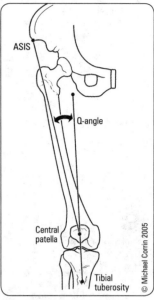

Figure 44. Q-angle
The angle between a vertical line through the patella and tibial tuberosity and a line from the ASIS to the middle patella; the larger the angle the greater the amount of lateral force on the knee (normal <20°)

J-sign: associated with patella alta, increased lateral translation in extension which pops into groove as the patella engages the trochlea early in flexion

Patellofemoral Syndrome (Chondromalacia Patellae)

- syndrome of anterior knee pain associated with idiopathic articular changes of patella

Risk Factors
- malalignment causing patellar maltracking (Q angle ≥20°, genu valgus)
- post-trauma
- deformity of patella or femoral groove
- recurrent patellar dislocation, ligamentous laxity
- excessive knee strain (athletes)

Mechanism
- softening, erosion and fragmentation of articular cartilage, predominantly medial aspect of patella
- commonly seen in active young females

Clinical Features
- deep, aching anterior knee pain
  - exacerbated by prolonged sitting (theatre sign), strenuous athletic activities, stair climbing, squatting or kneeling
- insidious onset and vague in nature
- sensation of instability, pseudolocking
- pain with extension against resistance through terminal 30-40°
- pain with compression of patella with knee ROM or resisted knee extension
- swelling rare, minimal if present
- palpable crepitus

Pain with firm compression of patella into medial femoral groove is pathognomonic of patellofemoral syndrome

Investigations
- x-ray: AP, lateral, skyline – may find chondrosis, lateral patellar tilt, patella alta/baja, or shallow sulcus
- CT-scan
- MRI – best to assess articular cartilage

Treatment
- non-operative
  - continue non-impact activities; rest and rehabilitation
  - NSAIDs
  - physiotherapy: vastus medialis and core strengthening
- operative
  - indication: failed non-operative treatment
  - tibial tubercle elevation
  - arthroscopic shaving/debridement
  - lateral release of retinaculum

Tibia

Tibial Plateau Fracture

Mechanism
- varus/valgus load ± axial loading (e.g. fall from height)
- femoral condyles driven into proximal tibia
- can result from minor trauma in osteoporotics

Clinical Features
- frequency: lateral > bicondylar > medial
- medial fractures require higher energy – often have concomitant vascular injuries
- knee effusion
- inability to bear weight
- swelling
- associated with compartment syndrome, ACL injury and meniscal tears
- Schatzker classification

Investigations
- x-ray: AP, lateral, oblique
- CT: pre-operative planning, identify articular depression and comminution
- ABI if any differences in pulses between extremities

Treatment

Approach #1 (based on amount of depression seen on x-ray)	**Non-operative indication** (if depression on x-ray is <3 mm): straight leg immobilization x 4-6 wk with progressive ROM weight bearing **Operative indication** (if depression is >3 mm): ORIF often requiring bone grafting to elevate depressed fragment
Approach #2 (based on varus/ valgus instability)	**Non-operative indication** (if minimal varus/valgus instability [<15°]): straight leg immobilization x 4-6 wk with progressive ROM weight bearing **Operative indication** (if significant varus/valgus instability [>15°]): ORIF often requiring bone grafting to elevate depressed fragment

Specific Complications (see *General Fracture Complications*, OR6)
- ligamentous injuries
- meniscal lesions
- AVN
- infection
- OA

Tibial Shaft Fracture

- most common long bone fracture and open fracture

Mechanism
- low energy pattern: torsional injury
- high energy: including MVC, falls, sporting injuries

Clinical Features
- pain, inability to weight bear
- open vs. closed
- neurovascular compromise

Investigations
- x-ray: AP, lateral
- full length, plus knee and ankle

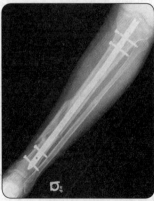

Figure 45. Tibial shaft fracture treated with IM nail and screws

Treatment
- non-operative
    - indication: closed and minimally displaced or adequate closed reduction
        - long leg cast x 8-12 wk, functional brace after
- operative
    - indication: displaced or open
        - if displaced and closed: ORIF with IM nail, plate and screws, or external fixator
        - if open: antibiotics, I&D, external fixation or IM nail, and vascularized coverage of soft tissue defects

Specific Complications (see *General Fracture Complications*, OR6)
- high incidence of neurovascular injury and compartment syndrome
- poor soft tissue coverage (critical to outcome)

Tibial shaft fractures have high incidence of compartment syndrome and are often associated with soft tissue injuries

Ankle

Evaluation of Ankle and Foot Complaints

Special Tests
- anterior drawer: examiner attempts to displace the foot anteriorly against a fixed tibia
- talar tilt: foot is stressed in inversion and angle of talar rotation is evaluated by x-ray

X-Ray
- AP, lateral
- mortise view: ankle at 15° of internal rotation
    - gives true view of ankle joint
    - joint space should be symmetric with no talar tilt
- Ottawa Ankle Rules should guide x-ray use (see <u>Emergency Medicine</u>, ER17); nearly 100% sensitivity
- ± CT to better characterize fractures

Ottawa Ankle Rules (see <u>Emergency Medicine</u>, ER17)
X-rays are only required if:
Pain in the malleolar zone AND bony tenderness over the distal 6cm of the posterior aspect of the medial or lateral malleolus OR inability to weight bear both immediately after injury and in the ER

Ankle Fracture

Mechanism
- pattern of fracture depends on the position of the ankle when trauma occurs
- generally involves
    - ipsilateral ligamentous tears or transverse bony avulsion
    - contralateral shear fractures (oblique or spiral)
- classification systems
    - Danis-Weber
    - Lauge-Hansen: based on foot's position and motion relative to leg

Treatment
- non-operative
    - indication: non-displaced, no history of dislocation, usually lateral sided injury only
    - below knee cast, NWB
- operative
    - indications
        - any fracture-dislocation: restore vascularity, minimize articular injury, reduce pain and skin pressure
        - most of type B, and all of type C
        - trimalleolar (medial, posterior, lateral) fractures
        - talar tilt >10°
        - medial clear space on x-ray greater than superior clear space
        - open fracture/open joint injury
    - ORIF

Complications
- high incidence of post-traumatic arthritis

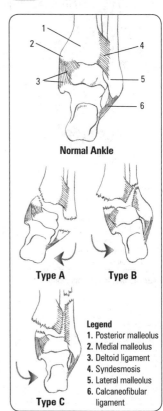

Figure 46. Ring principle of the ankle and Danis-Weber classification

Legend
1. Posterior malleolus
2. Medial malleolus
3. Deltoid ligament
4. Syndesmosis
5. Lateral malleolus
6. Calcaneofibular ligament

Ankle Ligamentous Injuries

- see Figure 47 for ankle ligaments

Medial Ligament Complex (deltoid ligament)
- eversion injury
- usually avulses medial or posterior malleolus and strains syndesmosis

Lateral Ligament Complex (Anterior Talofibular, Calcaneofibular, Posterior Talofibular)
- inversion injury, >90% of all ankle sprains
- ATF most commonly and severely injured if ankle is plantar flexed
- swelling and tenderness anterior to lateral malleolus
- ++ ecchymoses
- positive ankle anterior drawer
- may have significant medial talar tilt on inversion stress x-ray

Treatment
- non-operative
  - microscopic tear (Grade I)
    - rest, ice, compression, elevation
  - macroscopic tear (Grade II)
    - strap ankle in dorsiflexion and eversion x 4-6 wk
    - physiotherapy: strengthening and proprioceptive retraining
  - complete tear (Grade III)
    - below knee walking cast x 4-6 wk
    - physiotherapy: strengthening and proprioceptive retraining
    - surgical intervention may be required if chronic symptomatic instability develops

Foot

Talar Fracture

Mechanism
- axial loading or hyperdorsiflexion (MVC, fall from height)
- 60% of talus covered by articular cartilage
- talar neck is most common fracture of talus (50%)
- tenuous blood supply runs distal to proximal along talar neck
  - high risk of AVN with displaced fractures

Investigations
- x-ray: AP, lateral, Canale view
- CT to better characterize fracture
- MRI can clearly define extent of AVN

Treatment
- non-operative
  - indication: non-displaced
  - NWB, below knee cast x 6 wk
- operative
  - indication: displaced
  - ORIF (high rate of nonunion, AVN)
  - neck fracture: Pin (nondisplaced) or ORIF

Calcaneal Fracture

- most common tarsal fracture

Mechanism
- high energy, axial loading: fall from height onto heels
- 10% of fractures associated with compression fractures of thoracic or lumbar spine (rule out spine injury)
- 75% intra-articular and 10% are bilateral

Clinical Features
- marked swelling, bruising on heel/sole
- wider, shortened, flatter heel when viewed from behind
- varus heel

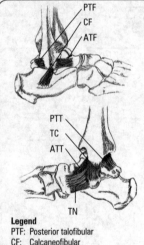

Legend
PTF: Posterior talofibular
CF: Calcaneofibular
ATF: Anterior talofibular
PTT: Posterior tibiotalar
TC: Tibiocalcaneal
ATT: Anterior tibiotalar
TN: Tibionavicular

Figure 47. Ankle ligament complexes

Investigations
- x-rays: AP, lateral, oblique (Broden's view) Harris axial
- loss of Bohler's angle
- CT: gold-standard, assess intra-articular extension

Treatment
- closed vs. open reduction is controversial
- NWB cast x 3 mo with early ROM and strengthening

Calcaneal Fracture Treatment Principles
- Avoid wound complications (10-25%)
- Restore articular congruity
- Restore normal calcaneal width and height
- Maximum functional recovery may take longer than 12 mo

Achilles Tendonitis

Mechanism
- chronic inflammation from activity or poor-fitting footwear
- may also develop heel bumps (retrocalcaneobursitis or Haglund deformity)

Clinical Features
- pain, stiffness, and crepitus with ROM
- thickened tendon, palpable bump

Haglund Deformity: an enlargement of the posterior-superior tuberosity of the calcaneus

Investigations
- x-ray: lateral, evaluate bone spur and calcification; U/S, MRI (to assess degenerative change)

Treatment
- non-operative
  - rest, NSAIDs, shoe wear modification (orthotics, open back shoes)
  - heel sleeves and pads are mainstay of non-operative treatment
  - gentle gastrocnemius-soleus stretching, eccentric training with physical therapy, deep tissue calf massage
  - shockwave therapy in chronic tendonitis
  - DO NOT inject steroids (risk of tendon rupture)

Achilles Tendon Rupture

Mechanism
- loading activity, stop-and-go sports (e.g. squash, tennis, basketball)
- secondary to chronic tendonitis, steroid injection

Clinical Features
- audible pop, sudden pain with push off movement
- pain or inability to plantar flex
- palpable gap
- apprehensive toe off when walking
- weak plantar flexion strength
- Thompson test: with patient prone, squeeze calf, normal response is plantar flexion
  - no passive plantar flexion is positive test = ruptured tendon

The most common site of Achilles tendon rupture is 2-6 cm from its insertion where the blood supply is the poorest

Investigations
- x-ray (to rule out other pathology), U/S or MRI (for partial vs complete ruptures)

Treatment
- non-operative
  - indication: low athletic demand or elderly
  - cast foot in plantar flexion (to relax tendon) x 8-12 wk
- operative
  - indication: high athletic demand
  - surgical repair, then cast as above x 6-8 wk

Complications of Achilles Tendon Rupture
- Infection
- Sural nerve injury
- Re-rupture: surgical repair decreases likelihood of re-rupture compared to non-operative management

Plantar Fasciitis (Heel Spur Syndrome)

- inflammation of plantar aponeurosis at calcaneal origin
- common in athletes (especially runners, dancers)
- also associated with obesity, DM, seronegative and seropositive arthritis

Mechanism
- repetitive strain injury causing microtears and inflammation of plantar fascia
- common in athletes (especially runners, dancers)
- also associated with obesity, DM, seronegative and seropositive arthritis

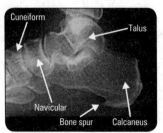

Figure 48. X-ray of bony heel spur

Foot

Clinical Features
- insidious onset of heel pain, pain when getting out of bed and stiffness
- intense pain when walking from rest that subsides as patient continues to walk, worse at end of day with prolonged standing
- swelling, tenderness over sole
- greatest at medial calcaneal tubercle and 1-2 cm distal along plantar fascia
- pain with toe dorsiflexion (stretches fascia)

Investigations
- plain radiographs to rule out fractures
- often see bony exostoses (heel spurs) at insertion of fascia into medial calcaneal tubercle
- spur is secondary to inflammation, not the cause of pain

Treatment
- non-operative
  - pain control and stretching programs are first line
  - rest, ice, NSAIDs, steroid injection
  - physiotherapy: Achilles tendon and plantar fascia stretching, extracorporeal shockwave therapy
  - orthotics with heel cup – to counteract pronation and disperse heel strike forces
- operative
  - indication: failed non-operative treatment
  - endoscopic surgical release of fascia
  - spur removal is not required

Bunions (Hallux Valgus)

- bony deformity characterized by medial displacement of first metatarsal and lateral deviation of hallux

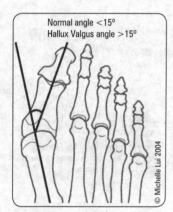

Normal angle <15°
Hallux Valgus angle >15°

© Michelle Lui 2004

Figure 49. Hallux valgus

Mechanism
- valgus alignment on 1st MTP (hallux valgus) causes eccentric pull of extensor and intrinsic muscles
- many associated deformities in foot from altered mechanics
- reactive exostosis forms with thickening of the skin creating a bunion
- most often associated with poor-fitting footwear (high heel and narrow toe box)
- can be hereditary (70% have family history)
- 10x more frequent in women

Clinical Features
- painful bursa over medial eminence of 1st MT head
- pronation (rotation inward) of great toe
- numbness over medial aspect of great toe

Investigations
- x-ray: standing AP/lateral/sesamoid view, NWB oblique

Treatment
- indications: painful corn or bunion, overriding 2nd toe
- non-operative (first line)
  - properly fitted shoes (low heel) and toe spacer
- operative: goal is to restore normal anatomy, not cosmetic reasons alone
  - osteotomy with realignment of 1st MTP joint (Chevron Procedure)
  - arthrodesis

Metatarsal Fracture

- as with the hand, 1st, 4th, 5th MT are relatively mobile, while the 2nd and 3rd are fixed
- use Ottawa Foot Rules to determine need for x-ray

Table 22. Types of Metatarsal Fractures

Fracture Type	Mechanism	Clinical	Treatment
Avulsion of Base of 5th MT	Sudden inversion followed by contraction of peroneus brevis	Tender base of 5th MT	Requires ORIF if displaced
Midshaft 5th MT (Jones Fracture)	Stress injury	Painful shaft of 5th MT	*NWB BK cast x 6 wk ORIF if athlete
Shaft 2nd, 3rd MT (March Fracture)	Stress injury	Painful shaft of 2nd or 3rd MT	Symptomatic
1st MT	Trauma	Painful 1st MT	ORIF if displaced otherwise *NWB BK cast x 3 wk then walking cast x 2 wk
Tarso-MT Fracture – Dislocation (Lisfranc Fracture)	Fall onto plantar flexed foot or direct crush injury	Shortened forefoot prominent base	ORIF

*NWB BK = Non weight bearing, below knee

Ottawa Ankle and Foot Rules
(see Emergency Medicine, ER17)
X-rays only required if:
Pain in the midfoot zone AND bony tenderness over the navicular or base of the fifth metatarsal OR inability to weight bear both immediately after injury and in the ER

Pediatric Orthopedics

Fractures in Children

- type of fracture
  - thicker, more active periosteum results in pediatric specific fractures: greenstick (one cortex), torus (i.e. 'buckle', impacted cortex) and plastic (bowing)
  - distal radius fracture most common in children (phalanges second), the majority are treated with closed reduction and casting
  - adults fracture through both cortices
- epiphyseal growth plate
  - weaker part of bone, susceptible to fractures
  - plate often mistaken for fracture on x-ray and vice versa (x-ray opposite limb for comparison), especially in elbow
  - tensile strength of bone < ligaments in children, therefore clinician must be confident that fracture and/or growth plate injury have been ruled out before diagnosing a sprain
  - intra-articular fractures have worse consequences in children because they usually involve the growth plate
- anatomic reduction
  - gold standard with adults
  - may cause limb length discrepancy in children (overgrowth)
  - accept greater angular deformity in children (remodelling minimizes deformity)
- time to heal
  - shorter in children
- always be aware of the possibility of child abuse
  - make sure stated mechanism compatible with injury
  - high index of suspicion with fractures in non-ambulating children (<1 yr); look for other signs, including x-ray evidence of healing fractures at different sites and different stages of healing

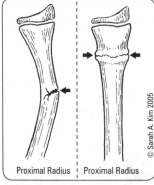

Proximal Radius   Proximal Radius

Figure 50. Greenstick (left) and torus (right) fractures

Greenstick fractures are easy to reduce but can redisplace while in cast due to intact periosteum

Stress Fractures

Mechanism
- insufficiency fracture
  - stress applied to a weak or structurally deficient bone
- fatigue fracture
  - repetitive, excessive force applied to normal bone
- most common in adolescent athletes
- tibia is most common site

Diagnosis
- localized pain and tenderness over the involved bone
- plain films may not show fracture for 2 wk
- bone scan positive in 12-15 d

Treatment
- rest from strenuous activities to allow remodelling (can take several months)

Epiphyseal Injury

Table 23. Salter-Harris Classification of Epiphyseal Injury

SALT(E)R–Harris Type	Description	Treatment
I (Straight through; Stable)	Transverse through growth plate	Closed reduction and cast immobilization (except SCFE – ORIF); heals well, 95% do not affect growth
II (Above)	Through metaphysis and along growth plate	Closed reduction and cast if anatomic; otherwise ORIF
III (Low)*	Through epiphysis to plate and along growth plate	Anatomic reduction by ORIF to prevent growth arrest, avoid fixation across growth plate
IV (Through and through)*	Through epiphysis and metaphysis	Closed reduction and cast if anatomic; otherwise ORIF
V (Ram)*	Crush injury of growth plate	High incidence of growth arrest; no specific treatment

* Types III – IV are more likely to cause growth arrest and progressive deformity

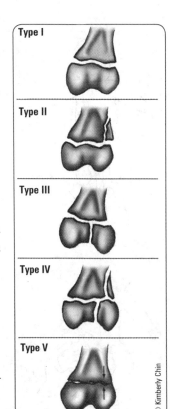

Type I

Type II

Type III

Type IV

Type V

Figure 51. Salter-Harris classification

Slipped Capital Femoral Epiphysis

- type I Salter-Harris epiphyseal injury at proximal hip
- most common adolescent hip disorder, peak incidence at pubertal growth spurt
- risk factors: male, obese (#1 factor), hypothyroid (risk of bilateral involvement)

Etiology
- multifactorial
  - genetic: autosomal dominant, black children at highest risk
  - cartilaginous physis hypertrophies too rapidly under growth hormone effects
  - sex hormone secretion, which stabilizes physis, has not yet begun
  - overweight: mechanical stress
  - trauma: causes acute slip

Clinical Features
- acute: sudden, severe pain with limp
- chronic (typically): groin and anterior thigh pain, may present with knee pain
  - positive Trendelenburg sign on affected side, due to weakened gluteal muscles
- tender over joint capsule
- restricted internal rotation, abduction, flexion
  - Whitman's sign: obligatory external rotation during passive flexion of hip
- Loder classification: stable vs. unstable (provides prognostic information)
  - unstable means patient cannot ambulate even with crutches

Investigations
- x-ray: AP, frog-leg, lateral radiographs both hips
  - posterior and medial slip of epiphysis
  - disruption of Klein's line
  - AP view may be normal or show widened/lucent growth plate compared with opposite side

Treatment
- operative
  - mild/moderate slip: stabilize physis with pins in current position
  - severe slip: ORIF or pin physis without reduction and osteotomy after epiphyseal fusion

Complications
- AVN (roughly half of unstable hips), chondrolysis (loss of articular cartilage, resulting in narrowing of joint space), pin penetration, premature OA, loss of ROM

Developmental Dysplasia of the Hip

- abnormal development of hip resulting in dysplasia and subluxation/dislocation of hip
- most common orthopedic disorder in newborns

Etiology
- due to ligamentous laxity, muscular underdevelopment, and abnormal shallow slope of acetabular roof
- spectrum of conditions
  - dislocated femoral head completely out of acetabulum
  - dislocatable head in socket
  - head subluxates out of joint when provoked
  - dysplastic acetabulum, more shallow and more vertical than normal
- painless (if painful suspect septic dislocation)

Physical Exam
- diagnosis is clinical
  - limited abduction of the flexed hip (<50-60°)
  - affected leg shortening results in asymmetry in skin folds and gluteal muscles, wide perineum
  - Barlow's test (for dislocatable hip)
    - flex hips and knees to 90° and grasp thigh
    - fully adduct hips, push posteriorly to try to dislocate hips
  - Ortolani's test (for dislocated hip)
    - initial position as above but try to reduce hip with fingertips during abduction
    - positive test: palpable clunk is felt (not heard) if hip is reduced
  - Galeazzi's sign
    - knees at unequal heights when hips and knees flexed
    - dislocated hip on side of lower knee
    - difficult test if child <1 yr
    - Trendelenburg test and gait useful if older (>2 yr)

Bilateral involvement occurs in about 25%

Klein's Line
On AP view, line drawn along supero-lateral border of femoral neck should cross at least a portion of the femoral epiphysis. If it does not, suspect SCFE

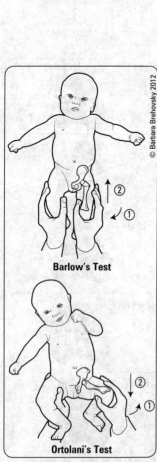

© Barbara Brehovsky 2012

Barlow's Test

Ortolani's Test

Figure 52. Barlow's test (checks if hips are dislocatable) and **Ortolani's test** (checks if hips are dislocated)

Investigations
- U/S in first few months to view cartilage (bone is not calcified in newborns until 4-6 mo)
- follow up radiograph after 3 mo
- x-ray signs (at 4-6 mo): false acetabulum, acetabular index >25°, broken Shenton's line, femoral neck above Hilgenreiner's line, ossification centre outside of inner lower quadrant (quadrants formed by intersection of Hilgenreiner's and Perkin's line)

Treatment
- 0-6 mo: reduce hip using Pavlik harness to maintain abduction and flexion
- 6-18 mo: reduction under GA, hip spica cast x 2-3 mo (if Pavlik harness fails)
- >18 mo: open reduction; pelvic and/or femoral osteotomy

Complications
- redislocation, inadequate reduction, stiffness
- AVN of femoral head

5 Fs that Predispose to Developmental Dysplasia of the Hip
Family history
Female
Frank breech
First born
LeFt hip

Legg-Calvé-Perthes Disease (Coxa Plana)

- idiopathic AVN of femoral head, presents at 4-8 yr of age
- 12% bilateral, M>F = 5:1, 1/1,200
- associations
  - family history
  - low birth weight
  - abnormal pregnancy/delivery
  - ADHD in 33% of cases, delayed bone age in 89%
  - second-hand smoke exposure
  - Asian, Inuit, Central European
- key features
  - AVN of proximal femoral epiphysis, abnormal growth of the physis, and eventual remodelling of regenerated bone

Clinical Features
- child with antalgic or Trendelenburg gait ± pain
- intermittent knee, hip, groin, or thigh pain
- flexion contracture (stiff hip): decreased internal rotation and abduction of hip
- limb length discrepancy (late)

Investigations
- x-ray: AP pelvis, frog leg laterals
- may be negative early (if high index of suspicion, move to bone scan or MRI)
- eventually, characteristic collapse of femoral head (diagnostic)

Treatment
- goal is to preserve ROM and keep femoral head contained in acetabulum
- non-operative
  - physiotherapy: ROM exercises
  - brace in flexion and abduction x 2-3 yr (controversial)
- operative
  - femoral or pelvic osteotomy (>8 yr of age or severe)
    - prognosis better in males, <5 yr, <50% of femoral head involved, abduction >30°
- 60% of involved hips do not require operative intervention
- natural history is early onset OA and decreased ROM

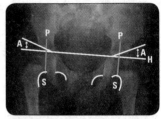

Figure 53. Pelvic x-ray and reference lines and angles for assessment of DDH
Triradiate Cartilage
y-shaped epiphyseal plate at junction of ilium, ischium and pubis
Hilgenreiner's Line
Line running between triradiate cartilages
Perkin's Line
Line through lateral margin of acetabulum, perpendicular to Hilgenreiner's Line
Shenton's Line
Arced line along inferior border of femoral neck and superior margin of obturator foramen
Acetabular Index
Angle between Hilgenreiner's Line and line from triradiate cartilage to point on lateral margin of acetabulum

Most common in adolescent athletes, especially jumping/sprinting sports

Children diagnosed with coxa plana <6 yr of age have improved prognosis

Osgood-Schlatter Disease

- inflammation of patellar ligament at insertion point on tibial tuberosity
- M>F
- age of onset: boys 12-15 yr; girls 8-12 yr

Mechanism
- repetitive tensile stress on insertion of patellar tendon over the tibial tuberosity causes minor avulsion at the site and subsequent inflammatory reaction (tibial tubercle apophysitis)

Clinical Features
- tender lump over tibial tuberosity
- pain on resisted leg extension
- anterior knee pain exacerbated by jumping or kneeling, relieved by rest

Investigations
- x-ray: lateral knee: fragmentation of the tibial tubercle, ± ossicles in patellar tendon

Treatment
- benign, self-limited condition, does not resolve until growth halts
- non-operative (majority)
  - may restrict activities such as basketball or cycling
  - NSAIDs, rest, flexibility, isometric strengthening exercises
  - casting if symptoms do not resolve with conservative management
- operative: ossicle excision in refractory cases (patient is skeletally mature with persistent symptoms)

Congenital Talipes Equinovarus (Club Foot)

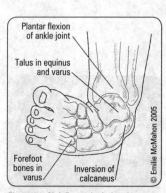

Plantar flexion
of ankle joint

Talus in equinus
and varus

Forefoot
bones in
varus

Inversion of
calcaneus

© Emilie McMahon 2005

Figure 54. Club Foot - depicting the gross and bony deformity

CAVE deformity
- midfoot **C**avus
- forefoot **A**dductus
- hindfoot **V**arus
- hindfoot **E**quinus

- congenital foot deformity
- muscle contractures resulting in CAVE deformity
- bony deformity: talar neck medial and plantar deviated; varus calcaneus and rotated medially around talus; navicular and cuboid medially displaced
- 1-2/1,000 newborns, 50% bilateral, occurrence M>F, severity F>M

Etiology
- intrinsic causes (neurologic, muscular, or connective tissue diseases) vs. extrinsic (intrauterine growth restriction), may be idiopathic, neurogenic, or syndrome-associated
- fixed deformity

Physical Exam
- examine hips for associated DDH
- examine knees for deformity
- examine back for dysraphism (unfused vertebral bodies)

Treatment
- largely non-operative via Ponseti Technique (serial manipulation and casting)
  - correct deformities in CAVE order
    - change strapping/cast q1-2wk
    - surgical release in refractory case (rare)
      - delayed until 3-4 mo of age
- 3 yr recurrence rate = 5-10%
- mild recurrence common; affected foot is permanently smaller/stiffer than normal foot with calf muscle atrophy

Scoliosis

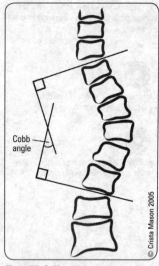

Cobb
angle

© Crista Mason 2005

Figure 55. Cobb angle – used to monitor the progression of the scoliotic curve

Scoliosis screening is not recommended in Canada (Grieg A, et al. 2010; Health Canada, 1994)

In structural or fixed scoliosis, bending forwards makes the curve more obvious

- lateral curvature of spine with vertebral rotation
- age: 10-14 yr
- more frequent and more severe in females

Etiology
- idiopathic: most common (90%)
- congenital: vertebrae fail to form or segment
- neuromuscular: UMN or LMN lesion, myopathy
- postural: leg length discrepancy, muscle spasm
- other: osteochondrodystrophies, neoplastic, traumatic

Clinical Features
- ± back pain
- primary curve where several vertebrae affected
- secondary curves above and below fixed 1° curve to try and maintain normal position of head and pelvis
- asymmetric shoulder height when bent forward
- Adam's test: rib hump when bent forward
- prominent scapulae, creased flank, asymmetric pelvis
- associated posterior midline skin lesions in neuromuscular scolioses
  - café-au-lait spots, dimples, neurofibromas
  - axillary freckling, hemangiomas, hair patches
- associated pes cavus or leg atrophy
- apparent leg length discrepancy

Investigations
- x-ray: 3-foot standing, AP, lateral
  - measure curvature: Cobb angle
  - may have associated kyphosis

Treatment
- based on Cobb angle
  - <25°: observe for changes with serial radiographs
  - >25° or progressive: bracing (many types) that halt/slow curve progression but do NOT reverse deformity
  - >45°, cosmetically unacceptable or respiratory problems: surgical correction (spinal fusion)

Postural scoliosis can be corrected by correcting the underlying problem

Bone Tumours

- primary bone tumours are rare after 3rd decade
- metastases to bone are relatively common after 3rd decade

Clinical Features
- malignant (primary or metastasis): local pain and swelling (wk – mo), worse on exertion and at night, ± soft tissue mass
- benign: usually asymptomatic
- minor trauma often initiating event that calls attention to lesion

Red Flags
- Persistent skeletal pain
- Localized tenderness
- Spontaneous fracture
- Enlarging mass/soft tissue swelling

Table 24. Distinguishing Benign from Malignant Bone Lesions on X-Ray

Benign	Malignant
No periosteal reaction	Acute periosteal reaction • Codman's triangle • "Onion skin" • "Sunburst"
Thick endosteal reaction	Broad border between lesion and normal bone
Well developed bone formation	Varied bone formation
Intraosseous and even calcification	Extraosseous and irregular calcification

Adapted from: Buckholtz RW, Heckman JD. Rockwood and Green's Fractures in Adults. Volume 1. Philadephia: Lippincott Williams & Wilkins, 2001. p558

Diagnosis
- malignancy is suggested by rapid growth, warmth, tenderness, lack of sharp definition
- staging should include
  - blood work including liver enzymes
  - CT chest
  - bone scan
  - bone biopsy
    - should be referred to specialized centre prior to biopsy
    - classified into benign, benign aggressive, and malignant
  - MRI of affected bone

X-ray Findings
- lytic, lucent, sclerotic bone
- involvement of cortex, medulla, soft tissue
- radiolucent, radiopaque, or calcified matrix
- periosteal reaction
- permeative margins
- pathological fracture
- soft tissue swelling

Benign Active Bone Tumours

BONE-FORMING TUMOURS

Osteoid Osteoma
- bone tumour arising from osteoblasts
- peak incidence in 2nd and 3rd decades, M:F = 2:1
- proximal femur and tibia diaphysis most common locations
- not known to metastasize
- radiographic findings: small, round radiolucent nidus (<1.5 cm) surrounded by dense sclerotic bone ("bull's-eye")
- symptoms: produces severe intermittent pain from prostaglandin secretion and COX1/2 expression, mostly at night (diurnal prostaglandin production), thus is characteristically relieved by NSAIDs
- treatment: NSAIDs for night pain; surgical resection of nidus

FIBROUS LESIONS

Fibrous Cortical Defect
- or non-ossifying fibroma; fibrous bone lesion
- most common benign bone tumour in children, typically asymptomatic and an incidental finding
- occur in as many as 35% of children, peak incidence between 2-25 yr old, higher prevalence in males
- femur and proximal tibia most common locations, 50% of patients have multiple defects usually bilateral, symmetrical
- radiographic findings: diagnostic, metaphyseal eccentric 'bubbly' lytic lesion near physis; thin smooth/lobulated well-defined sclerotic margin
- treatment: most lesions resolve spontaneously

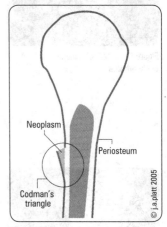

Neoplasm

Periosteum

Codman's triangle

© j.a.platt 2005

Figure 56. Codman's triangle – a radiographic finding in malignancy, where the partially ossified periosteum is lifted off the cortex by neoplastic tissue

Osteochondroma
- cartilage capped bony tumour
- 2nd and 3rd decades, M:F = 1.8:1
- most common of all benign bone tumours – 45%
- 2 types: sessile (broad based and increased risk of malignant degeneration) vs. pedunculated (narrow stalk)
- metaphysis of long bone near tendon attachment sites (usually distal femur, proximal tibia, or proximal humerus)
  - radiographic findings: cartilage-capped bony spur on surface of bone ("mushroom" on x-ray)
  - may be multiple (hereditary, autosomal dominant form) – higher risk of malignant change
- generally very slow growing and asymptomatic unless impinging on neurovascular structure ('painless mass')
  - growth usually ceases when skeletal maturity is reached
- malignant degeneration occurs in 1-2% (becomes painful or rapidly grows)
- treatment: typically observation; surgical excision if symptomatic

Enchondroma
- hyaline cartilage tumour; majority asymptomatic, presenting as incidental finding or pathological fracture
- 2nd and 3rd decades
- 60% occur in the small tubular bones of the hand and foot; others in femur (20%), humerus, ribs
- benign cartilagenous growth, an abnormality of chondroblasts, develops in medullary cavity
  - single/multiple enlarged rarefied areas in tubular bones
  - lytic lesion with sharp margination and irregular central calcification (stippled/punctate/popcorn appearance)
- malignant degeneration to chondrosarcoma occurs in 1-2% (pain in absence of pathologic fracture is an important clue)
- not known to metastasize
- treatment: observation with serial x-rays; surgical curettage if symptomatic or lesion grows

CYSTIC LESIONS

Unicameral/Solitary Bone Cyst
- most common cystic lesion; serous fluid filled lesion
- children and young adults, peak incidence during first 2 decades, M:F = 2:1
- proximal humerus and femur most common
- symptoms: asymptomatic, or local pain; complete pathological fracture (50% presentations) or incidental detection
- radiographic findings: lytic translucent area on metaphyseal side of growth plate, cortex thinned/expanded; well defined lesion
- treatment: aspiration followed by steroid injection; curettage ± bone graft indicated if re-fracture likely

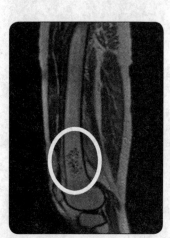

Figure 57. T1MRI of femoral enchondroma

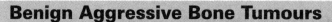

Benign Aggressive Bone Tumours

Giant Cell Tumours/Aneurysmal Bone Cyst/Osteoblastoma
- affects patients of skeletal maturity, peak 3rd decade
- osteoblastoma: found in the distal femur, proximal tibia, distal radius, sacrum, tarsal bones, spine
- giant cell tumour: pulmonary metastases in 3%
- aneurysmal bone cysts: either solid with fibrous/granular tissue, or blood-filled
- radiographic findings
  - giant cell tumour: eccentric lytic lesions, in epiphyses adjacent to subchondral bone; may break through cortex; T2 MRI enhances fluid within lesion (hyper-intense signal)
  - aneurysmal bone cyst: expanded with honeycomb shape
  - osteoblastoma: often nonspecific; calcified central nidus (>2 cm) with radiolucent halo and sclerosis
- symptoms: local tenderness and swelling, pain may be progressive (giant cell tumours), ± symptoms of nerve root compression (osteoblastoma)
- 15% recur within 2 yr of surgery

Treatment
- intralesional curettage + bone graft or cement
- wide local excision of expendable bones

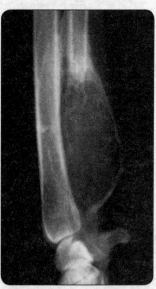

Figure 58. X-ray of aneurysmal bone cyst
Note the aggressive destruction of bone

Malignant Bone Tumours

Table 25. Most Common Malignant Tumour Types for Age

Age	Tumour
<1	Neuroblastoma
1-10	Ewing's of tubular bones
10-30	Osteosarcoma, Ewing's of flat bones
30-40	Reticulum cell sarcoma, fibrosarcoma, periosteal osteosarcoma, malignant giant cell tumour, lymphoma
>40	Metastatic carcinoma, multiple myeloma, chondrosarcoma

Osteosarcoma
- malignant bone tumour
- most frequently diagnosed in 2nd decade of life (60%), 2nd most common primary malignancy in adults
- history of Paget's disease (elderly patients), previous radiation treatment
- predilection for sites of rapid growth: distal femur (45%), proximal tibia (20%), and proximal humerus (15%)
  - invasive, variable histology; frequent metastases without treatment (lung most common)
- painful symptoms: progressive pain, night pain, poorly defined swelling, decreased ROM
- radiographic findings
  - characteristic periosteal reaction: Codman's triangle (see Figure 56) or "sunburst" spicule formation (tumour extension into periosteum)
  - destructive lesion in metaphysis may cross epiphyseal plate
- management: complete resection (limb salvage, rarely amputation), neo-adjuvant chemo; bone scan – rule out skeletal metastases, CT chest – rule out pulmonary metastases
- prognosis: 70% (high-grade); 90% (low-grade)

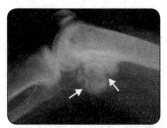

Figure 59. X-ray of osteosarcoma of distal femur

Chondrosarcoma
- malignant chondrogenic tumour
- primary (2/3 cases)
  - previous normal bone, patient >40 yr; expands into cortex to give pain, pathological fracture, flecks of calcification
- secondary (1/3 cases)
  - malignant degeneration of pre-existing cartilage tumour such as enchondroma or osteochondroma
  - age range 25-45 yr and better prognosis than primary chondrosarcoma
- symptoms: progressive pain, uncommonly palpable mass
- radiographic findings: in medullary cavity, irregular "popcorn" calcification
- treatment: unresponsive to chemotherapy, treat with aggressive surgical resection + reconstruction; regular follow-up x-rays of resection site and chest
- prognosis: 10-yr survival 90% low-grade, 20-40% high-grade

Ewing's Sarcoma
- malignant small round cell sarcoma
- most occur between 5-25 yr old
- florid periosteal reaction in metaphyses of long bone with diaphyseal extension
- metastases frequent without treatment
- signs/symptoms: presents with pain, mild fever, erythema and swelling, anemia, increased WBC, ESR, LDH (mimics an infection)
- radiographic findings: moth-eaten appearance with periosteal lamellated pattern ("onion-skinning")
- treatment: resection, chemotherapy, radiation
- prognosis – 70%, worst prognostic factor is distant metastases

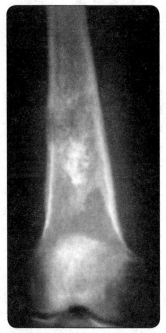

Figure 60. X-ray of femur chondrosarcoma

Multiple Myeloma
- proliferation of neoplastic plasma cells
- most common primary malignant tumour of bone in adults (~43%)
- 90% occur in people >40 yr old, M:F = 2:1, African-Americans (twice as common)
- signs/symptoms: localized bone pain (cardinal early symptom), compression/pathological fractures, renal failure, nephritis, high incidence of infections (e.g. pyelonephritis/pneumonia), systemic (weakness, weight loss, anorexia)
- labs: anemia, thrombocytopenia, increased ESR, hypercalcemia, increased Cr
- radiograpic findings: multiple, "punched-out" well-demarcated lesions, no surrounding sclerosis, marked bone expansion
- diagnosis
  - serum/urine immunoelectrophoresis (monoclonal gammopathy)
  - CT-guided biopsy of lytic lesions at multiple bony sites
- treatment: chemotherapy, bisphosphonates, radiation, surgery for symptomatic lesions or impending fractures – debulking, internal fixation
- prognosis: 5 yr survival 30%; 10 yr survival 11%
- see Hematology, H49

Signs of Hypercalcemia
"Bones, Stones, Moans, Groans, Psychiatric overtones"
CNS: headache, confusion, irritability, blurred vision
GI: N/V, abdominal pain, constipation, weight loss
MSK: fatigue, weakness, unsteady gait, bone and joint pain
GU: nocturia, polydipsia, polyuria, UTIs

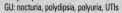

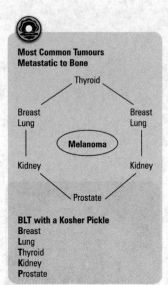

Most Common Tumours Metastatic to Bone

Thyroid

Breast Lung   Breast Lung

Melanoma

Kidney   Kidney

Prostate

BLT with a Kosher Pickle
Breast
Lung
Thyroid
Kidney
Prostate

Bone Metastases

- most common cause of bone lesions in adults; typically age >40
- 2/3 from breast or prostate; also consider thyroid, lung, kidney
- usually osteolytic; prostate occasionally osteoblastic
- may present with mechanical pain and/or night pain, pathological fracture, hypercalcemia
- bone scan for MSK involvement, MRI for spinal involvement may be helpful
- treatment: pain control, bisphosphonates, stabilization of impending fractures if Mirel's Critera >8 (ORIF, IM rod, bone cement)

Table 26. Mirel's Criteria for Impending Fracture Risk and Prophylactic Internal Fixation

Variable	Number Assigned		
	1	2	3
Site	Upper arm	Lower extremity	Peritrochanteric
Pain	Mild	Moderate	Severe
Lesion	Blastic	Mixed	Lytic
Size	<1/3 bone diameter	1/3-2/3 diameter	>2/3 diameter

Common Medications

Table 27. Common Medications

Drug Name	Dosing Schedule	Indications	Comments
cefazolin (Ancef®)	1-2 g IV q8h	Prophylactically before orthopedic surgery	First generation cephalosporin; do not use with penicillin allergy
heparin	5000 IU SC q12h	To prevent venous thombosis and pulmonary emboli	Monitor platelets, follow PTT which should rise 1.5-2x
LMWH dalteparin (Fragmin®) enoxaparin (Lovenox®) fondaparinux (Arixtra®)	5000 IU SC OD 30-40 mg SC bid 2.5 mg SC OD	DVT prophylaxis especially in hip and knee surgery	Fixed dose, no monitoring, improved bioavailability, increased bleeding rates
oral anticoagulants dabigatran (Pradaxa®) rivaroxaban (Xarelto®) apixaban	110 mg PO x1 then 220 mg PO OD 10 mg PO OD 2.5 mg PO bid	DVT prophylaxis especially TKA and THA	Predictable, no monitoring, oral administration; no antidote
midazolam (Versed®)	0.02-0.04 mg/kg IV	Conscious sedation for short procedures	Medication used during fracture reduction – monitor for respiratory depression
fentanyl (Sublimaze®)	0.5-3 μg/kg IV	Conscious sedation for short procedures	Short acting anesthetic used in conjunction with midazolam (Versed®)
triamcinolone (Aristocort®) – an injectable steroid	0.5-1 mL of 25 mg/mL	Suspension (injected into inflamed joint or bursa); amount varies by joint size	Potent anti-inflammatory effect;increased pain for 24 h, rarely causes fat necrosis and skin depigmentation
naproxen (Aleve®, Naprosyn®)	250-500 mg bid	Pain due to inflammation, arthritis, soft tissue injury	NSAID, may cause gastric erosion and bleeding
misoprostol (Cytotec®)	200 μg qid	Prophylaxis of HO after THA	Use with indomethacin
indomethacin (Indocid®)	25 mg PO tid	Prophylaxis of HO after THA	Use with misoprostol
ibuprofen (Advil®, Motrin®)	200-400 mg tid	Pain (including post-operative), inflammation (including arthritis)	NSAID, may cause gastric erosion and bleeding
propofol (Diprivan®)	1-2 mg/kg IV maintenance 0.5 mg/kg	Conscious sedation for short procedures	Short acting anesthetic often used in conjunction with fentanyl (Sublimaze®)

References

AAOS. The treatment of distal radius fractures: summary of recommendations. 2009. Available from: http://www.aaos.org/research/guidelines/DRFguideline.asp.
Adams JC, Hamblen DL. Outline of fractures: including joint injuries, 11th ed. Toronto: Churchill Livingstone, 1999.
Adkins SB. Hip pain in athletes. Am Fam Phys 2000;61:2109-2118.
Armagan OE, Shereff MJ. Injuries of the toes and metatarsals. Orthop Clin North Am 2001;32:1-10.
Barei DP, Bellabarba C, Sangeorzan BJ, et al. Fractures of the calcaneus. Orthop Clin North Am 2001;33:263-285.
Barrett SL. Plantar fasciitis and other causes of heel pain. Am Fam Phys 1999;59:2200-2206.
Blackbourne LH (editor). Surgical recall, 3rd ed. Philadelphia: Lippincott Williams & Wilkins, 2002.
Brand DA, Frazier WH, Kohlhepp WC, et al. A protocol for selecting patients with injured extremities who need x-rays. NEJM 1982;306:833-839.
Brinker MR. Review of orthopedic trauma. Toronto: WB Saunders, 2001.
Brinker M, Miller M. Fundamentals of orthopedics. Philadelphia: WB Saunders, 1999.
Canadian CT Head and C-Spine (CCC) Study Group. Canadian c-spine rule study for alert and stable trauma patients: background and rationale. CJEM 2002;4:84-90.
Canale ST, Beaty JH. Campbell's operative orthopaedics, 12th ed. Philadelphia: Elsevier Mosby, 2013.
Carek PJ. Diagnosis and management of osteomyelitis. Am Fam Phys 2001;63:2413-2420.
Dee R, Hurst LC, Gruber MA, et al. (editors). Principles of orthopedic practice, 2nd ed. Toronto: McGraw-Hill, 1997.
Donatto KC. Ankle fractures and syndesmosis injuries. Orthop Clin North Am 2001;32:79-90.
Duane TM, Wilson SP, Mayglothling J, et al. Canadian cervical spine rule compared with computed tomography: a prospective analysis. J Trauma 2011;71:352-355.
Fernandez M. Discitis and vertebral osteomyelitis in children: an 18-year review. Pediatrics 2000;105:1299-1304
Flyn JM. Orthopaedic Knowledge Update 10. Rosemont IL: American Academy of Orthopaedic Surgeons, 2011.
Fortin PT. Talus fractures: evaluation and treatment. J Am Acad Orthop Surg 2001;9:114-127.
French B, Tornetta III P. High energy tibial shaft fractures. Orthop Clin North Am 2002;33:211-230.
Gable H, Nunn D. Image Interpretation Course. 2009. Available from: http://www.imageinterpretation.co.uk.
Geerts WH, Heit JA, Clagett GP, et al. Prevention of venous thromboembolism. Chest 2001;119(1 Suppl):132S-175S.
Goldbloom RB. Screening for idiopathic adolescent scoliosis. Ottawa: Health Canada. Canadian Task Force on the Periodic Health Examination, Canadian Guide to Clinical Preventive Health Care, 1994. 346-353.
Gosselin RA, Roberts I, Gillespie WJ. Antibiotics for preventing infection in open limb fractures. Cochrane DB Syst Rev.2004;1:CD003764.
Greig A, Constantin E, Carsley S, et al. Preventive health care visits for children and adolescents aged six to 17 years: the Greig health record – executive summary. Ped Child Health 2010;15:157-159.
Grover R. Clinical assessment of scaphoid injuries and the detection of fractures. J Hand Surg Br 1996;21:341-343.
Gustilo RB, Mendoza RM, Williams DN. Problems in the management of type III (severe) open fractures: a new classification of type III open fractures. J Trauma 1984;24:742-746.
Hamilton H, McIntosh G, Boyle C. Effectiveness of a low back classification system. Spine J 2009;9:648-657.
Harty MP. Imaging of pediatric foot disorders. Radiol Clin North Am 2001;39:733-748.
Hermans J, Luime JL, Meuffels DE, et al. Does this patient with shoulder pain have rotator cuff disease? The rational clinical examination systematic review. JAMA 2013;310:837-847.
Irrgang JJ. Rehabilitation of multiple ligament injured knee. Clin Sports Med 2000;19:545-571.
Kao LD. Pre-test surgery. Toronto: McGraw-Hill, 2002.
Karachalios T, Hantes M, Zibis AH, et al. Diagnostic accuracy of a new clinical test (the Thessaly test) for early detection of meniscal tears. J Bone Joint Surg Am 2005;87:955-962.
Lawrence LL. The limping child. Emerg Med Clin North Am 1998;169:911-929.
Litaker D, Pioro M, El Bilbeisi H, et al. Returning to the bedside: using the history and physical examination to identify rotator cuff tears. J Am Geriat Soc 2000;48:1633-1637.
Lo IK, Nonweiler B, Woolfrey M, et al. An evaluation of the apprehension, relocation, and surprise tests for anterior shoulder instability. American Journal of Sports Medicine 2004;32:301-7.
Magee DJ. Orthopedic physical assessment, 5th ed. St. Louis: WB Saunders Elsevier, 2008.
Margaretten ME, Kohlwes J, Moore D, et al. Does this adult patient have septic arthritis? JAMA 2007;297:1478-1488.
Mathews CJ, Coakley G. Septic arthritis: current diagnostic and therapeutic algorithm. Curr Opin Rheumatol 2008;20:457-462.
Mazzone MF. Common conditions of the Achilles tendon. Am Fam Phys 2000;65:1805-1810.
Miller MD, Thompson SR, Hart J. Review of Orthopaedics, 6th ed. Philadelphia: Elsevier, 2012.
Miller SL. Malignant and benign bone tumours. Radiol Clin North Am 2000;39:673-699.
Murrell GA, Walton JR. Diagnosis of rotator cuff tears. Lancet 2001;357:769-770.
Ochiai DH. The orthopedic intern pocket survival guide. McLean: International Medical Publishing, 2007.
Okike K, Bhattacharyya T. Trends in the management of open fractures: a critical analysis. J Bone Joint Surg Am 2006;88:2739-2748.
Oudjhane K. Imaging of osteomyelitis in children. Radiol Clin North Am 2001;39:251-266.
Patel DR. Sports injuries in adolescents. Med Clin North Am 2000;84:983-1007.
Roberts DM, Stallard TC. Emergency department evaluation and treatment of knee and leg injuries. Emerg Med Clin North Am 2000;18:67-84.
Rockwood CA, Williams GR, Young DC. Disorders of the acromioclavicular joint. Rockwood CA, Masten FA II (editors). The shoulder. Philadelphia: Saunders, 1998. 483-553.
Rockwood CA Jr, Greene DP, Bucholz RU, et al. (editors). Rockwood and Green's fractures in adults, 4th ed. Philadelphia: Lippincott Raven, 1996.
Russell GV Jr. Complicated femoral shaft fractures. Orthop Clin North Am 2002;33:127-142.
Ryan SP, Pugliano V. Controversies in initial management of open fractures. Scan J Surg 2014;103(2):132-7.
Skinner HB. Current diagnosis and treatment in orthopedics, 4th ed. New York: McGraw-Hill, 2006.
Solomon DH, Simel DL, Bates DW, et al. The rational clinical examination: does this patient have a torn meniscus or ligament of the knee? Value of the physical examination. JAMA 2001;286:1610-1620.
Solomon L, Warwick DJ, Nayagam S. Apley's system of orthopedics and fractures, 8th ed. New York: Hodder Arnold, 2001.
St Pierre P. Posterior cruciate ligament injuries. Clin Sports Med 1999;18:199-221.
Steele PM, Bush-Joseph C, Bach Jr B. Management of acute fractures around the knee, ankle, and foot. Clin Fam Pract 2000;2:661-705.
Stewart DG Jr, Kay RM, Skaggs DL. Open fractures in children. Principles of evaluation and management. JBJS Am 2005;87:2784-2798.
Swenson TM. The dislocated knee: physical diagnosis of the multiple-ligament-injured knee. Clin Sports Med 2000;19:415-423.
Testroote M, Stigter WA, Janssen L, et al. Low molecular weight heparin for prevention of venous thromboembolism in patients with lower-leg immobilization. Cochrane DB Syst Rev 2014;4:CD006681.
Thompson JC. Netter's concise atlas of orthopedic Anatomy. USA: Elsevier, 2001.
Wong M. Pocket orthopedics: evidence-based survival guide. Sudbury: Jones and Bartlett Publishers, 2010.
Zhang Y. Clinical Epidemiology of Orthopedic Trauma. New York: Thieme Medical Publishers, 2012.
Zollinger PE, Tuinebreijer WE, Kreis RW, et al. Effect of vitamin C on frequency of reflex sympathetic dystrophy in wrist fractures: a randomized trial. Lancet 1999;354:2025-2058.

Notes

Otolaryngology – Head & Neck Surgery

Terence Fu, Ragavan Ganeshathasan, and **Rebecca Stepita**, chapter editors
Dhruvin Hirpara and **Sneha Raju**, associate editors
Valerie Lemieux and **Simran Mundi**, EBM editors
Dr. Jonathan C. Irish and **Dr. Evan J. Propst**, staff editors

Acronyms

ABR	auditory brainstem response	EBV	Epstein-Barr virus	HPV	human papillomavirus	SCC	squamous cell carcinoma
AC	air conduction	FAP	familial adenomatous polyposis	INCS	intranasal corticosteroids	SCM	sternocleidomastoid
AOM	acute otitis media	FESS	functional endoscopic sinus surgery	MEE	middle ear effusion	SNHL	sensorineural hearing loss
BAHA	bone anchored hearing aid	FNA	fine needle aspiration	MEI	middle ear inflammation	SRT	speech reception threshold
BC	bone conduction	GERD	gastroesophageal reflux disease	OE	otitis externa	TEF	tracheoesophageal fistula
CHL	conductive hearing loss	GPA	granulomatosis with polyangiitis	OME	otitis media with effusion	TM	tympanic membrane
CPA	cerebellopontine angle	H&N	head and neck	OSA	obstructive sleep apnea	TNM	tumour, node, metastases
EAC	external auditory canal	HL	hearing loss	RA	rheumatoid arthritis	URTI	upper respiratory tract infection

Basic Anatomy Review

Ear

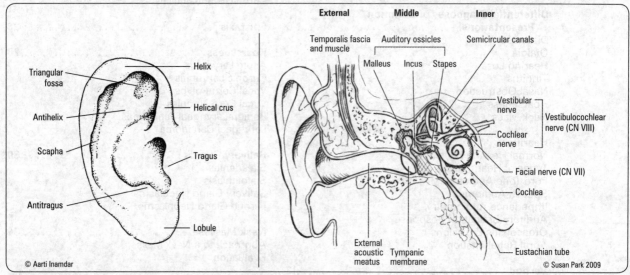

Figure 1. Surface anatomy of the external ear; anatomy of ear

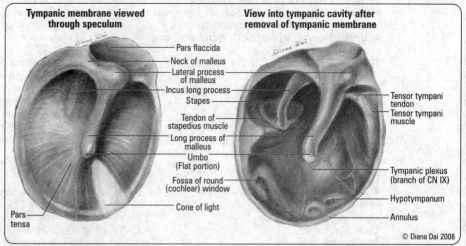

Figure 2. Normal appearance of right tympanic membrane on otoscopy

Nose

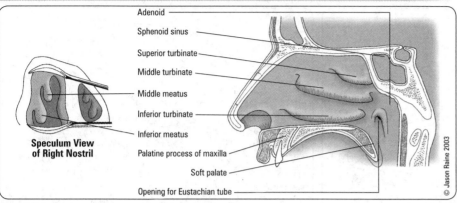

Figure 3. Nasal anatomy

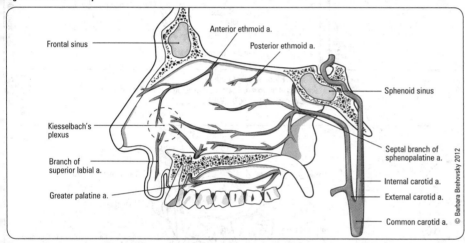

Figure 4. Nasal septum and its arterial supply (see *Epistaxis*, OT26 for detailed blood supply)

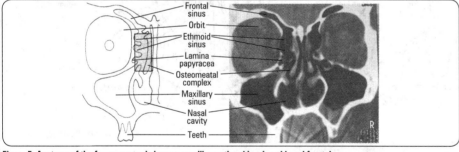

Figure 5. Anatomy of the four paranasal sinuses: maxillary, ethmoid, sphenoid, and frontal
Reprinted from: Dhillon RS, East CA. Ear, Nose and Throat and Head and Neck Surgery, 2nd ed. Copyright 1999, with permission from Elsevier

Throat

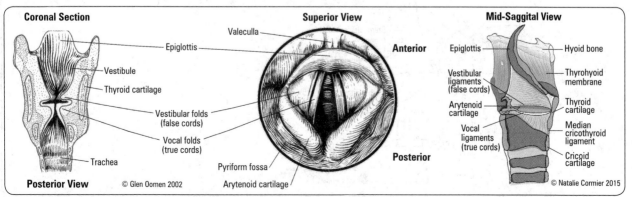

Figure 6. Anatomy of a normal larynx; superior view of larynx on indirect laryngoscopy

Head and Neck

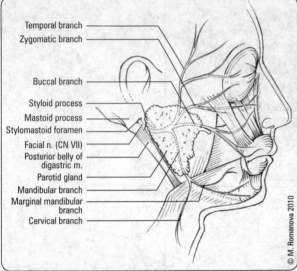

Temporal branch
Zygomatic branch
Buccal branch
Styloid process
Mastoid process
Stylomastoid foramen
Facial n. (CN VII)
Posterior belly of digastric m.
Parotid gland
Mandibular branch
Marginal mandibular branch
Cervical branch

© M. Romanova 2010

Figure 7. Extratemporal segment of facial nerve
Branches of facial nerve (in order from superior to inferior)
To Zanzibar By Motor Car

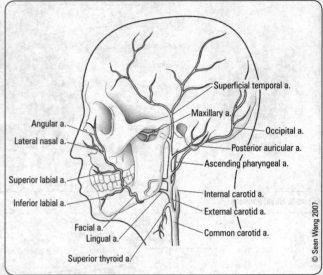

Superficial temporal a.
Maxillary a.
Angular a.
Lateral nasal a.
Occipital a.
Posterior auricular a.
Ascending pharyngeal a.
Superior labial a.
Inferior labial a.
Internal carotid a.
External carotid a.
Facial a.
Common carotid a.
Lingual a.
Superior thyroid a.

© Sean Wang 2007

Figure 8. Blood supply to the face
Branches of the external carotid artery (in order from inferior to superior)
Some Angry Lady Figured Out PMS

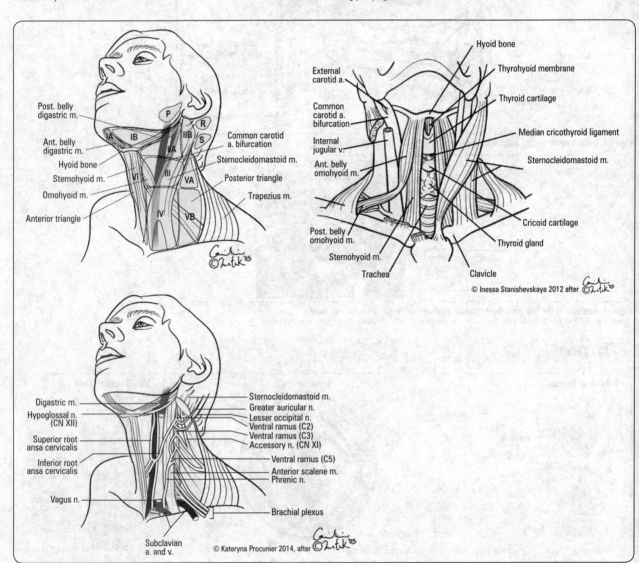

Post. belly digastric m.
Ant. belly digastric m.
Hyoid bone
Sternohyoid m.
Omohyoid m.
Anterior triangle

Common carotid a. bifurcation
Sternocleidomastoid m.
Posterior triangle
Trapezius m.

Hyoid bone
Thyrohyoid membrane
Thyroid cartilage
External carotid a.
Common carotid a. bifurcation
Internal jugular v.
Ant. belly omohyoid m.
Median cricothyroid ligament
Sternocleidomastoid m.
Post. belly omohyoid m.
Sternohyoid m.
Cricoid cartilage
Thyroid gland
Trachea
Clavicle

© Inessa Stanishevskaya 2012 after

Digastric m.
Hypoglossal n. (CN XII)
Superior root ansa cervicalis
Inferior root ansa cervicalis
Vagus n.

Sternocleidomastoid m.
Greater auricular n.
Lesser occipital n.
Ventral ramus (C2)
Ventral ramus (C3)
Accessory n. (CN XI)
Ventral ramus (C5)
Anterior scalene m.
Phrenic n.
Brachial plexus

Subclavian a. and v.

© Kateryna Procunier 2014, after

Figure 9. Anatomy of the neck

Anatomical Triangles of the Neck

Anterior triangle
- bounded by anterior border of SCM, midline of neck, and lower border of mandible
- divided into
  - **submental triangle:** bounded by both anterior bellies of digastric and hyoid bone
  - **digastric triangle:** bounded by anterior and posterior bellies of digastric and inferior border of mandible
  - **carotid triangle:** bounded by sternocleidomastoid, anterior belly of omohyoid, and posterior belly of digastric
    - contains: tail of parotid, submandibular gland, hypoglossal nerve, carotid bifurcation, and lymph nodes

Posterior triangle
- bounded by posterior border of sternocleidomastoid, anterior border of trapezius, and middle third of clavicle
- divided into
  - **occipital triangle:** superior to posterior belly of the omohyoid
  - **subclavian triangle:** inferior to posterior belly of omohyoid
- contains: spinal accessory nerve and lymph nodes

Table 1. Lymphatic Drainage of Nodal Groups and Anatomical Triangles of Neck

Nodal Group/Level	Location	Drainage
1. Suboccipital (S)	Base of skull, posterior	Posterior scalp
2. Retroauricular (R)	Superficial to mastoid process	Scalp, temporal region, external auditory meatus, posterior pinna
3. Parotid-preauricular (P)	Anterior to ear	External auditory meatus, anterior pinna, soft tissue of frontal and temporal regions, root of nose, eyelids, palpebral conjunctiva
4. Submental (Level IA)	Anterior bellies (midline) of digastric muscles, tip of mandible, and hyoid bone	Floor of mouth, anterior tongue, anterior mandibular alveolar ridge, lower lip
5. Submandibular (Level IB)	Anterior belly of digastric muscle, stylohyoid muscle, body of mandible	Oral cavity, anterior nasal cavity, soft tissues of the mid-face, submandibular gland
6. Upper jugular (Levels IIA and IIB)	Skull base to inferior border of hyoid bone along SCM muscle	Oral cavity, nasal cavity, naso/oro/hypopharynx, larynx, parotid glands
7. Middle jugular (Level III)	Inferior border of hyoid bone to inferior border of cricoid cartilage along SCM muscle	Oral cavity, naso/oro/hypopharynx, larynx
8. Lower jugular* (Level IV)	Inferior border of cricoid cartilage to clavicle along SCM muscle	Hypopharynx, thyroid, cervical esophagus, larynx
9. Posterior triangle** (Levels VA and VB)	Posterior border of SCM, anterior border of trapezius, from skull base to clavicle	Nasopharynx and oropharynx, cutaneous structures of the posterior scalp and neck
10. Anterior compartment*** (Level VI)	Hyoid bone (midline) to suprasternal notch between the common carotid arteries	Thyroid gland, glottic and subglottic larynx, apex of piriform sinus, cervical esophagus

*Virchow node: left lower jugular (level IV) supraclavicular node
**Includes some supraclavicular nodes
***Includes pretracheal, precricoid, paratracheal, and perithyroidal nodes

Paired Parasympathetic Ganglia of the Head and Neck
- **Ciliary:** pupillary constriction
- **Pterygopalatine:** lacrimal gland, nasal mucosa
- **Submandibular:** submandibular, sublingual glands
- **Otic:** parotid gland

Function of Facial Nerve

"Ears, Tears, Face, Taste"
Ears: stapedius muscle
Tears: lacrimation (lacrimal gland) and salivation (parotid)
Face: muscles of facial expression
Taste: sensory anterior 2/3 of tongue (via chorda tympani)

- **Left-sided** enlargement of a supraclavicular node (Virchow's node) may indicate an abdominal malignancy
- **Right-sided** enlargement may indicate malignancy of the mediastinum, lungs, or esophagus
- Occipital and/or posterior auricular node enlargement may indicate rubella

4 Strap Muscles of the Neck
- Thyrohyoid
- Omohyoid
- Sternohyoid
- Sternothyroid

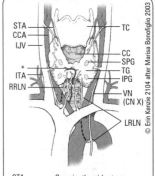

STA	— Superior thyroid artery
CCA	— Common carotid artery
IJV	— Internal jugular vein
ITA	— Inferior thyroid artery
RRLN	— Right recurrent laryngeal nerve
TC	— Thyroid cartilage
CC	— Cricoid cartilage
SPG	— Superior parathyroid gland
TG	— Thyroid gland
IPG	— Inferior parathyroid gland
VN (CN X)	— Vagus nerve (CN X)
LRLN	— Left recurrent laryngeal nerve

*Thyroidea ima artery: present in 3% of population, arises from aortic arch or innominate artery

Figure 10. Anatomy of the thyroid gland

Differential Diagnoses of Common Presentations

Dizziness

True nystagmus and vertigo caused by a peripheral lesion will never last longer than a couple of weeks because of compensation from the cerebellum (unless there is a history of cerebellar ischemia/stroke). Central lesions do not compensate, hence nystagmus and vertigo will persist

5 "D"s of Vertebrobasilar Insufficiency
Drop attacks
Diplopia
Dysarthria
Dizziness
Dysphagia

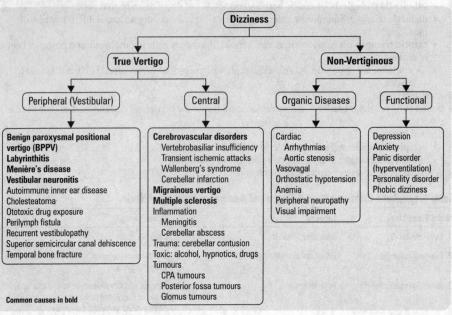

Figure 11. Differential diagnosis of dizziness

Otalgia

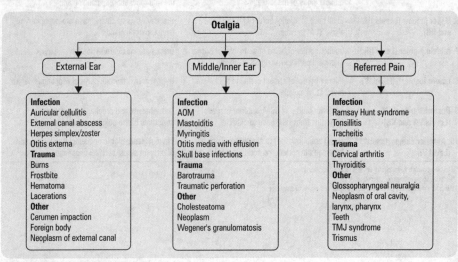

Figure 12. Differential diagnosis of otalgia

Hearing Loss

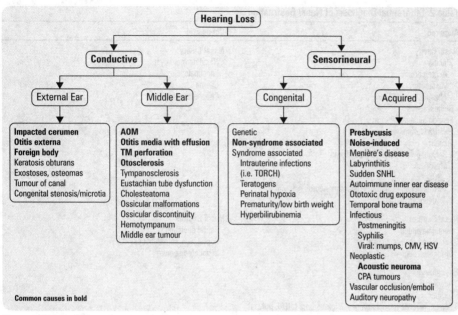

Figure 13. Differential diagnosis of hearing loss

Tinnitus

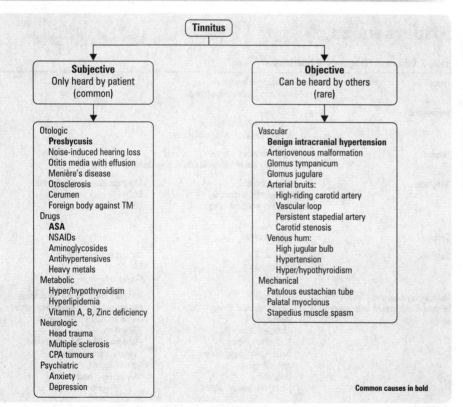

Figure 14. Differential diagnosis of tinnitus

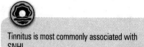

Tinnitus is most commonly associated with SNHL

Glomus Tympanicum/Jugulare Tumour Signs and Symptoms
- Pulsatile tinnitus
- Hearing loss
- Blue mass behind TM
- Brown's sign (blanching of the TM with pneumatic otoscopy)

Nasal Obstruction

Table 2. Differential Diagnosis of Nasal Obstruction

Acquired	Congenital
Nasal Cavity	**Nasal Cavity**
Rhinitis	Nasal dermoid cyst
Acute/chronic	Encephalocele
Vasomotor	Glioma
Allergic	Choanal atresia
Rhinosinusitis	
Foreign bodies	
Enlarged turbinates	
Tumour	
Benign: polyps, inverting papilloma	
Malignant	
SCC	
Esthesioneuroblastoma (olfactory neuroblastoma)	
Adenocarcinoma	
Nasal Septum	**Nasal Septum**
Septal deviation	Septal deviation
Septal hematoma/abscess	Septal hematoma/abscess
Dislocated septum	Dislocated septum
Nasopharynx	
Adenoid hypertrophy	
Tumour	
Benign: juvenile nasopharyngeal angiofibroma (JNA), polyps	
Malignant: nasopharyngeal carcinoma	
Systemic	
Granulomatous diseases, diabetes, vasculitis	

Hoarseness

Lung malignancy is the most common cause of extralaryngeal vocal cord paralysis

Table 3. Differential Diagnosis of Hoarseness

Infectious	Acute/chronic laryngitis	
	Laryngotracheobronchitis (croup)	
Inflammatory	GERD	
	Vocal cord polyps/nodules	
	Lifestyle: smoking, chronic EtOH use	
Trauma	External laryngeal trauma	
	Endoscopy and endotracheal tube (e.g. intubation granuloma)	
Neoplasia	Benign tumour	Malignant tumours (e.g. thyroid)
	Papillomas (HPV infection)	SCC
	Minor salivary gland tumours	Other
	Other	
Cysts	Retention cysts	
Systemic	Endocrine	Connective tissue disease
	Hypothyroidism	RA
	Virilization	SLE
Neurologic (vocal cord paralysis due to superior ± recurrent laryngeal nerve injury)	Central lesions	Iatrogenic injury: thyroid, parathyroid surgery, carotid endarterectomy, patent ductus arteriosus (PDA) ligation
	Cerebrovascular accident (CVA)	Bilateral
	Head injury	Iatrogenic injury: bilateral thyroid
	Multiple sclerosis (MS)	surgery, forceps delivery
	Skull base tumours	Neuromuscular
	Arnold-Chiari malformation	Myasthenia gravis
	Peripheral lesions	
	Unilateral	
	Lung malignancy	
Functional	Psychogenic aphonia (hysterical aphonia)	
Congenital	Laryngomalacia	
	Laryngeal web	
	Laryngeal atresia	

Neck Mass

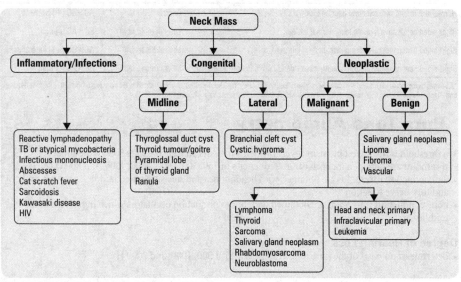

Figure 15. Differential diagnosis of a neck mass

Hearing

Normal Hearing Physiology

- **conductive pathway** (EAC to cochlea): air conduction of sound down the EAC → vibration of TM → sequential vibration of middle ear ossicles (malleus, incus, stapes) → transmission of amplified vibrations from stapes footplate to the oval window of the cochlea → transmitted vibrations via cochlear fluid create movement along the basilar membrane within the cochlea
- **neural pathway** (nerve to brain): basilar membrane vibration stimulates overlying hair cells in the organ of Corti → stimulation of bipolar neurons in the spiral ganglion of the cochlear division of CN VIII → cochlear nucleus → superior olivary nucleus → lateral lemniscus → inferior colliculus → Sylvian fissure of temporal lobe

Order of the Neural Pathway (with corresponding waves on ABR)

E COLI
Eighth cranial nerve (I – II)
Cochlear nucleus (III)
Superior Olivary nucleus
Lateral leminiscus (IV – V)
Inferior colliculus

Types of Hearing Loss

1. Conductive Hearing Loss
- conduction of sound to the cochlea is impaired
- can be caused by external and middle ear disease

2. Sensorineural Hearing Loss
- defect in the conversion of sound into neural signals or in the transmission of those signals to the cortex
- can be caused by disease of the inner ear (cochlea), acoustic nerve (CN VIII), brainstem, or cortex

3. Mixed Hearing Loss
- combination of conductive and sensorineural hearing loss

Auditory Acuity
- whispered-voice test: mask one ear and whisper into the other
- tuning fork tests (see Table 4; audiogram is of greater utility)
  - Rinne test
    - 512 Hz tuning fork is struck and held firmly on mastoid process to test BC; the tuning fork is then placed beside the pinna to test AC
  - If AC >BC → positive Rinne (normal)
  - Weber test
    - 512 Hz tuning fork is held on vertex of head and patient states whether it is heard centrally (Weber negative) or is lateralized to one side (Weber right, Weber left)
    - can place vibrating fork on patient's chin while they clench their teeth, or directly on teeth to elicit more reliable response
    - will only lateralize if difference in hearing loss between ears is >6 dB

Weber Test lateralization = ipsilateral conductive hearing loss or contralateral sensorineural hearing loss

The Weber test is more sensitive in detecting conductive hearing loss than the Rinne test

Frequency of Tuning Fork (Hz)	Minimum Hearing Loss for Rinne to Reverse (BC>AC, NEGATIVE Rinne) (dB)
256	15
512	30
1024	45

Range of Frequencies Audible to Human Ear
- 20 to 20000 Hz
- Most sensitive frequencies: 1000 to 4000 Hz
- Range of human speech: 500 to 2000 Hz

Hearing loss most often occurs at higher frequencies. Noise-induced (occupational) HL is classically seen at 4000 Hz. HL associated with otosclerosis is seen at 2000 Hz (Carhart's notch)

Table 4. The Interpretation of Tuning Fork Tests

Examples	Weber	Rinne
Normal or bilateral sensorineural hearing loss	Central	AC>BC (+) bilaterally
Right-sided conductive hearing loss, normal left ear	Lateralizes to right	BC>AC (−) right
Right-sided sensorineural hearing loss, normal left ear	Lateralizes to left	AC>BC (+) bilaterally
Right-sided severe sensorineural hearing loss or dead right ear, normal left ear	Lateralizes to left	BC>AC (−) right*

*A vibrating tuning fork on the mastoid stimulates the cochlea bilaterally, therefore in this case the left cochlea is stimulated by the Rinne test on the right (e.g. a false negative test). These tests are not valid if the ear canals are obstructed with cerumen (e.g. will create conductive loss)

Pure Tone Audiometry

- a threshold is the lowest intensity level at which a patient can hear the tone 50% of the time
- thresholds are obtained for each ear at frequencies of 250, 500, 1000, 2000, 4000, and 8000 Hz
- air conduction thresholds are obtained with headphones and measure outer, middle, inner ear, and auditory nerve function
- bone conduction thresholds are obtained with bone conduction oscillators which bypass the outer and middle ear

Degree of Hearing Loss
- determined on basis of the pure tone average (PTA) at 500, 1000, and 2000 Hz

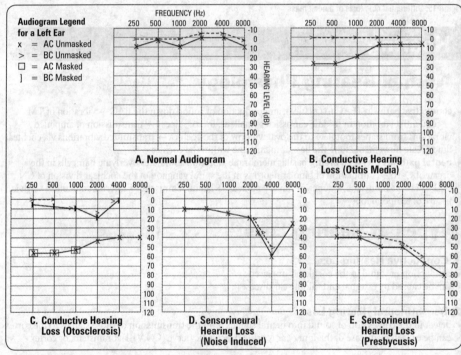

Figure 16. Types of hearing loss and associated audiograms of a left ear

PURE TONE PATTERNS

1. Conductive Hearing Loss (Figure 16B and 16C)
- BC in normal range
- AC outside of normal range
- gap between AC and BC thresholds >10 dB (an air-bone gap)

2. Sensorineural Hearing Loss (Figure 16D and 16E)
- both air and bone conduction thresholds below normal
- gap between AC and BC <10 dB (no air-bone gap)

3. Mixed Hearing Loss
- both air and bone conduction thresholds below normal
- gap between AC and BC thresholds >10 dB (an air-bone gap)

Speech Audiometry

Speech Reception Threshold
- lowest hearing level at which patient is able to repeat 50% of two syllable words which have equal emphasis on each syllable (spondee words)
- SRT and best pure tone threshold in the 500 to 2000 Hz range (frequency range of human speech) usually agree within 5 dB; if not, suspect a retrocochlear lesion or functional hearing loss
- used to assess the reliability of the pure tone audiometry

Speech Discrimination Test
- percentage of words the patient correctly repeats from a list of 50 monosyllabic words
- tested at 40 dB above the patient's SRT, therefore degree of hearing loss is taken into account
- patients with normal hearing or conductive hearing loss score >90%
- rollover effect: a decrease in discrimination as sound intensity increases; typical of a retrocochlear lesion (e.g. acoustic neuroma)
- investigate further if scores differ more than 20% between ears as asymmetry may indicate a retrocochlear lesion
- best predictor of hearing aid response: a poor discrimination score indicates significant neural degeneration and hearing aids may not be the best option for the patient

Impedance Audiometry

Tympanogram
- the Eustachian tube equalizes the pressure between the external and middle ear
- tympanograms graph the compliance of the middle ear system against a pressure gradient ranging from to −400 to +200 mmH$_2$O
- tympanogram peak occurs at the point of maximum compliance: where the pressure in the external canal is equivalent to the pressure in the middle ear
- normal range: −100 to +50 mmH$_2$O

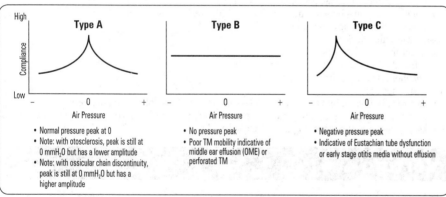

Figure 17. Tympanograms

Static Compliance
- volume measurement reflecting overall stiffness of the middle ear system
- normal range: 0.3-1.6 cc
- negative middle ear pressure and abnormal compliance indicate middle ear pathology
- in a type B curve, ear canal volumes of >2 cc in children and 2.5 cc in adults indicate TM perforation or presence of a patent ventilation tube

Acoustic Stapedial Reflexes
- stapedius muscle contracts in response to loud sound
- **acoustic reflex threshold** = 70-100 dB greater than hearing threshold; if hearing threshold >85 dB, reflex likely absent
- stimulating either ear causes bilateral and symmetrical reflexes
- for reflex to be present, CN VII must be intact and no conductive hearing loss in monitored ear
- if reflex is absent without conductive or severe sensorineural loss, suspect CN VII lesion
- **acoustic reflex decay test** = ability of stapedius muscle to sustain contraction for 10 s at 10 dB
- normally, little reflex decay occurs at 500 and 1000 Hz
- with cochlear hearing loss, acoustic reflex thresholds are 25-60 dB
- with retrocochlear hearing loss (acoustic neuroma), absent acoustic reflexes or marked reflex decay (>50%) within 5 s

Auditory Brainstem Response

- measures neuroelectric potentials (waves) in response to a stimulus in five different anatomic sites (see *Order of Neural Pathway* sidebar on OT9; this test can be used to determine the site of lesion
- delay in brainstem response suggests cochlear or retrocochlear abnormalities
- does not require volition or co-operation of patient (therefore of value in children and malingerers)

Otoacoustic Emissions

- objective test of hearing where a series of clicks is presented to the ear and the cochlea generates an echo which can be measured
- often used in newborn screening
- can be used to uncover normal hearing in malingering patients
- absence of emissions can be due to hearing loss or fluid in the middle ear

Aural Rehabilitation

- dependent on degree of hearing loss, communicative requirements, motivation, expectations, and physical and mental abilities
- negative prognostic factors
  - poor speech discrimination
  - narrow dynamic range (recruitment)
  - unrealistic expectations
- types of hearing aids
  - BTE: behind-the-ear (with occlusive mould or open fit which allows natural sound to pass – for milder hearing losses)
  - ITE: in-the-ear, placed in concha
  - ITC: in-the-canal, placed entirely in ear canal
  - CIC: contained-in-canal, placed deeply in ear canal
  - bone conduction – bone-anchored hearing aid (BAHA): attached to the skull
  - contralateral routing of signals (CROS)
- assistive listening devices
  - direct/indirect audio output
  - infrared, FM radio, or induction loop systems
  - telephone, television, or alerting devices
- cochlear implants
  - electrode is inserted into the cochlea to allow direct stimulation of the auditory nerve
  - for profound bilateral sensorineural hearing loss not rehabilitated with conventional hearing aids
  - established indication: post-lingually deafened adults, pre- and post-lingually deaf children

Pre-lingually deaf infants are the best candidates for aural rehabilitation because they have maximal benefit from ongoing developmental plasticity

Bone Anchored Hearing Aids (BAHA)
BAHAs function based on bone conduction and are indicated primarily for patients with conductive hearing loss, unilateral hearing loss, and mixed hearing loss who cannot wear conventional hearing aids. BAHAs consist of a titanium implant, an external abutment, and a sound processor. The sound processor transmits vibrations through the external abutment to the titanium implant and then directly to the cochlea

Pre-lingual deafness: deafness occurring before speech and language are acquired
Post-lingual deafness: deafness occurring after speech and language are acquired

Vertigo

Evaluation of the Dizzy Patient

- vertigo: illusion of rotational, linear, or tilting movement of self or environment
- vertigo is produced by peripheral (inner ear) or central (brainstem-cerebellum) stimulation
- it is important to distinguish vertigo from other potential causes of "dizziness" (see Figure 11, OT6)

Table 5. Peripheral vs. Central Vertigo

Symptoms	Peripheral	Central
Imbalance	Moderate-severe	Mild-moderate
Nausea and Vomiting	Severe	Variable
Auditory Symptoms	Common	Rare
Neurologic Symptoms	Rare	Common
Compensation	Rapid	Slow
Nystagmus	Unidirectional Horizontal or rotatory	Bidirectional Horizontal or vertical

Table 6. Differential Diagnosis of Vertigo Based on History

Condition	Duration	Hearing Loss	Tinnitus	Aural Fullness	Other Features
Benign Paroxysmal Positional Vertigo (BPPV)	Seconds	–	–	–	
Ménière's Disease	Minutes to hours Precedes attack	Uni/bilateral, fluctuating	+	Pressure/warmth	
Labyrinthitis/Vestibular Neuronitis	Hours to days	Unilateral	± Whistling	–	May have recent AOM
Acoustic Neuroma	Chronic	Progressive	+	–	Ataxia CN VII palsy

Table 7. Differential Diagnosis of Vertigo Based on Time Course

Time Course	Condition
Recurrent, lasting	BPPV
Single episode, lasting minutes to hours	Migraine, transient ischemia of the labyrinth or brainstem
Recurrent to hours	Ménière's
Prolonged	Vestibular neuritis, MS, brainstem/cerebellum infarct
Acoustic neuroma	Chronic

Benign Paroxysmal Positional Vertigo

Definition
- acute attacks of transient rotatory vertigo lasting seconds to minutes initiated by certain head positions, accompanied by torsional (i.e. rotatory) nystagmus (geotropic = fast phase towards the floor)
- most common form of positional vertigo (50% of patients with peripheral vestibular dysfunction)

Etiology
- due to canalithiasis (migration of free floating otoliths within the endolymph of the semicircular canal) or cupulolithiasis (otolith attached to the cupula of the semicircular canal)
  - can affect each of the 3 semicircular canals, although the posterior canal is affected in >90% of cases
  - causes: head injury, viral infection (URTI), degenerative disease, idiopathic
  - results in slightly different signals being received by the brain from the two balance organs resulting in sensation of movement

Diagnosis
- history (time course, provoking factors, associative symptoms)
- positive Dix-Hallpike maneuver (sensitivity 82%, specificity 71%)

Dix-Hallpike Positional Testing (see website for video and illustrations)
- the patient is rapidly moved from a sitting position to a supine position with the head hanging over the end of the table, turned to one side at 45° and neck extended 20° holding the position for 20 s
- onset of vertigo and rotary nystagmus indicate a positive test for the dependent side
- other diagnostic testing is not indicated in posterior canal BPPV

Treatment
- reassure patient that process resolves spontaneously
- particle repositioning maneuvers
  - Epley maneuver (performed by MD or by patient with the help of devices such as the DizzyFIX™)
  - Brandt-Daroff exercises (performed by patient)
- surgery for refractory cases
- anti-emetics for N/V
- drugs to suppress the vestibular system delay eventual recovery and are therefore not used

Ménière's Disease (Endolymphatic Hydrops)

Definition
- episodic attacks of tinnitus, hearing loss, aural fullness, and vertigo lasting minutes to hours

Proposed Etiology
- inadequate absorption of endolymph leads to endolymphatic hydrops (over accumulation) that distorts the membranous labyrinth

Epidemiology
- peak incidence 40-60 yr
- bilateral in 35% of cases

BPPV is the most common cause of episodic vertigo; patients often are symptomatic when rolling over in bed or moving their head to a position of extreme posterior extension such as looking up at a tall building or getting their hair washed at the hairdresser

Signs of BPPV seen with Dix-Hallpike Maneuver
- Latency of ~20 s
- Crescendo/decrescendo vertigo lasting 20 s
- Geotropic rotatory nystagmus (nystagmus MUST be present for a positive test)
- Reversal of nystagmus upon sitting up
- Fatigability with repeated stimulation

Diagnostic Criteria for Ménière's Disease (must have all three):
- Two spontaneous episodes of rotational vertigo ≥20 minutes
- Audiometric confirmation of SNHL (often low frequency)
- Tinnitus and/or aural fullness

Clinical Features
- episodic vertigo, fluctuating low frequency SNHL, tinnitus, and aural fullness
- ± drop attacks (Tumarkin crisis), ± N/V
- vertigo disappears with time (min to h), but hearing loss remains
- early in the disease: fluctuating SNHL
- later stages: persistent tinnitus and progressive hearing loss
- attacks come in clusters and can be debilitating to the patient
- triggers: high salt intake, caffeine, stress, nicotine, and alcohol

Treatment
- acute management may consist of bed rest, antiemetics, antivertiginous drugs (e.g. betahistine [Serc®] meclizine, dimenhydramine), and anticholinergics (e.g. scopolamine)
- long-term management may include
  - medical
    - low salt diet, diuretics (e.g. hydrochlorothiazide, triamterene, amiloride)
    - Serc® prophylactically to decrease intensity of attacks
    - intratympanic gentamicin to destroy vestibular end-organ, results in complete SNHL
    - intratympanic glucocorticoids (e.g. dexamethasone) may improve vertigo symptoms
  - surgical
    - selective vestibular neurectomy or labyrinthectomy
    - potential benefit for endolymphatic sac decompression or sacculotomy
- must monitor opposite ear as bilaterality occurs in 35% of cases

Vestibular Neuronitis (Labyrinthitis)

Definition
- acute onset of disabling vertigo often accompanied by N/V and imbalance without hearing loss that resolves over days leaving a residual imbalance that lasts **days to weeks**
- vestibular neuronitis: inflammation of the vestibular portion of CNVIII
- labyrinthitis: inflammation of both vestibular and cochlear portions

Etiology
- thought to be due to a viral infection (e.g. measles, mumps, herpes zoster) or post-viral syndrome
- only ~30% of cases have associated URTI symptoms
- labyrinthitis may occur as a complication of acute and chronic otitis media, bacterial meningitis, cholesteatoma, and temporal bone fractures

Drop Attacks (Tumarkin's Otolithic Crisis) are sudden falls occurring without warning and without LOC, where patients experiences feeling of being pushed down into the ground

Clinical Features
- acute phase
  - severe vertigo with N/V and imbalance lasting 1-5 d
  - irritative nystagmus (fast phase towards the offending ear)
  - ataxia: patient tends to veer towards affected side
  - tinnitus and hearing loss in labyrinthitis
- convalescent phase
  - imbalance and motion sickness lasting days to weeks
  - spontaneous nystagmus away from affected side
  - gradual vestibular adaptation requires weeks to months

Before proceeding with gentamicin treatment, perform a gadolinium enhanced MRI to rule out CPA tumour as the cause of symptoms

Treatment
- acute phase
  - bed rest, antivertiginous drugs
  - corticosteroids (methylprednisolone) ± antivirals
  - bacterial infection: treat with IV antibiotics, drainage of middle ear, ± mastoidectomy
- convalescent phase
  - progressive ambulation especially in the elderly
  - vestibular exercises: involve eye and head movements, sitting, standing, and walking

Acoustic Neuroma (Vestibular Schwannoma)

Definition
- schwannoma of the vestibular portion of CN VIII

Pathogenesis
- starts in the internal auditory canal and expands into cerebellopontine angle (CPA), compressing cerebellum and brainstem
- when associated with type 2 neurofibromatosis (NF2): bilateral acoustic neuromas, juvenile cataracts, meningiomas, and ependymomas

Acoustic neuroma is the most common intracranial tumour causing SNHL and the most common cerebellopontine angle tumour

In the elderly, unilateral tinnitus or SNHL is acoustic neuroma until proven otherwise

Clinical Features
- usually presents with unilateral SNHL (chronic) or tinnitus
- dizziness and unsteadiness may be present, but true vertigo is rare as tumour growth occurs slowly and thus compensation occurs

- facial nerve palsy and trigeminal (V1) sensory deficit (corneal reflex) are late complications
- risk factors: exposure to loud noise, childhood exposure to low-dose radiation, history of parathyroid adenoma

Diagnosis
- MRI with gadolinium contrast (gold standard)
- audiogram (to assess SNHL)
- poor speech discrimination relative to the hearing loss
- stapedial reflex absent or significant reflex decay
- ABR: increase in latency of the 5th wave
- vestibular tests: normal or asymmetric caloric weakness (an early sign)

Treatment
- expectant management if tumour is very small, or in elderly
- definitive management is surgical excision
- other options: gamma knife, radiation

Tinnitus

Definition
- an auditory perception in the absence of an acoustic stimuli, likely related to loss of input to neurons in central auditory pathways and resulting in abnormal firing

History
- subjective vs. objective (see Figure 14, OT7)
- continuous vs. pulsatile (vascular in origin)
- unilateral vs. bilateral
- associated symptoms: hearing loss, vertigo, aural fullness, otalgia, otorrhea

Investigations
- audiology
- if unilateral
  - ABR, gadolinium enhanced MRI to exclude a retrocochlear lesion
  - CT to diagnose glomus tympanicum (rare)
  - MRI or angiogram to diagnose AVM
- if suspect metabolic abnormality: lipid profile, TSH, zinc levels

Treatment
- if a cause is found, treat the cause (e.g. drainage of middle ear effusion, embolization or excision of AVM)
- with no treatable cause: 50% will improve, 25% worsen, 25% remain the same
- avoid loud noise, ototoxic meds, caffeine, smoking
- tinnitus clinics
- identify situations where tinnitus is most bothersome (e.g. quiet times), mask tinnitus with soft music or "white noise"
- hearing aid if coexistent hearing loss
- tinnitus instrument: combines hearing aid with white noise masker
- trial of tocainamide

Diseases of the External Ear

Cerumen Impaction

Etiology
- ear wax: a mixture of secretions from ceruminous and pilosebaceous glands, squames of epithelium, dust, and debris

Risk Factors
- hairy or narrow ear canals, in-the-ear hearing aids, cotton swab usage, osteomata

Clinical Features
- hearing loss (conductive)
- ± tinnitus, vertigo, otalgia, aural fullness

Treatment
- water or ceruminolytic drops (bicarbonate solution, olive oil, glycerine, Cerumenol®, Cerumenex®)
- manual debridement (by MD)

Cerumen impaction is the most common cause of conductive hearing loss for those aged 15-50 yr

Syringing

Indications
- Totally occlusive cerumen with pain, decreased hearing, or tinnitus

Contraindications
- Active infection
- Previous ear surgery
- Only hearing ear
- TM perforation

Complications
- Otitis externa
- TM perforation
- Trauma
- Pain
- Vertigo
- Tinnitus
- Otitis media

Method
- Establish that TM is intact
- Gently pull the pinna superiorly and posteriorly
- Using lukewarm water, aim the syringe nozzle upwards and posteriorly to irrigate the ear canal

Diseases of the External Ear

Exostoses

Definition
• bony protuberances in the external auditory canal composed of lamellar bone

Etiology
• possible association with swimming in cold water

Clinical Features
• usually an incidental finding
• if large, they can cause cerumen impaction or otitis externa

Treatment
• no treatment required unless symptomatic

Otitis Externa

Etiology
• bacterial (90% of OE): *Pseudomonas aeruginosa*, *Pseudomonas vulgaris*, *E. coli*, *S. aureus*
• fungal: *Candida albicans*, *Aspergillus niger*

Risk Factors
• associated with swimming ("swimmer's ear")
• mechanical cleaning (Q-tips®), skin dermatitis, aggressive scratching
• devices that occlude the ear canal: hearing aids, headphones, etc.
• allergic contact dermatitis, dermatologic conditions (psoriasis, atopic dermatitis)

Clinical Features
• acute
  ▪ pain aggravated by movement of auricle (traction of pinna or pressure over tragus)
  ▪ otorrhea (sticky yellow purulent discharge)
  ▪ conductive hearing loss ± aural fullness 2° to obstruction of external canal by swelling and purulent debris
  ▪ posterior auricular lymphadenopathy
  ▪ complicated OE exists if the pinna and/or the periauricular soft tissues are erythematous and swollen
• chronic
  ▪ pruritus of external ear ± excoriation of ear canal
  ▪ atrophic and scaly epidermal lining, ± otorrhea, ± hearing loss
  ▪ wide meatus but no pain with movement of auricle
  ▪ tympanic membrane appears normal

Pulling on the pinna is extremely painful in otitis externa, but is usually well tolerated in otitis media

Treatment
• clean ear under magnification with irrigation, suction, dry swabbing, and C&S
• bacterial etiology
  ▪ antipseudomonal otic drops (e.g. ciprofloxacin) or a combination of antibiotic and steroid (e.g. Cipro HC®)
  ▪ do not use aminoglycoside if the tympanic membrane (TM) is perforated because of the risk of ototoxicity
  ▪ introduction of fine gauze wick (pope wick) if external canal edematous
  ▪ ± 3% acetic acid solution to acidify ear canal (low pH is bacteriostatic)
  ▪ systemic antibiotics if either cervical lymphadenopathy or cellulitis is present
• fungal etiology
  ▪ repeated debridement and topical antifungals (gentian violet, Mycostatin® powder, boric acid, Locacorten®, Vioform® drops)
• ± analgesics
• chronic otitis externa (pruritus without obvious infection) → corticosteroid alone (e.g. diprosalic acid)

Malignant (Necrotizing) Otitis Externa (Skull Base Osteomyelitis)

Definition
• osteomyelitis of the temporal bone

Epidemiology
• occurs in elderly diabetics and immunocompromised patients

Etiology
• rare complication of otitis externa
• *Pseudomonas* infection in 99% of cases

Clinical Features
- otalgia and purulent otorrhea that is refractory to medical therapy
- granulation tissue on the floor of the auditory canal

Complications
- cranial nerve palsy (most commonly CN VII>CN X>CN XI)
- systemic infection, death

Management
- imaging: high resolution temporal bone CT scan, gadolinium enhanced MRI, technetium scan
- requires hospital admission, debridement, IV antibiotics, hyperbaric O_2
- may require OR for debridement of necrotic tissue/bone

Gallium and Technetium Scans
Gallium scans are used to show sites of active infection. Gallium is taken up by PMNs and therefore only lights up when active infection is present. It will not show the extent of osteomyelitis. Technetium scans provide information about osteoblastic activity and, as a result, are used to demonstrate sites of osteomyelitis. Technetium scans help with diagnosis whereas gallium scans are useful in follow-up

Diseases of the Middle Ear

Acute Otitis Media and Otitis Media with Effusion

- see *Pediatric Otolaryngology*, OT38

Chronic Otitis Media

Definition
- an ear with TM perforation in the setting of recurrent or chronic ear infections

Benign
- dry TM perforation without active infection

Chronic Serous Otitis Media
- continuous serous drainage (straw-coloured)

Chronic Suppurative Otitis Media
- persistent purulent drainage through a perforated TM

Cholesteatoma

Definition
- a cyst composed of keratinized desquamated epithelial cells occurring in the middle ear, mastoid, and temporal bone
- two types: congenital and acquired

Congenital
- presents as a "small white pearl" behind an intact tympanic membrane (anterior and medial to the malleus) or as a conductive hearing loss
- believed to be due to aberrant migration of external canal ectoderm during development
- not associated with otitis media/Eustachian tube dysfunction

Acquired (more common)
- primary cholesteatoma
  - frequently associated with retraction pockets in the pars flaccida (may lead to attic cholesteatomas which are difficult to visualize)
  - often has crusting or desquamated debris on lateral surface
- secondary cholesteatoma
  - pearly mass evident behind TM, frequently associated with marginal perforation
  - may appear as skin that have replaced the mucosa of the middle ear
- the associated chronic inflammatory process causes progressive destruction of surrounding bony structures

Mechanisms of Cholesteatoma Formation
- Epithelial migration through TM perforation (2° acquired)
- Invagination of TM (1° acquired)
- Metaplasia of middle ear epithelium or basal cell hyperplasia (congenital)

Clinical Features
- history of otitis media (especially if unilateral), ventilation tubes, ear surgery
- symptoms
  - progressive hearing loss (predominantly conductive although may get sensorineural hearing loss in late stage)
  - otalgia, aural fullness, fever
- signs
  - retraction pocket in TM, may contain keratin debris
  - TM perforation
  - granulation tissue, polyp visible on otoscopy
  - malodourous, unilateral otorrhea

Complications

Table 8. Complications of Cholesteatoma

Local	Intracranial
Ossicular erosion: conductive hearing loss	Meningitis
Inner ear erosion: SNHL, dizziness, and/or labyrinthitis	Sigmoid sinus thrombosis
Temporal bone infection: mastoiditis, petrositis	Intracranial abscess (subdural, epidural, cerebellar)
Facial paralysis	

Investigations
- audiogram and CT scan

Treatment
- there is no conservative therapy for cholesteatoma
- surgical: mastoidectomy ± tympanoplasty ± ossicular reconstruction

Mastoiditis

Definition
- infection (usually subperiosteal) of mastoid air cells, most commonly seen approximately two weeks after onset of untreated or inadequately treated acute suppurative otitis media
- more common in children than adults

Etiology
- acute mastoiditis caused by the same organisms as AOM: *S. pneumoniae*, *H. influenzae*, *M. catarrhalis*, *S. pyogenes*, *S. aureus*, *P. aeruginosa*

Clinical Features
- otorrhea
- tenderness to pressure over the mastoid
- retroauricular swelling with protruding ear
- fever, hearing loss, ± TM perforation (late)
- CT radiologic findings: opacification of mastoid air cells by fluid and interruption of normal trabeculations of cells (coalescence)

Classic Triad
- Otorrhea
- Tenderness to pressure over the mastoid
- Retroauricular swelling with protruding ear

Treatment
- IV antibiotics with myringotomy and ventilation tubes – usually all that is required acutely
- cortical mastoidectomy
- debridement of infected tissue allowing aeration and drainage
- indications for surgery
- failure of medical treatment after 48 h
- symptoms of intracranial complications
- aural discharge persisting for 4 wk and resistant to antibiotics

Complications of AOM are rare due to rapid and effective treatment of AOM with antibiotics

Otosclerosis

Definition
- fusion of stapes footplate to oval window so that it cannot vibrate

Etiology
- autosomal dominant, variable penetrance approximately 40%
- F>M, progresses during pregnancy (hormone responsive)

Otosclerosis is the 2nd most common cause of conductive hearing loss in 15-50 yr old (after cerumen impaction)

Clinical Features
- progressive conductive hearing loss first noticed in teens and 20s (may progress to sensorineural hearing loss if cochlea involved)
- ± pulsatile tinnitus
- tympanic membrane normal ± pink blush (Schwartz's sign) associated with the neovascularization of otosclerotic bone
- characteristic dip at 2000 Hz (Carhart's notch) on audiogram (see Figure 16C, OT10)

Treatment
- monitor with serial audiograms if coping with loss
- hearing aid (air conduction, bone conduction, BAHA)
- stapedectomy or stapedotomy (with laser or drill) with prosthesis is definitive treatment

Diseases of the Inner Ear

Congenital Sensorineural Hearing Loss

Hereditary Defects
- non-syndrome associated (70%)
  - often idiopathic, autosomal recessive
  - connexin 26 (GJB2) most common
- syndrome associated (30%)
  - Waardenburg: white forelock, heterochromia iridis (each eye different colour), wide nasal bridge, and increased distance between medial canthi
  - Pendred: deafness associated with thyroid gland disorders, SLC26A4 gene, enlarged vestibular aqueducts
  - Treacher-Collins: first and second branchial cleft anomalies
  - Alport: hereditary nephritis

Prenatal TORCH Infections
- toxoplasmosis, others (e.g. HIV, syphilis), rubella, CMV, HSV

Perinatal
- Rh incompatibility
- anoxia
- hyperbilirubinemia
- birth trauma (hemorrhage into inner ear)

Postnatal
- meningitis, mumps, measles

High Risk Factors (for hearing loss in newborns)
- low birth weight/prematurity
- perinatal anoxia (low APGARs)
- kernicterus: bilirubin >25 mg/dL
- craniofacial abnormality
- family history of deafness in childhood
- 1st trimester illness: TORCH infections
- neonatal sepsis
- ototoxic drugs
- perinatal infection, including post-natal meningitis
- consanguinity
- 50-75% of newborns with SNHL have at least one of the above risk factors and 90% of these have spent time in the NICU

Treatment
- presence of any risk factor: ABR study performed before leaving NICU and at 3 mo adjusted age
- early rehabilitation improves speech and school performance

Presbycusis

Definition
- SNHL associated with aging (starting in 5th and 6th decades)

Presbycusis is the most common cause of SNHL

Etiology
- hair cell degeneration
- age related degeneration of basilar membrane, possibly genetic etiology
- cochlear neuron damage
- ischemia of inner ear

Clinical Features
- progressive, bilateral hearing loss initially at high frequencies, then middle frequencies
- loss of discrimination of speech especially with background noise present – patients describe people as mumbling
- recruitment phenomenon: inability to tolerate loud sounds
- tinnitus

Treatment
- hearing aid if patient has difficulty functioning, hearing loss >30-35 dB, and good speech discrimination
- ± lip reading, auditory training, auditory aids (doorbell and phone lights)

Sudden Sensorineural Hearing Loss

Clinical Features
- presents as a sudden onset of significant SNHL (usually unilateral) ± tinnitus, aural fullness
- usually idiopathic, rule out other causes
- autoimmune causes (e.g. ESR, rheumatoid factor, ANA)
- MRI to rule out tumour and/or CT to rule out ischemic/hemorrhagic stroke if associated with any other focal neurological signs (e.g. vertigo, ataxia, abnormality of CN V or VII, weakness)

Treatment
- Intratympanic or oral corticosteroids within 3 d of onset: prednisone 1 mg/kg/d for 10-14 d

Prognosis
- depends on degree of hearing loss
- 70% resolve within 10-14 d
- 20% experience partial resolution
- 10% experience permanent hearing loss

Sudden SNHL may easily be confused with ischemic brain events. It is important to keep a high index of suspicion especially with elderly patients presenting with sudden SNHL as well as vertigo

Autoimmune Inner Ear Disease

Etiology
- idiopathic
- may be associated with systemic autoimmune diseases (e.g. rheumatoid arthritis, SLE), vasculitides (e.g. GPA, polyarteritis nodosa), and allergies

Epidemiology
- most common between ages 20-50

Clinical Features
- rapidly progressive or fluctuating bilateral SNHL
- ± tinnitus, aural fullness, vestibular symptoms (e.g. ataxia, disequilibrium, vertigo)

Investigations
- autoimmune workup: CBC, ESR, ANA, rheumatoid factor

Treatment
- high-dose corticosteroids: treat early for at least 30 d
- consider cytotoxic medication for steroid non-responders

Drug Ototoxicity

Aminoglycosides
- streptomycin and gentamicin (vestibulotoxic), kanamycin, and tobramycin (cochleotoxic)
- toxic to hair cells by any route: oral, IV, and topical (if the TM is perforated)
- destroys sensory hair cells: outer first, inner second (therefore otoacoustic emissions are lost first)
- high frequency hearing loss develops earliest
- ototoxicity occurs days to weeks post-treatment
- must monitor with peak and trough levels when prescribed, especially if patient has neutropenia and/or history of ear or renal problems
- q24h dosing recommended (with amount determined by creatinine clearance)
- aminoglycoside toxicity displays saturable kinetics, therefore, once daily dosing presents less risk than divided daily doses
- duration of treatment is the most important predictor of ototoxicity
- treatment: immediately stop aminoglycosides

Salicylates
- hearing loss with tinnitus, reversible if discontinued

Antimalarials (Quinines)
- hearing loss with tinnitus
- reversible if discontinued but can lead to permanent loss

Others
- many antineoplastic agents are ototoxic (weigh risks vs. benefits)
- loop diuretics

Noise-Induced Sensorineural Hearing Loss

Pathogenesis
- 85-90 dB over months or years or single sound impulses >135 dB can cause cochlear damage
- bilateral SNHL initially and most prominently at 4000 Hz (resonant frequency of the temporal bone), known as "boilermaker's notch" on audiogram, extends to higher and lower frequencies with time (see Figure 16D, OT10)
- speech reception not altered until hearing loss >30 dB at speech frequency, therefore considerable damage may occur before patient complains of hearing loss
- difficulty with speech discrimination, especially in situations with competing noise

Phases of Hearing Loss
- dependent on: intensity of sound and duration of exposure
  - temporary threshold shift
  - when exposed to loud sound, decreased sensitivity or increased threshold for sound
  - may have associated aural fullness and tinnitus
  - with removal of noise, hearing returns to normal
- permanent threshold shift
  - hearing does not return to previous state

Treatment
- hearing aid
- prevention
  - ear protectors: muffs, plugs
  - limit exposure to noise with frequent rest periods
  - regular audiologic follow-up

Temporal Bone Fractures

Table 9. Features of Temporal Bone Fractures

	Transverse (1)	Longitudinal (2)
Extension	Into bony labyrinth and internal auditory meatus	Into middle ear
Incidence	10-20%	70-90%
Etiology	Frontal/occipital trauma	Lateral skull trauma
CN Pathology	CN VII palsy (50%)	CN VII palsy (10-20%)
Hearing Loss	SNHL due to direct cochlear injury	CHL secondary to ossicular injury
Vestibular Symptoms	Sudden onset vestibular symptoms due to direct semicircular canal injury (vertigo, spontaneous nystagmus)	Rare
Other Features	Intact external auditory meatus, TM ± hemotympanum Spontaneous nystagmus CSF leak in Eustachian tube to nasopharynx ± rhinorrhea (risk of meningitis)	Torn TM or hemotympanum Bleeding from external auditory canal Step formation in external auditory canal CSF otorrhea Battle's sign = mastoid ecchymoses Raccoon eyes = periorbital ecchymoses

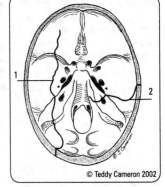

© Teddy Cameron 2002

Figure 18. Types of temporal bone fractures

- characterized as longitudinal or transverse relative to the long axis of the petrous temporal bone
- temporal bone fractures are rarely purely transverse or longitudinal (often a mixed picture)

Diagnosis
- otoscopy
- do not syringe or manipulate external auditory meatus due to risk of inducing meningitis via TM perforation
- CT head
- audiology, facial nerve tests (for transverse fractures), Schirmer's test (of lacrimation), stapedial reflexes if CN VII palsy
- if suspecting CSF leak: look for halo sign, send fluid for β-2 transferrin or β trace protein (prostaglandin D synthase)

Treatment
- ABCs
- medical: expectant, prevent otogenic meningitis
- surgical: explore temporal bone, indications
  - CN VII palsy (immediate and complete)
  - gunshot wound
  - depressed fracture of external auditory meatus
  - early meningitis (mastoidectomy)
  - bleeding intracranially from sinus
  - CSF otorrhea (may resolve spontaneously)

Hemotympanum can be indicative of temporal bone trauma

Signs of Basilar Skull Fracture
Battle's Sign: ecchymosis of the mastoid process of the temporal bone

Racoon Eyes

CSF Rhinorrhea/Otorrhea

Cranial Nerve Involvement: facial palsy → CN VII, nystagmus → CN VI, facial numbness → CN V

Complications
- AOM ± labyrinthitis ± mastoiditis
- meningitis/epidural abscess/brain abscess
- post-traumatic cholesteatoma

Facial Nerve (CN VII) Paralysis

Peripheral Facial Paralysis (PFP)
- mononeuropathy of the facial nerve where there is weakening in the facial muscles, which alter the facial symmetry and functions
- can have a detectable cause (secondary facial nerve palsy) or may be idiopathic (primary)

Etiology
- supranuclear and nuclear (MS, poliomyelitis, cerebral tumours)
- infranuclear

Treatment
- treat according to etiology plus provide corneal protection with artificial tears, nocturnal lid taping, tarsorrhaphy, gold weighting of upper lid
- facial paralysis that does not resolve with time or with medical treatment will often be referred for possible reanimation techniques to restore function
  - common reanimation techniques include
    - direct facial nerve anastomosis
    - interpositional grafts
    - anastomosis to other motor nerves
    - muscle transpositions

Table 10. Differential Diagnosis of Peripheral Facial Paralysis (PFP)

Etiology	Incidence	Findings	Investigations	Treatment, Follow-up, and Prognosis (Px)
Bell's Palsy Idiopathic, (HSV) infection of the facial nerve Diagnosis of exclusion	80-90% of PFP **Risk Factors:** DM Pregnancy Viral prodrome (50%)	**Hx** Acute onset Numbness of ear Schirmer's test Recurrence (12%) + FHx (14%) Hyperacusis (30%) **P/E** Paralysis or paresis of all muscle groups on one side of the face Absence of signs of CNS disease Absence of signs of ear or CPA diseases	Stapedial reflex absent Audiology normal (or baseline) EMG – best measure for prognosis Topognostic testing MRI with gadolinium – enhancement of CN VII and VIII High resolution CT	**Rx** Protect the eye to prevent exposure keratitis with patching or tarsorraphy Systemic steroids may lessen degeneration and hasten recovery Consider antiviral (acyclovir) **F/U** Spontaneous remission should begin within 3 wk of onset Delayed (3-6 mo) recovery portends at least some functional loss **Px** ENoG testing between day 3-14 of onset: <90% degeneration=high likelihood of recovery >90% + no voluntary EMG motor unit potentials= surgical decompression Poorer if hyperacusis, >60 yr, DM, HTN, severe pain
Ramsay Hunt Syndrome (Herpes Zoster Oticus) Varicella zoster infection of CN VII/VIII	4.5-9% of PFP **Risk Factors:** >60 yr Impaired immunity Cancer Radiotherapy Chemotherapy	**Hx** Hyperacusis SNHL Severe pain of pinna, mouth, or face **P/E** Vesicles on pinna, external canal (errupt 3-7 d after onset of pain) Associated herpes zoster ophthalmicus (uveitis, keratoconjunctivitis, optic neuritis, or glaucoma)	Stapedial reflex absent Audiology – SNHL Viral ELISA studies to confirm MRI with gadolinium (86% of facial nerves enhance)	**Rx** Avoid touching lesions to prevent spread of infection Systemic steroids can relieve pain, vertigo, avoid postherpetic neuralgia Acyclovir may lessen pain, aid healing of vesicles **F/U:** 2-4 wk **Px** Poorer prognosis than Bell's palsy; 22% recover completely, 66% incomplete paralysis, 10% complete paralysis
TEMPORAL BONE FRACTURE *rarely a patient has a single type of fracture				
Longitudinal (90%)	20% have PFP	**Hx** Blow to side of head **P/E** Trauma to side of head Neuro findings consistent with epidural/subdural bleed	Skull x-rays CT head	**Px** Injury usually due to stretch or impingement; may recover with time
Transverse (10%)	40% have PFP	**Hx** Blow to frontal or occipital area **P/E** Trauma to front or back of head	Skull x-rays CT head	**Px** Nerve transection more likely
Iatrogenic		Variable (depending on level of injury)	Wait for lidocaine to wear off EMG	**Rx** Exploration if complete nerve paralysis No exploration if any movement present Source: Paul Warrick, MD

Rhinitis

Definition
- inflammation of the lining (mucosa) of the nasal cavity

Table 11. Classification of Rhinitis

Inflammatory	Non-Inflammatory

Perennial non-allergic
  Asthma, ASA sensitivity
Allergic
  Seasonal
  Perennial
Atrophic
  Primary: *Klebsiella ozena* (especially in elderly)
  Acquired: post-surgery if too much mucosa or turbinate has
  been resected
Infectious
  Viral: e.g. rhinovirus, influenza, parainfluenza, etc.
  Bacterial: e.g. *S. aureus*
  Fungal
  Granulomatous: TB, syphilis, leprosy
Non-infectious
  Sarcoidosis
  GPA
Irritant
  Dust
  Chemicals
  Pollution
	Rhinitis medicamentosa
	  Topical decongestants
	Hormonal
	  Pregnancy
	  Estrogens
	  Thyroid
	Idiopathic vasomotor

Rhinitis medicamentosa: rebound congestion due to the overuse of intranasal vasoconstrictors; for prevention, use of these medications for only 5-7 d is recommended

Table 12. Nasal Discharge: Character and Associated Conditions

Character	Associated Conditions
Watery/mucoid	Allergic, viral, vasomotor, CSF leak (halo sign)
Mucopurulent	Bacterial, foreign body
Serosanguinous	Neoplasia
Bloody	Trauma, neoplasia, bleeding disorder, hypertension/vascular disease

Allergic Rhinitis (i.e. Hay Fever)

Definition
- rhinitis characterized by an IgE-mediated hypersensitivity to foreign allergens
- acute-and-seasonal or chronic-and-perennial
- perennial allergic rhinitis often confused with recurrent colds

Etiology
- when allergens contact the respiratory mucosa, specific IgE antibody is produced in susceptible hosts
- concentration of allergen in the ambient air correlates directly with the rhinitis symptoms

Congestion reduces nasal airflow and allows the nose to repair itself (i.e. washes away the irritants)

Treatment should focus on the initial insult rather than target this defense mechanism

Epidemiology
- age at onset usually <20 yr
- more common in those with a personal or family history of allergies/atopy

Clinical Features
- nasal: obstruction with pruritus, sneezing
- clear rhinorrhea (containing increased eosinophils)
- itching of eyes with tearing
- frontal headache and pressure
- mucosa: swollen, pale, "boggy"
- seasonal (summer, spring, early autumn)
  - pollens from trees
  - lasts several weeks, disappears, and recurs following year at same time
- perennial
  - inhaled: house dust, wool, feathers, foods, tobacco, hair, mould
  - ingested: wheat, eggs, milk, nuts
  - occurs intermittently for years with no pattern or may be constantly present

Complications
- chronic sinusitis/polyps
- serous otitis media

Diagnosis
- history
- direct exam
- allergy testing

Treatment
- education: identification and avoidance of allergen
- nasal irrigation with saline
- antihistamines (e.g. diphenhydramine, fexofenadine)
- oral decongestants (e.g. pseudoephedrine, phenylpropanolamine)
- topical decongestant (may lead to rhinitis medicamentosa)
- other topicals: steroids (fluticasone), disodium cromoglycate, antihistamines, ipratropium bromide
- oral steroids if severe
- desensitization by allergen immunotherapy

Vasomotor Rhinitis

- neurovascular disorder of nasal parasympathetic system (vidian nerve) affecting mucosal blood vessels
- nonspecific reflex hypersensitivity of nasal mucosa
- caused by
  - temperature change
  - alcohol, dust, smoke
  - stress, anxiety, neurosis
  - endocrine: hypothyroidism, pregnancy, menopause
  - parasympathomimetic drugs
  - beware of rhinitis medicamentosa: reactive vasodilation due to prolonged use (>5 d) of nasal drops and sprays (Dristan®, Otrivin®)

Clinical Features
- chronic intermittent nasal obstruction, varies from side to side
- rhinorrhea: thin, watery
- mucosa and turbinates: swollen
- nasal allergy must be ruled out

Treatment
- elimination of irritant factors
- parasympathetic blocker (Atrovent® nasal spray)
- steroids (e.g. beclomethasone, fluticasone)
- surgery (often of limited lasting benefit): electrocautery, cryosurgery, laser treatment, or removal of inferior or middle turbinates
- vidian neurectomy (rarely done)
- symptomatic relief with exercise (increased sympathetic tone)

Rhinosinusitis

Pathogenesis of Rhinosinusitis
- ostial obstruction or dysfunctional cilia permit stagnant mucous and, consequently, infection
- all sinuses drain to a common prechamber under the middle meatus called the osteomeatal complex

Definition
- inflammation of the mucosal lining of the sinuses and nasal passages

Classification
- acute: <4 wk
- subacute: 4-8 wk
- chronic: >8-12 wk

Table 13. Etiologies of Rhinosinusitis

Ostial Obstruction	Inflammation	URTI
		Allergy
	Mechanical	Septal deviation
		Turbinate hypertrophy
		Polyps
		Tumours
		Adenoid hypertrophy
		Foreign body
		Congenital abnormalities (e.g. cleft palate)
	Immune	PA
		Lymphoma, leukemia
		Immunosuppressed patients (e.g. neutropenics, diabetics, HIV)
Systemic		Cystic fibrosis
		Immotile cilia (e.g. Kartagener's
Direct Extension	Dental	Infection
	Trauma	Facial fractures

Acute Bacterial Rhinosinusitis

Definition
- bacterial infection of the paranasal sinuses and nasal passages lasting >7 d
- clinical diagnosis requiring ≥2 major symptoms, at least one of the symptoms is either nasal obstruction or purulent/discoloured nasal discharge
  - **major symptoms**
    - ◆ facial pain/pressure/fullness
    - ◆ nasal obstruction
    - ◆ purulent/discoloured nasal discharge
    - ◆ hyposmia/anosmia
  - **minor symptoms**
    - ◆ headache
    - ◆ halitosis
    - ◆ fatigue
    - ◆ dental pain
    - ◆ cough
    - ◆ ear pain/fullness

Etiology
- bacteria: *S. pneumoniae* (35%), *H. influenzae* (35%), *M. catarrhalis*, *S. aureus*, anaerobes (dental)
- children are more prone to a bacterial etiology, but viral is still more common
- maxillary sinus most commonly affected
- must rule out fungal causes (mucormycosis) in immunocompromised hosts (especially if painless, black or pale mucosa on examination)

Clinical Features
- sudden onset of
  - nasal blockage/congestion and/or purulent nasal discharge/posterior nasal drip
  - ± facial pain or pressure, hyposmia, sore throat
- persistent/worsening symptoms >5-7 d or presence of purulence for 3-4 d with high fever
- speculum exam: erythematous mucosa, mucopurulent discharge, pus originating from the middle meatus
- predisposing factors: viral URTI, allergy, dental disease, anatomical defects
- differentiate from acute viral rhinosinusitis (course: <10 d, peaks by 3 d)

Diagnosis
- along with clinical criteria, can confirm radiographically and/or endoscopically using antral puncture for bacterial cultures

Management
- depends on symptom severity (i.e. intensity/duration of symptoms, impact on quality of life)
- mild-moderate: INCS
  - if no response within 72 h, add antibiotics
- severe: INCS + antibiotics
- antibiotics
  - 1st line: amoxicillin x 10 d (TMP-SMX or macrolide if penicillin allergy)
- if no response to 1st line antibiotics within 72 h, switch to 2nd line
  - 2nd line: fluoroquinolones or amoxicillin-clavulanic acid inhibitors
- adjuvant therapy (saline or HOCL (pediatric sinusitis) irrigation, analgesics, oral/topical decongestant) may provide symptomatic relief
- CT indicated only if complications are suspected

Acute Rhinosinusitis Complications
Consider hospitalization if any of the following are suspected
- Orbital (Chandler's classification)
  • Preseptal cellulitis
  • Postseptal cellulitis
  • Subperiosteal abscess
  • Orbital abscess
  • Cavernous sinus thrombosis
- Intracranial
  • Meningitis
  • Abscess
- Bony
  • Subperiosteal frontal bone abscess ("Pott's Puffy tumour")
  • Osteomyelitis
- Neurologic
  • Superior orbital fissure syndrome (CN III/IV/VI palsy, immobile globe, dilated pupils, ptosis, V1 hypoesthesia)
  • Orbital apex syndrome (as above, plus neuritis, papilledema, decreased visual acuity)

Chronic Rhinosinusitis

Definition
- inflammation of the mucosa of paranasal sinuses and nasal passages >8-12 wk
- diagnosis requiring ≥2 major symptoms for >8-12 wk and ≥1 objective finding of inflammation of the paranasal sinuses (CT/endoscopy)

Etiology
- unclear etiology but the following may contribute or predispose
  - inadequate treatment of acute rhinosinusitis
  - bacterial colonization/biofilms
    - *S. aureus*, enterobacteriaceae, *Pseudomonas, S. pneumoniae, H. influenzae*, β-hemolytic streptococci
  - fungal infection (e.g. *Aspergillus, Zygomycetes, Candida*)
  - anatomic abnormality (e.g. lost ostia patency, deviated septum – predisposing factors)
  - allergy/allergic rhinitis
  - ciliary disorder (e.g. cystic fibrosis, Kartagener syndrome)
  - chronic inflammatory disorder (e.g. GPA)
  - untreated dental disease

Allergic fungal rhinosinusitis is a chronic sinusitis affecting mostly young, immunocompetent, atopic individuals
Treatment options include FESS
± intranasal topical steroids, antifungals, and immunotherapy

Clinical Features (similar to acute, but less severe)
- chronic nasal obstruction
- purulent anterior/posterior nasal discharge
- facial congestion/fullness
- facial pain/pressure
- hyposmia/anosmia
- halitosis
- chronic cough
- maxillary dental pain

Management
- identify and address contributing or predisposing factors
- obtain CT or perform endoscopy
- if polyps present: INCS, oral steroids ± antibiotics (if signs of infection), refer to otolaryngologist/H&N surgeon
- if polyps absent: INCS, antibiotics, saline irrigation, oral steroids (severe cases)
- antibiotics for 3-6 wk
  - amoxillin-clavulanic acid inhibitors, fluoroquinolone (moxifloxacin), macrolide (clarithromycin), clindamycin, Flagyl® (metronidazole)
- surgery if medical therapy fails or fungal sinusitis: FESS, balloon sinoplasty

FESS = Functional Endoscopic Sinus Surgery
Opening of the entire osteomeatal complex in order to facilitate drainage while sparing the sinus mucosa

Complications
- same as acute sinusitis, mucocele

Epistaxis

Blood Supply to the Nasal Septum (see Figure 4, OT3)
1. Superior posterior septum
   - internal carotid → ophthalmic → anterior/posterior ethmoidal
2. Posterior septum
   - external carotid → internal maxillary → sphenopalatine artery → nasopalatine
3. Lower anterior septum
   - external carotid → facial artery → superior labial artery → nasal branch
   - external carotid → internal maxillary → descending palatine → greater palatine
- these arteries all anastomose to form Kiesselbach's plexus, located at Little's area (anterior-inferior portion of the cartilaginous septum)
- bleeding from above middle turbinate is internal carotid, and from below is external carotid

90% of nose bleeds occur in Little's area

Table 14. Etiology of Epistaxis

Type	Causes	

Local	Trauma (most common)
	  Fractures: facial, nasal
	  Self-induced: digital, foreign body
		Tumours
		  Benign: polyps, inverting papilloma, angiofibroma
		  Malignant: SCC, esthesioneuroblastoma (olfactory neuroblastoma)

	Iatrogenic: nasal, sinus, orbit surgery	Inflammation
		  Rhinitis: allergic, non-allergic
		  Infections: bacterial, viral, fungal

	Barometric changes	
	Nasal dryness: dry air ± septal deformities	Idiopathic
	Septal perforation	
	Chemical: cocaine, nasal sprays, ammonia, etc.	

Systemic	Coagulopathies
	  Meds: anticoagulants, NSAIDs
	  Hemophilias, von Willebrand's
	  Hematological malignancies
	  Liver failure, uremia	

	Vascular: HTN, atherosclerosis, Osler-Weber-Rendu (hereditary hemorrhagic telangectasia)	
	Others: GPA, SLE	

Special Cases
- Adolescent male with unilateral recurrent epistaxis - consider juvenile nasopharyngeal angiofibroma (JNA); this is the most common benign tumour of the nasopharynx
- Thrombocytopenic patients: use resorbable packs to avoid risk of re-bleeding caused by pulling out the removable pack

Investigations
- CBC, PT/PTT (if indicated)
- x-ray, CT as needed

Treatment
- locate bleeding and achieve hemostasis

1. ABCs
- lean patient forward to minimize swallowing blood and avoid airway obstruction
- apply constant firm pressure for 20 min on cartilaginous part of nose (not bony pyramid)
- if significant bleeding, assess vitals for signs of hemorrhagic shock ± IV NS, cross-match blood

2. Determine Site of Bleeding
- anterior/posterior hemorrhage defined by location in relationship to bony septum
- visualize nasal cavity with speculum
- use cotton pledget with topical lidocaine ± topical decongestant (i.e. Otrivin®) to help identify area of bleeding (often anterior septum)
- if suspicious bleeding disorder, coagulation workup (platelet number and platelet function assay)

3. Control the Bleeding
- first line topical vasoconstrictors (Otrivin®)
- if first line fails and bleeding adequately visualized, cauterize with silver nitrate
- **do not cauterize both sides of the septum** at one time due to risk of septal perforation from loss of septal blood supply

  A. Anterior hemorrhage treatment
  - if failure to achieve hemostasis with cauterization
    - place anterior pack* with half inch Vaseline®-soaked ribbon gauze strips layered from nasal floor toward nasal roof extending to posterior choanae or lubricated absorbable packing (i.e. Gelfoam wrapped in Surgicel®) for 2-3 d
    - can also attempt packing with Merocel® or nasal tampons of different shapes
    - can also apply Floseal® (hemostatic matrix consisting of topical human thrombin and cross-linked gelatin) if other methods fail

  B. Posterior hemorrhage treatment
  - if unable to visualize bleeding source, then usually posterior source
    - place posterior pack* using a Foley catheter, gauze pack, or Epistat® balloon
    - subsequently, layer anterior packing bilaterally
    - admit to hospital with packs in for 3-5 d
    - watch for complications: hypoxemia (naso-pulmonic reflex), toxic shock syndrome (Rx: remove packs immediately), pharyngeal fibrosis/stenosis, alar/septal necrosis, aspiration

  C. If anterior/posterior packs fail to control epistaxis
  - ligation or embolization of culprit arterial supply by interventional radiology
  - ± septoplasty

*antibiotics for any posterior pack or any pack left for >48 h because of risk of toxic shock syndrome

4. Prevention
- prevent drying of nasal mucosa with humidifiers, saline spray, or topical ointments
- avoidance of irritants
- medical management of HTN and coagulopathies

Hoarseness

Hoarseness

If hoarseness present for >2 wk in a smoker, laryngoscopy must be done to rule out malignancy

Definitions
- hoarseness: change in voice quality, ranging from voice harshness to voice weakness; reflects abnormalities anywhere along the vocal tract from oral cavity to lungs
- dysphonia: a general alteration in voice quality
- aphonia: no sound emanates from vocal folds

Acute Laryngitis

Definition
- <2 wk inflammatory changes in laryngeal mucosa

Etiology
- viral: influenza, adenovirus, HSV
- bacterial: Group A *Streptococcus*
- mechanical acute voice strain → submucosal hemorrhage → vocal cord edema → hoarseness
- environmental: toxic fume inhalation

Clinical Features
- URTI symptoms, hoarseness, aphonia, cough attacks, ± dyspnea
- true vocal cords erythematous/edematous with vascular injection and normal mobility

Treatment
- usually self-limited, resolves within ~1 wk
- voice rest
- humidification
- hydration
- avoid irritants (e.g. smoking)
- treat with antibiotics if there is evidence of coexistent bacterial pharyngitis

Vocal Cord Paralysis

Unilateral: affected cord lies in the paramedian position, inadequate glottic closure during phonation → weak, breathy voice. Usually medializes with time whereby phonation and aspiration improve. Treatment options include voice therapy, injection laryngoplasty (Radiesse), medialization using silastic block

Bilateral: cords rest in midline therefore voice remains good but respiratory function is compromised and may present as stridor. If no respiratory issues, may monitor closely and wait for improvement. If respiratory issues, intubate and will likely require vocal cord lateralization, arytenoidectomy, posterior costal cartilage graft or tracheotomy

Chronic Laryngitis

Definition
- >2 wk inflammatory changes in laryngeal mucosa

Etiology
- repeated attacks of acute laryngitis
- chronic irritants (dust, smoke, chemical fumes)
- chronic voice strain
- chronic rhinosinusitis with postnasal drip
- chronic EtOH use
- esophageal disorders: GERD, Zenker's diverticulum, hiatus hernia
- systemic: allergy, hypothyroidism, Addison's disease

Clinical Features
- chronic dysphonia: rule out malignancy
- cough, globus sensation, frequent throat clearing 2° to GERD
- laryngoscopy: cords erythematous, thickened with ulceration/granuloma formation, and normal mobility

Treatment
- remove offending irritants
- treat related disorders (e.g. antisecretory therapy for GERD)
- speech therapy with voice rest
- ± antibiotics ± steroids to decrease inflammation
- laryngoscopy to rule out malignancy

Vocal Cord Polyps

Definition
- structural manifestation of vocal cord irritation
- acutely, polyp forms 2° to capillary damage in the subepithelial space during extreme voice exertion

Etiology
- most common benign tumour of vocal cords
- voice strain (muscle tension dysphonia)
- laryngeal irritants (GERD, allergies, tobacco)

Epidemiology
- 30-50 yr of age
- M>F

Clinical Features
- hoarseness, aphonia, cough attacks ± dyspnea
- pedicled or sessile polyp on free edge of vocal cord
- typically polyp asymmetrical, soft, and smooth
- more common on the anterior 1/3 of the vocal cord
- intermittent respiratory distress with large polyps

Treatment
- avoid irritants
- endoscopic laryngeal microsurgical removal if persistent or if high risk of malignancy

Vocal Cord Nodules

Definition
- vocal cord callus
- i.e. "screamer's or singer's nodules"

Etiology
- early nodules occur 2° to submucosal hemorrhage
- mature nodules result from hyalinization which occurs with long-term voice abuse
- chronic voice strain
- frequent URTI, smoke, EtOH

Epidemiology
- frequently in singers, children, bartenders, and school teachers
- F>M

Clinical Features
- hoarseness worst at end of day
- on laryngoscopy
  - often bilateral
  - at the junction of the anterior 1/3 and posterior 2/3 of the vocal cords – point of maximal cord vibration
- chronic nodules may become fibrotic, hard, and white

Treatment
- voice rest
- hydration
- speech therapy
- avoid irritants
- surgery rarely indicated for refractory nodules

Benign Laryngeal Papillomas

Etiology
- HPV types 6, 11
- possible hormonal influence, possibly acquired during delivery

Epidemiology
- biphasic distribution: 1) birth to puberty (most common laryngeal tumour) and 2) adulthood

Clinical Features
- hoarseness and airway obstruction
- can seed into tracheobronchial tree
- highly resistant to complete removal
- some juvenile papillomas resolve spontaneously at puberty
- may undergo malignant transformation
- laryngoscopy shows wart-like lesions in supraglottic larynx and trachea

Treatment
- microdebridement or CO_2 laser
- adjuvants under investigation: interferon, cidofovir, acyclovir
- HPV vaccine may prevent/decrease the incidence but more research is needed

Laryngeal Carcinoma

- see *Neoplasms of the Head and Neck*, OT34

Vocal Cords: Polyps vs. Nodules	
Polyps	**Nodule**
Unilateral, asymmetric	Bilateral
Acute onset	Gradual onset
May resolve spontaneously	Often follow a chronic course
Subepithelial capillary breakage	Acute: submucosal hemorrhage or edema Chronic: hyalinization within submucosal lesion
Soft, smooth, fusiform, pedunculated mass	Acute: small, discrete nodules Chronic: hard, white, thickened fibrosed nodules
Proton pump inhibitor	Voice rest but no whispering, hydration, speech therapy if refractory to therapy
Surgical excision if persistent or in presence of risk factors for laryngeal cancer	Surgical excision as last resort

Salivary Glands

Sialadenitis

Definition
- inflammation of salivary glands

Etiology
- viral most common (mumps)
- bacterial causes: *S. aureus, S. pneumoniae, H. influenzae*
- obstructive vs. non-obstructive
- obstructive infection involves salivary stasis and bacterial retrograde flow

Bilateral enlargement of the parotid glands may be a manifestation of a systemic disease, such as Mumps, HIV, Sjögren's or an eating disorder (i.e. anorexia, bulimia)

Predisposing Factors
- HIV
- anorexia/bulimia
- Sjögren's syndrome
- Cushing's, hypothyroidism, DM
- hepatic/renal failure
- meds that increase stasis: diuretics, TCAs, β-blockers, anticholinergics, antibiotics
- sialolithiasis (can cause chronic sialadenitis)

Mumps usually presents with bilateral parotid enlargement ± SNHL ± orchitis

Clinical Features
- acute onset of pain and edema of parotid or submandibular gland that may lead to marked swelling
- ± fever
- ± leukocytosis
- ± suppurative drainage from punctum of the gland

Investigations
- U/S imaging to differentiate obstructive vs. non-obstructive sialadenitis

Treatment
- bacterial: treat with cloxacillin ± abscess drainage, sialogogues
- viral: no treatment

Sialolithiasis

Definition
- ductal stone (mainly hydroxyapatite) in adults, sand/sludge in children, leading to chronic sialadenitis
- 80% in submandibular gland, <20% in parotid gland, ~1% in sublingual gland

Risk Factors
- any condition causing duct stenosis or a change in salivary secretions (e.g. dehydration, diabetes, EtOH, hypercalcemia, psychiatric medication)

Clinical Features
- pain and tenderness over involved gland
- intermittent swelling related to meals
- digital palpation reveals presence of calculus

Investigations
- U/S ± sialogram

Treatment
- may resolve spontaneously
- encourage salivation to clear calculus
- massage, analgesia, antibiotics, sialogogues (e.g. lemon wedges, sour lemon candies), warm compresses
- remove calculi endoscopically, by dilating duct or orifice, or by excision through floor of the mouth
- gland preserving surgery has long-term symptom improvement and favourable gland retention rates

Salivary Gland Neoplasms

Etiology
- anatomic distribution
- parotid gland: 70-85%
- submandibular gland: 8-15%
- sublingual gland: 1%
- minor salivary glands, most concentrated in hard palate: 5-8%
- malignant (see Table 15, OT31 and Table 16, OT35)
- benign

- benign mixed (pleomorphic adenoma): 80%
- Warthin's tumour (5-10% bilateral, M>F): 10%
- cysts, lymph nodes and adenomas: 10%
- oncocytoma: <1%

Epidemiology
- 3-6% of all head and neck neoplasms in adults
- mean age at presentation: 55-65
- M=F

Parotid Gland Neoplasms

Clinical Features
- 80% benign (pleomorphic adenoma: most common), 20% malignant (mucoepidermoid: most common)
- if bilateral, suggests benign process (Warthin's tumour, Sjögren's, bulimia, mumps) or possible lymphoma
- facial nerve involvement (i.e. facial paralysis): increases risk of malignancy

Investigations
- FNA biopsy
- CT, U/S, or MRI to determine extent of tumour

Treatment
- treatment of choice is surgery for all salivary gland neoplasms – benign and malignant
- pleomorphic adenomas are excised due to risk of malignant transformation (5% risk over prolonged period of time)
- superficial tumour
  - superficial parotidectomy above plane of CN VII ± radiation
  - incisional biopsy contraindicated
- deep lesion
  - near-total parotidectomy sparing as much of CN VII as possible
  - if CN VII involved then it is removed and cable grafted
- complications of parotid surgery
  - hematoma, infection, salivary fistula, temporary facial paresis, Frey's syndrome (gustatory sweating)

Prognosis
- benign: excellent, <5% of pleomorphic adenomas may recur
- malignant: dependent on stage and type of malignancy (see Table 16, OT35)

Neck Masses

Approach to a Neck Mass

- ensure that the neck mass is not a normal neck structure (hyoid, transverse process of C1 vertebra, prominent carotid bulb)
- any neck mass persisting for >2 wk should be investigated for possible neoplastic causes

Table 15. Acquired Causes of Neck Lumps According to Age

Age (yr)	Possible Causes of Neck Lump		
<20	1. Congenital	2. Inflammatory/Infectious	3. Neoplastic
20-40	1. Inflammatory	2. Congenital	3. Neoplastic
>40	1. Neoplastic	2. Inflammatory	3. Congenital

Differential Diagnosis
- congenital
  - lateral (branchial cleft cyst, lymphatic/venous/venolymphatic malformation)
  - midline (thyroglossal duct cyst, dermoid cyst, laryngocele, thyroid/thymus anomaly, vascular malformation)
- infectious/inflammatory
  - reactive lymphadenopathy (20 to tonsillitis, pharyngitis)
  - infectious mononucleosis
  - Kawasaki, Kikuchi, Kimura, Cat Scratch, Castleman's
  - HIV
  - salivary gland calculi, sialadenitis
  - thyroiditis
- granulomatous disease
  - mycobacterial infections
  - sarcoidosis

A mass sitting above an imaginary line drawn between the mastoid process and angle of the mandible is a parotid neoplasm until proven otherwise

DDx Parotid Tumour

Benign
- Pleomorphic adenoma
- Warthin's tumour (more common in men)
- Benign lymphoepithelial cysts (viral eitiology e.g. HIV)
- Oncocytoma

Malignant
- Mucoepidermoid carcinoma
- Adenoid cystic carcinoma
- Acinic cell carcinoma

Frey's syndrome is a post-operative complication characterized by gustatory sweating. It is due to aberrant innervation of cutaneous sweat glands by parasympathetic nerve fibres that are divided during surgery

- neoplastic
  - lymphoma
  - salivary gland tumours
  - thyroid tumours
  - metastatic malignancy ("unknown primary")

Evaluation

Investigations
- history and physical (including nasopharynx and larynx)
- all other investigations and imaging are dependent upon clinical suspicion following history and physical
- laboratory investigations
  - WBC: infection vs. lymphoma
  - Mantoux TB test
  - thyroid function tests and scan
- imaging
  - neck U/S
  - CT scan
  - angiography: vascularity and blood supply to mass
- biopsy: for histologic examination
  - FNA: least invasive
  - needle biopsy
  - open biopsy: for lymphoma
- identification of possible primary tumour (rule out a metastatic lymph node from an "unknown primary")
  - panendoscopy: nasopharyngoscopy, laryngoscopy, esophagoscopy, bronchoscopy with washings, and biopsy of suspicious lesions
  - biopsy of normal tissue of nasopharynx, tonsils, base of tongue, and hypopharynx
  - primary identified 95% of time → stage and treat
  - primary occult 5% of time: excisional biopsy of node for histologic diagnosis → manage with radiotherapy and/or neck dissection (squamous cell carcinoma)

Inflammatory vs. Malignant Neck Masses

	Inflammatory	Neoplastic
History		
Painful	Y	N
H&N infection	Y	N
Fever	Y	N
Weight loss	N	Y
CA risk factors	N	Y
Age	Younger	Older
Physical		
Tender	Y	N
Rubbery	Y	Occ.
Rock hard	N	Y
Mobile	Y	± fixed

Congenital Neck Masses

Brachial Cleft Cysts/Sinuses/Fistulae

Embryology
- at the 6th wk of development, the 2nd branchial arch grows over the 3rd and 4th arches and fuses with the neighbouring caudal pre-cardial swelling forming the cervical sinus
- 3 types of malformations
  1. branchial fistula: persistent communication between skin and GI tract
  2. branchial sinus: blind-ended tract opening to skin
  3. branchial cyst: persistent cervical sinus with no external opening

Clinical Features
- 2nd branchial cleft malformations most common
  - sinuses and fistulae present in infancy as a small opening anterior to the sternocleidomastoid muscle
  - cysts present as a smooth, painless, slowly enlarging lateral neck mass, often following a URTI
- 1st branchial cleft malformations present as sinus/fistula or cyst in preauricular area or on face over angle of mandible
- 3rd branchial cleft malformations present as recurrent thyroiditis or thyroid abscess and have a tract leading usually to the left pyriform sinus. Air on CT scan in or near the thyroid gland is pathognomonic for this anomaly.
- there is controversy whether or not 4th branchial cleft anomalies exist, as they may be remnants of the thyrothymic axis

Treatment
- surgical removal of cyst or fistula tract
- if infected: allow infection to settle before removal (antibiotics may be required)

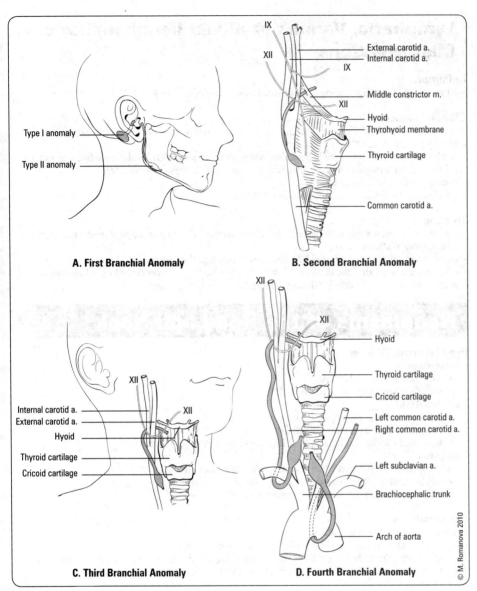

Figure 19. Branchial cleft cysts

Thyroglossal Duct Cysts

Embryology
- thyroid originates as ventral midline diverticulum at base of tongue caudal to junction of 3rd and 4th branchial arches (foramen cecum) and migrates down to inferior aspect of neck
- thyroglossal duct cysts are vestigial remnants of tract

Clinical Features
- usually presents in childhood or during 20-40s as a midline cyst that enlarges with URTI and elevates with swallowing and tongue protrusion

Treatment
- pre-operative antibiotics to reduce inflammation (infection before surgery is a well described cause of recurrence)
- small potential for neoplastic transformation so complete excision of cyst and tissue around tract up to foramen cecum at base of tongue with removal of central portion of hyoid bone (Sistrunk procedure) recommended

Lymphatic, Venous or Mixed Venolymphatic Malformations

Definition
- lymphatic malformation arising from vestigial lymph channels of neck

Clinical Features
- commonly identified in many fetuses but regress before birth and never cause a clinical problem
- usually present by age 2
- can be macrocystic (composed of large thin-walled cysts, usually below level of mylohyoid muscle) or microcystic (composed of minute cysts, usually above level of mylohyoid muscle)
- usually painless, soft, compressible
- infection or trauma causes a sudden increase in size

Treatment
- can regress spontaneously after bacterial infection, therefore do not plan surgical intervention until several months after infection
- macrocystic lesions can be treated by sclerotherapy or surgical excision
- microcystic lesions are difficult to treat, but can be debulked if it will not cause loss of function of normal structures, or injected with sclerotherapy in surrounding tissues

Neoplasms of the Head and Neck

All patients presenting with a head and neck mass should be asked if they are experiencing the following obstructive, referred, or local symptoms:
- Dyspnea or stridor (positional vs. non-positional)
- Hoarseness or dysphonia
- Otalgia
- Non-healing oral ulcer
- Dysphagia
- Hemoptysis, hematemesis

Detection of cervical lymph nodes on physical exam:
False negative rate: 15-30%
False positive rate: 30-40%

Pathological lymphadenopathy defined radiographically as:
- A jugulodigastric node >1.5 cm in diameter, or a retropharyngeal node >1 cm in diameter
- A node of any size which contains central necrosis

Common sites of distant metastases for head and neck neoplasms:
lungs > liver > bones

Pre-Malignant Disease
- **leukoplakia**
  - hyperkeratosis of oral mucosa
  - risk of malignant transformation 5-20%
- **erythroplakia**
  - red superficial patches adjacent to normal mucosa
  - commonly associated with epithelial dysplasia
  - associated with carcinoma in situ or invasive tumour in 40% of cases
- **dysplasia**
  - histopathologic presence of mitoses and prominent nucleoli
  - involvement of entire mucosal thickness = carcinoma in situ
  - associated progression to invasive cancer in 15-30% of cases

Investigations
- initial metastatic screen includes CXR
- scans of liver, brain, and bone only if clinically indicated
- CT scan is superior to MRI for the detection of pathologic nodal disease and bone cortex invasion
- MRI is superior to discriminate tumour from mucus and to detect bone marrow invasion
- ± PET scans

Treatment
- treatment depends on
  - histologic grade of tumour
  - stage
  - physical and psychological health of patient
  - facilities available
  - expertise and experience of the medical and surgical oncology team
- in general
  - 1° surgery for malignant oral cavity tumours with radiotherapy reserved for salvage or poor prognostic indicators
  - 1° radiotherapy for nasopharynx, oropharynx, hypopharynx, larynx malignancies with surgery reserved for salvage
  - palliative chemotherapy for metastatic or incurable disease
  - concomitant chemotherapy increases survival in advanced disease
  - chemotherapy has a role as induction therapy prior to surgery and radiation
  - panendoscopy to detect primary disease when lymph node metastasis is identified
  - anti-EGFR treatment (cetuximab, panitumumab) has a role as concurrent therapy with radiation for SCC of the head and neck (for advanced local and regional disease)

Prognosis
- synchronous tumours occur in 9-15% of patients
- late development of 2nd primary most common cause of post-treatment failure after 36 mo

Table 16. Quick Look-Up Summary of Head and Neck Malignancies – Etiology and Epidemiology

Etiology	Epidemiology	Risk Factors
Oral Cavity		
95% SCC others: sarcoma, melanoma, minor salivary gland tumour	Mean age: 50-60 yr M>F Most common site of H&N cancers 50% on anterior 2/3 of tongue	Smoking/EtOH Poor oral hygiene Leukoplakia, erythroplakia Lichen planus, chronic inflammation Sun exposure – lip HPV infection
Nose and Paranasal Sinus		
75-80% SCC Adenocarcinoma (2nd most common) and mucoepidermoid 99% in maxillary/ethmoid sinus 10% arise from minor salivary glands	Mean age: 50-70 yr Rare tumours ↓ incidence in last 5-10 yr	Wood/shoe/textile industry Hardwood dust (nasal/ethmoid sinus) Nickel, chromium (maxillary sinus) Air pollution Chronic rhinosinusitis
Carcinoma of the Pharynx – Subtypes (Nasopharynx, Oropharynx, Hypopharynx, and Larynx)		
Nasopharynx		
90% SCC ~10% lymphoma	Mean age: 50-59 yr M:F= 2.4:1 Incidence 0.8 per 100,000 100x increased incidence in Southern Chinese	Epstein-Barr virus (EBV) Salted fish Nickel exposure Poor oral hygiene Genetic – Southern Chinese
Oropharynx		
95% SCC – poorly differentiated Up to 70% of oropharyngeal cancer (OPC) attributable to HPV	Mean age: 50-70 yr Patients with HPV+ OPC are approximately 10 yrs younger Prevalence of HPV+ OPC has increased by 225% from 1988 to 2004. M:F = 4:1	Smoking/EtOH HPV 16 infection: increased sexual encounters, specifically oral sex
Hypopharynx		

95% SCC
3 sites
  1. pyriform sinus (60%)
  2. post-cricoid (30%)
  3. post pharyngeal wall (10%)
	Mean age: 50-70 yr
	M>F
	8-10% of all H&N cancer
		Smoking/EtOH

Larynx		

SCC most common
3 sites
  1. supraglottic (30-35%)
  2. glottic (60-65%)
  3. subglottic (1%)
	Mean age: 45-75 yr
	M:F = 10:1
	45% of all H&N cancer
		Smoking/EtOH
		HPV 16 infection strongly associated
		with the risk of laryngeal squamous cell
		cancers

Salivary Gland		
40% mucoepidermoid 30% adenoid cystic 5% acinic cell 5% malignant mixed 5% lymphoma	Mean age: 55-65 yr M=F 3-6% of all H&N cancer Rate of malignancy: Parotid 15-25% Submandibular 37-43% Minor salivary >80%	
Thyroid (90% benign – 10% malignant)		
>80% papillary 5-15% follicular 5% medullary <5% anaplastic 1-5% hürthle cell 1-2% metastatic	Children Adults <30 or >60 yr Nodules more common in females Malignancy more common in males	Radiation exposure Family history – papillary CA or multiple endocrine neoplasia – MEN II Older age Male Papillary – Gardner's, Cowden's, familial adenomatous polyposis (FAP)
Parathyroid		
	Mean age: 44-55 yr Rare tumour	

Risk Factors for Head and Neck Cancer include
- Smoking
- EtOH (synergistic with smoking)
- Radiation
- Occupational/environmental exposures
- Oral HPV infection (independent of smoking and EtOH exposure)

The smaller the salivary gland, the greater the likelihood that a mass in the gland is malignant

Table 17. Quick Look-Up Summary of Head and Neck Malignancies – Diagnosis and Treatment

Clinical Features	Investigations	Treatment	Prognosis
Oral Cavity			

Asymptomatic neck mass (30%)
Non-healing ulcer ± bleeding
Dysphagia, sialorrhea, dysphonia
Oral fetor, otalgia, leukoplakia, or erythroplakia (pre-malignant changes or CIS)
	Biopsy
	CT
		1° surgery
		  local resection
		  ± neck dissection
		  ± reconstruction
		2° radiation
			5 yr survival
			T1/T2: 75%
			T3/T4: 30-35%
			Poor prognostic indicators
			  Depth of invasion, close surgical margins location (tongue worse than floor of mouth)
			  Cervical nodes, extra-capsular spread

Nose and Paranasal Sinus			
Early symptoms: Unilateral nasal obstruction Epistaxis, rhinorrhea **Late symptoms:** 2o to invasion of nose, orbit, nerves, oral cavity, skin, skull base, cribriform plate	CT/MRI Biopsy	Surgery and radiation Chemoradiotherapy	5 yr survival: 30-60% Poor prognosis 2o to late presentation
Nasopharynx			
Cervical nodes (60-90%) Nasal obstruction, epistaxis Unilateral otitis media ± hearing loss CN III to VI, IX to XII (25%) Proptosis, voice change, dysphagia	Nasopharyngoscopy Biopsy CT/MRI	1° radiation, chemoradiation Surgery for limited or recurrent disease	5 yr survival T1: 79% T2: 72% T3: 50-60% T4: 36-42%
Oropharynx			

Odynophagia, otalgia
Ulcerated/enlarged tonsil
Fixed tongue/trismus/dysarthria
Oral fetor, bloody sputum
HPV+ OPC predominantly arises at base of tongue or tonsillar region
Cervical lymphadenopathy (60%)
Distant mets: lung/bone/liver (7%)
	Biopsy
	Determine HPV status via RT=PCR: positive if presence of HPV DNA and p16 overexpression
	CT
		1° radiation
		2° surgery
		  local resection
		  ±neck dissection
		  ±reconstruction
			5 year overall survival
			Stratified by TMN stage (I, II, III, IV)
			  HPV negative OPC (70%, 58%, 50%, 30%)
			  HPV positive OPC (88%, 78%, 71%, 74%)
			HPV positive OPC further stratified by stage, age and smoking pack years (PY)
			  group I (T1-3N0-N2c, ≤20 PY): 89%
			  group II (T1-3N0-N2c, >20 PY): 64%
			  group III (T4 or N3, age ≤70): 57%
			  group IVA (T4 or N3, age >70): 40%

Hypopharynx			
Dysphagia, odynophagia Otalgia, hoarseness Cervical lymphadenopathy	Pharyngoscopy Biopsy CT	1° radiation 2° surgery	5 yr survival T1: 53% T2/T3: 36-39% T4: 24%
Larynx			
Dysphagia, odynophagia, globus Otalgia, hoarseness Dyspnea/stridor Cough/hemoptysis Cervical nodes (rare with glottic CA)	Laryngoscopy CT/MRI	1° radiation 2° surgery 1° surgery for bulky T4 disease	5 yr survival T4: >40% (surgery with radiation) Control rate early lesions >90% (radiation) 10 to 12% of small lesions fail radiotherapy
Salivary Gland			

Painless mass (occ. pain is possible)
CN VII palsy
Cervical lymphadenopathy
Rapid growth
Invasion of skin
Constitutional signs/symptoms
	FNA
	MRI/CT/U/S
		1° surgery ± neck dissection
		Post-operative radiotherapy
		Chemotherapy if unresectable
			Parotid
			  10 yr survival: 85, 69, 43, and 14% for stages T1 to T4
			Submandibular
			  2 yr survival: 82%, 5 yr: 69%
			Minor salivary gland
			  10 yr survival: 83, 52, 25, 23% for stages T1 to T4

Thyroid			
Thyroid mass, cervical nodes Vocal cord paralysis Hyper/hypothyroidism Dysphagia	FNA U/S	1° surgery I¹³¹ for intermediate and high risk well differentiated thyroid cancer	Recurrences occur within 5 yr Need long-term follow-up: clinical exam, thyroglobulin
Parathyroid			
Increased serum Ca²⁺ Neck mass Bone disease, renal disease Pancreatitis	Sestamibi	Wide surgical excision Post-operative monitoring of serum Ca²⁺	Recurrence rates 1 yr: 27% 5 yr: 82% 10 yr: 91% Mean survival: 6-7 yr

Thyroid Carcinoma

Table 18. Bethesda Classification of Thyroid Cytology

Category	Risk of Malignancy
Non-diagnostic or unsatisfactory	Unknown
Benign	0-3%
Follicular lesion of undetermined significance/ Atypia of undetermined significance	5-15%
Follicular/hürthle cell neoplasms	15-30%
Suspicious for malignancy	60-75%
Malignant	97-99%

Table 19. Thyroid Carcinoma

	Papillary	Follicular	Medullary	Anaplastic	Lymphoma
Incidence (% of all thyroid cancers)	70-80%	10-15%	1 to 2% (90% sporadic, 10% familial – test for RET germline mutation)	<2%	<1%
Route of Spread	Lymphatic	Hematogenous	Lymphatic and hematogenous		
Histology	Orphan Annie nuclei Psammoma bodies Papillary architecture	Capsular/vascular invasion Invasion influences prognosis	Amyloid May secrete calcitonin, prostaglandins, ACTH, serotonin, kallikrein, or bradykinin	Giant cells Spindle cells	
Other	**P**s – **P**apillary cancer **P**opular (most common) **P**alpable lymph nodes **P**ositive I131 uptake **P**ositive prognosis **P**ost-operative I131 scan to guide treatments	**F**s – **F**ollicular cancer **F**ar away mets **F**emale (3:1) NOT **F**NA (cannot be diagnosed by **F**NA) **F**avourable prognosis	**M**s – **M**edullary cancer **M**ultiple endocrine neoplasia (**M**EN IIa or IIb) a**M**yloid **M**edian node dissection	More common in elderly 70% in women 20-30% have Hx of differentiated thyroid Ca (mostly papillary) or nodular goitre mass Rapidly enlarging neck Rule out lymphoma	Usually non-Hodgkin's lymphoma Rapidly enlarging thyroid mass Hx of Hashimoto's thyroiditis increases risk 60x 4:1 female predominance dysphagia, dyspnea, stridor, hoarseness, neck pain, facial edema, accompanied by "B" symptoms*
Prognosis	98% at 10 yr	92% at 10 yr	50% at 10 yr 20% at 10 yr if detected when clinically palpable	20-35% at 1 yr 13% at 10 yr	5 yr survival Stage IE 55%-80% Stage IIE 20%-50% Stage IIE/IV 15%-35%
Treatment	Small tumours: Near total thyroidectomy or lobectomy Diffuse/bilateral: Total thyroidectomy ± neck dissection ± post-operative I131 treatment	Small tumours: Near total thyroidectomy/lobectomy/ isthmectomy Large/diffuse tumours: Total thyroidectomy	Total thyroidectomy Median and/or lateral compartment node neck dissection (based on serum calcitonin) Modified neck dissection Post-operative thyroxine, radiotherapy Tracheostomy Screen relatives	Radiation and chemotherapy Small tumours: Total thyroidectomy ± external beam	Non-surgical Combined radiation Chemotherapy (CHOP**)

*B symptoms = fever, night sweats, chills, weight loss >10% in 6 mo   ** CHOP = cyclophosphamide, adriamycin, vincristine, prednisone

Approach to Thyroid Nodule

- all patients with thyroid nodules require evaluation of serum TSH and ultrasound
- intermediate-high suspicion nodule >1 cm and low suspicion nodule >1.5 cm should undergo FNA
- nodules <1 cm with clinical symptoms or lymphadenopathy may require further evaluation
- when performing repeat FNA on initially non-diagnostic nodules, U/S-guided FNA should be employed
- nuclear scanning has minimal value in the investigation of the thyroid nodule

Table 20. Management of the Thyroid Nodule

Treatment	Indications
Radioiodine therapy	For the treatment of hyperthyroidism or as adjuvant treatment after surgery in the treatment of intermediate-high risk papillary or follicular carcinoma
Chemotherapy and/or radiotherapy	Recurrent/residual Medullary CA, Anaplastic CA or thyroid lymphoma
Surgical excision	Nodule that is suspicious on FNA cytology Malignancy other than anaplastic CA or thyroid lymphoma Mass that on FNA is benign but increasing in size on serial imaging and/or >3-4 cm in size Hyperthyroidism not amenable to medical therapy

*U/S findings: cystic: risk of malignancy <1%; solid: risk of malignancy ~10%; solid with cystic components: risk of malignancy same as if solid

Indications for Post-Operative Radioactive Iodine Ablation – I131
Adjuvant therapy: decrease recurrent disease
RAI therapy: treat persistent cancer

Pediatric Otolaryngology

Acute Otitis Media

Definition
- all of: presence of middle ear effusion (MEE); presence of middle ear inflammation (MEI); acute onset of symptoms of MEE and MEI

Epidemiology
- most frequent diagnosis in sick children visiting clinicians' offices and most common reason for antibiotic administration
- peak incidence between 6-15 mo; ~85% of children have >1 episode by 3 yr old
- seasonal variability: peaks in winter

Etiology
- primary defect causing AOM: Eustachian tube dysfunction/obstruction → stasis/colonization by pathogens
- bacterial: *S. pneumoniae*, non-typable *H. influenzae*, *M. catarrhalis*, Group A *Streptococcus, S. aureus*
- viral: RSV, influenza, parainfluenza, adenovirus
- commonly due to bacterial/viral co-infection

Predisposing Factors
- Eustachian tube dysfunction/obstruction
  - swelling of tubal mucosa
    - ◆ upper respiratory tract infection (URTI)
    - ◆ allergic rhinitis
    - ◆ chronic rhinosinusitis
  - obstruction/infiltration of Eustachian tube ostium
    - ◆ tumour: nasopharyngeal carcinoma (adults)
    - ◆ adenoid hypertrophy (not due to obstruction but by maintaining a source of infection)
    - ◆ barotrauma (sudden changes in air pressure)
  - inadequate tensor palati function: cleft palate (even after repair)
  - abnormal Eustachian tube
    - ◆ Down syndrome (horizontal position of Eustachian tube), Crouzon syndrome, cleft palate, and Apert syndrome
- disruption of action of
  - cilia of Eustachian tube: Kartagener's syndrome
  - mucus secreting cells
  - capillary network that provides humoral factors, PMNs, phagocytic cells
- immunosuppression/deficiency due to chemotherapy, steroids, DM, hypogammaglobulinemia, cystic fibrosis

Risk Factors
- non-modifiable: young age, family history of OM, prematurity, orofacial abnormalities, immunodeficiencies, Down syndrome, race, and ethnicity
- modifiable: lack of breastfeeding, day care attendance, household crowding, exposure to cigarette smoke and air pollution, pacifier use

Pathogenesis
- obstruction of Eustachian tube → air absorbed in middle ear → negative pressure (an irritant to middle ear mucosa) → edema of mucosa with exudate/effusion → infection of exudate from nasopharyngeal secretions

Clinical Assessment of AOM in Pediatrics
JAMA 2010;304:2161-2169
In assessment of AOM in pediatrics, ear pain is the most useful symptom with a likelihood ratio (LR) between 3.0-7.3. Useful otoscopic signs include erythematous (LR 8.4, 95% CI 7-11), cloudy (LR 34, 95% CI 28-42), bulging (LR 51, 95% CI 36-73), and immobile tympanic membrane (LR 31, 95% CI 26-37) on pneumatic otoscopy.

Clinical Features
  - triad of otalgia, fever (especially in younger children), and conductive hearing loss
  - rarely tinnitus, vertigo, and/or facial nerve paralysis
  - otorrhea if tympanic membrane perforated
  - infants/toddlers
  - ear-tugging (this alone is not a good indicator of pathology)
  - hearing loss, balance disturbances (rare)
  - irritable, poor sleeping
  - vomiting and diarrhea
  - anorexia
- otoscopy of TM
  - hyperemia
  - bulging, pus may be seen behind TM
  - loss of landmarks: handle and long process of malleus not visible

Diagnosis

- history
  - acute onset of otalgia or ear tugging in a preverbal child, otorrhea, decreased hearing
  - unexplained irritability, fever, upper respiratory symptoms, poor sleeping, anorexia, N/V, and diarrhea
- physical
  - febrile
  - MEE on otoscopy: immobile tympanic membrane, acute otorrhea, loss of bony landmarks, opacification of TM, air-fluid level behind TM
  - MEI on otoscopy: bulging TM with marked discolouration (hemorrhagic, red, grey, or yellow)

Management

- supportive care and symptom management: maintain hydration, analgesic and antipyretic (acetaminophen, ibuprofen)
- watchful waiting: in a generally healthy child >6 mo of age with unilateral non-severe suspected AOM
  - without MEE, OR with MEE but non-bulging or mildly erythematous TM
    - consider viral etiology
    - reassess in 24-48h if not clinically improved (or earlier if worsening)
  - mildly ill (alert, responsive, no rigors, mild otalgia, fever <39 ºC, <48h illness) with MEE present AND bulging TM
    - recommend analgesia
    - observe and follow-up in 24-48h – if not improved or worsening, treat with antimicrobials
- antimicrobials indicated: infants <6 mo of age, or in a generally healthy child >6 mo of age with suspected AOM and the following features
  - moderately or severely ill (irritable, difficulty sleeping, poor antipyretic response, severe otalgia) OR fever ≥39 ºC OR >48h of symptoms
    - treat with antimicrobials: 10d course if 6mo to 2yr old, 5d if ≥2yr old
  - perforated TM with purulent drainage
    - treat with antimicrobials for 10d
- referral to otolaryngology for myringotomy and tympanostomy tubes may be warranted for recurrent infections

Treatment

- antimicrobial agents for AOM
  - 5 day course of appropriate dose antimicrobial recommended for most ≥ 2 yr old with uncomplicated AOM. 10d course for 6-23 mo, and perforated TM or recurrent AOM
  - 1st line treatment (no penicillin allergy)
    - amoxicillin: 5 day course of 45mg/kg/d to 60mg/kg/d divided 3x/d, or 75 mg/kg/d to 90 mg/kg/d divided 2x/d
  - 2nd line treatment
    - cefprozil: 30 mg/kg/d divided 2x/d
    - cefuroxime axetil: 30 mg/kg/d divided 2-3x/d (also is 1st line for penicillin allergy)
    - ceftriaxone: 50 mg/kg IM (or IV) x 3 doses (also is 1st line for penicillin allergy)
    - azithromycin: 10 mg/kg OD x 1 dose, then 5 mg/kg OD x 4 doses
    - clarithromycin: 15 mg/kg/d divided 2x/d
  - if initial therapy fails (i.e. no symptomatic improvement after 2-3 d)
    - amoxicillin-clavulanate: : 45mg/kg/d to 60mg/kg/d (7:1 formulation, 400mg/5mL suspension) for 10 d for child weighing ≤35kg, or 500mg tablets 3x/d for 10 d for child weighing >35kg
- if AOM-related symptoms do not resolve with amoxicillin/clavulanate, a course of ceftriaxone 50 mg/kg/d intramuscularly (or intravenously) 1/d x 3 doses could be considered

Complications

- extracranial
  - hearing loss and speech delay (secondary to persistent MEE), TM perforation, extension of suppurative process to adjacent structures (mastoiditis, petrositis, labyrinthitis), cholesteatoma, facial nerve palsy, middle ear atelectasis, ossicular necrosis, vestibular dysfunction, persistent effusion (often leading to hearing loss)
- intracranial
  - meningitis, epidural and brain abscess, subdural empyema, lateral and cavernous sinus thrombosis, carotid artery thrombosis, facial nerve paralysis
- other
  - mastoiditis, labyrinthitis, sigmoid sinus thrombophlebitis

Otitis Media with Effusion

Definition

- presence of fluid in the middle ear without signs or symptoms of ear infection

Epidemiology

- most common cause of pediatric hearing loss
- not exclusively a pediatric disease
- follows AOM frequently in children
- middle ear effusions have been shown to persist following an episode of AOM for 1 mo in 40% of children, 2 mo in 20%, and >3 mo in 10% (i.e. 90% of children clear the fluid within 3 mo – observe for 3 mo before considering myringotomy and tubes)

Antibiotics for Acute Otitis Media in Children
Cochrane DB Syst Rev 2013;1:CD000219
Study: Meta-analysis of Randomized Controlled Trials (RCTs) on children (1-15 mo) with acute otitis media comparing any antibiotic regime to placebo and expectant observation.
Data Sources: Cochrane Central Register of Controlled Trials (2012 issue 10), MEDLINE (1966 to October 2012), OLDMEDLINE (1958 to 1965), EMBASE (January 1990 to November 2012), Current Contents (1966 to November 2012), CINAHL (2008 to November 2012) and LILACS (2008 to November 2012) without language restrictions.
Main Outcomes: 1) Pain at 24 h, 2-3 d, and 4-7 d; 2) Abnormal tympanometry findings; 3) TM perforation; 4) Contralateral otitis; 5) AOM recurrences; 6) Serious complications from AOM; 7) Adverse effects from antibiotics.
Results: Treatment with antibiotics had no significant impact on pain at 24 h. However, pain at 2-3 d and 4-7 d was lower in the antibiotic groups with a NNT of 20. Antibiotics had no significant effect on tympanometry findings, number of AOM recurrences, or severity of complications. Antibiotic treatment led to a significant reduction in TM perforations (NNT 33) and halved contralateral AOM (NNT 11). Adverse events (vomiting, diarrhea, or rash) occurred more often in children taking antibiotics.
Conclusion: The role of antibiotics is largely restricted to pain control at 2-7 d, but most (82%) settle without antibiotics. This can also be achieved by analgesics. However, antibiotic treatment can reduce risk of TM perforation and contralateral AOM episodes. These benefits must be weighed against risks of adverse events from antibiotics.

Risk Factors
- same as AOM

Clinical Features
- conductive hearing loss ± tinnitus
    - confirm with audiogram and tympanogram (flat) (see Figure 16B, OT10 and Figure 17B, OT11)
- fullness – blocked ear
- ± pain, low grade fever
- otoscopy of tympanic membrane
    - discolouration – amber or dull grey with "glue" ear
    - meniscus fluid level behind TM
    - air bubbles
    - retraction pockets/TM atelectasis
    - most reliable finding with pneumotoscopy is immobility

Treatment
- expectant: 90% resolve by 3 mo
    - watchful waiting for 3 mo from onset, or 3 mo from diagnosis if onset unknown
- document hearing loss with audiogram
- no clinical evidence that antihistamines, decongestants, or antibiotics clear disease faster
    - recommend **against** intranasal or systemic steroids, systemic antibiotics, antihistamines, decongestants for OME treatment
- surgery: myringotomy ± ventilation tubes (tympanostomy tubes recommended) ± adenoidectomy (not recommended in <4yr old unless nasal obstruction, chronic adenoiditis; recommended in ≥ 4yr old)
- ventilation tubes to equalize pressure and drain ear

Complications of Otitis Media with Effusion
- hearing loss, speech delay, learning problems in young children
- chronic mastoiditis
- ossicular erosion
- cholesteatoma especially when retraction pockets involve pars flaccida
- retraction of tympanic membrane, atelectasis, ossicular fixation

Adenoid Hypertrophy

- size peaks at age 5 and resolves by age 12
- increase in size with repeated URTI and allergies

Clinical Features
- nasal obstruction
    - adenoid facies (open mouth, high arched palate, narrow midface, malocclusion)
    - history of hypernasal voice and snoring
    - long-term mouth breather; minimal air escape through nose
- choanal obstruction
    - chronic rhinosinusitis/rhinitis
    - obstructive sleep apnea
- chronic inflammation
    - nasal discharge, post-nasal drip, and cough
    - cervical lymphadenopathy

Diagnosis
- enlarged adenoids on nasopharyngeal exam (usually with flexible nasopharyngoscope)
- enlarged adenoid shadow on lateral soft tissue x-ray

Complications
- Eustachian tube obstruction leading to serous otitis media
- interference with nasal breathing, necessitating mouth-breathing
- malocclusion
- sleep apnea/respiratory disturbance
- orofacial developmental abnormalities

Adenoidectomy

Indications for Adenoidectomy
- chronic upper airway obstruction with sleep disturbance/apnea ± cor pulmonale
- chronic nasopharyngitis resistant to medical treatment
- chronic serous otitis media and chronic suppurative otitis media (with 2nd set of tubes)
- recurrent acute otitis media resistant to antibiotics
- suspicion of nasopharyngeal malignancy
- persistent rhinorrhea secondary to nasal obstruction

Indications for Myringotomy and Tympanostomy Tubes in Recurrent AOM (RAOM) and OME
- Chronic bilateral OME and documented hearing difficultues >3 mo
- Unilateral of bilateral OME >3 mo and symptoms likely attributable to OME (e.g. balance problems, poor school performance, ear discomfort, etc.)
- At-risk children (permanent hearing loss, speech/language delay, autism-spectrum disorder, syndromes/craniofacial disorders, blindness, cleft palate, developmental delay) with unilateral or bilateral OME with type B tympanogram or persistent effusion > 3 mo
- RAOM (>3 episodes in 6 mo or >4 in 12 mo) with unilateral or bilateral middle ear effusion

Clinical practice guidelines: Tympanostomy tubes in children. Otolaryng Head Neck 2013;149:S1-S35

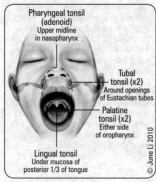

Figure 20. Waldeyer's ring
An interrupted circle of protective lymphoid tissue at the upper ends of the respiratory and alimentary tracts

Pharyngeal tonsil (adenoid) Upper midline in nasopharynx

Tubal tonsil (x2) Around openings of Eustachian tubes

Palatine tonsil (x2) Either side of oropharynx

Lingual tonsil Under mucosa of posterior 1/3 of tongue

Contraindications
- uncontrollable coagulopathy
- recent pharyngeal infection
- conditions that predispose to velopharyngeal insufficiency (cleft palate, impaired palatal function, or enlarged pharynx)

Complications
- bleeding, infection
- velopharyngeal insufficiency (hypernasal voice or nasal regurgitation)
- scarring of Eustachian tube orifice

Sleep-Disordered Breathing in Children

Definition
- spectrum of sleep-related breathing abnormalities ranging from snoring to OSA

Epidemiology
- peak incidence between 2-8 yr when tonsils and adenoids are the largest relative to the pharyngeal airway

Etiology
- due to a combination of anatomic and neuromuscular factors
  - adenotonsillar hypertrophy
  - craniofacial abnormalities
  - neuromuscular hypotonia (i.e. cerebral palsy, Down syndrome)
  - obesity

Clinical Features
- heavy snoring, mouth breathing, pauses or apnea, enuresis, excessive daytime sleepiness, behavioural/learning problems, diagnosis of ADHD, morning headache, failure to thrive, sleeping with neck hyperextended, cyanosis

Investigations
- flexible nasopharyngoscopy for assessment of nasopharynx and adenoids
- polysomnography (apnea-hypopnea index >1/h considered abnormal)
  - children: Mild OSA≥1to <5/hr; Moderate OSA≥5/hr to <10/hr; Severe OSA≥10/hr
  - adults: Mild OSA 5.1/hr to 15/hr; Moderate OSA 15.1/hr to 30/hr; Severe OSA>30.1/hr

Treatment
- nonsurgical: CPAP, BiPAP, sleep hygiene, weight loss in overweight/obese child with OSA
- surgical: bilateral tonsillectomy and adenoidectomy is first surgery of choice
  - if persistent obstructive sleep apnea following tonsillectomy and adenoidectomy, consider adenoid regrowth
  - if these fail and not tolerant of PAP therapy, consider lingual tonsillectomy, midline glossectomy, or other surgeries targeting areas of resistance as required (STAR surgery); surgery may be guided by Drug-Induced Sleep Endoscopy (DISE) or CINE-MRI to localize site of resistance

Acute Tonsillitis

- see Pediatrics, P57

Peritonsillar Abscess (Quinsy)

Definition
- cellulitis of space behind tonsillar capsule extending onto soft palate leading to abscess

Etiology
- bacterial: Group A strep (GAS) (50% of cases), *S. pyogenes*, *S. aureus*, *H. influenzae*, and anaerobes

Epidemiology
- can develop from acute tonsillitis with infection spreading into plane of tonsillar bed
- unilateral
- most common in 15-30 yr age group

Clinical Features
- trismus (due to irritation and reflex spasm of the medial pterygoid) is the most reliable indicator of peritonsillar abscess
- fever and dehydration
- sore throat, dysphagia, and odynophagia
- extensive peritonsillar swelling but tonsil may appear normal

Quinsy Triad
- Trismus
- Uvular deviation
- Dysphonia ("hot potato voice")

- edema of soft palate
- uvular deviation
- dysphonia (edema → failure to elevate palate) 2° to CN X involvement
- unilateral referred otalgia
- cervical lymphadenitis

Complications
- aspiration pneumonia 2° to spontaneous rupture of abscess
- airway obstruction
- lateral dissection into parapharyngeal and/or carotid space
- bacteremia
- retropharyngeal abscess

Treatment
- secure airway
- surgical drainage (incision or needle aspiration) with C&S
- warm saline irrigation
- IV penicillin G x 10 d if cultures positive for GAS
- add PO/IV metronidazole or clindamycin x 10 d if culture positive for *Bacteroides*
- consider tonsillectomy after second episode

Other Sources of Parapharyngeal Space Infections
- pharyngitis
- acute suppurative parotitis (see *Salivary Glands*, OT30)
- AOM
- mastoiditis (Bezold's abscess)
- odontogenic infection

Tonsillectomy

Absolute Indications
- most common indication: sleep-disordered breathing
- 2nd most common indication: recurrent throat infections
- tonsillar hypertrophy causing upper airway obstruction, obstructive sleep apnea, severe dysphagia, or cardiopulmonary complications such as cor pulmonale
- suspicion of malignancy (e.g. lymphoma, squamous cell carcinoma)
- orofacial/dental deformity
- hemorrhagic tonsillitis

Relative Indications (To Reduce Disease Burden)
- recurrent throat infection with a frequency of at least 7 episodes in the past year, at least 5 episodes per year for 2 yr, or at least 3 episodes per year for 3 yr, with documentation in the medical record for each episode of sore throat and 1 or more of the following: temperature >38.3°C, cervical adenopathy, tonsillar exudate, or positive test for Group A β-hemolytic *Streptococcus* (Paradise Criteria)
- chronic tonsillitis with halitosis (bad breath) or sore throat ± tonsilloliths (clusters of material that form in the crevices of the tonsils)
- complications of tonsillitis: quinsy/peritonsillar abscess, parapharyngeal abscess, retropharyngeal abscess
- failure to thrive

Relative Contraindications
- velopharyngeal insufficiency: overt or submucous/covert cleft of palate, impaired palatal function due to neurological or neuro-muscular abnormalities
- hematologic: coagulopathy, anemia
- infectious: active local infection without urgent obstructive symptoms

Complications
- hemorrhage: primary (within 24 h); secondary (within first 7-10 d)
- odynophagia and/or otalgia; dehydration 20 to odynophagia
- infection
- atlantoaxial subluxation (Grisel's syndrome) - rare

Airway Problems in Children

DIFFERENTIAL DIAGNOSIS BY AGE GROUP

Neonates (Obligate Nose Breathers)
- extralaryngeal
  - choanal atresia (e.g. CHARGE syndrome)
  - nasopharyngeal dermoid, glioma, encephalocele
  - glossoptosis: Pierre-Robin sequence, Down syndrome, lymphatic malformation, hemangioma

- laryngeal
  - laryngomalacia: most common cause of stridor in children
  - vocal cord palsy (due to trauma or Arnold-Chiari malformation)
  - glottic web
  - subglottic stenosis
  - laryngeal cleft
  - laryngocele
- tracheal
  - tracheoesophageal fistula
  - tracheomalacia
  - vascular rings
  - complete tracheal rings

2-3 Months
- congenital
  - laryngomalacia
  - vascular: subglottic hemangioma (more common), innominate artery compression, double aortic arch
  - laryngeal papilloma
- acquired
  - subglottic stenosis: post-intubation
  - tracheal granulation: post-intubation
  - tracheomalacia: post-tracheotomy and TEF repair

Infants – Sudden Onset
- foreign body aspiration
- croup
- bacterial tracheitis
- caustic ingestion
- epiglottitis

Children and Adults
- infection
  - Ludwig's angina
  - peritonsillar/parapharyngeal abscess
  - retropharyngeal abscess
- neoplastic
  - squamous cell carcinoma (SCC) (adults): larynx, hypopharynx
  - retropharyngeal: lymphoma, neuroblastoma
  - nasopharyngeal: carcinoma, rhabdomyosarcoma
- allergic
  - angioneurotic edema
  - polyps (suspect cystic fibrosis in children)
- trauma
  - laryngeal fracture, facial fracture
  - burns and lacerations
  - post-intubation
  - caustic ingestion
- congenital
  - lingual thyroglossal duct cyst
  - lingual tonsil hypertrophy
  - lingual thyroid

Signs of Airway Obstruction

Stridor
- note quality, timing (inspiratory or expiratory)
- body position important
  - lying prone: double aortic arch
  - lying supine: laryngomalacia, glossoptosis
- site of stenosis
  - vocal cords or above: inspiratory stridor
  - subglottis and extrathoracic trachea: biphasic stridor
  - distal tracheobronchial tree: expiratory stridor

Respiratory Distress
- nasal flaring
- supraclavicular and intercostal indrawing
- sternal retractions
- use of accessory muscles of respiration
- tachypnea
- cyanosis
- altered LOC

Feeding Difficulty and Aspiration
- supraglottic lesion
- laryngomalacia
- vocal cord paralysis
- laryngeal cleft → aspiration pneumonia
- TEF

Acute Laryngotracheobronchitis (Croup)

- inflammation of tissues in subglottic space ± tracheobronchial tree
- swelling of mucosal lining and associated with thick, viscous, mucopurulent exudate which compromises upper airway (subglottic space narrowest portion of upper airway)
- normal function of ciliated mucous membrane impaired

Etiology
- viral: parainfluenzae I (most common), II, III, influenza A and B, RSV

Clinical Features

Signs of Croup

The 3 Ss
Stridor
Subglottic swelling
Seal bark cough

- age: 4 mo-5 yr
- preceded by URTI symptoms
- generally occurs at night
- biphasic stridor and croupy cough (loud, sea-lion bark)
- appear less toxic than epiglottitis
- supraglottic area normal
- rule out foreign body and subglottic stenosis
- "steeple-sign" on AP x-ray of neck
- if recurrent croup, think subglottic stenosis

Treatment
- racemic epinephrine via MDI q1-2h, prn (only if in respiratory distress)
- systemic corticosteroids (e.g. dexamethasone 0.5 mg/kg, prednisone)
- adequate hydration
- close observation for 3-4 h
- intubation if severe (use smaller endotracheal tube than expected for age)
- hospitalize if poor response to steroids after 4 h and persistent stridor at rest
- consider alternate diagnosis if poor response to therapy (e.g. bacterial tracheitis)
- if recurrent episodes of croup-like symptoms, perform high kv croup series xray AP and LAT when well to rule out underlying subglottic stenosis and consider bronchoscopy for definitive diagnosis

Acute Epiglottitis

Acute epiglottitis is a medical emergency

- acute inflammation causing swelling of supraglottic structures of the larynx without involvement of vocal cords

Etiology
- *H. influenzae* type b
- relatively uncommon condition due to Hib vaccine

Clinical Features
- any age, most commonly 1-4 yr
- rapid onset
- toxic-looking, fever, anorexia, restlessness
- cyanotic/pale, inspiratory stridor, slow breathing, lungs clear with decreased air entry
- prefers sitting up ("tripod" posture), open mouth, drooling, tongue protruding, sore throat, dysphagia

When managing epiglottitis, it is important not to agitate the child, as this may precipitate complete obstruction

Investigations and Management
- investigations and physical exam may lead to complete obstruction, thus preparations for intubation or tracheotomy must be made prior to any manipulation
- stat ENT/anesthesia consult(s)
- WBC (elevated), blood and pharyngeal cultures after intubation
- lateral neck radiograph (only done if patient stable)

Thumb sign: cherry-shaped epiglottic swelling seen on lateral neck radiograph

Treatment
- secure airway
- IV access with hydration
- antibiotics: IV cefuroxime, cefotaxime, or ceftriaxone
- moist air
- extubate when leak around tube occurs and afebrile
- watch for meningitis

Subglottic Stenosis

Congenital
- diameter of subglottis <4 mm in neonate (due to thickening of soft tissue of subglottic space or maldevelopment of cricoid cartilage)

Acquired
- following prolonged, repeated, or traumatic intubation
  - most commonly due to endotracheal intubation; nasal intubation is less traumatic and preferred in long-term intubation as it puts less pressure on the subglottis (tube sits at different orientation) and there is less movement
  - subglottic stenosis is related to duration of intubation and pressure of the endotracheal tube cuff
- can also be due to foreign body, infection (e.g. TB, diphtheria, syphilis), or chemical irritation

Clinical Features
- biphasic stridor
- respiratory distress
- recurrent/prolonged croup

Diagnosis
- rigid laryngoscopy and bronchoscopy

Treatment
- if soft stenosis: divide tissue with knife or laser, dilate with balloon ± steroids
- if firm stenosis: laryngotracheoplasty

Laryngomalacia

- short aryepiglottic folds, omega-shaped epiglottis, pendulous mucosa
- caused by indrawing of supraglottis on inspiration leading to laryngopharyngeal reflux of acid

Clinical Features
- high-pitched inspiratory stridor at 1-2 wk
- constant or intermittent and more pronounced supine and following URTI
- usually mild but when severe can be associated with cyanosis or feeding difficulties, leading to failure to thrive

Laryngomalacia is the most common cause of stridor in infants

Treatment
- observation ± proton pump inhibitor (to break the acid reflux cycle that leads to edema and worse airway obstruction) is usually sufficient as symptoms spontaneously subside by 12-18 mo in >90% of cases
- if severe, division of the aryepiglottic folds (supraglottoplasty) provides relief

Foreign Body

Ingested
- usually stuck at cricopharyngeus
- coins, toys, batteries (emergency)
- presents with drooling, dysphagia, stridor if very large

Aspirated
- usually stuck at right main bronchus
- peanuts, carrot, apple core, popcorn, balloons
- presentation
  - stridor if lodged in trachea
  - unilateral "asthma" if bronchial, therefore often misdiagnosed as asthma
  - if totally occludes airway: cough, lobar pneumonia, atelectasis, mediastinal shift, pneumothorax, death

Foreign body inhalation is the most common cause of accidental death in children

Diagnosis and Treatment
- sudden onset, not necessarily febrile or elevated WBC
- any patient with suspected foreign body should be kept NPO immediately
- older patient: inspiratory-expiratory chest x-ray (if patient is stable)
- younger patient: right and left decubitus chest x-rays. Lack of lung deflation while resting on dependent side suggests foreign body blocking bronchus.
- bronchoscopy or esophagoscopy with removal

Batteries MUST be ruled out as a foreign body (vs. coins) as they are lethal and can erode through the esophagus. Batteries have a halo sign around the rim on AP x-ray and a step deformity on lateral x-ray

Deep Neck Space Infection

- most commonly arise from an infection of the mandibular teeth, tonsils, parotid gland, deep cervical lymph nodes, middle ear, or the sinuses
- often a rapid onset and may progress to fatal complications

Etiology
- usually mixed aerobes and anaerobes that represent the flora of the oral cavity, upper respiratory tract, and certain parts of the ears and eyes

Clinical Features
- sore throat or pain and trismus
- dysphagia and odynophagia
- stridor and dyspnea
- late findings may include dysphonia and hoarseness
- swelling of the face and neck, erythema
- asymmetry of the oropharynx with purulent oral discharge
- lymphadenopathy

Diagnosis
- lateral cervical view plain radiograph
- CT
- MRI

Treatment
- secure the airway
- surgical drainage
- maximum doses of IV systemic antimicrobials regimens according to the site of infection

These investigations should be obtained carefully and the surgeon should consider accompanying the patient as the worst place to lose an airway is during imaging

Ludwig's angina is the prototypical infection of the submandibular and sublingual space

Common Medications

Table 21. Antibiotics

Generic Name (Brand Name)	Dose	Indications	Notes
amoxicillin (Amoxil®, Amoxi®, Amox®)	Adult: 500 mg PO tid Children: 75-90 mg/kg/d in 2 divided doses	*Streptococcus, Pneumococcus, H. influenzae, Proteus* coverage	May cause rash in patients with infectious mononucleosis
piperacillin with tazobactam (Zosyn®)	3 g PO q6h	Gram-positive and negative aerobes and anaerobes plus Pseudomonas coverage	May cause pseudomembranous colitis
ciprofloxacin (Cipro®, Ciloxan®)	500 mg PO bid	Pseudomonas, Streptococci, MRSA, and most Gram-negative; no anaerobic coverage	Animal studies suggest that systemic quinolones may cause cartilage necrosis in children
erythromycin (Erythrocin®, EryPed®, Staticin®, T-Stat®, Erybid®, Novorythro Encap®)	500 mg PO qid	Alternative to penicillin	Ototoxic

Table 22. Otic Drops

Generic Name (Brand Name)	Dose	Indications	Notes
ciprofloxacin (Ciprodex®)	4 gtt in affected ear bid	For otitis externa and complications of otitis media *Pseudomonas, Streptococci,* MRSA, and most Gram-negative; no anaerobic coverage	
neomycin, polymyxin B sulfate, and hydrocortisone (Cortisporin Otic®)	5 gtt in affected ear tid	For otitis externa Used for inflammatory conditions which are currently infected or at risk of bacterial infections	May cause hearing loss if placed in inner ear
hydrocortisone and acetic acid (VoSol HC®)	5-10 gtt in affected ear tid	For otitis media	Bactericidal by lowering pH
tobramycin and dexamethasone (TobraDex®)	5-10 gtt in affected ear bid	For chronic suppurative otitis media	Risk of vestibular or cochlear toxicity

Table 23. Nasal Sprays

Generic Name (Brand Name)	Indications	Notes
Steroid		
flunisolide (Rhinalar®) budesonide (Rhinocort®) triamcinolonoe (Nasacort®) beclomethasone (Beconase®) mometasone furoate, monohydrate (Nasonex®) fluticasone furoate (Avamys®)	Allergic rhinitis Chronic sinusitis	Requires up to 4 wk of consistent use to have effect Long-term use Dries nasal mucosa; may cause minor bleeding Patient should stop if epistaxis May sting Flonase® and Nasonex® not absorbed systemically
Antihistamine		
levocarbastine (Livostin®)	Allergic rhinitis	Immediate effect If no effect by 3 d then discontinue Use during allergy season
Decongestant		
xylometazoline (Otrivin®) oxymetazoline (Dristan®) phenylephrine (Neosynephrine®)	Acute sinusitis Rhinitis	Careful if patient has hypertension Short-term use (<5 d) If long-term use, can cause decongestant addiction (i.e. rhinitis medicamentosa)
Antibiotic/Decongestant		
framycetin, gramicidin, phenylephrine (Soframycin®)	Acute sinusitis	
Anticholinergic		
ipratropium bromide (Atrovent®)	Vasomotor rhinitis	Careful not to spray into eyes as can cause burning or precipitation of narrow angle glaucoma Increased rate of epistaxis when combined with topical nasal steroids
Lubricants		
saline, NeilMed®, Rhinaris®, Secaris®, Polysporin®, Vaseline®	Dry nasal mucosa	Use prn Rhinaris® and Secaris® may cause stinging

Source: Dr. MM Carr

References

Bailey BJ. Head and neck surgery-otolaryngology, 2nd ed. Philadelphia: Lippincott Williams and Wilkins, 1998.

Baugh RF, Archer SM, Mitchell RB, et al. Clinical practice guideline: Tonsillectomy in children. Otolaryngol Head Neck Surg 2011; 144(1S):S1-S30.

Becker W, Naumann HH, Pfaltz CR. Ear, nose, and throat diseases, 2nd ed. New York: Thieme Medical Publishers, 1994.

Berman S. Current concepts: otitis media in children. NEJM 1995;332:1560-1565.

Bonner JA, Harari PM, Giralt J, et al. Radiotherapy plus cetuximab for squamous-cell carcinoma of the head and neck. NEJM 2006;354:567-568.

Casey JR, Pichichero ME. Changes in frequency and pathogens causing acute otitis in 1995-2003. Pediatr Infect Dis J 2004;23(9):824-828.

Chang WH, Tseng HC, Chao TK, et al. Measurement of hearing aid outcome in the elderly: comparison between young and old elderly. Otolaryngol Head Neck Surg 2008;138:730.

Cho, H.-J., Min, H. J., Chung, H. J., Park, D.-Y., Seong, S. Y., Yoon, J.-H., Lee, J.-G. and Kim, C.-H. (2016), Improved outcomes after low-concentration hypochlorous acid nasal irrigation in pediatric chronic sinusitis. The Laryngoscope, 126: 791–795. doi: 10.1002/lary.25605

Coker TR, Chan LS, Newberry SJ, et al. Diagnosis, microbial epidemiology, and antibiotic treatment of acute otitis media in children: a systemic review. JAMA 2010;304:2161-169.

Cooper DS, Doherty GM, Haugen BR, et al. Revised American Thyroid Association management guidelines for patients with thyroid nodules and differentiated thyroid cancer. Thyroid 2009;19:1167-1214.

Deschler DG, Richmon JD, Khariwala SS, et al. The "new" head and neck cancer patient - young, nonsmoker, nondrinker, and HPV positive. Otolaryngol Head Neck Surg 2014; 151(3): 375-380

Dhillon RS, East CA. Ear, nose, and throat, and head and neck surgery: an illustrated colour text, 2nd ed. New York: Churchill & Livingston, 1999.

D'Souza G, Kreimer AR, Viscidi R, et al. Case-control study of human papillomavirus and oropharyngeal cancer. NEJM 2007;356:1944-1956.

Fakhry C, Westra WH, Li S, et al. Improved survival of patients with human papillomavirus-positive head and neck squamous cell carcinoma in a prospective clinical trial. J Natl Cancer Inst 2008;100:261-269.

Finn DG, Buchalter IH, Sarti E, et al. First branchial cleft cysts: clinical update. Laryngoscope 1987;97:136-140.

Forastiere A, Koch W, Trotti A, et al. Head and neck cancer. NEJM 2001;345:1890-1900.

Frisina A, Piazza F, Pasanisi E, et al. Cleft palate and dysfunction of the Eustachian tube. Acta Biomed Ateneo Parmense 1998;69(5-6):129-132.

Furman JM, Cass SP. Benign paroxysmal positional vertigo. NEJM 1999;341:1590-1596.

Gillespie, M. B., O'Connell, B. P., Rawl, J. W., McLaughlin, C. W., Carroll, W. W. and Nguyen, S. A. (2015), Clinical and quality-of-life outcomes following gland-preserving surgery for chronic sialadenitis. The Laryngoscope, 125: 1340–1344. doi: 10.1002/lary.25062

Grégoire V, Maignon P. Intensity modulated radiation therapy in head and neck squamous cell carinoma: state of the art and future challenges. Cancer Radiother 2005;9:42-50.

Haugen BR, Alexander EK, Bible KC, et al. 2015 American Thyroid Association management guidelines for adult patients with thyroid nodules and differentiated thyroid cancer: The American Thyroid Association guidelines task force on Thyroid nodules and differentiated thyroid cancer. Thyroid, 2016; 26(1): 1-133.

Hilton M, Pinder D. The Epley (canalith repositioning) maneuver for benign paroxysmal positional vertigo. Cochrane ear, nose, and throat disorders group. Cochrane DB Syst Rev 2004;Issue 4.

Huang SH, Xu W, Waldron J, et al. Refining American Joint Committee On Cancer/Union for International Cancer Control TMN stage and prognostic groups for Human Papillomavirus-related oropharyngeal carcinomas. JCO 2015; 33(8): 836-845.

Jackson CG, von Doersten PG. The facial nerve: current trends in diagnosis, treatment, and rehabilitation. Otolaryngol for Internist 1999;83:179-195.

Jafek BW, Murrow BW. ENT secrets, 2nd ed. Philadelphia: Hanley & Belfus, 2001.

Kaselas CH, Tsikopoulos G, Chortis CH, et al. Thyroglossal duct cyst's inflammation. When do we operate? Pediatr Surg Int 2005;21(12):991.

Kotecha S, Bhatia P, Rout PG. Diagnostic ultrasound in the head and neck region. Dent Update 2008;35(8):529.

Layland MK (editor). Washington manual otolaryngology survival guide. Philadelphia: Lippincott Williams and Wilkins, 2003.

Le Saux N, Robinson JL. Management of acute otitis media in children six months of age and older. Canadian Pediatrics Society, 2016.

Lee KJ (editor). Essential otolaryngology: head and neck surgery, 8th ed. New York: McGraw-Hill, 2003.

Li X, Gao L, Li H, et al. Human papillomavirus infection and laryngeal cancer risk: a systemic review and meta-analysis. J Infect Dis 2013;207:479-488.

Lieberthal AS, Carroll AE, Chonmaitree T, et al. The diagnosis and treatment of acute otitis media. Pediatrics 2013;e964-e999.

Lucente FE, Har-El G (editors). Essentials of otolaryngology, 4th ed. Philadelphia: Lippincott Williams and Wilkins, 1999.

MacCallum PL, Parnes LS, Sharpe MD, et al. Comparison of open, percutaneous and translaryngeal tracheostomies. Otolaryngol Head Neck Surg 2000;122:686-690.

Marcus CL, Brooks LJ, Draper KA, et al. Clinical practice guideline: Diagnosis and management of childhood obstructive sleep apnea syndrome. American Academy of Pediatrics, 2012.

McIsaac WJ, Coyte PC, Croxford R, et al. Otolaryngologists' perceptions of the indications for typanostomy tube insertion in children. CMAJ 2000;162:1285-1288.

Mehanna H, Beech T, Nicholson T, et al. Prevalence of human papillomavirus in oropharyngeal and nonoropharyngeal head and neck cancer - systematic review and meta-analysis of trends by time and region. Head & Neck 2013; 35(5): 747-755

Pasha R. Otolaryngology head and neck surgery clinical reference guide, 3rd ed. San Diego: Plural Publishing, 2010.

Patel ND, van Zante A, Eisele DW, et al. Oncocytoma: the vanishing parotid mass. AJNR Am J Neuroradiol 2011;32(9):1703-1706.

Pohar S, Gay H, Rosenbaum P, et al. Malignant parotid tumors: presentation, clinical/pathologic prognostic factors, and treatment outcomes. Int J Radiat Oncol Biol Phys 2005;61(1):112-118.

Prasad HK, Bhojwani KM, Shenoy V, et al. HIV manifestations in otolaryngology. Am J Otolaryngol 2006;27(3):179.

Quesnel AM, Lindsay RW, Hadlock TA. When the bell tolls on Bell's palsy: finding occult malignancy in acute-onset facial paralysis. AM J Otolaryngol 2010;31(5):339-342.

Ramqvist T, Grun N, Dalianis T. Human papillomavirus and tonsillar and base of tongue cancer. Viruses 2015; 7(3): 1332-1343.

Rosenfield RM, Schwartz SR, Pynnonen MA, et al. Clinical practice guideline: tympanostomy tubes in children. Otolaryngol Head Neck Surg 2013;49:S1-S33.

Rosenfeld FM, Shin JJ, Schwartz SR, et al. Clinical practice guideline: Otitis media with effusion (update). Otolaryngol Head Neck Surg 2016; 154(1S):S1-S41.

Schularick, N. M., Mowry, S. E., Soken, H. and Hansen, M. R. (2013), Is electroneurography beneficial in the management of Bell's palsy?. The Laryngoscope, 123: 1066–1067. doi: 10.1002/lary.23560

Smith, S. S., Ference, E. H., Evans, C. T., Tan, B. K., Kern, R. C. and Chandra, R. K. (2015), The prevalence of bacterial infection in acute rhinosinusitis: A Systematic review and meta-analysis. The Laryngoscope, 125: 57–69. doi: 10.1002/lary.24709

Srafford ND, Wilde A. Parotid cancer. Surg Oncol 1997;6:209-213.

Valenzuela, C. V., Newbill, C. P., Johnston, C. and Meyer, T. K. (2016), Proliferative laryngitis with airway obstruction in an adult: Consider herpes. The Laryngoscope, 126: 945–948. doi: 10.1002/lary.25555

Venekamp RP, Sanders S, Glasziou PP, et al. Antibiotics for acute otitis media in children. Cochrane DB Syst Rev 2013;1:CD000219.

Wells SA, Henning Dralle SL, Elisei R, et al. Revised American Thyroid Association guidelines for the management of medullary thyroid carcinoma: The American Thyroid Association guidelines task force on medullary thyroid carcinoma. Thyroid 2015; 25(6): 567-610.

P

Pediatrics

Daniel Axelrod, Paige Burgess, and **Nicholas Light,** chapter editors
Narayan Chattergoon and **Desmond She,** associate editors
Arnav Agarwal and **Quynh Huynh,** EBM editors
Dr. Nirit Bernhard, Dr. Sharon Naymark, and **Dr. Angela Punnett,** staff editors

P Pediatrics

Acronyms

AAP	American Academy of Pediatrics	DS	Down syndrome	IUGR	intra-uterine growth restriction
ABG	arterial blood gas	DSD	disorder of sexual differentiation	IVH	intraventricular hemorrhage
ACE	angiotensin converting enzyme	EBV	Epstein-Barr virus	IVIg	intravenous immunoglobulin
ALL	acute lymphoblastic leukemia	Echo	echocardiogram	JIA	juvenile idiopathic arthritis
ALPS	autoimmune lymphoproliferative syndrome	EMG	electromyography	LAH	left atrial hypertrophy
AML	acute myelogenous leukemia	FAS	fetal alcohol syndrome	LGA	large for gestational age
ANA	antinuclear antibody	FASD	fetal alcohol spectrum disorder	LH	luteinizing hormone
AOM	acute otitis media	FISH	fluorescent in situ hybridization	LLSB	lower left sternal border
ARB	angiotensin receptor blocker	FSH	follicle stimulating hormone	LOC	level of consciousness
ARBD	alcohol-related birth defects	FTT	failure to thrive	LP	lumbar puncture
ARND	alcohol-related neurodevelopmental disorder	G6PD	glucose-6-phosphate dehydrogenase	LRTI	lower respiratory tract infection
ASD	atrial septal defect	GA	gestational age	LVH	left ventricular hypertrophy
ASOT	antistreptolysin-o titre	GBM	glomerular basement membrane	MAS	meconium aspiration syndrome
ATN	acute tubular necrosis	GBS	group B Streptococcus	MCAD	medium-chain acyl-CoA dehydrogenase
AVM	arteriovenous malformation	GERD	gastroesophageal reflux disease	MCD	minimal change disease
BRUE	brief resolved unexplained events	GH	growth hormone	MDI	metred dose inhaler
CAH	congenital adrenal hyperplasia	GN	glomerulonephritis	MSUD	maple syrup urine disease
CAS	Children's Aid Society	GSD	glycogen storage disease	NCS	nerve conduction study
CF	cystic fibrosis	HDNB	hemorrhagic disease of the newborn	NEC	necrotizing enterocolitis
CHD	congenital heart defect	Hib	Haemophilus influenzae type b	NF	neurofibromatosis
CML	chronic myelogenous leukemia	HIDA	hepatobiliary iminodiacetic acid	NICU	neonatal intensive care unit
CMV	cytomegalovirus	HIE	hypoxic ischemic encephalopathy	NS	normal saline
CP	cerebral palsy	HPA	human platelet antigen	OCP	oral contraceptive pill
CPS	Canadian Pediatric Society	HRV	human rotavirus	ORT	oral rehydration therapy
DDAVP	1-desamino-8-D-arginine vasopressin	HSP	Henoch-Schönlein purpura	PAC	premature atrial contraction
DI	diabetes insipidus	HUS	hemolytic uremic syndrome	PDA	patent ductus arteriosus
DIC	disseminated intravascular coagulation	IBW	ideal body weight	PKU	phenylketonuria
DKA	diabetic ketoacidosis	ICH	intracranial hemorrhage	PPHN	persistent pulmonary hypertension of newborn
DMARD	disease modifying antirheumatic drug	ITP	immune thrombocytopenic purpura		

PPV	positive pressure ventilation
PUVA	psoralen + UVA
RAD	right axis deviation
RAS	renal artery stenosis
RBBB	right bundle branch block
RDS	respiratory distress syndrome
RF	rheumatoid factor
RL	Ringer's lactate
RSV	respiratory syncytial virus
RUSB	right upper sternal border
RVH	right ventricular hypertrophy
RVOTO	right ventricular outflow tract obstruction
SEM	systolic ejection murmur
SGA	small for gestational age
SIADH	syndrome of inappropriate antidiuretic hormone
SVT	supraventricular tachycardia
TEF	tracheo-esophageal fistula
TM	tympanic membrane
TPN	total parenteral nutrition
TTN	transient tachypnea of the newborn
UMN	upper motor neuron
URTI	upper respiratory tract infection
UVA	ultraviolet A
VCUG	voiding cystourethrogram
VSD	ventricular septal defect
VUR	vesicoureteral reflux
WPW	Wolff-Parkinson-White

Pediatric Quick Reference Values

Table 1. Average Vitals at Various Ages

Age (years)	Pulse (bpm)	Respiratory Rate (br/min)	sBP (mmHg)
<1	110-160	30-40	70-90
1-2	100-150	25-35	80-95
2-5	95-140	25-35	80-100
5-12	80-120	20-25	90-110
>12	60-100	15-20	110-120

Primary Care

Visit Overview

- schedule
  - newborn (within 1 wk post-discharge), 1, 2, 4, 6, 9, 12, 15, 18, 24 mo
  - annually between age 2-5; every 1-2 years between age 6-18
- content
  - history and physical exam including growth, development, and nutrition
  - routine immunizations
  - counselling and anticipatory guidance

Routine Immunization

Table 2. Publicly Funded Immunization Schedule for Ontario, August 2011

Age	DTaP-IPV-Hib	dTaP-IPV	Pneu-C-13	Rot-1	Men-C-C	MMR	Var	MMRV	Men-C-ACYW	HepB	HPV-4	Tdap	Inf
2 mo	✓IM		✓IM	✓PO									
4 mo	✓IM		✓IM	✓PO									
6 mo	✓IM												
12 mo			✓IM		✓IM	✓SC							
15 mo							✓SC						
18 mo	✓IM												
4-6 yr		✓IM						✓SC					
Grade 7									✓IM	✓IM 3 doses (0,1,6 mo)	✓IM 3 doses (0,2,6 mo)		
14-16 yr												✓IM	
Every autumn													✓IM

IM = intramuscular; PO = per oral; SC = subcutaneous

Vaccine	Adverse Reaction	Contraindication
DTaP-IPV	Prolonged crying Hypotonic unresponsive state (rare) Seizure on day of vaccine (rare)	Evolving unstable neurologic disease Hyporesponsive/hypotonic following previous vaccine Anaphylactic reaction to neomycin or streptomycin
Rot-1	Cough Diarrhea, vomiting	History of intussusception Immunocompromised Abdominal disorder (e.g. Meckel's diverticulum) Received blood products (e.g. immunoglobulin) within 42 d
MMR	Measle-like rash (7-14 d) Lymphadenopathy, arthralgia, arthritis Parotitis (rare) Especially painful injection Transient thrombocytopenia (1/30,000)	Pregnancy Immunocompromised infants (except healthy HIV positive children) Anaphylactic reaction to gelatin
Var	Mild varicella-like papules or vesicles; 2 weeks may get local or generalized rash	Pregnant or planning to get pregnant within 3 mo Anaphylactic reaction to gelatin
HepB		Anaphylactic reaction to Baker's yeast
MMRV	Same as MMR and Var vaccines	Same as MMR and Var vaccines
dTAP		1st trimester pregnancy
Inf	Malaise, myalgia Febrile seizure when given with Pneu-C 13 or DTap Hypersensitivity reaction	<6 months of age Immunocompromised Egg-allergic individuals – Live attenuated influenza vaccine is not recommended for those with an egg allergy. In these individuals, trivalent or quadrivalent vaccine can be given in environment where anaphylaxis can be managed
HPV-4	Pruritis	
MenB*		Anaphylactic reaction to MenB vaccine or its components in the past

* Currently only publicly funded for select groups (asplenia, antibody/complement deficiencies, cochlear implant recipients, HIV, close contacts with infected individuals)

dTAP = diphtheria, tetanus, acellular pertussis vaccine; DTaP-IPV = diphtheria, tetanus, acellular pertussis, inactivated polio vaccine (i.e. Pentacel®, Pentavax®);
HepB = hepatitis B vaccine; Hib = Haemophilus influenzae type b conjugate vaccine; HPV-4 = human papillomavirus vaccine; Inf = influenza vaccine;
MMR = measles, mumps, rubella vaccine; Men = multicomponent meningococcal B vaccine; Men-C-C = meningococcal c conjugate vaccine;
MMRV = measles, mumps, rubella, varicella vaccine; Pneu-C-13 = pneumococcal 13-valent conjugate vaccine; Rot-1 = rotavirus oral vaccine; Var = varicella vaccine

Canadian Immunization Guide
National Advisory Committee on Immunization. Canadian Immunization Guide (CIG). Last Modified 2014. Public Health Agency of Canada, 2006. Available at: http://www.phac-aspc.gc.ca/publicat/cig-gci/

According to the CDC, the weight of currently available scientific evidence does not support the hypothesis that MMR vaccine causes either autism or IBD. The landmark paper linking autism to the MMR vaccine (*Lancet* 1998;351:637-641) was retracted due to false claims in the article (*Lancet* 2010;375:445)

Any Vaccine

Adverse Reactions
Local: induration, tenderness, redness, swelling
Systemic: fever, rash, irritability
Allergic: urticaria, rhinitis, anaphylaxis

Contraindications
Moderate/severe illness ± fever
Allergy to vaccine component
No need to delay vaccination for mild URTI

Vaccination in Cases of Asplenia or Hyposplenia (such as Sickle Cell Disease)
• Should receive all routine immunizations, including the yearly influenza vaccine
• No vaccines are contraindicated
• Susceptible to infection by encapsulated bacteria ("SHiNE KISS" – *S. pneumoniae, H. influenzae, N. meningitidis, E. coli, Klebsiella, Salmonella,* Group B *Strep*), so must add:
  • Meningococcal-C-Conjugate at age ≥2 yr + Quadravalent Men-P-ACYW at least 2 wk later
  • Booster of Men-P-ACYW q2-5yr
  • Pneumococcal polysaccharide vaccine (Pneu-P-23) at age ≥2 yr
  • Single booster of Pneu-P-23 at age ≥3 yr
  • Consider single booster HiB at age >5 yr

Injection site
Infants (<12 mo): anterolateral thigh

Growth and Development

Growth
• growth is not linear
  ▪ most rapid growth during first 2 yr and at puberty
  ▪ tissues grow at different times
    ♦ first 2 yr = CNS; mid-childhood = lymphoid tissue; puberty = gonads
• measurement of growth
  ▪ premature infants (<37 wk) use corrected GA until age 2
  ▪ body proportion = upper/lower segment ratio (use symphysis pubis as midpoint)
    ♦ newborn = 1.7, adult male = 0.9, adult female = 1.0

Average Growth Parameters

Table 3. Parameter of Average Growth at Birth

	Normal	Growth	Comments
Birth Weight	3.25 kg (7 lbs)	Gain 20-30 g/d (term neonate) 2 x birth wt by 4-5 mo 3 x birth wt by 1 yr 4 x birth wt by 2 yr	Weight loss (up to 10% of birth weight) in first 7 d of life is normal Neonate should regain birth weight by ~10-14 d of age
Length/Height	50 cm (20 in)	25 cm in 1st yr 12 cm in 2nd yr 8 cm in 3rd yr then 4-7 cm/yr until puberty 1/2 adult height at 2 yr	Measure supine length until 2 yr of age, then measure standing height
Head Circumference	35 cm (14 in)	2 cm/mo for 1st 3 mo 1 cm/mo at 3-6 mo 0.5 cm/mo at 6-12 mo	Measure around occipital, parietal, and frontal prominences to obtain the greatest circumference

Safety and Efficacy of an Attenuated Vaccine Against Severe Rotavirus Gastroenteritis
NEJM 2006;354:11-22
Study: Randomized, double-blind, phase 3 trial.
Patients: 63,225 healthy infants from Latin America and Finland.
Intervention: Two oral doses of HRV vaccine vs. placebo at 2 and 4 mo of age.
Outcome: Episodes of gastroenteritis and severity.
Results: The vaccine is 85% efficacious against severe rotavirus gastroenteritis and hospitalizations associated with gastroenteritis and 100% efficacious against more severe gastroenteritis.

Reflexes

Table 4. Reflexes

Reflex	Maneuver to Elicit Reflex	Appropriate Reflex Response
Moro	Infant placed semi-upright, head supported by examiner's hand, sudden withdrawal of supported head with immediate return of support	Abduction and extension of the arms, opening of the hands, followed by flexion and adduction of arms
Galant	Infant held in ventral suspension and one side of back is stroked along paravertebral line	Pelvis will move in the direction of stimulated side
Grasp	Placement of examiner's finger in infant's palm	Flexion of infant's fingers
ATNR	Turn infant's head to one side	"Fencing" posture (extension of ipsilateral leg and arm and flexion of contralateral arm)
Placing	Dorsal surface of infant's foot placed touching edge of table	Flexion followed by extension of ipsilateral limb up onto table (resembles primitive walking)
Rooting	Tactile stimulus near mouth	Infant turns head and opens mouth to suck on same side that cheek was stroked
Parachute	Tilt infant to side while in sitting position	Ipsilateral arm extension, present by 6-8 mo

ATNR = asymmetric tonic neck reflex

Abnormal Reflex Response
- Absence may suggest CNS abnormality
- Persistence after 4-6 mo may indicate abnormality (e.g. cerebral palsy)
- Asymmetry suggests focal motor lesions (e.g. brachial plexus injury)
- Upgoing plantar reflex (Babinski's sign) normal in infants up to age 2 yr

Developmental Milestones

Table 5. Developmental Milestones

Age*	Gross Motor	Fine Motor	Speech and Language	Adaptive and Social Skills
1 mo	Turns head side to side when supine	Hands fisted, thumb in fist	Cries, startles to loud noises	Calms when comforted
2 mo	Briefly raises head when prone, holds head erect when upright	Pulls at clothes	Variety of sounds (e.g. coos, gurgles)	Smiles responsively, recognizes and calms down to familiar voice, follows movement with eyes
4 mo	Lifts head and chest when prone, holds head steady when supported sitting, rolls prone to supine	Briefly holds object when placed in hand, reaches for midline objects	Turns head towards sounds	Laughs responsively, follows moving toy or person with eyes, responds to people with excitement (e.g. leg movement)
6 mo	Tripod sit, pivots in prone position	Ulnar or raking grasp, transfers objects from hand to hand, brings objects to mouth	Babbles	Stranger anxiety, beginning of object permanence
9 mo	Sits well without support, crawls, pulls to stand, stands with support	Early pincer grasp with straight wrist	"Mama, dada" – appropriate, imitates 1 word, responds to "no" regardless of tone	Plays games (e.g. peek-a-boo), reaches to be picked up
12 mo	Gets into sitting position without help, stands without support, walks while holding on	Neat pincer grasp, releases ball with throw	2 words, follows 1-step command, uses facial expression, sounds, actions to make needs known	Responds to own name, separation anxiety begins

*Use corrected GA until 2 yr

Developmental Red Flags
- Gross motor: not walking at 18 mo rolling too early at <3 mo
- Fine motor: hand preference at <18 mo
- Speech: <10 words at 18 mo
- Social: not smiling at 3 mo; not pointing at 15-18 mo
- See the Nipissing District Developmental Screen for a checklist of important 18 mo milestones: www.ndds.ca

Table 5. Developmental Milestones (continued)

Age*	Gross Motor	Fine Motor	Speech and Language	Adaptive and Social Skills
15 mo	Walks without support, crawls up stairs/steps	Picks up and eats finger foods, scribbles, stacks 2 blocks	4-5 words, points to needs/wants	Looks to see how others react (e.g. after falling)
18 mo	Runs, walks forward pulling toys or carrying objects	Tower of 3 cubes, scribbling, eats with spoon	10 words, follows simple commands	Shows affection towards others, points to show interest in something
24 mo	Climbs up and down steps with 2 feet per step, runs, kicks ball	Tower of 6 cubes, undresses	2-3 word phrases, uses "I, me, you", 50% intelligible, understands 2-step commands	Parallel play, helps to dress
3 yr	Rides tricycle, climbs up 1 foot per step, down 2 feet per step, stands on one foot briefly	Copies a circle, turns pages one at a time, puts on shoes, dress/undress fully except buttons	Combines 3 or more words into sentence, recognizes colours, prepositions, plurals, counts to 10, 75% intelligible	Knows sex and age, shares some of the time, plays make-believe games
4 yr	Hops on 1 foot, climbs down 1 foot per step	Copies a cross, uses scissors, buttons clothes	Speech 100% intelligible, uses past tense, understands 3-part directions	Cooperative play, fully toilet-trained by day, tries to comfort someone who is upset
5 yr	Skips, rides bicycle	Copies a triangle and square, prints name, ties shoelaces	Fluent speech, future tense, alphabet, retells sequence of a story	Cooperates with adult requests most of the time, separates easily from caregiver

*Use corrected GA until 2 yr

Nutrition

Dietary Requirements

Weight	<10 kg	10-20 kg		>20 kg
Needs	100 kcal/kg/d	1,000 cal + 50 kcal/kg/d for each kg >10		1,500 cal + 20 kcal/kg/d for each kg >20

Dietary Recommendations
- 0-6 mo: breast milk or formula
  - exclusive breast milk during first 6 mo recommended over formula unless contraindicated
  - breastfed infants require supplements: vitamin D (400-800 IU/d), fluoride (after 6 mo if not sufficient in water), iron (6-12 mo, only if not receiving fortified cereals/meat/meat alternatives)
- >6 mo: solid food introduction – do not delay beyond 9 mo
  - 2-3 new foods per wk with a few days in between each food to allow time for adverse reaction identification
  - suggested order of introduction
    - meat, meat alternatives, and iron-enriched cereal (rice cereal is least allergenic)
    - pureed vegetables
    - fruit
- 9-12 mo: finger foods and switch to homogenized (3.25%) milk
  - feed child based on hunger/satiety cues; encourage self-feeding and introduce open cup
  - foods to avoid
    - honey until past 12 mo (risk of botulism)
    - added sugar, salt
    - excessive milk (i.e. no more than 16 oz/d after 1 yr)
    - juice (not nutritious, too much sugar) maximum 4-6 oz (1/2 cup) daily
    - anything that is a choking hazard (chunks, round foods like grapes)

2 yrs: switch to 2% milk
- content of breast milk
  - colostrum (first few days): clear, rich in nutrients (i.e. high protein, low fat), immunoglobulin
  - mature milk: 70:30 whey:casein ratio, fat from dietary butterfat, carbohydrate from lactose
- advantages
  - easily digested, low renal solute load
  - immunologic
    - contains IgA, macrophages, active lymphocytes, lysozymes, lactoferrin (which inhibits *E. coli* growth in intestine)
    - lower pH promotes growth of *Lactobacillus* in GI tract
  - parent-child bonding
  - economical, convenient

Peanut Allergies in Children
NEJM 2015;372(9):803-813
Study: 640 children identified as "at risk to peanut allergy" due to severe eczema, egg allergy, or both were split into two cohorts depending on their pre-existing sensitivity to peanut extract on skin-prick test. These two cohorts were randomized to peanut consumption or avoidance up until 60 mo of age.
Results: In the cohort with negative skin-prick test at start of study, prevalence of peanut allergy at 60 mo of age was 13.7% in peanut avoidance and 1.9% in the peanut consumption group. In cohort with positive skin-prick test at start of study, prevalence of peanut allergy at 60 mo of age was 35.3% in peanut avoidance and 10.6% in peanut consumption group.
Conclusion: Early introduction of peanuts significantly decreased prevalence of peanut allergies in children deemed "at risk to peanut allergy".

Dietary Exposures and Allergy Prevention in High-Risk Infants
Paediatr Child Health 2013;18(10):545-549
There is no evidence that restriction of highly allergenic foods is beneficial in the first year of life. Later introduction of peanut, fish, or egg does not prevent, and may increase the risk of developing food allergy. There is also no evidence that dietary restrictions during pregnancy or breastfeeding are protective to the child.

- maternal contraindications
  - chemotherapy or radioactive compounds
  - HIV/AIDS, active untreated TB, herpes in breast region
  - >0.5 g/kg/d of alcohol or illicit drugs
  - medications known to cross to breast milk
  - OCPs are *not* a contraindication to breastfeeding (estrogen may decrease lactation, but is not dangerous to infant)
  - MotherRisk™ Program – valuable research and counselling on reproductive risk or safety of drugs and chemicals
  - breastfeeding jaundice (first 1-2 wk): due to lack of maternal milk production and subsequent infant dehydration (see *Jaundice*, P69)
  - breast milk jaundice (0.5% of newborns, persists up to 4-6 mo): rare, glucuronyl transferase inhibitor in breast milk inhibits conjugation of bilirubin, increases enterohepatic circulation of bilirubin
    - baby presents healthy and thriving, and jaundice (secondary to unconjugated bilirubin) resolves
  - poor weight gain: consider dehydration or FTT
  - oral candidiasis (thrush): treat baby with antifungal such as nystatin; can occur in breast or bottle-fed infants

Medications that Cross into Breast Milk
- Antimetabolites
- Bromocriptine
- Chloramphenicol
- High dose diazepam
- Ergots
- Gold
- Metronidazole
- Tetracycline
- Lithium
- Cyclophosphamide

Table 6. Common Formulas Compared to Breast Milk

Type of Nutrition	Indications	Content (as compared to breast milk)
Cow's Milk-Based (Enfamil®, Similac®)	Prematurity Transition into breastfeeding Contraindication to breastfeeding	Lower whey:casein ratio Plant fats instead of dietary butterfat
Fortified Formula	Low birth weight Prematurity	Higher calories and vitamins A, C, D, K May only be used in hospital due to risk of fat-soluble vitamin toxicity
Soy Protein (Isomil®, Prosobee®)	Galactosemia Desire for vegetarian/vegan diet*	Corn syrup solids or sucrose in place of lactose
Partially Hydrolyzed Proteins (Good Start®)	Delayed gastric emptying Risk of cow milk protein allergy	Protein is 100% whey with no casein
Protein Hydrolysate (Nutramigen®, Alimentum®, Pregestimil®, Portagen®)	Malabsorption Food allergy	Protein is 100% casein with no whey Corn syrup solids, sucrose, or tapioca starch instead of lactose Expensive
Amino Acid (Neocate®, PurAminoTM)	Food allergy Short gut	Free amino acids (no protein) Corn syrup solids instead of lactose Very expensive
Metabolic	Inborn errors of metabolism	Various different compositions for children with galactosemia, propionic acidemia, etc.

* 10-35% of children with cow's milk protein allergy also have reactions to soy-based formula

Signs of Inadequate Intake
- <6 wet diapers/d after first wk
- <7 feeds/d
- Sleepy or lethargic, sleeping throughout the night <6 wk
- Weight loss >10% of birth weight
- Jaundice

- 1 wet diaper per/d of age for first week
- 1-2 black or dark green stools/d on Day 1 & 2
- 3+ brown/green/yellow stools/d on Day 3 & 4
- 3+ yellow, seedy stools/d on Day 5+

Injury Prevention Counselling

- injuries are the leading cause of death in children >1 yr of age
- main causes: motor vehicle crashes, burns, drowning, falls, choking, infanticide

Table 7. Injury Prevention Counselling

0-6 mo	6-12 mo	1-2 yr	2-5 yr
Do not leave alone on bed, on changing table, or in tub	Install stair barriers	Never leave unattended	Bicycle helmet
Keep crib rails up	Discourage use of walkers	Keep pot handles turned to back of stove	Never leave unsupervised at home, driveway, or pool
Check water temperature before bathing	Avoid play areas with sharp-edged tables and corners	Caution with whole grapes, nuts, raw carrots, hotdogs, etc. due to choking hazard	Teach bike safety, stranger safety, and street safety
Do not hold hot liquid and infant at the same time	Cover electrical outlets	No running while eating	Swimming lessons (>4 yr), sunscreen (from 6 mo), fences around pools
Check milk temperature before feeding	Unplug appliances when not in use	Appropriate car seats	Appropriate car seats
Appropriate car seats are required before leaving hospital	Keep small objects, plastic bags, cleaning products, and medications out of reach		
	Supervise during feeding		
	Appropriate car seats		

Note: This list is not exhaustive. For more details, see Rourke Baby Record (http://www.rourkebabyrecord.ca/pdf/RBR20110nt_Eng.pdf)

Common Complaints

Breath Holding Spells

- epidemiology: 0.1-5% of healthy children 6 mo-4 yr of age, usually start during first year of life
- etiology: child is provoked (usually by anger, injury, or fear) → holds breath and becomes silent → spontaneously resolves or loses consciousness
- types
  - cyanotic (more common), usually associated with anger/frustration
  - pallid, usually associated with pain/surprise
- management
  - usually resolves spontaneously and rarely progresses to seizure
  - help child control response to frustration and avoid drawing attention to spell
  - commonly associated with iron deficiency anemia, improves with supplemental iron

Circumcision

Circumcision
Sorokan, S. Todd, Jane C. Finlay, and Ann L. Jefferies. "Newborn male circumcision." *Paediatrics & Child Health* 20.6 (2015): 1.

- elective procedure
  - not covered by OHIP in Ontario, but recent evidence shows show risks vs benefit → not clearly different; no clear position by CPS in 2015 statement
  - often for religious or culture reasons
- benefits: prevention of phimosis and slightly reduced incidence of UTI, STI, balanitis, cancer of the penis
- complications (<1%): local infection, bleeding, urethral injury
- contraindications: presence of genital abnormalities (e.g. hypospadias) or known bleeding disorder

Crying/Fussing Child

- history
  - description of baseline feeding, sleeping, crying patterns
  - infectious symptoms: fever, tachypnea, rhinorrhea, ill contacts
  - feeding intolerance: gastroesophageal reflux with esophagitis, N/V, diarrhea, constipation
  - trauma
  - recent immunizations (vaccine reaction) or medications (drug reactions), including maternal drugs taken during pregnancy (neonatal withdrawal syndrome) and drugs that may be transferred via breast milk
  - inconsistent history, pattern of numerous emergency department visits, high-risk social situations all raise concern of maltreatment

Table 8. Physical Exam and Differential Diagnosis

Organ System	Possible Examination Findings	Possible Diagnosis
HEENT	Bulging fontanelle, bulging and erythematous TM Blepharospasm, tearing Retinal hemorrhage Oropharyngeal infections	Meningitis, shaken baby syndrome, hydrocephalus Corneal abrasion, glaucoma Shaken baby syndrome Thrush, gingivostomatitis, herpangina, otitis media
Neurological	Irritability or lethargy	Meningitis, shaken baby syndrome
Cardiovascular	Poor perfusion Tachycardia	Sepsis, anomalous coronary artery, meningitis, myocarditis, CHF
Respiratory	Tachypnea Grunting	Pneumonia, CHF Respiratory disease, response to pain
Abdominal	Mass, empty RLQ	Intussusception
Genitourinary	Scrotal swelling Penile/clitoral swelling	Incarcerated hernia, testicular torsion Hair tourniquet
Rectal	Anal fissure Hemoccult positive stool	Constipation or diarrhea Intussusception, NEC, volvulus
Musculoskeletal	Point tenderness or decreased movement	Fracture, syphilis, osteomyelitis, toe/finger hair tourniquet

Infantile Colic

- definition: unexplained paroxysms of irritability and crying for >3 h/d, >3 d/wk for >3 wk in an otherwise healthy, well-fed baby (rule of 3s)
- epidemiology: 10% of infants; usual onset 10 d to 3 mo of age with peak at 6-8 wk
- etiology: lag in development of normal peristaltic movement in gastrointestinal tract; other theories suggest a lack of self-soothing mechanisms or extreme of normal

- management
  - parental relief, rest, and reassurance
  - hold baby, soother, car ride, music, vacuum, check diaper
  - medications (Ovol° drops, gripe water) have no proven benefit, some evidence for probiotics
  - if breastfeeding, elimination of cow's milk protein from mother's diet (effective in very small percentage of cases)
  - check for otitis media, cow's milk intolerance, GI problem, fracture
  - try casein hydrolysate formula (Nutramigen°)
  - time – all resolve, most in the first 2-3 mo of life

Dentition and Caries

Dentition
- primary dentition (20 teeth)
  - first tooth at 5-9 mo (lower incisor), then 1/mo
  - 6-8 central teeth by 1 yr
  - assessment by dentist 6 mo after eruption of first tooth and certainly by 1 yr of age (Grade B recommendation)
- secondary dentition (32 teeth)
  - first adult tooth is 1st molar at 6 yr, then lower incisors

Caries
- milk caries: decay of superior front teeth and back molars in first 4 yr of life
- cause: often due to prolonged feeding (e.g. put to bed with bottle, prolonged breastfeeding)
- prevention
  - no bottle at bedtime, clean teeth after last feed
  - minimize juice and sweetened pacifier
  - clean teeth with soft damp cloth or toothbrush and water
  - water fluoridation

Enuresis

Definition
- involuntary urinary incontinence by day and/or night in child >5 yr

General Approach
- should be evaluated if dysuria, change in colour, odour, stream, secondary or diurnal, change in gait, stool incontinence

Primary Nocturnal Enuresis
- definition: involuntary loss of urine at night, bladder control has never been attained
- epidemiology: boys > girls; 10% of 6 yr olds, 3% of 12 yr olds, 1% of 18 yr olds
- etiology: developmental disorder or maturational lag in bladder control while asleep
- management
  - time and reassurance (~20% resolve spontaneously each yr)
  - behaviour modification (limiting fluids, voiding prior to sleep), bladder retention exercises, scheduled toileting overnight has limited effectiveness
  - conditioning: "wet" alarm wakes child upon voiding (70% success rate)
  - medications (considered second line therapy, may be used for sleepovers/camp): DDAVP oral tablets (high relapse rate, costly), imipramine (Tofranil°) (rarely used, lethal if overdose, cholinergic side effects)

Secondary Enuresis
- definition: involuntary loss of urine at night, develops after child has sustained period of bladder control (>6 mo)
- etiology: inorganic regression due to stress or anxiety (e.g. birth of sibling, significant loss, family discord), focused on other activities, secondary to organic disease (UTI, DM, DI, neurogenic bladder, CP, seizures, pinworms)
- management: treat underlying cause

Diurnal Enuresis
- definition: daytime wetting (60-80% also wet at night)
- etiology: micturition deferral (holding urine until last minute) due to psychosocial stressor (e.g. shy), structural anomalies (e.g. ectopic ureteral site, neurogenic bladder), UTI, constipation, CNS disorders, DM
- management: treat underlying cause, behavioural (scheduled toileting, double voiding, good bowel program, sitting backwards on toilet, charting/incentive system, relaxation/biofeedback), pharmacotherapy

Treatment for primary nocturnal enuresis should not be considered until 7 yr of age due to high rate of spontaneous cure

Antidiuretic Hormone Regulation in Primary Nocturnal Enuresis
Arch Dis Child 1995;73(6):508-11
Treatment of primary nocturnal enuresis using DDAVP is based upon the hypothesis that ADH secretion is insufficient at night. The known efficacy of the treatment on the one hand, and persisting doubts about its theoretical basis on the other, formed the background of the present study. Ten children (mean age 10.5 yr) with primary nocturnal enuresis were compared with a corresponding control group of eight patients. Diurnal and nocturnal urine production, ADH secretion, and plasma osmolality were determined.
No differences between the two groups were found for urine production, ADH levels during day and night, or plasma osmolality. However, in order to regulate plasma osmolality the enuretic children required a markedly greater output of ADH: 2.87 pg/ml/mmol/kg compared with 0.56 in the controls (p < 0.01). The results are consistent with the established fact that ADH secretion is a function of plasma osmolality, and they contradict the hypothesis that urine production is increased at night in enuretics because of lower ADH secretion.

Encopresis

- definition: fecal incontinence in a child >4 yr old, at least once per mo for 3 mo
- prevalence: 1-1.5% of school-aged children (rare in adolescence); M:F = 6:1 in school-aged children
- causes: chronic constipation (retentive encopresis), Hirschsprung disease, hypothyroidism, hypercalcemia, spinal cord lesions, anorectal malformations, bowel obstruction

Retentive Encopresis
- definition: child holds bowel movement, develops constipation, leading to fecal impaction and seepage of soft or liquid stool (overflow incontinence)
- etiology
  - physical: painful stooling often secondary to constipation
  - emotional: disturbed parent-child relationship, coercive toilet training, social stressors
- clinical presentation
  - history
    - crosses legs or stands on toes to resist urge to defecate
    - distressed by symptoms, soiling of clothes
    - toilet training coercive or lacking in motivation
    - may show oppositional behaviour
    - abdominal pain
  - physical exam
    - digital rectal exam: large fecal mass in rectal vault
    - anal fissures (result from passage of hard stools)
  - palpable stool in LLQ
- management
  - complete clean-out of bowel: PEG 3350 given orally is most effective, enemas and suppositories may be second line therapies, but these are invasive and often less effective
  - maintenance of regular bowel movements (see *Constipation Treatment*, P36)
  - assessment and guidance regarding psychosocial stressors
  - behavioural modification
- complications: recurrence, toxic megacolon (requires >3-12 mo to treat), bowel perforation

Toilet Training

- 90% of children attain bladder control before bowel control
- generally, females train earlier than males
- 25% by 2 yr (in North America), 98% by 3 yr have daytime bladder control
- signs of toilet readiness
  - ambulating independently, stable on potty, desire to be independent or to please caregivers (i.e. motivation), sufficient expressive and receptive language skills (2-step command level), can stay dry for several hours (large enough bladder), can recognize need to go, able to remove clothing

Failure to Thrive

Mid-Parental Height
- Boys target height = (father ht + mother ht + 13) / 2
- Girls target height = (father ht + mother ht – 13) / 2

Note: height should be taken in cm

- definition
  - weight <3rd percentile, falls across two major percentile curves, or <80% of expected weight for height and age
  - inadequate caloric intake most common factor in poor weight gain
  - may have other nutritional deficiencies (e.g. protein, iron, vitamin D)
  - factors affecting physical growth: genetics, intrauterine factors, nutrition, endocrine hormones, chronic infections/diseases, psychosocial factors
- clinical presentation
  - history
    - nutritional intake
    - current symptoms
    - past illnesses
    - family history: growth, puberty, parental height and weight including mid-parental height
    - psychosocial history
  - physical exam
    - growth parameters, plotted: height, weight, head circumference, arm span
    - vital signs
    - complete head to toe exam
    - dysmorphic features or evidence of chronic disease
    - upper to lower segment ratio
    - sexual maturity staging
    - signs of maltreatment or neglect
- investigations (as indicated by clinical presentation)
  - CBC, blood smear, electrolytes, T4, TSH
  - bone age x-ray
  - chromosomes/karyotype
  - chronic illness: chest (CXR, sweat Cl-), cardiac (CXR, ECG, Echo), GI (celiac screen, inflammatory markers, malabsorption), renal (urinalysis), liver (enzymes, albumin)

Clinical Signs of FTT

SMALL KID
Subcutaneous fat loss
Muscle atrophy
Alopecia
Lethargy
Lagging behind normal
Kwashiorkor
Infection (recurrent)
Dermatitis

Table 9. Failure to Thrive Patterns

Growth Parameters			Suggestive Abnormality	
Decreased Wt	Normal Ht	Normal HC	Caloric insufficiency Decreased intake	Hypermetabolic state Increased losses
Decreased Wt	Decreased Ht	Normal HC	Structural dystrophies Endocrine disorder	Constitutional growth delay (BA < CA) Familial short stature (BA = CA)
Decreased Wt	Decreased Ht	Decreased HC	Intrauterine insult	Genetic abnormality

BA = bone age; CA = chronological age; HC = head circumference; Ht = height; Wt = weight

Non-Organic FTT (90%)
- most common cause of FTT
- results from complex factors in parent-child relationship
  - dietary intake, knowledge about feeding, improper mixing of formula, economic factors
  - feeding environment
  - parent-child interaction, attachment
  - child behaviours, hunger/satiety cues
  - social factors: stress, poverty
- management
  - most as outpatient using multidisciplinary approach: primary care physician, dietitian, psychologist, social work, CAS
  - medical: oromotor problems, iron-deficiency anemia, gastroesophageal reflux
  - nutritional: educate about age-appropriate foods, calorie boosting, mealtime schedules and environment; goal to reach 90-110% IBW, correct nutritional deficiencies, and promote catch-up growth/development
  - behavioural: positive reinforcement, mealtime environment

Organic FTT (10%)
- inadequate intake: non-organic, vomiting, oromotor dysfunction, anorexia
- excessive consumption: CHD, CF, hyperthyroidism
- abnormal utilization: inborn errors of metabolism
- excessive output: IBD, celiac, malabsorption
- management: treat specific cause

Energy Requirements
- see *Nutrition*, P6

Obesity

- definition: BMI >95th percentile for age and height
- risk factors: genetic predisposition (e.g. both parents obese – 80% chance of obese child)
- etiology: organic causes are rare (<5%), but may include Prader-Willi, Carpenter, Turner, Cushing syndromes, hypothyroidism
- complications: association with HTN, dyslipidemia, slipped capital femoral epiphysis, type 2 DM, asthma, obstructive sleep apnea, gynecomastia, polycystic ovarian disease, early menarche, irregular menses, psychological trauma (e.g. bullying, decreased self-esteem, unhealthy coping mechanisms, depression)
- childhood obesity often persists into adulthood
- management
  - encouragement and reassurance; engagement of entire family
  - diet: qualitative changes (do not encourage weight loss, but allow for linear growth to catch up with weight), special diets used by adults and very low calorie diets are not encouraged
  - behaviour modification: increase activity, change eating habits/meal patterns
  - education: multidisciplinary approach, dietitian, counselling
  - surgery and pharmacotherapy are rarely used in children
  - increase physical activity (30 min/day), reduce screen time

Poison Prevention

- keep all types of medicines, vitamins, and chemicals locked up in a secure container
- potentially dangerous: medications, illicit drugs, drain cleaners, furniture polish, insecticides, cosmetics, nail polish remover, automotive products
- do not store any chemicals in juice, soft drink, or water bottles
- keep alcoholic beverages out of reach: 3 oz hard liquor can kill a 2 yr old
- always read labels before administering medicine to ensure correct medication drug and dose and/or speak with a pharmacist or healthcare provider

Upper to Lower Segment Ratio
- **Increased** in achondroplasia, short limb syndromes, hypothyroid, storage diseases
- **Decreased** in Marfan's, Klinefelter's, Kallman's syndromes, and testosterone deficiency
- **Calculation:** upper segment/lower segment
  - Upper segment: top of head to pubic symphysis
  - Lower segment: pubic symphysis to floor

Perinatal and Early Childhood Factors for Overweight and Obesity in Young Canadian Children
Can J Public Health 2013;104(1):e69-74
Background: This study assessed potential early-life factors and their interrelationships with obesity among young Canadian children.
Methods: Data from a nationally representative sample of children aged 6-11 yr in the Canadian Health Measures Survey were analyzed. The associations of perinatal and early childhood behaviours and socioeconomic factors with overweight or obesity were evaluated using multivariate logistic regression models.
Results: Of 968 term-born children, 21% were overweight and another 13% were obese. Maternal smoking during pregnancy was positively associated with obesity. This association was mediated by birth weight and once controlled, the strength of the association between smoking and child obesity increased by 12%. Birth weight per 100 g (1.05; 1.005-1.09) was significantly associated with obesity. Exclusive breastfeeding for 6 mo, adequate sleep hours, and being physically active were found to be protective. Breastfeeding, whether exclusive or not, significantly reduced obesity risk among children whose mothers never smoked in pregnancy.
Conclusions: This study identified multiple perinatal and childhood factors associated with obesity in young Canadian children. Effective prevention strategies targeting four modifiable maternal and child risk factors may reduce childhood obesity by up to 54% in Canada.

Screen Time Guidelines (Canadian Society for Exercise Physiology)
- Screen time is not recommended for children under 2 yr
- <1 h/d screen time is appropriate for children aged 2-5 yr
- <2 h/d screen time is appropriate for children 5-17 yr

Rashes

Table 10. Common Pediatric Rashes

Type of Rash	Differential	Appearance	Management
Diaper Dermatitis			
	Irritant contact dermatitis	Shiny, red macules/patches, no skin fold involvement	Eliminate direct skin contact with urine and feces, allow periods of rest without a diaper, frequent diaper changes, topical barriers (petrolatum, zinc oxide or paste), short-term low-potency topical corticosteroids (severe cases)
	Seborrheic dermatitis	Yellow, greasy macules/plaques on erythema, scales	Short-term, low-potency topical corticosteroids
	Candidal dermatits	Erythematous macerated papules/plaques, satellite lesions, involvement of skin folds	Antifungal agents (e.g. clotrimazole, nystatin)
Other Dermatitis			
	Atopic dermatitis	Erythematous, papules/plaques, oozing, excoriation, lichenification, classic areas of involvement	Eliminate exacerbating factors, maintain skin hydration, corticosteroids, topical calcineurin inhibitor, daily baths
	Nummular dermatitis	Annular erythematous plaques, oozing, crusting	Avoid irritant if identified, potent topical steroid in emollient base, short-term systemic steroids ± antibiotics (severe)
	Allergic contact dermatitis	Red papules/plaques/vesicles/bullae, only in area of allergen	Mild: soothing lotion (e.g. calamine lotion) Moderate: low-to-intermediate potency topical corticosteroids Severe: systemic corticosteroids and antihistamine
	Irritant contact dermatitis	Morphology depends on irritant	Avoid skin contact
	Dyshidrotic dermatitis	Papulovesicular, cracking/fissuring, hands and feet ("tapioca pudding")	Mild/moderate: medium/potent topical corticosteroids Severe: systemic corticosteroids, local PUVA or UVA treatments
Infectious			
	Scabies	Polymorphic (red excoriated papules/nodules, burrows), in web spaces/folds, very pruritic Often affects multiple family members	Permethrin (Nix®) 5% cream for patient and family (2 applications, 1 wk apart)
	Impetigo	Honey-coloured crusts or superficial bullae	Oral antibiotics (e.g. cephalexin/erythromycin) Topical if mild: fucidic acid or mupirocin cream
	Tinea corporis	Round erythematous plaques, central clearing and scaly border	Topical anti-fungal for skin, systemic anti-fungals for nails/head

Pediatric Exanthems (see *Infectious Pediatric Exanthems*, P55)

Drug Reactions (see Dermatology, D21)

 Acne (see Dermatology, D11)

Sleep Disturbances

Daily Sleep Requirement
- <6 mo 16 h
- 6 mo   14.5 h
- 12 mo 13.5 h
- 2 yr   13 h
- 4 yr   11.5 h
- 6 yr   9.5 h
- 12 yr   8.5 h
- 18 yr   8 h

Nap Patterns
- 2/d at 1 yr
- 1/d at 2 yr: 2-3 h
- 0.5/d at 5 yr: 1.7 h

Types of Sleep Disturbances
- insufficient sleep quantity
  - difficulty falling asleep (e.g. limit setting sleep disorder)
    - preschool and older children
    - bedtime resistance
    - due to caregiver's inability to set consistent bedtime rules and routines
    - often exacerbated by child's oppositional behaviours
- poor sleep quality
  - frequent arousals (e.g. sleep-onset association disorder)
    - infants and toddlers
    - child learns to fall asleep only under certain conditions or associations (e.g. with parent, held, rocked or fed, with light on, in front of television), and loses ability to self-soothe
    - during the normal brief arousal periods of sleep (q90-120 min), child cannot fall back asleep because same conditions are not present

- obstructive sleep apnea
  - epidemiology: 1-5% of preschool aged children, more common in African American children
  - definition: partial or intermittent complete airway obstruction during sleep causing disrupted ventilation and sleep pattern
  - features: snoring/gasping/noisy breathing during sleep and irritable/tired/hyperactive during the day
  - sequelae: cardiovascular (HTN/LV remodelling due to sympathetic activation), growth, cognitive, and behavioural deficitis
  - risk factors: adenotonsillar hypertrophy, obesity
  - management: watchful waiting, weight reduction, airway pressure devices, or surgery depending on the cause
  - adenotonsillectomy does not improve executive function or attention but reduces symptoms and improves behaviour, quality of life, and polysomnographic findings
- parasomnias
  - episodic nocturnal behaviours (e.g. sleepwalking, sleep terrors, nightmares)
  - often involves cognitive disorientation and autonomic/skeletal muscle disturbance

Management of Sleep Disturbances
- set strict bedtimes and "wind-down" routines
- do not send child to bed hungry
- positive reinforcement for: limit setting sleep disorder
- always sleep in own bed, in a dark, quiet, and comfortable room
- do not use bedroom for timeouts
- systematic ignoring and gradual extinction for: sleep-onset association disorder

Nightmares
- epidemiology: common in boys, 4-7 yr old
- associated with REM sleep (anytime during night)
- features: upon awakening, child is alert and clearly recalls frightening dream ± associated with daytime stress/anxiety
- management: reassurance

Night Terrors
- epidemiology: 15% of children have occasional episodes
- abrupt sitting up, eyes open, screaming
- clinical features: occurs in early hours of sleep, stage 4 of sleep; signs of panic and autonomic arousal, no memory of event, inconsolable, stress/anxiety can aggravate them
- course: remits spontaneously at puberty
- management: reassurance for parents, ensure child is safe (e.g. if sleepwalks)

Sudden Infant Death Syndrome

Definition
- sudden and unexpected death of an infant <12 mo of age in which the cause of death cannot be found by history, examination, or a thorough postmortem and death scene investigation

Epidemiology
- 0.5/1,000 (leading cause of death between 1-12 mo of age); M:F = 3:2
- more common in children placed in prone position
- in full term infants, peak incidence is 2-4 mo, 95% of cases occur by 6 mo
- increase in deaths during peak RSV season
- most deaths occur between midnight and 8 AM

Risk Factors
- prematurity, smoking in household, socially disadvantaged, higher incidence in Aboriginals and African Americans
- risk of SIDS is increased 3-5x in siblings of infants who have died of SIDS
- bedsharing: sleeping on a sofa, sleeping with an infant after consumption of alcohol/street drugs or extreme fatigue,sleeping on a surface with a fixed wall (couch/sofa), infant sleeping with someone other than primary caregiver

Prevention
- "Back to Sleep, Front to Play" (place infant on back when sleeping)
- allow supervised play time daily in prone position ("tummy time")
- alarms, monitors not recommended – increase anxiety, do not prevent life-threatening events
- avoid overheating and overdressing
- appropriate infant bedding (firm mattress; avoid loose bedding, pillows, stuffed animals, and crib bumper pads)
- no smoking
- pacifiers appear to have a protective effect; do not reinsert if falls out during sleep

Brief Resolved Unexplained Events (BRUE)
A group of conditions often marked by an episode of apnea, cyanosis, change in tone, or change in mental status occurring in a child, where an observer fears the child may be dying. There is no clear connection between most BRUEs and SIDS. Evaluating for a cause of the BRUE (e.g. infection, cardiac, neurologic) is guided by history, physical exam, and period of observation

Child Abuse and Neglect

Definition
- an act of commission (physical, sexual, or psychological abuse) or omission (neglect) by a caregiver that harms a child

Legal Duty to Report
- upon reasonable grounds to suspect abuse and/or neglect, physicians are required by legislation to contact the CAS to personally disclose all information relevant to the child safety concern
- duty to report overrides patient confidentiality; physician is protected against liability

Ongoing Duty to Report
- if there are additional reasonable grounds to suspect abuse and/or neglect, a further report to the CAS must be made

Risk Factors
- environmental factors: social isolation, poverty, domestic violence
- caregiver factors: personal history of abuse, psychiatric illness, substance abuse, single parent family, poor social and vocational skills, below average intelligence
- child factors: difficult temperament, disability, special needs (e.g. developmental delay), premature

Management of Physical Abuse, Child Abuse, and Neglect
- report all suspicions to CAS; request emergency visit if imminent risk to child or any siblings in the home
- acute medical care: hospitalize for medical evaluation or treatment of injuries if indicated
- arrange consultation to social work and appropriate follow-up
- may need to discharge child directly to CAS or to responsible guardian under CAS supervision

Physical Abuse

CPS position statement – 2013: Ward, Michelle GK, et al. "The medical assessment of bruising in suspected child maltreatment cases: A clinical perspective." *Paediatrics & child health* 18.8 (2013): 1.

History
- history that is not compatible with physical findings, or history not reproducible
- delay in seeking medical attention that is unexplained by other factors

Physical Exam
- physical findings not explained by underlying medical condition
- growth parameters (weight, height, head circumference)
- recurrent or multiple injuries not explained by accidental injury or child's development level
- patterned skin injuries: belt buckle, hand prints, burns that do not match provided history
- injury location: bruises on areas with abundant soft-tissue cushioning, such as abdomen, buttocks, genitalia, fleshy part of cheek; bruises on ears, neck or feet; posterior rib/metaphyseal/scapular/vertebral/sternal fractures (more suspicious for non-accidental injuries); bruises that do not fit described cause; immersion burns (e.g. hot water)
- altered mental status: head injury, poisoning
- head trauma is the leading cause of death in child maltreatment (e.g. acceleration-deceleration forces [shaking], direct force application [blow or impact])

"If no cruising, no bruising"

Investigations
- document all injuries on a body diagram: type, location, size, shape, colour, pattern
  - photography of skin injuries is ideal (police or hospital photography preferred; do not use physician's personal camera)
- rule out medical causes of bruising/fracture with appropriate investigations:
  - if fractures evident: Ca^{2+}, Mg^{2+}, PO_4^{3-}, ALP, PTH, Vitamin D, renal function, and bone density
  - if bruising present: CBC, INR, PTT, von Willebrand factor, factors VII/IX/X/XIII
- screen for abdominal trauma (transaminases and amylase): if increased, abdo CT recommended
- skeletal survey in children <2 yr
  - bone scan can be beneficial for assessing rib fractures (not helpful for skull or metaphyseal region due to active bone growth) – consider bone scan if equivocal findings on initial skeletal survey
  - dilated eye examination by pediatric ophthalmologist to rule out retinal hemorrhage
  - be aware of "red herrings" (e.g. Mongolian blue spots vs. bruises)
  - neuroimaging: CT and/or MRI

Sexual Abuse

Epidemiology
- peak ages at 2-6 yr and 12-16 yr
- most perpetrators are male and known to child
  - in decreasing order: family member, non-relative known to victim, stranger

History
- diagnosis usually depends on child disclosing to someone or forensic interview done by a trained individual
- psychosocial: specific or generalized fears, depression, nightmares, social withdrawal, lack of trust, low self-esteem, school failure, sexually aggressive behaviour, advanced sexual knowledge, sexual preoccupation or play

Physical Exam
- recurrent UTIs, pregnancy, STIs, vaginitis, vaginal bleeding, pain, genital injury, enuresis

Investigations
- depend on presentation, age, sex, and pubertal development of child
  - sexual assault examination kit within 24 h if prepubertal, within 72 h if pubertal
  - rule out STI, UTI, pregnancy (consider STI prophylaxis or emergency contraception)
  - rule out other injuries (vaginal/anal/oral penetration, fractures, head trauma)
  - investigations to rule out drug and alcohol screen e.g. Rohypnol, 'Liquid G,' etc.

Neglect

History
- from child and each caregiver separately (if possible)

Physical Exam
- head to toe (do not force), growth parameters, nutrition status
- dental care
- emotional state

Investigations
- blood tests to rule out medical conditions (e.g. thrombocytopenia or coagulopathy)

> **Presentation of Neglect**
> - FTT, developmental delay
> - Inadequate or dirty clothing, poor hygiene
> - Child exhibits poor attachment to parents, no stranger anxiety

Adolescent Medicine

Adolescent History (HEEADSSS)
- tailor your history according to the clinical context

Home: Who do you live with? What kind of place do you live in?

Education/Employment: What grade are you in? What are your favourite subjects? What was your average on your last report card? Who are your favourite teachers?

Eating: Tell me about your meals/snacks in a typical day. Have you ever gone on a diet? What are your favourite and least favourite foods? (see _Psychiatry, Eating Disorders_, PS30)

Activities: What do you do after school? On the weekends? How much time do you spend on the computer/watching TV every day? Do you use social media (i.e. Facebook, Twitter, Instagram, etc.)? What do you do with your friends outside of school?

Drugs: Which seems to be more popular at your school, alcohol or drugs? How often do you drink/smoke marijuana/take other drugs? Do you smoke cigarettes? When you drink, do you usually get drunk? Have you ever passed out or not been able to remember what happened while you were drinking? Has anything bad ever happened to you while you were drunk or stoned? (see _Psychiatry, Substance Abuse_, PS21)

Sexuality: Are you romantically interested in anyone? When you think about having sex with someone, do you think about girls, boys, or both? Have you ever had sex with anyone? Whether the answer is yes or no, the next question is: What activities would you include in the term 'having sex'? What do you do to prevent getting a STI/getting pregnant/getting someone pregnant? Has anyone ever given you money, drugs, or other stuff in exchange for sex? (see _Gynecology, Sexually Transmitted Infections_, GY27)

Suicidality/Depression: On a scale of 1 to 10, where 1 is so sad that you might kill yourself and 10 is the happiest you could be, where are you most days? Do you often have trouble sleeping? Is there a difference between school days and the weekend? Have you ever thought seriously about suicide? Did you make a plan? (see _Psychiatry, Depression/Suicide_, PS10, PS4)

Safety/Violence: Do you ever get into a car with a driver who has been drinking? Do you always wear a seatbelt/bicycle helmet? Are you being bullied at school? Has anyone ever touched you in an unwanted way?

See _Normal and Abnormal Pubertal Development_, P30

> **Adolescent Psychosocial Assessment**
>
> **HEEADSSS**
> Home
> Education/Employment
> Eating
> Activities
> Drugs
> Sexuality
> Suicide and depression
> Safety/violence

> Rates of drug use in high school students who have used in the past year: alcohol (58.2%), cannabis (25.6%), tobacco (11.7%)

> Date rape comprises 80% of sexual assault in teenagers

> Prevalence of depression: 1-2% in pre-pubertal children and 6-8% in adolescents

Cardiology

Congenital Heart Disease

PRENATAL CIRCULATION

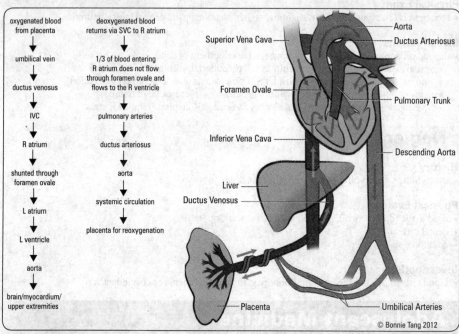

oxygenated blood from placenta
↓
umbilical vein
↓
ductus venosus
↓
IVC
↓
R atrium
↓
shunted through foramen ovale
↓
L atrium
↓
L ventricle
↓
aorta
↓
brain/myocardium/upper extremities

deoxygenated blood returns via SVC to R atrium
↓
1/3 of blood entering R atrium does not flow through foramen ovale and flows to the R ventricle
↓
pulmonary arteries
↓
ductus arteriosus
↓
aorta
↓
systemic circulation
↓
placenta for reoxygenation

© Bonnie Tang 2012

Figure 1. Prenatal circulation

Fetal circulation is designed so that oxygenated blood is preferentially delivered to the brain and myocardium

Before Birth
- shunting deoxygenated blood
  - ductus arteriosus: connection between pulmonary artery and aorta
- shunting oxygenated blood
  - foramen ovale: connection between right and left atria
  - ductus venosus: connection between umbilical vein and inferior vena cava

At Birth
- with first breath, lungs open up → pulmonary resistance decreases → pulmonic blood flow increases
- separation of low resistance placenta → systemic circulation becomes a high resistance system → ductus venosus closure
- increased pulmonic flow → increased left atrial pressures → foramen ovale closure
- increased oxygen concentration in blood after first breath → decreased prostaglandins → ductus arteriosus closure
- closure of fetal shunts and changes in vascular resistance → infant circulation assumes normal adult flow

Epidemiology
- 8/1,000 live births have CHD, which may present as a heart murmur, heart failure, or cyanosis; VSD is the most common lesion

Investigations
- Echo, ECG, CXR
- pre and postductal oxygen saturations, 4 limb BPs, hyperoxia test

CYANOTIC VS. ACYANOTIC CONGENITAL HEART DISEASE
- cyanosis: blue mucous membranes, nail beds, and skin secondary to an absolute concentration of deoxygenated hemoglobin of at least 30 g/dL
- acyanotic heart disease (i.e. L to R shunt, obstruction occurring beyond lungs): blood passes through pulmonic circulation → oxygenation takes place → low levels of deoxygenated blood in systemic circulation → no cyanosis
- cyanotic heart disease (i.e. R to L shunt): blood bypasses the lungs → no oxygenation occurs → high levels of deoxygenated hemoglobin enters the systemic circulation → cyanosis

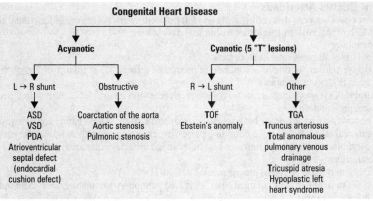

Figure 2. Common congenital heart diseases

Characteristic CXR Findings in CHD
- Boot-shaped heart: tetralogy of Fallot, tricuspid atresia
- Egg-shaped heart: transposition of great arteries
- "Snowman" heart: total anomalous pulmonary venous return

Acyanotic Congenital Heart Disease

1. LEFT-TO-RIGHT SHUNT LESIONS
- extra blood is displaced through a communication from the left to the right side of the heart → increased pulmonary blood flow → increased pulmonary pressures
- shunt volume is dependent upon three factors: (1) size of defect, (2) pressure gradient between chambers or vessels, and (3) peripheral outflow resistance
- untreated shunts can result in pulmonary vascular disease, left ventricular dilatation and dysfunction, right ventricular HTN and RVH, and ultimately R to L shunts

Atrial Septal Defect
- 3 types: *ostium primum* (common in DS), *ostium secundum* (most common type, 50-70%), *sinus venosus* (defect located at entry of superior vena cava into right atrium)
- epidemiology: 6-8% of congenital heart lesions
- natural history
  - 80-100% spontaneous closure rate if ASD diameter <8 mm
  - if remains patent, CHF and pulmonary HTN can develop in adult life
- clinical presentation
  - history: often asymptomatic in childhood
  - physical exam: grade 2-3/6 pulmonic outflow murmur, widely split and fixed S2
  - children with large ASDs may have signs of heart failure (tachypnea, FTT, hepatomegaly, pulmonary rales/retractions)
- investigations
  - ECG: RAD, mild RVH, RBBB
  - CXR: increased pulmonary vasculature, cardiac enlargement
  - Echo: test of choice
- management: elective surgical or catheter closure between 2-5 yr of age

Ventricular Septal Defect
- most common congenital heart defect (30-50%)
- small VSD (majority)
  - clinical presentation
    - history: asymptomatic, normal growth and development
    - physical exam: early systolic to holosystolic murmur, best heard at LLSB, thrill
  - investigations: ECG and CXR are normal; Echo to confirm diagnosis
  - management: most close spontaneously
- moderate-to-large VSD
  - epidemiology: CHF by 2 mo; late secondary pulmonary HTN if left untreated
  - clinical presentation
    - history: delayed growth, decreased exercise tolerance, recurrent URTIs or "asthma" episodes
    - physical exam: holosystolic murmur at LLSB, mid-diastolic rumble at apex, size of VSD is inversely related to intensity of murmur
  - investigations
    - ECG: LVH, LAH, RVH
    - CXR: increased pulmonary vasculature, cardiomegaly, CHF
    - Echo: diagnostic
  - management: treatment of CHF and surgical closure by 1 yr old

Moderate-to-Large VSD
Size of VSD is inversely related to intensity of murmur

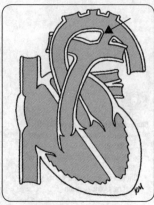

Figure 3. Patent duct arteriosus

Physical Exam for PDA
(in term infant)
- Heavy "machinery" murmur
- High pulse rate
- Wide pulse pressure
- Hyperactive precordium
- Big bounding pulse

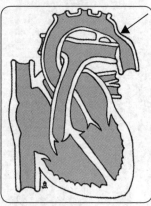

Figure 4. Coarctation of the aorta

Patent Ductus Arteriosus

- patent vessel between descending aorta and left pulmonary artery (normally, functional closure within first 15 h of life, anatomical closure within first days of life)
- epidemiology
  - 5-10% of all congenital heart defects
  - delayed closure of ductus is common in premature infants (1/3 of infants <1,750 g); this is different from PDA in term infants
- natural history: spontaneous closure common in premature infants, less common in term infants
- clinical presentation
  - history: asymptomatic, or have apneic or bradycardic spells, poor feeding, accessory muscle use, CHF
  - physical exam: tachycardia, bounding pulses, hyperactive precordium, wide pulse pressure, continuous "machinery" murmur best heard at left infraclavicular area
- investigations
  - ECG: may show left atrial enlargement, LVH, RVH
  - CXR: normal to mildly enlarged heart, increased pulmonary vasculature, prominent pulmonary artery
  - Echo: diagnostic
- management
  - indomethacin (Indocid®): antagonizes prostaglandin E2, which maintains ductus arteriosus patency; only effective in premature infants
  - catheter or surgical closure if PDA causes respiratory compromise, FTT, or persists beyond 3rd mo of life

2. OBSTRUCTIVE LESIONS

- present with decreased urine output, pallor, cool extremities and poor pulses, shock, or sudden collapse

Coarctation of the Aorta

- definition: narrowing of aorta (almost always at the level of the ductus arteriosus)
- epidemiology: commonly associated with bicuspid aortic valve (50%); Turner syndrome (35%)
- clinical presentation
  - history: often asymptomatic
  - physical exam
    - blood pressure discrepancy between upper and lower extremities (increased suspicion/severity if >20 mmHg difference)
    - diminished or delayed femoral pulses relative to brachial (i.e. brachial-femoral delay)
    - possible systolic murmur with late peak at apex, left axilla, and left back
    - if severe, presents with shock in the neonatal period when the ductus arteriosis closes
- investigations: ECG shows RVH early in infancy, LVH later in childhood; Echo or MRI for diagnosis
- prognosis: can be complicated by HTN; if associated with other lesions (e.g. PDA, VSD) can lead to CHF
- management: give prostaglandins to keep ductus arteriosus patent for stabilization and perform surgical correction in neonates; for older infants and children balloon arterioplasty may be an alternative to surgical correction

Aortic Stenosis

- 4 types: valvular (75%), subvalvular (20%), supravalvular, and idiopathic hypertrophic subaortic stenosis (5%)
- clinical presentation
  - history: often asymptomatic, but may be associated with CHF, exertional chest pain, syncope, or sudden death
  - physical exam: SEM at RUSB with aortic ejection click at the apex (only for valvular stenosis)
- investigations: Echo for diagnosis
- management: valvular stenosis is usually treated with balloon valvuloplasty, patients with subvalvular or supravalvular stenosis require surgical repair, exercise restriction required

Pulmonary Stenosis

- 3 types: valvular (90%), subvalvular, or supravalvular
- definition of critical pulmonary stenosis: inadequate pulmonary blood flow, dependent on ductus for oxygenation, progressive hypoxia and cyanosis
- natural history: may be part of other congenital heart lesions (e.g. Tetralogy of Fallot) or in association with syndromes (e.g. congenital rubella, Noonan syndrome)
- clinical presentation
  - history: spectrum from asymptomatic to CHF
  - physical exam: wide split S2 on expiration, SEM at LUSB, pulmonary ejection click (for valvular lesions)
- investigations
  - ECG: RVH
  - CXR: post-stenotic dilation of the main pulmonary artery
  - Echo: diagnostic
- management: surgical repair if critically ill or if symptomatic in older infants/children

Cyanotic Congenital Heart Disease

- systemic venous return re-enters systemic circulation directly
- most prominent feature is cyanosis (O_2 sat <75%)
- hyperoxic test differentiates between cardiac and other causes of cyanosis
  - obtain preductal, right radial ABG in room air, then repeat after the child inspires 100% O_2
  - if PaO_2 improves to greater than 150 mmHg, cyanosis less likely cardiac in origin
- pre-ductal and post-ductal pulse oximetry
  - >5% difference suggests R to L shunt

1. RIGHT-TO-LEFT SHUNT LESIONS

Tetralogy of Fallot
- epidemiology: 10% of all CHD, most common cyanotic heart defect diagnosed beyond infancy with peak incidence at 2-4 mo of age
- pathophysiology
  - embryological defect due to anterior and superior deviation of the outlet septum leading to: VSD, RVOTO (i.e. pulmonary stenosis ± subpulmonary valve stenosis), over-riding aorta, and RVH
    - infants may initially have a L → R shunt (therefore no cyanosis); however, RVOTO is progressive, leading to increasing R → L shunting with hypoxemia and cyanosis
    - degree of RVOTO determines the direction and degree of shunt and, therefore, the extent of clinical cyanosis and degree of RVH
- clinical presentation
  - history: hypoxic "tet" spells
    - during exertional states (crying, exercise) the increasing pulmonary vascular resistance and decrease in systemic resistance causes an increase in right-to-left shunting
    - clinical features include paroxysms of rapid and deep breathing, irritability and crying, increasing cyanosis, decreased intensity of murmur (decreased flow across RVOTO)
    - if severe, can lead to decreased level of consciousness, seizures, death
  - physical exam
    - single loud S2 due to severe pulmonary stenosis (i.e. RVOTO), SEM at LSB
- investigations
  - ECG: RAD, RVH
  - CXR: boot-shaped heart, decreased pulmonary vasculature, right aortic arch (in 20%)
  - Echo: diagnostic
- management of spells: O_2, knee-chest position, fluid bolus, morphine sulfate, propranolol
- treatment: surgical repair at 4-6 mo of age; earlier if marked cyanosis or "tet" spells

2. OTHER CYANOTIC CONGENITAL HEART DISEASES

Transposition of the Great Arteries (TGA)
- epidemiology: 3-5% of all congenital cardiac lesions, most common cyanotic CHD in neonates
- pathophysiology: parallel pulmonary and systemic circulations
  - systemic: body → RA → RV → aorta → body
  - pulmonary: lungs → LA → LV → pulmonary artery → lungs
  - survival is dependent on mixing through PDA, ASD, or VSD
- physical exam
  - neonates: ductus arteriosus closure causes rapidly progressive severe hypoxemia unresponsive to oxygen therapy, acidosis, and death
  - VSD present: cyanosis is not prominent; CHF within first weeks of life
  - VSD absent: no murmur
- investigations
  - ECG: RAD, RVH, or may be normal
  - CXR: egg-shaped heart with narrow mediastinum ("egg on a string")
  - Echo: diagnostic
- management
  - symptomatic neonates: prostaglandin E1 infusion to keep ductus open until balloon atrial septostomy
  - surgical repair: arterial switch performed in the first two weeks in those without a VSD while LV muscle is still strong

Total Anomalous Pulmonary Venous Return
- epidemiology: 1-2% of CHD
- pathophysiology
  - all pulmonary veins drain into right-sided circulation (systemic veins, RA)
  - no direct oxygenated pulmonary venous return to left atrium
  - often associated with obstruction at connection sites
  - ASD must be present for oxygenated blood to shunt into the LA and systemic circulation
- management: surgical repair in all cases and required urgently for severe cyanosis

Causes of Cyanotic Heart Disease – 5T's
Truncus arteriosus
Transposition of the great vessels
Tricuspid atresia
Tetralogy of Fallot
Total anomalous pulmonary venous return

Tetralogy of Fallot
1. VSD
2. RVOTO
3. Aortic root "overriding" VSD
4. RVH

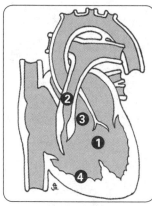

Figure 5. Tetralogy of Fallot

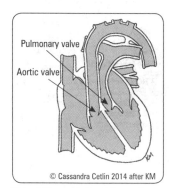

© Cassandra Cetlin 2014 after KM

Figure 6. Transportation of the great arteries

Ebstein's Anomaly
- Septal and posterior leaflets of tricuspid valve are malformed and displaced into the RV
- Potential for RV dysfunction, tricuspid stenosis, tricuspid regurgitation, or functional pulmonary atresia if RV unable to open pulmonic valves
- Accessory conduction pathways (e.g. WPW) are often present

Etiology
- Unknown, associated with maternal lithium and benzodiazepine use in 1st trimester

Treatment
- Newborns: consider closure of tricuspid valve + aortopulmonary shunt, or transplantation
- Older children: tricuspid valve repair or valve replacement + ASD closure

Truncus Arteriosus
- pathophysiology
  - single great vessel gives rise to the aorta, pulmonary, and coronary arteries
  - truncal valve overlies a large VSD
  - potential for coronary ischemia with fall in pulmonary vascular resistance
- management: surgical repair within first 6 wk of life

Hypoplastic Left Heart Syndrome
- epidemiology: 1-3% of CHD; most common cause of death from CHD in first month of life
- pathophysiology: LV hypoplasia may include atretic or stenotic mitral and/or aortic valve, small ascending aorta, and coarctation of the aorta with resultant systemic hypoperfusion
- systemic circulation is dependent on ductus patency; upon closure of the ductus, infant presents with circulatory shock and metabolic acidosis
- management
  - intubate and correct metabolic acidosis
  - IV infusion of prostaglandin E1 to keep ductus open
  - surgical palliation (overall survival 50% to late childhood) or heart transplant

4 Features of Hypoplastic Left Heart Syndrome
- Hypoplastic LV
- Narrow mitral/aortic valves
- Small ascending aorta
- Coarctation of the aorta

Congestive Heart Failure

- see <u>Cardiology and Cardiac Surgery</u>, C34

Etiology
- CHD
- cardiomyopathy (primary or secondary)
- high output circulatory states (e.g. anemia, AVMs, cor pulmonale, hyperthyroidism)
- non-cardiac (e.g. sepsis, renal failure)
- pressure overload (e.g. aortic stenosis/co-arctation, pulmonary stenosis, HTN)
- volume overload (e.g. L to R shunt, valve insufficiency)

History
- infant: weak cry, irritability, feeding difficulties, early fatigability, diaphoresis while sleeping or eating, respiratory distress, lethargy, FTT
- child: decreased exercise tolerance, fatigue, decreased appetite, respiratory distress, frequent URTIs or "asthma" episodes
- orthopnea, paroxysmal nocturnal dyspnea, pedal/dependent edema are all uncommon in children

Physical Findings
- 4 key features: tachycardia, tachypnea, cardiomegaly, hepatomegaly
- FTT
- alterations in peripheral pulses, four limb blood pressures (in some CHDs)
- dysmorphic features associated with congenital syndromes

4 Key Features of CHF

2 Tachy's and 2 Megaly's
- Tachycardia
- Tachypnea
- Cardiomegaly
- Hepatomegaly

Investigations
- CXR: cardiomegaly, pulmonary venous congestion
- ECG: sinus tachycardia, signs of underlying cause (heart block, atrial enlargement, hypertrophy, ischemia/infarct)
- Echo: structural and functional assessment
- blood work: CBC, electrolytes, BUN, Cr, LFTs

Management
- general: sitting up, O₂, sodium and water restriction, increased caloric intake
- pharmacologic: diuretics, afterload reduction (e.g. ACEI), β-blockers; digoxin rarely used
- curative: correction of underlying cause

Dysrhythmias

- see <u>Cardiology and Cardiac Surgery</u>, C16
- can be transient or permanent, congenital (structurally normal or abnormal), or acquired (toxin, infection, infarction)

Sinus Arrhythmia
- phasic variations with respiration (present in almost all normal children)

Sinus Tachycardia
- rate of impulses arising from sinus node is elevated (>150 bpm in infants, >100 bpm in older children)
- characterized by: beat-to-beat heart rate variability with changes in activity, P waves present/normal, PR constant, QRS narrow
- etiology: HTN, fever, anxiety, sepsis, anemia/hypoxia, PE, drugs, etc.
- differentiate from SVT (see below) by slowing the sinus rate (vagal massage, β-blockers) to identify sinus P waves

Pediatric vs. Adult ECG
Pediatric ECG findings that may be normal:
- HR >100 bpm
- Shorter PR and QT intervals and QRS duration
- Inferior and lateral small Q waves
- RV larger than LV in neonates, so normal to have:
  - RAD
  - Large precordial R waves
  - Upright T waves
  - Inverted T waves in the anterior precordial leads from early infancy to teen years

Premature Atrial Contractions
• may be normal variant or can be caused by electrolyte disturbances, hyperthyroidism, cardiac surgery, digitalis toxicity

Premature Ventricular Contractions
• common in adolescents
• benign if single, uniform, disappear with exercise, and no associated structural lesions
• if not benign, may degenerate into more severe dysrhythmias

Supraventricular Tachycardia
• abnormally rapid heart rhythm originating above the ventricles – most frequent sustained dysrhythmia in children
• no beat-to-beat HR variability, >220 bpm (infants) or >180 bpm (children), P waves absent/abnormal, PR indeterminable, QRS usually narrow
• pre-excitation syndromes (subset of SVT): WPW syndrome, congenital defect (see Cardiology and Cardiac Surgery, C21)

Complete Heart Block
• congenital heart block can be caused by maternal anti-Ro or anti-La (e.g. mother with SLE)
• often diagnosed in utero (may lead to development of fetal hydrops)
• clinical symptoms related to level of block (the lower the block, the slower the heart rate and greater the symptoms of inadequate cardiac output)
• symptomatic patients need a pacemaker

Heart Murmurs

• 50-80% of children have audible heart murmurs at some point in their childhood
• most childhood murmurs are functional (e.g. "innocent") without associated structural abnormalities and have normal ECG and radiologic findings
• in general, murmurs can become audible or accentuated in high output states (e.g. fever, anemia)

Table 11. Differentiating Heart Murmurs

	Innocent	Pathological
History and Physical	Asymptomatic	Symptoms and signs of cardiac disease (FTT, exercise intolerance)
Timing	SEM	All diastolic, pansystolic, or continuous (except venous hum)
Grade/Quality	<3/6; soft/blowing/vibratory	≥3/6 (palpable thrill); harsh
Splitting	Physiologic S2	May have fixed split or single S2
Extra Sounds/Clicks	None	May be present
Change of Position	Murmur varies	Unchanged

Table 12. Five Innocent Heart Murmurs

Type	Etiology	Location	Description	Age	Differential Diagnosis
Peripheral Pulmonic Stenosis	Flow into pulmonary branch arteries from main, larger, artery	Left upper sternal border	Neonates, low-pitched, radiates to axilla and back	Neonates, usually disappears by 3-6 mo	PDA Pulmonary stenosis
Still's Murmur	Flow across the pulmonic valve leaflets	Left lower sternal border	High-pitched, vibratory, LLSB or apex, SEM	3-6 yr	Subaortic stenosis Small VSD
Venous Hum	Altered flow in veins	Infraclavicular (R>L)	Infraclavicular hum, continuous, R>L	3-6 yr	PDA
Pulmonary Ejection	Flow through the pulmonic valve	Left upper sternal border	Soft, blowing, LUSB, SEM	8-14 yr	ASD Pulmonary stenosis
Supraclavicular Arterial Bruit	Turbulent flow in the carotid arteries	Supraclavicular	Low intensity, above clavicles	Any age	Aortic stenosis Bicuspid aortic valve

Infective Endocarditis

• see Infectious Diseases, ID16

Development

Approach to Global Developmental Delay

- also known as Early Developmental Impairment

Definition
- performance significantly below average in two or more domains of development (gross motor, fine motor, speech/language, cognitive, social/personal, activities of daily living) in a child <5 yr of age
- predict a diagnosis of intellectual disability in the future

Epidemiology
- 5-10% of children have neurodevelopmental delay
- careful evaluation can reveal a cause in 50-70% of cases

Etiology
- CNS abnormalities (meningitis/encephalitis, brain malformation, trauma, etc.)
- sensory deficits (hearing, vision)
- environmental (psychosocial neglect, lead exposure, antenatal drug or alcohol exposure, etc.)
- genetic/chromosomal disorders (DS, Fragile X, etc.)
- metabolic disorders (inborn errors of metabolism, hypothyroidism, iron deficiency, etc.)
- obstetrical (prematurity, HIE, TORCH infections, etc.)
- sleep disorders
- seizures

Clinical Presentation
- history
    - intrauterine exposures, perinatal events
    - detailed developmental milestones: rate of acquisition, regression of skills
    - associated problems: feeding, seizures, behaviour, sleep
    - family history, consanguinity
    - social history
- physical exam
    - dysmorphic features, hepatosplenomegaly, neurocutaneous markers, growth parameters, detailed neurological examination
- investigations (guided by history and physical examination)
    - neurodevelopmental assessment, neuroimaging, vision and hearing test, EEG, sleep study
    - OT, PT, and/or SLP assessments
    - psychosocial evaluation
    - blood work (lead, CBC, ferritin, TSH)
    - genetics consultation (microarray, Fragile X testing, testing for inborn errors of metabolism)

Management
- dependent on specific area of delay
- therapy services (e.g. speech and language therapy for language delay, OT and/or PT for motor delay), early intervention services (e.g. infant development services, Ontario Early Years Centres)

Intellectual Disability

Definition
- state of functioning that begins in childhood and is characterized by limitations in both intelligence and adaptive skills
- historically defined as an IQ <70
- often preceded by diagnosis of global developmental delay

Epidemiology
- 1% of general population; M:F = 1.5:1

Clinical Presentation
- history
    - well below average general intellectual functioning
    - significant deficits in adaptive functioning in at least 2 of: communication, self-care, home-living, social skills, self-direction, academic skills, work, leisure, health, safety
- physical exam
    - check growth, dysmorphic features, complete physical exam
- investigations
    - standardized psychology assessment (includes IQ test and measure of adaptive functioning)
    - vision, hearing, and neurologic assessment
    - genetic and metabolic testing as indicated

Classification of Intellectual Disability

Severity	% Cases	IQ
Mild	85	50-70
Moderate	10	35-49
Severe	3-4	20-34
Profound	1-2	<20

Management
- main objective: enhance adaptive functioning level
- requires an interprofessional team with strong case coordination
- emphasize community-based treatment and early intervention
- individual/family therapy, behaviour management services, therapy services (e.g. OT, SLP), medications for associated conditions
- education: life skills, vocational training, communication skills, family education
- psychosocial support for individual and family; respite care

Prognosis
- higher rates of sensory deficits, motor impairment, behavioural/emotional disorders, seizures, psychiatric illness

Language Delay

Definition
- no universally accepted definition, but often identified around 18 mo of age with enhanced well baby visit
- if formally tested, performance on a standardized assessment of language is at least one standard deviation below mean of age
- can be expressive (ability to produce or use language), receptive (ability to understand language), or both

Epidemiology
- M>F
- ~10-15% of 2 yr old children have a language delay, but only 4-5% remain delayed after 3 yr of age
- ~6-8% of school-aged children have specific language impairment (many of whom were not identified before school entry)

Etiology
- cognitive disability
- constitutional language delay
- genetic/metabolic: DS, Fragile X syndrome, Williams syndrome, hypothyroidism, PKU, etc.
- hearing impairment
- mechanical problems: cleft palate, cranial nerve palsy
- medical condition: seizure disorder (includes acquired epileptic aphasia), CP, TORCH infection, iron deficiency, lead poisoning, etc.
- autism spectrum disorder
- psychosocial: neglect or abuse
- selective mutism

Risk Factors for Sensorineural Hearing Loss
- Genetic syndromes/family history
- Congenital (TORCH) infections
- Craniofacial abnormalties
- <1,500 g birthweight
- Hyperbilirubinemia/kernicterus
- Asphyxia/low APGAR scores
- Bacterial meningitis, viral encephalitis

Clinical Presentation
- history
  - concerns about hearing, delay in language development or regression in previously normal language development
  - delayed language milestones, presence of red flags, regression
  - must determine if language delay is expressive, receptive, or mixed
  - risk factors for hearing loss (hereditary, recurrent AOM) and language delay
- physical exam
  - guided by history: look for abnormal growth, dysmorphisms, unusual social interactions (lack of eye contact, not pointing)
  - include full exam of the external/internal ear (e.g. TM scarring), oral pharynx (e.g. cleft palate), and neurologic system (including tone)
- investigations
  - use of language specific screens in primary care setting: The Early Language Milestone, CAT/CLAMS, MCHAT, etc.
  - all children with suspected language delay MUST be referred to an audiologist for a hearing assessment
  - CBC (to rule out anemia), venous blood lead levels, genetic/metabolic workup as indicated

Bilingual exposure generally does NOT explain a frank delay in language development

Management
- specific to etiology
- often multidisciplinary and requires appropriate referrals: early intervention services, special education services, SLP, OHNS and dental professionals, general support services
- prevention: parents can read aloud to their child, engage in dialogic reading, avoid baby talk, narrate daily activities, etc.

Primary care physicians should suspect a receptive language delay in any young child with an expressive language delay

Prognosis
- depends on etiology
- if language delay persists beyond 5 yr old, more likely to have difficulties in adulthood
- persistent language delay is associated with poor academic performance, behavioural problems, social isolation

Specific Learning Disorder

Definition
- specific and persistent failure to acquire academic skills despite conventional instruction, adequate intelligence, and sociocultural opportunity
- a significant discrepancy between a child's intellectual ability and their academic performance
- types: reading (dyslexia), writing, mathematics (dyscalculia)

Epidemiology
- prevalence: 10%
- high incidence of psychiatric comorbidity: anxiety, dysthymia, conduct disorder, major depressive disorder, oppositional defiant disorder, ADHD

Etiology
- pathogenesis is unknown, likely genetic factors involved
- learning disabilities may be associated with a number of conditions:
  - genetic/metabolic: Turner syndrome, Klinefelter syndrome
  - perinatal: prematurity, low birth weight, birth trauma/hypoxia
  - postnatal: CNS damage, hypoxia, environmental toxins, FAS, psychosocial deprivation (understimulation), malnutrition
- poor visual acuity is NOT a cause

Risk Factors
- positive family history, prematurity, other developmental and mental health conditions, neurologic disorders (e.g. seizure disorders, neurofibromatosis), history of CNS infection/irradiation/traumatic injury

Clinical Presentation
- history and physical exam
  - school difficulties (academic achievement, behaviour, attention, social interaction)
  - development of negative self-concept → reluctance to participate even in areas of strength
  - social issues: overt hostility towards parents/teachers; difficulties making friends, bullying, and anxiety
  - look for dysmorphisms, complete physical exam
- investigations
  - standardized tests for IQ
  - individual scores on achievement tests in reading, mathematics, or written expression (WISC III, WRAT) >2 SD below that expected for age, education, and IQ

Management
- provide quality instruction for specific learning disability
- support student by modifying the curriculum and/or providing accommodations (e.g. scribe for writing, extra time for tests, photocopied notes, etc.)
- consider grade retention in certain students (no guidelines exist, very rare in Ontario)
- specialized education placements that can provide educational remediation

Prognosis
- limited information available about persistence of learning disabilities over time
- low self-esteem, poor social skills, 40% school drop-out rate

Fetal Alcohol Spectrum Disorder

Definition
- term describing the range of effects of prenatal exposure to alcohol, including physical, mental, behavioural, and learning disabilities
- no "safe" level of alcohol consumption during pregnancy has been established
- spectrum includes: FAS, partial FAS, ARBD, and ARND

Epidemiology
- prevalence of FAS and FASD is 0.1% and 1.0%, respectively
- most common preventable cause of intellectual disability

Pathogenesis
- specific mechanism of FASD is unknown, but hypotheses include nutritional deficits, toxic effects of acetaldehyde, alteration of placental transport, abnormal protein synthesis, and altered cerebral neurotransmission

Diagnosis

- often misdiagnosed or missed entirely
- diagnosis of FAS, ARBD, and ARND all require evidence of maternal drinking during pregnancy
- criteria for diagnosis of FAS
    - growth deficiency: low birth weight and/or decelerating weight over time not due to nutrition
    - characteristic pattern of facial anomalies: short palpebral fissures, flattened philtrum, thin upper lip, flat midface
    - CNS dysfunction: microcephaly and/or neurobehavioural dysfunction (hyperactivity, fine motor problems, attention deficits, learning disabilities, cognitive disabilities, difficulties in adaptive functioning, etc.)
- criteria for diagnosis of ARBD
    - congenital anomalies, including malformations and dysplasias of the cardiac, skeletal, renal, ocular, and auditory systems
- criteria for diagnosis of ARND
    - CNS dysfunction (similar to FAS)
    - complex pattern of behavioural or cognitive abnormalities inconsistent with developmental level that cannot be explained by familial background or environment alone

Management

- early diagnosis is essential to prevent secondary disabilities
- no cure, but individuals with FASD and their families should be linked to community resources and services to improve outcome

Prognosis

- secondary disabilities include unemployment, mental health problems, difficulties with the law, inappropriate sexual behaviour, disrupted school experience, peer problems

Attention Deficit Hyperactivity Disorder

- see Psychiatry, *Neurodevelopmental Disorders*, PS37

Autism Spectrum Disorder

- see Psychiatry, *Neurodevelopmental Disorders*, PS37

Motor Delay

- see *Cerebral Palsy*, P83 and *Muscular Dystrophy*, P43

Endocrinology

Antidiuretic Hormone

Diabetes Insipidus

- see Endocrinology, E18 and Nephrology, NP11

Syndrome of Inappropriate Antidiuretic Hormone

- see Endocrinology, E18 and Nephrology, NP10

Diabetes Mellitus

DIABETES MELLITUS TYPE 1

- see Endocrinology, *Disorders of Glucose Regulation*, E6

Epidemiology

- most common form of DM in children, M=F
- variable prevalence internationally, affects ~1:4,000 children in Canada
- can present at any age, but bimodal peaks at 5-7 yr old and at puberty

Clinical Presentation

- can present as polyuria (often manifested as nocturia or secondary enuresis), polydipsia, weight loss (lack of insulin leading to a catabolic state), polyphagia, DKA (~20%) (see Endocrinology, E11)

Management

- patients and families are best managed with a family-centred pediatric multidisciplinary team able to provide education, ongoing care, and psychosocial support surrounding survival skills, meal plans, and insulin injections as a cornerstone of treatment
- blood glucose monitoring is especially important in children as they are more susceptible to hypoglycemia
- if DKA present: ABCs, admit, monitors, correct fluid losses, administer insulin and restore glucose gradually, correct electrolyte disturbances, identify/treat precipitating event, avoid complications (i.e. cerebral edema)
  - low threshold to investigate (CT/MRI) and treat DKA, as cerebral edema is a major concern
  - see Endocrinology, E11
- screen for micro- and macrovascular complications (regular ophthalmology assessments, BP, microalbuminuria), concurrent autoimmune diseases (thyroiditis, celiac disease, etc.), and mental health issues (depression, eating disorders)

Prognosis

- no cure currently
- short-term complications
  - hypoglycemia
  - due to missed/delayed meals, excess insulin or exercise, illness
  - can lead to seizures and/or coma
  - reversed with PO/IV glucose or IM glucagon
  - hyperglycemia
  - due to intercurrent illness, diet-to-insulin mismatch
  - risk of end-organ damage
  - DKA: due to missed insulin doses, infection; most common cause of death
- long-term complications
  - microvascular: retinopathy, nephropathy, neuropathy
  - macrovascular: metabolic syndrome, CVD, CAD, PVD
  - increased risk of other autoimmune diseases

DIABETES MELLITUS TYPE 2

- see Family Medicine, FM21, Endocrinology, E7
- impaired glucose metabolism due to increased peripheral insulin resistance
- rare before 10 yr of age, but more common in older children/adolescents
- prevalence is rising mainly due to the increased incidence of childhood obesity
- risk factors: obesity, positive family history, female gender, certain ethnic groups
- clinical presentation may be similar to that of type 1 DM, though most children are asymptomatic
- may present in DKA or hyperglycemic hyperosmotic nonketotic state
- management
  - initiate lifestyle modification program, including diet, weight loss, physical activity (moderate-to-vigorous activity for at least 60 min/d; screen time less than 2 h/d)
  - glycemic target: HbA1c ≤7%
  - if glycemic targets not achieved within 3-6 mo from diagnosis with lifestyle intervention alone, either metformin, glimepiride, or insulin should be initiated
  - monitor HbA1c every 3 mo
  - advise patient to monitor finger-stick blood glucose levels if on medication with risk of hypoglycemia, are changing medication regimen, have not met treatment goals, or have intercurrent illness
- prognosis: includes microvascular and macrovascular complications similar to type 1 DM

Growth

APPROACH TO SHORT STATURE

Definition

- short stature: height <3rd percentile
- poor growth evidenced by growth deceleration (height crosses major percentile lines, growth velocity <25th percentile)

Epidemiology

- ~2.5% of the population by definition

Etiology

- see sidebar

Blood Glucose Targets by Age

Age range	Pre-meal blood glucose target	HbA1c target
<6	6-10	<8%
6-12	6-10	<7.5%
>12	4-7	<7%

Management of Newly Diagnosed Type 2 DM in Children and Adolescents
Pediatrics 2013;131(2):364-82
Key Action Statements
1. Clinicians should ensure that insulin therapy is initiated for children and adolescents with type 2 DM who are ketotic or in DKA and in whom the distinction between types 1 and 2 DM is unclear and, in usual cases, should initiate insulin therapy for patients
    a. who have random venous or plasma BG concentrations 14 mmol/L; or
    b. whose HbA1c is >9%.
2. Clinicians should initiate a lifestyle modification program, including nutrition and physical activity, and start metformin as first-line therapy for children and adolescents at the time of diagnosis of type 2 DM.
3. The committee suggests that clinicians monitor HbA1c concentrations every 3 mo and intensify treatment if treatment goals for finger-stick BG and HbA1c concentrations are not being met.
4. Clinicians should advise patients to monitor finger-stick BG concentrations in patients who
    a. are taking insulin or other medications with a risk of hypoglycemia; or
    b. are initiating or changing their diabetes treatment regimen; or
    c. have not met treatment goals; or
    d. have intercurrent illnesses.
5. Clinicians should incorporate the Academy of Nutrition and Dietetics' Pediatric Weight Management Evidence-Based Nutrition Practice Guidelines in their dietary or nutrition counselling of patients with type 2 DM at the time of diagnosis and as part of ongoing management.
6. Clinicians should encourage children and adolescents with type 2 DM to engage in moderate-to-vigorous exercise for at least 60 min daily and to limit nonacademic "screen time" to less than 2 h/d.

Clinical Presentation

- history and physical exam
  - plot on growth curve (special growth charts available for Turner syndrome, achondroplasia, DS)
  - assess for dysmorphic features, disproportionate short stature
  - risk factors for GH deficiency: previous head trauma, history of intracranial bleed or infection, head surgery or irradiation, positive family history, breech delivery
  - decreased growth velocity may be more worrisome than actual height
- investigations
  - calculate mid-parental height: children are usually in a percentile between their parents' height
  - AP x-ray of left hand and wrist for bone age
  - remaining investigations guided by history and physical (e.g. TSH, sweat chloride, etc.)

Short Stature DDx

ABCDEFG
Alone (neglected infant)
Bone dysplasias (rickets, scoliosis, mucopolysaccharidoses)
Chromosomal (Turner, Down)
Delayed growth (constitutional)
Endocrine (low GH, Cushing, hypothyroid)
Familial
GI malabsorption (celiac, Crohn's)

Management

- depends on severity of problem as perceived by parents/child
- no treatment for non-pathological short stature, except for idiopathic short stature
- GH therapy: if administered at an early age, can help patients achieve adult height
- requirements
  - GH shown to be deficient by 2 different stimulation tests
  - growth velocity <3rd percentile or height <<3rd percentile
  - bone age x-rays show unfused epiphyses/delayed bone age
- support and management of resultant self-image issues, social anxiety, etc.

4 Questions to Ask when Evaluating Short Stature
- Was there IUGR?
- Is the growth proportionate?
- Is the growth velocity normal?
- Is bone age delayed?

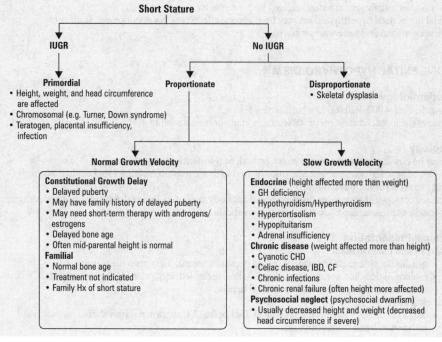

Figure 7. Approach to the child with short stature

To check for proportionality, measure upper to lower segment ratio (U/L) using the pubic symphysis as your landmark. Normals are 1.7 for newborn, 1.4 for young child, 0.9 for adult male, 1.0 for adult female

TALL STATURE

- height greater than two SD above the mean for a given age, sex, and race

Etiology

- constitutional/familial
- endocrine: Beckwith-Wiedemann syndrome, hyperthyroidism, hypophyseal gigantism, precocious puberty
- genetic: homocystinuria, Klinefelter syndrome, Marfan syndrome, Sotos syndrome

Hypercalcemia/Hypocalcemia/Rickets

- see Endocrinology, E37

Hyperthyroidism and Hypothyroidism

- may be congenital or acquired (for acquired causes, see Endocrinology, E22)

CONGENITAL HYPERTHYROIDISM

- also known as neonatal Graves' disease

Epidemiology
- ~1:25,000 neonates, M=F

Etiology
- results from transplacental passage of maternal thyroid stimulating antibodies from mother with a history of Graves' disease

Clinical Presentation
- history and physical exam
    - clinical manifestations may be masked if mother on antithyroid treatment
    - may present with tachycardia with CHF, heart murmur, goitre, craniosynostosis, irritability, poor feeding, FTT
- investigations:
    - serum levels of TSH and free T4 in all infants with suspected congenital hyperthyroidism or infants born to mothers with Graves' disease

Management
- methimazole until antibodies cleared
- symptomatic treatment as needed (e.g. β-blockers to control tachycardia)

Prognosis
- if prompt and adequate treatment given, most neonates improve rapidly
- antibodies usually spontaneously cleared by 2-3 mo of life
- fetal or neonatal hyperthyroidism may have adverse effects on CNS development, leading to developmental and behaviour problems

CONGENITAL HYPOTHYROIDISM

Epidemiology
- incidence: 1:4,000-1:20,000 newborn births; F:M = 2:1
- one of the most common preventable causes of intellectual disability

Etiology
- may be classified as permanent primary, central, or transient hypothyroidism
- ~85% of primary cases are sporadic (mostly thyroid dysgenesis), remaining 15% hereditary (mostly inborn errors of thyroid synthesis)
- causes of transient hypothyroidism: maternal antibody-mediated, iodine deficiency (rare in developed countries), prenatal exposure to antithyroid medications

Clinical Presentation
- history and physical exam
    - usually asymptomatic in neonatal period because maternal T4 crosses the placenta
    - prolonged jaundice, constipation, sluggish, hoarse cry, lethargy, poor feeding, macroglossia, coarse facial features, large fontanelles, umbilical hernia
- investigations
    - diagnosis through newborn screening of TSH or free T4; abnormal results should be confirmed with serum levels from venipuncture

Management
- thyroxine replacement

Prognosis
- excellent outcome if treatment started within 1-2 mo of birth
- if treatment started after 3-6 mo of age, may result in permanent developmental delay and/or disability (mild to profound)

Sexual Development

AMBIGUOUS GENITALIA

Definition
- newborn or child whose gender is difficult to assign based on the appearance of genitalia
- subtype of DSD: a condition in which development of chromosomal, gonadal, or anatomic sex is atypical
- subtypes: 46,XX DSD, 46,XY DSD, ovotesticular DSD (true hermaphrodite)

Epidemiology
- incidence of genital abnormalities at birth is as high as 1:300
- prevalence of complex anomalies with true sexual ambiguity much lower at ~1:5,000

Etiology
- 46,XY DSD
  - inborn error of testosterone biosynthesis or Leydig cell hypoplasia
  - 5-α-reductase deficiency, androgen receptor deficiency or insensitivity
  - LH/hCG unresponsiveness
- 46,XX DSD
  - virilizing CAH (most common)
  - maternal source: virilizing ovarian or adrenal tumours, untreated maternal CAH, placental aromatase deficiency
- ovotesticular DSD
  - both ovarian follicles and seminiferous tubules in the same patient with a 46,XX karyotype
  - mixed gonadal dysgenesis

Risk Factors
- parental consanguinity, positive family history of ambiguous genitalia, early childhood illness/death, or primary amenorrhea, maternal medications during pregnancy (e.g. androgens, progesterones, danazol, phenytoin, aminoglutethimide, endocrine disruptors)

Clinical Presentation
- history
  - thorough obstetrical history, including prenatal screens and maternal medications
  - family history: autosomal recessive pattern may suggest CAH, X-linked recessive pattern may suggest androgen insensitivity syndrome
- physical exam
  - male pseudohermaphrodite (XY): small phallus, hypospadias, undescended testicles
  - female pseudohermaphrodite (XX): clitoral hypertrophy, labioscrotal fusion
  - look for concurrent midline defects, dysmorphic features, and congenital abnormalities
- investigations
  - karyotype and genetic workup as indicated
  - blood work: electrolytes and renin (evidence of salt-wasting in CAH); 17-OH-progesterone, androgens, FSH, and LH
  - imaging: abdominal U/S to look for uterus, testicles, ovaries

Management
- avoid announcement of probable sex or use of personal pronouns until all tests are complete
- continuous psychosocial support for parents and child during development
- elective surgical reconstruction of genitalia is sometimes possible

CONGENITAL ADRENAL HYPERPLASIA

Definition
- autosomal recessive disorder characterized by the partial or total defect of various synthetic enzymes of the adrenal cortex required for cortisol and aldosterone production

Epidemiology
- occurs in ~1:15,000 live births
- most common cause of ambiguous genitalia

Etiology
- for biosynthetic pathways of adrenal cortex, see Endocrinology, E29
- 21-OH responsible for ~95% of CAH cases
- results in ↓ cortisol and aldosterone production with shunting toward ↑↑ androgens
- cortisol deficiency leads to elevated ACTH, which causes adrenal hyperplasia
- rarer causes include deficiencies in 11-OH, cholesterol desmolase, 17-OH, and 3-HSD

Clinical Presentation
- depends on which enzyme in cortisol synthesis pathway is defective
- presentation of 21-OH deficiency can be divided into
  - classic deficiency with salt wasting: inadequate aldosterone resulting in FTT, hyperkalemia, hyponatremia, hypoglycemia, acidosis
  - classic deficiency without salt wasting: simple virilizing type
  - non-classic: signs/symptoms of androgen excess (e.g. amenorrhea, precocious puberty, etc.)
- 21-OH deficiency screening is part of many newborn screening programs across North America
- high serum levels of 17-OH progesterone in random blood sample diagnostic for 21-OH deficiency

Management
- correct any abnormalities in fluids, electrolytes, or serum glucose
- provide glucocorticoids/mineralocorticoids as necessary, extra glucocorticoids in times of stress
- psychosocial support

Prognosis
- complications if untreated include virilization, acne, salt wasting, hypotension

NORMAL PUBERTAL DEVELOPMENT

Physiology
- puberty occurs with the maturation of the HPG axis
- ↑ pulsatile release of GnRH → ↑ release of LH and FSH → maturation of gonads, release of sex steroids → secondary sexual characteristics
- adrenal production of androgens also required

Females
- onset: age 8-13 yr old (may start as early as 7 yr in girls of African descent)
- usual sequence
  1. thelarche: breast budding
  2. pubarche: axillary hair, body odour, mild acne
  3. growth spurt
  4. menarche: mean age 12.5 yr; indicates that growth spurt is almost complete; menses may be irregular in duration and length of cycle
- early puberty is common and often constitutional, late puberty is rare (rule out organic causes)

Males
- onset: age 9-14 yr old
- usual sequence
  1. testicular enlargement
  2. penile enlargement
  3. pubarche: axillary and facial hair, body odour, mild acne
  4. growth spurt: occurs later in boys
- early puberty is uncommon (rule out organic causes), late puberty is common and often constitutional
- gynecomastia (transient development of breast tissue) is a common self-limited condition seen in 50% of males during puberty (but any discharge from nipple or fixed mass should be investigated)

Tanner Staging
- scale used in pediatrics that defines physical measurements of development based on external primary and secondary sex characteristics

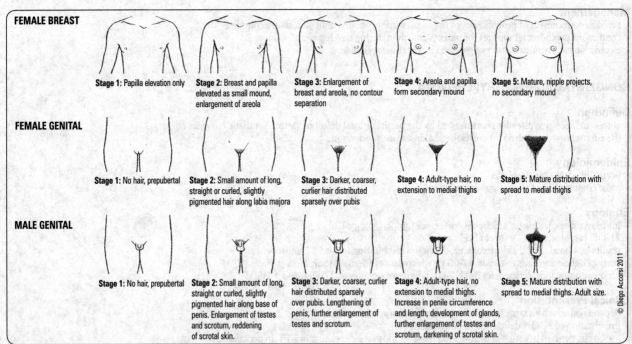

FEMALE BREAST
- Stage 1: Papilla elevation only
- Stage 2: Breast and papilla elevated as small mound, enlargement of areola
- Stage 3: Enlargement of breast and areola, no contour separation
- Stage 4: Areola and papilla form secondary mound
- Stage 5: Mature, nipple projects, no secondary mound

FEMALE GENITAL
- Stage 1: No hair, prepubertal
- Stage 2: Small amount of long, straight or curled, slightly pigmented hair along labia majora
- Stage 3: Darker, coarser, curlier hair distributed sparsely over pubis
- Stage 4: Adult-type hair, no extension to medial thighs
- Stage 5: Mature distribution with spread to medial thighs

MALE GENITAL
- Stage 1: No hair, prepubertal
- Stage 2: Small amount of long, straight or curled, slightly pigmented hair along base of penis. Enlargement of testes and scrotum, reddening of scrotal skin.
- Stage 3: Darker, coarser, curlier hair distributed sparsely over pubis. Lengthening of penis, further enlargement of testes and scrotum.
- Stage 4: Adult-type hair, no extension to medial thighs. Increase in penile circumference and length, development of glands, further enlargement of testes and scrotum, darkening of scrotal skin.
- Stage 5: Mature distribution with spread to medial thighs. Adult size.

© Diego Accorsi 2011

Figure 8. Tanner staging

PRECOCIOUS PUBERTY

Definition
- development of secondary sexual characteristics 2-2.5 SD before population mean
- <8 yr old for females, <9 yr old for males

Epidemiology
- 1/10,000; F>M

Etiology
- usually idiopathic in females (90%), more suggestive of pathology in males (50%)
- central (GnRH dependent)
  - hypergonadotropic hypergonadism; hormone levels as in normal puberty
  - premature activation of the HPG axis
  - differential diagnosis: idiopathic or constitutional (most common in females), CNS disturbances (tumours, hamartomas, post-meningitis, increased ICP, radiotherapy), NF, primary severe hypothyroidism
- peripheral (GnRH independent)
  - hypogonadotropic hypergonadism
  - differential diagnosis: adrenal disorders (CAH, adrenal neoplasm), testicular/ovarian tumour, gonadotropin/hCG secreting tumour (hepatoblastoma, intracranial teratoma, germinoma), exogenous steroid administration, McCune-Albright syndrome, aromatase excess syndrome, rarely hypothyroidism (Van Wyk-Grumbach syndrome)

Clinical Presentation
- history
  - symptoms of puberty, family history of precocious puberty, medical illness
- physical exam
  - growth velocity
  - prepubertal: 4 to 6 cm/yr
  - growth spurt: boys 8-10 cm/yr, girls 6-8 cm/yr
  - complete physical exam, including Tanner staging and neurological assessment
- investigations
  - initial screening tests: bone age, serum hormone levels (estradiol, testosterone, LH, FSH, TSH, free T4, DHEA-S, 17-OH-progesterone)
  - secondary tests: MRI head, pelvic U/S, β-hCG, GnRH, and/or ACTH stimulation test

A child with proven central precocious puberty should receive an MRI of the brain

Management
- indications for medical intervention to delay progression of puberty: rapid advancement of puberty, early age, risk of compromise of final adult height, psychological
- central causes: goals are to preserve height and alleviate psychosocial stress; GnRH agonists (e.g. leuprolide) most effective
- peripheral causes: goal is to limit effects of elevated sex steroids; treat underlying cause; medications that decrease the production of a specific sex steroid or block its effects (e.g. ketoconazole, spironolactone, tamoxifen, anastrozole), surgical intervention

DELAYED PUBERTY

Definition
- failure to develop secondary sex characteristics by 2-2.5 SD beyond the population mean
  - for males: lack of testicular enlargement by 14 yr old
  - for females: lack of breast development by 13 yr old OR absence of menarche by 16 yr old or within 5 yr of pubertal onset

Epidemiology
- M>F

Etiology
- usually constitutional delay in males, more suggestive of pathology in females
- central causes
  - constitutional delay in activation of HPG axis (most common)
  - hypogonadotropic hypogonadism
- peripheral causes
  - hypergonadotropic hypogonadism (e.g. primary gonadal failure, gonadal damage, Turner syndrome, hormone deficiency, androgen insensitivity syndrome, etc.)

Clinical Presentation
- history: weight loss, short stature, family history of puberty onset, medical illness, high performance athletes (females)
- physical exam: growth velocity (minimum 4 cm/yr), Tanner staging, neurological exam, complete physical exam
- investigations
  - initial screening tests: bone age, serum hormone levels (estradiol, testosterone, LH, FSH, TSH, free T4, IGF-1), CBC, electrolytes, BUN, Cr, LFTs, liver enzymes, ESR, CRP, urinalysis
  - secondary tests: MRI head, pelvic U/S, karyotype, IBD panel, celiac disease panel, LH levels following GnRH agonist

Management
- identify and treat underlying cause
- hormonal replacement: cyclic estradiol and progesterone for females, testosterone for males

Gastroenterology

Vomiting

Vomiting: forceful expulsion of stomach contents through the mouth
Regurgitation: the return of partially digested food from the stomach to the mouth

History
- characteristic of emesis (e.g. projectile, bilious, bloody)
- pattern of emesis (e.g. association with feeds, cyclic, morning)
- associated symptoms (e.g. anorexia, diarrhea, etc.)
- red flags: bilious or bloody emesis, projectile vomit, abdominal distension and tenderness, high fever, signs of dehydration
- note that vomiting without diarrhea is most likely not gastroenteritis.
  - post tussive vomiting is also common with coughing fits in children

Physical Findings
- vital signs to determine clinical status and hydration state

Investigations
- CBC, electrolytes, BUN, Cr, amylase, lipase, glucose done routinely
- in sick child, add: ESR, venous blood gases, C&S (blood, stool), imaging

Pyloric Stenosis 3 Ps
Palpable mass
Peristalsis visible
Projectile vomiting (2-4 wk after birth)

Table 13. Common Differential Diagnosis, Associated Findings, and Diagnostic Approach Based on Age

Cause	Suggestive Findings	Diagnostic Approach
NEONATES – NON-BILIOUS		
Tracheoesophageal Fistula	Vomiting, excessive secretions soon after birth (e.g. drooling, choking, respiratory distress), inability to feed, inability to advance NG tube	Inability to advance NG tube, CXR, upper GI series with water-soluble contrast
Pyloric stenosis	Projectile vomiting immediately after feeding, dehydrated, palpable "olive" in RUQ, decreased stools, hunger	U/S of pylorus, upper GI study (if U/S not diagnostic) Electrolytes, ABG (hypokalemic, hypochloremic metabolic alkalosis)
GERD	Fussiness after feeds, spit ups, arching of back, poor weight gain	Empiric trial of acid suppression, pH monitoring study, upper GI study, endoscopy
Sepsis	Fever, lethargy, tachycardia, tachypnea, widening pulse pressure	CBC, cultures (blood, urine, CSF), CXR
Inborn error of metabolism	Poor feeding, FTT, jaundice, hepatosplenomegaly, cardiomyopathy, dysmorphia, developmental delay	Electrolytes, ABG (hyponatremic, hyperkalemic metabolic acidosis), lactate, ammonia, LFTs, BUN, Cr, serum glucose, bilirubin, PT/PTT, CBC
NEONATES – BILIOUS		
Malrotation with volvulus	Bilious emesis, abdominal distension, pain, bloody stool, shock	AXR, upper GI series, contrast enema
Duodenal atresia	Bilious emesis, abdominal distension, often seen in DS, jaundice, polyhydramnios during pregnancy. Hypokaelmic, hypochloremic metabolic alkalosis.	AXR, upper GI series ('double bubble' sign)
Hirschsprung's disease	Bilious emesis, abdominal distension, pain, failure to pass stool	AXR, upper GI series, contrast enema, rectal biopsy
CHILDREN AND ADOLESCENTS		
Gastroenteritis	Diarrhea, fever, sick contact, recent travel	CBC, stool culture
Appendicitis	Periumbilical discomfort that later localizes to RLQ, fever, anorexia	Abdominal U/S
Intussusception	Colicky progressive abdominal pain, drawing of legs up to chest, lethargy, bloody "red currant jelly" stool (Triad)	Abdominal U/S
Non-GI infection (e.g. meningitis)	Fever, localized findings depending on cause	Cultures (CSF, blood, urine), brain imaging, CXR
Increased ICP	Nocturnal wakening, progressive recurrent headache worse with Valsalva, nuchal rigidity	Brain CT without contrast Therapeutic LP in idiopathic intracranial HTN
Toxic ingestion	Finding possibly varying by substance- toxidrome, often a history of ingestion	Qualitative and sometimes quantitative levels (urine, blood)
Pregnancy	Amenorrhea, morning sickness, bloating, breast tenderness	Urine β-hCG
Cyclic vomiting	At least 3 self-limited episodes of vomiting lasting 12 h, 7 d between episodes, no organic cause of vomiting	Diagnosis of exclusion

Management
- rehydration (see *Fluids and Electrolytes*, P74)
- treat underlying cause

Gastroesophageal Reflux

Epidemiology
- extremely common in infancy (up to 50%)

Clinical Presentation
- vomiting typically soon after feeding, non-bilious, rarely contains blood, small volume (<30 mL)

Investigations
- thriving baby requires no investigation
- investigations required if concomitant FTT, feeding aversion, recurrent cough, pneumonia or bronchospasm, GI blood loss or symptoms persist after 18 mo

Management
- conservative: thickened feeds, frequent and smaller feeds, elevation of head
- medical
  - short-term parenteral feeding to enhance weight gain
  - ranitidine, PPI: decreases gastric acidity, decreases esophageal irritation
  - domperidone, metoclopramide: improves gastric emptying and GI motility; safety concerns and limited efficacy, should be reserved for children with gastroparesis contributing to GERD
- surgical: indicated for failure of medical therapy (Nissen fundoplication)

Complications
- esophagitis, strictures, Barrett's esophagus, FTT, aspiration, oral feeding aversion

Tracheoesophageal Fistula

- see General Surgery, GS64

Pyloric Stenosis

- see General Surgery, GS62

Duodenal Atresia

- see General Surgery, GS63

Malrotation of the Intestine

- see General Surgery, GS63

Diarrhea

- definition of diarrhea varies with diet and age (stool normalcy difficult to define in children)
- infants → increase in stool frequency to twice as often per day; older children → 3+ loose or watery stools/d
- duration: acute: <2 wk; chronic: >2 wk

Diarrhea is defined as an increase in frequency and/or decreased consistency of stools compared to normal

Normal stool volume
Infants: 5-10 g/kg/d
Children: 200 g/d

Pathophysiology
- osmotic: due to non-absorbable solutes in GI tract (e.g. lactose intolerance)
- secretory: increased secretion of Cl⁻ ions and water in intestinal lumen (e.g. bacterial toxin)
- malabsorption: less time for absorption due to increased motility or less villi to absorb (e.g. short bowel syndrome)

History
- frequency, duration, quality of diarrhea
- associated symptoms (e.g. fever, abdominal pain, hematochezia, etc.)
- recent antibiotic use or recent travel
- elements of diet

Diarrhea Red Flags
Bloody stool, fever, petechiae or purpura, signs of severe dehydration, weight loss/FTT

Physical Findings
- vital signs to determine clinical status and hydration state

Investigations
- acute diarrhea
  - stool for C&S, O&P, electron microscopy for viruses, *C. difficile* toxin, microscopy (leukocytes suggestive of invading pathogen), blood and urine cultures, blood work
- chronic diarrhea
  - serial heights, weights, growth percentiles
  - if child growing well and thriving, workup is limited (stool cultures as above, stool reducing substances)
  - red flags: poor growth, chronic rash, other serious infections, hospitalizations for dehydration
  - require full workup (as per below)
  - stool: consistency, pH, reducing substances, microscopy, occult blood, O&P, C&S, *C. difficile* toxin, 3 d fecal fat, α-1-antitrypsin clearance, fecal elastase
  - urinalysis, urine culture
  - CBC, differential, ESR/CRP, smear, electrolytes, total protein, albumin, carotene, Ca^{2+}, PO_4^{3-}, Mg^{2+}, Fe, ferritin, folate, fat-soluble vitamins, PTT, INR
  - sweat chloride, celiac screen, thyroid function tests, urine VMA and HVA, HIV test, lead levels
  - CXR, upper GI series and follow-through
  - specialized tests: endoscopy, small bowel biopsy

Differential Diagnosis

Table 14. Differential Diagnosis of Diarrhea

	Infectious			Non-infectious
Acute	**Viral** Rotavirus Norwalk Enteric adenovirus	**Bacterial** *Salmonella* *Campylobacter* *Shigella* Pathogenic *E. coli* *Yersinia* *C. difficile*	**Parasitic** *Giardia lamblia* *Entamoeba histolytica*	Antibiotic-induced Non-specific: associated with systemic infection Hirschsprung's disease Toxin ingestion Primary disaccharidase deficiency
Chronic	**0 – 3 mo**	**3 mo – 3 yr**	**3 – 18 yr**	**Uncommon**
No FTT	GI infection	GI infection Toddler's diarrhea	GI infection Lactase deficiency Irritable bowel syndrome	Drug-induced Chronic constipation UTI
FTT	Disaccharidase deficiency Cow's milk protein intolerance CF	Celiac disease	IBD Endocrine (thyrotoxicosis, Addison's) Neoplastic (pheochromocytoma, lymphoma)	Short bowel syndrome Schwachman-Diamond syndrome

Gastroenteritis

History
- non-specific: diarrhea, vomiting, fever, anorexia, headache, myalgias, abdominal cramps
- bacterial and parasitic agents more common in older children (2-4 yr)
- recent infectious contacts: symptoms usually begin 24-48 h after exposure

Physical Exam
- febrile
- dehydrated: must assess extent (see *Approach to Infant/Child with Dehydration*, P74)

Investigations
- not usually necessary in young children
- stool analysis: leukocytes/erythrocytes suggests bacterial or parasitic etiology; pH <6 and presence of reducing substances suggests viral etiology

Complications
- viral gastroenteritis usually self-limiting (lasts 3-7 d in most cases)
- adverse effects related to hypovolemia, shock, tissue acidosis, and rapid onset and over-correction of electrolyte imbalances
- death in severe dehydration (rare in developed countries)

Table 15. Gastroenteritis

	Viral Infection	Bacterial Infection
Etiology	Most common cause of gastroenteritis Commonly: rotaviruses (most common), enteric adenovirus, norovirus (typically older children)	*Salmonella, Campylobacter, Shigella*, pathogenic *E. coli, Yersinia, C. difficile*
Clinical Presentation	Associated with URTIs Resolves in 3-7 d Slight fever, malaise, vomiting, vague abdominal pain	Severe abdominal pain High fever Bloody diarrhea
Risk Factors	Day care, young age, sick contacts, immunocompromised Bacterial infection: travel, poorly cooked meat, poorly refrigerated foods, antibiotics	
Management	Prevention and treatment of dehydration most important (see Dehydration, P74) Early refeeding advisable, with age-appropriate diet upon completion of rehydration Ondansetron for suspected gastroenteritis with mild to moderate dehydration or failed ORT and significant vomiting Antibiotic or antiparasitic therapy when indicated, antidiarrheal medications not indicated Notify Public Health authorities if appropriate Promote regular hand-washing and return to school 24 h after last diarrheal episode to prevent transmission Rotavirus vaccine	

Toddler's Diarrhea

Epidemiology
- most common cause of chronic diarrhea during infancy
- onset between 6-36 mo of age, ceases spontaneously between 2-4 yr

Clinical Presentation
- diagnosis of exclusion in thriving child
- 4-6 bowel movements per day
- diet history (e.g. excess juice intake overwhelms small bowel resulting in disaccharide malabsorption)
- stool may contain undigested food particles
- excoriated diaper rash

Management
- reassurance that it is self-limiting
- 4Fs (adequate Fibre, normal Fluid intake, 35-40% Fat, discourage excess Fruit juice)

Lactase Deficiency (Lactose Intolerance)

Clinical Presentation
- chronic, watery diarrhea and abdominal pain, bloating associated with dairy intake
- primary lactose intolerance: crampy abdominal pain with loose stool (older children, usually of East Asian and African descent)
- secondary lactose intolerance: older infant, persistent diarrhea (post viral/bacterial infection, celiac disease, or IBD)

Diagnosis
- trial of lactose-free diet
- watery stool, acid pH, positive reducing sugars
- positive breath hydrogen test if >6 yr

Management
- lactose-free diet, soy formula
- lactase-containing tablets/capsules/drops (e.g. Lacteeze®, Lactaid®)

Irritable Bowel Syndrome

- see Gastroenterology, G23

Celiac Disease

- see Gastroenterology, G18
- in children: presents at any age, usually 6-24 mo with the introduction of gluten in the diet
- FTT with poor appetite, irritability, apathy, rickets, wasted muscles, flat buttocks, rarely distended abdomen
- GI symptoms: anorexia, N/V, edema, anemia, abdominal pain
- non-GI manifestations: iron-deficiency anemia, dermatitis herpetiformis, dental enamel hypoplasia, osteopenia/osteoporosis, short stature, delayed puberty, behavioural changes
- associated with other autoimmune disorders

Celiac disease is associated with an increased prevalence of IgA deficiency. Since tTG is an IgA-detecting test, you must order an accompanying IgA level

A Celiac disease diet must avoid gluten present in "**BROW**" foods
Barley
Rye
Oats (controversial)
Wheat

Milk Protein Allergy

Pathophysiology
- immune-mediated mucosal injury (IgE- and non-IgE-mediated)

Clinical Presentation
- up to 50% of children intolerant to cow's milk may be intolerant to soy protein as well
- often history of atopy
- can present as
  - proctocolitis: mild diarrhea, small amounts of bloody stools (common presentation in young infant)
  - enterocolitis: vomiting, diarrhea, anemia, hematochezia
  - enteropathy: chronic diarrhea, hypoalbuminemia

Management
- casein hydrolysate formula (dairy-free e.g. Nutramigen®, Pregestimil®) or mother may remove all milk protein from diet and continue breastfeeding (with adequate calcium and vit D intake)
- often outgrow by 1 yr of age

Inflammatory Bowel Disease

- see <u>Gastroenterology</u>, G19

Cystic Fibrosis

- see *Respirology*, P84

Constipation

- decreased stool frequency (<3 stools/wk) and/or stool fluidity (hard, pellet-like)

FUNCTIONAL CONSTIPATION
- 99% of cases of constipation
- Rome III criteria; ≥2 of the following
  - ≤2 defecations in the toilet/wk
  - ≥1 episode of fecal incontinence/wk
  - history of retentive posturing or excessive volitional stool retention
  - history of painful or hard bowel movements
  - large fecal mass in rectum
  - history of large diameter stools that may obstruct toilet

Pathophysiology
- lack of fibre in diet or change in diet, poor fluid intake, behavioural
  - infants: often occurs when introducing cow's milk after breast milk due to high fat and solute content, lower water content
  - toddlers/older children: can occur during toilet training, or due to pain on defecation, leading to withholding of stool
  - two crucial time periods: toilet training and starting school

Management
- education: explanation of mechanism of functional constipation for parents/older children
- clean out: PEG 3350 flakes (1-1.5 g/kg/d, max 100 g/d), picosalax, PEGlyte®
- maintenance: adequate fluid intake (if <6 mo, 150 mL/kg/d), adequate dietary fibre (fruit, vegetables, whole grains), stool softening (PEG 3350, mineral oil), appropriate toilet training technique (dedicated time for defecation: 3-10 min, 1-2 x/d)
- children should be treated for at least 6 mo, and should not be weaned from maintenance therapy until they are having regular bowel movements without difficulty
- regular follow-up with ongoing support and encouragement is essential

Complications
- pain retention cycle: anal fissures + pain withhold passing stool chronic dilatation ± overflow incontinence

HIRSCHSPRUNG'S DISEASE (Congenital Aganglionic Megacolon)
- see <u>General Surgery</u>, GS64

OTHER ORGANIC DISORDERS CAUSING CONSTIPATION
- endocrine: hypothyroidism, DM, hypercalcemia
- neurologic: spinal cord abnormalities/trauma, NF
- anatomic: bowel obstruction, anus (imperforate, atresia, stenosis, anteriorly displaced)
- drugs: lead, chemotherapy, opioids
- others

Abdominal Pain

ACUTE ABDOMINAL PAIN

History
- description of pain (location, radiation, duration, constant vs. colicky, relation to meals)
- associated symptoms: N/V, diarrhea, fever

Physical Exam
- abdominal exam, rectal exam, rash

Investigations
- CBC, differential, urinalysis to rule out UTI

Table 16. Differential Diagnosis of Acute Abdominal Pain

Gastrointestinal	Hepatobiliary Tract	Genitourinary	Hematologic	Miscellaneous
Gastroenteritis	Cholecystitis	UTI	Henoch-Schönlein purpura	DKA
Appendicitis	Pancreatitis	Nephrolithiasis	Sickle cell crisis	Pneumonia
Meckel's diverticulum		Testicular torsion		Somatization
Mesenteric adenitis		Ovarian torsion		
Ileus		Ectopic pregnancy		
Intestinal obstruction		PID		
(incarcerated hernia,		Endometriosis		
intussusception, volvulus)		Menstruation		
Malabsorption				
IBS				
Constipation				

APPENDICITIS

- see General Surgery, GS27
- most common cause of acute abdomen after 5 yr of age
- clinical features: low grade fever, abdominal pain, anorexia, N/V (after onset of pain), peritoneal signs (generalized peritonitis is a common presentation in infants/young children)
- treatment: surgical
- complications: perforation (common in young children), abscess

INTUSSUSCEPTION

- telescoping of segment of bowel into distal segment causing ischemia and necrosis

Epidemiology
- 90% idiopathic, children with CF or GJ tube at significantly increased risk; M:F = 3:1
- 50% between 3-12 mo, 75% before 2 yr of age

Pathophysiology
- usual site: ileocecal junction; jejunum in children with GJ tubes
- lead point of telescoping segment may be swollen Peyer's patches, Meckel's diverticulum, polyp, malignancy, HSP, structural abnormalities

Clinical Presentation
- "classic triad" (<25% patients) - abdominal pain, palpable mass, red currant jelly stools
- often preceded by URTI
- sudden onset of recurrent, paroxysmal, severe periumbilical pain with pain-free intervals
- later vomiting (may be bilious) and rectal bleeding (late finding)
- shock and dehydration; lethargy may be only presenting symptom

Diagnosis
- U/S, air enema

Management
- air enema can be therapeutic (reduces intussusception in 75% of cases), reduction under hydrostatic pressure, surgery rarely needed
- recurrence rate 10-15%, need to consider pathologic lead point

Intussusception – Classic Triad
- Abdominal pain
- Palpable mass
- Red currant jelly stools

Chronic Abdominal Pain

Epidemiology
- prevalence: 10% of school children (peak at 8-10 yr), F>M

Etiology
- organic (<10%)
  - gastrointestinal
    - constipation (cause vs. effect), infectious
    - IBD, esophagitis, peptic ulcer disease, lactose intolerance
    - anatomic anomalies, masses
    - pancreatic, hepatobiliary
    - celiac disease
  - genitourinary causes: recurrent UTI, nephrolithiasis, chronic PID, Mittelschmerz
  - neoplastic
- functional abdominal pain (90%): can be diagnosed when there are no alarm symptoms or signs, physical exam is normal, and stool sample tests are negative for occult blood; no further testing is required, unless high suspicion for organic cause

Clinical Presentation
- clustering episodes of vague, crampy periumbilical/epigastric pain, vivid pain description
- seldom awakens child from sleep, less common on weekends
- aggravated by exercise, alleviated by rest
- psychological factors related to onset and/or maintenance of pain, school avoidance
- psychiatric comorbidity: anxiety, somatoform, mood, learning disorders, sexual abuse, eating disorders, elimination disorders
- diagnosis of exclusion

Investigations
- fecal occult blood and others based on clinical suspicion (CBC, ESR, urinalysis, etc.)

Management
- continue to attend school
- manage any emotional or family problems, counselling, CBT
- trial of high fibre diet, trial of lactose-free diet
- possible role for amitriptyline
- reassurance

Prognosis
- pain resolves in 30-50% of children within 2-6 wk of diagnosis
- 30-50% of children with functional abdominal pain have functional pain as adults (e.g. IBS)

Chronic Abdominal Pain

Rule of 3s
3 episodes of severe pain
Child >3 yr old
Over 3 mo period

Red Flags for Organic Etiology of Chronic Abdominal Pain
- Age <5 yr old
- Fever
- Localizes pain away from midline
- Anemia
- Evidence of GI blood loss
- Rash
- Pain awakens child at night
- Travel history
- Prominent vomiting, diarrhea
- Weight loss or failure to gain weight
- Deceleration in linear growth
- Joint pain
- Family history of IBD
- Abnormal or unexplained physical exam findings

Abdominal Mass

Table 17. Differential Diagnosis for Abdominal Mass

	Benign	Malignant
Renal (note: 50% of abdominal masses in newborn are renal in origin)	Hydronephrosis Polycystic kidney disease Hamartoma	Nephroblastoma (Wilms' tumour) Renal cell carcinoma
Adrenal		Neuroblastoma
Ovarian	Ovarian cysts	Ovarian tumours
Other	Hepatomegaly/splenomegaly Pyloric stenosis Abdominal hernia Teratoma Fecal impaction	Lymphoma Rhabdomyosarcoma Retroperitoneal sarcoma

Upper Gastrointestinal Bleeding

- see <u>Gastroenterology</u>, G25

Lower Gastrointestinal Bleeding

- see Gastroenterology, G27

Etiology
- acute
  - infectious (bacterial, parasitic)
  - antibiotic-induced (*C. difficile*)
  - NEC in preterm infants
  - anatomic
  - malrotation/volvulus, intussusception
  - Meckel's diverticulitis
  - anal fissures, hemorrhoids
  - vascular/hematologic
  - HSP
  - HUS
  - coagulopathy
- chronic
  - anal fissures (most common)
  - colitis
  - IBD
  - allergic (milk protein)
  - structural
  - polyps (most are hamartomas)
  - neoplasms (rare)
  - coagulopathy

Physical Exam
- hemodynamic status, evidence of FTT, fever
- anal and rectal exam: tags, fissures, anal fistulas, polyps, foreign body, blood per rectum
- stool appearance
- NG aspirate
- lower GI bleed may present as melena (if it involves the small bowel) or hematochezia

Investigations
- stool cultures (C&S, *C. difficile* toxin)
- urinalysis and microscopy
- CBC, smear, differential, ESR, CRP, electrolytes, urea, Cr, INR, PTT, albumin, iron studies, amoeba titers
- radiologic investigations (including abdominal x-ray to rule out obstruction)
- Meckel's radionuclide scan

Management
- acute stabilization: ABCs, volume and blood replacement, bowel rest (NPO, NG tube)
- once stable, endoscopy and/or surgery as indicated

Genetics, Dysmorphisms, and Metabolism

Genetics

MECHANISMS OF INHERITANCE

Mendelian Inheritance
- disorders caused by mutation of one or both copies (alleles) of a gene, inherited in one of two patterns
  - autosomal: encoded by genes on one of 22 pairs of autosomes (chromosomes 1-22)
  - X-linked: encoded by a gene on the X chromosome

Triplet Repeat Expansions
- disorder in which trinucleotide repeats in certain genes exceed the normal number and result in altered gene expression or production of an abnormal protein (e.g. Fragile X syndrome, spinocerebellar ataxias, myotonic dystrophy, Huntington disease)

Imprinting Disorders
- imprinting: epigenetic process that involves methylation or acetylation of DNA, affecting gene expression
- imprinted genes are expressed entirely from either the maternal or paternal alelle, depending on the gene (parent-of-origin gene expression)
- occur when a mutation disrupts the normally expressed allele of imprinted gene (e.g. Prader-Willi syndrome, Angelman syndrome, Beckwith-Wiedemann syndrome)

Mitochondrial Inheritance
- disorders caused by mutations of the DNA present in mitochondria
- inheritance pattern: mother passes on the defect to all her children; father can not pass on defect since embryo only receives mitochondria from the mother (in the egg)

Whole-Genome Sequencing Expands Diagnostic Utility and Improves Clinical Management in Paediatric Medicine
Genomic Med 1:15012
While the standard of care for neurodevelopmental and congenital malformations is chromosome microarray analysis for copy-number variations, whole exome sequencing allows the identification of sequence-level mutations across all known coding genes. Whole genome sequencing has been previously associated with a diagnostic yield of ~25% for neurological disorders or congenital anomalies. A recent study published in Genomic Medicine has demonstrated that whole genome sequencing exceeds other technologies in detecting genetic variants with a 34% diagnostic yield, a four-fold increase in molecular diagnosis relative to chromosome microarray analysis and a two-fold increase relative to all genetic testing protocols. These results suggest that whole genome sequencing may be used as a first-tier molecular test in individuals with development delays and congenital abnormalities, with a higher diagnostic yield than conventional genetic testing and decreased time to genetic diagnosis.

VACTERL Association
V   Vertebral dysgenesis
A   Anal atresia (imperforate anus)
        ± fistula
C   Cardiac anomalies
T-E TracheoEsophageal fistula
        ± esophageal atresia
R   Renal anomalies
L   Limb anomalies

METHODS OF GENETIC TESTING
- microarray analysis
  - a microarray is a collection of DNA probes attached to a solid surface
  - microarray analysis can identify small deletions or duplications of genetic material anywhere in the genome
  - indicated when there is developmental delay + one or more major malformations
- FISH: usually to identify a gain or loss of chromosomal material
- karyotype: microscopic analysis of all 46 chromosomes with a special stain that shows large changes in the number or structure of chromosomes
  - sanger sequencing: the 'gold-standard' method for identfication of single nucleotide variants in short DNA sequences (e.g. the exons of the gene(s) known to cause suspected syndrome)
  - next generation sequencing: high-throughput method to sequence exomes or whole-genomes; useful when genetic syndrome is suspected, but diagnosis is unclear

Genetic Anomalies

Minor and Major Anomalies
- minor anomaly: an unusual anatomic feature that is of no serious medical or cosmetic consequence to the patient
- major anomaly: anomaly that creates significant medical, surgical, or cosmetic problems for the patient

Mechanism for Anomalies
- malformation: results from an intrinsically abnormal developmental process (e.g. polydactyly)
- disruption: results from the extrinsic breakdown of, or interference with, an originally normal developmental process (e.g. amniotic band disruption sequence)
- deformation: alteration of the final form of a structure by mechanical forces (e.g. Potter deformation sequence)
- dysplasia: abnormal development that results in abnormal organization of cells into tissues (e.g. bone dysplasia)

Multiple Anomalies
- association: non-random occurrence of multiple independent anomalies that appear together more than would be predicted by chance but are not believed to have a single etiology (e.g. VACTERL)
- sequence: related anomalies that come from a single initial major anomaly or precipitating factor that changes the development of other surrounding or related tissues or structures (e.g. Potter sequence)
- syndrome: a pattern of anomalies that occur together and are caused by a single known or unknown cause (e.g. Down syndrome)

Approach to the Dysmorphic Child

- genetic disorders are the most common cause of infant death in developed countries

General Approach to the Dysmorphic Child
- Are the anomalies major or minor?
- What is the mechanism underlying the anomaly?
- Do the anomalies fit as part of an association, sequence, or syndrome?

History
- prenatal/obstetrical history (see <u>Obstetrics</u>, OB6) with particular attention to potential teratogenic exposures
- complete 3 generation family pedigree: consanguinity, stillbirths, neonatal deaths, specific illnesses, intellectual disability, multiple miscarriages, ethnicity

Physical Exam

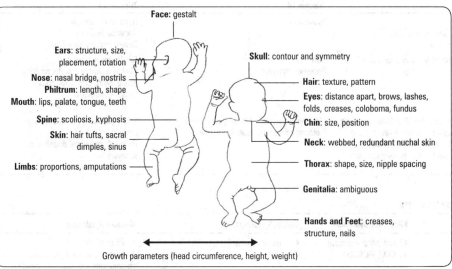

Figure 9. Physical exam of the dysmorphic child

Investigations

- screening for TORCH infections
- serial photographs if child is older
- x-rays for bony abnormalities
- cytogenetic studies
  - karyotype if recognized syndrome
  - chromosome microarray analysis (array comparative genomic hybridization) if developmental delay with one or more congenital anomalies
  - FISH if microdeletion syndrome or trisomy suspected
- biochemistry: specific enzyme assays
- single gene testing

Check the umbilical cord for 2 arteries and 1 vein. The presence of a single umbilical artery may be associated with other congenital anomalies

Management

- prenatal counselling and assessing risk of recurrence
- referral for specialized pediatric or genetic care

Genetic Syndromes

Table 18. Common Genetic Syndromes

	Trisomy 21	Trisomy 18	Trisomy 13
Disease	Down syndrome	Edwards' syndrome	Patau syndrome
Incidence	1:600-800 births Most common abnormality of autosomal chromosomes Rises with advanced maternal age from 1:1,500 at age 20 to 1:20 by age 45	1:6,000 live births F:M = 3:1	1:10,000 live births
Cranium/Brain	Mild microcephaly, flat occiput, 3rd fontanelle, brachycephaly	Microcephaly, prominent occiput	Microcephaly, sloping forehead, occipital scalp defect, holoprosencephaly
Eyes	Upslanting palpebral fissures, inner epicanthal folds, speckled iris (Brushfield spots), refractive errors (myopia), acquired cataracts, nystagmus, strabismus	Microphthalmia, hypotelorism, iris coloboma, retinal anomalies	Microphthalmia, corneal abnormalities
Ears	Low-set, small, overfolded upper helix, frequent AOM, hearing loss	Low-set, malformed	Low-set, malformed
Facial Features	Protruding tongue, large cheeks, low flat nasal bridge, small nose	Cleft lip/palate Small mouth, micrognathia	60-80% cleft lip and palate
Skeletal/MSK	Short stature Excess nuchal skin Joint hyperflexibility (80%) including dysplastic hips, vertebral anomalies, atlantoaxial instability	Short stature Clenched fist with overlapping digits, hypoplastic nails, clinodactyly, polydactyly	Severe growth retardation Polydactyly, clenched hand
Cardiac Defect	50%, particularly atrioventricular septal defect	60% (VSD, PDA, ASD)	80% (VSD, PDA, ASD)
GI	Duodenal/esophageal/anal atresia, TEF, Hirschsprung's disease, chronic constipation	Hernia, TEF	
GU	Cryptorchidism, rarely fertile	Polycystic kidneys, cryptorchidism	Polycystic kidneys

Table 18. Common Genetic Syndromes (continued)

	Trisomy 21	Trisomy 18	Trisomy 13
CNS	Hypotonia at birth Low IQ, developmental delay, hearing problems Onset of Alzheimer's disease in 40s	Hypertonia	Hypo- or hypertonia Seizures, deafness Severe developmental delay
Other Features	Transverse palmar crease, clinodactyly, and absent middle phalanx of the 5th finger 1% lifetime risk of leukemia Polycythemia Hypothyroidism	SGA Rocker-bottom feet	Single umbilical artery Midline anomalies: scalp, pituitary, palate, heart, umbilicus, anus Rocker-bottom feet
Prognosis/ Management	Prognosis: long-term management per AAP Guidelines (Health Supervision of Children with Down syndrome), recommend chromosomal analysis, CBC, Echo, yearly thyroid test, atlanto-occipital x-ray at 2 yr, sleep study, hearing test, and ophthalmology assessment	13% 1-year survival, 10% ten-year survival Profound intellectual disability in survivors	20% 1-year survival, 13% ten-year survival Profound intellectual disability in survivors

Table 19. Most Common Sex Chromosome Disorders

	Fragile X Syndrome	Klinefelter Syndrome	Turner Syndrome	Noonan Syndrome
Genotype	X-linked Genetic anticipation CGG trinucleotide repeat on X chromosome measurable by molecular analysis	47,XXY (most common) 48,XXXY, 49,XXXXY	45,X (most common)	46,XX or 46,XY Autosomal dominant (not a sex chromosome disorder) with variable expression PTPN11 mutation most common cause Higher transmission of affected maternal gene
Incidence	1:3,600 males, 1:6,000 females Most common heritable cause of intellectual disability in boys	1:1,000 live male births Increased risk with advanced maternal age	1:4,000 live female births Risk not increased with advanced maternal age	1:2,000 male and female live births
Phenotype	Overgrowth: prominent jaw, forehead, and nasal bridge with long and thin face, large protuberant ears, macroorchidism, hyperextensibility, and high arched palate Complications: seizures, scoliosis, mitral valve prolapse	Tall, slim, underweight No features prepuberty Postpuberty: male may suffer from developmental delay, long limbs, gynecomastia, lack of facial hair	Short stature, short webbed neck, low posterior hair line, wide carrying angle Broad chest, widely spaced nipples Lymphedema of hands and/or feet, cystic hygroma in newborn with polyhydramnios, lung hypoplasia Coarctation of aorta, bicuspid aortic valve Renal and cardiovascular abnormalities, increased risk of HTN Less severe spectrum with mosaic	Certain phenotypic features similar to females with Turner syndrome; therefore, sometimes called the "male Turner syndrome", although it affects both males and females Short stature, webbed neck, triangular facies, hypertelorism, low set ears, epicanthal folds, ptosis Pectus excavatum Right-sided CHD, pulmonary stenosis Increased risk of hematological cancers
IQ and Behaviour	Mild to moderate intellectual disability, 20% of affected males have normal IQ ADHD and/or autism Female carriers may show intellectual impairment Male carriers may demonstrate tremor/ataxia syndrome in later life	Mild intellectual disability Behavioural or psychiatric disorders – anxiety, shyness, aggressive behaviour, antisocial acts	Mild intellectual disability to normal intelligence	Moderate intellectual disability in 25% of patients
Gonad and Reproductive Function	Premutation carrier females at risk of developing premature ovarian failure	Infertility due to hypogonadism/hypospermia	Streak ovaries with deficient follicles, infertility, primary amenorrhea, impaired development of secondary sexual characteristics	Delayed puberty
Diagnosis/ Prognosis/ Management	Molecular testing of FMR1 gene: overamplification of the trinucleotide repeat, length of segment is proportional to severity of clinical phenotype (genetic anticipation)	Increased risk of germ cell tumours and breast cancer Management: testosterone in adolescence	Normal life expectancy if no complications Increased risk of X-linked diseases Management: Echo, ECG to screen for cardiac malformation GH therapy for short stature Estrogen replacement at time of puberty for development of secondary sexual characteristics	Molecular testing of PTPN11 gene Management: affected males may require testosterone replacement therapy at puberty Echo, ECG

Table 20. Other Genetic Syndromes

	DiGeorge Syndrome	Prader-Willi Syndrome	Angelman Syndrome	CHARGE Syndrome
Genotype	Microdeletions of chromosome region 22q11	Lack of expression of genes on paternal chromosome 15q11-13 due to deletion, maternal uniparental disomy of chromosome 15, or imprinting defect	Lack of expression of genes on maternal chromosome 15q11-13 due to deletion or inactivation or paternal uniparental disomy	2/3 of children with CHARGE have been found to have a *CHD7* mutation on chromosome 8
Incidence	1:4000; Second most common genetic diagnosis (next to DS)	1:15,000	1:10,000	1:10,000
Clinical Features	**"CATCH 22"** **C**yanotic CHD **A**nomalies: craniofacial anomalies typically micrognathia and low set ears **T**hymic hypoplasia: "immunodeficiency" recurrent infections **C**ognitive impairment **H**ypoparathyroidism, hypocalcemia **22**q11 microdeletions High risk for psychiatric disorders	**"H₃O"**: **H**ypotonia and weakness, **H**ypogonadism, obsessive **H**yperphagia, **O**besity Short stature, almond-shaped eyes, small hands and feet with tapering of fingers Developmental delay (variable) Hypopigmentation, type 2 DM	Ataxia with severe intellectual disability, seizures, tremulousness, hypotonia Midface hypoplasia, fair hair, uncontrollable laughter	**"CHARGE"** **C** **C**oloboma **H** congenital **H**eart disease **A** choanal **A**tresia **R** mental **R**etardation **G** **G**U anomalies **E** **E**ar anomalies

DUCHENNE MUSCULAR DYSTROPHY

Epidemiology
- 1:4,000 males

Etiology
- one type of muscular dystrophy characterized by progressive skeletal and cardiac muscle degeneration
- X-linked recessive: 1/3 spontaneous mutations, 2/3 inherited mutations
- missing structural protein (dystrophin) → muscle fibre fragility → fibre breakdown → necrosis and regeneration

Gower's Sign
Child uses hands to "climb up" the legs to move from a sitting to a standing position

Clinical Presentation
- proximal muscle weakness by age 3, positive Gower's sign, waddling gait, toe walking
- pseudohypertrophy of calf muscles (muscle replaced by fat) and wasting of thigh muscles
- decreased reflexes
- non-progressive delayed motor and cognitive development (dysfunctional dystrophin in brain)
- cardiomyopathy

Diagnosis
- molecular genetic studies of dystrophin gene (DMD) (first line)
- family history (pedigree analysis)
- increased CK (50-100x normal) and lactate dehydrogenase
- elevated transaminases
- muscle biopsy, EMG

Management
- supportive (e.g. physiotherapy, wheelchairs, braces), prevent obesity
- cardiac health monitoring and early intervention
- bone health monitoring and intervention (vitamin D, bisphosphonates)
- steroids (e.g. prednisone or deflazacort)
- surgical (for scoliosis)
- gene therapy trials underway

Complications
- patient usually wheelchair-bound by 12 yr of age
- early flexion contractures, scoliosis, osteopenia of immobility, increased risk of fracture
- death due to pneumonia/respiratory failure or CHF in 2nd-3rd decade

Metabolic Diseases

Metabolic disease must be ruled out in any newborn who becomes acutely ill after a period of normal behaviour and development or with a family history of early infant death even if the newborn screen is negative

- inherited disorders of metabolism; often autosomal recessive
- infants and older children may present with FTT or developmental delay
- universal newborn screening in Ontario includes metabolic disorders

Table 21. Metabolic Disorders

	Organic and Amino Acid Disorders	Carbohydrate Disorders	Fatty Acid Disorders	Organelle Disorders
Examples of Conditions	PKU Tyrosinemia Homocystinuria MSUD Alkaptonuria Urea cycle defects	Galactosemia GSDs: von Gierke's, Pompe's, Cori's, Andersen, McArdle	MCAD deficiency Carnitine deficiency	Mucopolysaccharidosis Congenital disorders of glycosylation Lysosomal storage diseases: Hurler's, Niemann-Pick, Tay-Sachs, Gaucher, Fabry, Krabbe
Clinical Manifestations	Irritability, lethargy, poor feeding Seizures Intellectual disability Vomiting and acidosis after feeding initiation Sweet-smelling urine (MSUD)	Vomiting and acidosis after feeding initiation Growth retardation, FTT	Lethargy, poor feeding Seizures, coma Symptoms triggered by fasting Liver dysfunction Sudden infant death	Seizures/early-onset severe epilepsy Acute and chronic encephalopathy Developmental delay Bone crises (Gaucher) Deafness, blindness
Laboratory Findings	Hypoglycemic hyperammonemia, high anion gap (organic acidemia) Normoglycemic hyperammonemia, normal anion gap (urea cycle defects)	Hypoglycemia, hyperlipidemia (GSD)	Hypoketotic hypoglycemia Elevated free fatty acids	Elevated urine oligosaccharides (oligosaccharidoses) and glycosaminoglycans (mucopolysaccharidoses)
Physical Exam	Hypotonia/hypertonia Microcephaly, musty odour, eczema, hypopigmentation (PKU) Dark urine, pigmented sclerae, arthralgias (alkaptonuria) Lens subluxation, marfanoid appearance (homocystinuria)	Infantile cataracts (galactosemia) Hepatomegaly Muscle weakness/cramping	Hepatomegaly Hypotonia	Dysmorphic facial features Macrocephaly (Tay-Sachs, Hurler's) Hepatosplenomegaly (not Tay-Sachs) Cherry-red spot on macula (Niemann-Pick, Tay-Sachs, Gaucher's) Corneal clouding (Hurler's) Infantile cataract (Fabry) Peripheral neuropathy (Fabry, Krabbe) Spasticity

Initial Investigations
- important to send lab studies at initial presentation in order to facilitate immediate diagnosis and treatment
- check newborn screening results
- electrolytes, ABGs (calculate anion gap, rule out acidosis)
- CBC with differential and smear
- blood glucose (hypoglycemia seen with organic acidemia, fatty acid oxidation defects, and GSDs)
- lactate, ammonium (hyperammonemia with urea cycle defects), plasma Ca2+ and Mg2+
- routine urinalysis: ketonuria must be investigated
- carnitine levels with acylcarnitine profile
- others: urate, urine nitroprusside, plasma amino acid screen, urine organic acids, CSF glycine, free fatty acids (3-β-hydroxybutyrate ratio >4 in fatty acid oxidation defect)
- storage diseases: urine mucopolysaccharide and oligosaccharide screen

Treatment
- varies according to inborn error of metabolism
- dietary restrictions, supplementation, enzyme replacement therapy, gene therapy, liver transplant, stem cell transplant

PHENYLKETONURIA

Epidemiology
- 1:10,000; autosomal recessive disease

Etiology
- deficiency of phenylalanine hydroxylase prevents conversion of phenylalanine to tyrosine leading to build up of toxic metabolites
- mothers who have PKU may have infants with congenital abnormalities

Clinical Presentation
- baby is normal at birth, then develops a musty odour, eczema, hypertonia, tremors, and mental retardation
- hypopigmentation due to low tyrosine (fair hair, blue eyes)

Management
- PKU screening at birth
- dietary restriction of phenylalanine starting within the first 10 d of life
- duration of dietary restriction controversial – lifelong or until end of puberty; should be resumed during pregnancy to maintain normal phenylalanine levels
- large neutral amino acid (tyrosine) replacement, BH4 enzyme treatment, phenylalanine lyase treatment are other options

GALACTOSEMIA

Epidemiology
- 1:60,000; autosomal recessive disease

Etiology
- most commonly due to deficiency of galactose-1-phosphate uridyltransferase leading to an inability to process lactose/galactose

Clinical Presentation
- signs of liver and renal failure, jaundice, FTT, and cataracts with ingestion of lactose/galactose

Management
- elimination of galactose from the diet (e.g. dairy, breast milk)
- most infants are fed a soy-based diet

Complications
- increased risk of sepsis, especially *E. coli*
- if the diagnosis is not made at birth, liver and brain damage may become irreversible

Hematology

Approach to Anemia

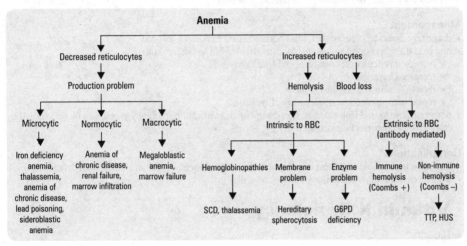

Figure 10. Approach to anemia

Physiologic Anemia

- high Hb (>170 g/L) and reticulocyte count at birth is caused by a hypoxic environment in utero
- after birth, levels start to fall due to shorter fetal RBC lifespan, decreased RBC production (during first 6-8 wk of life, there is virtually no erythropoiesis due to new O_2 rich environment), and increasing blood volume secondary to growth
- lowest levels about 100 g/L at 8-12 wk age (earlier and more exaggerated in premature infants); levels rise spontaneously with activation of erythropoiesis
- usually no treatment required

Iron Deficiency Anemia

- most common cause of childhood anemia
- full term infants exhaust iron reserves by 6 mo of age
- premature infants have lower reserves, therefore exhausted by 2-3 mo of age
- common diagnosis between 6 mo-3 yr and 11-17 yr due to periods of rapid growth and increased iron requirements; adolescents also have poor diet and menstrual losses

Etiology
- children at risk (premature, LBW, low SES, etc.)
- dietary risk factors: whole cow milk in first year of life
- age >6 mo: <2 servings/d of iron-fortified cereal, red meat, or legumes
- age <12 mo: use of low-iron formula (<10 mg/L), primary diet of cow, goat, or soy milk

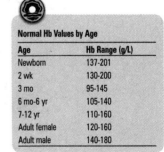

Normal Hb Values by Age	
Age	Hb Range (g/L)
Newborn	137-201
2 wk	130-200
3 mo	95-145
6 mo-6 yr	105-140
7-12 yr	110-160
Adult female	120-160
Adult male	140-180

- age 1-5 yr: >16-20 oz/d of non-fortified milk
- blood loss
  - iatrogenic: repeated blood sampling (especially in hospitalized neonates)
  - allergic: cow milk protein-induced colitis

Clinical Manifestation
- usually asymptomatic until marked anemia, pallor, fatigue, pica (eating non-food materials), tachycardia, systolic murmur, angular cheilitis, koilonychias

Investigations
- CBC: low Hb, MCV, and MCH, reticulocyte count normal or high (absolute number low)
- Mentzer index (MCV/RBC) can help distinguish iron deficiency anemia from thalassemia
  - ratio <13 suggests thalassemia; ratio >13 suggests iron deficiency
- blood smear: hypochromic, microcytic RBCs, pencil shaped cells, poikylocytosis
- iron studies: low ferritin, other (low iron, high total iron binding capacity, high transferrin, low transferrin saturation)
- initial therapy: trial of iron

Prevention
- breastfed term infants: begin iron supplementation (1 mg/kg/d) at 4-6 mo, continuing until able to eat ≥2 feeds/d of iron-rich foods
- non-breastfed (<50% of diet) term infants: give iron-fortified formula from birth
- premature infants: give iron supplements from 1 mo through to 1 yr of age
- no cow's milk until 9-12 mo, early introduction of red meat and iron-rich vegetables: total daily iron should be 11 mg (age 6-12 mo), 7 mg (age 1-3 yr)
- universal screening of Hb levels recommended at 9 mo

Management
- encourage diverse, balanced diet, limit homogenized milk to 16-20 oz/d
- oral iron therapy: 6 mg/kg/d elemental iron, divided bid to tid, for 3 mo
  - increased reticulocyte count in 2-3 d (peaks day 5-7)
  - increased hemoglobin in 4-30 d
  - repletion of iron stores in 1-3 mo
  - repeat hemoglobin levels after 1 mo of treatment
- poor response to oral iron therapy: non-compliance, medication intolerance, ongoing blood loss, IBD, celiac disease, incorrect diagnosis

Complications
- can cause irreversible effects on development if untreated (behavioural and intellectual deficiencies)
- angular cheilitis, glossitis, koilonychia (spoon nails)

Vitamin K Deficiency

Etiology
- hemorrhagic disease of the newborn due to relative deficiencies of vitamin K-dependent coagulation factors
  - generalized bleeding; GI/intracranial hemorrhage
- IM injection at birth, can also be given orally (3 doses: at birth, 2-4 wk, 6-8 wk) but infants at higher risk of HDNB
- reason for administration at birth:
  - human milk contains small amounts of vitamin K, and infants require ingestion of large volumes of human milk to promote GI bacterial colonization
  - until few days after birth, susceptible to vitamin K deficiency

Anemia of Chronic Disease

- see Hematology, H13

Sickle Cell Disease

- see Hematology, H20

Thalassemia

- see Hematology, H18

MCV in childhood varies with age
Rule of thumb: lower normal limit of MCV = 70 + age (yr) until 80 fL (adult standard)

Ferritin is an acute phase reactant, therefore, normal or high ferritin does not exclude iron deficiency anemia during an infection

Iron deficiency is rare in children <6 mo in the absence of blood loss or prematurity

Hereditary Spherocytosis

- see Hematology, H22

Glucose-6-Phosphate Dehydrogenase Deficiency

- see Hematology, H23

G6PD deficiency protects against parasitism of RBCs (i.e. malaria)

Bleeding Disorders

- see Hematology, H27

Table 22. Evaluation of Abnormal Bruising/Bleeding

	PFA	PT	PTT	VIII:C	vWF	Platelets	Fibrinogen
Hemophilia A	N	N	↑	↓	N	N	N
Hemophilia B	N	N	↑	N	N	N	N
von Willebrand Disease	↑	N	N or ↑	↓	↓	N	N
DIC	N or ↑	↑	↑	↓	N	↓	↓
Vitamin K Deficiency	N	↑	↑	N	N	N	N
Thrombocytopenia	↑	N	N	N	N	↓	N

DIC = disseminated intravascular coagulation; PFA = platelet function assay; VIII:C = Factor VIII coagulant activity; vWF = von Willebrand Factor

Extensive bruising in the absence of lab abnormalities: consider child maltreatment

Immune Thrombocytopenic Purpura

Epidemiology
- most common cause of thrombocytopenia in childhood
- peak age: 2-6 yr, M=F
- incidence 5:100,000 children per year

Etiology
- caused by autoantibodies that bind to platelet membranes → Fc-receptor mediated splenic uptake → destruction of platelets

Clinical Presentation
- 50% present 1-3 wk after viral illness (URTI, chicken pox)
- sudden onset of petechiae, purpura, epistaxis in an otherwise well child
- clinically significant bleed in only 3% (severe bleed more likely with platelet count <10) with <0.5% risk of intracranial bleed
- no lymphadenopathy, no hepatosplenomegaly
- labs: thrombocytopenia with normal RBC, WBC
- bone marrow aspirate only if atypical presentation (≥1 cell line abnormal, hepatosplenomegaly)
- differential diagnosis: leukemia, drug-induced thrombocytopenia, HIV, infection (viral), autoimmune (SLE, ALPS)

Management
- observation vs. pharmacologic intervention highly debated; spontaneous recovery in >70% of cases within 3 mo
- treatment with IVIg or prednisone if mucosal or internal bleeding, platelets <10, or at risk of significant bleeding (surgery, dental procedure, concomitant vasculitis or coagulopathy)
- life-threatening bleed: additional platelet transfusion ± emergency splenectomy
- persistent (>3-12 mo) or chronic (>12 mo): re-evaluate; treat if symptoms persist
- supportive: avoid contact sports and ASA/NSAIDs

The American Society of Hematology 2011 Evidence-Based Practice Guideline for Immune Thrombocytopenia
Blood 2011;117(16):4190-207
Recommendations
- Bone marrow examination is unnecessary in children and adolescents with the typical features of ITP.
- Bone marrow examination is not necessary in children who fail IVIg therapy (grade 1B).
- Children with no bleeding or mild bleeding (defined as skin manifestations only, such as bruising and petechiae) may be managed with observation alone regardless of platelet count.
- For pediatric patients requiring treatment, a single dose of IVIg (0.8-1 g/kg) or a short course of corticosteroids may be used as first-line treatment.
- IVIg can be used if a more rapid increase in the platelet count is desired.
- Anti-D therapy is not advised in children with a hemoglobin concentration that is decreased due to bleeding, or with evidence of autoimmune hemolysis.

Suggestions
- Bone marrow examination is also not necessary in similar patients prior to initiation of treatment with corticosteroids or before splenectomy.
- Testing for antinuclear antibodies is not necessary in the evaluation of children and adolescents with suspected ITP.
- A single dose of anti-D can be used as first-line treatment in Rh-positive, nonsplenectomized children requiring treatment.

Hemophilia

- see Hematology, H31

von Willebrand's Disease

- see Hematology, H30

Oncology

- cancer is the second most common cause of death after injuries in children after 1 yr of age
- cause is rarely known, but increased risk for children with: chromosomal syndromes (e.g. Trisomy 21), cancer predisposition syndromes (e.g. Li-Fraumeni syndrome), prior malignancies, neurocutaneous syndromes, immunodeficiency syndromes, family history, exposure to radiation, chemicals, biologic agents
- leukemias are the most common type of pediatric malignancy (30%) followed by brain tumours (25%), and lymphomas (15%)
- some malignancies are more prevalent in certain age groups
  - newborns: neuroblastoma, Wilms' tumour, retinoblastoma
  - infancy and childhood: leukemia, neuroblastoma, CNS tumours, Wilms' tumour, retinoblastoma
  - adolescence: lymphoma, gonadal tumours, germ cell tumours, bone tumours
- unique treatment considerations in pediatrics because radiation, chemotherapy, and surgery can impact growth and development, endocrine function, and fertility
- good prognosis: treatments have led to remarkable improvements in overall survival and cure rates for many pediatric cancers (>80%)

Lymphadenopathy

Clinical Presentations
- features of malignant lymphadenopathy: firm, discrete, non-tender, enlarging, immobile ± suspicious mass/imaging findings ± constitutional symptoms
- fluctuance, warmth, or tenderness are more suggestive of benign nodes (infection)

Differential Diagnosis
- infection
  - viral: URTI, EBV, CMV, adenovirus, HIV
  - bacterial: *S. aureus*, GAS, anaerobes, *Mycobacterium* (e.g. TB), cat scratch disease (*Bartonella*)
  - other: fungal, protozoan, *Rickettsia*
- autoimmune: rheumatoid arthritis, SLE, serum sickness
- malignancy: lymphoma, leukemia, metastatic solid tumours
- storage diseases: Niemann-Pick, Gaucher's
- other: sarcoidosis, Kawasaki disease, histiocytoses

Most common cause of acute bilateral cervical LAD is viral illness

Investigations
- generalized lymphadenopathy
  - CBC and differential, blood culture
  - uric acid, LDH
  - ANA, RF, ESR
  - EBV/CMV/HIV serology
  - toxoplasma titre
  - fungal serology
  - CXR
  - TB tests
  - biopsy
- regional lymphadenopathy
  - period of observation if asymptomatic
  - trial of oral antibiotics
  - ultrasound
  - biopsy (especially if persistent >6 wk and/or constitutional symptoms)

Leukemia

- see <u>Hematology</u>, H37

Epidemiology
- mean age of diagnosis 2-5 yr but can occur at any age
- heterogeneous group of diseases
  - ALL (80%)
  - AML (15%)
  - CML (<5%)
- children with DS are 15x more likely to develop leukemia

Clinical Presentation
- infiltration of leukemic cells into bone marrow results in bone pain and bone marrow failure (anemia, neutropenia, thrombocytopenia)
- infiltration into tissues results in lymphadenopathy, hepatosplenomegaly, CNS manifestations, testicular disease
- fever, fatigue, weight loss, bruising, and easy bleeding
- hyperleukocytosis (total WBC >100 x 10^9/L) is a medical emergency
  - presents clinically with respiratory or neurological distress caused by hyperviscosity of blood and leukostasis
  - risk of ICH, pulmonary leukostasis syndrome, tumour lysis syndrome
  - management: fluids, allopurinol/rasburicase, fresh frozen plasma/platelets to correct thrombocytopenia, induction chemotherapy, avoid transfusing RBCs unless symptomatic (and then use very small volumes)

Management
- combination chemotherapy using non-cross resistant chemotherapy agents, allogeneic stem cell transplantation for high-grade or recurrent disease
- supportive care and management of treatment complications
    - febrile neutropenia: see Infectious Diseases, ID45
    - tumour lysis syndrome: see Hematology, H52

Prognosis
- 80-90% 5 yr event-free survival for ALL, 50-60% 5-yr survival for AML
- patients are stratified into standard risk and high risk based on WBC and age; other prognostic factors include presence of CNS/testicular disease, immunophenotype, cytogenetics, and initial response to therapy (most important prognostic variable)

Lymphoma

- see Hematology, H45

Epidemiology
- Hodgkin lymphoma: incidence is bimodal, peaks at ages 15-34 and >50 yr old
- non-Hodgkin lymphoma: incidence peaks at 7-11 yr

Clinical Presentation
- Hodgkin lymphoma
    - most common presentation is persistent, painless, firm, cervical or supraclavicular lymphadenopathy
    - can present as persistent cough or dyspnea (secondary to mediastinal mass) or less commonly as splenomegaly, axillary, or inguinal lymphadenopathy
    - constitutional symptoms in 30% of children
    - lymph nodes become sequentially involved as disease spreads
- non-Hodgkin lymphoma
    - generally categorized into lymphoblastic, large cell, and Burkitt's/Burkitt's-like lymphoma
    - rapidly growing tumour with distant metastases (unlike adult non-Hodgkin lymphoma)
    - signs and symptoms related to disease site: most commonly abdomen, chest (mediastinal mass), head and neck region

Back pain in children must always be investigated!
Unlike adults, back pain in children often points to a pathological process

Management
- Hodgkin lymphoma
    - combination chemotherapy and radiation
    - aimed at limiting cumulative doses of anthracyclines (toxic to heart) and alkylators (risk of second malignancy, infertility) and limiting dose and field of radiation
    - increasing role for use of PET scanning to assess early disease response and plan therapy
- non-Hodgkin lymphoma
    - combination chemotherapy
    - no added benefit of radiation in pediatric protocols

Constitutional symptoms = fever, chills, night sweats, unexplained weight loss

Prognosis
- Hodgkin lymphoma: >90% 5 yr survival
- non-Hodgkin lymphoma: 75-90% 5 yr survival

Brain Tumours

- see Neurosurgery, NS11

Wilms' Tumour (Nephroblastoma)

Epidemiology
- usually diagnosed between 2-5 yr; M=F
    - most common primary renal neoplasm of childhood
    - 5-10% of cases both kidneys are affected (simultaneously or in sequence)

Differential Diagnosis
- hydronephrosis, polycystic kidney disease, renal cell carcinoma, neuroblastoma

Clinical Presentation
- 80% present with asymptomatic, unilateral abdominal mass
- may also present with HTN, gross hematuria, abdominal pain, vomiting
- may have pulmonary metastases at time of diagnosis (respiratory symptoms)

Oncology

Associated Congenital Abnormalities
- **WAGR** syndrome (**W**ilms' tumour, **A**niridia, **G**enital anomalies, mental **R**etardation) with 11p13 deletion
- Beckwith-Wiedemann syndrome:
  - characterized by enlargement of body organs (especially tongue), hemihypertrophy, renal medullary cysts, and adrenal cytomegaly
  - also at increased risk for developing hepatoblastoma, and less commonly adrenocortical tumours, neuroblastomas, and rhabdomyosarcomas
- Denys-Drash syndrome: characterized by gonadal dysgenesis and nephropathy leading to renal failure

Management
- staging ± nephrectomy
- chemotherapy, radiation for higher stages

Prognosis
- 90% long-term survival

Neuroblastoma

Epidemiology
- most common cancer occurring in first year of life
- neural crest cell tumour arising from sympathetic tissues (neuroblasts)

Clinical Presentation
- can originate from any site in sympathetic nervous system, presenting as mass in neck, chest, or abdomen (most common site is adrenal gland)
- signs and symptoms of disease vary with location of tumour
  - thoracic: dyspnea, Horner's syndrome
  - abdomen: palpable mass
  - spinal cord compression
- metastases are common at presentation (>50% present with advanced stage disease):
  - usually to bone or bone marrow (presents as bone pain, limp)
  - can also present with periorbital ecchymoses, abdominal pain, emesis, fever, weight loss, anorexia, hepatomegaly, "blueberry muffin" skin nodules
- paraneoplastic: HTN, palpitations, sweating (from excessive catecholamines), diarrhea, FTT (from vasoactive intestinal peptide secretion), opsomyoclonus

Management
- depends on prognostic factors and may include combination of: surgery, radiation, chemotherapy, autologous stem cell transplantation, immunotherapy

Prognosis
- prognosis is often poor due to late detection
- good prognostic factors
  - "age and stage" are important determinants of better outcome: <18 mo, stage I, II, IV-S disease ("S" designates a "Special" classification only pertaining to infants)
  - primary site: posterior mediastinum and neck
  - low serum ferritin
  - more differentiated histology
  - tumour cell markers: aneuploidy, absent *MYCN* oncogene amplification

Bone Tumours

- see Orthopedics, OR45

Cancer Predisposition Syndromes

- suspected in cases of multiple primary neoplasms, especially early onset for cancer type and/or family history consistent with known cancer predisposition syndrome (critical to obtain family history and refer if syndrome suspected)
- cancer predisposition syndromes with pediatric onset include Li-Fraumeni syndrome (soft tissue sarcomas, osteosarcoma, CNS tumours and adrenal cortical carcinoma), hereditary retinoblastoma and Fanconi anemia (leukemias)

Infectious Diseases

Fever

Definition
- fever: a practical definition is >38°C/100.4°F oral or rectal
- fever without a source/focus: acute febrile illness (typically <10 d duration) with no cause of fever even after careful history and physical
- fever of unknown origin: daily or intermittent fevers for at least 2 consecutive weeks of uncertain cause after careful history and physical, and initial laboratory assessment

Etiology
- infectious: anatomic approach (CNS, ears, upper and lower respiratory tract, GI, GU, skin, soft tissue, bones and joints, etc.)
- inflammatory: mainly autoimmune (Kawasaki disease, JIA, IBD, SLE, etc.)
- malignancy: childhood cancers (leukemia, lymphoma, neuroblastoma, etc.)
- miscellaneous: dehydration, drugs and toxins, post-immunization, familial dysautonomia, factitious disorder, etc.

Diagnosis
- history: duration, height and pattern of fever, associated symptoms, exposures, constitutional symptoms, recent antipyretic use, ethnic or genetic background, day care, sick contacts, travel, tick bites, age of child
- physical exam: toxic vs. non-toxic, vitals, growth, complete exams of the skin, HEENT, chest, abdomen, lymph nodes, genitalia
- investigations: guided by history, physical exam, and clinical suspicion

Evaluation of Neonates and Infants with Fever
- several protocols exist that attempt to identify neonates and young infants at low risk of serious bacterial infection (e.g. Rochester Criteria)
  - such protocols are not as sensitive in the 1-28 d age group; therefore, febrile neonates should be considered high risk regardless of clinical presentation and laboratory findings

Management
- admit to hospital if appropriate
- treat the source if known
- replace fluid losses (e.g. from vomiting, diarrhea, etc.); maintenance fluid needs are higher in febrile child
- reassure parents that most fevers are benign and self-limited
- antipyretics (acetaminophen and/or ibuprofen) are not necessary in most cases, but can be given if child is uncomfortable

Rochester Criteria – Developed to Identify Infants ≤60 d of Age with Fever at Low Risk of Serious Bacterial Infection

Clinically	Well
WBC Count	5-15 x 10⁹/L
Bands	<1.5 x 10⁹/L
Urinalysis	<10 WBC/HPF
Stool (if diarrhea)	<5 WBC/HPF
Past Health	Born >37 wk
	Home with/before mom
	No hospitalizations
	No prior antibiotic use
	No prior treatment for unexplained hyperbilirubinemia
	No chronic disease

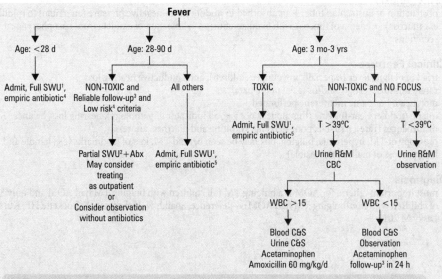

NOTES
1. SWU = Septic Workup
2. Partial Septic Workup – blood C&S, CBC and differential, urine R&M, C&S, LP, CXR if respiratory symptoms, stool C&S if GI symptoms
3. Follow-up is crucial – if adequate follow-up is not assured, a more aggressive diagnostic and therapeutic approach may be indicated
4. Low-risk (Rochester) criteria
5. Considerable practice variation exists in terms of empiric antibiotic treatment
6. Important principles – the younger the child, the greater the difficulty to clinically assess the degree of illness

Figure 11. Approach to the febrile child

Clinical Assessment of AOM in Pediatrics
JAMA 2010;304:2161-2169
In assessment of AOM in pediatrics, ear pain is the most useful symptom with a LR between 3.0 and 7.3. Useful otoscopic signs include erythematous (LR 8.4, 95% CI 7-11), cloudy (LR 34, 95% CI 28-42), bulging (LR 51, 95% CI 36-73), and immobile tympanic membrane on pneumatic otoscopy (LR 31, 95% CI 26-37).

The Diagnosis and Management of Acute Otitis Media
Pediatrics 2013;131:e964-e999
Recommendations
• Management of AOM should include an assessment of pain; if pain is present, the clinician should recommend treatment to reduce pain.
• Prescribe antibiotic therapy for AOM (bilateral or unilateral) in children 6 mo and older with severe signs or symptoms (i.e. moderate or severe otalgia or otalgia for at least 48 h or temperature 39°C [102.2°F] or higher).
• For bilateral or unilateral AOM in children 6 mo through 23 mo of age without severe signs or symptoms (i.e. mild otalgia for less than 48 h and temperature less than 39°C [102.2°F]) either prescribe antibiotic therapy or offer observation with close follow-up based on joint decision-making with the parent(s)/caregiver(s). With observation ensure follow-up and begin antibiotic therapy if the child worsens or fails to improve within 48-72 h of onset of symptoms.
• Do NOT prescribe prophylactic antibiotics to reduce the frequency of episodes of AOM in children with recurrent AOM.
• Recommend annual influenza vaccine and pneumococcal conjugate vaccine to all children according to vaccination schedule.
Option
• Offer tympanostomy tubes for recurrent AOM (3 episodes in 6 mo or 4 episodes in 1 yr with 1 episode in the preceding 6 mo).

Acute Otitis Media

All of:
1. presence of middle ear effusion
2. presence of middle ear inflammation
3. acute onset of symptoms of middle ear effusion and inflammation

Epidemiology
• 60-70% of children have at least 1 episode of AOM before 3 yr of age
• 18 mo-6 yr most common age group
  ▪ 22% of children in this age range will develop AOM in the first week of a viral URI
• one third of children have had ≥3 episodes by age 3; peak incidence January to April

Etiology
• *S. pneumoniae*: 32% of cases (decreasing since the introduction of PCV7 and PCV 13)
  ▪ *H. influenzae* (non-typeable): >50% of refractory AOM
• *M. catarrhalis*: 14% of cases - less virulent
• GAS
• viral – more likely to spontaneously resolve
• less common - anaerobes (newborns) , Gram-negative enterics (infants)

Predisposing Factors
• Eustachian tube dysfunction/obstruction
  ▪ swelling of tubal mucosa: URTI, allergic rhinitis, chronic rhinosinusitis
  ▪ obstruction/infiltration of Eustachian tube ostium: adenoid hypertrophy (not due to obstruction but by maintaining a source of infection), barotrauma (sudden changes in air pressure)
  ▪ inadequate tensor palatini function: cleft palate (even after repair)
• abnormal Eustachian tube: gentic syndromes such as DS, Crouzon, Apert
• disruption of action of cilia of Eustachian tube: Kartagener's syndrome, CF
• immunosuppression/deficiency due to chemotherapy, steroids, DM, hypogammaglobulinemia, CF

Risk Factors
• prolonged bottle feeding, while laying down and/or shorter duration of breast feeding
  ▪ pacifier use
• second-hand smoke
• crowded living conditions (day care/group child care facilities) or sick contacts
• family history of otitis media
• orofacial abnormalities
• immunideficiency
• ethnicity – First Nations and Inuit
  ▪ FOR recurrent AOM: lower levels of secretory IgA or persistent biofilms in the middle ear

Pathogenesis
• obstruction of Eustachian tube → air absorbed in middle ear → negative pressure (an irritant to middle ear mucosa) → edema of mucosa with exudate/effusion → infection of exudate from nasopharyngeal secretions

Clinical Features
• triad of otalgia, fever (especially in younger children), and conductive hearing loss
• rarely tinnitus, vertigo, and/or facial nerve paralysis
• otorrhea if tympanic membrane perforated
• infants/toddlers: ear-tugging (this alone is not a good indicator of pathology), hearing loss, balance disturbances (rare), irritable, poor sleeping, vomiting and diarrhea, anorexia
• otoscopy of TM: hyperemia, bulging, pus may be seen behind TM, loss of landmarks (e.g. handle and long process of malleus not visible)

Diagnosis
• most important criteria for AOM is a bulging TM (all children with bulging TM had AOM and only 8% of children with non-bulging TM had AOM) – Reference: Shaikh N, Hoberman A, Rockette HE, Kurs-Lasky M 2012

Management

- 1st line
  - amoxicillin 75-90 mg/kg/d divided into two doses: safe, effective, and inexpensive. Use high doses to overcome MIC for penicillin binding proteins (method of resistance)
  - if penicillin allergic: macrolide (clarithromycin, azithromycin – high resistance), trimethoprim-sulphamethoxazole (Bactrim®)
- 2nd line
  - amoxicillin-clavulanic acid (Clavulin®)
  - cephalosporins: cefuroxime axetil (Ceftin®), ceftriaxone (Rocephin®), cefaclor (Ceclor®), cefixime (Suprax®)
  - AOM deemed unresponsive if clinical signs/symptoms and otoscopic findings persist beyond 48 h of antibiotic treatment
  - use second line treatment for otitis-conjunctivitis syndrome (AOM with bacterial conjunctivitis) because *H. influenzae* and *M. catarrhalis* are more likely pathogens which are Beta lactamase producing, so Amoxil is ineffective
- symptomatic therapy: antipyretics/analgesics (e.g. acetaminophen), decongestants (may relieve nasal congestion but does not treat AOM)
- prevention: parent education about risk factors, pneumococcal and influenza vaccines, surgery (e.g. tympanostomy tubes)
  - choice of surgical therapy for recurrent AOM depends on whether local factors (Eustachian tube dysfunction) are responsible (use ventilation tubes), or regional disease factors (tonsillitis, adenoid hypertrophy, sinusitis) are responsible

Complications

- extracranial: hearing loss and speech delay (secondary to persistent middle ear effusion), TM perforation, extension of suppurative process to adjacent structures (mastoiditis, petrositis, labyrinthitis), cholesteatoma, facial nerve palsy, middle ear atelectasis, ossicular necrosis, vestibular dysfunction
- intracranial: meningitis, epidural and brain abscess, subdural empyema, lateral and cavernous sinus thrombosis, carotid artery thrombosis

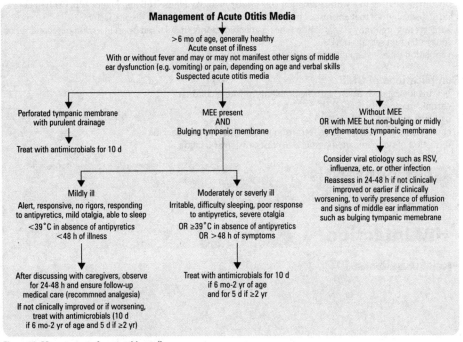

Figure 12. Management of acute otitis media
Flow diagram for the management of children with suspected and confirmed acute otitis media – from CPS statement Feb 2016

Otitis Media with Effusion

Definition
• presence of fluid in the middle ear without signs or symptoms of ear infection

Epidemiology
• most common cause of pediatric hearing loss
• not exclusively a pediatric disease
• follows AOM frequently in children
• middle ear effusions have been shown to persist following an episode of AOM for 1 mo in 40% of children, 2 mo in 20%, and >3 mo in 10%

Risk Factors
• same as AOM

Clinical Features
• conductive hearing loss ± tinnitus
• fullness – blocked ear
• ± pain, low grade fever
• otoscopy of TM
    ▪ discolouration – amber or dull grey
    ▪ meniscus fluid level behind TM
    ▪ air bubbles
    ▪ retraction pockets/TM atelectasis
    ▪ flat tympanogram
    ▪ most reliable finding with pneumatic otoscopy is immobility

Treatment

• expectant: 90% resolve by 3 mo
• document hearing loss with audiogram (see <u>Otolaryngology</u> Figure 16B and Figure 17B, OT10-11)
• no statistical proof that antihistamines, decongestants, antibiotics clear disease faster
• surgery: myringotomy ± ventilation tubes ± adenoidectomy (if enlarged or on insertion of second set of tubes after first set falls out)
• ventilation tubes to equalize pressure and drain ear

Complications of OME
• hearing loss, speech delay, learning problems in young children
• chronic mastoiditis
• ossicular erosion
• cholesteatoma especially when retraction pockets involve pars flaccida
• retraction of tympanic membrane, atelectasis, ossicular fixation

Gastroenteritis

• see *Gastroenterology*, P34

HIV Infection

• see <u>Infectious Diseases</u>, ID27

Infectious Pediatric Exanthems

Table 23. Common Infectious Pediatric Exanthems

Disease	Pathogen(s)	Incubation Period	Communicability	Mode of Transmission	Rash	Associated Features	Management	Outcomes and Complications
Erythema Infectiosum (i.e. Fifth Disease/ Slapped Cheek)	Parvovirus B19	4-14 d	Low risk of transmission once symptomatic	Respiratory secretions or infected blood	Appearance: uniform, erythematous maculopapular 'lacy' rash; Timing: 10-17 d after symptoms (immune response); Distribution: bilateral cheeks ('slapped cheeks') with circumoral sparing; may affect trunk and extremities	Initial 7-10 d of flu-like illness and fever; Rash may be warm, non-tender, and pruritic; Less common presentations include 'gloves and socks syndrome' or STAR complex (sore throat, arthritis, rash)	Supportive	Rash fades over days to week, but may reappear months later with sunlight, exercise; Aplastic crisis
Gianotti-Crosti Syndrome (i.e. Papular Acrodermatitis)	EBV and Hep B (majority)	Variable	None	—	Appearance: asymptomatic symmetric papules; Distribution: face, cheeks, extensor surfaces of the extremities, spares trunk	Viral prodrome; May have lymphadenopathy and/or hepatosplenomegaly	Supportive; Pain control	Resolves in 3-12 wk
Hand, Foot, and Mouth Disease	Coxsackie group A	3-5 d	Likely 1-7 d after symptoms but may be up to months	Direct and indirect contact with infected bodily fluids, fecal-oral	Appearance: vesicles and pustules on an erythematous base; Distribution: acral, but may exetend up the extremity	Enanthem: vesicles in the POSTERIOR oral cavity (pharynx, tongue)	Supportive	Mainly dehydration
Herpes Simplex	HSV 1,2	1-26 d		Direct contact, often through saliva for HSV-1 and sexual contact for HSV-2	Grouped vesicles on an erythematous base	Enanthem: vesicles/erosions in the ANTERIOR oral cavity (buccal mucosa, tongue); May present with herpetic whitlow (autoinoculation)	Mainly supportive; Consider oral or topical antivirals	Local: secondary skin infections, keratitis, gingivostomatitis; CNS: encephalitis; Disseminated hepatitis, DIC; Eczema herpeticum
Kawasaki Disease	See P92							
Measles	Morbillivirus	8-13 d	4 d before and after rash	Airborne	Appearance: erythematous maculopapular; Timing: 3 d after start of symptoms; Distribution: starts at hairline and spreads downwards with sparing of palms and soles	Prodome of cough, coryza, conjunctivitis (3 Cs); Enanthem: Koplik's spots 1-2 d before rash; Desquamation; Positive serology for measles IgM	Infected: supportive; Unimmunized contacts: measles vaccine within 72 h of exposure or IgG within 6 d of exposure; Respiratory isolation, report to Public Health; Prevention: MMR vaccine	Secondary bacterial infections: AOM, sinusitis, pneumonia; Encephalitis; Rare: myocarditis, pericarditis, thrombocytopenia, Stevens-Johnson syndrome, GN, subacute sclerosing panencephalitis

Table 23. Common Infectious Pediatric Exanthems (continued)

Disease	Pathogen(s)	Incubation Period	Communicability	Mode of Transmission	Rash	Associated Features	Management	Outcomes and Complications
Non-Specific Enteroviral Exanthems	Enteroviruses	Variable	Variable	Direct and indirect contact with infected bodily fluids	Polymorphous rash (macules, papules, vesicles, petechiae, urticaria)	Systemic involvement is rare, but possible	Supportive. Diagnosis confirmed using viral cultures (NP and rectal swabs)	Self-limiting
Roseola	HHV 6	5-15 d	Unknown	—	Appearance: blanching, pink, maculopapular. Timing: appears once fever subsides. Distribution: starts at the neck and trunk and spreads to the face and extremities	High grade fever. Common: irritability, anorexia, lymphadenopathy, erythematous TM and pharynx, Nagayama spots (erythematous papules on soft palate and uvula). Less common: cough, coryza, bulging fontanelles	Supportive	CNS: febrile seizures (10-25%), aseptic meningitis. Thrombocytopenia
Rubella	Rubivirus	14-21 d	7 d before and after eruptions	Droplet	Appearance: pink, maculopapular. Timing: 1-5 d after start of symptoms. Distribution: starts on face and spreads to neck and trunk	Prodrome of low grade fever and occipital/retroauricular nodes. STAR complex (sore throat, arthritis, rash). Positive serology for rubella IgM. Caution to pregnant women with exposure	Infected: supportive. Prevention: MMR vaccine. Report to Public Health	Excellent prognosis with acquired disease. Arthritis may last days to weeks. Encephalitis. Irreversible defects in congenitally infected patients (i.e. congenital rubella syndrome)
Scarlet Fever	See P58							
Varicella	Varicella zoster virus	0-21 d	1-2 d pre-eruptions and 5 d post-eruption	Mainly airborne, but also through direct contact with vesicle fluid	Appearance: groups of skin lesions, polymorphic, from macules to papules to vesicles to crusts. Timing: 1-3 d after start of symptoms. Distribution: generalized	Significant pruritus. Enanthem: vesicular lesions which may become pustular or ulcerate. Caution to pregnant women	Supportive. Avoid salicylates (due to risk of Reye syndrome). Consider antivirals. Respiratory and contact isolation, report to Public Health. Prevention: varicella vaccine	Skin: bacterial suprainfection, necrotizing fasciitis. CNS: acute encephalitis and cerebellar ataxia. Systemic: hepatitis, DIC. Congenital varicella syndrome if intrapartum infection

Infectious Mononucleosis

Definition
- systemic viral infection caused by EBV with multivisceral involvement; often called "the great imitator"

Epidemiology
- peak incidence between 15-19 yr old
- ~50% of children in developed countries have a primary EBV infection by 5 yr old, but <10% of children develop clinical infection

Etiology
- EBV: a member of herpesviridae
- transmission is mainly through infected saliva ("kissing disease") and sexual activity (less commonly); incubation period of 1-2 mo

Risk Factors
- infectious contacts, sexually active, multiple sexual partners in the past

History
- prodrome: 2-3 d of malaise, anorexia
- infants and young children: often asymptomatic or mild disease
- older children and adolescents: malaise, fatigue, fever, sore throat, abdominal pain (often LUQ), headache, myalgia

Physical Exam
- classic triad: febrile, generalized non-tender lymphadenopathy, pharyngitis/tonsillitis (exudative)
- ± hepatosplenomegaly
- ± periorbital edema, ± rash (urticarial, maculopapular, or petechial) – more common after inappropriate treatment with β-lactam antibiotics
- any "-itis" (including arthritis, hepatitis, nephritis, myocarditis, meningitis, encephalitis, etc.)

Investigations
- heterophil antibody test (Monospot® test)
  - 85% sensitive in adults and older children, but only 50% sensitive if <4 yr of age
  - false positive results with HIV, SLE, lymphoma, rubella, parvovirus
- EBV titres
- CBC and differential, blood smear: reactive lymphocytes, lymphocytosis, Downey cells ± anemia ± thrombocytopenia
- throat culture to rule out streptococcal pharyngitis

Management
- supportive: adequate rest, hydration, saline gargles, and analgesics for sore throat
- splenic enlargement is often not clinically apparent so all patients should avoid contact sports for 6-8 wk
- if airway obstruction secondary to nodal and/or tonsillar enlargement is present (especially younger children), admit for steroid therapy
- acyclovir does NOT reduce duration of symptoms or result in earlier return to school/work

Prognosis
- most acute symptoms resolve in 1-2 wk, though fatigue may last for months
- short-term complications: splenic rupture, Guillain-Barré syndrome

Infectious Pharyngitis/Tonsillitis

Definition
- inflammation of the pharynx, especially the tonsils if present, causing a sore throat

Etiology
- viral (~80%): adenoviruses, enteroviruses, coxsackie, upper respiratory tract viruses, EBV, CMV
- bacterial (~20%): mainly GAS, *M. pneumoniae* (older children), *N. gonorrhoeae* (sexually active), *C. diphtheriae* (unvaccinated), *Fusobacterium necrophorum* (anaerobe causing Lemierre syndrome)
- fungal: *Candida*

Epidemiology
- season: GAS pharyngitis more common in late winter or early spring; viral all year long
- age: GAS pharyngitis peak incidence at 5-12 yr of age and uncommon <3 yr; viral pharyngitis affects all ages

History
- GAS: sore throat (may be severe), fever, malaise, headache, abdominal pain, N/V, absence of other URTI symptoms
- viral: sore throat (often mild), conjunctivitis, cough, rhinorrhea, hoarseness, diarrhea, flu-like symptoms (fever, malaise, myalgias)

Physical Exam
- GAS: febrile, pharyngeal/tonsillar erythema and exudates, enlarged (>1 cm) and tender anterior cervical lymph nodes, palatal petechiae, strawberry tongue, scarlatiniform rash
- viral: afebrile, absent/mild tonsillar exudates, minor and non-tender adenopathy, viral exanthems

Investigations
- no single sign or symptom reliably identifies GAS as the causative organism in children with sore throat
- scores are used to predict if throat culture will be positive (e.g. McIsaac Criteria)
    - these score systems have not been found to be sensitive or specific enough to diagnose GAS in children and adolescents with sore throat
- suspected diagnosis of GAS pharyngitis should be confirmed with a rapid streptococcal antigen test and a follow-up throat culture if the rapid test is negative

Management
- antibiotics (for GAS/*S. pyogenes*)
    - penicillin V or amoxicillin or erythromycin (if penicillin allergy) x 10 d
    - can prevent rheumatic fever if given within 9 d of symptoms; does NOT alter risk of post-streptococcal GN
- supportive: hydration and acetaminophen for discomfort due to pain and/or fever
- follow-up: if uncomplicated course, no follow-up or post-antibiotic throat cultures needed
- prophylaxis: consider tonsillectomy for proven, recurrent streptococcal tonsillitis

Complications
- preventable with antibiotics: AOM, sinusitis, cervical adenitis, mastoiditis, retropharyngeal/peritonsillar abscess, sepsis
- immune-mediated complications: scarlet fever, acute rheumatic fever, post-streptococcal GN, reactive arthritis, pediatric autoimmune neuropsychiatric disorder associated with group A streptococci (i.e. PANDAS)

McIsaac Criteria (if >3 yr old)

HOT LACE
HOT – Fever >38°C
Lymphadenopathy (anterior cervical, tender)
Age 3-14 yr
No Cough
Erythematous, exudative tonsils
CMAJ 1998;158(1):75-83

SCARLET FEVER
- diffuse erythematous eruption
- delayed-type hypersensitivity reaction to pyrogenic exotoxin produced by GAS
- acute onset of fever, sore throat, strawberry tongue
- 24-48 h after pharyngitis, rash begins in the groin, axillae, neck, antecubital fossa; Pastia's lines may be accentuated in flexural areas
- within 24 h, sandpaper rash becomes generalized with perioral sparing, non-pruritic, non-painful, blanchable
- rash fades after 3-4 d, may be followed by desquamation
- treatment is penicillin, amoxicillin, or erythromycin x 10 d

RHEUMATIC FEVER
- inflammatory disease due to antibody cross-reactivity following GAS infection
- affects ~1:10,000 children in developed world; much more prevalent in developing nations; peak incidence at 5-15 yr of age
- mainly a clinical diagnosis based on Jones Criteria (revised)
    - requires 2 major OR 1 major and 2 minor PLUS evidence of preceding strep infection (history of scarlet fever, GAS pharyngitis culture, positive rapid Ag detection test, ASOTs)
- treatment: penicillin or erythromycin for acute course x 10 d, prednisone if severe carditis
- secondary prophylaxis with daily penicillin or erythromycin
- complications
    - acute: myocarditis, conduction system aberrations (sinus tachycardia, atrial fibrillation), valvulitis (acute MR), pericarditis
    - chronic: valvular heart disease (mitral and/or aortic insufficiency/stenosis), infectious endocarditis ± thromboembolic phenomenon
    - onset of symptoms usually after 10-20 yr latency from acute carditis of rheumatic fever

POST-STREPTOCOCCAL GLOMERULONEPHRITIS
- most common in children aged 4-8 yr old; M>F
- antigen-antibody mediated complement activation with diffuse, proliferative GN
- occurs 1-3 wk following initial GAS infection (skin or throat)
- clinical presentation varies from asymptomatic, microscopic and macroscopic hematuria (cola-coloured urine) to all features of nephritic syndrome (see *Nephritic Syndrome*, P77)
- diagnosis is confirmed with elevated serum antibody titres against streptococcal antigens (ASOT, anti-DNAse B), low serum complement (C3)
- management
    - symptomatic: fluid and sodium restrictions; loop diuretics for HTN and edema
    - in severe cases, may require dialysis if renal function significantly impaired
    - treat with penicillin or erythromycin if evidence of persistent GAS infection
- 95% of children recover completely within 1-2 wk; 5-10% have persistent hematuria

Meningitis

Definition
- inflammation of the meninges surrounding the brain and spinal cord

Epidemiology
- peak age: 6-12 mo; 90% of cases occur in children <5 yr old

Etiology
- viral: enteroviruses, HSV
- bacterial: age-related variation in specific pathogens
- fungal and parasitic meningitis also possible
- most often due to hematogenous spread or direct extension from a contiguous site

Risk Factors
- unvaccinated
- immunocompromised: asplenia, DM, HIV, prematurity
- recent or current infections: AOM, sinusitis, orbital cellulitis
- neuroanatomical: congenital defects, dermal sinus, neurosurgery, cochlear implants, recent head trauma
- exposures: day care centres, household contact, recent travel

History
- signs and symptoms variable and dependent on age, duration of illness, and host response to infection
- infants: fever, lethargy, irritability, poor feeding, vomiting, diarrhea, respiratory distress, seizures
- children: fever, headache, photophobia, N/V, confusion, back/neck pain/stiffness, lethargy, irritability

Physical Exam
- infants: toxic, hypothermia, bulging anterior fontanelle, respiratory distress, apnea, petechial/purpuric rash, jaundice
- children: toxic, ↓ LOC, nuchal rigidity, Kernig's and Brudzinski's signs, focal neurologic findings, petechial/purpuric rash

Investigations
- blood work: CBC, electrolytes, Cr, BUN, glucose, C&S
- LP required for definitive diagnosis
  - Gram stain, bacterial C&S, WBC count and differential, RBC count, glucose, protein concentration
  - acid-fast stain if suspect TB
  - PCR for specific bacteria if available (helpful if already treated with antibiotics)
  - urinalysis and urine C&S in infants, Gram stain and culture of petechial/purpuric lesions
  - HSV and enterovirus PCR if suspected

Table 24. CSF Findings of Meningitis

Component	Normal Child	Normal Newborn	Bacterial Meningitis	Viral Meningitis	Herpes Meningitis
WBC (/μL)	0-6	0-30	>1,000 (cloudy, xanthochromic)	100-500*	10-1,000
Neutrophils (%)	0	2-3	>50	<40	<50
Glucose (mmol/L)	2.2-4.4	1.8-6.7	<1.66	>1.66	>1.66
Protein (mg/dL)	0.2-0.3	0.19-1.49	>1.0	0.50-1.0	>0.75
RBC (/μL)	0-2	0-2	0-10	0-2	10-50

*Lymphocytes predominate   Modified from *Peds in Review* 1993;14:11-18 and *Ped Inf Dis J* 1996;15:298-303

Management
- supportive care
  - preservation of adequate cerebral perfusion by maintaining normal BP and managing ↑ ICP
  - close monitoring of fluids, electrolytes, glucose, acid-base disturbances, coagulopathies
- bacterial meningitis
  - if suspected or cannot be excluded, commence empiric antibiotic therapy while awaiting cultures or if LP contraindicated or delayed
  - isolation with appropriate infection control procedures until 24 h after culture-sensitive antibiotic therapy
  - fluid restrict if any concern for SIADH
  - hearing test
  - report to Public Health; prophylactic antibiotics for close contacts of Hib and *N. meningitidis* meningitis

Table 25. Antibiotic Management of Bacterial Meningitis

Age	Main Pathogens	Antibiotics
0 to 28 d	GBS, *E. coli*, *Listeria* Other: Gram-negative bacilli	Ampicillin + cefotaxime
28 to 90 d	Overlap of neonatal pathogens and those seen in older children	Cefotaxime + Vancomycin (+ Ampicillin If immunocompromised)
>90 d	*S. pneumoniae*, *N. meningitidis*	Ceftriaxone ± vancomycin If Penicillin allergic: Vancomycin + Rifampin

- viral meningitis
  - mainly supportive (except for HSV)
  - acyclovir for HSV meningitis
  - report to Public Health
- prophylaxis: appropriate vaccinations significantly decrease incidence of bacterial meningitis (see *Routine Immunization*, P4)

Complications
- mortality: neonate 15-20%, children 4-8%; pneumococcus > meningococcus > Hib
- acute: SIADH, subdural effusion/empyema, brain abscess, disseminated infection (osteomyelitis, septic arthritis, abscess), shock/DIC
- chronic: hearing loss, neuromotor/cognitive delay, learning disabilities, neurological deficit, seizure disorder, hydrocephalus

Mumps

Definition
- acute, self-limited viral infection that is most commonly characterized by adenitis and swelling of the parotid glands

Epidemiology
- incidence in Ontario has declined since introduction of two-dose MMR vaccination schedule
- average of 25 reported cases per yr
- majority of reported cases in children between 5-10 yr of age

Etiology
- mumps virus (RNA virus of the genus *Rubulavirus* in the *Paramyxoviridae* family)
- transmission via respiratory droplets, direct contact, fomites
- incubation period: 14-25 d
- infectivity period: 7 d pre-parotitis to 5 d post-parotitis
- upper respiratory tract lymph nodes salivary glands, gonads, pancreas, meninges, kidney, heart, thyroid

History
- non-specific prodome of fever, headache, malaise, myalgias (especially neck pain)
- usually followed within 48 h by parotid swelling secondary to parotitis (bilateral, preauricular, ear pushed up and out)
- parotid gland is tender and pain worsened with spicy or sour foods
- one third of infections do not cause clinically apparent salivary gland swelling and may simply present as an URTI

Investigations
- clinical diagnosis, but may be confirmed with IgM positive serology within 4 wk of acute infection
  - may also use PCR or viral cultures from oral secretions, urine, blood, and CSF
  - blood work: CBC (leukopenia with relative lymphocytosis), serum amylase (elevated)

Management
- mainly supportive: analgesics, antipyretics, warm or cold packs to parotid may be soothing
- admit to hospital if serious complications (meningitis, pancreatitis)
- droplet precautions recommended until 5 d after onset of parotid swelling
- prophylaxis: routine vaccination (see *Routine Immunization*, P4)

Complications
- common: aseptic meningitis, orchitis/oophoritis
- less common: encephalitis, pancreatitis, thyroiditis, myocarditis, arthritis, GN, ocular complications, hearing impairment

Pertussis

Definition
- prolonged respiratory illness characterized by paroxysmal coughing and inspiratory "whoop"

Epidemiology
- ~10 million children <1 yr old affected worldwide, causes up to 400,000 deaths/yr
- greatest incidence among children <1 yr (not fully immunized) and adolescents (waning immunity)

Etiology
- *Bordetella pertussis*: Gram negative pleomorphic rod
- highly contagious; transmitted via respiratory droplets released during intense coughing
- incubation period: 6-20 d; most contagious during catarrhal phase but may remain contagious for weeks after

History
- prodromal catarrhal stage
  - lasts 1-7 d; URTI symptoms (coryza, mild cough, sneezing) with NO or LOW-GRADE fever
- paroxysmal stage
  - lasts 4-6 wk; characterized by paroxysms of cough ("100 day cough"), sometimes followed by inspiratory whoop ("whooping cough")
  - infants <6 mo may present with post-tussive apnea, whoop is often absent
  - onset of attacks precipitated by yawning, sneezing, eating, physical exertion
  - ± post-tussive emesis, may become cyanotic before whoop
  - vomiting after whooping episodes
- convalescent stage;
  - lasts 1-2 wk; characterized by occasional paroxysms of cough, but decreased frequency and severity
  - non-infectious but cough may last up to 6 mo

Investigations
- NP specimen using aspirate or NP swab
  - gold standard: culture using special media (Regan-Lowe agar)
  - PCR to detect pertussis antigens
- blood work: CBC (lymphocytosis) and serology (antibodies against *B. pertussis*)

Management
- admit if paroxysms of cough are associated with cyanosis and/or apnea and give O_2
- supportive care
- antimicrobial therapy indicated if B. pertussi isolated, or symptoms present for <21 d
  - use macrolide antibiotics (azithromycin, erythromycin, or clarithromycin)
- droplet isolation until 5 d of treatment and report to Public Health
- prophylaxis
  - macrolide antibiotics for all household contacts
  - prevention with vaccination in infants and children (Pentacel*), and booster in adolescents (Adacel*) (see *Routine Immunization*, P4)

Complications
- pressure-related from paroxysms: subconjunctival hemorrhage, rectal prolapse, hernias, epistaxis
- respiratory: sinusitis, pneumonia, aspiration, atelectasis, pneumomediastinum, pneumothorax, alveolar rupture
- neurological: seizures (~3%), encephalopathy, ICH
- mortality: ~0.3%; highest risk in infants <6 mo old

Pneumonia

- see *Respirology*, P85

Periorbital (Preseptal) and Orbital Cellulitis

- see <u>Ophthalmology</u>, OP9

Sexually Transmitted Infections

- see <u>Family Medicine</u>, FM42 and <u>Gynecology</u>, GY27

Cardinal Signs of Orbital Cellulitis
- Ophthalmoplegia/diplopia
- Decreased visual acuity
- Pain with extraocular eye movement

Sinusitis

- see Family Medicine, FM44
- complication of ≤10% of URTIs in children
- clinical diagnosis
- diagnostic imaging is NOT required to confirm diagnosis in children
  - routine CT not recommended, but consider if suspect complications of sinusitis, persistent/recurrent disease, need for surgery
- antibiotic therapy for all children (although nearly half resolve spontaneously within 4 wk)
- complications: preseptal/orbital (preseptal/orbital cellulitis, orbital abscess, osteomyelitis, etc.), intracranial (meningitis, abscess, etc.), Pott's Puffy tumour

Urinary Tract Infection

Definition
- infection of the urinary bladder (cystitis) and/or kidneys (pyelonephritis)

Epidemiology
- overall prevalence in infants and young children presenting with fever is 7%
- <4-6 wk old: more common in boys
- >1 yr old: females have two- to four-fold higher prevalence

Etiology
- majority (>95%) have a single cause (~70% *E. coli*)
- Gram-negative bacilli: *E. coli, Klebsiella, Proteus, Enterobacter, Pseudomonas*
- Gram-positive cocci: *S. saprophyticus, Enterococcus*

Risk Factors
- non-modifiable: female gender, Caucasian, previous UTIs, family history
- modifiable: urinary tract abnormalities (VUR, neurogenic bladder, obstructive uropathy, posterior urethral valve), dysfunctional voiding, repeated bladder catheterization, uncircumcised males, labial adhesions, sexually active, constipation, toilet training

History
- infants and young child: often just fever or non-specific symptoms (poor feeding, irritability, FTT, jaundice if <28 d old, vomiting)
- older child: fever, urinary symptoms (dysuria, urgency, frequency, incontinence, hematuria), abdominal and/or flank pain

Physical Exam
- infants and young child: toxic vs non-toxic, febrile, FTT, jaundice; look for external genitalia abnormalities (phimosis, labial adhesions) and lower back signs of occult myelodysplasia (e.g. hair tufts), which may be associated with neurogenic bladder
- older child: febrile, suprapubic and/or CVA tenderness, abdominal mass (enlarged bladder or kidney); may present with short stature, FTT, or HTN secondary to renal scarring from previously unrecognized or recurrent UTIs

Features Suggestive of Pyelonephritis
- High-grade fever
- Flank or high abdominal pain
- CVA tenderness on palpation

Bagged urine specimen not useful for ruling in UTI (high false positive rate >85%), but useful for ruling out UTI (high sensitivity)

Investigations
- sterile urine specimen
  - clean catch, catheterization, suprapubic aspiration or 'Tap and Rub' technique
  - urinalysis (leukocyte esterase, nitrites, erythrocytes, hemoglobin), microscopy (bacteria and leukocytes, erythrocytes), C&S
- diagnosis established if urinalysis suggests infection AND if ≥50,000 colony-forming units per mL of a uropathogen cultured

Management
- admit if: <2 mo old, urosepsis, persistent vomiting, inability to tolerate oral medication, moderate-severe dehydration, immunocompromised, complex urologic pathology, inadequate follow-up, failure to respond to outpatient therapy
- supportive care: maintenance of hydration and adequate pain control
- antibiotics
  - base on local antimicrobial susceptibility patterns
  - commence broad empiric therapy until results of urine C&S known, and then tailor as appropriate
  - neonates: IV ampicillin and gentamicin
  - infants and older children: oral antibiotics (based on local *E. coli* sensitivity) if outpatient; IV ampicillin and gentamicin if inpatient
  - duration 7-10 d
- imaging
  - renal and bladder U/S for all febrile infants (<2 yr) with UTIs looking for anatomical abnormalities, hydronephrosis, abscess
  - VCUG not recommended after 1st febrile UTI unless U/S reveals hydronephrosis, obstructive uropathies or other signs suggestive of high-grade VUR

Prophylaxis After First Febrile Urinary Tract Infection in Children? A Multicentre, Randomized Controlled, Noninferiority Trial
Pediatrics 2008;122:1064-1071
Study: Randomized, controlled, open-label, 2 armed, noninferiority trial.
Patients: 338 patients aged 2 mo to <7 yr who had a first episode of febrile UTI.
Intervention: No prophylaxis vs. prophylaxis.
Outcome: Recurrence rate of febrile UTI and rate of renal scarring.
Results: No significant difference in recurrence rate or in the rate of renal scarring between the prophylaxis and no prophylaxis group.

- follow-up: outpatients to return in 24-48 h if no clinical response and seek prompt medical evaluation for future febrile illnesses
- prophylaxis: generally not recommended unless higher grades of VUR

Complications
- long-term morbidity: focal renal scarring develops in 8% of patients; long-term significance unknown

Neonatology

Gestational Age and Size

Definitions
- classification by GA
  - preterm: <37 wk
  - near-term: 35-37 wk
  - term: 37-42 wk
  - post-term: >42 wk
- classification by birth weight
  - SGA: 2 SD < mean weight for GA or <10th percentile
  - AGA: within 2 SD of mean weight for GA
  - LGA: 2 SD > mean weight for GA or >90th percentile

Dubowitz/Ballard Scores
GA can be determined after birth using Dubowitz/Ballard scores:
- Assessment at delivery of physical maturity (e.g. plantar creases, lanugo, ear maturation) and neuromuscular maturity (e.g. posture, arm recoil) translates into a score from -10 to +50
- Higher score means greater maturity (increased GA)
- -10 = 20 wk; +50 = 44 wk
- Ideal = 35-40, which corresponds to GA 38-40 wk
- Only accurate ± 2 wk

Table 26. Abnormalities of Gestational Age and Size

Features	Causes	Problems
Pre-Term Infants <37 wk	Spontaneous: cause unknown Maternal disease: HTN, DM, cardiac and renal disorders Fetal conditions: multiple pregnancy, congenital abnormalities, macrosomia, red blood cell isoimmunization, fetal infection Pregnancy issues: placental insufficiency, placenta previa, uterine malformations, previous preterm birth, infection, placental abruption Behavioural and psychological contributors: smoking, EtOH, drug use, psychosocial stressors Sociodemographic factors: age, socioeconomic conditions	RDS, apnea of prematurity, chronic lung disease, bronchopulmonary dysplasia Feeding difficulties, NEC Hypocalcemia, hypoglycemia, hypothermia Anemia, jaundice Retinopathy of prematurity ICH/IVH PDA
Post-Term Infants >42 wk Leathery skin Meconium staining	Most cases unknown Increased in first pregnancies Previous post-term birth Genetic factors	Increased risk of stillbirth or neonatal death Increased birthweight Fetal "postmaturity syndrome": impaired growth due to placental dysfunction Meconium aspiration
SGA Infants <10th percentile Asymmetric (head-sparing): late onset, growth arrest	Extrinsic causes: placental insufficiency, poor nutrition, HTN, multiple pregnancies, drugs, EtOH, smoking	Perinatal hypoxia Hypoglycemia, hypocalcemia, hypothermia, hyperviscosity (polycythemia), jaundice, hypomotility
Symmetric: early onset, lower growth	Intrinsic causes: maternal infections (TORCH), congenital abnormalities, syndromal, idiopathic	PDA
LGA Infants >90th percentile	Maternal DM Racial or familial factors Increasing parity Previous LGA infant, high BMI, large pregnancy weight gain Certain syndromes	Birth trauma, perinatal depression (meconium aspiration) RDS, TTN Jaundice, polycythemia Hypoglycemia, hypocalcemia

Routine Neonatal Care

1. erythromycin ointment: applied to both eyes for prophylaxis of ophthalmia neonatorum (of questionable efficacy)
2. vitamin K IM: prophylaxis against HDNB
3. newborn screening tests in Ontario
   - in Ontario, newborn screening tests for
   - metabolic disorders (amino acid disorders, organic acid disorders, fatty acid oxidation defects, biotinidase deficiency, galactosemia)
   - blood disorders (SCD, other hemoglobinopathies)
   - endocrine disorders (CAH, congenital hypothyroidism)
   - others (CF, severe combined immunodeficiency)
   - congenital hearing loss
4. if mother Rh negative: send cord blood for blood group and direct antiglobulin test
5. if mother hepatitis B surface antigen positive: HBIg and start hepatitis B vaccine series

Neonatal Resuscitation

- assess Apgar score at 1 and 5 min
- if <7 at 5 min then reassess q5min, until >7
- do not wait to assign Apgar score before initiating resuscitation

Table 27. Apgar Score

Sign	0	1	2
Heart Rate	Absent	<100/min	>100/min
Respiratory Effort	Absent	Slow, irregular	Good, crying
Irritability	No response	Grimace	Cough/cry
Tone	Limp	Some flexion of extremities	Active motion
Colour	Blue, pale	Body pink, extremities blue (acrocyanosis)	Completely pink

Initial Resuscitation
- anticipation: know maternal history, history of pregnancy, labour, and delivery
- steps to take for all infants
  - warm (radiant heater, warm blankets) and dry the newborn (remove wet blankets)
  - position and clear airway ("sniffing" position)
  - stimulate infant: rub lower back gently or flick soles of feet EXCEPT if meconium present (in which case tracheal suction first)
  - assess breathing and heart rate

Table 28. Interventions Used in Neonatal Resuscitation

Intervention	Schedule	Indications	Comments
Epinephrine (adrenaline)	0.1-0.3 mL/kg/dose of 1:10,000 (0.01-0.03 mg/kg) IV 0.5-1 mL/kg/dose of 1:10,000 (0.05-0.1 mg/kg) endotracheally can be considered while awaiting IV access (IV preferred) Can be repeated q3-5 min prn	HR <60 and not rising	Side effects: tachycardia, HTN, cardiac arrhythmias
Fluid Bolus (NS, whole blood, Ringer's lactate)	10 mL/kg May need to be repeated Avoid giving too rapidly as large volume rapid infusions can be associated with IVH	Evidence of hypovolemia	

Approach to the Depressed Newborn
- a depressed newborn lacks one or more of the following characteristics of a normal newborn
  - pulse >100 bpm
  - cries when stimulated
  - actively moves all extremities
  - has a good strong cry
- approximately 10% of newborn babies require assistance with breathing after delivery

Table 29. Etiology of Respiratory Depression in the Newborn

Etiology	Examples
Respiratory Problems	RDS/hyaline membrane disease Pulmonary hypoplasia CNS depression MAS Pneumonia Pneumothorax Pleural effusions Congenital malformations
Anemia (severe)	Erythroblastosis fetalis Secondary hydrops fetalis
Maternal Causes	Drugs/anesthesia (opiates, magnesium sulphate) DM Maternal myasthenia gravis
Congenital Malformations/Birth Injury	Nuchal cord, perinatal depression Bilateral phrenic nerve injury Potter's sequence
Shock	Antepartum hemorrhage
CHD	Transposition of the great arteries with intact ventricular septum
Other	Hypothermia Hypoglycemia Infection

Apgar Score
Appearance (colour)
Pulse (heart rate)
Grimace (irritability)
Activity (tone)
Respiration (respiratory effort)
Or: "How Ready Is This Child?"

Use of 100% Oxygen in Neonatal Resuscitation
Wyckoff MH, Aziz K, Escobedo MB, Kapadia VS, Kattwinkel J, Perlman JM, Simon WM, Weiner GM, Zaichkin, JG. Part 13: neonatal resuscitation: 2015 American Heart Association Guidelines Update for Cardiopulmonary Resuscitation and Emergency Cardiovascular Care. *Circulation* 2015;132(suppl 2):S543–S560.

Findings from animal and theoretical studies have suggested potential adverse effects with the administration of 100% oxygen. However, given available data is limited in general and only obtained from newborn samples, the 2015 neonatal resuscitation guidelines have provided the following recommendation: "Since an oxygen saturation of 100% may correspond to a PaO₂ anywhere between ~80 and 500 mm Hg, in general it is appropriate to wean the FIO₂ for a saturation of 100%, provided the oxyhemoglobin saturation can be maintained ≥94%." (Class IIb, LOE C).

Corrective Actions for PPV in Neonatal Resuscitation

MR SOPA
Mask readjustment
Reposition airway
Suction mouth and nose
Open mouth
Pressure increase
Alternative airway

Targeted Preductal SpO₂ After Birth
1 min — 60-65%
2 min — 65-70%
3 min — 70-75%
4 min — 75-80%
5 min — 80-85%
10 min — 85-95%

Diagnosis

- vital signs
- detailed maternal history: include prenatal care, illnesses, use of drugs, labour, previous high risk pregnancies, infections during pregnancy, current infections, duration of ruptured membranes, blood type and Rh status, amniotic fluid status, GA, meconium, Apgar scores
- clinical findings (observe for signs of respiratory distress such as cyanosis, tachypnea, retractions, grunting, temperature instability)
- laboratory results (CBC, ABG, blood type, glucose)
- transillumination of chest to evaluate for pneumothorax
- CXR

Management

- see *Neonatal Resuscitation*, identify and treat underlying cause

Common Conditions of Neonates

Apnea

Definition

- "periodic breathing": normal respiratory pattern seen in newborns in which periods of rapid respiration are alternated with pauses lasting 5-10 s
- "apnea": absence of respiratory gas flow for >20 s (or less if associated with bradycardia or desaturation)
  - 3 types
    - central: no chest wall movement, no signs of obstruction
    - obstructive: chest wall movement continues against obstructed upper airway, no airflow
    - mixed: combination of central and obstructive apnea

Differential Diagnosis

- in term infants, apnea requires full workup as it can be associated with sepsis
- other causes
  - CNS
  - apnea of prematurity (<34 wk): combination of CNS immaturity and obstructive apnea; resolves by 36 wk GA; diagnosis of exclusion
  - seizures
  - ICH
  - hypoxic injury
  - infectious: sepsis, meningitis, NEC
  - GI: GERD, aspiration with feeding
  - metabolic: hypoglycemia, hyponatremia, hypocalcemia, inborn error of metabolism
  - cardiovascular: anemia, hypovolemia, PDA, heart failure
  - medications: morphine

Management

- O_2, ventilatory support, maintain normal blood gases
- tactile stimulation
- correct underlying cause
- medications: methylxanthines (caffeine) stimulate the CNS and diaphragm and are used for apnea of prematurity (not in term infants)

Bleeding Disorders in Neonates

Clinical Presentation

- oozing from the umbilical stump, excessive bleeding from peripheral venipuncture/heel stick sites/IV sites, large caput succedaneum, cephalohematomas (in absence of significant birth trauma), subgaleal hemorrhage and prolonged bleeding following circumcision

Etiology

- 4 major categories
  - increased platelet destruction: maternal ITP or SLE, infection/sepsis, DIC, neonatal alloimmune thrombocytopenia, autoimmune thrombocytopenia
  - decreased platelet production/function: pancytopenia, bone marrow replacement, Fanconi anemia, Trisomy 13 and 18
  - metabolic: congenital thyrotoxicosis, inborn error of metabolism
  - coagulation factor deficiencies (see Hematology, H31): hemophilia A/B, HDNB

NEONATAL ALLOIMMUNE THROMBOCYTOPENIA

Epidemiology
• 1 per 4,000-5,000 live births

Pathophysiology
• platelet equivalent of Rh disease of the newborn
• occurs when mother is negative for HPA and fetus is positive
• development of maternal IgG antibodies against HPA antigens on fetal platelets

Clinical Presentation
• petechiae, purpura, thrombocytopenia in otherwise healthy neonate
• severe disease can lead to intracranial bleeding

Diagnosis
• maternal and paternal platelet typing and identification of platelet alloantibodies

Treatment
• IVIg to mother prenatally starts in second trimester ± steroids ± fetal platelet transfusions
• treat neonate with IVIg
• if transfusion required should be with washed maternal platelets or donor HPA negative platelets

AUTOIMMUNE THROMBOCYTOPENIA

Pathophysiology
• caused by antiplatelet antibodies from maternal ITP or SLE
• passive transfer of antibodies across placenta

Clinical Presentation
• similar presentation to neonatal alloimmune thrombocytopenia, but thrombocytopenia usually less severe

Treatment
• steroids to mother for 10-14 d prior to delivery or IVIg to mother before delivery
• treat neonate with IVIg (usually if platelets <60,000)
• transfusion of infant with maternal/donor platelets only in severe cases, as antibodies will destroy transfused platelets

HEMORRHAGIC DISEASE OF THE NEWBORN

Pathophysiology
• caused by vitamin K deficiency
• factors II, VII, IX, X are vitamin K-dependent, therefore both PT and PTT are abnormal

Etiology and Clinical Presentation
• neonates at risk of vitamin K deficiency if: vitamin K poorly transferred across the placenta; maternal use of antiepileptics; insufficient bacterial colonization of colon at birth to synthesize vitamin K; breastfed (vitamin K intake inadequate in breastfed infants)
• neonate may present with hematomas, ICH (causing apnea or seizures), internal bleeding, hematuria, bruising, prolonged bleeding (often from mucous membranes, umbilicus, circumcision, and venipunctures)

Prevention
• vitamin K IM administration at birth to all newborns

Bronchopulmonary Dysplasia

Definition
• also known as chronic lung disease
• clinically defined as O_2 requirement for >28 d plus persistent need for oxygen and/or ventilatory support at 36 wk corrected GA
• damage to developing lungs with prolonged intubation/ventilation, high levels O_2, infections

Investigations
• CXR findings may demonstrate decreased lung volumes, areas of atelectasis, signs of inflammation, and hyperinflation

Treatment
- no good treatments
- gradual wean from ventilator, optimize nutrition
- dexamethasone may help decrease inflammation and encourage weaning, but use of dexamethasone is associated with increased risk of adverse neurodevelopmental outcomes

Prognosis
- chronic respiratory failure may lead to pulmonary HTN, poor growth, and right-sided heart failure
- patients with bronchopulmonary dysplasia may continue to have significant impairment and deterioration in lung function late into adolescence
- some lung abnormalities may persist into adulthood including airway obstruction, airway hyper-reactivity, and emphysema
- associated with increased risk of adverse neurodevelopmental outcomes

Cyanosis

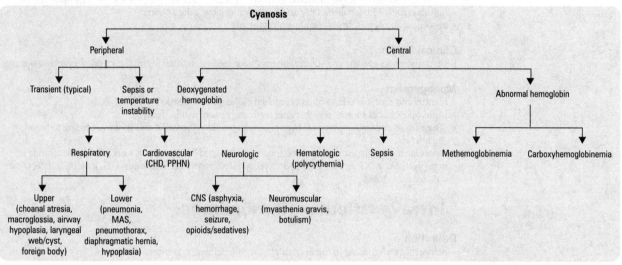

Figure 13. Approach to neonatal cyanosis

Management
- ABGs
  - elevated CO_2 suggests respiratory cause
  - hyperoxia test (to distinguish between cardiac and respiratory causes of cyanosis): get baseline PaO_2 in room air, then PaO_2 on 100% O_2 for 10-15 min
    - PaO_2 <150 mmHg: suggests cyanotic CHD or possible PPHN (see *Cardiology*, P16)
    - PaO_2 >150 mmHg: suggests cyanosis likely due to respiratory or non-cardiac cause
- CXR: look for respiratory abnormalities (respiratory tract malformations, evidence of shunting, pulmonary infiltrates) and cardiac abnormalities (cardiomegaly, abnormalities of the great vessels)

Diaphragmatic Hernia

- see General Surgery, GS62

Definition
- developmental defect of the diaphragm with herniation of abdominal organs into thorax
- associated with pulmonary hypoplasia and PPHN

Clinical Presentation
- respiratory distress, cyanosis
- scaphoid abdomen and barrel-shaped chest
- affected side dull to percussion and breath sounds absent, may hear bowel sounds instead
- heart sounds shifted to contralateral side
- asymmetric chest movements, trachea deviated away from affected side
- may present outside of neonatal period
- often associated with other anomalies (cardiovascular, CNS, chromosomal abnormalities)
- CXR: bowel loops in thorax (usually left side), displaced mediastinum

Carboxyhemoglobinemia (secondary to carbon monoxide poisoning) results in impaired binding of oxygen to hemoglobin but does not discolour the blood. Therefore it may not register on pulse oximetry and cyanosis may not be evident clinically

Methemoglobinemia typically reads higher on pulse oximetry than the true level of oxyhemoglobin. Methemoglobin alters the absorption of red light at the two wavelengths that pulse oximetry uses to predict oxygen saturation

Treatment
- immediate intubation required at birth: DO NOT bag mask ventilate because air will enter stomach and further compress lungs
- place large bore orogastric tube to decompress bowel
- initial stabilization and management of pulmonary hypoplasia and PPHN, hemodynamic support and surgery when stable

Hypoglycemia

Definition
- glucose <2.6 mmol/L

Etiology
- decreased carbohydrate stores: premature, SGA, RDS, maternal HTN
- endocrine: hormonal deficiencies (GH, cortisol, epinephrine), insulin excess (infant of diabetic mother, Beckwith-Wiedemann syndrome/islet cell hyperplasia), HPA axis suppression (panhypopituitarism)
- inborn errors of metabolism: fatty acid oxidation defects, galactosemia
- miscellaneous: sepsis, hypothermia, polycythemia

Clinical Findings
- signs often non-specific and subtle: lethargy, poor feeding, irritability, tremors, apnea, cyanosis, seizures

Management
- identify and monitor infants at risk (pre-feed blood glucose checks)
- begin oral feeds as soon as possible after birth and ensure regular feeds
- if significant and/or symptomatic hypoglycemia, provide glucose IV and titrate according to blood sugar levels
- if persistent hypoglycemia or no predisposing cause, send "critical blood work" during an episode of hypoglycemia: ABG, ammonia, β-hydroxybutyrate, cortisol, free fatty acids, GH, insulin, lactate, urine dipstick for ketones

Intraventricular Hemorrhage

Definition
- hemorrhage originating in the periventricular subependymal germinal matrix

Epidemiology
- incidence and severity inversely proportional to GA
- 50% of IVH occurs within 8 h of birth; 90% occurs by day 3

Risk Factors
- prematurity (<32 wk), BW <1,500 g, need for vigorous resuscitation at birth, pneumothorax, ventilated preterm infants, hemodynamic instability, RDS, coagulopathy

Clinical Presentation
- many infants with IVH are asymptomatic
- subtle signs: apnea, bradycardia, changes in tone or activity, altered LOC
- catastrophic presentation: bulging fontanelle, sudden drop in hematocrit, acidosis, seizures, hypotension

Papile Classification
Grade I: germinal matrix hemorrhage
Grade II: IVH without ventricular dilatation
Grade III: IVH with ventricular dilatation
Grade IV: IVH with parenchymal extension

Classification
- Papile classification
- parenchymal hemorrhage may also occur in the absence of IVH
- routine head U/S screening of all preterm infants <32 wk or <1,500 g gestation throughout NICU stay
- consider MRI at term for extremely LBW infants

Management of Acute Hemorrhage
- supportive care to maintain blood volume and acid-base status
- avoid fluctuations in blood pressure and cerebral blood flow
- follow-up with serial imaging

Prognosis
- outcome depends on grade of IVH
- short-term sequelae for severe IVH: mortality, extension of bleed, posthemorrhagic hydrocephalus, posthemorrhagic infarction, cyst formation
- possible long-term major neurological sequelae: CP, cognitive deficits, motor deficits, visual and hearing impairment
- Grades I and II hemorrhages have a relatively favourable prognosis
- greatest morbidity and mortality is seen with Grade IV hemorrhage and posthemorrhagic hydrocephalus requiring ventriculoperitoneal shunt placement

Jaundice

Clinical Presentation
- jaundice is visible at serum bilirubin levels of 85-120 µmol/L; visual assessment is often misleading
- look at sclera, tip of nose in natural light
- jaundice more severe/prolonged (due to increased retention of bilirubin in the circulation) with: prematurity, acidosis, hypoalbuminemia, dehydration, hemolysis

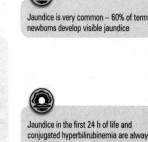

Jaundice is very common – 60% of term newborns develop visible jaundice

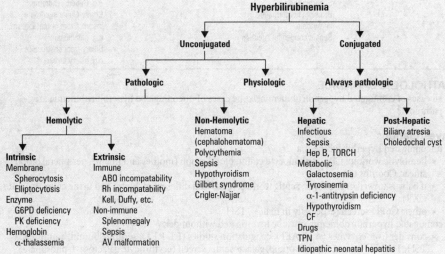

Figure 14. Approach to neonatal hyperbilirubinemia

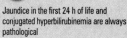

Jaundice in the first 24 h of life and conjugated hyperbilirubinemia are always pathological

Jaundice must be investigated if
- It occurs within 24 h of birth
- Conjugated hyperbilirubinemia is present
- Unconjugated bilirubin rises rapidly or is excessive for patient's age and weight
- Persistent jaundice lasts beyond 1-2 wk of age

PHYSIOLOGIC JAUNDICE

Epidemiology
- term infants: onset 3-4 d of life, resolution by 10 d of life
- premature infants: higher peak and longer duration

Pathophysiology
- increased hematocrit and decreased RBC lifespan
- immature glucuronyl transferase enzyme system (slow conjugation of bilirubin)
- increased enterohepatic circulation

Breastfeeding Jaundice
- common; due to a lack of milk production → dehydration → exaggerated physiologic jaundice

Breast Milk Jaundice
- 1 per 200 breastfed infants
- glucuronyl transferase inhibitor found in breast milk
- onset 7 d of life, peak at 2-3 wk of life, usually resolved by 6 wk

Table 30. Risk Factors for Jaundice

Maternal Factors	Perinatal Factors	Neonatal Factors
Ethnic group (e.g. Asian, native American) Complications during pregnancy (infant of diabetic mother, Rh or ABO incompatibility) Breastfeeding Family history/previous child required phototherapy	Birth trauma (cephalohematoma, ecchymoses) Prematurity	Difficulty establishing breastfeeding Infection (sepsis, hepatitis) Genetic factors Polycythemia Drugs TPN

Table 31. Causes of Neonatal Jaundice by Age

<24 h	24-72 h	72-96 h	Prolonged (>1 wk)
ALWAYS PATHOLOGIC Hemolytic Rh or ABO incompatibility Sepsis Congenital infection (TORCH) Severe bruising/hemorrhage	Physiologic, polycythemia Dehydration (breastfeeding jaundice) Hemolysis G6PD deficiency Pyruvate kinase deficiency Spherocytosis Bruising, hemorrhage, hematoma Sepsis/congenital infection	Physiologic ± breastfeeding Sepsis	Breast milk jaundice Prolonged physiologic jaundice in preterm Hypothyroidism Neonatal hepatitis Conjugation dysfunction e.g. Gilbert syndrome, Crigler-Najjar syndrome Inborn errors of metabolism e.g. galactosemia Biliary tract obstruction e.g. biliary atresia

PATHOLOGIC JAUNDICE
- all cases of conjugated hyperbilirubinemia; some cases of unconjugated hyperbilirubinemia are pathologic

Investigations
- unconjugated hyperbilirubinemia
  - hemolytic workup: CBC, reticulocyte count, blood group (mother and infant), peripheral blood smear, Coombs test
  - if baby is unwell or has fever: septic workup (CBC and differential, blood and urine cultures ± LP, CXR)
  - other: G6PD screen (especially in males), TSH
- conjugated hyperbilirubinemia must be investigated without delay
  - consider liver enzymes (AST, ALT), coagulation studies (PT, PTT), serum albumin, ammonia, TSH, TORCH screen, septic workup, galactosemia screen (erythrocyte galactose-1-phosphate uridyltransferase levels), metabolic screen, abdominal U/S, HIDA scan, sweat chloride

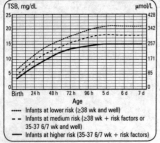

"Bronzed" Baby in Infants with Conjugated Hyperbilirubinemia
Phototherapy results in the production and accumulation of a toxic metabolite which also imparts a bronze hue on the baby's skin

TREATMENT OF UNCONJUGATED HYPERBILIRUBINEMIA
- to prevent kernicterus
- breastfeeding does not usually need to be discontinued, ensure adequate feeds and hydration
- lactation consultant support, mother to pump after feeds
- treat underlying causes (e.g. sepsis)
- phototherapy (blue-green wavelength, not UV light)
  - insoluble unconjugated bilirubin is converted to excretable form via photoisomerization
  - serum bilirubin should be monitored during and immediately after therapy (risk of rebound because photoisomerization reversible when phototherapy discontinued)
  - contraindicated in conjugated hyperbilirubinemia: results in "bronzed" baby
  - side effects: skin rash, diarrhea, eye damage (eye shield used routinely for prevention), dehydration
  - use published guidelines and nomogram for initiation of phototherapy
- exchange transfusion
  - indications: high bilirubin levels as per published graphs based on age, weeks gestation
  - most commonly performed for hemolytic disease and G6PD deficiency
  - use of IVIg in case of severe hyperbilirubinemia (DAT+) becoming evidence-based practice

Figure 15. Gold standard in deciding when to initiate phototherapy for unconjugated hyperbilirubinemia

KERNICTERUS

Etiology
- unconjugated bilirubin concentrations exceed albumin binding capacity and bilirubin is deposited in the brain resulting in permanent damage (typically basal ganglia or brainstem)
- incidence increases as serum bilirubin levels increase above 340 μmol/L
- can occur at lower levels in presence of sepsis, meningitis, hemolysis, hypoxia, acidosis, hypothermia, hypoglycemia, and prematurity

Clinical Presentation
- up to 15% of infants have no obvious neurologic symptoms
- early stage: lethargy, hypotonia, poor feeding, emesis (bilirubin encephalopathy)
- mid stage: hypertonia, high pitched cry, opisthotonic posturing (back arching), bulging fontanelle, seizures, pulmonary hemorrhage
- late stage (first year and beyond)
  - hypotonia, delayed motor skills, extrapyramidal abnormalities (choreoathetoid CP), gaze palsy, mitral regurgitation, sensorineural hearing loss

Prevention
- exchange transfusion, IVIg if indicated

BILIARY ATRESIA

Definition
- atresia of the extrahepatic bile ducts which leads to cholestasis and increased conjugated bilirubin after the first week of life
- progressive obliterative cholangiopathy

Epidemiology
- incidence: 1:10,000-15,000 live births
- associated anomalies in 10-35% of cases: situs inversus, congenital heart defects, polysplenia

Clinical Presentation
- dark urine, pale stool, jaundice (persisting for >2 wk), abdominal distension, hepatomegaly

Diagnosis
- conjugated hyperbilirubinemia, abdominal U/S, operative cholangiogram
- HIDA scan (may be bypassed in favour of biopsy if timing of diagnosis is critical)
- liver biopsy

Treatment
- surgical drainage procedure
- hepatoportoenterostomy (Kasai procedure; most successful if <8 wk of age)
- two-thirds will eventually require liver transplantation
- vitamins A, D, E, and K; diet should be enriched with medium-chain triglycerides to ensure adequate fat ingestion

Necrotizing Enterocolitis

Definition
- intestinal inflammation associated with focal or diffuse ulceration and necrosis
- primarily affecting terminal ileum and colon

Epidemiology
- affects 1-5% of preterm newborns admitted to NICU

Pathophysiology
- postulated mechanism of bowel ischemia: mucosal damage and enteral feeding → bacterial growth → bowel necrosis/gangrene/perforation

Risk Factors
- prematurity (immature defenses)
- asphyxia, shock (poor bowel perfusion)
- hyperosmolar feeds
- enteral feeding with formula (breast milk can be protective)
- sepsis

Clinical Presentation
- usually presents at 2-3 wk of age
- distended abdomen
- increased amount of gastric aspirate/vomitus with bile staining
- frank or occult blood in stool
- feeding intolerance
- diminished bowel sounds
- signs of bowel perforation (sepsis, shock, peritonitis, DIC)

Investigations
- AXR: pneumonitis intestinalis (intramural air is a hallmark of NEC), free air, fixed loops, ileus, thickened bowel wall, portal venous gas
- CBC, ABG, lactate, blood culture, electrolytes
- high or low WBC, low platelets, hyponatremia, acidosis, hypoxia, hypercapnea

Treatment
- NPO (7-10 d), vigorous IV fluid resuscitation, decompression with NG tube, supportive therapy
- TPN
- antibiotics (usually ampicillin, gentamicin ± metronidazole if risk of perforation x 7-10 d)
- serial AXRs detect early perforation (40% mortality in perforated NEC)
- peritoneal drain/surgery if perforation
- surgical resection of necrotic bowel and surgery for complications (e.g. perforation, strictures)

Influence of Enteral Nutrition on Occurrences of Necrotizing Enterocolitis in Very-Low-Birth-Weight Infants
J Pediatr Gastroenterol Nutr 2015; 61(4):445-50
Study: Case-control study of very-low-birth-weight (VLBW) infants and occurrences of NEC within 30 days of life.
Population: 1028 VLBW infants in neonatal intensive care unit Jan 2003-May 2008.
Main Outcome: NEC defined using stage ≥2 of modified Bell criteria.
Results: 55 infants developed NEC within 30 days of life (5.4%). Those with NEC had higher odds of having been fed breast milk <7days (OR: 4.02), not having achieved full enteral feeding during the first month (OR: 3.50), and having had parenteral feeding (OR: 2.70).
Conclusions: Occurrence of NEC can be reduced with breast milk feeding beyond 7 days and early full enteral feeding.

Persistent Pulmonary Hypertension of the Newborn

Definition
- persistence of fetal circulation as a result of persistent elevation of pulmonary vascular resistance
- classified as primary (absence of risk factors) or secondary

Epidemiology
- incidence 1.9/1,000 live births

Clinical Presentation
- usually presents within 12 h of birth with severe hypoxemia/cyanosis; may have only mild respiratory distress

Pathophysiology
- elevated pulmonary pressures cause R → L shunt through PDA, foramen ovale → decreased pulmonary blood flow and hypoxemia → further pulmonary vasoconstriction

Risk Factors
- secondary PPHN: asphyxia, MAS, RDS, sepsis, pneumonia, structural abnormalities (e.g. diaphragmatic hernia, pulmonary hypoplasia)
- more common in term or post-term infants

Investigations
- measure pre- and post-ductal oxygen levels
- hyperoxia test to exclude CHD
- ECG (RV strain)
- Echo reveals increased pulmonary arterial pressure and a R → L shunt across PDA and patent foramen ovale; also used to rule out other cardiac defects

Treatment
- maintain good oxygenation (SaO_2 >95%) in at-risk infants
- O_2 given early and tapered slowly, minimize stress and metabolic demands, maintain normal blood gases, circulatory support
- mechanical ventilation, high frequency oscillation in a sedated muscle-relaxed infant
- nitric oxide, surfactant
- extracorporeal membrane oxygenation used in some centres when other therapy fails

Respiratory Distress in the Newborn

Clinical Presentation
- tachypnea: RR >60/min; tachycardia: HR >160/min
- grunting, subcostal/intercostal indrawing, nasal flaring
- duskiness, central cyanosis
- decreased air entry, crackles on auscultation

Differential Diagnosis of Respiratory Distress
- pulmonary: RDS (Respiratory Distress Syndrome), TTN (Transient Tachypnea of the Newborn), MAS (Meconium Aspiration Syndrome), pleural effusion, pneumothorax, congenital lung malformations
- infectious: sepsis, pneumonia
- cardiac: CHD (cyanotic, acyanotic), PPHN
- hematologic: blood loss, polycythemia
- anatomic: TEF, congenital diaphragmatic hernia, mucous or meconium plug, upper airway obstruction (see Otolaryngology, OT41)
- metabolic: hypoglycemia, inborn errors of metabolism
- neurologic: CNS damage (trauma, hemorrhage), drug withdrawal syndromes

Investigations
- CXR, ABG (or venous blood gas from umbilical venous line)
- CBC, blood cultures, blood glucose
- ECG if indicated

Table 32. Distinguishing Features of RDS, TTN, MAS

	RDS	TTN	MAS
Etiology	Surfactant deficiency → poor lung compliance due to high alveolar surface tension → atelectasis → ↓ surface area for gas exchange → hypoxia + acidosis → respiratory distress "Hyaline membrane disease"	Delayed resorption of fetal lung fluid → accumulation of fluid in peribronchial lymphatics and vascular spaces → tachypnea "Wet lung syndrome"	Meconium is sterile but causes airway obstruction, chemical inflammation, and surfactant inactivation leading to chemical pneumonitis
Gestational Age	Preterm	Usually term and late preterm	Term and post-term
Risk Factors	Maternal DM Preterm delivery Male sex LBW Acidosis, sepsis Hypothermia Second born twin	Maternal DM Maternal asthma Male sex Macrosomia (>4,500 g) Elective Cesarean section or short labour Late preterm delivery	Meconium-stained amniotic fluid Post-term delivery
Clinical Presentation	Respiratory distress within first few hours of life, worsens over next 24-72 h Hypoxia Cyanosis	Tachypnea within the first few hours of life ± retractions, grunting, nasal flaring Often NO hypoxia or cyanosis	Respiratory distress within hours of birth Small airway obstruction, chemical pneumonitis tachypnea, barrel chest with audible crackles Hypoxia
CXR Findings	Homogenous infiltrates Air bronchograms Decreased lung volumes May resemble pneumonia (GBS) If severe, "white-out" with no differentiation of cardiac border	Perihilar infiltrates "Wet silhouette"; fluid in fissures	Hyperinflation Patchy atelectasis Patchy and coarse infiltrates 10-20% have pneumothorax
Prevention	Prenatal corticosteroids (e.g. Celestone® 12 mg q24h x 2 doses) if risk of preterm delivery <34 wk Monitor lecithin:sphingomyelin (L/S) ratio with amniocentesis, L/S >2:1 indicates lung maturity	Where possible, avoidance of elective Cesarean delivery, particularly before 38 wk GA	If infant is depressed at birth, intubate and suction below vocal cords Avoidance of factors associated with in utero passage of meconium (e.g. post term delivery)
Treatment	Resuscitation Oxygen Ventilation Surfactant (decreases alveolar surface tension, improves lung compliance, and maintains functional residual capacity)	Supportive Oxygen if hypoxic Ventilator support (e.g. CPAP) IV fluids and NG tube feeds if too tachypneic to feed orally	Resuscitation Oxygen Ventilatory support Surfactant Inhaled nitric oxide Extracorporeal membrane oxygenation for PPHN
Complications	In severe prematurity and/or prolonged ventilation, increased risk of bronchopulmonary dysplasia	Hypoxemia Hypercapnea Acidosis PPHN	Hypoxemia Hypercapnea Acidosis PPHN Pneumothorax Pneumomediastinum Chemical pneumonitis Secondary surfactant inhibition Respiratory failure
Prognosis	Dependent on GA at birth and severity of underlying lung disease; long-term risks of chronic lung disease	Recovery usually expected in 24-72 h	Dependent on severity, mortality up to 20%

PNEUMONIA

- see *Respirology*, P85
- consider in infants with prolonged or premature rupture of membranes, maternal fever, or if mother is GBS positive
- suspect if infant exhibits respiratory distress, temperature instability, or WBC is low, elevated, or left-shifted
- symptoms may be non-specific
- CXR: hazy lung and/or distinct infiltrates (may be difficult to differentiate from RDS)

Retinopathy of Prematurity

- see Ophthalmology, OP38

Sepsis in the Neonate

Table 33. Sepsis Considerations in the Neonate

Early Onset (<72 h)	Late Onset (72 h – 28 d)

Vertical transmission, 95% present within 24 h after birth
Risk factors:
  Maternal infection: UTI, GBS positive, previous child with GBS sepsis or meningitis
  Maternal fever/leukocytosis/chorioamnionitis
  Prolonged rupture of membranes (>18 h)
  Preterm labour
Pathogens: GBS, *E. coli*, *Listeria* most common
Pneumonia more common with early onset sepsis
	Acquired after birth
	Most common in preterm infants in NICU (most commonly due to coagulase negative *Staphylococcus*)
	Other pathogens implicated include GBS, anaerobes, *E. coli*, *Klebsiella*

Signs of Sepsis
- no reliable absolute indicator of occult bacteremia in infants <3 mo, most specific result has been WBC <5
- temperature instability (hypo/hyperthermia)
- respiratory distress, cyanosis, apnea
- tachycardia/bradycardia
- lethargy, irritability
- poor feeding, vomiting, abdominal distension, diarrhea
- hypotonia, seizures, lethargy
- jaundice, hepatomegaly, petechiae, purpura

Skin Conditions of the Neonate

Table 34. Common Neonatal Skin Conditions

Neonatal Skin Condition	Description
Vasomotor Response (Cutis Marmorata, Acrocyanosis)	Transient mottling when exposed to cold; usually normal, particularly if premature
Vernix Caseosa	Soft, creamy, white layer covering baby at birth
Congenital Dermal Melanocytosis ('Mongolian Spots')	Slate grey macules over lower back and buttocks (may look like bruises); common in dark skinned infants
Capillary Hemangioma	Raised red lesion, which increases in size after birth and involutes; 50% resolved by 5 yr, 90% by 9 yr
Erythema Toxicum	Yellow-white papules/pustules surrounded by erythema, eosinophils within the lesions; common rash, resolves by 2 wk
Milia	Lesions 1-2 mm firm white pearly papules on nasal bridge, cheeks, and palate; self-resolving
Transient Pustular Melanosis	Brown macular base with pustules, seen more commonly in African American infants; may be present at birth
Nevus Simplex (Salmon Patch)	Transient macular vascular malformation of the eyelids and/or neck ("Angel Kiss" or "Stork Bite"); most lesions disappear by 1 yr of life
Neonatal Acne	Inflammatory papules and pustules mainly on face; self-resolving usually within 4 mo

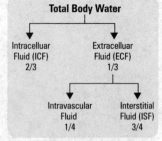

Figure 16. Body fluid compartments

Fluids and Electrolytes

Approach to Infant/Child with Dehydration

Etiology
- decreased intake: poor oral intake during acute illness, breastfeeding difficulties, eating disorders
- increased losses: common sites include GI tract (diarrhea, vomiting, bleeding), skin/mucous membranes (fever, burns, hemorrhage, stomatitis), urine (osmotic diuresis [e.g. hyperglycemia, DKA], diuretic therapy, DI, post-obstructive/post ATN recovery diuresis), and respiratory tract (tachypnea, bronchiolitis, pneumonia)

Management
- if suspect dehydration based on history (acute illness, decreased number of wet diapers, lethargy, changes in mental status, increased thirst, etc.), you must:

1) Determine degree of extracellular volume contraction

Table 35. Assessment of Degree of Extracellular Volume Contraction Based on Physical Exam

	Mild	Moderate	Severe
<2 yr	5%*	10%*	15%*
>2 yr	3%*	6%*	9%*
Pulse	Normal, full	Rapid	Rapid, weak
Blood Pressure	Normal	Low to normal	Decreased in shock (very late finding in pediatrics and very dangerous)
Urine Output	Decreased	Markedly decreased	Anuria
Oral Mucosa	Slightly dry	Dry	Parched
Anterior Fontanelle	Normal	Sunken	Markedly sunken
Eyes	Normal	Sunken	Markedly sunken
Skin Turgor	Normal	Decreased	Tenting
Capillary Refill	Normal (<3 s)	Normal to increased	Increased (>3 s)

* Note that percentages refer to percent loss of pre-illness body weight

2) Determine the likely electrolyte disturbance
- dependent on etiology of dehydration and type of fluid loss (isotonic vs. hypertonic vs. hypotonic)

Table 36. Electrolyte Content of Various Bodily Fluids

Bodily Fluid	Na^+ (mmol/L)	K^+ (mmol/L)	Cl^- (mmol/L)	HCO_3^- (mmol/L)
Saliva	30-80	20	70	30
Gastric Juice	60-80	15	100	0
Pancreatic Juice	140	5-10	60-90	40-100
Bile	140	5-10	100	40
Small Bowel	140	20	100	25-50
Large Bowel	75	30	30	0
Sweat	20-70	5-10	40-60	0

- for moderate and severe dehydration, initial investigations should include urinalysis and blood work examining electrolyte (Na^+, K^+, Cl^-), glucose, and acid-base (blood pH, pCO_2, HCO_3^- disturbances), and impaired renal function (creatinine, BUN)

3) Determine if the child requires PO or IV rehydration
- dehydrated child must receive adequate fluid management, including replacement of ongoing losses and maintenance fluids
- ORT indication: mild to moderate dehydration caused by diarrhea
  - advantages: ↓ cost, no IV needed, no increase in incidence of iatrogenic hyper/hyponatremia, parental involvement in therapy
- IV rehydration indications: indications for IV rehydration therapy: severe dehydration requiring close monitoring and frequent assessment of electrolytes, inability to tolerate ORT (e.g. vomiting, alteration in mental status, ileus, monosaccharide malabsorption, etc.), inability to provide ORT, failure of ORT in providing adequate rehydration (e.g. persistent diarrhea or vomiting)

4) Return the child to a normal volume and electrolyte status by replacing current deficits and ongoing losses

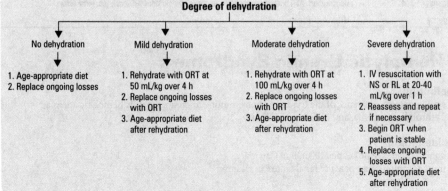

Figure 17. Algorithm for deficit replacement and replacement of ongoing losses in the dehydrated child

Assessment of Severity of Dehydration

C BASE H₂0
Capillary refill
BP
Anterior fontanelle
Skin turgor
Eyes sunken
HR
Oral mucosa
Output of urine

Special Consideration – SIADH
Clinical Signs: hyponatremia and excretion of concentrated urine
Risk Factors: certain medications (e.g. morphine), post-operative, pain, N/V, pulmonary disease (e.g. pneumonia), CNS disease (e.g. meningitis)
Caution: acute hyponatremia is associated with rapid administration of hypotonic IV fluids, this can lead to cerebral edema and brain herniation or central pontine myelinolysis

5) Provide the appropriate fluid and electrolyte maintenance daily requirements

Table 37. Maintenance Fluid Requirements

Body Weight	100:50:20 Rule (24 h maintenance fluids)	4:2:1 Rule (hourly rate of maintenance fluids)
1-10 kg	100 cc/kg/d	4 cc/kg/h
11-20 kg	1000 cc + 50 cc/kg/d for every kg >10 kg	40 cc + 2 cc/kg/h for every kg >10 kg
>20 kg	1500 cc + 20 cc/kg/d for every kg > 20 kg	60 cc + 1 cc/kg/h for every kg > 20 kg

- in children, all maintenance fluids should have a dextrose component due to their higher risk of hypoglycemia, especially if they are NPO
- common IV fluid combinations used in pediatrics
  - newborn: D10W
  - first month of life: D5W/0.45 2 NS + KCl 20 mEq/L (only add KCl if voiding well)
  - children: D5W/NS + KCl 20 mEq/L or D5W/0.45 NS + KCl 20 mEq/L; NS bolus for dehydration
- most important thing to remember when correcting Na aberrations due to fluid deficits
  - risk of cerebral edema with rapid rehydration with hypotonic or isotonic solutions (i.e. NS), therefore replace fluid slowly with close monitoring; aim to adjust (increase or decrease) plasma [Na$^+$] by no more than 12 mmol/L/d
  - management depends on etiology, severity of symptoms, and timing (acute vs. chronic)

6) Continue to monitor fluid and electrolyte status
- accurate monitoring of daily fluid intake (PO and IV) and ongoing losses (urine output, diarrhea, emesis, drains)
- if child receiving >50% of maintenance fluids through IV, serum electrolyte values should be monitored daily and therapy adjusted accordingly
- avoid iatrogenic hyper/hyponatremia, keep the possibility of SIADH in mind

Nephrology

Common Pediatric Renal Diseases

Table 38. Common Manifestations of Renal Disease

Neonate	Common Causes
Flank Mass	Hydronephrosis, polycystic disease (autosomal dominant or recessive subtypes), tumour
Hematuria	Renal vein thrombosis, asphyxia, malformation, trauma
Anuria/Oliguria	Bilateral renal agenesis, obstruction, asphyxia
Child and Adolescent	
Cola/Red-Coloured Urine	Acute GN (post-streptococcal, HSP, IgA nephropathy, etc.), hemoglobinuria (hemolysis), myoglobinuria (rhabdomyolysis)
Gross Hematuria	Urologic disease (nephrolithiasis, trauma, etc.), UTI, acute GN
Edema	Nephrotic syndrome, nephritis, acute/chronic renal failure, consider cardiac or liver disease
HTN	GN, renal failure, dysplasia (consider coarctation, drugs, endocrine causes)
Polyuria	DM, central and nephrogenic DI, renal Fanconi's syndrome (genetic/metabolic/acquired causes), hypercalcemia, polyuric renal failure (renal dysplasia)
Proteinuria	Orthostatic, nephrotic syndrome (MCD, etc.), GN
Oliguria	Dehydration, ATN, interstitial nephritis, acute or chronic kidney disease (i.e. renal failure)
Urgency	UTI, vulvovaginitis

Hemolytic Uremic Syndrome

Definition
- simultaneous occurrence of the triad of 1) non-immune microangiopathic hemolytic anemia, 2) thrombocytopenia, and 3) acute renal injury

Epidemiology
- annual incidence of 1-2 per 100,000 in Canada
- most common cause of acute renal failure in children

Etiology
- diarrhea positive HUS: 90% of pediatric HUS from *E. coli* O157:H7, shiga toxin, or verotoxin
- diarrhea negative HUS: other bacteria, viruses, drugs, familial/genetic

Pathophysiology
- toxin binds, invades, and destroys colonic epithelial cells, causing bloody diarrhea
- toxin enters the systemic circulation, attaches to, and injures endothelial cells (especially in kidney), causing a release of endothelial products (e.g. von Willebrand factor, platelet aggregating factor)
- platelet/fibrin thrombi form in multiple organ systems (e.g. kidney, pancreas, brain, etc.) resulting in thrombocytopenia
- RBCs are forced through occluded vessels, resulting in fragmented RBCs (schistocytes) that are removed by the reticuloendothelial system (hemolytic anemia)

History and Physical Exam
- history: initial presentation of abdominal pain and diarrhea, followed by bloody diarrhea; within 5-7 d begins to show signs of anemia, thrombocytopenia, and renal insufficiency
- physical exam: pallor, jaundice (hemolysis), edema, petechiae, HTN

Investigations
- CBC (anemia, thrombocytopenia), blood smear (schistocytes), electrolytes, renal function, urinalysis (microscopic hematuria), stool cultures, and verotoxin/shigella toxin assay

Management
- mainly supportive: nutrition, hydration, ventilation (if necessary), blood transfusion for symptomatic anemia
- monitor electrolytes and renal function: dialysis if electrolyte abnormality (hyperkalemia) cannot be corrected, fluid overload, or uremia
- steroids are not helpful
- antibiotics are contraindicated because death of bacteria leads to increased toxin release and worse clinical course

Prognosis
- <5% mortality, 5-25% long-term renal damage (HTN, proteinuria, decreased renal function)

Nephritic Syndrome

Definition
- acute or chronic syndrome affecting the kidney, characterized by glomerular injury and inflammation, and defined by hematuria (>5 RBCs per high-powered microscope field) and the presence of dysmorphic RBCs and RBC casts on urinalysis
- often accompanied by at least one of proteinuria (<50 mg/kg/d), edema, HTN, azotemia, and oliguria

Epidemiology
- highest incidence in children aged 5-15 yr old

Etiology
- humoral immune response to a variety of etiologic agents → immunoglobulin deposition → complement activation, leukocyte recruitment, release of growth factors/cytokines → glomerular inflammation and injury → porous podocytes → hematuria + RBC casts ± proteinuria
- HTN secondary to fluid retention and increased renin secretion by ischemic kidneys

Nephritic Syndrome

PHAROH
Proteinuria (<50 mg/kg/d)
Hematuria
Azotemia
RBC casts
Oliguria
HTN

Table 39. Major Causes of Nephritic Syndrome

	Decreased C3	Normal C3

Primary (idiopathic)	Post-infectious GN (most common cause of acute GN in pediatrics)
	Membranoproliferative
	  Type I (50-80%)
	  Type II (>80%)
		IgA nephropathy
		Idiopathic rapidly progressive GN
		Anti-GBM disease

Secondary (systemic disease)	SLE Bacterial endocarditis Abscess or shunt nephritis Cryoglobulinemia	HSP (very common) Polyarteritis nodosa Granulomatosis with polyangiitis Goodpasture's syndrome

History and Physical Exam
- often asymptomatic; some overlap in clinical findings for nephritic and nephrotic syndrome
- gross hematuria, mild-moderate edema, oliguria, HTN
- signs and symptoms suggestive of underlying systemic causes (e.g. fever, arthralgias, rash, dyspnea, pulmonary hemorrhage)

Investigations
- urine
  - dipstick (hematuria, 0 to 2+ proteinuria) and microscopy (>5 RBCs per high-powered microscope field, acanthocytes, RBC casts)
  - first morning urine protein/creatinine ratio (<200 mg/mmol)

- blood work
  - impaired renal function (↑ Cr and BUN) resulting in ↓ pH and electrolyte abnormalities (hyperkalemia, hyperphosphatemia, hypocalcemia)
  - mild anemia on CBC (secondary to hematuria)
  - hypoalbuminemia (secondary to proteinuria)
  - appropriate investigations to determine etiology: C3/C4 levels, serologic testing for recent streptococcal infection (ASOT, anti-hyaluronidase, anti-streptokinase, anti-NAD, anti-DNAse B), ANA, anti-DNA antibodies, ANCA, serum IgA levels, anti-GBM antibodies
- renal biopsy should be considered only in the presence of acute renal failure, no evidence of streptococcal infection, normal C3/C4

Management
- treat underlying cause
- symptomatic
  - renal insufficiency: supportive (dialysis if necessary), proper hydration
  - HTN: salt and fluid restriction (but not at expense of renal function), ACEI or ARBs for chronic persistent HTN (not acute cases because ACEI or ARBs may decrease GFR further)
  - edema: salt and fluid restriction, possibly diuretics (avoid if significant intravascular depletion)
- corticosteroids if indicated: IgA nephropathy, lupus nephritis, etc.

Prognosis
- dependent on underlying etiology
- complications include HTN, heart failure, pulmonary edema, chronic kidney injury (requiring renal transplant)

Nephrotic Syndrome

Definition
- clinical syndrome affecting the kidney, characterized by significant proteinuria, peripheral edema, hypoalbuminemia, and hyperlipidemia

Epidemiology
- highest incidence in children 2-6 yr old, M>F

Etiology
- primary (idiopathic): nephrotic syndrome in the absence of systemic disease (most common cause in pediatrics)
  - glomerular inflammation ABSENT on renal biopsy: MCD (85%), focal segmental glomerular sclerosis
  - glomerular inflammation PRESENT on renal biopsy: membranoproliferative GN, IgA nephropathy
- secondary: nephrotic syndrome associated with systemic disease or due to another process causing glomerular injury (<10% in pediatrics)
  - autoimmune: SLE, DM, rheumatoid arthritis
  - genetic: sickle cell disease, Alport syndrome
  - infections: hepatitis B/C, post-streptococcal, infective endocarditis, HUS, HIV
  - malignancies: leukemia, lymphoma
  - medications: captopril, penicillamine, NSAIDs, antiepileptics
  - vasculitides: HSP, granulomatosis with polyangiitis
- congenital: congenital nephropathy of the Finnish type, Denys-Drash syndrome, etc.

History and Physical Exam
- non-specific symptoms such as irritability, malaise, fatigue, anorexia, or diarrhea
- edema
  - often first sign; detectable when fluid retention exceeds 3-5% of body weight
  - starts periorbital and often pretibial → edematous areas are white, soft, and pitting
  - gravity dependent: periorbital edema ↓ and pretibial edema ↑ over the day
  - anasarca may develop (i.e. marked periorbital and peripheral edema, ascites, pleural effusions, scrotal/labial edema)
- decrease in effective circulating volume (e.g. tachycardia, HTN, oliguria, etc.)
- foamy urine is a possible sign of proteinuria

PALE
Proteinuria (>50 mg/kg/d)
Hypo**A**lbuminemia (<20 g/L)
Hyper**L**ipidemia
Edema

Daily protein excretion can be estimated from a random urine protein/creatinine ratio

Investigations
- urine
  - urine dipstick (3 to 4+ proteinuria, microscopic hematuria) and microscopy (oval fat bodies, hyaline casts)
  - first morning urine protein/creatinine ratio (>200 mg/mmol)
- blood work
  - diagnostic: hypoalbuminemia (<25 g/L), hyperlipidemia/hypercholesterolemia (total cholesterol >5 mmol/L)
  - secondary: electrolytes (hypocalcemia, hyperkalemia, hyponatremia), renal function ($\uparrow$ BUN and Cr), coagulation profile ($\downarrow$ PTT)
  - appropriate investigations to rule out secondary causes: CBC, blood smear, C3/C4, ANA, hepatitis B/C titres, ASOT, HIV serology, etc.
- consider renal biopsy if: HTN, gross hematuria, renal function, low serum C3/C4, no response to steroids after 4 wk of therapy, frequent relapses (>2 in 6 mo), presentation before first year of life (high likelihood of congenital nephrotic syndrome), presentation ≥12 yr (rule out more serious renal pathology than MCD)

Management
- MCD: oral prednisone 2 mg/kg/d (or equivalent) for up to 12 wk → varicella status should be known before starting
- consider cytotoxic agents, immunomodulators, or high-dose pulse corticosteroid if steroid resistant
- symptomatic
  - edema: salt and fluid restriction, possibly diuretic (avoid if significant intravascular depletion); furosemide + albumin for anasarca
  - hyperlipidemia: generally resolves with remission; limit dietary fat intake; consider statin therapy if persistently nephrotic
  - hypoalbuminemia: IV albumin and furosemide not routinely given; consider if refractory edema
  - abnormal BP: control BP; fluid resuscitation if severe intravascular depletion; ACEI or ARBs for persistent HTN
- diet: no added salt; monitor caloric intake and supplement with Ca^{2+} and Vit D if on corticosteroids
- daily weights and BP to assess therapeutic progress
- secondary infections: treat with appropriate antimicrobials; antibiotic prophylaxis not recommended; pneumococcal vaccine at diagnosis and varicella vaccine after remission; varicella Ig + acyclovir if exposed while on corticosteroids
- secondary hypercoagulability: mobilize, avoid hemoconcentration due to hypovolemia, prompt sepsis treatment; heparin if thrombi occur

Side Effects of Long-Term Steroid Use
- Increased appetite
- Weight gain
- Dorsal hump
- Impaired growth
- Behavioural changes
- Risk of infection
- Salt and water retention
- HTN
- Bone demineralization
- Skin striae

Prognosis
- generally good: 80% of children responsive to corticosteroids
- up to 2/3 experience relapse, often multiple times; sustained remission with normal kidney function usually by adolescence
- complications: $\uparrow$ risk of infections (spontaneous peritonitis, cellulitis, sepsis); hypercoagulability due to decreased intravascular volume and antithrombin III depletion (PE, renal vein thrombosis); intravascular volume depletion, leading to hypotension, shock, renal failure; side effects of drugs

Hypertension in Childhood

Definition
- HTN: sBP and/or dBP ≥95th percentile for sex, age, and height on ≥3 occasions
- pre-HTN: sBP and/or dBP ≥90th percentile but <95th percentile OR BP ≥120/80 irrespective of age, gender, and height

Table 40. 95th Percentile Blood Pressures (mmHg)

Age (Yr)	Female		Male	
	50th Percentile for Height	75th Percentile for Height	50th Percentile for Height	75th Percentile for Height
1	104/58	105/59	103/56	104/57
6	111/74	113/74	114/74	115/75
12	123/80	124/81	123/81	125/82
17	129/84	130/85	136/87	138/87

Adapted from: the Fourth report on the diagnosis, evaluation, and treatment of high blood pressure in children and adolescents. National Heart, Lung and Blood Institute. National Institutes of Health. May 2004.

Epidemiology
- prevalence: 3-5% for HTN, 7-10% for pre-HTN; M>F
- increasing prevalence of pre-HTN over the last 25+ years

Etiology
- primary HTN
  - diagnosis of exclusion
  - most common in older children (≥10 yr), especially if positive family history, overweight, and only mild HTN
  - responsible for ~90% of cases of HTN in adolescents, rarely in young children
- secondary HTN
  - identifiable cause of HTN (most likely etiology depends on age)
  - responsible for majority of childhood HTN
- always consider white coat HTN for all ages

Table 41. Etiology of Secondary HTN by Age Group

System	Neonates	1 mo-6 yr	7-12 yr	>13 yr
Endocrine/Metabolic	CAH	Wilms' tumour (↑ renin) Neuroblastoma (↑ catecholamines)	Endocrinopathies*	Endocrinopathies*
Renal	Congenital renal disease	Renal parenchymal disease	Renal parenchymal disease	Renal parenchymal disease
Vascular	Coarctation of the aorta Renal artery thrombosis	Coarctation of the aorta RAS	Renovascular abnormalities	
Drugs		Corticosteroids Cyclosporine and tacrolimus	Corticosteroids OCP Cyclosporine and tacrolimus	Corticosteroids OCP Cyclosporine and tacrolimus Recreational drugs (amphetamines, cocaine, etc.)

*Note: may include hyperthyroidism, hyperparathyroidism, Cushing's syndrome, primary hyperaldosteronism/Conn's syndrome, pheochromocytoma

Risk Factors
- primary HTN: male gender, positive family history, obesity, obstructive sleep apnea, African American, prematurity/LBW
- secondary HTN: history of renal disease, abdominal trauma, family history of autoimmune diseases, umbilical artery catheterization

Signs of Secondary HTN
- Edema (renal parenchymal disease)
- Abdominal or renal bruit (RAS)
- Differential 4 limb BP/diminished femoral pulses (coarctation)
- Abdominal mass (Wilms', neuroblastoma)
- Goitre/skin changes (hyperthyroidism)
- Ambiguous genitalia (CAH)

History
- often asymptomatic, but can include FTT, fatigue, epistaxis
- symptoms of hypertensive emergency
  - neurologic: headache, seizures, focal complaints, change in mental status, visual disturbances
  - cardiovascular: symptoms of MI or heart failure (chest pain, palpitations, cough, SOB)
- symptoms of secondary HTN: guided by etiology; ask about medications and recreational drugs (current and past)

Physical Exam
- BP measurement (make sure correct cuff size is used), plot on growth chart, BMI
- look for signs of hypertensive emergency (e.g. full neurologic exam, ophthalmoscopy, precordial exam, peripheral pulses, perfusion status)
- look for signs of secondary HTN

Investigations
- laboratory
  - urine dipstick for hematuria and/or proteinuria (renal disease), urine catecholamines (pheochromocytoma, neuroblastoma)
  - blood work: renal function tests (electrolytes, Cr, BUN), consider renin and aldosterone levels (RAS, Conn's syndrome, Wilms' tumour)
  - other specific hormones if indicated on history and physical
- imaging: Echo (coarctation, heart function), abdominal U/S (RAS, abdominal mass), renal radionucleide imaging (renal scarring)

Management
- treat underlying cause
- non-pharmacologic: modify concurrent cardiovascular risk factors (weight reduction, exercise, salt restriction, smoking cessation)
- pharmacologic: gradual lowering of BP using thiazide diuretics; no antihypertensives have been formally studied in children; if hypertensive emergencies use hydralazine, labetalol, sodium nitroprusside
- management of end-organ damage (e.g. retinopathy, LVH)
- consider referral to specialist

Pediatric BP Calculation
sBP = age x 2 + 90
dBP = 2/3 x sBP

Prognosis
- end-organ damage (similar to adults) including LVH, CHF, cerebrovascular insults, renal disease, retinopathy

Neurology

Seizure Disorders

- see Neurology, N18

Differential Diagnosis of Seizures in Children
- benign febrile seizure
- CNS: infection, tumour, HIE, trauma, hemorrhage
- metabolic: hypoglycemia, hypocalcemia, hyponatremia
- idiopathic epilepsy and epileptic syndromes
- others: neurocutaneous syndromes, AVM, drug ingestions/withdrawal
- seizure mimics

Investigations
- lab tests: CBC, electrolytes, calcium, magnesium, glucose
- toxicology screen if indicated
- EEG
- CT/MRI, if indicated (focal neurological deficit or has not returned to baseline several hours after seizure)
- consider LP if first-time non-febrile seizure (not indicated for determining recurrence risk of benign febrile seizures or to determine seizure type or epileptic syndrome)

Heart problems, such as long QT syndrome and hypertrophic cardiomyopathy, are often misdiagnosed as epilepsy. Include cardiac causes of syncope in your differential diagnosis, particularly when the episodes occur during physical activity

CHILDHOOD EPILEPSY SYNDROMES

Infantile Spasms
- brief, repeated symmetric contractions of neck, trunk, extremities (flexion and extension) lasting 10-30 s
- occur in clusters; often associated with developmental delay; onset 4-8 mo
- 20% unknown etiology (usually good response to treatment); 80% due to metabolic or developmental abnormalities, encephalopathies, or are associated with neurocutaneous syndromes (usually poor response to treatment)
- can develop into West syndrome (infantile spasms, psychomotor developmental arrest, and hypsarrhythmia) or Lennox-Gastaut (see below)
- typical EEG: hypsarrhythmia (high voltage slow waves, spikes and polyspikes, background disorganization)
- management: ACTH, vigabatrin, benzodiazepines

Seizure Mimics
- Benign paroxysmal vertigo
- Breath holding
- Hypoglycemia
- Narcolepsy
- Night terror
- Pseudoseizure
- Syncope
- TIA
- Tic

Lennox-Gastaut
- characterized by triad of 1) multiple seizure types, 2) diffuse cognitive dysfunction, and 3) slow generalized spike and slow wave EEG
- onset commonly 3-5 yr of age
- seen with underlying encephalopathy and brain malformations
- management: valproic acid, benzodiazepines, and ketogenic diet; however, response often poor

Juvenile Myoclonic Epilepsy (Janz Syndrome)
- myoclonus particularly in morning; frequently presents as generalized tonic-clonic seizures
- adolescent onset (12-16 yr of age); autosomal dominant with variable penetrance
- typical EEG: 3.5-6 Hz irregular spike and wave, increased with photic stimulation
- management: lifelong treatment (valproic acid); excellent prognosis

Childhood Absence Epilepsy
- multiple daily absence seizures lasting <30 s without post-ictal state that may resolve spontaneously or become generalized in adolescence
- peak age of onset 6-7 yr, F>M, strong genetic predisposition
- typical EEG: 3 Hz spike and wave
- management: valproic acid or ethosuximide

Benign Focal Epilepsy of Childhood with Rolandic/Centrotemporal Spikes
- focal motor seizures involving tongue, mouth, face, upper extremity usually occuring in sleep-wake transition states; remains conscious, but aphasic post-ictally
- onset peaks at 5-10 yr of age; 16% of all non-febrile seizures; remits spontaneously in adolescence without sequelae
- typical EEG: repetitive spikes in centrotemporal area with normal background
- management: frequent seizures controlled by carbamazepine, no medication if infrequent seizures

Ketogenic Diet and other Dietary Treatments for Epilepsy
Cochrane DB Syst Rev 2012;3:CD001903
Study: Systematic review of all studies of ketogenic and related diets. Included the review of 4 RCTs, 6 prospective studies, and 5 retrospective studies.
Population: Adults and children with diagnosed epilepsy of any type.
Intervention: Ketogenic diet, control (placebo diet, any treatment with known antiepileptic properties).
Main Outcome Measure: Seizure control at 3, 6, 12 mo.
Results: Studies showed a response rate of at least 38-50% seizure reduction at 3 mo. This response was maintained for up to a year. A range of side effects were reported. The most frequent were gastrointestinal effects (30%).
Conclusion: The ketogenic diet is a valid option for people with medically-intractable epilepsy.

General Approach to Treatment
- education for patient and parents including education and precautions in daily life (e.g. buddy system, showers instead of baths)
- medication
  - initiate: treatment with drug appropriate to seizure type; often if >2 unprovoked afebrile seizures within 6-12 mo
  - optimize: start with one drug and increase dosage until seizures controlled
  - if no effect, switch over to another before adding a second antiepileptic drug
  - continue antiepileptic drug therapy until patient free of seizures for >2 yr, then wean over 4-6 mo
- ketogenic diet (high fat diet): used in patients who do not respond to polytherapy or who do not wish to take medication (valproic acid contraindicated in conjunction with ketogenic diet because may increase hepatotoxicity)
- legal obligation to report to Ministry of Transportation if patient wishes to drive

Generalized and Partial Seizures
- see Neurology, N18

Febrile Seizures

Epidemiology
- most common cause of seizure in children (3-5% of children)
- M>F; age 6 mo-6 yr

Clinical Presentation
- often with associated illness or fever and family history
- no evidence of CNS infection/inflammation before or after seizure; no history of non-febrile seizures

Table 42. Comparison of Typical and Atypical Febrile Seizures

Simple/Typical (70-80%)	Complex/Atypical (20-30%)
All of the following: Duration <15 min (95% <5 min) Generalized tonic-clonic No recurrence in 24 h period No neurological impairment or developmental delay before or after seizure	At least one of the following: Duration >15 min Focal onset or focal features during seizure Recurrent seizures (>1 in 24 h period) Previous neurological impairment or neurological deficit after seizure

Workup
- history: determine focus of fever, description of seizure, medications, trauma history, development, family history
- physical exam: LOC, signs of meningitis, neurological exam, head circumference, focus of infection
- septic workup including LP if suspecting meningitis (strongly consider if child <12 mo; consider if child is 12-18 mo; only if meningeal signs present if child >18 mo)
- if typical febrile seizure, investigations only for determining focus of fever
- EEG/CT/MRI brain not warranted unless atypical febrile seizure or abnormal neurologic findings

Management
- counsel and reassure patient and parents
  - febrile seizures do not cause brain damage
  - very small risk of developing epilepsy: 9% in child with multiple risk factors; 2% in child with typical febrile seizures compared to 1% in general population
  - 33% chance of recurrence (mostly within 1 yr of first seizure and in children <1 yr old)
- antipyretics and fluids for comfort (though neither prevent seizure)
- prophylaxis with antiepileptic drugs not recommended
- if high risk for recurrent or prolonged seizures, have rectal or sublingual lorazepam at home
- treat underlying cause of fever

Recurrent Headache

Headache – Red Flags
- First and worst headache of their life
- Sudden onset
- Focal neurological deficits
- Constitutional symptoms
- Worse in morning
- Worse with bending over, coughing, straining
- Change in LOC
- Sudden mood changes
- Pain that wakes patient
- Fatigue
- Affecting school attendance

- see Neurology, N44

Differential Diagnosis
- primary headache: tension, migraine, cluster
- secondary headache: see Neurology, N44

General Assessment
- if unremarkable history and neurological and general physical exam is negative, most likely diagnosis is migraine or tension headache
- CT or MRI if history or physical reveals red flags
- inquire about level of disability, academic performance, after-school activities

Hypotonia

- decreased resistance to passive movements – "floppy baby"

Differential Diagnosis

- central: chromosomal (DS, Prader-Willi, Fragile X syndrome), metabolic (hypoglycemia, kernicterus), perinatal problems (asphyxia, ICH), endocrine (hypothyroidism, hypopituitarism), systemic illness (TORCH infection, sepsis, dehydration), CNS malformations, dysmorphic syndromes
- peripheral: motor neuron (spinal muscular atrophy, polio), peripheral nerve (Charcot-Marie-Tooth syndrome) neuromuscular junction (myasthenia gravis), muscle fibre (mitochondrial myopathy, muscular dystrophy, myotonic dystrophy)

History and Physical Exam

- proper assessment of tone requires accurate determination of GA
- differentiate between UMN and LMN lesion: spontaneous posture (spontaneous movement, movement against gravity, frog-leg position); muscle weakness; joint mobility (hyperextensibility); muscle bulk; presence of fasciculations
- postural maneuvers
  - traction response: pull to sit, look for flexion of arms to counteract traction and head lag
  - axillary suspension: suspend infant by holding at axilla and lifting; hypotonic babies will slip through grasp because of low shoulder girdle tone
  - ventral suspension: infant is prone and supported under the abdomen by one hand; infant should be able to hold up extremities; inverted "U" posturing demonstrates hypotonia
- dysmorphic features, cognitive ability, reflexes, strength

Causes of hypotonia that respond to rapid treatment: hypokalemia, hypermagnesemia, acidemia, toxins, drugs, hypoglycemia, seizure, infection, intracranial bleeding, hydrocephalus

Investigations

- rule out systemic disorders (e.g. electrolytes, ABG, blood glucose, CK, and serum/urine investigations for multiple etiologies including mitochondrial causes)
- neuroimaging: MRI/MRA when indicated
- EMG, muscle biopsy/NCS
- chromosome analysis, genetic testing, metabolic testing, neuromuscular testing

Treatment

- depends on etiology: some treatments available for specific diagnosis
- counsel parents on prognosis and genetic implications
- refer patients for specialized care, refer for rehabilitation, OT, PT, assess feeding ability

Cerebral Palsy

Definition

- a symptom complex, not a disease
- non-progressive central motor impairment syndrome due to insult to or anomaly of the immature CNS
- incidence: 1.5-2.5/1,000 live births (industrialized nations)
- life expectancy is dependent on the degree of mobility and intellectual impairment, not on severity of CNS lesion

Etiology

- often obscure, no definite etiology identified in 1/3 of cases
- 10% related to intrapartum asphyxia; 10% due to postnatal insult (infections, asphyxia, prematurity with IVH and trauma)
- association with LBW babies

Clinical Presentation

- general signs: delay in motor milestones, developmental delay, learning disabilities, visual/hearing impairment, seizures, microcephaly, uncoordinated swallow (aspiration)

Table 43. Types of Cerebral Palsy

Type	% of Total	Characteristics	Area of Brain Involved
Spastic	70-80%	Truncal hypotonia in first yr Increased tone, increased reflexes, clonus Can affect one limb (monoplegia), one side of body (hemiplegia), both legs (diplegia), or both arms and legs (quadriplegia)	UMN of pyramidal tract Diplegia associated with periventricular leukomalacia in premature babies Quadriplegia associated with HIE (asphyxia), higher incidence of intellectual disability
Athetoid/ Dyskinetic	10-15%	Athetosis (involuntary writhing movements) ± chorea (involuntary jerky movements) Can involve face, tongue (results in dysarthria)	Basal ganglia (may be associated with kernicterus)
Ataxic	<5%	Poor coordination, poor balance (wide based gait) Can have intention tremor	Cerebellum
Mixed	10-15%	More than one of the above motor patterns	

Investigations
- may include metabolic screen, chromosome studies, serology, neuroimaging (MRI), EMG, EEG (if seizures), ophthalmology assessment, audiology assessment

Treatment
- maximize potential through multidisciplinary services such as primary care physician, OT, PT, SLP, school supports, etc.
- orthopedic management (e.g. dislocations, contractures, rhizotomy)
- management of symptoms: spasticity (baclofen, Botox®), constipation (stool softeners)

Neurocutaneous Syndromes

In neurocutaneous syndromes, the younger the child at presentation, the more likely they are to develop mental retardation

- characterized by tendency to form tumours of the CNS, PNS, viscera, and skin

NEUROFIBROMATOSIS TYPE I
- autosomal dominant but 50% are the result of new mutations
- also known as von Recklinghausen disease
- incidence 1:3,000, mutation in NF1 gene on 17q11.2 (codes for neurofibromin protein)
- learning disorders, abnormal speech development, and seizures are common
- diagnosis of NF-1 requires 2 or more of
  - ≥6 café-au-lait spots (>5 mm if prepubertal, >1.5 cm if postpubertal)
  - ≥2 neurofibromas of any type or one plexiform neurofibroma
  - ≥2 Lisch nodules (hamartomas of the iris)
  - optic glioma
  - freckling in the axillary or inguinal region
  - a distinctive bony lesion (e.g. sphenoid dysplasia, cortical thinning of long bones)
  - a first degree relative with confirmed NF-1

NEUROFIBROMATOSIS TYPE II
- autosomal dominant
- incidence 1:33,000
- characterized by predisposition to form intracranial, spinal tumours
- diagnosed when bilateral vestibular schwannomas are found, or a first-degree relative with NF-2 and either unilateral vestibular schwannoma, or any two of the following: meningioma, glioma, schwannoma, neurofibroma, posterior subcapsular lenticular opacities.
- treatment consists of monitoring for tumour development and surgery

Respirology

Approach to Dyspnea

- determine if patient is sick or not sick; ABCs
- history: onset, previous episodes, precipitating events, associated symptoms, past medical/family history of respiratory disease
- physical exam: vitals, SpO₂, evidence of cyanosis, respiratory, cardiovascular
- investigations: CBC and differential, electrolytes, BUN, Cr, NP swab, ABG, CXR, ECG (based on clinical findings)

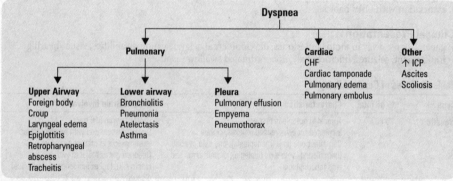

Figure 18. Approach to dyspnea in childhood

Upper Respiratory Tract Diseases

- see Otolaryngology, OT40
- diseases above the thoracic inlet characterized by inspiratory stridor, hoarseness, and suprasternal retractions
- differential diagnosis of stridor: croup, bacterial tracheitis, epiglottitis, foreign body aspiration, subglottic stenosis (congenital or iatrogenic), laryngomalacia/tracheomalacia (collapse of airway cartilage on inspiration)

Table 44. Common Upper Respiratory Tract Infections in Children

	Croup (Laryngotracheobronchitis)	Bacterial Tracheitis	Epiglottitis
Anatomy	Subglottic laryngitis	Subglottic tracheitis	Supraglottic laryngitis
Epidemiology	Common in children <6 yr, with peak incidence between 7-36 mo Common in fall and early winter	Rare All age groups	Very rare – due to Hib vaccination Usually older (2-6 yr)
Etiology	Parainfluenza (75%) Influenza A and B RSV Adenovirus	S. aureus H. influenzae α-hemolytic strep Pneumococcus M. catarrhalis	H. influenzae β-hemolytic strep
Clinical Presentation	Common prodrome: rhinorrhea, pharyngitis, cough ± low-grade fever Hoarse voice Barking cough Stridor Worse at night	Similar symptoms as croup, but more rapid deterioration with high fever Toxic appearance Does not respond to croup treatments	Toxic appearance Rapid progression 4 Ds – drooling, dysphagia, dysphonia, distress Stridor Tripod position Sternal recession Anxious Fever (>39°C)
Investigations	Clinical diagnosis CXR in atypical presentation: "steeple sign" from subglottic narrowing	Clinical diagnosis Endoscopy: definitive diagnosis	Clinical diagnosis Avoid examining the throat to prevent further respiratory exacerbation
Treatment	Stridor at rest is an EMERGENCY No evidence for humidified O_2 Dexamethasone: PO 1 dose Racemic epinephrine: nebulized, 1-3 doses, q1-2h Intubation if unresponsive to treatment	Usually requires intubation IV antibiotics	Intubation Antibiotics Prevented with Hib vaccine

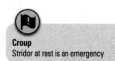

Croup
Stridor at rest is an emergency

Lower Respiratory Tract Diseases

- obstruction of airways below thoracic inlet, produces more expiratory sounds
- classic symptom: wheezing

Differential Diagnosis of Wheezing

- common: asthma (recurrent wheezing episodes, identifiable triggers, typically over 6 yr), bronchiolitis (first episode of wheezing, usually under 1 yr), recurrent aspiration (often neurological impairment), pneumonia (fever, cough, malaise)
- uncommon: foreign body (acute unilateral wheezing and coughing), CF (prolonged wheezing, unresponsive to therapy), bronchopulmonary dysplasia (often develops after prolonged ventilation in the newborn)
- rare: CHF, mediastinal mass, bronchiolitis obliterans, tracheobronchial anomalies

Pneumonia

Etiology
- inflammation of pulmonary tissue, associated with consolidation of alveolar spaces

Clinical Presentation
- incidence is greatest in first year of life with viral causes being most common in children <5 yr
- fever, cough, tachypnea
- CXR: diffuse, streaky infiltrates bilaterally
- bacterial causes may present with cough, fever, chills, dyspnea, more dramatic CXR changes (e.g. lobar consolidation, pleural effusion)

Management

- supportive therapy: hydration, antipyretics, humidified O_2

Table 45. Common Causes and Treatment of Pneumonia at Different Ages

Age	Bacterial	Viral	Atypical Bacteria	Treatment
Neonates	GBS *E. coli* *Listeria*	CMV Herpes virus Enterovirus	*Mycoplasma hominis* *Ureaplasma urealyticum*	Ampicillin + gentamicin / tobramycin (add erythromycin if suspect *Chlamydia*)
1-3 mo	*S. aureus* *H. influenzae* *S. pneumoniae* *B. pertussis*	CMV, RSV Influenza Parainfluenza	*Chlamydia trachomatis* *Ureaplasma urealyticum*	Cefuroxime OR ampicillin ± erythromycin OR clarithromycin
3 mo-5 yr	*S. pneumoniae* *S. aureus* *H. influenzae* GAS	RSV Adenovirus Influenza	*Mycoplasma pneumoniae* TB	Amoxicillin (if mild) OR ampicillin OR cefuroxime
>5 yr	*S. pneumoniae* *H. influenzae* *S. aureus*	Influenza Varicella Adenovirus	*Mycoplasma pneumoniae* *Chlamydia pneumoniae* TB *Legionella pneumophila*	Erythromycin OR clarithromycin (1st line) OR ampicillin OR cefuroxime

Bronchiolitis

Definition
- LRTI, usually in children <2 yr, that has wheezing and signs of respiratory distress

Epidemiology
- the most common LRTI in infants, affects 50% of children in first 2 yr of life; peak incidence at 6 mo, winter or early spring
- increased incidence of asthma in later life

Etiology
- RSV (>50%), parainfluenza, influenza, rhinovirus, adenovirus, *M. pneumoniae* (rare)

Clinical Presentation
- prodrome of URTI with cough and/or rhinorrhea, possible fever
- feeding difficulties, irritability
- wheezing, crackles, respiratory distress, tachypnea, tachycardia, retractions, poor air entry; symptoms often peak at 3-4 d

Investigations
- CXR (only in severe disease, poor response to therapy, chronic episode): air trapping, peribronchial thickening, atelectasis, increased linear markings
- NP swab: direct detection of viral antigen (immunofluorescence)
- WBC can be normal

Treatment
- self-limiting disease with peak symptoms usually lasting 2-3 wk
- mild to moderate distress
  - supportive: PO or IV hydration, antipyretics for fever, regular or humidified high flow O_2
- severe distress
  - as above ± intubation and ventilation as needed
  - consider rebetol (Ribavirin®) in high risk groups: bronchopulmonary dysplasia, CHD, congenital lung disease, immunodeficient
- monthly RSV-Ig or palivizumab (monoclonal antibody against the F-glycoprotein of RSV) is protective against severe disease in high risk groups; case fatality rate <1%
- antibiotics have no therapeutic value unless there is secondary bacterial pneumonia
- indications for hospitalization
  - hypoxia: O_2 saturation <92% on initial presentation
  - persistent resting tachypnea >60/min and retractions after several salbutamol masks
  - past history of chronic lung disease, hemodynamically significant cardiac disease, neuromuscular problem, immunocompromised
  - young infants <6 mo old (unless extremely mild)
  - significant feeding problems
  - social problem (e.g. inadequate care at home)

Bronchodilators for Bronchiolitis
Cochrane DB Syst Rev 2010;12:CD001266
Study: Meta-analysis of prospective, randomized, double-blinded, placebo-controlled trials.
Patients: 1,912 infants (28 trials) up to 24 mo old with bronchiolitis.
Intervention: Bronchodilators (including albuterol, salbutamol, terbutaline, ipratropium bromide, and adrenergic agents) given oral, subcutaneous, or nebulized vs. placebo.
Main Outcome: Oxygen saturation.
Results: No clinically significant difference for infants treated with bronchodilators vs. placebo for bronchiolitis. Given the costs and side effects, it is not recommended to use bronchodilators as management for bronchiolitis in infants.

Children with bronchiolitis do not respond to ipratropium bromide (Atrovent®) or steroids

Asthma

Definition
- see Respirology, R7
- inflammatory disorder of the airwarys characterized by recurrent episodes of reversible small airway obstruction, resulting from airway hyperresponsiveness to endogenous and exogenous stimuli
- very common, presents most often in early childhood
- associated with other atopic diseases such as allergic rhinitis or atopic dermatitis

Clinical Presentation
- episodic bouts of wheezing, dyspnea, tachypnea, cough (usually at night/early morning, with activity, or cold exposure)
- physical exam may reveal hyper-resonant chest, prolonged expiration, wheeze

Triggers
- URTI (viral or *Mycoplasma*), weather (cold exposure, humidity changes), allergens (pets), irritants (cigarette smoke), exercise, emotional stress, drugs (ASA, β-blockers)

Classification
- mild: occasional attacks of wheezing or coughing (<2/wk); symptoms respond quickly to inhaled bronchodilator; never needs systemic corticosteroids
- moderate: more frequent episodes with symptoms persisting and chronic cough; decreased exercise tolerance; sometimes needs systemic corticosteroids
- severe: daily and nocturnal symptoms; frequent ED visits and hospitalizations; usually needs systemic corticosteroids

Management
- acute
  - O_2 (keep O_2 saturation >94%) and fluids if dehydrated
  - β2-agonists: salbutamol (Ventolin®) MDI + spacer (nebulized or IV in very severe episodes with impending respiratory failure), 5 puffs (<20 kg) or 10 puffs q20min for first hour (>20 kg)
  - ipratropium bromide (Atrovent®) if severe: MDI + spacer, 3 puffs (<20 kg) or 6 puffs (>20 kg) q20min with salbutamol, or add to first 3 salbutamol masks (0.25 mg if <20 kg, 0.5mg if >20 kg)
  - steroids: prednisone (1-2 mg/kg x 5 d) or dexamethasone (0.3 mg/kg/d x 5 d or 0.6 mg/kg/d x 2 d); in severe disease, use IV steroids
  - continue to observe; can discharge patient if asymptomatic for 2-4 h after last dose
- chronic
  - education, emotional support, avoid allergens or irritants, develop an "action plan"
  - exercise program (e.g. swimming)
  - monitor respiratory function with peak flow meter (improves self-awareness of status)
  - PFTs for children >6 yr
  - reliever therapy: short acting β2-agonists (e.g. salbutamol)
  - controller therapy (first line therapy for all children): low dose daily inhaled corticosteroids
  - second line therapy for children <12 yr: moderate dose of daily inhaled corticosteoroids
  - second line therapy for children >12 yr: leukotriene receptor antagonist OR long acting β2-agonist in conjunction with low dose inhaled corticosteroids; leukotriene receptor antagonist monotherapy may be considered an alternative second line therapy
  - severe asthma unresponsive to first and second line treatments: injection immunotherapy
  - aerochamber for children using daily inhaled corticosteroids
- indications for hospitalization
  - ongoing need for supplemental O_2
  - persistently increased work of breathing
  - β2-agonists are needed more often than q4h after 4-8 h of conventional treatment
  - patient deteriorates while on systemic steroids

Cystic Fibrosis

- see Respirology, R12

Etiology
- 1 per 3,000 live births, mostly Caucasians
- autosomal recessive, *CFTR* gene found on chromosome 7 (ΔF508 mutation in 70%, but >1,600 different mutations identified) resulting in a dysfunctional chloride channel on the apical membrane of cells
- leads to relative dehydration of airway secretions, resulting in impaired mucociliary transport and airway obstruction

Updated guidance for palivizumab prophylaxis among infants and young children at increased risk of hospitalization for respiratory syncytial virus infection.
Pediatrics 2014 Aug;134(2):415-20.
Erratum in: *Pediatrics* 2014 Dec;134(6):1221.

Palivizumab prophylaxis is recommended for the first year of life for infants born before 29 weeks gestation, and preterm infants with chronic lung disease of maturity (born at <32 weeks gestation and requiring >21% oxygen for at least 28 days after birth). Such prophylaxis may be administered in the first year of life to infants with hemodynamically significant heart disease, and a maximum of 5 monthly 15 mg/kg doses may be administered during the RSV season to infants requiring it; infants born during the RSV season may need fewer doses. Prophylaxis may be considered in the first year of life for children with pulmonary abnormalities or neuromuscular disease impairing the ability to clear secretions from the upper airway, and may be considered for children younger than 24 months who are profoundly immunocompromised during the RSV season. Palivizumab prophylaxis is only recommended in the second year of life for children who required at least 28 days of supplemental oxygen after birth with ongoing medical intervention needs.
Monthly prophylaxis should be discontinued in children experiencing breakthrough RSV hospitalizations. Insufficient evidence exists to support the use of prophylaxis for children with cystic fibrosis or Down's syndrome.

Canadian Pediatric Asthma Consensus Guidelines for Assessing Adequate Control of Asthma
- Daytime symptoms <4 d/wk
- Night time symptoms <1 night/wk
- Normal physical activity
- Mild and infreqeunt exacerbations
- No work/school absenteeism
- Need for β-agonist <4 doses/wk
- FEV1 or peak expiratory flow ≥90% of personal best
- Peak expiratory flow diurnal variation <10-15%

Clinical Presentation
- neonatal: meconium ileus, prolonged jaundice, antenatal bowel perforation
- infancy: pancreatic insufficiency with steatorrhea and FTT (despite voracious appetite), anemia, hypoproteinemia, hyponatremia
- childhood: heat intolerance, wheezing or chronic cough, recurrent chest infections (*S. aureus, P. aeruginosa, H. influenzae*), hemoptysis, nasal polyps, distal intestinal obstruction syndrome, rectal prolapse, clubbing of fingers
- older patients: COPD, infertility (males), decreased fertility (female)

Investigations
- sweat chloride test x 2 (>60 mEq/L)
  - false positive tests: malnutrition, atopic dermatitis, hypothyroidism, hypoparathyroidism, GSD, adrenal insufficiency, G6PD, Klinefelter syndrome, technical issues, autonomic dysfunction, familial cholestasis syndrome
  - false negative tests: technical problem with test, malnutrition, skin edema, mineralocorticoids

Management
- nutritional counselling: high calorie diet, pancreatic enzyme replacements, fat soluble vitamin supplements
- management of chest disease: physiotherapy, postural drainage, exercise, bronchodilators, aerosolized DNAase and inhaled hypertonic saline, antibiotics (e.g. cephalosporin, cloxacillin, ciprofloxacin, inhaled tobramycin depending on sputum C&S), lung transplantation
- genetic counselling

Complications
- respiratory failure, pneumothorax (poor prognostic sign), cor pulmonale (late), pancreatic fibrosis with DM, gallstones, cirrhosis with portal HTN, infertility (male)
- early death (current median survival in Canada is 46.6 yr)

CF Presenting Signs

CF PANCREAS
Chronic cough and wheezing
FTT
Pancreatic insufficiency (symptoms of malabsorption such as steatorrhea)
Alkalosis and hypotonic dehydration
Neonatal intestinal obstruction (meconium ileus)/Nasal polyps
Clubbing of fingers/Chest radiograph with characteristic changes
Rectal prolapse
Electrolyte elevation in sweat, salty skin
Absence or congenital atresia of vas deferens
Sputum with *S. aureus* or *P. aeruginosa* (mucoid)
- Pancreatic dysfunction – determined by 3 d fecal fat collection
- Genetics – useful where sweat chloride test is equivocal

Rheumatology

Evaluation of Limb Pain

Table 46. Differential Diagnosis of Limb Pain

Cause	<3 yr	3-10 yr	>10 yr
Trauma	x	x	x
Infectious			
Septic arthritis	x	x	x
Osteomyelitis	x	x	x
Inflammatory			
Transient synovitis	x	x	
JIA	x	x	x
Spondyloarthritis		x	x
SLE		x	x
Dermatomyositis		x	x
HSP		x	x
Anatomic/Orthopedic			
Legg-Calvé-Perthes disease		x	x
Slipped capital femoral epiphysis			x
Osgood-Schlatter disease			x
Neoplastic			
Leukemia	x	x	x
Neuroblastoma	x	x	x
Bone tumour		x	x
Hematologic			
Hemophilia (hemarthrosis)	x	x	x
Sickle cell anemia	x	x	x
Pain Syndromes			
Growing pains		x	x
Fibromyalgia		x	x
Complex regional pain syndrome			x

- must rule out infection, malignancy, and acute orthopedic conditions

History
- demographics (age, gender)
- pattern of onset and progression of symptoms (including acuity and chronicity)
- morning stiffness, limp/weight-bearing status, night pain
- joint involvement (type, distribution) ± spine (axial) involvement
- extra-articular manifestations and systemic symptoms
- functional status – activities of daily living
- family history (arthritis, IBD, psoriasis, spondyloarthropathies, uveitis, bleeding disorders, sickle cell anemia)
- past medical illness, intercurrent infection, travel, sick contact history, joint injury

Red Flags for Limb Pain
Fever, pinpoint pain/tenderness, pain out of proportion to degree of inflammation, night pain, weight loss, erythema

Physical Exam
- growth parameters
- screening examination (pediatric gait, arms, legs, spine exam)
- joint exam: inspection/palpation (swelling, erythema, warmth, tenderness, deformity), ROM
- adjacent structures (bone, tendon, muscle, skin)
- leg length
- neurologic exam

Investigations
- basic: CBC and differential, blood smear, ESR, CRP, x-ray
- as indicated: blood (ANA, RF, culture, viral/bacterial serology, CK, PTT, sickle cell screen, immunoglobulins, complement), urinalysis, synovial fluid (cell count, Gram stain, culture), TB skin test, imaging, bone marrow aspiration, slit lamp exam

Growing Pains

Epidemiology
- age 2-12 yr, M=F

Clinical Presentation
- diagnosis of exclusion
- intermittent, non-articular pain in childhood with normal physical exam findings
- pain at night, often bilateral and limited to the calf, shin, or thigh; typically short-lived
- relieved by heat, massage, mild analgesics
- child is well, asymptomatic during the day, no functional limitation
- possible family history of growing pains

Management
- lab investigations not necessary if typical presentation; reassurance and supportive management

Transient Synovitis of the Hip

- benign, self-limited disorder, usually occurs after URTI, pharyngitis, AOM

Epidemiology
- age 3-10 yr, M>F

Clinical Presentation
- afebrile or low-grade fever, pain typically occurs in hips, knees (referred from hip); painful limp but full ROM (pain not as pronounced as in joint or bone infections)
- symptoms resolve over 7-10 d

Investigations
- WBC within normal limits; ESR and CRP may be mildly elevated
- joint effusions may be seen on imaging
- diagnosis of exclusion (rule out septic arthritis and osteomyelitis)

Treatment
- symptomatic and anti-inflammatory medications

Septic Arthritis and Osteomyelitis

- **MEDICAL EMERGENCY**
- see Orthopedics, OR9

Table 47. Microorganisms and Treatment Involved in Septic Arthritis/Osteomyelitis

Age	Pathogens	Treatment
Neonate	GBS, *S. aureus*, Gram negative bacilli	cloxacillin + aminoglycoside or cefotaxime
Infant (1-3 mo)	*Strep.* spp., *Staph.* spp., *H. influenzae* Pathogens as per neonate	cloxacillin + cefotaxime
Child	*S. aureus*, *S. pneumoniae*, GAS	cefazolin
Adolescent	As above; also *N. gonorrhoeae*	cefazolin
Sickle cell disease	As above; also *Salmonella*	cefotaxime

GAS = group A *Strep*; GBS = group B *Strep*   Adapted from Tse SML, Laxer RM. *Pediatrics in Review* 2006;27:170-179

Juvenile Idiopathic Arthritis

- a heterogenous group of conditions characterized by persistent arthritis in children <16 yr
- diagnosis: arthritis in ≥1 joint(s); duration ≥6 wk; onset age <16 yr old; exclusion of other causes of arthritis; classification defined by features/number of joints affected in the first 6 mo of onset

Systemic Arthritis (Still's Disease)
- onset at any age, M=F
- once or twice daily fever spikes (>38.5°C) ≥2 d/wk; children usually acutely unwell during fever episodes
- extra-articular features: erythematous "salmon-coloured" maculopapular rash, lymphadenopathy, hepatosplenomegaly, leukocytosis, thrombocytosis, anemia, serositis
- arthritis may occur weeks to months later
- high ESR, CRP, WBC, platelet count

Oligoarticular Arthritis (1-4 joints)
- onset early childhood, F>M
- persistent: affects no more than 4 joints during the disease course
- extended: affects more than 4 joints after the first 6 mo
- typically affects large joints: knees > ankles, elbows, wrists; hip involvement unusual
- ANA positive ~60-80%, RF negative
- screening eye exams for asymptomatic anterior uveitis (occurs in ~30%)
- complications: knee flexion contracture, quadriceps atrophy, leg-length discrepancy, growth disturbances

Polyarticular Arthritis (5 or more joints)
- uveitis is present in 10% of patients
- RF negative
  - onset: 2-4 yr and 6-12 yr, F>M
  - symmetrical involvement of large and small joints of hands and feet, TMJ, cervical spine
- RF positive
  - onset: late childhood/early adolescence, F>M
  - similar to the aggressive form of adult rheumatoid arthritis
  - severe, rapidly destructive, symmetrical arthritis of large and small joints
  - may have rheumatoid nodules at pressure points (elbows, knees)
  - unremitting disease, persists into adulthood

Enthesitis-Related Arthritis
- onset: late childhood/adolescence, M>F
- arthritis and/or enthesitis (inflammation at the site where tendons or ligaments attach to the bone)
- weight bearing joints, especially hip and intertarsal joints
- risk of developing ankylosing spondylitis in adulthood

Psoriatic Arthritis
- onset: 2-4 yr and 9-11 yr, F>M
- arthritis and psoriasis OR arthritis and at least two of:
  - dactylitis, nail pitting or other abnormalities, or family history of psoriasis in a 1st degree relative
  - asymmetric or symmetric small or large joint involvement

Management
- goals of therapy: eliminate inflammation, prevent joint damage, promote normal growth and development as well as normal function, minimize medication toxicity
- exercise to maintain ROM and muscle strength
- multidisciplinary approach: OT/PT, social work, orthopedics, ophthalmology, rheumatology
- 1st line drug therapy: NSAIDs, intra-articular corticosteroids
- 2nd line drug therapy: DMARDs (methotrexate, sulfasalazine, leflunamide), corticosteroids (acute management of severe arthritis, systemic symptoms of JIA, topical eye drops for uveitis), biologic agents

Reactive Arthritis

- see Rheumatology, RH23
- arthritis (typically the knee) follows bacterial infection, especially with *Salmonella, Shigella, Yersinia, Campylobacter, Chlamydia*, and most commonly *Streptococcus* (post-streptococcal reactive arthritis)
- typically resolves spontaneously
- may progress to chronic illness or Reiter's syndrome (urethritis, conjunctivitis)

Lyme Arthritis

- see Infectious Diseases, ID23
- caused by spirochete *Borrelia burgdorferi*
- incidence highest among 5-10 yr olds
- do not treat children <8 yr old with doxycycline (may cause permanent tooth discolouration)

Systemic Lupus Erythematosus

- see Rheumatology, RH11
- autoimmune illness affecting multiple organ systems
- incidence 1/1,000, more commonly age >10, F:M = 10:1
- childhood-onset SLE vs. adult-onset SLE: children have more active disease, are more likely to have renal disease, and children receive more intensive drug therapy and have a poorer prognosis

Vasculitides

HENOCH-SCHÖNLEIN PURPURA
- most common vasculitis of childhood, peak incidence 4-10 yr, M:F = 2:1
- vasculitis of small vessels
- often have history of URTI 1-3 wk before onset of symptoms

Clinical Presentation
- clinical triad: 1) palpable purpura, 2) abdominal pain, 3) arthritis
- skin: palpable, non-thrombocytopenic purpura in lower extremities and buttocks, edema, scrotal swelling
- joints: arthritis/arthralgia involving large joints associated with painful edema
- GI: abdominal pain, GI bleeding, intussusception
- renal: microscopic hematuria, IgA nephropathy, proteinuria, HTN, renal failure in <5%

Management
- mainly supportive
- anti-inflammatory medications for joint pain, corticosteroids for select patients
- monitor for protein on urinalysis every month for 6 mo, checking for renal disease, which may develop late (immunosuppressive therapy if severe)

Prognosis
- self-limited, resolves within 4 wk
- recurrence in about one-third of patients
- long-term prognosis dependent on severity of nephritis

Diagnostic Criteria for Kawasaki Disease

Warm **CREAM**
Fever ≥5 d with ≥4 of:
Conjunctivitis
Rash
Edema/Erythema (hands and feet)
Adenopathy
Mucosal involvement

KAWASAKI DISEASE
- acute vasculitis of unknown etiology (likely triggered by infection)
- medium-sized vasculitis with predilection for coronary arteries
- most common cause of acquired heart disease in children in developed countries
- peak age: 3 mo-5 yr; Asians > Blacks > Caucasians

Diagnostic Criteria
- fever persisting ≥5 d AND ≥4 of the following features
  1. bilateral, non-exudative conjunctival injection
  2. oral mucous membrane changes (fissured lips, strawberry tongue, injected pharynx)
  3. changes of the peripheral extremities
     - acute phase: extremity changes including edema of hands and feet or erythema of palms or soles
     - subacute phase: periungual desquamation
  4. polymorphous rash
  5. cervical lymphadenopathy >1.5 cm in diameter (usually unilateral)
- exclusion of other diseases (e.g. scarlet fever, measles)
- atypical Kawasaki disease: fever persisting ≥5 d and 2-3 of the above criteria
  - further evaluation dictated by CRP, ESR, and supplemental laboratory criteria

Management
- initial therapy: IVIG (2g/kg) and high (anti-inflammatory) dose of ASA
- once afebrile >48 hours: low (anti-platelet) dose of ASA until platelets normalize, or longer if coronary artery involvement
- IVIg within 10 d of onset reduces risk of coronary aneurysm formation
- baseline 2D-Echo and follow up periodic 2D-Echo (usually at 2, 6 wk)

Complications
- coronary artery vasculitis with aneurysm formation occurs in 20-25% of untreated children, <5% if receive IVIg within 10 d of fever
- 50% of aneurysms regress within 2 yr
- anticoagulation for multiple or large coronary aneurysms
- risk factors for coronary disease: male, age <1 or >9 yr, fever >10 d, Asian or Hispanic ethnicity, thrombocytopenia, hyponatremia

Common Medications

Table 48. Commonly Used Medications in Pediatrics

Drug Name	Dosing Schedule	Indications	Comments
acetaminophen	10-15 mg/kg/dose PO q4-6h prn	Analgesic, antipyretic	Not to exceed 60 mg/kg/d in neonates or 75 mg/kg/d in older children to a max of 4 g/d. Causes hepatotoxicity at high doses
amoxicillin	80-90 mg/kg/d PO divided q8h	Otitis media	
dexamethasone	0.6 mg/kg PO x 1 / 0.6 mg/kg/d PO for 2 d	Croup / Acute asthma	
fluticasone (Flovent®)	Moderate dose – 250-500 μg/d divided bid / High dose – >500 μg/d divided bid	Asthma	
ibuprofen	5-10 mg/kg/dose PO q6-8h	Analgesic, antipyretic	Cautious use in patients with liver impairment, history of GI bleeding or ulcers
iron	6 mg/kg/d elemental iron OD or divided tid	Anemia	SE: dark stool, constipation, dark urine
omeprazole	0.7-3.3 mg/kg/d (max dose 20 mg/d) OD or divided bid/tid	GERD	SE: headache, diarrhea, nausea, abdominal pain
ondansetron	0.15 mg/kg/dose (max dose 16 mg) q4-8h up to 3x	Post-operative N/V, Gastroenteritis, Cyclic vomiting	SE: QTc prolongation, orally disintegrating tablets contain phenylalanine (caution in PKU patients)
phenobarbital	3-5 mg/kg/d PO OD or bid	Seizures	SE: CNS depression
polyethylene glycol 3350 (PEG)	Disimpaction: 1-1.5 g/kg/d x 3 d / Maintenance: starting dose at 0.4-1 g/kg		
prednisone/prednisilone	1-2 mg/kg/d PO x 5 d / 3-4 mg/kg/d PO then taper to 1-2 mg/kg/d PO once platelet count >30 x 109/L / 60 mg/m²/d PO	Asthma / ITP / Nephrotic syndrome	Oral prednisone is bitter tasting, consider using prednisilone
salbutamol (Ventolin®)	0.01-0.03 mL/kg/dose in 3 mL NS via nebulizer q0.5-4h prn / 100-200 μg/dose prn, max 4-8 puffs frequency q4h	Acute asthma / Maintenance treatment for asthma	Can cause tachycardia, hypokalemia, restlessness

Source: Lau E. (2009) The 2010-2011 Formulary – The Hospital for Sick Children

References

Cardiology
Bhandar A, Bhandari V. Pitfalls, problems, and progress in bronchopulmonary dysplasia. Pediatrics 2009;123;1562-1573.
Ganz L. Sinus tachycardia. Rose BD (editor). Waltham: UpToDate. 2012.
National Heart, Lung, and Blood Institute (Bethesda, Maryland). Task force on blood pressure control in children: report of the second task force on blood pressure control in children. Pediatrics 1987;79:1-2.
Silversides CK, Kiess M, Beauchesne L, et al. Canadian Cardiovascular Society 2009 Consensus Conference on the management of adults with congenital heart disease: outflow tract obstruction, coarctation of the aorta, tetralogy of Fallot, Ebstein anomaly and Marfan's syndrome. Can J Cardiol 2010; 26:e80.
Singh RK, Singh TP. Etiology and diagnosis of heart failure in infants and children. Rose BD (editor). Waltham: UpToDate. 2013.
Vick GW, Bezold LI. Classification of atrial septal defects (ASDs), and clinical features and diagnosis of isolated ASDs in children. Rose BD (editor). Waltham: UpToDate. 2014.

Endocrinology
Lenhard MJ, Reeves GD. Continuous subcutaneous insulin infusion: a comprehensive review of insulin pump therapy. Arch Int Med 2001;161:2293-3000.
Muir A. Precocious puberty. Pediatr Rev 2006;27:373-380.
Panagiotopoulos C, Riddell MC, Sellers EAC. Canadian Diabetes Association 2013 Clinical Practice Guidelines for the Prevention and Management of Diabetes in Canada: Type 2 diabetes in children and adolescents. Can J Diabetes 2013;37(suppl 1):S163-S167.
Silverstein J, Kilgensmith G, Copeland K, et al. Care of children and adolescents with type 1 diabetes: a statement of the American Diabetes Association. Diabetes Care 2005;28:186-208.
Styne DM, Glaser NS. Nelson's essentials of pediatrics, 4th ed. Philadelphia: WB Saunders, 2002. Endocrinology. 711-766.
Wherrett D, Huot C, Mitchell B, et al. Canadian Diabetes Association 2013 Clinical Practice Guidelines for the Prevention and Management of Diabetes in Canada: Type 1 diabetes in children and adolescents. Can J Diabetes 2013;37(suppl 1):S153-S162.

Gastroenterology
American Academy of Pediatrics Subcommittee on Chronic Abdominal Pain. Chronic abdominal pain in children. Pediatrics 2005;115:812.
Foisy M, Ali S, Geist R, et al. The Cochrane Library and the treatment of chronic abdominal pain in children and adolescents: an overview of reviews. Evid-Based Child Health 2011;6:1027-1043.
Friedman JN. Risk of acute hyponatremia in hospitalized children and youth receiving maintenance intravenous fluids. Canadian Pediatric Society, 2013.
Kirshner BS, Black DD. Nelson's essentials of pediatrics, 3rd ed. Philadelphia: WB Saunders, 1998. The gastrointestinal tract. 419-458.
Rowan-Legg A. Oral health care for children: a call for action. Canadian Pediatric Society, 2013.
Rowan-Legg A. Canadian Pediatric Society, Community Pediatrics Committee. Managing functional constipation in children. Pediatr Child Health 2011;16(10):661-665.
Scott RB. Recurent abdominal pain during childhood. Can Fam Phys 1994;40:539-547.

General Topics
Albright EK. Pediatric history and physical examination, 4th ed. Current Clinical Strategies Publishing, 2003.
American Academy of Pediatrics Task Force on Circumcision. Circumcision policy statement. Pediatrics 2012;130(3):585-6.
Blank S, Brady M, Buerk E, et al. Male circumcision. Pediatrics 2012;130(3):e756-85.
Canadian Task Force on Preventive Health Care. Recommendations for growth monitoring, and prevention and management of overweight and obesity in children and youth in primary care. CMAJ 2015;187(6):411-21.
Chan ES, Cummings C. Dietary exposures and allergy prevention in high-risk infants. Paediatr Child Health 2013:18(10):545-549.
Critch JN. Nutrition for healthy term infants, birth to six months: an overview. Canadian Pediatric Society, 2013.
D'Augustine S, Flosi T. Tarascon pediatric outpatient pocketbook, 1st ed. Tarascon Publishing, 2008.
Dipchand A, Friedman J, Bismilla Z, et al.The Hospital for Sick Children handbook of pediatrics, 11th ed. Toronto: Elsevier Canada, 2009.
Greer FR, Sicherer SH, Burks AW, et al. Effects of nutritional interventions on the development of atopic disease in infants and children: the role of maternal dietary restriction, breastfeeding, timing of introduction of complementary foods, and hydrolyzed formulas. Pediatrics 2008;129:183-191.
Hospital for Sick Children. Clinical Practice Guidelines: fluid and electrolyte administration in children, 2011.
Hospital for Sick Children handbook of pediatric emergency medicine. Sudbury: Jones and Bartlett, 2008.
Klemola T, Vanto T, Juntunen-Backman K,et al. Allergy to soy formula and to extensively hydrolyzed whey formula in infants with cows' milk allergy: a prospective, randomized study with a follow-up to the age of 2 years. J Pediatr 2002;140:219-224.
Lau E. 2010-2011 Drug handbook and formulary. Toronto: Hospital for Sick Children Department of Pharmacy, 2009.
McGahren ED, Wilson WG. Pediatrics recall, 3rd ed. Baltimore: Lippincott Williams & Wilkins, 2008.
Nelson essentials of pediatrics, 5th ed. Philadelphia: Elsevier Saunders, 2006.
Pediatric Emergency Medicine. Apparent life-threatening events. Saunders Elsevier, 2008. 269-272.
Publicly funded immunization schedules for Ontario. August 2011.
Scruggs K, Johnson MT. Pediatrics 5-minute reviews. Current Clinical Strategies Publishing, 2001-2002.
Shields M. Measured obesity: overweight Canadian children and adolescents. Nutrition findings from the Canadian Community Health Survey. Statistics Canada, 2005.

Genetic Disorders and Developmental Disorders
Amato RSS. Nelson's essentials of pediatrics, 4th ed. Philadelphia: WB Saunders, 2002. Human genetics and dysmorphology. 129-146.
Blake KD, Prasad C. CHARGE syndrome, orphanet. J Rare Diseases 2006;1.
Biggar W. Duchenne muscular dystrophy. Pediatr Rev 2006;27:83-88.
Chudley AE, Conry J, Cook JL, et al. Fetal alcohol spectrum disorder: Canadian guidelines for diagnosis. CMAJ 2005;172(5 Suppl):S1-21.
Moeschler JB, Shevell M. Committee on Genetics. Comprehensive evaluation of the child with intellectual disability or global developmental delays. Pediatrics 2014 Sep;134(3):e903-18. doi:10.1542/peds.2014-1839.
Nicholson JF. Nelson's essentials of pediatrics, 4th ed. Philadelphia: WB Saunders, 2002. Inborn errors of metabolism. 153-178.
Vissers LE, van Ravenswaaij CM, Admiraal R, et al. Mutations in a new member of the chromodomain gene family cause CHARGE syndrome. Nat Genet 2004;36:955-957.

Hematology
Baker RD, Greer FR. Committee on Nutrition American Academy of Pediatrics. Diagnosis and prevention of iron deficiency and iron-deficiency anemia in infants and young children (0-3 yr of age). Pediatrics 2010;126:1040-1050.
Corrigan J, Boineau F. Hemolytic-uremic syndrome. Pediatr Rev 2001;22:365-369.
Pearce JM, Sills RH. Childhood leukemia. Pediatr Rev 2005;26:96-102.
Provan D, Stasi R, Newland AC, et al. International consensus report on the investigation and management of primary immune thrombocytopenia. Blood 2010;115:168-186.
Segel GB. Anemia. Pediatr in Rev 1988;10:77-88.

Infectious Disease and Immunizations
Advisory Committee Statement National Advisory Committee on Immunization. Volume 28. ACS-2.
American Academy of Pediatrics. Committee on quality improvement: subcommittee on urinary tract infection. Practice parameter: the diagnosis, treatment, and evaluation of the initial urinary tract infection in febrile infants and young children. Pediatrics 1999;103(4pt1):843.
American Academy of Pediatrics. Red Book, 28th ed. 2009. Haemophilus influenzae infections: 2009 report of the committee on infectious diseases. 324.
American Academy of Pediatrics. Red Book, 28th ed. 2009. Pertussis (whooping cough) 2009 report of the committee on infectious diseases. 504.
Baraff LJ, Lee SI, Schriger DL. Outcomes of bacterial meningitis in children: a meta-analysis. Pediatr Infect Dis J 1993;12:389.
Forgie S, Zhanel G, Robinson J. Canadian Paediatric Society Infectious Diseases and Immunization Committee, 2009. Position statement on management of acute otitis media. Available from: http://www.cps.ca/documents/position/acute-otitis-media.
National Advisory Committee on Immunization. Canadian Immunization Guide (CIG), 7th edition. Public Health Agency of Canada, 2006. Last modified 2014. Available at: http://www.phac-aspc.gc.ca/publicat/cig-gci/
Special Writing Group of the Committee. Rheumatic fever, endocarditis, and Kawasaki disease of the council on cardiovascular disease in the young of the American Heart Association. Guidelines for the diagnosis of rheumatic fever – Jones criteria, 1992 update. JAMA 1992;268:2069.
Tiwari T, Murphy TV, Moran J, et al. National Immunization Program, CDC. Recommended antimicrobial agents for the treatment and postexposure prophylaxis of pertussis: 2005 CDC guidelines. MMWR Recomm Rep 2005;54(RR-14):1.
Wubbel L, McCracken D, McCracken GH. Management of bacterial meningitis. Pediatr Rev 1998;19(3):78-84.
Zorc JJ, Kiddoo DA, Shaw KN. Diagnosis and management of pediatric urinary tract infections. Clin Microbiol Rev 2005;18:417.

Neonatology

Barrington KJ, Sankaran K. Guidelines for detection, management and prevention of hyperbilirubinemia in term and late preterm newborn infants. Pediatr Child Health 2007;12:1B-12B.

Gomella TL, Cunningham MD, Eyal FG, et al. Neonatology: management, procedures, on-call problems, diseases and drugs, 5th ed. New York: McGraw-Hill, 2004. Assessment of gestational age. 21-28, 491-6, 559-62.

Jain L, Douglas E. Physiology of fetal lung fluid clearance and the effect of Labor. Seminars in Perinatology, 2006.

Joseph J, Zorc ZK. A cyanotic infant: true blue or otherwise? Pediatr Ann 2001;30(10):597-601.

Meinzen-Derr J, Poindexter B, Wrage L, et al. Role of human milk in extremely low birth weight infants' risk of necrotizing enterocolitis or death. J Perinatol 2009;29:57-62.

Niermeyer S, Kattwinkel J, Van Reempts P, et al. International guidelines for neonatal resuscitation: an excerpt from the guidelines 2000 for cardiopulmonary resuscitation and emergency cardiovascular care: international consensus on science. Pediatrics 2000;106:E29.

Nephrology

Diven SC, Luther BT. A practical primary care approach to hematuria in children. Pediatr Nephrol 2000;14:65-72.

Hogg RJ, Portman RJ, Milliner D, et al. Evaluation and management of proteinuria and nephrotic syndrome in children: recommendations from a pediatric nephrology panel established at the National Kidney Foundation Conference on proteinuria, albuminuria, risk assessment, detection and elimination (PARADE). Pediatrics 2000;105:1242-1249.

Michael RS. Toilet training. Pediatr Rev 1999;20(7):240-245.

Neurology

Bergman I, Painter MJ. Nelson's essentials of pediatrics, 4th ed. Philadelphia: WB Saunders, 2002. Neurology. 767-820.

Hirtz D, Ashwal S, Berg A, et al. Practice parameter: evaluation of a first nonfebrile seizure in children. Report of the quality standards subcommittee of the American Epilepsy Academy of Neurology. The Child Neurology Society and The American Epilepsy Society. Neurology 2000;55:616-623.

Levy RG, Cooper PN, Giri P. Ketogenic diet and other dietary treatments for epilepsy. Cochrane DB Syst Rev 2012;3:CD001903.

Lewis DW, Ashawal S, Dahl G, et al. Report of the Quality Standards Subcommittee of the American Academy of Neurology and the Practice Committee of the Child Neurology Society. Practice parameter: evaluation of children and adolescents with recurrent headaches. Neurology 2002;59:490-498.

Lewis D, Ashwal S, Hershey A, et al. American Academy of Neurology. Practice parameter: pharmacological treatment of migraine headache in children and adolescents. Neurology 2004;63:2215-24.

Tenembaum S. Clinical neurology and neurosurgery. Elsevier, November 2007. Disseminated encephalomyelitis in children.

Oncology

SEER Cancer Statistics Review, National Cancer Institute. Bethesda, MD. Available at: http://seer.cancer.gov/faststats/selections.php?#Output (Accessed on April 04, 2016).

Strahm B, Malkin D. Hereditary cancer predisposition In children: Genetic basis and clinical implications. International Jounral of Cancer 2006;119,2001-2006.

Respirology

Canadian cystic fibrosis patient data registry report. Canadian Cystic Fibrosis Foundation, 2008.

Ducharme FM, Dell SD, Radhakrishnan D, et al., Diagnosis and management of asthma in preschoolers: A Canadian Thoracic Society and Canadian PaediatricSociety position paper. Paediatr Child Health. 2015 Oct;20(7):353-71.

Gadomski AM, Brower M. Bronchodilators for bronchiolitis. Cochrane DB Syst Rev 2010;12:CD001266.

Garrison MM, Christakis DA, Harvey E, et al. Systemic corticosteroids in infant bronchiolitis: a meta-analysis. Pediatrics 2000;105:e44.

Lougheed MD, Lemiere C, Dell SD, et al. Canadian Thoracic Society Asthma Management Continuum: 2010 consensus symmary for children six yr of age and over, and adults. Can Respir J 2010;17:15-24.

Ortiz-Alvarez O, Mikrogianakis A, Canadian Pediatric Society Acute Care Committee. Managing the pediatric patient with an acute asthma exacerbation. Pediatr Child Health 2012;17(5):251-255.

Summary of recommendations from the Canadian Asthma Consensus Guidelines, 2003 and Canadian Pediatric Asthma Consensus Guidelines, 2003 (updated to December 2004) CMAJ 2005;173(suppl):S1-56.

Rheumatology

Minich LL, Sleeper LA, Atz AM, et al, Pediatric Heart Network Investigators. Delayed diagnosis of Kawasaki disease: what are the risk factors? Pediatrics 2007;120(6):e1434.

Newburger JW, Takahashi M, Gerber MA, et al. Diagnosis, treatment, and long-term management of Kawasaki disease: a statement for health professionals from the Committee on Rheumatic Fever, Endocarditis and Kawasaki Disease, Council on Cardiovascular Disease in the Young, American Heart Association. Circulation 2004;110:2747-71.

Olson JC. Nelson's essentials of pediatrics, 3rd ed. Philadelphia: WB Saunders, 1998. Rheumatic diseases of childhood. 299-314.

Wormser GP, Dattwyler RJ, Shapiro ED, et al. The clinical assessment, treatment, and prevention of Lyme disease, human granulocytic anaplasmosis, and babesiosis: clinical practice guidelines by the Infectious Diseases Society of America. Clin Infect Dis 2006;43:1089.

Web-Based Resources

http://www.medscape.com/home/topics/pediatrics.
http://www.icondata.com/health/pedbase.
http://www.cda-adc.ca.
http://www.aboutkidshealth.ca.
http://www.healthychildren.org.
http://www.publichealth.gc.ca.
http://www.cps.ca.
www.uptodate.com.

PL Plastic Surgery

Matthew Lee, **Daniel Jeffrey Low**, and **Janelle Yu**, chapter editors
Dhruvin Hirpara and **Sneha Raju**, associate editors
Valerie Lemieux and **Simran Mundi**, EBM editors
Dr. Melinda A. Musgrave, **Dr. Kyle R. Wanzel**, and **Dr. Michael J. Weinberg**, staff editors

Acronyms

ABI	ankle-brachial index	DM	diabetes mellitus	IP	interphalangeal	RL	Ringer's lactate
ABG	arterial blood gas	EMG	electromyography	IVIg	intravenous immunoglobulin	ROM	range of motion
APL	abductor pollicis longu	ENT	ear, nose, throat	MC	metacarpal	SGAP	superior gluteal artery perforator
ARDS	acute respiratory distress syndrome	EOM	extraocular movement	MCP	metacarpal phalangeal joint	SIADH	syndrome of inappropriate antidiuretic
ATLS	advanced trauma life support	EPB	extensor pollicis brevis	NCV	nerve conduction velocity		hormone
BMR	basal metabolic rate	FDP	flexor digitorum profundus	NS	normal saline	SIEA	superficial inferior epigastric artery
CHF	congestive heart failure	FDS	flexor digitorum superficialis	NSAIDs	nonsteroidal anti-inflammatory drugs	SLP	speech language pathology
CMC	carpo-metacarpal	FTSG	full thickness skin graft	OM	otitis media	SOF	superior orbital fissure
CO	carbon monoxide	GBS	group B *Streptococcus*	OR	operating room	STSG	split thickness skin graft
CSF	cerebrospinal fluid	HTN	hypertension	ORIF	open reduction internal fixation	TBSA	total body surface area
CVD	cerebrovascular disease	I&D	incision and drainage	PIP	proximal interphalangeal joint	TMJ	temporomandibular joint
CXR	chest x-ray	ICP	intracranial pressure	PMN	polymorphonuclear	TRAM	transverse rectus abdominus myocutaneous
D5W	5% dextrose in water	ICU	intensive care unit	PVD	peripheral vascular disease	UCL	ulnar collateral ligament
DIEP	deep inferior epigastric perforator	IGAP	inferior gluteal artery perforator	RA	rheumatoid arthritis	UV	ultraviolet
DIP	distal interphalangeal joint						

Basic Anatomy Review

Skin

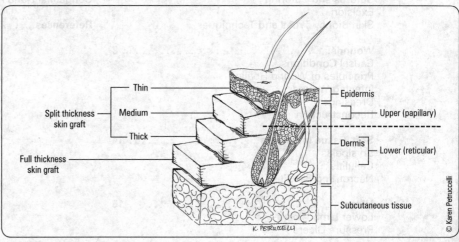

Figure 1. Split and full thickness skin grafts

Hand

BONES AND NERVES

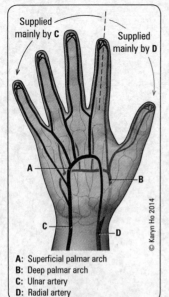

A: Superficial palmar arch
B: Deep palmar arch
C: Ulnar artery
D: Radial artery

Figure 2. Arterial supply in the hand

1. Radius
2. Scaphoid
3. Trapezium
4. Trapezoid
5. Capitate
6. Ulna
7. Lunate
8. Pisiform
9. Triquetrum
10. Hamate
11. Metacarpal bones

Figure 3. Carpal bones

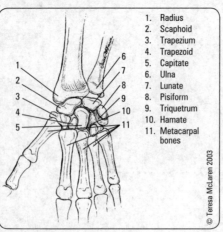

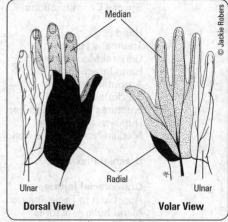

Figure 4. Sensory distribution in the hand

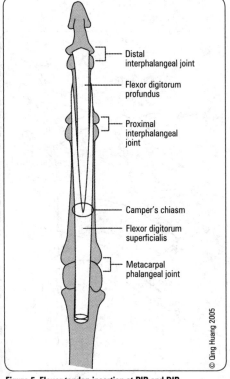

Distal interphalangeal joint

Flexor digitorum profundus

Proximal interphalangeal joint

Camper's chiasm

Flexor digitorum superficialis

Metacarpal phalangeal joint

© Qing Huang 2005

Figure 5. Flexor tendon insertion at PIP and DIP

Lateral bands — DIP

Central slip

Extensor hood
— Oblique fibres
— Sagittal fibres — PIP

Lumbrical

Interosseous muscles — MCP

Extensor digitorum communis

© Crista Mason 2005

Figure 6. Extensor mechanism of digits

© Ashley Hui 2016

1. Hyponychium	6. Eponychium
2. Sterile matrix	7. Dorsal root
3. Germinal matrix	8. Distal phalanx
4. Ventral floor	9. Extensor tendon
5. Lunula	10. Flexor tendon

Nail anatomy

Flexor Tendons
All require OR repair

Extensor Tendons
ER repair unless proximal/multiple tendons

Carpal Bone Mnemonic

So Long to Pinky. Here Comes The Thumb.
Scaphoid
Lunate
Triquetrum
Pisiform
Hamate
Capitate
Trapezoid
Trapezium

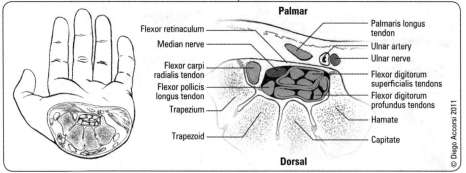

Palmar

Flexor retinaculum

Median nerve

Flexor carpi radialis tendon

Flexor pollicis longus tendon

Trapezium

Trapezoid

Palmaris longus tendon

Ulnar artery

Ulnar nerve

Flexor digitorum superficialis tendons

Flexor digitorum profundus tendons

Hamate

Capitate

Dorsal

© Diego Accorsi 2011

Figure 7. Carpal tunnel

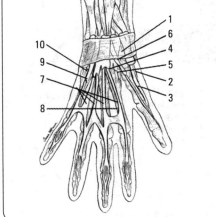

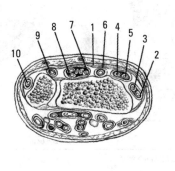

1. Extensor retinaculum

Compartment 1
2. Abductor pollicis longus
3. Extensor pollicis brevis

Compartment 2
4. Extensor carpi radialis brevis
5. Extensor carpi radialis longus

Compartment 3
6. Extensor pollicis longus
(EPL tendon passes around Lister's tubercle)

Compartment 4
7. Extensor digitorum
8. Extensor indicis

Compartment 5
9. Extensor digiti minimi

Compartment 6
10. Extensor carpi ulnaris

Figure 8. Extensor compartment of the wrist (dorsal view and cross-sectional view)

Brachial Plexus

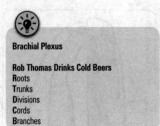

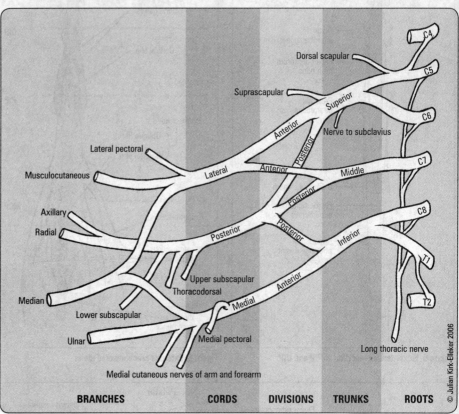

Figure 9. Brachial plexus anatomy

Face

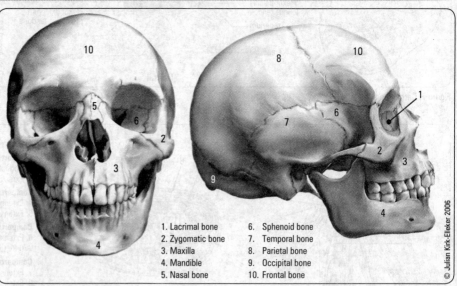

1. Lacrimal bone
2. Zygomatic bone
3. Maxilla
4. Mandible
5. Nasal bone
6. Sphenoid bone
7. Temporal bone
8. Parietal bone
9. Occipital bone
10. Frontal bone

Figure 10. Skull and facial bones

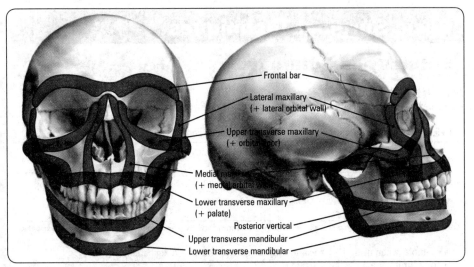

Figure 11. Craniofacial horizontal and vertical buttresses

Skin Lesions and Masses

Differential Diagnosis of Skin Lesions/Masses

- for background information and medical management (see Dermatology, D5)
- for biopsy techniques, see *Skin Biopsy Types and Techniques*, PL7

Surgical Management of Malignant Skin Lesions

- surgical treatment for all malignant skin lesions involve total excision of the primary lesion
- excision margin of lesion depends on the type of lesion, the lesion diameter and (for melanoma) the lesion depth
- for decisions regarding reconstruction using flaps or skin grafts, see *Reconstruction*, PL11

Precursors of Malignant Lesions

Table 1. Precursors

Basal Cell Carcinoma	Squamous Cell Carcinoma	Malignant Melanoma
Nevus sebaceous of Jadassohn	Actinic keratosis	Lentigo maligna
	Bowen's disease	Giant congenital nevus
	Bowenoid papulosis	
	Paget's disease	
	Leukoplakia	
	Erythroplasia	

Surgical Margins

Table 2. Surgical Margins for Basal Cell Carcinoma

Type of Lesion	Surgical Margins
Low Risk (<20 mm trunk; < 6 mm face, hands, feet)	3 mm
High Risk (>20 mm trunk; >6 mm face, hands, feet)	3-5 mm

Table 3. Surgical Margins for Squamous Cell Carcinoma

Diameter or Location of Lesion	Surgical Margins
≤2 cm	1-2 cm
>2 cm	2 cm
High risk (facial)	1 cm
Low risk (elsewhere)	1-2 cm

Table 4. Surgical Margins for Malignant Melanoma

Depth of Lesion	Surgical Margins
In situ	0.5 cm
<1 mm	1 cm
1.01-1.99 mm	1-2 cm
≥2 mm	2 cm

Basic Surgical Techniques

Sutures and Suturing

ANESTHESIA
- irrigate before injecting anesthetic, followed by debridement and more vigorous irrigation

Traumatic tattoos are permanent discolourations resulting from new skin growth over foreign material or dirt left behind in the dermis. Copious irrigation and debridement should be done ASAP in order to prevent traumatic tattoos as they are very difficult to treat later

Table 5. Toxic Limit and Duration of Action (1 cc of 1% solution contains 10 mg lidocaine)

	Without Epinephrine	With Epinephrine (vasoconstrictor, limits bleeding)
Lidocaine (Xylocaine®)*	5 mg/kg, lasts 45-60 min	7 mg/kg, lasts 2-6 h
Bupivicaine (Marcaine®) for longer analgesic effect	2 mg/kg, lasts 2-4 h	3 mg/kg, lasts 3-7 h

* Lidocaine toxicity symptoms include circumoral numbness, light-headedness and drowsiness followed by tremors and seizures. Cardiac and respiratory signs are late findings

- for example, when using 1% lidocaine without epinephrine in a 70 kg patient:
  - toxic limit = 5 mg x 70 kg = 350 mg
  - max bolus injection = 350 mg ÷ 10 mg/cc = 35 cc (may add more after 30 min)

IRRIGATION AND DEBRIDEMENT
- irrigate copiously with a physiologic solution such as Ringer's lactate or normal saline to remove surface clots, foreign material, and bacteria
- use a 19 gauge needle and 35 cc syringe to generate ~18 psi when irrigating
- debride all obviously devitalized tissue; irregular or ragged wounds must be excised to produce sharp wound edges that will assist healing when approximated
- wounds left unapproximated ≥8 h should be debrided to ensure wound edges are optimized for healing

SUTURES
- use of a particular suture material is highly dependent on surgeon preference; however, skin should be closed with a non absorbable material when traumatic mechanisms are involved

Table 6. Suture Materials: Absorbable vs. Non-absorbable and Monofilmaent vs. Multifilament

Suture Materials	Uses	Examples	Notes
Absorbable	Deep sutures under short-term tension Skin closure in children	Plain gut®, Vicryl®, Polysorb®, chromic gut, fast absorbing gut	Loses at least 50% of their strength in 4 wk; eventually absorbed
Non-absorbable	Skin closure Sites of long-term tension	Nylon, polypropylene (Prolene), stainless steel, silk, ticron, ethibond	Lower likelihood of wound dehiscence, more difficult to tie, makes track marks
Monofilament	Everyday use and optimal for contaminated and infected wounds (lower likelihood of bacterial trapping in suture material)	Monosof®, Monocryl®, Biosyn®, Prolene	Slides through tissue with less friction; more memory/stiffness
Multifilament	AVOID in contaminated wounds (increased likelihood of bacterial trapping)	Vicryl® and Silk, Ticron, Ethibond	Less memory/stiffness thus easier to work with

BASIC SUTURING TECHNIQUES

Basic Suture Methods
- simple interrupted: can be used in almost all situations
- sub-cuticular: good cosmetic result but weak, used in combination with deep sutures; not used in trauma
- vertical mattress: for areas difficult to evert (e.g. solar palm of the hand)
- horizontal mattress: everting, time saving
- continuous over and over (i.e. "running", "baseball stitch"): time saving, good for hemostasis

Other Skin Closure Materials
- tapes: may be indicated for superficial wounds and those with opposable edges. Tape cannot be used on actively bleeding wounds. When placed across the incision, will prevent surface marks and can be used primarily or after surface sutures have been removed
- skin adhesives: e.g. 2-octylcyanoacrylate (e.g. Dermabond®) works well on small areas without much tension or shearing; may cause irreversible tattooing
- staples: steel-titanium alloys that incite minimal tissue reaction (healing is comparable to wounds closed by suture)

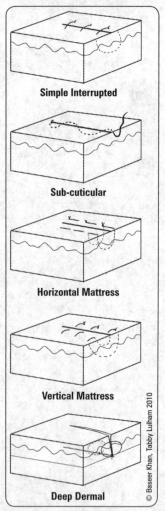

Simple Interrupted

Sub-cuticular

Horizontal Mattress

Vertical Mattress

© Baseer Khan, Tabby Lulham 2010

Deep Dermal

Figure 12. Basic suture methods

Steps to Ensuring Good Suturing Cosmesis
- Incisions should be made along relaxed skin tension lines
- Attain close apposition of wound edges
- Minimize tension on skin by closing in layers
- Evert wound edges
- Use appropriately sized suture for skin closure (5-0, 6-0 on face; 3-0, 4-0 elsewhere)
- Ensure equal width and depth of tissue on both sides
- Remove sutures within 5-7 d from the face, 10-14 d from scalp/torso/extremities

Excision

- plan your incision along relaxed skin tension lines to minimize appearance of scar
- use elliptical incision to prevent "dog ears" (heaped up skin at end of incision) so the length of the ellipse should be approximately 3x the width
- if needed, undermine skin edges to decrease wound tension
- use layered closure including dermal sutures when wound is deeper than superficial (decreases tension)

Skin Biopsy Types and Techniques

SHAVE BIOPSY
- used for superficial lesions where sampling of the full thickness of the dermis is not necessary or practical
- most suitable lesions for shave biopsies are either elevated above the skin or have pathology confined to the epidermis (e.g. seborrheic or actinic keratoses, skin tags, warts, and superficial basal cell or squamous cell carcinomas)
- rapid, requires little training, and does not require sutures for closure
- heals by secondary intent (moist dressings should be used)
- should not be used for pigmented lesions – an unsuspected melanoma cannot be properly staged if partially removed

NEEDLE BIOPSY
- 21 G for lymph node biopsy
- Trucut needle biopsy for breast masses suspected for carcinoma

INCISIONAL BIOPSY
- can either be a punch biopsy or can be an ellipse within the lesion
- gives pathologists a portion of the lesion and the border with normal skin too
- punch biopsies involves the removal of a core-shaped piece of tissue to allow sampling of the deep dermis, performed with round, disposable knives ranging in diameter from 2-10 mm
- punch biopsies can be used for the diagnosis and treatment of small pigmented lesions and atypical moles
- punch biopsy wounds can be closed with suture or left to heal by secondary intention. Punches greater than 3 mm may produce scarring and are best closed with one or two sutures
- punch biopsies have a low incidence of infection, bleeding, nonhealing, significant scarring

EXCISIONAL BIOPSY
- performed for lesions that require complete removal for diagnostic or therapeutic purposes
- performed for lesions that cannot be adequately punch biopsied due to size, depth, or location
- best for small lesions that are easily removed and primarily closed
- requires the greatest amount of expertise and time
- always requires sutures for closure

TECHNIQUE

General
- all shave and punch biopsies performed in clinic are done using aseptic technique, but are not sterile
- sterile gloves are indicated for biopsies and excisions in all patients

Preparing the Site
- common skin antiseptics (betadine, chlorhexidine) can be used to prepare the biopsy site
- chlorhexidine is used in concentrations ranging from 0.5-4%. The higher concentration cannot be used on the face as it could get into the eyes or ears and may burn or cause damage. Most chlorhexidine preps also do contain alcohol which can be flammable, so allow to dry before the biopsy and certainly before using any cautery
- Betadine® (7.5% povidone – iodine) may be safer for the head and neck (as to avoid the above problems with chlohexidene/alcohol) around the eyes and ears
- mark the intended lesion and surgical margins with a surgical marker since they may be temporarily obliterated following injection of the anesthetic
- for all biopsies, a sterile drape technique is indicated. A fenestrated surgical drape is placed around the biopsy site after the area is cleansed and anesthetized

Anesthesia
- most commonly used local anesthetic is 1% or 2% lidocaine (with epinephrine)
- small amounts of epinephrine are added to constrict blood vessels, decrease bleeding, prolong anesthesia, and limit lidocaine toxicity. The local with epinephrine can be injected directly into the lesion
- local anesthetics with epinephrine may be used anywhere in the body (including the digits – except if the digits have been significantly injured and could have vascular compromise – e.g. saw injury)
- epinephrine should be avoided in patients with history of vascular compromise

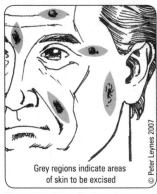

Grey regions indicate areas of skin to be excised

© Peter Leynes 2007

Figure 13. Incision of lesions along relaxed skin tension lines

Wounds

Causal Conditions

- laceration: cut or torn tissue
- abrasion: superficial skin layer is removed, variable depth
- contusion: injury caused by forceful blow to the skin and soft tissue; entire outer layer of skin intact yet injured
- avulsion: tissue/limb forcefully separated from surrounding tissue, either partially or fully; "de-gloving"
- puncture wounds: cutaneous opening relatively small as compared with depth (e.g. needle)
- includes bite wounds
- crush injuries: caused by compression
- thermal and chemical wounds

Principles of Wound Healing

- wound: disruption of the normal anatomical relationships of tissue as a result of injury

FACTORS INFLUENCING WOUND HEALING

Local (reversible/controllable)
- mechanical (local trauma, significant crush, avulsion, tension)
- blood supply (ischemia/circulation)
- temperature
- technique and suture materials
- retained foreign body
- infection
- venous HTN
- peripheral vascular disease
- PVD
- hematoma/seroma (↑ infection rate)

General (often irreversible)
- age
- nutrition (protein, vitamin C, O_2)
- smoking
- chronic illness (e.g. DM, cancer, CVD)
- immunosuppression (steroids, chemo)
- collagen vascular disease
- tissue irradiation

STAGES OF WOUND HEALING

- growth factors released by tissues play an important role
- scar is mature once it has completed the final stage, usually after 1-2 yr

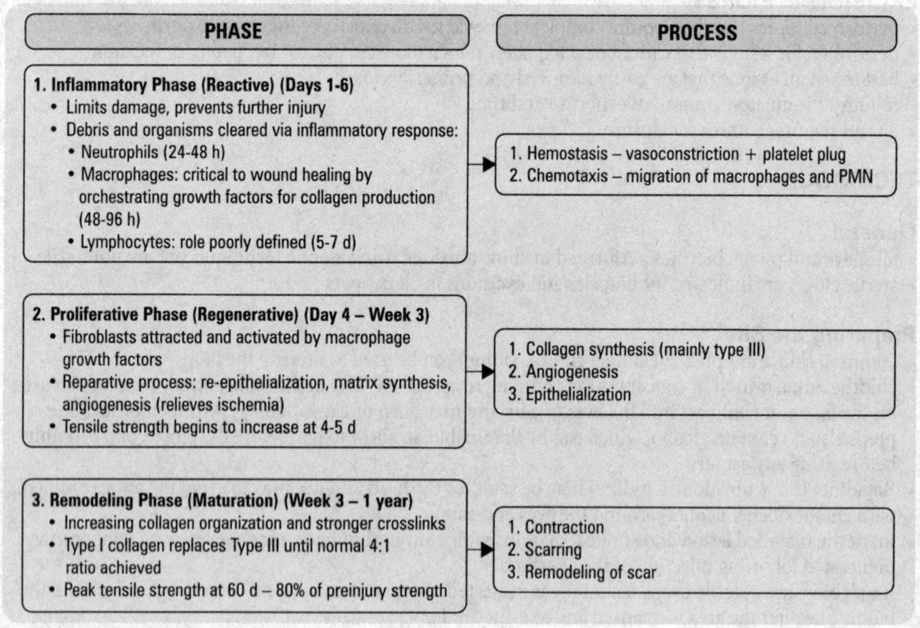

PHASE	PROCESS

1. Inflammatory Phase (Reactive) (Days 1-6)
• Limits damage, prevents further injury
• Debris and organisms cleared via inflammatory response:
  • Neutrophils (24-48 h)
  • Macrophages: critical to wound healing by orchestrating growth factors for collagen production (48-96 h)
  • Lymphocytes: role poorly defined (5-7 d)
	1. Hemostasis – vasoconstriction + platelet plug
	2. Chemotaxis – migration of macrophages and PMN

2. Proliferative Phase (Regenerative) (Day 4 – Week 3) • Fibroblasts attracted and activated by macrophage growth factors • Reparative process: re-epithelialization, matrix synthesis, angiogenesis (relieves ischemia) • Tensile strength begins to increase at 4-5 d	1. Collagen synthesis (mainly type III) 2. Angiogenesis 3. Epithelialization
3. Remodeling Phase (Maturation) (Week 3 – 1 year) • Increasing collagen organization and stronger crosslinks • Type I collagen replaces Type III until normal 4:1 ratio achieved • Peak tensile strength at 60 d – 80% of preinjury strength	1. Contraction 2. Scarring 3. Remodeling of scar

Figure 14. Stages of wound healing

ABNORMAL HEALING

Hypertrophic Scar
- definition: scar remains roughly within boundaries of original scar
- red, raised, widened, frequently pruritic
- common sites: back, shoulder, sternum

- treatment: scar massage, pressure garments, silicone gel sheeting, corticosteroid injection, surgical excision if other options fail (however, may still recur)
- will often improve slowly over time

Keloid Scar
- definition: scar grows outside boundaries of original scar
- red, raised, widened, frequently pruritic
- caused by 1. genetic factors (highest rates in African Americans, Asians), 2. endocrine factors and/or 3. excess tension on wound or delayed closure (as in burn wounds)
- common sites: back, shoulders, deltoid, ear, andle, angle of mandible
- treatment: multimodal therapy, including pressure garments, silicone gel sheeting, corticosteroid injection, surgical excision with post-surgical management if other options fail (however, there is a high chance of recurrence), fractional carbon dioxide ablative laser, radiation

Spread Scar
- characterized by having the exactly same order of collagen fibers as normal scars
- clinically, a typical spread scar is flat, wide and often dented
- treatment: surgical excision and closure

Chronic Wound
- fails to achieve primary wound healing within 4-6 wk
- common chronic wounds include diabetic, pressure and venous stasis ulcers
- treatment: may heal with meticulous wound care; may also require surgical intervention
- Marjolin's ulcer: squamous cell carcinoma arising in a chronic wound secondary to genetic changes caused by chronic inflammation → always consider biopsy of chronic wound

WOUND HEALING

Healing (First Intention)
- definition: wound closure by direct approximation of edges within hours of wound creation (i.e. with sutures, staples, skin graft, etc.)
- indication: recent (<6 h, longer with facial wounds), clean wounds
- contraindications: animal/human bites (except on face), crush injuries, infection, long time lapse since injury (>6-8 h), retained foreign body

Spontaneous Healing (Second Intention)
- definition: wound left open to heal spontaneously (epithelialization 1 mm/d from wound margins in concentric pattern), contraction (myofibroblasts) and granulation – maintained in inflammatory phase until wound closed; requires dressing changes; inferior cosmetic result
- indication: when 1° closure not possible or indicated (see *Primary Healing*)

Myofibroblasts are the cells responsible for wound contraction; they do this at a rate of less than 0.75 mm/d

Delayed Primary Healing (Third Intention)
- definition: intentionally interrupt healing process (e.g. with packing), then wound can be closed at 4-10 d post-injury after granulation tissue has formed and there is <10^5 bacteria/gram of tissue
- indication: contaminated (high bacterial count), long time lapse since initial injury, severe crush component with significant tissue devitalization, closure of fasciotomy wounds
- prolongation of inflammatory phase decreases bacterial count and lessens chance of infection after closure

Infected Wounds

Definitions
- contamination: the presence of nonreplicating microorganisms within a wound
- colonization: the presence of replicating microorganisms within a wound
- infection: greater than 10^5 microorganisms in a wound without intact epithelium, a wound may also be infected with small amounts of a very virulent organism (e.g. GBS)

Risk Factors for Infection
- Virulence of the infecting microorganism
- Amount of bacteria present
- Host resistance

Management of Acute Contaminated Wound (<24 h)
- cleanse and irrigate open wound with physiologic solution (NS or RL) using sufficient pressure
- evaluate for injury to underlying structures (vessels, nerve, tendon and bone)
- control active bleeding; previously closed wounds may require suture removal in order to drain any pus and allow for thorough irrigation and debridement
- debridement: removal of foreign material, devitalized tissue, old blood
  - surgical debridement: blade and irrigation if indicated
- systemic antibiotics are commonly indicated for obvious infection. Risk factors include wound older than 8 h, severely contaminated, human/animal bites, immunocompromised, involvement of deeper structures (e.g. joints, fractures)
- ± tetanus toxoid 0.5 mL IM ± tetanus immunoglobulin 250 U deep IM (see Table 7 and Table 8)
- ± post-exposure treatment of
  - hepatitis B, HIV, hepatitis C (if titres confirmed at 6 mo)

- re-evaluate in 24-48 h for signs of superficial or deep infection
    - if evidence of infection, open infected portion of wound by removing sutures (i.e. erythema, warmth, pain, discharge), swab sample for culture and sensitivity, irrigate wound and allow healing secondary intention

Table 7. Risks for Tetanus

Wound Characteristics	Tetanus-Prone	Not Tetanus-Prone
Time since injury	>6 h	<6 h
Depth of injury	>1 cm	<1 cm
Mechanism of Injury	Crush, burn, gunshot, frostbite, puncture through clothing, farming injury	Sharp cut (e.g. clean knife, clean glass)
Devitalized tissue	Present	Not present
Contamination (e.g. soil, dirt, saliva, grass)	Yes	No
Retained foreign body	Yes	No

Table 8. Tetanus Immunization Recommendations

History of Tetanus Immunization	Clean, Minor Wounds		All Other Wounds	
	Td or Tdap*	Tig**	Td or Tdap	Tig
Uncertain or <3 doses of immunization	Yes	No	Yes	Yes
3 doses received in immunization series	No~	No	No§	No¶

* 0.5 mL of combined tetanus and diptheria toxoids ± acellular pertussis   ~ Yes, if >10 yr since last booster   ¶ Yes, if immunocompromised
** Tetanus immune globulin, 250 U given at a separate site from Td/Tdap   § Yes, if >5 yr since last booster

Management of Contaminated Wounds (>24 h, including ulcers)
- irrigation and debridement
    - traumatic tattooing can occur if foreign materials left in wound
- systemic antibiotics indicated if there is concern of infection (e.g. redness, swelling, pain, clinically unwell)
- topical antimicrobials: beneficial for minor wounds, but no additional benefit for wounds requiring systemic antibiotics. May aid in healing of chronic wounds
- closure: final closure via secondary intention (most common), delayed wound closure (3° closure), skin graft or flap; successful closure depends on bacterial count of ≤10^5/cm³ prior to closure and frequent dressing changes

BITES

- see Emergency Medicine, ER47

Dog and Cat Bites
- pathogens: *Pasteurella multocida, S. aureus, S. viridans*
- **investigations**
    - radiographs prior to therapy to rule out foreign body (e.g. tooth) or fracture
    - culture for aerobic and anaerobic organisms, Gram stain
- **treatment**: Clavulin® (500 mg PO q8h started immediately – amoxicillin + clavulanic acid)
    - consider rabies prophylaxis if animal has symptoms of rabies or unknown animal
        - ± rabies Ig (20 IU/kg around wound, or IM) and 1 of the 3 types of rabies vaccines (1.0 mL IM in deltoid, repeat on days 3, 7, 14, 28)
- aggressive irrigation with debridement
- healing by secondary intention is mainstay of treatment
- only consider primary closure for bite wounds on the face; otherwise primary closure is contraindicated
- contact Public Health if animal status unknown

Human Bites
- pathogens: *Staphylococcus* > β-hemolytic *Streptococcus* > *Eikenella corrodens* > *Bacteroides*
- mechanism: most commonly over dorsum of MCP from a punch in mouth; "fight-bite"
- serious, as mouth has 10^9 microorganisms/mL, which get trapped in joint space when fist unclenches and overlying skin forms an air-tight covering ideal for anaerobic growth – can lead to septic arthritis
- **investigations**
    - radiographs prior to therapy to rule out foreign body (e.g. tooth) or fracture
    - culture for aerobic and anaerobic organisms, Gram stain
- **treatment**
    - urgent surgical exploration of joint, drainage and debridement of infected tissue
    - wound must be copiously irrigated
    - Clavulin® 500 mg PO q8h or (if penicillin allergy) clindamycin 300 mg PO q6h + ciprofloxacin 500 mg PO q12h + secondary closure
    - splint

Dressings

- dressing selection depends on the wound characteristics and surgeon preference
  - as the wound progresses through healing it will require different types of dressings, therefore, routine inspection is recommended
  - principles of dressing may want to add that the old principle of wound healing was to dry it if it was wet and wet it if it was dry but now we choose the principle of moist interactive wound healing we also need. A basic classification of dressings like films foams alginates etc.
    - ◆ clean vs. infected wounds
      - clean wounds can be dressed with non-adherent dressing (which is non-adhering to epithelializing tissue); requires secondary dressing
      - infected wounds may need debridement and antibiotics and can be dressed with iodine gauze, silver-containing, or antimicrobial dressings
    - ◆ wide-based vs. cavitary/tunnelling wounds
      - cavitary or tunnelling wounds (i.e. through a fascial layer) can be packed with saline-soaked (non-infected)
      - infected wounds require irrigation and debridement prior to appropriate dressing care (e.g. betadine-soaked (infected) ribbon gauze, or other easily retrievable one-piece moisture providing dressing

Negative-pressure wound therapy uses sealed vacuum dressings that remove wound fluid and promote increased blood flow to enhance the healing process

Table 9. Recommended Dressings for Wound Type

Wound Depth	Exudate Level	Dressing Material
Superficial	Lightly exuding	Films (Opsite®) , hydrogels (Intrasite®, Nu-gel®, Duoderm®)
	Any exudate level	Contact layers
Superficial to Deep	Light to moderately exuding wounds	Amorphous gels, hydrogels, hydrocolloids (Duoderm®, Tegaderm®), collagen, hypertonic saline gauze (Mesalt®)
	Moderately to heavily exuding wounds	Foams (Mepilex®, Allevyn®), alginates (Sorbsan®, Kalto-stat®), hypertonic saline gauze, hydrofibre (Aquacel®)

Table adapted from Grabb & Smith's Plastic Surgery, 6th ed. Chapter 3, Table 3.3

Reconstruction

RECONSTRUCTION LADDER

Definition
- an approach to wound management with successively more complex methods of treatment
- surgeons should start with the least complex method and progressively increase in complexity as appropriate

SKIN GRAFTS

Definition
- skin that is harvested from a donor site and transferred to the recipient site and that does not carry its own blood supply. Survival requires the generation of new blood vessels from the recipient site bed; they are classified according to the depth of dermis they contain: full thickness (entire epidermis + dermis) vs. split-thickness (epidermis + partial dermis)

Donor Site Selection
- must consider size, hair pattern, texture, thickness of skin, and colour (facial grafts best if taken from "blush zones" above clavicle e.g. pre/post auricular or neck)
- partial thickness grafts usually taken from inconspicuous areas (e.g. buttocks, lateral thighs, etc.)

Partial Thickness Skin Graft Survival
- 3 phases of skin graft "take"
  1. plasmatic imbibition: diffusion of nutrition from recipient site (first 48 h)
  2. inosculation: vessels in graft connect with those in recipient bed (day 2-3)
  3. neovascular ingrowth: graft revascularized (day 3-5)
- requirements for survival
  - well-vascularized bed (unsuitable beds include: bone, tendon, heavily irradiated, infected wounds)
  - good contact between graft and recipient bed. Staples, sutures, splinting and pressure dressings are used to prevent movement of the graft and hematoma/seroma formation
- bed: well-vascularized (unsuitable: bone, tendon, heavily irradiated, infected wounds, etc.)
  - contact between graft and recipient bed: fully immobile (decreased shearing and hematoma formation)
  - staples, sutures, splinting, and appropriate dressings (pressure) are used to prevent movement of graft and hematoma or seroma formation
  - site: low bacterial count ($<10^5/cm^3$, to prevent infection)

Reconstruction Ladder (in the order of increasing complexity of treatment)
- Healing by secondary intention
- Primary closure
- Delayed closure
- Split thickness graft
- Full thickness graft
- Random pattern flap
- Pedicle flap
- Tissue expansion
- Free flap

Classification of Skin Grafts

1. by species
   - autograft: from same individual
   - allograft (homograft): from same species, different individual
   - xenograft (heterograft): from different species (e.g. porcine)
2. by thickness: see Table 10

Table 10. Skin Grafts

	Split Thickness Skin Graft	Full Thickness Skin Graft
Definition	Epidermis and part of dermis	Epidermis and all of dermis
Donor Site	More sites	Donor sites limited by the ability to use primary closure
Healing of Donor Site	Re-epithelialization via dermal appendages in graft and wound edges	Primary closure
Re-Harvesting	~10 d (faster on scalp)	N/A
Graft Take	More reliable and better survival; shorter nutrient diffusion distance	Lower rate of survival (thicker, slower vascularization)
Contraction*	Less 1° contraction, greater 2° contraction (less with thicker graft)	Greater 1° contraction, less 2° contraction
Aesthetic	Poor	Good
Comments	Can be meshed for greater area Allows for extravasation of blood/serum	May use on face and fingers
Advantages	Takes well in less favourable conditions Can cover a larger area Can be meshed for greater area Allows for extravasation of blood/serum Potential for healing in less favourable environment Large number of donor sites	Resists contraction, better colour match May use on face and fingers
Disadvantages	Contracts significantly, abnormal pigmentation, high susceptibility to trauma	Requires well vascularized bed Must remove fat from graft before application
Uses	Large areas of skin, granulating tissue beds	Face (colour match), site where thick skin or decreased contracture is desired (e.g. finger)

*Primary: immediate reduction in size upon harvesting; Secondary: reduction in size once graft placed on wound bedand healing has occurred.

- meshed grafts (split thickness grafts can be meshed after harvest by a mesher to either 1.5:1 or 3:1)
- **advantages**
  - prevents accumulation of fluids (e.g. hematoma, seroma)
  - covers a larger area
  - best for contaminated recipient site
- **disadvantages**
  - poor cosmesis ("alligator hide" appearance)
  - has significant contraction
- common reasons for graft loss: hematoma/seroma, infection, mechanical force (e.g. shearing, pressure)

OTHER GRAFTS

Table 11. Various Tissue Grafts

Graft Type	Use	Preferred Donor Site
Bone	Repair rigid defects	Cranial, rib, iliac, fibula
Cartilage	Restore contour of ear and nose	Ear, nasal septum, costal cartilage
Tendon	Repair or replace a damaged tendon	Palmaris longus, plantaris (present in 85% population)
Nerve	Conduit for regeneration across nerve gap	Sural, antebrachial cutaneous, medial brachial cutaneous
Vessel	Bridge vascular gaps	Forearm or foot vessels for small vessels, saphenous vein for larger vessels
Dermis	Contour restoration (± fat for bulk)	Thick skin of buttock or abdomen
Fat	Contour restoration	Abdomen, any area with fat available
Nipple	To create a new nipple on a reconstructed breast	Nipple

FLAPS

- **definition**: tissue transferred from one site to another with a known blood supply (random, pedicled or named); not dependent on neovascularization, unlike a graft
- **may consist of**: skin, subcutaneous tissue, fascia, muscle, tendon, bone, other tissue (e.g. omentum)
- **classification**: based on blood supply to skin (random, axial) and anatomic location (local, regional, distant)
- **indications for flaps**
  - replaces tissue loss due to trauma or surgery (reconstruction)
  - provides skin and temporary soft tissue coverage through which surgery can be carried out later
  - to aid healing or treatment of infection by providing vascularized tissue to a poorly vascularized bed
- **complications**: flap loss due to hematoma, seroma, infection, poor flap design, extrinsic compression (dressing too tight) or vascular failure/thrombosis, fat necrosis (in free and pedicled flaps)

Random Pattern Flaps

- blood supply by dermal and subdermal plexus to skin and subdermal tissue with random vascular supply
- limited length:width ratio to ensure adequate blood supply (typically 3:1 in the head and neck, 1-2:1 elsewhere)
- flap choice is often a combination of available tissue, type of tissue needed, location of reconstruction site with respect to donor site, and surgeon preference
- types
  - **rotation**: semicircular tissue rotated around a pivot point for defect closure; commonly used on sacral pressure sores, scalp and cheek defects
  - **transposition**: tissue is transposed (ie. Lifted up from its native location and brought into the defect) around a pivot point from one location to another; commonly used on certain areas of the face using adjacent areas of excess skin laxity
  - **Z-plasty**: two triangular flaps are repositioned; used to reorient a scar, lengthen the line of a scar or to break up a scar
  - **advancement flaps (V-Y, Y-V)**: defect is closed with unidirectional tissue advancement
    - single/bipedicle V-Y flaps: wounds with lax surrounding tissue; the pedicle is the deep tissue underlying the flap

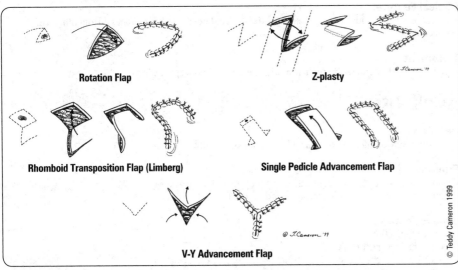

Rotation Flap

Z-plasty

Rhomboid Transposition Flap (Limberg)

Single Pedicle Advancement Flap

V-Y Advancement Flap

© Teddy Cameron 1999

Figure 15. Wound care flaps – random pattern

Axial Pattern Flaps (Arterialized)

- flap contains a well defined artery and vein
- allows greater length:width ratio (5-6:1)
- types
  - **peninsular flap**: skin and vessel intact in pedicle
  - **island flap**: vessel intact, pedicle is better defined
  - **free flap**: vascular supply anastomosed at recipient site by microsurgical techniques
- can be sub-classified according to tissue content of flap
  - e.g. musculocutaneous/myocutaneous (e.g. transverse rectus abdominal myocutaneous) vs. fasciocutaneous

Free Flaps

- transplanting expendable donor tissue from one part of the body to another by isolating and dividing a dominant artery and vein to a flap and performing a microsurgical anastomosis between these and the vessels in the recipient wound
- survival rates >95%
- types: muscle and skin (common), bone, jejunum, omentum, fascia
- e.g. radial forearm, scapular, latissimus dorsi

Table 12. Characteristics of Healthy Free Flap

Characteristic	Normal	Arterial Insufficiency	Venous Insufficiency
Colour	Pink	Pale	Purple or blue
Temperature	Warm	Cool	Warm or cool
Arterial Pulse (Doppler)	+	–	±
Turgor	Soft, but with some firmness	Decreased tissue firmness	Increased (tissue firmness with tissue stiffness)
Capillary Refill	2-5 seconds	> 5 seconds	<2 seconds

Soft Tissue Infections

Table 13. Classification of Soft Tissue Infections by Depth

Erysipelas	Superficial with upper dermis and superficial lymphatics involvement
Cellulitis	Full thickness of skin with subcutaneous tissue involvement
Fasciitis	Fascia
Myositis	Muscle

Erysipelas

Definition
• acute skin infection that is more superficial than cellulitis

Etiology
• typically caused by Group A β-hemolytic *Streptococcus*

Clinical Features
• intense erythema, induration, and **sharply demarcated borders** (differentiates it from other skin infections)

Treatment
• penicillin or first generation cephalosporin (e.g. cefazolin or cephalexin)

Cellulitis

Definition
• non-suppurative infection of skin and subcutaneous tissues

Etiology
• skin flora most common organisms: *S. aureus*, β-hemolytic *Streptococcus*
• immunocompromised: Gram-negative rods and fungi

Clinical Features
• source of infection
  ▪ trauma, recent surgery
  ▪ PVD, DM – cracked skin in feet/toes
  ▪ foreign bodies (IV, orthopedic pins)
• systemic symptoms (fever, chills, malaise)
• pain, tenderness, edema, erythema with poorly defined margins, regional lymphadenopathy
• can lead to ascending lymphangitis (visible red streaking in skin proximal to area of cellulitis)

Investigations
• CBC, blood cultures
• culture and Gram stain a collection/aspirate from wound if open wound
• plain radiographs show soft tissue edema only

Treatment
• antibiotics: first line – cephalexin 500 mg PO q6h or cloxacillin 500 mg PO q6h x 7 d; if complicated (e.g. lymphangitis, DM, severe infection, oral antibiotic therapy failure) consider IV cefazolin 1-2 g q8h or IV cloxacillin, IV penicillin. All patients should have reassessment in 48 hours for resolution if on a oral antibiotic
• outline area of erythema to monitor success of treatment
• immobilize and splint (hands)

Necrotizing Fasciitis

Definition
- rapidly spreading, very painful infection of the fascia with necrosis of surrounding tissues
- some bacteria create gas that can be felt as crepitus and can be seen on x-rays
- infection spreads rapidly along deep fascial plane and is limb and life threatening

Etiology
- Type I: polymicrobial (less aggressive)
- Type II: monomicrobial, usually β-hemolytic *Streptococcus*

Clinical Features
- **pain out of proportion to clinical findings and beyond border of erythema**
    - edema, tenderness, ± crepitus (subcutaneous gas from anaerobes)
- overlying skin changes including blistering and ecchymoses
- disorganized physiology
- patients may look deceptively well at first, but may rapidly become very sick/toxic
- late findings
    - skin turns dusky blue and black (secondary to thrombosis and necrosis)
    - induration, formation of bullae
    - cutaneous gangrene, subcutaneous emphysema

Investigations
- a clinical diagnosis
- CT scan only if suspect it is not necrotizing fasciitis (looking for abscess, gas collection, myonecrosis and possible source of infection)
- severely elevated CK: usually means myonecrosis (late sign)
- bedside incision, exploration, and incisional biopsy when ruling out conditions, clinical presentation is not supportive or difficult exam
- during incisional biopsy, often see "dish water pus" (Group A infection) and a hemostat easily passed along fascial plane (fascial biopsy to rule out in equivocal situations)

Treatment
- vigorous resuscitation (ABCs)
- urgent surgical debridement: remove all necrotic tissue, copious irrigation with plans for repeat surgery in 24-48 hours
- IV antibiotics: as appropriate for clinical scenario; consider penicillin 4 million IU IV q4h and/or clindamycin 900 mg IV q6h until final cultures available (the combination can be synergistic if Group A strep)
- urgent consultation with infectious disease specialist is recommended

Ulcers

Lower Limb Ulcers

Traumatic Ulcers (Acute)
- failure of wound to heal, usually due to compromised blood supply and unstable scar, secondary to pressure or bacterial colonization/infection
- usually over bony prominence ± edema ± pigmentation changes ± pain
- treatment: involvement of vascular surgery. Any debridement of ulcer and compromised tissues must be preceded by ABIs and vascular Doppler. Ulcers or compromised tissues left to heal via secondary intention with dressings, may need reconstruction with local or distant flap in select cases, vascular status of limb must be assessed clinically and via vascular studies (i.e. ABI, duplex doppler)

Non-Traumatic Ulcers (Chronic)

Table 14. Venous vs. Arterial vs. Diabetic Ulcers

Characteristic	Venous (70% of vascular ulcers)	Arterial	Diabetic
Cause	Valvular incompetence Venous HTN	2° to small and/or large vessel disease (be aware of risk factors)	Peripheral neuropathy: decreased sensation Atherosclerosis: microvascular disease
History	Dependent edema, trauma Rapid onset ± thrombophlebitis, varicosities	Arteriosclerosis, claudication Usually >45 yr Slow progression	DM Peripheral neuropathy Trauma/pressure
Common Distribution	Medial malleolus ("Gaiter" locations)	Distal locations (e.g. lower limb, feet)	Pressure point distribution (more likely metatarsal headsheads)

Table 14. Venous vs. Arterial vs. Diabetic Ulcers (continued)

Characteristic	Venous (70% of vascular ulcers)	Arterial	Diabetic
Appearance	Yellow exudates Granulation tissue Varicose veins Brown discolouration of surrounding skin	Pale/white, necrotic base ± dry eschar covering	Necrotic base
Wound Margins	Irregular	Even ("punched out")	Irregular or "punched out" or deep
Depth	Superficial	Deep	Superficial/deep
Surrounding Skin	Venous stasis discolouration (brown)	Thin shiny dry skin, hairless, cool	Thin dry skin ± hyperkeratotic border Hypersensitive/ischemic
Pulses	Normal distal pulses	Decreased or no distal pulses	Decreased pulses likely (Take caution in calcified vessels)
Vascular Exam	ABI >0.9 Doppler; abnormal venous system	ABI <0.9 Pallor on elevation, rubor on dependency Delayed venous filling	ABI is inaccurately high (due to PVD) Usually associated with arterial disease (microvascular/macrovascular disease)
Pain	Moderately painful Increased with leg dependency, decreased with elevation No rest pain	Extremely painful Decreased with dependency, increased with leg elevation and exercise (claudication) Rest pain	Painless (if neuropathy) No claudication or rest pain Associated paresthesia, anesthesia
Treatment	Leg elevation, rest Compression at 30 mmHg (stockings or elastic bandages) Moist wound dressings ± topical, systemic antibiotics if infected ± skin grafts	Rest, no elevation, no compression Moist wound dressing ± topical and/or systemic antibiotics if infected Modify risk factors (smoking, diet, exercise, etc.) Vascular surgical consultation (angioplasty or bypass) Treat underlying conditions (DM, proximal arterial occlusion, etc.)	Control DM Careful wound care Foot care Orthotics, off loading Early intervention for infections (topical and/or systemic antibiotics if infected) Vascular surgical consultation

ABI in diabetics can be falsely normal due to incompressible arteries secondary to plaques/calcification

All chronic ulcers require vascular studies, and a vascular consult, to assess for venous insufficiency, to rule in/out arterial pathology and to find out the potential role of vascular surgical management

Pressure Ulcers

Common Sites
• over bony prominences; 95% on lower body

Stages of Development
1. hyperemia: disappears 1 h after pressure removed
2. ischemia: follows 2-6 h of pressure
3. necrosis: follows >6 h of pressure
4. ulcer: necrotic area breaks down – N.B. skin is like tip of an iceberg

Classification (National Pressure Ulcer Advisory Panel 2014)
• Stage I: nonblanchable erythema present >1 h after pressure relief, skin intact
• Stage II: partial-thickness skin loss
• Stage III: full-thickness skin loss into subcutaneous tissue
• Stage IV: full-thickness skin loss into muscle, bone, tendon, or joint
  ▪ if an eschar is present, must fully debride before staging possible

Prevention
• good nursing care (clean dry skin, frequent repositioning), special beds or pressure relief surface, proper nutrition, activity, early identification of individuals at risk (e.g. immobility, incontinence, paraplegia, immunocompromised, DM, etc.)

Treatment
• depends on individual patient and condition
• treat underlying medical issues including nutrition
• continue with preventative measures (pressure relief, assess for pressure points e.g. wheelchairs, manage continence issues, divert contaminants e.g. urine and feces)
• wound debridement, moisture retentive or antimicrobial dressing, regular reassessment
• systemic antibiotics for infections
• assess for possible reconstruction

Complications
• cellulitis, osteomyelitis, sepsis, gangrene

Burns

Burn Injuries

Causal Conditions
- thermal (flame contact, scald)
- chemical
- radiation (UV, medical/therapeutic)
- electrical

Most Common Etiology
- children: scald burns
- adults: flame burns

Table 15. Skin Function and Burn Injury

Skin Function	Consequence of Burn Injury	Intervention Required
Thermoregulation	Prone to lose body heat	Must keep patient covered and warm
Control of fluid loss	Loss of large amounts of water and protein from the skin and other body tissues	Adequate fluid resuscitation is imperative
Mechanical barrier to bacterial invasion and immunological organ	High risk of infection	Antimicrobial dressings (systemic antbiotics if signs of specific infection present) Tetanus prophylaxis if not already administered

Pathophysiology of Burn Wounds

- amount of tissue destruction is based on temperature, time of exposure, and specific heat of the causative agent
- zone of hyperemia: vasodilation from inflammation; entirely viable, cells recover within 7 d; contributes to systemic consequences seen with major burns
- zone of stasis (edema): decreased perfusion; microvascular sludging and thrombosis of vessels results in progressive tissue necrosis → cellular death in 24-48 h without proper treatment
  - factors favouring cell survival: moist, aseptic environment, rich blood supply
  - zone where appropriate early intervention has most profound effect in minimizing injury
- zone of coagulation (ischemia): no blood flow to tissue → irreversible cell damage → cellular death/necrosis

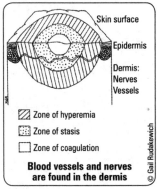

Figure 16. Zones of thermal injury

Diagnosis and Prognosis

- burn size
  - % of TBSA burned: rule of 9s for 2° and 3° burns only (children <10 yr old use Lund-Browder chart)
  - for patchy burns, surface area covered by patient's palm (fingers closed) represents approximately 1% of TBSA
- age: more complications if <3 or >60 yr old
- depth: difficult to assess initially – history of etiologic agent and time of exposure helpful (see Table 16)
- location: face and neck, hands, feet, perineum are critical areas requiring special care of a burn unit (see *Indications for Transfer to Burn Centre*, PL19)
- inhalation injury: can severely compromise respiratory system, affect fluid requirement estimation (underestimate), mortality secondary to ARDS
- associated injuries (e.g. fractures)
- comorbid factors (e.g. concurrent disability, alcoholism, seizure disorders, chronic renal failure) can exacerbate extent of injury, other trauma)

Prognosis best determined by burn size (TBSA), age of patient, presence/absence of inhalation injury

Circumferential burns can restrict respiratory excursion and/or blood flow to extremities and require escharotomy

TBSA does not include areas with 1° burns

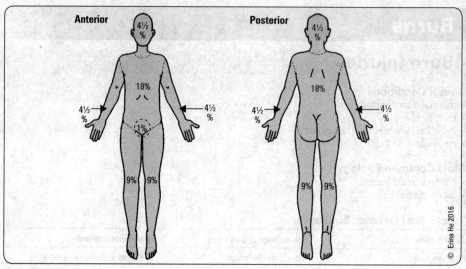

Figure 17. Rule of 9s for TBSA

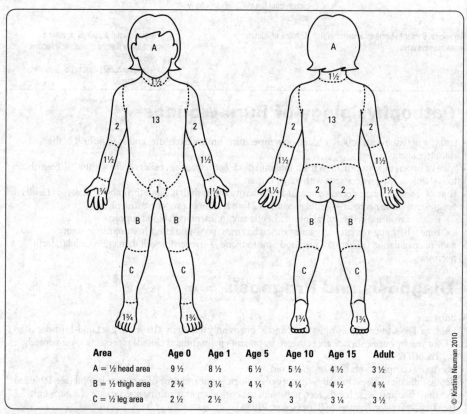

Area	Age 0	Age 1	Age 5	Age 10	Age 15	Adult
A = ½ head area	9 ½	8 ½	6 ½	5 ½	4 ½	3 ½
B = ½ thigh area	2 ¾	3 ¼	4 ¼	4 ¼	4 ½	4 ¾
C = ½ leg area	2 ½	2 ½	3	3	3 ¼	3 ½

Figure 18. Lund-Browder diagram

Table 16. Burn Depth (1st, 2nd, 3rd degree)

Nomenclature	Traditional Nomenclature	Depth	Clinical Features
Erythema/Superficial	First degree	Epidermis	Painful, sensation intact, erythema, blanchable
Superficial-Partial Thickness	Second degree	Into superficial dermis	Painful, sensation intact, erythema, blisters with clear fluid, blanchable, hair follicles present
Deep-Partial Thickness	Second degree	Into deep (reticular) dermis	Insensate, difficult to distinguish from full thickness, does not blanch, some hair follicles still attached, softer than full thickness burn
Full Thickness	Third degree / Fourth degree	Through epidermis and dermis / Injury to underlying tissue structures (e.g. muscle, bone)	Insensate (nerve endings destroyed), hard leathery eschar that is black, grey, white, or cherry red in colour, hairs do not stay attached, may see thrombosed veins

Indications for Transfer to Burn Centre

American Burn Association Criteria

- patients with partial or full-thickness burns that involve the hands, feet, genitalia, face, eyes, ears, and/or major joints or perineum
- partial thickness burns ≥20% TBSA in patients aged 10-50 yr old
- partial thickness burns ≥10% TBSA in children aged ≤10 or adults aged ≥50 yr old
- full thickness burns ≥5% TBSA in patients of all ages
- electrical burns, including lightening (internal injury underestimated by TBSA), and chemical burns
- inhalation injury (high risk of mortality and may lead to respiratory distress)
- burn injuries in patients with medical comorbidities, could complicate management and recovery
- any patient with simultaneous trauma plus burns should be stabilized for trauma first, then triaged appropriately to burn centre
- any patients with burn injury and who will require special emotional, social, and rehabilitation intervention
- children with burns in a hospital not equipped with pediatric care specialists

Acute Care of Burn Patients

- adhere to ATLS protocol
- resuscitation using Parkland formula to restore plasma volume and cardiac output, Parkland formula is a starting estimate and patients may require more volume. Other formulas exist but the Parkland formula is predominately used in North America
  - 4 cc/kg X %TBSA (greater than first degree) X wt(kg) (1/2 within first 8 h of sustaining burn, 1/2 in next 16 h)
- extra fluid administration required if
  - burn >80% TBSA
  - 4° burns
  - associated traumatic injury
  - electrical burn
  - inhalation injury
  - delayed start of resuscitation
  - pediatric burns
- monitor resuscitation
  - urine output is best measure: maintain at >0.5 cc/kg/h (adults) and 1.0 cc/kg/h
  - (children <12 yr)
  - maintain a clear sensorium, HR <120/min, MAP >70 mmHg
- burn specific care
  - relieve respiratory distress: intubation and/or escharotomy
  - Escharotomy in circumferential extremity burn including digits
  - prevent and/or treat burn shock: 2 large bore IVs for fluid resuscitation
  - insert Foley catheter to monitor urine output
  - identify and treat immediate life-threatening conditions (e.g. inhalation injury, CO poisoning)
  - determine TBSA affected first, since depth is difficult to determine initially (easier to determine after 24 h)
- tetanus prophylaxis if needed
  - all patients with burns >10% TBSA, or deeper than superficial partial thickness, need 0.5 cc tetanus toxoid
  - also give 250 U of tetanus Ig if prior immunization is absent/unclear, or the last booster >10 yr ago
- baseline laboratory studies (Hb, U/A, BUN, CXR, electrolytes, Cr, glucose, CK ECG, cross-match if traumatic injury, ABG, carboxyhemoglobin)
- cleanse, debride, and treat the burn injury (antimicrobial dressings)
- early excision and grafting important for outcome

Respiratory Problems

- 3 major causes
  - burn eschar encircling chest
    - distress may be apparent immediately
    - perform escharotomy to relieve constriction
  - CO poisoning
    - may present immediately or later
    - treat with 100% O_2 by facemask (decreases half-life of carboxyhemoglobin from 210 to 59 min) until carboxyHb <10%
  - smoke inhalation leading to pulmonary injury
    - chemical injury to alveolar basement membrane and pulmonary edema (insidious onset)
    - risk of pulmonary insufficiency (up to 48 h) and pulmonary edema (48-72 h)
    - watch for secondary bronchopneumonia (3-25 d) leading to progressive pulmonary insufficiency
    - intubate patient with any signs of inhalation injuries

Inhalation Injuries 101
- Indicators of inhalation injury
- Injury in a closed space
- Facial burn
- Singed nasal hair/eyebrows
- Soot around nares/oral cavity
- Hoarseness
- Conjunctivitis
- Tachypnea
- Carbon particles in sputum
- Elevated blood CO levels (i.e. brighter red)
- Suspected inhalation injury requires immediate intubation due to impending airway edema; failure to diagnose inhalation injury can result in airway swelling and obstruction, which, if untreated, can lead to death
- Neither CXR or ABG can be used to rule out inhalation injury
- Direct bronchoscopy now used for diagnosis
- Signs of CO poisoning (headache, confusion, coma, arrhythmias)

Burn Wound Healing

Table 17. Burn Shock Resuscitation (Parkland Formula)

Hour 0-24	4 cc RL/kg/% TBSA with 1/2 of total in first 8 h from time of injury and 1/2 of total in next 16 h from time of injury
Hour 24-30	0.35-0.5 cc plasma/kg/%TBSA
>Hour 30	D5W at rate to maintain normal serum sodium

*Do not forget to add maintenance fluid to resuscitation

Table 18. Burn Wound Healing

Depth	Healing
First degree	No scarring; complete healing
Second degree (Superficial partial)	Spontaneously re-epithelialize in 7 to 14 d from retained epidermal structures ± residual skin discolouration Hypertrophic scarring uncommon; grafting rarely required
Deep second degree (Deep partial)	Re-epithelialize in 14-35 d from retained epidermal structures Hypertrophic scarring frequent Grafting recommended to expedite healing
Third degree (Full thickness)	Re-epithelialize from the wound edge Grafting/flap necessary to replace dermal integrity, limit hypertrophic scarring
Fourth degree	Often results in amputations If not requiring amputation, needs flap for coverage after debridement (do not re-epithelialize – cannot graft)

Treatment

- 3 stages
    1. assessment: depth determined
    2. management: specific to depth of burn and associated injuries
    3. rehabilitation
- first degree
    - treatment aimed at comfort
        - topical creams (pain control, keep skin moist) ± aloe
        - oral NSAIDs (pain control)
- superficial second degree/partial thickness
    - daily dressing changes with topical antimicrobials (such as polysporin); leave blisters intact unless circulation impaired or unless over joint inhibiting motion
- deep second degree/deep partial thickness and third degree/full thickness
    - prevent infection and sepsis (significant complication and cause of death in patients with burns)
        - most common organisms: *S. aureus, P. aeruginosa,* and *C. albicans*
            - day 1-3 (rare): Gram-positive
            - day 3-5: Gram-negative (*Proteus, Klebsiella*)
        - topical antimicrobials: treat colonized wounds (from skin flora, gut flora or caregiver)
    - remove dead tissue
        - surgically debride necrotic tissue, excise to viable (bleeding) tissue

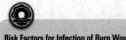

Risk Factors for Infection of Burn Wounds

Patient Related
- Extent >30% TBSA
- Depth: full-thickness and deep partial-thickness
- Patient age (higher risk with very young and very old)
- Comorbidities
- Wound dryness
- Wound temperature
- Secondary impairment of blood flow to wound
- Acidosis

Microbial Factors
- Density >10^5 organisms per gram tissue
- Motility
- Virulence and metabolic products (endotoxin, exotoxin, permeability factors, other factors)
- Antimicrobial resistance

Table 19. Antimicrobial Dressings for Burns

Antibiotic	Pain with Application	Penetration	Adverse Effects
Silver nitrate (0.5% solution)	None	Minimal	May cause methemoglobinemia, stains (black), leaches sodium from wounds
Nanocrystalline silver-coated dressing (Acticoat®)	None or transient	Medium, does not penetrate eschar	May stain, producing a pseudoeschar or facial discolouration (argyria-like symptoms); raised liver enzymes
Silver sulfadiazine (cream) (Flamazine®, Silvadene®)	Minimal	Medium, penetrates eschar poorly Most commonly used	Slowed healing, leukopenia, mild inhibition of epithelialization
Mafenide acetate (solution/cream)			
(Sulfamylon®)	Moderate	Well, penetrates eschar	Mild inhibition of epithelialization, may cause metabolic acidosis with wide application

- early excision and grafting is the mainstay of treatment for deep/full thickness burns
- initial dressing should decrease bacterial proliferation
- prevention of wound contractures: pressure dressings, joint splints, early physiotherapy

Other Considerations in Burn Management

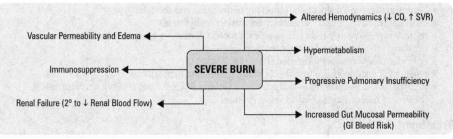

Figure 19. Systemic effects of severe burns

- nutrition
  - hypermetabolism: TBSA >40% have BMR 2-2.5x predicted
  - consider nutritional supplementation e.g. calories, vitamin C, vitamin A, Ca^{2+}, Zn^{2+}, Fe^{2+}
- immunosuppression and sepsis
  - must keep bacterial count $<10^5$ bacteria/g of tissue (blood culture may not be positive)
  - signs of sepsis: sudden onset of hyper/hypothermia, unexpected CHF or pulmonary edema, development of ARDS, ileus >48 h post-burn, mental status changes, azotemia, thrombocytopenia, hypofibrinogenemia, hyper/hypoglycemia (especially if burn >40% TBSA)
- GI bleed may occur with burns >40% TBSA (usually subclinical)
  - treatment: tube feeding or NPO if there is a GI bleed, antacids, H_2 blockers (preventative)
- renal failure secondary to under resuscitation, drugs, myoglobin, etc.
- progressive pulmonary insufficiency
  - can occur after: smoke inhalation, pneumonia, cardiac decompensation, sepsis
- wound contracture and hypertrophic scarring (outcomes optimized with timely wound closure, splinting, pressure garments) and physiotherapy

Special Considerations

CHEMICAL
- major categories: acid burns, alkaline burns, phosphorous burns, chemical injection injuries
- common agents: cement, hydrofluoric acid, phenol, tar
- mechanism of injury: chemical solutions coagulate tissue protein leading to necrosis
  - acids → coagulation necrosis
  - alkalines → saponification followed by liquefactive necrosis
- severity related to: type of chemical (alkali worse than acid), temperature, volume, concentration, contact time, site affected, mechanism of chemical action, degree of tissue penetration
- burns are deeper than they initially appear and may progress with time

Treatment (General)
- ABCs, monitoring
- remove contaminated clothing and brush off any dry powders before irrigation
- irrigation with water for 1-2 h under low pressure (contraindicated in heavy metal burns, such as sodium, potassium, magnesium, and lithium; in these cases soak in mineral oil instead)
- inspect eyes, if affected: wash with saline and refer to ophthalmology
- inspect nails, hair and webspaces
- correct metabolic abnormalities and tetanus prophylaxis if necessary
- contact poison control line if necessary
- local wound care 12 h after initial dilution (debridement)
- wound closure same as for thermal burn
- beware of underestimated fluid resuscitation, renal, liver, and pulmonary damage

Special Burns and Treatments

Acid Burn	Water irrigation, followed by dilute solution of sodium bicarbonate
Hydrofluroic Acid	Water irrigation; clip fingernails to avoid acid trapping; topical calcium gel ± subcutaneous injection of calcium gluconate ± 10% calcium gluconate IV depending on amount of exposure and pain
Sulfuric Acid	Treat with soap/lime prior to irrigation, as direct water exposure produces extreme heat
Tar	Remove with repeated application of petroleum-based antibiotic ointments (e.g. Polysporin®)

ELECTRICAL BURNS
- depth of burn depends on voltage and resistance of the tissue (injury more severe in tissues with high resistance)
- often presents as small punctate burns on skin with extensive deep tissue damage which requires debridement
- electrical burns require ongoing monitoring as latent injuries can occur

Tissue Resistance to Electrical Current
nerve < vessel/blood < muscle < skin < tendon < fat < bone

- watch for system specific damages and abnormalities
  - abdominal: intraperitoneal damage
  - bone: fractures and dislocations especially of the spine and shoulder
  - cardiopulmonary: anoxia, ventricular fibrillation, arrhythmias
  - muscle: myoglobinuria indicates significant muscle damage → compartment syndrome
  - neurological: seizures and spinal cord damage
  - ophthalmology: cataract formation (late complication)
  - renal: ATN resulting from toxic levels of myoglobin and hemoglobin
  - vascular: vessel thrombosis → tissue necrosis (increased Cr, K^+ and acidity), decrease in RBC (beware of hemorrhages/delayed vessel rupture)

Treatment
- ABCs, primary and secondary survey, treat associated injuries
- beware of cardiac arrhythmias (continue cardiac monitoring)
- monitor: hemochromogenuria, compartment syndrome, urine output
- wound management: topical agent with good penetrating ability (silver sulfadiazine or mafenide acetate)
- debride nonviable tissue early and repeat prn (every 48 h) to prevent sepsis
- amputations frequently required

FROSTBITE
- see Emergency Medicine, ER46

Hand

Traumatic Hand

Compartment Syndrome
Watch out for these signs with a closed or open injury: tense, painful extremity (worse on passive stretch), parasthesia/paralysis, pallor, distal pulselessness (often late in process), and contracture (irreversible ischemia) Intracompartmental pressures can be measured (normal pressure = up to 12 mmHg), (abnormal is 30-40 mmHg), but a clinical diagnosis is an indication for an emergent fasciotomy; if untreated, end result is ischemic contracture of the extremity (Volkmann's contracture)

Approach to Hand Lacerations

TIN AX
Tetanus prophylaxis
Irrigate with NS (copious irrigation and debridement in a timely manner)
NPO (NPO if you are considering replanting or an urgent OR, otherwise most operations are done as elective procedures)
Antibiotic prophylaxis (controversial – most require no ABx, mainly needed for animal bites and dirty wounds)
X-rays

Allen's Test: You need to exsanguinate the hand by having the patient open and close the hand. Then, while patient's hand is firmly closed, occlude both radial and ulnar arteries. Once fist is open, release either artery and assess collateral flow

High pressure injection injury, e.g. pain gun, is deceptively benign-looking (small pinpoint hole on finger pad) often with few clinical signs. Intense pain and tenderness, along the course the foreign material travelled, is present a few hours after the injury. Definitive treatment is exposure and removal of foreign material

Table 20. Key Features of the History and Physical Exam of the Injured Hand

HISTORY		
Key Questions	Age	Time and place of accident
	Hand dominance	Mechanism of injury
	Occupation	Tetanus status
PHYSICAL EXAM		
Observation	Position of finger	Abnormal cadence (fingers normally slightly flexed), scissoring
	Deformity	Bony protrusions or specific deformities (e.g. mallet, boutonniere, and swan neck deformity)
	Bruising or swelling	May indicate underlying skeletal injury
	Sweating pattern (usually felt more so than from observation)	May indicate denervation
	Anatomical structures beneath	If open laceration, need to explore within wound (under sterile conditions)
	Structure	**Examination**
Vascular Status	Radial and ulnar arteries	Allen's Test
	Digital arteries	Hard to palpate but you can assess capillary refill (<2-3 s) Oxygen saturation monitor to verify perfusion
	Temperature and skin turgor	For each test, need to compare both sides
Sensory (see Figure 4)	Median nerve	Volar radial tip of index finger
	Ulnar nerve	Volar ulnar tip of little finger
	Radial nerve	Dorsal web space of the thumb
	Digital nerves	2 point discrimination on both the radial and ulnar side of the DIPJ creases (static or moving 2 point discrimination)
Motor Function	Median nerve	Flex DIP of index finger to test the anterior interosseus (AIN) branch of the median nerve Touch the tip of the index finger to the thumb trying to break through ("OK sign") Thumb to ceiling with palm up
	Ulnar nerve	Extrinsic muscles: flex DIP of little finger Intrinsic muscles: abduct index finger ("Peace sign") or patient able to hold piece of paper between adducted fingers and resist pulling ("Fromment's sign")
	Radial nerve	Extrinsic muscles: extend thumb ("thumb's up") and wrist
Range of Motion	Tendons, bones, joints, nerves	Assess active and passive range of motion of wrist extension/flexion/ulnar/radial deviation, finger abduction/adduction/flexion/extension, thumb flexion/extension/abduction/adduction/circumflexion
Tendons	FDP	Stabilize PIP in extension, ask patient to flex fingers (at DIP)
	FDS	Stabilize non-exam fingers in extension (neutralizes FDP) and ask patient to flex examination finger
Palpation	Bones	Focal tenderness or abnormal alignment
	Joints	Instability may indicate ligamentous injury or dislocation

General Management

Nerves
- **test the nerve function BEFORE putting in local anesthesia**
- direct repair for a clean injury within 14 d and without concurrent major injuries → otherwise secondary repair
- epineural repair of all digital nerves with minimal tension
- post-operative: dress wound, elevate hand and immobilize
- Tinel's sign (cutaneous percussion over the repaired nerve) produces paresthesias and defines level of nerve regeneration
  - Wallerian degeneration occurs in the first 2 wk, which is why there is no Tinel's sign till after this time period
  - a peripheral nerve regenerates at 1 mm/d
  - paresthesias felt at area of percussion because regrowth of myelin (Schwann cells) is slower than axonal regrowth → percussion on exposed free-end of axon generates paresthesia

Vessels
- often associated with nerve injury (anatomical proximity)
- control bleeding with direct pressure and hand elevation
- if digit devascularized, optimal repair within 6 h
- close skin then dress, immobilize, and splint hand with fingertips visible
- monitor colour, capillary refill, skin turgor, fingertip temperature post-revascularization

Tendons
- most tendon lacerations require primary repair
- many extensors are repaired in the emergency room, flexors are repaired in the operating room within 2 wk
- avoid excessive immobilization after repair (specific protocols for flexors to minimize stiffness and facilitate rehabilitation

Bones
- see *Fractures and Dislocations*, PL26

Nailbed
- subungal hematomas >50% of the nail surface area need to be drained. done so under a digital block by puncturing nail plate
- is suspicous, remove nail to examine underlying nailbed under digital block anesthesia
- irrigate wound and nail thoroughly
- suture repair of nailbed with chromic suture
- replace cleaned nail, which acts as splint for any underlying distal phalangeal fracture and prevents adhesion formation between nail fold and nailbed

Hand Exam
- Never blindly clamp a bleeding vessel as nerves are often found in close association with vessels
- Never explore any volar hand wound in the ER
- Arterial bleeding from a volar digital laceration is likely associated with a nerve laceration (nerves in digits are superficial to arteries)

Hand Infections

Principles
- trauma is most common cause
- 5 cardinal signs: rubor (red), calor (hot), tumour (swollen), dolor (painful) and functio laesa (loss of function)
- 90% caused by Gram-positive organisms
- most common organisms (in order) – *S. aureus, S. viridans,* Group A *Streptococcus, S. epidermidis,* and *Bacteroides melaninogenicus* (MRSA is becoming more common)

TYPES OF INFECTIONS

Deep Palmar Space Infections
- uncommon, there are 9 spaces in the hand, the most commonly involved are thenar or mid-palm space

Felon
- **definition**: subcutaneous abscess in the fingertip that commonly occurs following a puncture wound into the pad of digit; may be associated with osteomyelitis (akin to compartment syndrome and can lead to skin necrosis)
- **treatment**: elevation, warm soaks, cloxacillin 500 mg PO q6h (if in early stage); if obvious abscess or pressure on the overlying skin or failure to resolve with conservative measures, then needs I&D; take cultures/gram stain and PO cloxacillin

Flexor Tendon Sheath Infection
- *Staphylococcus* > *Streptococcus* > Gram-negative rods
- **definition**: acute tenosynovitis commonly caused by a penetrating injury and can lead to tendon necrosis and rupture if not treated; it is often suppurative; however, early on there can be very little pus

- **clinical features**: Kanavel's 4 cardinal signs
  1. point tenderness along flexor tendon sheath
  2. severe pain on passive extension of DIP
  3. fusiform swelling of entire digit
  4. flexed posture (increased comfort)
- **treatment**
  - OR incision and drainage, irrigation, IV antibiotics, and resting hand splint until infection resolves

Herpetic Whitlow
- HSV-1, HSV-2
- **definition**: painful vesicle(s) around fingertip
  - often found in medical/dental personnel and children
- **clinical features**: can be associated with fever, malaise and lymphadenopathy
  - patient is infectious until lesion has completely healed
- **treatment**: routine culture and viral prep protection (cover), consider oral acyclovir; do not break blisters

Paronychia
- acute = *Staphylococcus*; chronic = *Candida*
- **definition**: infection (granulation tissue) of soft tissue around fingernail (within the paronychium and/or beneath eponychial fold)
- **etiololgy**
  - acute paronychia: a "hangnail", artificial nails, and nail biting
  - chronic paronychia: prolonged exposure to moisture
- **treatment**
  - acute paronychia: warm compresses and cephalexin 500 mg PO q6h if caught early and drainage if abscess present – can usually drain with a #11 blade directed into the abscess from underneath the paronychial fold
  - chronic paronychia: anti-fungals with possible debridement and marsupialization, removal of nail plate

Amputations

Hand or Finger
- emergency management: injured patient and amputated part require attention
  - **patient**: x-rays (stump and amputated part), NPO, clean wound and irrigate with NS, dress stump with nonadherent, cover with dry sterile dressing, tetanus and antibiotic prophylaxis (cephalosporin/erythromycin)
  - **amputated part**: x-rays, gently irrigate with RL, wrap amputated part in a NS/RL soaked sterile gauze and place inside waterproof plastic bag, place in a container, then place container on ice
- **indications for replantation**
  - **age**: children often better results than adults
  - **level of injury**: thumb and multiple digit amputations are higher priority
  - **nature of injury**: clean cut injuries have greater success; avulsion and crush injuries are relative contraindications to replant
- if replant contraindicated manage stump with revision amputation
  - involves deriding amputating end, trimming back the bone and nerve endings and gently closing the skin)
  - commonly done in the emerge under digital block

Tendons

Common Extensor Tendon Deformities
Table 21. Extensor Tendon Deformities

Injury	Definition	Zone	Etiology/Clinical Features	Treatment
Mallet Finger	DIP flexed with loss of active extension	1	There are bony and non-bony mallets Bony: Fracture of distal phalanx distal to tendon insertion Non-bony: Forced flexion of the extended DIP leading to extensor tendon rupture at DIP (e.g. sudden blow to tip of the finger)	Splint DIP in extension for 6 wk followed by 2 wk of night splinting; if inadequate improvement after 6 wk, check splinting routine and recommend 4 more wk of continuous splinting. If there is a bony component that is displaced the patient may require ORIF
Boutonniere Deformity	PIP flexed, DIP hyperextended	3	Injury or disease affecting the extensor tendon insertion into the dorsal base of the middle phalanx Associated with RA or trauma (laceration, volar dislocation, acute forceful flexion of PIP)	Splint PIP in extension and allow active DIP motion
Swan Neck Deformity	PIP hyperextended, DIP flexed	3	Trauma (PIP volar plate injury) Associated with RA and old, untreated mallet deformity Splint to prevent PIP hyperextension or DIP flexion	Corrective procedures involve tendon rebalancing or arthrodesis/arthroplasty

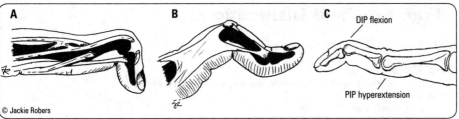

Figure 20. (A) Mallet finger deformity (B) Boutonniere deformity (C) Swan neck deformity

Tenosynovitis (zone 7; most common cause of radial wrist pain)
- **definition**: inflammation of the tendon and/or its sheath. Most common is DeQuervain tenosynovitis (inflammation of the extensor tendons in the 1st dorsal compartment [APL and EPB])
- **clinical features**
  - +ve Finkelstein's test (pain over the radial styloid induced by making fist, with thumb in palm, and ulnar deviation of wrist)
  - pain localized to the 1st extensor compartment
  - tenderness and crepitation over radial styloid may be present
  - differentiate from CMC joint arthritis (CMC joint arthritis will have a positive grind test, whereby crepitus and pain are elicited by axial pressure to the thumb)
- **treatment**
  - mild: NSAIDs, splinting and steroid injection into the tendon sheath (successful in over 60% of cases) severe: surgical release of stenotic tendon sheaths (APL and EPB); ganglion cyst

Ganglion Cyst
- **definition**
  - fluid-filled synovial lining that protrudes between carpal bones or from a tendon sheath; most commonly carpal in origin
  - most common soft tissue tumour of hand and wrist (60% of masses)
- **clinical features**
  - most common around scapholunate ligament junction
  - 3 times more common in women than in men
  - more common in younger individuals
  - can be large or small – may drain internally so size may wax and wane
  - often non-tender although tenderness increased when cyst smaller (from increased pressure within smaller cyst sac)
- **treatment**
  - conservative treatment: do nothing
  - aspiration (recurrence rate 65%)
  - consider operative excision of cyst and stalk (recurrence rate 5.9% for dorsal wrist ganglion, 30% for volar)
  - steroids if painful (done in combination with aspiration as results are no better than aspiration alone

Common Flexor Tendon Deformities
- flexor tendon zones (important for prognosis of tendon lacerations)
- "no-man's land"
- between distal palmar crease and mid-middle phalanx
- zone where superficialis and profundus lie ensheathed together
- recovery of glide very difficult after injury

Stenosing Tenosynovitis (trigger finger/thumb)
- **definition**: inflammation of synovium causes size discrepancy between tendon and sheath/pulley (most commonly at A-1 pulley) = locking of thumb or finger in flexion/extension
- **etiology**: idiopathic or associated with RA, DM, hypothyroidism, gout, and pregnancy
- **clinical features**
  - thumb, ring and long fingers most commonly affected
  - patient complains of catching, snapping or locking of affected finger
  - tenderness to palpation/nodule at palmar aspect of MCP over A-1 pulley
  - women are 4 times more likely than men to be affected
- **nonsurgical treatment**
  - NSAIDs
  - steroid injection
  - injections less likely to be successful in patients with DM or symptoms greater than 6 mo
  - splint
- **surgical treatment**
  - indicated if no relief of symptoms or minimal relief with steroids
  - incise A-1 flexor pulley to permit unrestricted, full active finger motion

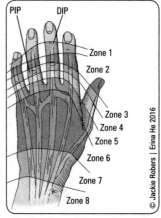

Figure 21. Zone of extensor tendon injury (odd numbered zones fall over a joint)

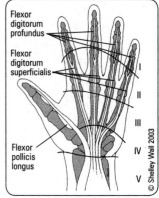

Figure 22. Zones of the flexor tendons

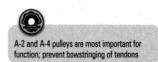

A-2 and A-4 pulleys are most important for function; prevent bowstringing of tendons

Fractures and Dislocations

- for fracture principles, see <u>Orthopedics</u>, OR4

FRACTURES
- about 90% of hand fractures are stable in flexion (splint to prevent extension)
- **position of safety**
  - wrist extension 0-30°
  - MCP flexion 70-90°
  - IP full extension
  - this is done if you want to immobilize a fracture but are not sure whether there are other injuries
- stiffness secondary to immobilization is the most important complication; Tx = early motion

Distal Phalanx Fractures
- most commonly fractured bone in the hand
- usual mechanism is crush injury and thus accompanied by soft tissue injury
- subungual hematoma is common and must be decompressed if there is involvement of >50% of the nail surface area
- injury involving >50% of the nail surface area often suggests a nail bed laceration, in which the patient would benefit from surgery
- treatment consists of 3 wk of digital splinting (immobilize the DIPJ with a STAX splint)

Proximal and Middle Phalanx Fractures
- check for: rotation, scissoring (overlap of fingers on making a fist), shortening of digit
- undisplaced or minimally displaced: closed reduction (if extra-articular) buddy tape to neighbouring stable digit, elevate hand, motion in guarded fashion early, splinted for **2-3 wk**
- displaced, nonreducible, not stable with closed reduction, or rotational or scissoring deformity: percutaneous pins (K-wires) or ORIF, and splint

Metacarpal Fractures
- generally accept varying degrees of deviation before reduction required: up to 10° (D2), 20° (D3), 30° (D4), or 40° (D5)
- **Boxer's fracture**: acute angulation of the neck of the 5th metacarpal into palm
  - mechanism: blow on the distal-dorsal aspect of closed fist
  - loss of prominence of metacarpal head, volar displacement of head
  - up to 30-40° angulation may be acceptable
  - if greater angulation, closed reduction should be considered to decrease the angle
  - if stable ulnar gutter splint for **4-6 wk**
- **Bennett's fracture**: two-piece fracture/dislocation of the base of the thumb metacarpal
  - unstable fracture
  - abductor pollicis longus pulls MC shaft proximally and radially causing adduction of thumb
  - treat with percutaneous pinning or ORIF followed by, thumb spica x 6 wk
- **Rolando fracture**: T- or Y-shaped fracture of the base of the thumb metacarpal T- or Y-shaped fracture of the base of the thumb metacarpal
  - treated like a Bennett's fracture

DISLOCATIONS
- must be reduced as soon as possible
- dislocation vs. subluxation
  - dislocation: severe injury where articular surfaces of a joint are no longer in contact with one another
  - subluxation: articular surfaces of a joint are partially out of place (i.e. "partial dislocation" – often unstable and requires reduction)

PIP and DIP Dislocations (PIP more common than DIP)
- usually dorsal dislocation (commonly from hyperextension)
- if closed dislocation: closed reduction and splinting (ideally in full extension if stable, or PIPJ in flexion if unstable) oror buddy taping and early mobilization (prolonged immobilization causes stiffness)
- open injuries are treated with wound care, closed or open reduction, irrigation and debridement, and antibiotics

MCP Dislocations (relatively rare)
- dorsal dislocations much more common than volar dislocations
- dorsal dislocation of proximal phalanx on metacarpal head; most commonly index finger (hyperextension)
- two types of dorsal dislocation
  - simple (reducible with manipulation): treat with closed reduction and splting for 2-4 wk at 60-70° MCP flexion
  - complex (irreducible - most commonly due to volar plate blocking the reduction): treat with open reduction

Ulnar Collateral Ligament (UCL) Injury
- forced abduction of thumb (e.g. ski pole injury)
- **Skier's thumb**: acute UCL injury – if stable treated with splint x **6-8 wk**, if unstable patient may have stener lesion
- **Gamekeeper's thumb**: chronic UCL injury, often requires open repair and tendon graft for stabilization
- **Stener Lesion**: the distal portion of the UCL can detach and flip superficial to the adductor aponeurosis and will not appropriately heal – requires open repair
- **evaluation**: radially deviate thumb MCP joint in full extension and at 30° flexion and compare with noninjured hand. UCL rupture is presumed if injured side deviates more than 30° in full extension or more than 15° in flexion

Dupuytren's Disease

Definition
- contraction of longitudinal palmar fascia, forming nodules (usually painless), fibrous cords and flexion contractures at the MCP and interphalangeal joints
- flexor tendons not involved
- Dupuytren's diathesis: early age of onset, strong family history, involvement of multiple digits, and nvolvement of sites other than palmar aspect of hand, including the plantar fascia (Ledderhose's) and the penis (Peyronie's) – (see Urology, U30)

Epidemiology
- genetic disorder, unusual in patients from African and Asian countries, high incidence in northern Europeans, men > women, often presents in 5th-7th decade of life, associated with but not caused by alcohol use and DM

Clinical Features
- order of digit involvement (most common to least common): ring > little > long > thumb > index

Treatment
- stages
  1. palmar pit or nodule: no surgery
  2. palpable band/cord with no limitation of extension of either MCP or PIP: no surgery
  3. lack of extension at MCP or PIP: treatment includes needle aponeurotomy, collagenase injection or surgical fasciectomy
  4. irreversible periarticular joint changes/scarring: surgical treatment possible but poorer prognosis compared to stage 3

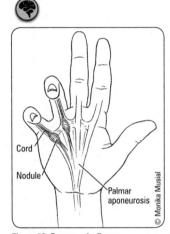

Cord

Nodule

Palmar aponeurosis

© Monika Musial

Figure 23. Dupuytren's disease

Median Nerve Compression

Definition
- median nerve compression at the level of the flexor retinaculum

Etiology
- median nerve entrapment at wrist
- primary cause is idiopathic
- secondary causes: space occupying lesions (tumours, hypertrophic synovial tissue, fracture callus, and osteophytes), metabolic and physiological (pregnancy, hypothyroidism, acromegaly, and RA)
- job/hobby related repetitive trauma, especially forced wrist flexion

Epidemiology
- female:male = 4:1, **most common entrapment neuropathy**

Clinical Features
- sensory loss in median nerve distribution (see Figure 4)
- discriminative touch often lost first
- classically, patient awakened at night with numb/painful hand, relieved by shaking/dangling/rubbing
- decreased light touch and 2point discrimination, especially fingertips
- advanced cases: thenar wasting/weakness due to involvement of the motor branch of the nerve
- ± Tinel's sign (tingling sensation on percussion of nerve)
- ± Phalen's sign (wrist flexion induces symptoms)

Investigations
- clinical diagnosis
- NCV and EMG may confirm, but do not exclude, the diagnosis

Treatment
- avoid repetitive wrist and hand motion, wrist splints at night and when repetitive wrist motion required
- conservative: night time splinting to keep wrist in neutral position
- medical: NSAIDs, local corticosteroids injection, oral corticosteroids
- surgical decompression: transverse carpal ligament incision to decompress median nerve
- indications for surgery: persistent signs and symptoms of median nerve compression not relieved by conservative management

Brachial Plexus

Etiology
- common causes of brachial plexus injury: complication of childbirth and trauma
- other causes of injury: compression from tumours, ectopic ribs

Common Palsies

Table 22. Named Neonatal Palsies of the Brachial Plexus

Palsy	Location of Injury	Mechanism of Injury	Features
Duchenne-Erb Palsy	Upper brachial plexus (C5-C6)	Head/shoulder distraction (e.g. motorcycle)	"Waiter's tip deformity" (shoulder internal rotation, elbow extension, wrist flexion)
Klumpke's Palsy	Lower brachial plexus (C7-T1)	Traction on abducted arm	"Claw hand" May include Horner's syndrome

Differential Diagnosis of Adult Acquired Brachial Plexus Palsies
- trauma (blunt, penetrating)
- thoracic outlet syndrome
  - neurogenic: associated with cervical rib; compression of C8/T1
  - vascular: pain or sensory symptoms without cervical rib; cessation of radial pulse with provocative maneuvers
- tumour
  - schwannoma: well-defined margins makes it easier for total resection
  - neurofibromas: associated with neurofibromatosis type I
  - other: e.g. Pancoast syndrome (apical lung tumour)
- neuropathy (compressive, post-irradiation, viral, diabetic, idiopathic)

Investigations
- EMG
- MRI: gold standard for identifying soft tissue masses and nerve roots
- CT myelogram: controversial, although some people think that it is better than MRI for identification of nerve root avulsion
- closed injuries: initially, CT myelogram or MRI (and follow recovery of function); may require additional imaging 6-12 weeks after initial imaging for potential surgical management (nerve transfer, tendon transfer, etc)
- open injuries: OR for immediate exploration

Management

Table 23. Management of Brachial Plexus Injuries

	Type	Treatment
Closed Injuries	Concussive/compressive	Usually improves (unless expanding mass, e.g. hematoma)
	Traction/stretch	If no continued insult, follow for 3-4 mo for improvement
	Obstetric palsy	Surgery if no significant improvement and/or residual paresis at 6 mo of age
Open Injuries	Sharp or vascular injury	Explore immediately in OR

Craniofacial Injuries

- low velocity vs. high velocity injuries determine degree of damage
- fractures cause bruising, swelling and tenderness → loss of function
- management: most can wait ~5 d for swelling to decrease before ORIF required

Approach to Facial Injuries

- ATLS protocol
- inspect, palpate, clinical assessment for injury to underlying structures (e.g. facial nerve, bony injuries, septal hematoma, ocular involvement, etc)
- tetanus prophylaxis
- radiological evaluation: CT scan with fine cuts through the orbit
- wound irrigation with NS/RL and remove foreign materials
- conservative debridement of detached or nonviable tissue
- repair when patient's general condition allows (for significant soft tissue injury: <8 h preferable)
- consider intracranial trauma; rule out skull fracture

Patients with major facial injuries are at risk of developing upper airway obstruction (displaced blood clots, teeth or fracture fragments; swelling of pharynx and larynx; loss of support of hyomandibular complex → retroposition of tongue); also at risk of ocular injury

Investigations
- CT (gold standard)
  - axial and coronal (specifically request 1.5 mm cuts): for fractures of upper and middle face, as well as mandible
  - indicated for significant head trauma, suspected facial fractures, pre-operative assessment
- panorex radiograph: shows entire upper and lower jaw; best for isolated mandible fracture but patient must be able to sit; however, if high clinical suspicion and negative panorex, CT should be done

Signs of Basal Skull Fracture
- Battle's sign (bruised mastoid process)
- Hemotympanum
- Raccoon eyes (periorbital bruising)
- CSF otorrhea/rhinorrhea

Treatment Goals
- consultation when indicated (dentistry, ophthalmology)
- re-establish normal occlusion if occlusion is an issue
- normal eye function (extraocular eye movements and vision)
- restore stability of face and appearance

Mandibular Fractures

- often two points of injury since it is a ring structure (includes fractures and dislocations)
- commonly at sites of weakness (condylar neck, angle of mandible,

Etiology
- anterior force: bilateral fractures
- lateral force: ipsilateral subcondylar and contralateral angle or body fracture
- note: classified as open if fracture into tooth bearing area (alveolus)

Clinical Features
- pain, swelling, difficulty opening mouth ("trismus")
- malocclusion, asymmetry of dental arch
- damaged, loose, or lost teeth
- palpable "step" along mandible
- numbness in V3 distribution
- intra-oral lacerations or hematoma (sublingual)
- chin deviating toward side of a fractured condyle

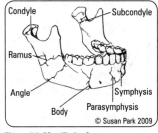

Figure 24. Mandibular fracture

Classification

Table 24. Mandibular Fracture Classifications by Anatomic Region

	Areas/Boundaries
Symphysis	Midline of the mandible; between the central incisors from the alveolar process through the inferior border of the mandible
Body	From the symphysis to the distal alveolar border of the third molar
Angle	Triangular region between the anterior border of the masseter and the posterosuperior insertion of the masseter distal to the third molar
Ramus	Part of the mandible that extends posteriosuperiorly into the condylar and coronoid processes
Condylar*	Area of condylar process of mandible
Subcondylar	Area below the condylar neck (i.e. sigmoid notch) of the mandible
Coronoid Process	Area of the coronoid process of mandible

*Most common mandibular fracture type

Treatment
- maxillary and mandibular arch bars wired together (intramaxillary fixation) or ORIF ideally managed within 24hr
- antibiotics from initial presentation to fracture reduction

Maxillary Fractures

Table 25. Le Fort Classification

	Le Fort I	Le Fort II	Le Fort III
Alternative Name	Guérin fracture	Pyramidal fracture	Craniofacial dysjunction
Type of Fracture	Horizontal	Pyramidal	Transverse
Structures Involved	Piriform aperture Maxillary sinus Pterygoid plates	Nasal bones Medial orbital wall Maxilla Pterygoid plates	Nasofrontal suture Zygomatofrontal suture Zygomatic arch Pterygoid plates
Anatomical Result	Maxilla divided into 2 segments	Maxillary teeth and midsection of the maxilla separated from upper face	Detach entire midfacial skeleton from cranial base

Nasal Fractures

Etiology
- lateral force → more common, good prognosis
- anterior force → can produce more serious injuries
- most common facial fracture

Clinical Features
- epistaxis/hemorrhage, deviation/flattening of nose, swelling, periorbital ecchymosis, tenderness over nasal dorsum, crepitus, septal hematoma, respiratory obstruction, subconjunctival hemorrhage

Treatment
- treated for airway or cosmetic issues
- always inspect for and drain septal hematoma as this is a cause of septal necrosis and perforation – completed in the ER with small incision in the septal mucosa followed by packing
- closed reduction with Asch or Walsham forceps under anesthesia, pack nostrils with petroleum or nonadhesive gauze packing, nasal splint for 7 d
- best reduction immediately (<6 h) or when swelling subsides (5-7 d)
- rhinoplasty may be necessary later for residual deformity (30%)

Zygomatic Fractures

Classification
1. fracture restricted to zygomatic arch
2. depressed fracture of zygomatic complex (zygoma)
3. unstable fracture of zygomatic complex (tetrapod fracture) – separations occur at maxilla, frontal bone, temporal bone and orbital rim

Clinical Features
- flattening of malar prominence (view from above)
- pain over fractures on palpation
- numbness in V2 distribution (infraorbital and superior dental nerves)
- palpable step deformity in bony orbital rim (especially inferiorly)
- often associated with fractures of the orbital floor
- ipsilateral epistaxis; trismus

Treatment
- if undisplaced, stable and no symptoms, then soft diet; no treatment necessary
- ophthalmologic evaluation if suspected globe injury
- undisplaced zygomatic arch fractures can be elevated using Gillies approach (leverage on the anterior part of the zygomatic arch via a temporal incision) or Keane approach (elevation through upper buccal sulcus incision); stabilization often unnecessary
- ORIF for displaced or unstable fractures of zygomatic complex

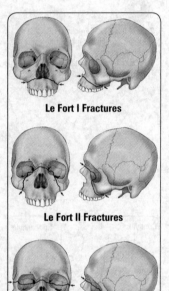

Le Fort I Fractures

Le Fort II Fractures

Le Fort III Fractures
©Rio Sakay 2007

Figure 25. Le Fort fractures

Frontozygomatic
Zygomatic arch
Zygomatico-maxillary
© Susan Park 2009

Figure 26. Zygomatic fractures

Orbital Floor Fractures

- see Ophthalmology, OP40

Definition
- fracture of floor of orbit: may be a "pure blow out fracture" which has an intact orbital rim or can be associated with other fractures (orbital rim fracture and/or zygoma)

Etiology
- blunt force to eyeball → sudden increase in intraorbital pressure (e.g. baseball or fist)

Clinical Features
- **check visual fields and visual acuity for injury to globe**
- periorbital edema and bruising, subconjunctival hemorrhage
- ptosis, exophthalmos, exorbitism, enophthalmos, or hypoglobus
- orbital rim step-offs with possible infraorbital nerve anesthesia
- vertical dystopia (abnormal displacement of the entire orbital cone in the vertical plane) – assessed by comparing the symmetry of the two pupils by a horizontal line running through the pupil of the unaffected eye
- orbital entrapment
  - clinical diagnosis that is a surgical emergency
  - diplopia with vertical gaze: diplopia looking up or down (entrapment of inferior rectus), limited EOM
  - severe pain or nausea and vomiting with upward globe movement
  - requires urgent ophthalmology evaluation if there are associated visual acuity changes

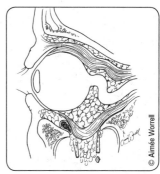

Figure 27. Blow-out fracture

Investigations
- CT (diagnostic): axial and coronal views – with fine cuts through orbit
- diagnostic maneuver for entrapment is forced duction test (pulling on inferior rectus muscle with forceps to ensure full ROM) under local anesthesia in the ER or OR

Treatment
- surgical repair indicated if: for entrapment (urgent), floor defect >1 cm, any size defect with enophthalmos or persistent diplopia (>10 d)
- reconstruction of orbital floor with bone graft or alloplastic material
- after repair, assess for diploplia: may require additional surgery for strabismus

Complications
- persistent diplopia
- enophthalmos

Superior Orbital Fissure Syndrome
- fracture of SOF causing ptosis, proptosis, anesthesia in V1 distribution, and painful ophthalmoplegia (paralysis of CN III, IV, VI)
- uncommon complication seen in Le Fort II and III fractures (1/130)
- recovery time reported as 4.8-23 wk following operative reduction of fractures

Orbital Apex Syndrome
- fracture through optic canal with involvement of CN II at apex of orbit
- symptoms are the same as SOF syndrome plus vision loss
- treatment is urgent decompression of fracture in optic canal (posterior craniotomy for decompression) or steroids

Breast

Anatomy

Vascular Supply

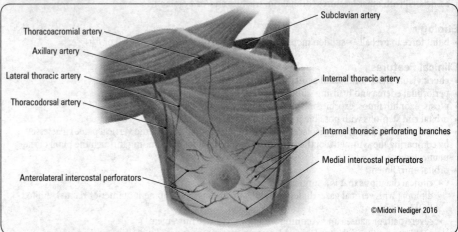

Figure 28. Breast Vasculature

- innervated in a dermatomal pattern from branches of the thoracic intercostal nerves (T3-6)
  - medially innervated from anterior cutenous branches of I-VI intercostal nerves
  - lateral innervated from lateral cutaneous nerve branches II-VII intercostal nerves
- lateral and upper portions of the breast innervated by lower fibres of the cervical plexus (C3, C4)
- nipple areolar complex (NAC)
  - supplied by anterior and lateral cutaneous branches of intercostal nerve IV
  - additional innervation by cutaneous branches of intercostal nerves III and VI

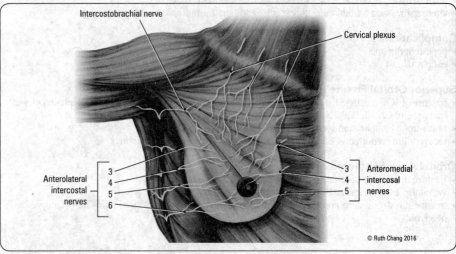

Figure 29. Innervation of the breast

Breast Reduction

Indications
- symptomatic (general symptoms)
  - musculoskeletal pain (back, strap, neck), chronic headache, paresthesia in upper limb, rashes under the breast, breast discomfort and physical impairment
- breast reduction methods can be classified based on pedicle (i.e. blood supply to the nipple/areolar complex) and skin resection pattern (i.e. the resultant scar)

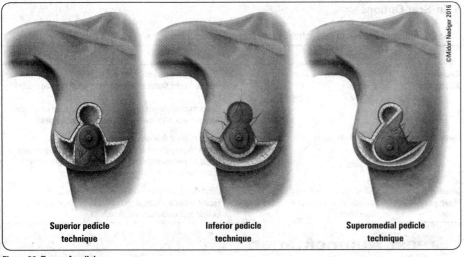

Figure 30. Types of pedicles

Table 26. Types of Pedicles

	Pedicle Description
Inferior Pedicle	Most commonly used technique; versatile use in small to large breast reduction Critiqued for boxy shape breast along with more extensive scarring (wise pattern skin resection) Recommended pedicle width 6-8 cm, 8-10 cm in large breasts
Superior Pedicle	Pedicle derived from the internal mammary perforator of the second intercostal space Pedicle must be thinned to permit inset
Central Pedicle	Modified from the inferior pedicle Blood supply derived from flow through glandular component rather than dermal component
Medial Pedicle	Modified from horizontal bipedicle (Strombeck) techniques Blood supplied from internal mammary perforator from third intercostal and potentially fourth intercostal space
Superomedial Pedicle	Incorporate the descending artery from second intercostal space as medial pedicle base extended superolaterally to breast meridian
Lateral Pedicle	Supplied by perforators from lateral thoracic artery

Table 27. Type of Skin Resections/Scar Options

	Indications	Description
Inverted T Pattern	Large breasts Breasts with poor quality skin that are challenging to remodel	Commonly used in associated with inferior pedicle Large portion of skin removed in horizontal and vertical direction Skin integrity important to shape and hold breast parenchyma
Vertical Pattern	Skin must be healthy and easy to remodel	Used in association with superior or medial pedicle Parenchyma needed to shape skin No horizontal scar Small to moderate reductions

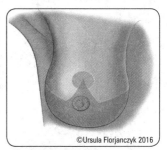

Figure 31. Inverted T shape

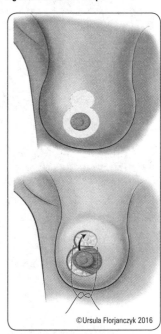

Figure 32. Vertical T shape

Mastopexy (Breast Lift)

Definition
- aesthetic procedure of the breast used to correct for breast ptosis by modifying the contour and size of the breast along with elevating the position of the nipple

Clinical Grading of Ptosis (Regnault Ptosis Grade Scale)
1. minor ptosis (1st degree)
   - nipple at inframammary fold
2. moderate ptosis (2nd degree)
   - nipple below inframammary fold, but above lower breast contour
3. severe ptosis (3rd degree)
   - nipple below inframammary fold and at lower breast contour
4. glandular ptosis
   - nipple above inframammary fold, but breast hangs below fold
5. pseudoptosis
   - nipple above inframammary fold, but breast is hypoplastic and hangs below the fold

Skin/Scar Options

Table 28. Timing of immediate reconstruction vs. delayed reconstruction

	Indications	Description
Circumareolar Mastopexy	Nipple located 1-2.5 cm too low	Originally described as "donut mastopexy" Reduce areolar diameter while simultaneously raising nipple (<2 cm) Can correct nipple position asymmetry when used unilaterally Also increase infra-areolar skin display in ptotic breasts
Vertical Mastopexy	Grade I - III ptosis	Larger removal than circumareolar Raises nipple position and reduce circumareolar skin tension Larger angle between vertical limb and limb length increase with more lower pole skin
Inverted T Mastopexy	Most effective in grade II to III ptosis caused by skin excess attributed to large weight loss	Large removal of skin in return for greater scar burden Facilitate nipple elevation and parenchymal redistribution, fixation and autoaugmentation techniques

Breast Augmentation

Definition
- procedure designed to increase the size of the breast

Choice of Incision
- position of incision individualized since no single incision is best for all
- 3 commonly used types of incision: periareolar, inframammary crease, axillary

Type of Implant
- silicone or saline-filled implants
- subclassified into
  - surface (smooth or textured)
  - shape (round or anatomic with varying projections)
  - can also be classified as having higher or low profile

Location of Implant
- implants are commonly placed in the following positions
  1. submuscular positions
     - implant placed below pectoralis major muscle
  2. subglandular position
     - implant placed deep to glandular breast tissue but superficial to muscle
  3. subfascial
     - implant placed below the fascia

Gynecomastia

Definition
- benign enlargement of the male breast due to proliferation of the glandular tissue

Clinical Classification
- gynecomastia can be further classified into
  1. idiopathic
  2. physiologic
     - neonatal: circulating maternal estrogens via placenta
     - pubertal: relative excess of plasma estradiol versus testosterone
     - elderly: decrease circulating testosterone, peripheral aromatization of testosterone to estrogen
  3. pathologic
     - excess estrogen, androgen deficiency, deficient production or action of testesterone (i.e. Klinefelter's syndrome, androgen resistance)
  4. pharmacologic
     - drugs that may interefere with estrogen-testosterone balance include: estrogens, estrogen-like compounds (marijuana, heroin), gonadotropins, inhibitors of testosterone
  5. congenital breast deformity
  6. massive weight loss gynecomastia

Surgical Options
- surgery is the accepted management for gynecomastia
- surgery addresses the three components (breast, fat, skin)
- often involves a combination of liposuction (to remove the fatty portion) and surgical excision through a small periareolar incision (to remove the glandular component)
- patients with significant skin excess may also require skin excision as well

Breast Reconstruction

- reconstruction of the breast after cancer or trauma to recreate the breast which is similar to the contralateral breast
- reconstruction can be completed immediately (at the same time as mastectomy), or delayed (as a separate surgery days, months or years after initial surgery)
- there are alloplastic and autogenous methods of reconstruction each with its advantages and disadvantages

Table 29. Timing of immediate reconstruction vs delayed reconstruction

	Advantages	Disadvantages
Immediate Reconstruction	Generally best aesthetic outcome and can preserve nipple Does not require creation of additional skin	Skin viability assessment may be compromised Increased post-op complications compared to delayed reconstruction
Delayed Reconstruction	Allows patient to receive adjuvant radiotherapy before definitive reconstruction	Loss of skin, volume, lateral border or breast, and natural landmarks including IMF Likely requires more stages for completion

Table 30. Alloplastic reconstruction vs autogenous reconstruction

		Advantages	Disadvantages
Alloplastic Reconstruction	One stage reconstruction with implant	Single surgery	Size restriction in reconstruction
	Two stage reconstruction with expander and implant	Less tension on mastectomy flaps compared to single stage reconstruction with implants	Requires post surgical procedures (requires patient to come to clinic for inflations) Risk of skin dehisenceclinical inflation
Autogenous Reconstruction	Latissimus Dorsi Flap	Reliable pedicle, provides skin and muscles(thoracodorsal artery) Provides good amount of skin and muscle for reconstruction	May also require implants for adequate volume
	TRAM (Transverse Rectus Abdominis Muscle) Flap	Volume generally sufficient for complete reconstruction, spares fascia	Higher incidence of long term donor site morbidity compared to DIEP (weakness in rectus abdominis, hernia, etc)
	DIEP (Deep Inferior Epigastric Perforator) Flap	Method spares rectus abdominis muscle and fascia Decreased donor site morbidity compared to TRAM flap	High technical skill required - meticulous dissection of flap, poor perforator choice may lead to flap death Requires microsurgical technique

Nipple Reconstruction
- final step of breast reconstruction
- nipple reconstruction is usually done as the final step when the patient is satisfied with breast mound creation
- reconstruction can be conducted with local anesthetic
- it can be done by either a flap or a graft

Skate Flap
- pedicle is elevated above breast mound, and the lateral most aspects of the flap are wrapped around the central aspect of flap
- defect is mainly closed by skin graft

CV Flap
- utilizes a C flap and two V flaps for nipple reconstruction
- diameter of C flap becomes the diameter of reconstructed nipple
- width of V flaps dictate projection of reconstructed nipple
- CV closed with primary closure

Nipple Graft from Contralateral Breast
- two methods for nipple graft
  1. distal aspect of nipple removed transversely, and defect closed with purse string suture
  2. nipple divided in half longitudinally, and folded over and closed with primary closure

Areolar Reconstruction
- tattooing vs. skin grafts
- tattooing: conducted 3-4 months after nipple reconstruction, after projection has stabilized
- skin grafts: full thickness skin grafts commonly taken from inner aspect of thigh

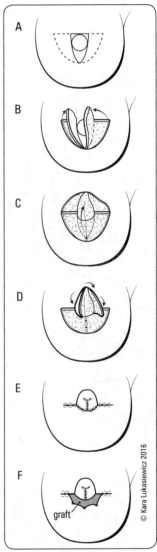

© Kara Lukasiewicz 2016

Figure 33. Skate flap
A-C, skate flap with primary closure of donor site. D-F, with skin graft

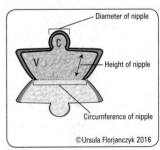

©Ursula Florjanczyk 2016

Figure 34. CV flap

Aesthetic Surgery

Aesthetic Procedures

Table 31. Aesthetic Procedures

Location	Procedure	Description
Head/Neck	Hair transplants	Aesthetic improvement of hair growth patterns using hair follicle grafts or flaps
	Otoplasty	Surgical correction of protruding ears
	Forehead/Brow lift	Surgical procedure to lift the forehead and eyebrows
	Rhytidectomy	Surgical procedure to reduce wrinkling and sagging of the face and neck; "face lift"
	Blepharoplasty	Surgical procedure to shape or modify the appearance of eyelids by removing excess eyelid skin ± fat pads
	Rhinoplasty	Surgical reconstruction of the nose ± nasal airway
	Genioplasty	Chin augmentation via osteotomy or synthetic implant to improve contour
	Lip augmentation	Procedure to create fuller lips and to reduce wrinkles around the mouth using fillers or fat
Skin	Chemical peel	Application of one or more exfoliating agents to the skin resulting in destruction of portions of the epidermis and/or dermis with subsequent tissue regeneration
	Dermabrasion	Skin resurfacing with a rapidly rotating abrasive tool; often used to reduce scars, irregular skin surfaces and fine lines
	Laser resurfacing	Application of laser to the skin which ultimately results in collagen reconfiguration and subsequent skin shrinking and tightening; often used to reduce scars and wrinkles
	Injectable fillers	An injectable substance is used to decrease frown lines, wrinkles, and nasolabial folds; substances include collagen, fat, hyaluronic acid, and calcium hydroxyapatite (most common substances include hyaluronic acid and fat)
Other	Abdominoplasty	Removal of excess skin and repair of rectus muscle laxity (rectus diastasis); "tummy tuck"
	Calf augmentation	Augmentation of calf muscle with implants
	Liposuction	Surgical removal of adipose tissue for body contouring (not a weight loss procedure)

Pediatric Plastic Surgery

Craniofacial Anomalies

Table 32. Pediatric Craniofacial Anomalies

	Definition	Epidemiology	Clinical Features	Treatment
Cleft Lip	Failure of fusion of maxillary and medial nasal processes	1 in 1000 live births (1 in 800 Caucasians, increased in Asians, decreased in Blacks) M:F = 2:1	Classified as incomplete/complete and uni/bilateral 2/3 cases: unilateral, left-sided, male	Surgery (3 mo): Millard Tennison-Randall, or Fisher (additional correct surgeries usually required later on - especially for nasal deformity)
Cleft Palate	Failure of fusion of lateral palatine/median palatine processes and nasal septum	Isolated cleft palate: 0.5 per 1000 (no racial variation) F>M	Classified as incomplete/complete and uni/bilateral Isolated (common in females) or in conjunction with cleft lip (common in males)	Special bottles for feeding Speech pathologist Surgery (6-9 mo): Von Langenbeck or Furlow Z-Plasty ENT consult – often recurrent otitis media, requiring myringotomy tubes
Craniosynostosis	Premature fusion of ≥1 cranial sutures	1 in 2000 live newborns; M:F = 52:48 Syndromes include: Crouzon's, Apert's, Saethre-Chotzen, Carpenter's, Pfeiffer's Jackson-Weiss and Boston-type syndromes	Primary (no known cause), or secondary (associated with a known cause or syndrome)	Multidisciplinary team (including neurosurgery, ENT, genetics, dentistry, pediatrics, SLP) The type, timing and procedure are dependent on which sutures (lambdoid, saggital etc.) are involved Early surgery prevents secondary deformities ↑ ICP is an indication for emergent surgery

Congenital Hand Anomalies

Table 33. American Society for Surgery of the Hand (ASSH) Classification of Congenital Hand Anomalies

Classification	Example	Features	Treatment
Failure of Formation	Transverse absence (congenital amputation)	At any level (often below elbow/wrist)	Early prosthesis
	Longitudinal absence (phocomelia)	Absent humerus Thalidomide association	
	Radial deficiency (radial club hand)	Radial deviation Thumb hypoplasia M>F	Physiotherapy + splinting Soft tissue release if splinting fails Distraction osteogenesis (Ilizarov) ± wedge osteotomy Tendon transfer Pollicization
	Thumb hypoplasia	Degree ranges from small thumb with all components to complete absence	Depends on degree – may involve no treatment, webspace deepening, tendon transfer, or pollicization of index finger
	Ulnar club hand	Rare, compared to radial club hand Stable wrist	Splinting and soft tissue stretching therapies Soft tissue release (if above fails) Correction of angulation (Ilizarov distraction)
	Cleft hand	Autosomal dominant Often functionally normal (depending on degree)	First web space syndactyly release Osteotomy/tendon transfer of thumb (if hypoplastic)
Failure of Differentiation/ Separation	Syndactyly	Fusion of ≥2 digits 1/3,000 live births M:F = 2:1 Classified as partial/complete Simple (skin only) vs. complex (osseous or cartilaginous bridges)	Surgical separation before 6-12 mo of age May require a skin graft to cover the fingers Usually good result
	Symbrachydactyly	Short fingers with short nails at fingertips	Digital separation Webspace deepening
	Camptodactyly	Congenital flexion contracture (usually at PIP, especially 5th digit)	Early splinting Volar release Arthroplasty (rarely)
	Clinodactyly	Radial or ulnar deviation Often middle phalanx	None (usually); if severe, osteotomy with grafting
Duplication	Polydactyly	Congenital duplication of digits May be radial (increased in Aboriginals and Asians) or central or ulnar (increased in Blacks)	Amputation of least functional digit Usually >1 yr of age (when functional status can be assessed)
Overgrowth	Macrodactyly	Rare	None (if mild) Soft tissue/bony reduction
Undergrowth	Brachydactyly	Short phalanges	Removal of nonfunctional stumps Osteotomies/tendon transfers Distraction osteogenesis Phalangeal/free toe transfer
	Symbrachydactyly Brachysyndactyly	Short webbed fingers	As above + syndactyly release
Constriction Band Syndrome	i.e. amniotic (annular) band syndrome	Variety of presentations	Urgent release for acute, progressive edema distal to band in newborn Other reconstruction is case specific
Generalized Skeletal Abnormality	Achondroplasia, Marfan's, Madelung's	Variety of presentations	Treatment depends on etiology

References

American Society for Surgery of the Hand. The hand: examination and diagnosis, 3rd ed. Philadelphia: Churchill Livingston, 1990.
Beredjiklian PK, Bozenika DJ. Review of hand surgery. Philadelphia: WB Saunders, 2004.
Britt LD, Trunkey DD, Feliciano DV. Acute care surgery: principles and practice. New York: Springer, 2007.
Borges AF. The rhombic flap. Plast Reconstr Surg 1981;67:458-466.
Bray DA. Clinical applications of the rhomboid flap. Arch Otolaryngol 1983;109:37-42.
Brown DL, Borschel GH. Michigan manual of plastic surgery. Philadelphia: WB Saunders, 2004.
Centers, B. Guidelines for the operation of burn centers. Resources for Optimal Care of the Injured Patient, 2006.
Daver BM, Antia NH, Furnas DW. Handbook of plastic surgery for the general surgeon, 2nd ed. New Delhi: Oxford University Press, 1995.
Department of Health, Western Australia. Guidelines for use of nanocrystalline silver dressing – Acticoat™. Perth: Health Networks Branch, Department of Health, Western Australia, 2011.
Diehr S, Hamp A, Jamieson B. Clinical inquiries: do topical antibiotics improve wound healing? J Fam Pract 2007;56:140-144.
Fee WE Jr, Gunter JP, Carder HM. Rhomboid flap principles and common variations. Laryngoscope 1976;86:1706-1711.
Georgiade GS, Riefkohl R, Levin LS. Georgiade plastic, maxillofacial and reconstructive surgery, 3rd ed. Baltimore: Williams & Wilkins, 1997.
Gourgiotis S, Villias C, Germanos S, et al. Acute limb compartment syndrome: a review. J Surg Educ 2007;64:178-186.
Graham B, Regehr G, Naglie G, et al. Development and validation of diagnostic criteria for carpal tunnel syndrome. J Hand Surg 2006;31:919.e1-919.e7.
Greene FL, Page DL, Fleming ID, et al. AJCC cancer staging handbook: from the AJCC cancer staging manual, 6th ed. Springer, 2002.
Gulleth Y, Goldberg N, Silverman R, et al. What is the best surgical margin for a basal cell carcinoma: a meta-analysis of the literature. Plast Reconstr Surg 2010;126:1222-1231.
Huang CC, Boyce SM. Surgical margins of excision for basal cell carcinoma and squamous cell carcinoma. Seminars In Cutaneous Med and Surg 2004;23:167-173.
Hunt TK, Doherty GM, Way LW (editors). Current surgical diagnosis and treatment, 12th ed. Norwalk: McGraw-Hill, 2006. Chapter: wound healing.
Janis JE. Essentials of plastic surgery: a UT Southwestern Medical Center handbook. St. Louis: Quality Medical, 2007.
Khalifian S, Brazio PS, Mohan R, et al. Facial transplantation: the first 9 years. Lancet 2014; S0140-6736(13)62632-X.
Larrabee WF Jr, Trachy R, Sutton D, et al. Rhomboid flap dynamics. Arch Otolaryngol 1981;107:755-757.
Lavigne E, Holowaty EJ, Pan SY, et al. Breast cancer detection and survival among women with cosmetic breast implants: systematic review and meta-analysis of observational studies. BMJ 2013;346:f2399
Muangman P, Chuntrasakul C, Silthram S, et al. Comparison of efficacy of 1% silver sulfadiazine and acticoat for treatment of partial thickness burn wounds. J Med Assoc Thailand 2006;89:953-958.
Noble J. Textbook of primary care medicine, 3rd ed. St. Louis: Mosby, 2001.
Ong YS, Samuel M, Song C. Meta-analysis of early excision of burns. Burns 2006;32:145-150.
Plastic Surgery Educational Foundation. Plastic and reconstructive surgery essentials for students. Arlington Heights: Plastic Surgery Educational Foundation, 2007. Available from: http://www.plasticsurgery.org/medical_professionals/publications/Essentials-for-Students.cfm.
Richards AM. Key notes in plastic surgery. Great Britain: Blackwell Science, 2002.
Salzberg CA, Ashikari AY, Koch RM, et al. An 8-year experience of direct-to-implant immediate breast reconstruction using human acellular dermal matrix (Allo Derm). Plast Reconstr Surg 2011;127:514-524.
Sermer NB. Practical plastic surgery for nonsurgeons. Philadelphia: Hanley & Belfus, 2001.
Smith DJ, Brown AS, Cruse CW, et al. Plastic and reconstructive surgery. Chicago: Plastic Surgery Educational Foundation, 1987.
Stone C. Plastic surgery: facts. London: Greenwich Medical Media, 2001.
Thorne CH. Grabb & Smith's plastic surgery, 6th ed. Lippincott Williams & Wilkins, 2007.
Townsend CM. Sabiston textbook of surgery – the biological basis of modern surgical practice, 16th ed. Philadelphia: WB Saunders, 2001. Chapter: plastic and reconstructive surgery.
Wolff K, Johnson RA. Fitzpatrick's color atlas and synopsis of clinical dermatology, 6th ed. McGraw-Hill, 2009.
Weinzweig J. Plastic surgery secrets. Philadelphia: Hanley and Belfus, 1999.

Population Health and Epidemiology

Nicholas A. Howell and Yasmin Nasirzadeh, chapter editors
Narayan Chattergoon and Desmond She, associate editors
Arnav Agarwal and Quynh Huynh, EBM editors
Dr. Katherine Bingham and Dr. Allison Chris, staff editors

For more detail on topics covered in this chapter, use website http://phprimer.afmc.ca/ as a resource

Acronyms

AR	attributable risk	FN	false negatives	NNT	number needed to treat	RR	relative risk
CAS	Children's Aid Society	IMR	infant mortality ratio	NPV	negative predictive value	SMR	standardized mortality ratio
CBA	cost benefit analysis	ITT	intention to treat analysis	OR	odds ratio	SN	sensitivity
CEA	cost effectiveness analysis	LICO	low income cut-off	PHAC	Public Health Agency of Canada	SP	specificity
CFR	case fatality rate	LR	likelihood ratio	PP	per protocol analysis	TP	true positives
CPHO	Chief Public Health Officer	MHO	Medical Health Officer	PPV	positive predictive value	TN	true negatives
DALY	disability adjusted life years	MOH	Medical Officer of Health	PYLL	potential years of life lost	WHMIS	Workplace Hazardous Materials
EBM	evidence based medicine	MMR	maternal mortality ratio	QALY	quality adjusted life years		Information System
HC	Health Canada	MSDS	Material Safety Data Sheets	QI	quality improvement	WHO	World Health Organization
FP	false positives	NNH	number needed to harm	RCT	randomized controlled trial	WSIB	Workplace Safety and Insurance Board

Preparing for the LMCC
The AFMC Primer on Population Health is the core text for the LMCC and is available as an online resource on the AFMC website (http://phprimer.afmc.ca)
For the LMCC exam, it is recommended that you also read Chapter 15 in Shah CP. Public health and preventive medicine in Canada, 5th ed. Toronto: *Elsevier*, 2003

Historical Perspective
Over the last century, Public Health has evolved through three main epidemiological phases:
- Infectious diseases: controlled in the more developed world but an issue in less developed countries (e.g. polio, malaria)
- Chronic diseases: chronic diseases and other noncommunicable conditions have increased morbidity and mortality (e.g. heart disease and cancer due to risk factors and/or exposures)
- Re-emerging infectious diseases: new or re-emergent infections emerge due to unfamiliar or new pathogens, inefficient or inappropriate antibiotic use, travel, and global warming (e.g. HIV, drug resistant TB and malaria)

CPHO of Canada
- Responsible for the PHAC and reports to the Minister of Health
- As the federal government's lead public health professional, provides advice to the Minister of Health and Government of Canada on health issues
- Collaborates with other governments, jurisdictions, agencies, organizations, and countries on health matters
- Communicates public health information to health professionals, stakeholders, and the public
- In an emergency, such as an outbreak or natural disaster, provides direction to PHAC staff, including medical professionals, scientists, and epidemiologists, as they plan and respond to the emergency
Source: Public Health Agency of Canada. http://www.phac-aspc.gc.ca/cpho-acsp/cpho-acsp-role-eng.php

Public Health Context

- see Ethical, Legal, and Organizational Medicine, ELOM2 *Overview of Canadian Healthcare System* for the organization of health care in Canada including the legal foundation and historical context

Definitions
- **population health**
  - refers to the health of defined groups of people, their health determinants, trends in health, and health inequalities
  - influenced by: physical, biological, social, environmental, and economic factors; personal health behaviours; health care services
  - broader scope vs. public health, accounts for socio-economic, policy, historical issues
- **public health**
  - "efforts organized by society to protect, promote, and restore the peoples' health" and prevent morbidity and mortality
  - refers to the practices, programs, policies, institutions, and disciplines required to achieve the desired state of population health
- **epidemiology**
  - "study of the distribution [...] of determinants of disease, health-related states, and events in populations"
- **public health and preventive medicine** (formerly called community medicine)
  - the postgraduate study of health and disease in the population or a specified community
  - 5 year Royal College specialty training
  - goal: to identify and address health problems and evaluate the extent to which health services and others address these issues

Sources: Shah, CP. Chapter 2 Measurement and Investigation. Public Health and Preventive Medicine in Canada, 5e. Toronto: Elsevier, 2003.
Shah, CP. Chapter 15 Community Health Services. Public Health and Preventive Medicine in Canada, 5e. Toronto: Elsevier, 2003.

Public Health Services in Canada

Mission: to promote and protect the health of Canadians through leadership, partnership, innovation, and action in public health" (Public Health Agency of Canada)
- local public health units and services within regional health authorities (in most provinces except Ontario, where local public health units are either autonomous or within local government) provide programs and activities for health protection, promotion, and disease prevention at local and regional levels
- catchment-area populations range widely (100s–1,000,000s), covering areas of 15 km^2 to 1.5 million km^2
- the "core functions" of public health include six essential activities (The Organization of Health Services in Canada. AFMC Primer on Population Health, Accessed: March 25 2016)
  1. **health protection**: take measures to address potential risks to health at the population level, including through regulation and advising government (e.g. safe water & food supply)
  2. **health surveillance**: monitoring and predict health outcomes and determinants with systematic, longitudinal data collection
  3. **disease and injury prevention**: address infectious disease through preventive (e.g. vaccination, droplet protection) and control (e.g. quarantine) measures; reduce morbidity through lifestyle improvement
  4. **population health assessment**: studying and engaging with a community to understand their needs and produce better policies and services
  5. **health promotion**: positively advocate for health through broad community and government measures (e.g. policy, interventions, community organizing)
  6. **emergency preparedness and response**: developing protocols and infrastructure for natural (e.g. hurricane) and man-made (e.g. toxic waste spill) disasters

Sources: Shah, CP. Chapter 15 Community Health Services. Public Health and Preventive Medicine in Canada, 5e. Toronto: Elsevier, 2003.
The Association of Faculties of Medicine of Canada Public Health Educators' Network. The Organization of Health Services in Canada. AFMC Primer on Population Health.

Legislation and Public Health in Canada

Table 1. Legislation and Public Health in Canada

Federal	Provincial	Municipal (Ontario)
Health Canada • Provides health services to First Nations, Aboriginal peoples, the Canadian military, and veterans • Approves new drugs and medical devices Canadian Food Inspection Agency • Monitors food products • Deals with animal-related infections • Regulates food labeling Public Health Agency of Canada (main Government of Canada agency responsible for public health) • An independent body created to strengthen public health capacity • Focuses on preventing chronic diseases, preventing injuries, and responding to public health emergencies and infectious disease outbreaks • Oversees immigration screening, protects Canadian borders (e.g. airport health inspection) • Liaises with the World Health Organization (WHO) on global health issues	Legislation is in the form of Acts and Regulations Each province has its own Public Health Act or equivalent (e.g. *the Health Protection and Promotion Act* in Ontario) • Designates the creation of geographic areas for the provision of public health services • Gives powers to the Chief Medical Officer of Health to control public health hazards • Specifies infectious diseases to be reported to public health units by physicians, laboratories, and hospitals (see *Appendix*, PH24) • Has the ability to mandate programs that address public health issues, environmental health, and chronic disease prevention	Local boards of health deliver programs mandated by provincial and municipal or regional legislation Boards of health are responsible for the delivery of most public health services, such as: • Infectious disease control, including the follow-up of reported diseases and management of outbreaks • Inspection of food premises including those in hospitals, nursing homes, and restaurants • Family health services including pre-conception, preschool, school-aged, and adult health programs • Tobacco control legislation enforcement • Assessment and management of local environmental health risks • Collection and dissemination of local health status reports • Public dental health services to children • By-laws may be approved by municipal governments to facilitate public health issues

Medical Officer of Health (MOH) (Ontario)
- May be called "Medical Health Officer" (MHO) in other provinces
- Appointed to each public health unit by the board of health
- Held by a licensed physician with public health training
- Responsibilities include:
- Collection and analysis of epidemiological data
- Occupational and environmental health surveillance
- Implementation of health programs, including:
- Counselling
- Family planning services
- Parenting programs, prenatal courses
- Preschool and school health services
- Disease screening programs
- Tobacco use prevention programs
- Nutrition services to schools and seniors' centres
- The Medical Officer of Health can require an individual/premise/agency to take or refrain from any action due to a public health hazard

Determinants of Health

Concepts of Health

- **wellness**: "state of dynamic physical, mental, social, and spiritual well-being that enables a person to achieve full potential and have an enjoyable life"
- **disease**: "abnormal, medically-defined changes in the structure or function of the human body"
- **illness**: "an individual's experience or subjective perception of a lack of physical or mental well-being and consequent inability to function normally in social roles"
- **illness behaviour**: an individual's actions resulting from and responding to their illness, including their interactions or avoidance of the health care system
- **sickness**: views the individual and their society hold towards a health condition, affecting their thoughts and actions
- **impairment**: "any loss or abnormality of psychological, physiological, or anatomical structure or function"
- **disability**: "any restriction or lack of ability to perform an activity within the range considered normal for a human being"
- **handicap**: a the disadvantage for an individual arising due to impairment and disability
    - "limits or prevents the fulfillment of an individual's normal role as determined by society and depends on age, sex, social, and cultural factors"
- **health equity**: when all people have "the opportunity to attain their full health potential" and no one is "disadvantaged from achieving this potential because of their social position or other socially determined circumstance." Health inequities are systematic differences in the health of individuals/groups which are considered unjust
- **health equality**: defined as where populations have equal or similar health status. Health inequalities are systematic differences in the health of groups that do not necessarily carry a moral judgement

Determinants of Health

- 1974: the Honourable Marc Lalonde, federal Minister of Health, publishes A New Perspective on the Health of Canadians which outlines four factors that determine health: "human biology, environment, lifestyle, and health care organizations." The idea of determinants of health has since been expanded and refined to include many additional factors

Sources: Shah, CP. Concepts, Determinants, and Promotion of Health. Public Health and Preventive Medicine in Canada, 5e. Toronto: Elsevier, 2003.
The Association of Faculties of Medicine of Canada Public Health Educators' Network. Concepts of Health and Illness. AFMC Primer on Population Health.

Definitions of Health
- First multidimensional definition of health, as defined by the WHO in 1948: "state of complete physical, mental and social well-being and not merely the absence of disease or infirmity"
- WHO updated the definition (socio-ecological definition) of health in 1986: "The ability to identify and to realize aspirations, to satisfy needs, and to change or cope with the environment. Health is therefore a resource for everyday life, not the objective of living. Health is a positive concept emphasizing social and personal resources, as well as physical capacities" (Ottawa Charter for Health Promotion)
- Other definitions of health have since been proposed that incorporate other dimensions of health (e.g. "Health is a social, economic, and political issue and above all a fundamental human right" – The People's Charter for Health)

Determinants of Health
- Income and social status
- Social support networks
- Education and literacy
- Employment and working conditions
- Social and work environments
- Physical environment
- Personal health practices and coping skills
- Healthy child development
- Biology, genetics, and epigenetics
- Health services
- Gender
- Culture

Source: Public Health Agency of Canada www.phac-aspc.gc.ca/ph-sp/determinants/determinants-eng.php

Social Determinants: Indigenous People's Health in Canada
- Colonization: subjugation of Indigenous peoples by the Europeans, leading to the loss of lands, cultural practices, and self-government
- Residential schools: placement of children from Indigenous groups in church-run, government-funded schools for the purpose of assimilation, resulting in loss of identity, alienation, and abuse, with long-lasting consequences of higher rates of addictions, abusive relationships, and suicide
- Treaties and Land Claims: inadequate services for those living on reserves leading to poverty and poor quality infrastructure, reflected in disproportionate burden of infectious diseases (e.g. pertussis, Chlamydia, hepatitis, shigellosis)
- Traditional Approach to Healing: restoring balance in the four realms of spiritual, emotional, mental and physical health of a person acting as an individual, as well as a member of a family, community and nation
- Ideas represented by medicine wheel of First Nations peoples, the Learning Blanket of Inuit peoples, and the Metis tree model of Holistic Lifelong Learning
- Contrast to Western medicine focus of treating illness, leading to challenges for practitioners of Western medicine to meet Aboriginal patients' needs
- National Aboriginal Health Organization (NAHO) offers 8 guidelines on practicing culturally safe health care for Aboriginal patients including need to allow Aboriginal patients access to ceremony, song, and prayer; the need for information and for family support; guidelines for the appropriate disposal of body parts and for handling death

New Immigrants to Canada
- Mandatory medical exams on entry to Canada by a designated medical practitioner:
- Complete medical examination for all persons of all ages
- Chest x-ray and report for persons 11 yr of age and over
- Urinalysis for persons 5 yr of age and over
- Syphilis serology for persons 15 yr of age and over
- HIV testing for applicants 15 yr of age and over, as well as for those children who have received blood or blood products, have a known HIV-positive mother, or have an identified risk. An ELISA HIV screening test should be done for HIV 1 and HIV 2
- Serum creatinine if the applicant has hypertension (resting blood pressure greater than 140/90 mmHg), a history of treated hypertension, DM, autoimmune disorder, persistent proteinuria, or kidney disorder

Citizenship and Immigration Canada Handbook http://www.cic.gc.ca/english/resources/publications/dmp-handbook/

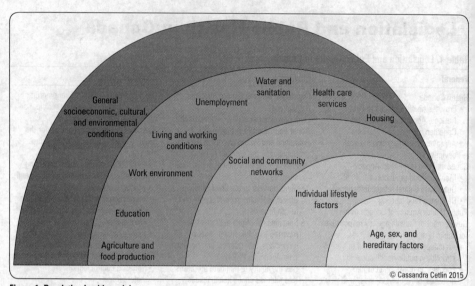

Figure 1. Population health model
Adapted from Dahlgreen G, Whitehead M. European strategies for tackling social inequities in health: Leveling up Part 2. World Health Organization, 2006.

Cultural Safety
- **cultural safety:** "interactions with people from different cultures that treat them respectfully in a manner that acknowledges relevant differences but does not create a sense of discrimination"
- **cultural sensitivity:** "being aware of (and understanding) the characteristic values and perceptions of your own culture and the way in which this may shape your approach to patients from other cultures"

Sources: The Association of Faculties of Medicine of Canada Public Health Educators' Network. Glossary. AFMC Primer on Population Health.

Vulnerable Populations

Table 2. Health Determinants of Vulnerable Populations

Definition	Psychosocial/ Socioeconomic	Physical	Environment	Individual Behaviour	Population-Specific Interventions
Aboriginal Peoples	Four specific groups: First Nations Status Indians (registered under the *Indian Act*), non-Status Indians, Métis, and Inuit	Low income Family violence Low education status Unemployment Homelessness Longer length of disability	Crowded housing Inefficient ventilation Environmental toxins (botulism) TB declining but prevalence higher than rest of population	Smoking Substance misuse Excessive gambling Poor nutrition Sedentary lifestyle High BMI Higher risk of suicide	Mental health awareness Aboriginal-specific DM initiatives Substance abuse treatment programs
Isolated Seniors	Individuals >65 yr	Elder abuse Lack of emotional support Isolation	Low hazard tolerance Institutionalization Mobility issues	Inactivity Polypharmacy Medical comorbidities	Aging in place of choice Falls and injury prevention Mental health promotion Preventing abuse and neglect
Children in Poverty	Based on Low Income Cut Offs (LICO) LICO is an income threshold below which a family will likely devote a larger share of its income on the necessities of food, shelter and clothing than the average family	Low income Family dysfunction Lack of educational opportunities	Housing availability Unsafe housing Lack of recreational space	Poor supervision Food insecurity High risk behaviours	Improvements in family income most significant Early childhood education

Table 2. Health Determinants of Vulnerable Populations (continued)

Definition	Psychosocial/ Socioeconomic	Physical	Environment	Individual Behaviour	Population-Specific Interventions
People with Disabilities	Includes impairments, activity limitations, and participation restrictions	Low income Low education status Discrimination Stigma	Institutionalization Barriers to access Transportation challenges	Substance misuse Poor nutrition Inactivity Dependency for ADLs	Transportation support Multidisciplinary care Unique support for individuals with specific disabilities (e.g. Trisomy 21)
New Immigrants	Person born outside of Canada who has been granted the right to live in Canada permanently by immigration authorities	Access to community services Cultural perspectives (including reliance on alternative health practices)	Exposure to diseases and conditions in country of origin (e.g. smoke from wood fires, incidence of TB, etc.)	Employment, ESL Healthy Newcomer Effect (health worsens over time to match that of the general population) Cultural or religious expectations	Women's health Mental health Infectious diseases (syphilis blood test, CXR, HIV) Dental and vision screening Vaccinations Cancer screening
Homeless Persons	An individual who lacks permanent housing	Low income Food insecurity Mental illness	Exposure to temperature extremes Infections such as West Nile Virus	Substance misuse Violence	Safe housing Addictions support Mental health
Refugee Health	Forced to flee country of origin because of a well-founded fear of persecution and given protection by the Government of Canada Refugee claimant: Arrive in Canada and ask to be considered refugee	Post-traumatic stress disorders Depression Adjustment problems Partial health coverage via Interim Federal Health Program	Diseases and conditions in country of origin (e.g. malaria, TB, onchocerciasis, etc.) Direct and indirect effects of war	Employment ESL Longstanding prior lack of access to health care (chronically neglected problems) Cultural or religious expectations	Vaccinations Women's health Mental health Infectious diseases Dental and vision screening Political advocacy

Note: this chart delineates the major challenges faced by each group, but the issues listed are not unique to each population
Sources: Shah, CP. The Health of Vulnerable Groups. Public Health and Preventive Medicine in Canada, 5e. Toronto: Elsevier, 2003.

Disease Prevention

Natural History of Disease
- course of a disease from onset to resolution
    1. pathological onset
    2. presymptomatic stage: from onset to first appearance of symptoms/signs
    3. clinically manifest disease: may regress spontaneously, be subject to remissions and relapses, or progress to death

Disease Prevention Strategies
- measures aimed at preventing the occurrence, interrupting through early detection and treatment, or slowing the progression of disease/mitigating the sequelae

Table 3. Levels of Disease Prevention

Level of Prevention	Goal	Sample Strategies
Primary	Protect health and prevent disease onset	Immunization programs (e.g. measles, diphtheria, pertussis, tetanus, polio, see Pediatrics, P4) Smoking Cessation Seatbelt use
Secondary	Early detection of disease to minimize morbidity and mortality	Mammography Routine Pap smears
Tertiary	Treatment and rehabilitation of disease to prevent progression, permanent disability, and future disease	DM monitoring with HbA1c, eye exams, foot exams Medication

Basic Concepts in Prevention, Surveillance, and Health Promotion. AFMC Primer on Population Health (http://phprimer.afmc.ca/Part1-TheoryThinkingAboutHealth Chapter4BasicConceptsInPreventionSurveillanceAndHealthPromotion/Thestagesofprevention)

Passive prevention, measures that operate without the person's active involvement (e.g. airbags in cars) are more effective than active prevention, measures that a person must do on their own (e.g. wearing a seatbelt)

Example of Primary Prevention Gardasil Vaccine and Its Efficacy in the Prevention of Cervical Cancer
Gardasil® is a quadrivalent HPV vaccine covering strains 6,11,16,18. The efficacy of Gardasil® was studied in 4 randomized, double-blind, placebo controlled trials on females between 16 and 26 yr of age and was found to prevent nearly 100% of precancerous cervical changes for up to 4 yr after vaccination

Ottawa Charter for Health Promotion (1986)
- Health promotion: the process of enabling people to increase control over and improve their health
- The charter states that governments and health care providers should be involved in a health promotion process that includes:
    1. Building healthy public policy
    2. Creating supportive environments
    3. Strengthening community action
    4. Developing personal skills
    5. Re-orienting health services

Screening (Secondary Prevention)

- "presumptive identification of unrecognized disease or defect by the application of tests, examinations, or other procedures which can be applied rapidly"
- **types of screening**
  - mass screening: screening all members of a population for a disease (e.g. phenylketonuria (PKU) and hypothyroidism in all newborns)
  - selective screening: screening of targeted subgroups of the population at risk for a disease (e.g. mammography in women >50 yr old)
  - multiphasic screening: the use of many measurements and investigations to look for many disease entities (e.g. periodic health exam)
- **bias in screening**
  - **lead-time**: false improvement in survival time caused by changing the starting point of measurement (lead time), as opposed to real improvements measured from the original starting point (e.g. due to better therapy)
  - **lead-time bias**: overestimation of survival time 'from diagnosis' when the estimate is made from the time of screening, instead of the later time when the disease would have been diagnosed without screening
  - **length-time bias**: overestimation of the survival time due to screening at one time point including more stable cases than aggressive cases of disease, who may have shorter survival times

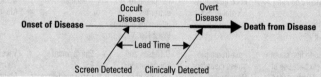

Figure 2. Lead-time bias

Table 4. Ideal Criteria for Screening Tests

Disease	Test	Health Care System
Causes significant suffering and/or death	High specificity and sensitivity	Adequate capacity for reporting, follow-up, and treatment of positive screens
Natural history must be understood	Safe, rapid, easy, relatively inexpensive	
Must have an asymptomatic stage that can be detected by a test	Acceptable to providers and to population	Cost effective
Early detection and intervention must result in improved outcomes		Sustainable program
Incidence is not too high or too low		Clear policy guidelines

Adapted from: Shah CP. Public Health and Preventive Medicine in Canada, 5th ed. Toronto: Elsevier, 2003

Sources: Shah, CP. Concepts, Determinants, and Promotion of Health. Public Health and Preventive Medicine in Canada, 5e. Toronto: Elsevier, 2003
Shah, CP. Measurement and Investigation. Public Health and Preventive Medicine in Canada, 5e. Toronto: Elsevier, 2003
The Association of Faculties of Medicine of Canada Public Health Educators' Network. Concepts of Health and Illness. AFMC Primer on Population Health

Health Promotion Strategies

Table 5. Disease Prevention vs. Health Promotion Approach

Disease Prevention	Health Promotion
Health = absence of disease	Health = positive and multidimensional concept
Medical model (passive role)	Participatory model of health
Aimed mainly at high-risk groups in the population	Aimed at the population in its total environment
One-shot strategy, aimed at a specific pathology	Diverse and complementary strategies aimed at a network of issues/determinants
Directive and persuasive strategies enforced in target groups	Facilitating and enabling approaches by incentives offered to the population
Focused mostly on individuals and groups of subjects	Focused on a person's health status and environment
Led by professional groups from health disciplines	Led by non-professional organizations, civic groups, local, municipal, regional, and national governments

Source: Shah CP. Public Health and Preventive Medicine in Canada, 5th ed. Toronto: Elsevier, 2003

Healthy Public Policy

- characterized by an explicit concern for health and equity in all areas of policy and by an accountability for health impact
- main aim: to create a supportive environment to enable people to lead healthy lives, thereby making healthy choices easier for citizens
- government sectors must take into account health as an essential factor when formulating policy and should be accountable for the health consequences of their policy decisions
- methods
  - fiscal: imposing additional costs (e.g. taxes on tobacco and alcohol)
  - legislative: implementing legal deterrents (e.g. smoking bans, legal alcohol drinking age)
  - social: improving health beyond providing universally funded health care (e.g. providing affordable housing)

Source: International Conference on Health Promotion, Adelaide, South Australia (1998)

Example of Harm Reduction Strategies: Tobacco Harm Reduction And The Case for the Electronic Cigarette
Harm Reduct J 2013 Oct 4;10:19.
Conventional smoking cessation strategies such as nicotine replacement therapy, buproprion or varenicline pharmacotherapy have demonstrated low uptake and poor overall efficacy despite garnering some increase in quit rates. Alternative sources of nicotine, such as the electronic cigarette, deliver nicotine vapor without combustion products responsible for most of the damaging effects experienced by traditional smoking methods, and without the emission of traditional cigarette toxins. Therefore, the electronic cigarette represents a harm reduction strategy with health risks similar to smokeless tobacco, with approximately 1% of the mortality risk associated with traditional cigarette smoking. Electronic cigarettes have also been associated with other benefits, such as improved exercise tolerance, decreased cough symptoms, decreased odourous breath, relief from withdrawal and craving symptoms of traditional cigarettes, relatively lower expenses and increased likelihood of smoking abstinence.

Behaviour Change

- health education serves to
  - increase knowledge and skills
  - encourage positive behaviour changes and discourage unhealthy choices
- health education is an important component of eliciting behaviour change
- behaviour is a result of three factors
  1. predisposing factors: knowledge, attitude, beliefs, values, intentions
  2. enabling factors: skills, supports
  3. reinforcing factors: health care professionals and the social context of family and community
- **Health Belief Model** (1975)
  - "behaviours undertaken by individuals in order to remain healthy [...] are a function of a set of interacting beliefs"
  - beliefs include: (i) individual's perception of their susceptibility to a disease, (ii) severity of the disease, (iii) efficacy of proposed change/action, (iv) benefits and costs of health-related actions
  - beliefs are modified by socio-demographic and psychosocial variables
  - individuals must be in a state of readiness
  - behaviour can be stimulated by cues to action, which are triggers that can encourage preventive health decisions and actions (e.g. physician recommendation, public advertising)
- **Stages of Change Model**
  - provides a framework in which the Health Belief Model is applied to facilitating behaviour change (e.g. quitting smoking)

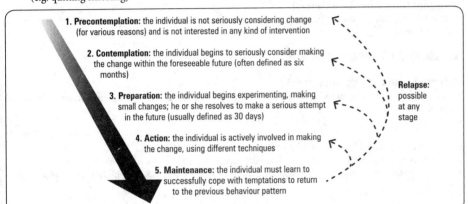

Figure 3. Stages of change model
Source: Prochaska JO, DiClemente CC, and Norcross JC. In Search of How People Change. Applications to Addictive Behaviours. *Am Psychol* 1992;47:1102-1114

Risk Reduction Strategies

- **risk reduction**: lower the risk to health without eliminating it (e.g. avoiding sun to lower risk of skin cancer)
- **harm reduction**: tolerance of some degree of risk behaviour, while aiming to minimize the adverse outcomes associated with these behaviours (e.g. needle exchange programs)
Source: Shah, CP. Concepts, Determinants, and Promotion of Health. Public Health and Preventive Medicine in Canada, 5e. Toronto: Elsevier, 2003

Measurements of Health and Disease in a Population

MEASURES OF DISEASE OCCURRENCE

Incidence Rate

- number of new cases in a population per unit of person-time

Prevalence

- *total number* of cases in a population over a defined period of time
- two forms of prevalence
  - **point prevalence**: assessed at one point in time
  - **period prevalence**: as above, but all cases over defined time window (including 'incident' ones) are included
- depends on **incidence rate** and disease duration from onset to termination (cure or death)
- favours the inclusion of chronic over acute cases and may underestimate disease burden if those with short disease duration are missed
- prevalence studies are cross-sectional and provide weak evidence for causal inferences
- prevalence figures are useful for determining the extent of a disease and can aid in the planning of facilities and services

Example of Harm Reduction Strategy
Summary of Findings from the Evaluation of a Pilot Medically Supervised Safer Injecting Facility
CMAJ 2006;175:1399-1404
Background: This study discusses the outcomes among a population of illicit injection drug users (IDUs) after initiating a supervised safe injecting facility in Vancouver, September 2003. Legal exemption by the Canadian government was granted such that an evaluation of its results be conducted over a 3 yr period.
Study Population: IDUs of the Vancouver area were allowed to inject previously obtained illicit drugs under the supervision of nurses and physicians. IDUs were offered addiction counselling and supports for appropriate community resources. A random sample of 670 IDUs was recruited and monitored from Dec 2003-July 2004.
Results: Characteristics of IDUs who used the safe injecting facility included age <30 yr, history of public drug use, homelessness, daily heroin and/or cocaine injection, and recent history of overdose. Mean measures of public order problems were taken 6 wk before and 12 wk after initiation of the safer injection facility. It was found that the mean number of IDUs injecting daily in public, along with the mean number of publically discarded syringes were reduced by approximately half.
Conclusions: Overall it has been found that the safer injecting facility in Vancouver has been successful in attracting IDUs at increased risk of HIV, overdose, and public injection of substances. This has resulted in lower incidences of public drug use, publically discarded syringes and sharing of needles. Other studies associated with this one have demonstrated that there has been no increase in the drug dealing, drug related crimes, or rates of new IDUs in the area surrounding the safer injection facility.

Incidence and Prevalence

$$\text{Incidence} = \frac{\text{\# of new cases in a time interval}}{\text{total person-time at risk}}$$
(measures the rate of new infections)

$$\text{Prevalence} = \frac{\text{\# of existing cases at a point in time}}{\text{total person-time at risk}}$$
(measures the frequency of disease at a point in time)

e.g. For Canada in 2011:
HIV incidence rate is 9.5 per 100,000 people
HIV prevalence is 213 per 100,000 people

Top 5 Causes of Mortality in Canada, 2012, by Sex
Female
- Cancer
- Heart disease
- Stroke
- COPD/chronic lower respiratory disease
- Alzheimer's
Male
- Cancer
- Heart disease
- Accidents
- Stroke
- COPD/chronic lower respiratory disease
Source: Statistics Canada. CANSIM, 2012. Table 102-0561 and 102-0562 and catalogue no.84-215-X

Age Standardized Rate
- adjustment of the crude rate of a health-related event using a "standard" population
- standard population is one with a known number of persons in each age and sex group
- standardization prevents bias which could be made by comparing crude rates from two dissimilar populations (e.g. crude death rates over a number of decades are not comparable as the population age distribution has changed with time)

MEASURES OF MORTALITY

Life Expectancy
- "the expected number of years to be lived by a newborn based on age-specific mortality rates at a selected time"
- usually qualified by country, gender, and age

Crude Death Rate
- mortality from all causes of death per 1,000 in the population

Infant Mortality Rate (IMR)
- number of deaths among children under 1 yr of age reported during a given time period divided by the number of live births reported during the same time period and expressed per 1,000 live births per year

Maternal Mortality Rate (MMR)
- "number of deaths of women during pregnancy and due to puerperal causes […] per 1000 live births in the same year"

MEASURES OF DISEASE BURDEN

Potential Years of Life Lost (PYLL)
- calculated for a population using the difference between the actual age at death and a standard/expected age at death
- increased weighting of mortality at a younger age

Disability Adjusted Life Year (DALY)
- life expectancy weighted by amount of disability experienced
- both premature death and time spent with disability accounted for; these disabilities can be physical or mental

Quality Adjusted Life Year (QALY)
- years of life weighted by utility (similar to quality of life), ranging from 0 to 1 assigned to a year of life based on perceived quality of life; a yr in "perfect" health is considered equal to 1 QALY, the value of a year in ill health would be lowered based on the burden of disease
- it is possible to have "states worse than death" for example QALY <0 for extremely serious conditions

For additional rate calculations see *Outbreak of Infectious Diseases*, PH19

Consult the Public Health Agency of Canada for examples and latest statistics
http://www.phac-aspc.gc.ca/cphorsphc-respcacsp/2008/fr-rc/cphorsphc-respcacsp06b-eng.php

Sources: Shah, CP. Health Indicators and Data Sources. Public Health and Preventive Medicine in Canada, 5e. Toronto: Elsevier, 2003
The Association of Faculties of Medicine of Canada Public Health Educators' Network. Methods: Measuring Health. AFMC Primer on Population Health.

Epidemiology

Population
- a defined collection of individuals/regions/institutions/etc (e.g. individuals defined by geographic region, sex, age)

Sample
- a selection of individuals from a population
- types
  - random: all members are equally likely to be selected
  - systematic: an algorithm is used to select a subset
  - stratified: population is divided into subgroups that are each sampled
  - cluster: grouped in space/time to reduce costs
  - convenience: non-random inclusion, usually volunteers

Sample Size
- sample size contributes to the statistical precision of the observed estimate
- increasing the sample size decreases the probability of type I and type II errors
- increasing sample size does not reduce bias/confounding

Bias

- systematic error causing results to differ from correct values/inferences
- can occur at any point in study execution (e.g. collection, analysis, interpretation, publication, or review of data)
    - **sampling bias**: occurs with the selection of a sample that does not truly represent the population
        - sampling procedures should be chosen to prevent or minimize bias
    - **measurement bias**: systematic error arising from inaccurate measurements of subjects
    - **recall bias**: bias in individuals' responses when reporting on past exposures/events
        - e.g. individuals with disease may be more likely to incorrectly recall/believe they were exposed to a possible risk factor than those who are free of disease

SPIN: use a **SP**ecific test to rule **IN** a hypothesis. Note that specific tests have very few false positives. If you get a positive test, it is likely a true positive
SNOUT: use a **SEN**sitive test to rule **OUT** a hypothesis. Note that sensitive tests have very few false negatives. If you get a negative test, it is likely a true negative

Confounder

- a variable that is related to both the exposure and outcome but is not a mediator in the exposure-outcome relationship
- distorts the estimated effect of an exposure if not accounted for in the study design/analysis (e.g. late maternal age could be a confounder in an investigation of birth order >4 and risk of developing Trisomy 21)
- randomization, stratification, matching, and regression modelling can help minimize confounder effects

Source: The Association of Faculties of Medicine of Canada Public Health Educators' Network. Assessing Evidence and Information. AFMC Primer on Population Health.

Interpreting Test Results

TP = True positive   TN = True negative   FP = False positive   FN = False negative

		Disease	
		Present	Negative
Test Result	Positive	TP	FP
	Negative	FN	TN

Sensitivity = TP/(TP+FN)
Specificity = TN/(TN+FP)

Likelihood Ratio (LR)

- Likelihood that a given test result would be expected in a patient with disease compared with the likelihood that the same result would be expected in a patient without disease
- LR+ indicates how much the probability of disease increases if the test is positive
- LR- indicates how much the probability of disease decreases if the test is negative

$$\mathbf{LR+} = \frac{Sensitivity}{1 - Specificity} = \frac{[TP/TP+FN)]}{[FP/(TN+FP)]} \qquad \mathbf{LR-} = \frac{1 - Sensitivity}{Specificity} = \frac{[FN/(TP+FN)]}{[TN/(TN+FP)]}$$

Positive Predictive Value (PPV)

- Proportion of people with a positive test who have the disease

$$\mathbf{PPV} = \frac{TP}{TP + FP}$$

Negative Predictive Value (NPV)

- Proportion of people with a negative test who are free of disease

$$\mathbf{NPV} = \frac{TN}{TN + FN}$$

		Advanced Neoplasia	
		Present	Negative
Test Result	Positive	68	147
	Negative	216	2234
	Total	284	2381

Sensitivity = 68/284 = 23.9%
Specificity = 2234/2381 = 93.8%

$$LR+ = \frac{0.239}{1 - 0.938} = 3.85$$

$$LR- = \frac{1 - 0.239}{0.938} = 0.81$$

$$PPV = \frac{68}{(68+147)} = 31.6\%$$

$$NPV = \frac{2234}{(2234+216)} = 91.2\%$$

Figure 5. Interpreting test results: Practical example using FOBT testing in advanced colon cancer
Source: Numbers from Collins J, Lieberman D, Durbin T, et al. Accuracy of screening for fecal occult blood on a single stool sample obtained by digital rectal examination: a comparison with recommended sampling practice. Ann Intern Med 2005;142:81-85

Sensitivity

- proportion of people with disease who have a positive test

Specificity

- proportion of people without disease who have a negative test

Pre-Test Probability

- the probability a particular patient has a given disease before a test/assessment results are known

Figure 4. Understanding sensitivity and specificity

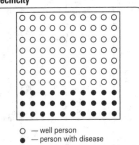

○ — well person
● — person with disease

Figure 4a. Hypothetical population

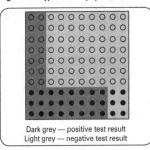

Dark grey — positive test result
Light grey — negative test result

Figure 4b. Results of diagnostic test on hypothetical population

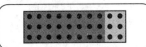

Figure 4c. Sensitivity of test (e.g. 24/30 = 80% sensitive)

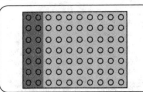

Figure 4d. Specificity of test (e.g. 56/70 = 80% specific)

Source: Loong TW. Understanding sensitivity and specificity with the right side of the brain.
BMJ 2003;327:716-719

Post-Test Probability

- a revision of the probability of disease after a patient has been interviewed/examined/tested
- calculation process can be explicit using results from epidemiologic studies, knowledge of the accuracy of tests, and a nomogram/Bayes' theorem
- the post-test probability from clinical examination is the basis of consideration when ordering diagnostic tests or imaging studies
  - after each iteration the resultant post-test probability becomes the pre-test probability when considering new investigations

Effectiveness of Interventions

Effectiveness, Efficacy, Efficiency

- three measurements indicating the relative value (beneficial effects vs. harmful effects) of an intervention
  - **efficacy**: the extent to which a specific intervention produces a beneficial result under ideal conditions (e.g. RCT)
    - ideal conditions include adherence, close monitoring, access to health resources, etc.
  - **effectiveness**: measures the benefit of an intervention under usual conditions of clinical care
    - considers both the efficacy of an intervention and its actual impact on the real world, taking into account access to the intervention, whether it is offered to those who can benefit from it, its proper administration, acceptance of intervention, and degree of adherence to intervention
  - **efficiency**: a measure of economy of an intervention with known effectiveness
    - considers the optimal use of resources (e.g. money, time, personnel, equipment, etc.)

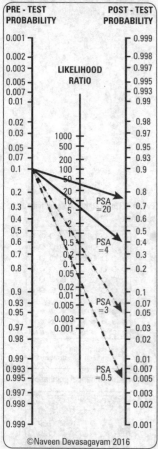

Figure 6. Fagan's likelihood ratio nomogram: Practical example using PSA levels to calculate post-test probability of prostate cancer
Source: Modified from Holmstrom B, Johansson M, Bergh A, et al. Prostate specific antigen for early detection of prostate cancer: longitudinal study. BMJ 2009;339:b3537

		Disease (e.g. lung CA)		
		Present	Absent	Total
Exposure (e.g. smoking)	Present	A	B	A + B
	Absent	C	D	C + D
	Total	A + C	B + D	A + B + C + D

Case-Control Study

$$\text{odds ratio (OR)*} = \frac{A \times B}{C \times D} = \frac{A \times D}{B \times C}$$

Cohort Study

$$\frac{A}{A + B} = \text{incidence rate of health outcome in exposed} \qquad \frac{C}{C + D} = \text{incidence rate of health outcome in non-exposed}$$

$$\text{relative risk (RR)**} = \frac{A}{A + B} \div \frac{C}{C + D} \qquad \text{attributable risk (AR)***} = \frac{A}{A + B} - \frac{C}{C + D}$$

*Ratio of the odds in favour of the health outcome among the exposed to the odds in favour among the unexposed
**Ratio of the risk of a health outcome among exposed to the risk among the unexposed
***Rate of health outcome in exposed individuals that can be attributed to the exposure

Figure 7. Measures of effect by study type

Number Needed to Treat (NNT)

- number of patients who need to be treated to achieve one additional favourable outcome
- only one of many factors that should be taken into account in clinical or health system decision making (e.g. must take into account cost, ease, feasibility of intervention)
  - a condition with death as a potential outcome can have a higher NNT (and be acceptable), as compared to an intervention to prevent an outcome with low morbidity, in which a low NNT would be necessary

Number Needed to Harm (NNH)

- number of patients who, if they received the experimental treatment, would lead to one additional patient being harmed, compared with patients who received the control treatment

Adherence (formerly compliance)

- degree to which a patient follows a treatment plan

Coverage

- extent to which the services rendered cover the potential need for these services in a community
Sources: Shah, CP. Health Indicators and Data Sources. Public Health and Preventive Medicine in Canada, 5e. Toronto: Elsevier, 2003
The Association of Faculties of Medicine of Canada Public Health Educators' Network. Assessing Evidence and Information. AFMC Primer on Population Health.

Sensitivity and specificity are characteristics of the test
LR depends on the test characteristics, not the prevalence
PPV and NPV depend on the prevalence of the disease in the population

Equations to Assess Effectiveness
CER = control group event rate
EER = experimental group event rate
RR = EER/CER
ARR = CER – EER
NNT = 1/ARR

Beware
Do not be swayed by a large RR or odds ratio, as it may appear to be large if event rate is small to begin with. In these cases AR is more important (e.g. a drug which lowers an event which occurs in 0.1% of a population to 0.05% can boast a RR of 50%, and yet the AR is only 0.05%, which is not nearly as impressive)

NNT
Consult http://www.thennt.com for quick summaries of evidence-based medicine (includes NNT, LR, and risk assessments)

Types of Study Design

Qualitative vs. Quantitative

Table 6. Qualitative vs. Quantitative Study Designs

Qualitative	Quantitative
Often used to generates hypothesis (Why? What does it mean?)	Often tests hypothesis (What? How much/many?)
"Bottom up" approach Observation → pattern → tentative hypothesis → theory	"Top down" approach Theory → hypothesis → observation → confirmation
Sampling approach to obtain representative coverage of ideas , concepts, or experiences	Sampling approach to obtain representative coverage of people in the population
Narrative: rich, contextual, and detailed information from a small number of participants	Numeric: frequency, severity, and associations from a large number of participants

Source: Adapted from http://phprimer.afmc.ca
Source: The Association of Faculties of Medicine of Canada Public Health Educators' Network. Assessing Evidence and Information. AFMC Primer on Population Health.

Quantitative Research Methods

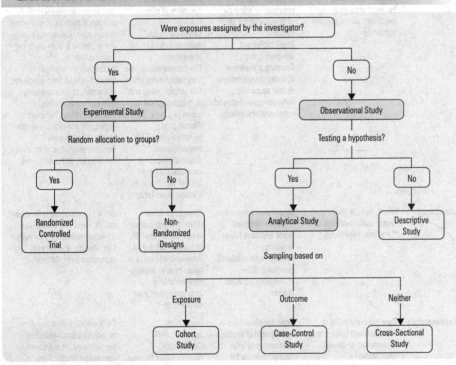

Figure 8. Quantitative study designs
Source: Adapted from http://phprimer.afmc.ca

Formulating a Research Question

PICO
Population/**P**atient Characteristics
Intervention/Exposure of Interest
Comparison Group or Control Group
Outcome that you are trying to prevent or achieve

Observational Study Designs

- observational studies involve neither the manipulation of the exposure of interest nor randomization of the study subjects
- there are two main subtypes of observational studies: descriptive and analytic studies

Descriptive Studies
- describe the events and rates of disease with respect to person, place and time and to estimate disease frequency and time trends
- can be used to generate an etiologic hypothesis and for policy planning

Analytic Studies
- observational studies used to test a specific hypothesis
- includes ecological studies, cohort studies, case-control studies, and cross-sectional studies

An example of an ecological fallacy would be concluding that red wine drinking leads to lower risk of death from CVS disease after an ecological study shows that countries with a higher rate of red wine consumption have a lower rate of death from CVS causes

Types of Study Design

Table 7. Observational Study Designs

Type of Study	Ecological	Cross-Sectional	Case-Control	Cohort
Definition	Units of analysis are populations or groups of people, rather than individuals	Use individual data on exposures and outcomes gathered at the same time	Samples a group of people who already have a particular outcome (cases) and compares them to a similar sample group without that outcome (controls)	Subjects are sampled and, as a group, classified on the basis of presence or absence of exposure to a particular risk factor
Subjects	Aggregated groups (e.g. cities)	Sample of a population	Two or more samples of individuals with and without the outcome(s) of interest (i.e. cases and controls)	One or more cohorts Cohort: group of people with common characteristics (e.g. year of birth, region of residence) Divided into measured exposed vs. non-exposed groups
Methods	Descriptions of the average exposure or risk of disease for a population Can use regression models to test associations between area-level predictors and aggregate outcomes	Collect information from each person at one particular time Tabulate the numbers in groups (e.g. by presence or absence of disease/factor of interest) Make tables and compare groups Estimate prevalence Use regression models to test associations between predictors and outcomes of interest	Select sample of cases of a specific disease during a specific time frame Representative of spectrum of clinical disease Select control(s) Represent the general population To minimize risk of bias, may select more than one control group and/or match controls to cases (e.g. age, gender) Assess past exposures (e.g. EMR, questionnaire) Association can be concluded between the risk factor and the disease (odds ratio)	Collect information on factors from all persons at the beginning of the study Subjects are followed for a specific period of time to determine development of disease in each exposure group Prospective: measuring from the exposure at present to the future outcomes Retrospective: measuring forward in time from exposures in the past to later outcomes Use statistical models to test associations between exposures and disease or other measured outcomes Provides estimates of incidence, relative risk, attributable risk
Advantages	Quick, easy to do Uses readily available data Generates hypothesis	Determines association between variables Quick and uses fewer resources Surveys with validated questions allows comparison between studies	Often used when disease in population is rare (less than 10% of population) due to increased efficiency or when time to develop disease is long Less costly and time consuming	Shows an association between risk factor(s) and outcome(s) Stronger evidence for causation Can consider a variety of exposures and outcomes
Disadvantages	Poor generalizability to individual level (not direct assessment of causal relationship) Ecological fallacy: an incorrect inference from groups to individuals Confounding	Does not allow for assessment of temporal relationship or offer strong evidence for causation between variables Confounding Selection bias Recall bias (see *Bias*, PH9)	Recall bias (see *Bias*, PH9) Confounding Selection bias for cases and controls Only one outcome can be measured	Confounding may occur due to individuals self-selecting the exposure, or unknown/unmeasured factors are associated with the measured exposure and outcome Cost and duration of time needed to follow cohort Selection bias
Examples	A study looking at the association between smoking rates and lung cancer rates in different countries at the population level without individual data on both factors	A study that examines the distribution of BMI by age in Ontario at a particular point in time	A famous case control study published by Sir Richard Doll demonstrated the link between tobacco smoking exposure and lung cancer cases at the individual level	A famous cohort study is the Framingham Heart Study, which assessed the long-term cardiovascular risks of diet, exercise, medications such as ASA, etc.

Sources: Shah, CP. Measurement and Investigation. Public Health and Preventive Medicine in Canada, 5e. Toronto: Elsevier, 2003.
The Association of Faculties of Medicine of Canada Public Health Educators' Network. Assessing Evidence and Information. AFMC Primer on Population Health.
Rothman KJ, Greenland SG, Lash TL. Modern Epidemiology, 3e. Philadelphia: Wolters Kluwer, 2012.

Experimental Study Designs

- not discussed here are non-randomized control trials (e.g. allocation by clinic or other non-random basis – performed when randomization is not possible)

RANDOMIZED CONTROLLED TRIAL (RCT)

Definition
- subjects are assigned by random allocation to two or more groups, one of which is the control group, the other group(s) receive(s) an intervention

Subjects
- individuals are selected using explicit inclusion/exclusion criteria with recruitment targets guided by sample size calculations

Methods
- random allocation of individuals into two or more treatment groups through a centralized concealed process
- method of assessment to reduce bias
    - **single-blind**: subject does not know group assignment (intervention or placebo)
    - **double-blind**: subject and observer both unaware of group assignment
    - **triple-blind**: subject, observer, and analyst unaware of group assignment
- one group receives placebo or standard therapy
- one or more groups receive(s) the intervention(s) under study
- baseline covariates and outcome(s) are measured and the groups are compared
- all other conditions are kept the same between groups

Advantages
- "gold standard" of studies, upon which the practice of EBM is founded
- provides the strongest evidence for effectiveness of intervention
- with sufficient sample size and appropriate randomization, threats to validity are minimized
- randomization is one of few methods that can address selection bias and confounding (including unmeasured confounders)
- allows prospective assessment of the effects of intervention

Disadvantages
- some exposures are not amenable to randomization (e.g. cannot randomize subjects to poverty/wealth or to harmful exposures such as smoking) due to ethical or feasibility concerns
- can be difficult to randomly allocate groups (e.g. communities, neighbourhoods)
- difficult to study rare events, since RCTs would require extremely large sample sizes
- contamination, co-intervention, and loss to follow up can all limit causal inferences
- can have poor generalizability
- costly

Sources: Shah, CP. Measurement and Investigation. Public Health and Preventive Medicine in Canada, 5e. Toronto: Elsevier, 2003.
The Association of Faculties of Medicine of Canada Public Health Educators' Network. Assessing Evidence and Information. AFMC Primer on Population Health.

Summary Study Designs

META-ANALYSIS

Definition
- a form of statistical analysis that synthesizes the results of independent studies addressing a common research question, as identified through systematic review

Subjects
- all the studies identified through the review (or all subjects used in original studies for individual-level meta-analysis)

Methods
- selection of relevant studies from the published literature which meet quality criteria
- statistical models used to combine the results of each independent study
- provides a summary statistic of overall results as well as graphic representation of included studies (forest plot)

Advantages
- attempts to overcome the problem of reduced power due to small sample sizes of individual studies
- ability to control for inter-study variation
- can address questions (e.g. subgroup analyses) that the original studies were not powered to answer

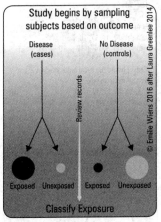

Figure 9. Case-control study
Adapted from http://phprimer.afmc.ca

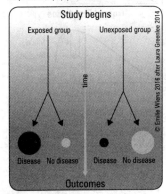

Figure 10. Cohort study
Adapted from http://phprimer.afmc.ca

Analysis
Per-Protocol Analysis (PP)
Strategy of analysis in which only patients who complete the entire study are counted towards the results

Intention-to-Treat Analysis (ITT)
When groups are analyzed exactly as they existed upon randomization (i.e. using data from all patients, including those who did not complete the study)

An example of an RCT is the SPARCL trial, which demonstrated intense lipid-lowering with atorvastatin reduces the risk of cerebro- and cardiovascular events in patients with and without carotid stenosis when compared to placebo

An example of a meta-analysis is one that compares the effects of ACE inhibitors, CCBs, and other antihypertensive agents on mortality and major cardiovascular events by compiling and analyzing data from a full set of reported RCTs

Consult the Cochrane Library of Systematic Reviews (http://www.cochranelibrary.com) for high-quality systematic reviews and meta-analyses

Example Calculation
Data set: 17, 14, 17, 10, 7
Mean = (17 + 14 + 17 + 10 + 7)
        ÷ 5 = 13
Median (write the list in order, median is the number in the middle)
= 7, 10, 14, 17, 17 = 14
Mode (number repeated more often) = 17
Range = 17- 7 = 10
Variance = [(17 – 13)² + (14 – 13)²
        + (17 – 13)² + (10 – 13)²
        + (7 – 13)²] ÷ 4 = 19.5
Standard Deviation = √variance = √19.5
= 4.42

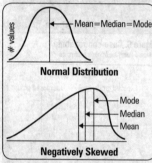

Figure 11. Distribution curves

Type I (α) Error
"There Is An Effect" where in reality there is none

Disadvantages
- sources of bias may not be controlled for
- reliance on published studies may increase the potential conclusion of an effect as it can be difficult to publish studies that show no significant results (publication bias)
- the decision to include/reject a particular study is subjective

Sources: Shah, CP. Measurement and Investigation. Public Health and Preventive Medicine in Canada, 5e. Toronto: Elsevier, 2003.
The Association of Faculties of Medicine of Canada Public Health Educators' Network. Assessing Evidence and Information. AFMC Primer on Population Health.

Methods of Analysis

Distributions

- distribution describes the probability of events
- normal (Gaussian) or non-normal (binomial, gamma, skewed, etc.)
- characteristics of the normal distribution
  - mean = median = mode
  - 67% of observations fall within one standard deviation of the mean
  - 95% of observations fall within two standard deviations of the mean
- measures of central tendency
  - **mean**: sum of each observations' data (e.g. ages) divided by total number of observations
  - **median**: value at the 50th percentile, this is a better reflection of the central tendency for a skewed distribution
  - **mode**: most frequently observed value in a series
- measures of dispersion
  - **range**: the largest value minus the smallest value
  - **variance**: a measure of the spread of data
  - **standard deviation**: the average distance of data points from the mean (the positive square root of variance)
- given the mean and standard deviation of a normal or binomial distribution curve, a description of the entire distribution of data is obtained

Data Analysis

Statistical Hypotheses
- null (H_0)
  - the default hypothesis , often that there is no relationship between two variables
- alternative (H_1)
  - the hypothesis that we are interested in, often that there is a relationship between two variables
  - we can find evidence against H_0 but we can never 'prove' H_1

Type I Error (α Error)
- the null hypothesis is falsely rejected (i.e. concluding an intervention X is effective when it is not, or declaring an observed difference to be real rather than by chance)
- the probability of this error is denoted by the p-value
- studies tend to be designed to minimize this type of error, since a type I error can have larger clinical significance than a type II error

Type II Error (β Error)
- the null hypothesis is falsely accepted (i.e. stating intervention X is not effective when it is, or declaring an observed difference/effect to have occurred by chance when it is present)
- by convention a higher level of error is often accepted for most studies
- can also be used to calculate statistical power

Power
- probability of correctly rejecting a null hypothesis when it is in fact false (i.e. the probability of finding a specified difference to be statistically significant at a given p-value)
- power increases with an increase in sample size
- power = $1 – \beta$, and is therefore equal to the probability of a true positive result

Statistical Significance
- the probability that the statistical association found between the variables is due to random chance alone (i.e. that there is no association)
- the preset probability is set sufficiently low that one would act on the result; frequently $p<0.05$
- when statistical tests result in a probability less than the preset limit, the results are said to be statistically significant (denoted by the α-value)

Clinical Significance
- measure of clinical usefulness (e.g. 1 mmHg BP reduction may be statistically significant, but may not be clinically significant)
- depends on factors such as cost, availability, patient compliance, and side effects in addition to statistical significance

Confidence Interval (CI)
- provides a range of values within which the true population result (e.g. the mean) lies
- frequently reported as 95% CI (i.e. 95% chance that the true value is within this data range)
- bounded by the upper and lower confidence limits

A wider confidence interval implies more variance than a tighter confidence interval given the same critical value

Data
- information collected from a sample of a population
- there are 4 overall levels of measurement for quantitative data listed with examples
  - **categorical** (e.g. gender, marital status)
  - **ordinal** (e.g. low, medium, high)
  - **interval** (e.g. °C, time of day)
  - **ratio** (e.g. serum cholesterol, hemoglobin, age)

Validity/Accuracy (of a measurement tool)
- how closely a measurement reflects the entity it claims to measure

Reliability/Precision
- how consistent multiple measurements are when the underlying subject of measurement has not changed
- may be assessed by different observers at the same time (inter-rater reliability) or by the same observer under different conditions (test-retest reliability)

Internal Validity
- degree to which the findings of the sample truly represent the findings in the study population
- dependent on the reliability, accuracy, and absence of other biases

External Validity (i.e. Generalizability)
- degree to which the results of the study can be generalized to other situations or populations

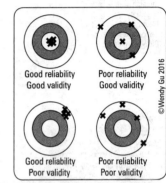

Figure 12. Validity vs. reliability

Common Statistical Tests

Table 8. Statistical Tests

	Two-sample Z-Test	Analysis of Variance (ANOVA)	Chi-Squared Test (χ^2)	Linear Regression	Logistic Regression	Pearson product-moment correlation (Pearson's r)
What are you trying to show?						
	Compare the mean values of an outcome variable between two groups (e.g. difference in average BP between men and women)	Compare the mean values of an outcome variable between two or more groups (e.g. difference in average BP between persons in three towns)	Test the correspondence between a theoretical frequency distribution and an observed frequency distribution (e.g. if one sample of 20 patients is 30% hypertensive and another comparison group of 25 patients is 60% hypertensive, a chi-squared test determines if this variation is more than expected due to chance alone)	Looks at associations between two or more variables (e.g. age and blood pressure)	Shows how a change in one explanatory variable affects the status (e.g. ill vs. non-ill) of the outcome variable	Assesses the strength of the linear relationship between two variables. Ranges from -1 (negative association, ie. Increases in one variable are associated with decreases in another) to 1 (positive association, increases in one variable are associated with increases in the other). A correlation of 0 indicates no relationship
What kind of variables do you measure?						
Dependent Variable	Continuous data	Continuous data	Categorical (2 or more) /ordinal	Continuous	Categorical (outcomes usually dichotomous)	Continuous
Independent Variable	Dichotomous	Categorical/Ordinal (2 or more)	Categorica/Ordinall (2 or more)	Continuous/Ordinal/ Categorical	Continuous/Ordinal/ Categorical	Continuous
Assumptions	Data follow a normal/t-distribution Equal variances Data are independent	"Normal" distribution of dependent variable's error term Data are independent	Expected counts must be at least 5 for all cells in n x n table Data are independent	Dependent variable's error term has "normal" distribution Linear relationship between variables Homoskedasticity No influential values Data are independent	Linearity (on logit scale) No influential values Model has adequate goodness-of-fit Data are independent	Underlying relationship is linear Data for both variables are Normally distributed Data are independent

What's the difference between Pearson and Spearman correlation?
Different types of correlation are used for different levels of measurement. Pearson is for continuous and Normal data, Spearman is for ordinal or non-Normal data. There are other forms of correlation for other levels of measurement (e.g. Tetrachoric/polychoric)

Beware
Correlation ≠ Causation
e.g. There is evidence of a direct correlation between the amount of ice cream sold and the amount of deaths in swimming pools. Of course, ice cream does not cause drowning, rather, they both increase in the summer

Criteria for Causation

ACCESS PTB
Analogy
Consistency
Coherence
Experimental evidence
Strength of association
Specificity
Plausibility
Temporal relationship
Biological gradient

Causation

Criteria for Causation (Sir Bradford Hill)

1. **strength of association**: the frequency with which the factor is found in the disease and the frequency with which it occurs in the absence of disease
2. **consistency**: is it the same relationship seen with different populations or study design?
3. **specificity**: is the association particular to your intervention and measured outcome?
4. **temporal relationship**: did the exposure occur before the onset of the disease?
5. **biological gradient**: finding a dose response relationship between the exposure-outcome
6. **biological plausibility**: does the association/causation make biological sense?
7. **coherence**: can the relationship be explained/accounted for based on what we know about science, logic, etc.?
8. **experimental evidence**: does experimental evidence support the association (e.g. is there improvement?)
9. **analogy**: do other established associations provide a model for this type of the relationship?

Note: Not all criteria must be fulfilled to establish scientific causation, and the modern practice of EBM emphasizes 'experimental evidence' as superior to other criteria for experimental causation review. However many causation questions in health cannot be answered with experimental methods.

Source: Bradford Hill A. The environment and disease: association or causation. *Proc R Soc Med* 1965; 58(5): 295-300.

Assessing Evidence

Validity
• The degree to which the outcome observed in the study can be attributed to the intervention

5 Questions About the Validity of Primary Studies
• Were the patients randomized?
• Was the follow-up of patients sufficiently long and complete?
• Were all patients analyzed in the groups to which they were randomized?
• Were the groups treated equally except for the intervention?
• Were the patients and clinicians kept blind to treatment?

Other Questions to Consider
• Were the groups similar (i.e. demographics, prognostic factors) at the start of the trial?
• Were the appropriate and valid exposure and outcome measures obtained?
• Were outcome assessors aware of group allocation?
• Was contamination reported?
• Were ethical issues continuously upheld?
Source: The Association of Faculties of Medicine of Canada Public Health Educators' Network. Assessing Evidence and Information. AFMC Primer on Population Health.

• critical appraisal is the process of systematically examining research evidence to assess validity, results, and relevance before using it to inform a decision

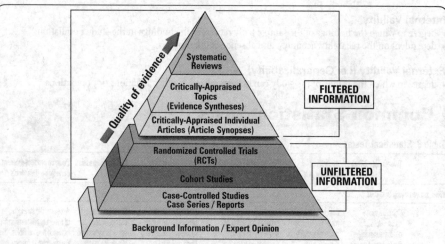

Figure 13. Pyramid of pre-appraised evidence

A. Are the results of the study valid?
  ▪ see below for classifications of evidence that has already been assessed; see sidebar for assessing primary studies

B. What are the results?
  ▪ what was the impact of the treatment effect?
  ▪ how precise was the estimate of treatment effect?
  ▪ what were the confidence intervals and power of the study?

C. Will the results help me in caring for my patients?
  ▪ are the results clinically significant?
  ▪ can I apply the results to my patient population?
  ▪ were all clinically important outcomes considered?
  ▪ are the likely treatment benefits worth the potential harm and costs?

Levels of Evidence: Classifications Cited in Guidelines/Consensus Statements

Level I evidence: based on RCTs (or meta-analysis of RCTs) big enough to have low risk of incorporating FP or FN results

Level II evidence: based on RCTs too small to provide Level I evidence; may show positive trends that are non-significant, or have a high risk of FN results

Level III evidence: based on non-randomized, controlled or cohort studies; case series; case-controlled; or cross-sectional studies

Level IV evidence: based on opinion of respected authorities or expert committees, as published consensus conferences/guidelines

Level V evidence: opinions of the individuals who have written/reviewed the guidelines (i.e. Level IV evidence), based on experience/knowledge of literature/peer discussion

Notes: These 5 levels of evidence are not direct evaluations of evidence quality or credibility; they reflect the nature of the evidence. While RCTs tend to be most credible (with <III), level III evidence gains credibility when multiple studies from different locations and/or time periods report consistent findings. Level IV and V evidence reflects decision-making that is necessary but in the absence of published evidence.

Figure 14. Levels of evidence classifications
Note: This is only one method of classifying evidence. Various systems exist, but operate within the same premise that certain types of evidence carry more weight than others

Health Services Research

Continuous Quality Improvement

Quality Improvement (QI)
- a means of evaluating and improving processes; focusing more on systems and systematic biases, which are thought to cause variation in quality
- measures to increase efficiency of action with the purpose of achieving optimal quality

Quality Assurance
- process to guarantee the quality of health care through improvement and attainment of set standards
- "five-stage process of quality assurance" (Public Health and Preventative Medicine in Canada, Shah)
    1. formulation of working goals
    2. procedural changes to implement those goals
    3. regular comparison of current performance with original goals
    4. development of solutions to bring performance closer to goals
    5. documentation of quality assurance activities

Quality Control
- a process of surveying the quality of all factors involved in the process to maintain standards

Continuous Quality Improvement
- the process of ongoing service/product refinement via the vigilant review of expectant issue detrimental to the system and regular incorporation of improvements

Quality Management
- combination of several process (assurance, control, improvement) to maintain consistent quality

Total Quality Management
- management principle for advancing quality while minimizing additional expenditures
- focuses on the entire system rather than discrete elements

Audit
- methodical analysis of a quality system by quality auditors
- to determine whether quality processes and results comply with goals, and whether processes have been implemented effectively

Systems Analyses Tools
1. **5 Whys**: brainstorming to simplify the process of change; continue asking 'why' until the root of the problem is discovered
2. **Ishikawa Diagrams (i.e. Fishbone Diagrams)**: identify generic categories of problems that have an overall contribution on the effect

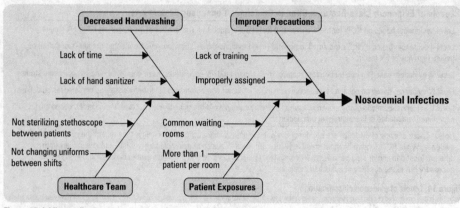

Figure 15. Ishikawa diagram

3. **Defect check sheets**: consider all defects and tally up the number of times the defect occurs
4. **Pareto Chart**: x vs. y chart; x-axis = defect categories, y-axis = frequency; plot cumulative frequency on the right y-axis
    - purpose is to highlight most important among large set of factors contributing to defects/poor quality

Precede-Proceed Model
- tool for designing, implementing, and evaluating health interventions/programs

Table 9. Precede-Proceed Model

PRECEDE Phase	PROCEED Phase
Phase 1 – Identify the ultimate desired result	Phase 5 – Implementation (design and conduct the intervention)
Phase 2 – Identify health issues and their behavioural and environmental determinants. Set priorities among them.	Phase 6 – Process Evaluation (determine if the program is implemented as planned)
Phase 3 – Identify the predisposing, enabling, and reinforcing factors that affect the behaviours and environmental determinants	Phase 7 – Impact Evaluation (measure intermediate objectives – predisposing, enabling, and reinforcing factors)
Phase 4 – Identify the administrative and policy factors that influence what can be implemented	Phase 8 – Outcome Evaluation (measure desired result)

Cost Analysis

Cost Benefit Analysis (CBA)
- an analysis which compares the total expected costs with the total expected benefits of actions in order to choose the most profitable or beneficial options
- costs are controlled for inflation and market changes so that the effect of the change is evaluated over a consistent, preset financial value

Cost Effectiveness Analysis (CEA)
- ratio of the change in cost (numerator) to change in effect (denominator) in response to a new strategy or practice
    - some examples of changes in effect (denominator) could be years of life gained or sight-years gained
    - the numerator highlights the cost of the health gain
    - the most commonly used outcome measure is quality-adjusted life years (QALY) (see *Quality Adjusted Life Year*, PH8)
- can be used where an extensive cost benefit analysis is not applicable or appropriate

Outbreak of Infectious Diseases

Definitions

Endemic
- consistent existence of infectious agent or disease in a given population or area (i.e. usual rate of disease)

Outbreak
- incidence of new cases beyond the usual frequency of disease in a particular population or community over a given period of time
- an epidemic that is in a confined location, has a short duration, or begins acutely

Epidemic
- an outbreak or excessive rate of disease that rapidly spreads to a large number of individuals (e.g. SARS epidemic)

Pandemic
- epidemic over a wide area, crossing international boundaries, and affecting an even larger number of people

Attack Rate
- cumulative incidence of infection within a defined group observed during a specific period of time in an epidemic
- calculated by dividing the total number of people who develop clinical disease by the population at risk, usually expressed as a percentage

Secondary Attack Rate
- the proportion of individuals who develop disease as a result of exposure to primary contacts during the incubation period
- infectiousness reflects the ease of disease transmission and is usually measured by the secondary attack rate

Virulence
- extent of sickness caused in host by a disease-causing agent
- ratio comparing those with the disease who are critically affected over the total number of individuals in the population who have the disease

Case-Fatality Rate (CFR)
- proportion of individuals with the disease who perish as a result of the illness
- most frequently applied to a specific outbreak of acute disease in which all patients have been followed for an adequate period of time to include all attributable deaths
- must be clearly differentiated from the mortality rate

Mortality Rate/Crude Death Rate
- estimation of the portion of the population that dies during a specified period from all causes of death

Steps to Control an Outbreak

Adopted from AFMC Primer on Population Health

1. Determine whether an outbreak

2. Develop case definitions and identify outbreak cases
- consider history, signs, symptoms, test results, and timing to balance sensitivity and specificity in case definition
- consider engaging in active surveillance to identify additional cases

3. Develop hypotheses regarding outbreak cause/source and implement initial control measures
- identify source, population at risk
- manage cases, including appropriate isolation
- reinforce importance of routine and additional precautions

4. Test hypotheses using surveillance data or special studies
- describe cases by person, place, and time to create a line listing
- plot an epidemic curve:
  - histogram with time on the x-axis and number of cases on the y-axis
  - often follows a characteristic pattern based on the nature of the exposure and/or infectious agent:
    - point source epidemic: exposure is brief and not continuous or propagated (e.g. single contaminated dish at a picnic)
    - extended source epidemic: exposure may be continuous (or intermittent if peaks are irregular) and lasts for days or weeks (e.g. ongoing or intermittent contamination of drinking water)
    - propagated epidemic: series of peaks demonstrating only a few cases initially, but then ongoing person-to-person transmission (e.g. influenza virus)

5. Re-evaluate hypothesis and adjust control measures

6. Create and implement plans for future prevention and control
- examples include prevention of transmission in the environment (e.g. handwashing and sterilization techniques), immunization of hosts, and education of health care professionals and the public

Infection Control Precautions
(see Family Medicine, FM49)
Contact (impetigo, chicken pox, warts)
- Wash hands
- Gloves
- Gown
- Wipe equipment after use
Airborne (TB)
- Contact precautions PLUS
- N95 mask (fit tested)
- Negative pressure room
Droplet (influenza, mumps, pneumonia)
- Contact precautions PLUS
- Goggles/face shield
- Surgical mask
Source: Public Health Ontario. http://www.publichealthontario.ca/en/eRepository/IPAC_Clinical_Office_Practice_2013.pdf
http://www.oahpp.ca/resources/documents/pidac/Routine%20Practices%20and%20Additional%20Precautions.pdf

For specific examples, see "Communicable Diseases" section in: Shah CP. Public Health and Preventive Medicine in Canada Toronto: Elsevier, 5th edition, 2003

Active Surveillance
Outreach such as visits or phone calls by the public health/surveillance authority to detect unreported cases (e.g. an infection control nurse goes to the ward and reviews temperature charts to see if any patient has a nosocomial infection)
Passive Surveillance
A surveillance system where the public health/surveillance authority depends on others to submit standardized forms or other means of reporting cases (e.g. ward staff notify infection control when new cases of nosocomial infections are discovered)

Figure 16. Epidemic curves

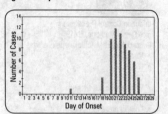

Figure 16a. Point source epidemic curve

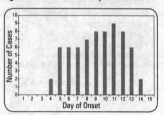

Figure 16b. Extended continuous source epidemic curve

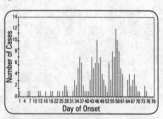

Figure 16c. Propagated source epidemic curve

Infection Control Targets

- interventions should target host, agent, environment, and their interactions

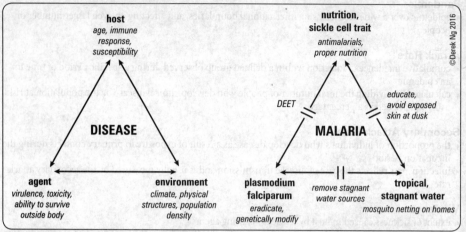

Figure 17. Epidemiology triad as framework for infection control interventions: Practical example using malaria

Environmental Health

Definition

- study of the association between environmental factors, both constructed and natural, and health
- environmental exposures
  - four common hazards: chemical, biological, physical, and radiation
  - four main reservoirs: air, food, water, and soil
  - three main routes: inhalation, ingestion, or absorption (skin)
  - usually divided into two main settings
    - workplace (including schools): may see high level exposure in healthy individuals (see *Occupational Health*, PH23)
    - non-workplace: lower levels of exposure over longer period of time. Affects vulnerable populations more severely, such as at extremes of age, immuno-suppressed. May be teratogenic.
- health impacts of the environment also include factors such as urban planning and how individuals interact with the built environment (e.g. safe pedestrian and bicycle paths can facilitate more active lifestyles)

Table 10. Environmental Health Jurisdiction

Public Health Unit	Enforcement of water and food safety regulations (including restaurant food safety) Sanitation Assessment of local environmental risks Monitoring and follow-up of reportable diseases
Municipal Government	Waste disposal Recycling Water and sewage treatment/collection/distribution
Provincial and Territorial Government	Water and air quality standards Industrial emission regulation Toxic waste disposal
Federal Government	Designating and regulating toxic substances Regulating food products (e.g. Health Canada) Setting policy for pollutants that can travel across provincial boundaries
International	Multilateral agreements (e.g. Kyoto Protocol, UN Convention on Climate Change, International Joint Commission)

Environmental Health Jurisdiction
Taking an Environmental Health History

CH₂OPD₂
Community
Home
Hobbies
Occupation
Personal habits
Diet
Drugs

Marshall L, Weir E, Abelsohn A, Sanborn MD. Identifying and managing adverse environmental health effects: 1. Taking an exposure history. *CMAJ* 2002 Apr 16;166(8):1049-1055.

Risk Assessment

Adopted from p.250, Sixth Edition of "A Dictionary of Epidemiology" by Miquel Porta

Hazard Identification
- what is the hazard involved?
- assess potential hazards by taking environmental health history

Risk Characterization
- is the identified agent likely to elicit the patient's current symptoms?
- review known health impacts of the hazard and identify specific properties that contribute to or diminish adverse effects (e.g. evaluate threshold levels)

Exposure Assessment
- is the patient's exposure to the environmental agent sufficient to have caused the current symptoms?
- quantify exposure through direct measurement or by reviewing frequency and nature of contact with hazard

Air

Biological Hazards
- moulds thrive in moist areas; 10-15% of the population allergic
- bacteria survive as spores and aerosols, can be distributed through ventilation systems (e.g. *Legionella*)
- dust mites (year-round) and pollens (seasonal) can trigger upper and lower-airway symptoms

Chemical Hazards
- ground-level ozone
  - main component of smog with levels increasing in major cities
  - worsens asthma, irritates upper airway
- carbon monoxide (fossil fuel-related, common byproduct of combustion)
  - aggravates cardiac disease at low levels
  - headache, nausea, dizziness at moderate levels
  - fatal at high levels
- sulphur dioxide (fossil fuel-related), nitrogen oxides
  - contribute to acid rain and exacerbate breathing difficulties
- organic compounds at high levels (e.g. benzene, methylene chloride, tetrachloroethylene)
  - tend to be fat-soluble, easily absorbed through skin and difficult to excrete
- heavy metal emissions (e.g. nickel, cadmium, chromium)
  - variety of health effects: upper airway disease, asthma, decreased lung function
- second-hand tobacco smoke
  - respiratory problems, increase risk of lung cancer
  - particulates associated with decreased lung function, asthma, upper airway irritation

Radiation Hazards
- sound waves
  - ionizing radiation
  - radon is naturally produced by soil containing uranium or radium, can contaminate indoor air and is associated with a small proportion of lung cancers
- ultraviolet radiation is increasing due to ozone layer destruction and increases risk of skin cancer
  - non-ionizing radiation
  - visible light, infrared, microwave

Water

Biological Hazards
- mostly due to human and animal waste
- Aboriginal Canadians, rural Canadians at higher risk
- bacteria: *Escherichia coli* (e.g. Walkerton, ON), *Salmonella*, *Pseudomonas*, *Shigella*
- protozoa: *Giardia*, *Cryptosporidium* (e.g. North Battleford, SK)

Chemical/Industrial Hazards
- chlorination by-products (e.g. chloroform can cause cancer at high levels)
- volatile organic compounds, heavy metals, pesticides, and other industrial waste products can be present in groundwater
- fluoride at high levels (greater than that of municipal fluoridation) can cause skeletal fluorosis

BPA, the Toxin Concern of 2009
Bisphenol A (BPA) is a chemical compound found in some hard, clear, lightweight plastics and resins. According to the NIH, animal studies suggest that ingested BPA may imitate estrogen and other hormones. In October 2008, Canada became the first country in the world to ban the import and sale of polycarbonate baby bottles containing BPA, stating that although exposure levels are below levels that cause negative effects, current safety margins need to be higher. The US FDA does not consider normal exposure to BPA to be a hazard, however the NIH has some concern that fetuses, infants, and children exposed to BPA may be at increased risk for early-onset puberty, prostate, and breast cancer

Particulate Matter Air Pollution and Cardiovascular Disease: An Update to the Scientific Statement from the American Heart Association
Circulation 2010 Jun 1;121(21):2331-78
A scientific statement by the American Heart Association in 2004 reported that exposure to particulate matter air pollution contributes to cardiovascular morbidity and mortality. An updated American Heart Association statement in 2010 confirmed a causal relationship between particulate matter exposure and cardiovascular morbidity and mortality. The statement reported that such an exposure over several hours to weeks may trigger cardiovascular disease-related mortality and non-fatal events, whereas longer exposures over several years may further increase cardiovascular mortality risk and reduce life expectancy within highly-exposed populations by several months to years.

The Walkerton Tragedy
In May 2000, the drinking water system in the town of Walkerton, ON, became contaminated with *Escherichia coli* O157:H7 and *Campylobacter jejuni*.
Over 2,300 individuals became ill; 27 people developed hemolytic uremic syndrome and 7 individuals died in the outbreak
Source: Ministry of the Attorney General. Report of the Walkerton inquiry. Ontario, 2002

To Fluoridate or Not
At the recommended concentration of 0.8-1.0 mg/L, fluoride reduces cavities by 18-40%, and there is little risk of fluorosis unless other exposures (e.g. toothpaste, rinses, mouthwash, etc.) are swallowed. Opposition raises concerns that the intake is not easily controlled, and that children, and others may be more susceptible to health problems. However, public health experts strongly support fluoridation as an effective measure to prevent dental caries at the community level and reduce dental health inequities

Soil

Biological Hazards
- biological contamination: tetanus, *Pseudomonas*

Chemical Hazards
- contamination sources: rupture of underground storage tanks, use of pesticides and herbicides, percolation of contaminated water runoffs, leaching of wastes from landfills, dust from smelting and coal burning power plants, residue of industrial waste/development (e.g. urban agriculture), lead deposition, leakage of transformers
- most common chemicals: petroleum hydrocarbons, solvents, lead, pesticides, motor oil, other industrial waste products
- infants and toddlers at highest risk of exposure due to hand-mouth behaviours
- dependent on contaminant: leukemia, kidney damage, liver toxicity, neuromuscular blockade, developmental damage to the brain and nervous system, skin rash, eye irritation, headache, nausea, fatigue

Food

Biological Hazards

Honey and Botulism
Although exceedingly rare, infant botulism has been documented as a form of food poisoning from *C. botulinum* found in honey. When an infant swallows spores of this bacterium, they grow and produce a toxin in the baby's intestine. By the time an infant is 1, its gut has a healthy colony of "good" bacteria that prevents this from occurring

Table 11. Comparison of Select Biological Contaminants of Food and Effects on Human Health

	Source	Effects
Salmonella	Raw eggs, poultry, meat	GI symptoms
Campylobacter	Raw poultry, raw milk	Joint pain, GI symptoms
Escherichia coli	Various including meat, sprouts Primarily undercooked hamburger meat	Watery or bloody diarrhea Hemolytic uremic syndrome (especially children)
Listeria monocytogenes	Unpasteurized cheeses, prepared salads, cold cuts	Listeriosis: nausea, vomiting, fever, headache, rarely meningitis or encephalitis
Clostridium botulinum	Unpasteurized honey, canned foods	Dizziness, weakness, respiratory failure, GI symptoms: thirst, nausea, constipation
Prion (BSE*)	Beef and beef products	Creutzfeldt-Jakob disease

*BSE = bovine spongiform encephalopathy

Organic Foods
- Foods designated as "organic" in Canada must conform to the Organic Products Regulations enforced by the Canadian Food Inspection Agency
- Organic foods are not free of synthetic pesticide residues but typically contain smaller amounts compared to conventionally grown foods
- Currently, there has not been strong evidence to suggest that eating organic foods is safer or more nutritious compared to eating conventionally grown food
Source: Organic foods. *Ann Intern Med* 2012;157:348-66. Health Canada. Pesticides and food, 2011. UpToDate. Organic foods and children, 2009

- other biological food contaminants include
  - viruses, mould toxins (e.g. aflatoxin has been associated with liver cancer), parasites (e.g. Toxoplasmosis, tapeworm), paralytic shellfish poisoning (rare), genetically modified organisms (controversial as to health risks/benefits)

Chemical Hazards
- many persistent organic pollutants are fat-soluble and undergo bioamplification
- drugs (antibiotics, hormones)
- inadequately prepared herbal medications
- food additives and preservatives
  - nitrites highest in cured meats; can be converted to carcinogenic nitrosamines
  - sulphites commonly used as preservatives; associated with sulphite allergy (hives, nausea, shock)
- pesticide residues
  - older pesticides (e.g. DDT) have considerable human health effects
- polychlorinated biphenyls (PCBs)
  - effects (severe acne, numbness, muscle spasm, bronchitis) much more likely to be seen in occupationally exposed individuals than in the general population
- dioxins and furans
  - levels highest in fish and marine mammals, also present in breast milk can cause immunosuppression, liver disease, respiratory disease

Occupational Health

- a field involved in the prevention of illness or injury and the promotion of health in the work environment
- services encompass "health promotion and protection (primary prevention), disease prevention (secondary prevention), and treatment and rehabilitation (tertiary prevention)" (Shah)
- occupational disease may be more difficult to recognize than occupational injury

Taking an Occupational Health History

- current and previous duties at place of employment
- exposures
  - identification: screen for chemical, metal, dust, biological, and physical hazards as well as psychological stressors; review relevant workplace MSDS
  - assessment: duration, concentration, route, exposure controls (e.g. ventilation, personal protective equipment)
- temporal relationship: changes in symptoms in relationship to work environment
- presence of similar symptoms in co-workers
- non-work exposures: home, neighbourhood, hobbies

Occupational Hazards

Table 12. Occupational Hazards

Physical	Chemical	Biological	Psychosocial

• Trauma (e.g. fractures, lacerations)
• Noise (e.g. hearing loss)
• Temperature
  • Heat cramps, heat exhaustion, heat stroke
  • Hypothermia, frostbite
• Air pressure (barotrauma, decompression sickness)
• Ergonomic
  • Repetitive use/overuse injuries, excessive force, awkward postures, poorly designed physical work environment
  • Tenosynovitis, bursitis, carpal tunnel syndrome
• Radiation
  • Non-ionizing: visible light, infrared
  • Ionizing: UV, x-rays, γ rays
• Electricity
	• Organic solvents (e.g. benzene, methyl alcohol; most toxic is carbon tetrachloride)
	• Mineral dusts (e.g. silica leads to silicosis and predisposition to TB, asbestos leads to diffuse fibrosis and mesothelioma, coal leads to pneumoconiosis)
	• Heavy metals (e.g. nickel, cadmium, mercury, lead)
	• Gases (e.g. halogen gases, sulphur dioxide, carbon monoxide, nitrogen oxides)
	• Second-hand smoke (causal factor for lung cancer, lung disease, heart disease, asthma exacerbations; may be linked to miscarriage)
	• Skin diseases (major portion of compensations, e.g. contact dermatitis, occupational acne, pigmentation disorders)
		• Exposure to bacteria, viruses, fungi, protozoa, Rickettsia
		• Blood should be considered a potentially toxic substance due to blood-borne infectious diseases (e.g. HIV, hepatitis B)
		• Consider exposure to disease in endemic countries, travellers from endemic countries, or recent travel history in the setting of acute onset of symptoms (e.g. malaria, SARS, TB)
			• Workload stressors
			  • Responsibility
			  • Fear of job loss
			  • Geographical isolation
			  • Shift work
			  • Bullying
			  • Harassment (sexual/non-sexual)
			• Incurs high cost from absenteeism, poor productivity, mental illness (e.g. post-traumatic stress disorder)

Workplace Legislation

- universal across Canada for corporate responsibility in the workplace: due diligence, application of Workplace Hazardous Materials Information System (WHMIS), existence of joint health and safety committees in the workplace with representatives from workers and management
- jurisdiction in Canada is provincial (90% of Canadian workers), except for 16 federally regulated industries (e.g. airports, banks, highway transport) under the *Canada Labour Code*
- Ontario's *Occupational Health and Safety Act*
  - sets out rights of workers and duties of employers, procedures for workplace hazards, and law enforcement
  - workers have the right to
    - **participate** (e.g. have representatives on joint health and safety committees)
    - **know** (e.g. be trained and have information about workplace hazards)
    - **refuse work** (e.g. workers can decline tasks they feel are overly dangerous)
      - note: For some occupations, this right is restricted if, for example, danger/risk is normal part of work or refusal would endanger others (e.g. police, firefighters, some health care workers)
    - **stop work** (e.g. 'certified' workers can halt work they feel is dangerous to other workers)

Taking an Occupational Health Hx WHACS
What do you do?
How do you do it?
Are you concerned about any particular exposures on or off the job?
Co-workers or others with similar problems?
Satisfied with your job?
J Occup Environ Med 1998;40:680-684

Most Effective

Elimination
Physically remove hazard

e.g. driverless car

Substitution
Replace Hazard

e.g. replace with train

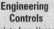

Engineering Controls
Isolate from Hazard

e.g. airbags

Administrative Controls
Change the way people work

e.g. traffic laws

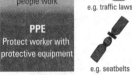

PPE
Protect worker with protective equipment

e.g. seatbelts

Least Effective ©Kristen Browne 2016

Figure 18. Hierarchy of controls for reduction of occupational exposures
Source: Modified from CDC. 2015. Hierarchy of controls.
http://www.cdc.gov/niosh/topics/hierarchy/

Ontario's *Workplace Safety and Insurance Act* (Each province will have their own similar legislation)
- Establishes Workplace Safety and Insurance Board (WSIB), an autonomous government agency that oversees workplace safety training and administers insurance for workers and employers
- WSIB decides benefits for workers, which may include reimbursement for
- Loss of earned income
- Non-economic loss (e.g. physical, functional, or psychological loss extending beyond the workplace)
- Loss of retirement income
- Health care expenses (e.g. first-aid, medical treatment)
- Survivor benefits (e.g. dependents and spouses can receive benefits)
- Employers pay for costs (e.g. no government funding)
- No-fault insurance (e.g. worker has no right to sue the employer) in return for guaranteed compensation for accepted claims
- Negligence is not considered a factor
- Physicians are required to provide the WSIB with information about a worker's health without a medical waiver once a claim is made
For more information: http://www.wsib.on.ca/en/community/WSIB

Occupational Health Statistics
- 1 in 68 employed workers in 2010 received workers compensation due to injury or harm on the job
- 4,405 fatal work injuries in the United States in 2013; rate = 3.2/100,000 workers

Source: Employment and Social Development Canada. Work-related injuries, 2015
U.S. Bureau of Labour Statistics. Census of Fatal Occupational Injuries Charts, 1992-2013, 2014

Information about worker's compensation at: http://www.awcbc.org/en/index.asp

- employers must take precautions to protect the health and safety of employees and investigate concerns
  - enforced by Ministry of Labour via inspectors
- *Health Protection and Promotion Act* (HPPA) (Ontario)
  - Medical Officer of Health has right to investigate and manage health hazards where workplace exposures may impact non-workers (e.g. community members living close to the work site)

Workplace Health Promotion and Protection

- pro-active preventative health measures can reduce workplace illness or injury
  - identifying workplace hazards (e.g. through material safety data sheets [MSDS])
  - assessing risk
  - reducing exposure : changes to work environment including elimination, substitution, and isolation of hazard (e.g. engineering controls) more effective than changes to how people work (e.g. administrative controls) and personal protective equipment

Workplace Disease Prevention and Identification

- avoid the development of disease with pro-active worker health surveillance
  - periodic examinations to facilitate diagnosis before symptoms develop
    - PFT for asthma (e.g. occupational dust exposure)
    - audiograms for hearing loss (e.g. occupational noise exposure)
  - substance misuse screening useful if concern surrounds decreased employee functioning

Workplace Treatment and Rehabilitation

- treatment of the disease or injury to facilitate safe and timely return to the workforce
- may require rehabilitation, retraining, change in job duties, and/or workers' compensation (WSIB)
- advise relevant authorities if necessary (e.g. report notifiable diseases to public health, conditions impeding driving to Ministry of Transportation, see *Other Reportable Conditions*, PH25)

Appendix – Mandatory Reporting

Reportable Diseases

As an essential part of the health system, physicians in Canada are required by law to report certain diseases to public health for the following reasons
1. to control the outbreak
   - if the disease presents an outbreak threat (e.g. measles, Salmonella, respiratory diseases in institutions)
2. to prevent spread
   - if the disease presents a significant threat to individuals or a subset of the population (e.g. Lassa Fever)
3. for surveillance
   - if the disease is preventable with immunization (e.g. polio, diphtheria, congenital rubella)
4. if infected individuals require education, treatment and/or partner notification (e.g. gonorrhea, TB)
5. reporting details (website, office etc.)
   - some are more urgent than others (must contact MOH)
   - physicians should also report unlisted diseases that appear in clusters

The following list is based on the reportable diseases in Ontario for 2015. Each province will have similar legislation

Note: Diseases marked * (and Influenza in institutions) should be reported immediately to the Medical Officer of Health by either telephone (24 hours a day, 7 days a week) or fax (Mon-Fri, 8:30 am – 4:30 pm only). Other diseases can be reported the next working day by fax, phone or mail.
Source: Health Protection and Promotion Act, O. Reg. 559/91, amended to O. Reg.49/07 (update)

Acquired Immunodeficiency
Syndrome (AIDS)
Acute flaccid paralysis <15 yr
Amoebiasis
Anthrax*

Botulism*
Brucellosis*

Campylobacter enteritis
Chancroid
Chickenpox (Varicella)
Chlamydia trachomatis infections
Cholera*
Clostridium difficile* associated disease (CDAD)
outbreaks in public hospitals
Creutzfeldt-Jakob Disease, all types
Cryptosporidiosis*
Cyclosporiasis*
Diphtheria*

Encephalitis*, including:
1. Primary, viral*
2. Post-infectious
3. Vaccine-related
4. Subacute sclerosing panencephalitis
5. Unspecified

Food poisoning, all causes*

Gastroenteritis, institutional outbreaks*
Giardiasis, except asymptomatic cases*
Gonorrhea

Haemophilus influenzae b disease, invasive*
Hantavirus pulmonary syndrome*
Hemorrhagic fevers*, including:
1. Ebola virus disease*
2. Marburg virus disease*
3. Other viral causes*
Hepatitis, viral*:
1. Hepatitis A*
2. Hepatitis B
3. Hepatitis C
Hep D is not listed in 2015 update

Herpes (neonatal) and HIV removed

Influenza

Lassa Fever*
Legionellosis*
Leprosy
Listeriosis*
Lyme Disease

Malaria
Measles*
Meningitis, acute*:
1. Bacterial*
2. Viral*
3. Other*
Meningococcal disease, invasive*
Mumps

Ophthalmia neonatorum

Paralytic shellfish poisoning
Paratyphoid fever*
Pertussis (whooping cough)
Plague*
Pneumococcal disease, invasive
Poliomyelitis, acute*
Psittacosis/Ornithosis

Q Fever*

Rabies*
Respiratory infection outbreaks in institutions*
Rubella*
Rubella, congenital syndrome

Salmonellosis
Severe Acute Respiratory Syndrome (SARS)*
Shigellosis*
Smallpox*
Streptococcal infections, Group A invasive*
Streptococcal infections, Group B neonatal
Syphilis

Tetanus
Trichinosis
Tuberculosis, active and latent
Tularemia*
Typhoid Fever*

Verotoxin-producing *E. coli* infection indicator conditions,
including Hemolytic Uremic Syndrome (HUS)*

West Nile Virus illness*, including:
1. West Nile fever*
2. West Nile neurological manifestations *

Yellow Fever*
Yersiniosis

Other Reportable Conditions

- in addition to reporting diseases, physicians have a legal responsibility to report certain conditions. The list below highlights some reportable conditions for Ontario, but is not exhaustive. See your jurisdiction's regulatory body for the full list

Child Abuse – to local Children's Aid Society (CAS)
- all child abuse and neglect where reasonable grounds to suspect exist (including physical harm, emotional harm, sexual harm, and neglect)
- duty to report is ongoing: if additional reasonable grounds are suspect, a further report to CAS is necessary

Unfit to Drive – to provincial Ministry of Transportation
- all patients with a medical condition (e.g. dementia, untreated epilepsy) that may impede their driving ability
- if a physician does not report and the driver gets into an accident, the physician may be held liable

Unfit to Fly – to federal Ministry of Transportation
- all patients believed to be flight crew members or air traffic controller with a medical or optometric condition that is likely to constitute a hazard to aviation safety

Gunshots Wounds – to local police service
- all patients with a gunshot or stab wounds
- self-inflicted knife wounds are not reportable

Source: CPSO. Mandatory and Permissive Reporting. 2012. Available from: http://www.cpso.on.ca/policies-publications/policy/mandatory-and-permissive-reporting

References

AFMC Primer on Population Health. Available from: http://phprimer.afmc.ca/.

Associated Faculties of Medicine of Canada (AFMC). Primer on public health (internet). AFMC, 2011. Virtual textbook available at: http://phprimer.afmc.ca.

Association of Workers' Compensation Boards of Canada. Available from: http://www.awcbc.org.

BMJ Updates Plus. Available from: http://plus.mcmaster.ca/evidenceupdates.

Braveman PA. Monitoring equity in health and health care: a conceptual framework. J Health Popul Nutr 2003;21:181-192.

Bureau of Labor Statistics. Available from: http://www.bls.gov.

Canada's National Occupational Health and Safety. Available from: http://www.canoshweb.org.

Canadian Centre for Occupational Health and Safety. Available from: http://www.ccohs.ca.

Canadian Food Inspection Agency. Available from: http://www.inspection.gc.ca.

Canadian Institute for Health Information. Available from: http://www.cihi.ca.

Canadian Medical Association. Available from: http://www.cma.ca.

Canadian Public Health Association. Available from: http://www.cpha.ca.

Canadian Public Health Association and WHO. Ottawa charter for health promotion. Ottawa: Health and Welfare Canada, 1986.

Canadian Society for International Health. Available from: http://www.csih.org.

Canadian Task Force on Preventative Health Care. Available from: http://www.canadiantaskforce.ca.

Center for Disease Control and Prevention. Available from: http://www.cdc.gov.

Clinical Evidence. Available from: http://www.clinicalevidence.com.

Hamilton N, Bhatti T. Integrated model of population health and health promotion. Ottawa: Health Promotion and Programs, 1996.

Health Canada. Available from: http://www.hc-sc.gc.ca.

Health Canada. Health and environment: partners for life. Ottawa: Minister of Public Works and Government Services Canada, 1997.

Health Protection and Promotion Act, R.S.O. 1990, c. H.7.

Health Protection and Promotion Act, R.S.O. 1990., c.H.7; O. Reg. 559/91, amended to O. Reg. 49/07.

Hennekens C, Buring J. Epidemiology in medicine. Philidelphia: Lippincott, Williams & Wilkins, 1987.

Hill AB. The environment and disease: association or causation? Proc Royal Soc Med 1965;58:295-300.

Hully SB, Cummings SR. Designing clinical research: an epidemiologic approach. Baltimore: Williams & Wilkins, 1988.

Institute for Population and Public Health, Canadian Institutes for Health Research. Available from: http://www.cihr-irsc.gc.ca/e/13970.html.

Intergovernmental Panel on Climate Change. Available from: http://www.ipcc.ch.

Kass NE. An ethics framework for public health. Am J Public Health 2001;91:1776-1782.

Kelsey JL, Whittemore AS, Evans AS, et al. Methods in observational epidemiology, 2nd ed. Oxford University Press, 1996.

Last JM. A dictionary of epidemiology, 4th ed. Oxford University Press, 2001.

McCurdy SA, Morrin LA, Memmott MM. Occupational history collection by third-year medical students during internal medicine and surgery inpatient clerkships. J Occup Environ Med 1998;40:680-684.

Medical Council of Canada. Available from: http://www.mcc.ca.

MedTerms. Available from: http://www.medterms.com.

National Advisory Committee on Immunization. Available from: http://www.phac-aspc.gc.ca/naci-ccni/.

O'Connor DR. Report of the Walkerton Inquiry: Part one and two. 2002.

Ontario Medical Association. Available from: https://www.oma.org/HealthPromotion/Pages/default.aspx.

Ontario Ministry of Labour Health and Safety. Available from: http://www.labour.gov.on.ca/english/hs/.

OVID EBM Reviews. Available from: http://gateway.ovid.com/ovidweb.cgi.

Pan-American Health Organization. Available from: http://www.paho.org/index.php.

Pier (ACP). Available from: http://www.pier.acponline.org.

Public Health Agency of Canada. Available from: http://www.phac-aspc.gc.ca/about_apropos/index-eng.php.

PubMed – Clinical Queries. Available from: http://www.ncbi.nlm.nih/gov/pubmed.

Sackett DL, Strauss SE, Richardson WS, et al. Evidence-based medicine: how to practice and teach EBM. 2nd ed. Toronto: Churchill, Livingstone, 2002.

Shah CP. Public health and preventive medicine in Canada, 5th ed. Toronto: Elsevier Canada, 2003.

Smith-Spangler C, Brandeau ML, Hunter GE, et al. Are organic foods safer or healthier than conventional alternatives?: a systematic review. Ann Intern Med 2012;157:348-366.

UpToDate. Available from: http://www.uptodate.com.

Users' Guide Series. Available from: http://www.jamaevidence.com/edguides.

WHO. World Health Report 2006. Available from: http://www.who.int/whr/2006/en/index.html.

Workplace Safety and Insurance Board. Available from: http://www.wsib.on.ca.

World Bank. Available from: http://www.worldbank.org.

PS Psychiatry

Ka Sing Paris Lai and **Cieran Tran**, chapter editors
Narayan Chatergoon and **Desmond She**, associate editors
Arnav Agarwal and **Quynh Huynh**, EBM editors
Dr. Chloe Leon, **Dr. Mary Preisman**, and **Dr. Oshrit Wanono**, staff editors

Diagnostic Criteria reprinted with permission from the
Diagnostic and Statistical Manual of Mental Disorders,
Fifth Edition. © 2013 American Psychiatric Association

Acronyms

5-HT	serotonin	DBT	dialectical behavioural therapy	MDD	major depressive disorder	ODD	oppositional defiant disorder
ACh	acetylcholine	DZ	dizygotic	MDE	major depressive episode	PD	personality disorder
ACT	assertive community treatment	ECT	electroconvulsive therapy	MET	motivational enhancement therapy	PDD	pervasive developmental disorder
ADHD	attention deficit hyperactivity disorder	EPS	extrapyramidal symptoms	MSE	mental status examination	PTSD	post-traumatic stress disorder
AN	anorexia nervosa	ERP	exposure with response	MST	magnetic stimulation therapy	rTMS	repetitive transcranial magnetic stimulation
ASD	autism spectrum disorder		prevention	MZ	monozygotic	SGA	second generation antipsychotics
ASPD	antisocial personality disorder	EtOH	ethanol/alcohol	NA	Narcotics Anonymous	SNRI	serotonin and norepinephrine reuptake inhibitors
BN	bulimia nervosa	GAD	generalized anxiety disorder	NMS	neuroleptic malignant syndrome	SS	serotonin syndrome
CBT	cognitive behavioural therapy	GMC	general medical condition	NOS	not otherwise specified	SSRI	selective serotonin reuptake inhibitor
CD	conduct disorder	IPT	interpersonal therapy	OCD	obsessive-compulsive disorder	TCA	tricyclic antidepressant
CRA	community reinforcement approach	MAOI	monoamine oxidase inhibitor	OCPD	obsessive-compulsive personality disorder	TD	tardive dyskinesia
CT	cognitive therapy						
CTO	community treatment order						
DA	dopamine						

Psychiatric Assessment

History

Identifying Data
- necessary: name, sex, age, ethnicity, marital status, occupation/source of financial support, place and type of residency
- adjunct: makeup of household, religion, education, referral source, known or unknown to treatment team

Reliability of Patient as a Historian
- indicate if, and for what content; utilize collateral source (e.g. parent, teacher) if patient unable/unwilling to cooperate

Chief Complaint
- in patient's own words, duration

History of Present Illness
- reason for seeking help (that day), current symptoms (onset, duration and course), stressors, supports, functional status, relevant associated symptoms (pertinent positives and negatives)
- safety screen: is the patient endangering self or others? dependents at home (e.g. children, pets), ability to drive safely, ability to care for self (e.g. eating, hygiene, taking medications)

Psychiatric Functional Inquiry
- mood: depression, mania
- anxiety: worries, panic attacks, phobias, history of trauma
- obsessive-compulsive: obsessions, compulsions
- psychosis: hallucinations, delusions
- risk assessment: suicidal ideation, plan, intent, history of attempts (see *Suicide*, PS4)
- organic: EtOH/drug use or withdrawal, illness, dementia

Past Psychiatric History
- all previous psychiatric diagnoses, psychiatric contacts, treatments (pharmacological and non-pharmacological), and hospitalizations
- include past suicide attempts, substance use/abuse, and problems/encounters with the legal system

Past Medical/Surgical History
- all medical, surgical, neurological (e.g. head trauma, seizures), and psychosomatic illnesses
- current medications, allergies

Family Psychiatric/Medical History
- family members: ages, occupations, personalities, medical or genetic illnesses and treatments, relationships with parents/siblings
- family psychiatric history: any past or current psychiatric illnesses and hospitalizations, suicide, substance abuse

Past Personal/Developmental History (as relevant)
- prenatal and perinatal history (desired vs. unwanted pregnancy, maternal and fetal health, domestic violence, maternal substance use and exposures, complications of pregnancy/delivery)
- early childhood to age 3 (developmental milestones, activity/attention level, family stability, attachment figures)
- middle childhood to age 11 (school performance, peer relationships, fire-setting, stealing, incontinence)
- late childhood to adolescence (drugs/alcohol, legal problems, peer and family relationships)
- history of physical or sexual abuse
- adulthood (education, occupations, relationships)
- personality before current illness, recent changes in personality
- psychosexual history (puberty, first sexual encounter, romantic relationships, gender roles, sexual dysfunction)

Mental Status Exam

General Appearance

- dress, grooming, posture, gait, physical characteristics, body habitus, apparent vs. chronological age, facial expression (e.g. sad, suspicious), tattoos, piercings (if numerous or atypical), acute distress or relaxed

Behaviour

- psychomotor activity (agitation, retardation), abnormal movements or lack thereof (tremors, akathisia, tardive dyskinesia, paralysis), attention level and eye contact, attitude toward examiner (ability to interact, level of cooperation)

Speech

- rate (e.g. pressured, slowed), rhythm/fluency, volume, tone, articulation, quantity, spontaneity

Mood and Affect

- mood: subjective emotional state (in patient's own words)
- affect: objective emotional state inferred from emotional responses to stimuli; described in terms of
  - quality (euthymic, depressed, elevated, anxious, irritable)
  - range (full, restricted, flat, blunted)
  - stability (fixed, labile)
  - mood congruence (inferred by reader by comparing mood and affect descriptions)
  - appropriateness to thought content
- some clinicians use 0-10 scales when rating mood to help get a subjective norm for each patient that can help establish changes over time and with treatment

Thought Process/Form

- coherence (coherent, incoherent)
- logic (logical, illogical)
- stream
  - goal-directed: clearly answers questions in a linear, organized, logical fashion
  - circumstantial: speech that is indirect and delayed in reaching its goal; eventually comes back to the point
  - tangential: speech is oblique or irrelevant; does not come back to the original point
  - loosening of associations/derailment: illogical shifting between topics
  - flight of ideas: quickly skipping from one idea to another where the ideas are marginally connected, usually associated with mania
  - word salad: jumble of words lacking meaning or logical coherence
- perseveration: repetition of the same verbal or motor response to stimuli
- echolalia: repetition of phrases or words spoken by someone else
- thought blocking: sudden cessation of flow of thought and speech
- clang associations: speech based on sound such as rhyming or punning
- neologism: use of novel words or of existing words in a novel fashion

Thought Content

- suicidal ideation/homicidal ideation
  - frequency and pervasiveness of thoughts, formulation of plan, means to plan, intent, active vs. passive, protective factors
- preoccupations, ruminations: reflections/thoughts at length, not fixed or false
- obsession: recurrent and persistent thought, impulse, or image which is intrusive or inappropriate and unwanted
  - cannot be stopped by logic or reason
  - causes marked anxiety and distress
  - common themes: contamination, orderliness, sexual, pathological doubt/worry/guilt
- magical thinking: belief that thinking something will make it happen; normal in children and certain cultures
- ideas of reference: similar to delusion of reference, but less fixed (the reality of the belief is questioned)
- overvalued ideas: unusual/odd beliefs that are not of delusional proportions
- first rank symptoms of schizophrenia: thought insertion/withdrawal/broadcasting
- delusion: a fixed false belief that is out of keeping with a person's cultural or religious background and is firmly held despite incontrovertible proof to the contrary

Perception

- hallucination: sensory perception in the absence of external stimuli that is similar in quality to a true perception
  - auditory (most common), visual, gustatory, olfactory, tactile
- illusion: misperception of a real external stimulus (such as mistaking a coat on a rack as a person late at night)
- depersonalization: change in self-awareness such that the person feels unreal, distant, or detached from his or her body, and/or unable to feel emotion
- derealization: feeling that the world/outer environment is unreal

Mental Status Exam

ASEPTIC
Appearance and behaviour
Speech
Emotion (mood and affect)
Perception
Thought content and process
Insight and judgment
Cognition

The MSE is analogous to the physical exam. It focuses on current signs, affect, behaviour, and cognition

Spectrum of Affect
Full > Restricted > Blunted > Flat

There is poor correlation between clinical impression of suicide risk and frequency of attempts

Cognitive Assessment
Use MMSE to assess
- Orientation (time and place)
- Memory (immediate and delayed recall)
- Attention and concentration
- Language (comprehension, reading, writing, repetition, naming)
- Spatial ability (intersecting pentagons)
Gross screen for cognitive dysfunction:
Total score is out of 30; <26 abnormal, 20-26 mild, 10-19 moderate, <10 severe

The key to differentiating obsessions and delusions is that obsessions are usually ego dystonic, meaning unwanted and not fitting in with a person's goals and self-image, while delusions are ego syntonic

Delusions
- Persecutory: belief that others are trying to cause harm to you
- Reference: interpreting publicly known events/celebrities as having direct reference to you
- Erotomania: belief that another is in love with you
- Grandiose: belief that he or she has special powers, talents or abilities
- Religious: belief of receiving instructions/ powers from a higher being; of being a higher being
- Somatic: belief that you have a physical disorder/defect
- Nihilistic: belief that things do not exist; a sense that everything is unreal

Cognition
- level of consciousness (alert, reduced, obtunded)
- orientation: time, place, person
- memory: immediate, recent, remote
- global evaluation of intellect (below average, average, above average, in keeping with person's education)
- intellectual functions: attention, concentration, calculation, abstraction (proverb interpretation, similarities test), language, communication
- MMSE/MOCA useful as standard screening assessments of cognition

Insight
- patient's ability to realize that he or she has a physical or mental illness and to understand its implications (none limited, partial, full)

Judgment
- patient's ability to understand relationships between facts and draw conclusions that determine one's actions

Assessing Insight and Judgment

Insight
- Do you think that you have a mental illness?
- Why are you taking this medication?
- Why are you in the hospital?

Judgment
Can be observed from collected history and patient's appearance and actions
- Is he/she dressed appropriately for the weather?
- Is he/she acting appropriately in the given situation?
- Is he/she taking care of self and/or dependents?

Assessment and Plan

Historical Multiaxial Model
- since DSM-5, this Model is no longer used for psychiatric diagnosis. Instead, relevant psychiatric and medical diagnoses are simply listed. Nevertheless, we offer it here as a possible framework for psychiatric patient assessment, as many physicians still employ it

Multiaxial Assessment
- Axis I: differential diagnosis of DSM-5 clinical disorders
- Axis II: personality disorders, developmental disability
- Axis III: general medical conditions potentially relevant to understanding/management of the mental disorder
- Axis IV: psychosocial and environmental issues
- Axis V: Global Assessment of Functioning (GAF, 0 to 100) incorporating effects of axes I to IV

After History and MSE, the assessment and plan is recorded

Assessment/Problem Formulation
- identify predominant symptom cluster (mood, anxiety, psychosis, organic) causing the most distress/interference, persist when other symptom categories not present (e.g. psychosis in the absence of mood symptoms)
- dominating symptoms will direct differential
- consider current issues as they relate to an individual's factors in three domains: biological, psychological, and social
- for each category: predisposing, precipitating, perpetuating, and protecting factors are considered

Always rule out substance use and organic causes before considering psychiatric causes

Approach to Management
- consider short-term and long-term, and three types: biological (e.g. pharmacotherapy), psychological (e.g. CBT), and social (e.g. support group)

Suicide

Importance
- must be screened for in every encounter; part of risk assessment along with violent/homicidal ideation

Approach
- <u>ask every patient</u> – e.g. "Have you had any thoughts of wanting to harm or kill yourself?"
- classify ideation
  - passive ideation: would rather not be alive but has no active plan for suicide
    - e.g. "I'd rather not wake up" or "I would not mind if a car hit me"
  - active ideation
    - e.g. "I think about killing myself"
- assess risk
  - plan: "Do you have a plan as to how you would end your life?"
  - intent: "Do you think you would actually carry out this plan?" "If not, why not?"
  - past attempts: highest risk if previous attempt in past year
    - ask about lethality, outcome, medical intervention
- assess suicidal ideation
  - onset and frequency of thoughts: "When did this start?" or "How often do you have these thoughts?"
  - control over suicidal ideation: "How do you cope when you have these thoughts?" "Could you call someone for help?"
  - intention: "Do you want to end your life?" or "Do you wish to kill yourself?"
  - intended lethality: "What do you think would happen if you actually took those pills?"
  - access to means: "How will you get a gun?" or "Which bridge do you think you would go to?"
  - time and place: "Have you picked a date and place? Is it in an isolated location?"
  - provocative factors: "What makes you feel worse (e.g. being alone)?"

- protective factors: "What keeps you alive (e.g. friends, family, pets, faith, therapist)?"
- final arrangements: "Have you written a suicide note? Made a will? Given away your belongings?"
- practiced suicide or aborted attempts: "Have you ever put the gun to your head?" "Held the medications in your hand?" "Stood at the bridge?"
- ambivalence: "I wonder if there is a part of you that wants to live, given that you came here for help?"

Assessment of Suicide Attempt
- setting (isolated vs. others present/chance of discovery)
- planned vs. impulsive attempt, triggers/stressors
- substance use/intoxication
- medical attention (brought in by another person vs. brought in by self to ED)
- time lag from suicide attempt to ED arrival
- expectation of lethality, dying
- reaction to survival (guilt/remorse vs. disappointment/self-blame)

Epidemiology
- attempted:completed = 20:1
- M:F = 1:4 for attempts, 3:1 for completed

Risk Factors
- epidemiologic factors
  - age: increases after age 14, second most common cause of death for ages 15-24, highest rates of completion in persons >65 yr
  - sex: male
  - race/ethnic background: white or Native Canadians
  - marital status: widowed/divorced
  - living situation: alone; no children <18 yr old in the household
  - other: stressful life events, access to firearms
- psychiatric disorders
  - mood disorders (15% lifetime risk in depression; higher in bipolar)
  - anxiety disorders (especially panic disorder)
  - schizophrenia (10-15% risk)
  - substance abuse (especially alcohol – 15% lifetime risk)
  - eating disorders (5% lifetime risk)
  - adjustment disorder
  - conduct disorder
  - personality disorders (borderline, antisocial)
- past history
  - prior suicide attempt
  - family history of suicide attempt/completion

Clinical Presentation
- symptoms associated with suicide
  - hopelessness
  - anhedonia
  - insomnia
  - severe anxiety
  - impaired concentration
  - psychomotor agitation
  - panic attacks

Management
- proper documentation of the clinical encounter and rationale for management is essential
- higher risk (hospitalization needs to be strongly considered)
  - patients with a plan and intention to act on the plan, access to lethal means, recent social stressors, and symptoms suggestive of a psychiatric disorder
  - do not leave patient alone; remove potentially dangerous objects from room
  - if patient refuses to be hospitalized, complete form for involuntary admission (Form 1)
- lower risk
  - patients who are not actively suicidal, with no plan or access to lethal means
  - discuss protective factors and supports in their life, remind them of what they live for, promote survival skills that helped them through previous suicide attempts
  - make a safety plan that could include an agreement that they will:
    - not harm themselves
    - avoid alcohol, drugs, and situations that may trigger suicidal thoughts
    - follow-up with you at a designated time
    - contact a health care worker, call a crisis line, or go to an emergency department if they feel unsafe or if their suicidal feelings return or intensify
- depression: consider hospitalization if symptoms severe or if psychotic features are present; otherwise outpatient treatment with good supports and SSRIs/SNRIs
- alcohol-related: usually resolves with abstinence for a few days; if not, suspect depression
- personality disorders: crisis intervention, may or may not hospitalize
- schizophrenia/psychosis: hospitalization might be necessary
- parasuicide/self-mutilation: long-term psychotherapy with brief crisis intervention when necessary

Suicide Risk Factors

SAD PERSONS
Sex (male)
Age >60 yr old
Depression
Previous attempts
Ethanol abuse
Rational thinking loss (delusions, hallucinations, hopelessness)
Suicide in family
Organized plan
No spouse (no support systems)
Serious illness, intractable pain

Suicidal Ideation Assessment
- Asking patients about suicide will not give them the idea or the incentive to commit suicide
- The best predictor of completed suicide is a history of attempted suicide
- The most common psychiatric disorders associated with completed suicide are mood disorders and alcohol abuse

Psychotic Disorders

Definition

- characterized by a significant impairment in reality testing
- delusions or hallucinations (with/without insight into their pathological nature)
- behaving in a disorganized way so that it is reasonable to infer that reality testing is disturbed

Delusions: fixed, false beliefs
Hallucinations: perceptual experiences without an external stimulus

Duration of Time Differentiates the following 3 Psychotic Disorders

Brief Psychotic Disorder <1 month	Schizophreniform Disorder 1-6 months	Schizophrenia >6 months

Figure 1. Differentiating psychotic disorders with duration

Differential Diagnosis of Psychosis

Approach

- differentiate among psychotic disorders and distinguish them from other primary diagnoses with psychotic features
- consider symptoms, persistence, and time
- symptoms: what symptoms exist? The primary diagnosis needs full criteria to be met
  - mood: depressive episodes with psychotic features, manic episodes with psychotic features
  - psychotic: consider symptoms in Criterion A of schizophrenia, such as delusions, hallucinations, disorganized speech, grossly disorganized/catatonic behaviour, negative symptoms (i.e. diminished emotional expression or avolition)
- persistence: is there a time when certain symptom clusters are present without other clusters?
  - e.g. if there is a period of time with mood symptoms but not psychotic symptoms, consider mood disorder
  - e.g. if two weeks where psychotic symptoms persist in the absence of mood symptoms, consider schizoaffective disorder
- time: how long have the symptoms been present?

Differential

- Primary psychotic disorders: schizophrenia, schizophreniform, brief psychotic, schizoaffective, delusional disorder
- Mood disorders: depression with psychotic features, bipolar disorder (manic or depressive episode with psychotic features)
- Personality disorders: schizotypal, schizoid, borderline, paranoid, obsessive-compulsive
- General medical conditions: tumour, head trauma, dementia, delirium, metabolic, infection, stroke, temporal lobe epilepsy
- Substance-induced psychosis: intoxication or withdrawal, prescribed medications, toxins

Table 1. Differentiating Psychotic Disorders

Disorder	Psychotic Symptoms	Duration
Brief Psychotic Disorder	≥1 positive symptoms of criterion A	<1 mo
Schizophreniform Disorder	Criterion A	1-6 mo
Schizophrenia	Criterion A	>6 mo
Schizoaffective Disorder	Criterion A + major mood episode, but ≥2 wk psychotic without mood symptoms	>1 mo
Delusional Disorder	Non-bizarre delusions, hallucinations	>1 mo
2° to Substance Intoxication/Withdrawal	Delusions or hallucinations	During intoxication/withdrawal, not >1 mo without use
2° to Mood Disorder	Mood symptoms dominant + delusions/hallucinations (mood congruent)	Psychosis may be present for the duration of the mood episode

Schizophrenia

Management of Acute Psychosis and Mania

- Ensure safety of self, patient, and other patients
- Have an exit strategy
- Decrease stimulation
- Assume a non-threatening stance
- IM medications (benzodiazepine + antipsychotic) often needed as patient may refuse oral medication
- Physical restraints may be necessary
- Do not use antidepressants or stimulants

DSM-5 Diagnostic Criteria for Schizophrenia

Reprinted with permission from the Diagnostic and Statistical Manual of Mental Disorders, 5th ed. 2013. American Psychiatric Association

A. two (or more) of the following, each present for a significant portion of time during a 1 mo period (or less if successfully treated). At least one of these must be (1), (2), or (3)
   1. delusions
   2. hallucinations
   3. disorganized speech (e.g. frequent derailment or incoherence)
   4. grossly disorganized or catatonic behaviour
   5. negative symptoms (i.e. diminished emotional expression or avolition)
B. decreased level of function: for a significant portion of time since onset, one or more major areas affected (e.g. work, interpersonal relations, self-care) is markedly decreased (or if childhood/adolescent onset, failure to achieve expected level)
C. at least 6 mo of continuous signs of the disturbance. Must include at least 1 mo of symptoms (or less if successfully treated) that meet Criterion A (i.e. active-phase symptoms) and may include periods of prodromal or residual symptoms (during which, disturbance may manifest by only negative symptoms or by two or more Criterion A symptoms present in an attenuated form (e.g. odd beliefs, unusual perceptual experiences)
D. rule out schizoaffective disorder and depressive or bipolar disorder with psychotic features because either 1) no major depressive or manic episodes have occurred concurrently with the active-phase symptoms, or 2) if mood episodes have occurred during active-phase symptoms, they have been present for a minority of the total duration of the active and residual periods of the illness
E. rule out other causes: GMC, substances (e.g. drug of abuse, medication)
F. if history of autism spectrum disorder or communication disorder of childhood onset, the additional diagnosis of schizophrenia is made only if prominent delusions or hallucinations are also present for at least 1 mo (or less if successfully treated)

- **specifiers:** type of episode (e.g. first episode, multiple episodes, continuous), with catatonia, current severity based on quantitative assessment of primary symptoms of psychosis (in acute episode, in partial remission, in full remission)

Disorganized Behaviours in Schizophrenia

- Catatonic stupor: fully conscious, but immobile, mute, and unresponsive
- Catatonic excitement: uncontrolled and aimless motor activity, maintaining bizarre positions for a long time
- Stereotypy: repeated but non-goal-directed movement (e.g. rocking)
- Mannerisms: goal-directed activities that are odd or out of context (e.g. grimacing)
- Echopraxia: imitates movements and gestures of others
- Automatic obedience: carries out simple commands in robot-like fashion
- Negativism: refuses to cooperate with simple requests for no apparent reason
- Inappropriate affect, neglect of self-care, other odd behaviours (random shouting)

Epidemiology
- prevalence: 0.3-0.7%, M:F = 1:1
- mean age of onset: females late-20s; males early- to mid-20s
- suicide risk: 10% die by suicide, 30% attempt suicide

Etiology
- multifactorial: disorder is a result of interaction between both biological and environmental factors
  - genetic: 40% concordance in monozygotic (MZ) twins; 46% if both parents have schizophrenia; 10% of dizygotic (DZ) twins, siblings, children affected; vulnerable genes include Disrupted-in-Schizophrenia 1 (DISC1); neuregulin 1 (NRG 1); dystrobrevin binding protein / dysbindin (DTNBP1); catechol-O-methyltransferase (COMT); d-amino acid oxidase activator (DAOA); metabotropic glutamate receptor 3 (GRM3); and brain-derived neurotrophic factor (BDNF)
  - neurochemistry ("dopamine hypothesis"): excess activity in the mesolimbic dopamine pathway may mediate the positive symptoms of psychosis, while decreased dopamine in the prefrontal cortex may mediate negative and cognitive symptoms. GABA, glutamate, and ACh dysfunction are also thought to be involved
  - neuroanatomy: decreased frontal lobe function; asymmetric temporal/limbic function; decreased basal ganglia function; subtle changes in thalamus, cortex, corpus callosum, and ventricles; cytoarchitectural abnormalities
  - neuroendocrinology: abnormal growth hormone, prolactin, cortisol, and ACTH
  - neuropsychology: global defects seen in attention, language, and memory suggest disrupted connectivity of neural networks
  - environmental: indirect evidence of cannabis use, geographical variance, winter season of birth, obstetrical complications, and prenatal viral exposure

Pathophysiology
- neurodegenerative theory: natural history may be a rapid or gradual decline in function and ability to communicate
  - glutamate system may mediate progressive degeneration by excitotoxic mechanism which leads to production of free radicals
- neurodevelopmental theory: abnormal development of the brain from prenatal life
  - neurons fail to migrate correctly, make inappropriate connections, and apoptose in later life

Comorbidity
- substance-related disorders
- anxiety disorders
- reduced life expectancy secondary to medical cormobidities (e.g. obesity, diabetes, metabolic syndrome, CV/pulmonary disease)

Management of Schizophrenia
- biological / somatic
  - acute treatment and maintenance: antipsychotics (haloperidol, risperidone, olanzipine, paliperidone; clozapine if refractory); often regiments of IM q2-4 wk used in severe cases to ensure compliance
  - adjunctive: ± mood stabilizers (for aggression/impulsiveness - lithium, valproate, carbamazepine) ± anxiolytics ± ECT
  - treat for at least 1-2 years after the first episode, at least 5 years after multiple episodes (relapse causes severe deterioration)
- psychosocial
  - psychotherapy (individual, family, group), supportive, CBT (see Table 14, PS41)
  - ACT (Assertive Community Treatment): mobile mental health teams that provide individualized treatment in the community and help patients with medication adherence, basic living skills, social support, job placements, resources
  - social skills training, employment programs, disability benefits
  - housing (group home, boarding home, transitional home)

Course and Prognosis
- majority of individuals display some type of prodromal phase
- course is variable: some individuals have exacerbations and remissions while others remain chronically ill; accurate prediction of the long-term outcome is not possible
- negative symptoms may be prominent early in the illness and may become more prominent and more disabling later on; positive symptoms appear and typically diminish with treatment
- over time: 1/3 improve, 1/3 remain the same, 1/3 worsen

Relationship Between Duration of Untreated Psychosis (DUP) and Outcome in First-Episode Schizophrenia
Am J Psychiatry 2005;162:1785-1804
Purpose: To review the association between DUP and symptom severity at first treatment contact, and between DUP and treatment outcomes.
Study Characteristics: Critical review and meta-analysis of 43 studies with 4,177 patients.
Participants: Patients with non-affective psychotic disorders at or close to first treatment.
Results: Shorter DUP was associated with greater response to antipsychotic treatment, as measured by global psychopathology, positive symptoms, negative symptoms, and functional outcomes. At the time of treatment initiation, longer DUP was associated with the severity of negative symptoms but not with the severity of positive symptoms, global psychopathology, or neurocognitive function.
Conclusions: DUP may be a potentially modifiable prognostic factor.

Good Prognostic Factors
- Acute onset
- Shorter duration of prodrome
- Female gender
- Good cognitive functioning
- Good premorbid functioning
- No family history
- Presence of affective symptoms
- Absence of structural brain abnormalities
- Good response to drugs
- Good support system

Schizophreniform Disorder

Diagnosis
- criteria A, D, and E of schizophrenia are met; an episode of the disorder lasts for at least 1 mo but less than 6 mo
- if the symptoms have extended past 6 mo the diagnosis becomes schizophrenia
- **specifiers:** with/without good prognostic features (e.g. acute onset, confusion, good premorbid functioning, absence of blunt/flat affect), with catatonia, current severity based on quantitative assessment of primary symptoms of psychosis

Treatment
- similar to acute schizophrenia

Prognosis
- better than schizophrenia; begins and ends more abruptly; good pre- and post-morbid function

Brief Psychotic Disorder

Diagnosis
- criteria A1-A4, D, and E of schizophrenia are met; an episode of the disorder lasts for at least 1 d, but less than 1 mo with eventual full return to premorbid level of functioning
- **specifiers:** with/without marked stressors, with postpartum onset, with catatonia, current severity
- can occur after a stressful event or postpartum (see *Postpartum Mood Disorders*, PS12)

Treatment
- secure environment, antipsychotics, anxiolytics

Prognosis
- good, self-limiting, should return to pre-morbid function within 1 mo

Schizoaffective Disorder

DSM-5 Diagnostic Criteria for Schizoaffective Disorder
Reprinted with permission from the Diagnostic and Statistical Manual of Mental Disorders, 5th ed. 2013. American Psychiatric Association
A. concurrent psychosis (criterion A of schizophrenia) and major mood episode - uninterrupted period of illness
B. delusions or hallucinations for 2 or more wk in the absence of a major mood episode during the lifetime duration of the illness
C. major mood episode symptoms are present for the majority of the total duration of the active and residual periods of the illness
D. the disturbance is not attributable to the effects of a substance or another medical condition
- **specifiers:** bipolar type, depressive type, with catatonia, type of episode, severity

Epidemiology
- one-third as prevalent as schizophrenia; schizoaffective disorder bipolar type more common in young adults, schizoaffective disorder depressive type more common in older adults
- depressive symptoms correlated with higher suicide risk

Treatment
- antipsychotics, mood stabilizers, antidepressants

Prognosis
- between that of schizophrenia and of mood disorder

Non-bizarre delusions involve situations that could occur in real life (e.g. being followed, poisoned, loved at a distance)

Delusional Disorder

DSM-5 Diagnostic Criteria for Delusional Disorder
Reprinted with permission from the Diagnostic and Statistical Manual of Mental Disorders, 5th ed. 2013. American Psychiatric Association
A. the presence of one (or more) delusions with a duration of 1 mo or longer
B. criterion A for schizophrenia has never been met
  Note: hallucinations, if present, are not prominent and are related to the delusional theme
C. apart from the impact of the delusion(s) or its ramifications, functioning is not markedly impaired, and behaviour is not obviously bizarre or odd
D. if manic or major depressive episodes have occurred, these have been brief relative to the duration of the delusional periods
E. the disturbance is not attributable to the physiological effects of a substance or another medical condition and is not better explained by another mental disorder
- **subtypes:** erotomanic, grandiose, jealous, persecutory, somatic, mixed, unspecified
- **further specify:** bizarre content, type of episode (e.g. first episode, multiple episode), severity

Treatment
- psychotherapy, antipsychotics, antidepressants

Prognosis
- chronic, unremitting course but high level of functioning; a portion will progress to schizophrenia

Mood Disorders

Definitions
- accurate diagnosis of a mood disorder requires a careful past medical and psychiatric history to detect past mood episodes and to rule out whether these episodes were secondary to substance use, a medical condition, a loss, etc
- mood episodes represent a combination of symptoms comprising a predominant mood state that is abnormal in quality or duration (e.g. major depressive, manic, mixed, hypomanic). DSM-5 Criteria for mood episodes are listed below
- types of mood disorders include
  - depressive (major depressive disorder, persistent depressive disorder)
  - bipolar (bipolar I/II disorder, cyclothymia)
  - secondary to general medical condition, substances, medications, other psychiatric issue

Medical Workup of Mood Disorder
- routine screening: physical exam, CBC, thyroid function test, extended electrolytes, urinalysis, drug screen, medications list
- additional screening: neurological consultation, chest X-ray, ECG, CT head

Mood Episodes

DSM-5 Diagnostic Criteria for Major Depressive Episode
Reprinted with permission from the Diagnostic and Statistical Manual of Mental Disorders, 5th ed. 2013. American Psychiatric Association

A. ≥5 of the following symptoms have been present during the same 2 wk period and represent a change from previous functioning; at least one of the symptoms is either 1) depressed mood or 2) loss of interest or pleasure (anhedonia)
   Note: do not include symptoms that are clearly attributable to another medical condition
   - depressed mood most of the day, nearly every day, as indicated by either subjective report or observation made by others
   - markedly diminished interest or pleasure in all, or almost all, activities most of the day, nearly every day
   - significant and unintentional weight loss/weight gain, or decrease/increase in appetite nearly every day
   - insomnia or hypersomnia nearly every day
   - psychomotor agitation or retardation nearly every day
   - fatigue or loss of energy nearly every day
   - feelings of worthlessness or excessive or inappropriate guilt (which may be delusional) nearly every day (not merely self-reproach or guilt about being sick)
   - diminished ability to think or concentrate, or indecisiveness, nearly every day
   - recurrent thoughts of death (not just fear of dying), recurrent suicidal ideation without a specific plan, or a suicide attempt or a specific plan for committing suicide
B. the symptoms cause clinically significant distress or impairment in social, occupational, or other important areas of functioning
C. the episode is not attributable to the direct physiological effects of a substance or a GMC

Criteria for Depression (≥5)

MSIGECAPS
Mood: depressed
Sleep: increased/decreased
Interest: decreased
Guilt
Energy: decreased
Concentration: decreased
Appetite: increased/decreased
Psychomotor: agitation/retardation
Suicidal ideation

DSM-5 Criteria for Manic Episode
Reprinted with permission from the Diagnostic and Statistical Manual of Mental Disorders, 5th ed. 2013. American Psychiatric Association

A. a distinct period of abnormally and persistently elevated, expansive, or irritable mood and abnormally and persistently increased goal-directed activity or energy, lasting ≥1 wk and present most of the day, nearly every day (or any duration if hospitalization is necessary)
B. during the period of mood disturbance and increased energy or activity, ≥3 of the following symptoms have persisted (4 if the mood is only irritable) and have been present to a significant degree and represent a noticeable change from usual behaviour
   - inflated self-esteem or grandiosity
   - decreased need for sleep (e.g. feels rested after only 3 h of sleep)
   - more talkative than usual or pressure to keep talking
   - flight of ideas or subjective experience that thoughts are racing
   - distractibility (i.e. attention too easily drawn to unimportant or irrelevant external stimuli)
   - increase in goal-directed activity (either socially, at work or school, or sexually) or psychomotor agitation
   - excessive involvement in pleasurable activities that have a high potential for painful consequences (e.g. engaging in unrestrained shopping sprees, sexual indiscretions, or foolish business investments)
C. the mood disturbance is sufficiently severe to cause marked impairment in social or occupational functioning or to necessitate hospitalization to prevent harm to self or others, or there are psychotic features
D. the episode is not attributable to the physiological effects of a substance or another medical condition

Criteria for Mania (≥3)

GST PAID
Grandiosity
Sleep (decreased need)
Talkative
Pleasurable activities, Painful consequences
Activity
Ideas (flight of)
Distractible

Note: A full manic episode that emerges during antidepressant treatment but persists at a fully syndromal level beyond the physiological effect of that treatment is sufficient evidence for a manic episode, and therefore, a bipolar I diagnosis
Note: Criteria A-D constitute a manic episode. At least one lifetime manic episode is required for the diagnosis of bipolar I disorder

Hypomanic Episode
- criterion A and B of a manic episode is met, but duration is ≥4 d
- episode associated with an uncharacteristic change in functioning that is observable by others but not severe enough to cause marked impairment in social or occupational functioning or to necessitate hospitalization
- absence of psychotic features (if these are present the episode is, by definition, manic)

Mixed Features
- an episode specifier in bipolar or depression that indicates the presence of both depressive and manic symptoms concurrently, classified by the disorder and primary mood episode component (e.g. bipolar disorder, current episode manic, with mixed features)
- clinical importance due to increased suicide risk
- if found in patient diagnosed with major depression, high index of suspicion for bipolar disorder
- while meeting the full criteria for a major depressive episode, the patient has on most days ≥3 of criteria B for a manic episode
- while meeting the full criteria for a manic/hypomanic episode, the patient has on most days ≥3 of criteria A for a depressive episode (the following criterion A cannot count: psychomotor agitation, insomnia, difficulties concentrating, weight changes)

Depressive Disorders

MAJOR DEPRESSIVE DISORDER

DSM-5 Diagnostic Criteria for Major Depressive Disorder (MDD)
Reprinted with permission from the Diagnostic and Statistical Manual of Mental Disorders, 5th ed. 2013. American Psychiatric Association
A. presence of a MDE
B. the MDE is not better accounted for by schizoaffective disorder and is not superimposed on schizophrenia, schizophreniform disorder, delusional disorder, or psychotic disorder NOS
C. there has never been a manic episode or a hypomanic episode
   Note: This exclusion does not apply if all of the manic-like, or hypomanic-like episodes are substance or treatment-induced or are due to the direct physiological effects of another medical condition
- **specifiers:** with anxious distress, mixed features, melancholic features, atypical features, mood-congruent psychotic features, mood-incongruent psychotic features, catatonia, peripartum onset, seasonal pattern
- single vs. recurrent is an episode descriptor that carries prognostic significance. Recurrent is classified as the patient having two or more distinct MDE episodes; to be considered separate the patient must have gone 2 consecutive months without meeting criteria

Epidemiology
- lifetime prevalence: 12%
- peak prevalence age 15-25 yr (M:F = 1:2)

Etiology
- biological
  - genetic: 65-75% MZ twins; 14-19% DZ twins, 2-4 fold increased risk in first-degree relatives
  - neurotransmitter dysfunction: decreased activity of 5-HT, NE, and DA at neuronal synapse; changes in GABA and glutamate; various changes detectable by fMRI
  - neuroendocrine dysfunction: excessive HPA axis activity
  - neuroanatomy and neurophysiology: decreased hippocampal volume, increased size of ventricles; decreased REM latency and slow-wave sleep; increased REM length
  - immunologic: increased pro-inflammatory cytokines IL-6 and TNF
  - secondary to medical condition, medication, substance use disorder
- psychosocial
  - psychodynamic (e.g. low self-esteem, unconscious aggression towards self or loved ones, disordered attachment)
  - cognitive (e.g. distorted schemata, Beck's cognitive triad: negative views of the self, the world, and the future)
  - environmental factors (e.g. job loss, bereavement, history of abuse or neglect, early life adversity)
  - comorbid psychiatric diagnoses (e.g. anxiety, substance abuse, developmental disability, dementia, eating disorder)

Risk Factors
- sex: F>M, 2:1
- family history: depression, alcohol abuse, suicide attempt or completion
- childhood experiences: loss of parent before age 11, negative home environment (abuse, neglect)
- personality: neuroticism, insecure, dependent, obsessional
- recent stressors: illness, financial, legal, relational, academic
- lack of intimate, confiding relationships or social isolation
- low socioeconomic status

Antidepressants for Depression in Medical Illness
Cochrane DB Syst Rev 2010; Issue 3
This systematic review and meta-analysis of 51 RCTs (3,603 patients) compared antidepressants to placebo in patients with a physical disorder (e.g. cancer, MI) who have been diagnosed as depressed (including major depression, adjustment disorder, and dysthymia).
Conclusions: Antidepressants, including SSRIs and TCAs, cause a significant improvement in patients with a physical illness, as compared to placebo.

Depression in the Elderly

- affects about 15% of community residents >65 yr old; up to 50% in nursing homes
- high suicide risk due to social isolation, chronic medical illness, decreased independence
- suicide peak: males aged 80-90; females aged 50-65
- dysphoria may not be a reliable indicator of depression in those >85 yr
- often present with somatic complaints (e.g. changes in weight, sleep, energy) or anxiety symptoms
- may have prominent cognitive changes after onset of mood symptoms (dementia syndrome of depression)
- see Table 3, PS21, for a comparison of delirium and dementia

Treatment

- lifestyle: increased aerobic exercise, mindfulness-based stress reduction, zinc supplementation
- biological: SSRIs, SNRIs, other antidepressants, somatic therapies (see *Pharmacotherapy*, PS42, and *Somatic Therapies*, PS49)
  - 1st line pharmacotherapy: sertraline, escitalopram, venlafaxine, mirtazapine
  - for partial or non-response can change class or add augmenting agent: buproprion, quetiapine-XR, aripiprazole, lithium
  - typical response to antidepressant treatment: physical symptoms improve at 2 wk, mood/cognition by 4 wk, if no improvement after 4 wk at a therapeutic dosage alter regimen
  - ECT: currently fastest and most effective treatment for MDD. Consider in severe, psychotic, or treatment-resistant cases
  - rTMS: early data support efficacy equivalent to ECT with good safety and tolerability
  - phototherapy: especially if seasonal component, shift work, sleep dysregulation
- psychological
  - individual therapy (interpersonal, CBT), family therapy, group therapy
- social: vocational rehabilitation, social skills training
- experimental: magnetic seizure therapy, deep brain stimulation, vagal nerve stimulation, ketamine

Prognosis

- one year after diagnosis of MDD without treatment: 40% of individuals still have symptoms that are sufficiently severe to meet criteria for MDD, 20% continue to have some symptoms that no longer meet criteria for MDD, 40% have no mood disorder

PERSISTENT DEPRESSIVE DISORDER

DSM-5 Diagnostic Criteria for Persistent Depressive Disorder

Note: in DSM-IV-TR this was referred to as Dysthymia
Reprinted with permission from the Diagnostic and Statistical Manual of Mental Disorders, 5th ed. 2013. American Psychiatric Association

A. depressed mood for most of the day, for more days than not, as indicated either by subjective account or observation by others, for ≥2 yr
   Note: in children and adolescents, mood can be irritable and duration must be at least 1 yr
B. presence, while depressed, of ≥2 of the following
   - poor appetite or overeating
   - insomnia or hypersomnia
   - low energy or fatigue
   - low self-esteem
   - poor concentration or difficulty making decisions
   - feelings of hopelessness
C. during the 2 yr period (1 yr for children or adolescents) of the disturbance, the person has never been without the symptoms in criteria A and B for more than 2 mo at a time
D. criteria for a major depressive disorder may be continuously present for 2 yr
E. there has never been a manic episode or a hypomanic episode, and criteria have never been met for cyclothymic disorder
F. the disturbance is not better explained by a persistent schizoaffective disorder, schizophrenia, delusional disorder, or other specified or unspecified schizophrenia spectrum and other psychotic disorder
G. the symptoms are not due to the direct physiological effects of a substance or another medical condition
H. the symptoms cause clinically significant distress or impairment in social, occupational, or other important areas of functioning

Epidemiology

- lifetime prevalence: 2-3%; M=F

Treatment

- psychological
  - traditionally psychotherapy was the principal treatment for persistent depressive disorder; recent evidence suggests some benefit but generally inferior to pharmacological treatment. Combinations of the two may be most efficacious
- biological
  - antidepressant therapy: SSRIs (e.g. sertraline, paroxetine), TCAs (e.g. imipramine) as an outpatient

St. John's Wort for Major Depression
Cochrane DB Syst Rev 2008;4:CD000448
Study: Systematic review of trials that were (1) randomized, double-blinded (2) with patients with major depression (3) comparing St. John's wort (hypericum extracts) with placebo or standard antidepressants and (4) included clinical outcomes.
Patients: 5,489 patients with major depression.
Outcomes: 1. Effectiveness: treatment response measured by a depression scale 2. Safety: the proportion of patients who dropped out due to adverse effects.
Intervention: St. John's wort vs. placebo; St. John's wort vs. standard antidepressants.
Results: 29 trials, 5,489 patients, with 18 comparisons with placebo and 17 with antidepressants. St John's wort is more effective than placebo (response rate ratio = 1.87), and similarly effective as antidepressants (RRR = 1.02). Less adverse effects with hypericum extracts. However, the effect size is dependent on the country of origin.

Cognitive Therapy vs. Medications in the Treatment of Moderate to Severe Depression
Arch Gen Psychiatry 2005;62:409-416
Study: Randomized control trial.
Patients: 240 outpatients with moderate to severe MDD, aged 18-70.
Intervention: 16 wk of paroxetine with or without augmentation with lithium carbonate or desipramine hydrochloride (n=120) versus cognitive behavioural therapy (n=60). Response up to 8 wk was controlled by pill placebo (n=60).
Main Outcomes: The Hamilton Depression Rating scale was used to determine response to treatment.
Results: At 8 wk, 50% (95%CI 41-59%) of patients on medication and 43% (95%CI 31-56%) of patients on CBT had responded in comparison to 25% (95%CI 16-38%) of patients on pill placebo. There was no significant difference between medication and CBT. At 16 wk, 46% of patients on medication and 40% of patients on CBT achieved remission.
Summary: There is no difference in efficacy between CBT vs. paroxetine in the treatment of moderate to severe depression.

Selective Serotonin Reuptake Inhibitors in Pregnancy and Infant Outcomes
Paediatr Child Health 2011;16:562-563
Study: Canadian Paediatric Society (CPS) Clinical practice guidelines.
Recommendations: It is important to treat depression in pregnancy. There is no evidence that SSRIs increase the risk of major malformations. There is conflicting evidence concerning the association of paroxetine and cardiac malformations. SSRIs are not contraindicated while breast-feeding.

Postpartum Mood Disorders

Postpartum "Blues"
- transient period of mild depression, mood instability, anxiety, decreased concentration; considered to be normal changes in response to fluctuating hormonal levels, the stress of childbirth, and the increased responsibilities of motherhood
- occurs in 50-80% of mothers; begins 2-4 d postpartum, usually lasts 48 h, can last up to 10 d
- does not require psychotropic medication
- usually mild or absent: feelings of inadequacy, anhedonia, thoughts of harming baby, suicidal thoughts

MAJOR DEPRESSIVE DISORDER WITH PERIPARTUM ONSET (POSTPARTUM DEPRESSION)

Clinical Presentation
- MDD with onset during pregnancy or within 4 wk following delivery
- typically lasts 2-6 mo; residual symptoms can last up to 1 yr
- may present with psychosis (rare, 0.2%), usually associated with mania, but also with MDE
- severe symptoms include extreme disinterest in baby, suicidal and infanticidal ideation

Epidemiology
- occurs in 10% of mothers, risk of recurrence 50%

Risk Factors
- previous history of a mood disorder (postpartum or otherwise), family history of mood disorder
- psychosocial factors: stressful life events, unemployment, marital conflict, lack of social support, unwanted pregnancy, colicky or sick infant

Treatment
- psychotherapy (CBT or IPT)
- short-term safety of maternal SSRIs for breastfeeding infants established; long-term effects unknown
- if depression severe or psychotic symptoms present, consider ECT

Prognosis
- impact on child development: increased risk of cognitive delay, insecure attachment, behavioural disorders
- treatment of mother improves outcome for child at 8 mo through increased mother-child interaction

Bipolar Disorders

BIPOLAR I / BIPOLAR II DISORDER

Definition
- Bipolar I Disorder
  - disorder in which at least one manic episode has occurred
  - if manic symptoms lead to hospitalization, or if there are psychotic symptoms, the diagnosis is BP I
  - commonly accompanied by at least 1 MDE but not required for diagnosis
  - time spent in mood episodes: 53% asymptomatic, 32% depressed, 9% cycling/mixed, 6% hypo/manic
- Bipolar II Disorder
  - disorder in which there is at least 1 MDE, 1 hypomanic and no manic episodes
  - while hypomania is less severe than mania, Bipolar II is not a "milder" form of Bipolar I
  - time spent in mood episodes: 46% asymptomatic, 50% depressed, 1% cycling/mixed, 2% hypo/manic
  - Bipolar II is often missed due to the severity and chronicity of depressive episodes and low rates of spontaneous reporting and recognition of hypomanic episodes

Bipolar II is quite often missed and many patients are symptomatic for up to a decade before accurate diagnosis and treatment

Classification
- classification of bipolar disorder involves describing the disorder (I or II) and the current or most recent mood episode as either manic, hypomanic, or depressed
- **specifiers:** with anxious distress, depressed with mixed features, hypo/manic with mixed features, melancholic features, atypical features, mood-congruent or -incongruent psychotic features, catatonia, peripartum onset, seasonal pattern, rapid cycling (4+ mood episodes in 1 yr)

Epidemiology
- lifetime prevalence: 1% BPI, 1.1% BPII, 2.4% Subthreshold BPD; M:F = 1:1
- age of onset: teens to 20s, usually MDE first, manic episode 6-10 years after, average age of first manic episode 32 yr

Patients with bipolar disorder are at higher risk for suicide when they switch from mania to depression, especially as they become aware of consequences of their behaviour during the manic episode

Risk Factors
- genetic: 60-65% of bipolar patients have family history of major mood disorders, especially bipolar disorders
- clinical features of MDE history favouring bipolar over unipolar diagnosis: early age of onset (<25 yr), increased number of MDEs, psychotic symptoms, postpartum onset, anxiety disorders (especially separation, panic), antidepressant failure due to early "poop out" or hypomanic symptoms, early impulsivity and aggression, substance abuse, cyclothymic temperament

Treatment

- **lifestyle:** psychoeducation regarding cycling nature of illness, ensure regular check ins, develop early warning system, "emergency plan" for manic episodes, promote stable routine (sleep, meals, exercise)
- **biological:** lithium, anticonvulsants, antipsychotics, ECT (if refractory); monotherapy with antidepressants should be avoided
  - mood stabilizers vary in their ability to "treat" (reduce symptoms acutely) or "stabilize" (prevent relapse and recurrence) manic and depressive symptoms; multi-agent therapy is common
  - treating mania: lithium, valproate, carbamazepine (2nd line), SGA, ECT, benzodiazepines (for acute agitation)
  - preventing mania: same as above but usually at lower dosages, minus benzodiazepines
  - treating depression: lithium, lurasidone, quetiapine, lamotrigine, antidepressants (only with mood stabilizer), ECT
  - preventing depression: same as above plus aripiprazole, valproate (note: quetiapine first line in treating bipolar II depression)
  - mixed episode or rapid cycling: multi-agent therapy, lithium or valproate + SGA (lurasidone, aripiprazole, olanzapine)
- **psychological:** supportive or psychodynamic psychotherapy, CBT, IPT or interpersonal social rhythm therapy, family therapy
- **social:** vocational rehabilitation, consider leave of absence from school/work, assess capacity to manage finances, drug and EtOH cessation, sleep hygiene, social skills training, education and recruitment of family members

Course and Prognosis

- high suicide rate (15% mortality from suicide), especially in mixed states
- BP I and II are chronic conditions with a relapsing and remitting course featuring alternating manic and depressive episodes; depressive symptoms tend to occur more frequently and last longer than manic episodes
- can achieve high level of functioning between episodes
- may switch rapidly between depression and mania without any period of euthymia in between
- high recurrence rate for mania – 90% will have a subsequent episode in the next 5 yr
- long term follow up of BP I – 15% well, 45% well with relapses, 30% partial remission, 10% chronically ill

CYCLOTHYMIA

Diagnosis

- presence of numerous periods of hypomanic and depressive symptoms (not meeting criteria for full hypomanic episode or MDE) for ≥2 yr; never without symptoms for >2 mo
- never have met criteria for MDE, manic or hypomanic episodes
- symptoms are not due to the direct physiological effects of a substance or GMC
- symptoms cause clinically significant distress or impairment in social, occupational, or other important areas of functioning

Treatment

- similar to Bipolar I: mood stabilizer ± psychotherapy, avoid antidepressant monotherapy, treat any comorbid substance use disorder

Anxiety Disorders

Definition

- anxiety is a universal human characteristic involving tension, apprehension, or even terror which serves as an adaptive mechanism to warn about an external threat
- manifestations of anxiety are a result of the activation of the sympathetic nervous system and can be described through
  - physiology: main brain structure involved is the amygdala (fear conditioning); neurotransmitters involved include 5-HT, cholecystokinin, epinephrine, norepinephrine, DA
  - psychology: one's perception of a given situation is distorted which causes one to believe it is threatening in some way
  - behaviour: once feeling threatened, one responds by escaping or facing the situation, thereby causing a disruption in daily functioning
- anxiety becomes pathological when:
  - fear is greatly out of proportion to risk/severity of threat
  - response continues beyond existence of threat or becomes generalized to other similar or dissimilar situations
  - social or occupational functioning is impaired
  - often comorbid with substance use and depression

Lithium is among few agents with proven efficacy in preventing suicide attempts and completions

Monotherapy with antidepressants should be avoided in patients with bipolar depression as patients can switch from depression into mania

The 4 L's for Bipolar Depression
Lithium, Lamotrigine, Lurasidone, SeroqueL

A Randomized Controlled Trial of Cognitive Therapy for Bipolar Disorder: Focus on Long-Term Change
J Clin Psychiatry 2006;67:277-286
Study: Randomized, blinded clinical trial.
Patients: 52 patients with DSM-IV bipolar 1 or 2 disorder.
Intervention: Patients allocated to either a 6 mo trial of cognitive therapy (CT) with emotive techniques or treatment as usual. Both groups received mood stabilizers.
Main Outcomes: Relapse rates, dysfunctional attitudes, psychosocial functioning, hopelessness, self-control, medication adherence. Patients were assessed by independent raters blinded to treatment group.
Results: At 6 mo, CT patients experienced fewer depressive symptoms and fewer dysfunctional attitudes. There was a non-significant (p=0.06) trend to greater time to depressive relapse. At 12 mo follow-up, CT patients had lower Young Mania Rating scores and improved behavioural self-control. At 18 mo, CT patients reported less severity of illness.
Conclusions: CT appears to provide benefits in the 12 mo after completion of therapy.

Differential Diagnosis

Table 2. Differential Diagnosis of Anxiety Disorders

Cardiovascular	Post-MI, arrhythmia, congestive heart failure, pulmonary embolus, mitral valve prolapse
Respiratory	Asthma, COPD, pneumonia, hyperventilation
Endocrine	Hyperthyroidism, pheochromocytoma, hypoglycemia, hyperadrenalism, hyperparathyroidism
Metabolic	Vitamin B_{12} deficiency, porphyria
Neurologic	Neoplasm, vestibular dysfunction, encephalitis
Substance-Induced	Intoxication (caffeine, amphetamines, cocaine, thyroid preparations, OTC for colds/decongestants), withdrawal (benzodiazepines, alcohol)
Other Psychiatric Disorders	Psychotic disorders, mood disorders, personality disorders (OCPD), somatoform disorders

Medical Workup of Anxiety Disorder
- routine screening: physical exam, CBC, thyroid function test, electrolytes, urinalysis, urine drug screening
- additional screening: neurological consultation, chest X-ray, ECG, CT head

Panic Disorder

DSM-5 Diagnostic Criteria for Panic Disorder
Reprinted with permission from the Diagnostic and Statistical Manual of Mental Disorders, 5th ed. 2013. American Psychiatric Association

A. recurrent unexpected panic attacks - a panic attack is an abrupt surge of intense fear or intense discomfort that reaches a peak within minutes, and during which time four (or more) of the following symptoms occur
- palpitations, pounding heart, or accelerated heart rate
- sweating
- trembling or shaking
- sensations of shortness of breath or smothering
- feelings of choking
- chest pain or discomfort
- nausea or abdominal distress
- feeling dizzy, unsteady, light-headed, or faint
- chills or heat sensations
- paresthesias (numbness or tingling sensations)
- derealization (feelings of unreality) or depersonalization (being detached from oneself)
- fear of losing control or "going crazy"
- fear of dying

B. 1 mo (or more) of "anxiety about panic attacks" - at least one of the attacks has been followed by one or both of the following:
- persistent concern or worry about additional panic attacks or their consequences
- a significant maladaptive change in behaviour related to the attacks

C. the disturbance is not attributable to the physiological effects of a substance or another medical condition

D. the disturbance is not better explained by another mental disorder

Epidemiology
- prevalence: 2-5% (one of the top five most common reasons to see a family doctor); M:F = 1:2-3
- onset: average early-mid 20s, familial pattern

Treatment
- psychological
  - CBT: interoceptive exposure (eliciting symptoms of a panic attack and learning to tolerate the symptoms without coping strategies); cognitive restructuring (addressing underlying beliefs regarding the panic attacks), relaxation techniques (visualization, box-breathing)
- pharmacological
  - SSRIs: fluoxetine, citalopram, paroxetine, fluvoxamine, sertraline
  - SNRI: venlafaxine
  - with SSRI/SNRIs start with low doses, titrate up slowly
  - anxiety disorders often require treatment at higher doses for a longer period of time than depression (i.e. full response may take up to 12 wk)
  - treat for up to 1 year after symptoms resolve to avoid relapse
  - to prevent non-compliance due to physical side effects, explain symptoms to expect prior to initiation of therapy
  - other antidepressants (mirtazapine, MAOIs)
  - consider avoiding bupropion or TCAs due to stimulating effects (exacerbate anxious symptoms)
  - benzodiazepines (short-term, low dose, regular schedule, long half-life, avoid prn usage)

Prognosis
- 6-10 yr post-treatment: 30% well, 40-50% improved, 20-30% no change or worse
- clinical course: chronic, but episodic with psychosocial stressors

Situational trigger → Panic attack
Increased anxiety and generalization to other situations ← Mentally associated with situation
Figure 2. Panic attack

Criteria for Panic Disorder (≥4)

STUDENTS FEAR the 3 Cs
Sweating
Trembling
Unsteadiness, dizziness
Depersonalization, **D**erealization
Excessive heart rate, palpitations
Nausea
Tingling
Shortness of breath
Fear of dying, losing control, going crazy
3 Cs: Chest pain, Chills, Choking

Panic Attack vs. Panic Disorder
Panic disorder consists of panic attacks + other criteria
Panic attack is not a codable disorder and can occur in the context of many different disorders

Starting Medication for Anxiety
Start low, go slow, aim high and explain symptoms to expect prior to initiation of therapy to prevent non-compliance due to physical side effects

Agoraphobia

DSM-5 Diagnostic Criteria for Agoraphobia
Reprinted with permission from the Diagnostic and Statistical Manual of Mental Disorders, 5th ed. 2013. American Psychiatric Association

A. marked fear or anxiety about two (or more) of the following five situations:
- using public transportation
- being in open spaces
- being in enclosed places
- standing in line or being in a crowd
- being outside of the home alone

B. the individual fears or avoids these situations because of thoughts that escape might be difficult or help might not be available in the event of developing panic-like symptoms or other incapacitating or embarrassing symptoms

C. the agoraphobic situations almost always provoke fear or anxiety

D. the agoraphobic situations are actively avoided, require the presence of a companion, or are endured with intense fear or anxiety

E. the fear or anxiety is out of proportion to the actual danger posed by the agoraphobic situations and to the sociocultural context

F. the fear, anxiety, or avoidance is persistent, typically lasting ≥6 mo

G. the fear, anxiety, or avoidance causes clinically significant distress or impairment in social, occupational, or other important areas of functioning

H. if another medical condition is present, the fear, anxiety, or avoidance is clearly excessive

I. the fear, anxiety, or avoidance is not better explained by the symptoms of another mental disorder and are not related exclusively to obsessions, perceived defects or flaws in physical appearance, reminders of traumatic events, or fear of separation

Note: agoraphobia is diagnosed irrespective of the presence of panic disorder. If an individual's presentation meets criteria for panic disorder and agoraphobia, both diagnoses should be assigned

Treatment
- as per panic disorder

Generalized Anxiety Disorder

DSM-5 Diagnostic Criteria for Generalized Anxiety Disorder
Reprinted with permission from the Diagnostic and Statistical Manual of Mental Disorders, 5th ed. 2013. American Psychiatric Association

A. excessive anxiety and worry (apprehensive expectation), occurring more days than not for at least 6 mo, about a number of events or activities (such as work or school performance)

B. the individual finds it difficult to control the worry

C. the anxiety and worry are associated with three (or more) of the following six symptoms (with at least some symptoms having been present for more days than not for the past 6 mo)
  1. restlessness or feeling keyed up or on edge
  2. being easily fatigued
  3. difficulty concentrating or mind going blank
  4. irritability
  5. muscle tension
  6. sleep disturbance (difficulty falling or staying asleep, or restless, unsatisfying sleep)

D. the anxiety, worry, or physical symptoms cause clinically significant distress or impairment in social, occupational, or other important areas of functioning

E. the disturbance is not attributable to the physiological effects of a substance or another medical condition

F. the disturbance is not better explained by another mental disorder

Criteria for GAD (≥3)

C-FIRST
Concentration issues
Fatigue
Irritability
Restlessness
Sleep disturbance
Tension (muscle)

Epidemiology
- 1 yr prevalence: 3-8%; M:F = 1:2
  - if considering only those receiving inpatient treatment, ratio is 1:1
- most commonly presents in early adulthood

Treatment
- lifestyle: caffeine and EtOH avoidance, sleep hygiene
- psychological: CBT including relaxation techniques, mindfulness
- biological
  - SSRIs and SNRIs are 1st line (paroxetine, escitalopram, sertraline, venlafaxine XL)
  - 2nd line: buspirone (tid dosing), bupropion (caution due to stimulating effects),
  - add-on benzodiazepines (short-term, low dose, regular schedule, long half-life, avoid prn usage)
  - β-blockers not recommended

Prognosis
- chronically anxious adults become less so with age
- depends on pre-morbid personality functioning, stability of relationships, work, and severity of environmental stress
- difficult to treat

Phobic Disorders

Specific Phobia
- definition: marked and persistent (> 6 mo) fear that is excessive or unreasonable, cued by presence or anticipation of a specific object or situation
- lifetime prevalence 12-16%; M:F ratio variable
- types: animal/insect, environment (heights, storms), blood/injection/injury, situational (airplane, closed spaces), other (loud noise, clowns)

Social Phobia (Social Anxiety Disorder)
- definition: marked and persistent (> 6 mo) fear of social or performance situations in which one is exposed to unfamiliar people or to possible scrutiny by others; fearing he/she will act in a way that may be humiliating or embarrassing (e.g. public speaking, initiating or maintaining conversation, dating, eating in public)
- 12-month prevalence rate may be as high as 7%; M:F ratio approximately equal

Diagnostic Criteria for Phobic Disorders
- exposure to stimulus almost invariably provokes an immediate anxiety response; may present as a panic attack
- person recognizes fear as excessive or unreasonable
- situations are avoided or endured with anxiety/distress
- significant interference with daily routine, occupational/social functioning, and/or marked distress

Treatment
- psychological
  - cognitive behaviour therapy (focusing on both *in vivo* and virtual exposure therapy, gradually facing feared situations)
  - behavioural therapy is more efficacious than medication
- biological
  - SSRIs/SNRIs (e.g. fluoxetine, paroxetine, sertraline, venlafaxine), MAOIs
  - β-blockers or benzodiazepines in acute situations (e.g. public speaking)

Prognosis
- chronic

Obsessive-Compulsive Disorder

DSM-5 Diagnostic Criteria for Obsessive-Compulsive Disorder
Reprinted with permission from the Diagnostic and Statistical Manual of Mental Disorders, 5th ed. 2013. American Psychiatric Association
A. presence of obsessions, compulsions, or both
  - obsessions are defined by (1) and (2)
    1. recurrent and persistent thoughts, urges, or images that are experienced, at some time during the disturbance, as intrusive and unwanted, and cause marked anxiety or distress in most individuals
    2. the individual attempts to ignore or suppress such thoughts, urges, or images, or to neutralize them with some other thought or action (i.e. by performing a compulsion; see below)
  - compulsions are defined by (1) and (2)
    1. repetitive behaviours (e.g. hand washing, ordering, checking) or mental acts (e.g. praying, counting, repeating words silently) that the individual feels driven to perform in response to an obsession or according to rules that must be applied rigidly
    2. behaviours mental acts are aimed at preventing or reducing anxiety or distress, or preventing some dreaded event or situation; however, these behaviours or mental acts are not connected in a realistic way with what they are designed to neutralize or prevent, or are clearly excessive
B. the obsessions or compulsions are time-consuming (e.g. take >1 h/d) or cause clinically significant distress or impairment in social, occupational, or other important areas of functioning
C. the obsessive-compulsive symptoms are not attributable to the physiological effects of a substance or another medical condition
D. the disturbance is not better explained by the symptoms of another mental disorder

Epidemiology
- 12 mo prevalence 1.1-1.8%; females affected at slightly higher rates than males
- rate of OCD in first-degree relatives is higher than in the general population

Treatment
- CBT: exposure with response prevention (ERP) – involves exposure to feared situations with the addition of preventing the compulsive behaviours; cognitive strategies include challenging underlying beliefs
- pharmacotherapy: SSRIs/SNRIs (12-16 week trials, higher doses vs. depression), clomipramine; adjunctive antipsychotics (risperidone)

Prognosis
- tends to be refractory and chronic

Trauma- and Stressor-Related Disorders

Post-Traumatic Stress Disorder

DSM-5 Diagnostic Criteria for Post-Traumatic Stress Disorder

Reprinted with permission from the Diagnostic and Statistical Manual of Mental Disorders, 5th ed. 2013. American Psychiatric Association.

A. exposure to actual or threatened death, serious injury, or sexual violence in one (or more) of the following ways
  1. directly experiencing the traumatic event(s)
  2. witnessing, in person, the event(s) as it occurred to others
  3. learning that the traumatic event(s) occurred to a close family member or close friend. In cases of actual or threatened death of a family member or friend, the event(s) must have been violent or accidental
  4. experiencing repeated or extreme exposure to aversive details of the traumatic event(s) (e.g. first responders collecting human remains: police officers repeatedly exposed to details of child abuse)
B. presence of one (or more) of the following intrusion symptoms associated with the traumatic event(s), beginning after the traumatic event(s) occurred
  1. recurrent, involuntary, and intrusive distressing memories of the traumatic event(s)
  2. recurrent distressing dreams in which the content and/or affect of the dream are related to the traumatic event(s)
  3. dissociative reactions (e.g. flashbacks) in which the individual feels or acts as if the traumatic event(s) were recurring
  4. intense or prolonged psychological distress at exposure to internal or external cues that symbolize or resemble an aspect of the traumatic event(s)
  5. marked physiological reactions to internal or external cues that symbolize or resemble an aspect of the traumatic event(s)
C. persistent avoidance of stimuli associated with the traumatic event(s), beginning after the traumatic event(s) occurred, as evidenced by one or both of the following
  1. avoidance of or efforts to avoid distressing memories, thoughts, or feelings about or closely associated with the traumatic event(s)
  2. avoidance of or efforts to avoid external reminders (people, places, conversations, activities, objects, situations) that arouse distressing memories, thoughts, or feelings about or closely associated with the traumatic event(s)
D. negative alterations in cognitions and mood associated with the traumatic event(s), beginning or worsening after the traumatic event(s) occurred, as evidenced by two (or more) of the following
  1. inability to remember an important aspect of the traumatic event(s)
  2. persistent and exaggerated negative beliefs or expectations about oneself, others, or the world
  3. persistent, distorted cognitions about the cause or consequences of the traumatic event(s) that lead the individual to blame himself/herself or others
  4. persistent negative emotional state (e.g. fear, horror, anger, guilt, or shame)
  5. markedly diminished interest or participation in significant activities
  6. feelings of detachment or estrangement from others
  7. persistent inability to experience positive emotions
E. marked alterations in arousal and reactivity associated with the traumatic event(s), beginning or worsening after the traumatic event(s) occurred, as evidenced by two (or more) of the following
  1. irritable behaviour and angry outbursts (with little or no provocation) typically expressed as verbal or physical aggression toward people or objects
  2. reckless or self-destructive behaviour
  3. hypervigilance
  4. exaggerated startle response
  5. problems with concentration
  6. sleep disturbance (e.g. difficulty falling or staying asleep or restless sleep)
F. duration of the disturbance (criteria B, C, D, and E) is more than 1 mo
G. the disturbance causes clinically significant distress or impairment in social, occupational, or other important areas of functioning
H. the disturbance is not attributable to the physiological effects of a substance or another medical condition

Epidemiology
- prevalence of 7% in general population
- men's trauma is most commonly combat experience/physical assault; women's trauma is usually physical or sexual assault

Treatment
- psychotherapy, CBT
  - ensure safety and stabilize: emotional regulation techniques (e.g. breathing, relaxation)
  - once coping mechanisms established, can explore/mourn trauma - challenge dysfunctional beliefs, etc.
  - reconnect and integrate - exposure therapy, etc.

Criteria for Post-Traumatic Stress Disorder

TRAUMA
Traumatic event
Re-experience the event
Avoidance of stimuli associated with the trauma
Unable to function
More than a Month
Arousal increased
+ negative alterations in cognition and mood

Acute Stress Disorder
- May be a precursor to PTSD
- Similar symptoms to PTSD
- Symptoms persist 3 d after a trauma until 1 mo after the exposure

- biological
  - SSRIs (e.g. paroxetine, sertraline)
  - prazosin (for treating disturbing dreams and nightmares)
  - benzodiazepines (for acute anxiety)
  - adjunctive atypical antipsychotics (risperidone, olanzapine)
- eye movement desensitization and reprocessing (EMDR): an experimental method of reprocessing memories of distressing events by recounting them while using a form of dual attention stimulation such as eye movements, bilateral sound, or bilateral tactile stimulation (its use is controversial because of limited evidence)

Complications
- substance abuse, relationship difficulties, depression, impaired social and occupational functioning disorders, personality disorders

Adjustment Disorder

Definition
- a diagnosis encompassing patients who have difficulty coping with a stressful life event or situation and develop acute, often transient, emotional or behavioural symptoms that resemble less severe versions of other psychiatric conditions

DSM-5 Diagnostic Criteria for Adjustment Disorder
Reprinted with permission from the Diagnostic and Statistical Manual of Mental Disorders, 5th ed. 2013. American Psychiatric Association

A. the development of emotional or behavioural symptoms in response to an identifiable stressor(s) occurring within 3 mo of the onset of the stressor(s)
B. these symptoms or behaviours are clinically significant as evidenced by either of the following:
  - marked distress that is in excess of what would be expected from exposure to the stressor
  - significant impairment in social or occupational (academic) functioning
C. the stress-related disturbance does not meet criteria for another mental disorder and is not merely an exacerbation of a pre-existing mental disorder
D. the symptoms do not represent normal bereavement
E. once the stressor (or its consequences) has terminated, the symptoms do not persist for more than an additional 6 mo
  - **specifiers:** with depressed mood, with anxiety, with mixed anxiety/depression, with conduct disturbance, with mixed disturbance of conduct/emotions, unspecified

Classification
- types of stressors
  - single (e.g. termination of romantic relationship)
  - multiple (e.g. marked business difficulties and marital problems)
  - recurrent (e.g. seasonal business crises)
  - continuous (e.g. living in a crime-ridden neighbourhood)
  - developmental events (e.g. going to school, leaving parental home, getting married, becoming a parent, failing to attain occupational goals, retirement)

Epidemiology
- F:M 2:1, prevalence 2-8% of the population

Treatment
- brief psychotherapy: individual or group (particularly useful for patients dealing with unique and specific medical issues; e.g. colostomy or renal dialysis groups), crisis intervention
- biological
  - benzodiazepines may be used for those with significant anxiety symptoms (short-term, low-dose, regular schedule)

Bereavement

Clinical Presentation
- bereavement is a normal psychological and emotional reaction to a significant loss, also called grief or mourning
- length and characteristics of "normal" bereavement are variable between individuals/cultures
- normal response: *protest → searching and acute anguish → despair and detachment → reorganization*
- presence of the following symptoms may indicate abnormal grief/presence of MDD
  - guilt about things other than actions taken or not taken by the survivor at the time of death
  - thoughts of death other than the survivor feeling that they would be better off dead or should have died with the deceased person; morbid preoccupation with worthlessness
  - marked psychomotor retardation; prolonged and marked functional impairment
  - hallucinatory experiences other than thinking that the survivor hears the voice of or transiently sees the image of the deceased person
  - dysphoria that is pervasive and independent of thoughts or triggers of the deceased, absence of mood reactivity

Risk Factors for Poor Bereavement Outcome
- Poor social supports
- Unanticipated death or lack of preparation for death
- Highly dependent relationship with deceased
- High initial distress
- Other concurrent stresses and losses
- Death of a child
- Pre-existing psychiatric disorders, especially depression and separation anxiety

- after 12 mo, if patient continues to yearn/long for the deceased, experience intense sorrow/emotional pain in response to the death, remain preoccupied with the deceased or with their circumstance of death, then may start to consider a diagnosis of "persistent complex bereavement disorder"
- if a patient meets criteria for MDD, even in the context of a loss or bereavement scenario, they are still diagnosed with MDD

Treatment
- support and watchful waiting should be first line, as well as education and normalization of the grief process
- screen for increased alcohol, cigarette and drug use
- normal grief should not be treated with antidepressant or antianxiety medication, as it is important to allow the person to experience the whole mourning process to achieve resolution
- psychosocial: for those needing additional support, complex grief/bereavement, or significant MDD, grief therapy (individual or group) is indicated
- pharmacotherapy: if MDD present, past history of mood disorders, severe or autonomous symptoms

Bereavement is associated with a significant increase in morbidity and mortality acutely following the loss, with effects seen up to 1 yr after

Loneliness is the most common symptom that continues to persist in normal bereavement and may last several years

Neurocognitive Disorders

Delirium

- see Neurology, N20 and Geriatric Medicine, GM4

DSM-5 Diagnostic Criteria for Delirium
Reprinted with permission from the Diagnostic and Statistical Manual of Mental Disorders, 5th ed. 2013. American Psychiatric Association

A. attention and awareness: disturbance in attention (i.e. reduced ability to direct, focus, sustain, and shift attention) and awareness (reduced orientation to the environment)
B. acute and fluctuating: disturbance develops over short period of time (usually hours to days), represents a change from baseline attention and awareness, and tends to fluctuate in severity during the course of a day
C. cognitive changes: an additional disturbance in cognition (e.g. memory deficit, disorientation, language, visuospatial ability, or perception)
D. not better explained: disturbances in criteria A and C are not better explained by another neurocognitive disorder (pre-existing, established, or evolving) and do not occur in the context of a severely reduced level of arousal (e.g. coma)
E. direct physiological cause: evidence that disturbance is a direct physiological consequence of another medical condition, substance intoxication or withdrawal (i.e. due to a drug of abuse or medication), toxin, or is due to multiple etiologies
- **Note:** can have HYPERactive, HYPOactive, or MIXED presentation

Clinical Presentation and Assessment
- common symptoms
  - distractibility, disorientation (time, place, rarely person)
  - misinterpretations, illusions, hallucinations
  - speech/language disturbances (dysarthria, dysnomia, dysgraphia)
  - affective symptoms (anxiety, fear, depression, irritability, anger, euphoria, apathy)
  - shifts in psychomotor activity (groping/picking at clothes, attempts to get out of bed when unsafe, sudden movements, sluggishness, lethargy)
- Folstein Mini Mental Status Exam or Montreal Cognitive Assessment are helpful to assess baseline of altered mental state (i.e. score will improve as symptoms resolve)

Risk Factors
- hospitalization (incidence 10-56%)
- previous delirium
- nursing home residents (incidence 60%)
- polypharmacy (e.g. anticholinergics)
- old age (especially males)
- severe illness (e.g. cancer, AIDS)
- recent anesthesia or surgery
- substance abuse
- pre-existing cognitive impairment, brain pathology, psychiatric illness

Investigations
- standard: CBC and differential, electrolytes, Ca^{2+}, PO_4^{3-}, Mg^{2+}, glucose, ESR, LFTs, Cr, BUN, TSH, vitamin B_{12}, folate, albumin, urine C&S, R&M
- as indicated: ECG, CXR, CT head, toxicology/heavy metal screen, VDRL, HIV, LP, blood cultures, EEG (typically abnormal - generalized slowing or fast activity, can also be used to rule out underlying seizures or post-ictal states as etiology)
- indications for CT head: focal neurological deficit, acute change in status, anticoagulant use, acute incontinence, gait abnormality, history of cancer

Confusion Assessment Method (CAM) for Diagnosis of Delirium

Highly sensitive and specific method to diagnosis delirium
Part 1: an assessment instrument that screens for overall cognitive impairment

Part 2: includes four features found best able to distinguish delirium from other cognitive impairments

Need (1) + (2) + (3 or 4)
(1) Acute onset and fluctuating course
(2) Inattention
(3) Disorganized thinking
(4) Altered level of consciousness - hyperactive or hypoactive

Visual hallucinations are organic until proven otherwise

Etiology of Delirium
- Infectious (encephalitis, meningitis, UTI, pneumonia)
- Withdrawal (alcohol, barbiturates, benzodiazepines)
- Acute metabolic disorder (electrolyte imbalance, hepatic or renal failure)
- Trauma (head injury, post-operative)
- CNS pathology (stroke, hemorrhage, tumour, seizure disorder, Parkinson's)
- Hypoxia (anemia, cardiac failure, pulmonary embolus)
- Deficiencies (vitamin B_{12}, folic acid, thiamine)
- Endocrinopathies (thyroid, glucose, parathyroid, adrenal)
- Acute vascular (shock, vasculitis, hypertensive encephalopathy)
- Toxins: substance use, sedatives, opioids (especially morphine), anesthetics, anticholinergics, anticonvulsants, dopaminergic agents, steroids, insulin, glyburide, antibiotics (especially quinolones), NSAIDs
- Heavy metals (arsenic, lead, mercury)

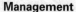

Management
- identify and manage underlying cause
  - identify and treat underlying cause immediately
  - stop all non-essential medications
  - maintain nutrition, hydration, electrolyte balance and monitor vitals
- optimize the environment
  - environment: quiet, well-lit, near window for cues regarding time of day
  - optimize hearing and vision
  - room near nursing station for closer observation; constant care if patient jumping out of bed, pulling out lines
  - family member present for reassurance and re-orientation
  - frequent orientation - calendar, clock, reminders
- pharmacotherapy
  - low dose, high potency antipsychotics: haloperidol has the most evidence; reasonable alternatives include risperidone, olanzapine (more sedating, less QT prolongation), quetiapine (if EPS), aripiprazole
  - benzodiazepines only to be used in alcohol withdrawal delirium; otherwise, can worsen delirium
  - try to minimize anticholinergic side effects
- physical restraints to maintain safety only if necessary

Prognosis
- up to 50% 1 yr mortality rate after episode of delirium

Major Neurocognitive Disorder (Dementia)

- see Neurology, N21

DSM-5 Diagnostic Criteria for Major Neurocognitive Disorder
Reprinted with permission from the Diagnostic and Statistical Manual of Mental Disorders, 5th ed. 2013. American Psychiatric Association

A. evidence of significant cognitive decline from a previous level of performance in one or more cognitive domains (complex attention, executive function, learning and memory, language, perceptual-motor, or social cognition) based on
  1. concern of the individual, a knowledgeable informant, or the clinician that there has been a significant decline in cognitive function; and
  2. substantial impairment in cognitive performance, preferably documented by standardized neuropsychological testing or, in its absence, another quantified clinical assessment
B. cognitive deficits interfere with independence in everyday activities (i.e. at a minimum, requiring assistance with complex instrumental activities of daily living such as paying bills or managing medications)
  - **Note:** if do not interfere in B, and impairments are mild-moderate in A, considered "mild neurocognitive disorder"; see Neurology, N21
C. cognitive deficits do not occur exclusively in the context of a delirium
D. cognitive deficits are not better explained by another mental disorder (e.g. major depressive disorder, schizophrenia)

Specify whether due to

Alzheimer's disease	Normal pressure hydrocephalus	Huntington's disease
Frontotemporal lobar degeneration	Substance/medication use	Another medical condition
Lewy body disease	HIV infection	Multiple etiologies
Vascular disease	Prion disease	Unspecified
Traumatic brain injury	Parkinson's disease	

Epidemiology
- prevalence increases with age: 10% in patients >65 yr of age; 25% in patients >85 yr of age
- prevalence is increased in people with Down's syndrome and head trauma
- Alzheimer's disease comprises >50% of cases; vascular causes comprise approximately 15% of cases (other causes of dementia neurocognitive disorder – see Neurology, N22)
- average duration of illness from onset of symptoms to death is 8-10 yr

Subtypes
- with or without behavioural disturbance (e.g. wandering, agitation)
- early-onset: age of onset <65 yr
- late-onset: age of onset >65 yr

Investigations (rule out reversible causes)
- standard: see Delirium, PS19
- as indicated: VDRL, HIV, SPECT, CT head in dementia
- indications for CT head: same as for delirium, plus: age <60, rapid onset (unexplained decline in cognition or function over 1-2 mo), dementia of relatively short duration (<2 yr), recent significant head trauma, unexplained neurological symptoms (new onset of severe headache/seizures)

Dosing for Haloperidol in Delirium
Typical dose 0.5-1 mg
Dosing schedule varies with clinical approach: PRN often used, but QHS or QHS and QAM also employed to account for hypoactive delirium, which is otherwise often missed

The 4 As of Dementia
Amnesia
Aphasia
Apraxia
Agnosia

The "Mini Cog" Rapid Assessment
- 3 word immediate recall
- Clock drawn to "10 past 11"
- 3 word delayed recall

Flags for Differentiating Most Common Causes of Dementia

Alzheimer's disease: predominantly memory and learning issues
Frontotemporal degeneration: language type (early preservation), behavioural type (apathy/disinhibition/self-neglect)
Lewy body disease: recurrent, soft visual hallucinations (e.g. rabbits), autonomic impairment (falls, hypotension), EPS, does not respond well to pharmacotherapy, fluctuating degree of cognitive impairment
Vascular disease: vascular risk factors, focal neurological signs, abrupt onset, stepwise progression
Normal pressure hydrocephalus: abnormal gait, early incontinence, rapidly progressive

Management
- see Neurology, N20 for further management
- treat underlying medical problems and prevent others
- provide orientation cues for patient (e.g. clock, calendar)
- provide education and support for patient and family (e.g. day programs, respite care, support groups, home care)
- consider long-term care plan (nursing home) and power of attorney/living will
- inform Ministry of Transportation about patient's inability to drive safely
- consider pharmacological therapy
  - cholinesterase inhibitors (e.g. donepezil [Aricept®], rivastigmine, galantamine) for mild to severe disease
  - NMDA receptor antagonist (e.g. memantine) for moderate to severe disease
  - low-dose neuroleptics (e.g. risperidone, quetiapine), antidepressants or trazodone if behavioural or emotional symptoms prominent – start low and go slow
  - reassess pharmacological therapy every 3 mo

Table 3. Comparison of Dementia, Delirium, and Pseudodementia of Depression

	Dementia/Major Neurocognitive Disorder	Delirium	Pseudodementia of Depression
Onset	Gradual/step-wise decline	Acute (h-d)	Subacute
Duration	Months-years	Days-weeks	Variable
Natural History	Progressive Usually irreversible	Fluctuating, reversible High morbidity/mortality in very old	Recurrent Usually reversible
Level of Consciousness	Normal	Fluctuating (over 24 h)	Normal
Attention	Not initially affected	Decreased (wandering, easy distraction)	Difficulty concentrating
Orientation	Intact initially	Impaired (usually to time and place), fluctuates	Intact
Behaviour	Disinhibition, impairment in ADL/IADL, personality change, loss of social graces	Severe agitation/retardation	Importuning, self-harm/suicide
Psychomotor	Normal	Fluctuates between extremes	Slowing
Sleep Wake Cycle	Fragmented sleep at night	Reversed sleep wake cycle	Early morning awakening
Mood and Affect	Labile but not usually anxious	Anxious, irritable, fluctuating	Depressed, stable
Cognition	Decreased executive functioning, paucity of thought	Fluctuating preceded by mood changes	Fluctuating
Memory Loss	Recent, eventually remote	Marked recent	Recent
Language	Agnosia, aphasia, decreased comprehension, repetition, speech (echolalia, palilalia)	Dysnomia, dysgraphia, speech rambling, irrelevant, incoherent, subject changes	Not affected
Delusions	Compensatory	Nightmarish and poorly formed	Nihilistic, somatic
Hallucinations	Variable	Visual common	Less common, auditory predominates
Quality of Hallucinations	Vacuous/bland	Frightening/bizarre	Self-deprecatory
Medical Status	Variable	Acute illness, drug toxicity	Rule out systemic illness, medications

Substance-Related and Addictive Disorders

Overview
- a neurobiological disorder involving compulsive drug seeking and drug taking, despite adverse consequences, with loss of control over drug use (think issues with the "3 Cs": compulsive, consequences, control)
- dependence is the hallmark of substance use disorders and comes in the following forms:
  - behavioural: substance-seeking activities and pathological use patterns
  - physical: physiologic withdrawal effects without use
  - psychological: continuous or intermittent cravings for the substance to avoid dysphoria or attain drug state
- abuse: drug use that deviates from the approved social or medical pattern, usually causing impairment or disruption to function in self or others
- these disorders are usually chronic with a relapsing and remitting course

Epidemiology
- 47% of those with substance abuse have mental health problems
- 29% of those with a mental health disorder have a substance use disorder
- 47% of those with schizophrenia and 25% of those with an anxiety disorder have a substance use disorder

Etiology
- almost all drugs (and activities) of abuse increase dopamine in the nucleus accumbens, an action that contributes to their euphoric properties and, with repeated use, to their ability to change signalling pathways in the brain's reward system
- substance use disorders arise from multifactorial interactions between genes (personality, neurobiology) and environment (low socioeconomic status, substance-using peers, abuse history, chronic stress)

Diagnosis
- substance use disorders are measured on a continuum from mild to severe based on the number of criteria met within 12 mo
    - mild: 2-3
    - moderate: 4-5
    - severe: 6 or more
- each specific substance is addressed as a separate use disorder and diagnosed utilizing the same overarching criteria (e.g. a single patient may have moderate alcohol use disorder, and a mild stimulant use disorder)
- criteria for substance use disorders (**PEC WITH MCAT**)
    - use despite **P**hysical or psychological problem (e.g. alcoholic liver disease or cocaine related nasal problems)
    - failures in important **E**xternal roles at work/school/home
    - **C**raving or a strong desire to use substance
    - **W**ithdrawal
    - continued use despite **I**nterpersonal problems
    - **T**olerance, needing to use more substance to get same effect
    - use in physically **H**azardous situations
    - **M**ore substance used or for longer period than intended
    - unsuccessful attempts to **C**ut down
    - **A**ctivities given up due to substance
    - excessive **T**ime spent on using or finding substance

Classification of Substances

	Drugs	Intoxication	Withdrawal
Depressants	Alcohol, opioids, barbiturates, benzodiazepines, GHB	Euphoria, slurred speech, disinhibition, confusion, poor coordination, coma (severe)	Anxiety, anhedonia, tremor, seizures, insomnia, psychosis, delirium, death
Stimulants	Amphetamines, methylphenidate, MDMA, cocaine	Euphoria, mania, psychomotor agitation, anxiety, psychosis (especially paranoia), insomnia, cardiovascular complications (stroke, MI, arrhythmias), seizure	'Crash', craving, dysphoria, suicidality
Hallucinogens	LSD, mescaline, psilocybin, PCP, ketamine, ibogaine, salvia	Distortion of sensory stimuli and enhancement of feelings, psychosis (++ visual hallucinations), delirium, anxiety (panic), poor coordination	Usually absent

General Approach to Assessment

- must be appropriate to the patient's current state of change (see <u>Population Health and Epidemiology</u>, *Health Promotion Strategies*, PH6, for Prochaska's Stages of Change Model)
- patients will only change when the pain of change appears less than the pain of staying the same
- provider can help by providing psychoeducation (emphasize neurobiologic model of addiction), motivation, and hope
- principles of motivational interviewing (see *Psychotherapy*, PS40)
    - non-judgmental stance
    - space for patient to talk and reflect
    - offer accurate empathic reflections back to patient to help frame issues

Questions to Characterize Substance Use and Risk Assessment
- When was the last time you used?
- How long can you go without using?
- By what route (oral ingestion, insufflation, smoking, IV) do you usually use?
- Are there any triggers that you know will cause you to use?
- How has your substance use affected your work, school, relationships?
- Substances can be very expensive, how do you support your drug use?
- Have you experienced medical or legal consequences of your use?
- Any previous attempts to cut down or quit, did you experience any withdrawal symptoms?

General Approach to Treatment
- encourage and offer referral to evidence based services
    - social: 12-step programs (alcoholics anonymous, narcotics anonymous), family education and support
    - psychological therapy: addiction counselling, motivational enhancement therapy (MET), CBT, contingency management, group therapy, family therapy, marital counselling
    - medical management (differs depending on substance): acute detoxification, pharmacologic agents to aid maintenance
- harm reduction whenever possible: safe-sex practices, avoid driving while intoxicated, avoiding substances with child care, safe needle practices/exchange, pill-testing kits, reducing tobacco use
- comorbid psychiatric conditions: many will resolve with successful treatment of the substance use disorder but patients who meet full criteria for another disorder should be treated for that disorder with psychological and pharmacologic therapies

Nicotine

- see Family Medicine, FM11

Alcohol

- see Family Medicine, FM12 and Emergency Medicine, ER54

History
- **CAGE:** validated screening questionnaire
  - C ever felt the need to Cut down on drinking?
  - A ever felt Annoyed at criticism of your drinking?
  - G ever feel Guilty about your drinking?
  - E ever need a drink first thing in morning (Eye opener)?
    - for men, a score of ≥2 is a positive screen; for women, a score of ≥1 is a positive screen
    - if positive CAGE, then assess further to distinguish between problem drinking and alcohol use disorder

Table 4. Canada's Low-Risk Alcohol Drinking Guidelines

Moderate Drinking		
Men: 3 or less/d (≤15/wk)	Women: 2 or less/d (≤10/wk)	Elderly: 1 or less/d

Alcohol Intoxication
- legal limit for impaired driving is 10.6 mmol/L (50 mg/dL) reached by 2-3 drinks/h for men and 1-2 drinks/h for women
- coma can occur with >60 mmol/L (non-tolerant drinkers) and 90-120 mmol/L (tolerant drinkers)

Alcohol Withdrawal
- occurs within 12-48 h after prolonged heavy drinking and can be life-threatening
- alcohol withdrawal can be described as having 4 stages, however not all stages may be experienced
  - stage 1 (onset 12-18 h after last drink): "the shakes" tremor, sweating, agitation, anorexia, cramps, diarrhea, sleep disturbance
  - stage 2 (onset 7-48 h): alcohol withdrawal seizures, usually tonic-clonic, non-focal and brief
  - stage 3 (onset 48 h): visual, auditory, olfactory or tactile hallucinations
  - stage 4 (onset 3-5 d): delirium tremens, confusion, delusions, hallucinations, agitation, tremors, autonomic hyperactivity (fever, tachycardia, HTN)
- course: almost completely reversible in young; elderly often left with cognitive deficits
- mortality rate 20% if untreated

Management of Alcohol Withdrawal
- monitor using the Clinical Institute Withdrawal Assessment for Alcohol (CIWA-A) scoring system
  - areas of assessment include
  - physical (5): nausea and vomiting, tremor, agitation, paroxysmal sweats, headache/fullness in head
  - psychological/cognitive (2): anxiety, orientation/clouding of sensorium
  - perceptual (3): tactile disturbances, auditory disturbances, visual disturbances
  - all categories are scored from 0-7 (except: orientation/sensorium 0-4), maximum score of 67
  - mild <10, moderate 10-20, severe >20

Table 5. CIWA-A Scale Treatment Protocol for Alcohol Withdrawal

Basic Protocol	Diazepam 20 mg PO q1-2h prn until CIWA-A <10 points Observe 1-2 h after last dose and re-assess on CIWA-A scale Thiamine 100 mg IM then 100 mg PO OD for 3 d Supportive care (hydration and nutrition)
History of Withdrawal Seizures	Diazepam 20 mg PO q1h for minimum of three doses regardless of subsequent CIWA scores
If age >65 or patient has severe liver disease, severe asthma or respiratory failure	Use a short acting benzodiazepine Lorazepam PO/SL/IM 1-4 mg q1-2h
If Hallucinations are present	Haloperidol 2-5 mg IM/PO q1-4h – max 5 doses/d or atypical antipsychotics (olanzapine, risperidone) Diazepam 20 mg x 3 doses as seizure prophylaxis (haloperidol lowers seizure threshold)
Admit to Hospital if	Still in withdrawal after >80 mg of diazepam Delirium tremens, recurrent arrhythmias, or multiple seizures Medically ill or unsafe to discharge home

Confabulations: the fabrication of imaginary experiences to compensate for memory loss

Make sure to ask about other alcohols: mouthwash, rubbing alcohol, methanol, ethylene glycol, aftershave (may be used as a cheaper alternative)

A "Standard Drink"
Spirit (40%): 1.5 oz. or 43 mL
Table Wine (12%): 5 oz. or 142 mL
Fortified Wine (18%): 3 oz. or 85 mL
Regular Beer (5%): 12 oz. or 341 mL
OR
1 pint of beer = 1.5 SD
1 bottle of wine = 5 SD
1 "mickey" = 8 SD
"26-er" = 17 SD
"40 oz." = 27 SD

**Delirium Tremens
(alcohol withdrawal delirium)**
- Autonomic hyperactivity (diaphoresis, tachycardia, increased respiration)
- Hand tremor
- Insomnia
- Psychomotor agitation
- Anxiety
- Nausea or vomiting
- Tonic-clonic seizures
- Visual/tactile/auditory hallucinations
- Persecutory delusions

Wernicke-Korsakoff Syndrome
- alcohol-induced amnestic disorders due to thiamine deficiency
- necrotic lesions: mammillary bodies, thalamus, brainstem
- Wernicke's encephalopathy (acute and reversible): triad of nystagmus (CN VI palsy), ataxia, and confusion
- Korsakoff's syndrome (chronic and only 20% reversible with treatment): anterograde amnesia and confabulations; cannot occur during an acute delirium or dementia and must persist beyond usual duration of intoxication/withdrawal
- management
  - Wernicke's: thiamine 100 mg PO OD x 1-2 wk
  - Korsakoff's: thiamine 100 mg PO bid/tid x 3-12 mo

Treatment of Alcohol Use Disorder
- non-pharmacological
  - see *General Approach to Treatment*, PS4
- pharmacological
  - naltrexone (Revia®): opioid antagonist, shown to be successful in reducing the "high" associated with alcohol, moderately effective in reducing cravings, frequency or intensity of alcohol binges
  - disulfiram (Antabuse®): prevents oxidation of alcohol (blocks acetaldehyde dehydrogenase); with alcohol consumption, acetaldehyde accumulates to cause a toxic reaction (vomiting, tachycardia, death); if patient relapses, must wait 48 h before restarting Antabuse®; prescribed only when treatment goal is abstinence. RCT evidence is generally poor or negative
  - acamprosate (Campral®): NMDA glutamate receptor antagonist; useful in maintaining abstinence and decreasing cravings

Opioids

- types of opioids: heroin, morphine, oxycodone, Tylenol #3® (codeine), hydromorphone, fentanyl
- major risks associated with the use of contaminated needles: increased risk of hepatitis B and C, bacterial endocarditis, HIV/AIDS

Acute Intoxication
- direct effect on receptors in CNS resulting in decreased pain perception, sedation, decreased sex drive, nausea/vomiting, decreased GI motility (constipation and anorexia), and respiratory depression

Toxic Reaction
- typical syndrome includes shallow respirations, miosis, bradycardia, hypothermia, decreased level of consciousness
- management
  - ABCs
  - IV glucose
  - naloxone hydrochloride (Narcan®): 0.4 mg up to 2 mg IV for diagnosis
  - treatment: intubation and mechanical ventilation, ± naloxone drip, until patient alert without naloxone (up to >48 h with long-acting opioids)
- caution with longer half-life; may need to observe for toxic reaction for at least 24 h

Withdrawal
- symptoms: depression, insomnia, drug-craving, myalgias, nausea, chills, autonomic instability (lacrimation, rhinorrhea, piloerection)
- onset: 6-12 h; duration: 5-10 d
- complications: loss of tolerance (overdose on relapse), miscarriage, premature labour
- management: long-acting oral opioids (methadone, buprenorphine), α-adrenergic agonists (clonidine)

Treatment of Opioid Use Disorder
- see *General Approach to Treatment*, PS4
- long-term treatment may include withdrawal maintenance treatment with methadone (opioid agonist) or buprenorphine (mixed agonist-antagonist)
- Suboxone® formulation includes naloxone in addition to buprenorphine, in an effort to prevent injection of the drug. When naloxone is injected, it will precipitate opiate withdrawal and block the opiate effect of buprenorphine; however, it will not have this antagonist action when taken sublingually

Opioid Antagonists
Naltrexone vs. Naloxone

Naltrexone (Revia®)
- Can be used for EtOH dependence (although not routinely used)
- Long half life (h)

Naloxone (Narcan®)
- Used for life-threatening CNS/respiratory depression in opioid overdose
- Short half life (<1 h)
- Very fast acting (min)
- High affinity for opioid receptor
- Induces opioid withdrawal symptoms

Maintenance Medication for Opiate Addiction: The Foundation of Recovery
J Addict Dis 2012;31:207-225
Study: Review.
Discussion: Maintenance treatment of opioid addiction with methadone or buprenorphine is associated with retention in treatment, reduction in illicit opiate use, decreased craving, and improved social function. Recently, studies showing extended release naltrexone injections have showed some promise.

Treatment of Cocaine Toxicity with Beta-Blockers and Alpha-Blockers
Medicine Forum. 2011;12(1):7
Ann Emerg Med. 2008 Mar;51(3 Suppl):S18-20. *

Patients treated with beta blockers and labetalol experience an unopposed alpha adrenergic effect, causing vasoconstriction and increased blood pressure. The use of beta blockers and labetalol is therefore contraindicated in the treatment of cocaine toxicity-related hypertension. Beta blockers are also contraindicated for patients with cocaine-precipitated STEMIs due to risk of exacerbating coronary spasms; several studies have demonstrated increased coronary vasoconstriction and decreased coronary sinus blood flow.

Based on cardiac catheterization laboratories demonstrating coronary artery vasodilation back to baseline with phentolamine, alpha-adrenergic antagonists have been recommended by most guidelines for the treatment of cocaine-associated acute coronary syndrome and cocaine-induced hypertension.

Cocaine

- street names: blow, C, coke, crack, flake, freebase, rock, snow
- alkaloid extracted from leaves of the coca plant; blocks presynaptic uptake of dopamine (causing euphoria), norepinephrine and epinephrine (causing vasospasm, HTN)
- self-administered by inhalation, insufflation, or intravenous route

Intoxication

- elation, euphoria, pressured speech, restlessness, sympathetic stimulation (e.g. tachycardia, mydriasis, sweating)
- prolonged use may result in paranoia and psychosis

Overdose

- medical emergency: HTN, tachycardia, tonic-clonic seizures, dyspnea, and ventricular arrhythmias
- treatment with IV diazepam to control seizures
- beta-blockers (incl. labetalol or propranolol) are not recommended because of risk from unopposed alpha-adrenergic stimulation

Withdrawal

- initial "crash" (1-48 h): increased sleep, increased appetite
- withdrawal (1-10 wk): dysphoric mood plus fatigue, irritability, vivid unpleasant dreams, insomnia or hypersomnia, psychomotor agitation or retardation
- complications: relapse, suicide (significant increase in suicide during withdrawal period)
- management: supportive management

Treatment of Cocaine Use Disorder

- see *General Approach to Treatment*, PS4
- no pharmacologic agents have widespread evidence or acceptance of use

Complications

- cardiovascular: arrhythmias, MI, CVA, ruptured AAA
- neurologic: seizures
- psychiatric: psychosis, paranoia, delirium, suicidal ideation
- other: nasal septal deterioration, acute/chronic lung injury "crack lung", possible increased risk of connective tissue disease

Amphetamines

- includes prescription medications for ADHD such as Ritalin® and Adderall®
- intoxication characterized by euphoria, improved concentration, sympathetic and behavioural hyperactivity and at high doses can mimic psychotic mania, can eventually cause coma
- chronic use can produce a paranoid psychosis which can resemble schizophrenia with agitation, paranoia, delusions and hallucinations
- withdrawal symptoms include dysphoria, fatigue, and restlessness
- treatment of amphetamine induced psychosis: antipsychotics for acute presentation, benzodiazepines for agitation, β-blockers for tachycardia, hypertension

Cannabis

- cannabis (marijuana) is the most commonly used illicit drug
- psychoactive substance: delta-9-tetrahydrocannabinol (Δ9-THC)
- intoxication characterized by tachycardia, conjunctival vascular engorgement, dry mouth, altered sensorium, increased appetite, increased sense of well-being, euphoria/laughter, muscle relaxation, impaired performance on psychomotor tasks including driving
- high doses can cause depersonalization, paranoia, anxiety and may trigger psychosis and schizophrenia if predisposed
- chronic use associated with tolerance and an apathetic, amotivational state, increases risk of later manic episodes
- cessation following heavy use produces a significant withdrawal syndrome: irritability, anxiety, insomnia, decreased food intake
- treatment of cannabis use disorder: see *General Approach to Treatment*, PS4

Common Presentations of Drug Use

System	Findings
General	Weight loss (especially cocaine, heroin)
	Injected conjunctiva (cannabis)
	Pinpoint pupils (opioids)
	Track marks (injection drugs)
MSK	Trauma
GI	Viral hepatitis (injection drugs)
	Unexplained elevations in ALT (injection drugs)
Behavioural	Missed appointments
	Non-compliance
	Drug-seeking (especially benzodiazepines, opioids)
Psychological	Insomnia
	Fatigue
	Depression
	Flat affect (benzodiazepines, barbiturates)
	Paranoia (cocaine)
	Psychosis (cocaine, cannabis, hallucinogens)
Social	Marital discord
	Family violence
	Work/school
	Absenteeism and poor performance

Cannabinoid Hyperemesis Syndrome
An interesting and relatively new clinical phenomenon associated with chronic cannabis use characterized by cyclical, recurrent severe nausea, vomiting, and colicky pain. Possibly due to increased potency of available THC products. Patients often present to ED in acute distress with no evidence of specific GI pathology. Many patients will successfully self-medicate with hot baths or showers

Medical Uses of Marijuana
- Anorexia-cachexia (AIDS, cancer)
- Spasticity, muscle spasms (multiple sclerosis, spinal cord injury)
- Levodopa-induced dyskinesia (Parkinson's Disease)
- Controlling tics and obsessive-compulsive behaviour (Tourette's syndrome)
- Reducing intra-ocular pressure (glaucoma)

Cannabis Use and Risk of Psychotic or Affective Mental Health Outcomes: A Systematic Review
The Lancet 2007;370:319-328
Purpose: To review the evidence for cannabis use and occurrence of psychotic or affective mental health outcomes.
Study Characteristics: A meta-analysis of 35 population-based longitudinal studies, or case-control studies nested within longitudinal designs.
Results: There was an increased risk of any psychotic outcome in individuals who had ever used cannabis (pooled adjusted odds ratio =1.41, 95% CI 1.20-1.65). Findings were consistent with a dose-response effect, with greater risk in people who used cannabis more frequently (2.09, 95% CI, 1.54-2.84). Findings for depression, suicidal thoughts, and anxiety outcomes were less consistent. In both cases (psychotic and affective outcomes), a substantial confounding effect was present.
Conclusions: The findings are consistent with the view that cannabis increases risk of psychotic outcomes independent of transient intoxication effects, although evidence is less strong for affective outcomes. Although cannabis use and the development of psychosis are strongly associated, it is difficult to determine causality and it is possible that the association results from confounding factors or bias. The authors did conclude that there is sufficient evidence to warn young people that using cannabis could increase their risk of developing a psychotic illness later in life.

Hallucinogens

- types of hallucinogens by primary action
  - 5-HT2A agonists: LSD, mescaline (peyote), psilocybin mushrooms, DMT (ayahuasca)
  - NMDA antagonists: PCP, ketamine
  - κ-opioid agonists: salvia divinorum, ibogaine
- 5-HT2A agonists are most commonly used; intoxication characterized by tachycardia, HTN, mydriasis, tremor, hyperpyrexia, and a variety of perceptual, mood and cognitive changes (rarely, if ever, deadly; treat vitals symptomatically)
- psychological effects of high doses: depersonalization, derealization, paranoia, and anxiety (panic with agoraphobia)
- tolerance develops rapidly (hours-days) to most hallucinogens so physical dependency is virtually impossible, although psychological dependency and problematic usage patterns can still occur
- no specific withdrawal syndrome characterized
- management of acute intoxication
  - support, reassurance, diminished stimulation; benzodiazepines or high potency antipsychotics seldom required (if used, use small doses), minimize use of restraints
- long term adverse effects: controversial role in triggering psychiatric disorders, particularly mood or psychosis, thought to be chiefly in individuals with genetic or other risk factors
- **Hallucinogen Persisting Perception Disorder:** DSM-5 diagnosis characterized by long lasting, spontaneous, intermittent recurrences of visual perceptual changes reminiscent of those experienced with hallucinogen exposure

"Club Drugs"

Table 6. The Mechanism and Effects of Common "Club Drugs"

Drug	Mechanism	Effect	Adverse Effects
MDMA ("Ecstasy", "X", "E")	Acts on serotonergic and dopaminergic pathways, properties of a hallucinogen and stimulant	Enhanced sensorium; feelings of well-being, empathy	Sweating, tachycardia fatigue, muscle spasms (especially jaw clenching), ataxia, hyperthermia, arrhythmias, DIC, rhabdomyolysis, renal failure, seizures, death
Gamma Hydroxybutyrate (GHB, "G", "Liquid Ecstasy")	Biphasic dopamine response (inhibition then release) and releases opiate-like substance	Euphoric effects, increased aggression, impaired judgment	Sweating, tachycardia, fatigue, muscle spasms (especially jaw clenching), ataxia, severe withdrawal from abrupt cessation of high doses: tremor, seizures, psychosis
Flunitrazepam (Rohypnol®, "Roofies", "Rope", "The Forget Pill")	Potent benzodiazepine, rapid oral absorption	Sedation, psychomotor impairment, amnestic effects, decreased sexual inhibition	CNS depression with EtOH
Ketamine ("Special K", "Kit-Kat")	NMDA receptor antagonist, rapid-acting general anesthetic used in pediatrics and by veterinarians	"Dissociative" state, profound amnesia/analgesia; hallucinations and sympathomimetic effects	Psychological distress, accidents due to intensity of experience and lack of bodily control, in overdose, decreased LOC, respiratory depression, catatonia
Methamphetamine ("speed", "meth", "chalk", "ice", "crystal")	Amphetamine stimulant, induces norepinephrine, dopamine, and serotonin release	Rush begins in min, effects last 6-8 h, increased activity, decreased appetite, general sense of well-being, tolerance occurs quickly, users often binge and crash	Short-term use: high agitation, rage, violent behaviour, occasionally hyperthermia and convulsions. Long-term use: addiction, anxiety, confusion, insomnia, paranoia, auditory and tactile hallucinations (especially formication), delusions, mood disturbance, suicidal and homicidal thoughts, stroke, may be contaminated with lead, and IV users may present with acute lead poisoning
Phencyclidine ("PCP", "angel dust")	Not understood, used by veterinarians to immobilize large animals	Amnestic, euphoric, hallucinatory state	Horizontal/vertical nystagmus, myoclonus, ataxia, autonomic instability (treat with diazepam IV), prolonged agitated psychosis (treat with haloperidol); high risk for suicide; violence towards others. High dose can cause coma

Date Rape Drugs
- GHB
- Flunitrazepam (Rohypnol®)
- Ketamine

Emerging Medical Uses of Hallucinogens
Many hallucinogens are currently under investigation for therapeutic benefit; LSD & Psilocybin for end of life anxiety, MDMA for PTSD, Ketamine for rapid treatment of depression, ibogaine derivatives for addiction

Formication
Tactile hallucination that insects or snakes are crawling over or under the skin (especially associated with crystal meth use)

Somatic Symptom and Related Disorders

General Characteristics
- physical signs and symptoms lacking objective medical support in the presence of psychological factors that are judged to be important in the initiation, exacerbation, or maintenance of the disturbance
- cause significant distress or impairment in functioning
- symptoms are produced unconsciously and are not the result of malingering or factitious disorder, which are disorders of voluntary "faking" of symptoms (or intentionally inducing, e.g. injecting feces) for secondary gain
- primary gain: somatic symptom represents a symbolic resolution of an unconscious psychological conflict; serves to reduce anxiety and conflict with no external incentive
- secondary gain: the sick role; external benefits obtained or unpleasant duties avoided (e.g. work)

Management of Somatic Symptom and Related Disorders
- brief, regular scheduled visits with GP to facilitate therapeutic relationship and help patient feel cared for
- limit number of physicians involved in care, minimize medical investigations; coordinate necessary investigations
- emphasis on what the patient can change and control; the psychosocial coping skills, not their physical symptoms (functional recovery > explanation of symptoms)
- do not tell patient it is "all in their head," emphasize these disorders are real entities or functional in nature
- psychotherapy: CBT, mindfulness interventions, biofeedback, conflict resolution
- minimize psychotropic drugs: anxiolytics in short-term only, antidepressants for comorbid depression and anxiety

> **Malingering:** intentional production of false or grossly exaggerated physical or psychological symptoms, motivated by external reward (e.g. avoiding work, obtaining financial compensation, or obtaining drugs)
>
> **Factitious Disorder:** intentional production or feigning of physical or psychological signs or symptoms

Somatic Symptom Disorder

DSM-5 Diagnostic Criteria for Somatic Symptom Disorder
Reprinted with permission from the Diagnostic and Statistical Manual of Mental Disorders, 5th ed. 2013. American Psychiatric Association

A. one or more somatic symptoms that are distressing or result in significant disruption of daily life
B. excessive thoughts, feelings, or behaviours related to the somatic symptoms or associated health concerns as manifested by at least one of the following
1. disproportionate and persistent thoughts about the seriousness of one's symptoms
2. persistently high level of anxiety about health or symptoms
3. excessive time and energy devoted to these symptoms or health concerns
C. although any one somatic symptom may not be continuously present, the state of being symptomatic is persistent (typically >6 mo)

- **specify: with predominant pain** (previously pain disorder) for those whose somatic symptom is primarily pain
- patients have physical symptoms and believe these symptoms represent the manifestation of a serious illness
- persistent belief despite negative medical investigations and may develop different symptoms over time
- lifetime prevalence may be around 5-7% in the general adult population
- females tend to report more somatic symptoms than males do, cultural factors may influence sex ratio
- complications: anxiety and depression commonly comorbid (up to 80%), unnecessary medications or surgery
- often a misdiagnosis for an insidious illness so rule out all organic illnesses (e.g. multiple sclerosis)

Illness Anxiety Disorder

- preoccupation with fear of having, or the idea that one has, a serious disease, to the point of causing significant impairment
- convictions persist despite negative investigations and medical reassurance
- somatic symptoms are mild or not present
- there is a high level of anxiety about health and the individual is easily alarmed about personal health status
- person engages in maladaptive behaviour such as excessive physical checking or total healthcare avoidance
- duration is ≥6 mo; onset in 3rd-4th decade of life
- a new diagnostic entity so epidemiology is not well known; however, it is likely less common than SSD
- possible role for SSRIs due to generally high level of anxiety

Conversion Disorder (Functional Neurological Symptom Disorder)

- one or more symptoms or deficits affecting voluntary motor or sensory function that mimic a neurological or GMC (e.g. impaired coordination, local paralysis, double vision, seizures, or convulsions)
- does not need to be preceded by a psychological event as per previous DSM criteria, however this is still worth exploring as many patients will present after such an event or related to a medical diagnosis in a first-degree relative
- 2-5/100,000 in general population; 5% of referrals to neurology clinics
- more common in rural populations and in individuals with little medical knowledge
- spontaneous remission in 95% of acute cases, 50% of chronic cases (>6 mo)
- incompatible findings detected from specific neurological testing can help differentiate between functional and neurological origin (e.g. Hoover's sign, dermatome testing)

Table 7. Differential of Somatic Symptom and Related Disorders

	Somatic Symptom Disorder	Illness Anxiety Disorder	Conversion Disorder	Factitious Disorder	Malingering
Somatic Symptoms	Present	Mild or absent	Neurologic, voluntary motor or sensory	Psychological or physical	Psychological or physical
Symptoms Produced	Unconsciously	Unconsciously	Unconsciously	Consciously	Consciously
Physical Findings	Absent	Absent	Incompatible	Possible, attempts to falsify	Possible, attempts to falsify

Dissociative Disorders

Definition
- severe dissociation resulting in breakdown of integrated functions of consciousness and perception of self
- differential diagnosis: PTSD, acute stress disorder, borderline personality disorder, somatic symptom disorder, substance abuse, GMC (various neurologic disorders including complex/partial seizures, migraine, Cotard syndrome)

Dissociative Identity Disorder

- disruption of identity characterized by two or more distinct personality states or an experience of possession
- can manifest as sudden alterations in sense of self and agency (ego-dystonic emotions, behaviours, speech)
- features recurrent episodes of amnesia (declarative or procedural)

Dissociative Amnesia

- inability to recall important autobiographical information, usually of a traumatic or stressful nature, that is inconsistent with normal forgetting and not attributable to a psychiatric disorder or medical illness
- localized/selective amnesia: failure to recall all/some events during a prescribed period of time
- generalized amnesia: (more rare) complete loss of memory for one's life history, ± procedural knowledge, ± semantic knowledge. Usually sudden onset. Often presents with perplexity, disorientation, aimless wandering

Depersonalization/Derealization Disorder

- persistent or recurrent episodes of one or both of:
  - **depersonalization:** experiences of detachment from oneself, feelings of unreality, or being an outside observer to one's thoughts, feelings, speech, and actions (can feature distortions in perception including time, as well as emotional and physical numbing)
  - **derealization:** experiences of unreality or detachment with respect to the surroundings (e.g. feeling as if in a dream, or that the world is not real, external visual world is foggy or distorted)
- transient (seconds-hours) experiences of this nature are quite common in the general population
- episodes can range from hours-years, patients are often quite distressed and verbalize concern of "going crazy"

Sleep Disorders

- for more information regarding normal sleep cycles and the illnesses described, see <u>Neurology</u>, *Sleep Disorders*, N46

Overview

- adequate sleep is essential to normal functioning; deprivation can lead to cognitive impairment and increased mortality
- circadian rhythms help regulate mood and cognitive performance
- neurotransmitters commonly implicated in psychiatric illnesses also regulate sleep
  - acetylcholine activity and decreased activity of monoamine neurotransmitters is associated with greater REM sleep
  - decreased adrenergic and cholinergic activity are associated with NREM sleep
- depression is associated with decreased Δ (deep, slow-wave) sleep, decreased REM latency, and increased REM density
- criteria
  - must cause significant distress or impairment in normal functioning
  - not due to a GMC or medications/drugs (unless specified)

Management

- pharmacological treatments are illness-specific
  - non-benzodiazepines preferable (e.g. trazodone, zoplicone, quetiapine), but benzodiazepines a short term option
  - medication should not be prescribed without having first made a diagnosis and considering major psychiatric illnesses (major depression and alcohol use disorders are common etiologies)
- sleep hygiene is a simple, effective, but often underutilized method for addressing sleep disturbances; recommendations include
  - waking up and going to bed at same time every day, including on weekends
  - avoiding long periods of wakefulness in bed
  - not using bed for non-sleep activities (reading, TV, work)
  - avoiding napping
  - discontinuing or reducing consumption of alcohol, caffeine, drugs
  - exercising at least 3-4x per week (but not in the evening, if this interferes with sleep)

Table 8. Major DSM-5 Sleep-Wake Disorders

Note: For more information regarding specific disorders, see: <u>Neurology</u>, *Sleep Disorders*, N46; <u>Family Medicine</u>, *Sleep Disorders*, FM45; and <u>Respirology</u>, *Sleep Apnea*, R31

Category	Disorder	Description
(Uncategorized)	Insomnia disorder	Difficulty sleeping
	Hypersomnolence disorder	Feeling sleepy throughout the day
	Narcolepsy	Recurrent attacks of irrepressible need to sleep
	Circadian rhythm sleep-wake disorders	Insomnia or excessive sleepiness due to misalignment or alteration in endogenous circadian rhythm
	Restless legs syndrome	Uncomfortable, frequent urge to move legs at night
	Substance/medication-induced sleep disorder	Disturbance in sleep (insomnia or daytime sleepiness) caused by substance/medication intoxication or withdrawal
Breathing-related sleep disorders	Obstructive sleep apnea hypopnea	Breathing issues due to obstruction
	Central sleep apnea	Breathing issues due to aberrant brain signaling
	Sleep-related hypoventilation	Breathing issues due to decreased responsiveness to carbon dioxide levels
Parasomnias	Non-rapid eye movement sleep arousal disorders	Incomplete awakening from sleep, complex motor behaviour without conscious awareness; amnesia regarding episodes; includes symptoms of **Sleepwalking:** rising from bed and walking about, blank face, unresponsive, awakened with difficulty **Sleep terrors:** recurrent episodes of abrupt terror arousals from sleep, usually beginning with a panicky scream, intense fear and autonomic arousal, relative unresponsiveness to comfort during episodes **Specifiers:** sleep-related sexual behaviour (sexsomnia) and sleep-related eating
	Nightmare disorder	Repeated extended, extremely dysphoric, often very vivid, well-remembered dreams that usually involve significant threats; rapid orientation and alertness on awakening with autonomic arousal
	Rapid eye movement sleep behaviour disorder	Arousal during sleep, associated with vocalization and/or complex motor behaviours; can cause violent injuries; rapid orientation and alertness on awakening

Sexuality and Gender

Gender Dysphoria

Definition
- the distress that may coincide with conflict between one's experienced/expressed gender and one's assigned gender

Typical Presentation
- strong and persistent cross-gender identification
- desire to be rid of primary/secondary sex characteristics and to gain the primary/secondary sex characteristics of their identified gender
- repeated stated desire or insistence that one is of the opposite sex
- preference for cross-dressing, cross-gender roles in make-believe play
- intense desire to participate in the stereotypical games and pastimes of the opposite sex
- strong preference for playmates of the opposite sex
- significant distress or impairment in functioning and persistent discomfort with his or her sex or gender role

Treatment
- psychotherapy
- hormonal therapy
- sexual reassignment surgery

Paraphilic Disorders

Definition
- intense and persistent sexual interest other than sexual interest in genital stimulation or preparatory fondling with phenotypically normal, physically mature, consenting human partners
- **paraphilic disorder:** paraphilia that causes distress or functional impairment to the individual, or a paraphilia whose realization entails personal harm, or risk of harm to others
- **subtypes:** voyeuristic, exhibitionistic, frotteuristic, sexual masochism, sexual sadism, pedophilic, fetishistic, transvestic, other specified paraphilic disorder, unspecified paraphilic disorder
- rarely self-referred; come to medical attention through interpersonal or legal conflict
- person usually has more than one paraphilia; 5% of paraphilias attributed to women
- typical presentation
- begins in childhood or early adolescence; increasing in complexity and stability with age
- chronic, decreases with advancing age but may increase with stress

Treatment
- anti-androgen drugs
- behaviour modification
- psychotherapy

SEXUAL DYSFUNCTION
- see <u>Gynecology</u>, GY33 and <u>Urology</u>, U34

Eating Disorders

Epidemiology
- anorexia nervosa (AN): 1% of adolescent and young adult females; onset 13-20 yr old
- bulimia nervosa (BN): 2-4% of adolescent and young adult females; onset 16-18 yr old
- F:M=10:1; mortality 5-10%

Etiology
- multifactorial: psychological, sociological, and biological associations
- individual: perfectionism, lack of control in other life areas, history of sexual abuse
- personality: obsessive-compulsive, histrionic, borderline
- familial: maintenance of weight equilibrium and control in dysfunctional family
- cultural factors: prevalent in industrialized societies, idealization of thinness in the media
- genetic factors
  - AN: 6% prevalence in siblings, with one study of twin pairs finding concordance in 9 of 12 monozygotic pairs versus concordance in 1 of 14 dizygotic pairs
  - BN: higher familial incidence of affective disorders than the general population

Risk Factors
- physical factors: obesity, chronic medical illness (e.g. DM)
- psychological factors: individuals who by career choice are expected to be thin, family history (mood disorders, eating disorders, substance abuse), history of sexual abuse (especially for BN), homosexual males, competitive athletes, concurrent associated mental illness (depression, OCD, anxiety disorder [especially panic and agoraphobia], substance abuse [specifically for BN])

Anorexia Nervosa

DSM-5 Diagnostic Criteria for Anorexia Nervosa
Reprinted with permission from the Diagnostic and Statistical Manual of Mental Disorders, 5th ed. 2013. American Psychiatric Association

A. intake and weight: restriction of energy intake relative to requirements, leading to a significantly low body weight in the context of age, sex, developmental trajectory, and physical health. Significantly low weight is defined as a weight that is less than minimally normal or, for children and adolescents, less than that minimally expected

B. fear or behaviour: intense fear of gaining weight or of becoming fat, or persistent behaviour that interferes with weight gain, even though at a significantly low weight

C. perception: disturbance in the way in which one's body weight or shape is experienced, undue influence of body weight or shape on self-evaluation, or persistent lack of recognition of the seriousness of the current low body weight

- **specifiers:** partial remission, full remission, severity based on BMI (mild = BMI >17 kg/m², moderate = BMI 16-16.99 kg/m², severe = BMI 15-15.99 kg/m², extreme = BMI <15 kg/m²), type (restricting = during last 3 mo no episodes of binge-eating or purging vs. binge-eating/purging type = in last 3 mo have participated in recurrent episodes of binge-eating/purging)

Athletic Triad
- Disordered eating
- Amenorrhea
- Osteoporosis

Some patients with insulin-dependent DM may stop their insulin in order to lose weight

Management
- psychotherapy: individual, group, family (gold standard): address food and body perception, coping mechanisms, health effects
- medications of little value
- outpatient and inpatient programs are available
- inpatient hospitalization for treatment of eating disorders is rarely on an acute basis (unless there is a concurrent psychiatric reason for emergent admission e.g. suicide risk)
- criteria to admit to medical ward for hospitalization: <65% of standard body weight (<85% of standard body weight for adolescents), hypovolemia requiring intravenous fluid, heart rate <40 bpm, abnormal serum chemistry, or if actively suicidal
- agree on target body weight on admission and reassure this weight will not be surpassed
- monitor for complications of AN (see Table 9, PS33)
- monitor for refeeding syndrome
  - potentially life-threatening metabolic response to refeeding in severely malnourished patients resulting in severe shifts in fluid and electrolyte levels
  - complications include hypophosphatemia, congestive heart failure, cardiac arrhythmias, delirium, and death
  - prevention: slow refeeding, gradual increase in nutrition, supplemental phosphorus, and close monitoring of electrolytes and cardiac status

Prognosis
- early intervention much more effective (adolescent onset has much better prognosis than adult onset)
- 1 in 10 adolescents continue to have anorexia nervosa as adults
- with treatment, 70% resume a weight of at least 85% of expected levels and about 50% resume normal menstrual function
- eating peculiarities and associated psychiatric symptoms are common and persistent
- long-term mortality: 10-20% of patients hospitalized will die in next 10-30 yr (secondary to severe and chronic starvation, metabolic or cardiac catastrophes, with a significant proportion committing suicide)

Bulimia Nervosa

DSM-5 Diagnostic Criteria for Bulimia Nervosa
Reprinted with permission from the Diagnostic and Statistical Manual of Mental Disorders, 5th ed. 2013. American Psychiatric Association

A. recurrent episodes of binge-eating; an episode of binge-eating is characterized by both of the following
  - eating, in a discrete period of time, an amount of food that is definitely larger than what most individuals would eat during a similar period of time and under similar circumstances
  - a sense of lack of control over eating during the episode

B. recurrent inappropriate compensatory behaviour in order to prevent weight gain, such as self-induced vomiting, misuse of laxatives, diuretics, enemas, or other medications, fasting, or excessive exercise

C. the binge-eating and inappropriate compensatory behaviours both occur, on average, at least once a week for 3 mo

D. self-evaluation is unduly influenced by body shape and weight

E. the disturbance does not occur exclusively during episodes of AN

- **specifiers:** partial remission, full remission, severity (measured in # of inappropriate compensatory behaviours/wk: mild = 1-3, moderate = 4-7, severe = 8-13, extreme = 14+)

Associated Features
- fatigue and muscle weakness due to repetitive vomiting and fluid/electrolyte imbalance
- tooth decay
- swollen appearance around angle of jaw and puffiness of eye sockets due to fluid retention
- reddened knuckles, Russell's sign (knuckle callus from self-induced vomiting)
- trouble concentrating
- weight fluctuation over time

Management
- admission for significant electrolyte abnormalities
- biological: treatment of starvation effects, SSRIs (fluoxetine most evidence) as adjunct
- psychological: develop trusting relationship with therapist to explore personal etiology and triggers, CBT, family therapy, recognition of health risks
- social: challenge destructive societal views of women, use of hospital environment to provide external patterning for normative eating behaviour

Prognosis
- relapsing/remitting disease
- good prognostic factors: onset before age 15, achieving a healthy weight within 2 yr of treatment
- poor prognostic factors: later age of onset, previous hospitalizations, individual and familial disturbance
- 60% good treatment outcome, 30% intermediate outcome, 10% poor outcome

Binge-Eating Disorder

Definition
- recurrent episodes of binge-eating (as defined by criteria A of BN) that are associated with eating much more rapidly than normal, eating until feeling uncomfortably full, eating large amounts when not physically hungry, eating alone because embarrassed by how much one is eating, feeling disgusted with self/depressed, very guilty afterwards at least once/wk x 3 mo
- not associated with any compensatory behaviours
- dieting usually follows binge-eating (vs. BN where dysfunctional dieting typically precedes binge-eating)
- associated with health consequences (e.g. increased risk of weight gain, obesity)

Epidemiology
- F:M = 2:1
- begins in adolescence or young-adulthood

Treatment
- CBT

Avoidant/Restrictive Food Intake Disorder

Definition
- eating/feeding disturbance to the extent of persistent failure to meet appropriate nutritional and/or energy needs, resulting in significant weight loss/growth failure and nutritional deficiencies. Patients experience disturbances in psychosocial functioning and may become dependent on enteral feeding/oral nutritional supplementation
  - does not occur during an episode of AN or BN
  - no evidence of distress in the way in which one's body weight or shape is experienced

Risk Factors
- temperament (e.g. anxiety disorders), environment (e.g. familial anxiety), genetic (e.g. history of GI conditions)
- begins in infancy and can persist into adulthood

Treatment
- watchful waiting
- behaviour modification
- psychotherapy

Points for Differentiating Between Eating Disorders
- AN of binge-eating/purging type (significantly low body weight) takes priority over a BN diagnosis (body weight not in criteria)
- BN requires compensatory behaviours
- Binge eating disorder does not involve compensatory behaviours
- Avoidant/restrictive food intake disorder does not involve disturbances in body image

Table 9. Physiologic Complications of Eating Disorders

System	Starvation/Restriction	Binge-Purge
General	Low BP, low HR, significant orthostatic changes ± syncopal episodes, low temperature, vitamin deficiencies	Russell's sign (knuckle callus) Parotid gland enlargement Perioral skin irritation Periocular and palatal petechiae Loss of dental enamel and caries Aspiration pneumonia Metabolic alkalosis secondary to hypokalemia and loss of acid
Endocrine	Primary or secondary amenorrhea, decreased T_3/T_4	
Neurologic	Seizure (decreased Ca^{2+}, Mg^{2+}, PO_4^{3-})	
Cutaneous	Dry skin, lanugo hair, hair loss or thinning, brittle nails, yellow skin from high carotene	
GI	Constipation, GERD, delayed gastric emptying	Acute gastric dilation/rupture, pancreatitis, GERD, hematemesis secondary to Mallory-Weiss tear
CVS	Arrhythmias, CHF	Arrhythmias, cardiomyopathy (from use of ipecac), sudden cardiac death (decreased K^+)
MSK	Osteoporosis secondary to hypogonadism	Muscle wasting
Renal	Pre-renal failure (hypovolemia), renal calculi	Renal failure (electrolyte disturbances)
Extremities	Pedal edema (decreased albumin)	Pedal edema (decreased albumin)
Lab Values	Starvation: decreased RBCs, decreased WBCs, decreased LH, decreased FSH, decreased estrogen, decreased testosterone, increased growth hormone, increased cholesterol Dehydration: increased BUN	Vomiting: decreased Na^+, decreased K^+, decreased Cl^-, decreased H^+, increased amylase; hypokalemia with metabolic alkalosis Laxatives: decreased Na^+, decreased K^+, decreased Cl^-, increased H^+; metabolic acidosis

 Important electrolytes in eating disorders: KPMg (potassium, phosphate, magnesium)

Personality Disorders

- in the literature, personality and its disorders are better understood using a trait-based dimensional approach (e.g. 5 major traits such as extraversion, agreeableness, conscientiousness, neuroticism, and openness to experiences rated on a continuum of dysfunctional effects) rather than discrete categories; however, the discrete categories still remain in the current DSM and will be referenced here

General Information
- an enduring pattern of inner experience and behaviour that deviates markedly from the expectations of the individual's culture; manifested in two or more of: cognition, affect, interpersonal functioning, impulse control
- inflexible and pervasive across a range of situations
- pattern is stable and well established by adolescence or early adulthood (vs. a sudden onset)
- associated with many complications, such as depression, suicide, violence, brief psychotic episodes, multiple drug use, and treatment resistance
- relationship building and establishing boundaries are important; focus should be placed on validating, finding things to be truly empathetic about, and speaking to the patient's strengths
- mainstay of treatment is psychotherapy, add pharmacotherapy to treat associated axis I disorders (i.e. depression, anxiety, substance abuse)

Classification
- personality disorders are divided into three clusters (A, B, and C), with shared features among disorders within each

 A flag for personality disorders in clinical setting is the reaction that a patient is eliciting in you

 Personality disorders with familial associations: Schizotypal, Antisocial, and Borderline

Table 10. Description and Diagnosis of Personality Disorders

Cluster A "Mad" Personality Disorders
- Patients seem odd, eccentric, withdrawn
- Familial association with psychotic disorders
- Common defense mechanisms: intellectualization, projection, magical thinking

Paranoid Personality Disorder (0.5-3%)
Pervasive distrust and suspiciousness of others, interpret motives as malevolent
Blame problems on others and seem angry and hostile
Diagnosis requires 4+ of: **SUSPECT**
1. **S**uspicious that others are exploiting or deceiving them
2. **U**nforgiving (bears grudges)
3. **S**pousal infidelity suspected without justification
4. **P**erceive attacks on character, counterattacks quickly
5. **E**nemies or friends? Preoccupied with acquaintance trustworthiness
6. **C**onfiding in others is feared
7. **T**hreats interpreted in benign remarks

Schizotypal Personality Disorder (3-5.6%)
Pattern of eccentric behaviours, peculiar thought patterns
Diagnosis requires 5+ of: **ME PECULIAR**
1. **M**agical thinking
2. **E**xperiences unusual perceptions (including body illusions)
3. **P**aranoid ideation
4. **E**ccentric behaviour or appearance
5. **C**onstricted or inappropriate affect
6. **U**nusual thinking/speech (e.g. vague, stereotyped)
7. **L**acks close friends
8. **I**deas of reference
9. **A**nxiety in social situations
(Note: Rule out psychotic/pervasive developmental disorders - this is not part of the criteria)

Schizoid Personality Disorder
Neither desires nor enjoys close relationships including being a part of a family; prefers to be alone
Lifelong pattern of social withdrawal
Seen as eccentric and reclusive with restricted affect
Diagnosis requires 4 of: **DISTANT**
1. **D**etached/flat affect, emotionally cold
2. **I**ndifferent to praise or criticism
3. **S**exual experiences of little interest
4. **T**asks done solitarily
5. **A**bsence of close friends (other than first-degree relatives)
6. **N**either desires nor enjoys close relationships (including family)
7. **T**akes pleasure in few (if any) activities

Cluster B "Bad" Personality Disorders
- Patients seem dramatic, emotional, inconsistent
- Familial association with mood disorders
- Common defense mechanisms: denial, acting out, regression (histrionic PD), splitting (borderline PD), projective identification, idealization/devaluation

Borderline Personality Disorder (2-4%)
Unstable moods and behaviour, feel alone in the world, problems with self-image. History of repeated suicide attempts, self-harm behaviours. Inpatients commonly report history of sexual abuse. Tends to fizzle out as patients age. DBT is the principal treatment (see *Psychotherapy*, PS40)
10% suicide rate
Diagnosis requires 5+ of: **IMPULSIVE**
1. **I**mpulsive (min. 2 self-damaging ways, e.g. sex/drugs/spending)
2. **M**ood/affect instability
3. **P**aranoia or dissociation under stress
4. **U**nstable self-image
5. **L**abile intense relationships
6. **S**uicidal gestures / self-harm
7. **I**nappropriate anger
8. a**V**oiding abandonment (real or imagined, frantic efforts to)
9. **E**mptiness (feelings of)

Narcissistic Personality Disorder (2%)
Sense of superiority, needs constant admiration, lacks empathy, but with fragile sense of self. Consider themselves "special" and will exploit others for personal gain
Diagnosis requires 5+ of: **GRANDIOSE**
1. **G**randiose
2. **R**equires excessive admiration
3. **A**rrogant
4. **N**eeds to be special (and associate with other specials)
5. **D**reams of success, power, beauty, love
6. **I**nterpersonally exploitative
7. **O**thers (lacks empathy, unable to recognize feelings/needs of)
8. **S**ense of entitlement
9. **E**nvious (or believes others are envious)

Antisocial Personality Disorder (M: 3%, F: 1%)
Lack of remorse for actions, manipulative and deceitful, often violate the law. May appear charming on first impression. Pattern of disregard for others and violation of others' rights must be present before age 15; however, for the diagnosis of ASPD patients must be at least 18. Strong association with Conduct Disorder, history of trauma/abuse common (see *Child Psychiatry*)
Diagnosis requires 3+ of: **CORRUPT**
1. **C**annot conform to law
2. **O**bligations ignored (irresponsible)
3. **R**eckless disregard for safety
4. **R**emorseless
5. **U**nderhanded (deceitful)
6. **P**lanning insufficient (impulsive)
7. **T**emper (irritable and aggressive)

Histrionic Personality Disorder (1.3-3%)
Attention-seeking behaviour and excessively emotional. Are dramatic, flamboyant, and extroverted. Cannot form meaningful relationships. Often sexually inappropriate
Diagnosis requires 5+ of: **ACTRESSS**
1. **A**ppearance used to attract attention
2. **C**entre of attention (else uncomfortable)
3. **T**heatrical
4. **R**elationships (believed to be more intimate than they are)
5. **E**asily influenced
6. **S**eductive behaviour
7. **S**hallow expression of emotions (which rapidly shift)
8. **S**peech (impressionistic and vague)

Table 10. Description and Diagnosis of Personality Disorders (continued)

Cluster C "Sad"
- Patients seem anxious, fearful
- Familial association with anxiety disorder
- Common defense mechanisms: isolation, avoidance, hypochondriasis

Avoidant Personality Disorder (0.5-1.6%)
Timid and socially awkward with a pervasive sense of inadequacy and fear of criticism. Fear of embarrassing or humiliating themselves in social situations so remain withdrawn and socially inhibited
Diagnosis requires 4+ of: **CRINGES**
1. **C**riticism or rejection preoccupies thoughts in social situations
2. **R**estraint in relationships due to fear of being shamed
3. **I**nhibited in new relationships due to fear of inadequacy
4. **N**eeds to be sure of being liked before engaging socially
5. **G**ets around occupational activities requiring interpersonal contact
6. **E**mbarrassment prevents new activity or taking risks
7. **S**elf-viewed as unappealing or inferior

Dependent Personality Disorder (1.6-6.7%)
Pervasive and excessive need to be taken care of, excessive fear of separation, clinging and submissive behaviours. Difficulty making everyday decisions. Useful to set regulated treatment schedule (regular, brief visits) and being firm about in between issues. Encourage patient to do more for themselves, engage in own problem-solving
Diagnosis requires 5 of: **RELIANCE**
1. **R**eassurance required for everyday decisions
2. **E**xpressing disagreement difficult
3. **L**ife responsibilities assumed by others
4. **I**nitiating projects difficult (because no confidence)
5. **A**lone (feels helpless and uncomfortable when alone)
6. **N**urturance (goes to excessive lengths to obtain)
7. **C**ompanionship sought urgently
8. **E**xaggerated fears of being left to care for self

Obsessive-Compulsive Personality Disorder (3-10%)
Preoccupation with orderliness, perfectionism, and mental and interpersonal control. Is inflexible, closed-off, and inefficient
Diagnosis requires 4+ of: **SCRIMPER**
1. **S**tubborn
2. **C**annot discard worthless objects
3. **R**ule/detail obsessed (to point of activity lost)
4. **I**nflexible in matters of morality, ethics, values
5. **M**iserly
6. **P**erfectionistic
7. **E**xcludes leisure due to devotion to work
8. **R**eluctant to delegate to others

Table 11. Key Differences Among Schizoid, Schizotypal, and Schizophrenia

	Schizoid	Schizotypal	Schizophrenia
Thought Form	Organized	Organized, but vague and circumstantial	Disorganized, tangiental, loosening of associations
Thought Content	No psychosis	No psychosis, may have ideas of reference, paranoid ideation, odd beliefs and magical thinking	Psychosis, hallucinations
Relationships	Solitary, NO desire for social relationships	Lacks close relationships, INTERESTED in relationships but socially inept	Socially marginalized, but not by choice

OCPD vs. OCD

	OCPD	OCD
Ego-Syntonic or Ego-Dystonic	Ego-syntonic	Ego-dystonic
Thought Content	Obsessional thinking, no compulsions, strict routine and rigidity in day-to-day matters, more perfectionistic and rigid	Obsessions and compulsions, rituals, anxiety provoking unwanted intrusive thoughts

Child Psychiatry

Developmental Concepts

- **temperament:** a child's innate psycho-physiological and behavioural characteristics (e.g. emotionality, activity, and sociability); spectrum from "difficult" to "slow-to-warm-up" to "easy temperament"
- **parental fit:** the congruence between parenting style (authoritative, permissive) and child's temperament
- **attachment:** special relationship between child and primary caretaker(s); develops during first year, the caretaker's attachment style is the best predictor of their child's attachment style, refer to Table 12
- **separation anxiety** (normal between 10-18 mo): where separation from attachment figure results in distress

Consider speaking to children alone. Always consider child abuse. See Pediatrics, P14

Table 12. Attachment Models

Parent/Caregiver	Attachment Type	Features in Child
Loving, consistently available, sensitive, and receptive	Secure	Freely explores and engages strangers well (as long as mother in close proximity), upset with caregiver's departure, happy with return
Rejecting, unavailable psychologically, insensitive responses	Insecure (avoidant)	Ignores caregiver, shows little emotion with arrival or departure, little exploration
Inconsistent, insensitive responses, role reversal	Insecure (ambivalent/resistant)	Clingy but inconsolable, often displays anger or helplessness, little exploration
Frightening, dissociated, sexualized, or atypical. Often history of trauma or loss	Disorganized	Simultaneous approach/avoidance and stress related straining behaviour

Tips for the Child Interview
- Use language the child will understand (i.e. don't ask about feeling of worthlessness, ask about whether they feel like they're a bad kid)
- Children in some cultures are taught to be quiet and avoid eye contact with adults who are authority figures (do not mistake with depression)
- Use developmentally-appropriate questions (i.e. don't ask about lack of interest in activities, ask children whether they feel bored)

HEADSSS Interview
Home environment
Education/Employment
Activities
Drugs/Diet
Sex
Safety
Suicide/depression

Mood Disorders

MAJOR DEPRESSIVE DISORDER

Epidemiology
- pre-pubertal 1-2% (no gender differences); post-pubertal 4-18% (F:M = 2:1)

Clinical Presentation
- see *Mood Disorders*, PS9
- only difference in diagnostic criteria is that irritable mood may replace depressed mood
- physical factors: insomnia (children), hypersomnia (adolescents), somatic complaints, substance abuse, decreased hygiene
- psychological factors: irritability, boredom, anhedonia, low self-esteem, deterioration in academic performance, social withdrawal, lack of motivation, listlessness
- comorbid diagnoses: anxiety, ADHD, ODD, conduct disorder, and eating disorders

Treatment
- majority never seek treatment
- individual (CBT, IPT)/family therapy and education, modified school program
- SSRIs (strongest evidence for fluoxetine)
- close follow-up for adolescents starting SSRIs to monitor for increased suicidal ideation or behaviour
- in severe depression, best evidence for combined pharmacotherapy and psychotherapy
- ECT: only in adolescents who have severe illness, psychotic features, catatonic features, persistently suicidal
- light therapy, self-help books

Prognosis
- prolonged episodes, up to 1-2 yr
- adolescent onset predicts chronic mood disorder; up to 2/3 will have another depressive episode within 5 yr
- complications: negative impact on family and peer relationships, school failure, significantly increased risk of suicide attempt (10%) or completion (however, suicide risk low for pre-pubertal children), substance abuse

DISRUPTIVE MOOD DYSREGULATION DISORDER

Clinical Presentation
- severe, developmentally inappropriate, recurrent verbal or behavioural temper outbursts at least 3x per wk
- mood is predominantly irritable or angry in between outbursts, as observable by others
- these symptoms occur before 10 yr, have been occurring for 12 mo, with no more than 3 consecutive mo free from symptoms
- high rates of comorbidities; ADHD, ODD, anxiety disorders, depressive disorders

BIPOLAR DISORDER

Clinical Presentation
- see *Bipolar Disorder*, PS12
- mixed presentation and psychotic symptoms (hallucinations and delusions) more common in adolescent population than adult population
- unipolar depression may be an early sign of adult bipolar disorder
- ~30% of psychotic depressed adolescents receive a bipolar diagnosis within 2 yr of presentation
- associated with rapid onset of depression, psychomotor retardation, mood-congruent psychosis, affective illness in family, pharmacologically-induced mania

Treatment
- pharmacotherapy: mood stabilizers and/or antipsychotics
- psychotherapy: CBT, Family Focused Therapy

Anxiety Disorders

- lifetime prevalence 10-20%; F:M = 2:1

Clinical Presentation
- children and adolescents rarely vocalize their anxiety but instead exhibit behavioural manifestations
- school problems, recurrent physical symptoms (abdominal pain, headaches) especially in mornings, social and relationship problems, social withdrawal and isolation, family conflict, difficulty with sleep initiation, temper tantrums, irritability and mood symptoms, alcohol and drug use in adolescent

Differential Diagnosis
- depressive disorders, ODD, truancy
- clinical judgment important to differentiate developmentally normal from pathological anxiety
- for school avoidance, differentiate fear of general performance and humiliation. Consider anxiety about separation, and rule out bullying and school refusal due to learning disorder

Course and Prognosis
- better prognosis with later age of onset, lower co-morbidities, early initiation of treatment, ability to maintain school attendance and peer relationships, absence of social anxiety disorder
- with treatment, up to 80% of children will not meet criteria for their anxiety disorder at 3 yr follow-up, but up to 30% will meet criteria for another psychiatric disorder

Treatment
- similar principles for most childhood anxiety disorders due to overlapping symptomatology and frequent comorbidity
- family psychotherapy, predictive and supportive environment
- CBT: child and parental education, relaxation techniques (e.g. deep breathing), exposure/desensitization, recognizing and correcting anxious thoughts
- pharmacotherapy: SSRIs (e.g. fluoxetine), benzodiazepines (alprazolam, clonazepam have evidence – use with caution due to addictive and abuse potential as well as disinhibiting effect, especially in neurodevelopmental delay)
    - fluvoxamine and sertraline also have good evidence, particularly for OCD

Attachment type can be assessed in infants 10-18 mo of age using the Strange Situation test, in which the child is stressed by the caregiver being removed from the situation and the stranger staying. Attachment style is measured by the child's behaviour during the reunion with the caregiver

SEPARATION ANXIETY DISORDER
- excessive and developmentally inappropriate anxiety on real, threatened, or imagined separation from primary caregiver or home, with physical or emotional distress for at least 4 wk (e.g. worries of something happening to parent or themselves if separated)
- school refusal (75%) and comorbid major depression common (2/3)
- persistent worry, refusal to sleep alone, clinging, nightmares involving separation, somatic symptoms

Attachment problems may present as a child who is difficult to soothe, has difficulty sleeping, problems feeding, tantrums, or behavioural problems

SOCIAL ANXIETY DISORDER (SOCIAL PHOBIA)
- anxiety, fear, and/or avoidance provoked by situations where child feels under the scrutiny of others
- must distinguish between shy child, child with issues functioning socially (e.g. autism), and child with social anxiety
    - diagnosis only if anxiety interferes significantly with daily routine, social life, academic functioning, or if markedly distressed. Must occur in settings with peers, not just adults
- features: temper tantrums, freezing, clinging behaviour, mutism, excessively timid, stays on periphery, refuses to be involved in group play
- significant implication for future quality of life if untreated; lower levels of satisfaction in leisure activities, higher rates of school dropout, poor workplace performance, increased rates of remaining single

The shy child is quiet and reluctant to participate but slowly 'warms up'

SELECTIVE MUTISM
- consistent failure to speak in specific social situations where speaking is expected, despite speaking in other situations
- the disturbance interferes with educational or occupational achievement or with social communication

GENERALIZED ANXIETY DISORDER
- diagnostic criteria same as adults (see *Generalized Anxiety Disorder*, PS15)
    - **note:** only 1 item is required in children for Criteria C
- often redo tasks, show dissatisfaction with their work, and tend to be perfectionistic
- often fearful in multiple settings and expect more negative outcomes when faced with academic or social challenges, and require reassurance and support to take on new tasks

SPECIFIC PHOBIA
- common phobias in childhood: fear of heights, small animals, doctors, dentists, darkness, loud noises, thunder, and lightning

Fluoxetine, Cognitive-Behavioural Therapy and Their Combination for Adolescents with Depression: Treatment for Adolescents with Depression Study (TADS) Randomized Controlled Trial
JAMA 2004;292:807-820
Study: Randomized controlled trial at 13 US academic and community clinics between spring 2000-summer 2003.
Patients: 439 patients ages 12-17 with a primary DSM IV diagnosis of major depressive disorder.
Outcomes: Children's Depression Rating Scale-Revised (CDRSR) total score.
Interventions: 12 wk of (1) fluoxetine (10-40 mg/d), (2) CBT, (3) CBT + fluoxetine (10-40 mg/d), or (4) placebo.
Results: Fluoxetine with CBT had a statistically significant CDRSR score as compared to placebo (p=0.001) with a 71% response rate. This combination was greater than fluoxetine alone (p=0.02), and CBT alone (p=0.01). Fluoxetine alone was greater than CBT alone (p=0.01).

Neurodevelopmental Disorders

Autism Spectrum Disorder

Diagnosis
- persistent deficits in social communication and interaction, manifested in three areas
    - <u>social-emotional reciprocity</u>, ranging, for example, from abnormal social approach and failure of normal back-and-forth conversation, to reduced sharing of interests, emotions, or affect, to failure to initiate or respond to social interactions
    - <u>nonverbal communicative behaviours</u>, ranging, for example, from poorly integrated verbal and nonverbal communication, to abnormalities in eye contact and body language or deficits in understanding and use of gestures, to a total lack of facial expressions and nonverbal communication
    - <u>developing, maintaining, and understanding relationships</u>, ranging, for example, from difficulties adjusting behaviour to suit various social contexts, to difficulties in sharing imaginative play or in making friends, to absence of interest in peers
- restricted, repetitive patterns of behaviour, interests, or activities. Two or more of: stereotyped or repetitive motor movements, insistence on sameness, highly restricted fixated interests, hyper-/hypo-reactivity to sensory input

Newer Generation Antidepressants for Depressive Disorders in Children and Adolescents
Cochrane DB Syst Rev 2012;11:CD004851
Study: Meta-analysis of 19 trials containing 3,335 participants (including RCTs, cross-over trials, and cluster trials).
Population: Children and adolescents aged 6-18 yr with diagnosed depressive disorder.
Interventions: Antidepressants, placebo.
Main Outcome Measure: Depression severity score.
Results: Children treated with an antidepressant had lower depression severity score and higher rates of response/remission. Children on antidepressants were also found to be at increased risk (58%) of suicide-related outcome (RR 1.58; 95% CI 1.02-2.45).
Conclusions: In children and adolescents, antidepressants are effective at treating depression, yet may cause a higher chance of suicide-related outcomes.

- symptoms must be present in early developmental period
- symptoms cause clinically significant impairment in social, occupational, or other important areas of current functioning
- not better explained by intellectual disability or global developmental delay
- **specifiers**
  - current severity: requiring very substantial support, requiring substantial support, requiring support
  - ± language impairment, ± intellectual impairment
  - associated with known medical or genetic condition or environmental factors (i.e. Rett's disorder)

Differential Diagnosis
- developmental disability, childhood schizophrenia, social phobia, OCD, communication disorder, non-verbal learning disorder, ADHD, abuse, hearing or visual impairment, seizure disorder, motor impairment

Management
- hearing and vision test to rule out impairment
- psychological testing to assess intellectual functioning and learning
- chromosomal analysis to rule out abnormalities (e.g. Trisomy 21, Fragile X syndrome)
- rule out psychotic disorders, social problems, depression, anxiety, abuse

Treatment
- team-based: school, psychologist, occupational therapist, physiotherapist, speech and language therapy, pediatrics, psychiatry
- psychosocial: family education and support, school programming, behaviour management, social skills training
- treat concomitant disorders such as ADHD, tics, OCD, anxiety, depression, and seizure disorder
- pharmacotherapy: atypical antipsychotics (for irritability, aggression, agitation, self-mutilation, tics), SSRIs (for anxiety, depression), stimulants (for associated inattention and hyperactivity)

Prognosis
- variable, but improves with early intervention
- better if IQ >60 and able to communicate

Attention Deficit Hyperactivity Disorder

- prevalence: 5-12% of school-aged children; M:F = 4:1, although girls may be under-diagnosed
- girls tend to have inattentive/distractible symptoms; boys have impulsive/hyperactive symptoms

Observe child for "ATENTION" features
Annoying
Temperamental
Energetic
Noisy
Task incompletion
Inattentive
Oppositional
Negativism

Etiology
- genetic: 75% heritability, dopamine candidate genes DAT1, DRD4
- neurobiology: decreased catecholamine transmission, low prefrontal cortex (PFC) activity, increased beta activity on EEG
- cognitive: developmental disability, poor inhibitory control, and other errors of executive function

Diagnosis
- differential: learning disorders, hearing/visual defects, thyroid, atopic conditions, congenital problems (fetal alcohol syndrome, Fragile X), lead poisoning, history of head injury, traumatic life events (abuse)
- diagnosis requires: onset before age 12, persistent symptoms >6 mo, symptoms present in at least two settings (i.e. home, school, work), interferes with academic, family, and social functioning, and is divided into 3 subtypes
  - **combined type:** 6 or more symptoms of inattention and "≥6 symptoms of hyperactivity-impulsivity
  - **predominantly inattentive type:** "≥6 symptoms of inattention
  - **predominantly hyperactive-impulsive type:** "≥6 symptoms of hyperactivity-impulsivity
  - for older adolescents (>17 yr) or adults, 5 symptoms required
  - does not occur exclusively during the course of another psychiatric disorder

Treatment with stimulant medications of ADHD in childhood does not increase the likelihood of substance abuse later in life, contrary to the concerns of many parents and health care providers

Table 13. Core Symptoms of ADHD (DSM-5)

Inattention	Hyperactivity	Impulsivity
Careless mistakes	Fidgets, squirms in seat	Blurts out answers before questions completed
Cannot sustain attention in tasks or play	Leaves seat when expected to remain seated	Difficulty awaiting turn
Does not listen when spoken to directly	Runs and climbs excessively	Interrupts/intrudes on others
Fails to complete tasks	Cannot play quietly	
Disorganized	"On the go", driven by a motor	
Avoids, dislikes tasks that require sustained mental effort	Talks excessively	
Loses things necessary for tasks or activities		
Distractible		
Forgetful		

Features
- difficult to differentiate from highly variable normative behaviour before age 4, but often identified upon school entry
- rule out developmental delay, sensory impairments, genetic syndromes, encephalopathies or toxins (alcohol, lead)
- increased risk of substance abuse, depression, anxiety, academic failure, poor social skills, comorbid CD and/or ODD, adult ASPD
- associated with family history of ADHD, difficult temperamental characteristics

Treatment
- non-pharmacological: parent management, anger control strategies, positive reinforcement, social skills training, individual/family therapy, behaviour therapy, tutors, classroom intervention, exercise routines, extracurricular activities, omega-3 fatty acids
- pharmacological: first line: stimulants (methylphenidate, amphetamine salts); second line: atomoxetine; third line/adjunct: nonstimulants (α-agonists; clonidine, guanfacine, NDRI; buproprion)
- for comorbid symptoms: antidepressants, antipsychotics

Prognosis
- 70-80% continue into adolescence, but hyperactive symptoms usually abate
- 65% continue into adulthood; secondary personality disorders and compensatory anxiety disorders are identifiable

Disruptive, Impulse Control, and Conduct Disorder

Oppositional Defiant Disorder

- prevalence: 2-16%, M=F after puberty

Diagnosis
- pattern of negativistic/hostile and defiant behaviour for ≥6 mo with ≥4 of
  - angry/irritable mood: easily loses temper, touchy or easily annoyed, often angry and resentful
  - argumentative/defiant: argues with adults/authority figure, defies requests/rules, deliberately annoys, blames others for their own mistakes or misbehaviour
  - vindictiveness: spiteful or vindictive twice in past 6 mo
- behaviour causes significant impairment in social, academic, or occupational functioning
- behaviours do not occur exclusively during the course of a psychotic or mood disorder
- criteria not met for conduct disorder (CD); if ≥18 yr, criteria not met for ASPD
- may progress to CD, differentiated by an absence of destructive or physically aggressive behaviour
- features that typically differentiate ODD from transient developmental stage: onset <8 yr, chronic duration (>6 mo), frequent intrusive behaviour
- impact of ODD: poor school performance, few friends, strained parent/child relationships, risk of later mood disorders

Treatment
- parent: management training, psychoeducation and family therapy to reduce punitive parenting and parent-child conflict
- behavioural therapy: to teach, practice, and reinforce prosocial behaviour
- social: school/day-care interventions
- pharmacotherapy for comorbid disorders

Conduct Disorder

- prevalence: 1.5-3.4% (M:F = 4-12:1)

Etiology
- parental/familial factors: parental psychopathology (e.g. ASPD, substance abuse), child-rearing practices (e.g. child abuse, discipline), low socioeconomic status (SES), family violence
- child factors: difficult temperament, ODD, learning problems, neurobiology

A Systematic Review and Analysis of Long-Term Outcomes in Attention Deficit Hyperactivity Disorder: Effects of Treatment and Non-Treatment
BMC Med 2012;10:99
Study: Systematic review of 351 studies.
Purpose: To determine the long-term outcomes of ADHD and whether there is an effect on long-term outcomes with treatment.
Population: Patients with diagnosed or symptomatic presentation of ADHD.
Interventions: No treatment (control), treatment (pharmacological, non-pharmacological, and multi-modal).
Outcome Groups: Drug use/addictive behaviour, academic outcomes, antisocial behaviour, social function, occupation, self-esteem, driving outcomes, services use, obesity.
Results: Untreated participants with ADHD had poorer outcomes vs. non-ADHD participants in 74% (n=244) of studies, while 26% (n=89) showed similar outcomes. 72% (n=37) of studies showed a benefit from ADHD treatment vs. untreated ADHD and 28% (n=15) showed no benefit. Treatment of ADHD was found to be beneficial in studies looking at driving (100%), obesity (100%), self-esteem (90%), social function (83%), academic outcomes (71%), drug use/addictive behaviour (67%), antisocial behaviour (50%), and occupation (33%).
Conclusions: Overall, people with ADHD have poorer long-term outcomes than controls (those without ADHD). For those with ADHD, treatment improves long-term outcomes.

ODD kids "ARE BRATS"
Annoying
Resentful
Easily annoyed
Blames others
Rule breaker
Argues with adults
Temper
Spiteful/vindictive

Diagnosis

Conduct Disorder Diagnosis

TRAP
Theft: breaking and entering, deceiving, non-confrontational stealing
Rule breaking: running away, skipping school, out late
Aggression: people, animals, weapons, forced sex
Property destruction

- differential: ADHD, depression, head injury, substance abuse
- diagnosis: use multiple sources (Achenbach Child Behavioural Checklist, Teacher's Report Form)
  - pattern of behaviour that violates rights of others and age appropriate social norms with ≥3 criteria noted in past 12 mo and ≥1 in past 6 mo
    - <u>aggression to people and animals</u>: bullying, initiating physical fights, use of weapons, forced sex, cruel to people and/or animals, stealing while confronting a person (e.g. armed robbery)
    - <u>destruction of property</u>: arson, deliberately destroying others' property
    - <u>deceitfulness or theft</u>: breaking and entering, conning others, stealing nontrivial items without confrontation
    - <u>violation of rules</u>: out all night before age 13, often truant from school before age 13, runaway ≥2 times at least overnight or for long periods of time
  - disturbance causes clinically significant impairment in social, academic, or occupational functioning
  - if ≥18 yr, criteria not met for ASPD
- diagnostic types
  - childhood onset: at least one criterion prior to age 10
    - poor prognosis: associated with ODD, aggressiveness, impulsiveness
  - adolescent onset: absence of any criteria until age 10
    - better prognosis; least aggressive, gang-related delinquency
  - mild, moderate, severe

Treatment

- early intervention necessary and more effective; long-term follow-up required
- psychosocial: parent management training, anger replacement training, CBT, family therapy, education/employment programs, social skills training,
- pharmacotherapy: for comorbid disorders

Prognosis

- poor prognostic indicators include early-age onset, high frequency, variety of behaviours, pervasiveness (i.e. in home, school, community), comorbid ADHD, early sexual activity, substance abuse
- 50% of CD children become adult ASPD

Intermittent Explosive Disorder

Diagnosis

- recurrent behavioural outbursts representing a failure to control aggressive impulses in children >6 yr, manifested as either
  - verbal or physical aggression that does not damage others or property, occurring 2+ times per wk for 3 mo
  - 3 outbursts involving physical damage to another person, animal or piece of property in the last 12 mo
- outbursts are out of proportion to triggers or provocation, are not premeditated, and not for primary gain
- outbursts cause clinically significant impairment in social, academic, or occupational functioning

See <u>Pediatrics</u>

- Child Abuse, P14
- Chronic Abdominal Pain, P37
- Developmental Delay, P22
- Intellectual Disability, P22
- Learning Disabilities, P24
- Sleep Disturbances, P12

See <u>Neurology</u>

- Tic Disorders, N33
- Tourette's Syndrome, N34

Psychotherapy

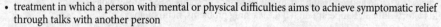

- treatment in which a person with mental or physical difficulties aims to achieve symptomatic relief through talks with another person
- psychotherapy is delivered by a specially trained social worker, nurse, psychologist, psychiatrist, counsellor or general practitioner
- various types of therapy exist because of diverse theories of human psychology and mental illness etiology

Common Factors of Psychotherapy

Freudian Psyche
id: instinctual drives, unconscious
superego: person's conscience, formed by societal/parental norms
ego: latin "I", sense of self, conscious actions, attempts to satisfy drives of id within confines of reality and demands of superego

- good evidence that effective psychotherapy creates observable changes in brain circuitry and connectivity, similar to those observed with successful pharmacologic and other treatment modalities
- studies suggest that up to 30-70% of therapy outcome is due to common factors with only 10-40% from specific factors
- common factors are: warmth (unconditional positive regard), accurate empathy, genuineness, goodness of fit

Table 14. Summary of Psychotherapeutic Modalities

Type	Indications	Approach, Technique and Theory	Ideal Candidates	Duration
Psychoanalytic/ Psychodynamic	Psychoneuroses; anxiety, obsessional thinking, compulsive or conversion disorders, sexual dysfunction, depressive states	Theory: Exploration of meaning of early experiences and how they affect emotions and patterns of behaviour Recollection (remembering), repetition (reliving with the analyst), working through (gaining insight) Techniques: free association, dream interpretation, transference analysis	Psychologically minded, highly motivated, wish to understand selves and not just relieve symptoms Able to withstand difficult emotions without fleeing or self-destructive acts High level of function	Time intensive: -Classically: 4-5 times/wk for 3-7 yr Psychodynamically oriented therapy: 2-3 times/wk for fewer years
Supportive	Adjustment disorders, psychosomatic disorders, severe psychotic or personality disorders	Ameliorate symptoms through behavioural or environmental restructuring to aid adaptation and facilitate coping Help patients feel safe, secure, and encouraged	Individuals in crisis or with severe symptoms in acute or chronic settings Low insight, low motivation, "weak" ego systems	Variable (single session to years, though often short-intermittent)
Interpersonal	Mood disorders, bulimia nervosa	Focuses on how interpersonal relationships impact symptoms 4 key problem areas addressed: grief and loss, role transitions, conflict, interpersonal deficits Break the interpersonal cycle: depression, self-esteem, social withdrawal	Individuals with depression or bipolar disorder with some insight and difficult social functioning Absence of severe psychotic process, personality disorder, or comorbid substance abuse	12-20 wk
Behavioural	Most mental health disorders benefit from specific application of behavioural therapy (e.g. behavioural activation for depression; exposure therapy for phobias; contingency management for anorexia nervosa, substance use disorder)	Systematic Desensitization: mastering anxiety-provoking situations by approaching them gradually and in a relaxed state that limits anxiety Flooding: confronting feared stimulus for prolonged periods until it is no longer frightening Positive Reinforcement: strengthening behaviour and causing it to occur more frequently by rewarding it Negative Reinforcement: causing behaviour to occur more frequently by removing a noxious stimulus when desired behaviour occurs Extinction: causing a behaviour to diminish by not rewarding it Punishment (aversion therapy): causing a behaviour to diminish by applying a noxious stimulus	Individuals with motivation to change and specific symptoms that are amenable to change Global areas of dysfunction such as personality disorder are difficult to treat with behavioural therapy	Usually short term (weeks-months)
Cognitive Therapy	Depression, anxiety, panic disorder, personality disorders, and somatoform disorders	Moods/emotions are influenced by one's thoughts and psychiatric disturbances are often caused by habitual errors in thinking Therapy helps patient make explicit their inaccurate automatic thoughts and correct assumptions with a more balanced perspective Uses thought records (often charts with column headings including "situation," "feeling," "thought," "cognitive distortion") to help monitor thoughts, the situations they occur in, and the feelings they might provoke due to their underlying cognitive errors	Motivated patients who will comply with homework, openness to changing core beliefs	First course - usually 15 - 25 wk Maintenance therapy can be carried out over years
Cognitive Behavioural Therapy	Most mental health disorders including; mood, anxiety, OCD, personality, eating, substance use, psychotic disorders	Combines theory and method from Cognitive and Behavioural therapies to teach the patient to change connections between thinking patterns, habitual behaviours, and mood/anxiety problems	Individuals with motivation to change and are able to participate in homework	Typically 6-18 wk, 1 hr sessions Maintenance sessions can be added over time
Dialectical Behavioural Therapy	Borderline Personality Disorder	Therapy that combines CBT techniques with Buddhist Zen mindfulness practices and dialectical philosophy Focuses on 4 types of skills: mindfulness, emotion regulation, interpersonal effectiveness, and distress tolerance Involves 4 components: individual therapy, group skills training, phone consultations, and a consultation team	Patients with severe problems of emotional dysregulation, impulsivity, and self-harm Patients with borderline personality disorder or borderline personality trait	Typically 1 yr
Motivational Interviewing Motivational Enhancement Therapy (MET)	Substance use disorders Techniques can be applied to facilitate behavioural change in most psychological problems	Spirit of MI (CAPE): Compassion, Acceptance, Partnership, Evocation Principles of MI (RULE): Resist "righting reflex", Understand client and their reasons for change, Listen, Empower by conveying hope and supporting autonomy Techniques of MI (OARS): Open-ended questions, Affirmations to validate client, Reflections (the skill of accurate empathy), Summaries to help client organize self	Patients with problematic substance use, maladaptive behaviour patterns (therapy disengagement, medication noncompliance, poor health habits)	Brief interventions (efficacy with as little as 15 min, single sessions), better result with more sessions Addiction is a chronic condition, often need boosters over time MET = 4 sessions

Two Year Randomized Controlled Trial and Follow-Up of Dialectical Behaviour Therapy vs. Therapy by Experts for Suicidal Behaviours and Borderline Personality Disorder
Arch Gen Psychiatry 2006;63:757-66
Objective: To determine how DBT compares with non-behavioural psychotherapy.
Study: One year randomized controlled trial followed by one year follow-up period.
Patients: 100 women with recent suicidal and self-injurious behaviours meeting DSM criteria and matched to various demographic data.
Intervention: One year of DBT or one year of non-behavioural therapy.
Outcomes: Trimester assessments of suicidal behaviour, emergency services use, general psychological well-being.
Results: Patients receiving DBT were half as likely to attempt suicide, required less hospitalization for suicidal ideation, had lower medical risk for suicide attempts, were less likely to drop out of therapy, and had fewer emergency room visits for suicidal ideation.
Conclusions: DBT is effective in reducing suicidal behaviour in patients with borderline personality disorder.

Dopamine Pathways Affected by Antipsychotics

Pathway	Effects	Associated Pathology
Mesolimbic	Emotion origination, reward	HIGH dopamine causes positive symptoms of schizophrenia (delusions, hallucinations)
Mesocortical	Cognition, executive function	LOW dopamine causes negative symptoms of schizophrenia
Nigrostriatal	Movement	LOW dopamine causes EPS
Tuberoinfundibular	Prolactin hormone release	LOW dopamine causes hyperprolactinemia

Typical (First Generation) vs. Atypical (Second Generation) Antipsychotics

	Typical	Atypical
Mechanism	Block postsynaptic dopamine receptors (D2)	Block postsynaptic dopamine receptors (D2) Block serotonin receptors (5-HT2) on presynaptic dopaminergic terminals, triggering dopamine release, and reversing dopamine blockade in some pathways
Pros	Inexpensive Plenty of injectable forms available	Fewer EPS Low risk of tardive syndromes Mood stabilizing effects
Cons	More EPS Tardive syndromes in long-term Not mood stabilizing	Expensive Few injectable forms available Metabolic side effects (weight gain, hyperglycemia, lipid abnormalities, metabolic syndrome) Exacerbation (or new onset) of obsessive behaviour

Other Therapies

- group psychotherapy
  - aims to promote self-understanding, acceptance, social skills
- family therapy
  - family system considered more influential than individual, especially for children
  - focus on here and now, re-establishing parental authority, strengthening normal boundaries, and rearranging alliances
- narrative psychotherapy
  - an integrative approach that attempts to understand the patient's experience as a whole
- hypnosis
  - mixed evidence for treatment of pain, phobias, anxiety, and smoking cessation
- mindfulness-based cognitive therapy (MBCT)/stress reduction (MBSR)
  - derived from Buddhist meditative and philosophical practices; aims to help people attend to thoughts, behviaours, and emotions in the moment and non-judgmentally using guided breathing exercises. Emerging evidence for treating adjustment disorder, MDD, anxiety, pain disorders, insomnia, substance relapse prevention

Pharmacotherapy

Antipsychotics

- "antipsychotics" and "neuroleptics" are terms used interchangeably
- overall mechanism of action: block, to varying degrees, dopamine activity in target brain pathways (see sidebar)
- indications: for managing agitation, sleep, psychosis and mania reduction, mood stabilizing - used in schizophrenia and other psychotic disorders, mood disorders with or without psychosis, violent behaviour, autism, Tourette's, somatoform disorders, dementia, OCD
- onset: immediate calming effect and decrease in agitation; thought disorder responds in 2-4 wk
- rational use
  - no reason to combine antipsychotics
  - choosing an antipsychotic
    - all antipsychotics are equally effective, except for clozapine (considered to be most effective in treatment-refractory psychosis)
    - atypical antipsychotics (SGA) are as effective as typical (first generation) antipsychotics but are thought to have better side effect profiles
    - choose a drug that the patient has responded to in the past or that was used successfully in a family member
- route: PO, short-acting or long-acting depot IM injections, sublingual
- if no response in 4-6 weeks, switch drugs; if response, titrate dose
- duration: minimum 6 mo, usually for life

Long-Acting Preparations
- antipsychotics formulated in oil for IM injection (see Table 15)
- received on an outpatient basis
- indications: individuals with schizophrenia or other chronic psychosis who relapse because of non-adherence
- dosing: start at low dosages, then titrate every 2-4 wk to maximize safety and minimize side effects
- should be exposed to oral form prior to first injection
- side effects: risk of EPS, parkinsonism, increased risk of NMS

Canadian Guidelines for the Treatment of Acute Psychosis in the Emergency Setting
- haloperidol 5 mg IM ± lorazepam 2 mg IM
- loxapine 25 mg ± lorazepam 2 mg IM
- olanzapine 2.5-10 mg (PO, IM, quick dissolve)
- risperidone 2 mg (M-tab, liquid)

Table 15. Common Antipsychotic Agents

	Starting Dose	Maintenance	Maximum	Relative Potency (mg)
Typicals (in order of potency from high to low)				
Haloperidol (Haldol®)	2-5 mg IM q4-8h 0.5-5 mg PO b/tid 0.2 mg/kg/d PO	Based on clinical effect	20 mg/d PO	2
Fluphenazine enanthate (Moditen®, Modecate® for IM formulation)	2.5-10 mg/d PO	1-5 mg PO qhs 25 mg IM/SC q1-3wk	20 mg/d PO	2
Zuclopenthixol HCl (Clopixol®)	20-30 mg/d PO	20-40 mg/d PO	100 mg/d PO	4
Zuclopenthixol acetate (Acuphase®)	50-150 mg IM q48-72h		400 mg IM (q2wk)	
Zuclopenthixol decanoate (Cloxipol Depot®)	100 mg IM q1-4wk	150-300 mg IM q2wk	600 mg IM/wk	
Perphenazine (Trilafon®)	8-16 mg PO b/tid	4-8 mg PO t/qid	64 mg/d PO	10
Loxapine HCl (Loxitane®)	10 mg PO tid 12.5-50 mg IM q4-6h	60-100 mg/d PO	250 mg/d PO	10
Chlorpromazine (Largactil®)	10-25 mg PO b/t/qid	400 mg/d PO	1000 mg/d PO	100
Atypicals (in order of potency from high to low)				
Risperidone (Risperdal®, Risperdal Consta® for IM long acting preparation, Risperdal® M-Tab for melting form – placed on tongue)	1-2 mg OD/bid	4-8 mg/d PO 25 mg IM q2wk	8 mg/d PO	2
Paliperidone (Invega®)	3 mg/d PO	3-12 mg /d PO	12 mg/d PO	4
Olanzapine (Zyprexa®, Zyprexa Zydis® for melting form – placed on tongue, Zyprexa Intramuscular®)	5 mg/d PO	10-20 mg/d PO	30 mg/d PO	5
Asenapine (Saphris®)	5 mg SL bid	5-10 mg SL bid	10 mg bid	5
Ziprasidone (Zeldox®)	20 mg bid PO	40-80 mg bid PO	160 mg/d PO	6
Aripiprazole (Abilify®)	10-15 mg/d PO	10-15 mg/d PO	30 mg/d PO	7.5
Quetiapine (Seroquel®, Seroquel XR® for extended release®)	25 mg PO bid	400-800 mg/d PO	800 mg/d PO	75
Clozapine (Clozaril®)	25 mg PO bid	300-600 mg/d PO	600 mg/d PO	100

Effectiveness of Antipsychotic Drugs in Patients with Chronic Schizophrenia
NEJM 2005;353:1209-23
Study: Randomized, double-blind, active-control trial with median follow-up of 6 mo.
Patients: 1,432 patients with a diagnosis of schizophrenia (as per DSM-IV criteria) and able to take antipsychotic medications (as determined by study doctors. Mean age 41, 74% male, 26% female.
Intervention: 1-4 capsules daily of olanzapine (20.1 mg), quetiapine (543.4 mg), risperidone (3.9 mg), perphenazine (20.8 mg), or ziprasidone (112.8 mg), with dosage at the discretion of the study doctor. Mean modal doses in parentheses.
Main Outcome: Discontinuation of treatment for any cause.
Results: Olanzapine group had statistically significant lower rate of discontinuation for any cause (64%) from all others (quetiapine – 82%, risperidone – 74%, perphenazine – 75%, ziprasidone – 79%). There were no significant differences in time until discontinuation due to intolerable side effects; however, olanzapine was associated with a significantly higher rate of metabolic side effects.

Note: high potency antipsychotics (e.g. haloperidol) have low doses, while low potency antipsychotics (e.g. chlorpromazine) have high doses

Anticholinergic Effects
Red	as a	beet
Hot	as a	hare
Dry	as a	bone
Blind	as a	bat
Mad	as a	hatter

Table 16. Commonly Used Atypical Antipsychotics

	Risperidone (Risperdal®)	Olanzapine (Zyprexa®, Zydis®)	Quetiapine (Seroquel®)	Clozapine (Clozaril®)	Aripiprazole (Abilify®)
Advantages	Lower incidence of EPS than typical antipsychotics at lower doses (<8 mg) Associated with less weight gain compared to clozapine and olanzapine	Better overall efficacy compared to haloperidol Well tolerated Low incidence of EPS and TD	Associated with less weight gain compared to clozapine and olanzapine Mood stabilizing	Most effective for treatment-resistant schizophrenia Does not worsen tardive symptoms; may treat them Approximately 50% of patients benefit, especially paranoid patients and those with onset after 20 yr	Less weight gain and risk of metabolic syndrome compared to olanzapine and a lower incidence of EPS compared to haloperidol.
Disadvantages	SE: insomnia, agitation, EPS, H/A, anxiety, prolactin, postural hypotension, constipation, dizziness, weight gain Highest risk of EPS among atypicals (still lower than high-potency typicals)	SE: mild sedation, insomnia, dizziness, minimal anticholinergic, early AST and ALT elevation, restlessness High risk of metabolic effects (weight gain, DM, hyperlipidemia)	SE: H/A, sedation, dizziness, constipation Most sedating of first line atypicals	SE: drowsiness/sedation, hypersalivation, tachycardia, myocarditis, cardiomyopathy, dizziness, EPS, NMS 1% agranulocytosis	SE: H/A, agitation, anxiety, insomnia, weight gain, decreased serum prolactin levels
Comments	Quick dissolve (M-tabs), and long-acting (Consta®) formulations available	Quick dissolve formulation (Zydis®) used commonly in ER setting for better compliance IM form available		Weekly blood counts for 6 mo, then q2wk Do not use with drugs which may cause bone marrow suppression due to risk of agranulocytosis	

Note: Risk of weight gain: Clozapine > Olanzapine > Quetiapine > Risperidone

Metabolic and Cardiovascular Adverse Effects Associated with Antipsychotic Drugs
Nat Rev Endocrinol 2012;8:114-126
Study: Review.
Conclusions: All antipsychotics can cause cardiovascular and metabolic side effects, such as obesity, dyslipidemia, hyperglycermia and metabolic syndrome. Olanzapine and clozapine are most likely to cause these side effects. The mechanism that underlies the metabolic and cardiovascular effects is not fully understood, however, the histamine, dopamine, serotonin, and muscarinic receptors are implicated.

Features of Neuroleptic Malignant Syndrome

FARM
Fever
Autonomic changes (e.g. increased HR/BP, sweating)
Rigidity of muscles
Mental status changes (e.g. confusion)

FARM symptoms are also seen in SS

SS can be distinguished from NMS by the following:

SS	NMS
Twitchy, shivering, restless	Severe global rigidity
Flushed, sweaty	Pallor
Vomiting, diarrhea, abdominal pain	No GI symptoms

QT Prolongation is an important side effect of antipsychotics; ECGs should be obtained prior to initiating a new medication and to monitor side effects

Typicals: chlorpromazine and haloperidol warrant cardiac monitoring

Atypicals: ziprasidone has the highest risk among atypicals, clozapine also warrants monitoring

Selective Serotonin Reuptake Inhibitors (SSRIs) vs. Other Antidepressants for Depression
Cochrane DB Syst Rev 2004; Issue 3
This systematic review of 98 RCTs compared the efficacy of SSRIs with other kinds of antidepressants in the treatment of patients with depressive disorders.
Conclusions: There is no significant difference in the effectiveness of SSRIs vs. TCAs. Consider relative patient acceptability, toxicity, and cost when choosing.

How Long to Treat?
6-12 mo: if first or second episode
2 yr-indefinitely: if third episode, elderly, psychotic features, refractory depression, >2 episodes in 5 yr

Table 17. Side Effects of Antipsychotics

System	Side Effects
Anticholinergic	Dry mouth, urinary retention, constipation, blurred vision, toxic-confusional states
α-adrenergic Blockade	Orthostatic hypotension, impotence, failure to ejaculate
Dopaminergic Blockade	Extrapyramidal syndromes, galactorrhea, amenorrhea, impotence, weight gain
Anti-histamine	Sedation
Hematologic	Agranulocytosis (clozapine)
Hypersensitivity Reactions	Liver dysfunction, blood dyscrasias, skin rashes, neuroleptic malignant syndrome, altered temperature regulation (hypothermia or hyperthermia)
Endocrine	Metabolic syndrome

Neuroleptic Malignant Syndrome
- psychiatric emergency
    - due to massive dopamine blockade; increased incidence with high potency and depot neuroleptics
- risk factors
    - medication factors: sudden increase in dosage, starting a new drug
    - patient factors: medical illness, dehydration, exhaustion, poor nutrition, external heat load, male, young adults
- clinical presentation
    - mental status changes (usually occur first), fever, autonomic reactivity, rigidity
    - develops over 24-72 h
    - labs: increased creatine phosphokinase, leukocytosis, myoglobinuria
- treatment: supportive - discontinue drug, hydration, cooling blankets, dantrolene (hydrantoin derivative, used as a muscle relaxant), bromocriptine (DA agonist)
- mortality: 5%

Extrapyramidal Symptoms
- incidence related to increased dose and potency
- acute (early-onset; reversible) vs. tardive (late-onset; often irreversible)

Table 18. Extrapyramidal Symptoms

	Dystonia	Akathisia	Pseudoparkinsonism	Dyskinesia
Acute or Tardive	Both	Both	Acute	Tardive
Risk Group	Acute: Young Asian and Black males	Elderly females	Elderly females	
Presentation	Sustained abnormal posture; torsions, twisting, contraction of muscle groups; muscle spasms (e.g. oculogyric crisis, laryngospasm, torticollis)	Motor restlessness; crawling sensation in legs relieved by walking; very distressing, increased risk of suicide and poor adherence	Tremor; rigidity (cogwheeling); akinesia; postural instability (decreased/absent arm-swing, stooped posture, shuffling gait, difficulty pivoting)	Purposeless, constant movements, involving facial and mouth musculature, or less commonly – the limbs
Onset	Acute: within 5 d Tardive: >90 d	Acute: within 10 d Tardive: >90 d	Acute: within 30 d	Tardive: >90 d
Treatment	Acute: benztropine or diphenhydramine	Acute: lorazepam, propranolol, or diphenhydramine; reduce or change neuroleptic to lower potency	Acute: benztropine (or benzodiazepine if side effects); reduce or change neuroleptic to lower potency	Tardive: no good treatment; may try clozapine; discontinue drug or reduce dose

Anticholinergic Agents
- types
    - benztropine (Cogentin®) 2 mg PO, IM, or IV OD (~1-6 mg)
    - amantadine (Symmetrel®) 100 mg PO bid (100-400 mg)
    - diphenhydramine (Benadryl®) 25-50 mg PO/IM qid
- do not always prescribe with neuroleptics
    - give anticholinergic agents only if at high risk for acute EPS or if acute EPS develops
- do not give these for tardive syndromes because they worsen the condition

Antidepressants

- onset of effect
    - relief of neurovegetative/physical symptoms: 1-3 wk
    - relief of emotional/cognitive symptoms: 2-6 wk
- taper TCAs slowly (over weeks-months) because they can cause withdrawal reactions
- tapering of any antidepressant is usually required and is based on the medication's half-life and the patient's individual sensitivity (e.g. fluoxetine does not require a slow taper due to long half life)

- must be vigilant over the first 2 wk of therapy; neurovegetative symptoms may start to resolve while emotional and cognitive symptoms may not (patients may be particularly at risk for suicidal behaviour during this time; in children/adolescents, paroxetine and venlafaxine increase restlessness and suicide ideation, so are not prescribed)
- treatment of bipolar depression
  - patients with bipolar disorder should only be treated with an antidepressant if combined with a mood stabilizer or antipsychotic; monotherapy with antidepressants is not advisable as the depression can turn into mania

Table 19. Common Antidepressants

Class	Drug	Daily Starting Dose (mg)	Therapeutic Dose (mg)	Comments
SSRI	fluoxetine (Prozac®)	20	20-80	Useful for anxiety states, OCD, eating disorders, seasonal depression, typical and atypical depression
	fluvoxamine (Luvox®)	50-100	150-300	
	paroxetine (Paxil®)	10	20-60	All SSRIs have similar effectiveness but consider side effect profiles and half-lives
	sertraline (Zoloft®)	50	50-200	Sertraline, citalopram, and escitalopram have the fewest drug-interactions and are sleep-wake neutral
	citalopram (Celexa®)	20	20-40	Fluoxetine and paroxetine are the most activating drugs (recommend taking in the AM)
	escitalopram (Cipralex®)	10	10-20	Fluoxetine does not require a taper due to long half-life and is the most used in children as it has most evidence
				Fluvoxamine is sedating (should be taken in PM)
SNRI	venlafaxine (Effexor®)	37.5-75	75-225	Useful for depression, anxiety disorders
	duloxetine (Cymbalta®)	40	40-60	
NDRI	bupropion (Wellbutrin®)	100	300-450	Useful for depression, seasonal depression
				Causes less sexual dysfunction (may reverse effects of SSRIs/SNRIs), weight gain, and sedation
				Increased risk of seizures at higher doses
				Contraindicated with history of seizure, stroke brain tumour, brain injury, closed head injury
				Not recommended for anxiety disorder treatment because of stimulating effects
				Important to specify formulation, as available in IR, SR, XL (longest)
TCA (3° Amines)	amitriptyline (Elavil®)	75-100	150-300	Useful for OCD (clomipramine), melancholic depression
	imipramine (Tofranil®)	75-100	150-300	
TCA (2° Amines)	nortriptyline (Aventyl®)	75-100	75-150	
	desipramine (Norpramin®)	100-200	150-300	
MAOI	phenelzine (Nardil®)	45	60-90	Useful for moderate/severe depression that does not respond to SSRI, atypical depression
	tranylcypromine (Parnate®)	30	10-60	
RIMA	moclobemide (Manerix®)	300	300-600	Useful for depression unresponsive to other therapies
NASSA	mirtazapine (Remeron®)	15	15-45	Useful in depression with prominent features of insomnia, agitation, or cachexia

MAOI = monoamine oxidase inhibitors; NASSA = noradrenergic and specific serotonin antagonists; NDRI = norepinephrine and dopamine reuptake inhibitors; RIMA = reversible inhibition of MAO-A; SNRI = serotonin and norepinephrine reuptake inhibitors; SSRI = selective serotonin reuptake inhibitors; TCA = tricyclic antidepressants

Treatment Approach for Depression

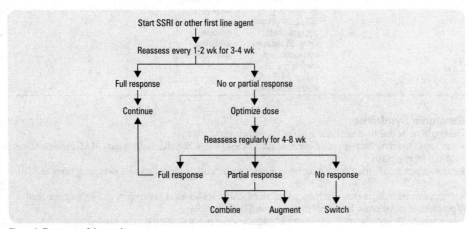

Figure 3. Treatment of depression

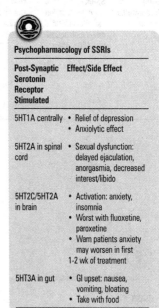

Psychopharmacology of SSRIs	
Post-Synaptic Serotonin Receptor Stimulated	Effect/Side Effect
5HT1A centrally	• Relief of depression • Anxiolytic effect
5HT2A in spinal cord	• Sexual dysfunction: delayed ejaculation, anorgasmia, decreased interest/libido
5HT2C/5HT2A in brain	• Activation: anxiety, insomnia • Worst with fluoxetine, paroxetine • Warn patients anxiety may worsen in first 1-2 wk of treatment
5HT3A in gut	• GI upset: nausea, vomiting, bloating • Take with food

- **optimization:** ensuring adequate drug doses for the individual
- **augmentation:** the addition of a medication that is not considered an antidepressant to an antidepressant regimen (e.g. thyroid hormone, lithium, atypical antipsychotics [specifically: olanzapine, risperidone, aripiprazole])
- **combination:** the addition of another antidepressant to an existing treatment regimen (e.g. the addition of bupropion to an SSRI or SNRI)
- **substitute:** change in the primary antidepressant (within or outside a class)
- note: it is important to fully treat depression symptoms in order to decrease relapse rates and severity

Table 20. Features of Commonly Used Antidepressant Classes

	SSRI	SNRI	TCA	MAOI	NDRI	RIMA	NASSA
Examples	Fluoxetine, Sertraline, Citalopram	Venlafaxine, Duloxetine	Amitriptyline, Clomipramine	Phenelzine	Buproprion	Moclobemide	Mirtazapine
Mode of Action	Block serotonin reuptake only	Block norepinephrine and serotonin reuptake	Block norepinephrine and serotonin reuptake	Irreversible inhibition of monoamine oxidase A and B Leads to norepinephrine and serotonin	Block norepinephrine and dopamine reuptake	Reversible inhibitor of monoamine oxidase A Leads to norepinephrine and serotonin	Enhance central noradrenergic and serotonergic activity by inhibiting presynaptic α-2 adrenergic receptors
Side Effects	Fewer than TCA, therefore increased compliance CNS: restlessness, tremor, insomnia, headache, drowsiness GI: N/V, diarrhea, abdominal cramps, weight loss Sexual dysfunction: impotence, anorgasmia CVS: increased HR, conduction delay, serotonin syndrome, EPS, SIADH	Low dose side effects include insomnia (serotonergic) Higher dose side effects include: tremors, tachycardia, sweating, insomnia, dose-dependent increase in diastolic BP (noradrenergic)	Anticholinergic effects: (see Table 17, PS44) Noradrenergic effects: tremors, tachycardia, sweating, insomnia, erectile and ejaculation problems α-1 adrenergic effects: orthostatic hypotension Antihistamine effects: sedation, weight gain CNS: sedation, stimulation, seizure threshold CVS: HR, conduction delay	Hypertensive crises with tyramine rich foods (e.g. wine, cheese), headache, flushes, palpitations, N/V, photophobia, dizziness, reflex tachycardia, postural hypotension, sedation, insomnia, weight gain, social dysfunction Energizing Minimal anticholinergic and antihistamine effects	CNS: dizziness, headache, tremor, insomnia CVS: dysrhythmia, HTN GI: dry mouth, N/V, constipation, appetite Other: agitation, anxiety, anaphylactoid reaction	CNS: dizziness, headache, tremor, insomnia CVS: dysrhythmia, hypotension GI: dry mouth, N/V, diarrhea, abdominal pain, dyspepsia GU: delayed ejaculation Other: diaphoresis	CNS: somnolence, dizziness, seizure (rare) Endocrine: cholesterol, triglycerides GI: constipation, ALT
Risk in Overdose	Relatively safe in OD	Tachycardia and N/V seen in acute overdose	Toxic in OD 3 times therapeutic dose is lethal Presentation: anticholinergic effects, CNS stimulation, then depression and seizures ECG: prolonged QT (duration reflects severity) Treatment: activated charcoal, cathartics, supportive treatment, IV diazepam for seizure, physostigmine salicylate for coma Do not give ipecac, as can cause rapid neurologic deterioration and seizures	Toxic in OD, but wider margin of safety than TCA	Tremors and seizures seen in acute overdose	Risk of fatal overdose when combined with citalopram or clomipramine	Mild symptoms with overdose
Drug Interactions	SSRIs inhibit P450 enzymes, therefore will affect levels of drugs metabolized by P450 system	MAOI, SSRI Does not seem to inhibit P450 system	MAOI, SSRI EtOH	EtOH Hypertensive crises with noradrenergic medications (e.g. TCA, decongestants, amphetamines) Serotonin syndrome with serotonergic drugs (e.g. SSRI, tryptophan, dextromethorphan)	MAOI Drugs that reduce seizure threshold: antipsychotics, systemic steroids, quinolone antibiotics, antimalarial drugs	MAOI, SSRI, TCA Opioids	MAOI, SSRI, SNRI, RIMA

Serotonin Syndrome
- thought to be due to over-stimulation of the serotonergic system
- can result from medication combinations such as SSRI+MAOI, SSRI+tryptophan, MAOI+meperidine, MAOI+tryptophan
- rare but potentially life-threatening adverse reaction to SSRIs, especially when switching from an SSRI to an MAOI
- symptoms include nausea, diarrhea, palpitations, chills, restlessness, confusion, and lethargy but can progress to myoclonus, hyperthermia, rigor and hypertonicity
- treatment: discontinue medication and administer emergency medical care as needed
- important to distinguish from NMS

Symptoms of Antidepressant Discontinuation

FINISH
Flu-like symptoms
Insomnia
Nausea
Imbalance
Sensory disturbances
Hyperarousal (anxiety/agitation)

Discontinuation Syndrome
- caused by the abrupt cessation of an antidepressant; most commonly with paroxetine, fluvoxamine, and venlafaxine (drugs with shortest half-lives)
- symptoms usually begin within 1-3 d and include: anxiety, insomnia, irritability, mood lability, nausea/vomiting, dizziness, headache, dystonia, tremor, chills, fatigue, lethargy, and myalgia
- treatment: symptoms may last between 1-3 wk, but can be relieved within 24 h by restarting antidepressant therapy at the same dose the patient was taking and initiating a slow taper over several weeks
- consider using a drug with a longer half-life such as fluoxetine

Mood Stabilizers
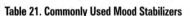

General Prescribing Information

- examples: lithium, lamotrigine, divalproex, carbamazepine
- used in conjunction with atypical antipsychotics for managing episodes of bipolar disorder - depression, mania, stabilization
- vary in their ability to "treat" (reduce symptoms acutely) or "stabilize" (prevent relapse and recurrence) manic and depressive symptoms; multi-agent therapy is common
- before initiating, get baseline: CBC, ECG (if patient >45 yr old or cardiovascular risk), urinalysis, BUN, Cr, electrolytes, TSH
- before initiating lithium: screen for pregnancy, thyroid disease, seizure disorder, neurological, renal, cardiovascular diseases
- full effects not for 2-4 wk, thus may need acute coverage with benzodiazepines or antipsychotics

Specific Prescribing Information

- detailed pharmacological guidelines available online from the Canadian Network for Mood and Anxiety Treatments (CANMAT) and International Society for Bipolar Disorders (ISBD)
- for clinical information for treating bipolar disorder (see *Mood Disorders*, PS9)

Sequenced Treatment Alternatives to Relieve Depression
Journal of Psychosocial Nursing 2008;46:21-24
Study: Prospective randomized anti-depressant treatment trial.
Patients: 4,000 patients with major depressive disorder.
Objective: To compare the efficacy and tolerability of various antidepressant therapies through four sequential treatment levels.
Intervention: Level 1-citalopram if relapse Level 2-citalopram + bupropion SR, sertraline, venlafaxine XR, or cognitive psychotherapy. Level 2A-switch to bupropion or venlafaxine XR. Level 3-either mirtazapine or nortriptyline + lithium, T3. Level 4-tranylcypromine or venlafaxine XR + mirtazapine.
Results: Remission rates were 28% for Level 1, 17% for Level 2, 12-25% for Level 3, and 7-14% for Level 4. When more treatment steps are required, there are lower remission rates, greater degrees of tolerance, and higher rates of relapse.

Table 21. Commonly Used Mood Stabilizers

	Lithium	Lamotrigine (Lamictal®)	Divalproex (Epival®)	Carbamazepine (Tegretol®)
Indications	**1st line** Acute mania (monotherapy or with adjunct SGA) Bipolar I depression (monotherapy or in combination with SSRI, divalproex, or bupropion) Bipolar disorder maintenance (monotherapy or with adjunct SGA) **Other uses** Bipolar II depression Augmentation of antidepressants in MDE and OCD Schizoaffective disorder Chronic aggression antisocial behaviour Recurrent depression	**1st line** Bipolar I depression (monotherapy) Bipolar disorder maintenance (limited efficacy in preventing mania, more effective when combined with lithium) **Other uses** Bipolar II depression Not recommended for: Acute mania as monotherapy	**1st line** Acute mania (monotherapy or with adjunct SGA) Bipolar I depression (combination with SSRI or lithium) Bipolar disorder maintenance (monotherapy or with adjunct SGA) **Other uses** Bipolar II depression Rapid cycling bipolar disorder Mixed phase/dysphoric mania	**2nd line** Acute mania (monotherapy) Bipolar disorder maintenance (monotherapy or in combination with lithium) **Other uses** Rapid cycling bipolar disorder
Mode of Action	Unknown Therapeutic response within 7-14 d	May inhibit 5-HT3 receptors May potentiate DA activity	Depresses synaptic transmission Raises seizure threshold	Depresses synaptic transmission Raises seizure threshold
Dosage	Adult: 600-1500 mg/d Geriatric: 150-600 mg/d Usually daily dosing	Starting: 12.5-15 mg/d Daily dose: 100-200 mg/d Dose adjusted in patients taking other anticonvulsants Note: very slow titration due to risk of Stevens-Johnson Syndrome	750-2500 mg/d Usually tid dosing	400-1600 mg/d Usually bid or tid dosing
Therapeutic Level	Adult: 0.8-1.0 mmol/L (1.0-1.25 mmol/L for acute mania) Geriatric: 0.5-0.8 mmol/L	Therapeutic plasma level not established Dosing based on therapeutic response	17-50 mmol/L Therapeutic levels are for seizure prophylaxis	350-700 µmol/L
Monitoring	Monitor serum levels until therapeutic (always wait 12 h after dose) Then monitor biweekly or monthly until a steady state is reached, then q2mo Monitor thyroid function q6mo, creatinine q6mo, urinalysis q1yr	Monitor for suicidality, particularly when initiating treatment	LFTs weekly x 1 mo, then monthly, due to risk of liver dysfunction Watch for signs of liver dysfunction: nausea, edema, malaise Monitor levels to confirm adherence	Weekly blood counts for first month, due to risk of agranulocytosis Watch for signs of blood dyscrasias: fever, rash, sore throat, easy bruising
Side Effects	GI: N/V, diarrhea, stomach pain GU: polyuria, polydipsia, GN, renal failure, nephrogenic DI CNS: fine tremor, lethargy, fatigue, headache Hematologic: reversible leukocytosis Other: teratogenic (Ebstein's anomaly), weight gain, edema, psoriasis, hypothyroidism, hair thinning, muscle weakness, ECG changes	GI: N/V, diarrhea CNS: ataxia, dizziness, diplopia, headache, somnolence Skin: rash (should discontinue drug because of risk of Stevens-Johnson syndrome), increased lamotrigine levels = increased risk of rash Other: anxiety	GI: liver dysfunction, N/V, diarrhea CNS: ataxia, drowsiness, tremor, sedation, cognitive blurring Other: hair loss, weight gain, transient thrombocytopenia, neural tube defects when used in pregnancy	GI: N/V, diarrhea, hepatic toxicity CNS: ataxia, dizziness, slurred speech, drowsiness, confusion, nystagmus, diplopia Hematologic: transient leukopenia (10%), agranulocytosis, aplastic anemia Skin: rash (5% risk; should discontinue drug because of risk of Stevens-Johnson syndrome) Other: neural tube defects when used in pregnancy
Interactions	NSAIDs decrease clearance		OCP	OCP

Long-term lithium use can lead to a nephropathy and diabetes insipidus in some patients

Lithium Toxicity
- clinical diagnosis as toxicity can occur at therapeutic levels
- **common causes:** overdose, sodium/fluid loss, concurrent medical illness
- **clinical presentation**
  - GI: severe nausea/vomiting and diarrhea
  - cerebellar: ataxia, slurred speech, lack of coordination
  - cerebral: drowsiness, myoclonus, tremor, upper motor neuron signs, seizures, delirium, coma
- **management**
  - discontinue lithium for several doses and begin again at a lower dose when lithium level has fallen to a non-toxic range
  - serum lithium levels, BUN, electrolytes
  - saline infusion
  - hemodialysis if lithium >2 mmol/L, coma, shock, severe dehydration, failure to respond to treatment after 24 h, or deterioration

Anxiolytics

- anxiolytics mask or alleviate symptoms; they do not cure them
- **indications**
- short-term treatment of transient forms of anxiety disorders, insomnia, alcohol withdrawal (especially delirium tremens), barbiturate withdrawal, organic brain syndrome (acute agitation in delirium), EPS and akathisia due to antipsychotics, seizure disorders, musculoskeletal disorders
- **relative contraindications**
- major depression (except as an adjunct to other treatment), history of drug/alcohol abuse, caution in pregnancy/breastfeeding
- **mechanism of action**
- benzodiazepines: potentiate binding of GABA to its receptors; results in decreased neuronal activity
- buspirone: partial agonist of 5-HT1A receptors

Benzodiazepines
- should be used for limited periods (weeks-months) to avoid dependence
- all benzodiazepines are sedating; be wary with use in the elderly
- have similar efficacy, so choice depends on half-life, metabolites and route of administration, OD or bid
- taper slowly over weeks-months because they can cause withdrawal reactions
  - low dose withdrawal: tachycardia, HTN, panic, insomnia, anxiety, impaired memory and concentration, perceptual disturbances
  - high dose withdrawal: hyperpyrexia, seizures, psychosis, death
- avoid alcohol because of potentiation of CNS depression; caution with drinking and driving/machinery use
- **side effects**
  - CNS: drowsiness, cognitive impairment, reduced motor coordination, memory impairment
  - physical dependence, tolerance
- **withdrawal**
  - symptoms: anxiety, insomnia, autonomic hyperactivity (less common)
  - onset: 1-2 d (short-acting), 2-4 d (long-acting)
  - duration: weeks-months
  - complications with above 50 mg diazepam/day: seizures, delirium, arrhythmias, psychosis
  - management: taper with long-acting benzodiazepine
  - similar to but less severe than alcohol withdrawal; can be fatal
- **overdose**
  - commonly used drug in overdose
    - overdose is rarely fatal
    - benzodiazepines are more dangerous and may cause death when combined with alcohol, other CNS depressants or TCAs

Benzodiazepine Antagonist – Flumazenil (Anexate®)
- use for suspected benzodiazepine overdose
- specific antagonist at the benzodiazepine receptor site

Table 22. Common Anxiolytics

Class	Drug	Dose Range (mg/d)	$t_{1/2}$ (h)	Appropriate Use
Benzodiazepines				
Long-acting	clonazepam (Rivotril®)	0.25-4	18-50	Akathisia, generalized anxiety, seizure prevention, panic disorder
	diazepam (Valium®)	2-40	30-100	Generalized anxiety, seizure prevention, muscle relaxant, alcohol withdrawal
	chlordiazepoxide (Librium®)	5-300	30-100	Sleep, anxiety, alcohol withdrawal
	flurazepam (Dalmane®)	15-30	50-160	Sleep
Short-acting	alprazolam (Xanax®)	0.25-4.0	6-20	Panic disorder, high dependency rate
	lorazepam (Ativan®)	0.5-6.0	10-20	Sleep, generalized anxiety, akathisia, alcohol withdrawal, sublingual available for very rapid action
	oxazepam (Serax®)	10-120	8-12	Sleep, generalized anxiety, alcohol withdrawal
	temazepam (Restoril®)	7.5-30	8-20	Sleep
	triazolam (Halcion®)	0.125-0.5	1.5-5	Shortest $t_{1/2}$, rapid sleep, but rebound insomnia
Azapirones				
	zopiclone (Imovane®)	5-7.5	3.8-6.5	Sleep

Benzodiazepines

LOT
Lorazepam
Oxazepam
Temazepam
Safe for patients with impaired liver function because not metabolized by liver

Benzodiazepines used for Alcohol Withdrawal
- Diazepam 20 mg PO/IV q1h prn
- Lorazepam 2-5 mg PO/IV/SL for patients with liver disease, chronic lung disease, or elderly

Somatic Therapies

Electroconvulsive Therapy

- various methodological improvements have been made since the first treatment in 1938 to reduce adverse effects
- modern ECT: induction of a generalized seizure using an electrical pulse through scalp electrodes while the patient is under general anesthesia with a muscle relaxant
- considerations: unilateral vs. bilateral electrode placement, pulse rate, dose, number and spacing of treatments
- usual course is 6-12 treatments, 2-3 treatments per wk
- **indications**
  - depression refractory to adequate pharmacological trial (MDD or Bipolar I depression)
  - high suicide risk
  - medical risk in addition to depression (dehydration, electrolytes, pregnancy)
  - previous good response to ECT
  - familial response to ECT
  - elderly
  - psychotic depression
  - catatonic features
  - marked vegetative features
  - acute schizophrenia unresponsive to medication
  - mania unresponsive to medications
  - OCD refractory to conventional treatment
- **side effects:** risk of anesthesia, memory loss (may be retrograde and/or anterograde, tends to resolve by 6-9 mo, permanent impairment controversial), headaches, myalgias
- unilateral ECT causes less memory loss than bilateral but may not be as effective
- **contraindications:** increased intracranial pressure, recent (<2 wk) MI (not absolute but requires special monitoring)

Magnetic Seizure Therapy (MST)
- seizure induction by magnetic current induction rather than direct stimulation
- early studies demonstrate efficacy for depression as well as anxiety, reduced memory side effects vs. ECT

Repetitive Transcranial Magnetic Stimulation (rTMS)

- noninvasive production of focal electrical currents in select brain areas using magnetic induction
- **indications:** strong evidence for treatment-resistant depression, pain disorders; possibly efficacious for anxiety disorders, eating disorders, substance use disorders
- **adverse effects:** common - transient local discomfort, hearing issues, cognitive changes; rare - seizure, syncope, mania induction

ECT in Society
Prior to the 1940's, ECT was performed without the use of muscle relaxants, resulting in seizures with full-scale convulsions and rare but serious complications such as vertebral and long-bone fractures. This practice may have led to negative societal perceptions of ECT, further perpetuated by barbaric depictions in popular culture. Despite ongoing stigmatization, ECT as it is practiced today is an effective and safe option for patients struggling with mental illness

Efficacy of ECT in Depression: A Meta-Analytic Review
J of ECT 2004; 20:13-20
Study: Meta-analysis of randomized and non-randomized control trials.
Patients: Individuals with unipolar and bipolar depression.
Methods: MEDLINE search for relevant papers from 1966-2003.
Main Outcomes: The Hamilton Depression Rating scale was used to determine response to treatment.
Results: ECT was found to be superior to simulated ECT, placebo, TCAs, MAOIs, and anti-depressants in general.
Summary: ECT is an efficacious treatment modality, particularly in severe and treatment-resistant depression.

Neurosurgical Treatments

Ablative/Lesion Procedures
- used for intractable MDD or OCD, efficacy ranges from 25-75% depending on procedure
- **adverse effects:** related to lesion location and size, high risk of suicide in those who are not helped by surgery

Deep Brain Stimulation
- placement of small electrode leads in specific brain areas to alter neuronal signaling, usually for intractable MDD
- response rates (>50% symptom reduction) of 40-70%, adverse effects related to surgical risks and poor treatment response

Vagus Nerve Stimulation
- direct, intermittent electrical stimulation of left cervical vagus nerve via implanted pulse generator
- used for chronic, recurrent MDD that has failed previous therapy and ECT; slow onset, approximately 30% response rate at 1 yr

Other Therapy Modalities

Phototherapy (Light Box Therapy)
- bright light source exposure, best in morning, for 30-60 minutes (usually 10 000 lux)
- proposed mechanisms: reverses pathological alterations in circadian rhythm through action on suprachiasmatic nucleus
- indications: SAD, non-seasonal depression (as augmentation), sleep disorders
- adverse effects: mania induction, reaction with photosensitizing drug or photosensitive eye or skin conditions

Aerobic Exercise
- moderate-intense aerobic exercise is associated with acute increased secretion of serotonin, phenethylamine, BDNF, endogenous opioids and cannabinoids (likely this combination is what contributes to the "runner's high")
- long term increases grey matter in multiple areas, as well as improvements in cognition, memory, and stress tolerance
- indications: ongoing research suggests efficacy as adjunctive treatment for MDD; may be helpful in PTSD, schizophrenia

Canadian Legal Issues

Common Forms

Form 1: Application for Psychiatric Assessment
- Filled out when a patient is suspected of being an imminent harm to themselves (suicide) or others (homicide) or when they are incapable of self-care (e.g. not dressed for freezing weather) and are suffering from an apparent mental disorder
- Based on any combination of the physician's own observations and facts communicated by others
- Box A or Box B completed
- **Box A:** Serious Harm Test
- The Past/Present Test assesses current behaviours/threats/attempts
- The Future Test assesses the likelihood of serious harm occurring as a result of the presenting mental disorder. In this section, one should document evidence of the mental disorder and concerning behaviour/thoughts
- **Box B:** Patients with a known mental disorder, who are incapable of consenting to treatment (substitute decision-maker needed), have previously received treatment and improved, and are currently at risk of serious harm due to the same mental disorder

Table 23. Common Forms Under the *Mental Health Act* (in Ontario)

Form	Who Signs	When	Expiration Date	Right of Patient to Review Board Hearing	Options Before Form Expires
Form 1: Application by physician to hospitalize a patient for psychiatric assessment against his/her will to a schedule 1 facility (Form 42 given to patient)	Any MD	Within 7 d after examination of the patient	72 h after hospitalization Void if not implemented within 7 d	No	Form 3 + 30 or voluntary admission or Send home ± follow-up
Form 2: Order for a psychiatric assessment against his/her will which is ordered by Justice of the Peace	Justice of the Peace	No statutory time restriction	7 d from when completed Purpose of form is complete once patient brought to hospital	No	Form 1 + 42 or Send home ± follow-up
Form 3: Certificate of involuntary admission to a schedule 1 facility (Form 30 given to patient, notice to rights advisor)	Attending MD (different than MD who completed Form 1)	Before expiration of Form 1 Any time to change status of a voluntary patient	14 d	Yes	Form 4 + 30 or Voluntary admission (Form 5)
Form 4: Certificate of renewal of involuntary admission to a schedule 1 facility (original Form 30 given to patient, notice to rights advisor)	Attending MD following patient on Form 3	Prior to expiration of Form 3	First: 1 mo Second: 2 mo Third: 3 mo (max)	Yes	Form 4 + 30 or Voluntary admission (Form 5)

Table 23. Common Forms Under the *Mental Health Act* (in Ontario) continued

Form	Who Signs	When	Expiration Date	Right of Patient to Review Board Hearing	Options Before Form Expires
Form 5: Change to informal/voluntary status	Attending MD following patient on Form 3/4	Whenever deemed appropriate	N/A	N/A	N/A
Form 30: Notice to patient that they are now under involuntary admission on either Form 3 or 4. Original to the patient, copy to chart	Attending MD	Whenever Form 3 or Form 4 filled	N/A	Yes	N/A
Form 33: Notice to patient that patient is incapable of consenting to treatment of mental disorder, and/or management of property and/or disclosure of health information (original copy to patient)	Attending MD	Whenever deemed appropriate	N/A	Yes	N/A

* Schedule 1 Facilities: Able to provide intensive inpatient and outpatient care

Consent

- see Ethical, Legal, and Organizational Medicine, ELOM6

Community Treatment Order (CTO)

- purpose: a CTO orders a person suffering from a serious mental disorder to receive treatment and supervision in the community. Based on a comprehensive plan outlining medications, appointments, and other care believed necessary to allow the person to live in the community (vs. in a psychiatric facility, where things are more restrictive)
- intended for those who
  - due to their serious mental disorder, experience a pattern of admission to a psychiatric facility where condition is usually stabilized
  - after being released, these patients often lack supervision and stop treatment, leading to destabilization
  - due to the destabilization of their condition, these patients usually require re-admission to hospital
  - if CTO violated (e.g. treatment not taken), patient brought in by police to hospital for treatment as per CTO
- criteria for a physician to issue a CTO
  - patient with a prior history of hospitalization
  - a community treatment plan for the person has been made
  - examination by a physician within the previous 72 h before entering into the CTO plan
  - ability of the person subject to the CTO to comply with it
  - consultation with a rights advisor and consent of the person or the person's substitute decision maker
- CTOs are valid for 6 mo unless they are renewed or terminated at an earlier date such as
  - where the person fails to comply with the CTO
  - when the person or his/her substitute decision-maker withdraws consent to the community treatment plan
- CTO process is consent-based and all statutory protections governing informed consent apply
- the rights of a person subject to a CTO include
  - the right to a review by the Consent and Capacity Board with appeal to the courts each time a CTO is issued or renewed
  - a mandatory review by the Consent and Capacity Board every second time a CTO is renewed
  - the right to request a re-examination by the issuing physician to determine if the CTO is still necessary for the person to live in the community
  - the right to review findings of incapacity to consent to treatment
  - provisions for rights advice

> **CTO Legislature**
> - Ontario passed CTO legislature on December 1, 2000 (known as "Brian's Law")
> - Similar CTOs have been implemented in Saskatchewan (1995), Manitoba (1997), and British Columbia (1999)

Duty to Inform/Warn

- see Ethical, Legal, and Organizational Medicine, ELOM6

References

Abel KM, Drake R, Goldstein JM. Sex differences in schizophrenia. Int Rev Psychiatr 2010;22:417-28.
American Psychiatric Association. Diagnostic and statistical manual of mental disorders, 5th ed. Washington: American Psychiatric Publishing, 2013.
American Psychiatric Association. Highlights of changes from DSM-IV-TR to DSM-5. Washington: American Psychiatric Publishing, 2013.
Ball JR, Mitchell PB, Corry JC, et al. A randomized controlled trial of cognitive therapy for bipolar disorder: focus on long-term change. J Clin Psychiat 2006;67:277-86.
Black and Andreasen, Introductory Textbook of Psychiatry, 6th Edition. American Psychiatric Pub, 2014
Caplan JP & Stern TA. Mnemonics in a mnutshell: 32 aids to psychiatric diagnosis. Current Psychiatry. 2008;7(10):27
Clarke MC, Harley M, Cannon M. The role of obstetric events in schizophrenia. Schizophr Bull 2006;32:3-8.
Clinical Practice Guidelines: treatment of schizophrenia. Can J Psychiat 2005;50(Suppl1):19-28.
Conley RR, Kelly DL. Pharmacologic treatment of schizophrenia, 1st ed. USA: Professional Communications, 2000.
Croxtall JD. Aripiprazole: a review of its use in the management of schizophrenia in adults. CNS Drugs 2012;26:155-83.
DeRubeis RJ, Hollon SD, Amsterdam JD, et al. Cognitive therapy vs. medications in the treatment of moderate to severe depression. Arch Gen Psychiat 2005;62:409-16.
Ditto KE. SSRI discontinuation syndrome: awareness as an approach to prevention. Postgrad Med 2003;114:79-84.
Firth J, Cotter J, Elliott R et al. A systematic review and meta-analysis of exercise interventions in schizophrenia patients. Psychol Med. 2015;45(7):1343-61.
Folstein MF, Folstein SE, McHugh PR. Mini-mental state: a practical method for grading the state of patients for the clinician. J Psychiatr Res 1975;12:189-98.
Food and Drug Administration. Latuda (Lurasidone) NDA 200603 Approval Package. http://www.accessdata.fda.gov/drugsatfda_docs/nda/2010/200603Orig1s000TOC.cfm. Accessed March 15, 2011.
Gliatto MF, Rai AK. Evaluation and treatment of patients with suicidal intention. Am Fam Physician 1999;59:1500-14.
Graham-Knight D, Karch AM. Pharm party. Am J Nurs 2007;107:79.
Hembree EA, Foa EB. Post traumatic stress disorder: psychological factors and psychosocial interventions. J Clin Psychiat 2000;61(Suppl7):33-9.
Herrmann N. Recommendations for the management of behavioural and psychological symptoms of dementia. Can J Neurol Sci 2001;28(Suppl1):96-107.
Howland RH. Sequenced treatment alternatives to relieve depression (STAR*D). Part 2: study outcomes. J Psychosoc Nurs Ment Health Serv 2008;46:21-4.
Judd LL, Schettler PJ, Akiskal HS, et al. Long-term symptomatic status of bipolar I vs. bipolar II disorders. Int J Neuropsychopharmacol. 2003;6(2):127-37
Kahan M, Wilson L. Managing alcohol, tobacco and other drug problems: a pocket guide for physicians and nurses. Toronto: Centre for Addiction and Mental Health, 2002.
Kapur S, Zipursky RB, Remington G. Clinical and theoretical implications of 5-HT2 and D2 receptor occupancy of clozapine, risperidone, and olanzapine in schizophrenia. Am J Psychiat 1999;156:286-93.
Kim SI, Swanson TA, Caplan JP, eds. Underground clinical vignettes step 2: psychiatry. 4th ed. Philadelphia, PA: Lippincott Williams & Wilkins; 2007:130
Koch T. A tour of the psychotropics, 4th ed. Toronto: Mental Health Service, St Michael's Hospital.
Krupnick JL, Sotsky SM, Simmens S, et al. The role of the therapeutic alliance in psychotherapy and pharmacotherapy outcome: findings in the National Institute of Mental Health treatment of depression collaborative research program. J Consult Clin Psychol 1996;64:532-39.
Kuepper R, van Os J, Lieb R, et al. Continued cannabis use and risk of incidence and persistence of psychotic symptoms: 10 year follow-up cohort study. BMJ 2011;342:d738.
Lieberman JA, Stroup TS, McEvoy JP, et al. Effectiveness of antipsychotic drugs in patients with chronic schizophrenia. NEJM 2005;353:1209-23.
Linde K, Berner MM, Kriston L. St John's wort for major depression. Cochrane DB Syst Rev 2008;4:CD000448.
Lineham MM, Comtois KA, Murray AM, et al. Two-year randomized controlled trial and follow-up of dialectical behaviour therapy vs. therapy by experts for suicidal behaviours and boderline personality disorder. Arch Gen Psychiat 2006;63:757-66.
Lopez M, Torpac MG. The Texas children's medication algorithm project: report of the Texas consensus conference panel on medication treatment of childhood attention-deficit/hyperactivity disorder. Part I. Am Acad Child Adolescent Psychiat 2000;39:908-19.
March J, Silva S, Petrycki S, et al. Fluoxetine, cognitive-behavioral therapy, and their combination for adolescents with depression: Treatment for Adolescents With Depression Study (TADS) randomized controlled trial. JAMA 2004;292:807-20.
Moore TH, Zammit S, Lingford-Hughes A, et al. Cannabis use and risk of psychotic or affective mental health outcomes: a systematic review. Lancet 2007;370:319-28.
Morishita T, Fayad SM, Higuchi MA, et al., Deep Brain Stimulation for Treatment-resistant Depression: Systematic Review of Clinical Outcomes. Neurotherapeutics eurotherapeutics : The Journal of the American Society NeuroThera-peutics, 2014;11(3), 475–84. http://doi.org/10.1007/s13311-014-0282-1
MTA Cooperative Group. A 14-month randomized clinical trial of treatment strategies for attention-deficit/hyperactivity disorder. Arch Gen Psychiat 1999;56:1073-86.
Nakamura M, Ogasa M, Guarino J, et al. Lurasidone in the treatment of acute schizophrenia: a double-blind, placebo-controlled trial. J Clin Psychiatry. 2009;70(6):829-36.
National Institute on Drug Abuse. Research report series: methamphetamine abuse and addiction. reprinted 2002 Jan. NIH Publication No.: 02-4210.
Noble J. Textbook of primary care medicine, 3rd ed. Mosby, 2000. 466-70.
Pagnin D, de Queiroz V, Pini S, et al. Efficacy of ECT in depression: a meta-analytic review. J ECT 2004;20:13-20.
Pail G, Huf W, Pjrek E, et al. Bright-light therapy in the treatment of mood disorders. Neuropsychobiology, 2011;64(3):152–62.
Patten SB, Wang JL, Williams JV, et al. Descriptive epidemiology of major depression in Canada. 2006;51:84-90.
Patterson CJ, Gauthier S, Bergman H, et al. Canadian Consensus Conference on Dementia: A Physician's Guide to Using the Recommendations. CMAJ 1999;160:1738-42.
Perkins DO, Gu H, Boteva K, et al. Relationship between duration of untreated psychosis and outcome in first-episode schizophrenia: a critical review and meta-analysis. Am J Psychiat 2005;162:1785-1804.
Pinkofsky HB. Mnemonics for DSM-IV personality disorders. Psychiatr Serv 1997;48(9):1197-8.
Pliszka SR, Greenhill LL, Crismon ML, et al. Textbook of psychiatry. London: Oxford University Press, 1997. 109.
Reinares M, Rosa AR, Franco C, et al. A systematic review on the role of anticonvulsants in the treatment of acute bipolar depression. Intl J Neuropsychopharm 2012;10:1-12.
Rosenbaum S, Sherrington C, & Tiedemann. A. Exercise augmentation compared with usual care for post-traumatic stress disorder : a randomized controlled trial. Acta Psychiatr Scand. 2015;131(5):350-9.
Sadock BJ, Sadock VA, & Ruiz P. Kaplan & Sadock's Synopsis of Psychiatry: Behavioral Sciences/Clinical Psychiatry, 11th ed. Wolters Kluwer, 2014.
Schneider LS, Dagerman KS, Insel P. Risk of death with atypical antipsychotic drug treatment for dementia: meta-analysis of randomized placebo-controlled trials. JAMA 2005;294:1934-43.
Schuch FB, Vasconcelos-moreno MP, Borowsky C, et al. Exercise and severe major depression : Effect on symptom severity and quality of life at discharge in an inpatient cohort. Journal of Psychiatric Research. 2015;61:25-32.
Senger HL. Borderline mnemonic. Am J Psychiatry 1997;154(9): 1321.
Stahl SM. Psychopharmacology of antipsychotics. London: Martin Dunitz, 1999.
Stoner SC, Pace HA. Asenapine: a clinical review of a second-generation antipsychotic. Clinical Therapeutics 2012;34:1023-40.
Stroebe M, Schut H, & Stroebe W. Health outcomes of bereavement. Lancet, 2007;370(9603), 1960-73.
Szewczyk M. Women's health: depression and related disorders. Primary Care 1997;24:83-101.
Troiden R. The formation of homosexual identities. J Homosexuality 1989;17:43-73.
Warneke L. Breaking the urges of obsessive-compulsive disorder. Can J Diag 1996;13:107-20.
Weller EB, Weller RA, Fristad MA. Bipolar disorder in children: misdiagnosis, underdiagnosis, and future directions. J Am Acad Child Adolescent Psychiat 1995;34:709-14.
Whittington CJ, Kendall T, Fonagy P, et al. Selective serotonin reuptake inhibitors in childhood depression: systematic review of published versus unpublished data. Lancet 2004;363:1341-45.
Yatham LN, Kennedy SH, Parikh SV, et al. Canadian Network for Mood and Anxiety Treatments (CANMAT) and International Society for Bipolar Disorders (ISBD) collaborative update of CANMAT guidelines for the management of patients with bipolar disorder: update 2013. Bipolar Disorders 2013: 15: 1-44.
Zimmerman M. Interview guide for evaluating DSM-IV psychiatric disorders and the mental status examination. East Greenwich: Psych Products Press, 1994.

Respirology

Benjamin Chin-Yee and **Cameron Williams**, chapter editors
Claudia Frankfurter and **Inna Gong**, associate editors
Brittany Prevost and **Robert Vanner**, EBM editors
Dr. Meyer Balter, Dr. Matthew Binnie, and **Dr. David Hall**, staff editors

Acronyms

A-a	alveolar-arterial	CO	cardiac output	LAAC	long-acting anti-cholinergic	PSV	pressure support ventilation
A-aDO₂	alveolar-arterial oxygen diffusion gradient	COP	cryptogenic organizing pneumonia	LABA	long-acting beta-agonist	PTH	parathyroid hormone
ABG	arterial blood gas	COPD	chronic obstructive pulmonary	LLN	lower limit of normal	PTT	partial thromboplastin time
ACEI	angiotensin converting enzyme inhibitor		disease	LMWH	low molecular weight heparin	PUD	peptic ulcer disease
ACV	assist-control ventilation	CPAP	continuous positive airway pressure	LTRA	leukotriene receptor antagonist	PVC	premature ventricular contraction
AECOPD	acute exacerbation of COPD	CSA	central sleep apnea	LV	left ventricle	RA	rheumatoid arthritis
AFB	acid-fast bacillus	CVD	cardiovascular disease	LVEDP	left ventricular end diastolic	RAD	right axis deviation
AFP	alpha-fetoprotein	CVP	central venous pressure		pressure	RAP	right atrial pressure
AHI	apnea hypopnea index	CWP	coal worker's pneumoconiosis	LVF	left ventricular failure	RBBB	right bundle branch block
ALS	amyotrophic lateral sclerosis	DIC	disseminated intravascular	MAC	*Mycobacterium avium* complex	RF	rheumatoid factor
ANA	antinuclear antibody		coagulation	MDI	metered dose inhaler	RV	residual volume
ANCA	anti-neutrophil cytoplasmic antibody	DLco	carbon monoxide diffusing	MEP	maximum expiratory pressure	RVEDV	right ventricular end diastolic volume
APTT	activated partial thromboplastin time		capacity of lung	MIP	maximum inspiratory pressure	RVH	right ventricular hypertrophy
ARDS	acute respiratory distress syndrome	EBUS	endobronchial ultrasound	MSA	mixed sleep apnea	RVSP	right ventricular systolic pressure
ASA	acetylsalicylic acid (Aspirin®)	ECMO	extracorporeal membrane	MSK	musculoskeletal	SCC	squamous cell carcinoma
ASD	atrial septal defect		oxygenation	NPPV	non-invasive positive pressure	SCLC	small cell lung cancer
AV	arteriovenous	EGPA	eosinophilic granulomatosis with		ventilation	ScvO₂	central venous oxygen saturation
AVM	arteriovenous malformation		polyangiitis	NSCLC	non-small cell lung cancer	SIMV	synchronous intermittent mandatory
AVN	avascular necrosis	EGDT	early goal-directed therapy	NTT	nasotracheal tube		ventilation
BG	blood glucose	ERV	expiratory reserve volume	OCP	oral contraceptive pill	SIRS	systemic inflammatory response
BiPAP	bilevel positive airway pressure	ETT	endotracheal tube	OSA	obstructive sleep apnea		syndrome
BOOP	bronchiolitis obliterans with organizing	FEF	forced expiratory flow rate	PA	posteroanterior	SV	stroke volume
	pneumonia	FEV₁	forced expiratory volume in 1	PaCO₂	arterial partial pressure of carbon	SVC	superior vena cava
BSA	body surface area		second		dioxide	SVRI	systemic vascular resistance index
CA	cancer	FiO₂	fraction of oxygen in inspired air	PaO₂	arterial partial pressure of oxygen	TB	tuberculosis
CCB	calcium channel blocker	FRC	functional residual capacity	PAO₂	alveolar partial pressure of oxygen	TCA	tricyclic antidepressant
CD	Crohn's disease	GBM	glomerular basement membrane	Patm	atmospheric pressure	TLC	total lung capacity
CF	cystic fibrosis	GERD	gastroesophageal reflux disease	PCP	*Pneumocystis carinii* pneumonia	TNM	tumour, node, metastasis
CHF	congestive heart failure	H/A	headache	PCV	pressure control ventilation	TPN	total parenteral nutrition
CI	cardiac index	HPA	hypothalamic-pituitary axis	PCWP	pulmonary capillary wedge pressure	UC	ulcerative colitis
		HRT	hormone replacement therapy	PDA	patent ductus arteriosus	URTI	upper respiratory tract infection
		IBD	inflammatory bowel disease	PE	pulmonary embolism	V/Q	ventilation-to-perfusion
		IC	inspiratory capacity	PEEP	positive end expiratory pressure	VATS	video-assisted thorascopic surgery
		ICP	intracranial pressure	PEF	peak expiratory flow	VC	vital capacity
		ICS	inhaled corticosteroid	PFT	pulmonary function tests	VSD	ventricular septal defect
		ILD	interstitial lung disease	PMNs	polymorphonuclear cells	VTE	venous thromboembolism
		IPF	idiopathic pulmonary fibrosis	PP	pulse pressure	VT	tidal volume

Respiration Pattern

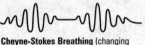

Normal

Obstructive (prolonged expiration)
• Asthma, COPD

Bradypnea (slow respiratory rate)
• Drug-induced respiratory depression
• Diabetic coma (nonketotic)
• Increased ICP

Kussmaul's Breathing (fast and deep)
• Metabolic acidosis
• Exercise
• Anxiety

Biot's/Ataxic
(irregular with long apneic periods)
• Drug-induced respiratory depression
• Increased ICP
• Brain damage (especially medullary)

Cheyne-Stokes Breathing (changing
rates and depths with apneic periods)
• Drug-induced respiratory depression
• Brain damage (especially cerebral)
• CHF
• Uremia

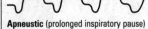

Apneustic (prolonged inspiratory pause)
• Pontine lesion

© Bonnie Tang 2012

**Figure 2. Respiration patterns in
normal and disease states**

Approach to the Respiratory Patient

Basic Anatomy Review

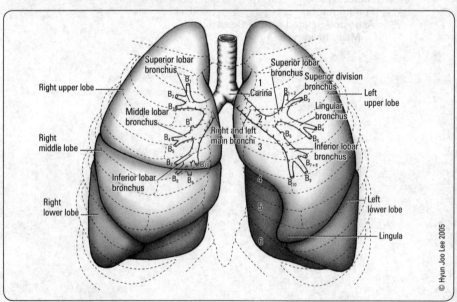

Figure 1. Lung lobes and bronchi

© Hyun Joo Lee 2005

Differential Diagnoses of Common Presentations

Table 1. Differential Diagnosis of Dyspnea

ACUTE DYSPNEA (MINUTES-HOURS)

Cardiac causes
- Ischemic heart disease
- CHF exacerbation
- Cardiac tamponade

Pulmonary causes
- Upper airway obstruction (anaphylaxis, foreign body)
- Airway disease (asthma, COPD exacerbation, bronchitis)
- Parenchymal lung disease (ARDS, pneumonia)
- Pulmonary vascular disease (PE, vasculitis)
- Pleural disease (pneumothorax, tension pneumothorax)
- Respiratory control (metabolic acidosis, ASA toxicity)

Psychiatric causes
- Anxiety/psychosomatic

CHRONIC DYSPNEA (WEEKS-MONTHS)

Cardiac causes
- Valvular heart disease
- Decreased CO

Respiratory causes
- Parenchymal lung disease (interstitial disease)
- Pulmonary vascular disease (pulmonary HTN, vasculitis)
- Pleural disease (effusion)
- Airway disease (asthma, COPD)

Metabolic causes
- Severe anemia
- Hyperthyroidism

Neuromuscular and chest wall disorders
- Deconditioning, obesity, pregnancy, neuromuscular disease

Table 2. Differential Diagnosis of Chest Pain
(see Cardiology and Cardiac Surgery C4 and Emergency Medicine ER21)

NONPLEURITIC	PLEURITIC
Pulmonary	**Pulmonary**
Pneumonia	Pneumonia
PE	PE
Neoplasm	Pneumothorax
Cardiac	Hemothorax
MI	Neoplasm
Myocarditis/pericarditis	TB
Esophageal	Empyema
GERD	**Cardiac**
Spasm	Pericarditis
Esophagitis	Dressler's syndrome
Ulceration	**GI**
Achalasia	Subphrenic abscess
Neoplasm	Pancreatitis
Esophageal rupture	**MSK**
Mediastinal	Costochondritis
Lymphoma	Fractured rib
Thymoma	Myositis
Subdiaphragmatic	Herpes zoster
PUD	
Gastritis	
Biliary colic	
Pancreatitis	
Vascular	
Dissecting aortic aneurysm	
MSK	
Costochondritis	
Skin	
Breast	
Ribs	

Table 3. Differential Diagnosis of Hemoptysis

Airway Disease
- Acute or chronic bronchitis
- Bronchiectasis
- Bronchogenic CA
- Bronchial carcinoid tumour

Parenchymal Disease
- Pneumonia
- TB
- Lung abscess

Vascular Disease
- PE
- Elevated pulmonary venous pressure:
  - LVF
  - Mitral stenosis
- Vascular malformation
- Vasculitis
  - Goodpasture's syndrome
  - Idiopathic pulmonary hemosiderosis

Miscellaneous
- Impaired coagulation
- Pulmonary endometriosis

Table 4. Differential Diagnosis of Cough

Airway Irritants
- Inhaled smoke, dusts, fumes
- Postnasal drip (upper airway cough syndrome)
- Aspiration
  - Gastric contents (GERD)*
  - Oral secretions
  - Foreign body

Airway Disease
- URTI including postnasal drip and sinusitis*
- Acute or chronic bronchitis
- Bronchiectasis
- Neoplasm
- External compression by node or mass lesion
- Asthma*
- COPD

Parenchymal Disease
- Pneumonia
- Lung abscess
- Interstitial lung disease

CHF

Drug-induced (e.g. ACEI)

*"Big Three" causes of chronic cough

Adapted from: Weinberger SE. Principles of pulmonary medicine, 5th ed. 2008. With permission from Elsevier

Signs of Respiratory Distress
- Tachypnea
- Central/peripheral cyanosis
- Inability to speak
- Nasal flaring
- Tracheal tug
- Accessory muscle use
- Intercostal indrawing
- Tripoding
- Abdominal breathing (paradoxical breathing)

Common Causes of Clubbing
- Pulmonary: Lung CA, bronchiectasis, pulmonary fibrosis, abscess, CF, empyema (NOT COPD)
- Cardiac: Cyanotic heart disease, endocarditis, A-V fistula
- GI: IBD, celiac, cirrhosis
- Endocrine: Graves'
- Other: Other malignancy, primary hypertrophic osteoarthropathy

Clubbing is not seen in COPD – if present, think malignancy

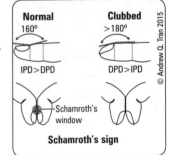

Figure 3. Signs of nail clubbing

Hemoptysis
- Most common cause is bronchitis
- 90% of massive hemoptysis is from the bronchial arteries
- Considered "massive" if >600 mL/24 h

Most Common Causes of Chronic Cough in the Non-smoking Patient (cough >3 mo with normal CXR)
- GERD
- Asthma
- Postnasal drip
- ACEI

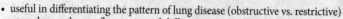

Pulmonary Function Tests

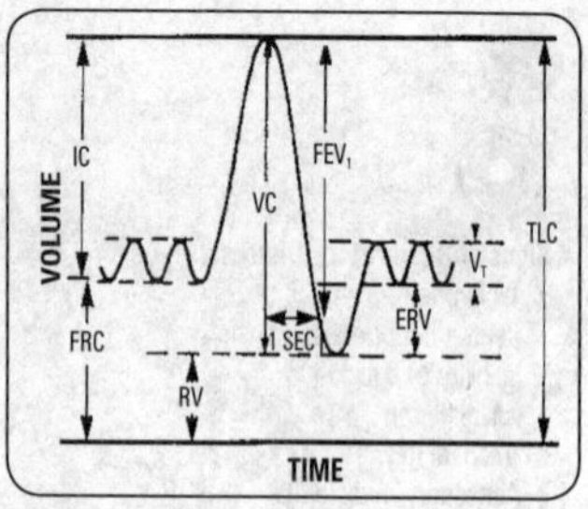

- useful in differentiating the pattern of lung disease (obstructive vs. restrictive)
- assess lung volumes, flow rates, and diffusion capacity (Figures 4A and 4B)
- note: normal values for FEV_1 are approximately ±20% of the predicted values (for age, sex, and height); ethnicity may affect predicted values

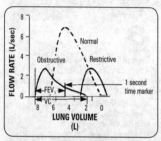

Figure 4A. Subcompartment of lung volumes

Figure 4B. Expiratory flow volume curves
Adapted with permission from Elsevier. Weinberger SE. Priniciples of pulmonary medicine, 5th ed. 2008

Lung Volumes
ERV – Expiratory Reserve Volume
FEF – Forced Expiratory Flow Rate
FEV_1 – Forced Expiratory Volume
(in one second)
FRC – Functional Residual Capacity
IC – Inspiratory Capacity
RV – Residual Volume
TLC – Total Lung Capacity
VC – Vital Capacity
V_T – Tidal Volume

Table 5. Comparison of Lung Flow and Volume Parameters in Lung Disease

	Obstructive	Restrictive
	Decreased flow rates (most marked during expiration)	Decreased lung compliance
	Air trapping (increased RV/TLC)	Decreased lung volumes
	Hyperinflation (increased FRC, TLC)	
DDx	Asthma, COPD, CF, bronchiolitis, bronchiectasis*	ILD, pleural disease, neuromuscular disease, chest wall disease
FEV_1/FVC	↓	↑ or N
TLC	↑ or N	↓
RV	↑ or N	↓
RV/TLC	↑ or N	N
DL_{CO}	↓/↑ or N	↓ or N

*Bronchiectasis can be obstructive or mixed

Table 6. Common Respirology Procedures

Technique	Purpose	Description
Plethysmography ("body box")	Measure FRC	After a normal expiration the patient inhales against a closed mouthpiece
		Resultant changes in the volume and pressure of the plethysmograph are used to calculate the volume of gas in the thorax
		Useful for patients with air trapping
He dilution	Measure FRC	A patient breathes from a closed circuit containing a known concentration and volume of helium
		Since the amount of helium remains constant, FRC is determined based on the final concentration of the helium in the closed system
		Only includes airspaces that communicate with the bronchial tree
Bronchoscopy	Diagnosis and therapy	A flexible or rigid bronchoscope is used for visualization of a patient's airways. Allows for:
		Bronchial and broncho-alveolar lavage (washings) for culture and cytology
		Endobronchial or transbronchial tissue biopsies
		Removal of secretions/foreign bodies/blood
		Laser resections
		Airway stenting
		Mediastinal lymph nodes can also be sampled using a special bronchoscope equipped with an U/S probe (EBUS)

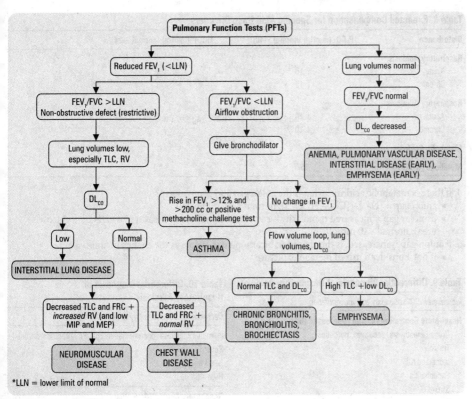

Figure 5. Interpreting PFTs

Chest X-Rays

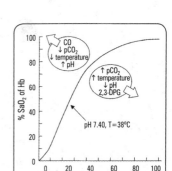

• see <u>Medical Imaging</u>, MI4

Table 7. CXR Patterns and Differential Diagnosis

Pattern	Signs	Common DDx
Consolidation ("Airspace disease")	Air bronchogram Silhouette sign Less visible blood vessels	Acute: water (pulmonary edema), pus (pneumonia), blood (hemorrhage) Chronic: neoplasm (lymphoma), inflammatory (eosinophilic pneumonia), infection (TB, fungal)
Reticular ("Interstitial disease")	Increased linear markings Honeycombing (IPF)	ILD (IPF, collagen vascular disease, asbestos, drugs)
Nodular	Cavitary vs. non-cavitary	Cavitary: neoplasm (primary vs. metastatic lung cancer), infectious (anaerobic or Gram negative, TB, fungal), inflammatory (RA, Granulomatosis with Polyangiitis [GPA])

Non-cavitary: above + sarcoid, Kaposi's sarcoma (in HIV), silicosis and other pneumoconioses

Arterial Blood Gases

• provides information on acid-base and oxygenation status
• see <u>Nephrology</u>, NP15

Approach to Acid-Base Status
1. Is the pH acidemic (pH <7.35), alkalemic (pH >7.45), or normal (pH 7.35-7.45)?
2. What is the primary disturbance?
   ▪ metabolic: change in HCO_3^- and pH in same direction
   ▪ respiratory: change in HCO_3^- and pH in opposite directions
3. Is there appropriate compensation? (see Table 8)
   ▪ metabolic compensation occurs over 2-3 d reflecting altered renal HCO_3^- production and excretion
   ▪ respiratory compensation through ventilatory control of P_aCO_2 occurs immediately
   ▪ inadequate compensation may indicate a second acid-base disorder

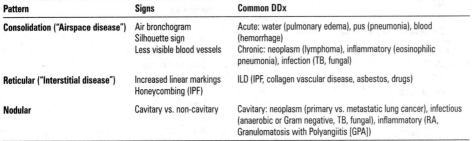

Figure 6. Oxygen-Hb dissociation curve

Factors that Shift the Oxygen-Hb Dissociation Curve to the Right

"CADET, face right!"
CO₂
Acid
2,3-DPG
Exercise
Temperature (increased)

ABG Normal Values
pH 7.35-7.45
HCO₃ 22-26 mEq/L
PₐCO₂ 35-45 mm Hg
PₐO₂ 80-100 mm Hg

Acidosis ⟷ Hyperkalemia
Alkalosis ⟷ Hypokalemia

Note: Mixed acid-base disturbances can still have a "normal" pH

Osmolar Gap = measured osmolarity – calculated osmolarity; for calculated osmolarity think "2 salts and a sticky BUN" (2Na + glucose + urea)

Anion Gap Metabolic Acidosis

MUDPILESCAT
Methanol
Uremia
Diabetic ketoacidosis/starvation ketoacidosis
Phenformin/Paraldehyde
Isoniazid, Iron, Ibuprofen
Lactate
Ethylene glycol
Salicylates
Cyanide, Carbon dioxide
Alcoholic ketoacidosis
Toluene, Theophylline

Table 8. Expected Compensation for Specific Acid-Base Disorders

Disturbance	PₐCO₂ (mmHg) (normal ~40)	HCO₃⁻ (mmHg) (normal ~24)
Respiratory Acidosis		
Acute	↑ 10	↑ 1
Chronic	↑ 10	↑ 3
Respiratory Alkalosis		
Acute	↓ 10	↓ 2
Chronic	↓ 10	↓ 5
Metabolic Acidosis	↓ 1	↓ 1
Metabolic Alkalosis	↑ 5-7	↑ 10

4. if there is metabolic acidosis, what is the anion gap and osmolar gap?
- anion gap = $[Na^+]-([Cl^-]+[HCO_3^-])$; normal ≤10-15 mmol/L
- osmolar gap = measured osmolarity – calculated osmolarity = measured – $(2[Na^+] + glucose + urea)$; normal ≤10 mmol/L

5. if anion gap is increased, is the change in bicarbonate the same as the change in anion gap?
- if not, consider a mixed metabolic picture

Table 9. Differential Diagnosis of Respiratory Acidosis

Increased PₐCO₂ secondary to hypoventilation

Respiratory Centre Depression (Decreased RR)
Drugs (anesthesia, sedatives, narcotics)
Trauma
Increased ICP
Encephalitis
Stroke
Central apnea
Supplemental O₂ in chronic CO₂ retainers (e.g. COPD)

Neuromuscular Disorders (Decreased Vital Capacity)
Myasthenia gravis
Guillain-Barré syndrome
Poliomyelitis
Muscular dystrophies
ALS
Myopathies
Chest wall disease (obesity, kyphoscoliosis)

Lung Disease
COPD
Asthma
Pulmonary edema
Pneumothorax
Pneumonia
ILD (late stage)
ARDS

Mechanical Hypoventilation (Inadequate Mechanical Ventilation)

Table 10. Differential Diagnosis of Respiratory Alkalosis

Decreased PₐCO₂ secondary to hyperventilation

Pulmonary disease (pneumonia, edema, PE, interstitial fibrosis)
Severe anemia
Heart failure
High altitude

Respiratory Centre Stimulation
Myasthenia gravis
Guillain-Barré syndrome
Poliomyelitis
Muscular dystrophies
ALS
Myopathies
Chest wall disease (obesity, kyphoscoliosis)

Lung Disease
CNS disorders
Hepatic failure
Pulmonary edema
Gram-negative sepsis
Drugs (ASA, progesterone, theophylline, catecholamines, psychotropics)
Pregnancy
Anxiety
Pain

Mechanical Hyperventilation (Excessive Mechanical Ventilation)

- see Nephrology, NP16 for differential diagnosis of metabolic acidosis and alkalosis

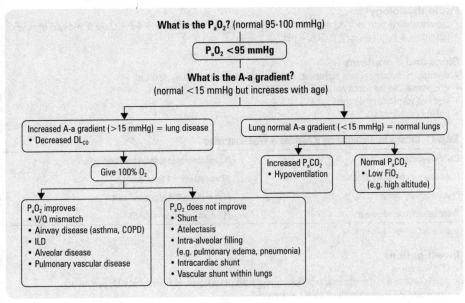

Figure 7. Approach to hypoxemia

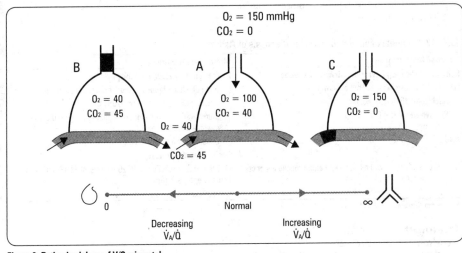

Figure 8. Pathophysiology of V/Q mismatch
Figure adapted from West – Respiratory Physiology: The Essentials. 9th Ed. 2012. Lippincott Williams & Wilkins, Philadelphia, PA.

Diseases of Airway Obstruction

Pneumonia

- see Infectious Diseases, ID7, ID34

Asthma

- see Family Medicine, FM16 and Pediatrics, P85

Definition
- chronic inflammatory disorder of the airways resulting in episodes of reversible bronchospasm causing airflow obstruction
- associated with reversible airflow limitation and airway hyper-responsiveness to endogenous or exogenous stimuli

Epidemiology
- common, 7-10% of adults, 10-15% of children
- most children with asthma significantly improve in adolescence
- often family history of atopy (asthma, allergic rhinitis, eczema)
- occupational asthma (organic allergies, isocyanates, animals, etc.)

At Sea Level on Room Air
$FiO_2 = 0.21$
$P_{atm} = 760$ mmHg
$PH_2O = 47$ mmHg
$RQ = 0.8$
Thus, A-aDO_2 Gradient on Room Air
$A\text{-}aDO_2 = (150 - 1.25\ [P_aCO_2]) - P_aO_2$

Diffusion Capacity for CO

DL_{CO} decreases with:
- Decreased surface area (e.g. emphysema)
- Decreased hemoglobin
- Interstitial lung disease
- Pulmonary vascular disease

DL_{CO} increases with:
- Asthma
- Pulmonary hemorrhage
- Polycythemia
- Increased pulmonary blood volume

Pulmonary Shunt
Occurs when the capillary networks of the alveoli are perfused, yet there is a lack of adequate ventilation (and thus oxygenation) in that alveolus or group of alveoli. Thus this blood enters the pulmonary venous system without being oxygenated

Airway Obstruction (decreased FEV₁)
- Asthma
- COPD (chronic bronchitis, emphysema)
- Bronchiectasis (obstructive or mixed)
- Cystic fibrosis (obstructive or mixed)

Red Flags
Severe tachypnea/tachycardia, respiratory muscle fatigue, diminished expiratory effort, cyanosis, silent chest, decreased LOC

Central cyanosis is not detectable until SaO_2 is <85%. It is more easily detected in polycythemia and less readily detectable in anemia

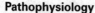

Pathophysiology

• airway obstruction → V/Q mismatch → hypoxemia → ↑ ventilation → ↓ P_aCO_2 → ↑ pH and muscle fatigue → ↓ ventilation, ↑ P_aCO_2/↓ pH

Signs and Symptoms

• dyspnea, wheezing, chest tightness, cough (especially nocturnal), sputum
• symptoms can be paroxysmal or persistent
• signs of respiratory distress
• pulsus paradoxus

Table 11. Criteria for Determining if Asthma is Well Controlled

Daytime symptoms <4 d/wk	No asthma-related absence from work/school
Night-time symptoms <1 night/wk	β2-agonist use <4 times/wk
Physical activity normal	FEV_1 or PEF >90% of personal best
Exacerbations mild, infrequent	PEF diurnal variation <10-15%

Adapted from: *Can Respir J* 2012; 19:127-164

Investigations

• O_2 saturation
• ABGs (consider in acute exacerbation, along with peak flows, in Emergency Department)
• decreased P_aO_2 during attack (V/Q mismatch)
• decreased P_aCO_2 in mild asthma (hyperventilation)
• normal or increased P_aCO_2 is an ominous sign: patient is no longer able to hyperventilate (worsened airway obstruction or respiratory muscle fatigue)
• PFTs (do when stable)

Table 12. Pulmonary Function Criteria for Diagnosis of Asthma

Preferred Measurement	Alternative Measurements
Spirometry Showing Reversible Airway Obstruction	**Peak Expiratory Flow Variability**
(1) ↓ FEV_1/FVC below lower limit of normal	(1) ↓ in PEF after a bronchodilator or course of controller therapy
Adults: <0.75 to 0.8 in adults	Adults: PEF ↑ 60 L/min (min. 20%) OR
Children age 6+: <0.8-0.9	Diurnal variation >8% for twice daily readings (20% for multiple daily readings)
AND	Children age 6+: PEF ↑ 20%
	Positive Challenge Test
(2) ↑ FEV_1 ≥12% (min. 200 mL in adults) after bronchodilator or controller therapy	(1) Methacholine challenge: PC20 <4 mg/mL (4-16 mg/mL is borderline; >16 mg/mL is negative) OR
	(2) Post-exercise: ↓ FEV_1 ≥10-15%

Adapted from: *Can Respir J* 2012; 19:127-164

Treatment

• environment: avoid triggers
• patient education: features of the disease, goals of treatment, self-monitoring
• pharmacological
• symptomatic relief in acute episodes: short-acting β2-agonist, anticholinergic bronchodilators, oral steroids, addition of a long acting β2-agonist
• long-term prevention: inhaled/oral corticosteroids, anti-allergic agents, long-acting β2-agonists, long-acting anticholinergics, methylxanthine, LTRA, anti-IgE antibodies (e.g. omalizumab)

Emergency Management of Asthma

• see Emergency Medicine, ER29
1. inhaled β2-agonist first line (MDI route and spacer device recommended)
2. systemic steroids (PO or IV if severe)
3. if severe add anticholinergic therapy ± magnesium sulphate
4. rapid sequence intubation in life-threatening cases (plus 100% O_2, monitors, IV access)
5. SC/IV adrenaline if caused by anaphylaxis, IV salbutamol if unresponsive
6. corticosteroid therapy at discharge

Guidelines for Asthma Management

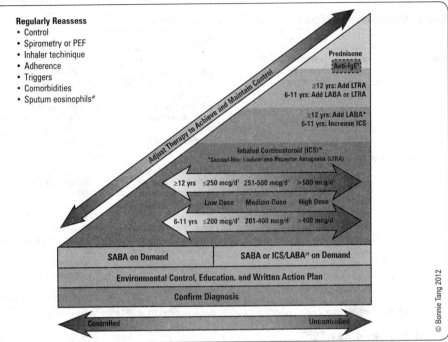

Figure 9. Guidelines for asthma management
†HFA Becolmethasone or equivalent; *Second-line: LTRA; ‡Approved for 12 yr and over; ¶Using a formulation approved for use as a reliever; #In adults 18 yr and older with moderate to severe asthma
Adapted from: *Can Respir J* 2012;19:127-164

LTRA in Addition to Usual Care for Acute Asthma in Adults and Children
Cochrane DB Syst Rev 2012;CD006100
Purpose: To determine if the addition of LTRA is beneficial to patients with acute asthma receiving inhaled bronchodilators and systemic corticosteroids.
Methods: RCTs in Cochrane Airway Group's Specialised Register of trials that compared LTRA and standard vs. placebo and standard in people with acute asthma of any age.
Results: 8 trials, 1,470 adults and 470 children. For oral treatment, no significant difference between LTRAs and control in hospital admission (RR 0.86; 95% CI 0.21-3.52) or requirement for additional care (RR 0.87; 95% CI 0.60-1.68). LTRAs improved FEV_1 in adults (mean difference 0.08; 95% CI 0.01-0.14) but not in children. No significant difference in adverse events between LTRAs and control (RR 0.81; 95% CI 0.22-2.99). Similar results were found for intravenous treatment.
Conclusions: Currently, there is no evidence to support routine use of LTRAs in acute asthma.

Chronic Obstructive Pulmonary Disease

- see Family Medicine, FM16

Definition
- progressive and irreversible condition of the lung characterized by chronic obstruction to airflow with many patients having periodic exacerbations, gas trapping, lung hyperinflation, and weight loss
- 2 subtypes: chronic bronchitis and emphysema (usually coexist to variable degrees)
- gradual decrease in FEV_1 over time with episodes of acute exacerbations

Natural Progression of COPD
40s	Chronic productive cough, wheezing occasionally
50s	1st acute chest illness
60s	Dyspnea on exertion, increasing sputum, more frequent exacerbations
Late Stage	Hypoxemia with cyanosis, polycythemia, hypercapnia (morning headache), cor pulmonale, weight loss

Table 13. Clinical and Pathologic Features of COPD*

Chronic Bronchitis	Emphysema
Defined Clinically	**Defined Pathologically**
Productive cough on most days for at least 3 consecutive months in 2 successive years	Dilation and destruction of air spaces distal to the terminal bronchiole without obvious fibrosis
Obstruction is due to narrowing of the airway lumen by mucosal thickening and excess mucus	Decreased elastic recoil of lung parenchyma causes decreased expiratory driving pressure, airway collapse, and air trapping
	2 Types
	1) **Centriacinar** (respiratory bronchioles predominantly affected)
	Typical form seen in smokers, primarily affects upper lung zones
	2) **Panacinar** (respiratory bronchioles, alveolar ducts, and alveolar sacs affected)
	Accounts for about 1% of emphysema cases
	α1-antitrypsin deficiency, primarily affects lower lobes

*Note that both chronic bronchitis and emphysema can exist without obstruction. Only if obstruction is also present is it termed COPD

Complications of COPD
- Polycythemia 2° to hypoxemia
- Chronic hypoxemia
- Pulmonary HTN from vasoconstriction
- Cor pulmonale
- Pneumothorax due to rupture of emphysematous bullae

CO_2 Retainers
On ABG, retainers have chronically elevated CO_2 levels with a normal pH. Maintain O_2 Sat between 88-92% to prevent Haldane effect, worsening V/Q mismatch, and decreased respiratory drive

Remember, first line therapy for COPD is smoking cessation

Risk Factors
- smoking is #1 risk factor
- others
- environmental: air pollution, occupational exposure, exposure to wood smoke or other biomass fuel for cooking
- treatable factors: α1-antitrypsin deficiency, bronchial hyperactivity
- demographic factors: age, family history, male sex, history of childhood respiratory infections, low socioeconomic status

α-1-Antitrypsin Deficiency
Inherited disorder of defective production of α1-antitrypsin, a protein produced by hepatocytes. Acts in the alveolar tissue by inhibiting the action of proteases from destroying alveolar tissue. When deficient, proteases can destroy lung alveoli resulting in emphysema

GOLD Classification of the Severity of COPD
GOLD 1 Mild $FEV_1 \geq 80\%$ of predicted
GOLD 2 Moderate $50\% \leq FEV_1$
    $<80\%$ of predicted
GOLD 3 Severe $30\% \leq FEV_1 <50\%$ of predicted
GOLD 4 Very Severe $FEV_1 <30\%$ of predicted

Remember to step down therapy to lowest doses which control symptoms/ signs of bronchoconstriction

Influenza Vaccine for Patients with Chronic Obstructive Pulmonary Disease
Cochrane DB Syst Rev 2006;1:CD002733
Study: Cochrane Systematic Review. 11 RCTs included, 6 specifically in COPD patients.
Population: Six of the studies were done on COPD patients in particular, while the others were on elderly and high-risk individuals. Asthma patients were excluded.
Intervention: Live or inactivated virus vaccines vs. placebo.
Outcome: Exacerbation rates, hospitalizations, mortality, lung function and adverse effects.
Results: In patients with COPD, inactive vaccine correlated with fewer exacerbations per vaccinated subject than placebo (weighted mean difference (WMD) -0.37, 95% CI -0.64 to -0.11). Inactivated vaccine resulted in fewer influenza-related infections than placebo (WMD 0.19, 95% CI 0.07-0.48). There was also an increased risk of local mild, transient adverse reactions with the vaccine.
Conclusions: There appears to be a reduction in influenza-related infections, as well as exacerbations in patients with COPD receiving the vaccine.

Systemic Corticosteroids for Acute Exacerbations of Chronic Obstructive Pulmonary Disease
Cochrane DB Syst Rev 2014: CD001228
Study: Cochrane systematic review 16 studies.
Population: 1,787 patients with acute COPD exacerbations.
Intervention: Oral or parenteral corticosteroids vs. placebo.
Outcome: treatment failure, risk of relapse, time to next COPD exacerbation, likelihood of adverse event, length of hospital stay, and lung function at end of treatment.
Results: Systemic corticosteroids reduced the risk of treatment failure by over half compared with placebo in nine studies (n = 917) with median treatment duration 14 d, odds ratio (OR) 0.48 (95% CI 0.35-0.67). The evidence was graded as high quality and it would have been necessary to treat nine people (95% CI 7-14) with systemic corticosteroids to avoid one treatment failure. There was moderate-quality evidence for a lower rate of relapse by one month for treatment with systemic corticosteroid in two studies (n = 415) (hazard ratio (HR) 0.78; 95% CI 0.63-0.97). Mortality up to 30 d was not reduced by treatment with systemic corticosteroid compared with control in 12 studies (n = 1,319; OR 1.00; 95% CI 0.60-1.66). FEV_1, measured up to 72 hours, showed significant treatment benefits (7 studies; n = 649; mean difference (MD) 140 mL; 95% CI 90-200); however, this benefit was not observed at later time points. The likelihood of adverse events increased with corticosteroid treatment (OR 2.33; 95% CI 1.59-3.43). The risk of hyperglycemia was significantly increased (OR 2.79; 95% CI 1.86-4.19). For general inpatient treatment, duration of hospitalization was significantly shorter with corticosteroid treatment (MD -1.22 d; 95% CI -2.26 to -0.18), with no difference in length of stay in the intensive care unit (ICU) setting. Comparison of parenteral versus oral treatment showed no significant difference in the primary outcomes of treatment failure, relapse or mortality or for any secondary outcomes.
Conclusion: There is high-quality evidence to support treatment of exacerbations of COPD with systemic corticosteroid by the oral or parenteral route in reducing the likelihood of treatment failure and relapse by 1 mo, shortening length of stay in hospital inpatients not requiring assisted ventilation in ICU and giving earlier improvement in lung function and symptoms. There is no evidence of benefit for parenteral treatment compared with oral treatment with corticosteroid on treatment failure, relapse or mortality. There is an increase in adverse drug effects with corticosteroid treatment, which is greater with parenteral administration compared with oral treatment.

Signs and Symptoms

Table 14. Clinical Presentation and Investigations for Chronic Emphysema

	Symptoms	Signs	Investigations
Bronchitis (Blue Bloater*)	Chronic productive cough Purulent sputum Hemoptysis	Cyanosis ($2°$ to hypoxemia and hypercapnia) Peripheral edema from RVF (cor pulmonale) Crackles, wheezes Prolonged expiration if obstructive Frequently obese	**PFT:** $\downarrow FEV_1$, $\downarrow FEV_1/FVC$ N TLC, $\downarrow$ or N DL_{CO} **CXR:** AP diameter normal $\uparrow$ bronchovascular markings Enlarged heart with cor pulmonale
Emphysema (Pink Puffer*)	Dyspnea ($\pm$ exertion) Minimal cough Tachypnea Decreased exercise tolerance	Pink skin Pursed-lip breathing Accessory muscle use Cachectic appearance due to anorexia and increased work of breathing Hyperinflation/barrel chest, hyperresonant percussion Decreased breath sounds Decreased diaphragmatic excursion	**PFT:** $\downarrow FEV_1$, $\downarrow FEV_1/FVC$ $\uparrow$ TLC (hyperinflation) $\uparrow$ RV (gas trapping) $\uparrow DL_{CO}$ **CXR:** $\uparrow$ AP diameter Flat hemidiaphragm (on lateral CXR) $\downarrow$ heart shadow $\uparrow$ retrosternal space Bullae $\downarrow$ peripheral vascular markings

*Note that the distinction between "blue bloaters" and "pink puffers" is more of historical than practical interest as most COPD patients have elements of both

Table 15. Treatment of Stable COPD

Treatment	Details
PROLONG SURVIVAL	
Smoking cessation	Nicotine replacement, bupropion, varenicline
Vaccination	Influenza, pneumococcal vaccine
Home oxygen	Prevents cor pulmonale and decreases mortality if used >15h/d; indicated if (1) $P_aO_2 <55$ mmHg or (2) <60 mmHg with cor pulmonale or polycythemia
SYMPTOMATIC RELIEF (no mortality benefit)	
Bronchodilators (mainstay of current drug therapy, used in combination)	Short-acting anticholinergics (e.g. ipratropium bromide) and short-acting β2-agonists (e.g. salbutamol, terbutaline)
	SABAs: rapid onset but significant side effects at high doses (e.g. hypokalemia)
	Short-acting anticholinergics more effective than SABAs with fewer side effects but slower onset; take regularly rather than PRN
	LABAs (e.g. salmeterol, formoterol, indacaterol) and long-acting anticholinergics (e.g. tiotropium bromide, glycopyrronium bromide)
	More sustained effects for moderate to severe COPD
	Inhaled corticosteroid (ICS) + LABA combination (e.g. Advair®: fluticasone + salmeterol, Symbicort®: budesonide + formoterol)
	ICS/LABA increases effectiveness vs. LABA alone
	Theophylline: weak bronchodilator; limited evidence to suggest combination with bronchodilator
	Side effects: nervous tremor, nausea/vomiting/diarrhea, tachycardia, arrhythmias, sleep changes
	PDE4 inhibitor: roflumilast (Daxas®) anti-inflammatory medication useful in COPD with chronic bronchitis, severe airflow obstruction, frequent exacerbations
Corticosteroids	ICS monotherapy has been shown to increase the incidence of pneumonia in COPD; ICS should only be used with a LABA in combination in patients with a history of exacerbations
	Oral steroids are important when treating exacerbations; chronic systemic glucocorticoids are generally not recommended due to unfavourable benefit to risk ratio
Surgical	Lung volume reduction surgery (resection of emphysematous parts of lung, associated with higher mortality if $FEV_1 <20\%$), lung transplant
Other	Patient education, eliminate respiratory irritants/allergens (occupational/environmental), exercise rehabilitation to improve physical endurance

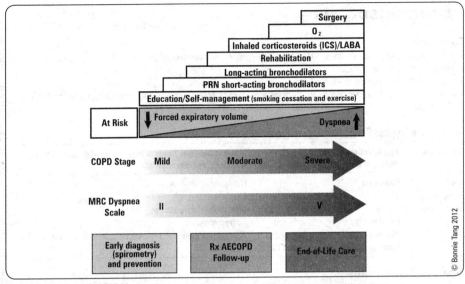

Figure 10. Guidelines for COPD Management
Adapted from: Canadian Thoracic Society recommendations for management of chronic obstructive pulmonary disease. *Can Respir J* 2008;(Suppl A):15

Acute Exacerbations of COPD
- definition
  - sustained (>48 h) worsening of dyspnea, cough, or sputum production leading to an increased use of medications
  - in addition, defined as either purulent or non-purulent (to predict need for antibiotic therapy)
- **etiology**: viral URTI, bacteria, air pollution, CHF, PE, MI must be considered
- **management**
  - ABCs, consider assisted ventilation if decreasing LOC or poor ABGs
  - O_2: target 88-92% SaO_2 for CO_2 retainers
  - bronchodilators by MDI with spacer or nebulizer
    - SABA + anticholinergic, e.g. salbutamol and ipratropium bromide via nebulizers × 3 back-to-back q15min
  - systemic corticosteroids: IV solumedrol or oral prednisone
  - antibiotics for exacerbations with increased sputum production and at least one of the following: increased dyspnea or sputum purulence
    - simple exacerbation (no risk factors): amoxicillin, 2nd or 3rd generation cephalosporin, macrolide, or TMP/SMX
    - complicated exacerbation (one of: FEV_1 ≤50% predicted, ≥4 exacerbations per year, ischemic heart disease, home O_2 use, chronic oral steroid use): fluoroquinolone or β-lactam + β-lactamase inhibitor (amoxicillin/clavulanate)
  - post exacerbation: rehabilitation with general conditioning to improve exercise tolerance
- ICU admission
  - for life threatening exacerbations
  - ventilatory support
    - non-invasive: NPPV, BiPAP
    - conventional mechanical ventilation

Prognosis in COPD
- prognostic factors
  - level of dyspnea is the single best predictor
  - development of complications, e.g. hypoxemia or cor pulmonale
- 5 yr survival
  - FEV_1 <1 L = 50%
  - FEV_1 <0.75 L = 33%
- **BODE** index for risk of death in COPD
  - greater score = higher probability the patient will die from COPD; score can also be used to predict hospitalization
  - 10 point index consisting of four factors
    - **B**ody mass index (BMI): <21 (+1 point)
    - **O**bstruction (FEV_1): 50-64% (+1), 36-49% (+2), <35% (+3)
    - **D**yspnea (MRC scale): walks slower than people of same age on level surface, stops occasionally (+1), stops at 100 yards or a few minutes on the level (+2), too breathless to leave house or breathless when dressing/undressing (+3)
    - **E**xercise capacity (6 minute walk distance): 250-349 m (+1), 150-249 m (+2), <149 m (+3)

Pulmonary Embolism in Patients with Unexplained Exacerbation of COPD: Prevalence and Risk Factors
Ann Intern Med 2006;144:390-396
Study: Prospective cohort study of 211 patients with COPD (all current and former smokers) admitted to hospital for severe COPD exacerbation of unknown origin.
Measurements: All patients received spiral CT angiogram (CTA) and venous compression ultrasonography of both legs.
Results: 25% of patients met diagnostic criteria for PE (+ CTA or + U/S).
Conclusions: Prevalence of PE in patients hospitalized for COPD exacerbation of unknown origin is 25%. Therefore, all patients presenting to hospital with COPD exacerbation without obvious cause require PE workup (leg dopplers or CTA – decision of which to use depends on pre-test probability of the patient).

Non-Invasive Positive Pressure Ventilation for Treatment of Respiratory Failure due to Exacerbations of COPD
Cochrane DB Syst Rev 2004;CD004104
Study: Cochrane Systematic Review. 14 RCTs.
Population: 758 adult patients with COPD and acute respiratory failure due to COPD exacerbation.
Intervention: Usual medical care (UMC) and Non-invasive positive pressure ventilation (NPPV) vs. UMC alone.
Primary Outcome: Treatment failure, mortality, and tracheal intubation.
Results: The risks for all primary outcomes were reduced with NPPV use: treatment failure (RR 0.48); mortality (RR 0.52); and intubation use (RR 0.61). Length of hospital stay was a significant mean 3.24 d shorter, but no difference between ICU length of stay. There is a small and significant improvement in pH (weight mean difference (WMD)=0.04), P_aCO_2 (WMD=0.40 kPa), and respiratory rate (WMD=-3.08 bpm) within 1 h post-treatment with NPPV. Complications associated with treatment were reduced in the NPPV treatment arm (RR 0.38).
Conclusion: For patients in respiratory failure due to a COPD exacerbation, NPPV is effective in reducing treatment failure, mortality, and need for intubation when used as a first line treatment adjunct to UMC.

Different Durations of Corticosteroid Therapy for Exacerbations of Chronic Obstructive Pulmonary Disease
Cochrane DB Syst Rev 2014;CD006897
Study: Cochrane systematic review. 8 studies.
Population: 582 patients, with severe or very severe COPD.
Intervention: Corticosteroids given at equivalent daily doses for 3-7 d (short duration) vs. 10-15 d (longer-duration).
Outcome: treatment failure, risk of relapse, time to next COPD exacerbation, likelihood of adverse event, length of hospital stay, and lung function at end of treatment.
Results: In four studies there was no difference in risk of treatment failure between short-duration and longer-duration systemic corticosteroid treatment (n = 457; odds ratio (OR) 0.72, 95% confidence interval (CI) 0.36 to 1.46)), which was equivalent to 22 fewer per 1000 for short-duration treatment (95% CI 51 fewer to 34 more). No difference in risk of relapse (a new event) was observed between short-duration and longer-duration systemic corticosteroid treatment (n = 457; OR 1.04, 95% CI 0.70 to 1.56), which was equivalent to nine fewer per 1,000 for short-duration treatment (95% CI 68 fewer to 100 more). Time to the next COPD exacerbation did not differ in one large study that was powered to detect non-inferiority and compared five days versus 14 d of systemic corticosteroid treatment (n = 311; hazard ratio 0.95, 95% CI 0.66 to 1.37). In five studies no difference in the likelihood of an adverse event was found between short-duration and longer-duration systemic corticosteroid treatment (n = 503; OR 0.89, 95% CI 0.46 to 1.69, or nine fewer per 1000 (95% CI 44 fewer to 51 more)). Length of hospital stay (n = 421; mean difference (MD) -0.61 days, 95% CI -1.51 to 0.28) and lung function at the end of treatment (n = 185; MD FEV1 -0.04 L; 95% CI -0.19 to 0.10) did not differ between short-duration and longer-duration treatment.
Conclusion: 5 d of oral corticosteroids is likely to be sufficient for treatment of adults with acute exacerbations of COPD, and this review suggests that the likelihood is low that shorter courses of systemic corticosteroids (of around five days) lead to worse outcomes than are seen with longer (10 to 14 d) courses.

Bronchiectasis

Definition
- irreversible dilatation of airways due to inflammatory destruction of airway walls resulting from persistently infected mucus
- usually affects medium sized airways
- *P. aeruginosa* is the most common pathogen; *S. aureus, H. influenzae*, and nontuberculous mycobacteria also common

Table 16. Etiology and Pathophysiology of Bronchiectasis

Obstruction	Post-Infectious (results in dilatation of bronchial walls)	Impaired Defenses (leads to interference of drainage, chronic infections, and inflammation)
Tumour	Pneumonia	Hypogammaglobulinemia
Foreign body	TB	CF
Thick mucus	Measles	Defective leukocyte function
	Pertussis	Ciliary dysfunction
	Allergic bronchopulmonary aspergillosis	(Kartagener's syndrome: bronchiectasis, sinusitis, situs inversus)
	Nontuberculous mycobacterium (NTM)	

Signs and Symptoms
- chronic cough, purulent sputum (but 10-20% have dry cough), hemoptysis (can be massive), recurrent pneumonia, local crackles (inspiratory and expiratory), wheezes
- clubbing
- may be difficult to differentiate from chronic bronchitis

Investigations
- PFTs: often demonstrate obstructive pattern but may be normal
- CXR
  - nonspecific: increased markings, linear atelectasis, loss of volume in affected areas
  - specific: "tram tracking" – parallel narrow lines radiating from hilum, cystic spaces, honeycomb like structures
- high-resolution thoracic CT (diagnostic, gold standard)
  - 87-97% sensitivity, 93-100% specificity
  - "signet ring": dilated bronchi with thickened walls where diameter bronchus > diameter of accompanying artery
- sputum cultures (routine + AFB)
- serum Ig levels
- sweat chloride if cystic fibrosis suspected (upper zone predominant)

Treatment
- vaccination: influenza and pneumococcal vaccination
- antibiotics (oral, IV, inhaled): routinely used for mild exacerbations, driven by sputum sensitivity; macrolides may be used chronically for an anti-inflammatory effect
- inhaled antibiotics (tobramycin) used chronically to suppress *Pseudomonas* and reduce exacerbations
- inhaled corticosteroids: decrease inflammation and improve FEV_1; however, may increase risk of exacerbations
- oral corticosteroids for acute, major exacerbations
- chest physiotherapy, breathing exercises, physical exercise
- pulmonary resection: in selected cases with focal bronchiectasis

Cystic Fibrosis

- see Pediatrics, P87

Pathophysiology
- chloride transport dysfunction: thick secretions from exocrine glands (lung, pancreas, skin, reproductive organs) and blockage of secretory ducts

Clinical Features
- results in severe lung disease, pancreatic insufficiency, diabetes, and azoospermia
- other manifestations: meconium ileus in infancy, distal ileal obstruction in adults, sinusitis, liver disease
- chronic lung infections
  - *S. aureus*: early
  - *P. aeruginosa*: most common
  - *B. cepacia*: worse prognosis but less common
  - *Aspergillus fumigatus*

Usually presents in childhood as recurrent lung infections that become persistent and chronic

Investigations
- sweat chloride test
  - increased concentrations of NaCl and K$^+$ ([Cl$^-$] >60 mmol/L is diagnostic in children)
    - heterozygotes have normal sweat tests (and no symptoms)
- PFTs
  - early: airflow limitation in small airways
  - late: severe airflow obstruction, hyperinflation, gas trapping, decreased DL$_{CO}$ (very late)
- ABGs
  - hypoxemia, hypercapnia later in disease with eventual respiratory failure and cor pulmonale
- CXR
  - hyperinflation, increased pulmonary markings (especially upper lobes)

Treatment
- chest physiotherapy and postural drainage
- bronchodilators (salbutamol ± ipratropium bromide)
- inhaled mucolytic (reduces mucus viscosity), hypertonic saline DNase
- inhaled antibiotics (tobramycin, colistin, aztreonam)
- antibiotics (e.g. ciprofloxacin)
- lung transplant
- pancreatic enzyme replacements, high calorie diet

Prognosis
- depends on: infections (cepacia colonization), FEV$_1$, acute pulmonary exacerbations, lung transplant vs. non-lung transplant

Interstitial Lung Disease

Definition
- a group of disorders which cause progressive scarring of lung tissue
- this scarring can eventually impair lung function and gas exchange

Pathophysiology
- inflammatory and/or fibrosing process in the alveolar walls → distortion and destruction of normal alveoli and microvasculature
- typically associated with
  - lung restriction (decrease in TLC and VC)
  - decreased lung compliance (increased or normal FEV$_1$/FVC)
  - impaired diffusion (decreased DL$_{CO}$)
  - hypoxemia due to V/Q mismatch (usually without hypercapnia until end stage)
  - pulmonary HTN and cor pulmonale occur with advanced disease secondary to hypoxemia and blood vessel destruction

Etiology
- >100 known disorders can cause ILD
- majority due to unknown agents or cause

In ILD think
FASSTEN and BAD RASH

Upper Lung Disease (FASSTEN)
Farmer's lung (hypersensitivity pneumonitis)
Ankylosing spondylitis
Sarcoidosis
Silicosis
TB
Eosinophilic granuloma (Langerhans-cell histiocytosis)
Neurofibromatosis

Lower Lung Disease (BADRASH)
Bronchiolitis obliterans with organizing pneumonia (BOOP)
Asbestosis
Drugs (nitrofurantoin, hydralazine, INH, amiodarone, many chemo drugs)
Rheumatologic disease
Aspiration
Scleroderma
Hamman Rich (acute interstitial pneumonia) and IPF

Table 17. Interstitial Lung Diseases

UNKNOWN ETIOLOGY	KNOWN ETIOLOGY		
Idiopathic interstitial pneumonias	**ILD Associated with Systemic Rheumatic Disorders**	**ILD Associated with Drugs or Treatments**	**Inherited Disorders**
UIP (usual interstial pneumonia e.g. IPF)	Scleroderma	Antibiotics (nitrofurantoin)	Familial IPF
NSIP (non-specific interstitial pneumonia)	Rheumatoid arthritis	Anti-inflammatory agents (methotrexate)	Telomerase mutations
LIP (lymphocytic interstitial pneumonia)	SLE	Cardiovascular drugs (amiodarone)	Neurofibromatosis
COP (cryptogenic organizing pneumonia e.g. BOOP)	Polymyositis/dermatomyositis	Antineoplastic agents (chemotherapy agents)	Tuberous sclerosis
DIP (desquamative interstitial pneumonia)	Anti-synthetase syndromes	Illicit drugs	Gaucher's disease
IPPFE (idiopathic pleuroparenchymal fibroelastosis)	Mixed connective tissue disease	Radiation	**Alveolar Filling Disorders**
AFOP (acute fibrinous and organizing pneumonia)	**Environment/Occupation Associated ILD**	**ILD Associated with Pulmonary Vasculitis**	Chronic eosinophilic pneumonia
Sarcoidosis	Hypersensitivity pneumonitis	Granulomatosis with Polyangiitis (GPA)	Pulmonary alveolar proteinosis
Langerhans-cell histiocytosis	(usually organic antigen)	Goodpasture's syndrome	
(eosinophilic granuloma)	Farmer's lung	Idiopathic pulmonary hemosiderosis	
Lymphangioleiomyomatosis	Air conditioner/humidifier lung		
	Bird breeder's lung		
	Pneumoconioses (inorganic dust)		
	Silicosis		
	Asbestosis		
	Coal worker's pneumoconiosis		
	Chronic beryllium disease		
	Pneumonitis from gases/fumes/vapour		

Signs and Symptoms

- dyspnea, especially on exertion
- nonproductive cough
- crackles (dry, fine, end-inspiratory)
- clubbing (especially in IPF and asbestosis)
- features of cor pulmonale
- note that signs and symptoms vary with underlying disease process
  - e.g. sarcoidosis is seldom associated with crackles and clubbing

Investigations

The CXR can be normal in up to 15% of patients with interstitial lung disease

- CXR/high resolution CT (see Medical Imaging, MI7)
  - usually decreased lung volumes
  - reticular, nodular, or reticulonodular pattern (nodular <3 mm)
  - hilar/mediastinal adenopathy (especially in sarcoidosis)
- PFTs
  - restrictive pattern: decreased lung volumes and compliance
  - normal or increased FEV_1/FVC (>70-80%), e.g. flow rates are often normal or high when corrected for absolute lung volume
  - DL_{CO} decreased due to V/Q mismatch (less surface area for gas exchange ± pulmonary vascular disease)
- ABGs
  - hypoxemia and respiratory alkalosis may be present with progression of disease
- other
  - bronchoscopy, bronchoalveolar lavage, lung biopsy
  - ESR, ANA (lupus), RF (RA), serum-precipitating antibodies to inhaled organic antigens (hypersensitivity pneumonitis), c-ANCA (GPA), anti-GBM (Goodpasture's)

Unknown Etiologic Agents

IDIOPATHIC PULMONARY FIBROSIS

Definition

- pulmonary fibrosis of unknown cause with usual interstitial pneumonia (UIP) pattern on biopsy (or inferred from CT)
- a progressive, irreversible condition
- commonly presents over age 50, incidence rises with age; males > females
- most cases associated with honeycomb lung on CT
- differential diagnosis includes NSIP, COP, desquamative interstitial pneumonitis (DIP), lymphocytic interstitial pneumonitis (LIP), Sjögren's disease

IPF Prevalence
- Age 35-44: 2-7 per 100,000
- Age >75: 175 per 100,000

Signs and Symptoms

- commonly presents over age 50, incidence rises with age; males > females
- dyspnea on exertion, nonproductive cough, constitutional symptoms, late inspiratory fine crackles at lung bases, clubbing

Investigations

- labs (nonspecific, autoimmune serology usually negative)
- CXR: reticular or reticulonodular pattern with lower lung predominance; may appreciate honeycombing in advanced disease
- high resolution CT: lower zone peripheral reticular markings, traction bronchiectasis, honeycombing; ground glass, consolidation, or nodules should not be prominent in IPF
- biopsy: rarely for UIP as honeycombing usually makes radiologic diagnosis possible

Treatment

- O_2
- pirfenidone and nintedanib can slow disease progression
- lung transplantation for advanced disease
- mean survival of 3-5 yr after diagnosis

SARCOIDOSIS

Definition

- idiopathic non-infectious granulomatous multi-system disease with lung involvement in 90%
- characterized pathologically by non-caseating granulomas
- numerous HLA antigens have been shown to play a role and familial sarcoidosis is now recognized

Epidemiology

- typically affects young and middle-aged patients
- higher incidence among people of African descent and from northern latitudes e.g. Scandinavia, Canada

Signs and Symptoms
- asymptomatic, cough, dyspnea, fever, arthralgia, malaise, erythema nodosum, chest pain
- chest exam often normal
- common extrapulmonary manifestations
  - cardiac (arrhythmias, sudden death)
  - eye involvement (anterior or posterior uveitis)
  - skin involvement (skin papules, erythema nodosum, lupus pernio)
  - peripheral lymphadenopathy
  - arthralgia
  - hepatomegaly ± splenomegaly
- less common extra-pulmonary manifestations involve bone, CNS, kidney
- two acute sarcoid syndromes
  - Lofgren's syndrome: fever, erythema nodosum, bilateral hilar lymphadenopathy, arthralgias
  - Heerfordt-Waldenstrom syndrome: fever, parotid enlargement, anterior uveitis, facial nerve palsy

Investigations
- CBC (cytopenias from spleen or marrow involvement)
- serum electrolytes, creatinine, liver enzymes, calcium (hypercalcemia/hypercalciuria due to vitamin D activation by granulomas)
- hypergammaglobulinemia, occasionally RF positive
- elevated serum ACE (non-specific and non-sensitive)
- CXR: predominantly nodular opacities especially in upper lung zones ± hilar adenopathy
- PFTs: normal, obstructive pattern, restrictive pattern with normal flow rates and decreased DLco, or mixed obstructive/restrictive pattern
- ECG: to rule out conduction abnormalities
- slit-lamp eye exam: to rule out uveitis

Diagnosis
- biopsy
  - transbronchial lung biopsy, transbronchial lymph node aspiration, endobronchial ultrasound guided surgical (EBUS) biopsy, or mediastinoscopic lymph node biopsy for granulomas
  - in ~75% of cases, transbronchial biopsy shows granulomas in the parenchyma even if the CXR is normal

Staging
- radiographic, based on CXR
  - Stage 0: normal radiograph
  - Stage I: bilateral hilar lymphadenopathy ± right paratracheal lymphadenopathy
  - Stage II: bilateral hilar lymphadenopathy and diffuse interstitial disease
  - Stage III: interstitial disease only (reticulonodular pattern or nodular pattern)
  - Stage IV: pulmonary fibrosis (honeycombing)

Treatment
- 85% of stage I resolve spontaneously
- 50% of stage II resolve spontaneously
- steroids for symptoms, declining lung function, hypercalcemia, or involvement of eye, CNS, kidney, or heart (not for abnormal CXR alone)
- methotrexate or other immunosuppressives occasionally used

Prognosis
- approximately 10% mortality secondary to progressive fibrosis of lung parenchyma

Known Etiologic Agents

HYPERSENSITIVITY PNEUMONITIS
- also known as extrinsic allergic alveolitis
- non-IgE mediated inflammation of lung parenchyma (acute, subacute, and chronic forms)
- caused by sensitization to inhaled agents, usually organic dust
- pathology: airway-centred, poorly formed granulomas and lymphocytic inflammation
- exposure usually related to occupation or hobby
  - Farmer's Lung (*Thermophilic actinomycetes*)
  - Bird Breeder's/Bird Fancier's Lung (immune response to bird IgA)
  - Humidifier Lung (*Aureobasidium pullulans*)
  - Sauna Taker's Lung (*Aureobasidium* spp.)

Signs and Symptoms
- acute presentation: (4-6 h after exposure)
  - dyspnea, cough, fever, chills, malaise (lasting 18-24 h)
  - CXR: diffuse infiltrates
  - type III (immune complex) reaction
- subacute presentation: more insidious onset than acute presentation

Most common presentation of sarcoidosis: asymptomatic CXR finding

Hilar adenopathy refers to enlargement of mediastinal lymph nodes which is most often seen by standard CXR as spherical/ellipsoidal and/or calcified nodes. If unilateral - think neoplasia, TB, or sarcoid. If bilateral - think sarcoid or lymphoma

Corticosteroids for Pulmonary Sarcoidosis
Cochrane DB Syst Rev 2005;CD001114
Study: Meta-analysis of 13 RCTs involving 1,066 participants examining the use of steroids (oral or inhaled) in sarcoidosis.
Results: Oral steroids demonstrated an improvement in CXR (RR 1.46, 95% CI 1.01-2.09). For inhaled corticosteroids, two studies showed no improvement in lung function and one study showed an improvement in diffusing capacity. No data on side-effects.
Conclusions: Oral steroids improve CXR findings and global scores of CXR, symptoms, and spirometry over 3-24 mo, but do not improve lung function or modify disease course. Oral steroids may be of benefit for patients with Stage 2 and 3 disease.

Calcified diaphragmatic plaques are highly suggestive of asbestosis, especially if bilateral

CXR Fibrotic Patterns
- Asbestosis: lower > upper lobes
- Silicosis: upper > lower lobes
- Coal: upper > lower lobes

- chronic presentation
  - insidious onset
  - dyspnea, cough, malaise, anorexia, weight loss
  - PFTs: progressively restrictive
  - CXR: predominantly upper lobe reticulonodular pattern
  - type IV (cell mediated, delayed hypersensitivity) reaction (see Rheumatology, RH2)
- in both acute and chronic reactions, serum precipitins may be detectable (neither sensitive nor specific)

Remember to involve occupational health and place of work for data collection and treatment plan.
Also counsel re: worker's insurance as per jurisdiction (e.g. Workers Safety Insurance Board [WSIB] in Ontario)

Treatment
- early diagnosis: avoidance of further exposure is critical as chronic changes are irreversible
- systemic corticosteroids can relieve symptoms and speed resolution

PNEUMOCONIOSES
- reaction to inhaled inorganic dusts 0.5-5 μm in size
- no effective treatment, therefore key is exposure prevention through the use of protective equipment
- smoking cessation, annual influenza and pneumococcal vaccination, rehabilitation, lung transplant for endstage disease

Table 18. Pneumoconioses

Diagnosis	Etiology	Symptoms	Investigations	Complications
Asbestosis	Exposure risks: insulation, shipyard, construction, brake linings, pipe fitters, plumbers Slowly progressive diffuse interstitial fibrosis induced by inhaled asbestos fibres Usually >10-20 yr of exposure; may develop with shorter but heavier exposure; typically prolonged interval (20-30 yr) between exposure and clinical disease	Insidious onset Dyspnea Cough: paroxysmal, non-productive Cough: paroxysmal, non-productive Clubbing (much more likely in asbestosis than silicosis or CWP)	CXR Lower > upper lobe Reticulonodular pattern, may develop IPF-like honeycombing Asbestos exposure can also cause pleural and diaphragmatic plaques (± calcification), pleural effusion, round atelectasis Microscopic examination reveals ferruginous bodies: yellow-brown rod-shaped structures which represent asbestos fibres coated in macrophages	Asbestos exposure increases risk of bronchogenic CA and malignant mesothelioma Risk of lung cancer dramatically increased for smokers
Silicosis	At risk population: sandblasters, rock miners, stone cutters, quarry and highway workers Generally requires >20 yr exposure; may develop with much shorter but heavier exposure	Dyspnea, cough, and wheezing	CXR Silicosis Upper > lower lobe Early: nodular disease (simple pneumoconiosis), lung function usually normal Late: nodules coalesce into masses (progressive massive fibrosis) Possible hilar lymph node enlargement (frequently calcified), especially "egg shell" calcification	Mycobacterial infection (e.g. TB)
Coal Worker's Pneumoconiosis (CWP)	At risk population: coal workers, graphite workers Coal and silica, coal is less fibrogenic than silica	Pathologic hallmark is coal macule Simple CWP No signs or symptoms, usually normal lung function Complicated CWP (also known as progressive massive fibrosis) Dyspnea Course: few patients progress to complicated CWP	Simple CWP CXR: multiple nodular opacities, mostly upper lobe Complicated CWP CXR: opacities larger and coalesce	Caplan's syndrome: rheumatoid arthritis and CWP present as larger nodules

INTERSTITIAL LUNG DISEASE ASSOCIATED WITH DRUGS OR TREATMENTS

Drug-Induced
- antineoplastic agents: bleomycin, mitomycin, busulfan, cyclophosphamide, methotrexate, chlorambucil, BCNU (carmustine)
- antibiotics: nitrofurantoin, penicillin, sulfonamide
- cardiovascular drugs: amiodarone, tocainide
- anti-inflammatory agents: methotrexate, penicillamine
- gold salts
- illicit drugs (heroin, methadone)
- rituximab, anti-TNF-α agents (infliximab, etanercept, adalimumab)

Radiation-Induced
- early pneumonitis: approximately 6 wk post-exposure
- late fibrosis: 6-12 mo post-exposure
- infiltrates conform to the shape of the radiation field

Pulmonary Vascular Disease

Pulmonary Hypertension

Definition
- mean pulmonary arterial pressure >25 mmHg at rest and >30 mmHg with exercise, or a systolic pulmonary artery pressure of >40 mmHg at rest
- in the past, pulmonary HTN was classified as primary or secondary pulmonary HTN, but this classification was modified to a more clinically useful, treatment based classification

Table 19. World Health Organization Classification of Pulmonary Hypertension

Classification	Some Causes	Treatment Options	Consider in All Patients with PH
I. Pulmonary Arterial HTN	Idiopathic Collagen vascular disease (scleroderma, SLE, RA) Congenital systemic-to-pulmonary shunts (Eisenmenger syndrome) Persistent pulmonary hypertension of the newborn (PPHN) Portopulmonary HTN HIV infection Drugs and toxins (e.g. anorexigens) Pulmonary veno-occlusive disease Schistosomiasis Pulmonary capillary hemangiomatosis Sickle cell disease	No effective treatment CCBs or advanced therapy often needed The latter includes: prostanoids, endothelin receptor antagonists, PDE5 inhibitors Lung transplantation	
II. Pulmonary HTN due to Left Heart Disease	Left-sided atrial or ventricular heart disease (e.g. LV dysfunction) Left-sided valvular heart disease (e.g. aortic stenosis, mitral stenosis) Congenital/acquired left heart inflow/outflow tract obstruction and congenital cardiomyopathies	Treat underlying heart disease	Oxygen therapy Exercise Consider anticoagulation
III. Pulmonary HTN due to Lung Disease and/or Hypoxia	Parenchymal lung disease (COPD, interstitial fibrosis, cystic fibrosis) Chronic alveolar hypoxia (chronic high altitude, alveolar hypoventilation disorders, sleep-disordered breathing)	Treat underlying cause of hypoxia and correct with supplemental oxygen (proven mortality benefit)	
IV. Chronic Thromboembolic Pulmonary HTN (CTEPH)	Thromboembolic obstruction of proximal pulmonary arteries Obstruction of distal pulmonary arteries – PE (thrombus, foreign material, tumour, in situ thrombosis)	Anticoagulation, thromboendarterectomy	
V. Pulmonary HTN with Unclear Multifactorial Mechanisms	Hematologic disorders Systemic disorders (e.g. sarcoidosis) Metabolic disorders Extrinsic compression of central pulmonary veins (tumour, adenopathy, fibrosing mediastinitis) Chronic hemolytic anemia Segmental pulmonary hypertension	Treat underlying cause	

Adapted from: Simonneau G, et al. *J Am Coll Cardio* 2013;62(25 Suppl):D34-D41

IDIOPATHIC PULMONARY ARTERIAL HYPERTENSION (PRIMARY PULMONARY HYPERTENSION)

Definition
- pulmonary HTN in the absence of a demonstrable cause
- exclude
  - left-sided cardiac valvular disease
  - myocardial disease
  - congenital heart disease
  - any clinically significant parenchymal lung disease
  - systemic connective-tissue disease
  - chronic thromboembolic disease

Epidemiology
- usually presents in young females (20-40 yr); mean age of diagnosis is 36 yr
- most cases are sporadic; familial predisposition in 10% of cases, some linked to mutations in BMPR2
- may be associated with the use of anorexic drugs (e.g. Aminorex®, Fenfluramine®), amphetamines, and cocaine

Guidelines for Vasodilator Response in Pulmonary Arterial HTN
- Patients with IPAH that respond to vasodilators acutely, have an improved survival with long-term use of CCBs
- Vasoreactivity testing: short-acting agent such as IV epoprostenol, IV adenosine, or inhaled NO
- Positive vasodilator response: mean PAP fall of at least 10 mmHg to ≤40 mmHg with an increased or unchanged cardiac output (European Society of Cardiology)
- Positive vasodilator response: should be considered as candidate for trial of oral CCB therapy

Medical Therapy for Pulmonary Arterial Hypertension. ACCP Evidence-Based Clinical Practice Guidelines. *Chest* 2004;(Suppl)06:126

Pulmonary arterial pressures are measured by pulmonary artery catheters (i.e. Swan-Ganz catheter) which are inserted into a large vein (often internal jugular). A balloon at the end of the catheter tip is inflated causing the catheter to advance through the right side of the heart and into the pulmonary artery. This allows for the measurement of RA, RV, PA, and pulmonary capillary wedge pressures as well as sampling of mixed venous blood. A thermistor near the end of the catheter also allows for assessment of cardiac output by thermodilution

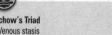

Virchow's Triad
- Venous stasis
- Endothelial cell damage
- Hypercoagulable states

Multidetector Computed Tomography for Acute Pulmonary Embolism (PIOPED II Trial)
NEJM 2006;354:2317-2327
Study: Multicentre, prospective study investigating accuracy of computed tomography angiography (CTA) alone and combined with venous phase imaging (CTA-CTV) for the diagnosis of PE.
Patients: 824 patients of several thousand eligible for study received reference diagnosis to confirm absence or presence of PE (V/Q scan, venous compression U/S of lower extremities, and pulmonary digital-subtraction angiography (DSA) if necessary). To confirm absence, patients in whom PE was excluded were telephoned 3-6 mo after enrollment. Any deaths were reviewed by an outcome committee. All patients enrolled also underwent clinical assessment of PE (including a Wells' score) prior to imaging.
Outcomes: Diagnosis of pulmonary embolism.
Results: 773 of 824 patients had adequate CTAs for interpretation. PE was diagnosed in 192 of the 824 patients. Sensitivity was 83% (150 of 181 patients, 95% CI 0.76-0.92) and specificity was 96% (567 of 592 patients, 95% CI 0.93-0.97). However, the predictive value of CTA-CTV varied when clinical pre-test probability was taken into account. PPV of CTA for high, intermediate and low clinical probability were 96% (95% CI 0.78-0.99), 92% (95% CI 0.84-0.96), and 58% (95% CI 0.40-0.73), respectively. NPV of CTA for high, intermediate and low clinical probability were 60% (95% CI 0.32-0.83), 89% (95% CI 0.82-0.93), and 96% (95% CI 0.92-0.98) respectively.
Conclusion: CTA is effective for diagnosing or excluding PE in accordance with assessment of clinical pretest probability. When clinical probability is inconsistent with imaging results, further investigations are required to rule out PE.

Signs and Symptoms

Table 20. Signs and Symptoms of Pulmonary Hypertension

Symptoms	Signs
Dyspnea	Loud, palpable P2
Fatigue	RV heave
Retrosternal chest pain	Right-sided S4 (due to RVH)
Syncope	Systolic murmur (tricuspid regurgitation [TR])
Symptoms of underlying disease	If RV failure: right sided S3, increased JVP, positive HJR, peripheral edema, TR
	Reynaud's phenomenon

Investigations
- CXR: enlarged central pulmonary arteries, cardiac changes due to RV enlargement (filling of retrosternal air space)
- ECG
  - RVH/right-sided strain (see <u>Cardiology and Cardiac Surgery</u>, C7)
- 2-D echo doppler assessment of right ventricular systolic pressure
- cardiac catheterization: direct measurement of pulmonary artery pressures (necessary to confirm diagnosis)
- PFTs to asses for underlying lung disease: DLco usually reduced; volumes and flows normal
- CT angiogram to assess lung parenchyma and possible PE
- V/Q scan ± pulmonary angiogram to rule out thromboembolic disease
- serology: ANA positive in 30% of patients with primary pulmonary HTN; other serologic markers can be used in the appropriate clinical setting

Treatment
- see Table 19

Prognosis
- 2-3 yr mean survival from time of diagnosis
- survival decreases to approximately 1 yr if severe pulmonary HTN or right-heart failure

Pulmonary Embolism

Definition
- lodging of a blood clot in the pulmonary arterial tree with subsequent increase in pulmonary vascular resistance, impaired V/Q matching, and possibly reduced pulmonary blood flow

Etiology and Pathophysiology
- one of the most common causes of preventable death in the hospital
- proximal leg thrombi (popliteal, femoral, or iliac veins) are the source of most clinically recognized pulmonary emboli
- thrombi often start in calf, but must propagate into proximal veins to create a sufficiently large thrombus for a clinically significant PE
- fewer than 30% of patients have clinical evidence of DVT (e.g. leg swelling, pain, or tenderness)
- always suspect PE if patient develops fever, sudden dyspnea, chest pain, or collapse 1-2 wk after surgery

Risk Factors
- stasis
  - immobilization: paralysis, stroke, bed rest, prolonged sitting during travel, immobilization of an extremity after fracture
  - obesity, CHF
  - chronic venous insufficiency
- endothelial cell damage
  - post-operative injury, trauma
- hypercoagulable states
  - underlying malignancy (particularly adenocarcinoma)
  - cancer treatment (chemotherapy, hormonal)
  - exogenous estrogen administration (OCP, HRT)
  - pregnancy, post-partum
  - prior history of DVT/PE, family history
  - nephrotic syndrome
  - coagulopathies: Factor V Leiden, Prothrombin 20210A variant, inherited deficiencies of antithrombin/protein C/protein S, antiphospholipid antibody, hyperhomocysteinemia, increased Factor VIII levels, and myeloproliferative disease
- increasing age

Investigations (if highly suspicious, go straight to CT angiogram)
- see Emergency Medicine, ER33

Table 21. Common Investigations for Pulmonary Embolism

Investigation	Purpose/Utility
Pulmonary Angiogram (Gold Standard)	Filling defect indicative of embolus; negative angiogram excludes clinically relevant PE More invasive, and harder to perform than CT, therefore done infrequently
D-Dimer	Highly sensitive D-dimer result can exclude DVT/PE if pretest probability is already low Little value if pretest probability is high If D-dimer positive, will need further evaluation with compression U/S (for DVT) and/or CT (for PE)
CT Angiogram	Both sensitive and specific for PE Diagnosis and management uncertain for small filling defects CT may identify an alternative diagnosis if PE is not present CT scanning of the proximal leg and pelvic veins can be done at the same time and may be helpful
Venous Duplex U/S or Doppler	With leg symptoms Positive test rules in proximal DVT Negative test rules out proximal DVT Without leg symptoms Positive test rules in proximal DVT Negative test does not rule out a DVT: patient may have non-occlusive or calf DVT
ECG	Findings not sensitive or specific Sinus tachycardia most common; may see non-specific ST segment and T wave changes RV strain, RAD, RBBB, S1-Q3-T3 with massive embolization
CXR	Frequently normal; no specific features Atelectasis (subsegmental), elevation of a hemidiaphragm Pleural effusion: usually small Hampton's hump: cone-shaped area of peripheral opacification representing infarction Westermark's sign: dilated proximal pulmonary artery with distal oligemia/decreased vascular markings (difficult to assess without prior films) Dilatation of proximal PA: rare

V/Q Scan	Very sensitive but low specificity
	Order scan if
	  CXR normal, no COPD
	  Contraindication to CT (contrast allergy, renal dysfunction, pregnancy)
	Avoid V/Q scan if
	  CXR abnormal or COPD
	  Inpatient
	  Suspect massive PE
	Results
	  Normal: excludes the diagnosis of PE
	  High probability: most likely means PE present, unless pre-test probability is low
	  60% of V/Q scans are nondiagnostic

Echocardiogram	Useful to assess massive or chronic PE Not routinely done
ABG	No diagnostic use in PE (insensitive and nonspecific) May show respiratory alkalosis (due to hyperventilation)

Treatment
- admit for observation (patients with DVT only are often sent home on LMWH)
- oxygen: supplemental O_2 if hypoxemic or short of breath
- pain relief: analgesics if chest pain – narcotics or acetaminophen
    - acute anticoagulation: therapeutic-dose SC LMWH or IV heparin – start ASAP
    - anticoagulation stops clot propagation, prevents new clots and allows endogenous fibrinolytic system to dissolve existing thromboemboli over months get baseline CBC, INR, aPTT ± renal function ± liver function
    - for SC LMWH: dalteparin 200 U/kg once daily, enoxaparin 1 mg/kg bid or 1.5mg/kg once daily, or tinzaparin 175 U/kg once daily – no lab monitoring – avoid or reduce dose in renal dysfunction
    - for IV heparin: bolus of 75 U/kg (usually 5,000 U) followed by infusion starting at 20 U/kg/h – aim for aPTT 2-3x control
    - rivaroxaban is accepted alternative for acute PE
- long-term anticoagulation
    - warfarin: start the same day as LMWH/heparin – overlap warfarin with LMWH/heparin for at least 5 d and until INR in target range of 2-3 for at least 2 d
    - LMWH instead of warfarin for pregnancy, active cancer, or high bleeding risk patients

D-dimer is elevated in patients with recent surgery, cancer, inflammation, infection, and severe renal dysfunction. It has good sensitivity and negative predictive value, but poor specificity and positive predictive value

Classic ECG finding of PE is S1-Q3-T3 (inverted T3), but most commonly see only sinus tachycardia

Clinical Prediction Rule for Pulmonary Embolism
J Thromb Hemost 2000;83:416-420
Wells' Criteria

Risk Factors	Points
Clinical signs of DVT	3.0
No more likely alternative diagnosis (using H&P, CXR, ECG)	3.0
Immobilization or surgery in previous 4 wk	1.5
Previous PE/DVT	1.5
HR >100 beats/min	1.5
Hemoptysis	1.0
Malignancy	1.0
Clinical Probability	
Low (0-2)	3%
Intermediate (3-6)	28%
High (>6)	78%

Modified Wells": >4 PE likely; ≤4 PE unlikely
JAMA 2006

PE Rule Out Criteria (PERC)
Prospective Multicentre Evaluation of the Pulmonary Embolism Rule Out Criteria
J Thromb Hemost 2008;6:772
- Age less than 50 yr
- Heart rate less than 100 bpm
- Oxyhemoglobin saturation ≥95 percent
- No hemoptysis
- No estrogen use
- No prior DVT or PE
- No unilateral leg swelling
- No surgery or trauma requiring hospitalization within the past 4 wk

Acute PE can probably be excluded without further diagnostic testing if the patient meets all PERC criteria AND there is a low clinical suspicion for PE, according to either the Wells' criteria or a low gestalt probability determined by the clinician prior to diagnostic testing for PE.

Evaluation of a Suspected Pulmonary Embolism
Low clinical probability of embolism
D-dimer (+ve) → CT scan (+ve) → ruled in
      (–ve) → ruled out (–ve) → ruled out
Intermediate or high probability
CT scan (–ve) → ruled out
      (+ve) → ruled in
Notes
- Use D-dimers only if low clinical probability, otherwise, go straight to CT
- If using V/Q scans (CT contrast allergy or renal failure):
- Negative V/Q scan rules out the diagnosis
- High probability V/Q scan only rules in the diagnosis if have high clinical suspicion
- Inconclusive V/Q scan requires leg U/S to look for DVT or CT

Workup for Idiopathic VTE
Thrombophilia Workup: recurrent or idiopathic DVT/PE, age <50, FHx, unusual location, massive
Malignancy Workup: 12% of patients with idiopathic VTE will have a malignancy

The Use of Unfractionated Heparin Should Be Limited to:
• Patients with severe renal dysfunction (CrCl <30 ml/min) in whom LMWH and novel oral anticoagulation should be avoided
• Patients at elevated risk of bleeding that may need rapid reversal of anticoagulation
• Patients who receive thrombolytic therapy

Extended Use of Dabigatran, Warfarin or Placebo in Venous Thromboembolism
NEJM 2013;368:709-718
Study: Two double blind, RCTs; one comparing against placebo, the other against active treatment.
Population: 4,199 patients (2,856 in active-control study, 1,343 in placebo-control study) with VTE who had completed at least 3 mo of therapy.
Intervention: In the active-control study, patients randomized to either 150 mg dabigatran or warfarin (INR 2.0-3.0). Patients in the placebo-control study received either 150 mg dabigatran or placebo.
Outcome: Recurrence of VTE, risk of major or clinically relevant bleed.
Results: In the active-control study, there was a hazard ratio (HR) of 1.44 (95% CI 0.78-2.64 for non-inferiority) of recurrent VTE with dabigatran vs. warfarin. HR of major or clinically relevant bleed was 0.54 (95% CI 0.41-0.71). In the placebo-control study, the HR of VTE with dabigatran vs. placebo was 0.08 (95% CI 0.02-0.25). HR of major or clinically relevant bleed was 2.92 (95% CI 1.52-5.60).
Conclusions: Dabigatran appears to be non-inferior to warfarin in the prevention of VTE recurrence. Dabigatran is associated with a lower risk of major or clinically relevant bleed than warfarin, but greater than placebo.

- direct thrombin inhibitors: can treat from outset with rivaroxaban; dabigatran has been shown to have lower bleeding risk than warfarin; no monitoring required, however agents not reversible, so avoid if bleeding concerns
- IV thrombolytic therapy
  - if patient has massive PE (hypotension or clinical right heart failure) and no contraindications
  - hastens resolution of PE but may not improve survival or long-term outcome and doubles risk of major bleeding
- interventional thrombolytic therapy
  - massive PE is preferentially treated with catheter-directed thrombolysis by an interventional radiologist
  - works better than IV thrombolytic therapy and fewer contraindications
- IVC filter: only if recent proximal DVT + absolute contraindication to anticoagulation
- duration of long-term anticoagulation: individualized, however generally
  - if reversible cause for PE (surgery, injury, pregnancy, etc.): 3-6 mo
  - if PE unprovoked: 6 mo to indefinite
  - if ongoing major risk factor (active cancer, antiphospholipid antibody, etc.): indefinite

Thromboprophylaxis
- mandatory for most hospital patients: reduces DVT, PE, all-cause mortality, cost-effective
- start ASAP
- continue at least until discharge or recommend extending for 35 d post-operatively, if major orthopedic surgery

Table 22. VTE Risk Categories and Prophylaxis (see <u>Hematology</u>, H35)

Risk Group	Prophylaxis Options
Low Thrombosis Risk	
Medical patients: fully mobile	No specific prophylaxis
Surgery: <30 min, fully mobile	Frequent ambulation
Moderate Thrombosis Risk	
Most general, gynecologic, urologic surgery	LMWH
Sick medical patients	Low dose unfractionated heparin
	Fondaparinux
High Thrombosis Risk	
Arthoplasty, hip fracture surgery	LMWH
Major trauma, spinal cord injury	Fondaparinux
	Warfarin (INR 2-3)
	Dabigatran
	Apixaban
	Rivaroxaban
	Low dose unfractionated heparin
High Bleeding Risk	
Neurosurgery, intracranial bleed	TED stockings, pneumatic compression devices
Active bleeding	LMWH or low dose heparin when bleeding risk decreases

Pulmonary Vasculitis

Table 23. Pulmonary Vasculitis

Disease	Definition	Pulmonary Features	Extra-pulmonary Features	Investigations	Treatment
Granulomatosis with Polyangiitis (GPA, previously Wegener's Granulomatosis) (see <u>Nephrology</u>, NP22)	Systemic vasculitis of medium and small arteries	Necrotizing granulomatous lesions of the upper and lower respiratory tract	Focal necrotizing lesions of arteries and veins; crescentic glomerulonephritis	CXR: nodules, cavities, and alveolar opacities c-ANCA Tissue confirmation	Corticosteroids and cyclophosphamide or rituximab
Eosinophilic Granulomatosis with Polyangiitis (EGPA, Churg-Strauss)	Multisystem disorder characterized by allergic rhinitis, asthma, and prominent peripheral eosinophilia	Asthma Infiltrates	Life-threatening systemic vasculitis involving the lungs, pericardium and heart, kidneys, skin, and PNS (mononeuritis multiplex)	Peripheral eosinophilia is the most common finding p-ANCA may be positive Biopsy involved tissue	Corticosteroids
anti-GBM Disease (Goodpasture's) (see <u>Nephrology</u>, NP24)	A disorder characterized by diffuse alveolar hemorrhage and glomerulonephritis caused by anti-GBM antibodies, which cross-react with basement membranes of the kidney and lung	Hemoptysis May follow an influenza infection	Anemia	CXR: may see alveolar infiltrates if hemorrhage is profuse ELISA test with anti-GBM antibodies Renal biopsy/indirect immunofluorescence shows linear staining	Acutely: corticosteroids, plasmapheresis Immunosuppressive therapy Severe cases: bilateral nephrectomy
Systemic Lupus Erythematosus, Rheumatoid Arthritis, Scleroderma	See <u>Rheumatology</u>, RH17				

Pulmonary Edema

- see Cardiology and Cardiac Surgery, C36

Diseases of the Mediastinum and Pleura

Mediastinal Masses

Definition
- mediastinum: bound by the thoracic inlet, diaphragm, sternum, vertebral bodies, and the pleura
- can be broken down into 3 compartments: anterior, middle, and posterior

Etiology and Pathophysiology
- diagnosis is aided by location and patient's age
- anterior compartment: more likely to be malignant
  - "Four Ts" (see sidebar), lymphoma, lipoma, pericardial cyst
- middle compartment
  - pericardial cyst, bronchogenic cyst/tumour, lymphoma, lymph node enlargement, aortic aneurysm
- posterior compartment
  - neurogenic tumours, meningocele, enteric cysts, lymphoma, diaphragmatic hernias, esophageal tumour, aortic aneurysm

Differential of an Anterior Compartment Mass

4 Ts
Thymoma
Thyroid enlargement (goitre)
Teratoma
Tumours
(lymphoma, parathyroid, esophageal, angiomatous)

Signs and Symptoms
- 50% asymptomatic (mainly benign); when symptomatic, 50% are malignant
- chest pain, cough, dyspnea, recurrent respiratory infections
- hoarseness, dysphagia, Horner's syndrome, facial/upper extremity edema (SVC compression)
- paraneoplastic syndromes (e.g. myasthenia gravis [thymomas])

Investigations
- CXR (compare to previous)
- CT with contrast (anatomic location, density, relation to mediastinal vascular structures)
- MRI: specifically indicated in the evaluation of neurogenic tumours
- U/S (best for assessment of structures in close proximity to the heart and pericardium)
- radionuclide scanning: ^{131}I (for thyroid), gallium (for lymphoma)
- biochemical studies: thyroid function, serum calcium, phosphate, PTH, AFP, β-hCG
- biopsy (mediastinoscopy, percutaneous needle aspiration)

Mediastinal Components
Anterior: sternum to pericardium and great vessels. Includes: thymus, extrapericardial aorta and branches, great veins, lymphatic tissues
Middle: pericardium (anteriorly) posterior pericardial reflection, diaphragm, thoracic inlet. Includes: heart, intrapericaridal great vessels, pericardium, trachea
Posterior: posterior pericardial reflection, posterior border of vertebral bodies, first rib to the diaphragm. Includes: esophagus, vagus nerve, thoracic duct, sympathetic chain, azygous venous system

Management
- excision if symptomatic enlarging benign masses or concerns of malignancy
- resect bronchogenic cysts and localized neurogenic tumours via minimally invasive video assisted procedures
- exploration via sternotomy or thoracotomy
- diagnostic biopsy rather than major operation if mass is likely to be a lymphoma, germ cell tumour, or unresectable invasive malignancy
- ± post-operative radiotherapy/chemotherapy if malignant

Horner's Syndrome
Ptosis, Miosis, Anhydrosis

Mediastinitis

- most common causes: post-operative complications of cardiovascular or thoracic surgical procedures

Acute
- etiology
- complication of endoscopy (e.g. esophageal perforation providing entry point for infection)
- esophageal or cardiac surgery
- tumour necrosis
- signs and symptoms
- fever, substernal pain
- pneumomediastinum, mediastinal compression
- Hamman's sign (auscultatory "crunch" during cardiac systole)
- treatment
- antibiotics, drainage, ± surgical closure of perforation

Chronic
- usually granulomatous process or fibrosis related to previous infection (e.g. histoplasmosis, TB, sarcoidosis, syphilis)

Pleural Effusions

Definition
- excess amount of fluid in the pleural space (normally up to 25 mL)

Etiology
- disruption of normal equilibrium between pleural fluid formation/entry and pleural fluid absorption/exit
- pleural effusions are classified as transudative or exudative
  - distinguish clinically using Light's Criteria, which has a sensitivity of 98% and specificity of 83% for identifying exudative pleural effusions

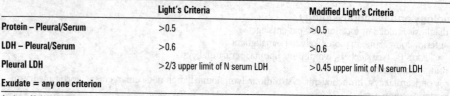

All criteria for transudate must be fulfilled to be considered a transudative effusion. If any one of the criteria for exudates is met – it is an exudate

Table 24. Laboratory Values in Transudative and Exudative Pleural Effusion

	Light's Criteria	Modified Light's Criteria
Protein – Pleural/Serum	>0.5	>0.5
LDH – Pleural/Serum	>0.6	>0.6
Pleural LDH	>2/3 upper limit of N serum LDH	>0.45 upper limit of N serum LDH
Exudate = any one criterion		

Ann Intern Med 1979;77:507-513   Chest 1997;111:970-980

Transudative Pleural Effusions
- pathophysiology: alteration of systemic factors that affect the formation and absorption of pleural fluid (e.g. increased capillary hydrostatic pressure, decreased plasma oncotic pressure)
- etiology
  - CHF: usually right-sided or bilateral
  - cirrhosis
  - nephrotic syndrome, protein losing enteropathy, cirrhosis
  - pulmonary embolism (may cause transudative but more often causes exudative effusion)
  - peritoneal dialysis, hypothyroidism, CF, urinothorax

Transudative effusions are usually bilateral, not unilateral

Exudative effusions can be bilateral or unilateral

Exudative Pleural Effusions
- pathophysiology: increased permeability of pleural capillaries or lymphatic dysfunction
- etiology (see Table 25)

Table 25. Exudative Pleural Effusion Etiologies

Etiology	Examples
Infectious	Parapneumonic effusion (associated with bacterial pneumonia, lung abscess) Empyema (bacterial, fungal, TB) TB pleuritis Viral infection
Malignancy	Lung carcinoma (35%) Lymphoma (10%) Metastases: breast (25%), ovary, kidney Mesothelioma
Inflammatory	Collagen vascular diseases: RA, SLE Pulmonary embolism Post-CABG Drug reaction
Intra-Abdominal	Subphrenic abscess Pancreatic disease (elevated pleural fluid amylase) Meigs' syndrome (ascites and hydrothorax associated with an ovarian fibroma or other pelvic tumour)
Intra-Thoracic	Esophageal perforation (elevated fluid amylase)
Trauma	Chylothorax: thoracic duct disrupted and chyle accumulates in the pleural space due to trauma, tumour Hemothorax: rupture of a blood vessel, commonly by trauma or tumours Pneumothorax (spontaneous, traumatic, tension)

Appearance of Pleural Fluid
- Bloody: trauma, malignancy
- White: empyema, chylous or chyliform effusion
- Black: aspergillosis, amoebic liver abscess
- Yellow-green: rheumatoid pleurisy
- Viscous: malignant mesothelioma
- Ammonia odour: urinothorax
- Food particles: esophageal rupture

Signs and Symptoms
- often asymptomatic
- dyspnea: varies with size of effusion and underlying lung function
- pleuritic chest pain
- inspection: trachea deviates away from effusion, ipsilateral decreased expansion
- percussion: decreased tactile fremitus, dullness
- auscultation: decreased breath sounds, bronchial breathing and egophony at upper level, pleural friction rub

Investigations

- CXR
  - must have >200 mL of pleural fluid for visualization on PA film
  - lateral: >50 mL leads to blunting of posterior costophrenic angle
  - PA: blunting of lateral costophrenic angle
  - dense opacification of lung fields with concave meniscus
  - decubitus: fluid will shift unless it is loculated
  - supine: fluid will appear as general haziness
- CT may be helpful in differentiating parenchymal from pleural abnormalities, may identify underlying lung pathology
- U/S: detects small effusions and can guide thoracentesis
- thoracentesis: indicated if pleural effusion is a new finding; be sure to send off blood work (LDH, glucose, protein) at the same time for comparison
  - risk of re-expansion pulmonary edema if >1.5 L of fluid is removed
  - inspect for colour, character, and odour of fluid
  - analyze fluid
- pleural biopsy: indicated if suspect TB, mesothelioma, or other malignancy (and if cytology negative)
- treatment depends on cause, ± drainage if symptomatic
- CT can be helpful in differentiating parenchymal from pleural abnormalities, assessing for pleural nodules and/or fluid loculation

Role of CT in Pleural Effusion
- To assess for fluid loculation, pleural thickening and nodules, parenchymal abnormalities and adenopathy
- Helps to distinguish benign from malignant effusion and transudative from exudative effusion
- May not distinguish empyema from parapneumonic effusion

Features of Malignant Effusion
- Multiple pleural nodules
- Nodular pleural thickening

Features of Exudative Effusion
- Loculation
- Pleural thickening
- Pleural nodules
- Extrapleural fat of increased density

Table 26. Analysis of Pleural Effusion

Measure	Purpose
Protein, LDH	Transudate vs. exudate
Gram stain, Ziehl-Nielsen stain (TB), culture	Looking for specific organisms
Cell count differential	Neutrophils vs. lymphocytes (lymphocytic effusion in TB, cancer, lymphoma, serositis)
Cytology	Malignancy, infection
Glucose (low)	RA, TB, empyema, malignancy, esophageal rupture
Rheumatoid factor, ANA, complement	Collagen vascular disease
Amylase	Pancreatitis, esophageal perforation, malignancy
pH	Empyema <7.2, TB, and mesothelioma <7.3
Blood	Mostly traumatic, malignancy, PE with infarction, TB
Triglycerides	Chylothorax from thoracic duct leakage, mostly due to trauma, lung CA, or lymphoma
Cholesterol	Distinguish between chylous and chyliform effusion (seen in inflammation, e.g. TB, RA)

Pleural Effusions
Simple Effusion
pH >7.2, LDH <1/2 serum, glucose >2.2

Complicated Effusion
pH <7.2, LDH >1/2 serum, glucose <2.2, positive Gram stain
Needs drainage

Treatment

- thoracentesis
- treat underlying cause
- consider indwelling pleural catheter or pleurodesis in refractory effusions

Complicated Effusion

- persistent bacteria in the pleural space but fluid is non-purulent
- neutrophils, pleural fluid acidosis (pH <7.00), and high LDH
- often no bacteria grown since rapidly cleared from pleural space
- fibrin layer leading to loculation of pleural fluid
- treatment: antibiotics and drainage, treat as an empyema

Empyema

Definition

- pus in pleural space or an effusion with organisms seen on a Gram stain or culture (e.g. pleural fluid is grossly purulent)
- positive culture is not required for diagnosis

Etiology

- contiguous spread from lung infection (most commonly anaerobes) or infection through chest wall (e.g. trauma, surgery)

Signs and Symptoms

- fever, pleuritic chest pain

Investigations
- CT chest
- thoracentesis
- PMNs (lymphocytes in TB) ± visible organisms on Gram stain

When possible, organism-directed therapy, guided by culture sensitivities or local patterns of drug resistance, should be utilized

Treatment
- antibiotic therapy for at least 4-6 wk (rarely effective alone)
- complete pleural drainage with chest tube
- if loculated, more difficult to drain – may require surgical drainage with video-assisted thorascopic surgery (VATS), or surgical removal of fibrin coating to allow lung re-expansion (decortication)

Atelectasis

- see General Surgery, GS10

Pneumothorax

Definition
- presence of air in the pleural space

Pathophysiology
- entry of air into pleural space raises intrapleural pressure causing partial lung deflation

Etiology
- traumatic: penetrating or non-penetrating chest injuries
- iatrogenic (central venous catheter, thoracentesis, mechanical ventilation with barotrauma)
- spontaneous (no history of trauma)
  - primary (no underlying lung disease)
    - spontaneous rupture of apical subpleural bleb of lung into pleural space
    - predominantly tall, healthy, young males
  - secondary (underlying lung disease)
    - rupture of subpleural bleb which migrates along bronchioalveolar sheath to the mediastinum then to the intrapleural space
    - necrosis of lung tissue adjacent to pleural surface (e.g. pneumonia, abscess, PCP, lung CA, emphysema)

Need to Rule Out Life-Threatening Tension Pneumothorax
If pneumothorax with:
- Severe respiratory distress
- Tracheal deviation to contralateral side
- Distended neck veins (↑ JVP)
- Hypotension

Do not perform CXR
Needs immediate treatment
See Emergency Medicine, ER11

Signs and Symptoms
- can be asymptomatic
- acute-onset pleuritic chest pain, dyspnea
- tachypnea, tachycardia
- tracheal deviation (contralateral deviation in tension pneumothorax)
- ipsilateral diminished chest expansion
- decreased tactile/vocal fremitus
- hyperresonance
- ipsilateral diminished breath sounds

Investigations
- CXR
  - small: separation of visceral and parietal pleura seen as fine crescentic line parallel to chest wall at apex
  - large: increased density and decreased volume of lung on side of pneumothorax
  - see Medical Imaging, MI8

Treatment
- small pneumothoraces (<20% with no signs of respiratory/circulatory collapse) resolve spontaneously; breathing 100% oxygen accelerates resorption of air
- small intercostal tube with Heimlich valve for most spontaneous pneumothoraces
- large pneumothoraces or those complicating underlying lung disease require placement of a chest tube connected to underwater seal ± suction
- for repeated episodes: pleurodesis with sclerosing agent or apical bullectomy and abrasion
- treat underlying cause (e.g. antibiotic for PCP)

Asbestos-Related Pleural Disease and Mesothelioma

Etiology and Pathophysiology
- benign manifestations of asbestos exposure:
  - "benign asbestos pleural effusion"
    - exudative effusion, typically ~10 yr after exposure, resolves
  - pleural plaques, usually calcified
    - marker of exposure; usually an asymptomatic radiologic finding

- mesothelioma
  - primary malignancy of the pleura
  - decades after asbestos exposure (even with limited exposure)
  - smoking not a risk factor, but asbestos and smoking synergistically increase risk of lung cancer

Signs and Symptoms
- persistent chest pain, dyspnea, cough, bloody pleural effusion, weight loss

Investigations
- biopsy (pleuroscopic or open)
- needle biopsy may seed needle tract with tumour

Treatment
- resection (extrapleural pneumonectomy) requires careful patient selection; rarely successful (average survival <1 yr)

Respiratory Failure

Definition
- failure of respiratory system to maintain normal blood gases
- hypoxemic (P_aO_2 <60 mmHg)
- hypercapnic (P_aCO_2 >50 mmHg)
- acute vs. chronic (compensatory mechanisms activated)

Signs and Symptoms
- signs of underlying disease
- hypoxemia: restlessness, confusion, cyanosis, coma, cor pulmonale
- hypercapnia: headache, dyspnea, drowsiness, asterixis, warm periphery, plethora, increased ICP (secondary to vasodilatation)

Investigations
- serial ABGs
- CXR and/or CT, bronchoscopy to characterize underlying cause if unclear

Hypoxemic Respiratory Failure

Definition
- P_aO_2 decreased, P_aCO_2 normal or decreased

Treatment
- reverse the underlying pathology
- oxygen therapy: maintain oxygenation (if shunt present, supplemental O_2 is less effective; see Anesthesia and Perioperative Medicine, A10, for oxygen delivery systems)
- ventilation, BiPAP, and PEEP/CPAP (see Anesthesia and Perioperative Medicine, A10): positive pressure can recruit alveoli and redistribute lung fluid
- improve cardiac output: ± hemodynamic support (fluids, vasopressors, inotropes), reduction of O_2 requirements

Table 27. Approach to Hypoxemia

Type of Hypoxemia	Settings	P_aCO_2	A-aDO₂	Oxygen Therapy	Ventilation, BiPAP and PEEP	Improved Cardiac Output
1. Low F_iO_2	Postop, high altitude	N or ↓	N	Improves	No change	No change
2. Hypoventilation	Drug overdose	↑	N	Improves	Improves with ventilation	No change
3a. Shunt (intrapulmonary)	ARDS, pneumonia	N or ↓	↑	No change	Improves (except if one-sided)	Improves
3b. Shunt (Right to Left)	Pulmonary HTN	N or ↓	↑	No change	Worsens	Worsens
4. Low Mixed Venous O₂ Content	Shock	↓	↑	Improves or no change	Worsens	Improves
5. V/Q Mismatch	COPD	N or ↑	↑	Improves (small amounts)	Often improves	Improves
6. Diffusion Impairment	ILD, emphysema	N	↑	Improves	Improves with positive pressure	No change or worsens

Reprinted with permission from Dr. Ian Fraser

Hypercapnic Respiratory Failure

- P_aCO_2 increased, P_aO_2 decreased

Pathophysiology
- increased CO_2 production: fever, sepsis, seizure, acidosis, carbohydrate load
- alveolar hypoventilation: COPD, asthma, CF, chest wall disorder, dead space ventilation (rapid shallow breathing)
  - inefficient gas exchange results in inadequate CO_2 removal in spite of normal or increased minute volume
- hypoventilation
  - central: brainstem stroke, hypothyroidism, severe metabolic alkalosis, drugs (opiates, benzodiazepines)
  - neuromuscular: myasthenia gravis, Guillain-Barré, phrenic nerve injury, muscular dystrophy, polymyositis, kyphoscoliosis
  - muscle fatigue

Treatment
- reverse the underlying pathology
- if P_aCO_2 >50 mmHg and pH <7.35 consider noninvasive or mechanical ventilation
- correct exacerbating factors
  - NTT/ETT suction: clearance of secretions
  - bronchodilators: reduction of airway resistance
  - antibiotics: treatment of infections
- maintain oxygenation (see above)
- diet: increased carbohydrate can increase P_aCO_2 in those with mechanical or limited alveolar ventilation; high lipids decrease P_aCO_2

Acute Respiratory Distress Syndrome

- clinical syndrome characterized by severe respiratory distress, hypoxemia, and noncardiogenic pulmonary edema
- The Berlin Criteria (*JAMA* 2012; 307:2526-2533) for ARDS
  - acute onset
    - within 7 d of a defined event, such as sepsis, pneumonia, or patient noticing worsening of respiratory symptoms
      - usually occurs within 72 h of presumed trigger
    - bilateral opacities consistent with pulmonary edema on either CT or CXR
    - not fully explained by cardiac failure/fluid overload, but patient may have concurrent heart failure
    - objective assessment of cardiac function (e.g. echocardiogram) should be performed even if no clear risk factors

Etiology
- direct lung injury
- airway: aspiration (**gastric contents**, drowning), **pneumonia**, inhalation injury (oxygen toxicity, nitrogen dioxide, smoke)
- circulation: embolism (fat, amniotic fluid), reperfusion injury
- indirect lung injury
- circulation: **sepsis, shock, trauma**, blood transfusion, pancreatitis
- neurogenic: head trauma, intracranial hemorrhage, drug overdose (narcotics, sedatives, TCAs)

Pathophysiology
- disruption of alveolar capillary membranes → leaky capillaries → interstitial and alveolar pulmonary edema → reduced compliance, V/Q mismatch, shunt, hypoxemia, pulmonary HTN

Clinical Course
A. Exudative Phase
- first 7 d of illness after exposure to ARDS precipitant
- alveolar capillary endothelial cells and type I pneumocytes are injured, resulting in loss of normally tight alveolar barrier
- patients develop dyspnea, tachypnea, increased work of breathing
  - these result in respiratory fatigue and eventually respiratory failure (see *Hypoxemic Respiratory Failure*, R25)
B. Fibroproliferative Phase
- after day 7
- may still experience dyspnea, tachypnea, fatigue, and hypoxemia
- most patients clinically improve and are able to wean off mechanical ventilation

Dead Space
- Ventilation without perfusion
- The opposite of shunt

Causes of Hypercapnia
- High Inspired CO_2
- Low Total Ventilation
- High Deadspace Ventilation
- High CO_2 Production

In chronic hypercapnia, supplemental O_2 may decrease the hypoxic drive to breathe, but do not deny oxygen if the patient is hypoxic

In COPD patients with chronic hypercapnia ("CO_2 retainers"), provide supplemental oxygen to achieve target SaO_2 from 88-92%

ALI vs. ARDS: Definition is the same, except ALI is a P_aO_2/F_iO_2 ≤300, while ARDS is a P_aO_2/F_iO_2 ≤200

Categorization of ARDS as Mild, Moderate or Severe – The Berlin Criteria

ARDS Severity	P_aO_2/FiO_2 (mmHg)*	Mortality (95% CI)#
Mild	200-300	27 (24-30)%
Moderate	100-200	32 (29-34)%
Severe	<100	45 (42-48)%

*on ≥5 cm H2O PEEP, #P<0.001
JAMA 2012;307:2526-2533

Risk Factors for Aspiration Pneumonia

Categories	Examples
Decreased level of consciousness	Alcoholism
Upper GI tract disorders	Dysphagia, esophageal disorders
Mechanical instrumentation	Intubation, nasogastric tube, feeding tubes
Neurologic conditions	Dementia, Parkinson disease
Others	Protracted vomiting

- some patients develop fibrotic lung changes that may require long-term support on supplemental oxygen or even mechanical ventilation
- if fibrosis present, associated with increased mortality

Treatment
- based on ARDS network (see *Landmark Respirology Trials*, R37)
- treat underlying disorder (e.g. antibiotics if infection present)
- mechanical ventilation using low tidal volumes (<6 mL/kg) to prevent barotrauma
  - use optimal amount of PEEP (positive end-expiratory pressure) to keep airways open and allow the use of lower F_iO_2
  - may consider using prone ventilation, ± inhaled nitric oxide, short term paralytics (<48 h) or ECMO (extracorpeal membrane oxygenation) if conventional treatment is failing
- fluids and inotropic therapy (e.g. dopamine, vasopressin) if cardiac output inadequate
- pulmonary-arterial catheter now seldom used for monitoring hemodynamics
- mortality: 30-40%, usually due to non-pulmonary complications
- sequelae of ARDS include residual pulmonary impairment, severe debilitation, polyneuropathy and psychologic difficulties, which gradually improve over time
- most survivors eventually regain near-normal lung function, often with mildly reduced diffusion capacity

Neoplasms

Lung Cancer

Classification
- lung tumours can be classified as primary or secondary, benign or malignant, endobronchial or parenchymal
- bronchogenic carcinoma (epithelial lung tumours) are the most common type of primary lung tumour (other types make up less than 1%)
  - small cell lung cancer (SCLC): 10-15%
  - non-small-cell lung cancer (NSCLC): 85-90%
    - squamous cell carcinoma: arise from the proximal respiratory epithelium
    - adenocarcinoma: incidence is increasing; most common subtype in nonsmokers
      - mucinous adenocarcinoma: grows along the alveolar wall in the periphery; may arise at sites of previous lung scarring
    - large cell undifferentiated cancer: diagnosis of exclusion
- benign epithelial lung tumours can be classified as papillomas or adenomas

Table 28. Characteristics of Bronchogenic Cancer

Cell Type	Incidence	Correlation with Smoking	Location	Histology	Metastasis	5 Yr Survival Rates
SCLC	10-15%	Strong	Central	Oat cell, neuroendocrine	Disseminated at presentation Origin in endobronchial cells	1% (poorest prognosis)
Adenocarcinoma	M: 35% F: 40%	Weak	Peripheral	Glandular, mucin producing	Early, distant	12% (60% for mucinous adenocarcinoma, a subtype, with a resectable solitary lesion)
Squamous Cell Carcinoma (SCC)	30%	Strong	Central	Keratin, intercellular bridges	Local invasion and distant spread, may cavitate	25%
Large Cell Carcinoma	10-15%	Strong	Peripheral	Anaplastic, undifferentiated	Early, distant	13%

Risk Factors
- cigarette smoking: the relative risk of developing lung cancer is 10-30 times higher for smokers than for nonsmokers
- other risk factors include cigar smoking, pipe smoking, second-hand smoke, asbestos without smoking (relative risk is 5), asbestos with smoking (relative risk is 92), metals (e.g. chromium, arsenic, nickel), radon gas, ionizing radiation, genetics

Signs and Symptoms
- may be due to primary lesion, metastasis, or paraneoplastic syndrome
- primary lesion
  - cough (75%): beware of chronic cough that changes in character
  - dyspnea (60%)

Summary of Recommendations on Screening for Lung Cancer

Canadian Task Force on Preventative Health Care (2016)
Screening with CXR (± sputum cytology) not recommended

Screening with low-dose CT recommended for high-risk patients (current or former smokers quit within last 15 yr, aged 55-74, ≥30 pack yr smoking Hx) for 3 consecutive years
Number needed to screen = 322

American College of Chest Physicians (2013)
Screening with CXR not recommended

Screening with low-dose CT recommended for high-risk patients (current or former smokers quit within last 15 yr, aged 55-74, ≥30 pack yr smoking Hx)

American Lung Association (2013)
Screening with CXR not recommended

Screening with low-dose CT recommended for high-risk patients (current or former smokers aged 55-74, ≥30 pack yr smoking Hx, no Hx of lung cancer)

Malignant lung tumours are the most common cause of cancer mortality throughout the world in both men and women

Horner has a MAP of the Coast
A Pancoast tumour compresses the cervical sympathetic plexus causing a **Horner's** syndrome:
Miosis
Anhydrosis
Ptosis

Reduced Lung Cancer Mortality with Low-Dose CT Screening
NEJM 2011;365:395-409
Study: Multicentre, RCT.
Methods: 53,454 participants at high risk for lung cancer (55-74 yr, >30 yr smoking, and smoking cessation for <5 y) were assigned to undergo three annual screenings with either low dose CT or single-view PA CXR.
Results: A relative reduction in mortality from lung cancer with low-dose CT screening of 20.0% (95% CI 6.8-26.7; p=0.004). Rate of death from any cause was reduced in the low-dose CT group as compared to the CXR group by 6.7% (95% CI 1.2-13.6; p=0.02).

	Low-dose CT	CXR
Rate of positive screening test	24.2%	6.9%
False positives	96.4%	94.5%
Incidence of lung cancer	645/100 K person yr	572/100 K person yr
Deaths from lung cancer	247/100 K person yr	309/100 K person yr

Conclusions: Screening with low-dose CT reduces mortality from lung cancer.

Endobronchial Ultrasound (EBUS)
• Allows visualization of peri-bronchial structures and distal peripheral lung lesions
• Provides detailed assessment of the airway wall layers
• Allows for guided biopsies of lymph nodes and tumours
• Used for diagnosis and staging

- chest pain (45%)
- hemoptysis (35%)
- other pain (25%)
- clubbing (21%)
- constitutional symptoms: anorexia, weight loss, fever, anemia
- metastasis
  - lung, hilum, mediastinum, pleura: pleural effusion, atelectasis, wheezing
  - pericardium: pericardial effusion, pericardial tamponade
  - esophageal compression: dysphagia
  - phrenic nerve: paralyzed diaphragm
  - recurrent laryngeal nerve: hoarseness
  - superior vena cava syndrome
    - obstruction of SVC causing neck and facial swelling, as well as dyspnea and cough
    - other symptoms: hoarseness, tongue swelling, epistaxis, and hemoptysis
    - physical findings: dilated neck veins, increased number of collateral veins covering the anterior chest wall, cyanosis, edema of the face, arms, and chest, Pemberton's sign (facial flushing, cyanosis, and distension of neck veins upon raising both arms above head)
    - milder symptoms if obstruction is above the azygos vein
  - lung apex (Pancoast tumour): Horner's syndrome, brachial plexus palsy (most commonly C8 and T1 nerve roots)
  - rib and vertebrae: erosion
  - distant metastasis to brain, bone, liver, adrenals
- paraneoplastic syndromes
  - a group of disorders associated with malignant disease, not related to the physical effects of the tumour itself
  - most often associated with SCLC

Table 29. Paraneoplastic Syndromes

System	Clinical Presentation	Associated Malignancy
Skeletal	Clubbing, hypertrophic pulmonary osteoarthropathy (HPOA)	Non-small cell lung cancer (NSCLC)
Dermatologic	Acanthosis nigricans Dermatomyositis	Bronchogenic cancer Bronchogenic cancer
Endocrine	Hypercalcemia (osteolysis or PTHrP) Hypophosphatemia Hypoglycemia Cushing's syndrome (ACTH) Somatostatinoma syndrome SIADH	Squamous cell cancer Squamous cell cancer Sarcoma Small cell lung cancer (SCLC) Bronchial carcinoid SCLC
Neuromyopathic	Lambert-Eaton syndrome Polymyositis Subacute cerebellar degeneration Spinocerebellar degeneration Peripheral neuropathy	SCLC
Vascular/Hematologic	Nonbacterial endocarditis Trousseau's syndrome (migratory thrombophlebitis) DIC	Bronchogenic cancer NSCLC
Renal	Nephrotic syndrome	

Investigations
- initial diagnosis
  - imaging: CXR, CT chest + upper abdomen, PET scan, bone scan
  - cytology: sputum
  - biopsy: bronchoscopy, EBUS, CT-guided percutaneous needle biopsy, mediastinoscopy
- staging workup
  - TMN staging system: T – primary tumour (size); N – regional lymph nodes; M – distant metastasis
  - blood work: electrolytes, LFTs, calcium, ALP
  - imaging: CXR, CT thorax and upper abdomen, bone scan, neuroimaging
  - invasive: bronchoscopy (EBUS), mediastinoscopy, mediastinotomy, thoracotomy
  - screen adenocarcinoma for EGFR and ALK mutations

Table 30. SCLC vs. NSCLC

	Stage	Definition	Treatment	Median Survival
SCLC	Limited stage	Confined to single radiation port (one hemithorax and regional lymph nodes)	Radiation ± chemotherapy ± prophylactic to brain	1-2 yr (12 wk without treatment)
	Extensive stage	Extension beyond a single radiation port	Chemotherapy	6 mo (5 wk without treatment)

	Stage	TNM	Treatment	5 Yr Survival (%)*
NSCLC	IA	T1a-1bN0M0	1st line is complete surgical resection with possible post-operative adjuvant chemotherapy with stage IB and stage II; radiotherapy for non-surgical candidates	50-73
	IB	T2aN0M0		43-58
	IIA	T1a-T2a,N1M0 or T2bN0M0		36-46
	IIB	T2bN1M0 or T3N0M0		25-36
	IIIA	T1a-T2bN2M0 or T3N1-2M0 or T4N0-1M0	Combined modality approach (concurrent chemotherapy followed by surgery)	19-24
	IIIB	T4N2M0 or T1-4N3M0		7-9
	IV	T1-4N0-3M1a-1b	Systemic therapy or molecularly targeted therapy or symptom-based palliative management (radiation); isolated metastasis may be resected	2-13

* Depends on clinical vs. pathologic stage
Refer to AJCC Cancer Staging Manual, 7th ed. 2010 for complete TNM classification

2/3 of primary lung cancer is found in the upper lung; 2/3 of metastases occur in the lower lung (hematogenous spread secondary to increased blood flow to the base of the lung)

Treatment
- options include surgery, radiotherapy, chemotherapy, and palliative care for end-stage disease
- surgery not usually performed for SCLC since it is generally non-curable
- contraindications for surgery
  - spread to contralateral lymph nodes or distant sites
    - patients with potentially resectable disease must undergo mediastinal node sampling since CT thorax is not accurate in 20-40% of cases
  - poor pulmonary status (e.g. unable to tolerate resection of lung)
- chemotherapy (used in combination with other treatments)
  - common agents: etoposide, platinum agents (e.g. cisplatinum), ifosfamide, vincristine, anthracyclines, paclitaxel, irinotecan, gefitinib (an endothelial growth factor receptor inhibitor)
  - complications
    - acute: tumour lysis syndrome, infection, bleeding, myelosuppression, hemorrhagic cystitis (cyclophosphamide), cardiotoxicity (doxorubicin), renal toxicity (cisplatin), peripheral neuropathy (vincristine)
    - chronic: neurologic damage, leukemia, additional primary neoplasms

Prevention
Smoking cessation
Avoidance of exposures
Early detection

Approach to the Solitary Pulmonary Nodule

- see Medical Imaging, MI7

Definition
- a round or oval, sharply circumscribed radiographic lesion up to 3 cm, which may or may not be calcified, and is surrounded by normal lung
- can be benign or malignant

Terminology
- "nodule" <3 cm
- "mass" >3 cm

Table 31. Differential Diagnosis for Benign vs. Malignant Solitary Nodule

Benign (70%)	Malignant (30%)	
Infectious granuloma (histoplasmosis, coccidiomycosis, TB, atypical mycobacteria)	**Bronchogenic carcinoma**	**Metastatic lesions**
Other infections (bacterial abscess, PCP, aspergilloma)	Adenocarcinoma	Breast
Benign neoplasms (hamartoma, lipoma, fibroma)	Squamous cell carcinoma	Head and neck
Vascular (AV malformation, pulmonary varix)	Large cell carcinoma	Melanoma
Developmental (bronchogenic cyst)	Small cell carcinoma	Colon
Inflammatory (granulomatosis with polyangiitis, rheumatoid nodule, sarcoidosis)		Kidney
Other (infarct, pseudotumour, rounded atelectasis, lymph nodes, amyloidoma)		Sarcoma
		Germ cell tumours
		Pulmonary carcinoid

Hamartomas
- 10% of benign lung lesions
- Composed of tissues normally present in lung (fat, epithelium, fibrous tissue, and cartilage), but they exhibit disorganized growth
- Peak incidence is age 60, more common in men
- Usually peripheral and clinically silent
- CXR shows clustered "popcorn" pattern of calcification (pathognomonic for hamartoma)

Pulmonary neoplasms may present as a solitary pulmonary nodule identified incidentally on a radiographic study (~10% of cases) or as symptomatic disease (most cases)

Adenocarcinoma present in a non-smoker may be due to endothelial growth factor receptor mutation

Corona Radiata Sign on Chest CT
• Fine striations that extend linearly from a nodule in a spiculated fashion
• Highly associated with malignancy

Carcinoids
• Early onset (40-60 yr)
• Most are central and can produce symptoms and signs of bronchial obstruction
• Hemoptysis is present in ~50% of cases

Investigations
• CXR: always compare with previous CXR
• CT densitometry and contrast enhanced CT of thorax
• sputum cytology: usually poor yield
• biopsy (bronchoscopic or percutaneous) or excision (thoracoscopy or thoracotomy): if clinical and radiographic features do not help distinguish between benign or malignant lesion
  ▪ if at risk for lung cancer, biopsy may be performed regardless of radiographic features
  ▪ if a biopsy is non-diagnostic, whether to observe, re-biopsy, or resect will depend on the level of suspicion
• watchful waiting: repeat CXR and/or CT scan at 3, 6, 12 mo
• PET scan can help distinguish benign from malignant nodules

Table 32. CXR Characteristics of Benign vs. Malignant Solitary Nodule

Parameters	Benign	Malignant
Size	<3 cm, round, regular	>3 cm, irregular, spiculated
Margins	Smooth margin	Ill-defined or notched margin
Features	Calcified pattern: central, "popcorn" pattern if hamartoma, usually no cavitation; if cavitating, wall is smooth and thin, no other lung pathology	Usually not calcified; if calcified, pattern is eccentric, no satellite lesions, cavitation with thick wall, may have pleural effusions, lymphadenopathy
Doubling Time	Doubles in <1 mo or >2 yr	Doubles in >1 mo or <2 yr

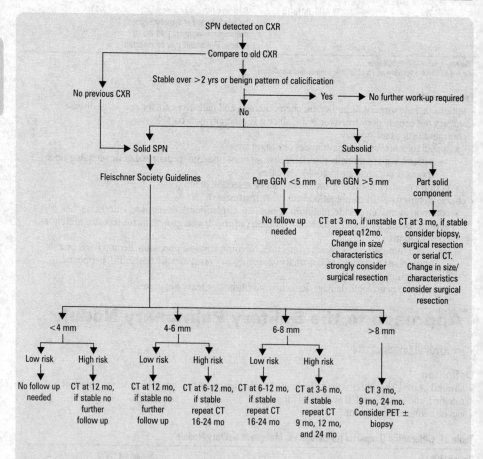

Figure 11. Evaluation of a solitary pulmonary nodule
Adapted from Patel et al 2013 & Fleischner Society 2005.

Sleep-Related Breathing Disorders

Hypoventilation Syndromes

- primary alveolar hypoventilation: idiopathic
- obesity-hypoventilation syndrome (Pickwickian syndrome)
- respiratory neuromuscular disorders

Sleep Apnea

Definition

- episodic decreases in airflow during sleep
- quantitatively measured by the Apnea/Hypopnea Index (AHI) = # of apneic and hypopneic events per hour of sleep
- sleep apnea generally accepted to be present if AHI >15

Classification

- obstructive (OSA)
- caused by transient, episodic obstruction of the upper airway
- absent or reduced airflow despite persistent respiratory effort
- central (CSA) (see Neurology, N47)
- caused by transient, episodic decreases in CNS drive to breathe
- no airflow because no respiratory effort
- Cheyne-Stokes Respiration: a form of CSA in which central apneas alternate with hyperpneas to produce a crescendo-decrescendo pattern of tidal volume; seen in severe LV dysfunction, brain injury, and other settings (see Figure 2)
- mixed (MSA)
- features of both OSA and CSA
- loss of hypoxic and hypercapnic drives to breathe secondary to "resuscitative breathing": overcompensatory hyperventilation upon awakening from OSA induced hypoxia

Risk Factors

- for OSA: obesity, upper airway abnormality, neuromuscular disease, hypothyroidism, alcohol/sedative use, nasal congestion, sleep deprivation
- for CSA: LV failure, brainstem lesions, encephalitis, encephalopathy, myxedema, high altitude

Signs and Symptoms

- obtain history from spouse/partner
- secondary to repeated arousals and fragmentation of sleep: daytime somnolence, personality and cognitive changes, snoring
- secondary to hypoxemia and hypercapnia: morning headache, polycythemia, pulmonary/systemic HTN, cor pulmonale/CHF, nocturnal angina, arrhythmias
- the typical presentation for OSA is a middle-aged obese male who snores
- CSA can be due to neurological disease

Investigations

- sleep study (polysomnography)
- evaluates sleep stages, airflow, ribcage movement, ECG, SaO_2, limb movements
- indications
  - excessive daytime sleepiness
  - unexplained pulmonary HTN or polycythemia
  - daytime hypercapnia
  - titration of optimal nasal CPAP
  - assessment of objective response to other interventions

Treatment

- modifiable factors: weight loss, decreased alcohol/sedatives, nasal decongestion, treatment of underlying medical conditions
- OSA or MSA: nasal CPAP, postural therapy (e.g. no supine sleeping), dental appliance, uvulopalatopharyngoplasty, tonsillectomy
- CSA or hypoventilation syndromes: nasal BiPAP/CPAP, respiratory stimulants, adaptive servoventilation (e.g. progesterone) in select cases
- tracheostomy rarely required and should be used as last resort for OSA

Complications

- depression, weight gain, decreased quality of life, workplace and vehicular accidents, cardiac complications (e.g. HTN), reduced work/social function

Normal Respiratory Changes during Sleep
- Tidal volume decreases
- Arterial CO_2 increases (due to decreased minute ventilation)
- Pharyngeal dilator muscles relax causing increased upper airway resistance

Apnea: absence of breathing for ≥10 s
Hypopnea: excessive decrease in rate or depth of breathing (>50% reduction in ventilation for >10 sec)
Hyperpnea: excessive increase in rate or depth of breathing

Continuous Positive Airways Pressure for Obstructive Sleep Apnea
Cochrane DB Syst Rev 2006;CD001106
Study: Pooled analysis of 36 RCTs (n=1,718) comparing nocturnal CPAP with an inactive control or oral appliances in adults with OSA.
Conclusions: The use of CPAP showed significant improvements in objective and subjective measures including cognitive function, sleepiness, measures of quality of life, and a lower average systolic and diastolic blood pressure. People who responded equally well to CPAP and oral appliances expressed a strong preference for oral appliances; however, participants on oral appliances were more likely to withdraw from therapy.

CPAP has been shown to reduce cardiovascular risk and cardiovascular related deaths in patients with obstructive sleep apnea

Introduction to Intensive Care

- goal is to provide stabilization for critically ill patients: hemodynamic, respiratory or cardiac instability, or need for close monitoring

Intensive Care Unit Basics

Lines and Catheters
- arterial lines
  - monitor beat-to-beat blood pressure variations, obtain blood for routine ABGs
  - common sites are the radial and femoral arteries
- central venous catheter (central line)
  - administer IV fluids, monitor CVP, insert pulmonary artery catheters
  - administer TPN and agents too irritating for peripheral line
  - common sites: internal jugular vein, subclavian vein, femoral vein
- pulmonary arterial catheter
- balloon guides the catheter from a major vein to the right heart
  - measures pulmonary capillary wedge pressure (PCWP) via a catheter wedged in distal pulmonary artery
  - PCWP reflects the LA and LV diastolic pressure (barring pulmonary venous or mitral valve disease)
  - indications (now used infrequently due to associated complications)
    - diagnosis of shock states, primary pulmonary HTN, valvular disease, intracardiac shunts, cardiac tamponade, PE
    - assessment of hemodynamic response to therapies
    - differentiation of high- versus low-pressure pulmonary edema
    - management of complicated MI, multiorgan system failure and/or severe burns, or hemodynamic instability after cardiac surgery
  - absolute contraindications
    - tricuspid or pulmonary valve mechanical prosthesis
    - right heart mass (thrombus or tumour)
    - tricuspid or pulmonary valve endocarditis

Intensive versus Conventional Glucose Control in Critically Ill Patients
NEJM 2009: 360;1283-1297
Purpose: To assess whether intensive glucose control improves mortality in critically ill patients.
Study: Prospective, randomized controlled trial.
Population: 6104 patients expected to require ICU treatment for 3 or more consecutive days.
Intervention: Patients were randomized to insulin therapy regimens with intensive (blood glucose 4.5-6 mM) or conventional (blood glucose 10 mM or less) glucose control targets. Intravenous insulin therapy was used to maintain blood glucose in target range.
Primary Outcome: Death from any cause within 90 days after randomization.
Results: The odds ratio for death in the intensive control group was 1.14 (95% CI 1.02-1.28; P=0.02) and this effect did not differ between surgical and medical patients. Severe hypoglycemia (blood glucose <2.2 mM) was significantly more common in the intensive management group (6.8% versus 0.5%; P<0.001).
Conclusion: Intensive insulin therapy in ICU patients increased mortality compared to blood glucose targeting of less than 10 mM with a number needed to harm of 38.

Table 33. Useful Equations and Cardiopulmonary Parameters

$BSA = [Ht\ (cm) + Wt\ (kg) - 60]/100$	$PCWP = LVEDP$
$SV = CO / HR$	$SVI = CI / HR$
$CI = CO / BSA$	$RV\ Ejection\ Fraction = SV / RVEDV$
$SVRI = [(MAP - RAP)\ 80]/CI$	$PP = sBP - dBP$
$P{:}F\ ratio = P_aO_2 / F_iO_2$	$MAP = 1/3\ sBP + 2/3\ dBP = dBP + 1/3\ PP$

BSA = body surface area; CI = cardiac index; CO = cardiac output; dBP = diastolic blood pressure; HR = heart rate; LVEDP = left ventricular end diastolic pressure; MAP = mean arterial pressure; PCWP = pulmonary capillary wedge pressure; PP = pulse pressure; RAP = right atrial pressure; RVEDV = right ventricular end diastolic volume; sBP = systolic blood pressure; SV = stroke volume; SVI = stroke volume index; SVRI = systemic vascular resistance index

Organ Failure

Table 34. Types of Organ Failure

Type of Failure	Clinical Presentation	Treatment
Respiratory Failure (see *Respiratory Failure*, R25)	Hypoxemia Hypercapnea	Treat underlying cause (e.g. lung disease, shunt, V/Q mismatch, drug-related, cardiac) Manage mechanical ventilation settings Supplemental oxygen
Cardiac Failure (see <u>Cardiology and Cardiac Surgery</u>, C24)	Hypotension Decreased urine output Altered mental status Arrhythmia Hypoxia	Treat underlying cause (e.g. bradycardia, tachycardia, blood loss, adrenal insufficiency) Volume resuscitation Vasopressors Inotropes Intra-aortic balloon pump
Coagulopathy (see <u>Hematology</u>, H55)	Increased INR or PTT Low platelet count Bleeding, bruising	Treat underlying cause (e.g. thrombocytopenia, drug-related, immune-related, DIC) Transfusion of blood products, clotting factors
Liver Failure (see <u>Gastroenterology</u>, G35)	Elevated transaminases, bilirubin Coagulopathy Jaundice Mental alteration (encephalopathy) Hypoglycemia	Treat underlying cause (e.g. viral hepatitis, drug related, metabolic) Liver transplant Lactulose
Renal Failure (see <u>Nephrology</u>, NP36)	Elevated creatinine Reduced urine output Signs of volume overload (e.g. CHF, effusions)	Treat underlying cause (e.g. shock, drug-related, obstruction) Correct volume and electrolyte status, eliminate toxins Diuretics Dialysis

Shock

- see Emergency Medicine, ER3
- inadequate tissue perfusion potentially resulting in end organ injury
  - categories of shock
    - hypovolemic: hemorrhage, dehydration, vomiting, diarrhea, interstitial fluid redistribution
    - cardiogenic: myopathic (myocardial ischemia ± infarction), mechanical, arrhythmic, pharmacologic
    - obstructive: massive PE (saddle embolus), pericardial tamponade, constrictive pericarditis, increased intrathoracic pressure (e.g. tension pneumothorax)
    - distributive: sepsis, anaphylactic reaction, neurogenic, endocrinologic, toxic

Causes of SHOCK
Spinal (neurogenic), Septic
Hemorrhagic
Obstructive (e.g. tension pneumothorax, cardiac tamponade, PE)
Cardiogenic (e.g. arrhythmia, MI)
AnaphylaKtic

Table 35. Changes Seen in Different Classes of Shock

	Hypovolemic	Cardiogenic	Obstructive	Distributive
HR	↑	↑, N, or ↓	↑	↑ or ↓
BP	↓	↓	↓	↓
JVP	↓	↑	↑	↓
Extremities	Cold	Cold	N or Cold	Warm
Other	Look for visible hemorrhage or signs of dehydration	Bilateral crackles on chest exam	Depending on cause, may see pulsus paradoxus, Kussmaul's sign, or tracheal deviation	Look for obvious signs of infection or anaphylaxis

Shock: Clinical Correlation

Hypovolemic: patients have cool extremities due to peripheral vasoconstriction
Cardiogenic: patients usually have signs of left-sided heart failure
Obstructive: varied presentation
Distributive: patients have warm extremities due to peripheral vasodilation

- treat underlying cause
- treatment goal is to return critical organ perfusion to normal (e.g. normalize BP)
- common treatment modalities include
  - fluid resuscitation
  - inotropes (e.g. dobutamine), vasopressors (e.g. norepinephrine), vasopressin
  - revascularization or thrombolytics for ischemic events

Sepsis

- the leading cause of death in noncoronary ICU settings is multi-organ failure due to sepsis
- the predominant theory is that sepsis is attributable to uncontrollable immune system activation

Systemic Inflammatory Response Syndrome (SIRS): generalized inflammatory reaction caused by infectious and noninfectious entities, manifested by two or more of:
- Body temperature >38°C or <36°C
- Heart rate >90/min
- Respiratory rate >20/min or P_aCO_2 <32 mmHg
- WBC >12,000 cells/mL or <4,000 cells/mL or >10% bands

Definitions
- the Third International Consensus Definition for Sepsis and Septic Shock (Singer et al. JAMA 2016: 315(8), 801-810) significantly revised sepsis definitions
- sepsis: life threatening organ dysfunction caused by dysregulated host response to infection (see Table 36)
- septic shock: a subset of sepsis, where sufficient circulatory and/or cellular/metabolic abnormalities substantially increase mortality. Clinically defined as sepsis with persisting hypotension requiring vasopressors to maintain MAP ≥65 mmHg and having a serum lactate ≥2 mmol/L (18 mg/dL) despite adequate fluid resuscitation

Signs and Symptoms
- new guidelines recommend the use of quick SOFA (qSOFA) criteria and SOFA score to replace SIRS criteria
- in patients with suspected infection, bedside application of qSOFA criteria identifies individuals with high likelihood of poor outcomes, including prolonged ICU stay and/or death
- a positive qSOFA (≥2 criteria) should prompt application of the SOFA score, and further evaluation of possible infection and organ dysfunction
- in the context of suspected infection, a SOFA score ≥2 reflects an overall morality risk of 10%
- the absence of ≥2 criteria on either qSOFA or SOFA score should not delay or defer investigation or treatment of infection or any other aspect of care deemed necessary by the practitioners

Quick SOFA (qSOFA) Criteria
- Respiratory rate ≥22/min
- Altered mentation
- Systolic blood pressure ≤100 mmHg

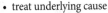

Goal-Directed Resuscitation for Patients with Early Septic Shock
NEJM 2014: 371;1496-1506
Study: Prospective, randomized controlled trial.
Population: 1600 patients in Australia and New Zealand presenting to the emergency department with early septic shock.
Intervention: patients were randomized to receive Early goal-directed therapy (EGDT) or usual care.
Outcome: The primary outcome was all-cause mortality within 90 days of randomization.
Results: The rate of death did not significantly differ between patients treated with EGDT or usual care (absolute risk difference EGDT versus usual care = -0.3%, 95% CI -4.1 to 3.6%; P=0.90). EGDT treated patients received more intravenous fluids, vasopressor infusions, red blood cell transfusions, and dobutamine (P<0.0001 for all). Survival time, in-hospital mortality, duration of organ support, and length of hospital stay did not significantly differ between patients randomized to EGDT or usual care.
Conclusions: EGDT did not improve all-cause mortality at 90 days in patients presenting to the emergency department with early septic shock.

Table 36. Sequential (Sepsis-Related) Organ Failure Assessment (SOFA) Score

System	Score				
	0	1	2	3	4
Respiratory					
P_aO_2/F_iO_2, mmHg (kPa)	≥400 (53.3)	<400 (53.3)	<300 (40)	<200 (26.7) with respiratory support	<100 (13.3) with respiratory support
Coagulation					
Platelets, x10³/μL	≥150	<150	<100	<50	<20
Liver					
Bilirubin, μmol/L (mg/dL)	<20 (1.2)	20-32 (1.2-1.9)	33-101 (2.0-5.9)	102-204 (6.0-11.9)	>204 (12.0)
Cardiovascular	MAP ≥70 mmHg	MAP <70 mmHg	Dopamine <5[a] or dobutamine (any dose)a	Dopamine 5.1-15[a] or epinephrine <0.1[a] or norepinephrine <0.1[a]	Dopamine >15a or epinephrine >0.1a or norepinephrine >0.1a
Central Nervous System					
Glasgow coma scale score	15	13-14	10-12	6-9	<6
Renal					
Creatinine, μmol/L (mg/dL)	<110 (1.2)	110-170 (1.2-1.9)	171-299 (2.0-3.4)	300-440 (3.5-4.9)	>440 (5.0)
Urine output, mL/d				<500	<200

[a]Catecholamine doses are given as μg/kg/min for at least 1hr
Table adapted from Singer et al. The Third International Consensus Definitions for Sepsis and Septic Shock (Sepsis-3). JAMA 2016; 315(8): 801-810

Glucocorticosteroids for sepsis: systematic review with meta-analysis and trial sequential analysis
Intsens Care Med 2015; 41(7): 1220–1234.
Study: Systematic review and trial sequential analysis of 35 randomized clinical trials.
Population: 4682 adult patients with SIRS, sepsis, severe sepsis or septic shock.
Results: 33 of 35 trials analyzed had a high risk of bias. There was no statistically significant effect on mortality of glucocorticosteroids given at any dose when compared to placebo (RR 0.89; TSA adjusted CI 0.74-1.08). No effect was identified in subgroup analysis based on high (>500 mg) or low (<500 mg) dosing or stratification by degree of sepsis. Serious adverse events besides mortality were not altered by glucocorticosteroid treatment (RR 1.02; TSA-adjusted CI 0.7-1.48).
Conclusions: There is no definitive evidence for or against the use of glucocorticosteroids in septic patients. Larger and better designed randomized controlled trials ongoing and in future are required.

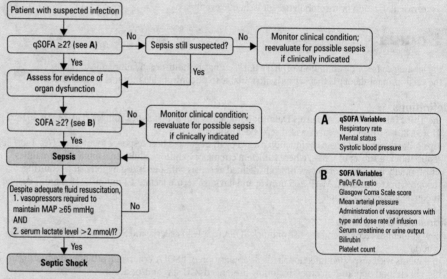

The baseline Sequential (sepsis-related) Organ Failure Assessment (SOFA) score should be assumed to be zero unless the patient is known to have pre-existing (acute or chronic) organ dysfunction before the onset of infection. qSOFA indicated quick SOFA; MAP, mean arterial pressure.

Figure 12. Approach to sepsis
Figure adapted from Singer et al. The Third International Consensus Definitions for Sepsis and Septic Shock (Sepsis-3). *JAMA* 2016; 315(8): 801-810.

Treatment
- identify the cause and source of infection: blood, sputum, urine Gram stain, and C&S
- initiate empiric antibiotic therapy
- monitor, restore, and maintain hemodynamic function

Surviving Sepsis (adapted from International Guidelines for Management of Severe Sepsis and Septic Shock 2012)
- adjustments of cardiac preload, afterload, and contractility to balance oxygen delivery with demand
- initial resuscitation (goals during first 6 hrs of resuscitation for sepsis induced hypotension persisting after initial fluid challenge or blood lactate ≥ 4 mmol/L)
- maintain CVP 8-12 mmHg with IV crystalloids/colloids
  - maintain MAP ≥ 65 mmHg with use of vasopressor agents, first line: norepinephrine
  - urine output ≥ 0.5 mL/kg/hr
  - central venous (SVC) or mixed oxygen saturation 70% or 65% respectively

- in patients with elevated lactate levels target resuscitation to normalize lactate
  - corticosteroid replacement therapy not indicated if adequate hemodynamic stability achieved with fluid resuscitation and vasopressor therapy
- infection control
  - prompt diagnosis of infection
    - cultures as clinically indicated prior to antibiotic therapy if no significant delay
    - imaging studies performed promptly to confirm possible infectious source
  - antibiotic therapy
- administer effective IV antimicrobials within first hour of recognition of sepsis
    - choice of anti-infective therapy should consider activity against all likely pathogens and penetrance of adequate concentration into tissue presumed to be source of infection
    - antimicrobial regimen should be reassessed daily for potential descalation
- surgical source control when appropriate
- supportive oxygenation and ventilation using lung-protective regimen
- early nutritional support: enteral route is used to preserve function of intestinal mucosal barrier
- DVT/PE prophylaxis
- advanced care planning, including the communication of likely outcome and realistic goals of treatment with patients and families

Common Medications

Table 37. Common Medications for Respiratory Diseases

	Drug	Typical Adult Dose	Indications	Side Effects
β2-AGONISTS				
Short-Acting	salbutamol/albuterol (Ventolin®, Airomir®) (light blue/navy MDI or diskus), terbutaline (Bricanyl®) (blue turbuhaler)	1-2 puffs q4-6h prn	Bronchodilator in acute reversible airway obstruction	CV (angina, flushing, palpitations, tachycardia, can precipitate atrial fibrillation), CNS (dizziness, H/A, insomnia, anxiety), GI (diarrhea, N/V), rash, hypokalemia, paroxysmal bronchospasm
Long-Acting	salmeterol (Serevent®) (green diskus), formoterol (Oxeze®, Foradil®) (blue/green turbuhalor or aerolizer) indacaterol (Onbrez®) (blue/white breezhaler)	1-2 puffs bid 1 puff daily	Maintenance treatment (prevention of bronchospasm) in COPD, asthma	
Combination Long-Acting β2- Agonist and Inhaled Corticosteroid	fluticasone and salmeterol (Advair®) (purple MDI or diskus) budesonide and formoterol (Symbicort®) (red turbuhaler) Mometasone and formoterol (Zenhale®) (blue MDI)	1 puff bid 2 puffs bid	COPD and asthma	Common: CNS, H/A, dizziness Resp: URTI, GI (N/V, diarrhea, pain/discomfort, oral candidiasis)
Combination Short-Acting β2- Agonist and Short-Acting Anti-Cholinergic	ipratropium/salbutamol (Combivent®, Respimat®) (orange respimat)	1 puff qid	Bronchodilator used in COPD, bronchitis and emphysema	Palpitations, anxiety, dizziness, fatigue, H/A, N/V, dry mucous membranes, urinary retention, increased toxicity in combination with other anticholinergic drugs
Combination Long-Acting β2- Agonist and Long-Acting Anti-Cholinergic	umeclidinium/vilanterol (Anoro®) (red ellipta) aclidinium/formoterol (Duaklir®) (yellow genuair) tiotropium/olodaterol (Inspiolto®) (green respimat) indacaterol/glycopyrronium (Ultibro®) (yellow breezhaler)	1 puff daily 1 puff bid 1 puff daily 1 puff daily	Bronchodilator used in COPD, bronchitis and emphysema	Palpitations, anxiety, dizziness, fatigue, H/A, N/V, dry mucous membranes, urinary retention, increased toxicity in combination with other anticholinergic drugs
ANTICHOLINERGICS				
Short-Acting Anti-Cholinergic	ipratropium bromide (Atrovent®) (clear/green MDI)	2-3 puffs qid	Bronchodilator used in COPD, bronchitis and emphysema	Palpitations, anxiety, dizziness, fatigue, H/A, N/V, dry mucous membranes, urinary retention, increased toxicity in combination with other anticholinergic drugs
Long-Acting Anti-Cholinergic	tiotropium bromide (Spiriva®) (green handihaler or respimat) glycopyrronium bromide (Seebri®) (orange breezhaler), umeclidinium (Incruse™) (green ellipta), aclidinium (Genuair®, Tudorza®) (green inhaler)	1 puff qam 1 puff daily	Bronchodilator used in COPD, bronchitis and emphysema	Palpitations, anxiety, dizziness, fatigue, H/A, N/V, dry mucous membranes, urinary retention, increased toxicity in combination with other anticholinergic drug

Table 37. Common Medications for Respiratory Diseases (continued)

	Drug	Typical Adult Dose	Indications	Side Effects
CORTICOSTEROIDS				
Inhaled	fluticasone (Flovent®) (orange/peach MDI or diskus)	2-4 puffs bid	Maintenance treatment of asthma	H/A, fever, N/V, MSK pain, URTI, throat irritation, growth velocity reduction in children/adolescents, HPA axis suppression, increased pneumonia risk in COPD
	budesonide (Pulmicort®) (brown turbuhaler)	2 puffs bid		
	ciclesonide (Alvesco®) (red MDI)	1 puff daily or bid		
	beclomethasone (QVAR®, Vanceril®) (brown MDI),	1-4 puffs bid		
	mometasone (Asmanex®) (pink/grey/brown twisthaler)	1 puff daily or bid		
	fluticasone furoate (Arnuity(®) (orange ellipta)	1 puff daily		
Systemic	prednisone (Apo-prednisone®, Deltasone®)	Typically 40-60 mg per day PO	Acute exacerbation of COPD; severe, persistent asthma, PCP Status asthmaticus	Endocrine (hirsutism, DM/glucose intolerance, Cushing's syndrome, HPA axis suppression), GI (increased appetite, indigestion), ocular (cataracts, glaucoma), edema, AVN, osteoporosis, H/A, psychiatric (anxiety, insomnia), easy bruising
	methylprednisolone (Depo-Medrol®, Solu-Medrol®)	125 mg q8h IV (sodium succinate) loading dose 2 mg/kg then 0.5-1 mg/kg q6h for 5 d		
ADJUNCT AGENTS				
	theophylline (Uniphyll®)	400-600 mg OD	Treatment of symptoms of reversible airway obstruction due to COPD	GI upset, diarrhea, N/V, anxiety, H/A, insomnia, muscle cramp, tremor, tachycardia, PVCs, arrhythmias Toxicity: persistent, repetitive vomiting, seizures
LEUKOTRIENE ANTAGONISTS				
	montelukast (Singular®) zafirlukast (Accolate®)	10 mg PO qhs, now only available as once daily slow release 20 mg bid	Prophylaxis and chronic treatment of asthma	H/A, dizziness, fatigue, fever, rash, dyspepsia, cough, flu-like symptoms
ANTI-IgE MONOCLONAL ANTIBODIES				
	omalizumab (Xolair®)	150-375 mg SC q2-4wk	Moderate-severe persistant asthma	H/A, sinusitis, pharyngitis, URTI, viral infection, thrombocytopenia, anaphylaxis
PDE-4 INHIBITORS				
	roflumilast (Daxas®)	500 μg PO OD	Severe emphysema, with frequent exacerbations	Weight loss, suicidal ideation
ANTIBIOTICS – COMMUNITY ACQUIRED PNEUMONIA				
Macrolide	erythromycin azithromycin	250-500 mg PO tid x 7-10 d 500 mg PO x 1 dose, then 250 mg OD x 4	Alternate to doxycycline or fluoroquinolone	GI (abdominal pain, diarrhea, N/V), H/A, prolonged QT, ventricular arrhythmias, hepatic impairment GI (diarrhea, N/V, abdominal pain), renal failure, deafness
	clarithromycin	1,000 mg od or 500 mg PO bid x 7-10 d		H/A, rash, GI (diarrhea, N/V, abnormal taste, heartburn, abdominal pain), increased urea
Doxycycline		100 mg PO bid x 7-10 d	Alternate to macrolide or fluoroquinolone	Photosensitivity, rash, urticaria, anaphylaxis, diarrhea, entercolitis, tooth discolouration in children
Fluoroquinolone	levofloxacin (Levaquin®) moxifloxacin (Avelox®)	500 mg PO OD x 7-10 d 400 mg PO OD x 7 d	Alternate to macrolide or doxycycline	CNS (dizziness, fever, H/A), GI (N/V, diarrhea, constipation), prolonged QT

Table 37. Common Medications for Respiratory Diseases (continued)

	Drug	Typical Adult Dose	Indications	Side Effects
ANTIBIOTICS – HOSPITAL ACQUIRED PNEUMONIA				
3rd gen Cephalosporin	ceftriaxone (Rocephin®)	1-2 g IV OD x 7-10 d	Combine with fluoroquinolone or macrolide	Rash, diarrhea, eosinophilia, thrombocytosis, leukopenia, elevated transaminases
Fluoroquinolone	levofloxacin moxifloxacin	750 mg PO OD x 5 d 400 mg PO OD x 7 d (5 d for AECOPD)	Combine with 3rd gen cephalosporin	See above
Piperacillin/Tazobactam (Tazocin®)		4.5 g IV q6-8h x 7-10 d	Suspect *Pseudomonas*	CNS (confusion, convulsions, drowsiness), rash Hematologic (abnormal platelet aggregation, prolonged PT, positive Coombs)
Vancomycin (Vancocin®)		1 g IV bid x 7-10 d	Suspect MRSA	CNS (chills, drug fever), hematologic (eosinophilia), rash, red man syndrome, interstitial nephritis, renal failure, ototoxicity
Macrolide	azithromycin clarithromycin	500 mg IV OD x 2 d, then 500 mg PO OD x 5 d 1,000 mg od or 500 mg PO bid x 7-10 d	Suspect *Legionella*	See above
ICU MEDICATIONS				
Pressors/Inotropes	norepinephrine (Levophed®) phenylephrine dobutamine	0.5-30 μg/min IV 0.5 μg/kg/min IV 2-20 μg/kg/min IV	Acute hypotension Severe hypotension Inotropic support	Angina, bradycardia, dyspnea, hyper/hypotension, arrhythmias See above See above
Sedatives/Analgesia	fentanyl (opioid class) propofol (anesthetic)	50-100 μg then 50-unlimited μg/h IV 1-3 mg/kg then 0.3-5 mg/kg/h IV	Sedation and/or analgesia Sedation and/or analgesia	Bradycardia, respiratory depression, drowsiness, hypotension Apnea, bradycardia, hypotension (good for ventilator sedation)

See Infectious Diseases, ID26 – for the management of pulmonary tuberculosis

Landmark Respirology Trials

Trial	Reference	Results
ARDS Network	*NEJM* 2000; 342:1301-8	Mortality decreased in ARDS patients ventilated with a low tidal volume strategy
Berlin Criteria	*JAMA* 2012; 307:2526-33	The new definition of ARDS, better predicts mortality
CPAP and Apnea	*NEJM* 2005; 353:2025-33	CPAP ameliorates symptoms of sleep apnea but does not affect mortality in CHF
EINSTEIN-PE	*NEJM* 2012; 366:1287-97	Fixed dose of rivoxabarin was non-inferior to standard therapy (Vit K antagonist) initial and long-term treatment of PE
Emphysema Treatment Trial	*NEJM* 2003; 348:2059-73	Lung volume reduction surgery benefits patients with upper lobe disease and low exercise capacity
IELCAP	*NEJM* 2006; 355:1763-71	High survival rate in patients with early stage lung cancer detected by low dose CT screening
Lung Health	*JAMA* 1994; 272:1497-505	Aggressive smoking intervention significantly decreases the age-related decline in FEV_1 in middle-aged smokers with mild airways obstruction
OSCILLATE	*NEJM* 2013; 368: 795-805	Early high-frequency oscillatory ventilation in patients with moderate to severe ARDS might increase in-hospital mortality
ILD	*NEJM* 1978; 298:801-9	Interstitial lung disease subsets have different prognoses and response to treatment (e.g. desquamative but not usual interstitial pneumonia respond well to corticosteroids)
POET-COPD	*NEJM* 2011; 364:1093-103	Tiotropium decreases the number of moderate-to-severe exacerbations in comparison to salmeterol
REDUCE	*JAMA* 2013; 309: 2223-2231	5 d course of glucocorticoids is non-inferior to a 14 d course for treatment of acute COPD exacerbations
ROFLUMILAST	*Lancet* 2009; 374:695-703	Phosphodiesterase-4 inhibitor improves FEV_1 when used as add-on therapy in COPD patients on tiotropium or salmeterol
TORCH	*NEJM* 2007; 356:775-89	Combination of inhaled steroids and long-acting β2-agonists improves COPD symptoms, reduces exacerbations, and shows a trend to lowers mortality
UPLIFT	*NEJM* 2008; 359:1543-54	Tiotropium improves symptoms of COPD with fewer exacerbations, but does not affect FEV_1 decline

References

Aaron SD, Vandemheen KL, Hebert P, et al. Outpatient oral prednisone after emergency treatment of chronic obstructive pulmonary disease. NEJM 2003;348:2618-2625.
Andreoli TE. Cecil essentials of medicine, 8th ed. Philadelphia: WB Saunders, 2010.
Annane D, Bellissant E, Bollaert PE, et al. Corticosteroids for treating severe sepsis and septic shock. Cochrane DB Syst Rev 2004;1:CD002243.
ARDS Definition Task Force. Acute respiratory distress syndrome: the Berlin definition. JAMA 2012;307:2526-2533.
Augustinos P, Ouriel K. Invasive approaches to treatment of venous thromboembolism. Circulation 2004;110(Suppl1):127-134.
Bach PB, Brown C, Gelfand SE, et al. Management of acute exacerbations of chronic obstructive pulmonary disease: a summary and appraisal of published evidence. Ann Int Med 2001;134:600-620.
Bach PB, Silvestri GA, Hanger M, et al. Screening for lung cancer: ACCP evidence-based clinical practice guidelines, 2nd ed. Chest 2007;132:695-775.
Badesch DB, Abman SH, Ahearn GS, et al. Medical therapy for pulmonary arterial hypertension. ACCP evidence-based clinical practice guidelines. Chest 2004;126(Suppl1):35S-62S.
Balk RA. Optimum treatment of severe sepsis and septic shock: evidence in support of the recommendations. Dis Mon 2004;50:168-213.
Bartlett JG, Dowell SF, Mandell LA, et al. Practice guidelines for the management of community-acquired pneumonia in adults. Clin Infect Dis 2000;31:347-382.
Bass JB Jr, Farer LS, Hopewell PC, et al. Treatment of tuberculosis and tuberculosis infection in adults and children. American Thoracic Society and The Centers for Disease Control and Prevention. Am J Respir Crit Care Med 1994;149:1359-1374.
Baumann MH. Treatment of spontaneous pneumothorax. Curr Opin Pulm Med 2000;6:275-280.
Boulet LP, Becker A, Berube D, et al. Canadian asthma consensus report. CMAJ 1999;161(Suppl11):S1-61.
Buller HR, Agnelli G, Hull RD, et al. Antithrombotic therapy for venous thromboembolic disease. Chest 2004;126:401S-428S.
Chunilal SD, Eikelboom JW, Attia J, et al. Does this patient have pulmonary embolism? JAMA 2003;290:2849-2858.
Crapo JD, Glassroth JL, Karlinsky JB, et al. Baum's textbook of pulmonary diseases, 7th ed. USA: Lippincott Williams & Wilkins, 2003.
Canadian Task Force on Preventative Health Care. Recommendations on screening for lung cancer. CMAJ 2016;188:425-432.
Dellinger RP, Carlet JM, Masur H, et al. Surviving sepsis campaign guidelines for management of severe sepsis and septic shock. Crit Care Med 2004;32:858-873.
Esteban A, Frutos F, Tobin M, et al. A comparison of four methods of weaning patients from mechanical ventilation. NEJM 1995;332:345-350.
Ferguson GT, Cherniack RM. Management of chronic obstructive pulmonary disease. NEJM 1993;328:1017-1022.
Ferri F. Ferri's clinical advisor. Mosby/Elsevier Health Sciences, 2002.
Ferri F. Practical guide to the care of the medical patient, 5th ed. St.Louis: Mosby/Elsevier Sciences, 2001.
File TM. The epidemiology of respiratory tract infections. Semin Respir Infect 2000;15:184-194.
Fine MJ, Auble TE, Yealy DM, et al. A prediction rule to identify low-risk patients with community-acquired pneumonia. NEJM 1997;336:243-250.
Gaine S. Pulmonary hypertension. JAMA 2000;284:3160-3168.
Garcia D, Ageno W, Libby E. Update on the diagnosis and management of pulmonary embolism. Brit J Haematol 2005;131:301-312.
Geerts WH, Pineo GF, Heit JA, et al. Prevention of venous thromboembolism. Chest 2004;126(Suppl3):338S-400S.
Giles TL, Lasserson TJ, Smith BJ, et al. Continuous positive airways pressure for obstructive sleep apnea in adults. Cochrane DB Syst Rev 2006;5:CD001106.
Górecka D, Gorzelak K, Sliwinski P, et al. Effect of long term oxygen therapy on survival in patients with chronic obstructive pulmonary disease with moderate hypoxaemia. Thorax 1997;52:674-679.
Gotfried M, Freeman C. An update on community-acquired pneumonia in adults. Compr Ther 2000;26:283-293.
Green DS, San Pedro GS. Empiric therapy of community-acquired pneumonia. Semin Respir Infect 2000;15:227-233.
Hershfield E. Tuberculosis: treatment. CMAJ 1999;161:405-411.
Holleman D, Simel D. Does the clinical examination predict airflow limitation? JAMA 1995;273:313-319.
Hotchkiss RS, Karl IE. The pathophysiology and treatment of sepsis. NEJM 2003;348:138-150.
Kasper DL, Braunwald E, Fauci AS, et al (editors). Harrison's principles of internal medicine, 16th ed. USA: McGraw-Hill Professional, 2004.
Kline JA, Courtney DM, Kabrhel C, et al. Prospective multicenter evaluation of the pulmonary embolism rule-out criteria. J Thromb Haemost 2008;6:772-780.
Light RW, Macgregor MI, Luchsinger PC, et al. Pleural effusions: the diagnostic separation of transudates and exudates. Ann Intern Med 1972;77:507-513.
Light RW. The management of parapneumonic effusions and empyema. Curr Opin Pulm Med 1998;4:227-229.
Light RW. Useful tests on the pleural fluid in the management of patients with pleural effusions. Curr Opin Pulm Med 1999;5:245-249.
Long R, Njoo H, Hershfield E. Tuberculosis: epidemiology of the disease in Canada. CMAJ 1999;160:1185-1190
Lougheed MD, Lemière C, Ducharme FM, et al. Canadian Thoracic Society 2012 guideline update: diagnosis and management of asthma in preschoolers, children and adults. Can Respir J 2012;19:127-164.
MacMahon H et al. Guidelines for management of small pulmonary nodules detected on CT scans: a statement from the Fleischner Society. Radiology. 2005 Nov;237(2):395-400.
Mansharamani NG, Koziel H. Chronic lung sepsis: lung abscess, bronchiectasis, and empyema. Cur Opin Pulmon Med 2003;9:181-185.
McLoud TC, Swenson SJ. Lung carcinoma. Clin Chest Med 1999;20:697-713.
McPhee SJ, Papadakis MA, Tierney LM. Current medical diagnosis and treatment 2007, 47th ed. USA: McGraw-Hill Professional, 2006.
National Lung Screening Trial Research Team. Reduced lung-cancer mortality with low-dose computed tomographic screening. NEJM 2011;365:395-409.
Nguyen HB, Rivers EP, Abrahamian FM, et al. Severe sepsis and septic shock: review of the literature and emergency department management guidelines. Ann Emerg Med 2006;48:28-54.
O'Donnell DE, Hernandez P, Kaplan A, et al. Canadian thoracic society recommendations for management of chronic obstructive pulmonary disease – 2008 update – highlights for primary care. Can Respir J 2008;15(Suppl A):1A-8A.
Ost D, Fein A. Evaluation and management of the solitary pulmonary nodule. Am J Respir Crit Care Med 2000;162:782-787.
Ost D, Fein AM, Feinsilver SH. The solitary pulmonary nodule. NEJM 2003;348:2535-4252.
Paramothayan NS, Lasserson TJ, Jones P. Corticosteroids for pulmonary sarcoidosis. Cochrane DB Syst Rev 2005;2:CD001114.
Parfrey H, Chilvers ER. Pleural disease – diagnosis and management. Practitioner 1999;243:412,415-421.
Patel VK. A practical algorithmic approach to the diagnosis and management of solitary pulmonary nodules: part 1: radiologic characteristics and imaging modalities. Chest. 2013 Mar;143(3):825-39.
Pauwels RA, Buist AS, Calverly PM. Global strategy for the diagnosis, management, and prevention of chronic obstructive pulmonary disease. NHLBI/WHO Global Initiative for Chronic Obstructive Lung Disease (GOLD) Workshop Summary. Am J Resp and Crit Care Med 2001;163:1256-1276.
Ram FSF, Picot J, Lightowler J, et al. Non-invasive positive pressure ventilation for treatment of respiratory failure due to exacerbations of chronic obstructive pulmonary disease. Cochrane DB Syst Rev 2004;3:CD004104.
Reimer LG. Community-acquired bacterial pneumonias. Semin Respir Infect 2000;15:95-100.
Rivers E, Nguyen B, Havstad S, et al. Early goal-directed therapy in the treatment of severe sepsis and septic shock. NEJM 2001;345:1368-1413.
Sabatine MS. Pocket medicine: the Massachusetts general hospital handbook of internal medicine. Philadelphia: Lippincott Williams and Wilkins, 2004. 6-1 and 5-2.
Scharschmidt, Bruce F. Pocket medicine: internal medicine pulmonary medicine. 2002. PocketMedicine.com.
Schidlow DV, Taussig LM, Knowles MR. Cystic fibrosis foundation consensus conference report on pulmonary complications of cystic fibrosis. Peds Pulmonol 1993;15:187-196.
Schulman S, Kearon C, Kakkar AK, et.al. Extended use of dabigatran, warfarin, or placebo in venous thromboembolism. NEJM 2013;368:709-718.
Simonneau G, Robbins IM, Beghetti M, et al. Updated clinical classification of pulmonary hypertension. J Am Coll Cardiol 2009;54(Suppl1):S43-54.
Singer M, Deutschman CS, Seymour CW, et al. The Third International Consensus Definitions for Sepsis and Septic Shock (Sepsis-3). JAMA;315:801-810.
Stein PD, Saltzman HA, Weg JG. Clinical characteristics of patients with acute pulmonary embolism. Am J Cardiol 1991;68:1723-1724.
Stein PD, Fowler SE, Goodman LR, et al. Multidetector computed tomography for acute pulmonary embolism. NEJM 2006;354:2317-2327.
The ARISE Investigators and ANZICS Clinical Trials Group. Goal-Directed Resuscitation for Patients with Early Septic Shock. New England Journal of Medicine 2014; 371: 1496-1506.
The NICE-SUGAR Study Investigators. Intensive versus Conventional Glucose Control in Critically Ill Patients. New England Journal of Medicine 2009; 360:1283-1297.
Thrombosis Interest Group of Canada. Clinical guides. 27 brief, evidence-based guides on thrombosis for general practitioners. Available from: www.tigc.org.
van den Berghe G, Wouters P, Weekers F, et al. Intensive insulin therapy in critically ill patients. NEJM 2001;345:1359-1367.
Volbeda M, Wetterslev J, Gluud C, et al. Glucocorticosteroids for sepsis: systematic review with meta-analysis and trial sequential analysis. Intensive Care Medicine 2015; 41: 1220-1234.
Walters JAE, Gibson PG, Wood-Baker R, et al. Systemic corticosteroids for acute exacerbations of chronic obstructive pulmonary disease. Cochrane DB Syst Rev 2009;1:CD001288
Watts K, Chavesse RJ. Leukotriene receptor antagonists in addition to usual care for acute asthma in adults and children. Cochrane DB Syst Rev 2012;5:CD006100.
West J. Respiratory Physiology: The Essentials. 9th Ed. 2012. Lippincott Williams & Wilkins, Philadelphia, PA.
Wongsurakiat P, Maranetra KN, Wasi C, et al. Acute respiratory illness in patints with COPD and the effectiveness of influenza vaccination: a randomized controlled study. Chest 2004;125:2011-2020.

Rheumatology

Ayan Dey, Mathew Nicholas, and Trang Vu, chapter editors
Claudia Frankfurter and Inna Gong, associate editors
Brittany Prevost and Robert Vanner, EBM editors
Dr. Arthur Bookman, Dr. Simon Carette, and Dr. Natasha Gakhal, staff editors

Acronyms

Ab	antibody	DIP	distal interphalangeal joint	ILD	interstitial lung disease	RBC	red blood cell
ACPA	anti-citrullinated protein antibodies	DM	diabetes mellitus	ITP	idiopathic thrombocytopenic	ReA	reactive arthritis
Ag	antigen	DMARD	disease-modifying		purpura	RF	rheumatoid factor
ANA	antinuclear antibody		anti-rheumatic drug	MCP	metacarpal phalangeal joint	ROM	range of motion
ANCA	antineutrophil cytoplasmic antibody	DMM	dermatomyositis	MCTD	mixed connective tissue disease	SI	sacroiliac
Anti-RNP	antiribonuclear protein	dsDNA	double stranded DNA	MHC	major histocompatibility complex	SLE	systemic lupus erythematosus
Anti-Sm	anti-Smith antibodies	EA	enteropathic arthritis	MPO	myeloperoxidase	SNRI	serotonin-norepinephrine
APLA	antiphospholipid antibody syndrome	ECASA	enteric-coated acetylsalicylic	MTP	metatarsal phalangeal joint		reuptake inhibitors
AS	ankylosing spondylitis		acid	MTX	methotrexate	SS	Sjögren's syndrome
AVN	avascular necrosis	ESR	erythrocyte sedimentation rate	OA	osteoarthritis	SSA	Sjögren's syndrome antigen A
BUN	blood urea nitrogen	GC	Neisseria gonorrhoeae gonococcus	PAN	polyarteritis nodosa	SSB	Sjögren's syndrome antigen B
CBC	complete blood count	GCA	giant cell arteritis	PIP	proximal interphalangeal joint	TNF	tumour necrosis factor
CCB	calcium channel blocker	GPA	granulomatosis with polyangiitis	PM	polymyositis	U/A	urinalysis
CCP	cyclic citrullinated peptide	H/A	headache	PMN	polymorphonuclear leukocyte	ULN	upper limit of normal
CMC	carpometacarpal joint	Hb	hemoglobin	PMR	polymyalgia rheumatica	U-SpA	undifferentiated
CNS	central nervous system	HLA	human leukocyte antigen	PsA	psoriatic arthritis		spondyloarthropathy
CTD	connective tissue disease	IA	intra-articular	PTT	partial thromboplastin time	VDRL	venereal disease research
CPPD	calcium pyrophosphate dihydrate	IBD	inflammatory bowel disease	PUD	peptic ulcer disease		laboratory
CRP	C-reactive protein	IE	infective endocarditis	RA	rheumatoid arthritis	WBC	white blood cell
DEXA	dual energy X-ray absorptiometry						

Terminology in Rheumatology

Arthritis
- Joint swelling: effusion/synovial thickening
- Decreased ROM
- Stress pain (pain at the end of ROM)
- Increased warmth

Arthralgia: perception of joint pain without obvious clinical findings

Active Joint: swollen joint, joint line tenderness, or stress pain

Innate Immune Cells
- **Neutrophil (PMN)**: circulate in blood and respond to inflammatory stimuli, kill invading organisms by phagocytosis, degranulation and neutrophil extracellular traps
- **Natural Killer Cell**: innate immunity against intracellular infections (especially viruses), killing function and produce cytokines
- **Macrophage**: arrive after PMNs, suppress PMN efflux and phagocytose PMN debris, secrete pro-inflammatory cytokines in response to microbial debris
- **Dendritic Cell**: actively phagocytic when immature, activated by signals from toll-like receptor (TLR), release pro-inflammatory cytokines, present antigens to T cells in lymph nodes
- **Eosinophil**: respond to inflammatory cytokines and degranulate releasing reactive oxygen species, and cytokines, associated with allergy, asthma and parasitic infection
- **Mast Cell**: present in connective tissue and mucosa, allergen cross-linking of IgE bound to mast cell triggers degranulation and release of inflammatory mediators

Key Cytokine Targets of Biologic Drugs
TNF
- **Source**: T cells, macrophages
- **Major Functions**: cachexia, induces other cytokines, T cell stimulation, induces metalloproteinases and prostaglandins, increases expression of adhesion molecules, increases vascular permeability leading to increased entry of IgG, complement and cells into tissues
IL-6
- **Source**: Many cells
- **Major Functions**: proliferation of B and T cells, acute phase reactant, induces natural protease inhibitor

Anatomy of Joint Pathology

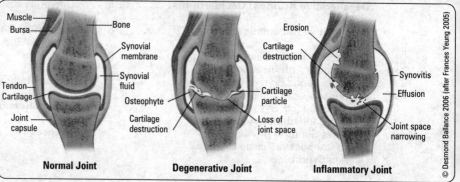

Figure 1. Structure of normal, degenerative, and inflammatory joint

© Desmond Ballance 2006 (after Frances Yeung 2005)

Basics of Immunology

Immune Mechanisms of Disease

Table 1. Mechanisms of Immunologically Mediated Disorders

Type	Pathophysiology	Examples
Immediate Hypersensitivity (Type I)	Formation of IgE → release of immunologic mediators from basophils/mast cells → diffuse inflammation	Asthma, Allergic rhinitis, Anaphylaxis
Cytotoxic (Type II)	Formation of Ab → deposit and bind to Ag on cell surface → phagocytosis or lysis of target cell	Autoimmune hemolytic anemia, Anti glomerular membrane disease (Goodpasture's syndrome), Graves' disease, pemphigus vulgaris, rheumatic fever, ITP
Immune Complex (Type III)	Formation and deposition of Ag-Ab complexes → activate complement → leukocyte recruitment and activation → tissue injury	SLE, PAN, post-streptococcal glomerulonephritis, serum sickness, viral hepatitis
Cell-Mediated/Delayed Hypersensitivity (Type IV)	Release of cytokines by sensitized T-cells and T-cell mediated cytotoxicity	Contact dermatitis, insect venom, mycobacterial proteins

Immunogenetics and Disease

- cell surface molecules called HLAs play a role in mediating immune reactions
- MHC are genes on the short arm of chromosome 6 that encode HLA molecules
- certain HLA haplotypes are associated with increased susceptibility to autoimmune diseases

Table 2. Classes of MHCs

MHC Class	Types	Location	Function
I	HLA-A, B, C	All cells	Recognized by CD8+ (cytotoxic) T-lymphocytes
II	HLA-DP, DQ, DR	Ag presenting cells (mononuclear phagocytes, B cells, etc.)	Recognized by CD4+ (helper) T-lymphocytes
III	Some components of the complement cascade	In plasma	Chemotaxis, opsonization, lysis of bacteria and cells

Table 3. HLA-Associated Rheumatic Disease

HLA Type	Associated Conditions	Comments
B27	Ankylosing Spondylitis (AS) Reactive Arthritis (ReA) Enteropathic arthritis (EA)	Relative risk 20x for developing AS and ReA
DR4, DR1	Rheumatoid Arthritis (RA)	In RA, relative risk = 2-10x; found in 93% of patients
DR3	Sjögren's syndrome (SS) Systemic Lupus Erythematosus (SLE)	DR3 is associated with the production of anti-Ro/SSA and anti-La/SSB antibodies

Adaptive Immune Cells
- **B Cell:** produce antibodies after activation by specific antigen and B-cell co-receptor, additional signals provided by CD4 T helper cells
- **Cytotoxic T Cell:** CD8, direct cytotoxicity of target cells at sites of infection, kill via lytic granules and FasL-Fas interaction, recognize specific antigen and MHC1
- **Helper T Cell:** subset of CD4 cells, activate and help other types of cells carry out immune defense (activate macrophages, help B cells, release cytokines)
- **Regulatory T Cell:** Subset of CD4 cells, suppress activation of naïve autoreactive T cells

Differential Diagnoses of Common Presentations

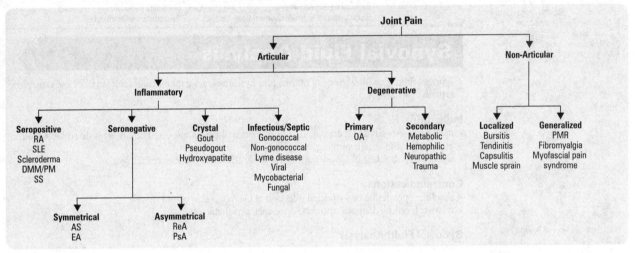

Figure 2. Clinical approach to joint pain

Table 4. Differential Diagnosis of Monoarthritis

ACUTE MONOARTHRITIS

Non-Inflammatory	Inflammatory		Infectious	Hemorrhagic
Trauma	**Crystal induced** Monosodium urate (MSU-gout) Calcium pyrophosphate dehydrate (CPPD) or pseudogout Hydroxyapatite (HA)	**Non-crystal induced** Seropositive Seronegative	*S. aureus*, GC	Trauma, fracture, blood dyscrasias and anticoagulants Congenital clotting disorders e.g. hemophilia

CHRONIC MONOARTHRITIS

Non-Inflammatory	Inflammatory	Infectious	Hemorrhagic
OA and osteonecrosis	serpositive and seronegative	TB and fungi	Tumour

Table 5. Differential Diagnosis of Oligoarthritis/Polyarthritis

ACUTE (<6 wk)	CHRONIC (>6 wk)		
Post-viral infection (parvovirus B19, HIV) Post bacterial Infection (GC and non-GC, rheumatic fever) Crystal induced Other (sarcoidosis, lyme disease)	**Seropositive inflammatory arthritis** RA SLE Scleroderma DMM/PM	**Seronegative inflammatory arthritis** AS EA PsA ReA Crystal (polyarticular gout)	**Degenerative** OA

Causes of Joint Pain

SOFTER TISSUE
Sepsis
OA
Fracture
Tendon/muscle
Epiphyseal
Referred
Tumour
Ischemia
Seropositive arthritides
Seronegative arthritides
Urate (gout)/other crystal
Extra-articular rheumatism (PMR/fibromyalgia)

Patterns of Joint Involvement
- Symmetrical vs. asymmetrical
- Small vs. large
- Mono vs. oligo (2-4 joints) vs. polyarticular (≥5 joints)
- Axial vs. peripheral

The presence of synovitis often indicates articular as opposed to non-articular joint pain; synovitis presents with: soft tissue swelling, effusion, warmth, and pain with movement

ESR
Advantages
- Much clinical information
- May reflect overall health status
Disadvantages
- Affected by age and gender
- Affected by RBC/morphology/anemia/polycythemia
- Reflects many plasma proteins
- Responds slowly to inflammatory stimulus
- Requires fresh sample

CRP
Advantages
- Unaffected by age/gender
- Rapid response to inflammatory stimulus
- Wide range of clinically relevant values
- Can be measured on stored sera
- Quantification precise/reproducible
Disadvantages
- More expensive

Most Important Tests of Synovial Fluid (3 Cs)
1. **C**ulture and gram stain
2. **C**ell count and differential
3. **C**rystal examination (protein, LDH, glucose less helpful)

Choosing Wisely Canada Recommendations
1. Do not order ANA as a screening test in patients without specific signs or symptoms of SLE or another CTD
2. Do not order an HLA-B27 unless spondyloarthritis is suspected based on specific signs or symptoms
3. Do not repeat DEXA scans more often than every 2 years
4. Do not prescribe bisphosphonates for patients at low risk of fracture
5. Do not perform whole body bone scans (e.g. scintigraphy) for diagnostic screening for peripheral and axial arthritis in the adult population

Table 6. Symptoms of Inflammatory Arthritis vs. Degenerative Arthritis

Inflammatory	Degenerative
Pain at rest, relieved by motion	Pain with motion, relieved by rest
Morning stiffness >1 h	Morning stiffness <½ h
Warmth, swelling, erythema	Joint instability, buckling, locking
Mal alignment/deformity	Bony enlargement, mal alignment/deformity
Extra-articular manifestations	Evening pain
Nighttime awakening	

Table 7. Seropositive vs. Seronegative Rheumatic Diseases

	Seropositive	Seronegative
Demographics	F>M	M>F
Peripheral Arthritis	Symmetrical Small (PIP, MCP) and medium joints (wrist, knee, ankle, elbow) common DIP less often involved	Usually asymmetrical Usually larger joints, lower extremities (exception: PsA) DIP in PsA Dactylitis ("sausage digit")
Pelvic/Axial Disease	No (except for C-spine)	Yes
Enthesitis	No	Yes
Extra-Articular	Nodules Vasculitis Sicca Raynaud's phenomenon Rashes, internal organ involvement (lung, cardiac)	Iritis (anterior uveitis) Oral ulcers Gastrointestinal Dermatologic features Genitourinary inflammation

Synovial Fluid Analysis

- synovial fluid is an ultrafiltrate of plasma plus hyaluronic acid; it lubricates joint surfaces and nourishes articular cartilage

Indications
- diagnostic tests advised if crystal arthritis or hemoarthritis is suspected or if there is unexplained joint, bursa or tendon sheath swelling
- therapeutic: drainage of blood, purulent or tense effusions; corticosteroid injection

Contraindications
- absolute: open lesion or suspected infection of overlying skin or soft tissue
- relative: bleeding diathesis, thrombocytopenia, prosthetic joint

Synovial Fluid Analysis
- most important to assess the 3C's: culture and order gram stain, cell count (WBC) and differential, and crystal analysis
- other parameters to consider are listed in Table 8

Table 8. Synovial Fluid Analysis

Parameter	Normal	Non-Inflammatory	Inflammatory	Infectious	Hemorrhagic
Colour	Pale yellow	Pale yellow	Pale yellow	Yellow to white	Red/brown
Clarity	Clear	Clear	Opaque	Opaque	Sanguinous
Viscosity	High (due to hyaluronic acid)	High	Low	Low or paradoxically high if purulent	Variable
WBC/mm³	<200	<2,000	≥2,000	Higher cell counts (particularly >50,000) suggestive	Variable
% PMN	<25%	<25%	≥25%	>75%	Variable
Culture/GrGram Stain	–	–	–	Usually positive	–
Examples		Trauma OA Neuropathy Hypertrophic – arthropathy	Seropositive Seronegative Crystal arthropathies	S. aureus Gram negative GC → difficult to culture	Trauma Hemophilia

Septic Arthritis

- septic arthritis is a medical emergency because it can lead to rapid joint destruction and has a 10-15% risk of mortality
- most commonly caused by bacterial infection (gram positive cocci > gram negative bacilli)
- consider empiric antibiotic therapy, until septic arthritis is excluded from history, physical examination and synovial fluid analysis
- poor prognostic factors include: older age, immunocompromised, delay in treatment, previously damaged joint, joint prosthesis
- see *Gonoccocal Arthritis*, Infectious Diseases, ID14 and Orthopedics, OR10
- most common method is hematogenous spreading from other infection such as skin infection or pneumonia
- knee and hip most common joints affected
- risk factors: very young, portal of entry, recent infection

Septic arthritis is a medical emergency; it leads to rapid joint destruction, and there is a 10-15% risk of mortality

Degenerative Arthritis: Osteoarthritis

Definition
- progressive deterioration of articular cartilage and surrounding joint structures caused by genetic, metabolic, biochemical, and biomechanical factors with secondary components of inflammation

OA of MCP joints can be seen in hemochromatosis or CPPD related disease (chondrocalcinosis)

Classification (based on etiology)
- primary (idiopathic)
  - most common, unknown etiology
- secondary
  - post-traumatic or mechanical
  - post-inflammatory (e.g. RA) or post-infectious
  - heritable skeletal disorders (e.g. scoliosis)
  - endocrine disorders (e.g. acromegaly, hyperparathyroidism, hypothyroidism)
  - metabolic disorders (e.g. gout, pseudogout, hemochromatosis, Wilson's disease, ochronosis)
  - neuropathic (e.g. Charcot joints)
    - atypical joint trauma due to peripheral neuropathy (e.g. diabetes mellitus, syphilis)
  - avascular necrosis (AVN)
  - other (e.g. congenital malformation)

Pathophysiology
- the process appears to be initiated by abnormalities in biomechanical forces and/or, less often, in cartilage
- elevated production of pro-inflammatory cytokines is important in OA progression
- tissue catabolism > repair
- genetics, alignment (bow-legged, knock-kneed), joint deformity (hip dysplasia), joint injury (meniscal or ligament tears), obesity, environmental, mechanical loading, age and gender factors contribute, but mechanism is unknown
- now considered to be a systemic musculoskeletal disorder rather than a focal disorder of synovial joints

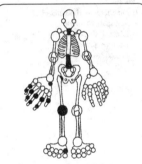

- Hand (DIP, PIP, 1st CMC)
- Hip
- Knee
- 1st MTP
- L-spine (L4-L5, L5-S1)
- C-spine
- Uncommon: ankle, shoulder, elbow, MCP, rest of wrist

© Linda Colati

Figure 3. Common sites of joint involvement in OA

Epidemiology
- most common arthropathy (accounts for ~75% of all arthritis)
- increased prevalence with increasing age (35% of 30 yr olds, 85% of 80 yr olds)

Risk Factors
- genetic predisposition, advanced age, obesity (for knee and hand OA), female, trauma

Signs and Symptoms
- localized to affected joints (not a systemic disease)
- pain is often insidious, gradually progressive, with intermittent flares and remissions, neuropathic pain may also be present
- fatigue, poor sleep, impact on mood (depression, anxiety)

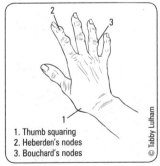

1. Thumb squaring
2. Heberden's nodes
3. Bouchard's nodes

© Tabby Lulham

Figure 4. Hand findings in OA

Table 9. Signs and Symptoms of OA

Signs	Symptoms
Joint line tenderness; stress pain ± joint effusion	Joint pain with motion; relieved with rest
Bony enlargement at affected joints	Short duration of stiffness (<1/2 h) after immobility
Malalignment/deformity (angulation)	Joint instability/buckling
Limited ROM	Joint locking due to "joint mouse" (bone or cartilage fragment)
Crepitus on passive ROM	Loss of function or other internal derangements (e.g. meniscal tear)
Inflammation (mild if present)	
Periarticular muscle atrophy	

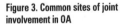

Differential Diagnosis of Elevated ESR
- Systemic inflammatory diseases
- Localized inflammatory diseases
- Malignancy
- Trauma
- Infection
- Tissue injury/ischemia

The Radiographic Hallmarks of OA
- Joint space narrowing
- Subchondral sclerosis
- Subchondral cysts
- Osteophytes

Joint Involvement
- generalized osteoarthritis: 3+ joint groups
- asymmetric (knees usually affected bilaterally)
- hand
  - DIP (Heberden's nodes = osteophytes → enlargement of joints)
  - PIP (Bouchard's nodes)
  - CMC (usually thumb squaring)
  - 1st MCP (other MCPs are usually spared)
- hip
  - usually presents as groin pain ± dull or sharp pain in the trochanteric area, internal rotation and abduction are lost first
  - pain can radiate to the anterior thigh, but generally does not go below the knee
- knee
  - initial narrowing of one compartment, medial > lateral; seen on standing x-rays, often patellar-femoral joint involved
- foot
  - common in first MTP and midfoot
- lumbar spine
  - very common, especially L4-L5, L5-S1
  - degeneration of intervertebral discs and facet joints
  - reactive bone growth can contribute to neurological impingement (e.g. sciatica, neurogenic claudication) or spondylolisthesis (forward or backward movement of one vertebra over another)
- cervical spine
  - commonly presents with neck pain that radiates to scapula, especially in mid-lower cervical area (C5 and C6)

Investigations
- blood work
  - normal CBC and ESR, CRP
  - negative RF and ANA
- radiology: 4 hallmark findings, see sidebar
- synovial fluid: non-inflammatory (see Table 8)

Treatment
- presently no treatment alters the natural history of OA
- prevention: prevent sports injury, healthy weight management
- **non-pharmacological therapy**
  - weight loss (minimum 5-10 lb loss) if overweight
  - physiotherapy: heat/cold, low impact exercise programs
  - occupational therapy: aids, splints, cane, walker, bracing
- **pharmacological therapy** (see Table 33)
  - oral: acetaminophen/NSAIDs, glucosamine ± chondroitin (nutraceuticals not proven)
  - treat neuropathic pain if present (anti-depressants, anti-epileptics, etc.)
  - joint injections: corticosteroid (effective for short term treatment), hyaluronic acid (evidence of long term benefits)
  - topical: capsaicin, NSAIDs
- **surgical treatment**
  - joint debridement, osteotomy, total and/or partial joint replacement, fusion (see Orthopedics, OR6)

Seropositive Rheumatic Disease

- diagnosis vs. classification in rheumatology
  - diagnostic criteria are often dependent on disease progression and evolution over time, as early objective measures are often unavailable
  - classification criteria are derived from studying patients with long-term diseases and clear diagnoses in order to determine which criteria have good specificity in the early prediction of certain diagnoses
- seropositive arthropathies are characterized by the presence of a serologic marker such as positive RF or ANA
- a small subset of the vasculitides, the small vessel ANCA-associated vasculitides, have a measurable serological component, but they are often considered a separate entity from seropositive disease by experts

Table 10. Autoantibodies and their Prevalence in Rheumatic Diseases

Autoantibody	Disease	Healthy Controls	Comments
RF	RA 80% SS 50% SLE 20%	<5% 10-20% >65	Autoantibodies directed against Fc domain of IgG Sensitive in RA (can be negative early in disease course), levels correlate with disease activity Present in most seropositive diseases Non-specific; may be present in IE, TB, hepatitis C, silicosis, sarcoidosis
Anti-CCP	RA 80%		Specific for RA (94-98%) May be useful in early disease and to predict aggressive disease
ANA	SLE 98% MCTD 100% SS 40-70% CREST 60-80%	High titers <5% Low titers Up to 30% (Often seen in other CTDs)	Ab against nuclear components (DNA, RNA, histones, centromere) Sensitive but not specific for SLE Given high false positive rate -only measure when high pre-test probability of CTD
Anti-dsDNA	SLE 50-70%	0%	Specific for SLE (95%) Levels correlate with disease activity (i.e. SLE flare)
Anti-Sm	SLE <30%	0%	Specific but not sensitive for SLE Does not correlate with SLE disease activity If positive, will remain positive through disease course
Anti-Ro (SSA)	SS 40-95% SSc 21% SLE 32% RA 15%	0.5%	Subacute cutaneous SLE (74%) May be only Ab present in ANA negative SLE Increases risk of having child with neonatal lupus syndrome
Anti-La (SSB)	SS 40% SLE 10%	0%	Usually occurs with anti-Ro Specific for SS and SLE when anti-Ro is also positive Increases risk of having child with neonatal lupus syndrome
Antiphospholipid Ab (LAC, aCLA, aB2GP)	APLS 100% SLE 31-40%	<5%	By definition present in APLS Only small subset of SLE patients develop clinical syndrome of APLA If positive, will often get a false positive VDRL test
Anti-Histone	Drug-induced SLE 95% SLE 30-80%	0% 0%	Highly specific for drug-induced SLE
Anti-RNP	MCTD SLE		High titres present in MCTD; present in many other CTD (especially SLE)
Anti-Centromere	CREST >80%	0%	Specific for CREST, cutaneous variant of systemic sclerosis
Anti-Topoisomerase I (formerly Scl-70)	Diffuse SSc 26-76%	0%	Specific for SSc Increased risk pulmonary fibrosis in SSc
Anti-Jo1	PM DMM	0%	Less frequent for DMM
c-ANCA	Active GPA >90%	0%	Specific and sensitive
p-ANCA	GPA 10% Other vasculitis	0%	Nonspecific and poor sensitivity (found in ulcerative colitis, PAN, microscopic polyangiitis, Churg-Strauss, rapidly progressive glomerulonephritis)
Anti-Mi-2	DMM 15-20%		Specific but not sensitive (not available in all centres)
Ab Against RBCs, WBCs, or Platelets	SLE		Perform direct Coomb's test Test Hb, reticulocyte, leukocyte and platelet count, antiplatelet Abs
Anti-mitochondria	Primary biliary cholangitis	0%	Sensitive and specific

- note: some individuals in the normal population test positive for RF and/or ANA, but do not have the conditions listed in Table 10

Connective Tissue Disorders

Table 11. Features of Seropositive Arthropathies

	RA	SLE	Scleroderma	Dermatomyositis
CLINICAL FEATURES				
History	Symmetrical polyarthritis (small joint involvement) Morning stiffness (>1 h)	Multisystemic disease: rash, photosensitivity, Raynaud's, alopecia, cardiac and pulmonary serositis, CNS symptoms, glomerulonephritis	Skin tightness, stiffness of fingers, Raynaud's, heartburn, dysphagia, pulmonary HTN, renal crisis with new onset HTN or hypertensive urgency/emergency, dyspnea on exertion	Heliotrope rash (periorbital), Gottron's papules (violaceous papules over knuckles and IP joints) ± poikiloderma Shawl sign: macular erythema over chest and shoulder Proximal muscle weakness ± pain Dyspnea on exertion
Physical Examination	Effused joints Tenosynovitis Subcutaneous nodules Joint deformities Bone-on-bone crepitus in advanced disease	Confirm historical findings (rash, serositis, renal, CVS, etc.) ± effused (typically small) joints (can be minimal, look for soft tissue swelling)	Skin tightness on dorsum of hand, facial skin tightening, telangiectasia, calcinosis, non-effused joint, inspiratory crackles	Rash, proximal muscle weakness, inspiratory crackles
LABORATORY				
Non-Specific	↑ ESR in 50-60% ↑ platelets ↓ Hb	↑ ESR ↓ platelets (autoimmune) ↓ Hb (autoimmune) ↓ WBC (leukopenia, lymphopenia)	↑ ESR ↓ Hb Normal WBC	Possible increased ESR ↓ Hb Normal WBC
Specific	RF +ve in ~80% Anti-CCP +ve in ~80%	ANA +ve in 98% Anti-dsDNA +ve in 50-70% Anti-SM +ve in 30% ↓ C3, C4, total hemolytic complement False positive VDRL (in SLE subtypes) ↑ PTT (in SLE subtypes, e.g. APLA)	ANA +ve in >90% Anti-topoisomerase 1 (diffuse) Anti-centromere (usually in *CREST*, see RH13)	CK elevated in 80% ANA +ve in 33% anti-Jo-1, anti-Mi-2 Muscle biopsy EMG MRI
Radiographs	Periarticular osteopenia Joint space narrowing Erosions Absence of bone repair Symmetric/concentric	Non-erosive ± osteopenia ± soft tissue swelling	± pulmonary fibrosis ± esophageal dysmotility ± calcinosis ± ILD	± esophageal dysmotility ± ILD ± calcifications

Rheumatoid Arthritis

RA is an independent risk factor for atherosclerosis and CV disease. RA is associated with increased overall mortality/ morbidity from all causes: CV disease, neoplasm (especially lymphoma), infection

Definition
- chronic, symmetric, erosive synovitis of peripheral joints (e.g. wrists, MCPs, MTPs)
- characterized by a number of extra-articular features

Table 12. 2010 ACR/EULAR Classification Criteria for RA

Criteria	Score	Comments
1. Joint involvement (swollen or tender)		
1 large joint (shoulders, elbows, hips, knees, and ankles)	0	
2-10 large joints	1	
1-3 small joints (MCPs, PIPs, wrists, 2nd-5th MTPs)	2	
4-10 small joints	3	
>10 joints (at least 1 small joint)	5	
2. Serology		Total score of ≥6: definite RA
Negative RF and negative Anti-CCP	0	Must have ≥1 joint with definite
Low-positive RF or low-positive Anti-CCP (<3x ULN)	2	clinical swelling, not better explained by other
High-positive RF or high-positive Anti-CCP (>3x ULN)	3	disease
3. Acute phase reactants		
Normal CRP and normal ESR	0	
Abnormal CRP and abnormal ESR	1	
4. Duration of symptoms		
<6 wk	0	
≥6 wk	1	

Arthritis Rheum 2010;62:2569-2581

Common Presentation
- Morning stiffness >1 h, improves with use
- Symmetric joint involvement
- Initially involves small joints of hands and feet
- Constitutional symptoms

Pathophysiology

- autoimmune disorder, unknown etiology
- complex interaction of genes and environment leading to breakdown of immune tolerance: many pathways result in autoreactivity leading to a final common pathway to synovial inflammation
  - genetic predisposition: HLA-DR4/DR1 association (93% of patients have either HLA type), cytokine promotors, T cell signaling
    - induction of enzymes that convert arginine to citrulline caused by environmental stress (cigarette smoking)
    - RA: propensity for immune reactivity to neoepitopes created by protein citrullination and production of anti-citrullinated protein antibodies
- once inflammatory process is established, synovium organizes itself into an invasive tissue that degrades cartilage and bone
- progressive bone destruction with absence of bone repair in response to inflammation
  - elevated TNF levels increases osteoclasts and decreases osteoblasts at the site of inflammation
  - upregulation of RANK ligand increases osteoclast-mediated destruction

Epidemiology

- most common inflammatory arthritis: prevalence 1% of population
- F:M = 3:1
- age of onset 20-40 yr

Signs and Symptoms

- variable course of exacerbations and remissions
- morning stiffness >1 h, improves with use, worsens with rest
- polyarthritis: symmetric joint involvement (tender, swollen), small joints affected, most commonly in hands and feet (MCP, PIP, MTP)
- extra-articular (systemic) symptoms: profound fatigue, depression, myalgia, weight loss
- limitation of function and decrease in global functional status
- complications of chronic synovitis
  - signs of mechanical joint damage: loss of motion, instability, deformity, crepitus, joint deformities
    - swan neck deformity, boutonnière deformity
    - ulnar deviation of MCP, radial deviation of wrist joint
    - hammer toe, mallet toe, claw toe
    - flexion contractures
  - atlanto-axial and subaxial subluxation
    - C-spine instability
    - neurological impingement (long tract signs)
    - difficult/dangerous intubation: risk of worsening subluxation and damage to spinal cord
- limited shoulder mobility, spontaneous tears of the rotator cuff leading to chronic spasm
- tenosynovitis → may cause rupture of tendons
- carpal tunnel syndrome
- ruptured Baker's cyst (outpouching of synovium behind the knee); presentation similar to acute DVT
- poor prognostic factors include: young age of onset, high RF titer, elevated ESR, activity of >20 joints, and presence of extra-articular features

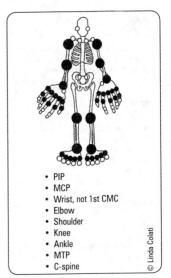

- PIP
- MCP
- Wrist, not 1st CMC
- Elbow
- Shoulder
- Knee
- Ankle
- MTP
- C-spine

Figure 5. Common sites of joint involvement in RA

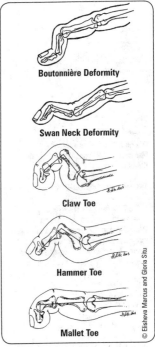

Boutonnière Deformity

Swan Neck Deformity

Claw Toe

Hammer Toe

Mallet Toe

Figure 6. Joint deformities

Table 13. Extra-Articular Features of RA Classified by Underlying Pathophysiology

System	Vasculitic	Lymphocytic Infiltrate
Skin	Periungual infarction, cutaneous ulcers, palpable purpura	Rheumatoid nodules (may have vasculitic component)
Ocular	Episcleritis, scleritis	Keratoconjunctivitis sicca
Head and Neck		Xerostomia, Hashimoto's thyroiditis (see Endocrinology, E27)
Cardiac		Peri-/myocarditis, valvular disease, conduction defects
Pulmonary		Pulmonary fibrosis, pleural effusion, pleuritis, pulmonary nodules
Neurologic	Peripheral neuropathy: sensory stocking-glove, mononeuritis multiplex	
Hematologic		Splenomegaly, neutropenia (Felty's syndrome)
Renal		Amyloidosis – caused by accumulation of abnormal proteins

Classification of Global Functional Status in RA

- **Class I:** able to perform usual ADLs (self-care, vocational, avocational)
- **Class II:** able to perform self-care and vocational activities, restriction of avocational activities
- **Class III:** able to perform self-care, restriction of vocational and avocational activities
- **Class IV:** limited ability to perform self-care, vocational, and avocational activities

Syndromes in RA
- SS (common): keratoconjunctivitis sicca and xerostomia (dry eyes and mouth)
- Caplan's syndrome (very rare): combination of RA + Pneumoconiosis that manifests as multiple intrapulmonary nodules
- Felty's syndrome (rare): arthritis, splenomegaly, neutropenia

Connective Tissue Disorders

Poor prognostic features of RA include: young age of onset, high RF titer, elevated ESR, activity of >20 joints, and presence of extra-articular features

Side Effects of Steroids
- Weight gain
- Osteoporosis
- AVN
- Cataracts, glaucoma
- PUD
- Susceptibility to infection
- Easy bruising
- Acne
- HTN
- Hyperlipidemia
- Hypokalemia, hyperglycemia
- Mood swings

DMARDs, prednisone and biologics alter the course of RA but not analgesics or NSAIDs

CRA Guidelines for Pharmacological Management of RA with Traditional and Biologic DMARDs
J Rheumatol 2011;39:1559-1582
CRA Recommendations of RA Pharmacologic Management
1. General Management: Remission is the goal of management and if not possible, minimal disease activity and quality of life improvement are desired. Poor prognostic factors should be assessed at baseline (RF, functional limitation, extra-articular features). Active RA patients should be monitored every 1-3 mo. A change in management should be considered where erosions are seen on x-ray despite clinical response.
2. Glucocorticoids: Should be used at the lowest possible dose and tapered as soon as possible. Can be added to initial DMARD therapy or used for managing flares, or symptom control if all other options have been exhausted.
3. Treatment with MTX or DMARD: MTX is the preferred DMARD and should be used unless contraindicated. DMARDs should be used rapidly in patients with persistent synovitis. CBC, LFT, renal function, and CXR should be assessed prior to MTX therapy. MTX requires individualized dosing. In patients with poor prognostic features or high disease activity, DMARD combinations where MTX is the anchor medication should be considered. Biologics are indicated for therapy in patients who continue to have moderate-high disease activity despite being treated with at least two DMARDs in therapeutic doses for 3 mo. Anti-TNFs are the first line recommended treatment after DMARDs. Addition of MTX to biologics improves efficacy.

Investigations
- blood work
  - RF: sensitivity 80% but non-specific; may not be present at onset of symptoms; levels **DO NOT** correlate with disease activity
    - can be associated with more erosions, more extra-articular manifestations, and worse function
  - anti-CCP: sensitivity 80% but more specific (94-98%); may precede onset of symptoms
  - increased disease activity is associated with decreased Hb (anemia of chronic disease), increased platelets, ESR, CRP, and RF
- imaging
  - x-rays may be normal at onset
  - first change is periarticular osteopenia, followed by erosions
  - U/S (with power doppler), MRI may be used to image hands to detect early synovitis and erosions
    - MRI T1 inflamed synovium is hypointense and hyperintense on T1; bone marrow edema can be seen as well as areas of increased uptake gadolinium contrast

Treatment
- goals of therapy: remission or lowest possible disease activity
  - key is early diagnosis and early intervention with DMARDs
  - "window of opportunity" = early treatment within first 3 mo of disease may allow better control/remission
  - assess poor prognostic factors at baseline (RF positive, functional limitations and extra-articular features)
- behavioural
  - exercise program (isometrics and active, gentle ROM exercise during flares, aquatic/aerobic/strengthening exercise between flares), assistive devices as needed
  - job modification may be necessary
- pharmacologic: alter disease progression
  - only DMARDs and biologics (not analgesics or NSAIDs) can alter the course of RA
  - DMARDs
    - methotrexate (MTX) is the gold standard and is first-line unless contraindicated
      - chest X-ray should be assessed prior to MTX therapy
      - if inadequate response (3-6 mo) → combine or switch
      - consider including add-on medications to MTX if patients have poor prognostic features or high disease activity
      - add-ons include: hydroxychloroquine, sulfasalazine, leflunomide
  - biologics
    - indicated if inadequate response to DMARDs
    - can be combined with DMARD therapy (initiating with combination therapy is associated with faster response rates)
    - anti-TNF is the first line therapy
    - options: infliximab, etanercept, adalimumab, abatacept, rituximab, tocilizumab
    - reassess every 3-6 mo and monitor disease severity
- pharmacologic: reduce inflammation and pain
  - NSAIDs
    - individualize according to efficacy and tolerability
    - contraindicated/cautioned in some patients (e.g. PUD, ischemic cardiac disease, pregnancy)
    - add acetaminophen ± opioid prn for synergistic pain control
  - corticosteroids
    - local: injections to control symptoms in a specific joint
    - systemic (prednisone)
      - low dose (5-10 mg/d) useful for short-term to improve symptoms if NSAIDs ineffective, to bridge gap until DMARDs take effect
      - severe RA: add low dose prednisone to DMARDs
      - do baseline DEXA bone density scan and consider bone supportive pharmacologic therapy if using corticosteroids >3 mo at 7.5mg/d
      - cautions/contraindications: active infection, TB, osteoporosis, HTN, gastric ulcer, DM

Follow-Up Management and Clinical Outcomes
- follow-up every 3-6 mo, then 6-12 mo after inflammation has been suppressed
- examine joints for active inflammation – if active, consider adjusting medications, PT/OT
- if assessment reveals joint damage – consider analgesia, referral to PT/OT, surgical options
- outcome depends on disease activity, joint damage, physical functional status, psychological health, and comorbidities
- functional capacity is a useful tool for determining therapeutic effectiveness: many tools for evaluation have been validated
- patients with RA have an increased prevalence of other serious illnesses: infection (e.g. pulmonary, skin, joint), renal impairment, lymphoproliferative disorders, cardiovascular disease (correlates with disease activity and duration)
- increased risk of premature mortality, decreased life expectancy (most mortality not directly caused by RA)

Surgical Therapy
- indicated for structural joint damage
- surgical options include: synovectomy, joint replacement, joint fusion, reconstruction/tendon repair

Systemic Lupus Erythematosus

- see Nephrology, NP24

Definition
- chronic inflammatory multi-system disease of unknown etiology
- characterized by production of autoantibodies and diverse clinical manifestations

Table 14. Diagnostic Criteria of SLE*

Criteria	Description
CLINICAL	
Malar rash	Classic "butterfly rash", sparing of nasolabial folds, no scarring
Discoid rash	May cause scarring due to invasion of basement membrane
Photosensitivity	Skin rash in reaction to sunlight
Oral/nasal ulcers	Usually painless
Arthritis	Symmetric, involving ≥2 small or large peripheral joints, non-erosive
Serositis	Pleuritis or pericarditis
Neurologic disorder	Seizures or psychosis
LABORATORY	
Renal disorder	Proteinuria (>0.5 g/d or 3+)
	Cellular casts (RBC, Hb, granular, tubular, mixed)
Hematologic disorder	Hemolytic anemia, leukopenia, lymphopenia, thrombocytopenia
Immunologic disorder	Anti-dsDNA or anti-Sm or antiphospholipid Ab (anticardiolipin Ab, SLE anticoagulant) or false positive VDRL with 6 mo confirmatory negative
ANA	Most sensitive test (98%), not specific

*Note: "4, 7, 11" rule → 4 (or more) out of 11 criteria (4 lab, 7 clinical) must be present, serially or simultaneously, for diagnosis
American College of Rheumatology, 1997 update

Etiology and Pathophysiology
- production of cytotoxic autoantibodies and immune complex formation
- multi-factorial etiology
- **genetics**
  - common association with HLA-B8/DR3; ~10% have positive family history
  - strong association with defects in apoptotic clearance → fragments of nuclear particles captured by antigen-presenting cells → develop anti-nuclear antibodies
  - cytokines involved in inflammatory process and tissue injury: B-lymphocyte stimulator (BlyS), IL-6, IL-17, IL-18, TNF-α
- **environment**
  - UV radiation, cigarette smoking, infection, vitamin D deficiency
- **estrogen**
  - increased incidence after puberty, decreased incidence after menopause
  - men with SLE have higher concentration of estrogenic metabolites
- **infection**
  - viral (non-specific stimulant of immune response)
- **drug-induced**
  - anti-hypertensives (hydralazine), anti-convulsants (phenytoin), anti-arrhythmics (procainamide), isoniazid, biologics, oral contraceptive pills
  - anti-histone Ab are commonly seen in drug-induced SLE
  - symptoms resolve with discontinuation of offending drug

Epidemiology
- prevalence: 0.05% overall
- F:M = 10:1
- age of onset in reproductive yr (13-40)
- more common and severe in African-Americans and Asians
- bimodal mortality pattern
  - early (within 2 yr)
    - active SLE, active nephritis, infection secondary to steroid use
  - late (>10 yr)
    - inactive SLE, inactive nephritis, atherosclerosis likely due to chronic inflammation

Signs and Symptoms
- characterized by periods of exacerbation and remission

Diagnostic Criteria of SLE

MD SOAP BRAIN

Malar rash	Blood
Discoid rash	Renal
Serositis	Arthritis
Oral ulcers	Immune
ANA	Neurologic
Photosensitivity	

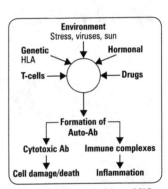

Figure 7. Multi-factorial etiology of SLE

Drug-Induced SLE
Often presents atypically with systemic features and serositis; usually associated with anti-histone Ab

Table 15. Symptoms of SLE

System	Symptoms
Systemic	Fatigue, malaise, weight loss, fever, lymphadenopathy
Renal	HTN, peripheral edema, glomerulonephritis, renal failure
Dermatologic	Photosensitivity, malar rash, discoid rash, oral ulcers, alopecia (hair loss), purpura, panniculitis (inflammation of subcutaneous fat and muscle tissue), urticaria
Musculoskeletal	Polyarthralgias, polyarthritis, myalgias, AVN; reducible deformities of hand = Jaccoud's arthritis
Ophthalmic	Keratoconjunctivitis sicca, episcleritis, scleritis, cytoid bodies (cotton wool exudates on fundoscopy = infarction of nerve cell layer of retina)
Cardiac	Pericarditis, CAD, non-bacterial endocarditis (Libman-Sachs), myocarditis Note: SLE is an independent risk factor for atherosclerosis and CAD
Vascular	Raynaud's phenomenon, livedo reticularis (mottled discolouration of skin due to narrowing of blood vessels, characteristic lacy or net-like appearance), thrombosis, vasculitis
Respiratory	Pleuritis, ILD, pulmonary HTN, PE, alveolar hemorrhage
Gastrointestinal	Pancreatitis, SLE enteropathy, hepatitis, hepatomegaly, splenomegaly
Neurologic	H/A, depression, psychosis, seizures, cerebritis, transverse myelitis, peripheral neuropathy, stroke
Life/Organ-Threatening	Cardiac: coronary vasculitis, malignant HTN, tamponade Hematologic: hemolytic anemia, neutropenia, thrombocytopenia, TTP, thrombosis Neurologic: seizures, CVA, stroke Respiratory: pulmonary hypertension, pulmonary hemorrhage, emboli

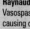

Raynaud's Phenomenon
Vasospastic disorder characteristically causing discolouration of fingers and toes (white → blue → red).
Classic triggers: cold and emotional stress

Investigations
- ANA (sensitivity 98%, but poor specificity → used as a screening test, ANA titres are not useful to follow disease course)
- anti-dsDNA and anti-Sm are specific (95-99%)
- anti-dsDNA titre and serum complement (C3, C4) are useful to monitor treatment response in patients who are clinically and serologically concordant (anti-dsDNA, C3, and C4 also fluctuates with disease acitivity)
- antiphospholipid Ab (anti-cardiolipin Ab, SLE anticoagulant, Anti-β2 glycoprotein-I Ab), may cause increased risk of clotting and increased aPTT

Consider SLE in a patient who has involvement of 2 or more organ systems

Treatment
- **goals of therapy**
  - treat early and avoid long-term steroid use, if unavoidable see Endocrinology, E41 for osteoporosis management
  - if high doses of steroids necessary for long-term control, add steroid-sparing agents and taper when possible
  - treatment is tailored to organ system involved and severity of disease
  - all medications used to treat SLE require periodic monitoring for potential toxicity
- **dermatologic**
  - sunscreen, avoid UV light and estrogens
  - topical steroids, hydroxychloroquine
- **musculoskeletal**
  - NSAIDs ± gastroprotective agent for arthritis (also beneficial for pleuritis and pericarditis)
  - hydroxychloroquine improves long-term control and prevents flares
  - bisphosphonates, calcium, vitamin D to combat osteoporosis
- **organ-threatening disease**
  - high-dose oral prednisone or IV methylprednisolone in severe disease
  - steroid-sparing agents: azathioprine, MTX, mycophenolate mofetil
  - IV cyclophosphamide for serious organ involvement (e.g. cerebritis or lupus nephritis) see Nephrology, NP24 for clinical features of lupus nephritis

The arthritis of SLE can be deforming but it is non-erosive (in contrast to RA)

Antiphospholipid Antibody Syndrome

Definition
- multi-system vasculopathy manifested by recurrent thromboembolic events, spontaneous abortions, and thrombocytopenia
- often presents with migraine-type H/As
- circulating antiphospholipid autoantibodies interfere with coagulation
- **primary APLS**: occurs in the absence of other disease
- **secondary APLS**: occurs in the setting of a connective tissue disease (including SLE), malignancy, drugs (hydralazine, procainamide, phenytoin, interferon, quinidine), and infections (HIV, TB, hepatitis C, infectious mononucleosis)
- **catastrophic APLS**: development within 1 wk of small vessel thrombotic occlusion in ≥3 organ systems with positive antiphospholipid Ab (high mortality)

Table 16. Classification Criteria of APLS*

Criteria	Description
CLINICAL	
Vascular thrombosis	Arterial: stroke/TIA, multi-infarct dementia, MI, valvular incompetence, limb ischemia Venous: DVT, PE, renal and retinal vein thrombosis Must be confirmed by imaging or histopathology
Pregnancy morbidity	Fetal death (>10 wk GA), recurrent spontaneous abortions (<10 wk GA) or premature birth (<34 wk GA)
LABORATORY	Labs must be positive on 2 occasions, at least 12 wk apart
SLE anticoagulant	Prolonged aPTT not corrected by the addition of normal plasma
Anti-cardiolipin Ab	IgG and/or IgM
Anti-β2 glycoprotein-I Ab	IgG and/or IgM
ANA	Most sensitive test (98%), not specific

* 1 clinical and 1 laboratory criteria must be present   *J Thromb Haemost* 2006;4:295-306

Manifestations of APLA
- Thromboembolic events
- Spontaneous abortions
- Thrombocytopenia
- Associated with livedo reticularis, migrane headaches

Arterial and venous thrombosis are usually mutually exclusive

Signs and Symptoms
- see clinical criteria in Table 16
- hematologic
    - thrombocytopenia, hemolytic anemia, neutropenia
- dermatologic
    - livedo reticularis, Raynaud's phenomenon, purpura, leg ulcers, and gangrene

Treatment
- thrombosis
    - lifelong anti-coagulation with warfarin
    - target INR 2.0-3.0 for first venous event, >3.0 for recurrent and/or arterial event
- recurrent fetal loss
    - heparin/low molecular weight heparin ± ASA during pregnancy
- catastrophic APLA
    - high-dose steroids, anti-coagulation, cyclophosphamide, plasmapheresis

Scleroderma (i.e. Systemic Sclerosis)

Definition
- a non-inflammatory autoimmune disorder characterized by widespread small vessel vasculopathy, production of autoantibodies, and fibroblast dysfunction causing fibrosis

CREST Syndrome
Calcinosis
Raynaud's phenomenon
Esophageal dysmotility
Sclerodactyly
Telangiectasia

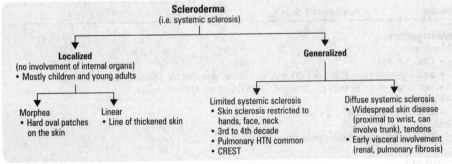

Figure 8. Forms of scleroderma

Table 17. The American College of Rheumatology (ACR)/European League Against Rheumatism (EULAR) Criteria for Scleroderma*

Item	Sub-item	Score
1. Skin thickening of fingers of both hands extending proximal to the MCP (sufficient criterion)		9
2. Skin thickening of the fingers	Puffy fingers Sclerodactyly	2 4
3. Fingertip lesions	Digital tip ulcers Fingertip pitting scars	2 3
4. Telengiectasia		2
5. Abnormal nailfold capillaries		2
6. Pulmonary arterial HTN ± ILD (max score 2)	Pulmonary arterial HTN ILD	2 2
7. Raynaud's phenomenon		3
8. Scleroderma related Ab	Anticentromere Anti-topoisomerase I Anti-RNA polymerase III	3

* Score of ≥9 is sufficient to classify a patient as having definite scleroderma (sensitivity 0.95, specificity 0.93) Arthritis & Rheum 2013;65(11):2737-2747

Scleroderma is the most common cause of secondary Raynaud's phenomenon

Etiology and Pathophysiology
- idiopathic vasculopathy (not vasculitis) leading to atrophy and fibrosis of tissues
  - intimal proliferation and media mucinous degeneration → progressive obliteration of vessel lumen → fibrotic tissue
  - resembles malignant HTN
  - lung disease is the most common cause of morbidity and mortality

Epidemiology
- F:M = 3-4:1, peaking in 5th and 6th decades
- associated with HLA-DR1
- associated with environmental exposure (silica, epoxy resins, toxic oil, aromatic hydrocarbons, polyvinyl chloride)
- limited systemic sclerosis has a higher survival prognosis (>70% at 10 yr) than diffuse systemic sclerosis (40-60% at 10 yr)

Signs and Symptoms

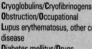

Raynaud's Phenomenon DDx

COLD HAND
Cryoglobulins/**C**ryofibrinogens
Obstruction/**O**ccupational
Lupus erythematosus, other connective tissue disease
Diabetes mellitus/**D**rugs
Hematologic problems (polycythemia, leukemia, etc.)
Arterial problems (atherosclerosis)/**A**norexia nervosa
Neurologic problems (vascular tone)
Disease of unknown origin (idiopathic)

Features of Pathologic Raynaud's Syndrome
- New onset
- Asymmetric
- Precipitated by stimuli other than cold or emotion
- Associated with distal pulp pitting or tissue reabsorption
- Digit ischemia
- Capillary dilatation by capillaroscopy

Table 18. Clinical Manifestations of Scleroderma

System	Features
Dermatologic	Painless non-pitting edema → skin tightening Ulcerations, calcinosis, periungual erythema, hypo/hyperpigmentation, pruritus, telangiectasias Characteristic face: mask-like facies with tight lips, beak nose, radial perioral furrows
Vascular	Raynaud's phenomenon → digital pits, gangrene
Gastrointestinal (~90%)	Distal esophageal hypomotility → dysphagia Loss of lower esophageal sphincter function → GERD, ulcerations, strictures Small bowel hypomotility → bacterial overgrowth, diarrhea, bloating, cramps, malabsorption, weight loss Large bowel hypomotility → wide mouth diverticuli are pathognomonic radiographic finding on barium study
Renal	Mild proteinuria, Cr elevation, HTN "Scleroderma renal crisis" (10-15%) may lead to malignant arterial HTN, oliguria, and microangiopathic hemolytic anemia
Pulmonary	Interstitial fibrosis, pulmonary HTN, pleurisy, pleural effusions
Cardiac	Left ventricular dysfunction, pericarditis, pericardial effusion, arrhythmias
Musculoskeletal	Polyarthralgias "Resorption of distal tufts" (radiological finding) Proximal weakness 2° to disuse, atrophy, low grade myopathy
Endocrine	Hypothyroidism

Investigations
- blood work
  - CBC, Cr, ANA
  - anti-topoisomerase 1/anti-Scl-70: specific but not sensitive for diffuse systemic sclerosis
  - anti-centromere: favours diagnosis of CREST (limited systemic sclerosis)
- PFT
  - assess for interstitial lung disease
- imaging
  - CXR for fibrosis, echo for pulmonary HTN

Treatment
- dermatologic
  - good skin hygiene
  - low-dose prednisone (>20 mg may provoke renal crisis if susceptible), MTX (limited evidence)
- vascular
  - patient education on cold avoidance
  - vasodilators (CCBs, local nitroglycerine cream, systemic PGE$_2$ inhibitors, PDE5 inhibitors)
- gastrointestinal
  - GERD: PPIs are first line, then H$_2$-receptor agonists
  - small bowel bacterial overgrowth: broad spectrum antibiotics (tetracycline, metronidazole)
- renal disease
  - ACEI for hypertensive crisis
  - see Nephrology, NP32 for scleroderma renal crisis

- pulmonary
  - early interstitial disease: cyclophosphamide
  - pulmonary HTN: vasodilators e.g. bosentan , epoprostenol, PDE5 inhibitors
- cardiac
  - pericarditis: systemic steroids
- musculoskeletal
  - arthritis: NSAIDs
  - myositis: systemic steroids

Idiopathic Inflammatory Myopathy

Definition
- autoimmune diseases characterized by proximal muscle weakness ± pain
- muscle becomes damaged by a non-suppurative lymphocytic inflammatory process

Classification
- PM/DMM
- adult and juvenile form
- associated with malignancy
  - increased risk of malignancy: age >50, DMM>PM, normal CK, refractory disease
- associated with other connective tissue disease, Raynaud's phenomenon, autoimmune disorders

Inclusion Body Myositis
- age >50, M>F, slowly progressive, vacuoles in cells on biopsy
- suspect when patient unresponsive to treatment
- distal as well as proximal muscle weakness
- muscle biopsy positive for inclusion bodies

POLYMYOSITIS/DERMATOMYOSITIS

Table 19. Classification Criteria for PM/DMM*

Criteria	Description
1. Symmetric proximal muscle weakness	Typical involvement of shoulder girdle and hip girdle
2. Elevated muscle enzymes	↑ CK, aldolase, LDH, AST, ALT
3. EMG changes	Short polyphasic motor units, high frequency repetitive discharge, insertional irritability
4. Muscle biopsy	Segmental fibre necrosis, basophilic regeneration, perivascular inflammation (DMM), endomysial inflammation (PM) and atrophy
5. Typical rash of dermatomyositis	Required for diagnosis of DMM (see below)

*Definite if 4 present, probable if 3 present   NEJM 1975;292:403-407

Etiology and Pathophysiology
- PM is CD8 cell-mediated muscle necrosis, found in adults
- DMM is B-cell and CD4 immune complex-mediated peri-fascicular vascular abnormalities

Signs and Symptoms
- progressive symmetrical proximal muscle weakness (shoulder and hip) developing over weeks to months
  - difficulty lifting head off pillow, arising from chair, climbing stairs
- dermatological
  - DMM has characteristic dermatological features (F>M, children and adults)
    - Gottron's papules
      - pink-violaceous, flat-topped papules overlying the dorsal surface of the interphalangeal joints
    - Gottron's sign
      - erythematous, smooth or scaly patches over the dorsal IPs, MCPs, elbows, knees, or medial malleoli
    - heliotrope rash: violaceous rash over the eyelids; usually with edema
    - shawl sign: poikilodermatous erythematous rash over neck, upper chest, and shoulders
    - mechanic's hands: dark, dry, thick scale on palmar and lateral surface of digits
    - periungual erythema
- cardiac
  - arrhythmias, CHF, conduction defect, ventricular hypertrophy, pericarditis
- gastrointestinal
  - oropharyngeal and lower esophageal dysphagia, reflux
- pulmonary
  - weakness of respiratory muscles, ILD, aspiration pneumonia

Investigations
- blood work: CK, ANA, anti-Jo-1 (DMM), anti-Mi-2, anti-SRP
- imaging: MRI may be used to localize biopsy site
- EMG, muscle biopsy

Signs of DMM
Gottron's papules and Gottron's sign are pathognomonic of DMM (occur in 70% of patients)

Malignancies Associated with DMM
- Breast
- Lung
- Colon
- Ovarian

Treatment

- non-pharmacological treatment
  - physical therapy and occupational therapy
- pharmacological treatment
  - high-dose corticosteroid (1-2 mg/kg/d) and slow taper
  - add immunosuppressive agents (azathioprine, MTX, cyclosporine)
  - IVIg if severe or refractory
  - hydroxychloroquine for DMM rash
- malignancy surveillance
  - detailed history and physical (breast, pelvic, and rectal exam)
  - CXR, abdominal and pelvic U/S, fecal occult blood, Pap test, mammogram ± CT scan (thoracic, abdominal, pelvic)

Sjögren's Syndrome

Definition

- autoimmune condition characterized by dry eyes (keratoconjunctivitis sicca/xerophthalmia) and dry mouth (xerostomia), caused by lymphocytic infiltration of salivary and lacrimal glands
- may evolve into systemic disorder with diminished exocrine gland activity in respiratory tract and skin
- primary and secondary form (associated with RA, SLE, DMM, and HIV)
- prevalence, F>>M, 40-60 yo
- increased risk of non-Hodgkin's lymphoma

Patients with Sjögren's syndrome are at higher risk of non-Hodgkin's lymphoma

Classic Triad (identifies 93% of Sjögren's patients)
- Dry eyes
- Dry mouth (xerostomia) → dysphagia
- Arthritis (small joint, asymmetrical, non-erosive) but may be associated with rheumatoid arthritis, in which case, the arthritis is erosive and symmetric

Table 20. American College of Rheumatology Classification for Sjögren's*

Criteria	Comments
1. Positive serum anti-SSA/Ro and/or anti-SSB/La or positive RF and ANA titer>1:320	
2. Labial salivary gland biopsy with focal lymphocytic sialadenitis with focus score ≥1 focus /4mm²	Focus scores are histopathologic grading systems Strongly associated with phenotypic ocular and serological component's of Sjögren's
3. Keratoconjunctivitis sicca with ocular staining score >3	Ocular staining score based on fluorescein dye examination of conjunctiva and cornea to determine clinical changes

*Classification criteria is met in patients with signs/symptoms of Sjögren's, who have at least 2 of the above features
1. *Arthritis Care & Research* 2012;64(4):475-487; 2. *Arthritis Rheum* 2011;63(7):2021-2030; 3. *Am J Ophthalmol* 2010;149(3):405-441

Signs and Symptoms

- "sicca complex": dry eyes (keratoconjunctivitis sicca/xerophthalmia), dry mouth (xerostomia)
- staphylococcal blepharitis
- dental caries, oral candidiasis, angular cheilitis (inflammation and fissuring at the labial commissures of the mouth)
- systemic complications
  - sinusitis
  - autoimmune thyroid dysfunction
  - arthralgias, arthritis
  - subclinical diffuse ILD, xerotrachea leading to chronic dry cough
  - renal disease, glomerulonephritis
  - palpable purpura, vasculitis
  - peripheral neuropathy
  - lymphoma risk greatly increased

Treatment

- ocular
  - artificial tears or surgical punctal occlusion for dry eyes
- oral
  - good dental hygiene, hydration
  - parasympathomimetic agents that stimulate salivary flow (e.g. pilocarpine)
  - topical nystatin or clotrimazole x 4-6 wk for oral candidiasis
- systemic, e.g. hydroxychloroquine, corticosteroids

Mixed Connective Tissue Disease

- syndrome with features of 3 different connective tissue diseases (e.g. SLE, scleroderma, PM)
- common symptoms: Raynaud's phenomenon, swollen fingers
- blood work: anti-RNP (see Table 10)
- treatment is generally guided by the severity of symptoms and organ system involvement
- prognosis
- 50-60% will evolve into SLE
- 40% will evolve into scleroderma
- only 10% will remain as MCTD for the rest of their lives
- cardiac involvement (arrhythmia) common, renal or lung involvement rare

Overlap Syndrome

- syndrome with sufficient diagnostic features of 2+ different connective tissue diseases

Vasculitides

- inflammation and subsequent necrosis of blood vessels leading to tissue ischemia or infarction of any organ system
- diagnosis
    - clinical suspicion: suspect in cases of unexplained multiple organ ischemia or systemic illness with no evidence of malignancy or infection; constitutional symptoms such as fever, weight loss, anorexia, fatigue
    - labs non-specific: anemia, increased WBC and ESR, abnormal U/A
    - investigations: biopsy if tissue accessible; angiography if tissue inaccessible
- treatment generally involves corticosteroids and/or immunosuppressive agents

Table 21. Classification of Vasculitis and Characteristic Features

Classification	Characteristic Features
SMALL VESSEL	
Non-ANCA-associated	Immune complex-mediated (most common mechanism)
Predominantly cutaneous vasculitis	Also known as hypersensitivity/leukocytoclastic vasculitis
IgA vasculitis (formerly Henoch-Schönlein purpura [HSP]) (see Pediatrics, P91)	Vascular deposition of IgA causing systemic vasculitis (skin, GI, renal), usually self-limiting; most common in childhood
Cryoglobulinemic vasculitis (CV)	Systemic vasculitis caused by circulating cryoproteins forming immune complexes; 60-80% of cases are due to Hepatitis C, 5-10% are due to a CTD (SLE, RA, SS), 5-10% are due to a lymphoproliferative disorder and the remaining 5-10% are idiopathic or "essential". CV may be associated with underlying infection (e.g. hepatitis C) or connective tissue disease
ANCA-associated (i.e. PR3-ANCA) Granulomatosis with polyangiitis (GPA, formerly Wegener's) pR3 (c-ANCA) > MPO (p-ANCA)	Granulomatous inflammation of vessels of respiratory tract and kidneys, initially have URTI symptoms; most common in middle age
Eosinophilic granulomatosis with polyangiitis (Churg-Strauss syndrome) (50% ANCA positive)	Granulomatous inflammation of vessels with hypereosinophilia and eosinophilic tissue infiltration, frequent lung involvement (asthma, allergic rhinitis), associated with MPO-ANCA in 40-50% of cases. Other manifestations include peripheral neuropathy (70%), GI involvement, myocarditis and rarely coronary arteritis; average age 40s
Microangiopathic polyangiitis (70% ANCA positive, usually MPO)	Pauci-immune necrotizing vasculitis, affecting kidneys (necrotizing glomerulonephritis), lungs (capillaritis and alveolar hemorrhage), skin,; most common in middle age
MEDIUM VESSEL	
Polyarteritis nodosa	Segmental, non-granulomatous necrotizing inflammation Unknown etiology in most cases, any age (average 40-50s), M>F
Kawasaki disease (see Pediatrics, P92)	Arteritis and mucocutaneous lymph node syndrome
LARGE VESSEL	
GCA/Temporal arteritis	Inflammation predominantly of the aorta and its branches >50 yr of age, F>M
Takayasu's arteritis	"Pulseless disease", unequal peripheral pulses, chronic inflammation, most often the aorta and its branches Usually young adults of Asian descent, F>M, risk of aortic aneurysm
OTHER VASCULITIDES	
Buerger's disease ("Thromboangiits Obliterans")	Inflammation and clotting of small and medium-sized arteries and veins of distal extremities, may lead to distal claudication and gangrene, most important etiologic factor is cigarette smoking. Most common in young Asian males
Behçet's disease	Multi-system disorder presenting with ocular involvement (uveitis), recurrent oral and genital ulceration, venous thrombosis, skin and joint involvement, more common in Mediterranean and Asia, average age 30 yr old, M>F
Vasculitis mimicry (i.e. pseudovasculitis)	Cholesterol emboli, atrial myxoma, bacterial endocarditis (SBE), APLS

Features of Small Vessel Vasculitis
- Palpable purpura
- Vesicles
- Chronic urticaria
- Superficial ulcers (erosions)

c-ANCA (i.e. pR3-ANCA): cytoplasmic anti-neutrophil cytoplasmic Ab associated with anti-pR3
p-ANCA (i.e. MPO-ANCA): perinuclear anti-neutrophil cytoplasmic Ab associated with multiple antigens, e.g. myeloperoxidase, lactoferrin (IBD), cathepsin, elastase etc. Of these only antibodies to myeloperoxidase have been associated with the development of vasculitis

Features of Medium Vessel Vasculitis
- Livedo reticularis
- Erythema nodosum
- Raynaud's phenomenon
- Nodules
- Digital infarcts
- Ulcers

Churg-Strauss Triad
- Allergic rhinitis and asthma (often quiescent at time of vasculitis)
- Eosinophilic infiltrative disease resembling pneumonia
- Systemic vasculitis often mononeuritis multiplex/peripheral neuropathy and peripheral eosinophilia

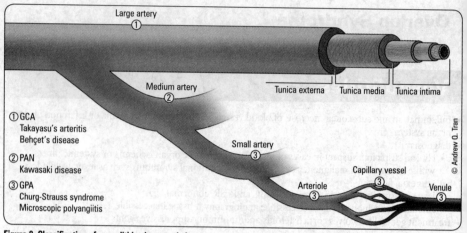

① GCA
Takayasu's arteritis
Behçet's disease

② PAN
Kawasaki disease

③ GPA
Churg-Strauss syndrome
Microscopic polyangiitis

© Andrew Q. Tran

Figure 9. Classification of vasculitides by vessel size

Small Vessel Non-ANCA Associated Vasculitis

CUTANEOUS VASCULITIS
- subdivided into
  - drug-induced vasculitis
  - serum sickness reaction
  - vasculitis associated with other underlying primary diseases (CTD, infections, malignancies-hematologic> solid tumours)

Etiology and Pathophysiology
- cutaneous vasculitis following
  - drug exposure (allopurinol, gold, sulfonamides, penicillin, phenytoin)
  - viral or bacterial infection
  - idiopathic causes
- small vessels involved (post-capillary venules most frequently)
- usually causes a leukocytoclastic vasculitis: debris from neutrophils around vessels
- sometimes due to cryoglobulins which precipitate in cold temperatures

Signs and Symptoms
- palpable purpura ± vesicles and ulceration, urticaria, macules, papules, bullae, subcutaneous nodules
  - renal or joint involvement may occur, especially in children

Investigations
- vascular involvement (both arteriole and venule) established by skin biopsy

Treatment
- stop possible offending drug
- NSAID, low dose corticosteroids
  - immunosuppressive agents in resistant cases
- usually self-limiting

Small Vessel ANCA-Associated Vasculitis

GRANULOMATOSIS WITH POLYANGIITIS
(GPA, formerly known as Wegener's Granulomatosis)

Definition
- granulomatous inflammation of vessels that may affect the upper airways (rhinitis, sinusitis), lungs (pulmonary nodules, infiltrates), and kidneys (glomerulonephritis, renal failure)
- highly associated with c-ANCA by indirect immunofluorescence (IIF) and pR3-ANCA by ELISA; however, changes in ANCA levels do not predict remission or relapse
- incidence 2-3 per 100,000; more common in Northern latitudes

Table 22. Classification Criteria for GPA*

Criteria	Description
1. Nasal or oral involvement	Inflammation, ulcers, epistaxis
2. Abnormal findings on CXR	Nodules, cavitations, etc.
3. Urinary sediment	Microscopic hematuria ± RBC casts
4. Biopsy of involved tissue	Lungs show granulomas, kidneys show necrotizing segmental glomerulonephritis

*Diagnosed if 2 or more of the above 4 criteria present   American College of Rheumatology, 1990

Classic Features of GPA
- Necrotizing granulomatous vasculitis of lower and upper respiratory tract
- Focal segmental glomerulonephritis

Etiology

- pathogenesis depends on genetic susceptibility and environmental triggers (e.g. infection)
  - dysregulated immune response due to loss of B and T-cell tolerance
  - acute vascular injury mediated by neutrophils and monocytes

Signs and Symptoms

- systemic
  - malaise, fever, weakness, weight loss
- HEENT
  - sinusitis or rhinitis, nasal crusting and bloody nasal discharge, nasoseptal perforation, saddle nose deformity
  - proptosis due to: inflammation/vasculitis involving extra-ocular muscles, granulomatous retrobulbar space occupying lesions or direct extension of masses from the upper respiratory tract
  - hearing loss due to involvement of CN VIII
- pulmonary
  - cough, hemoptysis, granulomatous upper respiratory tract masses
- renal
  - hematuria, proteinuria, elevated creatinine
- other
  - joint, skin, eye complaints, vasculitic neuropathy

Investigations

- blood work: anemia (normal MCV), increased WBC, increased Cr, increased ESR, elevated platelet count, ANCA (PR3 > MPO)
- urinalysis: proteinuria, hematuria, RBC casts
- CXR: pneumonitis, lung nodules, infiltrations, cavitary lesions
- biopsy: renal (segmental necrotizing glomerulonephritis), lung (granulomas, tracheobronchial erosion)
- c-ANCA and ESR often correlate with disease activity and used to monitor response to treatment in some patients

Treatment

- for severe, life or organ threatening disease disease
  - pulse methylprednisolone x 3 days followed by prednisone 1 mg/kg/d PO + cyclophosphamide 2 mg/kg/d PO for 36 mo OR rituximab 375 mg/m² followed by high dose MTX (20-25 mg PO/SC weekly) or azathioprine (2 mg/kg/d PO OD)
- consider plasmapheresis in patients with rapidly deteriorating renal failure or pulmonary hemorrhage

RAVE Trial
NEJM 2010;363:221-232
Rituximab equivalent or superior to cyclophosphamide in severe or relapsing disease

Medium Vessel Vasculitis

POLYARTERITIS NODOSA

Definition

- systemic, necrotizing vasculitis of medium sized vessels
- ANCA negative
- 5-10% associated with hepatitis B positivity
- incidence 0.7 per 100,000; affects individuals between 40-60 yr; M:F = 2:1

Table 23. Classification Criteria for PAN*

Criteria	Description
1. Weight loss	>4 kg, not due to dieting or other factors
2. Myalgias, weakness, or leg tenderness	Diffuse myalgias or weakness
3. Livedo reticularis	Mottled, reticular pattern over skin
4. Neuropathy	Mononeuropathy, mononeuropathy multiplex, or polyneuropathy
5. Testicular pain or tenderness	Not due to infection, trauma, or other causes
6. dBP >90 mmHg	Development of HTN with dBP >90 mmHg
7. Elevated Cr or BUN	Cr >130 μmol/L (1.5 mg/dL), BUN >14.3 mmol/L (40 mg/dL)
8. Hepatitis B positive	Presence of hepatitis B surface antigen or Ab
9. Arteriographic abnormality	Commonly aneurysms
10. Biopsy of artery	Presence of granulocytes and/or mononuclear leukocytes in the artery wall

*Diagnosed if 3 or more of the above 10 criteria present   American College of Rheumatology, 1990

Etiology and Pathophysiology

- focal panmural necrotizing inflammatory lesions in small and medium-sized arteries
- thrombosis, aneurysm, or dilatation at lesion site may occur
- healed lesions show proliferation of fibrous tissue and endothelial cells that may lead to luminal occlusion

Investigations
- blood work: CBC, ESR, Cr, BUN, p-ANCA, hepatitis B serology
- imaging: angiography
- arterial biopsy

Treatment
- prednisone 1 mg/kg/d PO and cyclophosphamide 2 mg/kg/d PO
- ± anti-viral therapy to enhance clearance of hepatitis B virus

Large Vessel Vasculitis

GCA/TEMPORAL ARTERITIS

Table 24. Classification Criteria for GCA*

Criteria	Description
1. Age at onset ≥50	
2. New H/A	Often temporal
3. Temporal artery abnormality	Temporal artery tenderness or decreased pulsations, not due to arteriosclerosis
4. Elevated ESR	ESR ≥50 mm/h
5. Abnormal artery biopsy	Mononuclear cell infiltration or granulomatous inflammation, usually with multinucleated giant cells

*Diagnosed if 3 or more of the above 5 criteria present   American College of Rheumatology, 1990

GCA Criteria
Presence of 3 or more criteria yields sensitivity of 94%, specificity of 91%

Epidemiology
- most frequent vasculitis in North America
- patients >50 yr
- F:M = 2:1
- North-South gradient (predominance in Northern Europe/US)
- affects extracranial arteries

Signs and Symptoms
- new onset temporal H/A ± scalp tenderness due to inflammation of involved portion of the temporal or occipital arteries
- sudden, painless loss of vision and/or diplopia due to narrowing of the ophthalmic or posterior ciliary arteries (PCA more common); can affect both eyes
- tongue and jaw claudication (pain in muscles of mastication on prolonged chewing)
- PMR (proximal myalgia, constitutional symptoms, elevated ESR) occurs in 30% of patients
- aortic arch syndrome (involvement of subclavian and brachial branches of aorta resulting in pulseless disease), aortic aneurysm ± rupture are late complications
- constitutional symptoms and shoulder/pelvic girdle pain and stiffness

Medical Emergency
Untreated, GCA can lead to permanent blindness in 20-25% of patients
Treat on clinical suspicion

Investigations
- diagnosis made by clinical suspicion, increased ESR, increased CRP, temporal artery biopsy, possible U/S or MRI

Treatment
- if suspect GCA, immediately start high dose prednisone 1 mg/kg in divided doses for approximately 4 wk, and then tapering prednisone as symptoms resolve; highly effective in treatment and in prevention of blindness and other vascular complications
- consider low dose ASA to help decrease visual loss

Prognosis
- increased risk of thoracic aortic aneurysm and aortic dissection
- yearly CXR ± abdominal U/S as screening

Seronegative Rheumatic Disease

Table 25. A Comparison of the Spondyloarthropathies*

Feature	Ankylosing Spondylitis (AS)	Psoriatic Arthritis (PsA)	Reactive Arthritis (ReA)	Enteropathic Arthritis (EA)
M:F	3:1	1:1	8:1	1:1
Age of Onset	20s	35-45	20s	Any
Peripheral Arthritis	25%	96%	90%	Common
Distribution	Axial, LE	Any	LE	LE
Sacroiliitis	100%	40%	80%	20%
Dactylitis	Uncommon	Common	Occasional	Uncommon
Enthesitis	Common	Common	Common	Less Common
Skin Lesions	Rare	100% Psoriasis eventually 70% at onset of arthritis	Occasional Keratoderma blennorrhagica	Occasional Pyoderma, erythema nodosum
Uveitis	Common	Occasional	20%	Rare
Urethritis	Rare	Uncommon	Common	Rare
HLA-B27	90-95%	40%	80%	30%

LE = lower extremities   *Spondylarthropathy: inflammatory joint disease of the vertebral column

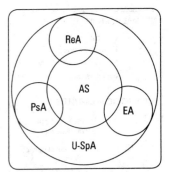

Figure 10. Spondyloarthropathy subsets

AS shares some features with the other three types of seronegative spondyloarthopathies such as ReA, EA, PsA and undifferentiated spondyloarthropathy (U-PSA)

Ankylosing Spondylitis

Definition
- chronic inflammatory arthritis involving the sacroiliac joints and vertebrae
- enthesitis is a major feature
- prototypical spondyloarthropathy

Table 26. ASAS Classification Criteria for Axial Spondyloarthritis*

Sacroiliitis on Imaging plus ≥1 AS Feature or HLA-B27 Positive plus ≥2 AS Features

AS Features	Sacroiliitis on Imaging
HLA-B27 positive	Active (acute) inflammation on MRI highly suggestive of sacroiliitis associated with AS
Inflammatory back pain	Definite radiographic sacroiliitis ≥ grade 2 bilaterally or grade 3-4 unilaterally
Arthritis	
Enthesitis (heel)	
Uveitis	
Dactylitis	
Psoriasis	
Crohn's disease/colitis	
Good response to NSAIDs	
Family history of AS	
Elevated CRP	

*For patients with ≥3 mo back pain and age at onset <45 yr

Enthesitis: inflammation of tendon or ligament at site of attachment to bone

Consider AS in the differential for causes of aortic regurgitation

Rule of 2s
AS occurs in
0.2% of the general population
2% of HLA-B27 positive individuals
20% of HLA-B27 positive individuals with affected family member

Etiology and Pathophysiology
- inflammation → osteopenia → erosion → ossification → osteoproliferation (syndesmophytes)

Epidemiology
- M:F = 3:1; females have milder disease which may be under-recognized and more peripheral arthritis and upper spine spondylitis
- 90-95% of patients have HLA-B27 (9% HLA-B27 positive in general population)

Table 27. Types of Back Pain

Parameter	Mechanical	Inflammatory
Past History	±	++
Family History	–	+
Onset	Acute	Insidious
Age	15-90 yr	<45 yr
Sleep Disturbance	±	++ (worse during 2nd half of night)
Morning Stiffness	<30 min	>1 h
Involvement of Other Systems	–	+
Exercise	Worse	Better
Rest	Better	Worse
Radiation of Pain	Anatomic (L5-S1)	Diffuse (thoracic, buttock)
Sensory Symptoms	+	–
Motor Symptoms	+	–

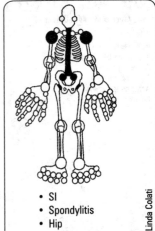

- SI
- Spondylitis
- Hip
- Shoulder

© Linda Colati

Figure 11. Common sites of involvement of AS

The **Bath Ankylosing Spondylitis Disease Activity Index (BASDAI)** is a self-reported scoring system that focuses on fatigue, axial pain, peripheral pain, enthesitis, and morning stiffness

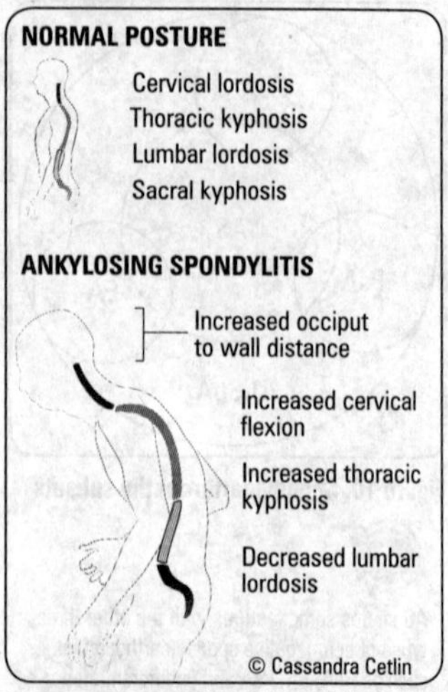

Figure 12. AS postural change

FABER (Flexion, ABduction, and External Rotation) Test
Passively flex, abduct, then gently externally rotate the leg. If pain is elicited during this movement, the location of the pain may help determine the location of the patient's pathology (e.g. hip joint, sacroiliac joint)

Modified Schöber Test
Patient must be standing erect with normal posture
Mark an imaginary line connecting both posterior superior iliac spines (close to the dimples of Venus)
The next mark is placed 10 cm above
The patient bends forward maximally: measure the difference
Report the increase (in cm to the nearest 0.1 cm)
The better of two tries is recorded

Extra-Articular Manifestations of AS

6 As
Atlanto-axial subluxation
Anterior uveitis
Apical lung fibrosis
Aortic incompetence
Amyloidosis (kidneys)
Autoimmune bowel disease (ulcerative colitis)

Both AS and EA feature symmetric sacroiliitis

Signs and Symptoms
- **axial**
  - mid and lower back stiffness, morning stiffness >1 h, night pain, persistent buttock pain, painful sacroiliac joint (+ FABER test)
  - spinal restriction (decreased ROM): lumbar (decreased Schöber), thoracic (decreased chest wall expansion, normal >5 cm at T4), cervical (global decrease, often extension first)
  - postural changes: decreased lumbar lordosis + increased thoracic kyphosis + increased cervical flexion = increased occiput to wall distance (>5 cm)
- **peripheral**
  - asymmetrical large joint arthritis, most often involving lower limb
  - enthesitis: tenderness over tibial tuberosity, or Achilles tendon and plantar fascia insertions into the calcaneus
- **extra-articular manifestations**
  - ophthalmic: acute anterior uveitis is common (25-30% patients)
  - renal: amyloidosis (late and rare), IgA nephropathy
  - gastrointestinal: IBD
  - cardiac: aortitis, aortic regurgitation, pericarditis, conduction disturbances, heart failure (rare)
  - respiratory: apical fibrosis (rare)
  - neurologic: cauda equina syndrome (rare)
  - skin: psoriasis

Investigations
- x-ray of SI joint: "pseudowidening" of joint due to erosion with joint sclerosis → bony fusion (late), symmetric sacroiliitis
- x-ray of spine: "squaring of edges" from erosion and sclerosis on corners of vertebral bodies (shiny corner sign) leading to ossification of outer fibres of annulus fibrosis (bridging syndesmophytes) → "bamboo spine" radiographically
- MRI of spine: assess activity in early disease; detection of cartilage changes, bone marrow edema, bone erosions, and subchondral bone changes. Best seen on T2 STIR (short tau inversion recovery) images (suppress fat and see bone edema)

Treatment
- **non-pharmacological therapy**
  - prevent fusion from poor posture and disability through: exercise (e.g. swimming), postural and deep breathing exercises, outpatient PT, smoking cessation
- **pharmalogical therapy**
  - NSAIDs (first line of treatment)
  - glucocorticoids (topical eye drops, local injections)
  - DMARDs only for peripheral arthritis (sulfasalazine, MTX)
  - anti-TNF agents for axial and peripheral involvement
  - manage extra-articular manifestations
- **surgical therapy**
  - hip replacement, vertebral osteotomy for marked deformity

Prognosis
- spontaneous remissions and relapses are common and can occur at any age
- function may be excellent despite spinal deformity
- favourable prognosis if female and age of onset >40 yr
- early onset with hip disease may lead to severe disability; may require arthroplasty

Enteropathic Arthritis

- see Gastroenterology, *Inflammatory Bowel Disease*, G19
- MSK manifestations in the setting of either ulcerative colitis or Crohn's disease include peripheral arthritis (large joint, asymmetrical), spondylitis, and hypertrophic osteoarthropathy
- non-arthritic MSK manifestations can occur 2° to steroid treatment of bowel inflammation (arthralgia, myalgia, osteoporosis, AVN)
- NSAIDs should be used cautiously as they may exacerbate bowel disease

Table 28. Comparing Features of Spondylitis vs. Peripheral Arthritis in EA

Parameter	Spondylitis	Peripheral Arthritis
HLA-B27 Association	Yes	No
Gender	M>F	M=F
Onset Before IBD	Yes	No
Parallels IBD Course	No	Yes
Type of IBD	UC=CD	CD

Psoriatic Arthritis

Definition
- arthritic inflammation associated with psoriasis

Etiology and Pathophysiology
- unclear but many genetic, immunologic, and some environmental factors involved (e.g. bacterial, viral, and trauma)

Epidemiology
- psoriasis affects 1% of population
- arthropathy in 15% of patients with psoriasis
- 15-20% of patients will develop joint disease before skin lesions appear

Signs and Symptoms
- **dermatologic**
  - well-demarcated erythematous plaques with silvery scale
  - nail involvement: pitting, transverse or longitudinal ridging, discolouration, subungual hyperkeratosis, onycholysis, and oil drops
- **musculoskeletal**
  - 5 general patterns
    - asymmetric oligoarthritis (most common – 70%)
    - arthritis of DIP joints with nail changes
    - destructive in small joints
    - symmetric polyarthritis (similar to RA)
    - sacroiliitis and spondylitis (usually older, male patients)
  - other findings: dactylitis, enthesopathy
- **ophthalmic**
  - conjunctivitis, iritis (anterior uveitis)
- **cardiac and respiratory** (late findings)
  - aortic insufficiency
  - apical lung fibrosis
  - neurologic
  - cauda equina syndrome
- **radiologic**
  - floating syndesmophytes
  - pencil-in-cup appearance at IP joints
  - osteolysis, periostitis

Check "hidden" areas for psoriatic lesions (ears, hair line, umbilicus, gluteal cleft, nails) TNF-α inhibitors are effective treatments for PsA with no important added risks associated with their short-term use

Treatment
- treat skin lesions (e.g. steroid cream, salicylic and/or retinoic acid, tar, UV light)
- NSAIDs or IA steroids
- DMARDs, biologic therapies to minimize erosive disease (use early if peripheral joint involvement)

Table 29. CASPAR Criteria for PsA*

Criterion	Description
1. Evidence of psoriasis	Current, past, or family history
2. Psoriatic nail dystrophy	Onycholysis, pitting, hyperkeratosis
3. Negative results for RF	
4. Dactylitis	Current or past history
5. Radiological evidence	Juxta articular bone formation on hand or foot x-rays

* To meet the CASPAR (ClASsification criteria for Psoriatic ARthritis) criteria, a patient must have inflammatory articular disease (joint, spine, or entheseal) with ≥3 points from the above 5 categories
Arthritis Rheum 2006 Aug;54(8):2665-73. Classification criteria for PsA: development

Reactive Arthritis

Definition
- one of the seronegative spondyloarthropathies in which patients have a peripheral arthritis (≥1 mo duration) accompanied by one or more extra-articular manifestations that appears shortly after certain infections of the GI or GU tracts
- this term should not be confused with rheumatic fever or viral arthritides.

Etiology
- onset following an infectious episode either involving the GI or GU tract
  - GI: *Shigella, Salmonella, Campylobacter, Yersinia, C. Difficile* species
  - GU: *Chlamydia* (isolated in 16-44% of ReA cases), *Mycoplasma* species

- acute clinical course
  - 1-4 wk post-infection
  - lasts weeks to years
  - often recurring
  - spinal involvement persists

Epidemiology
- in HLA-B27 patients, axial > peripheral involvement
- M>F

Clinical Triad of Reactive Arthritis
- Arthritis
- Conjunctivitis/uveitis
- Urethritis/cervicitis

"Can't see, can't pee, can't climb a tree"
Triad of conjunctivitis, urethritis, and arthritis is 99% specific (but 51% sensitive) for ReA

Signs and Symptoms
- **musculoskeletal**
  - peripheral arthritis, asymmetric pattern, spondylitis, Achilles tendinitis, plantar fasciitis, dactylitis
- **ophthalmic**
  - iritis (anterior uveitis), conjunctivitis
- **dermatologic**
  - keratoderma blennorrhagicum (hyperkeratotic skin lesions on palms and soles) and balanitis circinata (small, shallow, painless ulcers of glans penis and urethral meatus) are diagnostic
- **gastrointestinal**
  - oral ulcers, diarrhea
- **urethritis and cervicitis**
  - sterile pyuria; presence not related to site of initiating infection

Investigations
- diagnosis is clinical plus laboratory
- blood work: normocytic, normochromic anemia, and leukocytosis
- sterile cultures
- serology: HLA-B27 positive

Treatment
- antibiotics for non-articular infections
- NSAIDs, physical therapy, exercise
- local therapy
  - joint protection
  - IA steroid injection
  - topical steroid for ocular involvement
- systemic therapy
  - corticosteroids, sulfasalazine, MTX (for peripheral joint involvement only)
  - TNF-α inhibitors for spinal inflammation

Prognosis
- self-limited, typically 3-5 mo, varies based on pathogen and patient's genetic background
- chronic in 15-20% of cases

Crystal-Induced Arthropathies

Table 30. Gout vs. Pseudogout

Parameter	Gout	Pseudogout
Gender	M>F	M=F
Age	Middle-aged males	
Post-menopausal females	Age >60 yr	
Onset of Disease	Acute	Acute/insidious
Crystal Type	Monosodium urate	CPPD
	Negative birefringence (yellow when parallel to compensator filter), needle-shaped	Positive birefringence (blue when parallel), rhomboid-shaped
Distribution	First MTP classically; also midfoot, ankle, knee, or polyarticular	Knee, wrist; monoarticular, or polyarticular if chronic
Radiology (note findings are non-specific)	Erosions	Chondrocalcinosis OA (knee, wrist, 2nd and 3rd MCP)
Treatment	Acute: NSAIDs, corticosteroids, colchicine Chronic: ± allopurinol, fuboxostat	NSAIDs, corticosteroids

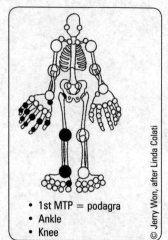

- 1st MTP = podagra
- Ankle
- Knee

Figure 13. Common sites of involvement of gout (asymmetric joint involvement)

© Jerry Won, after Linda Colati

Gout

Definition
- derangement in purine metabolism resulting in hyperuricemia; monosodium urate crystal deposits in tissues (tophi) and synovium (microtophi)

Etiology and Pathophysiology
- uric acid can be obtained from the diet or made endogenously by xanthine oxidase, which converts xanthine to uric acid
- an excess of uric acid results in hyperuricemia
- uric acid can deposit in the tissues (tophi), synovium (microtophi) and bones, where they can crystalize to form monsodium urate crystals that lead to gout
- both modifiable and non-modifiable risk factors contribute to gout
- non-modifiable risk factors include: genetic mutations, male gender and advanced age
- modifiable risk factors include: diet (alcohol, purine rich foods such as meats and seafoods, fructose/sugar sweetened foods (see list of precipitants below)
- other risk factors: renal failure, metabolic syndrome, diuretics

Clinical Features
- single episode progressing to recurrent episodes of acute inflammatory arthritis
- **acute gouty arthritis**
  - severe pain, redness, joint swelling, usually involving lower extremities
  - joint mobility may be limited
  - attack will subside spontaneously within several days to weeks; may recur
- **tophi**
  - urate deposits on cartilage, tendons, bursae, soft tissues, and synovial membranes
  - common sites: first MTP, ear helix, olecranon bursae, tendon insertions (common in Achilles tendon)
- **kidney**
  - gouty nephropathy
  - uric acid calculi

Investigations
- joint aspirate: >90% of joint aspirates show crystals of monosodium urate (negatively birefringent, needle-shaped)
- x-rays may show tophi as soft tissue swelling, punched-out lesions, erosion with "over-hanging"
- correlated with hyperuricemia in the blood
- may see elevated WBC and ESR (nonspecific)

Treatment
- **acute gout**
  - NSAIDs: high dose, then taper as symptoms improve
  - corticosteroids: IA, oral, or intra-muscular (if renal, cardiovascular, or GI disease and/or if NSAIDs contraindicated or failed)
  - colchicine within first 12 h but effectiveness limited by narrow therapeutic range
  - allopurinol can worsen an acute attack (do not start during acute flare)
- **chronic gout**
  - conservative
    - avoid foods with high purine content (e.g. visceral meats, sardines, shellfish, beans, peas)
    - avoid drugs with hyperuricemic effects (e.g. pyrazinamide, ethambutol, thiazide, alcohol)
  - medical
    - antihyperuricemic drugs (allopurinol and febuxostat): decrease uric acid production by inhibiting xanthine oxidase
    - uricosuric drugs (probenecid, sulfinpyrazone): very rarely used in combination with allopurinol or febuxostat in patients in whom hyperuricemia is not controlled with the latter
  - prophylaxis prior to starting antihyperuricemic drugs (colchicine/low-dose NSAID)
  - in renal disease secondary to hyperuricemia, use low-dose allopurinol and monitor Cr
- indications for treatment with antihyperuricemic medications include
  - recurrent attacks (more than 2-3/yr), tophi, bone erosions, urate kidney stones
  - perhaps in renal dysfunction with very high urate load (controversial)

Pseudogout (Calcium Pyrophosphate Dihydrate Disease)

Definition
- joint inflammation caused by calcium pyrophosphate crystals

Etiology and Pathophysiology
- acute inflammatory arthritis due to phagocytosis of IgG-coated CPPD crystals by neutrophils and subsequent release of inflammatory mediators within joint space
- more frequently polyarticular
- slower in onset in comparison to gout, lasts up to 3 wk but is self-limited

An acute gout attack may mimic cellulitis; however, joint mobility is usually preserved in cellulitis unless it overlaps a joint

Precipitants of Gout

Drugs are FACT
Furosemide
Aspirin® (low dose)/Alcohol
Cytotoxic drugs (cyclosporine)
Thiazide diuretics

Foods are SALT
Seafood
Alcohol (beer and spirits)
Liver and kidney
Turkey (meat)

The majority of people with hyperuricemia do not have gout
Normal or low uric acid levels do not rule out gout

10 Recommendations on the Diagnosis and Management of Gout
Ann of Rheum Dis 2013;73:328-335
1. Identification of monosodium urate crystals should be performed for a definitive diagnosis of gout.
2. Gout/hyperuricemia should prompt investigations of renal function and CV risk factors.
3. Acute gout should be treated with colchicine, NSAIDs, and/or glucocorticoids.
4. Patients should be counselled about lifestyle.
5. Allopurinol is first line for urate lowering therapy, with uricosurics as second line.
6. Patients should be informed about the risk of acute gout flare with initiation of urate lowering therapy; colchicine prophylaxis should be considered.
7. Allopurinol can be used in patients with mild/moderate renal impairment with slow titration and monitoring.
8. Treatment goal is urate <0.36 mM and absence of attacks and resolution of tophi.
9. Tophi should be treated medically by lowering serum urate to <0.3 mM. Surgery is only for select cases.
10. Prophylactic pharmacological management of asymptomatic hyperuricemia is not recommended.

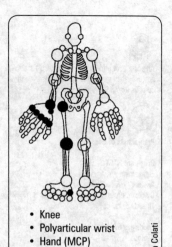

- Knee
- Polyarticular wrist
- Hand (MCP)
- Foot (1st MTP)
- Hip

© Linda Colati

Figure 14. Common sites of involvement of CCPD

Risk Factors
- old age, advanced OA, neuropathic joints
- other associated conditions: hyperparathyroidism, hypothyroidism, hypomagnesemia, hypophosphatasia (low ALP), DM, hemochromatosis

Signs and Symptoms
- affects knees, wrists, MCPs, hips, shoulders, elbows, ankles, big toe
- multiple manifestations
- asymptomatic crystal deposition (seen on radiograph only)
- acute crystal arthritis (self-limited flares of acute inflammatory arthritis resembling gout)
- pseudo-OA (progressive joint degeneration, sometimes with episodes of acute inflammatory arthritis)
- pseudo-RA (symmetrical polyarticular pattern with morning stiffness and constitutional symptoms)
- acute may be triggered by dehydration, acute illness, surgery, trauma

Investigations
- must aspirate joint to rule out septic arthritis, gout
- CPPD crystals: present in 60% of patients, often only a few crystals, positive birefringence (blue) and rhomboid shaped
- x-rays show chondrocalcinosis in 75%: radiodensities in fibrocartilaginous structures (e.g. knee menisci) or linear radiodensities in hyaline articular cartilage

Treatment
- joint aspiration, rest, and protection
- NSAIDs: also used for maintenance therapy
- prophylactic colchicine PO (controversial)
- IA or oral steroids to relieve inflammation

Non-Articular Rheumatism

Definition
- disorders that primarily affect soft tissues or periarticular structures
- includes bursitis, tendinitis, tenosynovitis, fibromyalgia, and PMR

Polymyalgia Rheumatica

Definition
- characterized by pain and stiffness of the proximal extremities (girdle area)
- closely related to GCA (15% of patients with PMR develop GCA)
- no muscle weakness

Table 31. PMR Classification Criteria Scoring Algorithm*

	Points without U/S (0-6)	Points with Abnormal U/S** (0-8)
Morning stiffness duration >45 min	2	2
Hip pain or limited ROM	1	1
Absence of RF or ACPA	2	2
Absence of other joint involvement	1	1
At least one shoulder with subdeltoid and/or biceps tenosynovitis and/or glenohumeral synovitis (either posterior or axillary) and at least one hip with synovitis and/or trochanteric bursitis on U/S	N/A	1
Both shoulders with subdeltoid bursitis, biceps tenosynovitis, or gleno-humeral synovitis on U/S	N/A	1

*Required criteria: age ≥50 yr, bilateral shoulder aching, and abnormal ESR/CRP
**A score of 4 or more is categorized as PMR in the algorithm without U/S and a score of 5 or more is categorized as PMR in the algorithm with U/S
**Optional U/S criteria
Ann Rheum Dis 2012;71:484-492

Epidemiology
- incidence 50 per 100,000 per year in those >50 yr
- age of onset typically >50 yr, F:M = 2:1

Signs and Symptoms
- constitutional symptoms prominent (fever, weight loss, malaise)
- pain and stiffness of symmetrical proximal muscles (neck, shoulder and hip girdles, thighs)
- gel phenomenon (stiffness after prolonged inactivity)
- physical exam reveals tender muscles, but no weakness or atrophy

Investigations

- blood work: often shows anemia, elevated platelets, elevated ESR and CRP, and normal CK; up to 5% of PMR reported with normal inflammatory markers

Treatment

- goal of therapy: symptom relief
- start with prednisone dose of 15-20 mg PO OD, reconsider diagnosis if no response within several days
- taper slowly over 1 yr period with closely monitoring
- relapses should be diagnosed and treated on clinical basis; do not treat a rise in ESR as a relapse
- treat relapses aggressively (50% relapse rate)
- monitor for steroid side effects, glucocorticoid-induced osteoporosis prevention, and follow for symptoms of GCA

Fibromyalgia

Definition

- chronic (>3 mo), widespread (axial, left- and right-sided, upper and lower segment), non-articular pain with characteristic tender points

Diagnosis

Table 32. 2010 ACR Preliminary Diagnostic Criteria for Fibromyalgia

Criteria	Comments

Widespread Pain Index = number of areas in which the patient had pain over the last week (max score = 19):
    L and R: shoulder girdle, upper arm, lower arm, hip, upper leg, lower leg, jaw
    One Area: chest, abdomen, upper back, lower back, neck
 	
 Symptom Severity Score = sum of:
  a) severity of fatigue
  b) waking unrefreshed
  c) cognitive symptoms over the past week
  d) extent of somatic symptoms (IBS, H/A, abdominal pain/cramps, dry mouth, fever, hives, ringing in ears, vomiting, heartburn, dry eyes, SOB, loss of appetite, rash, hair loss, easy bruising, etc.)
 all (a-d) rated on 0-3 scale: 0 = no problem, 1 = mild, 2 = moderate, 3 = severe
	A patient satisfies diagnostic criteria for fibromyalgia if the following 3 conditions are met:
	 1. Widespread Pain Index (WPI) ≥7 and Symptom Severity (SS) scale score ≥5 or WPI 3–6 and SS scale score ≥9
	 2. Symptoms have been present at a similar level for at least 3 mo
	 3. The patient does not have a disorder that would otherwise explain the pain

Arthritis Care and Research 2010;62(5):600-610

Epidemiology

- F:M = 3:1
- primarily ages 25-45 yr, some adolescents
- prevalence of 2-5% in general population
- overlaps with chronic fatigue syndrome and myofascial pain syndrome
- strong association with psychiatric illness

Signs and Symptoms

- widespread aching, stiffness
- easy fatigability
- sleep disturbance: non-restorative sleep, difficulty falling asleep, and frequent wakening
- symptoms aggravated by physical activity, poor sleep, emotional stress
- patient feels that joints are diffusely swollen although joint examination is normal
- neurologic symptoms of hyperalgesia, paresthesias
- associated with irritable bowel or bladder syndrome, migraines, tension H/As, restless leg syndrome, obesity, depression, and anxiety
- physical exam should reveal only tenderness with palpation of soft tissues, with no specificity for trigger/tender points

Investigations

- blood work: includes TSH and ESR; all typically normal unless unrelated, underlying illness present
- serology: do not order ANA or RF unless there is clinical suspicion for a connective tissue disease
- laboratory sleep assessment

Differential Diagnosis

- diagnosis of exclusion
- rule out other disorders by history and physical exam (RA, SLE, PMR, myositis, hypothyroidism, hyperparathyroidism, neuropathies)

Treatment
- **non-pharmacological therapy**
  - education
  - exercise program (walking, aquatic exercises), physical therapy (good posture, stretching, muscle strengthening, massage)
  - stress reduction, CBT
  - no evidence for alternative medicine such as biofeedback, meditation, acupuncture
- **pharmacological therapy**
  - low dose tricyclic antidepressant (e.g. amitriptyline)
    - ◆ for sleep restoration
    - ◆ select those with lower anticholinergic side effects
  - SNRI: duloxetine, milnacipran
  - anticonvulsant: pregabalin, gabapentin
  - analgesics may be beneficial for pain that interferes with sleep (NSAIDs, not narcotics)

Prognosis
- variable; usually chronic, unless diagnosed and treated early

Table 33. Clinical Features of Inflammatory Myopathy vs. Polymyalgia Rheumatica vs. Fibromyalgia

	Polymyositis	PMR	Fibromyalgia
Epidemiology	F > M, 40-50 yrs	F > M, > 50 yrs	F > M, 25-45 yrs
Muscle involvement	Proximal muscle	Proximal muscle	Diffuse
Weakness	Yes	No	No
Pain	Painless	Painful	Painful
Stiffness	Mild	Significant morning and gelling stiffness (shoulders, neck, hips)	None
Investigations	Muscle biopsy, CK, EMG, R/O malignancy	ESR/CRP, R/O giant cell arteritis	Sleep assessment, TSH
ESR/CRP	Usually normal	Markedly elevated	Normal
Treatment	High dose steroids, immuno-suppressants	Low dose steroids	Exercise, TCAs, SNRIs, anticonvulsants

Common Medications

Table 34. Common Medications for Osteoarthritis

Class	Generic Drug Name	Trade Name	Dosing (PO)	Indications	Contraindications	Adverse Effects
Analgesic	acetaminophen	Tylenol®	500 mg tid q4h (3 g daily max)	1st line		Hepatotoxicity Overdose Potentiates warfarin
NSAIDs	ibuprofen diclofenac diclofenac/misoprostol naproxen meloxicam	Advil®, Motrin® Voltaren® Arthrotec® Naprosyn®, Aleve® Mobicox®	200-600 mg tid 25-50 mg tid 50-75/200 mg tid 125-500 mg bid 7.5-15 mg OD	2nd line	GI bleed Renal impairment Allergy to ASA, NSAIDs Pregnancy (T3)	Nausea, tinnitus, vertigo, rash, dyspepsia, GI bleed, PUD, hepatitis, renal failure, HTN, nephrotic syndrome
COX-2 INHIBITORS						
	celecoxib	Celebrex®	200 mg OD	High risk for GI bleed: age >65 Hx of GI bleed, PUD	Renal impairment Sulfa allergy (celecoxib) Cardiovascular disease	Delayed ulcer healing Renal/hepatic impairment Rash

Other Treatments	Comments
Combination analgesics (acetaminophen + codeine, acetaminophen + NSAIDs)	Enhanced short-term effect compared to acetaminophen alone More adverse effects: sedation, constipation, nausea, GI upset
IA corticosteroid injection	Short-term (weeks-months) decrease in pain and improvement in function Used for management of an IA inflammatory process when infection has been ruled out
IA hyaluronic acid q6mo	Used for mild-moderate OA of the knees, however little supporting evidence, and not considered to be effective Precaution with chicken/egg allergy
Topical NSAIDs	25% wt/wt topical diclofenac (Pennsaid®) May use for patients who fail acetaminophen treatment and who wish to avoid systemic therapy
Capsaicin cream	Mild decrease in pain
Glucosamine sulfate ± chondroitin	Limited clinical studies. No regulation by Health Canada

Table 35. Disease Modifying Anti-Rheumatic Drugs (DMARDs)

Generic Drug Name	Trade Name	Dosing	Contraindications	Adverse Effects
COMMONLY USED				
hydroxychloroquine $	Plaquenil®	400 mg PO OD initially 200-400 mg PO OD maintenance (6.5 mg/kg ideal body weight per day)	Retinal disease, G6PD deficiency	GI symptoms, skin rash, macular damage, neuromyopathy Requires regular ophthalmological screening to monitor for retinopathy
sulfasalazine $	Salazopyrim® Azulfidine® (US)	1000 mg PO bid-tid	Sulfa/ASA allergy, kidney disease, G6PD deficiency	GI symptoms, rash, H/A, leukopenia
methotrexate $	Rheumatrex® Folex/Mexate®	7.5-25 mg PO/ IM/SC qweekly	Bone marrow suppression, liver disease, significant lung disease, immunodeficiency, pregnancy, EtOH abuse	Oral ulcers, GI symptoms, cirrhosis, myelosuppression, pneumonitis, tubular necrosis
leflunomide $$	Arava®	10-20 mg PO OD	Liver disease	Alopecia, GI symptoms, liver dysfunction, pulmonary infiltrates
NOT COMMONLY USED				
cyclosporine $$	Neoral®	2.5-3 mg/kg/d divided and given in 2 doses PO	Kidney/liver disease, infection, HTN	HTN, decreased renal function, hair growth, tremors, bleeding
gold (injectable) $	Solganal® Myocrysine®	50 mg IM q1wk after gradual introduction	IBD, kidney/liver disease	Rash, mouth soreness/ulcers, proteinuria, marrow suppression
azathioprine $	Imuran®	2/5 mg/kg/d PO once daily	Kidney/liver disease TPMT deficiency	Rash, pancytopenia (especially ↓ WBC, ↑ AST, ALT), biliary stasis, vomiting, diarrhea
cyclophosphamide $	Cytoxan®	1 g/m²/mo IV as per protocol	Kidney/liver disease	Cardiotoxicity, GI symptoms, hemorrhagic cystitis, nephrotoxicity, bone marrow suppression, sterility

Generic Drug Name	Trade Name	Dosing	Mechanism of Action
NEWER DMARDs (Biologics)			
etanercept $$$	Enbrel®	25 mg biweekly or 50 mg weekly SC	Fusion protein of TNF receptor and Fc portion of IgG
infliximab $$$	Remicade®	3-5 mg/kg IV q8wk	Chimeric mouse/human monoclonal anti-TNF
adalimumab $$$	Humira®	40 mg SC q2wk	Monoclonal anti-TNF
golimumab $$$	Simponi®	50 mg SC q mo	Monoclonal anti-TNF
certolizumab $$$	Cimzia®	400 mg SC q2wk x3 then 200 mg SC q4wk	PEGylated monoclonal anti-TNF
Apremilast $$$	Otezla®	Day 1: 10mg (AM), titrate up to 30mg BID by Day 6	Inhibitor of PDE4 which inhibits production of TNF alpha
abatacept $$$	Orencia®	IV infusion	Costimulation modulator of T-cell activation
rituximab $$$	Rituxan®	2 IV infusions, 2 wk apart	Causes B-cell depletion, binds to CD20
tocilizumab $$$	Actemra®	4-8 mg/kg IV q4wk	Interleukin-6 receptor antagonist
Tofacitinib	Xeljanz®	5mg BID	Inhibits the JAK enzyme and thus interferes with JAK-STAT signaling pathway

Risks of Biologics
Reactivation of TB or hepatitis B. Patients require negative TB skin test, chest x-ray and negative hepatitis B virus serology prior to starting any of these medications
Increased risk of: serious infections, worsening heart failure, multiple sclerosis, and positive auto-antibodies

Landmark Rheumatology Trials

Trial	Reference	Results
RHEUMATOID ARTHRITIS		
ATTEST	*Ann Rheum Dis* 2008; 67:1096-103	Abatacept and infliximab have similar efficacy in RA patients who have failed MTX
ATTRACT	*Lancet* 1999; 354:1932-9	Infliximab and MTX combined are more effective than MTX alone for patients with active RA
CIMESTRA	*Arthritis Rheum* 2006; 54:1401-9	Combination of MTX and sulfasalazine is superior to either alone
COMET	*Lancet* 2008; 372:375-82	Etanercept add-on therapy increases rates of remission in early RA
ERA	*NEJM* 2000; 343:1586-93	Etanercept more rapidly decreases symptoms in early RA compared to MTX
European Leflunomide Study Group	*Lancet* 1999; 353:259-66	Leflunomide is equal in efficacy to sulphasalazine and superior to placebo
FIN-RACo	*Lancet* 1999; 353:1568-73	Combination therapy with DMARDs improves remission rates in early RA
Infliximab and MTX	*NEJM* 2000; 343:1594-602	Infliximab combined with MTX reduces joint damage in RA
Leflunomide Rheumatoid Arthritis Investigators Group	*Arch Intern Med* 1999; 159:2542-50	Leflunomide is equivalent to MTX therapy and superior to placebo
PREMIER	*Arthritis Rheum* 2006; 54:26-37	Combination therapy with adalimumab and MTX is superior to either alone in patients with early RA
Swefot	*Lancet* 2009; 374:459-66	Anti-TNF agents are more effective second-line therapy than DMARDs in patients who fail MTX
OSTEOARTHRITIS		
GAIT	*NEJM* 2006; 354:795-808	Glucosamine, chondroitin, and the combination of both are no more effective than placebo in treatment of knee OA
Hyaluronan	*Ann Rheum Dis* 2010; 69:1097-102	Hyaluronan injections do not improve disease activity in patients with moderate-severe knee OA
SLE		
Belimumab	*Lancet* 2011; 377:721-31	Treatment with belimumab reduces the incidence of BILAG A and B flares in patients with SLE compared to placebo
BILAG open-RCT	*Rheumatology* 2010; 49:723-32	Low dose cyclosporine and azathioprine are equivalent in efficacy as maintenance therapy for SLE
Mycophenylate mofetil or intravenous cyclophosphamide	*NEJM* 2005; 353:2219-28	Mycophenylate mofetil is more efficacious than cyclophosphamide in inducing remission of SLE nephritis
CONNECTIVE TISSUE DISEASES		
Azathioprine or MTX maintenance for ANCA-associated vasculitis	*NEJM* 2008; 359:2790-803	MTX and azathioprine are equally safe and effective as maintenance agents in ANCA vasculitis
Cyclophosphamide in scleroderma lung disease	*NEJM* 2006; 354:2655-66	Cyclophosphamide therapy leads to transient improvements in lung function, skin scores, and overall health in patients with scleroderma
Etanercept plus standard therapy for granulomatosis with polyangiitis	*NEJM* 2005; 352:351-61	Etanercept is not effective in inducing remission in patients with ANCA vasculitis
Mycophenylate mofetil vs. azathioprine for maintenance in ANCA-associated vasculitis	*JAMA* 2010; 304:2381-8	Mycophenylate mofetil is less effective than azathioprine for maintaining disease in ANCA-associated vasculitis
Rituximab versus cyclophosphamide for ANCA-associated vasculitis	*NEJM* 2010; 363:221-32	Rituximab is not inferior to cyclophosphamide for induction of remission in ANCA vasculitis
GOUT		
Febuxostat vs. allopurinol	*NEJM* 2005; 353:2450-61	Febuxostat is more effective than allopurinol at lowering serum urate, and has similar effectiveness on flare reduction
ANKYLOSING SPONDYLITIS		
Adalimumab	*Arthritis Rheum* 2006; 54:2136-46	Adalimumab induced partial remission in 22% of AS patients
ASSERT (rituximab)	*Arthritis Rheum* 2005; 52:582-91	Sixty percent of patients treated with rituximab had a clinical response to the medication
ATLAS (adalimumab)	*J Rheumatol* 2008; 35:1346-53	Compared to placebo, adalimumab significantly reduces pain and fatigue in AS patients
Infliximab in AS	*Lancet* 2002; 359:1187-93	Infliximab induces regression of symptoms in 50% of patients and is superior to placebo
SPINE (etanercept)	*Ann Rheum Dis* 2011; 70:799-804	Etanercept has short-term efficacy for patients with advanced AS and reduces disease severity
Sulfasalazine	*Arthritis Rheum* 1995; 38:618-27	Sulfasalazine is superior to placebo in treatment of patients with seronegative spondyloarthropathy

References

ACR. Guidelines for the medical management of osteoarthritis of the hip. November 1995.

ACR. Guidelines for the medical management of osteoarthritis of the knee. November 1995.

ACR. Guidelines for referral and management of systemic lupus erythematosus in adults. September 1999.

ACR Subcommittee on Rheumatoid Arthritis Guidelines, 2002. Guidelines for the management of rheumatoid arthritis, 2002 Update.

Aletaha D, Neogi T, Silman AJ, et al. 2010 rheumatoid arthritis classification criteria. Arthritis Rheum 2010;62:2569-2581.

Arnett FC, Edworthy SM, Bloch DA, et al. The American Rheumatism Association 1987 revised criteria for the classification of rheumatoid arthritis. Arthritis Rheum 1988;31:315-324.

American College of Rheumatology Subcommittee on Rheumatoid Arthritis Guidelines. Guidelines for the management of rheumatoid arthritis: 2002 Update. Arthritis Rheum 2002;46:328-346.

Braun J, Bollow M, Remlinger G, et al. Prevalence of spondylarthropathies in HLA-B27 positive and negative blood donors. Arthritis Rheum. 1998 Jan; 41(1):58-67.

Bathon JM, Martin RW, Fleischmann RM, et al. A comparison of etanercept and methotrexate in patients with early rheumatoid arthritis. NEJM 2000;343:1586-1593.

Bohan A, Peter JB. Polymyositis and dermatomyositis (second of two parts). NEJM 1975;292:403-407.

Bombardier C, Laine L, Reicin A, et al. Comparison of upper gastrointestinal toxicity of rofecoxib and naproxen in patients with rheumatoid arthritis. The VIGOR Study Group. NEJM 2000;343:1520-1528.

Brady OH, Masri BA, Garbuz DS, et al. Joint replacement of the hip and knee – when to refer and what to expect. CMAJ 2000;163:1285-1291.

Brater DC, Harris C, Redfern JS, et al. Renal effects of COX-2-selective inhibitors. Amer J Nephrol 2001;21:1-15.

Bykrek VP, Akhavan P, Hazlewood GS. Canadian rheumatology association recommendations for pharmacological management of rheumatoid arthritis with traditional and biologic disease-modifying antirheumatic drugs. J Rheumatol 2011;39:1559-1582.

Cibere J. Acute monoarthritis. CMAJ 2000;162:1577-1583.

Clark BM. Physical and occupational therapy in the management of arthritis. CMAJ 2000;163:999-1005.

Ensworth S. Is it arthritis? CMAJ 2000;162:1011-1016.

Finkielman, JD, Merkel PA, Schroeder D, et al. Antiproteinase 3 Antineutrophil Cytoplasmic Antibodies and Disease Activity in Wegener Granulomatosis. Ann Intern Med 2007;147:611-619.

Healey LA. Long-term follow-up of polymyalgia rheumatica: evidence for synovitis. Semin Arthritis Rheum 1984;13:322-328.

Hochberg MC. Updating the American College of Rheumatology revised criteria for the classification of systemic lupus erythematosus [letter]. Arthritis Rheum 1997;40:1725.

Hunder GG, Bloch DA, Michel BA, et al. The American College of Rheumatology 1990 criteria for the classification of giant cell arteritis. Arthritis Rheum 1990;33:1122-1128.

Huang SHK. Basics of therapy. CMAJ 2000;163:417-423.

Klippel JH, Weyand CM, Wortmann RL. Primer on Rheumatic Diseases, 11th ed. Arthritis Foundation, 1997.

Klinkhoff A. Diagnosis and management of inflammatory polyarthritis. CMAJ 2000;162:1833-1838.

Kremer JM. Rational use of new and existing disease-modifying agents in rheumatoid arthritis. Ann Intern Med 2001;134:695-706.

Lacaille D. Advanced therapy. CMAJ 2000;163:721-728.

Leavitt RY, Fauci AS, Bloch DA, et al. The American College of Rheumatology 1990 criteria for the classification of Wegener's granulomatosis. Arthritis Rheum 1990;33:1101-1017.

Lightfoot RW Jr, Michel BA, Bloch DA, et al. The American College of Rheumatology 1990 criteria for the classification of polyarteritis nodosa. Arthritis Rheum 1990;33:1088-1093.

McAlindon TE, Bannuru RR, Sullivan MC, et al. OARSI guidelines for the non-surgical management of knee osteoarthritis. Osteoarthr Cartilage 2014;22:363-388.

Miyakis S, Lockshin MD, Atsumi T, et al. International consensus statement on an update of the classification criteria for definite antiphospholipid syndrome (APS). J Thromb Haemost 2006;4:295-306.

Puttick MPE. Evaluation of the patient with pain all over. CMAJ 2001;164:223-227.

Reid G, Esdaile JM. Getting the most out of radiology. CMAJ 2000;162:1318-1325.

Shojania K. What laboratory tests are needed? CMAJ 2000;162:1157-1163.

Sivera F, Andres M, Carmona L, et al. Recommendation: Multinational evidence-based recommendations for the diagnosis and management of gout: integrating systematic literature review and expert opinion of a broad panel of rheumatologists in the 3e initiative. Ann of Rheum Dis 2013;73:328-335.

Smetana GW, Shmerling RH. Does this patient have temporal arteritis? JAMA 2002;287:92-101.

Subcommittee for Scleroderma Criteria of the American Rheumatism Association Diagnostic and Therapeutic Criteria Committee. Preliminary criteria for the classification of systemic sclerosis (scleroderma). Arthritis Rheum 1980;23:581-590.

Taunton JE, Wilkinson M. Diagnosis and management of anterior knee pain. CMAJ 2001;164:1595-1601.

Tsang I. Pain in the neck. CMAJ 2001;164:1182-1187.

van der Linden S, Valkenburg HA, Cats A. Evaluation of diagnostic criteria for ankylosing spondylitis. A proposal for modification of the New York criteria. Arthritis Rheum 1984;27:361.

Vitali C, Bombardieri S, Jonsson R, et al. Classification criteria for Sjögren's syndrome: a revised version of the European criteria proposed by the American-European Consensus Group. Ann Rheum Dis 2002;61:554-558.

Wade JP. Osteoporosis. CMAJ 2001;165:45-50.

Wing PC. Minimizing disability in patients with low-back pain. CMAJ 2001;164:1459-1468.

Wolfe F, Smythe HA, Yunus MB, et al. The American College of Rheumatology 1990 criteria for the classification of fibromyalgia: report of the multicenter criteria committee. Arthritis Rheum 1990;33:160-172.

Wolfe F, Clauw DJ, Fitzcharles MA, et al. The American College of Rheumatology preliminary diagnostic criteria for fibromyalgia and measurement of symptom severity. Arthritis Care and Research 2010;62:600-610.

Notes

U

Urology

Matthew Da Silva, Ryan Sun, and **Weining Yang**, chapter editors
Dhruvin Hirpara and **Sneha Raju**, associate editors
Valerie Lemieux and **Simran Mundi**, EBM editors
Dr. Sender Herschorn and **Dr. Armando Lorenzo**, staff editors

Acronyms

β-hCG	beta-human chorionic gonadotropin	DSD	detrusor sphincter dyssynergia	MAG3	mercaptoacetyltriglycine	SUI	stress urinary incontinence
ABx	antibiotics	EBRT	external beam radiation therapy	MET	medical expulsive therapy	TMP/SMX	trimethoprim/sulfamethoxazole
AFP	alpha-fetoprotein	ED	erectile dysfunction	MS	multiple sclerosis	TRUS	transrectal ultrasound
ART	assisted reproductive technologies	EPS	expressed prostatic secretions	NSGCT	non-seminomatous germ cell tumour	TUIP	transurethral incision of the prostate
AUA	American Urology Association	ESWL	extracorporeal shockwave lithotripsy	PCKD	polycystic kidney disease	TUNA	transurethral needle ablation
BCG	Bacillus Calmette-Guérin	FNA	fine needle aspiration	PCNL	percutaneous nephrolithotomy	TURBT	transurethral resection of bladder tumour
BPH	benign prostatic hyperplasia	GA	general anesthesia	PDE	phosphodiesterase	TURP	transurethral resection of the prostate
CAH	congenital adrenal hyperplasia	GAG	glycosaminoglycan	PID	pelvic inflammatory disease	U/A	urinalysis
CaP	prostatic carcinoma	HIFU	high-intensity focused ultrasound	PMC	pontine micturition centre	U/O	urine output
CBI	continuous bladder irrigation	HPF	high power field	POD	post-obstructive diuresis	U/S	ultrasound
CFU	colony-forming unit	HPTA	hypothalamic-pituitary-testicular axis	PSA	prostate specific antigen	UCC	urothelial carcinoma
CHF	congestive heart failure	ICSI	intracytoplasmic sperm injection	PUV	posterior urethral valve	UMN	upper motor neuron
CIC	clean intermittent catheterization	IFN-α	interferon-alpha	PVD	peripheral vascular disease	UPJ	ureteropelvic junction
CIS	carcinoma *in situ*	IL-2	interleukin-2	PVR	post-void residual	URS	ureteroscopy
CMG	cystometrogram	IPSS	International Prostate Symptom Score	QOL	quality of life	UTI	urinary tract infection
CPPS	chronic pelvic pain syndrome	ISD	intrinsic sphincter deficiency	RCC	renal cell carcinoma	UVJ	ureterovesicular junction
CTU	CT urography	IUI	intrauterine insemination	RFA	radio-frequency ablation	VB1	voided bladder, initial (urethra)
CUA	Canadian Urological Association	IVF	*in vitro* fertilization	RP	radical prostatectomy	VB2	voided bladder, midstream (bladder)
CVA	costovertebral angle	IVP	intravenous pyelogram	RPLND	retroperitoneal lymph node dissection	VB3	voided bladder, post-massage/digital
d/c	discharge	KUB	kidneys, ureters, bladder	RTA	renal tubular acidosis		rectal exam
DHT	dihydrotestosterone	LFT	liver function test	RUG	retrograde urethrogram	VCUG	voiding cystourethrogram
DMSA	dimercaptosuccinic acid	LMN	lower motor neuron	SA	semen analysis	VIU	visual internal urethrotomy
DRE	digital rectal exam	LUTS	lower urinary tract symptoms	SCC	squamous cell carcinoma	VUR	vesicoureteral reflux

Basic Anatomy Review

- recall that the anatomical position of the penis is erect; therefore, the anatomical ventral side of the penis appears to be the dorsal side of the flaccid penis

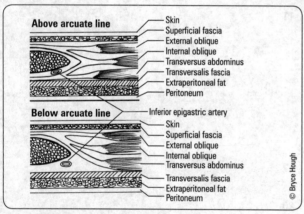

Figure 1. Midline cross-section of abdominal wall

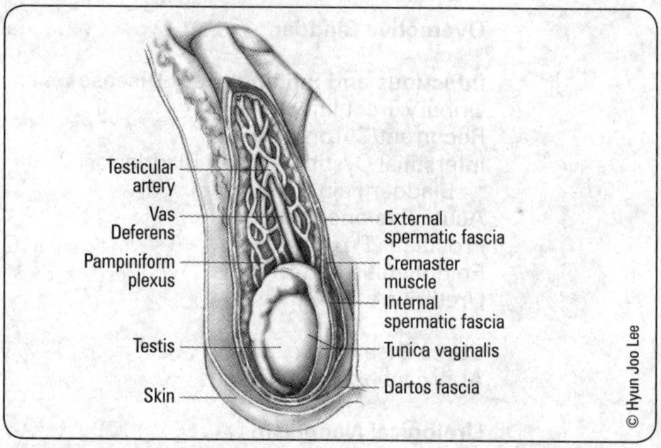

Figure 2. Anatomy of scrotum

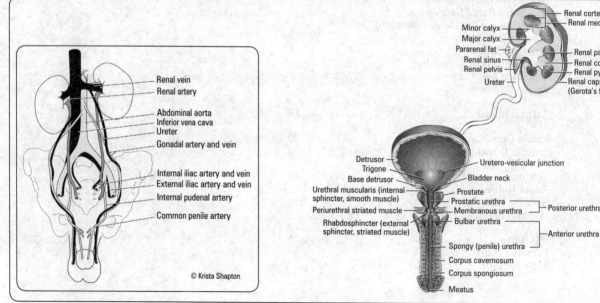

Figure 3. Essential male genitourinary tract anatomy

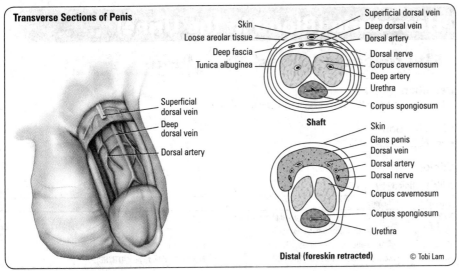

Figure 4. Cross section of the penis

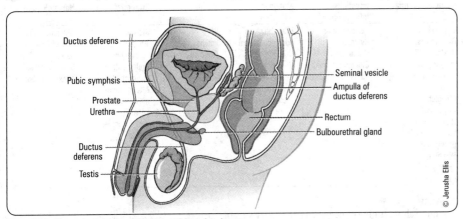

Figure 5. Median sagittal section of the male pelvis and perineum

Urologic History

- follow the OPQRSTUVW approach
  - note that pain may not be limited to the genital region (e.g. lower abdomen, CVA)
- inquire about risk factors: past urologic disease (e.g. UTI, stones, STI, cancers, anatomic abnormalities), family Hx, medications, lifestyle factors (smoking, alcohol, inactivity), trauma, previous surgical procedures
- urinary habits
  - frequency of voiding, incontinence, nocturia
  - specific urinary symptoms include
    - storage symptoms: frequency, nocturia, urgency, incontinence, urge (rush to toilet), stress (leak with cough/laugh)
    - voiding symptoms: straining, hesitancy, dysuria, intermittency, post-void dribbling, reduced stream, feeling of incomplete voiding
  - hematuria: blood clots, red/pink tinged urine
- sexual function
  - scrotal mass: see *Scrotal Mass*, U29
  - ED: see *Erectile Dysfunction*, U30
  - infertility: see *Infertility*, U34
- associated symptoms
  - N/V
  - bowel dysfunction
- constitutional symptoms
  - fever, chills, unintentional weight loss, night sweats, fatigue, malaise

Always ask about sexual function on history. Change in erectile function can be one of the first symptoms that there is concomitant vascular disease. If there is new onset ED, consider screening for DM and CAD risk factors

Hematuria (Blood in the Urine)

Macroscopic (Gross) Hematuria

> Gross, painless hematuria in adults is bladder cancer until proven otherwise

Definition
- blood in the urine that can be seen with the naked eye

Classification
- see Nephrology, NP21

Etiology

Table 1. Etiology by Age Group

Age (yr)	Etiology	
0-20	UTI, glomerulonephritis, congenital abnormalities	
20-40	UTI, stones, bladder tumour, exercise	
40-60	Male: bladder tumour, stones, UTI	Female: UTI, stones, bladder tumour
>60	Male: BPH, bladder tumour, UTI, RCC	Female: bladder tumour, UTI, RCC

Table 2. Etiology by Type

Pseudohematuria	Infectious/ Inflammatory	Malignancy	Benign	Structural	Hematologic
Vaginal bleeding	Pyelonephritis	RCC (mainly in adult population)	BPH	Stones	Anticoagulants
Dyes (beets, rhodamine B in candy and juices)	Cystitis	UCC	Polyps	Trauma	Coagulation defects
Hemoglobin (hemolytic anemia)	Urethritis	Wilms' tumour (mainly in pediatric population)	Exercise-induced	Foreign body	Sickle cell disease
Myoglobin (rhabdomyolysis)	Glomerulonephritis	Leukemia		Urethral stricture	Thromboembolism
Drugs (rifampin, phenazopyridine, phenytoin)	Interstitial nephritis			Polycystic kidneys	
Porphyria	Tuberculosis			Arteriovenous malformation	
Laxatives (phenolphthalein)				Infarct	
				Hydronephrosis	
				Fistula	

> **Common Urologic Causes of Hematuria can be Classified as:**
>
> **TICS**
> **T**rauma/**T**umour/**T**oxins
> **I**nfection/**I**nflammatory
> **C**alculi/**C**ysts
> **S**urgery/**S**ickle cell and other hematological causes

History
- inquire about timing of hematuria in urinary stream
  - initial: anterior urethra
  - terminal: bladder neck and prostatic urethra
  - total: bladder and/or above
- associated symptoms (storage and voiding)
  - pyuria, dysuria: UTI
  - flank pain, radiation: ureteral obstruction
- recent URTI: postinfectious glomerulonephrtis, IgA nephropathy

Investigations
- CBC (rule out anemia, leukocytosis), electrolytes, Cr, BUN, INR, PTT
- urine studies
  - U/A, C&S, cytology
- imaging
  - CT (with contrast) has largely replaced IVP to investigate upper tracts
  - consider contraindications: allergy, renal insufficiency, pregnancy
  - U/S alone may not be sufficient
  - cystoscopy to investigate lower tract (possible retrograde pyelogram)

> **Upper Tract Imaging Options**
> **CT Urography (CTU):** Optimal test for renal parenchyma, calculi, and infections. Involves exposure to radiation and IV contrast. Assess kidney function, allergies prior to use of contrast
> **U/S:** Superior to IVP for evaluation of renal parenchyma and renal cysts; limited sensitivity for UCC and small renal masses; U/S alone is not sufficient for upper tract imaging
> **Intravenous Pyelogram (IVP):** Traditional option but rarely used (replaced by CTU; reasonable sensitivity for UCC, but poor sensitivity for RCC

Acute Management of Severe Bladder Hemorrhage
- manual irrigation via catheter with normal saline to remove clots
- Continuous Bladder Irrigation (CBI) using large (22-26 Fr) 3-way Foley to help prevent clot formation
- cystoscopy if active bleeding
  - identify resectable tumours
  - coagulate obvious sites of bleeding
- refractory bleeding
  - intravesical agents
  - continuous intravesical irrigation with 1% aluminum potassium sulfate solution as needed
  - intravesical instillation of 1% silver nitrate solution
  - intravesical instillation of 1-4% formalin (requires GA and pre-procedure cystogram to rule out reflux)
  - embolization or ligation of iliac arteries
  - cystectomy and diversion (rarely performed)

Microscopic Hematuria

Definition
- blood in the urine that is not visible to the naked eye
- ≥2 RBCs/HPF on urinalysis of at least two separate samples

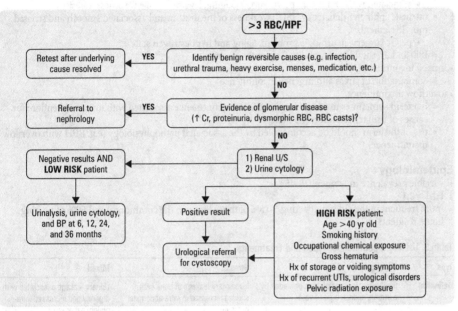

Figure 6. Workup of asymptomatic microscopic hematuria
Based on CUA Guidelines. Alternatively, the AUA recommends cystoscopy and CT urogram for all patients with confirmed microscopic hematuria; follow-up for negative workup is urinalysis yearly for two years, with repeat anatomic evaluation if microscopic hematuria persists

Lower Urinary Tract Dysfunction

- see Gynecology, GY46 for relevant female topics
- The lower urinary tract consists of the bladder and urethra. LUTD frequently involves both parts

Voiding

- two phases of lower urinary tract function
  1. storage phase (bladder filling and urine storage)
     - accommodation and compliance
     - no involuntary contraction(s)
  2. voiding phase (bladder emptying)
     - coordinated detrusor contraction
     - synchronous relaxation of outlet sphincters
     - no anatomic obstruction
- voiding dysfunction can therefore be classified as
  - failure to store: due to bladder or outlet
  - failure to void: due to bladder or outlet
- three types of symptoms
  - storage (formerly known as irritative)
  - voiding (formerly known as obstructive)
  - post-voiding

Urinary Incontinence

Definition
- involuntary leakage of urine

Etiology
- urgency incontinence
  - detrusor overactivity
    - CNS lesion, inflammation/infection (cystitis, stone, tumour), bladder neck obstruction (tumour, stone), BPH, idiopathic
  - decreased compliance of bladder wall (inability to store urine)
    - CNS lesion, fibrosis
    - sphincter/urethral problem

Lower Urinary Tract Symptoms (LUTS)

Storage (FUND)
Frequency
Urgency
Nocturia
Dysuria

Voiding (SHED)
Stream changes
Hesitancy
Incomplete Emptying
Dribbling

Causes of Reversible Urinary Incontinence

DIAPERS
Delirium
Inflammation/Infection
Atrophic vaginitis/urethritis
Pharmaceuticals/Psychological
Excess U/O
Restricted mobility/Retention
Stool impaction

Urgency is the symptom of a strong need to void; it is not necessarily associated with incontinence

- stress urinary incontinence (SUI)
  - common in women; seen in men after prostate cancer treatment or pelvic operations
  - urethral hypermobility
    - weakened pelvic floor and musculofascial urethral and vaginal supporting mechanisms allows bladder neck and urethra to descend with increased intra-abdominal pressure
    - urethra is pulled open by greater motion of posterior wall of outlet relative to anterior wall
    - associated with childbirth, pelvic surgery, aging, levator muscle weakness, obesity
  - intrinsic sphincter deficiency (ISD): weakness of the urethra and associated smooth and striated muscle elements
    - pelvic surgery, neurologic problem, aging and hypoestrogen state
  - ISD and urethral hypermobility frequently co-exist
- mixed incontinence
  - combination of stress and urgency incontinence
- overflow incontinence
  - is a term sometimes used to describe urinary incontinence associated with urinary retention; for causes of urinary retention see Table 4
  - use of the term should be accompanied by the associated pathophysiology (e.g. BPH with overflow incontinence)

Epidemiology
- variable prevalence in women: 25-45%
- F:M = 2:1
- more frequent in the elderly, affecting 5-15% of those living in the community and 50% of nursing home residents

Table 3. Urinary Incontinence: Types and Treatments

Type	Urgency	Stress	Mixed
Definition	Involuntary leakage of urine preceded by a strong, sudden urge to void	Involuntary leakage of urine with sudden increases in intra-abdominal pressure	Urinary leakage associated with urgency and increased intra-abdominal pressure
Etiology	Bladder (detrusor overactivity)	Urethra/sphincter weakness, post-partum pelvic musculature weakness	Combination of bladder and sphincter issues
Diagnosis	Hx Urodynamics	Hx Urodynamics Stress test (have patient bear down/cough)	Hx Urodynamics Stress test
Therapy	Lifestyle changes (fluid alterations, diet, etc.) Bladder habit training Anticholinergics Beta 3 agonist Botulinum toxin A Neuromodulation	Weight loss Kegel exercises Bulking agents Surgery (slings, tension-free vaginal tape, retropubic urethropexy, artificial sphincter)	Combination of management of urgency and stress incontinence

Urinary Retention

Table 4. Etiology of Urinary Retention

Outflow Obstruction	Bladder Innervation	Pharmacologic	Infection
Bladder neck or urethra: calculus, clot, foreign body, neoplasm, neurological (DSD) Prostate: BPH, prostate cancer Urethra: stricture, phimosis, traumatic disruption Miscellaneous: constipation, pelvic mass	Intracranial: CVA, tumour, Parkinson's, cerebral palsy Spinal cord: injury, disc herniation, MS DM Post-abdominal or pelvic surgery	Anticholinergics Narcotics Antihypertensives (ganglionic blockers, methyldopa) OTC cold medications containing ephedrine or pseudoephedrine Antihistamines Psychosomatic substances (e.g. ecstasy)	GU: UTI, prostatitis, abscess, genital herpes Infected foreign body Varicella zoster

Acute vs. Chronic Retention
Acute retention is a medical emergency characterized by suprapubic pain and anuria with normal bladder volume and architecture
Chronic retention can be painless with greatly increased bladder volume and detrusor hypertrophy followed by atony (late)

If a trauma patient is unable to void, has blood at urethral meatus, a scrotal hematoma, or a high riding prostate, there is urethral injury until proven otherwise so catheterization is CONTRAINDICATED unless performed by urology staff or resident

Patients with ascites may have a falsely elevated PVR measured by bladder scan

Clinical Features
- suprapubic pain, incomplete emptying, weak stream
- palpable and/or percussible bladder (suprapubic)
- possible purulent/bloody meatal discharge
- increased size of prostate or reduced anal sphincter tone on DRE
- neurological: presence of abnormal or absent deep tendon reflexes, reduced "anal wink", saddle anesthesia

Investigations
- CBC, electrolytes, Cr, BUN, U/A and urine C&S, U/S, cystoscopy, urodynamic studies, PVR

Treatment
- treat underlying cause
- catheterization
  - acute retention
    - ♦ immediate catheterization to relieve retention; leave Foley in to drain bladder; follow-up to determine cause; closely monitor fluid status and electrolytes (risk of POD)
  - chronic retention
    - ♦ intermittent catheterization by patient may be used; definitive treatment depends on etiology
- suprapubic catheter if obstruction precludes urethral catheter
- for post-operative patients with retention:
  - encourage ambulation
  - α-blockers to relax bladder neck outlet
  - may need catheterization
  - definitive treatment will depend on etiology

Benign Prostatic Hyperplasia

Definition
- periurethral hyperplasia of stroma and epithelium in prostatic transition zone
- prostatic smooth muscle cells play a role in addition to hyperplasia

Etiology
- etiology unknown
  - DHT required (converted from testosterone by 5-α reductase)
  - possible role of impaired apoptosis, estrogens, other growth factors

Epidemiology
- age-related, extremely common (50% of 50 yr olds, 80% of 80 yr olds)
- 25% of men will require treatment

Clinical Features
- result from outlet obstruction and compensatory changes in detrusor function
- voiding and storage symptoms
- DRE
  - prostate is smooth, rubbery, and may be symmetrically enlarged
- complications
  - retention
  - overflow incontinence
  - hydronephrosis
  - renal insufficiency
  - infection
  - gross hematuria
  - bladder stones

Investigations
- Hx, assessing LUTS and impact on QOL
  - may include self-administered questionnaires (IPSS or AUA symptom index for severity, progression, and treatment response)
- P/E, including DRE
- U/A to exclude UTI
- Cr to assess renal function
- renal U/S to assess for hydronephrosis
- PSA to rule out malignancy (see *Prostate Cancer Screening*, U26)
- uroflowmetry to measure flow rate (optional)
- PVR (optional)
- consider cystoscopy or bladder ultrasound prior to potential surgical management to evaluate outlet and prostate volume
- biopsy if suspicious for malignancy, i.e. elevated PSA or abnormal DRE

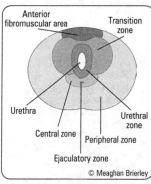

Figure 7. Cross-section of prostate

Prostate size does not correlate well with symptoms in BPH

Approximate Prostate Sizes
20 cc – chestnut
25 cc – plum
50 cc – lemon
75 cc – orange
100 cc – grapefruit

AUA BPH Symptom Score

FUNWISE
Frequency
Urgency
Nocturia
Weak stream
Intermittency
Straining
Emptying, incomplete feeling of

Each symptom graded out of 5
0-7: Mildly symptomatic
8-19: Moderately symptomatic
20-35: Severely symptomatic
Note: dysuria not included in score but is commonly associated with BPH

Initial alpha-adrenergic antagonist monotherapy for score <20, combination therapy for score >20

BPH Surgery

Absolute Indication
Renal failure with obstructive uropathy
Refractory urinary retention

Relative Indications
Recurrent UTIs
Recurrent hematuria refractory to medical treatment
Renal insufficiency (rule out other causes)
Bladder stones

Finasteride for Benign Prostatic Hyperplasia
Cochrane DB Syst Rev 2010;10:CD006015
Purpose: To examine the effectiveness and safety of finasteride versus placebo or other active controls for the treatment of urinary tract symptoms.
Summary of Findings:
1. Finasteride improved urinary symptoms more than placebo in trials >1 yr duration and significantly lowered the risk of BPH progression.
2. Compared with α-blockers, finasteride was less effective than either doxazosin or terazosin, but equally as effective as tamsulosin.
3. Symptom improvement with finasteride + doxazosin is equal to doxazosin alone.
4. Finasteride treatment resulted in an increased risk of ejaculation disorder, impotence and lowered libido compared with placebo.
5. Compared with doxazosin and terazosin, finasteride had a lower risk of asthenia, dizziness, and postural hypotension.

Microwave Thermotherapy for Benign Prostatic Hyperplasia
Cochrane DB Syst Rev 2012;9:CD004135
Purpose: To evaluate the efficacy and safety of microwave thermotherapy for the treatment of benign prostatic obstruction.
Selection Criteria: RCTs evaluating transurethral microwave therapy (TUMT) for men with symptomatic BPH with multiple comparison groups.
Results: 15 studies, 1,585 patients, mean age 66.8 yr, 3-60 mo duration. Mean urinary symptom scores decreased by 65% with TUMT and 77% with TURP. The pooled mean peak urinary flow increased by 70% with TUMT and 119% with TURP. Compared with TURP, TUMT was associated with decreased risks for retrograde ejaculation, treatment for strictures, hematuria, blood transfusions and transurethral resection syndrome, but increased risk for dysuria, urinary retention and retreatment for BPH symptoms.
Conclusions: Overall, microwave thermotherapy techniques are effective alternatives to TURP and α-blockers for treating symptomatic BPH, although less effective than TURP in improving symptom score and urinary flow.

Treatment

Table 5. Treatment of BPH

	Conservative	Medical	Surgical	Minimally Invasive Surgical Therapies
When to use	Asymptomatic patients or symptomatic without bother	Moderate to severe symptoms that are distressing for patient	Significant symptom burden, acute urinary retention, refractory hematuria, recurrent infections	Patients who wish to avoid or may not tolerate surgery
Options	Watchful waiting: 50% of patients improve spontaneously. Lifestyle modifications (e.g. evening fluid restriction, planned voiding)	α-adrenergic antagonists: reduce stromal smooth muscle tone; 5-α reductase inhibitor: block conversion of testosterone to DHT; act to reduce prostate size. Combination is synergistic. Anti-cholinergic agents or Beta-3 agonist (for storage LUTS, without elevated PVR)	TURP (see U41); Laser ablation; TUIP (prostate <30 g); Open prostatectomy	Microwave therapy; TUNA; Prostatic stent (not commonly used)

Urethral Stricture

Definition
- decrease in urethral calibre due to scar formation in urethra (may also involve corpus spongiosum)
- M>F

Etiology
- congenital
  - failure of normal canalization (i.e. posterior urethral valves)
- trauma
  - instrumentation/catheterization (most common)
  - external trauma (e.g. burns, straddle injury)
  - foreign body
- infection
  - long-term indwelling catheter
  - STI (gonococcal or chlamydial disease)
- inflammation
  - balanitis xerotica obliterans (BXO; lichen sclerosis or chronic progressive sclerosing dermatosis of the male genitalia) causing meatal and urethral stenosis

Clinical Features
- voiding and storage symptoms
- urinary retention
- hydronephrosis
- related infections: recurrent UTI, secondary prostatitis/epididymitis

Investigations
- laboratory findings
  - flow rates <10 mL/s (normal ~20 mL/s) on uroflowmetry
  - urine culture usually negative, but U/A may show pyuria
- radiologic findings
  - RUG and VCUG will demonstrate location
- cystoscopy

Treatment
- urethral dilatation
  - temporarily increases lumen size by breaking up scar tissue
  - healing will often reform scar tissue, recurrence of stricture
- visual internal urethrotomy (VIU)
  - endoscopically incise stricture
  - equal success rates to dilation with mid bulbar strictures <2 cm
  - high rate of recurrence (30-80%), avoid in younger patients
- open surgical reconstruction
  - complete stricture excision with anastomosis, ± urethroplasty depending on location and size of stricture

Neurogenic Bladder

Definition
- dysfunction of the urinary bladder due to deficiency in some aspect of its innervation

Neurophysiology

Table 6. Efferent Sympathetic, Parasympathetic, and Somatic Nerve Supply

Nerve Fibres	Nerve Roots	Neurotransmitter/Receptor	Target
Sympathetic	T10-L2	NA/Adrenergic	Trigone, internal sphincter, proximal urethra (Alpha receptors) Bladder body (Beta receptors)
Somatic (Pudendal)	S2-4	ACh/Nicotinic	External sphincter
Parasympathetic	S2-4	ACh/Muscarinic (M2, M3)	Detrusor

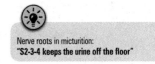

Nerve roots in micturition:
"S2-3-4 keeps the urine off the floor"

- stretch receptors in the bladder wall relay information to PMC and activate micturition reflex (normally inhibited by cortical input)
  - micturition
    - stimulation of parasympathetic neurons (bladder contraction)
    - inhibition of sympathetic and somatic neurons (internal and external sphincter relaxation, respectively)
    - urine storage
    - opposite of micturition
- voluntary action of external sphincter (pudendal nerve roots S2-S4) can inhibit urge to urinate
- cerebellum, basal ganglia, thalamus, and hypothalamus all have input at PMC in the brainstem

Examples of Neurologic Voiding Dysfunction
- neurogenic detrusor overactivity (NDO)(formerly termed detrusor hyperreflexia)
  - lesion above PMC (e.g. stroke, tumour, MS, Parkinson's disease)
  - loss of voluntary inhibition of voiding
  - intact pathway inferior to PMC maintains coordination of bladder and sphincter
- detrusor sphincter dyssynergia (DSD)
  - suprasacral lesion of spinal cord (e.g. trauma, MS, arteriovenous malformation, transverse myelitis)
  - loss of coordination between detrusor and sphincter (detrusor contracts on closed sphincter and vice versa)
  - component of detrusor overactivity as well
- detrusor atony/areflexia
  - lesion of sacral cord or peripheral efferents (e.g. trauma, DM, disc herniation, MS, congenital spinal cord abnormality, post abdominoperineal resection)
  - flaccid bladder which fails to contract
  - may progress to poorly compliant bladder with high pressures
- peripheral autonomic neuropathy
  - deficient bladder sensation → increasing residual urine → decompensation (e.g. DM, neurosyphilis, herpes zoster)
- muscular lesion
  - can involve detrusor, smooth/striated sphincter

"Spinal shock", initially manifests as atonic bladder

Neuro-Urologic Evaluation
- Hx and P/E (urologic and general neurologic)
- U/A, renal profile
- imaging
  - U/S to rule out hydronephrosis and stones; occasionally CT scanning with or without contrast
- cystoscopy
- urodynamic studies
  - uroflowmetry to assess flow rate, pattern
  - filling CMG to assess capacity, compliance, detrusor overactivity
  - voiding CMG (pressure-flow study) to assess bladder contractility and extent of bladder outflow obstruction
  - video study to visualize bladder/bladder neck/urethra during CMG using x-ray contrast
  - EMG and video ascertains presence of coordinated or uncoordinated voiding, allows accurate diagnosis of DSD

Treatment
- goals of treatment
  - prevent renal deterioration
  - prevent infections
  - achieve social continence
- clean intermittent catheterization (CIC)

- treatment options depend on status of bladder and urethra
  - bladder hyperactivity → anticholinergic medications to relax bladder (see *Urinary Incontinence*, U5)
    - if refractory
      - botulinum toxin injections into bladder wall
      - occasionally augmentation cystoplasty (enlarging bladder volume and improving compliance by grafting section of detubularized bowel onto the bladder)
      - occasionally urinary diversion (ileal conduit or continent diversion) in severe cases if bladder management unsuccessful
  - flaccid bladder → CIC

Dysuria

Definition
- painful urination

Etiology

Table 7. Differential Diagnosis of Dysuria

Infectious	Cystitis, urethritis, prostatitis, epididymitis/orchitis (if associated with lower tract inflammation), cervicitis, vulvovaginitis, perineal inflammation/infection, TB, vestibulitis
Neoplasm	Kidney, bladder, prostate, penis, vagina/vulva, BPH
Calculi	Bladder stone, urethral stone, ureteral stone
Inflammatory	Seronegative arthropathies (reactive arthritis: arthritis, uveitis, urethritis), drug side effects, autoimmune disorders, chronic pelvic pain syndrome (CPPS), interstitial cystitis
Hormonal	Endometriosis, hypoestrogenism
Trauma	Catheter insertion, post-coital cystitis (honeymoon cystitis)
Psychogenic	Somatization disorder, depression, stress/anxiety disorder
Other	Contact sensitivity, foreign body, radiation/chemical cystitis, diverticulum

Investigations
- focused Hx and P/E to determine cause (fever, d/c, conjunctivitis, CVA tenderness, back/joint pain)
  - any d/c (urethral, vaginal, cervical) should be sent for gonococcus/chlamydia testing; wet mount if vaginal d/c
  - U/A and urine C&S
  - if suspect infection, may start empiric ABx treatment (see Table 9, U12)
  - ± imaging of urinary tract (tumour, stones)

Hydronephrosis

- the upper urinary tract consists of the kidneys and ureters

Definition
- dilation of the renal pelvis and calyces caused by the impairment in antegrade urine flow

Etiology
- mechanical
  - congenital: see *Congenital Abnormalities*, U36
  - acquired
    - intrinsic: trauma, inflammation and bleeding, calculi, urologic neoplasms, BPH, urethral stricture, phimosis, previous urological surgery
    - extrinsic: trauma, neoplasms (uterine fibroid; colorectal, uterine, and cervical malignancies; lymphoma), aortic aneurysm, pregnancy (gravid uterus)
- functional
  - neuropathic: neurogenic bladder, diabetic neuropathy, spinal cord disease
  - pharmacologic: α-adrenergic agonists
  - hormonal: pregnancy (progesterone decreases ureteral tone)

Investigations
- focused Hx, inquiring about pain (flank, lower abdomen, testes, labia), U/O, medication use, pregnancy, trauma, fever, Hx of UTIs, calculi, PID, and urological surgery
- CBC, electrolytes, Cr, BUN, U/A, C&S
- imaging studies (U/S is >90% sensitive and specific)
  - MAG3 diuretic renogram: evaluates differential renal function and demonstrates if functional obstruction exists

Treatment
- hydronephrosis can be physiologic
- treatment should be guided at improving symptoms, treating infections, or improving renal function
- urgent treatment may require percutaneous nephrostomy tube or ureteral stenting to relieve pressure

Post-Obstructive Diuresis

Definition
- polyuria resulting from relief of severe chronic obstruction
- >3 L/24 h or >200 cc/h over each of two consecutive hours

Pathophysiology
- physiologic POD secondary to excretion of retained urea, Na^+, and H_2O (high osmotic load) after relief of obstruction
    - self-limiting; usually resolves in 48 h with PO fluids but may persist to pathologic POD
- pathologic POD is a Na^+-wasting nephropathy secondary to impaired concentrating ability of the renal tubules due to
    - decreased reabsorption of NaCl in the thick ascending limb and urea in the collecting tubule
    - increased medullary blood flow (solute washout)
    - increased flow and solute concentration in the distal nephrons

Management
- admit patient and closely monitor hemodynamic status and electrolytes (Na^+ and K^+ q6-12h and replace prn; follow Cr and BUN to baseline)
- monitor U/O q2h and ensure total fluid intake <U/O by replacing every 1 mL U/O with 0.5 mL 1/2 NS IV (PO fluids if physiologic POD)
- avoid glucose-containing fluid replacement (iatrogenic diuresis)

Overactive Bladder

Definition
- a symptom complex that includes urinary urgency with or without urgency incontinence, urinary frequency (voiding ≥8 times in a 24 hr period), and nocturia (awakening ONE or more times at night to void)

Etiology
- multiple etiologies proposed
- symptoms usually associated with involuntary contractions of the detrusor muscle. The overactivity of the muscle could be neurogenic, myogenic or idiopathic

Epidemiology
- F:M= 1:1
- prevalence increases with age. 42% in males 75 years old or older; 31% in females 75 years old or older

Diagnosis
- the diagnostic process should document symptoms that define overactive bladder and exclude other disorders that could cause of the patient's symptoms
- minimal requirements for the process consist of
    - focused history including past genitourinary disorders and conditions outlined in Table 8, questionnaires of LUTS for women and diaries of urination frequency, volume and pattern
    - P/E including genitourinary, pelvic and rectal examination
    - urinalysis to rule out hematuria and infection
- in some patients, the following investigations could be considered
    - bladder scan for residual urine in patients with risk factors of urinary retention
    - cystoscopy to rule out recurrent infections, carcinoma in situ and other intravesical abnormalities
        - urodynamics to rule out obstruction in older men

Treatment
- non-pharmacological: behaviour therapies such as bladder training, bladder control strategies, pelvic floor muscle training, fluid management, and avoidance of caffeine, alcohol
- pharmacological
    - anti-muscarinics such as oxybutynin hydrochloride, tolterodine, solifenacin, fesoterodine, or trospium
    - β3-adrenoceptor agonist such as mirabegron
- refractory patients may be treated with
    - neuromuscular-junction inhibition such as botulinum toxin bladder injection
- other interventional procedures include
    - percutaneous tibial nerve stimulation (not used commonly in Canada)
    - sacral neuromodulation

Table 8. Conditions that Could Contribute to Symptoms of Overactive Bladder

Lower Urinary Tract Conditions	UTI, obstruction, impaired bladder contractility
Neurological Conditions	Stroke, MS, dementia, diabetic neuropathy
Systemic Diseases	CHF, sleep disorders (primarily nocturia)
Functional and Behavioural	Excessive caffeine and alcohol, constipation, impaired mobility
Medication	Diuretics, anticholinergic agents, narcotics, calcium-channel blocker, cholinesterase inhibitors

Infectious and Inflammatory Diseases

Table 9. Antibiotic Treatment of Urological Infections

Condition	Drug	Duration
Urethritis	**Non-Gonococcal** azithromycin (1 g PO) OR doxycycline (100 mg PO bid) **Gonococcal** ceftriaxone (250 mg IM) AND treat for Chlamydia trachomatis	x 1 7 d x 1
Simple, Uncomplicated UTI	TMP-SMX (160 mg/800 mg PO bid) OR nitrofurantoin (100 mg PO bid)	3 d 5 d
Complicated UTI	ciprofloxacin (1 g PO daily OR 400 mg IV q12h) OR ampicillin (1 g IV q6h) + gentamicin (1 mg/kg IV q8h) (used for relatively short courses because of toxicity) OR ceftriaxone (1-2 g IV q24h)	up to 2-3 wk up to 2-3 wk up to 2-3 wk
Recurrent/Chronic Cystitis	**Prophylactic Treatment** Continuous: TMP-SMX (40 mg/200 mg PO qHS OR 3x/wk) OR nitrofurantoin (50-100 mg PO qHS) Post-Coital: TMP-SMX (40 mg/200 mg-80 mg/400 mg) OR nitrofurantoin (50-100 mg PO qd)	 6-12 mo 6-12 mo within 2 h of coitus within 2 h of coitus
Acute Prostatitis	ciprofloxacin (500-750 mg PO bid) OR TMP-SMX (160 mg/800 mg PO bid) OR IV therapy with gentamicin and ampicillin, penicillin with β-lactamase inhibitor, 3rd gen cephalosporin, OR a fluoroquinolone	2-4 wk 4 wk 4 wk (IV and oral step-down)
Chronic Prostatitis	ciprofloxacin (500 mg PO bid)	4-6 wk
Epididymitis/Orchitis	<35 yr ceftriaxone (200 mg IM) AND doxycycline (100 mg PO bid) ≥35 yr ofloxacin (300 mg PO bid)	 x 1 10 d 10 d
Acute Uncomplicated Pyelonephritis	ciprofloxacin (500 mg PO bid) ± ceftriaxone (1 g IV) OR ciprofloxacin (400 mg IV) OR IV therapy with a fluoroquinolone, gentamicin and ampicillin, extended spectrum cephalosporin, extended spectrum penicillin, OR a carbapenem	7 d x 1 14 d total (IV and oral step-down)

Antibiotic therapy should always be based on local resistance patterns and adjusted according to culture and sensitivity results

Cystitis: Common Pathogens

KEEPS
Klebsiella sp.
E. coli (90%), other Gram-negatives
Enterococci
Proteus mirabilis, Pseudomonas
S. saprophyticus

Acute uncomplicated pyelonephritis: suspected or confirmed *Enterococcus* infection requires treatment with ampicillin

Urinary Tract Infection

- for UTIs during pregnancy, see <u>Obstetrics</u>, OB28

Definition
- symptoms suggestive of UTI + evidence of pyuria and bacteriuria on U/A or urine C&S
  - if asymptomatic + 100,000 CFU/mL = asymptomatic bacteriuria; only requires treatment in certain patients (e.g. pregnancy)

Classification
- uncomplicated: lower UTI in a setting of functionally and structurally normal urinary tract
- complicated: structural and/or functional abnormality, male patients, immunocompromised, diabetic, iatrogenic complication, pregnancy, pyelonephritis, catheter-associated
- recurrent: see *Recurrent/Chronic Cystitis*

Risk Factors
- stasis and obstruction
  - residual urine due to impaired urine flow e.g. PUVs, reflux, medication, BPH, urethral stricture, cystocele, neurogenic bladder
- foreign body
  - introduce pathogen or act as nidus of infection e.g. catheter, instrumentation
- decreased resistance to organisms
  - DM, malignancy, immunosuppression, spermicide use, estrogen depletion, antimicrobial use
- other factors
  - trauma, anatomic abnormalities, female, sexual activity, menopause, fecal incontinence

Clinical Features
- storage symptoms: frequency, urgency, dysuria
- voiding symptoms: hesitancy, post-void dribbling
- other: suprapubic pain, hematuria, foul-smelling urine
- pyelonephritis – if present: typically presents with more severe symptoms (e.g. fever/chills, CVA tenderness, flank pain)

Organisms
- typical organisms: KEEPS (*E. coli* 75-95%)
- atypical organisms
  - tuberculosis (TB)
  - *Chlamydia trachomatis*
  - *Mycoplasma* (*Ureaplasma urealyticum*)
  - fungi (*Candida*)

Indications for Investigations
- pyelonephritis
- persistence of pyuria/symptoms following adequate antibiotic therapy
- severe infection with an increase in Cr
- recurrent/persistent infections
- atypical pathogens (urea splitting organisms)
- Hx of structural abnormalities/decreased flow

Investigations
- U/A, urine C&S
  - UA: leukocytes ± nitrites ± hematuria
  - C&S: midstream, catheterized, or suprapubic aspirate
- if hematuria present, retest post-treatment, if persistent need hematuria workup (see *Microscopic Hematuria*, U5)
- U/S, CT scan if indicated

Treatment
- see Table 9, U12, *Antibiotic Treatment of Urological Infections*
- if febrile, consider admission with IV therapy and rule out obstruction

Recurrent/Chronic Cystitis

Definition
- ≥3 UTIs/yr

Etiology
- bacterial reinfection (80%) vs. bacterial persistence (relapse)
  - bacterial reinfection
    - recurrence of infection with either 1) a different organism, 2) the same organism if cultured >2 wk following therapy, or 3) with any organism with an intermittent sterile culture
  - bacterial persistence
    - same organism cultured within 2 wk of sensitivity-based therapy

Investigations
- assess predisposing factors as described above
- investigations may include cystoscopy, U/S, CT

Prevention of UTIs
- Maintain good hydration (try cranberry juice)
- Wipe from front to back to avoid contamination of the urethra with feces from the rectum
- Avoid feminine hygiene sprays and scented douches
- Empty bladder immediately before and after intercourse

Treatment
- lifestyle changes (limit caffeine intake, increase fluid/H_2O intake)
- ABx: continuous vs. post-coital
- post-menopausal women: consider topical or systemic estrogen therapy
- no treatment for asymptomatic bacteriuria except in pregnant women or patients undergoing urinary tract instrumentation

Interstitial Cystitis (Painful Bladder or Bladder Pain Syndrome)

Definition
- bladder pain, chronic urgency and frequency without other reasonable causation

Classification
- non-ulcerative (more common)
- ulcerative

Etiology
- unknown
  - theories: increased epithelial permeability, autoimmune, neurogenic, defective GAG layer overlying mucosa

Epidemiology
- prevalence: 20/100,000
- 90% of cases are in females
- mean age at onset is 40 yr (non-ulcerative tends to affect a younger to middle-aged population, while ulcerative tends to be seen in middle-aged to older)

Clinical Features
- bladder pain, increase with filling and relief with emptying
- glomerulations (submucosal petechiae) or Hunner's lesions (ulcers) on cystoscopic examination
- urinary urgency
- negative U/A, urine C&S, and urine cytology

Differential Diagnosis
- UTI, vaginitis, bladder tumour
- radiation/chemical/eosinophilic/TB cystitis
- eosinophilic/TB cystitis
- bladder calculi

Investigations
- Hx, P/E, urinalysis with microscopy

Treatment
- first-line: patient empowerment (diet, lifestyle, stress management), pain management
- second-line
  - oral: pentosan polysulfate sodium, amitriptyline, cimetidine, hydroxyzine
  - intravesical: dimethylsulfoxide (DMSO), heparin, lidocaine
- third-line: cystoscopy with bladder hydrodistention (traditionally diagnostic) under GA, treat Hunner's lesions if present
- other: neuromodulation, cyclosporine A, intradetrusor botulinum toxin
- surgery (last resort): augmentation cystoplasty, or urinary diversion ± cystectomy

Acute Pyelonephritis

Definition
- infection of the renal parenchyma with local and systemic manifestations
- clinical diagnosis of flank pain, fever and elevated WBC

Etiology
- ascending (usually GN bacilli) or hematogenous route (usually GP cocci)
- causative microorganisms
  - gram positives: *Enterococcus faecalis*, *S. aureus*, *S. saphrophyticus*
  - gram negatives: *E. coli* (most common), *Klebsiella*, *Proteus*, *Pseudomonas*, *Enterobacter*
- common underlying causes of pyelonephritis
  - stones, strictures, prostatic obstruction, vesicoureteric reflux, neurogenic bladder, catheters, DM, sickle-cell disease, PCKD, immunosuppression, post-renal transplant, instrumentation, pregnancy

Cystoscopic evaluation is not necessary to make a diagnosis

Four Symptom Scores Exist to Evaluate and Monitor Patients with Interstitial Cystitis
- Interstitial Cystitis Symptom Index (ICSI)
- Interstitial Cystitis Problem Index (ICPI)
- Wisconsin Interstitial Cystitis (UW-IC) Scale
- Pain, Urgency and Frequency (PUF) Score

Clinical Features
- rapid onset (<24 h)
- LUTS including frequency, urgency, hematuria; NOT dysuria unless concurrent cystitis
- fever, chills, nausea, vomiting, myalgia, malaise
- CVA tenderness and/or exquisite flank pain

Investigations
- U/A, urine C&S
- CBC and differential: leukocytosis, left shift
- imaging indicated if suspicious of complicated pyelonephritis or symptoms do not improve with 48-72 h of treatment
    - abdominal/pelvic U/S
    - CT
- nuclear medicine: DMSA scan can be used to help secure the diagnosis
    - a photopenic defect indicates active infection or scar; if normal alternative diagnoses should be considered

Treatment
- hemodynamically stable
    - outpatient oral ABx treatment ± single initial IV dose (see Table 9, U12)
- severe or non-resolving
    - admit, hydrate, and treat with IV ABx (see Table 9, U12)
- emphysematous pyelonephritis
    - most patients receive nephrectomy after IV ABx started and patient stabilized
    - consider temporization with nephrostomy tubes
- renal obstruction
    - admit for emergent stenting or percutaneous nephrostomy tube

Cystoscopic evaluation is not necessary to make a diagnosis. Nitrofurantoin has poor tissue penetration and therefore is not used to treat pyelonephritis (requires post-renal uroconcentration)

Prostatitis/Prostatodynia

Epidemiology
- most common urologic diagnosis in men <50 yr
- prevalence 2-12%

Classification

Table 10. Comparison of the Three Types of Prostatitis

	Category I: Acute Bacterial Prostatitis	Category II: Chronic Bacterial Prostatitis	Category III: Chronic Pelvic Pain Syndrome (CPPS) (Abacterial)
Etiology	Ascending urethral infection with KEEPS: 80% E. coli Often associated with outlet obstruction, recent cystoscopy, prostatic biopsy Most infections occur in the peripheral zone (see Figure 7, U7)	Recurrent exacerbations of acute prostatitis-like signs and symptoms Recurrent UTI with same organism	Divided into inflammatory (IIIA) and non-inflammatory (IIIB) Intraprostatic reflux of urine ± urethral hypertonia Multifactorial (immunological, neuropathic, neuroendocrine, psychosocial)
Clinical Features	Acute onset fever, chills, malaise Rectal, lower back, and perineal pain LUTS	Pelvic pain, storage LUTS, ejaculatory pain, post-ejaculatory pain	Pelvic pain, storage LUTS, ejaculatory pain, post-ejaculatory pain
Investigations	P/E: abdomen, external genitalia, perineum, prostate U/A Blood CBC, C&S Transrectal U/S if non-resolving/suspect prostatic abscess	E: as per Category I + pelvic floor Urine C&S: 4-glass test VB1 (voided bladder): initial (urethra) P/VB2: midstream (bladder) EPS (expressed prostatic secretions): not usually performed VB3: post-massage/DRE	Same as per Category II NIH-CPSI score* Consider psychological assessment
Treatment	Supportive measures PO or IV ABx depending how sick (see Table 9, U12) May consider catheterization in patients with severe obstructive LUTS or retention Diagnose and treat if abscess is present	ABx (see Table 9, U12) Consider addition of an β-blocker	Supportive measures Trial of ABx therapy if newly diagnosed Multimodal treatment strategy may include: β-blocker Anti-inflammatories Phytotherapy (quercetin, cernilton)

*NIH-CPSI: National Institute of Health Chronic Prostatitis Symptom Index

Cystitis: Common Pathogens

KEEPS
Klebsiella sp.
E. coli (90%), other Gram-negatives
Enterococci
Proteus mirabilis, Pseudomonas
S. saprophyticus

4-Glass Test: Prostatic source is suggested when colony counts in EPS and VB3 exceed those of VB1 and VB2 by 10x

It is not recommended to do a serum PSA during acute bacterial prostatitis

Prostatic massage may cause extreme tenderness and increased risk of inducing sepsis, abscess, or epididymo-orchitis

Epididymitis and Orchitis

Etiology
- common infectious causes
  - <35 yr: *N. gonorrhoeae* or *Chlamydia trachomatis*
  - ≥35 yr or penetrative anal intercourse: GI organisms (especially *E. coli*)
- other causes
  - mumps infection may involve orchitis, post-parotitis
  - TB
  - syphilis
  - granulomatous (autoimmune) in elderly men
  - amiodarone (involves only head of epididymis)
  - chemical: reflux of urine into ejaculatory ducts

Risk Factors
- UTI
- unprotected sexual contact
- instrumentation/catheterization
- increased pressure in prostatic urethra (straining, voiding, heavy lifting) may cause reflux of urine along vas deferens → sterile epididymitis
- immunocompromise

Clinical Features
- sudden onset scrotal pain and swelling ± radiation along cord to flank
- scrotal erythema and tenderness
- fever
- storage symptoms, purulent d/c
- reactive hydrocele

Investigations
- U/A, urine C&S
- ± urethral d/c: Gram stain/culture
- if diagnosis uncertain, must do
  - colour-flow Doppler U/S to rule out testicular torsion

Treatment
- rule out torsion (see *Investigations* Table 24, U29)
- see Table 9, U12 for ABx therapy
- scrotal support, bed rest, ice, analgesia

Complications
- if severe → testicular atrophy
- 30% have persistent infertility problems

Prehn's Sign: pain may be relieved with elevation of testicles in epididymitis but not in testicular torsion (poor sensitivity, especially in children)

If unsure between diagnoses of epididymitis and torsion, always go to OR
Remember: torsion >6 h has poor prognosis

Inadequately treated acute epididymitis may lead to chronic epididymitis or epididymo-orchitis

Reactive Arthritis (formerly known as Reiter's syndrome)
Urethritis, uveitis (or conjunctivitis), and arthritis (can't pee, can't see, can't climb a tree)

If culture negative or unresponsive to treatment consider: *Ureaplasma urealyticum, Mycoplasma genitalium, Trichomonas vaginalis,* HSV, or adenovirus

Urethritis

Etiology
- infectious or inflammatory (e.g. reactive arthritis)

Table 11. Infectious Urethritis: Gonococcal vs. Non-Gonococcal

	Gonococcal	Non-Gonococcal
Causative Organism	*Neisseria gonorrhoeae*	Usually *Chlamydia trachomatis*
Diagnosis	Hx of sexual contact, thick, profuse, yellow-grey purulent d/c, LUTS. Gram stain (GN diplococci), urine PCR and/or culture from urethral specimen	Hx of sexual contact, mucoid whitish purulent d/c, ± storage LUTS. Gram stain demonstrates >4 PMN/oil immersion field, no evidence of *N. gonorrhoeae*, urine PCR and/or culture from urethral specimen
Treatment	See Table 9, U12	See Table 9, U12

Stone Disease

Epidemiology
- prevalence: ~8% and increasing
- M:F = 2:1
- peak incidence 30-50 yr of age
- recurrence rate: 10% at 1 yr, 50% at 5 yr, 60-80% lifetime

Risk Factors
- hereditary: RTA, Glucose-6-phosphate dehydrogenase deficiency, cystinuria, xanthinuria, oxaluria, etc.
- lifestyle: minimal fluid intake; excess vitamin C, oxalate, purines, calcium
- medications: loop diuretics (furosemide, bumetanide), acetazolamide, topiramate, zonisamide, indinavir, acyclovir, sulfadiazine, triamterene
- medical conditions: UTI (with urea-splitting organisms: *Proteus, Pseudomonas, Providencia, Klebsiella, Mycoplasma, Serratia, S. aureus*), myeloproliferative disorders, IBD, gout, DM, hypercalcemia disorders (hyperparathyroidism, tumour lysis syndrome, sarcoidosis, histoplasmosis), obesity (BMI >30)

Key Points in Stone Hx
- Diet (especially FLUID INTAKE)
- Predisposing medical conditions
- Predisposing medications
- Previous episodes/investigations/ treatments
- Family Hx (1st degree relative)

Clinical Features
- urinary obstruction → upstream distention → pain
  - flank pain from renal capsular distention (non-colicky)
  - severe waxing and waning pain radiating from flank to groin, testis, or tip of penis due to stretching of collecting system or ureter (ureteral colic)
- writhing, never comfortable, nausea, vomiting, hematuria (90% microscopic), diaphoresis, tachycardia, tachypnea
- occasionally symptoms of trigonal irritation (frequency, urgency)
- bladder stones result in: storage and voiding LUTS, terminal hematuria, suprapubic pain
- if fever, rule out concurrent pyelonephritis and/or obstruction

The four narrowest passage points for upper tract stones are:
- UPJ
- Pelvic brim
- Under vas deferens/broad ligament
- UVJ

Table 12. Differential Diagnosis of Renal Colic

GU	Abdominal	Neurological
Pyelonephritis	AAA	Radiculitis (L1): herpes zoster, nerve root compression
Ureteral obstruction from other cause: UPJ obstruction, clot colic secondary to gross hematuria, sloughed papillae	Bowel ischemia	
	Pancreatitis	
Gynecological: ectopic pregnancy, torsion/rupture of ovarian cyst, PID	Other acute abdominal crisis (appendicitis, cholecystitis, diverticulitis)	

Location of Stones
- calyx: may cause flank discomfort, persistent infection, persistent hematuria, or remain asymptomatic
- pelvis: tend to cause obstruction at UPJ, may cause persistent infection
- ureter: <5 mm diameter will pass spontaneously in 75% of patients

Stone Pathogenesis
- supersaturation of stone constituents (at appropriate temperature and pH)
- stasis, low flow, and low volume of urine (dehydration)
- crystal formation and stone nidus
- loss of inhibitory factors
  - citrate (forms soluble complex with calcium)
  - magnesium (forms soluble complex with oxalate)
  - pyrophosphate
  - Tamm-Horsfall glycoprotein

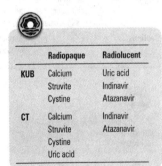

		Radiopaque	Radiolucent
KUB		Calcium	Uric acid
		Struvite	Indinavir
		Cystine	Atazanavir
CT		Calcium	Indinavir
		Struvite	Atazanavir
		Cystine	
		Uric acid	

Stone Disease

Approach to Renal Stones

Although hypercalciuria is a risk factor for stone formation, decreasing dietary calcium is NOT recommended to prevent stone formation. Low dietary calcium leads to increased GI oxalate absorption and higher urine levels of calcium oxalate

Stones and Infection
If septic, urgent decompression via ureteric stent or percutaneous nephrostomy is indicated. Definitive treatment of the stone should be delayed until the sepsis has cleared

Indications for PCNL
- Size >2 cm
- Staghorn
- UPJ obstruction with correction of obstruction
- Calyceal diverticulum
- Cystine stones (poorly fragmented with ESWL)
- Anatomical abnormalities
- Failure of less invasive modalities

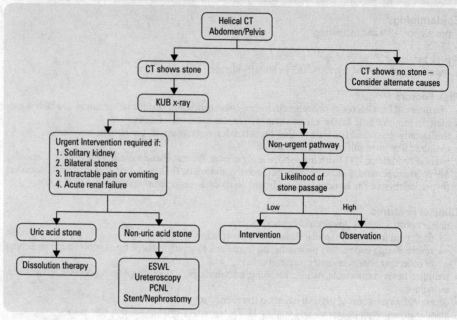

Figure 8. Approach to renal stone

Investigations

Table 13. Investigations for Renal Stones

	CBC, Uric Acid, U/A, Urine C&S	KUB x-ray	CT Scan	Abdominal Ultrasound	Cystoscopy	PTH, 24 h urine x 2 for volume, Cr, Ca^{2+}, Na$^+$, PO$_4$$^{3-}$, Mg^{2+}, oxalate, citrate, ± cystine
Who gets it?	Everyone	Most	First episode renal colic	Pediatric cases or those concerning for obstruction	± Those concerning for bladder stone	Recurrent Ca^{2+} stone formers ± pediatric cases
Why is it done?	May show signs of infection, ± sensitivities	90% of stones are radiopaque. Good for follow-up	Distinguish radiolucent stone from soft tissue filling defect. X-ray comparison	Identify and follow-up stone without radiation exposure. Visualize hydronephrosis	Visualize bladder	Need to rule out metabolic cause for stones
Cautions	—	Do not mistake phleboliths for stones!	Radiation (especially if female of child bearing age). Must be a non-contrast scan	—	—	—

24 h urine collections must be done AFTER discontinuing stone preventing/promoting medications

Indications for Admission to Hospital
- Intractable pain
- Intractable vomiting
- Fever (suggests infection)
- Compromised renal function (including single kidney, bilateral obstructing stone)
- Pregnancy

Detailed metabolic studies are NOT recommended unless complex patient (recurrent stone formers, pregnancy, pediatrics, strong family Hx, underlying kidney or systemic disease, etc.)

Treatment – Acute
- medical
  - analgesic ± antiemetic
  - NSAIDs help lower intra-ureteral pressure
  - medical expulsion therapy (MET)
    - α-blockers: increase rate of spontaneous passage in distal ureteral stones
  - ± Abx for bacteriuria
  - IV fluids if vomiting (note: IV fluids do NOT promote stone passage)
- interventional
  - required if obstruction endangers patient, e.g. sepsis, renal failure
  - first line: ureteric stent (via cystoscopy)
  - second line: image-guided percutaneous nephrostomy
- admit if necessary
  - *Indications for Admission to Hospital*

Treatment – Elective
- medical
  - likely conservative if ureteral stone <10 mm or kidney stone <5 mm and no complications/symptoms well controlled
    - stones <5 mm especially likely to pass spontaneously
  - PO fluids to increase urine volume to >2 L/d (3-4 L if cystine) and MET
  - specific to stone type (see Table 14)
  - periodic imaging to monitor stone position and assess for hydronephrosis
  - progress to interventional stone removal methods if symptoms worsen or fail to improve (indicating stone passage)

- interventional
  - kidney
    - may stent prior to ESWL if stone is 1.5-2.5 cm
    - ESWL if stone <2 cm
    - PCNL if stone >2 cm
  - ureteral stones >10 mm
    - ESWL and URS are both first line treatment modalities for all locations
      - URS has significantly greater stone-free rates for stones at all locations in ureter, but also has higher complication rates (ureter perforation, stricture formation, etc.)
    - PCNL is second line treatment
    - laparoscopic or open stone removal (very rare)
  - bladder
    - transurethral stone removal or cystolitholapaxy
    - remove outflow obstruction (TURP or stricture dilatation)

Prevention
- dietary modification
  - increase fluid (>2 L/d), K⁺ intake
  - reduce animal protein, oxalate, Na⁺, sucrose, and fructose intake
  - avoid high-dose vitamin C supplements
- medications
  - thiazide diuretics for hypercalciuria
  - allopurinol for hyperuricosuria
  - potassium citrate for hypocitraturia, hyperuricosuria

Alpha-blockers as Medical Expulsive Therapy for Ureteral Stones
Cochrane DB Syst Rev 2014;4:CD008509
Purpose: To determine whether or not alpha blockers compared with other pharmacological treatments or placebo improve stone clearance rates and other clinically relevant outcomes in patients presenting with symptoms of stones less than 10mm confirmed by imaging.
Results/Conclusions: 32 RCTs, 5,864 participants. Although patients using alpha-blockers were more likely to experience adverse effects compared to standard therapy, stone-free rates were significantly higher in the alpha-blocker group (RR 1.48, 95% CI 1.33-1.64), expulsion time was 2.91 days shorter, and there was a reduction in the number of pain episodes (MD -0.48, 95% CI -0.94 to -0.01), the need for analgesic medication (MD -38.17, 95% CI -74.93 to -1.41), and hospitalization (RR 0.35, 95% CI 0.13-0.97). Alpha blockers should therefore be offered as a primary treatment modality for ureteral stones.

Consideration must be given to monitoring stone formers with periodic imaging (i.e. at year 1 and then q2-4yr based on likelihood of recurrence)

Table 14. Stone Classification

Type of Stone	Calcium (75-85%)	Uric Acid (5-10%)	Struvite (5-10%)	Cystine (1%)
Etiology	Hypercalciuria Hyperuricosuria (25% of patients with Ca²⁺ stones) Hyperoxaluria (<5% of patients) Hypocitraturia (12% of patients) Other causes: Hypomagnesemia – associated with hyperoxaluria and hypocitraturia High dietary Na⁺ Decreased urinary proteins High urinary pH, low urine volume (e.g. GI water loss) Hyperparathyroidism, obesity, gout, DM	Uric acid precipitates in low volume, acidic urine with a high uric acid concentration: Hyperuricosuria alone Drugs (ASA, thiazides) Diet (purine rich red meats) Hyperuricosuria with hyperuricemia Gout High rate of cell turnover or cell death (leukemia, cytotoxic drugs)	Infection with urea-splitting organisms (*Proteus, Pseudomonas, Providencia, Klebsiella, Mycoplasma, Serratia, S. aureus*) results in alkaline urinary pH and precipitation of struvite (magnesium ammonium phosphate)	Autosomal recessive defect in small bowel mucosal absorption and renal tubular absorption of dibasic amino acids results in "COLA" in urine (cystine, ornithine, lysine, arginine)
Key Features	Radiopaque on KUB Reducing dietary Ca²⁺ is NOT an effective method of prevention/treatment	Radiolucent on KUB Radiopaque on CT Acidic urine, pH <5.5 (NOT necessarily elevated urinary uric acid)	Perpetuates UTI because stone itself harbours organism Stone and all foreign bodies must be cleared to avoid recurrence Associated with staghorn calculi Positive urine dip and cultures Note: *E. coli* infection does not cause struvite stones M:F = 3:1, UTI more common in female	Aggressive stone disease seen in children and young adults Recurrent stone formation, family Hx Often staghorn calculi Faintly radiopaque on KUB Positive urine sodium nitroprusside test, urine chromatography for cystine
Treatment Medical if stone <5 mm and no complications Procedural/Surgical treatment if stone >5 mm or presence of complications	Fluids to increase urine volume to >2 L/d For calcium stones: cellulose phosphate, orthophosphate for absorptive causes Calcium oxalate: thiazides, ± potassium citrate, ± allopurinol Calcium struvite: ABx (stone must be removed to treat infection)	Increased fluid intake Alkalinization of urine to pH 6.5 to 7 (bicarbonate, potassium citrate) ± allopurinol	Complete stone clearance ABx for 6 wk Regular follow-up urine cultures	Increased fluid intake (3-4 L of urine/d) Alkalinize urine (bicarbonate, potassium citrate), Penicillamine/α-MPG or Captopril (form complex with cystine) ESWL not effective

There is controversy over optimal management of small renal masses

Percutaneous needle biopsies of cystic renal masses may lead to peritoneal seeding

Tuberous Sclerosis
Syndrome characterized by mental retardation, epilepsy, and adenoma sebaceum. 45-80% of patients also present with angiomyolipomas which are often multiple and bilateral

Urological Neoplasms

Approach to Renal Mass

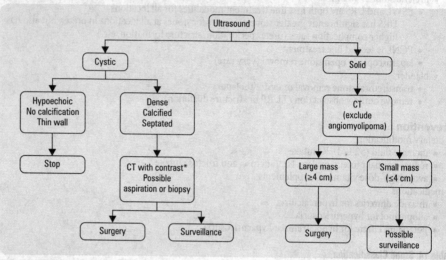

Figure 9. Workup of a renal mass
*Imaging modality may be different in cases of contrast allergy or elevated creatinine

Benign Renal Neoplasms

CYSTIC KIDNEY DISEASE
- simple cysts: usually solitary or unilateral
  - very common: up to 50% at age 50
  - usually incidental finding on abdominal imaging
  - Bosniak Classification is used to stratify for risk of malignancy based on cyst features from contrast CT
- polycystic kidney disease
  - autosomal recessive: multiple bilateral cysts, often leading to early renal failure in infants
  - autosomal dominant: progressive bilateral disease leading to HTN and renal failure, adult-onset
- medullary sponge kidney: cystic dilatation of the collecting ducts
  - usually benign course, but patients are predisposed to stone disease
- von Hippel-Lindau syndrome: multiple bilateral cysts or clear cell carcinomas (50% incidence of RCC)
  - renal cysts, cerebellar, spinal and retinal hemangioblastomas, pancreatic and epididymal cysts, pheochromocytomas

Table 15. Bosniak Classification of Renal Cysts

Class	Description	Features	Risk of Malignancy	Management Plan
I	Simple cyst	Round, no septations, no calcifications, no solid component	Near zero	Follow-up usually not required
II	Simple cyst	A few thin septa, no true enhancement, well-marginated, uniform high attenuation, <3 cm	Minimal	Follow-up usually not required
IIF	Minimally complex cyst with extra features that require follow-up	Still well-marginated and non-enhancing, but now multiple thin septa or some thickening/calcification of septa/wall, >3 cm	5-20%	Requires follow-up with imaging q6-12mo If the lesion evolves, may require surgical resection
III	Complex cyst	Thicker or more irregular walls with measurable enhancement	>50%	Requires surgical resection
IV	Clearly malignant	Class III + enhancing soft-tissue components	>90%	Requires surgical resection

Table 16. Benign Renal Masses

	Angiomyolipoma (Renal Hamartoma)	Renal Oncocytoma	Renal Adenoma
Epidemiology	<1% of adult renal tumours F>M 20% associated with tuberous sclerosis (especially if multiple, recurrent)	3-7% of renal tumours M>F Oncocytomas also found in adrenal, thyroid and parathyroid glands	Most common benign renal neoplasm M:F = 3:1 Incidence increases with age Found in 7-23% of all autopsies
Characteristics	Clonal neoplasm consisting of blood vessels (angio-), smooth muscle (-myo-), and fat (-lipoma) May extend into regional lymphatics and other organs and become symptomatic	Spherical, capsulated with possible central scar Histologically organized aggregates of eosinophilic cells originating from intercalated cells of collecting duct	Small cortical lesions <1 cm Majority are solitary but can be multifocal
Diagnosis	Incidental finding on CT Negative attenuation (-20 HU) on CT is pathognomonic Rare presentation of hematuria, flank pain, and palpable mass (same as RCC)	Incidental finding on CT Difficult to distinguish from RCC on imaging – treated as RCC until proven otherwise Biopsy may be performed to rule out malignancy	Incidental finding on CT Rarely symptomatic Controversy as to whether this represents benign or pre-malignant neoplasm
Management	May consider surgical excision or embolization if symptomatic (pain, bleeding) or higher risk of bleeding (e.g. pregnancy) Potential role for mTOR inhibitors in unresectable/metastatic disease Follow with serial U/S	Partial/radical nephrectomy for large masses HIFU or RFA for smaller masses	If mass >3 cm, likely not a benign adenoma; will require partial/radical nephrectomy due to increased likelihood of malignancy

Malignant Renal Neoplasms

RENAL CELL CARCINOMA

Etiology
- cause unknown
- originates from proximal convoluted tubule epithelial cells in clear cell subtype (most common)
- hereditary forms seen with von Hippel-Lindau syndrome and hereditary papillary renal carcinoma

Epidemiology
- 85% of primary malignant tumours in kidney
- M:F = 3:2
- peak incidence at 50-60 yr of age

Pathology
- histological subtypes: clear cell (75-85%), papillary (10-15%), chromophobic (5-10%), collecting duct
- sarcomatoid elements in any subtype is a poor prognostic factor

Risk Factors
- top 3 risk factors: smoking, HTN, obesity
- miscellaneous: horseshoe kidney, acquired renal cystic disease
- role of environmental exposures (aromatic hydrocarbons, etc.) remains an unproven risk factor for development of RCC

Clinical Features
- usually asymptomatic: frequently diagnosed incidentally by U/S or CT
- poor prognostic indicators: weight loss, weakness, anemia, bone pain
- classic "too late triad" found in 10-15%
  - gross hematuria 50%
  - flank pain <50%
  - palpable mass <30%
- was called the "internist's tumour" because of paraneoplastic symptomatology – now called the "radiologist's tumour" because of incidental diagnosis via imaging
- metastases: seen in a 1/3 of new cases; additional 20-40% will go on to develop metastases (mostly for late presentations or large tumours)
  - bone, brain, lung and liver most common site
  - may invade renal veins and inferior vena cava lumen. This may result in ascites, hepatic dysfunction, right atrial tumour, and pulmonary emboli

Investigations
- routine labs for paraneoplastic syndromes (CBC, ESR, LFTs, extended electrolytes)
- U/A
- renal U/S: solid vs. cystic lesion
- contrast-enhanced CT: higher sensitivity than U/S for detection of renal masses and for staging purposes
- MRI: useful for evaluation of vascular extension
- renal biopsy: to confirm diagnosis if considering observation or other non-surgical therapy

Staging
- involves CT, CXR, liver enzymes and LFTs, bone/head imaging (if symptoms dictate)

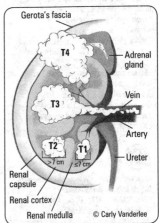

Figure 10. RCC staging

Role of environmental exposures (aromatic hydrocarbons, etc.) remains an unproven risk factor for development of RCC

RCC Systemic Effects: paraneoplastic syndromes (10-40% of patients)
- Hematopoietic disturbances: anemia, polycythemia, raised ESR
- Endocrinopathies: hypercalcemia (increased vitamin D hydroxylation), erythrocytosis (increased erythropoietin), HTN (increased renin), production of other hormones (prolactin, gonadotropins, TSH, insulin, and cortisol)
- Hepatic cell dysfunction or Stauffer syndrome: abnormal LFTs, decreased WBC count, fever, areas of hepatic necrosis; no evidence of metastases; reversible following removal of primary tumour
- Hemodynamic alterations: systolic HTN (due to AV shunting), peripheral edema (due to caval obstruction)

Tumour may invade renal veins and inferior vena cava lumen. This may result in ascites, hepatic dysfunction, right atrial tumour, and pulmonary emboli

Carcinoma: Final Efficacy of Safety Results of the Phase III Treatment Approaches in Renal Cancer Global Evaluation Trial
J Clin Oncol 2009; 27(20):3312-8.
Purpose: Phase III trial of renal cell carcinoma patients who were randomized to receive either sorafenib (n=451) or placebo (n=452).
Results: The overall survival was 17.8 months in the treatment group, compared to 15.2 months in the control group (HR = .88, p =.146). Following adjustment for crossover patients (from placebo to treatment), a significant difference was found in the overall survival (17.8 vs 14.3 months, HR = .78, p = .029). No difference was found in adverse events at 16 months.

Axitinib vs. Sorafenib as Second-Line Treatment for Advanced Renal Cell Carcinoma: Overall Survival Analysis and Updated Results from a Randomized Phase 3 Trial
Lancet Oncol 2013;14:552-562
Study: Phase 3 trial of patients with clear cell metastatic renal cell carcinoma randomized to receive axitinib 5 mg twice daily (n=361) or sorafenib 400 mg twice daily (n=362).
Results: Median overall survival was 20.1 mo with axitinib (16.7 -23.4) and 19.2 monwith sorafenib (17.5-22.3) (HR 0.969, 95% CI 0.800-1.174). Median progression-free survival was 8.3 months with axitinib (6.7-9.2) and 5.7 mo with sorafenib (4.7-6.5) (HR 0.656, 95% CI 0.552-0.779).
Conclusions: Axitinib should be a second-line treatment option for patients with metastatic renal cell carcinoma.

Radiotherapy With or Without Chemotherapy in Muscle-Invasive Bladder Cancer
NEJM 2012;366:1477-1488
Study: Phase 3 trial with random assignment of 360 patients with muscle-invasive bladder cancer to radiotherapy with or without chemotherapy.
Results: At 2 yr, rates of locoregional disease-free survival were 67% in the chemoradiotherapy group and 54% in the radiotherapy group (HR 0.68, 95% CI 0.48-0.96). Five year overall survival rates were 48% in the chemoradiotherapy group and 35% in the radiotherapy group (HR 0.82, 95% CI 0.63-1.09).
Conclusions: Chemotherapy with fluorouracil and mitomycin C in combination with radiotherapy improves locoregional control of bladder cancer compared to radiotherapy alone, with no significant increase in adverse events.

Differential Diagnosis of Filling Defect
- Urothelial carcinoma (differentiate via cytology and CT scan)
- Uric acid stone (differentiate via cytology and CT scan)
- Blood clot
- Pyelitis cystica
- Papillary necrosis
- Fungus ball
- Gas bubble from gas producing organisms

Table 17. 2010 TNM Classification of Renal Cell Carcinoma

T	N	M
T1: tumour <7 cm, confined to renal parenchyma	**N0**: no regional lymph node metastasis	**M0**: no evidence of metastasis
T1a: <4 cm	**N1**: metastasis in regional lymph nodes	**M1**: presence of distant metastasis
T1b: 4-7 cm		
T2: tumour >7 cm, confined to renal parenchyma		
T2a: 7-10 cm		
T2b: >10cm		
T3: tumour extends into major veins or perinephric tissues, but NOT into ipsilateral adrenal or beyond Gerota's fascia		
T3a: into renal vein or sinus fat		
T3b: into infradiaphragmatic IVC		
T3c: into supradiaphragmatic IVC		
T4: tumour extends beyond Gerota's fascia including extension into ipsilateral adrenal		

Treatment
- surgical
    - radical nephrectomy: en bloc removal of kidney, tumour, ipsilateral adrenal gland (in upper pole tumours) and intact Gerota's capsule and paraaortic lymphadenectomy
    - partial nephrectomy (parenchyma-sparing): small tumour (roughly <4 cm) or solitary kidney/bilateral tumours
    - surgical removal of solitary metastasis may be considered
- ablative techniques (cryoablation, RFA)
- palliative radiation to painful bony lesions
- therapy for advanced stage
    - tyrosine kinase inhibitors for metastatic disease (e.g. sunitinib, sorafenib)
    - anti-angiogenesis/anti-VEGF (e.g. bevacizumab)
    - mTOR inhibitors (e.g. temsirolimus, everolimus)
    - high-dose IL-2 (high toxicity but able to induce long-term cure in 5-7% of patients)
    - IFN-α: monotherapy has been largely replaced by molecularly targeted agents listed above

Prognosis
- stage at diagnosis most important prognostic factor
    - T1: 90-100% 5 yr survival
    - T2-T3: 60% 5 yr survival
    - metastatic disease: <5% 10 yr survival

Carcinoma of the Renal Pelvis and Ureter

Etiology
- risk factors include
    - smoking
    - chemicals/dietary exposures (industrial dyes and solvents; aristolochic acid)
    - analgesic abuse (acetaminophen, ASA, and phenacetin)
    - Balkan nephropathy

Epidemiology
- rare: accounts for 5% of all urothelial cancers
- frequently multifocal, 2-5% are bilateral
- M:F = 3:1
- relative incidence: bladder:renal:ureter = 100:10:1

Pathology
- 85% are papillary urothelial carcinoma; others include SCC and adenocarcinoma
- UCC of ureter and renal pelvis are histologically similar to bladder UCC

Clinical Features
- gross/microscopic hematuria
- flank pain
- storage or voiding symptoms (dysuria only if lower urinary tract involved)
- flank mass ± hydronephrosis (10-20%)

Investigations
- IVP/CT urogram
- cystoscopy and retrograde pyelogram

Treatment
- radical nephroureterectomy with cuff of bladder
- distal ureterectomy for distal ureteral tumours with concomitant ureteral reimplant
- emerging role for endoscopic laser ablation in patients with low grade disease, poor baseline renal health

Bladder Carcinoma

Etiology
- unknown, but environmental risk factors include
  - smoking (main factor – implicated in 60% of new cases)
  - aromatic amines: naphthylamines, benzidine, tryptophan, phenacetin metabolites
  - cyclophosphamide
  - prior Hx of radiation treatment to the pelvis
  - *Schistosoma hematobium* infection (associated with SCC)
  - chronic irritation: cystitis, chronic catheterization, bladder stones (associated with SCC)
  - aristolochic acid: associated with Balkan Nephropathy (renal failure, upper tract urothelial cancer) and Chinese Herbal Nephropathy

Epidemiology
- 2nd most common urological malignancy
- M:F = 3:1, more common among whites than blacks
- mean age at diagnosis is 65 yr

Pathology
- classification
  - urothelial carcinoma (UC) >90%
  - SCC 5-7%
  - adenocarcinoma 1%
  - others <1%
- stages and prognoses of urothelial carcinoma at diagnosis
  - non-muscle invasive (75%) → >80% overall survival
    - 15% of these will progress to invasive UCC
    - the majority of these patients will have recurrence
  - invasive (25%) → 50-60% 5 yr survival
    - 85% have no prior Hx of superficial UCC (i.e. *de novo*)
    - 50% have occult metastases at diagnosis, and most of these will develop overt clinical evidence of metastases within 1 yr – lymph nodes, lung, peritoneum, liver
- carcinoma *in situ* → flat, non-papillary erythematous lesion characterized by dysplasia confined to urothelium
  - more aggressive, worse prognosis
  - usually multifocal
  - may progress to invasive UCC

Clinical Features
- asymptomatic (20%)
- hematuria (key symptom: 85-90% at the time of diagnosis)
- pain (50%) → location determined by size/extent of tumour (i.e. flank, suprapubic, perineal, abdominal, etc.)
- clot retention (17%)
- storage urinary symptoms → consider carcinoma *in situ*
- palpable mass on bimanual exam → likely muscle invasion
- obstruction of ureters → hydronephrosis and uremia (nausea, vomiting, and diarrhea)

Investigations
- U/A, urine C&S, urine cytology
- U/S
- CT scan with contrast → look for filling defect
- cystoscopy with biopsy (gold standard)
- biopsy to establish diagnosis and to determine depth of penetration
- specific bladder tumour markers (e.g. NMP-22, BTA, Immunocyt, FDP)

Grading
- low grade: <=10% invasive, 60% recur
- high grade: 50-80% are invasive or should progress to invasive over time

Staging
- for invasive disease: CT or MRI, CXR, LFTs, extended electrolytes (Ca^{2+}, Mg^{2+}, PO_4^{3-}) (metastatic workup)

The "field defect" theory helps to explain why UCC has multiple lesions and has a high recurrence rate. The entire urothelium (pelvis to bladder) is bathed in carcinogens

The ENTIRE urinary tract must be evaluated in patients with hematuria unless there is clear evidence of glomerular bleeding (e.g. red cell casts, dysmorphic RBCs, etc.)

Cystoscopy is the initial procedure of choice for the diagnosis and staging of urothelial malignancy

Unexplained hematuria in any individual >40 yr old must be investigated to rule out a malignancy

Tumour grade is the single most important prognostic factor for progression

Neoadjuvant Chemotherapy plus Cystectomy Compared with Cystectomy Alone for Locally Advanced Bladder Cancer
NEJM 2003;349:859-866
Study: Randomized clinical trial.
Patients: 317 patients with transitional-cell carcinoma of the bladder (T2N0M0 to T4aN0M0).
Intervention: Randomized to undergo radical cystectomy or to receive three cycles of combined chemotherapy (methotrexate, vinblastine, doxorubicin, and cisplatin) followed by radical cystectomy.
Main Outcome: Survival. Secondary objective was to quantify down-staging of tumour following chemotherapy.
Results: At 5 yr after treatment initiation, 57% of the combination-therapy group vs. 43% of the cystectomy group were alive (p=0.06). In the combination-therapy group, 38% of the patients were pathologically free of cancer at the time of cystectomy vs. 15% of the cystectomy-only group at the time of surgery (p<0.001).
Conclusions: For locally advanced bladder carcinoma, neoadjuvant chemotherapy significantly reduces tumour volume and also improves survival.

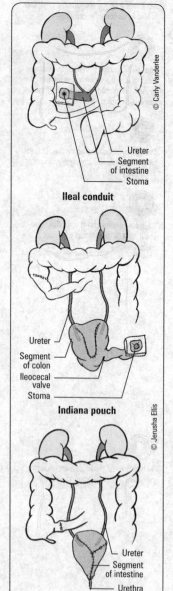

Figure 12. Ileal conduit, Indiana pouch, ileal neobladder

Table 18. 2010 TNM Classification of Bladder Carcinoma

T	N	M
TX: Primary tumour cannot be assessed	**NX**: Lymph nodes cannot be assessed	**M0**: No distant metastasis
T0: No evidence of primary tumour **Ta**: Noninvasive papillary carcinoma **Tis**: Carcinoma *in situ*: "flat tumour"	**N0**: No lymph node metastasis	**M1**: Distant metastasis
T1: Tumour invades subepithelial connective tissue	**N1**: Single regional lymph node metastasis in the true pelvis (hypogastric, obturator, external iliac, or presacral lymph node)	
T2: Tumour invades muscularis propria **pT2a**: Tumour invades superficial muscularis propria (inner half) **pT2b**: Tumour invades deep muscularis propria (outer half)	**N2**: Multiple regional lymph node metastasis in the true pelvis (hypogastric, obturator, external iliac, or presacral lymph node metastasis)	
T3: Tumour invades perivesical tissue **pT3a**: Microscopically **pT3b**: Macroscopically (extravesical mass)	**N3**: Lymph node metastasis to the common iliac lymph nodes	
T4: Tumour invades any of the following: prostatic stroma, seminal vesicles, uterus, vagina, pelvic wall, abdominal wall **T4a**: Tumour invades prostatic stroma, uterus, vagina **T4b**: Tumour invades pelvic wall, abdominal wall		

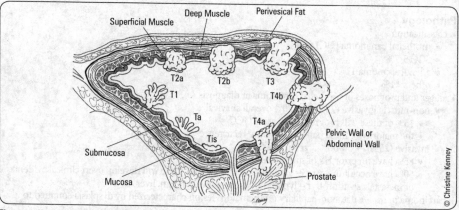

Figure 11. Urothelial carcinoma of bladder

Treatment
- superficial (non-muscle invasive) disease: Tis, Ta, T1
  - low-grade disease
    - single dose mitomycin C within 24 hours of resection reduces recurrence rates
  - high-grade
    - TURBT ± intravesical chemo/immuno-therapy (e.g. BCG, mitomycin C) to decrease recurrence rate
    - maintenance with intravesical chemotherapy with BCG for 3 cycles every 3 mo, may be continued for 2-3 yr
- invasive disease: T2a, T2b, T3
  - radical cystectomy + pelvic lymphadenectomy with urinary diversion (e.g. ileal conduit, Indiana pouch, ileal neobladder) or TURBT + chemo-radiation (bladder sparing) for small tumours with non-obstructed ureters
  - neo-adjuvant chemotherapy prior to cystectomy may also be done
  - use of adjuvant chemotherapy after definitive local treatment is controversial
- advanced/metastatic disease: T4a, T4b, N+, M+
  - initial combination of systemic chemotherapy ± irradiation ± surgery

Prognosis
- depends on stage, grade, size, number of lesions, recurrence and presence of CIS
  - T1: 90% 5 yr survival
  - T2: 55% 5 yr survival
  - T3: 30% 5 yr survival
  - T4/N+/M+: <5% 5 yr survival

Prostate Cancer

Etiology
- not known
- risk factors
  - increased incidence in persons of African descent
  - high dietary fat = 2x risk
  - family Hx
    - 1st degree relative = 2x risk
    - 1st and 2nd degree relatives = 9x risk

Epidemiology
- most prevalent cancer in males
- 3rd leading cause of male cancer deaths (following lung and colon)
- up to 50% risk of CaP at age 50
- lifetime risk of death from CaP is 3%
- 75% diagnosed between ages of 60 and 85; mean age at diagnosis is 72

Pathology
- adenocarcinoma
  - >95%, often multifocal
- urothelial carcinoma of the prostate (4.5%)
  - associated with UCC of bladder; does NOT follow TNM staging below; not hormone-responsive
- endometrial (rare)
  - carcinoma of the utricle

Anatomy (see Figure 7, U7)
- 60-70% of nodules arise in the peripheral zone
- 10-20% arise in the transition zone
- 5-10% arise in the central zone

Clinical Features
- usually asymptomatic
- most commonly detected by DRE, elevated PSA, or as an incidental finding on TURP
  - DRE: hard irregular nodule or diffuse dense induration involving one or both lobes
  - PSA: see *Prostate Cancer Screening*, U26
- locally advanced disease
  - storage and voiding symptoms, ED (all uncommon without spread)
- metastatic disease
  - bony metastases to axial skeleton common
  - visceral metastases are less common (liver, lung, and adrenal gland most common sites)
  - leg pain and edema with nodal metastases obstructing lymphatic and venous drainage

Methods of Spread
- local invasion
- lymphatic spread to regional nodes
  - obturator > iliac > presacral/para-aortic
- hematogenous dissemination occurs early

Investigations
- DRE
- PSA elevated in the majority of patients with CaP
- TRUS-guided needle biopsy
- bone scan may be omitted in untreated CaP with PSA <10 ng/mL
- CT scanning to assess metastases
- MRI: being investigated for possible role in detection, staging, MRI-guided biopsying and active surveillance

Table 19. 2010 TNM Classification of Prostate Carcinoma

T	N	M
T1: clinically undetectable tumour, normal DRE and TRUS **T1a**: tumour incidental histologic finding in <5% of tissue resected **T1b**: tumour incidental histologic finding in >5% of tissue resected **T1c**: tumour identified by needle biopsy (due to elevated PSA level)	**NX**: regional lymph nodes were not assessed **N0**: no regional lymph node metastasis	**M0**: no distant metastasis **M**: distant metastasis **M1a**: nonregional lymph nodes **M1b**: bone(s)
T2: palpable, confined to prostate **T2a**: tumour involving ≤ one half of one lobe **T2b**: tumour involving > one half of one lobe, but not both lobes **T2c**: tumour involving both lobes	**N1**: spread to regional lymph nodes	**M1c**: other site(s) with or without bone disease
T3: tumour extends through prostate capsule **T3a**: extracapsular extension (unilateral or bilateral) **T3b**: tumour invading seminal vesicle(s)		
T4: tumour invades adjacent structures (besides seminal vesicles)		

Table 20. Prostate Cancer Mortality Risk

	Low Risk	Intermediate Risk (if any of following)	High Risk (if any of following)
PSA	<10	10-20	>20
Gleason Score	<7	7	8-10
Stage	pT1-2a	pT2b-T2c	pT3/4

Radical Prostatectomy vs. Watchful Waiting in Early Prostate Cancer (Scandinavian Prostate Cancer Group Study)
NEJM 2011;364:1708-1717
Study: Randomized clinical trial comparing watchful waiting with radical prostatectomy for localized prostate cancer.
Methods: 695 men from 14 centres in Finland, Sweden, and Iceland with newly diagnosed, localized prostate cancer were included in this study.
Main Outcomes: Mortality, distant metastases, local progression.
Results: For men with low-risk prostate cancer (PSA<10, Gleason score<7), at 15 yr after treatment initiation, the relative risk of death due to prostate cancer in the radical prostatectomy group versus watchful waiting was 0.62 (p=0.01). The cumulative incidence of death from prostate cancer after radical prostatectomy was high as compared with other studies.
Conclusions: Radical prostatectomy was associated with reduced rate of death due to prostate cancer.

Radical Prostatectomy vs. Observation for Localized Prostate Cancer (Prostate Cancer Intervention vs. Observation Trial (PIVOT) Study Group)
NEJM 2012;367:203-213
Study: Randomized clinical trial comparing observation with radical prostatectomy for localized prostate cancer.
Methods: 731 men at 52 United States centres with localized prostate cancer participated.
Main Outcomes: Mortality, bone metastases, surgical morbidity.
Results: Radical prostatectomy did not reduce all-cause or prostate cancer mortality relative to observation (relative risk 0.60, p=0.09), through at least 12 yr of follow-up.
Conclusions: Observation is recommended for localized prostate cancer, especially in men with low PSA and low-risk disease.

Causes of Increased PSA
BPH, prostatitis, prostatic ischemia/infarction, prostate biopsy/surgery, prostatic massage, acute urinary retention, urethral catheterization, cystoscopy, TRUS, strenuous exercise, perineal trauma, ejaculation, acute renal failure, coronary bypass graft, radiation therapy

PSA is specific to the PROSTATE, but NOT to prostate cancer

Treatment
- T1/T2 (localized, low-risk)
  - if adequate life expectancy or no other significant comorbidities, consider active surveillance vs. definitive local treatment (RP, brachytherapy, or EBRT)
  - active surveillance for low risk, small volume Gleason 6 prostate cancer
  - no difference in cure rate between definitive treatment modalities
  - in older population: watchful waiting + palliative treatment for symptomatic progression
- T1/T2 (intermediate or high-risk)
  - definitive therapy over active surveillance
- T3, T4
  - EBRT + androgen deprivation therapy or RP + adjuvant EBRT
- N >0 or M >0
  - requires hormonal therapy/palliative radiotherapy for metastases; may consider combined androgen blockade
  - bilateral orchiectomy – removes 90% of testosterone
  - GnRH agonists (e.g. leuprolide, goserelin)
  - GnRH antagonist (e.g. degarelix)
  - estrogens (e.g. diethylstilbestrol [DES])
  - antiandrogens (e.g. bicalutamide)
  - local irradiation of painful secondaries or half-body irradiation
- hormone-refractory prostate cancer
  - chemotherapy: docetaxel, cabazitaxel, sipuleucel-T

Table 21. Treatment Options for Localized Prostate Cancer

Modality	Population Considered	Limitations
Watchful Waiting	Short life expectancy (<5-10 yr); will likely only receive non-curative hormonal therapy if disease progresses	Disease progression
Active Surveillance (serial PSA, DRE, and biopsies)	Low grade disease, good follow-up; is still considering more curative treatment if disease progresses	Disease progression; decrease in QOL associated with serial testing; risks associated with biopsies; no optimal monitoring schedule has been defined to date
Brachytherapy	Low volume, low PSA (<10), low grade	ED (50%), long-term effectiveness not well-established
EBRT	Locally advanced disease, older patients	Radiation proctitis (5%), ED (50%), risk of rectal cancer
RP	Young patients (<75 yr), high-risk disease	Incontinence (10%), ED (30-50%)

*Other options include cryosurgery, HIFU, hormonal ablation

Prognosis
- T1-T2: comparable to normal life expectancy
- T3-T4: 40-70% 10-yr survival
- N+ and/or M+: 4 % 5 yr survival
- prognostic factors: tumour stage, tumour grade, PSA value, PSA doubling time

Prostate Cancer Screening

Digital Rectal Exam
- should be included as part of initial screening
- suspicious findings: abnormal feeling, nodularity, focal lesion, discrete change in texture/fullness/symmetry

Prostate Specific Antigen
- glycoprotein produced by epithelial cells of prostate gland
- leaks into circulation in setting of disrupted glandular architecture
- value of <4 ng/mL traditionally considered as cut-off to differentiate normal from pathologic value, but no single justifiable cutpoint
- measured serum PSA is a combination of free (15%) and bound PSA (85%)
- PSA velocity, PSA density, and free:total PSA: all intended to increase sensitivity and specificity of serum PSA values
  - association of increased CaP rates with decreased free are total PSA, elevated PSA velocity and density

Screening Recommendations
- conflicting evidence regarding mortality reduction with PSA-based screening and debate regarding overdiagnosis/overtreatment
- Long-Term Care and United States Preventative Services Task Force all recommend against PSA testing as a population-wide screening tool

- however, serum PSA screening recommended in any man with >10 yr life-expectancy and any of the following
  - suspicious finding on DRE
  - moderate-severe LUTS
  - high risk individuals
  - investigating secondary carcinoma of unknown origin to rule out CaP as primary

Canadian Urological Association Guidelines (2011) re: CaP Screening
- harms and benefits of PSA testing must be explained to the patient and an informed, shared decision to test must be established
- initial screening should include both serum PSA and DRE
- all men should be offered screening at age 50 if >10 yr life-expectancy
- high-risk individuals (family Hx of CaP or African ancestry) should be offered screening at age 40 if >10 yr life-expectancy
- standard has been annual screening, but q2-4yr screening acceptable
- no strict cutpoint for when to biopsy; decision to biopsy should be based on more than a single PSA value
- AUA guidelines recommend against universal routine PSA screening for CaP

Screening for Prostate Cancer
Cochrane DB Syst Rev 2013;1:CD004720
Background: Screening for prostate cancer has an unclear benefit for reducing prostate cancer-specific mortality and morbidity.
Study: Systematic review of randomized clinical trials of screening vs no screening. A total of 31 trials were retrieved for this review.
Results: A meta-analysis of 5 RCTs with 341,342 participants was done. Collectively, there was no significant reduction in prostate cancer-specific mortality within 10 yr of follow-up. Screening procedures and biopsies were commonly associated with bleeding, bruising, and short-term anxiety; subsequent over-diagnosis and overtreatment resulted in additional harms, some severe.
Conclusions: Men who have a life expectancy less than 10-15 yr should be informed that screening for prostate cancer is unlikely to be beneficial. Significant harms are associated with screening, over-diagnosis, and overtreatment.

Testicular Tumours

Etiology/Risk Factors
- cryptorchidism, atrophy, sex hormones, HIV infection, infertility, family Hx, past Hx of testicular cancer

Epidemiology
- rare, but most common solid malignancy in young males 15-35 yr
- any solid testicular mass or acute hydrocoele in young patient – must rule out malignancy
- slightly more common in right testis (corresponds with slightly higher incidence of right-sided cryptorchidism)
- 2-3% bilateral (simultaneously or successively)

Pathology
- primary
  - 1% of all malignancies in males
  - cryptorchidism has increased risk (10-40x) of malignancy
  - 95% are germ cell tumours (all are malignant)
    - seminoma (35%) → classic, anaplastic, spermatocytic
    - NSGCT → embryonal cell carcinoma (20%), teratoma (5%), choriocarcinoma (<1%), yolk sac (<<1%), mixed cell type (40%)
  - 5% are non-germ cell tumours (usually benign) → Leydig (testosterone, precocious puberty), Sertoli (gynecomastia, decreased libido)
- secondary
  - male >50 yr
  - usually lymphoma or metastases (e.g. lung, prostate, GI)

Clinical Features
- painless testicular enlargement (painful if intratesticular hemorrhage or infarction)
- dull, heavy ache in lower abdomen, anal area or scrotum
- associated hydrocele (10%)
- coincidental trauma (10%)
- infertility (rarely presenting complaint)
- gynecomastia due to secretory tumour effects
- supraclavicular and inguinal lymphadenopathy
- abdominal mass (retroperitoneal lymph node mets)

Methods of Spread
- local spread follows lymphatics
  - right → medial, paracaval, anterior and lateral nodes
  - left → left lateral and anterior paraaortic nodes
  - "cross-over" metastases from right to left are fairly common, but no reports from left to right
- hematogenous most commonly to lung, liver, bones, and kidney

Investigations
- diagnosis is established by pathological evaluation of specimen obtained by radical inguinal orchidectomy
- tumour markers (β-hCG, LDH, AFP)
  - β-hCG and AFP are positive in 85% of non-seminomatous tumours
  - elevated marker levels return to normal post-operatively if no metastasis
  - β-hCG positive in 7% of pure seminomas, AFP never elevated with seminoma

Testes and scrotum have different lymphatic drainage, therefore trans-scrotal approach for biopsy or orchiectomy should be avoided

- testicular U/S (hypoechoic area within tunica albuginea = high suspicion of testicular cancer)
- evidence of testicular microlithiasis is not a risk factor for testicular cancer
- needle aspiration contraindicated

Staging
- clinical: CXR (lung mets), markers for staging (β-hCG, AFP, LDH), CT abdomen/pelvis (retroperitoneal lymphadenopathy)
  - Stage I: disease limited to testis, epididymis, or spermatic cord
  - Stage II: disease limited to the retroperitoneal nodes
  - Stage III: disease metastatic to supradiaphragmatic nodal or visceral sites

Table 22. 2010 TNM Classification of Testicular Carcinoma

T	N	M
Tis: intratubular germ cell neoplasia	**N0**: no regional lymph node metastasis	**M0**: no distant mets
T1: limited to testis and epididymis without vascular/lymphatic invasion	**N1**: Metastasis with a lymph node mass 2 cm or less in greatest dimension; or multiple lymph nodes, none more than 2 cm in greatest dimension	**M1**: distant mets
T2: limited to testis and epididymis with vascular/lymphatic invasion		**M1a**: nonregional lymph node(s) or pulmonary mets
T3: invasion of the spermatic cord ± vascular/lymphatics	**N2**: Metastasis with a lymph node mass more than 2 cm but not more than 5cm in greatest dimension	**M1b**: distant mets other than to regional lymph nodes and lung
T4: invasion of the scrotum ± vascular/lymphatics	**N3**: Metastasis with a lymph node mass more than 5 cm in greatest dimension	

Orchiopexy
Surgical descent (orchiopexy) of undescended testis does not eliminate the risk of malignancy, but allows for earlier detection by self-examination and reduces the risk of infertility

Management
- orchiectomy through inguinal ligament for all stages
- consider sperm banking, testicular prosthesis
- adjuvant therapies

Prognosis
- 99% cured with stage I and II disease
- 70-80% complete remission with advanced disease

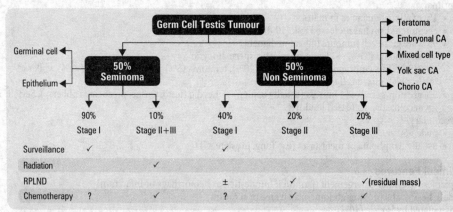

Figure 13. Adjuvant management of testicular cancer post-orchiectomy
Adapted from Dr. MAS Jewett

Penile Tumours

Epidemiology
- rare (<1% of cancer in males in U.S.)
- most common in 6th decade

Benign
- cyst, hemangioma, nevus, papilloma

Pre-Malignant
- balanitis xerotica obliterans, leukoplakia, Buschke-Lowenstein tumour (large condyloma)

Pre-invasive Cancer
- carcinoma *in situ*
  - Bowen's disease → crusted, red plaques on the shaft
  - erythroplasia of Queyrat → velvet red, ulcerated plaques on the glans
  - treatment options: local excision, laser, radiation, topical 5-fluorouracil

Malignant
- risk factors
  - chronic inflammatory disease
  - STI
  - phimosis
  - uncircumcised penis
- 2% of all urogenital cancers
- SCC (>95%), basal cell, melanoma, Paget's disease of the penis (extremely rare)
- definitive diagnosis requires full thickness biopsy of lesion
- lymphatic spread (superficial/deep inguinal nodes → iliac nodes) >> hematogenous

Treatment
- wide surgical excision with tumour-free margins (dependent on extent and area of penile involvement) ± lymphadenectomy
- consider less aggressive treatment modalities in CIS (cryotherapy, laser therapy, etc.) if available

Scrotal Mass

Table 23. Differentiating between Scrotal Masses

Condition	Pain	Palpation	Additional Findings
Torsion	+	Diffuse tenderness Horizontal lie of testicle	Absent cremaster reflex, negative Prehn's sign
Epididymitis (U16)	+	Epididymal tenderness	Present cremaster reflex, positive Prehn's sign
Orchitis (U16)	+	Diffuse tenderness	Present cremaster reflex, positive Prehn's sign
Hematocele	+	Diffuse tenderness	No transillumination
Hydrocele	–	Testis not separable from hydrocele, cord palpable	Transillumination, Hx of trauma
Spermatocele	–	Testis separable from spermatocele, cord palpable	Transillumination
Varicocele	–	Bag of worms	No transillumination, increases in size with Valsalva, decrease in size if supine
Indirect Inguinal	– (+ if strangulated)	Testis separable from hernia, cord not palpable, cough impulse may transmit, may be reducible	No transillumination
Tumour	– (+ if hemorrhagic)	Hard lump/nodule	
Generalized/ Dependant edema	–	Diffuse swelling	Often post-operative or immobilized, check for liver dysfunction
Idiopathic	–		

Varicocele Grading
- Grade 1: Palpable only with Valsalva manoeuvre
- Grade 2: Palpable without Valsalva
- Grade 3: Visible through scrotal skin

Suspect a Retroperitoneal Mass/Process in a Patient with a Varicocele if
- Acute onset
- Right sided (isolated)
- Palpable abdominal mass
- Does not reduce while supine

Indications for Treatment of Varicocele
- Impaired sperm quality or quantity
- Pain or dull ache affecting QOL
- Affected testis fails to grow in adolescents
- Cosmetic indications (especially in adolescents)

Table 24. Benign Scrotal Masses

Type	Varicocele	Spermatocele	Hydrocele	Testicular Torsion	Inguinal Hernia
Definition	Dilatation and tortuosity of pampiniform plexus	A benign, sperm filled epididymal retention cyst	Collection of serous fluid that results from a defect or irritation in the tunica vaginalis	Twisting of the testicle causing venous occlusion and engorgement as well as arterial ischemia and infarction	Protrusion of abdominal contents through the inguinal canal into the scrotum
Etiology	15% of men Due to incompetent valves in the testicular veins 90% left sided	Multiple theories, including: Distal obstruction Aneurysmal dilations of the epididymis Agglutinated germ cells	Usually idiopathic Found in 5-10% testicular tumours Associated with trauma/infection Communicating: patent processus vaginalis, changes size during day (peds) Non-communicating: non-patent processus vaginalis (adult)	Trauma Cryptorchidism "Bell clapper deformity" Many occur in sleep (50%) Necrosis of glands in 5-6 h	Indirect (through internal ring, often into scrotum): congenital Direct (through external ring, rarely into scrotum): abdominal muscle weakness
Hx/P/E	"Bag of worms" Often painless Pulsates with Valsalva	Non-tender, cystic mass Transilluminates	Non-tender, intrascrotal mass Cystic Transilluminates	Acute onset severe scrotal pain, swelling GI upsets cases Retracted and transverse testicle (horizontal lie) Negative Phren's sign Absent cremasteric reflex	A small bulge in the groin that may increase in size with Valsalva and disappear when lying down Can present as a swollen or enlarged scrotum Discomfort or sharp pain – especially when straining, lifting, or exercising
Investigations	P/E Valsava	P/E U/S to rule out tumour	U/S to rule out tumour	U/S with colour flow Doppler probe over testicular artery Decrease uptake on 99mTc-pertechnetate scintillation scan (doughnut sign)	Hx and P/E Invagination of the scrotum Valsalva
Treatment	Conservative Surgical ligation of testicular veins Percutaneous vein occlusion (balloon, sclerosing agents) Repair may improve sperm count/motility 50-75%	Conservative Avoid needle aspiration as it can lead to infection, reaccumulation and spilling of irritating sperm within scrotum Excise if symptomatic	Conservative Needle drainage Surgical	Emergency surgical exploration and bilateral orchiopexy Orchiectomy if poor prognosis	Surgical repair

Acute scrotal swelling/pain in young boys is torsion until proven otherwise

Transillumination refers to light being transmitted through tissue (i.e. due to excess fluid)

Differential of a Benign Scrotal Mass

HIS BITS
Hydrocele
Infection (epididymitis/orchitis)
Sperm (spermatocele)
Blood (hematocele)
Intestines (hernia)
Torsion
Some veins (varicocele)

TORSION OF TESTICULAR APPENDIX
- twisting of testicular/epididymal vestigial appendix

Signs and Symptoms
- clinically similar to testicular torsion, but vertical lie and cremaster reflex preserved
- "blue dot sign"
  - blue infarcted appendage seen through scrotal skin (can usually be palpated as small, tender lump)

Treatment
- analgesia – most will subside over 5-7 d
- surgical exploration and excision if refractory pain

HEMATOCELE
- trauma with bleed into tunica vaginalis
- U/S helpful to exclude fracture of testis which requires surgical repair

Treatment
- ice packs, analgesics, surgical repair

Penile Complaints

Table 25. Penile Complaints

Type	Peyronie's Disease	Priapism	Paraphimosis	Phimosis	Premature Ejaculation
Definition	Benign curvature of penile shaft secondary to fibrous thickening of tunica albuginea	Prolonged erection lasting >4 h in the absence of sexual excitement/desire	Foreskin caught behind glans leading to edema → inability to reduce foreskin	Inability to retract foreskin over glans penis	Ejaculation prior to when one or both partners desire it, either before or soon after penetration
Etiology	Etiology unknown Trauma/repeated inflammation Familial predisposition Associated with DM, vascular disease, autoimmunity, Dupuytren's contracture, erectile dysfunction	50% idiopathic **Ischemic (common)** Thromboembolic (sickle cell) **Non-Ischemic** Trauma Medications Neurogenic	Iatrogenic (post cleaning/ instrumentation) Trauma Infectious (balanitis, balanoposthitis)	Congential (90% natural separation by age 3) Balanitis Poor Hygiene	Psychological factors Primary: no period of acceptable control Secondary: symptoms after a period of control, not associated with general medical condition
Hx/P/E	Penile curvature/shortening Pain with erection Poor erection distal to plaque	Painful erection ± signs of necrosis	Painful, swollen glans penis, foreskin Constricting band proximal to corona Dysuria, decreased urinary stream in children	Limitation and pain when attempting to retract foreskin Balanoposthitis (infection of prepuce)	Ejaculatory latency ≥1 min Inability to control or delay ejaculation Psychological distress
Investigations	Hx and P/E	Hx and P/E Cavernosal blood gas analysis	Hx and P/E	Hx and P/E	Hx and P/E Testosterone levels if in conjunction with impotence
Treatment	Watchful waiting (spontaneous resolution in up to 50%) Intralesional or topical verapamil Incision/excision of plaque Shortening of less affected side ± penile prosthesis	Treat reversible causes **High-flow:** Self-limited Consider arterial embolization **Low-flow:** Needle aspirated decompression Phenylephrine intracorporeal injection q3-5min Surgical shunt no response within 1 h	Manual pressure (with analgesia) Dorsal slit Circumcision (urgent or electively to prevent recurrence)	Proper hygiene Topical corticiosterioids Dorsal slit Circumcision	Rule out medical condition Address psychiatric concerns, counselling **Medication:** SSRI or clomipramine Topical lidocaine, prilocaine

Erectile Dysfunction

Testosterone deficiency is an uncommon cause of ED

Definition
- consistent (>3 mo duration) or recurrent inability to obtain or maintain an adequate erection for satisfactory sexual performance

Physiology
- erection involves the coordination of psychologic, neurologic, hemodynamic, mechanical, and endocrine components
- nerves: sympathetic (T11-L2), parasympathetic (S2-4), somatic (dorsal penile/pudendal nerves [S2-4])
- erection ("POINT")
  - parasympathetics → NO release → increased cGMP within corpora cavernosa leading to:
    1. arteriolar dilatation
    2. sinusoidal smooth muscle relaxation → increased arterial inflow and compression of penile venous drainage (decreased venous outflow)

Erections POINT AND SHOOT
parasympathetics = **point**; and sympathetics/ somatics = **shoot**

- emission ("SHOOT")
  - sensory afferents from glans
  - secretions from prostate, seminal vesicles, and ejaculatory ducts enter prostatic urethra (sympathetics)
- ejaculation ("SHOOT")
  - bladder neck closure (sympathetic)
  - spasmodic contraction of bulbo-cavernosus and pelvic floor musculature (somatic)
- detumescence
  - sympathetic nerves, norepinephrine, endothelin-1 → arteriolar and sinusoidal constriction → penile flaccidity

Classification

Table 26. Classification of Erectile Dysfunction

	Psychogenic*	Organic*
Proportion	10%	90%
Onset	Sudden	Gradual
Frequency	Sporadic	All circumstances
Variation	With partner and circumstance	No
Age	Younger	Older
Organic Risk Factors (HTN, DM, dyslipidemia)	No organic risk factors	Risk factors present
Nocturnal/AM Erection	Present	Absent

*Combination can co-exist

Etiology ("IMPOTENCE")

- **I**atrogenic: pelvic surgery, pelvic radiation
- **M**echanical: Peyronie's, post-priapism
- **P**sychological: depression, stress, anxiety, PTSD, widower syndrome
- **O**cclusive: arterial HTN, DM, smoking, hyperlipidemia, PVD, impaired veno-occlusion
- **T**rauma: penile/pelvic, bicycling
- **E**xtra factors: renal failure, cirrhosis, COPD, sleep apnea, malnutrition
- **N**eurogenic: CNS (e.g. Parkinson's, MS, spinal cord injury, Guillain-Barré, spina bifida, stroke), PNS (e.g. DM, peripheral neuropathy)
- **C**hemical: antihypertensives, sedatives, antidepressants, antipsychotics, anxiolytics, anticholinergics, antihistamines, anti-androgens (including 5-α reductase inhibitors), statins, GnRH agonists, illicit drugs
- **E**ndocrine: DM, hypogonadism, hyperprolactinemia, hypo/hyperthyroid

Diagnosis

- complete Hx (include sexual, medical, and psychosocial aspects)
- self-administered questionnaires (e.g. International Index of Erectile Function, Sexual Health Inventory for Men Questionnaire, ED Intensity Scale, ED Impact Scale)
- focused P/E, including vascular and neurologic examinations, secondary sexual characteristics
- lab investigations, dependent on clinical picture
  - risk factor evaluation: fasting blood glucose or HbA1c, cholesterol profile
  - optional: TSH, CBC, U/A, testosterone (free and total), prolactin, LH
- specialized testing including nocturnal penile tumescence monitoring usually unnecessary
- evaluation of penile vasculature only relevant with past history of trauma (i.e. pelvic fracture)

Treatment

- can often be managed by family doctor, see sidebar for when to refer
- must fully inform patient/partner of options, benefits and complications
- non-invasive
  - lifestyle changes (alcohol, smoking), psychological (sexual counselling and education)
  - change precipitating medications
  - treat underlying causes (DM, CVD, HTN, endocrinopathies)
- minimally invasive
  - oral medication (see *Common Medications*, U42)
    - sildenafil, tadalafil, vardenafil, avanafil (not available in Canada): inhibits PDE-5 to increase intracavernosal cyclic GMP levels
      - all three have similar effectiveness, difference in onset of action is not clinically significant
      - tadalafil has longer half-life, no cyanopsia, and can be taken on empty or full stomach
  - vacuum devices: draw blood into penis via negative pressure, then put ring at base of penis
  - MUSE: male urethral suppository for erection – vasoactive substance (PGE1) capsule inserted into urethra
- invasive
  - intracavernous vasodilator injection/self-injection
    - triple therapy (papaverine, phentolamine, PGE1) or PGE1 alone
    - complications: priapism (overdose), thickening of tunica albuginea at site of repeated injections (Peyronie's plaque) and hematoma
- surgical
  - penile implant (last resort): malleable or inflatable
  - penile artery reconstruction (in young men with isolated vascular lesion – investigational)

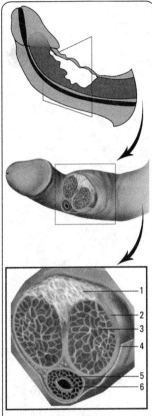

1. Fibrous plaque
2. Tunica albuginea
3. Corpus cavernosum
4. Buck's fascia
5. Corpus spongiosum
6. Urethra

© June Li

Figure 14. Peyronie's disease

Penile vascular abnormalities may be a marker of risk for CV disease. Young men with vascular ED have 50x higher risk of having a CV event

When to Consider Referral

FAT PEN
Failed medical therapy
penile **A**natomic abnormality
pelvic/perineal **T**rauma
Psychogenic cause
Endocrinopathy
vascular/**N**eurologic assessment

PDE-5 inhibitors are contraindicated in patients on nitrates/nitroglycerin due to severe hypotension

Initial trial of MUSE® or intracavernosal injection should be done under medical supervision

Trauma

- see Emergency Medicine, ER7

Renal Trauma

Classification According to Severity
- minor
  - contusions and superficial lacerations/hematomas: 90% of all blunt traumas, surgical exploration seldom necessary
- major
  - laceration that extends into medulla and collecting system, major renal vascular injury, shattered kidney

Etiology
- 80% blunt (MVC, assaults, falls) vs. 20% penetrating (stab wounds and gunshots)

Clinical Features
- mechanism of injury raises suspicion
- can be hemodynamically unstable secondary to renal vascular injury and/or other sustained injuries: ABCs
- upper abdominal tenderness, flank tenderness, flank contusions, lower rib/vertebral transverse process fracture

Investigations
- U/A
  - hematuria: requires workup but degree does not correlate with the severity of injury
- imaging
  - CT (contrast, triphasic) if patient stable: look for renal laceration, extravasation of contrast, retroperitoneal hematoma, and associated intra-abdominal organ injury

Staging (does not necessarily correlate well with clinical status)
- I: contusion/hematoma
- II: <1 cm laceration without urinary extravasation
- III: >1 cm laceration without urinary extravasation
- IV: laceration causing urinary extravasation and/or main arterial or vein injury with contained hematoma
- V: shattered kidney or avulsion of pedicle

Treatment
- microscopic hematuria + isolated well-staged minor injuries → no hospitalization
- gross hematuria + contusion/minor lacerations → hospitalize, bedrest, repeat CT if bleeding persists
- surgical intervention/minimally invasive angiography and embolization
  - absolute indications
    - hemorrhage and hemodynamic instability
  - relative indications
    - non-viable tissue and major laceration
    - urinary extravasation
    - vascular injury
    - expanding or pulsating peri-renal mass
    - laparotomy for associated injury
- follow-up with U/S or CT before discharge, and at 6 wk

Complications
- HTN in 5% of renal trauma

Bladder Trauma

Classification
- contusions: no urinary extravasation, damage to mucosa or muscularis
- intraperitoneal ruptures: often involve the bladder dome
- extraperitoneal ruptures: involve anterior or lateral bladder wall in full bladder

Etiology
- blunt (MVC, falls, and crush injury) vs. penetrating trauma to lower abdomen, pelvis, or perineum
- blunt trauma is associated with pelvic fracture in 97% of cases

Clinical Features
- abdominal tenderness, distention, peritonitis, and inability to void
- can be hemodynamically unstable secondary to pelvic fracture, other sustained injuries: ABCs
- suprapubic pain

Investigations
- U/A: gross hematuria in 90%
- imaging (including CT cystogram and post-drainage films for extravasation)

Treatment
- penetrating trauma → surgical exploration
- contusion → urethral catheter until hematuria completely resolves
- extraperitoneal bladder perforations → typically non-operative with foley insertion, and follow with cystograms
  - surgery if: infected urine, rectal/vaginal perforation, bony spike into bladder, laparotomy for concurrent injury, bladder neck involvement, persistent urine leak and failed conservative management
- intraperitoneal rupture usually requires surgical repair and suprapubic catheterization

Complications
- complications of bladder injury itself are rare
- mortality is around 20%, and is usually due to associated injuries rather than bladder rupture

Urethral Injuries

Etiology
- posterior urethra
  - common site of injury is junction of membranous and prostatic urethra due to blunt trauma, MVCs, pelvic fracture
  - shearing force on fixed membranous and mobile prostatic urethra
- anterior urethra
  - straddle injury can crush bulbar urethra against pubic rami
- other causes
  - iatrogenic (instrumentation, prosthesis insertion), penile fracture, masturbation with urethral manipulation
- always look for associated bladder rupture

Clinical Features
- blood at urethral meatus
- high-riding prostate on DRE
- swelling and butterfly perineal hematoma
- penile and/or scrotal hematoma
- sensation of voiding without U/O
- distended bladder

All patients with suspected urethral injury should undergo RUG

Investigations
- must perform RUG or cystoscopy prior to catheterization

Treatment
- simple contusions
  - no treatment
- partial urethral disruption
  - very gentle attempt at catheterization by urologist
  - with no resistance to catheterization → Foley x 2-3 wk
  - with resistance to catheterization → suprapubic cystostomy or urethral catheter alignment
- periodic flow rates/urethrograms to evaluate for stricture formation
- complete disruption
  - immediate repair if patient stable, delayed repair if unstable (suprapubic tube in interim)

Complications
- stricture

Infertility

Definition
- failure to conceive after one year of unprotected, properly timed intercourse
- incidence
  - 15% of all couples (35-40% female, 20% male, 25-30% combined)

Female Factors

- see Gynecology, GY23

Male Factors

Male Reproduction
- hypothalamic-pituitary-testicular axis (HPTA)
  - pulsatile GnRH from hypothalamus acts on anterior pituitary stimulating release of LH and FSH
  - LH acts on Leydig (interstitial) cells → testosterone synthesis and secretion
  - FSH acts on Sertoli cells → structural and metabolic support to developing spermatogenic cells
  - FSH and testosterone support germ cells (responsible for spermatogenesis)
  - sperm route: epididymis → vas deferens → ejaculatory ducts → prostatic urethra

Etiology
- idiopathic (40-50% infertile males)
- testicular
  - varicocele (35-40% infertile males)
  - tumour
  - congenital (Klinefelter's triad: small, firm testes, gynecomastia, and azoospermia)
  - post-infectious (epididymo-orchitis, STIs, mumps)
  - uncorrected torsion
  - cryptorchidism (<5% of cases)
- obstructive
  - iatrogenic (surgery: see below)
  - infectious (gonorrhea, chlamydia)
  - trauma
  - congenital (absence of vas deferens, CF)
  - bilateral ejaculatory duct obstruction, epididymal obstructions
  - Kartagener's syndrome (autosomal recessive disorder causing defect in action of cilia)
- endocrine (see Endocrinology, E45)
- HPTA (2-3%) e.g. Kallmann's syndrome (congenital hypothalamic hypogonadism), excess prolactin, excess androgens, excess estrogens
- other
  - retrograde ejaculation secondary to surgery
  - medications
  - drugs: marijuana, cocaine, tobacco, alcohol
  - increased testicular temperature (sauna, hot baths, tight pants or underwear)
  - chronic disease: e.g. liver, renal
  - unexplained infertility

History
- age of both partners
- medical: past illness, DM, trauma, CF, genetic syndromes, STIs, cryptorchidism
- surgical: vasectomy, herniorrhaphy, orchidopexy, prostate surgery
- fertility: pubertal onset, previous pregnancies, duration of infertility, treatments
- sexual: libido, erection/ejaculation, timing, frequency
- family Hx
- medications: cytotoxic agents, GnRH agonists, anabolic steroids, nitrofurantoin, cimetidine, sulfasalazine, spironolactone, α-blockers
- social Hx: alcohol, tobacco, cocaine, marijuana
- occupational exposures: radiation, heavy metals

Physical Exam
- general appearance: sexual development, gynecomastia, obesity
- scrotal exam: size, consistency, and nodularity of testicles; palpation of cord for presence of vas deferens; DRE; valsalva for varicocele

Investigations

- semen analysis (SA) at least 2 specimens, collected 1-2 weeks apart
- hormonal evaluation
  - indicated with abnormal SA (rare to be abnormal with normal SA)
  - testosterone and FSH
  - serum LH and prolactin are measured if testosterone or FSH are abnormal
- genetic evaluation
  - chromosomal studies (Klinefelter's syndrome – XXY)
  - genetic studies (Y-chromosome microdeletion, CF gene mutation)
- immunologic studies (antisperm antibodies in ejaculate and blood)
- testicular biopsy
- scrotal U/S (varicocele, testicular size)
- vasography (assess patency of vas deferens)

Treatment

- assessment of partner
- lifestyle
  - regular exercise, healthy diet
  - eliminate alcohol, tobacco and illicit drugs
- medical
  - endocrine therapy (see <u>Endocrinology</u>, E46)
  - treat retrograde ejaculation
  - discontinue anti-sympathomimetic agents, may start α-adrenergic stimulation (phenylpropanolamine, pseudoephedrine, or ephedrine)
  - treat underlying infections
- surgical
  - varicocelectomy (if indicated)
  - vasovasostomy (vasectomy reversal) or epididymovasostomy
  - transurethral resection of blocked ejaculatory ducts
- assisted reproductive technologies (ART)
  - refer to infertility specialist
  - sperm washing + intrauterine insemination (IUI)
  - *in vitro* fertilization (IVF)
  - intracytoplasmic sperm injection (ICSI) after CF screening of patient and partner in patients with congenital bilateral absence of vas deferens

Normal Semen Values
- Volume: 2-5 mL
- Concentration: >15 million sperm/mL
- Morphology: 30% normal forms
- Motility: >40% adequate forward progression
- Liquefaction: complete in 20 min
- pH: 7.2-7.8
- WBC: <10/HPF or <106 WBC/mL semen

Common Terminology on SA
- Teratospermia: Abnormal morphology
- Asthenospermia: Abnormal motility
- Oligospermia: Decreased sperm count
- Azoospermia: Absent sperm in semen
- Mixed types: i.e. oligoasthenospermia

Mutation of cystic fibrosis transmembrane conductance regulator (CFTR) gene is associated with congenital bilateral absence of vas deferens and epididymal cysts, even if patient manifests no symptoms of CF

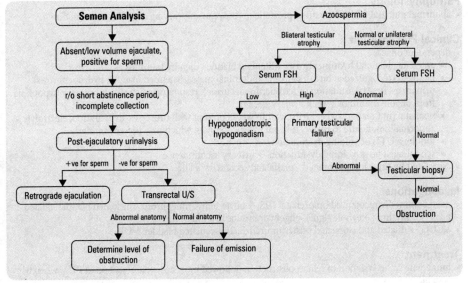

Figure 15. Infertility work up

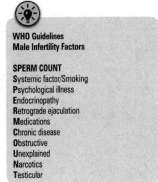

WHO Guidelines
Male Infertility Factors

SPERM COUNT
Systemic factor/Smoking
Psychological illness
Endocrinopathy
Retrograde ejaculation
Medications
Chronic disease
Obstructive
Unexplained
Narcotics
Testicular

Pediatric Urology

Congenital Abnormalities

- not uncommon; 1/200 have congenital abnormalities of the GU tract
- six common presentations of congenital urological abnormalities

1. ANTENATAL HYDRONEPHROSIS

Majority of antenatal hydronephroses resolve during pregnancy or within the first year of life

Epidemiology
- 1-5% fetal U/S, some detectable as early as first trimester
- most common urological consultation in perinatal period and one of most common U/S abnormalities of pregnancy

Differential Diagnosis
- UPJ or UVJ obstruction
- MCDS
- VUR
- PUVs (only in boys)
- duplication anomalies
- ureterocele
- ectopic ureter

Treatment
- antenatal *in utero* intervention rarely indicated unless evidence of lower urinary tract obstruction with oligohydramnios

2. POSTERIOR URETHRAL VALVES

Epidemiology
- the most common congenital obstructive urethral lesion in male infants

Pathophysiology
- abnormal mucosal folds at the distal prostatic urethra causing varying degrees of obstruction

Clinical Presentation
- dependent on age
  - antenatal: bilateral hydronephrosis, distended bladder, oligohydramnios
  - neonatal (recognized at birth): palpable abdominal mass (distended bladder, hydronephrosis), urinary ascites (transudation of retroperitoneal urine), respiratory distress (pulmonary hypoplasia from oligohydramnios), weak urinary stream
  - neonatal (not recognized at birth): within weeks present with urosepsis, dehydration, electrolyte abnormalities, failure to thrive; rule out pyloric stenosis, which may present similarly
  - toddlers: UTIs or voiding dysfunction
  - school-aged boys: voiding dysfunction → urinary incontinence
- associated findings include renal dysplasia and secondary VUR

Investigations
- most commonly recognized on prenatal U/S → bilateral hydronephrosis, thickened bladder, dilated posterior urethra ("keyhole sign"), oligohydramnios in a male fetus
- VCUG → dilated and elongated posterior urethra, trabeculated bladder, VUR

Treatment
- immediate catheterization to relieve obstruction, followed by cystoscopic resection of PUV when baby is stable
- if resection of PUV is not possible, vesicostomy is indicated

3. URETEROPELVIC JUNCTION OBSTRUCTION

Etiology
- unclear: adynamic ureteral segment, stenosis, strictures, extrinsic compression, aberrant blood vessels
- can rarely be secondary to tumour, stone, etc, in children

Epidemiology
- the most common congenital defect of the ureter
- M:F = 2:1
- up to 40% bilateral, which may be associated with worse prognosis

Clinical Presentation
- symptoms depend on severity and age at diagnosis (mostly asymptomatic finding on antenatal U/S)
  - infants: abdominal mass, urinary infection
  - children: pain, vomiting, failure to thrive
- some cases are diagnosed after puberty and into adulthood
  - in adolescents and adults, the symptoms may be triggered by episodes of increased diuresis, such as following alcohol ingestion (Dietl's crisis)

Investigations
- antenatal: serial U/S most common, and renal scan ± furosemide

Treatment
- surgical correction (pyeloplasty), consider nephrectomy if <15% differential renal function

4. VESICOURETERAL REFLUX

Definition
- retrograde passage of urine from the bladder, through the UVJ, into the ureter

Classification
- primary reflux: incompetent or inadequate closure of UVJ
  - lateral ureteral insertion, short submucosal segment
- secondary reflux: abnormally high intravesical pressure resulting in failure of UVJ closure
  - often associated with anatomic (PUV) or functional (neuropathic) bladder dysfunction

Epidemiology
- estimated ~1% of newborns, but not well known
- incidence and clinical relevance higher in children with febrile UTIs and prenatal hydronephrosis
- risk factors: race (white > black), female gender, age (<2 yr), genetic predisposition

Investigations
- focused Hx, particularly of voiding dysfunction (frequency, urgency, diurnal enuresis, constipation, encopresis)
  - also screen for infections (UTI, pyelonephritis, urosepsis) and renal failure (uremia, HTN)
- initial evaluation of renal status, growth parameters, and blood pressure is warranted in any child with VUR due to relatively high incidence of renal scarring
  - height, weight, blood pressure
  - serum Cr
  - U/A, C&S
  - renal U/S
  - DMSA renal scan if at high risk (greater sensitivity in detecting structural defects associated with dysplasia, renal scarring or pyelonephritis; entails radiation exposure)
  - sibling family screening is controversial

Treatment
- spontaneous resolution in 60% of primary reflux
  - in lower grades (I-III), goal is to prevent infection or renal damage via medical treatment
- medical treatment: daily ABx prophylaxis at half the treatment dose for acute infection (see Table 9, U12 - TMP/SMX, trimethoprim, amoxicillin, or nitrofurantoin)
- surgical treatment: ureteral reimplantation ± ureteroplasty, or subureteral injection with bulking agents (Deflux® or Macroplastique®)
  - indications include failure of medical management, renal scarring (e.g. renal insufficiency, HTN), breakthrough UTIs, persistent high grade (IV or V) reflux

5. HYPOSPADIAS

Definition
- a condition in which the urethral meatus opens on the ventral side of the penis, proximal to the normal location in the glans penis
- depending on severity, may result in difficulty directing urinary stream, having intercourse or depositing sperm in vagina

Epidemiology
- very common; 1/300 live male births
- distal hypospadias more common than proximal
- white >> black
- may be associated with ventral penile curvature, disorders of sexual differentiation, undescended testicles or inguinal hernia

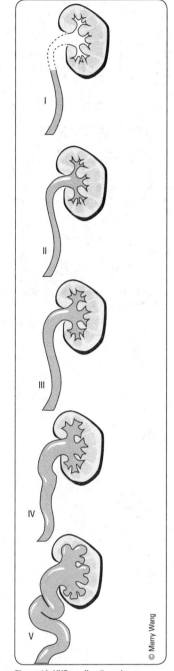

© Merry Wang

Figure 16. VUR grading (based on cystogram)

VUR Grading (based on cystogram)
- Grade I: ureters only fill
- Grade II: ureters and pelvis fill
- Grade III: ureters and pelvis fill with some dilatation
- Grade IV: ureters, pelvis, and calyces fill with significant dilatation
- Grade V: ureters, pelvis, and calyces fill with major dilatation and tortuosity

Defer circumcision in patients with hypospadias

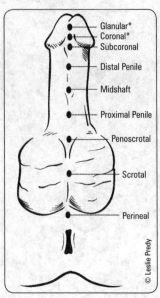

Figure 17. Classification of hypospadias
(*account for 75%)

Treatment
- early surgical correction; optimal repair before 2 yr
- neonatal circumcision should be deferred because the foreskin may be utilized in the correction

6. EXSTROPHY-EPISPADIAS COMPLEX

Definition
- a spectrum of defects depending on the timing of the rupture of the cloacal membrane
  - bladder exstrophy: congenital defect of a portion of lower abdominal and anterior bladder wall, with exposure of the bladder lumen
  - cloacal exstrophy
    - exposed bladder and bowel with imperforate anus
    - associated with spina bifida in >50%
  - epispadias (least severe)
    - urethra opens on dorsal aspect of the penis, often associated with penile curvature

Etiology
- represents failure of closure of the cloacal membrane, resulting in the bladder and urethra opening directly through the abdominal wall

Epidemiology
- rare: incidence 1/30,000, M:F = 3:1 predominance
- high morbidity → multiple reconstructive surgeries, incontinence, infertility, reflux

Treatment
- surgical correction at birth
- later corrections for incontinence, VUR, and low bladder capacity may be needed

Nephroblastoma (Wilms' Tumour)

Etiology
- arises from abnormal proliferation of metanephric blastema

Epidemiology
- 5% of all childhood cancers, 5% bilateral
- most common primary malignant renal tumour of childhood
- average age of incidence is 3 yr

Clinical Features
- abdominal mass: large, firm, unilateral (80%)
- HTN (25%)
- flank tenderness
- microscopic hematuria
- nausea/vomiting

Treatment
- always investigate contralateral kidney and renal vein (for tumour thrombus)
- unilateral disease: radical nephrectomy ± radiation ± chemotherapy
- bilateral disease: nephron-sparing surgery following neoadjuvant chemotherapy

Prognosis
- 5 yr survival 80%

Cryptorchidism/Ectopic Testes

Normal Testicular Development and Descent in Utero
2nd month: Testicle begins to form
4th month: Begins to take on its normal appearance and migrates from its origin at the kidney to the internal inguinal ring
7th month: The testis, surrounded in peritoneal covering, begins to descend through the internal ring, inguinal canal and external ring to terminate in the scrotum

Definition
- abnormal location of testes somewhere along the normal path of descent (external inguinal ring > inguinal canal > abdominal)
- Denis Browne pouch (between external oblique fascia and Scarpa's fascia) most common
- differential diagnosis:
  - retractile testes
  - atrophic testes
  - disorders of sexual differentiation (bilateral impalpable gonads)

Epidemiology
- 2.7% of full term newborns
- 0.7-0.8% at 1 yr

Treatment
- orchiopexy
- hormonal therapy not proven to be of benefit over standard surgical treatment

Prognosis
- reduction in fertility
  - untreated bilateral cryptorchidism: ~100% infertility
  - paternity rates: 53%, 90%, and 93% in formerly bilateral cryptorchid, formerly unilateral cryptorchid, and normal men, respectively
- increased malignancy risk
  - intraabdominal > inguinal
  - surgical correction facilitates testicular monitoring and may reduce malignancy risk
- increased risk of testicular torsion (reduced by surgical correction)

Disorders of Sexual Differentiation

Definition
- formerly known as intersex disorders: considered social emergency
- abnormal genitalia for chromosomal sex due to the undermasculinization of males or the virilization of females

Classification
1. 46 XY DSD
   - defect in testicular synthesis of androgens
   - androgen resistance in target tissues
   - palpable gonad
2. 46 XX DSD
   - most due to CAH (21-hydroxylase deficiency most common enzymatic defect) → shunt in steroid biosynthetic pathway leading to excess androgens
   - undiagnosed and untreated CAH can be associated with life-threatening electrolyte abnormalities in the newborn (salt-wasting CAH)
3. ovotesticular DSD
4. mixed gonadal dysgenesis (46 XY/45 XO most common karyotype)
   - presence of Y chromosome → partial testis determination to varying degrees

A phenotypic male newborn with bilateral non-palpable testicles should be considered 46XX with salt-wasting CAH and must undergo proper evaluation prior to discharge

Diagnosis
- thorough family Hx noting any consanguinity
- maternal Hx, especially medication/drug use during pregnancy (maternal hyperandrogenemia)
- P/E: palpable gonad (= chromosomal male), hyperpigmentation, evidence of dehydration, HTN, stretched phallus length, position of urethral meatus
- laboratory tests
  - plasma 17-OH-progesterone (after 36 h of life) → increased in CAH
  - plasma 11-deoxycortisol → increased in 11-β-hydroxylase deficiency
  - basal adrenal steroid levels
  - serum testosterone and DHT pre- and post-hCG stimulation (2,000 IU/d for 4 d)
  - serum electrolytes
  - chromosomal evaluation including sex karyotype
- U/S of adrenals, gonads, uterus, and fallopian tubes
- endoscopy and genitography of urogenital sinus

Treatment
- steroid supplementation as indicated (e.g. CAH)
- sex assignment after extensive family consultation
  - must consider capacity for sexually functioning genitalia in adulthood, fertility potential, and psychological impact
- reconstruction of external genitalia between 6 and 12 mo
- long-term psychological guidance and support for both patient and family

Enuresis

- see Pediatrics, P9

Selected Urological Procedures

Bladder Catheterization

- catheter size measured by the French (Fr) scale – circumference in mm
- each 1 mm increase in diameter = approximately 3 Fr increase (standard size 14-18 Fr)
- should be removed as soon as possible to reduce the risk of UTI

Continuous Catheterization
- indications
  - accurate monitoring of U/O
  - relief of urinary retention due to medication, neurogenic bladder, or intravesical obstruction
  - temporary therapy for urinary incontinence
  - perineal wounds
  - clot prevention (22-24 Fr) for CBI
  - post-operative

Alternatives to Continuous Catheterization
- intermittent catheterization
  - PVR measurement
  - to obtain sterile diagnostic specimens for U/A, urine C&S
  - management of neurogenic bladder or chronic urinary retention
- condom catheter
- suprapubic catheter

Causes of Difficult Catheterizations and Treatment
- patient discomfort → use sufficient lubrication (± xylocaine)
- collapsing catheter → lubrication as above ± firmer or larger catheter (silastic catheter)
- meatal/urethral stricture → dilate with progressively larger catheters/balloon catheter
- BPH → use coudé catheter as angled tip can help navigate around enlarged prostate
- urethral disruption/obstruction → filiform and followers or suprapubic catheterization
- anxious patient → anxiolytic medication

Complications of Catheterization
- infection: UTI
- meatal/urethral trauma

Contraindications
- trauma: blood at the urinary meatus, scrotal hematoma, pelvic fracture, and/or high riding prostate

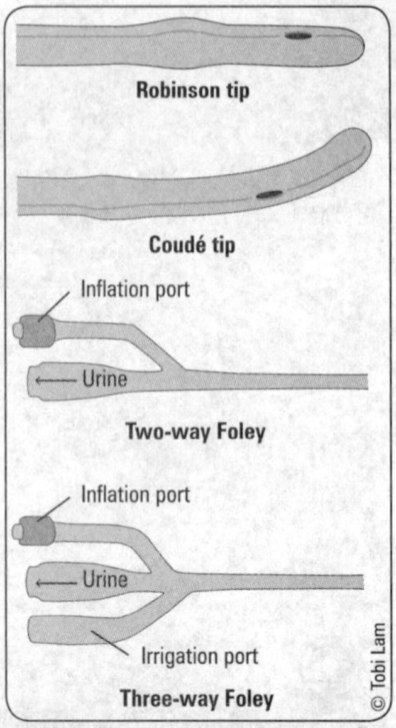

Circumcision

Definition
- removal of some or all of the foreskin from the penis

Epidemiology
- 30% worldwide
- frequency varies with geography, religious affiliation, socioeconomic status

Medical Indications
- phimosis and recurrent paraphimosis
- recurrent UTIs (particularly in infants and in association with other urinary abnormalities)
- balanitis xerotica obliterans or other chronic inflammatory conditions

Contraindications
- unstable or sick infant
- congenital genital abnormalities (hypospadias)
- family Hx of bleeding disorders warrants laboratory investigation prior to circumcision

Complications
- bleeding
- infection
- penile entrapment, skin bridges
- fistula
- glans injury
- penile sensation deficits

Robinson tip

Coudé tip

Inflation port

← Urine

Two-way Foley

Inflation port

← Urine

Irrigation port

Three-way Foley

© Tobi Lam

Figure 18. Transurethral (Foley) catheters

Male Circumcision for Prevention of Heterosexual Acquisition of HIV in Men
Cochrane DB Syst Rev 2009;2:CD003362
Purpose: To evaluate the effectiveness and safety of male circumcision for preventing acquisition of HIV in heterosexual men.
Methods: The analyzed data is from three randomized controlled trials to assess the efficacy of male circumcision for preventing HIV acquisition in men in Africa.
Results: Medical male circumcision reduces the acquisition of HIV by heterosexual men (38%-66% over 24 mo).

Circumcision Status and Risk of HIV and Sexually Transmitted Infections among Men who have Sex with Men: A Meta-Analysis
JAMA 2008;300:1674-1684
Purpose: To describe the association between male circumcision and HIV infection and other sexually transmitted infections (STIs) among men who have sex with men (MSM).
Methods: Meta-analysis of 15 studies (n=53,567)
Results: The associations between circumcision and HIV-positive and STIs were not statistically significant. Male circumcision had a protective association with HIV in studies of MSM conducted before the introduction of highly active anti-retroviral therapy.
Conclusions: There is insufficient evidence to support that male circumcision protects against HIV infection or other STIs.

Male Circumcision
Pediatrics 2012;130:e756-e785
Study: Guidelines by the American Academy of Pediatrics (AAP).
Recommendations: The American Academy of Pediatrics radically changed their position on male circumcision in 2012. The report from the AAP now states that the preventative health benefits outweigh the risks of the procedure and that the procedure is well-tolerated with adequate pain management and sterility. Stated benefits include the prevention of urinary tract infection, penile cancer, transmission of some sexually transmitted infections, including HIV. There is believed to be no effect on penile sexual function, sensitivity or sexual satisfaction. Acute complications are rare and more common if the procedure is done by an untrained provider.
Note: The Canadian Pediatric Society (CPS) has not yet updated their position on male circumcision since 1996, which stated that the CPS is opposed to routine circumcision. A new statement is expected soon.

Cystoscopy

Objective
- endoscopic inspection of the lower urinary tract (urethra, prostate, bladder, and ureteral orifices), samples for cytology
- scopes can be flexible or rigid

Indications
- gross hematuria
- LUTS (storage or voiding)
- urethral and bladder neck strictures
- bladder stones
- bladder tumour surveillance
- evaluation of upper tracts with retrograde pyelography (ureteric stents, catheters)

Complications
- during procedure
  - bleeding
  - anesthetic-related
  - perforation (rare)
- post-procedure (short-term)
  - infections, e.g. epididymo-orchitis (rare)
  - urinary retention
- post-procedure (long-term)
  - stricture

Radical Prostatectomy

Objective
- the removal of the entire prostate and prostatic capsule via a lower midline abdominal incision, laparoscopically or robotically
  - internal iliac and obturator vessel lymph nodes may also be dissected and sent for pathology (dependent on risk: clinical stage, grade, PSA)
  - seminal vesicle vessels are also partially or completely removed

Indications
- treatment for localized prostate cancer

Complications
- immediate (intraoperative)
  - blood loss
  - rectal injury (extremely rare)
  - ureteral injury (extremely rare)
- perioperative
  - lymphocele formation if concurrent pelvic lymphadenectomy performed)
- late
  - moderate to severe urinary incontinence (3-10%)
  - mild urinary incontinence (20%)
  - ED (~50%, depending on whether one, both, or neither of the neurovascular bundles are involved in extracapsular extension of tumour)

Retropubic, Laparoscopic, and Robot-Assisted Radical Prostatectomy: A Critical Review of Outcomes Reported by High-Volume Centres
J Endourology 2010;24:2003-2015
Study: A systematic review to compare perioperative outcomes, positive surgical margin (PSM) rates, and functional outcomes in retropubic radical prostatectomy (RRP) laparoscopic RP (LRP) and robot-assisted radical prostatectomy (RARP).
Methods: Medline database was searched. Weighted means (based on number of participants in each study) were calculated for all outcomes.
Results: 58 articles were reviewed. LRP and RARP were associated with better perioperative outcomes compared to RRP. RRP, LRP, and RARP had similar post-operative complication rates ranging from 10.3-10.98%. RARP had a lower overall PSM rate than LRP, and RRP. RARP had the highest continence rate and mean potency rates.
Conclusion: In high-volume centres, RRP, LRP and RARP are safe options for treating patients with localized prostate cancer. LRP and RARP are associated with better perioperative outcomes and RARP showed lower PSM rates, higher potency and continence compared to RRP and LRP.v

Transurethral Resection of the Prostate

Objective
- to partially resect the periurethral portion of the prostate (transition zone) to decrease symptoms of urinary tract obstruction
- accomplished via a transurethral (cystoscopic) approach using an electrocautery loop, irrigation (glycine), and illumination

Indications
- obstructive uropathy (large bladder diverticula, renal insufficiency)
- refractory urinary retention
- recurrent UTIs
- recurrent gross hematuria
- bladder stones
- intolerance/failure of medical therapy

Complications
- acute
  - intra- or extraperitoneal rupture of the bladder
  - rectal perforation
  - incontinence
  - incision of the ureteral orifice (with subsequent reflux or ureteral stricture)
  - hemorrhage
  - epididymitis
  - sepsis
  - transurethral resection syndrome (also called "post-TURP syndrome")
    - caused by absorption of a large volume of the hypotonic irrigation solution used, usually through perforated venous sinusoids, leading to a hypervolemic hyponatremic state
    - characterized by dilutional hyponatremia, confusion, nausea, vomiting, HTN, bradycardia, visual disturbances, CHF, and pulmonary edema
    - treat with diuresis and (if severe) hypertonic saline administration
- chronic
  - retrograde ejaculation (>75%)
  - ED (5-10% risk increases with increasing use of cautery)
  - incontinence (<1%)
  - urethral stricture
  - bladder neck contracture

Extracorporeal Shock Wave Lithotripsy

Objective
- to treat renal and ureteral calculi (proximal, middle or distal) which cannot pass through the urinary tract naturally
- shockwaves focused onto stone → fragmentation, allowing stone fragments to pass spontaneously and less painfully

Indications
- potential first-line therapy for renal and ureteral calculi <2.5 cm
- individuals with calculi in solitary kidney
- individuals with HTN, DM or renal insufficiency
*patient preference and wait-times play a large role in stone management

Contraindications
- acute UTI or urosepsis
- bleeding disorder or coagulopathy
- pregnancy
- obstruction distal to stone (ESWL can be used after stent or nephrostomy inserted)

Complications
- bacteriuria
- bacteremia
- post-procedure hematuria
- ureteric obstruction (by stone fragments)
- peri-nephric hematoma

A Comparison of Treatment Modalities for Renal Calculi Between 100 and 300 mm2: Are Shockwave Lithotripsy, Ureteroscopy, and Percutaneous Nephrolithotomy Equivalent?
J Endourol 2011;25:481-485
Purpose: To describe the outcomes of a series of patients who underwent shockwave lithotripsy (SWL), ureteroscopy (URS) or percutaneous nephrolithotomy (PCNL).
Methods: Patients treated for intermediate-sized upper tract calculi (100-300 mm2) at a single tertiary centre were included. Demographic and clinical data were collected from a prospectively maintained database.
Results: Of 137 patients, 38.7%, 29.9%, and 31.4% were treated with SWL, URS, and PCNL, respectively. Stone-free rate (95.3%) and single treatment success rate (95.3%) were highest for PCNL compared to SWL and URS (p<0.001). When allowing for up to two SWL treatments, success rates became equivalent for the three treatment groups (p=0.66). Auxiliary treatments were more frequent after SWL compared to URS and PCNL. Clavien grade complications did not differ between the three groups.
Conclusion: Up to two SWL treatments have equivalent success rate as compared to URS and PCNL. Hence, multiple SWL treatments may be a reasonable therapeutic option for patients who prefer SWL or who are not good candidates for alternative therapies.

Common Medications

Table 27. Erectile Dysfunction Medications

Drug	Class	Mechanism	Adverse Effects
sildenafil tadalafil vardenafil (PDE5s for use when some erection present)	Phosphodiesterase 5 inhibitor	Selective inhibition of PDE5 (enzyme which degrades cGMP) Leads to sinusoidal smooth muscle relaxation and erection	Severe hypotension (very rare) Contraindicated if Hx of priapism, or in conditions predisposing to priapism (leukemia, myelofibrosis, polycythemia, sickle cell disease) Contraindicated with nitrates
alprostadil (MUSE®), PGE_1 + phentolamine + papaverine mixture	Prostaglandin E_1	Activation of cAMP, relaxing sinusoidal smooth muscle Local release (urethral suppository)	Penile pain Presyncope
alprostadil, papaverine (intracavernosal injection) triple therapy also used: papaverine, phentolamine, PGE_1	See above	See above	Thickening of tunica albuginea at site of repeated injections (Peyronie's plaque) Painful erection Hematoma Contraindicated if Hx of priapism, or in high risk of priapism

Common Medications

Table 28. Benign Prostatic Hyperplasia Medications

Drug	Class	Mechanism	Adverse Effects
terazosin doxazosin	α_1 blockers	α-adrenergic antagonists reduce stromal smooth muscle tone Reduce dynamic component of bladder outlet obstruction	Presyncope Leg edema Retrograde ejaculation Headache Asthenia Nasal congestion
tamsulosin alfuzosin silodosin	α_{1A} selective		
finasteride dutasteride	5-α reductase inhibitor	Blocks conversion of testosterone to DHT Reduces static component of bladder outlet obstruction Reduces prostatic volume	Sexual dysfunction PSA decreases

Table 29. Prostatic Carcinoma Medications (N>0, M>0)

Drug	Class	Mechanism	Adverse Effects
leuprolide, goserelin	GnRH agonist	Initially stimulates LH, increasing testosterone and causing "flare" (initially increases bone pain) Later causes low testosterone	Hot flashes Headache Decreased libido
*diethylstilbestrol (DES)	Estrogens	Inhibit LH and cytotoxic effect on tumour cells	Increased risk of cardiovascular events (no longer available commercially in North America)
*cyproterone acetate	Steroidal antiandrogen	Competes with DHT for intracellular receptors: 1. Prevent flare produced by GnRH agonist 2. Use for complete androgen blockade 3. May preserve potency	
flutamide, bicalutamide	Non-steroidal antiandrogen	As above	Hepatotoxic: AST/ALT monitoring
*ketoconazole, spironolactone	Steroidogenesis inhibitors	Blocks multiple enzymes in steroid pathway, including adrenal androgens	GI symptoms Hyperkalemia Gynecomastia

*Very rarely used

Table 30. Continence Agents and Overactive Bladder Medications

Drug	Class	Mechanism	Indication	Adverse Effects
oxybutynin	Antispasmotic	Inhibits action of ACh on smooth muscle Decreases frequency of uninhibited detrusor contraction Diminishes initial urge to void	Overactive bladder Urge incontinence + urgency + frequency	Dry mouth Blurred vision Constipation Supraventricular tachycardia
oxybutynin, tolterodine, trospium, solifenacin, darifenacin fesoterodine	Anticholinergic	Muscarinic receptor antagonist Selective for bladder Increases bladder volume Decreases detrusor pressure	Overactive bladder Urge incontinence + urgency + frequency	As above
mirabegron	β_3 agonist	Beta sympathetic receptor blocker in the bladder; relaxes bladder during storage phase	Overactive bladder Urge incontinence + urgency + frequency	Blood pressure should be monitored
imipramine	Tricyclic antidepressant	Sympathomimetic effects: urinary sphincter contraction Anticholinergic effects: detrusor relaxation	Stress and urge incontinence	As above Weight gain Orthostatic hypotension Prolonged PR interval
Botulinum toxin A bladder injections	Neurotoxin	Prevents the release of neurotransmitters	Refractory OAB incontinence both neurogenic and non-neurogenic	Urinary retention, UTI

Note: All anti-cholinergics are equally effective and long-acting formulations are better tolerated. Newer muscarinic M3 receptor specific agents (solifenacin, darifenacin) are equally efficacious as older drugs, however, RCTs based on head-to-head comparison to long acting formulations are lacking

References

General Information
American Urological Association. Available from: http://www.auanet.org/guidelines/.
Canadian Urological Association. Available from: http://www.cua.org/guidelines_e.asp.
Ferri F. Practical guide to the care of the medical patient, 6th ed. St. Louis: Mosby, 2006.
Goldman L, Ausiello D. Cecil textbook of medicine, 23rd ed. Philadelphia: WB Saunders, 2007.
Macfarlane MT. House officer series: urology, 3rd ed. Philadelphia: Lippincott, 2001.
Montague DK, Jarow J, Broderick GA, et al. Guideline on the management of priapism. American Urological Association Education and Research, Inc. ©2003. Available from: http://www.auanet.org/education/guidelines/priapism.cfm.
Tanagho EA, McAninch JW. Smith's general urology, 17th ed. New York: McGraw-Hill, 2007.
Wein AJ, Kavoussi LR, Novick AC, et al. Campbell's urology, 10th ed. Philadelphia: WB Saunders, 2011.
Wieder JA. Pocket guide to urology, 4th ed. Oakland: Wieder, 2010.

Common Presenting Problems
Bremnor JD, Sadovsky R. Evaluation of dysuria in adults. Am Fam Phys 2002;65:1589-1597.
Cohen RA, Brown RS. Microscopic hematuria. NEJM 2003;348:2330-2338.
Morton AR, Iliescu EA, Wilson JWL. Nephrology: investigation and treatment of recurrent kidney stones. CMAJ 2002;166:213-218.
Teichman JMH. Acute renal colic from ureteral calculus. NEJM 2004;350:684-693.

Overactive Bladder
Ouslander JG. Management of overactive bladder. NEJM 2004: 250(8):786-799.

Benign Renal Neoplasm
Israel GM, Bosniak MA. An update of Bosniak renal cyst classification system, Urology 2005;66:484-488.

Urological Emergencies
Galejs LE. Diagnosis and treatment of the acute scrotum. Am Fam Phys 1999;5:817-824.

Medications
Bill-Axelson A, Holmberg L, Ruutu M, et al, SPCG-4 Investigators. Radical prostatectomy versus watchful waiting in early prostate cancer. NEJM 2011;364:1708-1717.
Compendium of Pharmaceuticals and Specialties. Available from: http://www.e-therapeutics.ca.
Micromedex health care series. Available from: http://www.micromedex.com.
Rini B, Halabi S, Rosenberg J, et. al. Bevacizumab plus interferon alfa compared with interferon alfa monotherapy in patients with metastatic renal cell carcinoma: CALGB 90206 trial. J Clin Oncol 2008;26:5422-5428.

EBM
Bill-Axelson A, Holmberg L, Ruutu M, et al. Radical prostatectomy versus watchful waiting in early prostate cancer. NEJM 2011;364:1708-1717.
Campschroer T, Zhu Y, Duijvesz D, et al. Alpha-blockers as medical expulsive therapy for ureteral stones. Cochrane DB Syst Rev 2014;4:CD008509.
Coelho RF, Rocco B, Patel MB, et al. Retropubic, laparoscopic, and robot-assisted radical prostatectomy: a critical review of outcomes reported by high-volume centers. J Endourol 2010;24:2003-2015.
Escudier B, Eisen T, Stadler WM, et al. Sorafenib in advanced clear-cell renal-cell carcinoma. NEJM 2007;356:125-134.
Grossman HB, Natale RB, Tangen CM, et al. Neoadjuvant chemotherapy plus cystectomy compared with cystectomy alone for locally advanced bladder cancer. NEJM 2003;349:859-866.
Hoffman RM, Monga M, Elliott SP, et al. Microwave thermotherapy for benign prostatic hyperplasia. Cochrane DB Syst Rev 2012;9:CD004135.
Ilic D, O'Connor D, Green S, et al. Screening for prostate cancer. Cochrane DB Syst Rev 2013;1:CD004720.
James ND, Hussain SA, Hall E, et al. Radiotherapy with or without chemotherapy in muscle-invasive bladder cancer. NEJM 2012;366:1477-1488.
Kim SC, Seo KK. Efficacy and safety of fluoxetine, sertraline and clomipramine in patients with premature ejaculation: a double-blind, placebo controlled study. J Urol 1998;159:425-427.
McDonnell JD, Roehrborn CG, Bautista OM, et al. The long-term effect of doxazosin, finasteride, and combination therapy on the clinical progression of benign prostatic hyperplasia. NEJM 2003;349:2387-2398.
Millett GA, Flores SA, Marks G, et al. Circumcision status and risk of HIV and sexually transmitted infections among men who have sex with men: a meta-analysis. JAMA 2008;300:1674-1684.
Motzer RJ, Escudier B, Tomczak P, et al. Axitinib versus sorafenib as second-line treatment for advanced renal cell carcinoma: overall survival analysis and updated results from a randomized phase 3 trial. Lancet Oncol 2013;14:552-562.
Outerbridge E, Canadian Paediatric Society, Fetus and Newborn Committee. Position statement: neonatal circumcision revisited. CMAJ 1996;154:769-780.
Parsons JK, Hergan LA, Sakamoto K, et al. Efficacy of alpha-blockers for the treatment of ureteral stones. J Urol 2007;177:983-987.
Schröder FH, Hugosson J, Roobol MJ, et al. Screening and prostate-cancer mortality in a randomized European study. NEJM 2009;360:1320-1328.
Siegfried N, Muller M, Deeks JJ, et al. Male circumcision for prevention of heterosexual acquisition of HIV in men. Cochrane DB Syst Rev 2009;2:CD003362.
Tacklind J, Fink HA, Macdonald R, et al. Finasteride for benign prostatic hyperplasia. Cochrane DB Syst Rev 2010;10:CD006015.
Wiesenthal JD, Ghiculete D, D'A Honey RJ, et al. A comparison of treatment modalities for renal calculi between 100 and 300 mm2: are shockwave lithotripsy, ureteroscopy, and percutaneous nephrolithotomy equivalent? J Endourol 2011;25:481-485.
Wilt TJ, Brawer MK, Jones KM, et al. Radical prostatectomy versus observation for localized prostate cancer. NEJM 2012;367:203-213.

VS

Vascular Surgery

Mohammed Firduouse, Dhruv Jain, and Jiayi Mary Tao, chapter editors
Dhruvin Hirpara and Sneha Raju, associate editors
Valerie Lemieux and Simran Mundi, EBM editors
Dr. John Byrne and Dr. George Oreopoulos, staff editors

Acronyms

AAA	abdominal aortic aneurysm	CCB	calcium channel blocker	EVAR	endovascular aortic aneurysm repair	PE	pulmonary embolism
ABI	ankle-brachial index	CLI	critical limb ischemia	EVLT	endovenous laser therapy	PT	prothrombin time
ACEI	angiotensin converting enzyme inhibitor	CTA	computed tomography angiography	GSV	greater saphenous vein	PTT	partial thromboplastin time (i.e. aPTT)
AFib	atrial fibrillation	CVD	cerebrovascular disease	HITT	heparin-induced thrombocytopenia	PVD	peripheral vascular disease
AKA	above-knee amputation	CVI	chronic venous insufficiency		with thrombosis	RIND	reversible ischemic neurologic deficit
AKI	acute kidney injury	CXR	chest x-ray	HTN	hypertension	SFA	superficial femoral artery
aPTT	activated partial thromboplastin time (i.e. PTT)	DIC	disseminated intravascular	IBD	inflammatory bowel disease	SVT	superficial venous thrombosis
ASA	acetylsalicylic acid (Aspirin®)		coagulation	INR	international normalized ratio	TAA	thoracic aortic aneurysm
AT	anterior tibial artery	DM	diabetes mellitus	LMWH	low molecular weight heparin	TEE	transesophageal echocardiography
BKA	below-knee amputation	DVT	deep vein thrombosis	LSV	lesser saphenous vein	TEVAR	thoracic endovascular aortic
BP	blood pressure	ECASA	enteric coated ASA	MCA	middle cerebral artery		aneurysm repair
CABG	coronary artery bypass graft	ECG	electrocardiogram	MRA	magnetic resonance angiography	TIA	transient ischemic attack
CAD	coronary artery disease	Echo	echocardiogram	MSK	musculoskeletal	TTE	transthoracic echocardiography
CBC	complete blood count	ET	essential thrombocythemia	OCP	oral contraceptive pill		

Peripheral Arterial Disease (PAD)

Acute Arterial Ischemia

Definition
- acute occlusion of a peripheral artery, usually without a history of claudication
- urgent management required
  - skeletal muscle can tolerate 6 h of ischemia before irreversible damage and myonecrosis; exception is in acute-on-chronic occlusion, where previously developed collaterals allow more time
- tends to be lower extremity > upper extremity; femoropopliteal > aortoiliac

Etiology and Risk Factors
- embolism vs. thrombosis
  - examples of conditions that predispose to embolism are: arrhythmias, endocarditis, and arterial aneurysms
  - existing atherosclerotic plaques (i.e. chronic PAD) can rupture causing thrombosis
  - previous vascular grafts/reconstructions can fail and thrombose leading to acute presentation
  - hypercoagulable states can contribute to arterial thrombosis

Clinical Features

Table 1. Arterial Embolism vs. Thrombosis

Presentation	Embolus	Thrombus
Onset	Acute	Progressive, acute-on-chronic
Loss of Function/Sensation	Prominent	Less profound (due to underlying collaterals)
Hx of Claudication	No	Maybe
Atrophic Changes	No	Maybe
Contralateral Limb Pulses	Classically normal	Decreased or absent

Investigations
- history and physical exam are essential: depending on degree of ischemia one may have to forego investigations and go straight to the operating room
- ABI: extension of physical exam, easily performed at bedside
- ECG, troponin: rule out recent MI or arrhythmia
- CBC: rule out leukocytosis, thrombocytosis or recent drop in platelets in patients receiving heparin (may suggest heparin induced thrombocytopenia syndrome or HITS)
- PT/INR, PTT: patient anticoagulated/sub-therapeutic INR
- Echo: identify wall motion abnormalities, intracardiac thrombus, valvular disease, aortic dissection (Type A)
- CT angiogram: underlying atherosclerosis, aneurysm, aortic dissection
- conventional catheter based angiography: can be obtained in OR; prelude to thrombolytics, as part of endovascular intervention or for planning treatment

Table 2. Clinical Categories of Acute Limb Ischemia

Grade	Category	Sensory Loss	Motor Deficit	Prognosis
I	Viable	None	None	No immediate threat
IIA	Marginally threatened	None or minimal (toes)	None	Salvageable if promptly treated
IIB	Immediately threatened	More than toes	Mild/moderate	Salvageable if promptly revascularized
III	Irreversible	Profound, anesthetic	Profound, paralysis (rigor)	Major tissue loss Amputation Permanent nerve damage inevitable

Symptoms of Acute Limb Ischemia
6 Ps – all may not be present
Pain: absent in 20% of cases
Pallor: within a few hours becomes mottled cyanosis
Paresthesia: light touch lost first then sensory modalities
Paralysis/Power loss: most important, heralds impending gangrene
Polar/Poikilothermia/'Perishing cold'
Pulselessness: not reliable

Treatment
- immediate heparinization with 5000 IU bolus (80 Units/kg) and continuous infusion to titrate PTT to 70-90s s
- if impaired neurovascular status: emergent revascularization
- if intact neurovascular status: time for work up (including angiogram-CTA)
- definitive treatment
- embolus: embolectomy
- thrombus: thrombectomy ± bypass graft ± endovascular therapy
- irreversible ischemia (complete loss of power or sensation, absent venous and arterial dopplers, rigor): primary amputation
- identify and treat underlying cause
- continue heparin post-operatively, start oral anticoagulant post-operative day 1 x 3 mo depending on underlying etiology

Complications
- compartment syndrome with prolonged ischemia; requires 4-compartment (anterior/lateral/superficial and deep posterior) fasciotomy
- risk of arrhythmia and death with reperfusion injury
- renal failure and multi-organ failure due to toxic metabolites from ischemic muscle

Prognosis
- 12-15% mortality rate
- 5-40% morbidity rate (amputation)

Chronic Arterial Occlusion/Insufficiency

Definition
- chronic ischemia due to inadequate arterial supply to meet cellular metabolic demands (during walking (claudication) or at rest (limb threat/critical limb ischemia)

Etiology and Risk Factors

- predominantly due to atherosclerosis (for pathogenesis, see Cardiology and Cardiac Surgery, C26); primarily occurs in the lower extremities
- major risk factors: smoking, DM, older age
- minor risk factors : HTN, hyperlipidemia, obesity, sedentary lifestyle, PMHx or FMHx CAD/CVD

Differential Diagnosis of Claudication
Vascular
- Atherosclerotic disease
- Vasculitis (e.g. Buerger's disease, Takayasu's arteritis)
- Diabetic neuropathy
- Popliteal entrapment syndrome
Neurogenic
- Neurospinal disease (e.g. spinal stenosis)
- Complex regional pain syndrome
MSK
- OA
- Rheumatoid arthritis/connective tissue disease
- Remote trauma

Clinical Features
- claudication: must differentiate vascular from neurogenic claudication or MSK (see Table 1)
    1. pain with exertion: usually in calves or any exercising muscle group
    2. relieved by short rest: 2-5 min, and no postural changes necessary
    3. reproducible: same distance or time to elicit pain, same location of pain, same amount of rest to relieve pain
- critical limb ischemia (CLI)
    1. includes rest pain, night pain, tissue loss (ulceration or gangrene)
    2. pain most commonly over the forefoot, waking person from sleep, and often relieved by hanging foot off bed
    3. ankle pressure <40 mmHg, toe pressure <30 mmHg, ABI <0.40
        - pulses may be absent at some locations, bruits may be present
        - signs of poor perfusion: hair loss, hypertrophic nails, atrophic muscle, ulcerations and infections, slow capillary refill, prolonged pallor with elevation and rubor on dependency, venous troughing (collapse of superficial veins of foot)

Investigations
- non-invasive
- routine blood work, fasting metabolic profile
- ABI: take highest brachial and highest ankle (dorsalis pedis artery or posterior tibial artery) pressures for each side generally (see Table 3) (may be falsely normal or elevated in those with calcified vessels e.g. diabetics)

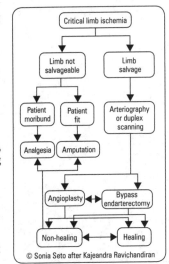

Figure 1. Treatment options for CLI
Modified from Beard JD. Chronic lower limb ischemia.
BMJ 2000;320:854-857

- CTA and MRA
  - excellent for large arteries (aorta, iliac, femoral, popliteal) but may have difficulty with tibial arteries (especially in the presence of disease)
  - **may have difficulty with tibial arteries (especially in the presence of disease)**
  - **require IV injection of nephrotoxic contrast (iodinated contrast for CT, gadolinium for MR)**
  - **used primarily for planning interventions**
- invasive
  - arteriography: superior resolution to CTA/MRA, better for tibial arteries, can be done intraoperatively or as part of endovascular intervention

Table 3. Ankle-Brachial Indices

ABI Recording	Degree of Ischemia
>1.20	Suspect wall calcification (most common in diabetics)
>0.95	Normal/no ischemia
0.50-0.80	Claudication range
<0.40	Possible critical ischemia

Treatment
- conservative
  - risk factor modification (smoking cessation, HbA1c control, treatment of HTN, hyperlipidemia (statin), antiplatelet therapy [ECASA])
  - exercise program (30 min 3x/wk): improves collateral circulation and oxygen extraction at the muscle level
  - foot care (especially in DM): keep wounds clean/dry, avoid trauma and pressure on wounds
- pharmacotherapy
  - antiplatelet agents (e.g. ECASA, clopidogrel)
  - cilostazol (cAMP-phosphodiesterase inhibitor with antiplatelet and vasodilatory effects): improves walking distance for some patients with claudication (not available in Canada)
- surgical/endovascular
  - indications: severe lifestyle impairment, vocational impairment, critical ischemia
  - revascularization
    - endovascular (angioplasty ± stenting)
    - endarterectomy: removal of plaque and repair with patch (usually distal aorta or common/profunda femoral)
    - bypass graft sites: aortofemoral, axillofemoral, femoropopliteal, distal arterial – graft choices: vein graft (reversed or *in situ*), synthetic (polytetrafluoroethylene graft (e.g. Gore-Tex®) or Dacron®)
    - amputation: if not suitable for revascularization, persistent serious infections/gangrene, unremitted rest pain poorly controlled with analgesics

Prognosis
- claudication: conservative therapy: 60-80% improve, 20-30% stay the same, 5-10% deteriorate, 5% will require intervention within 5 yr, <4% will require amputation
- for patients with CLI (rest pain, night pain, ulceration or gangrene): high risk of limb loss and predicts for increased mortality (carries 25% risk of death at 1 yr)

Aortic Disease

Aortic Dissection

Definition
- tear in aortic intima allowing blood to dissect into the media
- Stanford classification: Type A (involve the ascending aorta) vs. Type B (do not)
- acute <2 wk (initial mortality 1% per hour for Type A dissections)
- chronic >2 wk

Etiology
- most common: HTN → degenerative/cystic changes → damage to aortic media
- other: connective tissue disease (e.g. Marfan's, Ehlers-Danlos), cystic medial necrosis, atherosclerosis, congenital conditions (e.g. coarctation of aorta, bicuspid aortic valves, patent ductus arteriosus), infection (e.g. syphilis), trauma, arteritis (e.g. Takayasu's)

Hypercoagulable States

Congenital
- Group I (reduced anticoagulants)
- Antithrombin
- Protein C
- Protein S
- Group II (increased coagulants)
- Factor V Leiden
- Prothrombin
- Factor VIII
- Hyper-homocysteinemia

Acquired
- Immobility
- Cancer
- Pregnancy/Systemic hormonal contraceptives/HRT
- Antiphospholipid antibody syndrome
- Inflammatory disorders (e.g. IBD)
- Myeloproliferative disorders (e.g. ET)
- Nephrotic syndrome (acquired deficit in Protein C and S)
- DIC
- HITT

The Contemporary Safety and Effectiveness of Lower Extremity Bypass Surgery and Peripheral Endovascular Interventions in the Treatment of Symptomatic Peripheral Arterial Disease
Circulation 2015;132:1999-2011

Purpose: Compare the safety and effectiveness of lower extremity bypass surgery (LEB) to peripheral endovascular intervention (PVIs) in the treatment of symp-tomatic peripheral artery disease.
Methods/Results: Compared rates of revascularization in 883 patients treated with PVIs and 975 patients treated by LEB. Revascularization of target lesion and of critical limb ischemia were greater with PVI than LEB (12.3±2.7% and 19.0±3.5% at 1 and 3 years versus 5.2±2.4% and 8.3±3.1%, log-rank P<0.001 in target lesion; 19.1±4.8% and 31.6±6.3% at 1 and 3 years versus 10.8±2.5% and 16.0±3.2%, log-rankP<0.001 in limb ischemia). LEB was associated with significant in-creased rates of complications up to 30d after procedure (37.1% versus 11.9%,P<0.001). There were no differences in subsequent amputation rates between groups.
Conclusion: PVI is associated with higher revascularization rates, lower 30-day procedural complication rate, and no difference in subsequent amputations when compared to LEB in patients with symptomatic PAD.

Epidemiology
- M:F = 3.2:1
- small increased incidence in African-Canadians (related to higher incidence of HTN); lowest incidence in Asians
- peak incidence 50-65 yr old; 20-40 yr old with connective tissue diseases

Clinical Features
- sudden onset tearing chest pain that radiates to back with:
  - HTN (75-85% of patients)
  - asymmetric BPs and pulses between arms (>30 mmHg difference indicates poor prognosis)
  - ischemic syndromes due to occlusion of aortic branches: coronary (MI), carotids (ischemic stroke, Horner's syndrome), splanchnic (mesenteric ischemia), renal (AKI), peripheral (ischemic leg), intercostal vessels (spinal cord ischemia)
  - "unseating" of aortic valve cusps (new diastolic murmur in 20-30%) in Type A dissection
  - rupture into pleura (dyspnea, hemoptysis) or retroperitoneum (hypotension, shock) or pericardium (cardiac tamponade)
  - syncope
  - aortic dissection is 'the great imitator' thus increased risk to patient and MD (medicolegal)

Investigations
- CXR: pleural cap (pleural effusion in lung apices), widened mediastinum, left pleural effusion with extravasation of blood
- TEE: can visualize aortic valve and thoracic aorta but not abdominal aorta
- ECG: LVH ± ischemic changes, pericarditis, heart block
- CTA (gold standard), aortography, MRA: 100% sensitive and specific
- blood work: lactate (elevated in ischemic gut, shock), amylase (rule out pancreatitis), troponin (rule out MI)

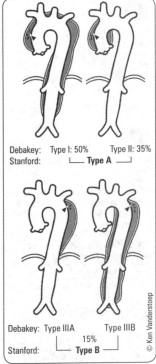

Debakey: Type I: 50%   Type II: 35%
Stanford: Type A

Debakey: Type IIIA   Type IIIB
              15%
Stanford: Type B

© Ken Vanderstoep

Figure 2. Classification of aortic dissection (black arrow indicates where the dissection begins)

Treatment
- Type A dissection needs referral to cardiac surgeon for urgent repair
  - Type B dissection is managed medically with selective intervention for complications or refractory symptoms/progression despite medical therapy – may be a subset of patients who could be well treated with early aortic stent-grafting after initial medical stabilization- evolving area of the literature
  - pharmacologic
  - acute therapy is typically with intravenous antihypertensives titrated to BP measured by arterial line in critical care setting
  - may transition to oral meds after initial control
  - β-blocker to lower BP and decrease cardiac contractility
  - use nondihydropyridine CCB if there is a clear contraindication to β-blockers
  - target sBP of 110 mmHg and HR <60 bpm- need to manage hypertension and pain-failure to do so is a relative indication for surgical intervention
  - ACEI and/or other vasodilators if insufficient BP or HR control
- surgical
  - urgent surgical consult if thoracic aortic dissection diagnosed or highly suspected
  - Type A to cardiac surgery, Type B to vascular surgery
  - resection of segment with intimal tear; reconstitution of flow through true lumen; replacement of the affected aorta with prosthetic graft
  - post-operative complications: renal failure, intestinal ischemia, stroke, paraplegia, persistent leg ischemia, death
  - 2/3 of patients die of operative or post-operative complications
  - Type A: requires emergent surgery with cardiopulmonary bypass;
    - initial mortality rate without surgery is 3% per h for first 24 h, 30% 1 wk, 80% 2 wk
  - Type B: managed medically in absence of spinal/mesenteric/limb malperfusion syndrome
    - <10-20% require urgent operation for complications or persistent symptoms (chest pain)
    - treatment can be surgical or endovascular (now more often endovascular)
    - require follow-up over time to monitor for aneurysmal degeneration
    - role for early endovascular intervention controversial (2013 INSTEAD trial)
- with treatment, 60% 5 yr survival, 40% 10 yr survival

Aortic Aneurysm

Definition of Aneurysm
- localized dilatation of an artery having a diameter at least 1.5x that of the expected normal diameter
- true aneurysm: involving all vessel wall layers (intima, media, adventitia)
- false aneurysm (also known as psuedo-aneurysm): disruption of the aortic wall or the anastomotic site between vessel and graft with containment of blood by a fibrous capsule made of surrounding tissue
- aneurysms can rupture, thrombose, embolize, erode, and fistulize

ACC/AHA 2005 Guidelines define an AAA when the minimum AP diameter of abdominal aorta ≥3.0 cm

Classification

• thoracic aortic aneurysm (TAA): ascending, transverse arch, descending
• thoracoabdominal
• abdominal aortic aneurysm (AAA): 90-98% are infrarenal
• suprarenal: involves one or more visceral arteries, but does not involve the chest
• pararenal: renal arteries arise from aneurysmal aorta, but the SMA origin is not aneurysmal
• juxtarenal: the renal arteries originate from normal aorta, but are immediately adjacent to aneurysmal aorta (there is no nonaneurysmal aorta distal to the origin of the renal arteries)
• infrarenal: the aneurysm originates distal to the renal arteries (there is nonaneurysmal aorta distal to the origins of the renal arteries)

Etiology and Risk Factors

• risk factors: smoking, HTN, PVD, CAD, CVD, age >70, family history
• degenerative
• traumatic
• mycotic (Salmonella, Staphylococcus, usually suprarenal aneurysms)
• connective tissue disorder (Marfan syndrome, Loeys-Dietz Syndrome, Ehlers-Danlos syndrome)
• vasculitis
• infectious (syphilis, fungal)
• ascending thoracic aneurysms are associated with bicuspid aortic valve

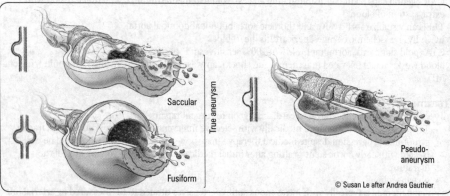

Figure 3. Classification of aneurysms

© Susan Le after Andrea Gauthier

Clinical Features

• most commonly in the abdominal aorta
• common presentation: due to acute expansion or rupture
  ▪ syncope
  ▪ pain (chest, abdominal, flank, back)
  ▪ hypotension
  ▪ palpable pulsatile mass above the umbilicus
  ▪ airway or esophageal obstruction, hoarseness (left recurrent laryngeal nerve paralysis), hemoptysis, or hematemesis (indicates thoracic or thoracoabdominal aortic aneurysm)
  ▪ distal pulses may be intact
• 75% asymptomatic (discovered incidentally)
• uncommon presentations
  ▪ ureteric obstruction and hydronephrosis (often with inflammatory aortic aneurysm)
  ▪ gastrointestinal bleed (duodenal mucosal hemorrhage, aortoduodenal fistula-most commonly a result of previous aortic surgery)
    ♦ aortocaval fistula
  ▪ distal embolization (blue toe syndrome) occurs in <1% of AAA's

Investigations

• blood work: CBC, electrolytes, urea, creatinine, PTT, INR, type and cross
• abdominal U/S (approaching 100% sensitivity, up to ±0.6 cm accuracy in size determination) – useful for screening and surveillance
• CT with contrast (accurate visualization, size determination, EVAR planning)
• peripheral arterial doppler/duplex (rule out aneurysms elsewhere, e.g. popliteal)

Treatment

• conservative (for asymptomatic aneurysms that do not meet the size threshold for repair)
  ▪ cardiovascular risk factor reduction: smoking cessation; control of HTN, DM, hyperlipidemia, regular exercise watchful waiting, U/S surveillance with frequency depending on size and location
• surgical
  ▪ indications
    ♦ ruptured
    ♦ symptomatic
    ♦ prophylaxis when risk of rupture is greater than risk of surgery (size >5.5 cm for AAA)

♦ ascending thoracic aortic aneurysms
  – symptomatic, enlarging, diameter >6 cm or >2x normal lumen size, >4.5 cm and aortic regurgitation (annuloaortic ectasia); ≥4.5-5 cm in Marfan syndrome
  ▪ risk of rupture depends on: size, family history of rupture, rate of enlargement (>1cm/yr in diameter), symptoms, and comorbidities (HTN, COPD, dissection), smoking
  ▪ elective AAA repair mortality 2-5% for open repair (1-2% for EVAR); elective TAA repair mortality <10% (highest with proximal aortic and thoracoabdominal repairs)
  ▪ surgical options
    ♦ open surgery (laparotomy or retroperitoneal) with graft replacement
      – complications
        • early: renal failure, spinal cord injury (paraparesis or paraplegia), impotence, arterial thrombosis, anastomotic rupture or bleeding, peripheral emboli
        • late: graft infection/thrombosis, aortoenteric fistula, anastomotic (pseudo) aneurysm
    ♦ endovascular aneurysm repair (EVAR)
      – newer procedure; high success rates in patients with suitable anatomy
      – advantages: preferred to open surgery in ruptured AAA for patients with suitable anatomy, decreased morbidity and mortality, procedure time, need for transfusion, ICU admissions, length of hospitalization, and recovery time
      – disadvantages: endoleak rates as high as 20-30%, device failure increasing as longer follow-up periods are achieved, re-intervention rates 10-30%, cost-effectiveness is an issue, radiation exposure (especially in younger patients due to need for life-long follow up)
      – complications
        • early: immediate conversion to open repair (<1%), groin hematoma, arterial thrombosis, iliac artery rupture, and thromboemboli
        • late: endoleak, graft kinking, migration, thrombosis, rupture of aneurysm

Carotid Stenosis

Definition
• narrowing of the internal carotid artery lumen due to atherosclerotic plaque formation, usually near common carotid bifurcation into internal and external carotids

Risk Factors
• for atherosclerosis: HTN, smoking, DM, CVD or CAD, dyslipidemia, older age

Clinical Features
• may be asymptomatic
• symptomatic stenosis may present as TIA, RIND, or stroke
• permanent or temporary retinal insufficiency or infarct (see Ophthalmology, OP22)

Investigations
• CBC, PT/INR, PTT (hypercoagulable states)
• fundoscopy: cholesterol emboli in retinal vessels (Hollenhorst plaques)
• auscultation over carotid bifurcation for bruits (do not correlate with degree of stenosis)
• carotid duplex: determines severity of disease (mild/moderate/severe stenosis or occlusion)
• catheter-based angiogram: "gold standard" but invasive and 1/200 risk of stroke (i.e. only used now during carotid angioplasty and stenting)
• MRA: safer than angiogram, may overestimate stenosis
• CTA

Treatment
• risk reduction - control of HTN, lipids, DM
• pharmacological - antiplatelet agents (ASA ± dipyridamole, clopidogrel) ~25% relative risk reduction
• surgical - carotid endarterectomy (generally if symptomatic and >70% stenosis)
• endovascular angioplasty ± stenting

Prognosis

Table 4. Symptomatic Carotid Stenosis: North American Symptomatic Carotid Endarterectomy Trial (NASCET)

% Stenosis on Angiogram	Risk of Major Stroke or Death	
	Medical Rx	Medical + Surgical Rx
70-99%	26% over 2 yr	9% over 2 yr
50-69%	22% over 5 yr	16% over 5 yr
<50%	Surgery has no benefit with 5% complication rate	

Endoleak Types
Definition: persistent blood flow into the aneurysm sac
Type I: ineffective seal at ends of graft
Type II: backflow from collateral vessels
Type III: ineffective seal of graft joints or rupture of graft fabric
Type IV: flow through pores of graft fabric
Type V: endotension, with continued expansion of the aneurysm without apparent flow into the sac

Long-Term Comparison of Endovascular and Open Repair of Abdominal Aortic Aneurysm
N Engl J Med 2012 Nov;367(21):1988-97.
Purpose: Determine if EVAR reduces long-term morbidity and mortality vs. open repair.
Methods: Randomly assigned patients (n=881) with asymptomatic AAA to EVAR vs. open repair and followed them for 9yrs.
Results: EVAR showed reduction in perioperative mortality at 2yrs (hazard ratio, 0.63; 95% CI, 0.40 to 0.98; P=0.04) and 3 yrs (hazard ratio, 0.72; 95% CI, 0.51 to 1.00; P=0.05). There was no significant difference in aneurysm-related deaths between groups (P=0.22). EVAR led to increased survival in pts <70yrs & open repair led to increased survival in pts ≥70yrs (P=0.006).
Conclusion: EVAR and open repair have similar long-term survival. EVAR has perioperative survival advantage that is sustained for several years. EVAR led to increased long-term survival among younger patients but not older patients.

Prevention of Disabling and Fatal Strokes by Successful Carotid Endarterectomy in Patients Without Recent Neurological Symptoms: Randomized Controlled Trial
Lancet 2004;363:1491-1502
Study: Asymptomatic Carotid Surgery Trial (ACST), a RCT with follow-up at 5 yr.
Patients: 3,120 asymptomatic patients with significant carotid artery stenosis were randomized equally between immediate carotid endarterectomy (CEA) and indefinite deferral of CEA and were followed for up to 5 yr (mean 3.4 yr).
Main Outcome: Any stroke (including fatal or disabling).
Conclusions: In asymptomatic patients with significant carotid artery stenosis, immediate CEA reduced the net 5-yr stroke risk from about 12% to about 6%. Half of this 5 yr benefit involved disabling or fatal strokes.

Table 5. Asymptomatic Carotid Stenosis:
Asymptomatic Carotid Atherosclerosis Study (ACAS) and Asymptomatic Carotid Surgery Trial (ACST)

% Stenosis on Angiogram	Risk of Major Stroke or Death	
	Medical Rx	Medical + Surgical Rx
70-99%	26% over 2 yr	9% over 2 yr
60-99%	11% over 5 yr	5.1% over 5 yr (ACAS)
50-69%	11.8% over 5 yr	6.4% over 5 yr (ACST)

Peripheral Venous Disease

Deep Venous Thromboembolism

• see Hematology, H35

Superficial Venous Thrombosis

Definition
• thrombosis of a superficial vein; usually spontaneous but can follow venous cannulation

Etiology
• infectious: suppurative phlebitis (complication of IV cannulation; associated with fever/chills)
• trauma
• inflammatory: varicose veins, migratory superficial thrombophlebitis, Buerger's disease, SLE
• hematologic: polycythemia, thrombocytosis
• neoplastic: occult malignancy (especially pancreatic)
• idiopathic

Migratory superficial thrombophlebitis is often a sign of underlying malignancy ("Trousseau's disease")

Clinical Features
• most common in greater saphenous vein and its tributaries
• pain and cord-like swelling along course of involved vein
• areas of induration, erythema, and tenderness correspond to dilated and often thrombosed superficial veins
• complications
  ▪ simultaneous DVT (up to 20% of cases), PE (rare unless DVT)
  ▪ recurrent superficial thrombophlebitis

Investigations
• non-invasive tests (e.g. Doppler) to exclude associated DVT

Treatment
• conservative
  ▪ moist heat, compression bandages, mild analgesic, anti-inflammatory and anti-platelet (e.g. ASA), ambulation
• surgical excision of involved vein
  ▪ indication: failure of conservative measures (symptoms that persist over 2 wk)
  ▪ suppurative thrombophlebitis: broad-spectrum IV antibiotics and excision

Varicose Veins

Definition
• distention of tortuous superficial veins resulting from incompetent valves in the deep, superficial, or perforator systems

Etiology
• primary (99% of cases) varicosities: venous valve incompetence or obstruction
  ▪ contributing factors: increasing age, systemic hormonal contraceptive use, prolonged standing, pregnancy, obesity
• secondary varicosities: DVT, malignant pelvic tumours with venous compression, congenital anomalies, arteriovenous fistulae, trauma

Epidemiology
• primary varicose veins are the most common form of venous disorder of lower extremity
• 65% of north American adult population gets some degree of venous insufficiency

Clinical Features (Not Correlated with Varicosity Size)
- diffuse aching, fullness/tightness, nocturnal cramping
  - aggravated by prolonged standing (end of day), premenstrual
- visible long, dilated and tortuous superficial veins along thigh and leg (greater or short saphenous veins and tributaries)
- ulceration, hyperpigmentation, and induration (ie-lipodermatosclerosis)
- Brodie-Trendelenburg test (valvular competence test)
  - with patient supine, raise leg and compress saphenous vein at thigh, have patient stand – if veins fill quickly from top down then incompetent valves; use multiple tourniquets to localize incompetent veins (can get same information with standing venous ultrasound looking for reflux)
- often the degree of symptoms do not correlate with the clinical findings

Complications
- recurrent superficial thrombophlebitis
- hemorrhage: external or subcutaneous
- ulceration, eczema, lipodermatosclerosis, and hyperpigmentation

Treatment
- largely a cosmetic problem
- conservative: elastic compression stockings
- surgical: high ligation and stripping of the long saphenous vein and its tributaries, ultrasound-guided foam sclerotherapy, endovenous laser therapy
- indications for surgery: symptomatic varix (pain, bleeding, recurrent thrombophlebitis), tissue changes (hyperpigmentation, ulceration), failure of conservative treatment, cosmetic

Prognosis
- benign course with predictable complications
- almost 100% symptomatic relief with treatment if varicosities are primary
- good cosmetic results with treatment
- significant post-operative recurrence

Chronic Venous Insufficiency

Definition
- venous insufficiency and skin damage

Etiology
- calf muscle pump dysfunction and valvular incompetence (reflux) due to phlebitis, varicosities, or DVT
- venous obstruction

Clinical Features
- pain (most common), ankle and calf edema – relieved by foot elevation
- pruritus, brownish hyperpigmentation (hemosiderin deposits)
- stasis dermatitis, subcutaneous fibrosis if chronic (lipodermatosclerosis)
- ulceration: shallow, above medial malleolus, weeping (wet), painless, irregular outline
- signs of DVT/varicose veins/thrombophlebitis

Investigations
- not required if conservative treatment only
- Doppler U/S (most commonly used in pre-operative assessment)
- venography or ambulatory venous pressure measurement (not often used)

Treatment
- conservative
  - elastic compression stockings, ambulation, periodic rest-elevation, avoid prolonged standing
  - ulcers: multilayer compression bandage, antibiotics prn
- surgical
  - if conservative measures fail, or if recurrent/large ulcers to reduce the risk of recurrence
  - surgical ligation of perforators in region of ulcer (GSV/LSV ligation and stripping)
- endovenous: laser or radiofrequency ablation, or foam sclerotherapy

Lymphedema

Definition
- obstruction of lymphatic drainage resulting in edema with high protein content

Etiology
- primary
  - Milroy's syndrome: congenital hereditary lymphedema
  - lymphedema praecox (75% of cases): starts in adolescence
  - lymphedema tarda: starts >35 yr
- secondary
  - infection: filariasis (#1 cause worldwide)
  - malignant infiltration: axillary, groin or intrapelvic
  - radiation/surgery (axillary, groin lymph node removal): #1 cause in North America

Clinical Features
- classically non-pitting edema
- impaired limb mobility, discomfort/pain, psychological distress

Treatment
- avoid limb injury (can precipitate or worsen lymphedema)
- skin hygiene
  - daily skin care with moisturizers
  - early medical assessment and treatment for infection (topical for fungal infection; systemic for bacterial infection)
- external support
  - intensive: compression bandages
  - maintenance: compression garment
- exercise
  - gentle daily exercise of affected limb, gradually increasing ROM
  - must wear a compression sleeve/bandages when doing exercises
- massage: manual lymph drainage therapy

Prognosis
- if left untreated becomes resistant to treatment due to subcutaneous fibrosis
- cellulitis causes rapid increase in swelling and worsening lymphedema (destruction of additional lymphatics)

References

Guidelines

ACC/AHA guidelines for percutaneous coronary intervention. Circulation 2001;103:3019-3041.

Beard JD. Chronic lower limb ischemia. BMJ 2000;320:854-857.

Bell AD, Roussin A, Cartier R, et al. The use of antiplatelet therapy in the outpatient setting: CCS guidelines. Can J Cardiol 2011;27:S1-S59.

Canadian Cardiovascular Society 2005 Consensus Conference Peripheral Arterial Disease (Draft). Available from: http:// www.ccs.ca.

CCS focused 2012 update of the CCS atrial fibrillation guidelines: recommendations for stroke prevention and rate/rhythm control. Can J Cardiol 2012;28:125-136.

European Stroke Organisation, Tendera M, Aboyans V, et al. ESC guidelines on the diagnosis and treatment of peripheral artery diseases: document covering atherosclerotic disease of extracranial carotid and vertebral, mesenteric, renal, upper and lower extremity arteries. Eur Heart J 2011;32(22):2851-2906.

Harrington RA, Becker RC, Ezekowitz M, et al. Antithrombotic therapy for coronary artery disease: the seventh ACCP conference on antithrombotic and thrombolytic therapy. Chest 2004;126(3 suppl):513s-584s.

May J, White GH, Harris JP. The complications and downside of endovascular therapies. Adv Surg 2001;35:153-172.

Rutherford RB. Vascular surgery, 4th ed. Toronto: WB Saunders, 1995. Chapter: Atherogenesis and the medical management of atherosclerosis. p222-234.

Schmieder FA, Comerota AJ. Intermittent claudication: magnitude of the problem, patient evaluation, and therapeutic strategies. Am J Card 2001;87(Suppl):3D-13D.

Task Force on the Diagnosis and Treatment of Peripheral Artery Diseases of the European Society of Cardiology (ESC). Eur Heart J 2011;32:2851-2906.

Way LW, Doherty GM (editors). Current surgical diagnosis and treatment, 11th ed. Lange Medical Books/McGraw-Hill, 2004.

Yang SC, Cameron DE (editors). Current therapy in thoracic and cardiovascular medicine. McGraw-Hill, 2004.

Vascular Surgery

Alexander P, Giangola G. Deep venous thrombosis and pulmonary embolism: diagnosis, prophylaxis, and treatment. Ann Vasc Surg 1999;13:318-327.

American College of Cardiology (clinical guidelines, etc). Available from: http://www.acc.org.

Beard JD. Chronic lower limb ischemia. BMJ 2000;320:854-857.

Bojar RM. Manual of perioperative care in cardiac surgery, 3rd ed. Massachusetts: Blackwell Science, 1999.

Cardiology Online (requires registration). Available from: http://www.theheart.org.

Cheng DCH, David TE. Perioperative care in cardiac anesthesia and surgery. Austin: Landes Bioscience, 1999.

Coulam CH, Rubin GD. Acute aortic abnormalities. Semin Roentgenol 2001;36:148-164.

Crawford ES, Crawford JL, Veith FJ, et al (editors). Vascular surgery: principles and practice, 2nd ed. Toronto: McGraw-Hill, 1994. Chapgter: Thoracoabdominal aortic aneurysm.

Cronenwett JL, Johnston W (editors). Rutherford's vascular surgery, 7th ed. Philadelphia: Saunders/Elsevier, 2014

Freischlag JA, Veith FJ, Hobson RW, et al (editors). Vascular surgery: principles and practice, 2nd ed. Toronto: McGraw-Hill, 1994. Chapter: Abdominal aortic aneurysms.

Fuchs JA, Rutherford RB (editors). Vascular surgery, 4th ed. Toronto: WB Saunders, 1995. Chapter: Atherogenesis and the medical management of atherosclerosis. p222-234.

Hallett JW Jr. Abdominal aortic aneurysm: natural history and treatment. Heart Dis Stroke 1992;1:303-308.

Hallett JW Jr. Management of abdominal aortic aneurysms. Mayo Clin Proc 2000;75:395-399.

Harlan BJ, Starr A, Harwin FM. Illustrated handbook of cardiac surgery. New York: Springer-Verlag, 1996.

Hiratzka LF, Bakris GL, Beckman JA, et al. 2010 ACCF/AHA/AATS/ACR/ASA/SCA/SCAI/SIR/STS/SVM guidelines for the diagnosis and management of patients with thoracic aortic disease. J Am Coll Cardiol 2010;55:e27-e129.

May J, White GH, Harris JP. The complications and downside of endovascular therapies. Adv Surg 2001;35153-35172.

Pitt MPI, Bonser RS. The natural history of thoracic aortic aneurysm disease: an overview. J Card Surg 1997;12(Suppl):270-278.

Powell JT, Brown LC. The natural history of abdominal aortic aneurysms and their risk of rupture. Adv Surg 2001;35:173-185.

Rabi D, Clement F, McAlister F, et al. Effect of perioperative glucose-insulin-potassium infusions on mortality and atrial fibrillation after coronary artery bypass grafting: a systematic review and meta-analysis. Can J Cardiol 2010;26;178-184.

Rosen CL, Tracy JA. The diagnosis of lower extremity deep venous thrombosis. Emerg Med Clin N Am 2001;19:895-912.

Schmieder FA, Comerota AJ. Intermittent claudication: magnitude of the problem, patient evaluation, and therapeutic strategies. Am J Cardiol 2001;87(Suppl):3D-13D.

Veith FJ, Hobson RW, Williams RA, et al. Vascular surgery: principles and practices, 2nd ed. Toronto: McGraw-Hill, 1994.

Verma S, Szmitko PE, Weisel RD, et al. Clinician update: should radial arteries be used routinely for coronary artery bypass grafting? Circulation 2004;110:e40-e46.

Way LW, Doherty GM. Current surgical diagnosis and treatment, 11th ed. Lange Medical Books/McGraw-Hill, 2004.

Yang SC, Cameron DE. Current therapy in thoracic and cardiovascular medicine. McGraw-Hill, 2004.

Notes

Index

A

α-Thalassemia; H20

Abdominal
- Computed Tomography; MI12
- Distention; G5
- Imaging; MI10
- Incisions; GS2
- Mass; GS5
- Pain; ER18, ER59, FM13, G4, GS4,P37
- Trauma; ER13
- X-Ray; MI10

Abnormal Pseudocholinesterase; A29

Abnormal Uterine Bleeding; GY6, GY11

Abruptio Placentae; OB14

Acalculous Cholecystitis; GS48

Achilles
- Tendonitis; OR39
- Tendon Rupture; OR39

Acid-Base Disorders; NP15

Acneiform Eruptions; D11

Acne Vulgaris; D11

Acoustic Neuroma; OT14

Acromioclavicular
- Joint Pathology; OR14

Actinic Keratosis; D33

Acute
- Abdominal Pain; GS4
- Arterial Ischemia; VS2
- Bacterial Rhinosinusitis; OT25
- Blood Transfusion Reactions; H54
- Cholangitis; GS49
- Cholecystitis; GS47
- Confusional State; N20
- Coronary Syndromes; C27, ER22, ER37
- Decompensated Heart Failure; ER32
- Diarrhea; G4, G15, ID11
- Epiglottitis; OT44
- Kidney Injury; NP18
- Laryngitis; OT28
- Laryngotracheobronchitis; OT44
- Liver Failure; G35
- Lymphoblastic Leukemia; H43
- Myeloid Leukemia; H37
- Otitis Media; FM50, OT17, OT38, P52
- Pain; A24
- Pancreatitis; G44, GS51
- Pelvic Pain; ER19
- Pericarditis; C47, ER22
- Psychosis; ER56
- Pyelonephritis; U14
- Respiratory Distress Syndrome; R26

Rhinitis; FM19, FM49

Viral Hepatitis; G28

Acyanotic Congenital Heart Disease; P17

Addictive Disorders; PS21

Addison's Disease; E33

Adenoidectomy; OT40

Adenoid Hypertrophy; OT40

Adenomyosis; GY15

Adhesive Capsulitis; OR15

Adjustment Disorder; PS18

Adolescent Medicine; P15

Adrenal Cortex; E29

Adrenal Gland; GS60

Adrenal Mass; MI17

Adrenal Medications; E52

Adrenal Medulla; E34

Adrenocortical
- Functional Workup; E30
- Hormones; E29
- Insufficiency; E33

Adrenocorticotropic Hormone; E29

Adult Polycystic Kidney Disease; NP35

Adverse Drug Reactions; CP9

Aesthetic Surgery; PL36

Age-Related Macular Degeneration; OP24

Agnosia; N28

Agoraphobia; PS15

Agranulocytosis; H11

AIDS; ID27, OP32

Airway Management; A7
- Difficult Airway; A9
- Oxygen Therapy; A10
- Ventilation; A10
- Airway Problems in Children; OT42

Airway Obstruction; R7

Alcohol; FM12, PS23

Alcohol Related Emergencies; ER54

Alcoholic Liver Disease; G34

Allergic Reactions; ER28

Allergic Rhinitis; FM14, OT23

Alopecia Areata; D38

Altered Level of Consciousness; ER19

Altered Sensation; N10

Alternative Medicine; FM48

Alzheimer's; N23

Amaurosis Fugax; OP35

Amblyopia; OP37

Amenorrhea; GY10

American Society of Anesthesiology
- Classification; A4

Amniocentesis; OB8

Amniotic Fluid Embolus; OB40

Amoebas; ID36

Amphetamines; PS25

Amputations; PL24

Amyotrophic Lateral Sclerosis; N35

Anagen Effluvium; D38

Anal Fissures; GS39

Analgesia; A19

Analgesic
- Nephropathies; NP30
- Techniques in Labour; OB33

Anal Neoplasms; GS42

Anaphylaxis; ER28

Anatomical Triangles of the Neck; OT5

Anatomy of the Eye; OP2

Anatomy of the Neck; OT4

Anatomy of the Thyroid Gland; OT5

Androgenetic Alopecia; D37

Androgen Regulation; E45

Anemia; H6, P45
- Folate Deficiency Anemia; OB25
- Hemolytic Anemia; H18
- Iron Deficiency Anemia; H15, OB25, P45
- Macrocytic Anemia; H23
- Microangiopathic Hemolytic Anemia; H22
- Microcytic Anemia; H13
- Normocytic Anemia; H17

Anemia of Chronic Inflammation; H16

Anesthesia
- Local Anesthesia; A22
- Monitoring; A6
- Obstetrical Anesthesia; A26
- Pediatric Anesthesia; A27
- Pre-Operative
  - Assessment; A2
  - Investigations; A4
  - Optimization; A4
- Regional Anesthesia; A20
- Types of Anesthesia; A2

Anesthetic Techniques in Labour; OB33

Angiodysplasia; GS36

Angioedema; D41

Angiography; MI27

Angiography of Gastrointestinal Tract; MI15

Angle-Closure Glaucoma; OP27

Ankle Fracture; OR37

Ankle Ligamentous Injuries; OR38

Ankylosing Spondylitis; RH21

Anorectal Abscess; GS40

Anorectum; GS38

Anorexia Nervosa; PS31

Antenatal Fetal Surveillance; OB12

Antepartum Care; OB4

Dysrhythmias; ER30
Tamponade; C48, ER22
Therapeutics; C49
Transplantation; C38
Cardinal Movements of Fetus, Delivery; OB32
Carotid Stenosis; VS7
Cataracts; OP20
Catecholamine Metabolism; E34
Catheter Ablation; C25
Cat Scratch Disease; ID24
Cauda Equina Syndrome; NS26
Cavernous Malformations; NS22
Celiac Disease; G18, P35
Cellulitis; D26, FM51, ID10, PL14
Central Retinal Artery Occlusion; OP22
Central Retinal Vein Occlusion; OP22
Central Venous Catheter; MI10
Cerebellar Ataxias; N35
Cerebellar Disorders; N34
Cerebral Abscess; NS14
Cerebral Hemorrhage; N52
Cerebral Palsy; P83
Cerebrospinal Fluid Fistulas; NS23
Cerebrovascular Disease; NS17
Cerumen Impaction; OT15
Cervical Cancer; FM5
Cervical Disc Syndrome; NS24
Cervical Spine; OR22
Cervical Spondylosis; NS24
Cervix; GY43, OB31
Cesarean Delivery; OB42
Cestodes; ID41
Chalazion; OP12
Chemical Burns; OP41
Chest Imaging; MI4
Chest Injuries; ER12
Chest Pain; C4, C31, ER21, FM18, R3
Chest Trauma; ER11
Chest Tube; MI10
Chest X-Rays; MI4, R5
Chiari Malformations; NS36
Child Abuse; ER60, P14
Chlamydia; FM51
Cholangiocarcinoma; GS50
Cholangitis; GS49
Cholecystitis; GS47
Choledocholithiasis; GS48
Cholelithiasis; GS46
Cholescintigraphy; MI26
Cholesteatoma; OT17
Chorioamnionitis; OB40
Chorionic Villus Sampling; OB8
Chronic Abdominal Pain; P38
Chronic Arterial Occlusion; VS3
Chronic Cystitis; U13
Chronic Diarrhea; G5, G16
Chronic Kidney Disease; NP33

Chronic Laryngitis; OT28
Chronic Lymphocytic Leukemia; H48
Chronic Myeloid Leukemia; H40
Chronic Obstructive Pulmonary
  Disease; ER31, FM16, GS17, R9
Chronic Pain; A26, NS38
Chronic Pancreatitis; G45, GS51
Chronic Rhinosinusitis; OT26
Chronic Stable Angina; C26
Chronic Venous Insufficiency; VS9
Circumcision; P8, U40
Cirrhosis; G35
Clavicle Fracture; OR14
Clinical Drug Testing; CP2
Clinical Nutrition; G47
Club Drugs; PS26
Club Foot; OR44
Coagulation Factors; H53
Cocaine; PS25
Cold Injuries; ER45
Collateral Ligament Tears; OR32
Colles' Fracture; OR20
Colorectal Cancer; FM4
Colorectal Carcinoma; GS34
Colorectal Neoplasms; GS33
Colorectal Polyps; GS33
Coma; NS33
Common Cold; FM19
Common Drug Endings; CP11
Common Statistical Tests; PH15
Compartment Syndrome; OR9
Complete Blood Count; H3
Complex Regional Pain Syndromes; N43
Complicated Effusion; R23
Complications of Pregnancy; OB25
Computed Tomography Chest; MI6
Concussion; FM19
Conduct Disorder; PS39
Condyloma Acuminata; D30
Confidentiality; ELOM5
Confusional State; N20
Congenital Abnormalities; U36
Congenital Diaphragmatic Hernias; GS62
Congenital Glaucoma; OP39
Congenital Hand Anomalies; PL37
Congenital Heart Disease; P16
Congenital Sensorineural Hearing Loss; OT19
Congenital Talipes Equinovarus; OR44
Congestive Heart Failure; C34, P20
Conjunctiva; OP13
Conjunctivitis; OP14
Connective Tissue Disorders; RH8
Consent; ELOM6
Constipation; G5, G24, GM3, P36
Constrictive Pericarditis; C48
Contact Dermatitis; D14
Contraception; FM19, GY16

Contrast Enhancement; MI4
Contrast Studies; MI13
Conversion Disorder; PS28
Cornea; OP16
Corneal Abrasion; OP16
Corneal Ulcer; OP17
Coronary Angiography; C15
Coronary Artery Disease; A5, E5
Coronary Circulation; C2
Coronary Revascularization; C31
Coronary Syndromes; C27, ER22, ER37
Cough; FM20, R3
Counselling of the Pregnant Woman; OB9
  Immunizations; OB11
  Lifestyle; OB10
  Medications; OB10
  Nutrition; OB9
  Radiation; OB11
Coxa Plana; OR43
Cranial Nerve Deficits; N11
Craniofacial Anomalies; PL36
Craniofacial Injuries; PL29
Craniosynostosis; NS36
Creutzfeldt-Jakob Disease; N27
Crohn's Disease; G19, G20, GS28
Cruciate Ligament Tears; OR32
Crying/Fussing Child; P8
Cryptococcus spp.; ID35
Cryptorchidism; GS64, U38
Cryptosporidium spp.; ID37
Crystal-Induced Arthropathies; RH24
CT Head; MI19
Cushing's Syndrome; E32
Cutaneous T-Cell Lymphoma; D36
Cyanosis; P67
Cyanotic Congenital Heart Disease; P19
Cystic Fibrosis; P87, R12
Cystoscopy; U41
Cysts; D5

D

Dacryoadenitis; OP11
Dacryocystitis; OP11
Dandy-Walker Malformation; NS35
Decompensated Heart Failure; ER32
Deep Neck Space Infection; OT46
Dehydration; P74
Delayed Blood Transfusion Reactions; H55
Delirium; GM4, N20, PS19
Delusional Disorder; PS8
Dementia; FM20, GM4
Dental Infections; FM50
Dentition and Caries; P9
Depression; FM20, GM4
Depressive Disorders; PS10

N

O